REPLACEMENT OF RENAL FUNCTION BY DIALYSIS

REPLACEMENT OF RENAL FUNCTION BY DIALYSIS

A textbook of dialysis

Edited by
WILLIAM DRUKKER, FRANK M. PARSONS AND JOHN F. MAHER

Second, revised and enlarged edition

1983 **MARTINUS NIJHOFF PUBLISHERS**
a member of the KLUWER ACADEMIC PUBLISHERS GROUP
BOSTON / THE HAGUE / DORDRECHT / LANCASTER

Distributors

for the United States and Canada: Kluwer Boston, Inc., 190 Old Derby Street, Hingham, MA 02043, USA
for all other countries: Kluwer Academic Publishers Group, Distribution Center, P.O. Box 322, 3300 AH Dordrecht, The Netherlands

Library of Congress Cataloging in Publication Data   CIP

```
Main entry under title:

Replacement of renal function by dialysis.

   Includes index.
   1. Hemodialysis.  2. Renal insufficiency--Treatment.
I. Drukker, William.  II. Parsons, Frank M.  III. Maher,
John F.  [DNLM: 1. Hemodialysis.  WJ 378 R425]
RC901.7.H45R46  1983     617'.461059     82-22271
```

ISBN 0-89838-553-9

Copyright

© 1983 by Martinus Nijhoff Publishers, Boston.

All rights reserved. No part of this publication may be reproduced, stored in a retrieval system, or transmitted in any form or by any means, mechanical, photocopying, recording, or otherwise, without the prior written permission of the publishers,
Martinus Nijhoff Publishers, 190 Old Derby Street, Hingham, MA 02043, USA.

PRINTED IN THE NETHERLANDS

It is difficult to say what is impossible, for the dream of yesterday is the hope of to-day and the reality of to-morrow.

ROBERT H. GODDARD

To Molly, Marjorie and Marge

FOREWORD TO THE SECOND EDITION

BELDING H. SCRIBNER

Since the Foreword to the First Edition was written, there have been important changes in the dialysis field. These developments are well represented in the additional material in the revised chapters and in the new chapters of the second edition of this book.

Specifically there has been an increasing interest in dialyzer re-use (Chapter 15). It is of historical interest that the technique of dialyzer re-use was first devised, not as a cost saving measure, but to reduce the work load of patients who were rebuilding their Kiil dialyzers at home (1). Re-use reduced this task from three times weekly to once every two weeks.

Continuous ambulatory peritoneal dialysis (CAPD) now has made peritoneal dialysis a more acceptable alternative to hemodialysis. It is my belief, however, that the ultimate role for CAPD will fall short of the current enthusiastic projections because of the tedium required of the patient by constant surveillance of sterile technique. In that regard, I particularly look forward to reading Charles Mion's new chapter 23. Mion and his colleagues have devised a filter system that protects the patient from infections that develop because of breaks in sterile technique. This system, if proven successful, should help to lower the current high drop-out rate among patients on CAPD.

Another new development (Chapter 48), the use of plasmapheresis to help prevent progression of antiglomerular basement membrane disease and possibly other conditions to end-stage renal disease, despite its obvious problems and limitations, represents a significant step toward the future development of new immunotherapeutic techniques to avoid the progression of glomerulonephritis to chronic renal failure.

For the dialysis patient, the most important development since the first edition of this book has been the recognition by Lundin and colleagues (2) and since confirmed by others (3–5), that control of hypertension can prevent the development of accelerated atherosclerosis. The pall of gloom raised by our 1974 publication (6) now has been lifted, and the prospects for long term survival on dialysis have been greatly enhanced. What emerges now is a whole new set of very difficult problems that deal with the more subtle factors which may interfere with long term survival, such as 30 years of exposure to plasticizers leached from blood tubing, or the possible longer term effects of mild aluminum intoxication which may result from the use of phosphate binders for half a lifetime (Chapter 42).

As I write this Foreword, very little progress has been made with the issue of priorities raised in the Foreword to the first edition. The difference now is that increasing fiscal austerity will force the issue sooner than expected and, particularly in the United States, we are still as ill-prepared as we were in 1977 to cope with this complex situation. The socioeconomic challenges must be met as vigorously as the medical and technological problems have been.

REFERENCES

1. Pollard TL, Barnett BMS, Eschbach JW, Scribner BH: A technique for storage and multiple re-use of the Kiil dialyzer and blood tubing. *Trans Am Soc Artif Intern Organs* 13:24, 1967
2. Lundin AP, Adler AJ, Feinroth MV: Maintenance hemodialysis. Survival beyond the first decade. *JAMA* 244:38, 1980
3. Scribner BH: The long-term Seattle hemodialysis and transplant survivors. *Proc Third Capri Uremia Conf: Pathobiology of Patients Treated for 10 Years or More,* edited by Giordano C, Friedman EA, Milan, New York NY, Wichtig Editore, 1981, p 32
4. Vincenti F, Amend WJ, Abele J, Feduska NJ, Salvatierra O Jr: The role of hypertension in hemodialysis-associated atherosclerosis. *Am J Med* 68:363, 1980
5. Charra B, Calemard E, Cuche M, Laurent G: Use of "long dialysis" to control hypertension and prolong survival among patients on maintenance hemodialysis. *Nephron,* (in press)
6. Lindner A, Charra B, Sherrard D, Scribner BH: Accelerated atherosclerosis in prolonged maintenance hemodialysis. *N Engl J Med* 290:697, 1974

FOREWORD TO THE FIRST EDITION

BELDING H. SCRIBNER

The year was 1942 and William Kolff was hard at work perfecting the device that would not only revolutionize the treatment of renal failure, but more importantly point the way to the development of the entire field of extracorporeal devices in general and cardiac bypass devices in particular.

The enormity of the impact that Kolff's contribution was to have on medicine was revealed retrospectively to me when I recalled that in that same year, 1942, I was a second year medical student at Stanford University, taking among other things, P.J. Hanzlik's required course in pharmacology. I have two memories of that course. One was the requirement that we students learn to recognize 64 old time drugs by appearance, smell and taste. For better or worse, almost all of the 64 have disappeared from the scene. The other memory is the more pertinent one. I can still visualize the scene in the small classroom in the attic of the old red brick Stanford Lane building at Webster and Sacramento Streets. Professor Hanzlik had a pigeon for a "patient" and had planned a dramatic demonstration. I can still hear him command one of my fellow students to "Seize the patient!", which the student did in fear and uncertainty as the poor bird struggled against its fate. Hanzlik then proceeded with great flair and ceremony to inject some drug intended for intravenous use into the poor pigeon, where upon the bird promptly expired and Hanzlik drove home the point that intravenous therapy of any kind was dangerous and should be avoided at all costs. This "conservative" attitude was quite consistent with that prevailing throughout the practice of medicine in that era. If intravenous therapy was dangerous, then a device for extracorporeal circulation must be an invention of the devil! Indeed, for the decade after the first clinical dialyses in Europe and Canada, acceptance was painfully slow and often resisted by all the usual techniques of those in power. During the early 60's, we encountered exactly the same kind of resistance to the concept of chronic dialysis. But as has happened over and over again in all of science, the heresy of one decade becomes the practice of the next—a phenomenon that the young heretics among the third generation readers of this volume should not forget.

And so, today Drukker, Parsons and Maher have successfully undertaken the very difficult task if bringing together in one volume all the diverse elements of dialysis therapy. The size of the volume reflects not only the magnitude of the interdisciplinary effort that brought about the technical and clinical advances, but also the many clinical and other ramifications of dialysis therapy.

In 1977, this therapy will cost the United States taxpayer nearly one billion dollars as the number of dialysis patients in the United States soars above 30,000, while the projection of the ultimate number increases from 40,000 to 60,000 and the cost projection to two billion per year by 1985. Concurrently, in the United States, the percentage of patients on home dialysis has dropped from a high of 41% in 1973 to just under 15%. This trend away from home dialysis cost the United States taxpayer an additional 150 million dollars in 1976. In an effort to control costs, the United Kingdom has increased the percentage of patients on home care to nearly 70%. In addition, the United Kingdom and perhaps other Western countries are beginning to exert subtle but effective cost control on dialyses by limiting the numbers of dialysis patients (1). In contrast, in the United States in 1977, there is no cost control on dialysis. What this contrast means to me is that dialysis is having an impact on Western medicine far beyond its significant impact on the patients, family physicians and staff who are directly involved.

The nature and enormity of this impact began to become apparent to me in 1962 when magazine writer Shana Alexander came to Seattle to do a story on the artificial kidney. I shall always remember how incredulous I was that she did not want to see or hear about the patients whose lives had been saved—no interest there. She wanted to find out all about the "life and death committee". As a result, her article on the Seattle Life and Death Committee appeared in *Life Magazine* that fall (2) and set off discussion and controversy that have persisted to the present (3); indeed, the current British versus American approach to chronic dialysis is but a dramatic extension to international medicine of the basic "who shall live" issue that was raised by the Seattle Life and Death Committee. I believe that what has happened is that dialysis has greatly accelerated the process of bringing to the forefront a basic issue in Western medicine that up to now has been kept hidden. That issue is *priorities*. Can the United States really afford to spend two billion dollars per year on dialysis? If not, who will decide to curtail expenses, and how will the decision be implemented? Significant curtailment already is being implemented in the United Kingdom by limiting the dialysis population (1). The question is how are they able to "get away with it", and if the real truth were known, could they get away with it?

To put this issue in a different context, I believe the rapid development of dialysis marks the beginning of the end for unrestrained expansion of expensive medical technology—just as surely as the energy crisis tells us that unlimited expansion of a petroleum based Western civilization is about to come to an end. I believe that the energy crisis poses the greatest threat to democracy that has ever been posed in peacetime because the basic inability of the democratic process to cope with decisions about priorities in times of crises. Does dialysis and other very expensive technology pose a similar threat to medical free enterprise as still practiced mainly in the United States? Unless we put our house in order, I believe it does.

Let us take a brief look at another example of costly medical technology that already has overtaken dialysis in terms of total cost. Coronary by-pass surgery is currently costing Americans nearly two billion dollars per year. Preston, in a just published critique of the operation (4), points out that not only is its efficacy unproven, but he makes a strong case for the point that the economic incentives of the free enterprise system rather than medical efficacy explain why in 1975 the operation was performed on 28 patients/100,000 population in the United States in contrast to 2.1 patients/100,000 population in Western Europe.

Dialysis doctors can take comfort in the fact that at least the question of efficacy is not an issue with our expensive technology. But important and unresolved issues nag at our conscience with respect to the cost-benefit ratio of dialysis. These issues are far too complex to be resolved during the life-time of the first generation of readers of this volume and pose the ultimate challenge to the younger generations. The clinical and technological aspects of dialysis must not remain static at the state of the art level described in this volume while the demand for costly services increases. Rather, we must build on the knowledge reviewed in this book to improve the cost-benefit ratio of our services. Meanwhile, we function as our technological advances create new social problems. And so my advice to all three generations is to try understand and cope with a new responsibility that dialysis, because of its high cost, has introduced into the basic doctor-patient relationship. How can each of us fulfill our basic responsibility to our patients while at the same time doing everything possible to reduce the overall cost to society of this very expensive treatment?

REFERENCES

1. Distribution of nephrological services for adults in Great Britain. Report of the Executive Committee of the Renal Association. *Br. Med J* 2:903, October 16, 1976
2. Alexander S: They decide who lives, who dies. *Life Magazine,* p. 102, November 9, 1962
3. Fox RC, Swazey JP: *The courage to fail—A social view of organ transplants and dialysis.* Chapters 8, 9 and 10. University of Chicago Press, 1974
4. Preston TA: *Coronary by-pass surgery: A critical review.* Raven Press, New York, 1977

PREFACE

More than 50 years after Haas' first human dialysis, and 40 years after Kolff's pioneering work, a book on the present state of the art cannot be written by one person: obviously it had to be a multi-authored volume. Therefore some overlap between chapters and even a few controversies between authors became unavoidable.

However we deliberately avoided editorial streamlining of manuscripts, leaving the authors' personal style and personal opinions unaltered as much as possible. This may make the book more vivid to read and may sometimes stimulate readers to study a subject in greater detail from the literature. Additionally, both British and American spellings have been kept because of the international nature of the book. To preserve space, though, the index uses only American spelling.

The first edition had to be reprinted within a year of initial publication and about one year later the publishers asked us to undertake the task of preparing a second edition.

In the 5 years since publication of the first edition much has changed. Not a single chapter remained unaltered. All were rewritten rather than simply reviewed and updated.

The number of authors and co-authors has increased from 64 to 78, 30 contributing for the first time. The number of chapters has been increased from 42 to 49, 16 being entirely new and written by new authors.

We are pleased that so many original contributors were anxious to participate again and that the newly invited contributors accepted the assignment of writing their chapters, starting from scratch.

It is, however, with deep sadness that we have to record the untimely death of two of our friends and colleagues. Dr. Arthur Gordon died suddenly in November 1979 and Dr. Reginald G. Mason died in October 1981 shortly after he had completed updating the chapter on thrombogenesis and anticoagulation for this new edition.

This second edition includes chapters on practical use of anticoagulants, on haemoperfusion, haemofiltration and plasmapheresis. Obviously, a few of them cover subjects which belong to fringe areas, not serving replacement of renal function. Nevertheless, they may be of interest to our readers. They have one important aspect in common with haemodialysis: they require a reliable angioaccess for repeated extracorporeal circulation.

Also included are new chapters on ophthalmological complications and aluminium intoxication in dialysis patients.

Peritoneal dialysis has received more emphasis in this second edition by incorporating chapters on its history and on the practical aspects.

The size of the book has almost doubled, partly by using more illustrations. The inclusion of a number of colour reproductions has been made possible by a supporting grant* of the National Kidney Foundation of the Netherlands, which the editors gratefully acknowledge.

We considered asking several authors to shorten their chapters. We resisted this as it would have delayed the publishing date and would possibly have removed much material besides being a painful task for our colleagues.

We are aware that there are some overlaps between chapters and observant readers may even note some controversies between authors. This, however, may stimulate further personal study of the literature.

Finally as the observant reader will notice, the sequence of chapters has been changed. Many chapters have been regrouped together in a more logical order.

The editors gratefully acknowledge the work of so many distinguished colleagues, who contributed to this second edition.

They again wish to thank Dr. Belding H. Scribner, the pioneer of chronic dialysis, for writing the Foreword to this second edition.

We reused the peak 7^c diagram of Dr. Jonas Bergström and Peter Fürst as a logogram, symbolising the uraemic toxins to be removed by dialysis and related techniques.

Again the editors want to acknowledge the invaluable help of Martinus Nijhoff's staff. In particular we thank Mr. Boudewijn F. Commandeur, chief of the Medical Division and his secretary Miss Judith van Arem and Mr. Frans B. van Schaik, without whose technical assistance the production of the book would have been impossible. We must pay tribute to the dedication and hard work of our secretaries: Mrs. Mabel Mary Lely, Amsterdam, The Netherlands, Mrs. Frances Haigh, Leeds, UK and Mrs. Barbara Fitzgerald, Bethesda, MD, USA. Finally without the tolerance, the support and devotion of Molly, Marjorie and Marge the editors' work would have been impossible.

Amsterdam, W.D.
Leeds, F.M.P.
Bethesda, Md, J.F.M.

March 1983.

---

* Grant no C80-279.

TABLE OF CONTENTS

Foreword to the second edition
    BELDING H. SCRIBNER VII
Foreword to the first edition
    BELDING H. SCRIBNER IX
Preface
    THE EDITORS XI
Contributors XVII

  1. Introduction
      THE EDITORS 1
  2. Haemodialysis: a historical review
      WILLIAM. DRUKKER 3
  3. Principles and biophysics of dialysis
      JOHN A. SARGENT and FRANK A. GOTCH 53
  4. Membranes
      DONALD J. LYMAN 97
  5. Dialysers
      NICHOLAS A. HOENICH and DAVID N. S. KERR 106
  6. Pretreatment and preparation of city water for hemodialysis
      CHRISTINA M. COMTY and FRED L. SHAPIRO 142
  7. The composition of dialysis fluid
      FRANK M. PARSONS and WILLIAM K. STEWART 148
  8. Angioaccess
      KHALID M. H. BUTT 171
  9. Extracorporeal thrombogenesis: mechanisms and prevention
      REGINALD G. MASON (deceased), HANSON Y.K. CHUANG and S. FAZAL MOHAM-
      MAD 186
10. Practical use of anticoagulants
      ROBERT M. LINDSAY 201
11. Haemodialysis monitors and monitoring
      PRAKASH R. KESHAVIAH and STANLEY SHALDON 223
12. Biophysics of ultrafiltration and hemofiltration
      LEE W. HENDERSON 242
13. Ultrafiltration and haemofiltration, practical applications
      EDUARD A. QUELLHORST 265
14. The polyacrylonitrile membrane; use in dialysis with the Rhodial system. Use in haemofiltration
      JEAN-LOUIS FUNCK-BRENTANO and NGUYEN-KHOA MAN 275
15. Multiple use of hemodialyzers
      NORMAN DEANE and JAMES A. BEMIS 286
16. Hemoperfusion
      JAMES F. WINCHESTER 305

XIV   *Table of contents*

17. Dialysate regeneration
    ANTONY J. WING, FRANK M. PARSONS and WILLIAM DRUKKER 323
18. Oral sorbents in uremia
    ELI A. FRIEDMAN 341
19. Uraemic toxins
    JONAS BERGSTRÖM and PETER FÜRST 354
20. Regular dialysis treatment (RDT)
    BARBARA G. DELANO 391
21. Peritoneal dialysis: a historical review
    WILLIAM DRUKKER 410
22. Peritoneal anatomy and transport physiology
    KARL D. NOLPH 440
23. Practical use of peritoneal dialysis
    CHARLES M. MION 457
24. Home dialysis
    ROSEMARIE A. BAILLOD 493
25. Paediatric dialysis
    RAYMOND A. DONCKERWOLCKE, CYRIL CHANTLER and MICHEL J.C. BROYER . 514
26. Acute renal failure
    CARL M. KJELLSTRAND, CESAR E. PRU, WILLIAM R. JAHNKE and THOMAS D.
    DAVIN 536
27. Nutrition in dialysis patients
    REINHOLD K.A. KLUTHE 569
28. Blood pressure control in chronic dialysis patients
    ROBERT P. WHITE and ALBERT L. RUBIN 575
29. Hyperlipidemia and atherosclerosis in chronic dialysis patients
    JOHN D. BAGDADE 588
30. Cardiac complications of regular dialysis therapy
    CHRISTINA M. COMTY and FRED L. SHAPIRO 595
31. Acute complications associated with hemodialysis
    CHRISTOPHER R. BLAGG 611
32. Hematologic problems of dialysis patients
    JOSEPH W. ESCHBACH 630
33. Host defenses and infectious complications in maintenance hemodialysis patients
    WILLIAM F. KEANE and LEOPOLDO R. RAIJ 646
34. Dialysis associated hepatitis
    SHEILA POLAKOFF 659
35. Renal osteodystrophy and maintenance dialysis
    JACK W. COBURN and FRANCISCO LLACH 679
36. Endocrine changes in patients on chronic dialysis
    JAMES P. KNOCHEL 712
37. Neurological aspects of dialysis patients
    FRANS G.I. JENNEKENS and AAGJE JENNEKENS-SCHINKEL 724
38. Ophthalmological complications associated with haemodialysis
    BETTINE C.P. POLAK 742
39. Pharmacological aspects of renal failure and dialysis
    JOHN F. MAHER 749
40. Anaesthesia and major surgery in patients with renal failure
    K. BRIAN SLAWSON 798
41. Trace metals and regular dialysis
    ALLEN C. ALFREY and W. RODMAN SMYTHE 804

42. Aluminium toxicity in renal failure
    MICHAEL K. WARD and IAN S. PARKINSON 811
43. Planning, developing and operating a dialysis programme
    ANTHONY J. F. d'APICE, NAPIER M. THOMSON, WALTER F. HEALE and PRISCILLA S. KINCAID-SMITH 820
44. Selection of patients and the integration between dialysis and transplantation, the quality of life of the patients
    TIMOTHY H. MATHEW, ANTHONY J. F. d'APICE and PRISCILLA S. KINCAID-SMITH   830
45. The quality of life of the chronic dialysis patient
    H. EARL GINN and PAUL E. TESCHAN 837
46. The social impact of chronic maintenance hemodialysis
    RICHARD B. FREEMAN 844
47. Comparative review between dialysis and transplantation
    ANTHONY J. WING, FELIX P. BRUNNER, HANS O. A. BRYNGER, CLAUDE JACOBS and PETER KRAMER 850
48. Plasma exchange: principles and practice
    ANDREW J. REES 872
49. Dialysis and haemofiltration for non-renal conditions
    HANS J. GURLAND, PETER KRAMER, NORBERT NEDOPIL, FRANK M. PARSONS, WALTER SAMTLEBEN, NEVILLE H. SELWOOD and ANTONY J. WING 884

Index of subjects 897

CONTRIBUTORS

Allen C. ALFREY, M.D.
Professor of Medicine University of Colorado
Chief of Renal Section
Denver Veterans Administration Medical Center
1055 Clermont, Denver, CO 80220, USA
Chapter 41

Anthony J. F. d'APICE, M.D., F.R.A.C.P., F.R.C.P.A.
Assistant Director Department of Nephrology
The Royal Melbourne Hospital
Senior Associate, Department of Medicine
The University of Melbourne,
Melbourne Vic. 3050, Australia
Chapters 43, 44

John D. BAGDADE, M.D.
Clinical Professor of Medicine
University of Washington
School of Medicine, Providence Medical Center
500 17th Ave, Seattle, WA 98124, USA
Chapter 29

Rosemarie A. BAILLOD, M.B., B.S., L.R.C.P., M.R.C.S.
First Assistant, Department of Nephrology and Transplantation
Renal Dialysis Unit, Royal Free Hospital
Pond Street, London NW3 2QG, England
Chapter 24

James A. BEMIS, Ph.D.
Microcal Inc., 320 North Pleasant Street
Amherst MA 01002, USA
Chapter 15

Jonas BERGSTRÖM, M.D.
Professor, Department of Renal Medicine
Huddinge University Hospital
S-141 86 Huddinge, Sweden
Chapter 19

Christopher R. BLAGG, M.D., F.R.C.P.
Professor of Medicine
University of Washington, Seattle, WA
Director North-West Kidney Center
700 Broadway, Seattle, WA 98122, USA
Chapter 31

Michel J.C. BROYER, M.D.
Professor of Paediatrics
Necker-Enfants Malades Hôpital
149 rue de Sèvres, 75730 Paris Cédex 15, France
Chapter 25

Felix P. BRUNNER, M.D.
Privatdozent, Department of Medicine
University of Basel, Kantonsspital,
CH-4031 Basel, Switzerland
Chapter 47

Hans O. A. BRYNGER, M.D.
Associate Professor of Surgery
Department of Surgery I, Sahlgren's Hospital
S-41345 Gothenburg, Sweden
Chapter 47

Khalid M. H. BUTT, M.D., F.R.C.S. (Eng.) F.A.C.S.
Professor of Surgery
Director of Transplantation
State University Hospital
Downstate Medical Center
450 Clarkson Ave, Box 40, Brooklyn.
New York, NY 11203, USA
Chapter 8

Cyril CHANTLER, M.A., M.D., F.R.C.P.
Professor of Paediatric Nephrology
Guy's Hospital Medical School
London SE1 9 RT, England
Chapter 25

Hanson Y. K. CHUANG, Ph.D.
Research Associate Professor
Department of Patholoy, School of Medicine
University of Utah, 50 N. Medical Drive
Salt Lake City, UT 84132, USA
Chapter 9

Jack W. COBURN, M.D.
Professor of Medicine, University of California Los Angeles
School of Medicine
Director of Nephrology Training Program
Veterans Administration Wadsworth Medical Center
Nephrology Section 691/111L
Wilshire and Sawtelle Blvd
Los Angeles, CA 90073, USA
Chapter 35

Christina M. COMTY, M.D., M.R.C.P.
Associate Professor of Medicine
University of Minnesota
Staff Nephrologist Hennepin County Medical Center
701 Park Avenue, Minneapolis, MN 55415, USA
Chapters 6, 30

Thomas D. DAVIN, M.D.
Assistant Professor of Medicine
University of Minnesota
St. Paul Ramsey Hospital, Division of Nephrology
640 Jackson Street, St. Paul, MN 55101, USA
Chapter 26

Norman DEANE, M.D.
Director Manhattan Kidney Center
Consulting Physician St Vincent's Hospital
and Medical Center
40 East 30th Street, New York, NY 10016, USA
Chapter 15

Barbara G. DELANO, B.A., M.D.
Associate Professor of Medicine
Downstate Medical Center, 450 Clarkson Ave
Brooklyn, New York, NY 11203, USA
Chapter 20

Raymond A. DONCKERWOLCKE, M.D.
Paediatrician, Queen Wilhelmina Children's Hospital
University of Utrecht
Nieuwe Gracht 137
3512 LK Utrecht, The Netherlands
Chapter 25

William DRUKKER, M.D.
Formerly Reader in Dialysis
Department of Medicine Queen Wilhelmina University
Hospital, Amsterdam
Emeritus Director Department of Nephrology and Dialysis
St. Lucas Hospital, Amsterdam
Present address: De Lairessestraat 75,
1071 NV Amsterdam, The Netherlands
Chapters 1, 2, 17, 21

Joseph W. ESCHBACH, M.D.
Clinical Professor of Medicine
University of Washington
Division of Nephrology, Box Rm-11
Department of Medicine, University of Washington
Seattle, WA 98195, USA
Chapter 32

Richard B. FREEMAN, M.D.
Head, Nephrology Unit
University of Rochester School of Medicine
601 Elmwood Ave, Rochester, NY 14642, USA
Chapter 46

Eli A. FRIEDMAN, M.D.
Professor of Medicine
State University Hospital
Department of Medicine, Division of Renal Diseases
Downstate Medical Center, 450 Clarkson Ave
Brooklyn, New York, NY 11203, USA
Chapter 18

Jean-Louis FUNCK-BRENTANO, M.D.
Professor of Nephrology
Director Research Laboratory INSERM
Department of Nephrology, Hôpital Necker
161 rue de Sèvres, 75015 Paris Cédex 15, France
Chapter 14

Peter FÜRST, M.D., Ph.D.
Professor and Chairman
Institute of Biological Chemistry and Nutrition
University of Hohenheim
30 Gargenstrasse, D 7000 Stuttgart 70, FRG
Chapter 19

H. Earl GINN, M.D.
Nephrologist
King Faisal Specialist Hospital and Research Centre
Adjunct Professor of Medicine
University of Riyadh Medical College
P.O. Box 3354, Riyadh, Saudi Arabia
Chapter 45

Frank A. GOTCH, M.D.
Dialysis Treatment and Research Center
Franklin Hospital, Castro and Buboce Streets
San Francisco, CA 94144, USA
Chapter 3

Hans J. GURLAND, M.D.
Professor, Director Nephrology Division
Medical Department I, Klinikum Grosshadern
University of Munich
P.O. Box 701 260, D 8000 München, FRG
Chapter 49

Walter F. HEALE, M.D., F.R.A.C.P.
Renal Physician, Renal Unit
Austin Hospital, Heidelberg
Melbourne, Vic. 3084, Australia
Chapter 43

Lee W. HENDERSON, M.D.
Professor of Medicine
University of California, San Diego and
Veterans Administration Medical Center
3350 La Jolla Village Drive
San Diego, CA 92161, USA
Chapter 12

Nicholas A. HOENICH, Ph.D.
Lecturer in Clinical Science
University of Newcastle upon Tyne
Department of Medicine, Royal Victoria Infirmary
Newcastle upon Tyne NE1 4LP, England
Chapter 5

Claude JACOBS, M.D.
Professor of Nephrology
Centre Pasteur-Valléry-Radot
26 rue des Peupliers, 75013 Paris, France
Chapter 47

William R. JAHNKE, M.D.
Fellow in Nephrology, University of Minnesota
121 Doctors Professional Building
280 North Smith
St. Paul, MN 55102, USA
Chapter 26

Frans G.I. JENNEKENS, M.D.
Senior Neurologist, Head of the Laboratory for Neuromuscular
Diseases
Department of Neurology
University Hospital Utrecht
Nicolaas Beetsstraat 24
3511 HE Utrecht, The Netherlands
Chapter 37

Aagje JENNEKENS-SCHINKEL, M.A.
Neuropsychologist, Department of Neuropsychology
University Hospital Leiden
Rijnsburgerweg 10
2333 AA Leiden, The Netherlands
Chapter 37

William F. KEANE, M.D.
Assistant Professor of Medicine
Department of Medicine, University of Minnesota
Regional Kidney Disease Program
at Hennepin County Medical Center
701 Park Avenue
Minneapolis, MN 55415, USA
Chapter 33

David N.S. KERR, M.D., M.Sc., F.R.C.P.
Professor of Medicine
University of Newcastle upon Tyne
Department of Medicine, Wellcome Research Laboratories
Royal Victoria Infirmary
Newcastle upon Tyne NE1 4LP, England
Chapter 5

Prakash R. KESHAVIAH, Ph. D.
Senior Research Associate
University of Minnesota, Department of Medicine
Manager of Bioengineering Regional Kidney Disease Program
Hennepin County Medical Center
701 Park Avenue
Minneapolis, MN 55415, USA
Chapter 11

Priscilla S. KINCAID-SMITH, D. Sc., M.D., B.Ch., F.R.A.C.P.,
F.R.C.P., F.R.C.P.A., D.C.P.
Professor of Medicine, University of Melbourne
Department of Medicine, Royal Melbourne Hospital
Grattan Street, Parkville, Vic. 3050, Australia
Chapters 43, 44

Carl M. KJELLSTRAND, M.D., F.A.C.P.
Professor of Medicine and Surgery
University of Minnesota
Regional Kidney Disease Program
Nephrology Division, Department of Medicine
Hennepin County Medical Center
701 Park Ave South
Minneapolis, MN 55415, USA
Chapter 26

Reinhold K.A. KLUTHE, M.D.
Professor of Medicine
Head, Division of Nutrition and Dietetics
Chief, Nutritional Laboratories and Dietetic Services
University Hospital
D 7800 Freiburg, FRG
Chapter 27

James P. KNOCHEL, M.D.
Professor and Vice-Chairman
Department of Internal Medicine, University of Texas,
Southwestern Medical School
5323 Harry Hines Boulevard, Dallas, TX 75235
Senior attending Physician,
Parkland Memorial Hospital, Dallas;
Chief, Medical Service
Veterans Administration Medical Center
Dallas, TX 75216, USA
Chapter 36

Peter KRAMER, M.D.
Professor of Internal Medicine
University Center for Internal Medicine
40 Robert Koch Strasse
D 34 Göttingen, FRG
Chapter 47

Robert M. LINDSAY, M.D., F.R.C.P.(E), F.R.C.P.(C), F.A.C.P.
Director Nephrology Section
Department of Medicine, Victoria Hospital
375 South Street
London, Ontario N6A 4G5, Canada
Chapter 10

Francisco LLACH, M.D.
Professor of Medicine
University of Oklahoma Health Sciences Center
Veterans Administration Hospital
Nephrology Section (111G)
Oklahoma City, OK 73104, USA
Chapter 35

Donald J. LYMAN, B.S., M.S., Ph.D.
Professor of Materials Science and Engineering
Professor of Bioengineering
Research Associate Professor of Surgery
Department of Materials Science and Engineering
University of Utah
Salt Lake City, UT 84112, USA
Chapter 4

John F. MAHER, M.D.
Professor of Medicine
Director, Nephrology Division
Uniformed Services University of the Health Sciences
School of Medicine
4301 Jones Bridge Road
Bethesda, MD 20814, USA
Chapters 1, 39

Nguyen-Khoa MAN, M.D.
Associate Professor of Nephrology
University of Paris
Department of Nephrology
Hôpital Necker, 161 rue de Sèvres
75015 Paris Cédex 15, France
Chapter 14

Reginald G. MASON, M.D., Ph.D. (deceased)
Professor and Chairman, Department of Pathology
School of Medicine, University of Utah
50 N. Medical Drive
Salt Lake City, UT 84132, USA
Chapter 9

Timothy H. MATHEW, M.B.B.S., F.R.A.C.P.
Director Renal Unit
Queen Elizabeth Hospital
Adelaide, S.A. 5011, Australia
Chapter 44

Charles M. MION, M.D.
Professor of Medicine, Head Division of Nephrology
University Hospital Montpellier
Service de Néphrologie, Hôpital Saint-Charles
34059 Montpellier, France
Chapter 23

S. Fazal MOHAMMAD, M.Sc., Ph.D.
Research Associate Professor
Department of Pathology, University of Utah
School of Medicine
Salt Lake City, UT 84132, USA
Chapter 9

Norbert NEDOPIL, M.D.
Staff Member, Department of Psychiatry
University of Munich,
7 Nussbaumstrasse, D 8000 München, FRG
Chapter 49

Karl D. NOLPH, M.D.
Professor of Medicine
Director, Division of Nephrology
Room M472
University of Missouri Health Sciences Center and
Harry S. Truman Memorial Veterans Administration
Hospital
Columbia, MO 65212, USA
Chapter 22

Ian S. PARKINSON, B.Sc. (Hons)
Research Associate, Wellcome Research Laboratories,
Department of Medicine
Royal Victoria Infirmary
Newcastle upon Tyne NE1 4LP, England
Chapter 42

Frank M. PARSONS, B.Sc., M.D., F.R.C.P. Ed.
Consultant Physician in Clinical Renal Physiology
The General Infirmary at Leeds
Renal Research Unit, Wellcome Wing
Leeds LS1 3EX
Senior Clinical Lecturer in Medicine
University of Leeds, England
Chapters 1, 7, 17, 49

Bettine C.P. POLAK, M.D.
Lecturer in Ophthalmology
Department of Ophthalmology, Erasmus University
Eye Hospital
Schiedamse Vest 180
3011 BH Rotterdam, The Netherlands
Chapter 38

Sheila POLAKOFF, M.D., M.F.C.M., D.P.H.
Consultant Epidemiologist
Epidemiological Research Laboratory
Central Public Health Laboratory
Colindale Avenue
London NW9 5HT, England
Chapter 34

Cesar E. PRU, M.D.
Renal Fellow, Regional Kidney Disease Program
Nephrology Division, Department of Medicine
Hennepin County Medical Center
701 Park Ave South
Minneapolis, MN 55415, USA
Chapter 26

Eduard A. QUELLHORST, M.D.
Professor of Medicine
Nephrological Centre Niedersachsen
D 3510 Hannover-München, FRG
Chapter 13

Leopoldo R. RAIJ, M.D.
Associate Professor of Medicine
Attending Physician University of Minnesota Hospitals
University of Minnesota
Department of Medicine
Mayo Memorial Building
Box 272, Minneapolis, MN 55455, USA
Chapter 33

Andrew J. REES, M.Sc., M.R.C.P.
Consultant Physician and Honorary Senior
Lecturer Royal Postgraduate Medical School,
Director, Department of Nephrology
Hammersmith Hospital
Ducane Road
London W12 OHS, England
Chapter 48

Albert L. RUBIN, M.D., F.A.C.P.
Professor of Biochemistry,
Medicine and Surgery
Director, Rogosin Kidney Center
The New York Hospital-Cornell Medical Center
525 East 68th Street
New York, NY 10021, USA
Chapter 28

Walter SAMTLEBEN, M.D.
Staff Member, Nephrology Division
Medical Department I, Klinikum Grosshadern
University of Munich
P.O. Box 701 260
D 8000 München, FRG
Chapter 49

John A. SARGENT, Ph.D.
Quantitative Medical Systems, Inc.
5901 Christie Ave, Suite 201
Emeryville, CA 94608, USA
Chapter 3

Belding H. SCRIBNER, M.D.
Professor of Medicine
Division of Nephrology Department of Medicine
University of Washington
Seattle, WA 98195, USA
Forewords to the First and the Second Edition

Neville H. SELWOOD, M.D.
UK Transplant Service
Southmead Hospital
Bristol BS10 5ND, England
Chapter 49

Stanley SHALDON, M.A., M.D., (Cantab), M.R.C.P.
Professor of nephrology
Université de Nîmes
Centre Hospitalier Régional, Service de Néphrologie
5 rue Hoche, 30006 Nîmes Cédex, France
Chapter 77

Fred L. SHAPIRO, M.D.
Professor of Medicine
University of Minnesota
School of Medicine and Chief of Nephrology
Hennepin County Medical Center
701 Park Ave
Minneapolis, MN 55415, USA
Chapters 6, 30

K. Brian SLAWSON, B.Sc., M.B., Ch.B., F.F.A.R.C.S.
Honorary Senior Lecturer
University of Edinburgh
Consultant Anaesthetist
Western General Hospital, Crewe Road
Edinburgh EH4 2XU, Scotland
Chapter 40

W. Rodman SMYTHE, Ph.D.
Professor of Physics
University of Colorado
Nuclear Physics Laboratory
Box 446
Boulder, CO 80309, USA
Chapter 41

William K. STEWART, M.D., Ph.D., F.R.C.P., F.R.C.P.E.
Senior Lecturer in Medicine
Consultant Physician, Tayside Health Board, Scotland
Department of Medicine
The University of Dundee
Dundee DD1 9SY, Scotland
Chapter 7

Paul E. TESCHAN, M.D.
Associate Professor of Medicine,
Urology and Biomedical Engineering
Vanderbilt University School of Medicine
Department of Medicine
Division of Nephrology, B-2214,
Medical Center North
Nashville, TN 37232, USA
Chapter 45

Napier M. THOMSON, M.B.B.S., M.D., F.R.A.C.P.
Senior Lecturer (Hon.). Department of Medicine
Monash University, Melbourne
Deputy Director, Department of Nephrology
Prince Henry's Hospital
St Kilda Road
Melbourne, Vic. 3004, Australia
Chapter 43

Michael K. WARD, M.B.B.S., M.R.C.P.
Senior Lecturer in Medicine
University of Newcastle upon Tyne
Consultant Physician
Royal Victoria Infirmary
Newcastle upon Tyne NE1 4LP, England
Chapter 42

Robert P. WHITE, M.D.
Clinical Assistant Professor of Medicine
Temple University School of Medicine
Philadelphia, PA.
Chief, Section of Nephrology.
Medical Director, Kidney Center, St. Luke's Hospital
801 Ostrum Street
Bethlehem, PA 18015, USA
Chapter 28

James F. WINCHESTER, M.D., M.B.Ch.B., M.R.C.P.
Associate Professor of Medicine
Georgetown University Medical Center
3800 Reservoir Road NW
Washington, DC 20007, USA
Chapter 16

Antony J. WING, M.A., D.M., F.R.C.P.
Consulting Physician,
St Thomas' Hospital
London SE1 7EH, England
Chapters 17, 47, 49

1
INTRODUCTION

The fate of the patient with irreversible terminal renal failure has changed dramatically in less than two decades.

Little more than 20 years ago, the patient in terminal renal failure if unresponsive to manipulations that sometimes restore renal function, had no alternative than to face death by uraemia. His relatives and his physician had to sit down at his bedside in frustration.

Much of the mental and physical suffering that characterised progressive and finally terminal renal failure as it led slowly to the end of life has nearly disappeared from our hospital wards. Currently, it is even difficult to expose our medical students to the clinical syndrome called uraemia and to teach them at the bedside the signs and symptoms of the end stage failing kidneys.

Newly acquired knowledge gained by the efforts of research scientists is usually rapidly accepted and absorbed by mankind. Panta rei: nothing is static, everything changes. Surprising and exciting medical progress of yesterday belongs today to the common daily medical practice. Twenty years ago, the patient in terminal renal failure and his relatives asked: 'Is there any chance of survival? Could my life be saved with dialysis? Is there any chance to survive with a transplant?' Today the preterminal renal failure patient asks his physician when he will start his chronic dialysis treatment which nowadays usually begins long before the patient has the onset of symptoms of uraemia and the second question is often: 'And what about holidays? What about travelling, swimming, camping or skiing when I am on that machine?' Presently, because of the availability of portable and sophisticated dialysis machinery, not only rehabilitation, gainful employment and leisure activities are achieved, but also travelling for holidays or business purposes is possible for maintenance dialysis patients. A wearable artificial kidney machine has been constructed and waits for miniaturisation and further perfection.

For many reasons, including the financial impact of thousands of patients treated for several years, there is a need to improve the technology and to prevent or delay when possible the occurrence of terminal renal failure.

The treatment of the patient in terminal renal failure can be complicated and difficult whilst an enormous, still fast growing literature about the technology and pathobiology of dialysis therapy has developed and is scattered over many journals, transactions, proceedings, monographs and manuals. The first generation nephrologists and internists, some of whom somewhat hesitatingly and even reluctantly, entered the field of replacement of renal function, started more or less from scratch and saw their knowledge grow. They could readily keep up with the modest volume of dialysis literature and learned from each other at meetings, symposia and congresses. They became a large family of enthusiastic, energetic physicians working in a new and fascinating field of medicine. However, the first generation is approaching, or even has already reached, the end of their careers. A second generation has taken over and a third generation of young physicians is entering the field. They face an abundant, often bewildering and widely scattered literature on dialysis and treatment of terminal renal failure in general. Because patients are kept alive by dialysis the opportunity has been afforded to elucidate the endocrine aspects of chronic renal failure, to study the neurological abnormalities of uraemia and to identify changes in various other organ systems. New subdisciplines have developed including trace metal homeostasis and pharmacokinetics in uraemia and the psychiatric aspects of life with renal substitution. It can be difficult, even frustrating for the novice in the field to sort out amongst so much information what is important from the past, what is useful at present and what should be disregarded in between. Unless one is especially gifted with mathematical and physical knowledge, it can be a difficult, even awesome or frightening task to assimilate the information in the treatises of physics of modern dialysers, the complicated electronics and hydraulics of modern monitoring and proportioning systems and the physics of sorbent and ion exchange regeneration systems for dialysis fluid. Therefore, a book offering an encyclopaedic review of the present state of the art seemed to be useful. The contributors to this text include many of the pioneers who laid the foundation for this discipline and others who contributed importantly to its rapid growth. Those who are presently newly entering the field may find this book a useful guide for the present treatment of the patient in terminal renal failure by haemodialysis or peritoneal dialysis and they will also find descriptions of the conservative methods of treatment which necessarily accompany dialysis treatment. Others, even those first and second generations of dialysis physicians and scientists, may find the book useful as a reference guide. Accordingly, we have attempted to offer in this manual full information and an extensive but critical review of the present concepts underlying this therapy. We have deemphasised or totally omitted, however, relatively unimportant details, outdated facts and descriptions of archaic techniques and machines.

In this second edition the reader will find new chapters on haemofiltration, haemoperfusion and plasma exchange, techniques which share with haemodialysis the need for extracorporeal circulation. They have been developed to a high degree of reliability thanks to haemodialysis. But, of these three, only haemofiltration is a new technique that primarily serves the purpose of the book: replacement of renal function. It has moved from the experimental to the point of practical application since the first edition was published. Haemoperfusion predominantly serves different purposes such as detoxification from exogenous poisons. Plasma-exchange is a method of treatment directed to (auto-)immune diseases mediated by antigen-antibody mechanisms and also serves to prevent permanent kidney disease leading to irreversible renal failure. Obviously there are some links with haemodialysis and we thought it justified to include chapters on these subjects, all written by experts in these relatively new fields. Since the first edition was published, there has been a resurgence of interest in peritoneal dialysis coincident with the introduction of the continuous ambulatory method and we have expanded this section. In addition the inclusion of a chapter on dialysis treatment of such divergent but non renal conditions as schizophrenia and psoriasis, still a somewhat controversial subject, seemed justified.

Dialysis interposes a semi-permeable membrane between a flowing stream of blood and an appropriate rinsing solution. By convective and diffusive transport, the composition of body fluids approaches that of the dialysis solution. Simultaneous ultrafiltration decreases body fluid volumes, ordinarily toward normal. Lower concentrations of toxic solutes in body fluids are generally associated with clinical improvement of the uraemic syndrome and hypertension and congestive heart failure usually recede as volume excess is corrected. But, as we cannot identify precisely and understand sufficiently the toxicity of the retained solutes, we deplete indiscriminately, removing toxic as well as useful solutes in proportions dictated by membrane permeability rather than according to their toxic potential. Further, we substitute poorly for the endocrine and metabolic aspects of renal regulation of body composition. Our therapy is a dramatic success compared to the natural history of progressive renal disease, but it is cumbersome, awkward and inefficient compared to the healthy kidney.

Following the initial successful dialysis for therapy of renal failure, numerous modifications in dialyser design and technique and in other aspects of therapy soon followed, improving the efficacy of therapy. It now appears that additional major improvements in therapy may await increased fundamental knowledge of renal failure and the biochemistry of uraemia. Accordingly, the complete reference work must review the basic concepts of mass transport, extracorporeal thrombogenesis, biochemical and metabolic abnormalities, organ pathophysiology and so forth, as well as present the pragmatic information of why, when and how to dialyse patients. We have striven for a balance of such practical and fundamental information.

The prophecy expressed in the introduction to the first edition of this book has become true; many segments of the first edition of the book have run out of date and we have been fortunate that so many previous authors, who were asked by us to update and completely revise their chapters, were willing to do so. We were also lucky to find so many new authors, with competence in the areas in which the book has expanded, who with their co-authors were willing to write a number of entirely new chapters. Hopefully the book will be as up-to-date when printed as the first edition was. But the science of the pathophysiology of terminal renal failure and the technology of its treatment continue to be in a stage of dynamic progress. Our knowledge in this field is far from petrified; it still shows dynamic progress. While we again have tried to be as current as possible, we have avoided, where appropriate, overemphasis on the current vogue or the dated hypothesis.

As we wrote before, the written word often stimulates criticism, even more than the oral presentation of facts or hypotheses. The authors and the editors are open for readers' criticisms and opinions. Recalling that sharing our clinical and investigative experiences helped our knowledge grow and remain current, we anticipate that such a dialogue will be helpful.

All generations of clinical nephrologists from the first to the third and those generations that follow, should be aware of the enormous responsibility for the quality of treatment offered to the terminal renal failure patient who puts his life in their hands, having virtually no other choice for survival. The quality of that treatment depends on the dedication and the knowledge, the training and professional skills of the physicians, their nurses and paramedical co-workers. We should never forget that a bad treatment often means a long period of disability, of misery and of suffering if not death. We are now not only capable of saving thousands of lives, but we are also able to attain the goal of offering those patients in terminal renal failure and their families a good and enjoyable quality of life.

For those patients who are suitable for transplantation and who have difficulties with being tied to a machine three times weekly or even to machine-free, but continuous ambulatory peritoneal dialysis, or who otherwise have difficulties in accepting dialysis treatment, the way to transplantation remains open; two chapters give additional information on the integration between dialysis and transplantation.

May this book contribute to the goal of improved treatment for those in terminal renal failure.

The Editors

2
HAEMODIALYSIS: A HISTORICAL REVIEW

WILLIAM DRUKKER

The invention of dialysis (1861)	3
The first 'artificial kidney' (1913)	3
The first human dialysis (october 1924)	7
The rotating drum dialyser, constructed by Kolff and Berk (1943)	12
Misfortunes, problems and unexpected support	13
Kolff's first survivor (September 1945)	16
Contributions of other investigators and criticism	16
The influence of Bull and coworkers in England and Borst in the Netherlands	17
Other dialysers	17
Parallel flow dialysers	19
The 'twin coil' dialyser (1955)	19
Access to the circulation (1960)	21
The Seattle dialysis system (1960)	24
The first successful chronic patients (1960)	28
Introduction of a central dialysate supply system (1964)	28
Another milestone: the start of regular dialysis treatment of terminal, irreversible renal failure (1960)	28
Home dialysis (1964)	28
The arteriovenous fistula (1966)	31
The roles of the ASAIO and the EDTA (founded in 1954 and 1964)	31
Further developments; the role of the industry	32
The square meter/hour and the middle molecule hypotheses (1965, 1971)	32
Short dialysis (1974)	33
The Seattle dialysis index	33
Progress in identification of middle molecules	33
Further progress in access to the circulation	34
Reuse of dialysis fluid (1969)	35
Sequential ultrafiltration and dialysis (1976)	35
Bicarbonate versus acetate	35
Haemoperfusion	35
Haemofiltration	36
Plasma exchange	36
Lipid abnormalities	37
Nephrogenic osteodystrophy and vitamin D	37
Aluminium toxicity in dialysis patients	38
Viral hepatitis	39
Dialysis treatment of 'non-renal' conditions	41
Some socio-economic considerations	41
A final word	42
Acknowledgments	43
References	44

THE INVENTION OF DIALYSIS

If somebody should be called the father of modern dialysis, the honour should go to a Scotsman, Thomas Graham (Figure 1), who lived from 1805-1869. He was appointed Professor of Chemistry at Anderson's University, Glasgow, in 1830 at the age of 25 (1), moving to the Chair of Chemistry at University College, London, in 1837 and was finally appointed Warden and Master Worker of the Mint, London, in 1855. Graham, an extraordinary genius, laid not only the foundation of what later became colloid chemistry, but also invented a method for separating gases by diffusion, which in later years was used for separating uranium 235 from the 238 isotope.

He demonstrated that vegetable parchment acted as a semipermeable membrane. After coating parchment with albumen to close defects, he stretched it over a wooden or guttapercha hoop, which he floated on water (Figure 2 [2]). Into this he placed, as on a seive, a fluid containing crystalloids and colloids and found that only the crystalloid material diffused through the parchment into the water. For this phenomenon Graham coined the name *dialysis*. In another experiment he used 0.5 l of urine and again demonstrated that crystalloid matter from the urine passed into the water which, after evaporation on a waterbath, yielded a white crystalloid mass which appeared to be mainly urea. Graham predicted that some of his findings, particularly those on osmosis, reported in 1854, might be applied to medicine.

THE FIRST 'ARTIFICIAL KIDNEY'

Graham's experiments conclusively demonstrated that this new dialysis procedure could remove solutes from fluids containing colloids and crystalloids. However, being a chemist, he did not proceed into the field of medicine and physiology. The next step, removing solutes through a semi-permeable membrane from the blood of an animal, did not take place for another fifty years and came from the United States. In 1913, John J. Abel (Figure 3) and his colleagues, Rowntree and Turner (3) of the Pharmacology Laboratory of the Johns Hopkins Medical School in Baltimore, described a method

... 'by which the blood of a living animal may be submitted to dialysis outside the body, and again returned to the natural circulation without exposure to air, infection by micro-organisms or any alteration which would necessarily be prejudicial to life'...

After making the animal's blood incoagulable with hirudin, they passed it from an arterial cannula through a series of tubes made of celloidin contained in a glass jacket filled with saline or artificial serum, returning

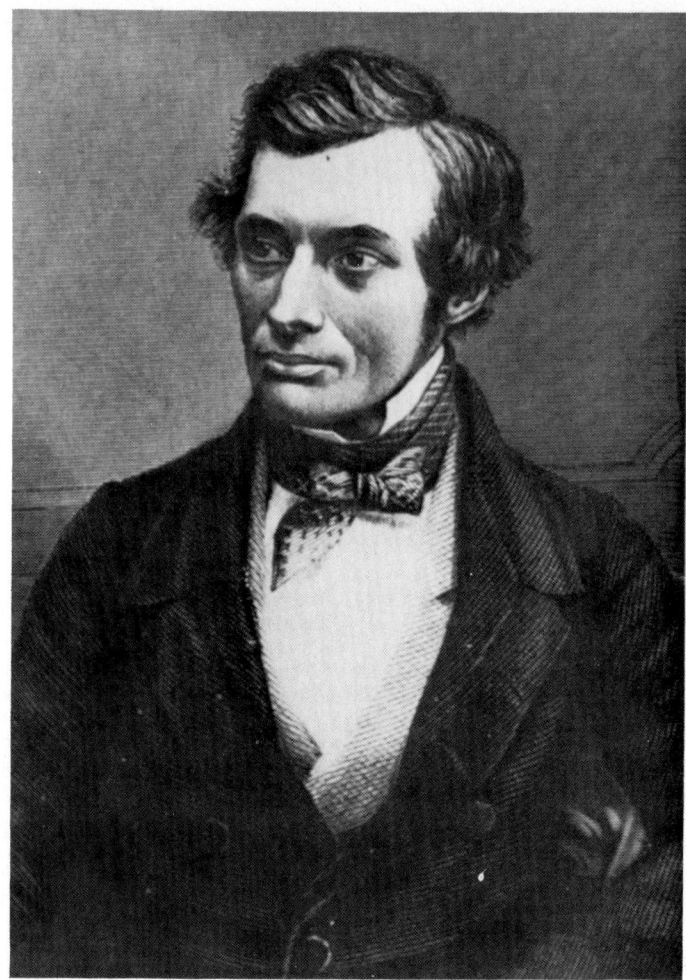

Figure 1. THOMAS GRAHAM (1805–1869), inventor of dialysis. (Engraving by C. Cook after a photograph by Claudet). From: J.S. Muspratt: *Chemistry theoretical, practical and analytical as applied and relating to the arts and manufactures*, vol. 1, Mackenzie 1853–1861.

the blood through another cannula into a vein of the animal.

Their dialyser, for which they coined the name *artificial kidney*, had a series of celloidin tubes of 8 mm diameter and 40 cm long fastened by tying with a string to a system of glass manifolds, branching dichotomously. Thus, the flow of blood took place horizontally, twice in each direction through 8 tubes in parallel (Figure 4). Abel and his co-workers soon became aware that only their most efficient apparatus (with 32 celloidin tubes) was suitable for larger animals of more than 20 kg weight. They suggested that flattening the tubes might improve the efficiency, more or less anticipating the flat tubing in today's coil dialysers. They mentioned also that ...'very small tubes would undoubtedly prove valuable when the necessary time and trouble are not prohibitive'... more or less predicting the hollow fiber type of dialysers in use today. With their apparatus, they removed from the dog either endogenous substances or foreign substances whose presence in excessive amounts endangered life. Subsequently, the investigators published in a series of articles (4–6) the results of dialysing nephrectomised dogs with their new '*vividiffusion*' apparatus, demonstrating that with a dialysing surface area of $0.32 \, m^2$ substantial quantities of non-protein nitrogen could be removed from the animals. However, the capacity of their dialyser was limited and insufficient for human application. The fragile and delicate celloidin tubes were also difficult to make and handle. They also encountered difficulties with clotting of blood since heparin was not available at that time. Hirudin, which they obtained by grinding up heads of leeches in solution (...'commercial preparations being too expensive'...), was also too toxic for human beings and was difficult to handle. However Abel and his associates developed a simple method of preparing a non-toxic hirudin solution (4) and they constructed several large surface area 'vividiffusion' devices, basically similar to

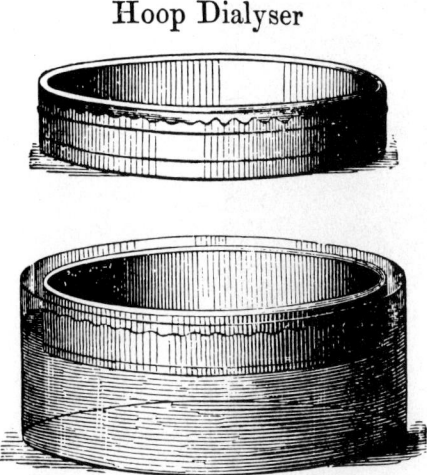

Figure 2. Hoop dialyser of Thomas Graham, with a 'dialytic septum' of parchment paper (1861 [2]).

their original apparatus but with 32 celloidin tubes instead of 16 and even with 192 tubes. The latter certainly must have had enough dialysing capacity for use in human patients (4).

Actually Abel was anxious to try his new invention in patients, as appears from the introductory paragraph of one of his papers, published in 1913 (4):

... 'There are numerous toxic states in which the eliminating organs of the body, more especially the kidneys, are incapable of removing from the body, at an adequate rate, the autochthonous or the foreign substances whose presence in excessive amount is detrimental to life processes. In the hope of providing a substitute in such emergencies, which might tide over a dangerous crisis ... we devised a method by which the blood ... may be submitted to dialysis outside the body'...

More than ten years later Abel wrote in a letter to Heinrich Necheles at Hamburg, Germany (see page 7) dated March 4, 1924:

... 'I personally also started out, quite contrary apparently to your conception of my purpose, with the view of relieving the kidney of human beings in certain pathological conditions'...

In a letter, dated December 16, 1930 to his previous co-worker Dr. Leonard Rowntree (then at the Mayo Clinic in Rochester, Minnesota) Abel refers to a paper published by Georg Haas of Gieszen, Germany, in Abderhalden's Handbuch (17) (see next section):

... 'You will see that he [*i.e. Haas*] has modified our method. He uses venous blood and circulates this blood in a dialysing apparatus and then returns it to the vein, taking about 500 ccs at a time from a human being'...

In his letter to Necheles, Abel writes (in 1924):

... 'My assistants and I had always hoped to try our apparatus on an appropriate case of kidney disease of mecurial [sic] poisoning and this was always in the backgrounds of our minds during the scientific work, which is represented in the paper reprints of which I am sending you. When the Great War came it was no longer possible for us to get leeches as these anilids ("Hirudo medicinalis") were imported by us in quantities of 1500 or more from Hungary. Shortly after the outbreak of the war indeed I had a consignment of 1500 leeches lieing [sic] at Copenhagen. The English Foreign Office ruled that this consignment was of "enemy origin" and the leeches were left to die at Copenhagen"...

As appears, however, from a letter, dated July 1, 1916 from the British Foreign Office, Abel could have had his leeches if he had applied to the British Government through the State Department at Washington for a transportation permit. He did not; however the unavoidable delay and the red tape would have resulted in the death of the leeches anyway... On the other hand, according to a footnote in the second article of Abel and his co-workers they could have obtained ... 'good medicinal leeches from France ... in lots of 100 or more from cupping barbers at the rate of $ 6 a hundred'..., which was rather cheap. According to the footnote there was also an American firm who hoped to be able to furnish the best leeches at $ 20-$ 25 a thousand. It remains unclear why Abel did not try to get leeches from 'non enemy origin' to continue his investigations.

In 1914 Abel stopped his work, because of the leeches problem, so never applied the 'vividiffusion apparatus' to a human being.

Even more than 15 years later Abel was still disappointed. In his letter to Rowntree (December 1930) he continues:

... 'As I read over the paper [*of Haas*] today I could not help thinking how unfortunate it was that our work was stopped by the World War when we were unable to obtain the supply of leeches. ... How would it be if a hospital such as yours would take up this whole subject again and train a special group of assistants and technicians to apply this venous method to chronic nephritics who are in the terminal stage of the disease and thus improve their condition and possibly prolong their life. I have always had the belief, and as I recall you agree with me, that something could be done by this method in cases of acute mercurial poisoning. If the blood could be washed every day, or every other day, in these cases at the time they become stuperous and unconscious, they might possibly recover. The kidney as I understood from the pathologists, has a great regenerative ability'...

It would be another 15 years until Abel's prediction became true: the first survivor from acute renal failure whose life was saved by an artificial kidney was dialysed by Kolff on the 3rd September 1945 (see page 16).

Interestingly, Dr. Leonard Rowntree witnessed one of the first clinical haemodialyses undertaken for acute poisoning about 40 years after Abel's letter at Georgetown, University Hospital in Washington, D.C.

Abel, Rowntree and Turner first demonstrated vividiffusion to their colleagues in Baltimore, on the 10th November 1912 and also demonstrated their invention in the summer of 1913 in London and at the Congress of Physiology in Groningen, The Netherlands. By coincidence a young Dutch doctor named Pim Kolff, working

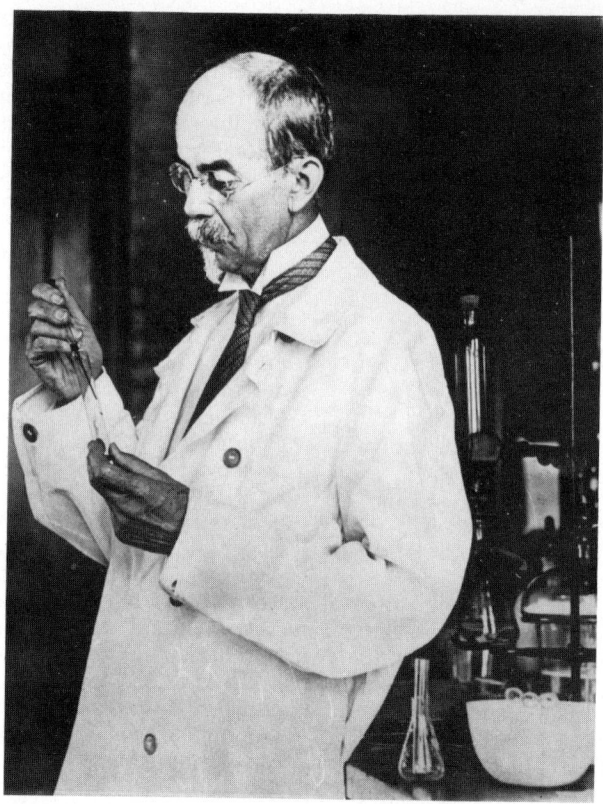

Figure 3. JOHN JACOB ABEL (1857–1938) 'a method has been devised by which the blood ... may be submitted to dialysis outside the body ...' (3).

in the Department of Medicine at the University Hospital also in Groningen started 25 years later his experiments, which led to the construction of an artificial kidney that was suitable for practical human application.

Various investigators attracted by the work from the Baltimore trio began using the new dialyser for experimental work. The two main problems, anticoagulation and a suitable membrane, remained major obstacles, however. In 1914 von Hess and McGuigan (7) used Abel's vividiffusion method in a series of experiments on the dog. They improved the apparatus by creating a pulsatile bloodflow through the celloidin tubes, which

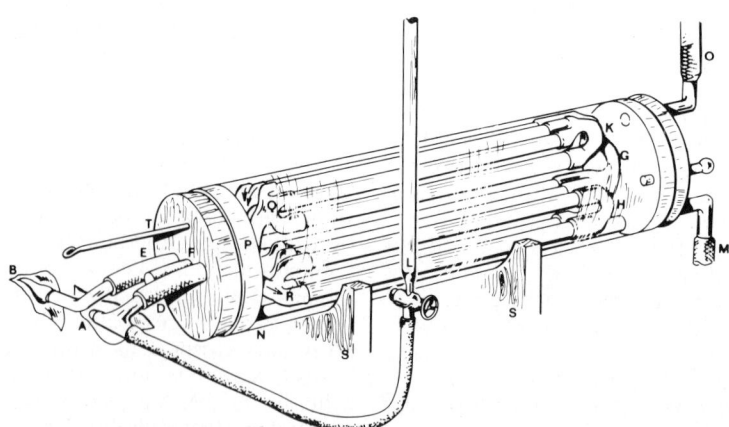

Figure 4. Vividiffusion apparatus of Abel, Rowntree and Turner with sixteen cellodin tubes (1913 [4]). (A) Arterial cannula; (B) Venous cannula; (L) Burette with hirudin solution; (M) Drain; (Q) and (R) Quadruple branch points; (O) Air outlet; (T) Thermometer.

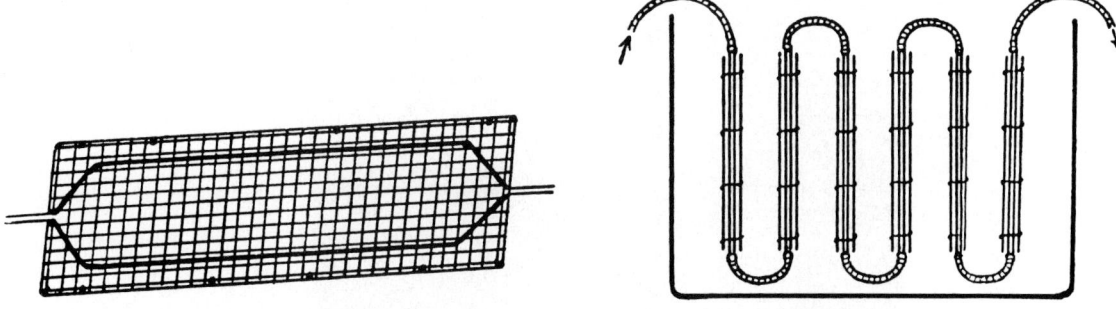

Figure 5a. Semipermeable conical tube prepared by Heinrich Necheles in 1925, compressed between metal wire grids (9, 10).

Figure 5b. Dialyser consisting of battery of 'gold-beater's skin' tubes in series constructed by Necheles (9, 10).

apparently helped inhibit clotting. They also enhanced the procedure by mixing the dialysate at short intervals or continuously, preventing formation of a stagnant layer of fluid around the dialysing tubes. This principle of turbulent dialysate flow was rediscovered some fifty years later and has found application in modern dialysers.

Several investigators on both sides of the Atlantic started preparing dialysis membranes from animal origin for dialysis purposes. Love (8) from Chicago used chicken intestines (1920). Necheles (9, 10) from Hamburg used semipermeable conical tubes made from visceral animal peritoneum (gold-beater's skin). These tubes were compressed between metal lattice screens in order to keep the blood volume small in relation to the dialysing surface area (1923). Necheles combined a number of his 'gold-beater's skin' tubes in series and was able to dialyse bilaterally nephrectomised uraemic dogs for several hours, using hirudin (Figures 5a and 5b). He noticed a striking improvement in their condition. Later working together with Lim (11) at the Peking Union Medical College in China, he continued his experiments with dogs, using heparin for the first time.

THE FIRST HUMAN DIALYSIS

The credit for the first human dialysis must go to Georg Haas (Figure 6) from Gieszen, Germany, who lived from 1886–1971 (12–17).

In 1911 Haas started working in Hofmeisters laboratory in Strassburg, Germany on amino acid synthesis *in vivo*; he wondered whether dialysis would help him in his so far negative experimental results, by separation of intermediate metabolic products from the blood. Therefore, he circulated blood from his animals through tubular membranes, which were prepared from reed stalks, by a procedure described by Philippson (18), who also worked in Hofmeisters laboratory, in 1902. These membranes apparently worked as dialysis membranes. Because of World War I Haas had to return to clinical work in 1914. Working in the Department of Medicine of the University Hospital at Gieszen and the local Military Hospital he was confronted with many cases of trench nephritis with rapid progression to fatal uraemia and Haas considered again a form of dialysis similar to his earlier animal experiments, instead of the customary procedures for uraemia like blood lettings, forced sweating sessions and dietary protein restriction.

... 'von der Annahme ausgehend, dass es sich bei der Urämie um der Retention von harnfähigen Stoffen handelt und dieselben wohl auch dialysabel seien, zog ich das dialysatorische Abtrennungsverfahren, das ich bei meinen intermediären Stofwechselstudien vorhatte durchzuführen, in Erwägung'... (16).*

Having no access to the literature which was published in the Allied countries during the war, Haas remained unaware of the work of the Baltimore trio which was published in 1913 shortly before the outbreak of World War I. He resumed his experimental work but soon encountered unsurmountable difficulties: trying again different membranes prepared from reed stalks, paper and animal peritoneum, which all proved unsuitable and having no other anticoagulants than crude and toxic hirudin, Haas abondoned the project in 1917 when he was sent to Rumania to combat epidemic typhus fever. Returning in 1919 to civil medical work in post war impoverished Germany, Haas had initially no facilities to resume his experimental work. However, the work on dialysis of uraemic dogs by his compatriot Heinrich Necheles (9, 10), published in 1923, rearoused Haas' interest in dialysis. He became aware of the work of an Austrian, Franz Pregl (19), who used celloidin tubes, similar to those made by Abel and his fellow workers, for dialysis purposes in his laboratory.

Haas acquired a great deal of skill in preparing long (1.20 m) tubes from this delicate material (Figure 7). He discovered that these tubes remained sterile when stored in 60% ethanol. He was able to construct a celloidin tube dialyser with a surface area of 1.5–2.1 m^2, which seemed suitable for human application (Figures 8 and 9).

---

* ... 'considering the hypothesis that uraemia is caused by retention of products which should be excreted in the urine and presumably can be removed by dialysis, I reconsidered my dialysis experiments from my previous metabolic studies'...

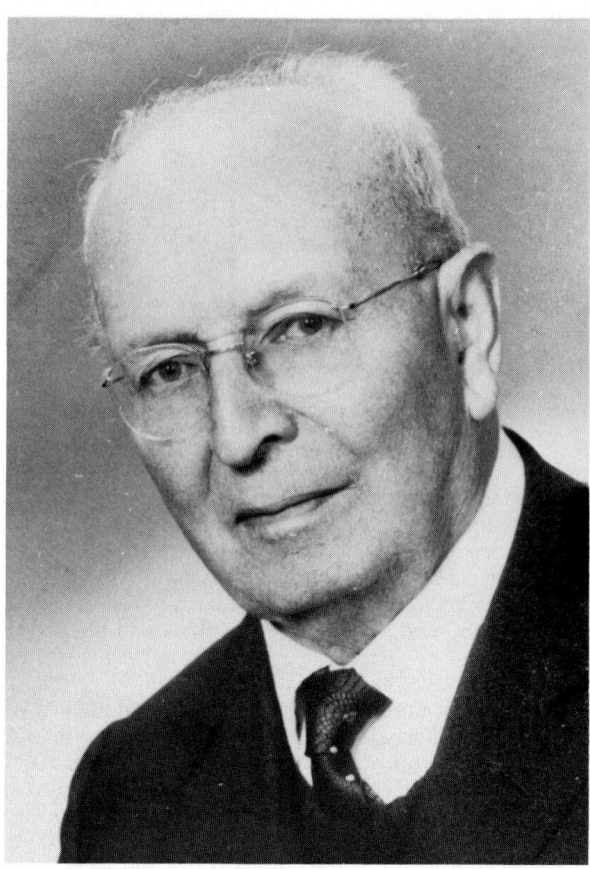

Figure 6. GEORG HAAS (1886–1971), who carried out the first human dialysis in 1924: '... because uraemia was a condition against which the doctor stands otherwise powerless ...' (15). Picture taken in 1968, at the age of 82.

The most serious obstacle was however to obtain a non-toxic and reliable anticoagulant, since heparin was not yet available for human application. He finally found a reasonably purified hirudin preparation of low toxicity. Using potassium iodide as a dialysable test substance, Haas performed a series of dialyses on the dog, most of them lasting ¾–1 hour. They were well tolerated and in an hour of dialysis complete removal of the iodide from the blood was apparently achieved.

Finally, he attempted dialysis in a patient with terminal uraemia: ...'because this was a condition against which the doctor stands otherwise powerless'... (13).

Assisted by a surgical colleague named von der Hütten, Haas performed the first human dialysis, according to Benedum (20, 21) in the autumn of 1924. This dialysis lasted 15 minutes. No complications occurred:

... 'Somit konnte zum ersten Mal gezeigt werden, dass eine Blutauswaschung durch Dialyse am Menschen

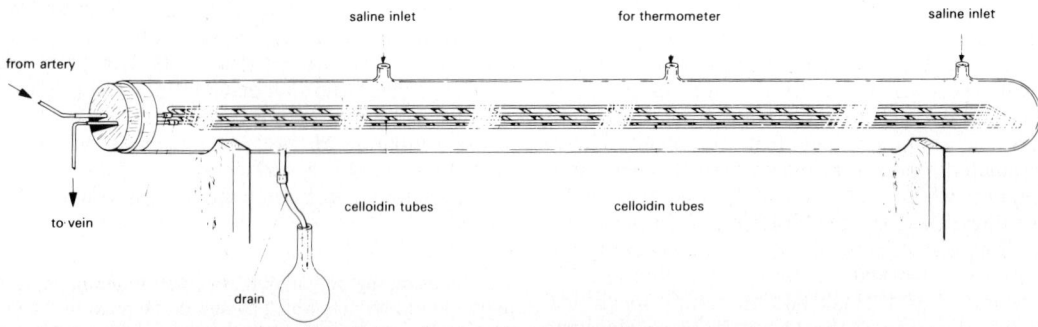

Figure 7. Glass container with pair of celloidin tubes, made by Georg Haas (1923 [17]).

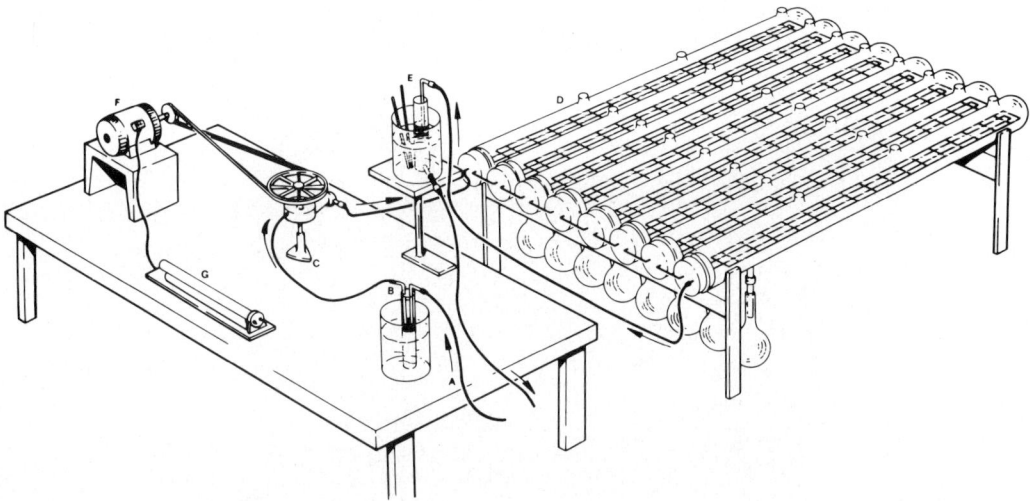

Figure 8. Battery of eight glass containers each with two celloidin dialysing tubes, used by Georg Haas in dog experiments (17). (A) Arterial bloodline; (B) Arterial blood container; (C) Blood pump; (D) Battery of dialysers with celloidin tubes; (E) venous blood collector.

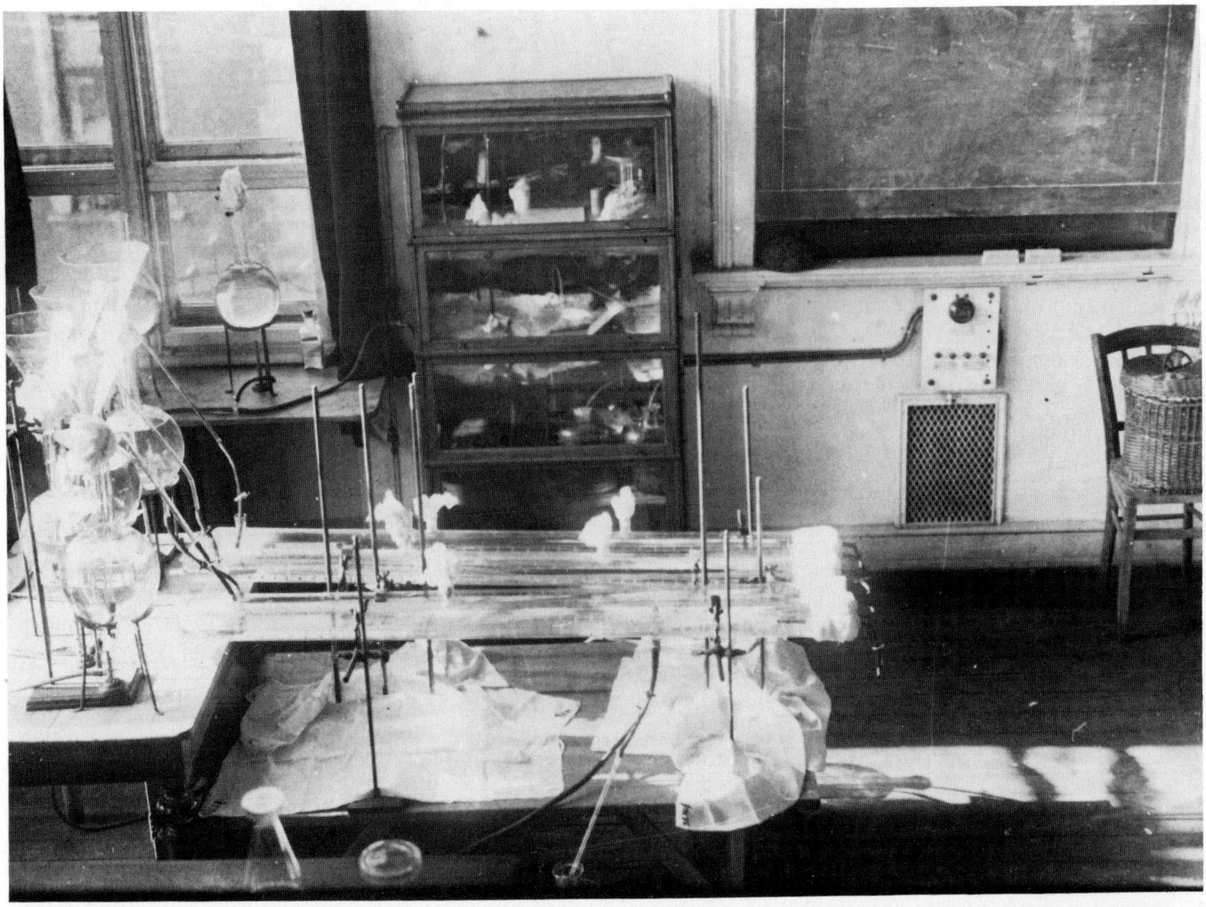

Figure 9. Battery of four glass containers with two celloidin dialysing tubes each ready, for use in a patient. Surface area appr. 2 m² (1926).

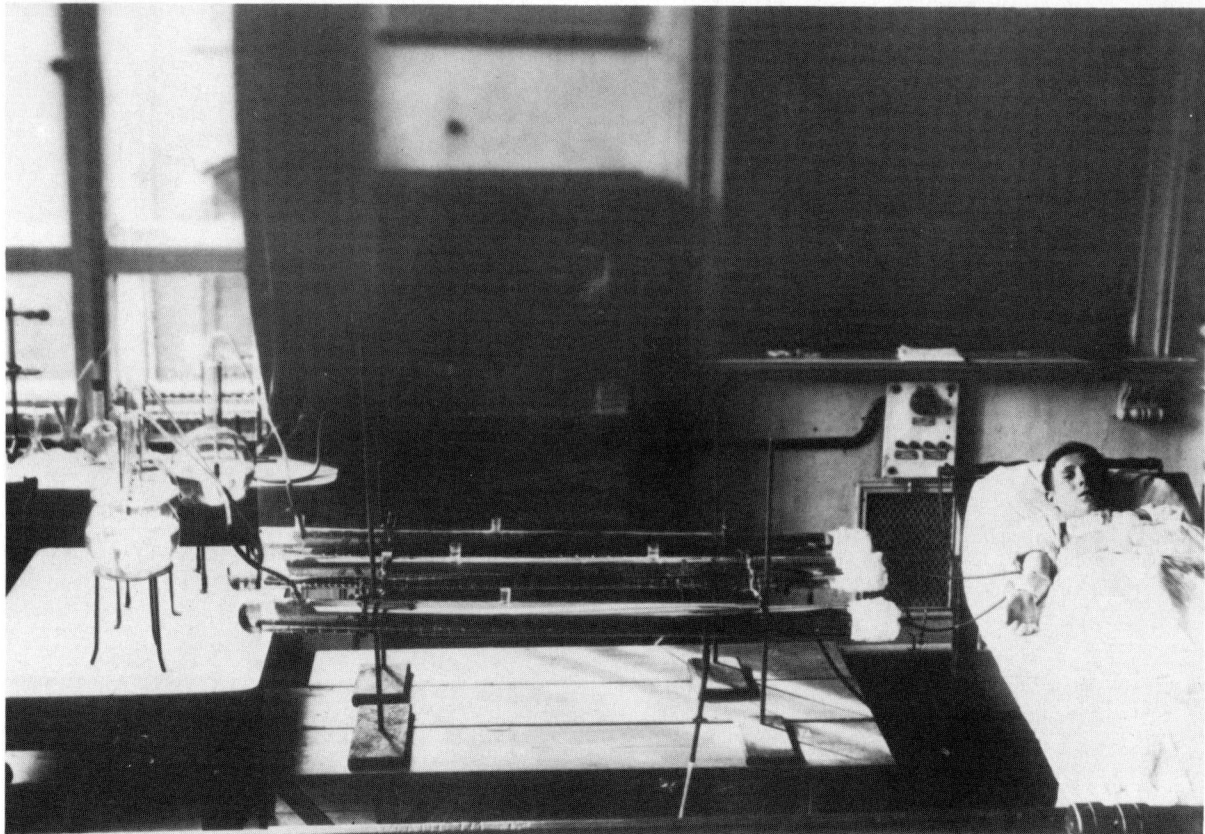

Figure 10. February 18, 1925: dialysis of a uraemic boy by Georg Haas in Gieszen with three glass containers each with two celloidin tubes. This was actually the second human dialysis recorded in literature (12-17, 21).

möglich und ohne jede Schädigung für den Patienten durchführbar ist'... (13).*

No further details of this dialysis have been recorded in literature, neither is a picture available.

The second dialysis occurred on the 18th of February 1925: Haas dialysed a youthful patient in the terminal stage of uraemia, using hirudin and a continuous circulation technique. The dialysis lasted 35 minutes and apart from a febrile reaction, the procedure was well tolerated, but of course had no therapeutic effect (Figure 10).

Subsequently, during 1926 Haas performed another four dialyses lasting from 30 to 60 minutes ([15, 21] Figure 11). Bleeding occurred from the surgical cannulation wounds and the gums, presumably caused by the anticoagulant.

Once a glass container had to be replaced because of rupture of a celloidin tube, which only took two minutes (21).

Some confusion has occurred from a personal statement of Haas in 1936 (17):

... 'Ohne Kenntnis der Abelschen Arbeiten versuchte ich aus therapeutischen Gesichtspunkten im Jahre 1915 zum ersten Mal die Blutwaschung am Lebenden mit Hilfe der Dialyse durchzuführen, und zwar beim Nierenkranken'...**

However neither case reports nor other particulars or results have been recorded in the literature. However according to Benedum (21) no practical attempt of a human dialysis was done in 1915; Haas apparently only *considered* such a procedure at that time.

Obviously Haas' dialysis procedures lasted too short for any significant therapeutic effect. The main drawback was the toxicity of the impure hirudin. This forced him to limit the dialysis sessions to 30-60 minutes: Haas always observed the basic principle of '*primum nil nocere*'.

Sometime elapsed before Haas again tried the new haemodialysis procedure for therapeutic purposes: in 1928 he reported on two cases (16): on the 13th January 1928 he treated a 55 kg uraemic man by fractionated dialysis, for the first time using a newly available, highly purified preparation of heparin and a dialyser of 1.5 m^2,

---

* ... 'This demonstrated for the first time that a purification of the blood by dialysis in a human being was possible without damaging the patient'...

** ... 'Without knowing of the work of Abel and collaborators I tried because of therapeutic considerations in 1915 for the first time a cleansing of the blood by means of dialysis in living individuals with kidney disease'...

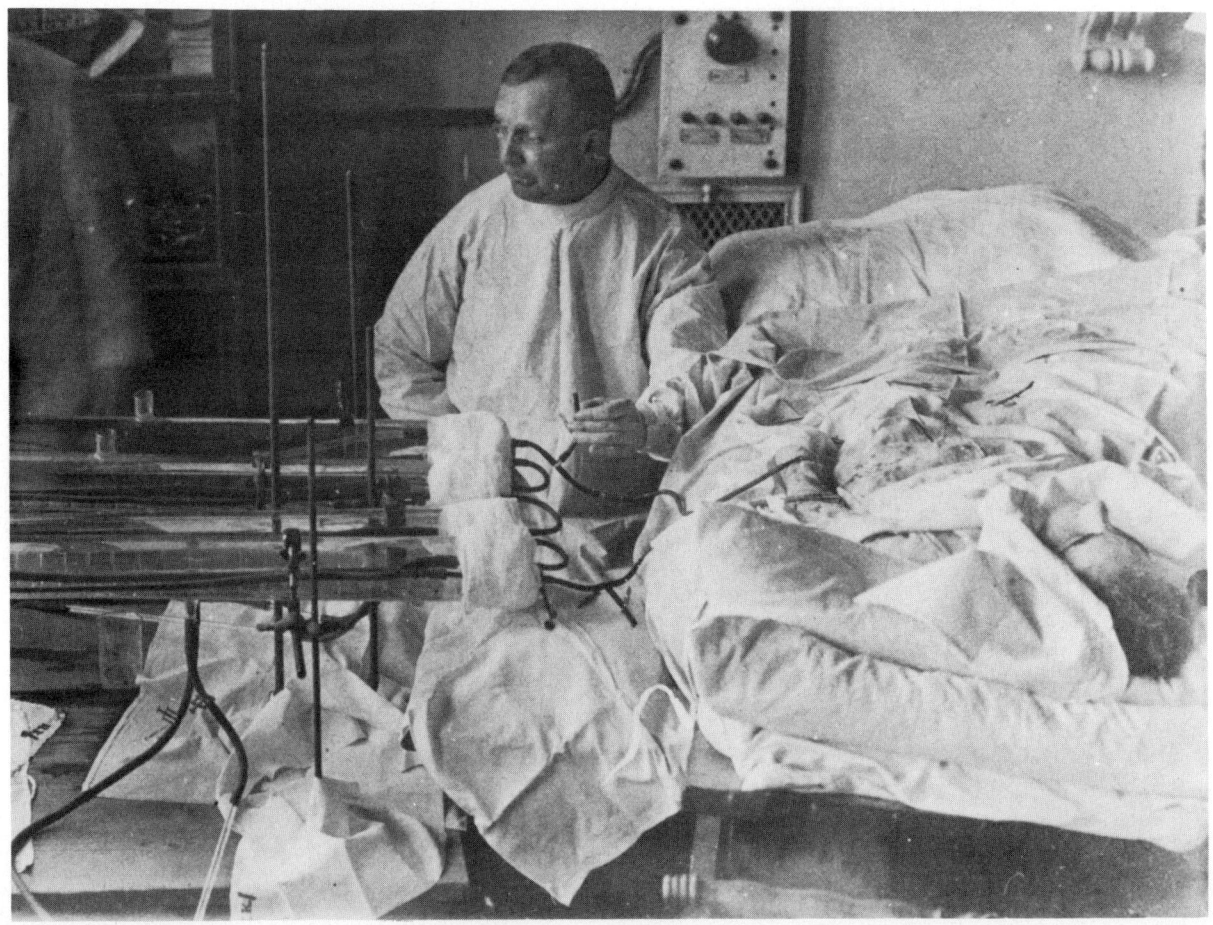

Figure 11. Georg Haas dialysing a uraemic girl. The apparatus consisted of four glass containers each provided with two celloidin dialysing tubes (1926). These experimental dialyses were performed in the lecture theatre of the Department of Medicine in Gieszen, Germany.

consisting of three pairs of celloidin tubes with a total length of 756 cm. Approximately 0.4 l of blood was taken, heparinised and circulated for half an hour through the dialyser, which was perfused with Ringer solution. The blood was reinfused into the same vein by means of a small funnel. The procedure was repeated nine times. The total removal of non-protein nitrogen was somewhat disappointing according to Haas; nevertheless the patient's clinical improvement was both subjectively and objectively impressive, lasting six days.

The second case was dialysed in a similar way on the 29th March 1928, the procedure being repeated after five weeks on 4th May 1928. After dialysing 500 ml of blood through a 2.1 m^2 celloidin dialyser, 2.5 g of non-protein nitrogen was removed with a gratifying symptomatic improvement. Blood pressure decreased from 205/100 to 145/95 mm Hg. Haas, who was obviously an astute observer, noted a temporary decrease in urine volume from 1000-1200 ml/24 h to 500 ml on the day after treatment. He offered several explanations for this phenomenon.

He also noted a decrease in the volume of the blood during the extracorporeal circulation. Actually, a loss of 100 ml from the 500 ml aliquot occurred during 30 min of dialysis. Haas discusses in his paper the explanation of this phenomenon, which actually was caused by ultrafiltration from positive pressure, not by osmotic fluid removal, because the dialysate was isotonic Ringer solution. He wondered whether this phenomenon could be of therapeutic value in cases of nephrotic oedema ... a cautious prophecy which later became true (22, 23).

At the end of one of his articles Haas, summarising his results, called them promising, but warns against overoptimism. His experience was only limited to a small number of experimental dialyses and Haas cautiously warned: 'one swallow does not make a summer'. His article published in 1928 (16) is a real classic in the field of dialysis.

Then follows a nine year interval of silence on the subject during which period two important advances were made: firstly purified heparin became readily available for human application and secondly a new cel-

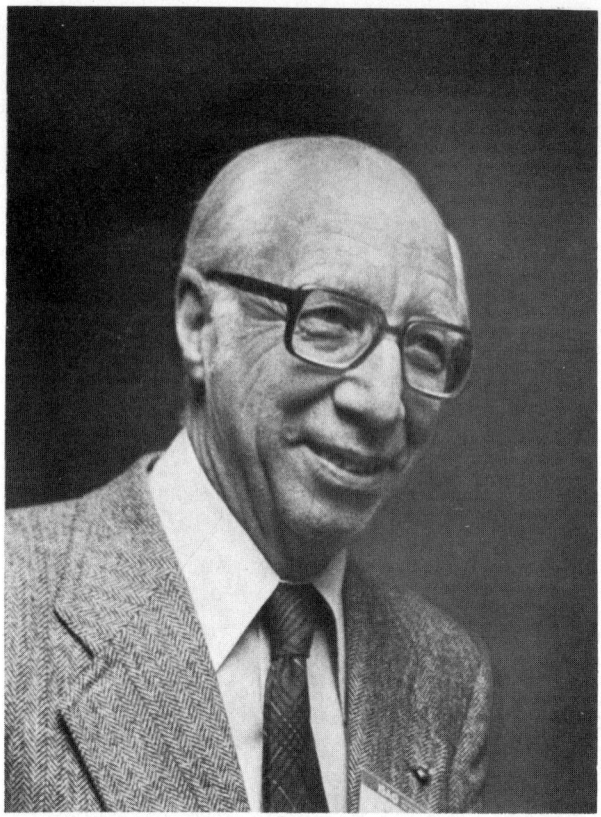

Figure 12. WILLEM ('PIM') JOHAN KOLFF M.D., Ph.D. (1979).

lulose product named cellophane was marketed, mainly for commercial use. In 1937, a short communication was published by William Thalhimer from New York (24), who had seen a demonstration of Abel's artificial kidney when he was a medical student at Johns Hopkins University. He initially did experimental work on the treatment of uraemia with exchange transfusions and then tried to use an artificial kidney for this purpose. He constructed a dialyser replacing Abel's celloidin tubes with cellophane sausage-tube made by Visking Casing Corporation in the United States, using heparin as an anticoagulant and dialysed nephrectomised dogs. He was, however, not very successful because the active surface of his dialyser was too small. Finally he turned again to exchange transfusions.

THE ROTATING DRUM DIALYSER, CONSTRUCTED BY KOLFF AND BERK

In the late 1930's, a young doctor named Willem ('Pim') Johan Kolff (Figure 12), entered the Department of Medicine at the Groningen University Hospital in the north of The Netherlands at the age of 27. What later could be called a definite break-through was a matter of chance and coincidence. It so happened that the young doctor Kolff had to treat Jan Bruning, a uraemic 22-year-old farmer's son, who died during Kolff's early training. His death made medical history. Kolff later described his feelings of frustration as a young and inexperienced physician. Feeling helpless and depressed by the terrible suffering of his patient, just as happened to Georg Haas ten years before, Kolff also began to think about an apparatus that could replace renal function and thereby save patients from death by uraemia (25). Unaware of previous publications, he met Dr. Brinkman, who was professor of biochemistry at Groningen University. He soon became young Kolff's stimulating adviser and showed him the 'wonders of cellophane'. At that time seamless cellophane tubing, used as sausage skin, had become commercially available and seemed to be an excellent material for dialysis. In order to determine how much cellophane was needed to construct an efficient artificial kidney for human use, Kolff took a 45 cm long piece of cellophane tubing, tied one end and filled it with 25 ml of water containing 0.1 g (1.6 mmol) of urea. The other end was also tied and the piece of tubing, fixed on a small wooden board, was rocked in saline (Figure 13). In 15 minutes all the urea had passed into the saline. Kolff repeated this experiment with 25 ml of blood, adding 400 mg (6.7 mmol) of urea and obtained similar results. By calculation, he deduced that at least 10 m of cellophane tubing were required to remove 2 g (33 mmol) of urea from 500 ml of blood in 15 min-

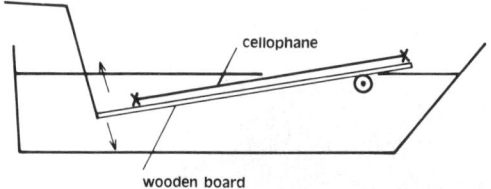

Figure 13. Kolff's first dialysis experiment: a piece of cellophane tubing filled with 'uraemic' blood and tied on a wooden board, rocked in saline (1938).

utes. Several types of apparatus were built, but not one appeared to be satisfactory.

On 10th May 1940, Hitler's armies invaded The Netherlands. Kolff's professor of medicine and his wife, who were Jews, committed suicide and a Dutch Nazi was appointed to the chair of medicine in Groningen. Kolff made an immediate decision. He left and found a job in the local hospital of the small town of Kampen. After settling in Kampen, Kolff started again to work on an artificial kidney. Eventually, he constructed, assisted by Hendrik Berk, who was an engineer and a managing director of Kampen's enamel factory (Figure 14), a 'dia-

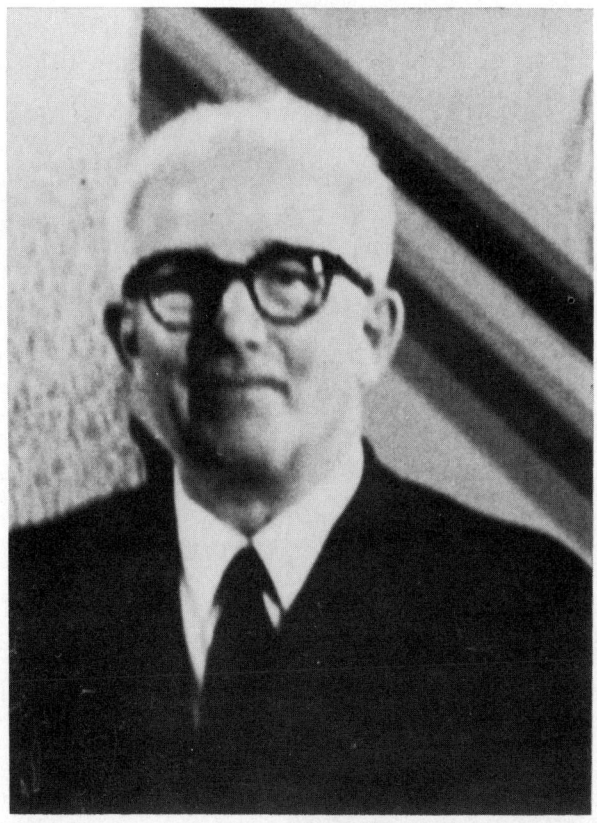

Figure 14. H.Th.J. (HENDRIK) BERK, who together with Kolff designed and constructed the rotating artificial kidney in Kampen in 1942–'43 (25–30). (Picture taken in 1968, at the age of 69).

lyser with a large surface area'. The apparatus consisted of a cylindrical drum (Figure 15a), originally made from an aluminium framework (Figure 15b). Later, drums were made from wooden laths as aluminium could no longer be obtained during the war (26–30). A 30 to 40 m length of $2\frac{1}{2}$ cm wide cellophane sausage tubing was wound on the cylinder to be perfused with the patient's blood through a rotating coupling which, according to Kolff, was copied from a Ford automobile waterpump (Figure 16). The lower half of the rotating drum was immersed in a stationary tank containing 70 l (later 100 l) of dialysis fluid.

It was actually Berk who suggested placing the drum horizontally instead of vertically, thereby making it possible to propel the blood along the cellophane tubing by rotation of the drum, eliminating the use of a bloodpump.

Meanwhile, purified heparin had become available and in February 1943 Kolff decided to dialyse the blood of an old gentlemen with endstage uraemia, caused by prostatic hypertrophy. He took 50 ml of blood from a vein, which was circulated through the rotating drum kidney machine and returned to a burette. By raising the burette the dialysed blood was reinfused in the patient through the same needle. When this was tolerated the procedure was repeated several times with increasing volumes of blood. No clinical effect was noted: the patient remained unconscious and died soon after the procedure (31). Kolff's next patient, Janny Schrijver, was a 29-year-old housemaid with contracted kidneys and malignant hypertension (26–30). Upon admission she had terminal uraemia and cardiac failure. Her blood pressure was 245/150 mm Hg. Initially fractionated dialysis was performed, beginning with dialysis of 50 ml of blood. The first day, actually the 17th March 1943, 0.5 l of blood was dialysed and during subsequent days, 1.5, 3.5, 4.5 and 5.5 l per day were dialysed. Six fractionated dialyses were performed and after each treatment Janny's condition improved remarkably. With the 7th treatment, Kolff changed to continuous dialysis, taking the blood from a femoral artery by needle puncture, circulating it through the kidney machine and reinfusing the 'washed' blood by puncture of a peripheral vein. Subsequently, he had to use a radial artery and surgical cutdowns into the vessels became necessary for access to the circulation. This frequently caused bleeding during heparinisation. Finally Kolff and his team experienced increasing difficulties with obtaining access to the circulation and when the 11th and 12th dialysis failed because no further arteriotomies and venesections were possible, further dialysis had to be abandoned. The patient died on the 26th day of treatment.

MISFORTUNES, PROBLEMS AND UNEXPECTED SUPPORT

Fate had it that the Kolff team had to struggle with a multitude of technical difficulties and problems such as membrane leaks, haemolysis, bloodline disconnections, haemorrhages and all kinds of other misfortunes. After this initial experience, they were not discouraged, how-

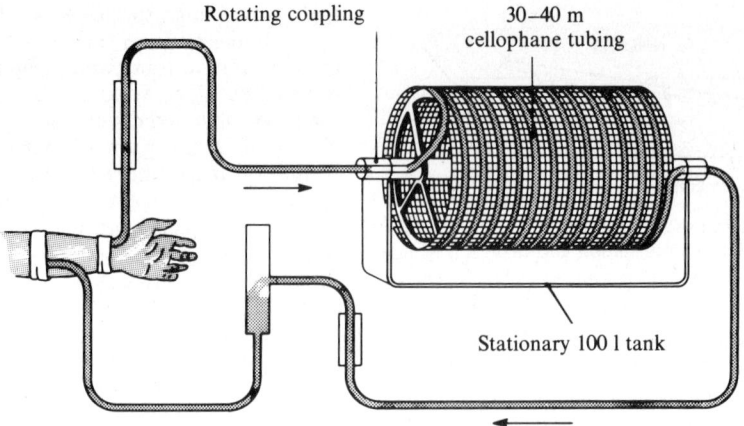

Figure 15a. Flow diagram of Kolff's rotating artificial kidney (25–30).

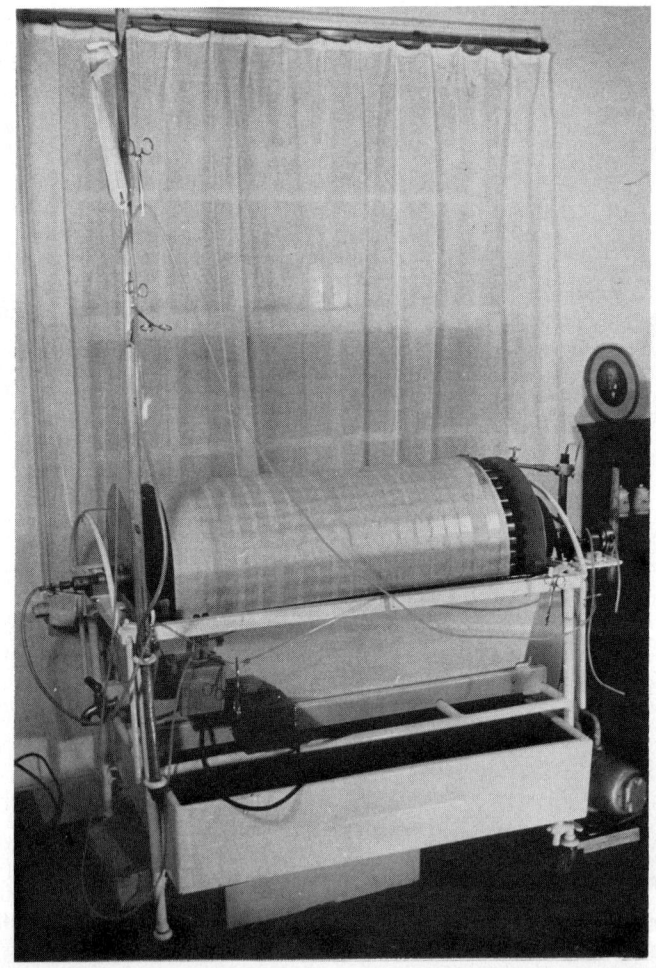

Figure 15b. Kolff's original rotating artificial kidney, used for dialysing his first patient at Kampen, The Netherlands (1943).

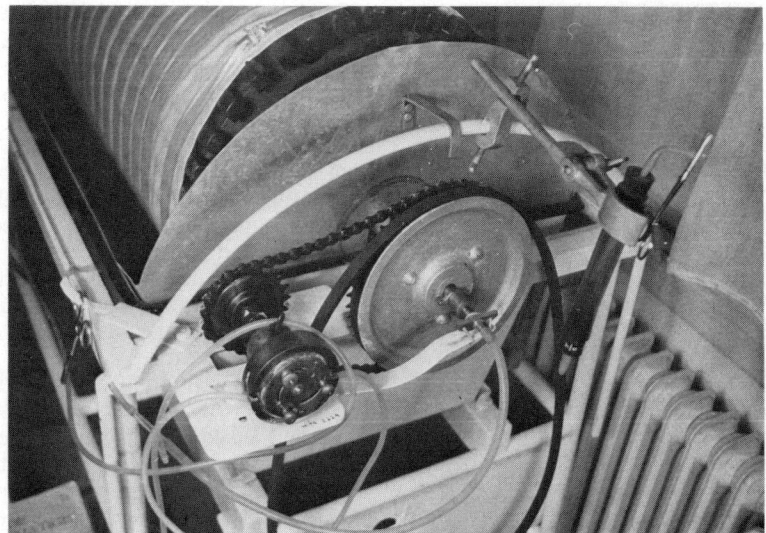
Figure 16. Rotating joint of the first rotating drum dialyser, copied from a Ford automobile waterpump (1943).

ever, and were resolute to continue their efforts. Kolff's tenacious character and his perseverance have been determinants of the further course of events. However, Kolff's initial ideal, the treatment of uraemic patients with irreversible chronic renal failure by repeated dialysis, seemed still far away. Obviously, the major obstacle was achieving repeated access to the bloodstream, a problem which had to wait for another 20 years before a new approach was made. In 1946, Kolff wrote in his thesis:
> ... 'in cases of chronic (irreversible) uraemia there is in general no indication for treatment with the artificial kidney. However temporary aggravation of chronic uraemia caused by intercurrent infection, diarrhoea or surgery could benefit from a dialysis to tide the patient over the critical period'...

Kolff tried, after these initial experiences, to limit his dialysis efforts to patients with reversible (acute) renal failure. Between the 17th March 1943 and the 27th July 1944, 15 patients were treated. Only one survived, a man treated with a sulpha drug for lobar pneumonia, who became anuric (a common complication of sulphonamide therapy in those days). One dialysis reduced his blood urea from 220 to 102 mg/dl (37 to 17 mmol/l). The next day his ureters were unblocked and cleared from sulphonamide crystals. Kolff wrote later:
> ... 'I never thought nor said that this man's life was saved by the artificial kidney, he might have survived without dialysis when the unblocking procedure had been done first'...

Interestingly Kolff got quite unexpected assistance for his clinical investigations with his new device. Located at Kampen was a state chemistry laboratory which did investigations for the Government in the new land reclaimed from the Zuiderzee. All important of course were sodium (and chloride) analyses of the soil drained from seawater. Sodium at that time was chemically analysed, a laborious and time consuming procedure with uranylacetate as major test substance. During World War II this compound soon became unavailable because uranium was precious war material both in Nazi Germany and in the Allied countries.

At that time Zeiss, the well-known optical firm in Germany, had constructed a flame emission photometer, which however was only suitable for potassium analysis.

The director of the soil laboratory was an agricultural engineer named W. R. Domingo (Figure 17). Domingo designed and built his own flame photometer which was suitable both for sodium and potassium analysis (32).

Kolff and Domingo met by coincidence at a house of a Domingo relative and started talking about their mutual fields of interest and electrolyte problems. Domingo offered to help Kolff with fast and accurate sodium and potassium analyses for his dialysis patients.

After the liberation of The Netherlands by the Allied armies Domingo constructed sodium/potassium flame photometers for the Hammersmith Hospital in London, England, the Queen Wilhelmina Hospital in Amsterdam, The Netherlands and several other hospitals.

During these war years, Kolff and his team had to fight an increasing number of other problems and misfortunes: as plastic tubing was not yet available, they had to use and to reuse rubber tubing over and over again, because it was often difficult or impossible to obtain fresh supplies. Pieces had to be put together by glass tubes (where cotting often started!), heparinisation was still a problem, penicillin had become available in the Allied armies but not in the occupied countries. New venipuncture needles were not available: the old ones had to be reused and resharpened, but they became rusty on the inside and clotted easily.

Finally, conditions in the Netherlands became increasingly difficult and transportation of seriously ill patients became virtually impossible so that suitable patients for dialysis treatment could no longer be sent to

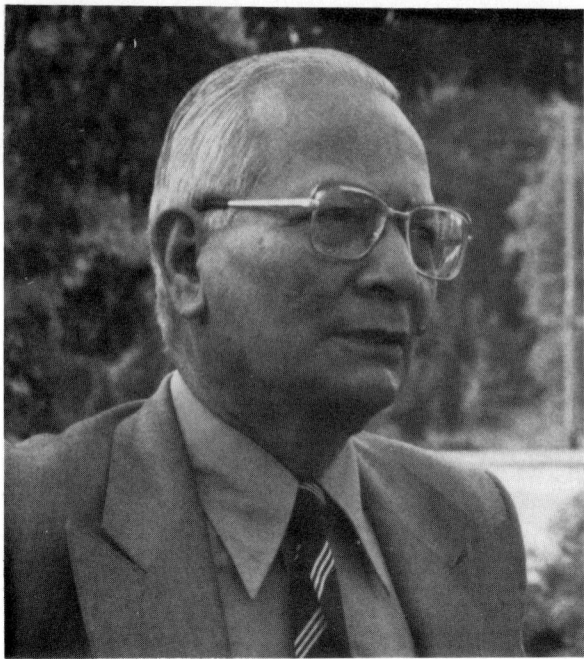

Figure 17. W.R. (RUUD) DOMINGO, who constructed the first flame photometer suitable for both sodium and potassium analysis (32) and who assisted Kolff with electrolyte chemistry.

Kampen, a town too small to provide an adequate number of patients locally. Kolff himself, however, was convinced that his machine was a workable device and that one day or another its value would be recognised. In later years, Kolff wondered what would have happened to his project had he not been working in occupied Holland under grim war conditions, but under more normal peaceful conditions after having treated 15 patients without a single definite therapeutic success. His coworkers and his nursing team were also convinced that one day or another the success would come and were prepared to work day and night to help Kolff with his efforts. Undoubtedly, the war and occupation made the Dutch extremely motivated to help each other and to save their sick compatriots.

During the last year of the war, conditions became critical. Aggressiveness of the Nazis against the Dutch population sharply increased and made further use of the artificial kidney impossible. Kolff had to interrupt his dialysis programme and had to wait for another suitable case to prove that his rotating dialyser could be life saving until a few months after the liberation of The Netherlands by the Allied armies.

KOLFF's FIRST SURVIVOR

Patient no. 17 was a 67-year-old female Nazi collaborator, who was after the liberation of The Netherlands imprisoned in the military barracks of the city of Kampen. She was admitted as an acute patient to the Kampen Hospital on 3rd September 1945, suffering from acute cholecystitis with jaundice and acute renal failure with anuria, presumably caused by the treatment with a sulphonamide drug. Her condition worsened, blood urea increased from 200 to 400 mg/dl (33-67 mmol/l) and finally the patient was transferred to Kolff's 'kidney room'. At that time she was unconscious and apparently in end stage uraemia. She was dialysed for 11 hours, regained consciousness and improved dramatically. Diuresis started within a week and the patient made a good recovery. She was the first patient who owed her life to treatment with an artificial kidney (30). She died six years later at the age of 73 from an unrelated disease.

After the liberation of The Netherlands, Kolff went to the office of the British Information Service at The Hague and asked the medical officer if he knew of an artificial kidney developed during the war in the free world. Apparently the man did not know and Kolff concluded that none had been constructed. Actually, he was wrong since Haas in Germany had already constructed a dialyser and used it clinically in 1924 (13-17) and at the Toronto General Hospital in Canada Murray, Delorme and Thomas (33), unaware of Kolff's work, constructed during World War II a coil type artificial kidney, incorporating small bore cellophane tubing, wound around a vertical, stationary drum. This dialyser was successfully used for patients at the end of 1946.

The dialysis equipment constructed in the pre-Kolff years by the Baltimore trio, by Georg Haas, Heinrich Necheles and by Thalhimer should be considered as precious relics of a period of experimental dialysis. It was Georg Haas who performed the first human dialysis, but it should be emphasised that Kolff's rotating dialyser was the first model that in practice was suitable for human application and it was in particular Kolff who made clinicians and experimentalists interested in the treatment of uraemia.

During the last year of World War II, when Kolff and his team had to interrupt their experimental work and had to put their machine temporarily out of use, they used their forced sparetime to make more artificial kidneys, receiving help from Dutch patriots wherever it was possible and even from Dutch Government officers who welcomed the opportunity to dodge or to circumvent the regulations and the supervision of the Nazi occupiers (25).

CONTRIBUTIONS OF OTHER INVESTIGATORS AND CRITICISM

When the war was over, Kolff gave these machines away to several hospitals, to make people familiar with the technology of dialysis. One machine went to the Royal Post Graduate School at Hammersmith Hospital in London, where a dialysis programme was promptly started by Bywaters and Joekes (34) who reported on their first series of 12 patients in 1948. Another was donated to the Mount Sinai Hospital in New York (Fishman et al [35]). One was sent to the Royal Victoria Hospital in Montreal and observations made with this dialyser were reported by DeLeeuw and Blaustein (36). Another machine was donated to professor Borst in Amsterdam, but was never used. Borst taught students that he never needed an artificial kidney machine and that the one he had was stored in the loft of his department in a somewhat rusty condition... Another rotating artificial kidney was sent to Poland. It went finally to the Department of Urology at the Jagiellonian University of Cracow, but was never extensively used for technical reasons and lack of trained personnel (Tadeusz Orlowski, personal communication to the author, 1977).

Others built their own machines, often with modifications and improvements. Darmady (37) a pathologist at Portsmouth and in the Isle of Wight built a rotating artificial kidney in 1946. He emphasised that it was important that the amount of blood which entered and left the machine should be controlled and provided his machine with synchronised inflow and outflow pumps. The system produced a certain amount of agitation and he pointed to the importance of turbulence which enhanced dialysis efficiency. This was later confirmed by several clinical investigators. His machine however was to bulky, therefore Darmady also constructed a machine of simpler design by passing a cellophane tube through a series of plates 1/16th inch (1,6 mm) apart. This provided a large dialysing surface and the flow of dialysing fluid passed along a number of small grooves in the plates, which allowed the dialysing fluid to flow from the centre outwards in either direction. Unfortunately, this machine for several reasons, did not produce as satisfactory dialysis as his rotating design.

Perhaps the most successful modification of the original rotating machine was that constructed in Boston, the Kolff-Brigham machine (38). It popularised dialysis in the United States and undoubtedly reduced mortality in acute renal failure during the Korean war. Above all it brought together teams of surgeons and physicians interested both in conservative and active methods of treating patients with acute reversible types of renal failure. Gradually, as experience grew, the complete natural history of the syndrome was established.

The Kolff-Brigham machine was improved by the French firm Usifroid for the Necker Hospital in Paris and was adopted by several other hospitals in Europe, the Middle East and even for the USSR. The team at the General Infirmary at Leeds, England increased its dialysing surface area to 3.2 m^2 (the Usifroid Model B) and still uses it occasionally for hypercatabolic patients with acute renal failure particularly in those with potential bleeding problems, for the blood is transported through the machine by friction, thereby preventing deposition of formed elements in the blood. Regional heparinisation is rarely required when the rotating model is used. (F. M. Parsons: personal communication).

THE INFLUENCE OF BULL AND CO-WORKERS IN ENGLAND AND BORST IN THE NETHERLANDS

Interest in the new way of treating uraemia slowly increased. But others, like Bull and co-workers (39) at the Hammersmith Hospital in London, who were acquainted with Kolff's dialysis technique, had other views: believing that dialysis treatment had to be avoided they preferred conservative treatment by feeding the patient a high calorie, protein free diet, with peanut oil and dextrose, given by stomach tube. On the continent, Borst (40) started from the same basic principles, feeding his uraemic patients sugar and butter balls and a gruel of custard powder, sugar, butter and water. Both groups claimed satisfactory results:

...'both starvation ... (and) injury of the erythrocytes by dialysis in the artificial kidney may be harmful'... (40)

...'Dialysis methods have their dangers and we believe that where this (peanut and oil regimen) is started, early dialysis should not be undertaken'... (39).

Both Borst and Bull were in their time and in their countries powerful and influential men. Both, at a time when pacemakers, respirators and artificial organs were still unknown, disliked medical machines and strongly opposed Kolff's 'gadgeteering'.

After the war, Kolff received little support and co-operation in Europe, but got more attention in America during a tour in 1947. He finally left The Netherlands in 1950, settling in the Cleveland Clinic, Cleveland, Ohio.

OTHER DIALYSERS

Soon after Kolff's (41) first series of publications, other dialysers were constructed, all based on the same principles and using cellophane tubing as a dialysing membrane. The goal now became to build a dialyser with a large active surface area and a limited blood volume. Therefore, in several designs the cellophane tubing was enclosed between screens or grids as Necheles had done in 1923 (9).

Nils Alwall, in Lund, Sweden (42–44) wrapped 10 to 11 m cellophane tubing around a metal screen and surrounded this in his first dialyser by a second screen, as a corset fitted around the body (Figure 18). The dialyser was placed in a glass tank, containing 25 l of dialysis fluid. In a later model, 20 m cellophane tubing was used with a dialysing area of about 1.6 m^2 and the inner

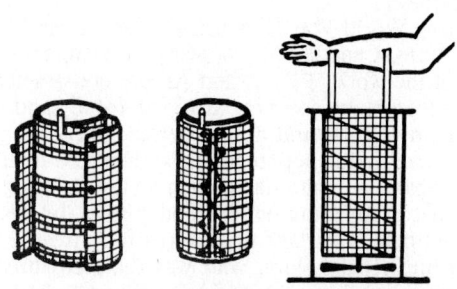

Figure 18. First Alwall dialyser (1946–1947): 10–11 m cellophane wrapped around a metal screen surrounded by a 'corset' (42).

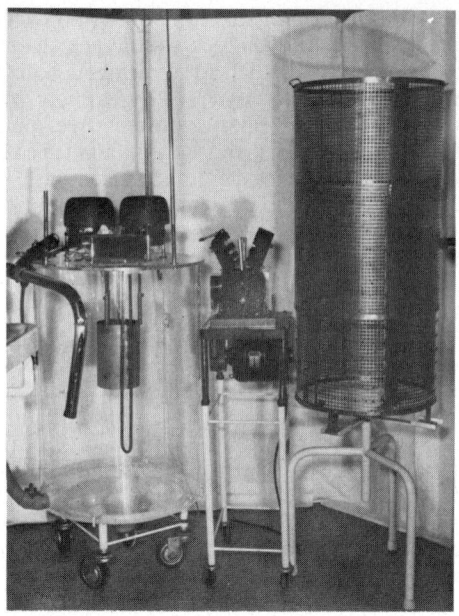

Figure 19. Alwall dialyser (1952 [44]). Glass tank, metal inner and outer screen. Centre: Sigma motor bloodpump.

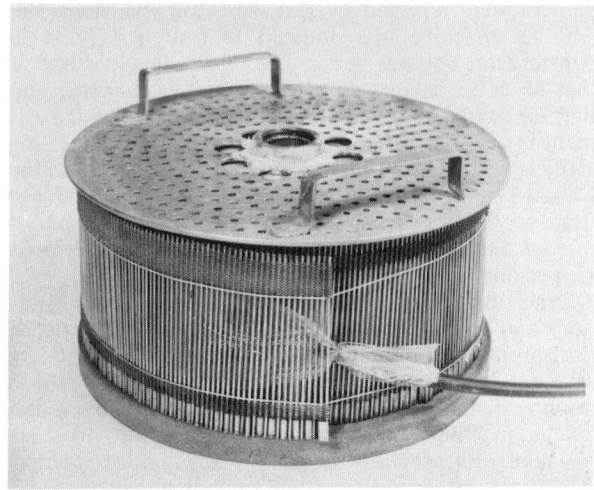

Figure 20. Stationary coil dialyser with cellophane tubing wrapped between a long strip with vertical stainless steel rods, constructed by Bodo von Garrelts, Stockholm, Sweden in 1947 (49). The surface area was later enlarged to 1.92 m^2; blood volume 675 ml (50). This device was a precursor of the pressure cooker dialyser constructed by Inouye and Engelberg in 1953 (51 [Figure 21]).

cylinder with the membrane was placed within a tight fitting metal screen outer jacket. The space between the two cylinders was so calculated that the cellophane tubing could only contain a thin layer of blood (Figure 19 [44]). This dialyser, marketed by a Swedish firm, had the advantage that a controllable ultrafiltration could be achieved. Nevertheless, it never gained very much popularity.

Alwall (45–47) pioneering like Kolff and having similar misfortunes and also a high mortality in his first series of patients, was criticised in a similar way. Even in his own hospital his colleagues invented a new-term: when a terminally ill patient died despite dialysis and came to autopsy, his critics talked about dialysis treatment as having been 'alwalled' ... (personal communication from Mrs. Alwall to the author, 1976).

Perhaps one of the most important aspects of Alwall's stationary coil type of dialyser is that it foreshadowed the construction of a new generation of coil type artificial kidneys.

During World War II, Murray, Delorme and Thomas in Toronto, Canada (33, 48, see p. 16) apparently unaware of the work of Kolff and Alwall, constructed independently a static coil type artificial kidney and started, after many efforts and a considerable period of experimenting, dialysing nephrectomised dogs and finally used their apparatus in human patients (1946), using a specially designed, atraumatic blood pump. In 1947 they reported details of their first successfully treated patient with acute renal failure, who was dialysed three times and recovered fully. Interestingly, they attached the patient to their machine by passing a catheter through a saphenous vein into the inferior vena cava and another catheter into the opposite femoral vein, a method which is still frequently used for access to the circulation in patients with acute renal failure (48).

In Sweden Von Garrelts (49, 50) constructed a rather compact coil dialyser by wrapping cellophane tubing together with a separating device like a rope-ladder with multiple vertical metal rods, not only supporting the membrane but also allowing the dialyser to be perfused by the dialysate solution (Figure 20). This dialyser was more or less a precursor of the *coil type* of artificial kidney constructed in 1953 by Inouye and Engelberg in Philadelphia, PA (51, 52 [Figure 21]). These investigators developed a coil type of artificial kidney, using cello-

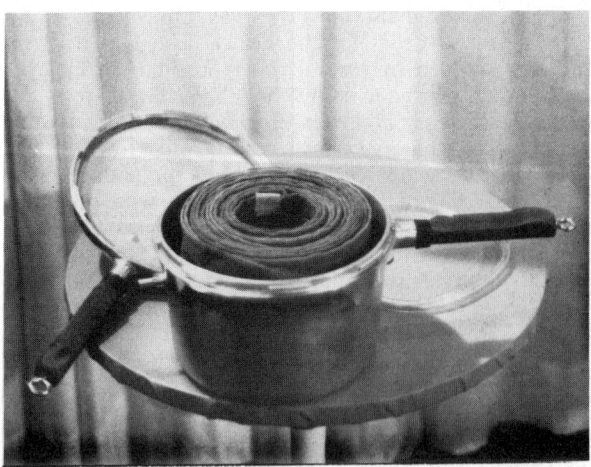

Figure 21. 'Pressure cooker' dialyser, developed by Inouye and Engelberg (51) in 1952–1953. This coil dialyser acted as a model for the ‚twin coil kidney' of Kolff and Watschinger.

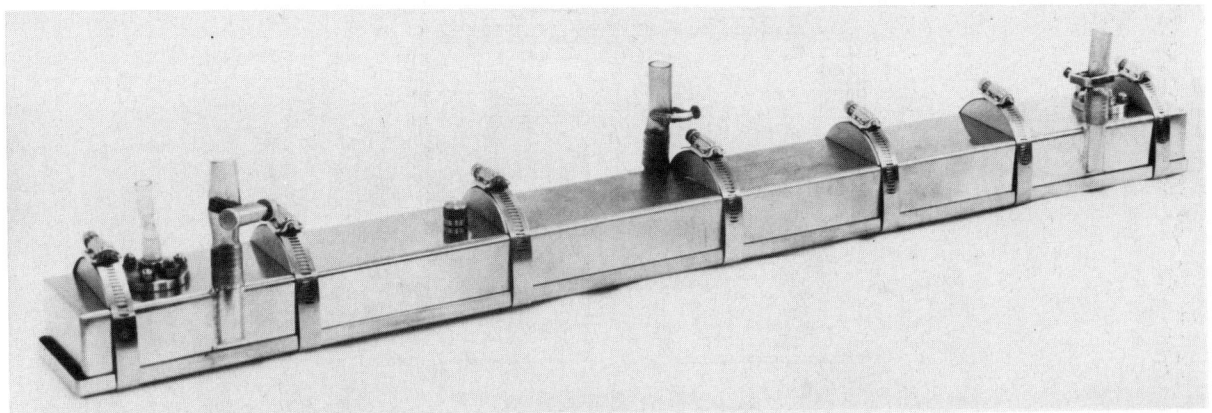

Figure 22. Plate dialyser constructed in 1947 by McNeill and associates, Buffalo NY (56–58). This dialyser was the prototype of a new generation parallel flow dialysers (see text).

phane tubing wound into a helix round a stainless steel core together with a strip of plastic mesh, acting as a spacer. The coil, having a surface area of $0.9\,m^2$ was placed in a cheap pressure cooker through which dialysis fluid was recirculated from a 50 l tank. The blood could be circulated either with or without a blood pump and ultrafiltration could be regulated by controlling the rate at which dialysing fluid was drawn into the dialyser by a waterpump. This coil dialyser acted as a model for the 'twin coil kidney' of Kolff and Watschinger (53, 54, see p. 20). This 'pressure cooker' design seems also a precursor of Michielsen's (55) Recirculating Single Pass (RSP) coil unit, developed about ten years later.

At that time, basically two types of artificial kidneys had been constructed: the rotating type with the cellophane tubing wrapped around a rotating drum and a stationary type like the Alwall model, the Murray dialyser and the Inouye and Engelberg coil dialyser.

PARALLEL FLOW DIALYSERS

Meanwhile, another type of stationary dialyser was developed. MacNeill and colleagues from Buffalo, N.Y. (56–58) constructed in 1947 a dialyser built from short lengths of flattened cellophane tubes, 28 of which were stacked together separated by specially prepared screens, made from nylon mesh. The appearance of the MacNeill dialyser (Figure 22) had much in common with the multiple layer Gambro dialyser, marketed 20 years later. The MacNeill dialyser was portable but not disposable and had to be rebuilt and sterilised for every dialysis procedure. In fact it was the prototype of a new generation of dialysers: *the parallel flow type.*

In 1948, Skeggs and Leonards of Western Reserve University, Cleveland, Ohio (59, 60) described a different type of parallel flow dialyser,
... 'consisting of a variable number of units, connected in parallel, each consisting of a single sheet of cellophane and two rubber pads (appr. $30 \times 45 \times 0.6$ cm), the inner surfaces of which were finely grooved'...

Later, they used two sheets of cellophane between the rubber pads, the blood flowing between the two cellophane membranes and the grooves in the pads carrying the dialysis fluid in the opposite direction on the outer surface of the cellophane. This was the first use of the *counter current principle.* As many units as desired could easily be assembled one above the other and clamped with a holder made of two flat steel plates. The dialyser could be steam sterilised and could be perfused by arterial pressure without the aid of a blood pump. The blood volume of the dialyser was relatively small compared with the dialysing surface area.

Claus Brun built in Copenhagen a $4\,m^2$ Skeggs-Leonard's machine which must have been the largest in the world. It was theoretically $4\,m^2$ but probably channelling gave a smaller effective area.

THE 'TWIN COIL' DIALYSER

In 1955, haemodialysis was still only available in a few hospitals and was applied only in exceptional cases. Many considered the procedure as experimental, laborious, expensive and dangerous. Many doubted its value.

At the first meeting of the American Society for Artificial Internal Organs on the 5th of June 1955, Watschinger and Kolff (53, 54) reported on further development of the artificial kidney of Inouye and Engelberg. To reduce the resistance in this coil dialyser, they used two cellophane tubes in parallel, each 10 m in length, giving a surface area of $1.8\,m^2$. Nevertheless, a blood-pump was necessary to obtain a blood flow of 200 ml/min from the radial artery. Both cellophane tubes and fibre glass screen with spacers were wound together around a metal core. During the initial experiments, several core sizes were tried: a beer can, a citrus can and a gallon can. The fruit juice can gave the most satisfactory results and the best pressure/flow relationship.

The urea clearance of this 'twin coil kidney' was

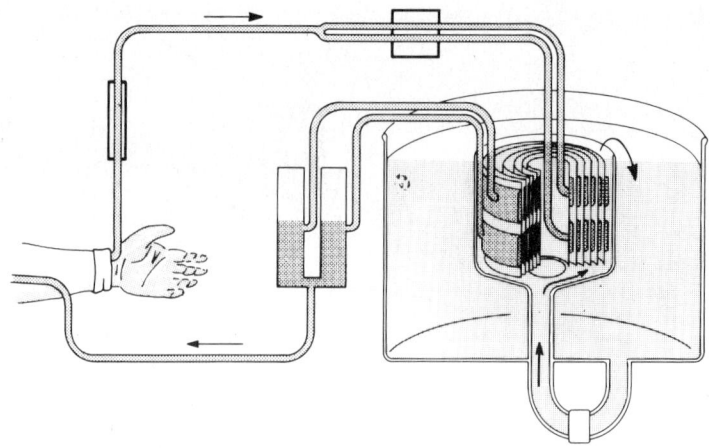

Figure 23a. 'Twin coil' artificial kidney (1955–1956 [53–54]). Flow diagram.

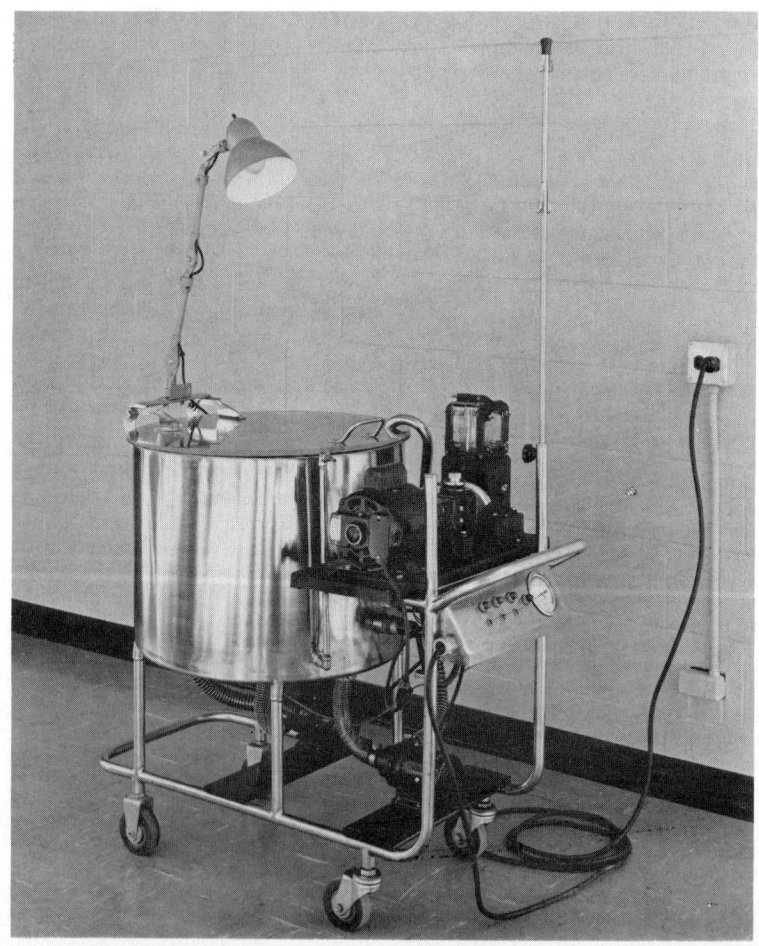

Figure 23b. 'Twin coil' artificial kidney developed by Kolff, Watschinger and Travenol Laboratories.

140 ml/min and considerable ultrafiltration took place. The amount of donor blood required to fill the two loops of cellophane tubing was about 750 ml. The dialyser itself was compact and in its original form, could be sterilised by steam or by ethylene oxide. It was disposable, relatively cheap and could be mass produced. For actual dialysis the coil was placed within a small open cannister in a 100 l dialysis fluid tank with the rinsing fluid pumped crosswise through the mesh of the fibre glass screening at 30 l/min overflowing back into the dialysis fluid tank (see Figure 23a). The system was commercially produced by Travenol Laboratories in the United States (Figure 23b) and rapidly gained popularity. Kidney centres which were opened in the early post war years, changed rapidly to the twin coil artificial kidney and new centres using this machine sprang up both in Europe and in America. Nephrologists and internists became familiar with the twin coil dialysis system and the treatment of acute renal failure: more or less a breakthrough in haemodialysis occurred. The decade after 1956, the year of the introduction of the twin coil kidney, may be called '*the period of acute renal failure*'.

However, several disadvantages of the twin coil kidney soon became apparent (61). It required a blood pump and had a high blood pressure in the extracorporeal circuit which carried the hazard of membrane ruptures. The necessity of priming the coil with several units of donor blood exposed the patient to the common risks of blood transfusion and made the system less suitable for repetitive dialysis as is required for chronic renal failure. In addition the bacterial contamination of the open tank system was high.

Nevertheless Maher, Schreiner and Waters (62) reported in April 1961 on five patients with acute renal failure and prolonged oliguria exceeding 60 days. They survived with multiple dialyses with the twin coil system for periods between 66 and 181 days.

Their longest survivor was maintained for 181 days. He received 11 haemodialyses which required multiple arterial and venous cut downs.

ACCESS TO THE CIRCULATION

A new and original approach to the latter problem came from the studies of Alwall et all (45), who during their experimental dialyses of anuric rabbits created an arterio-venous shunt between the carotid artery and jugular vein by siliconised glass tubes, which were joined together between treatments by a narrow glass capillary. Blood flow through the shunt was approximately 1 l/h. Heparin had to be injected every 4 to 6 h. Usually the device clotted after a week or so, but the concept of an arterio-venous cannula system for repeated haemodialysis was born. The application to humans was soon abandoned however, because of frequent clotting and local infection (47).

Several reports describing various techniques and devices, allowing repeated access to the circulation, appeared between 1950 and 1960. Some of them were simple, like cannulation of the iliac veins or the inferior vena cava with single or double lumen plastic catheters introduced by percutaneous puncture of a femoral vein. Others were quite ingenious like the indwelling 'permanent' vein cannulae described in 1963 by Giovannetti

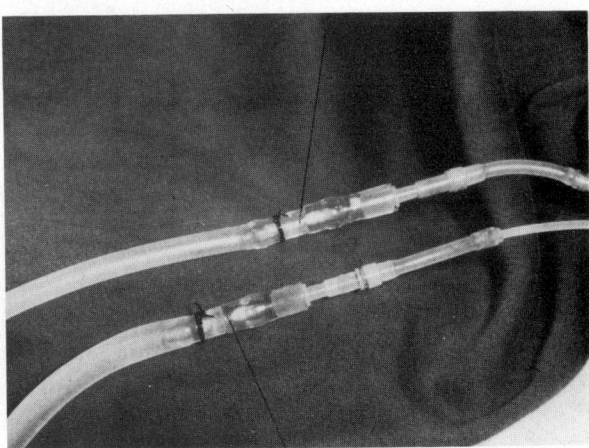

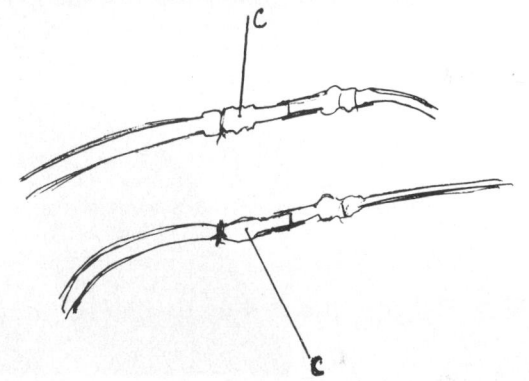

Figure 24a. Silastic heparin infusors connected to indwelling Teflon vena cava catheters used by Giovannetti and coworkers (1963 [63]) and Shaldon (64). The silastic tubing was closed at one end and filled with diluted heparin solution. This slowly perfused the catheters through the connectors which were provided with a capillary lumen (c).

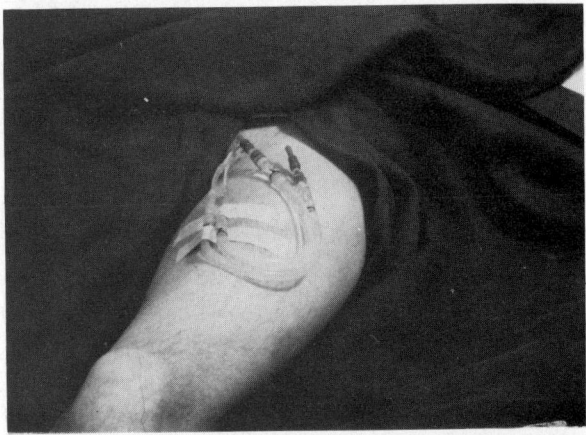

Figure 24b. Silastic heparin infusors in situ, fixed on upper leg.

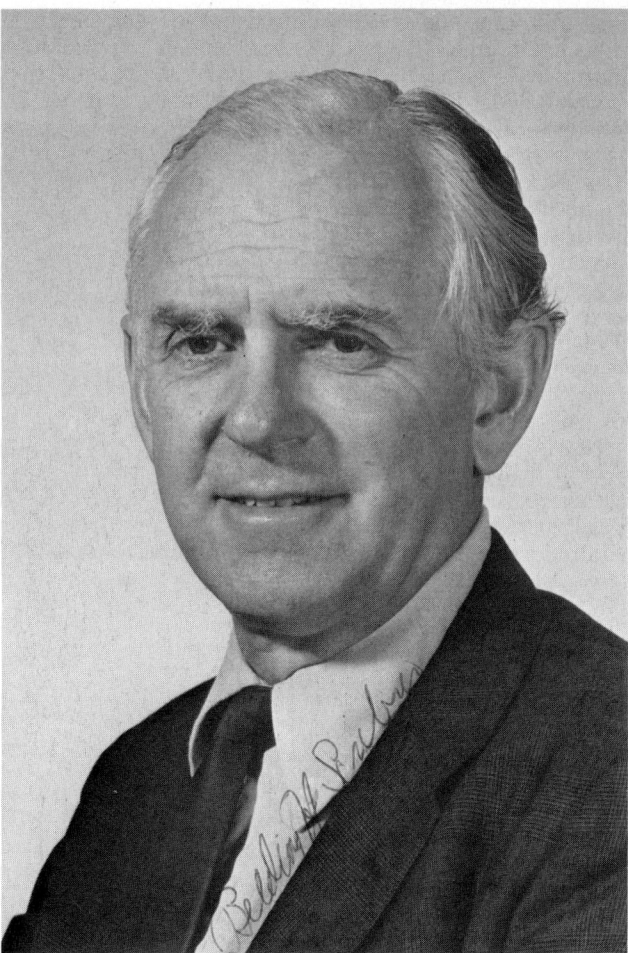

Figure 25. BELDING H. SCRIBNER, M.D. (1974).

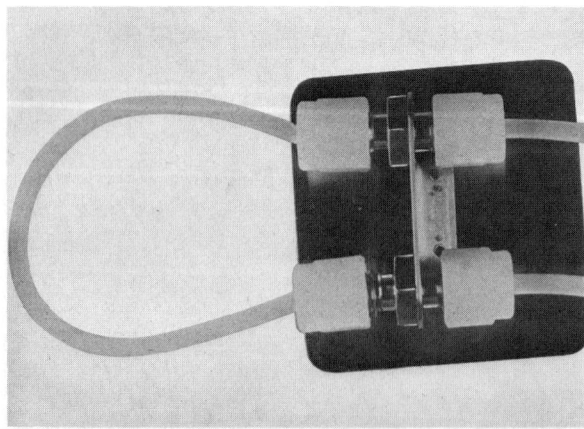

Figure 26. Prototype arterio-venous cannula system made from rigid Teflon with stainless steel armplate (Quinton, Dillard and Scribner, 1960 [65]). (Appr. actual size).

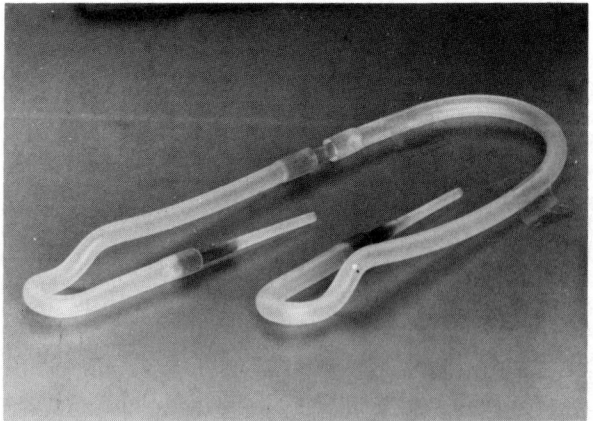

Figure 27. All Silastic, single break 'Scribner shunt' without metal parts. Teflon parts are etched to provide safe connections.

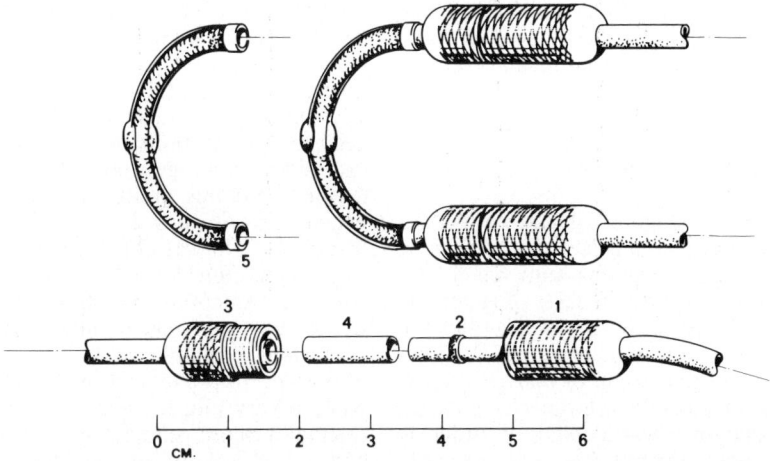

Figure 28. Edinburgh Teflon arterio-venous cannula system constructed by Sinclair, Henderson and Simpson (1961 [66]). (1) female end-piece; (2) metal collar; (3) male end-piece; (4) sleeve size-9 Teflon; (5) metal sleeve to protect U-shaped connecting segment.

and his co-workers from Pisa, Italy (63), somewhat modified by Shaldon and Rosen (64) in 1964 (Figures 24a and 24b). Obstacles such as local infection, septicaemia, recurrent clottings, clot-formations at the tip of the catheter even causing pulmonary emboli, made these devices dangerous and unsuitable for prolonged application.

Somewhat earlier, on 10th April 1960, Quinton, Dillard and Scribner ([65], Figure 25) reported at the Chicago meeting of the American Society for Artificial Internal Organs on an exteriorised bypass device made of Teflon which made the application of repeated haemodialysis for irreversible chronic renal failure a possibility. Their invention caused a major break-through and should be considered as a landmark in the history of dialysis. Two cannulae made from thin walled Teflon tubing with tapered ends were inserted, one in the radial artery and the other in the cephalic vein near the wrist of the patient, both cannulae being bent into a 180° turn beneath the skin. The external ends were connected to a curved Teflon bypass tube by means of two Swagelok couplings, which were fixed on a stainless steel armplate (Figure 26).

Shortly thereafter, a somewhat different arteriovenous shunt also made from Teflon was constructed in Edinburgh, Scotland by Sinclair, Henderson and Simpson (66) (and published as a new invention in the Lancet of the 19th August 1961 [Figure 28]). The credit for the first major step towards indefinite replacement of renal function by regular dialysis goes, however, to Scribner and his co-workers.

The first model with rigid Teflon cannulae had only a short life expectancy, which was attributed to either mechanical damage to the Teflon tubes or to the vascular wall. The Teflon tubing also had to be shaped while heated to fit the patient's needs. Therefore special preshaped cannulae made from flexible Silastic tubing were designed with vessel tips and extension tubes made from Teflon. The armplate was omitted and the parts were secured by special metal rings (67). Further modifications and improvements were made in the next few years, resulting in an all Silastic shunt system with a single break, a single short Teflon connector and Teflon vessel tips (60, 69). Those parts of the Teflon in contact with silicone rubber were etched to make safe connections without the use of metal rings (Figure 27). Several commercial firms made complete sets of various shaped cannulae systems available with different sizes of vessel tips and so called reverse and straight 'winged in line' cannulae, which were easier to declot (70). In recent years a new, small, somewhat different arteriovenous shunt was designed by Buselmeier and co-workers from Minneapolis (71), which has certain advantages in particular in paediatric patients (Figure 29). The clotting problems, however, and the frequency of infection,

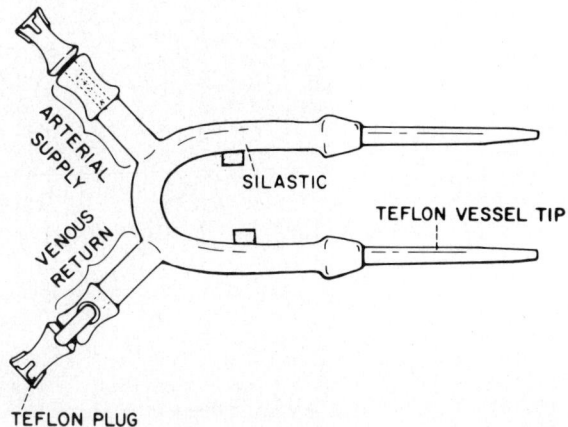

Figure 29. Buselmeier shunt (71).

which became apparent in 1961 (67), were not solved and still remain. Nevertheless, the 'Scribner shunt' and its modifications found wide application all over the world in every dialysis centre (72).

THE SEATTLE DIALYSIS SYSTEM

At the same time Scribner (Figure 25) and co-workers presented a fresh and more sophisticated approach to haemodialysis technique. Their original aim was to perform continuous, low flow dialysis in cases of acute renal failure, using an efficient, low resistance dialyser, which made a blood pump unnecessary (73). They started with a relatively large amount of dialysis fluid to make prolonged dialysis possible without changing the dialysis fluid. The dialysate was cooled in order to reduce the bacterial count (Figures 30a, 30b, 30c). Initially the MacNeill-Collins dialyser (56–58) was tried (see Figure 22, p. 19), which had a low resistance, but clotted repeatedly. Subsequently a six layer Skeggs-Leonards dialyser (59, 60) was tested. Clotting was less of a problem, but assembly was difficult. Either leaks occurred or compression of the rubber pads had to be excessive, resulting in poor flow characteristics. Finally, Scribner and his group changed to the Kiil dialyser, which was originally described in 1960 by Frederik Kiil from Oslo, Norway (74, 75 [Figures 31a, 31b and 31c]). The original four layer Kiil dialyser was modified into a two layer system and the flow path of the dialysis fluid was somewhat changed, maintaining however the counter current principle which was adopted by Kiil. An important improvement was the adoption of Cuprophan, a very thin membrane, more permeable than the original Viscose cellophane. The modified Kiil dialyser had a low volume of the blood compartment, which

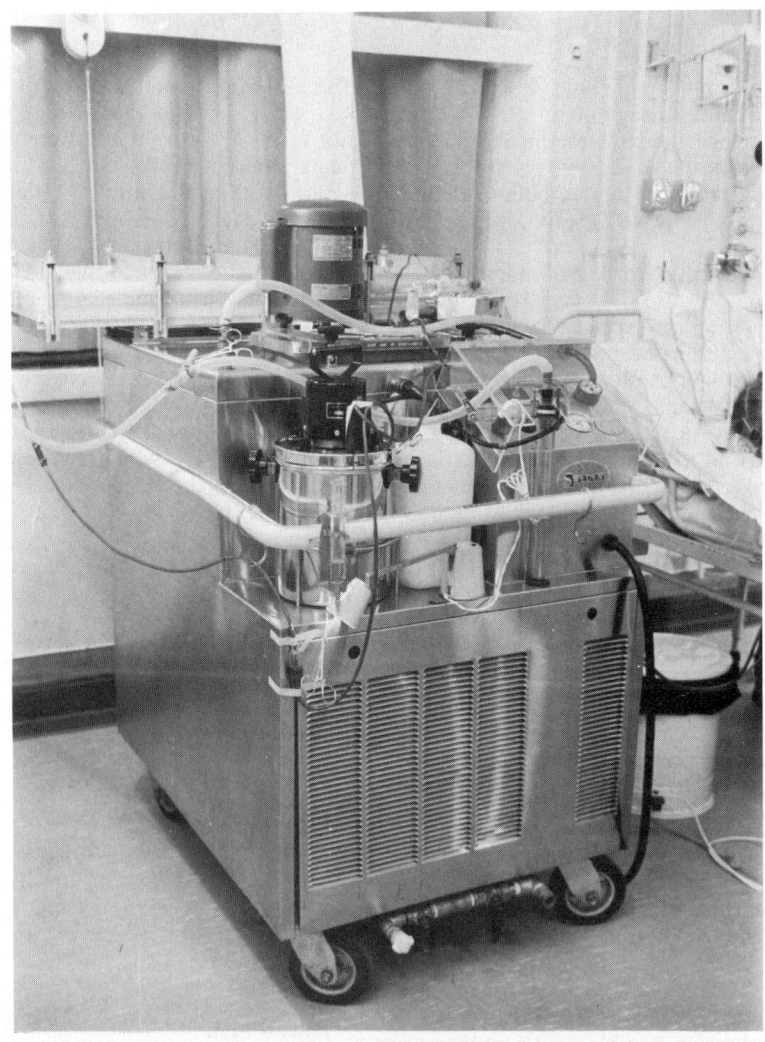

Figure 30a. The Seattle 'pumpless' haemodialysis system: 'Scribner tank' with modified two layer Kiil dialyser on top.

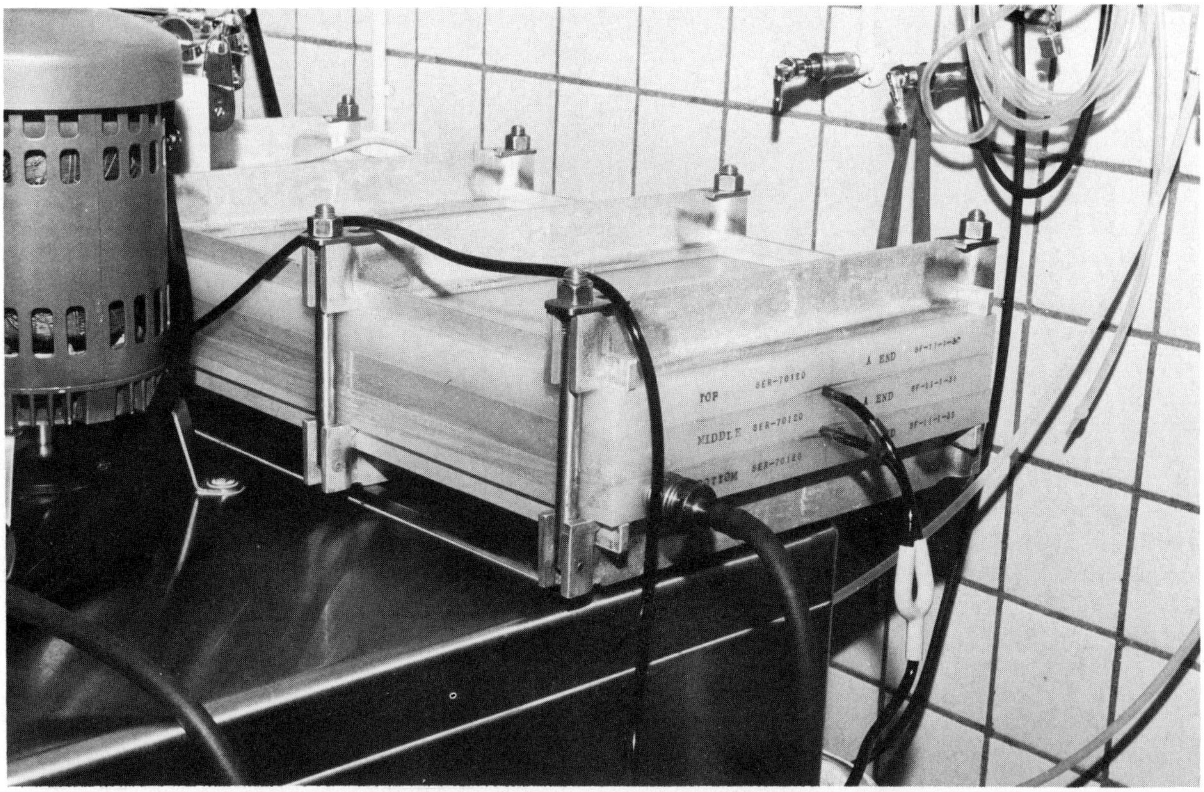

2: *Haemodialysis: a historical review* 25

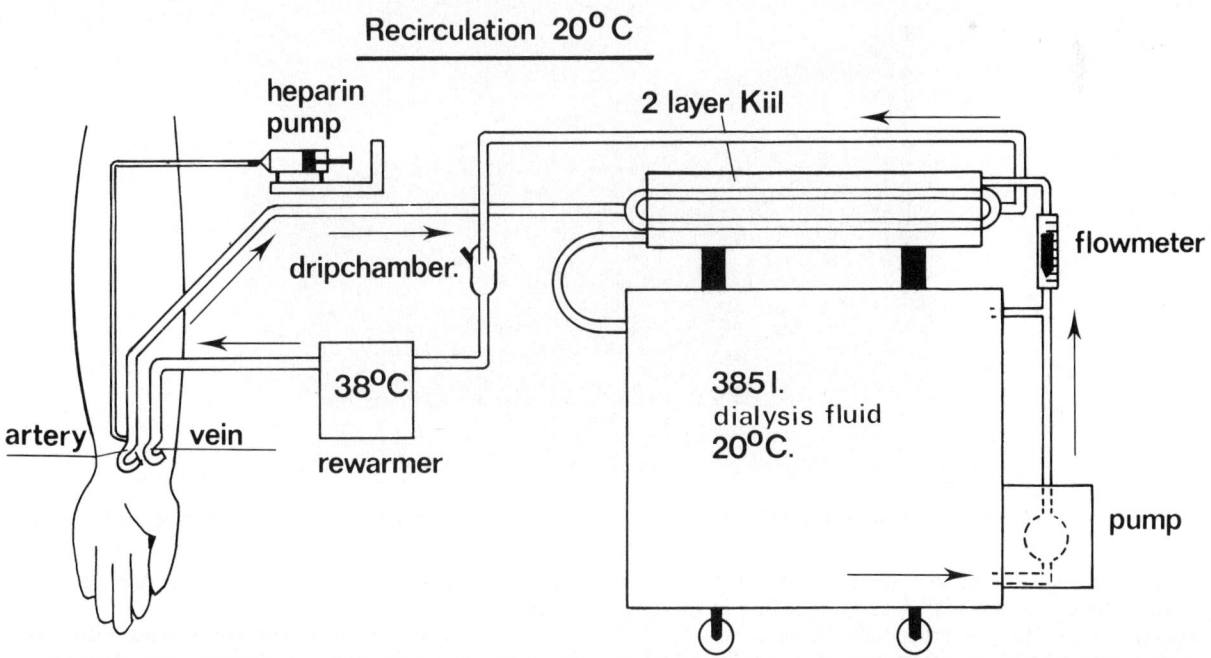

Figure 30b. Modified two layer Kiil dialyser during haemodialysis (1964).

Figure 30c. Flow diagram of the original Seattle 'pumpless' haemodialysis system. The dialysis fluid was cooled and recirculated through the dialyser (1960 [73, 77, 78]).

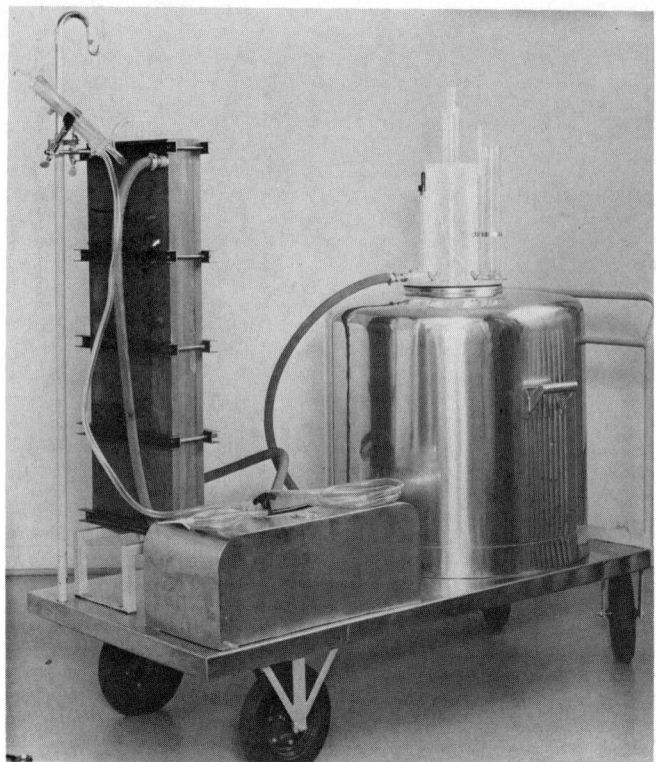

Figure 31a. Original Kiil dialyser (in vertical position) with stainless steel tank containing 300 l dialysis fluid and equipped with a open narrow overflow chimney, facilitating collection and measurement of ultrafiltrate (1960 [74, 75]).

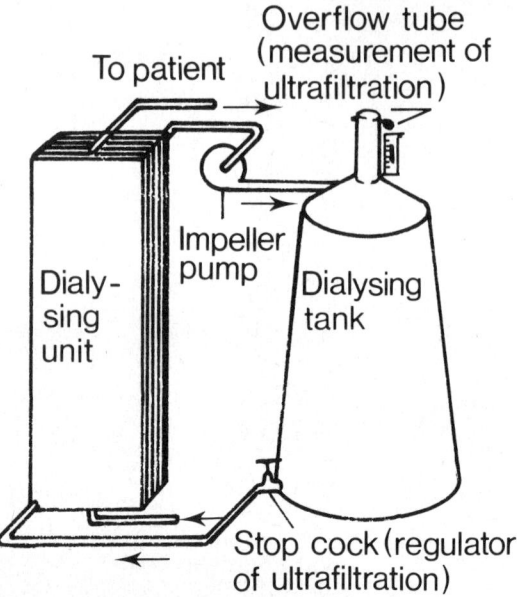

Figure 31b. Flow diagram of the original Kiil dialysis system (74, 75).

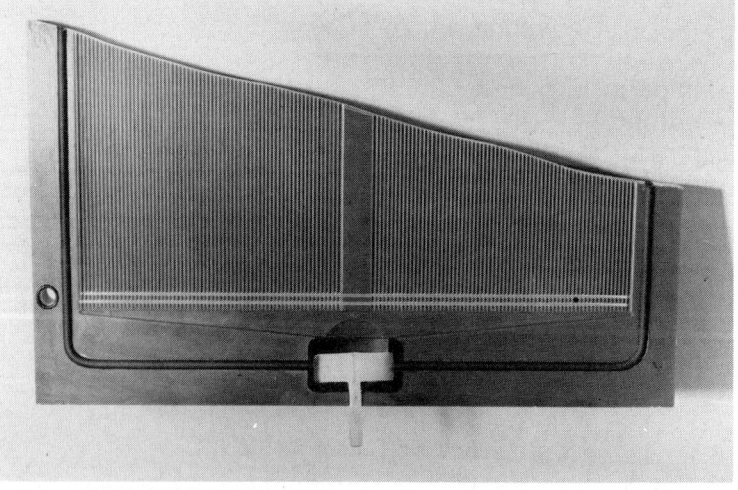

Figure 31c. End section of grooved plastic board of Kiil dialyser (made from Araldit, an epoxyresin compound [74, 75]).

made priming with donor blood unnecessary. The patient's blood was washed back, using saline at the conclusion of the dialysis procedure. In addition the flow resistance of the blood compartment was low and when an arterio-venous cannulae system was used a blood pump was unnecessary: the bloodflow through the dialyser could be maintained by the arterial pressure of the patient.

Despite numerous initial problems and difficulties, the new 'low temperature continuous flow dialysis system' finally worked satisfactorily, simplifying the technique of haemodialysis considerably.

2: Haemodialysis: a historical review   27

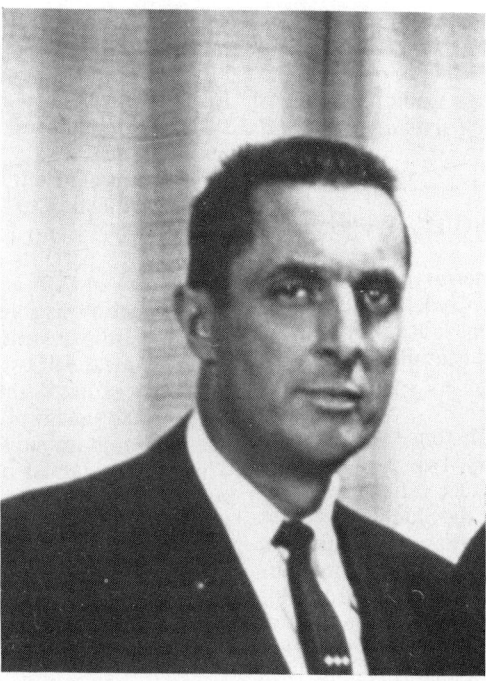

Figure 32. Mr. Clyde Shields (1921–1971), the first successful chronic dialysis patient. Picture taken in 1966 after 5 years of dialysis treatment.

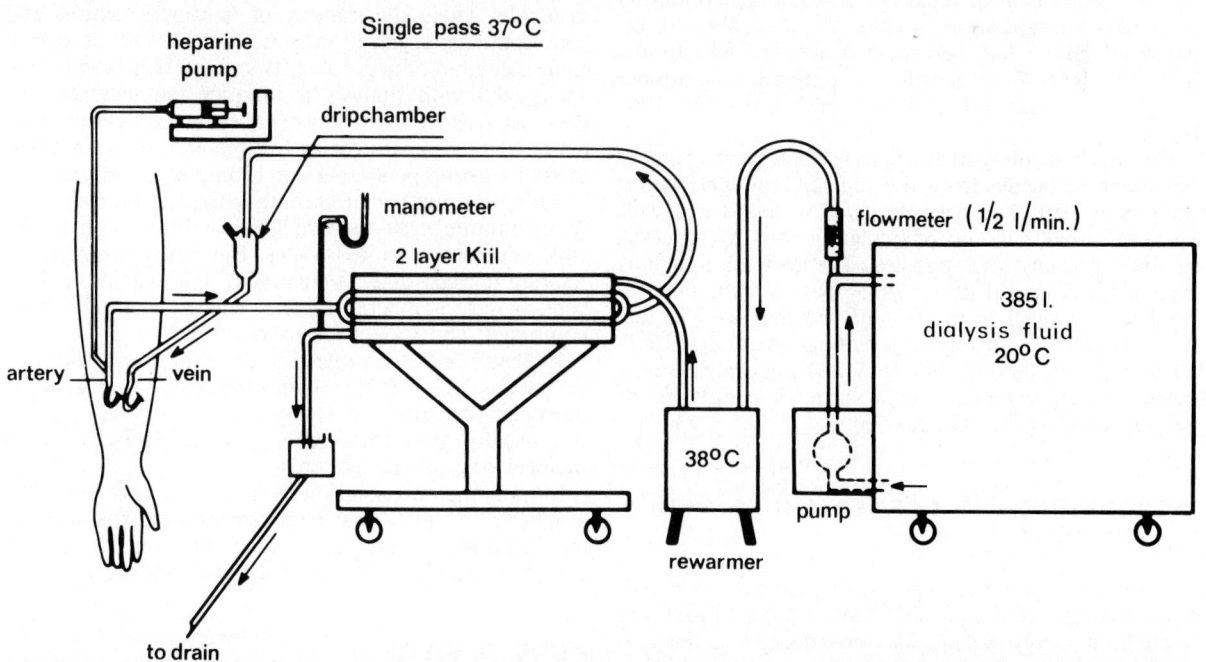

Figure 33. Flow diagram of the Seattle 'pumpless' haemodialysis system modified into a single pass system. The dialysis fluid was pumped from the tank, heated to 37 °C and discarded after a single passage through the dialyser (1964 [87]). See text.

The new technique for circulatory access by (semi-)permanent arterio-venous cannulation made it basically possible to perform an unlimited number of dialyses in a single patient and Scribner decided to study the application of his dialysis system in *chronic irreversible terminal renal failure patients*.

THE FIRST SUCCESSFUL CHRONIC PATIENTS

On 9th March 1960, a Teflon arterio-venous cannula system was inserted in the arm of Clyde Shields, a 39-year-old machinist in terminal renal failure (Figure 32) and on 23rd March, another pair of cannulae was placed in the right arm of Harvey Gentry, a 23-year-old shoe salesman.

The results of repeated (initially once, later twice weekly) haemodialyses in these first two patients were surprisingly good: both became successfully rehabilitated chronic dialysis patients. Clyde Shields lived for more than 11 years on intermittent dialysis and died in 1971 at the age of 50 from a myocardial infarction. Harvey Gentry received a successful transplant from his mother in 1968 and is still alive and well at the time of writing (March 1982). The Seattle dialysis system appeared to be so safe and reliable that patients with chronic uraemia could be haemodialysed entirely by nurses (76-78). In April 1962, the Seattle group reported on eight patients who were on the treatment programme for periods between four months and two years (79-81). Only one death occurred after 12 months of treatment.

Others, using different techniques, had more limited success (82-84), but it soon became apparent that successful replacement of renal function and rehabilitation by regular haemodialysis in cases of irreversible, terminal renal failure had become a reality (82, 83). In the Swedish Hospital in Seattle, an outpatient treatment centre was organised and activated early in 1962 (81, 85).

Obviously, cooling of the dialysis fluid, rewarming of the blood returning from the dialyser and performing dialysis at 20°C had been designed to avoid excessive bacterial growth in the recirculating tank system (86), but had certain disadvantages. The recirculating tank system was changed into a single pass circuit. Dialysis fluid was pumped from the tank, heated to 37°C and discarded after a single passage through the dialyser (87). This increased dialysis efficiency and appeared to be a significant improvement, while bacterial counts in the system remained low (Figure 33).

INTRODUCTION OF A CENTRAL DIALYSATE SUPPLY SYSTEM

The introduction of the single pass technique was actually the first step in the development of a centralised dialysate fluid supply system. The second step was the substitution of acetate for bicarbonate in the dialysis fluid (88), which was based on the discovery of Mudge, Manning and Gilman (89) in 1949, that sodium acetate could act as a source of fixed base. To realise a central multipatient dialysate supply system, a concentrated solution of salts and dextrose had to be diluted with (pretreated) tapwater by means of an accurate proportioning system to obtain a continuous supply of dialysis fluid. Sodium bicarbonate unlike sodium acetate cannot be mixed with concentrated calcium and magnesium salts without adjusting pH to 7.4 or less.

A central system for simultaneous supply of dialysis fluid for 15 patients was designed by Grimsrud, Cole, Lehman et al. (90) and built at the University of Washington. Dialysis solution 35 times normal strength was mixed in this system with the appropriate amount of water by means of two accurate pumps. This system significantly reduced the personnel requirement and the cost of dialysis. Surprisingly, an impressive reduction in bacterial contamination of the dialysis fluid was noted. This was explained by self sterilising properties of the concentrated bath solution (91), which, hower, from later investigations (92) and the author's own experience appeared to be non existent.

The use of concentrated solutions, containing acetate, for the preparation of dialysis fluid rapidly gained wide application, both for automatic proportioning systems and for manual preparation of dialysis fluid.

ANOTHER MILESTONE: THE START OF REGULAR DIALYSIS TREATMENT OF TERMINAL, IRREVERSIBLE RENAL FAILURE

Until the early 1960's, dialysis activities were limited to the treatment of acute renal failure. A few early attempts to treat patients with chronic renal failure by regular repeated dialyses failed until the Scribner shunt became available. Then, the number of treatment centres and hence patients began to increase, but because of lack of equipment and of nephrologists and internists, who were acquainted with dialysis techniques the increase was slow. In August 1965, however, some 160 chronic patients were on treatment in Europe and 40 centres had started treating patients with chronic renal failure (93).

Soon, the number of chronic patients requiring treatment outnumbered the available facilities, both in Europe and in the United States. But many hospitals intending to start dialysis treatment and existing dialysis centres were hampered at this stage by lack of money, equipment and trained personnel (93).

In Seattle, a patient selection procedure was instituted by means of a double committee (81, 85). Elsewhere however, patients were accommodated as well as possible, usually on a first come, first served basis for all medically acceptable patients.

Initially the only solution seemed to be to increase the number of hospital treatment centres and expand existing facilities. At that time, renal transplantation was even less established as a therapeutic procedure.

HOME DIALYSIS

In the next few years, a gradual increase of treatment facilities occurred both in America and in Europe (Table

Table 1. Regular dialysis treatment in Europe 1965–1968.

	1965	1966	1967	1968
No of centres	43	54	81	114
No of accepted patients	277	612	1163	2633
Alive and on regular dialysis	160	295	621	1281

(From Drukker et al. (82), with permission of Excerpta Medica, Amsterdam)

1 [94]). However, enormous problems of financing and training of doctors and nurses had to be faced and in an effort to achieve at least a partial solution of the dilemma Shaldon and co-workers of the Royal Free Hospital in London U.K. (95) introduced the concept of self dialysis in September 1964. From self dialysis in the hospital to home dialysis was the next step. This step had already been made by the Japanese in 1961, according to Nosé (96 [see Figures 34a and 34b]). In America, Merrill's group (97) in Boston had already initiated home dialysis in July 1964 and satisfactory results in three patients were soon reported.

The Seattle group started their home programme in September 1964 (98). The Royal Free team began home dialysis two months later (99), their first patient being a registered nurse. Her husband, an engineer, made the Kiil dialyser and the additional dialysis equipment himself.

Merrill and colleagues (97, 100) used the disposable twin coil dialyser with recirculating dialysate, a system which was popular in America at that time. The patient's own stored blood was used for priming the dialyser for the next dialysis. Curtis and coworkers (98) and Baillod et al. (99) used the non-disposable modified Kiil dialyser either with a 300 l static tank for dialysis fluid preparation or an automatic dialysis fluid supply system, based on the concept of the central supply machine, constructed in Seattle. These single patient proportioning systems were marketed at that time both in the United States and in England.

Home dialysis soon attracted both considerable interest and criticism. It took Scribner (101) several years 'to convince both patients and colleagues that home dialysis was the only way to go'. It soon became apparent that in the home more frequent dialysis was possible with better rehabilitation. Cost was considerably less compared to hospital dialysis (101). The self sufficiency and independence were considered more than adequate compensation for the extra burden on the patient and his family (98).

The construction of reliable proportioning machines has doubtless not only contributed to the safety of hospital dialysis, but in particular to the safety of self dialysis in the home setting.

Different systems have been developed. The simplest construction had motor driven pumps with a fixed dilution ratio (Figure 35).

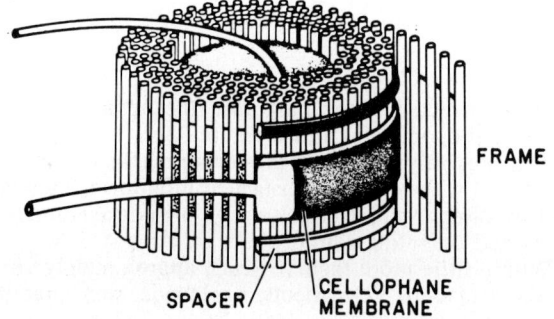

Figure 34a. Japanese coil dialyser used for home dialysis: 7 m cellophane sausage wound with a frame of plastic tubes laced with cords held on equal distance by spacers (Nosé, 1961 [96]). Surface area 0.63 m². This dialyser shows a striking similarity with the coil dialyser constructed by Bodo von Garrelts in Sweden in 1947 (see Figure 20).

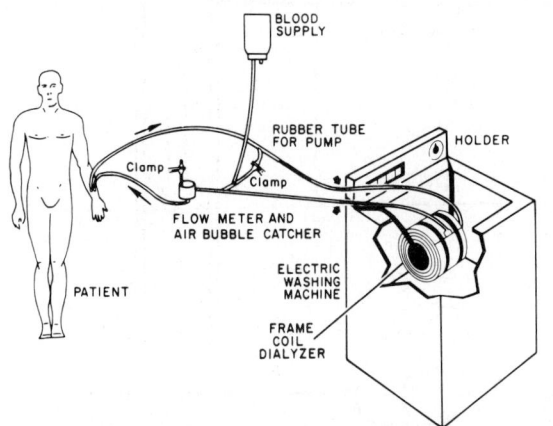

Figure 34b. Japanese home dialysis system with coil dialyser in ordinary domestic washing machine (1961 [96]).

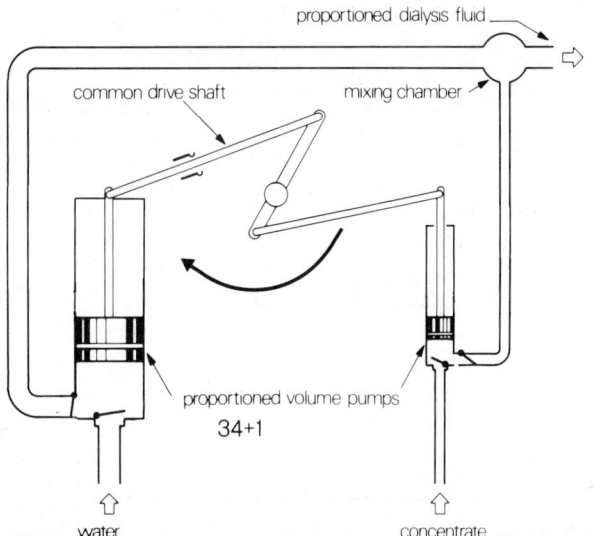

Figure 35. Motor driven piston pumps proportioning device with a fixed dilution ratio.

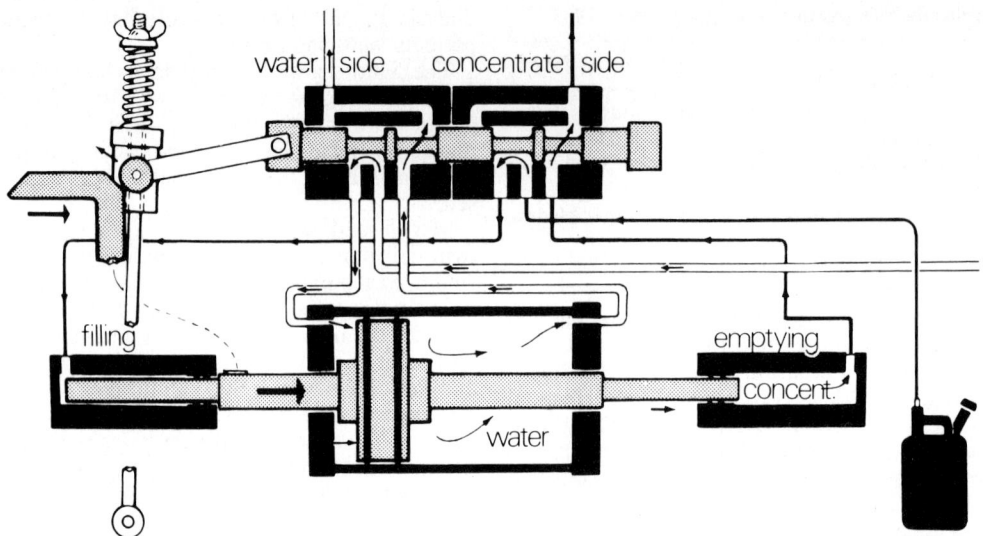

Figure 36. Proportioning device with water-driven pump system (carboy on bottom right contains concentrate). Two upper outlets, water and concentrate sides, unite in a mixing chamber. The open ended tube above the carboy is connected to the water supply. This system has also a fixed proportioning ratio.

In other systems a water driven proportioning device is used, also with a fixed dilution ratio (Figure 36).

In other systems also with motor driven proportioning pump systems the proportioning ratio can be varied between certain limits to adapt the dialysate sodium concentration to the individual requirements of the patients (Figure 37).

Later conductivity feed back proportioning systems were constructed. They have also the advantage of a variable proportioning ratio (Figure 38).

The presently marketed proportioning machines are combined with highly sophisticated monitoring systems and are often technical jewels with a high degree of reliability and operating comfort.

Within little more than 10 years, approximately 16% or more than 10 000 patients, worldwide, were practis-

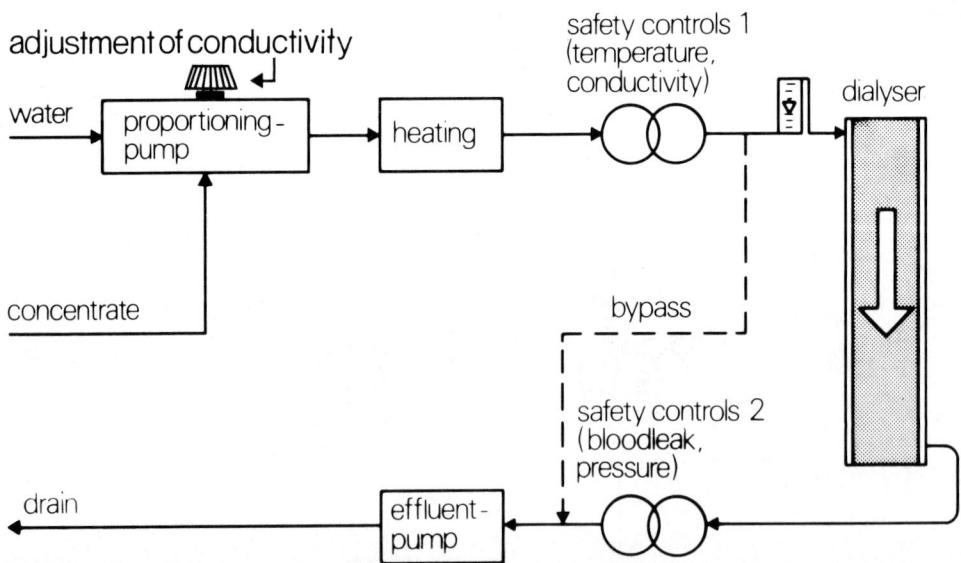

Figure 37. Proportioning system with motor driven pump. The proportioning ratio can be varied between certain limits to adapt dialysis fluid to individual requirement of the patient.

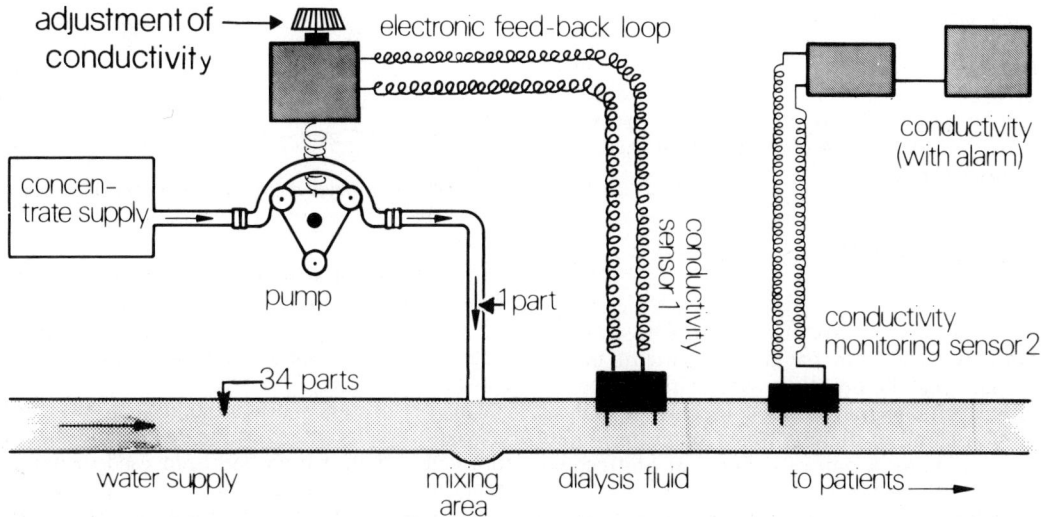

Figure 38. Proportioning system, with servo controlled speed of concentrate pump (so called electronic feed-back proportioning system) with variable proportioning ratio.

ing self dialysis in the home. In the U.K. the health authorities have traditionally been in favour of home dialysis. By the end of 1979 64% of the total haemodialysis population in that country dialysed at home (102, 103).

THE ARTERIOVENOUS FISTULA

It became obvious that the arterio-venous shunt was still the Achilles heel of chronic dialysis. Patients, doctors and nurses were plagued by episodes of clotting, infections and subsequent loss of shunts.

In 1966, a surgically created arterio-venous (A-V) fistula was introduced for access to the circulation by Brescia, Cimino, Appel and Hurwich (104): another landmark in the history of dialysis. In the same issue of the New England Journal of Medicine a now historical editorial comment was published (105):

'Whether or not this new internal shunt technic can be adapted for home use remains to be determined. Although such an adaptation seems to pose some formidable problems'...

The problems appeared to be neither insurmountable nor formidable. Shaldon (106) successfully began training patients to use the internal A-V fistula for overnight dialysis in the home and taught the patients self-needling (October 1967). The internal fistula became increasingly popular, soon dominating regular dialysis both in the home and in the hospital. In 1975, approximately 83% of all hospital and 88% of home dialysed patients in Europe had a subcutaneous A-V fistula for circulatory access (102). If newer fistula modifications were included, these figures were 88 and 91% respectively.

THE ROLE OF THE ASAIO AND THE EDTA

In the last 20 years, haemodialysis has been the subject of intensive investigations involving bio-engineering, membrane research, biochemistry, biophysics and evaluation of clinical experience (107, 108). In America, much of this research was initially supported by the John A. Hartford Foundation, and later by the Artificial Kidney-Chronic Uremia Program of the National Institutes of Health, directed by Dr. Benjamin Burton. In this period of initial turbulence, probably nothing has been more helpful to coordinate studies and to inform investigators and clinicians than the annual meetings of the American Society for Artificial Internal Organs (ASAIO) and its Transactions. The idea of founding an American Society for Artificial Organs came from the late Dr. Peter F. Salisbury from Los Angeles, in August 1954. The new Society had 47 founding members and held its first annual meeting in Atlantic City, on the 4th and 5th June 1955, in conjunction with the American Medical Association (109).

Salisbury (110) wrote in a chronicle on the occasion of the 5th anniversary of the Society, quoting the Holy Bible 'ever since Daniel described scientific meetings with the famous words ... "many shall run to and fro and knowledge shall be increased"...' (111).

In the first 15 years of its existence, the Society held its annual meetings in conjunction with the Federation of American Societies for Experimental Biology, usually on the east coast, in Atlantic City, sometimes in Chicago or Philadelphia. Then, they started to run to and fro, having their venues on the east and west coasts or in the midwest, and knowledge was increased immensely indeed... In less than 20 years the membership exceeded 1000.

A similar role was played in Europe by the European Dialysis and Transplant Associaton (EDTA), which was founded in Amsterdam on 25th September 1964 (112). Like the ASAIO, the EDTA has acted for many years as a forum where people could meet and could present and discuss the results of their investigations and clinical experience. Its annual statistical reports, which in 1980 included data on 107 004 patients treated by dialysis and transplantation (113), became highlights and derive from voluntary cooperation of 85-95% of all European dialysis centres. In 1980 1225 centres reported to the EDTA Registry (appr. 82% of all known European dialysis centres). In 1980 14 084 new patients started treatment in Europe (113).

FURTHER DEVELOPMENTS; THE ROLE OF THE INDUSTRY

The initial goal of the early investigators to develop methodology by which they could keep patients in terminal chronic renal failure alive was achieved before 1965. Further refinements included increasing dialysis efficiency, shortening of dialysis time, increasing safety and comfort, miniaturisation of equipment and economising.

Other investigations were directed to prevent and to heal complications and to improve the health rehabilitation and quality of life of chronic dialysis patients.

On the other hand, basic research focused on haemodynamics, kinetics of solute removal and development of new membranes. After 1965, industry became increasingly interested in dialysis and a growing number of proportioning machines, monitoring equipment, blood pumps and ancillary equipment was constructed and introduced. A plethora of different types of dialysers was made available, both disposable (coils or parallel flow dialysers) and nondisposable such as the standard two layer Kiil and its modification with multipoint membrane support (114-118, [see also chapter 5]).

Basic research directed to improving the performance of dialysers came, however, primarily from outside of the industry.

The efficiency of the coil dialyser was much improved by a new mesh support designed by Hoeltzenbein (119) in 1966. It was made from polyethylene and its geometry was derived from a certain type of fishing net. This membrane support (see Figure 39) eliminated spacers and increased turbulence of dialysate, decreasing the dialysing resistance of the stagnant film of dialysis fluid

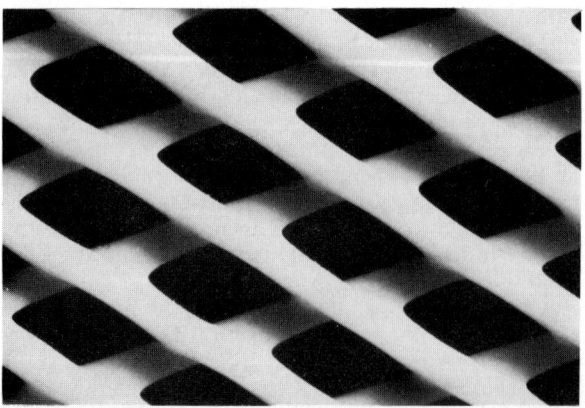

Figure 39. Hoeltzenbein mesh support used in coil dialysers (119). (See also figure 7 in chapter 5).

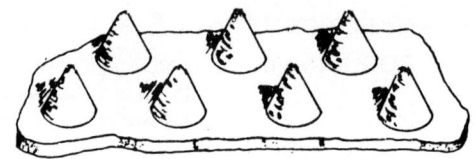

Figure 40. Multipoint membrane support (117). (See also figure 2 in chapter 5).

in direct contact with the membrane. In addition the Hoeltzenbein mesh improved the dialysis efficiency of the coil type dialyser by increasing the effective surface area of the membrane through reduced membrane contact.

The performance of coil dialysers was further improved by replacement of the cellophane membrane by thin Cuprophan, which had been used in Kiil type dialysers for several years.

The multicone membrane support was originally designed by investigators from New York, (E. F. Leonard) and from Philadelphia, (L. W. Bluemle Jr. and others) and was described in 1960 (114-118 [Figure 40, see also Figure 2 chapter 5, p. 109]). It serves the same purpose in parallel flow dialysers as the Hoeltzenbein mesh in coils. The pyramid membrane support improves the dialyser efficiency not only by increasing the effective membrane surface area (through reduced membrane support contact) but also through improved dialysate distribution (118). The advantages of the multiple cone support are particularly appreciable in situations with a low dialysate flow rate or (and) with a high transmembrane pressure for high ultrafiltration.

The multiple pyramid membrane support is employed in the non-disposable Meltec modification of the Kiil dialyser, which is still used in the United Kingdom and in a number of disposable flat plate dialysers (the reader is referred to chapter 5 for more detailed information).

Around 1965, when preferences were divided between Kiil and coil dialysers (120, 121) a new design, the hollow fiber artificial kidney, or capillary dialyser was introduced (122, 123). With a short length of the blood path, a thin blood film, a highly effective membrane surface area and excellent diffusive and convective capabilities this compact dialyser could control uraemia very well. Simultaneously, in Europe, the first disposable parallel flow dialyser was introduced by Alwall (124), soon to be followed by improved models produced in Sweden by Gambro Inc. The multitude of available systems soon became confusing, in particular to those who only recently entered the field of dialysis and confusion increased even more so when the traditional concepts were upset by new hypotheses which were derived from the reconsideration of old questions, i.e. what is toxic, what are uraemic toxins, what should be removed?

THE SQUARE METRE/HOUR AND MIDDLE MOLECULE HYPOTHESES

In the early years of regular peritoneal dialysis for chronic renal failure, Scribner (125) noted that patients on chronic peritoneal dialysis, which controls traditional plasma chemistries less than haemodialysis does, often felt better (1965). Despite a certain amount of 'underdialysis' with chronic peritoneal dialysis, peripheral neuropathy either did not occur or did not progress. Scribner presented the hypothesis that the peritoneum was more permeable and that peritoneal dialysis removed substances of higher molecular weight more efficiently than haemodialysis. Suspicion arose that the so called middle molecules played an important role in the toxicity of uraemia. Because of their size, it was suggested that they were very slowly removed compared to urea. The cellulose membranes used in haemodialysis (e.g. cellophane and Cuprophan) have according to Scribner's hypothesis a rather high diffusion resistance for these species of molecules.

This speculation correlated with the hypothesis that using a given membrane, prevention of peripheral neuropathy depends on a minimum number of hours of dialysis per week, rather than on maintaining specific levels of blood urea and creatinine. Further, it was suggested that larger toxic solutes permeated the peritoneum better than cellulose membranes. These considerations led to the square metre/hour hypothesis (126, 127) and to its modification, the middle molecule hypothesis (128). Both theories suggest that inadequate removal of the middle molecules (molecular weight between 300 and 2000) causes complications such as peripheral neuropathy, pericarditis and perhaps others.

Since the removal rate of middle molecules through a conventional haemodialysis membrane is slow, the diffusion gradient remains high throughout haemodialysis, unlike urea. Thus, the net removal rate of middle molecules remains rather constant during protracted dialysis and net removal is proportional to the total number of haemodialysis hours/week unlike urea which has a flow dependent removal which decreases with the decreasing plasma concentration as dialysis proceeds. Increasing the length of each dialysis may, therefore, arrest neuropathy. The Seattle group and others (127–133) presented indirect evidence that the so called middle molecules are the primary toxins causing uraemic neuropathy and other uraemic manifestations.

SHORT DIALYSIS

The square metre/hour and middle molecule hypotheses have profoundly influenced dialysis strategies, resulting in a confusing and conflicting array of various dialysis protocols (115, 134, 135). That does not alter the fact that isolation, identification and the toxicology of so called middle molecules are still in a process of highly active research. Several groups of investigators are active in this slippery field full of mantraps (136, see also chapter 19).

Nevertheless in many dialysis centres, protocols were changed according to the new theories, resulting in short dialysis schedules either with large surface area dialysers or with the same type of dialyser and increased frequency, but usually with less dialysis hours per week. Experimentally short dialysis has been performed with three hollow fibre artificial kidneys in series (131) with two 1.0 m² parallel flow dialysers in series (137) or with so called large surface area dialysers, which became commercially available in the early seventies (see chapter 5). Other clinical investigators simply shortened each dialysis, decreasing substantially total weekly hours of dialysis, without increasing surface area or membrane permeability (138). Sophisticated modifications of dialysis protocols made use of a special membrane with high clearances for molecules in the critical range of 300–2000 daltons (132, 133), but so far only one other special membrane has found limited practical application for dialysis (139–142).

Many early evaluations of short dialysis schedules did not take into account the fact that residual renal function contributes to removal of middle molecules (143, 144). Likewise the effect of ultrafiltration on convective removal of middle molecules (145) was often overlooked. Residual kidney function in haemodialysis patients should be measured (146) and considered in evaluating short dialysis schedules.

Dialysis protocols are usually still empirically determined. It appeared that in a period of 10 years (1968–1978), average dialysis treatment time was decreased more than 50% (147).

THE SEATTLE DIALYSIS INDEX

Babb and associates (148) introduced in 1975 the concept of the 'dialysis index', a theoretical number based on several parameters, i.e. the body surface and the residual creatinine clearance of the patient, the vitamin B12 clearance of the dialyser, the membrane used and the ultrafiltration rate. This dialysis index is considered as an estimate of adequate dialysis for an individual stable chronic dialysis patient.

Nomograms have been designed for easy estimation of dialysis indices and dialysis prescriptions for stable patients (149).

Until actual and accurate measurement of toxic plasma middle molecules and removal rates by dialysis are achieved, however, this index is not likely to be generally accepted and dialysis protocols will remain largely empirical. These studies may serve, however, as a warning against indiscriminate shortening of dialysis time in chronic patients on the one hand and against 'over-dialysis' on the other. *Over-dialysis,* previously considered as virtually nonexistent, may result from excessive duration of dialysis or too frequent dialysis and may affect the patient's well being adversely, possibly also causing post dialysis hangover. *Insufficient dialysis* may allow persistent hyperphosphataemia, acidaemia and abnormalities of mono- and divalent ions and excessive concentrations of urea, creatinine, uric acid and methylguanidine, which can contribute to signs and symptoms of the uraemic syndrome.

PROGRESS IN IDENTIFICATION OF MIDDLE MOLECULES

Despite the uncertainties mentioned above, the growing evidence that the accumulation of larger molecules is deleterious gave fresh impetus to the identification and isolation of such substances by modern analytical techniques, continuing the search for uraemic toxins which has gone on for more than 150 years (136, 150).

Dzúrik and co-workers in Bratislava (151, 152), using high voltage paper electrophoresis and Sephadex gel filtration, demonstrated peptides of 300-1500 daltons in uraemic sera which were not detectable in sera of normal individuals. The plasma concentration of these peptides correlated inversely with creatinine clearance and dialysis caused a transient decrease Dall'Aglio et al. (153) and Migone and coworkers (154), in Parma, Italy, confirmed the accumulation of peptides in uraemic sera and identified them in used dialysate, applying different techniques.

In Paris, Man et al. and Funck-Brentano and colleagues (132, 133; 155-158), using a new highly permeable polyacrylonitrile dialysis membrane with a middle molecule clearance twice that of Cuprophan, demonstrated that severe peripheral neuropathy could be reversed with improvement of the motor nerve conduction velocity even though plasma urea and creatinine concentrations remained high. These investigators identified the same chromatographic pattern and the same middle molecule peak in used dialysate as in normal urine. Toxicity tests with fibroblast cultures, sensitive for the toxic effects of middle molecules in the 300-1500 daltons range, showed a high activity with dialysate obtained with the polyacrylonitrile membrane dialyser in patients with neuropathy and a low activity when a Cuprophan membrane was used.

Bergström, Fürst and co-workers (150, 159-162), using advanced separation and analytical techniques (gel-chromatography, ion exchange chromatography, iso-tachophoresis) found abnormal UV absorption 'peaks' in uraemic plasma and in used dialysate from uraemic patients. Similar peaks were detected in normal urine. These peaks became measurable in plasma when the plasma creatinine concentration exceeded 400 mmol/l (4.5 mg/dl) or when creatinine clearance was below 12 ml/min. Ten or more different peaks were observed; one peak, number seven was present only in uraemic plasma and could be separated into seven or eight subfractions. Three of these fractions in the middle molecule range of 350-2000 daltons (which were called 7a, 7b and 7c) were obtained by ion exchange chromatography and could each be separated in at least two different subfractions with different mobility and UV absorption (163, 164). Recently (1980) the Swedish investigators demonstrated that fraction 7c contains glycine as the only amino-acid and further analysis suggested that the major compound of fraction 7c is a β-glucuronidated conjugate of ortho-hydroxy-benzoic acid and glycine (136, [see also chapter 19]).

Several other groups in Europe and Japan are involved in clarifying the structures and biological activities of middle molecule compounds. Several *in vitro* toxic effects of middle molecule fractions have been observed e.g. inhibition of glucose utilisation, of fibroblast proliferation, and of leukocyte phagocytosis (163). Direct evidence of *in-vivo* toxicity of middle molecules has still not been proven. But progress has been made towards the answer to the question 'what is really toxic?' At present however, no definite answer can be given yet. In future research, further purification, identification, determination, and if possible, synthesis of middle molecular substances should be the targets (163, 164).

Bergström and Fürst wrote in 1976 (150):
... 'In the light of our present knowledge there is virtually no justification for altering our current dialysis procedure in order to achieve preferential removal of middle molecules, except to carry out studies especially designed to challenge the middle molecule hypothesis'...

In spite of the progress made in recent years this statement is still valid, the middle molecule controversies are not yet solved: a break-through has not yet occurred. Consequently the optimal dialysis strategy, the optimal dialyser design and the optimal properties of dialysis membranes have yet to be determined.

FURTHER PROGRESS IN ACCESS TO THE CIRCULATION (see also chapter 8)

Circulatory access, *the conditio sine qua non* for successful dialysis, also can offer problems. Sometimes access difficulties still endanger the continuation of dialysis treatment (165), but many improvements and refinements have been achieved. The classical external Scribner-Quinton arteriovenous shunt, once called the achilles heel of chronic dialysis, has undergone many beneficial modifications, as have the surgical implantation techniques (166, 167).

Introduction of the straight 'winged' in line cannula by Ramirez and co-workers (168) in 1966 made possible a straight external shunt, which was easy to declot. Notwithstanding such improvements, the life span of external shunts remained limited to an average of 7 to 10 months (166).

The 'large vessel applique', introduced by Thomas (169) in 1969, consists of straight Silastic cannulae with a Dacron skirt attached. In the present model, the Dacron patches are sutured to the anterior wall of the superficial femoral artery and directly to the femoral vein at the origin of the long saphenous vein which is locally excised. The obvious advantage is that the cannulae do not interrupt the blood stream in both main vessels. Originally an unacceptably high percentage of infections occurred (166), often requiring shunt removal and occasionally causing loss of a leg or even death. However, these problems decreased with the improved model, introduced in 1973 (170). Presently, the life span of the Thomas shunt seems to be much longer.

Another ingenious device is the Buselmeier shunt (171, 172, introduced in 1973). This shunt consists essentially of a small U-shaped Silastic segment with two Teflon plugged outlets (see Figures 29). Implantation is done with standard vessel tips and the U-shaped portion is either partially or totally buried in the subcutaneous tissue, with the outlets remaining extracutaneous. The Buselmeier shunt is often preferred in paediatric dialysis.

Although a well created arteriovenous fistula functions for years, some patients have recurrent problems leading to obliteration of access vasculature. For these patients, other types of arteriovenous fistulas have been introduced. May and co-workers (173) introduced saphenous vein autographs as a bridge between an artery and a vein (1969). The saphenous vein can be fashioned as a loop in the forearm or as a straight bridge from the brachial artery to a distal vein. Several other modifications are possible. Chinitz and colleagues (174, 175) created bridged arteriovenous fistulae with bovine heterografts. Several others adopted this type of bridged fistula (176, 177). Others created bridged arteriovenous fistulae with mandril grown autografts (178) or with synthetic self sealing prosthetic material (179–181).

While they are very useful in special circumstances, so far none of these techniques has proved to be as satisfactory as a well created Brescia-Cimino type of arteriovenous fistula. However, the expanded polytetrafluoroethylene (PTFE) or Gore-Tex or Impra self sealing conduit seems to be an exceptable alternative (182).

Human umbilical cord allograft seems to be a less satisfactory material (183, 184).

REUSE OF DIALYSIS FLUID

As a rule haemodialysis requires large amounts of tap water, which must be pretreated with special equipment. Water and drain connections are required. Haemodialysis systems therefore, are in practice not portable and immobilise patients for their thrice weekly treatments. In addition in many areas in the world, city water is expensive and in short supply. To overcome these disadvantages, reuse of dialysis fluid has been tried, for example by activated carbon regeneration (185–188). Activated carbon, per se, has no effect on electrolytes, however, and only a limited absorption capacity for urea. Adapting a spaceflight technological approach, Gordon et al. (189–191) developed a system to regenerate 5.5 l of dialysate continuously by a multilayer disposable cartridge, containing urease, zirconium-derivatives and activated carbon. This 'Redy' system (also called 'Sorb System') became available around 1970 (192) and makes plumbing and fixed water and drain connections unnecessary. As the machine is semiportable, it makes travelling for holiday and business purposes possible for chronic dialysis patients (193, 194 [chapter 17]). Other portable and even wearable haemodialysis systems have been designed and constructed (195–199). They have, however, certain disadvantages and have found only limited practical application so far (see also chapter 17).

All these transportable and portable haemodialysis systems have in addition, when travelling, the disadvantage of a voluminous and heavy amount of accessories like dialysers, bags with sterile saline, regeneration cartridges etc., causing transportation problems.

SEQUENTIAL ULTRAFILTRATION AND DIALYSIS

Removal of fluid during haemodialysis by ultrafiltration, usually accomplished by negative pressure on the dialysate compartment, often causes arterial hypotension or muscle cramps or both, in particular when relatively large amounts of fluid have to be removed in brief periods of time. Bergström and co-workers (200) observed by chance that rapid ultrafiltration was much better tolerated (without significant fall in blood pressure) when performed without simultaneous dialysis, i.e. when negative pressure was applied with the dialysis fluid bypassing the dialyser. They successfully introduced a dialysis protocol of sequential ultrafiltration and dialysis: in this way even large amounts of fluid (e.g. 4 l or more in one hour) could be removed without discomfort to the patient and without a fall in bloodpressure. This was soon confirmed by other clinical investigators (201–203). Several dialysis machines are now provided with modifications to perform ultrafiltration without dialysis fluid passing through the dialyser.

BICARBONATE VERSUS ACETATE

With the construction of an on-line dialysate proportioning system by Grimstud, Cole and coworkers (90) in 1964, a concentrate was prepared with sodium acetate instead of sodium bicarbonate, which was the original alkalinising anion in dialysis fluid in the early years of haemodialysis (88). This was necessary to prevent precipitation of calcium carbonate.

In recent years suspicion arose that in acute, sick patients because of a reduced rate of conversion into bicarbonate, acetate could accumulate in the blood and tissues, leading to acetate toxicity with vascular instability and hypotension (204, 205). It was also suspected that undesirable side effects of acetate could occur in stable chronic dialysis patients during dialysis with large surface area dialysers, in particular in patients who were 'slow acetate metabolisers' (206). Rapid acetate infusion, exceeding maximum utilisation, could, under these circumstances, cause rising acetate levels, leading to discomfort of the patient and to 'dialysis hangover'. Simultaneous loss of bicarbonate from the blood through the dialyser may obviously contribute to these undesirable side effects.

Currently several clinical investigators have returned to bicarbonate containing dialysis fluid, instead of acetate as the alkalinising anion for selected patients as was done in the years before 1964. Several proportioning machines are presently marketed with special facilities for delivering bicarbonate containing dialysis fluid (207).

HAEMOPERFUSION

The principle of using sorbents in purification of blood dates back to 1948, when Muirhead and Reid (208) discovered that urea was adsorbed from animal blood by passing it through an ion exchange column. Sixteen years later, in 1964, Yatzidis from Athens, Greece (209) reported at the founding meeting of the European Dialysis and Transplant Association on the results of his attempts to treat uraemia by perfusing the blood of a heparinised patient over a column of activated charcoal.

It soon became apparent that activated charcoal is an effective sorbent for several 'uraemic' metabolites, e.g. creatinine and uric acid, but not for urea. Also charcoal perfusion does not correct water and electrolyte abnormalities. It also became obvious that charcoal had to be coated or micro-encapsulated to prevent charcoal particles from entering the bloodstream (210).

Haemoperfusion with coated activated charcoal or Amberlite resin is presently an effective treatment for severe hypnotic drug overdosage (with barbiturates, glutethimide, chlorpromazine, methaqualone and others [211–213]).

Haemoperfusion is used experimentally as an adjunct to dialysis treatment of chronic uraemia (214–216 [see also table 2]), but is not a complete alternative to haemo- or peritoneal dialysis therapy of end stage renal failure.

In recent years haemoperfusion with coated charcoal has been used for treatment of end stage hepatic failure (217, 218) with promising but yet inconsistent results (see also chapter 16).

HAEMOFILTRATION

Haemofiltration is a new form of replacement of renal function, introduced by Henderson and co-workers (219) in 1967, originally dating back to 1928 (Brull [220]).

It is presently an alternative to conventional dialysis (i.e. removal of solutes by diffusion) and has the advantage of removal of solutes by convection which mimics the performance of the human kidney better: small and large molecules are removed at the same rate (see table 2). The birth of the middle molecule hypothesis in the early seventies (125–128, 132–134, 149–164) stimulated practical application of haemofiltration and in several centres clinical trials were initiated (221–227).

Different filters with different membranes are presently used: the Amicon XM 50 membrane, which is a polysulfone membrane (222, 223 [see also chapter 12]), the polyacrylonitrile membrane, which is used in the Rhône-Poulenc RP6 dialyser (224, 226 [see also chapters 4 and 14]) and the Sartorius SM 40003 membrane, which is an asymmetric cellulose acetate membrane (226). To obtain adequate results rather large amounts of fluid have to be ultrafiltered (20–40 l three times weekly depending on body size). Approximately equal amounts of replacement fluids have to be added to the system either before ('predilution mode' [222, 223]) or after the ultrafilter ('postdilution mode' [224]), which is obviously one of the disadvantages of the method.

Haemofiltration is currently in a stage of practical evaluation; by the end of 1979 more than 890 European patients were exclusively treated with haemofiltration out of a total of some 48 000 haemodialysis patients (1.8% [113]). To avoid the need for large amounts of (expensive) sterile replacement fluid, sorbent regeneration and re-infusion of the ultrafiltrate has been attempted and seems to be feasible (227). This technique is still under investigation.

Present data indicate that haemofiltration is an effective method of replacement of renal function. Removal of small molecules (urea, creatinine and so forth) is somewhat less efficient, however, than with haemodialysis. Also, loss of protein through the membrane of the ultrafilter has been described (223, 228).

On the other hand, marked improvement of peripheral nerve function during treatment with haemofiltration has been observed; in addition better control of hyperphosphataemia and (in some patients) of hyperlipidaemia has been noted. Control of dialysis resistant hypertension has been described by several investigators (228, 229).

Haemofiltration seems to be a promising procedure for replacement of renal function in selected patients. However, at present it remains questionable if haemofiltration will become a serious competitor of 'classical' haemodialysis (230). For the time being haemofiltration is expensive and rather cumbersome.

Further evaluation is on its way (see chapters 12 and 13).

PLASMA EXCHANGE

A method of 'plasmaphaeresis' has been devised by Abel and colleagues (4, 231), as early as in 1914 with the purpose of 'using this method for the relief of toxemia'. Plasma exchange became feasable in the late sixties and early seventies, because technical facilities were developed and extracorporeal circulation technology had become available. Clinical investigators became interested

Table 2. Characteristics of different modes of blood cleansing (Reproduced from Manis and Friedman [230], slightly modified).

	Haemodialysis	Haemofiltration	Haemoperfusion (activated charcoal)
Fluid removal	Ultrafiltration	Ultrafiltration	None
Solute removal	Diffusion	Convection	Adsorption
Clearance of small molecules	High	Moderate to good	Variable
Clearance of 'middle' molecules (300-5000 d)	Low	High	High
Current use	Uraemia (Drugoverdose)	Uraemia	Drugoverdose Hepatic failure (Uraemia, adjunct therapy)

in plasma exchange as a method of treatment for a number of different rather divergent diseases, several of them having an 'auto-immune' pathogenesis (232–235).

Presently two different methods of plasma exchange are available. Until early in 1979 it was mainly performed by continuous flow separation (this method is now called *plasma separation*). Since then suitable membranes became available and membrane plasma separation, presently called *plasmapheresis,* seems to become the technique of choice (236, 237). Vascular access is usually achieved by means of an arteriovenous shunt.

During each treatment, which is initially performed daily or every other day, usually 4 to 5 l of plasma are removed and replaced by fresh frozen plasma or reconstituted dried plasma or PPF (Plasma Protein Fraction). Sometimes albumin-electrolyte solution is used (232, 233).

Recently a method has been described utilising two hollow fibre filters with different pore sizes. The first filter separates the plasma from the whole blood. This separated plasma is led through a second filter with smaller pores. The filtrate is, after removal of larger molecular substances, mixed with the cell rich residual blood from the first filter, returned to the patient (234). Other promising refinements and modifications have been published (e.g. selective plasma component removal [238] and plasma exchange with immuno-adsorption [239, 240]). Plasma exchange treatment is usually combined with intensive immunosuppressive therapy (steroids and cytotoxic drugs) and is now accepted as an effective and rational therapy for certain types of fulminating hypersensitivity glomerular disease, e.g. anti-GMB disease (Goodpasture's syndrome) and rapidly progressive nephritis. According to Peters, Rees and Lockwood (232) both free antibody and immune complexes are removed from the circulation and plasma exchange also depletes humoral mediators such as complement and fibrinogen.

In addition, plasma exchange therapy has been applied to other 'auto-immune' diseases (thrombotic thrombocytopenic purpura [241]), systemic lupus, myasthenia gravis, Guillain Barré syndrome and other disorders such as rheumatoid arthritis, scleroderma, Raynaud syndrome all with variable success: the therapeutic range of plasma exchange is presently under intensive investigation.

Technical aspects, therapeutic modalities and complications of plasma exchange have been extensively discussed and reviewed at recent international symposia in Cologne, West Germany (June 1980 [235]) and in Cleveland OH, USA (April 1982). (See chapter 48 for further details.)

LIPID ABNORMALITIES

In 1974, Lindner and co-workers (242) shocked the dialysis world by reporting an abnormally high premature mortality and morbidity due to atherosclerotic cardiovascular complications in Seattle dialysis patients. The incidence was much higer than for normal and hypertensive groups of comparable age. Although the group studied was rather small, the data supported the figures recorded in an early annual European statistical report (243). Recent European statistics, based on very large numbers of patients, indicate that the proportion of death due to cerebral vascular and cardiovascular causes in chronic haemodialysis patients is approximately 56% in the hospital haemodialysis population and approximately 60% in the home dialysis setting (244). Several studies have clarified certain pertinent metabolic abnormalities in dialysis patients. The investigations of Bagdade, Porte and Bierman (245) beginning in 1968, have shown a high incidence of plasma lipid abnormalities involving mainly the triglyceride rich very-low-density lipoproteins in patients with chronic renal failure, whether treated by dialysis or not. Bagdade and coworkers (246) and more recently Savdie and associates (247) demonstrated that the persistent hypertriglyceridaemia, a potential cardiovascular risk factor, is attributable to a delay of peripheral catabolism of very-low-density lipoproteins and impaired triglyceride removal due to a functional defect in lipoprotein lipase. This apparently results from the accumulation of uraemic toxins. Hypertriglyceridaemia also may be augmented by dialysate dextrose (248) and acetate (249).

NEPHROGENIC OSTEODYSTROPHY AND VITAMIN D

Substitution of renal function by dialysis not only opened up a new field of therapeutic potentialities, but also an enormous and still increasing area of research. Many studies, related to dialysis and uraemia, had their impact in much broader fields of nephrology and renal physiology.

For example, renal osteodystrophy, once infrequent, soon became a serious problem in many regular dialysis patients (250). Originally described as 'renal rickets' a series of observations brought new and exciting knowledge, clarifying vitamin D and calcium metabolism.

In 1935, Pappenheimer and Wilens (251, 252) noted parathyroid enlargement in cases of renal failure with bone disease. They could reproduce this syndrome by partial renal ablation in animals. A few years later, Liu and Chu (253) demonstrated calcium malabsorption in cases of nephrogenic osteodystrophy, which was resistant to vitamin D. However, renal osteodystrophy could be improved with unusually large doses of vitamin D or its derivative dihydrotachysterol (254). The observation of Bauer, Carlsson and Lindquist (255) that vitamin D also increased bone resorption, the demonstration of a long delay between intravenous administration of vitamin D in the rat and its physiological effects (256) and the ineffectiveness of the vitamin on resorption of bone *in vitro*, raised several questions. Although multiple interactions were apparent between the kidneys, the parathyroids, the skeleton and vitamin D, their interrelationship remained a mystery.

An important key to the understanding of the puzzle came from the studies of DeLuca and colleagues (256) who demonstrated that vitamin D had to be hydroxylated before any physiological effects could occur. The lag period of 10 to 12 h could be cut to approximately 3 to 4 h by administration of 25-hydroxyvitamin D_3 (25[OH]D_3) and the 25-hydroxy-derivative appeared to be active *in vitro* on cultures of bone (257).

The liver microsomes were shown to be the site of 25-hydroxylation of vitamin D_3, which was demonstrated to be a biofeedback regulated process (258, 259). It soon became evident that 25[OH]D_3 was not the final product in the metabolic chain of vitamin D: it had to be metabolised further before reaching full potency.

The next important key to the puzzle came when Fraser and Kodicek (260, 261) revealed that the kidney was the unique source of a very potent hormone, that stimulated intestinal calcium absorption and calcium resorption from bone. DeLuca and colleagues (262) then isolated from chickens given radioactive vitamin D_3, a highly active metabolite which was identified as 1,25-dihydroxy-vitamin D_3 (263).

The implications of these findings both for the renal patient and for further research and clarification of the metabolism of calcium, vitamin D and the skeleton have been enormous. Nephrogenic bone disease became a dilemma with prolongation of life of the uraemic patient by regular dialysis. This doubtless was an impetus for the research which led to the disentanglement of the mysteries of vitamin D metabolism:
... 'the unravelling of the interrelationships between vitamin D and its metabolites is one of the triumphs of recent medical research'... (J. Reeve [264]).

For the independent observer the completion of the jig-saw puzzle of vitamin D and its metabolites, the liver, the kidneys, the parathyroids and the skeleton by physiologists, clinical investigators and other scientists is highly impressive, even moving. Treatment of renal osteodystrophy and several other disorders with synthetic vitamin D metabolites and analogues is now available.

Calcitriol or 1,25-[OH]$_2$$D_3$ or 1α-[OH]D_3 (approved name alfacalcidol) which is easier to synthesise and which is converted in the liver to calcitriol by hydroxylation on the 25 position, usually provide a satisfactory response (264). Calcifedol, which is 25[OH]D_3 and which is the circulating form of vitamin D, is also effective but the effect may be less consistent because its full potency depends on the hydroxylation at the 1 position by the tubular cells of the kidney.

Nevertheless, recent observations which became possible after the introduction of methods for measuring 1-25-[OH]$_2$$D_3$ levels in plasma and results of longterm therapeutic trials with the new vitamin D derivatives have cast some doubt on the pathogenesis and therapy of osteomalacia either from renal or non-renal origin. With growing experience discrepancies have been observed: in some patients with osteomalacia blood levels of 1-25-[OH]$_2$$D_3$ were normal or even increased and, conversely, some patients with chronic renal failure had decreased or undetectable levels of 1-25-[OH]$_2$$D_3$ but no evidence of osteomalacia.

Also it turned out that the therapeutic results with the new vitamin D_3 derivatives in some patients with renal and non-renal osteomalacia were inexplicably disappointing (265). It has been suggested that the pathogenesis of nephrogenic osteomalacia is multifactorial. Recently this hypothesis gained support from observations from Newcastle upon Tyne, England, that under certain circumstances aluminium accumulation may occur in patients with chronic renal failure, the main source of aluminium uptake being the city water used for preparation of dialysis fluid (266, 267). Deposition of aluminium in bone may prevent calcification and may be responsible for at least some cases of osteomalacia resistant to therapeutic doses of vitamin D_3 derivatives (see below and chapter 42).

ALUMINIUM TOXICITY IN DIALYSIS PATIENTS

In 1972 Alfrey and associates (268) described a new and initially poorly understood clinical entity in a group of five patients, haemodialysed in Denver, Colorado, for three or more years. They developed a syndrome of dyspraxia, speech abnormalities, myoclonus, seizures, personality changes and disordered encephalograms. Without exception the disease progressed to death in 3–7 months (268). All patients received dialysis with untreated Denver city water. Trace element analysis was performed on brain tissue for a wide spectrum of elements; compared with uraemic patients who died without signs of encephalopathy and normals there were no impressive differences: rubidium and potassium concentrations in brain tissue were somewhat reduced (25–30%), in comparison with normal controls; tin (normally non detectable or less than 2 ppm [<1.7 nmol/100 g]) was the only element which was consistently increased in uraemic brain tissue, both in patients with and without the encephalopathy syndrome. The aluminium content was initially not analysed, probably because aluminium intoxication was considered highly unlikely.

Interestingly a syndrome of loss of memory, tremor, jerking movements and impaired coordination was described half a century before. In addition the patient was also suffering from chronic constipation, incontinence of urine and persistent vomiting (Spofforth, 1921 [269]).

The patient was a metalworker of 46 who had been dipping red-hot metal articles contained in an aluminium holder into concentrated nitric acid. His urine was analysed and reportedly contained a large amount of aluminium.

No data has been reported on renal function and on the analytical technique of aluminium determination in the urine sample, which obviously must have been rather crude in that time.

Between 1971 and 1976, 14 more cases in the Denver regular dialysis population (270) were observed. Suspicion rose that aluminium, which is toxic for the nervous system, was responsible for the dialysis encephalopathy syndrome. This hypothesis gained support by tissue aluminium studies in brain, bone and muscle: brain tissue aluminium values were four times higher than in dialysis patients who died from other causes and 10 times control values in non dialysed subjects. It appeared that the aluminium was predominantly localised in the gray matter of the brain. Aluminium concentrations in muscle and bone were also significantly higher than in controls (270).

Meanwhile similar cases were reported from Newcastle upon Tyne, England and from Ottawa, Canada. The tap water in these cities has a high aluminium content, an aluminium precipitation method being used to remove undesired colour from the water (271). In Eindhoven, The Netherlands, six cases were observed and at post mortem tissue analysis very high aluminium concentrations were found in brain, bone and other tissues. The aluminium contamination was brought into the water used for preparation of the dialysis fluid by aluminium electrodes in a heating tank (272, 273). In the west of Scotland in regions with a high aluminium content of tap water (mean 420 µg/l [16 µmol/l]) the dialysis encephalopathy syndrome occurred in 14 home dialysis patients, but no cases were observed in Glasgow itself, where the city water aluminium is less than 30 µg/l (1.1 µmol/l) (274). Obviously dialysis encephalopathy had a geographical distribution, related to the aluminium content of raw or inadequately treated city water, used for dialysis fluid preparation (275-277).

Other symptoms of chronic aluminium toxicity are vitamin D resistant osteomalacia, proximal muscle weakness (278), hypochromic microcytic anaemia (279) (see chapter 42).

Aluminium kinetics in dialysis patients are complex: aluminium entering the blood is eagerly bound to plasma protein and uptake from the dialysate may continue even when total plasma aluminium exceeds the dialysate aluminium concentration (280). Even when all plasma sides have been saturated, tissue deposition is likely to continue (in brain grey matter, skeleton and muscles).

In some cases a different aetiology of dialysis associated encephalopathy cannot be excluded, but the main source is doubtless aluminium intoxication from aluminium containing city water used for preparation of dialysis fluid, either untreated or inadequately treated.

However individual sensitivity for the toxic effects of aluminium varies.

Transfer of aluminium into the patient is highly promoted by alkalinity of the dialysate, either caused by high pH of the incoming raw water or by the use of bicarbonate instead of acetate in the dialysis fluid (281). A low pH (<6.5) has a similar effect (see also chapter 17).

So far dialysate pH has been routinely neglected; in this context it seems indicated to include pH monitoring and pH control of dialysis fluid in the parameters which are routinely checked.

Oral aluminium containing phosphate binders - routinely administered to dialysis patients - may also contribute to the aluminium load of the patients and the safety of these compounds is questionable (280, 282-284). According to data from Graf et al. (285) most of the intestinally absorbed aluminium is removed by dialysis if a dialysate with a very low aluminium content is used (0.1-0.3 µmol/l).

On the other hand Dewberry and associates (286) reported recently on 13 patients with dialysis associated encephalopathy who were dialysed with virtually aluminium free dialysis fluid, the only potential aluminium source being oral aluminium containing phosphate binders.

Dialysis encephalopathy may be precipitated in patients who have been dialysed with aluminium containing dialysate and who accumulated toxic amounts of aluminium, by catabolic events like surgery (also transplantation), immobilisation and cortocosteroid administration (287). This may be explained by mobilisation of aluminium from the skeleton and other depots.

Efficient aluminium free (and preferably also magnesium free) phosphate binders are not (yet) available.

It is still unknown if the practice of cooking in aluminium utensils and wrapping food in aluminium foil contribute to the aluminium load of renal failure patients (287-290).

The protein binding and tissue deposition of aluminium precludes its removal by dialysis with aluminium free dialysate: what is transferred into the patient cannot be taken out.

Nevertheless some opposite observations have recently been published (205, 287, 291, 292). In one case administration of desferrioxamine during dialysis apparently contributed to a successful outcome. According to Adhemar and colleagues (293) efficient removal of aluminium can be achieved with haemofiltration.

The maximum permissable aluminium content of water used for dilution of concentrated salt solutions for analysis has been somewhat arbitrarely set for 50 µg/l (1.9 µmol/l) but has recently been lowered to 15 µg/l (0.56 µmol/l) in the UK and to 10 µg/l (0.37 µmol/l) in the USA.

However according to Graf and associates (294) the ideal dialysis fluid aluminium concentration should be below 5,4 µg/l (0.2 µmol/l). This can be achieved by pretreatment of raw water used for preparation of dialysis fluid with reverse osmosis, preferable with spirally wound cartridges (see also chapters 6 and 7; for further reading the reader is referred to chapter 42). The aluminium concentration in the dialysis concentrate should not lead to an appreciable increase of aluminium in the dialysis fluid which is used to perfuse the dialyser (295).

Monitoring of aluminium levels in serum four to six times per year is recommended (295).

VIRAL HEPATITIS (see also chapter 34)

Chronic dialysis undoubtedly contributed indirectly to a totally different field of research: viral hepatitis. In 1964, Blumberg Alter and Visnich (296) found in the serum of a multitransfused haemophiliac (an Australian aborigine), an unusual new antigen which they named Australia antigen. The significance of the new antigen was obscure until a case of mild hepatitis was correlated with transient appearance of the Australia antigen in blood (297, 298). With the recognition that Australia antigen was found in the sera of about 10% of patients with viral hepatitis, notably those with serum hepatitis, a new era in hepatitis research began (298, 299).

About 1965, it became evident that serum hepatitis

was a danger in dialysis units, which at that time were rapidly proliferating. Serious hepatitis outbreaks occurred not only in several European centres (Manchester, Liverpool, London, Edinburgh, Stockholm) but also in the United States (300, 301). These hepatitis outbreaks were only the beginning of a serious danger: the major part of the iceberg was still under the surface. In the 1966 annual EDTA Report, Drukker et al. (301) identified 40 cases of viral hepatitis in 19 centres out of a total of 54 reporting, i.e. 35%. In 1965/1966, 14 cases with 4 deaths occurred in patients and there were 4 deaths out of 26 cases in dialysis personnel. Subsequently, an ever increasing incidence of hepatitis in patients and staff was reported annually. Further investigations showed that after mild hepatitis B infection, persistent Australia antigenaemia (HB$_s$Ag) may develop in individuals with a diminished immune response such as patients on maintenance dialysis (302). It became evident that those with persistent Australia antigenaemia could potentially infect others (303), endangering patients and staff of dialysis units. By 1971 there were 12 major outbreaks of hepatitis resulting in 357 cases with 18 (5%) deaths. In 1975, 870 of 927 dialysis centres in Europe (93%) reported on the incidence of hepatitis amongst their staff (243). The total number of infected members of staff was 748 with 8 deaths (1.1%). At present the tragedy is far from coming to an end. In 1980 2234 new cases of hepatitis were recorded in Europe in dialysis patients: 1800 hepatitis B, 52 A, 382 non A, non B (vide infra) and 566 in dialysis staff, with 11 deaths (1.9% [113]).

A series of committee recommendations among others in England and the Netherlands for prophylaxis (304, 305) were partly successful. But hepatitis continues to be a serious problem in dialysis communities in the majority of countries with dialysis facilities.

Further research on hepatitis continues. Subtypes of HB$_s$Ag have been discovered (298, 306) and in 1972 Magnius and Espmark (307) discovered a new antigen called the e determinant. The e antigen has been found exclusively in HB$_s$Ag-positive sera and apparently correlates with active liver disease and infectivity. Anti e antibodies occur in HB$_s$Ag-positive sera and in some anti-HB$_s$ (HB$_s$Ab) containing sera. This discovery is of considerable practical importance in dialysis units.

Recently Italian investigators identified a new hepatitis agent named delta (δ), which is invariably associated with progressive liver injury in human carriers.

The agent is obligatory associated with the hepatitis B virus and apparently cannot replicate without the help of HBV.

So far δ-Ag and its antibody anti-δ seems to be common (only simultaneously with HBV markers [HB$_s$Ag and anti-HB$_s$]) in drug addicts who take drugs parenterally (308, 309).

One of the structural forms bearing HB$_s$Ag consists of spherical double layered ultrastructures discovered by Dane, Camerone and Briggs (310) in 1970. The so called Dane particles represent the intact virus (311).

In contrast with the hepatitis B virus, the virus of hepatitis A has a short life and no carrier state has been defined (312), transmission can only occur during the acute phase of the disease. The reservoir of hepatitis B virus rests, however, in carriers. After the introduction of reliable serological tests for hepatitis B infection it became evident that with the exception of a rather small number of hepatitis cases caused by cytomegalovirus, the Epstein-Bar virus, yellow fever virus and drugs, dialysis associated hepatitis is predominantly caused by the hepatitis B virus (HBV).

Suspicion grew however that yet another type of viral hepatitis which was serologically HB$_s$Ag and HB$_s$Ab negative was responsible both for cases of post-transfusion hepatitis and dialysis associated hepatitis. This hypothesis was confirmed by Feinstone and Alter and associates (1975 [313, 314]). They observed eight hepatitis cases in a series of multiply-transfused open heart surgery patients, who were serologically not due to viral hepatitis A or B.

The aetiology of non-A, non-B hepatitis (NANB) remained initially obscure but soon it became apparent that the agent was transmissible from man to chimpanzee (315, 316) and recently Vitviski and co-workers (317) demonstrated a new antigen-antibody system distinct from HB$_s$Ag, which appeared specific for non-A, non-B acute hepatitis. The NANB antigen was also demonstrated in liver extract from patients with chronic NANB hepatitis.

The reservoir for NANB rests like the HBV in the so called carriers and according to the expectation NANB hepatitis is, like hepatitis B, a potential source for outbreaks in haemodialysis units.

The 1968-1970 outbreak of HB$_s$Ag negative acute hepatitis in the dialysis unit of the Fulham Hospital in London, appeared serologically unrelated to hepatitis A infection. In retrospection, nine years later, it was concluded that this epidemic had to be classified into the category of non-A, non-B hepatitis (318).

It is both of epidemiological and clinical importance that a significant number of affected dialysis patients remain NANB carriers and that 28% of the infected Fulham patients develop chronic liver disease (318).

Soon detection of NANB hepatitis became possible with specific serological tests, detecting the specific non-A, non-B antigen, called hepatitis C antigen (319).

Passive immunisation with gamma globulin is of temporary benefit for the prevention of hepatitis A in contacts with patients with viral hepatitis A and in subjects exposed to poor sanitary conditions (e.g. when travelling). The administration should be repeated at four to six months intervals (312, 320).

Hyperimmune, anti HB$_s$ gammaglobulin gives protection when administered within 48 hours of infection with HBV (e.g. needlestick injury with contaminated needle) and is efficacious injury with contaminated needle) and is efficacious in protection of new patients entering dialysis units with HB$_s$Ag positive patients. Routine use is however very expensive (312, 321): obviously there is an urgent need for active vaccination (322).

Attempts to prepare vaccines against HBV began in the early and mid 1970's (323, 324) and have given promising results.

From France, where the incidence of hepatitis B infection in dialysis units has been persistently high (113), the results of a two year study of a hepatitis B vaccine were published in 1978 by Maupas and co-workers (325, 326) and in 1981 Crosnier and colleagues reported on the results of a placebo controlled trial of a vaccine prepared at the Institut Pasteur at Paris. Both groups reported satisfactory results (327).

In 1980 Szmuness and colleagues (320) published the results of a large double blind trial of a hepatitis B vaccine in a large group of homosexual men in New York. The vaccine prepared in the Merck Institute for Therapeutic Research from HB_sAg virus particles by formalin inactivation appeared highly effective over a period of at least 8-18 months (329). It seems from the American study that the active immunisation even gives some protection after infection with the hepatitis B virus has occurred i.e. during the incubation period of the disease. The vaccine however induces a rather slow immune response and two booster injections (at 1 and 6 months) are required until satisfactory immunisation is obtained.

Recently (1981) Szmuness and colleagues (330) presented evidence that simultaneous administration of hepatitis B immunoglobulin and hepatitis B vaccine offered immediate protection. The passively acquired antibody did not interfere with the immuno-genecity of the vaccine and did not prevent development of antibody to the vaccine.

This opens not only possibilities for post exposure prophylaxis (330) but also offers immediate protection for susceptible persons (lacking detectable hepatitis B surface antigen and antibody to HB_sAg) working in (or entering) a HB_sAg positive dialysis unit.

A reduced immune response to the vaccine has been noted both the French and the American investigators in patients with naturally or artificially impaired immune response, e.g. in patients with advanced chronic renal failure and during immunosuppressive therapy (328, 331).

The results of further trials remain to be seen, but there is presently light at the end of the so far rather dark tunnel of hepatitis B prophylaxis. Many employees and patients in dialysis units are not only looking forward to effective vaccination against hepatitis B but also to a vaccine protective against non-A, non-B hepatitis.

Notwithstanding diagnostic tests for non-A, non-B hepatitis became available (317, 319), a vaccine has not yet been developed.

So far, the incidence of non-A, non-B hepatitis in dialysis units seems less than of hepatitis B, but the frequency may be on the increase: in the Netherlands, Sweden and the United Kingdom in 1979 more cases of non-A, non-B were reported than of hepatitis B (113).

In addition this form of hepatitis seems to be related to a high frequency of persistent hepatic dysfunction: 8 out of the 29 patients from the 1968-1970 outbreak at the Fulham renal unit in London reportedly had persistently elevated serum amino transferase activity (28%). Liver biopsy revealed chronic aggressive hepatitis in three and chronic persistent hepatitis in two (318).

Effective vaccination is urgently needed before the non-A, non-B type of hepatitis starts spreading in dialysis units.

In areas with a high frequency of primary hepatocellular carcinoma (e.g. Sub-Saharan Africa, Asia, Oceania and others) there is a close association between hepatitis B virus infection on one hand and postnecrotic cirrhosis of the liver and primary hepatocellular carcinoma on the other; primary livercarcinoma – in these areas responsible for 60% of the carcinoma deaths – commonly develops in livers with postnecrotic cirrhosis. In these areas hepatitis B virus carriers are also common.

This association supports the hypothesis that persistent hepatitis B virus infection is required for the development of most cases of primary hepatocellular carcinoma (331).

The next step in testing this hypothesis is by decreasing the frequency of hepatitis B infection by large scale vaccination, which should decrease the frequency of primary livercarcinoma in these affected areas (Blumberg and London [1981, 332]).

This hypothesis, if confirmed, would be another dialysis associated landmark in medical history.

DIALYSIS TREATMENT OF NON-RENAL CONDITIONS

In recent years psychiatrists, dermatologists, neurologists and dialysis physicians became interested in dialysis treatment of certain non-renal conditions. The idea of dialysis treatment of mental disorders (schizophrenia) and myasthenia gravis originated from Switzerland and dates back to 1960 (333). Interest was renewed by Cade and Wagemaker (334-336) in 1977/78. Cade started dialysing a schizophrenic patient with hypertension and kidney disease in 1971 on her own request and described remarkable improvement of her mental condition (334). Endorphin, identified as β-leucine-5-endorphin, was isolated from the dialysing fluid of several schizophrenic patients (337-339). This however was not confirmed by others. Ever since, a number of investigators reported both negative and positive results in schizophrenic patients: the matter is still under investigation and the issue is still undecided at the present time.

Other non-renal conditions experimentally treated with dialysis are psoriasis (339-342) and myasthenia gravis (333, 339, 343, 344). It has been suggested that other methods of blood purification (haemofiltration, haemoperfusion and plasma exchange) have become the methods of choice for treatment of these conditions; investigations are continuing. (For more detailed information the reader is referred to chapter 49.)

SOME SOCIO-ECONOMIC CONSIDERATIONS

For a few years after 1960 when treatment of end stage renal disease (ESRD) with dialysis began in Seattle, a closeted and anonymous committee decided which medically suitable patients would receive maintenance haemodialysis treatment; there were only a few machines and an overwhelming number of patients.

The costs were prohibitively high ($ 40 000 per patient/year) and financing of even a limited chronic dialysis programme raised insolvable dilemmas.

Nevertheless some 7000 American patients received regular dialysis treatment before legislation was passed in the American Congress in 1972 under which the Federal Government would pay for the cost of dialysis treatment. In the years that the new law has been effective, the number of patients on regular dialysis treatment in the USA showed a staggering growth to approximately 50 000 in 1980 (220 per million population). Since 1972 the mean annual increase of new dialysis patients in the USA has been 5000 to 7000 patients per year (345, 346).

The new legislation stimulated in the U.S. a great expansion of dialysis facilities and created a big dialysis industry: approximately 36% of the total number of dialysis patients are treated in 'for profit units' (347).

In addition the new law had several unexpected side-effects: the percentage of home dialysis patients in the U.S. decreased from 40% in 1972 to between 10 and 12% in 1979, because the new law provided economically much more attractive facilities for hospital dialysis, although home dialysis is much cheaper and survival rates and the rehabilitation figures are substantially better than with hospital dialysis (348). To reverse this highly undesirable side effect the law has been altered in 1980.

There is a remarkable variation of the number of regular dialysis patients in the U.S. from state to state (347) which can only partly be explained by the fact that patients are sometimes dialysed in a centre across the border of an adjacent state. The rate in the District of Columbia, Virginia and Maryland combined (because patients treated in the District of Columbia are often living in Virginia or Maryland) is 278 per million population. In Idaho on the contrary the rate is 67 and in Alaska 52 per million. All the other states showed considerable variations in between (347).

There was also a remarkable, geographical variation in the percentage of home dialysis (ranging from 0 to 59%) and in transplantation rates between the different states all over the U.S. continent. A similar phenomenon has recently been reported from England (349), and large variations also occur in Europe and adjacent countries: 1.2-260 patients per million population (as registered by the end of 1980 [113]). Correlation has been demonstrated between the total numbers of patients treated for ESRD and the gross national product (GNP) per capita (113, 350).

Some Western countries with relatively high GNP support however fewer patients than might have been expected and others treat substantially more (113, 350). It is obvious that both in the U.S. and in Europe important social, cultural and economic factors influence the numbers of patients offered treatment (351, 352). Other factors such as geographical differences in the prevalence of terminal uraemia may play a (probably minor) role. The total number of patients on dialysis treatment per million population is in Europe much less than in the U.S.: 89 against 220 per million population by the end of 1980, the total number of patients on regular dialysis treatment (including haemofiltration) in Europe was by the end of 1980 51 157 (113). The annual increase of the dialysis population is in Europe somewhat less than in the USA (approximately 4000 to 5500 against 5000 to 7000). The annual number of transplant operations (4000 in the USA and 3000 to 3500 in Europe) is more or less constant, further increase being limited by the lack of supply of cadaver grafts.

At the end of 1980 the total number of patients in the US with end stage kidney disease was 63 214 (353), an increase of 250% since 1974. It is expected that the number of patients on treatment in the US will increase to 87 000 in 1986.

The cost of the American ESRD programme rose fivefold between 1974 and 1980 to $ 1400 million and is expected to reach $ 1800 million in 1982 and $ 3000 million in 1986 as a result of expansion of the programme and inflation.

Figures of cost of dialysis in Europe are not readily available. In the Netherlands (population 14 million) in 1981 some 2000 patients were treated with regular dialysis. The annual increase of the dialysis population in this country is 450.

The cost of this national dialysis programme in 1981 was approximately $ 73 million (even with a substantial number of patients dialysed twice weekly) and is expected to increase to more than $ 390 million (for 8000 patients [354]) by the end of the century without correction for inflation.

In the climate of budget cutting the Reagan administration strives presently (1982) for greater efficiency of the ESRD programme, promoting (less expensive) home dialysis and reducing reimbursements both for hospital based dialysis and non hospital dialysis (in so called free standing units).

In the United Kingdom hospital haemodialysis has been limited by tight budgetary control and the majority (62%) of the patients practise home haemodialysis or peritoneal dialysis at home, which is cheaper.

On the other hand the group of transplanted patients in the UK continues to grow more rapidly which also helps in limiting the cost.

Nevertheless Manis and Friedman (355) were right with their statement that 'maintenance dialysis stands as an effective, costly – and incompletely understood – life sustaining regimen'. With continuing economical retrenchments we should anticipate a severe curtailment of dialysis facilities and ESRD programmes even in the 'rich' countries.

Hopefully it will not become necessary to turn the clock back to the early 1960's and to 'life committees'...

A FINAL WORD

So far the difficulties in establishing an all embracing dialysis system have been described. From Haas' faltering footsteps more than half a century ago progress has been meteoric, particularly during the past 20 years. The 'uraemic syndrome' is now a rarity having been replaced by a surprisingly good quality of life. That this has been achieved with an inanimate material such as cellophane or Cuprophan is almost incomprehensible for we still have incomplete knowledge as to the nature and biological importance of substances that pass through the membrane. It is also difficult to apportion effects on the patient between dialysis and the aftermath of physiopathological problems arising from a direct result of loss of normally functioning renal tissue. As a result a new series of clinical and pathological problems became manifest as the life of patients was usefully extended more and more. We are still hampered by the paucity of knowledge about the function of normal kidneys so it is not surprising that we are uncertain of the priorities required to build the most efficient type of artificial kidney. Treatment of patients one or more decades hence will rely not only on current knowledge and experience but also on future discoveries. Maybe in a short space of time, current major problems such as membrane design, vascular access, reuse of dialysers, hepatitis, metabolism of electrolytes, protein, carbohydrate and fat, the toxicology of aluminium, to mention a few, will be things of the past, only to be replaced, it is anticipated by more sophisticated problems. According to some clinical investigators it is 'reasonable to speculate that innovations in the conservative treatment of uraemia, may, within a decade, rival haemodialysis in both effectiveness and cost (355)'.

As the ideal of complete duplication of renal function by artificial and medical aids is approached perhaps one abnormality must be retained currently for patients with renal failure, They exhibit one deficit that is beneficial, namely the ability to retain patency of an arteriovenous shunt or fistula over prolonged periods of time by a process of 'natural anticoagulation'. Without this abnormality haemodialysis, as practised today, would be virtually impossible for it is common knowledge that arteriovenous shunts clot once recovery of renal function occurs after an episode of acute tubular necrosis and that arteriovenous fistulae frequently close after a succesful transplant.

The abnormal clinical states that bedevilled the well-being of past and present generations of patients have been mentioned briefly and will be described in detail in subsequent chapters of this book. That many problems have now been eradicated or reduced in severity, is a credit to those currently engaged in unravelling the complexities of the various physio-pathological processes that are involved. This should please the pioneers who grappled with the initial technical difficulties of establishing and maintaining intermittently an extracorporeal circulation.

In concluding this review it seems appropriate to repeat the question: 'Dialysis petrified or progressive?', which was the title of a round table discussion at the annual EDTA Congress in Tel-Aviv, Israel in 1974 (356). Considering the continuing progress made since the publication of the first edition of this book (August 1978) the answer is obvious.

ACKNOWLEDGMENTS

The author gratefully acknowledges the courtesy of Mrs. E. Frame, The Library, University of Strathclyde, Scotland for *Photograph 1*.

Figure 2 is reproduced with kind permission from the Editor of the Philosophical Transactions of the Royal Society of London.

Photograph 3 (John Jacob Abel) was kindly supplied by Mrs Doris Thibodeau, librarian, the Johns Hopkins University Institute of the History of Medicine, Baltimore MD, USA.

Figure 4 is redrawn from a figure in the Journal of Pharmacology and Experimental Therapy with permission from the Editor and Publishers.

A number of letters of John Jacob Abel and other historical material, which is kept at the Welch Medical Library of the Johns Hopkins University, Monumentstreet, Baltimore, MD, USA, were photocopied and made available to the author by Mr. David Hamilton, Ph D, FRCS, consultant surgeon at the Western Infirmary, University of Glasgow, Scotland.

Photograph 6 was kindly supplied by Prof. J. Benedum, Gieszen (DBR) (20, 21).

Figures 7 and 8 are redrawn from figures originally published in Abderhalden's Handbuch der biologischen Arbeitsmethoden, with permission from the Publishers.

The author gratefully acknowledges the courtesy of Prof. Jost Benedum, Gieszen (DBR), for the photographs which are reproduced in *figures 9, 10 and 11*. These figures are reproduced from originals kindly supplied by Dr. Med. Willi Haas, Erlensee/Krs. Hanau (DBR), who is a nephew of the late Dr. Georg Haas.

Figures 6, 9, 10 and 11 are reproduced with kind permission from the Editors and Publishers of the Medizin historisches Journal, Gustav Fisher Verlag, Stuttgart, New York.

Figure 13 is reproduced from Dr. Kolff's MD thesis, with permission.

Photographs 15b and 16 are by courtesy of the Municipal Museum of the City of Amsterdam.

Figure 18 is reproduced from the Acta Medica Scandinavica with permission from the Author and the Publishers.

Photograph 19 was kindly supplied by Dr. E.E. Twiss, St. Clara Hospital, Rotterdam, The Netherlands.

Figure 20 was kindly supplied by prof. Bodo von Garrelts, Stockholm, Sweden and is reproduced with his permission.

Photographs 21 and 22 were kindly supplied by Mr. Patrick T. McBride, author of Genesis of the Artificial Kidney (published by Travenol Laboratories Inc., Deerfield IL, USA, 1979), who's collection of antique dialysers and other material will be permanently displayed at the International Center for Artificial Organs and Transplantation, 8937 Euclid Avenue, Cleveland OH 44106, USA.

Photograph 23 by courtesy of Baxter-Tavenol Laboratories Inc., Morton Grove IL, USA.

Figure 28 was reproduced from the Lancet by kind permission from the Authors and the Editor of the Lancet.

Photographs 31a and 31c have been reproduced from original photographs kindly supplied by Dr. Frederik Kiil from Oslo, Norway.

Figure 31b is taken from a paper by Dr. Frederik Kiil in the Trans Am Soc Artif Intern Organs with permission from the Author and Editor (75).

Photograph 32 is reproduced from a photograph kindly supplied by Dr. Belding H. Scribner from Seattle, WA, USA.

Figures 34a and 34b are reproduced from a comment on a paper presented at an ASAIO meeting in 1965 by dr. Y. Nosé (96) with permission from Dr. Nosé and the Editor of the Trans Am Soc Artif Intern Organs.

Figures 35, 36, 37 are (slightly modified) reproduced from Chapter 15 (written by dr Shaldon en Mr Larson) in the 1st edition of this book.

Figure 40 is redrawn (slightly modified) from a diagram in a paper by Muldoon and Leonard in the Trans Am Soc Artif

Intern Organs (118). With permission from the Authors and the Editor.

Figures 4, 7, 8, 15a, 26 and 28 were prepared by Castado Illustrations Studio, Roermond, The Netherlands, Mr. P.R. Fraipont, Artist.

REFERENCES

1. Munro AC: Thomas Graham (1805–1869). *Phil J (Glasgow)* 8:30, 1971
2. Graham T: Liquid diffusion applied to analysis. *Phil Trans Roy Soc* London 151:183, 1861
3. Abell JJ, Rowntree LC, Turner BB: On the removal of diffusible substances from the circulating blood by means of dialysis. *Trans Ass Am Physicians* 28:51, 1913
4. Abel JJ, Rowntree LG, Turner BB: On the removal of diffusable substances from the circulating blood of living animals by dialysis. *J Pharmacol Exp Ther* 5:275, 1913–1914
5. Abel JJ, Rowntree LG, Turner BB: Some constituents of the blood. *J Pharmacol Exp Ther* 5:611, 1913–1914
6. Abel JJ, Rowntree LG, Turner BB: Plasma removal with return of corpuscles (plasmaphaeresis). *J Pharmacol Exp Ther* 5:625, 1913–1914
7. Hess CL von, McGuigan H: The condition of sugar in the blood. *J Pharmacol Exp Ther* 6:45, 1914–1915
8. Love GH: Vividiffusion with intestinal membranes. *Med Rec (NY)* 98:649, 1920
9. Necheles H: Ueber dialysieren des strömenden Blutes am Lebenden (On dialysis of the circulating blood in vivo). *Klin Wochenschr* 2:1257, 1923 (in German)
10. Necheles H: Erwiderung zu vorstehenden Bemerkungen (Comment on the previous remarks). *Klin Wochenschr.* 2:1888, 19123 (in German)
11. Lim RKS, Necheles H: Demonstration of a gastric secretory excitant in circulating blood by vividialysis. *Proc Soc Exp Biol Med* 24:197, 1926
12. Haas G: Dialysieren des strömenden Blutes am Lebenden (Dialysis of the circulating blood in vivo). *Klin Wochenschr* 2:1888, 1923 (in German)
13. Haas G: Versuche der Blutauswaschung am Lebenden mit Hilfe der Dialyse (Experiments on cleansing of blood in vivo by means of dialysis). *Klin Wochenschr* 4:13, 1925 (in German)
14. Haas G: Ueber Versuche der Blutauswaschung am Lebenden mit Hilfe der Dialyse (On experimental cleansing of blood in vivo with dialysis). *Naunyn Schmiedebergs Arch Pharmacol* 116:158, 1926 (in German)
15. Haas G: Ueber Versuche mit Blutwaschung am Lebenden mit Hilfe der Dialyse (On experimental cleansing of blood in vivo with dialysis). *Naunyn Schmiedebergs Arch Pharmacol* 120:371, 1927 (in German)
16. Haas G: Ueber Blutwaschung (On cleansing of blood). *Klin Wochenschr* 7:1356, 1928 (in German)
17. Haas G: Die Methoden der Blutauswaschung (Methods of cleansing of blood). *Abderhalden's Handb Biol Arbeitsmethoden V* 8:717, 1935 (in German)
18. Philipsson P: Ueber die Verwendbarkeit der Schilfschläuche zur Dialyse (The application of reed stalks to dialysis). *Beitr Chem Phys Path* 1:80, 1902 (in German)
19. Pregl F: Beitrage zur Methodik des Dialysierverfahrens von E. Abderhalden (Contribution to the methodology of the dialysis procedure of E. Abderhalden) *Ferm Forsch* 1:7, 1914 (in German)
20. Benedum J, Weise M: Georg Haas (1886–1971): Sein Beitrag zur Frühgeschichte der künstlichen Niere (Georg Haas: His contribution to the early history of the artificial kidney). *Dtsch Med Wochenschr* 103:1674, 1978 (in German)
21. Benedum J: Georg Haas (1886–1971) Pionier der Hämodialyse (Georg Haas: Pioneer of haemodialysis). *Med Hist J* 14:196, 1979 (in German)
22. Asaba H, Bergström J, Fürst P, Shaldon S, Wilkund S: Treatment of diuretic resistent fluid retention with ultrafiltration. *Acta Med Scand* 204:145, 1978
23. Verbanck J, Schelstraete J, De Paepe M, Hoenich N, Ringoir S: Pure ultrafiltration by repeated puncture of a peripheral armvein as treatment of refractory edema. *Int J Artif Organs* 3:342, 1980
24. Thalhimer W: Experimental exchange transfusion for reducing azotemia. Use of the artificial kidney for this purpose. *Proc Soc Exp Biol Med* 37:641, 1937
25. Kolff WJ: First clinical experience with the artificial kidney. *Ann Intern Med* 62:608, 1965
26. Kolff WJ, Berk HThJ: De kunstmatige nier: een dialysator met groot oppervlak (The artificial kidney: a dialyser with large surface area). *Ned Tijdschr Geneeskd* 87:1684, 1943 (in Dutch)
27. Kolff WJ, Berk HThJ, ter Welle M, van der Ley AJW, van Dijk EC, van Noordwijk J: De kunstmatige nier: een dialysator met groot oppervlak (The artificial kidney: a dialyser with large surface area. *Geneesk Gids* 21:409, 1943 (in Dutch)
28. Kolff WJ, Berk HThJ, ter Welle M, van der Ley AJW, van Dijk EC, van Noordwijk J: The artificial kidney, a dialyzer with a great area. *Acta Med Scand* 117:121, 1944
29. Kolff WJ: Le rein artificiel: un dialyseur à grande surface (The artificial kidney: a dialyser with large surface area). *Presse Méd* 52:103, 1944 (in French)
30. Kolff WJ: *De Kunstmatige Nier* (The artificial kidney), MD Thesis, University of Groningen, The Netherlands, Kampen, JH Kok NV, 1946 (in Dutch)
31. Thorwald J: *Die Patienten* (The Patients). München-Zürich, Droemer-Knauer Verlag 1975, p 99 (in German)
32. Domingo WR, Klijne W: A photoelectric flame photometer. *Biochem J* 45:400, 1949
33. Murray G, Delorme E, Thomas N: Development of an artificial kidney. *Arch Surg* 55:505, 1947
34. Bywaters EGL, Joekes BM: The artificial kidney: its clinical application in the treatment of traumatic anuria. *Proc R Soc Med* 41:411 and 420, 1948
35. Fishman AP, Kroop JG, Leiter HE, Hyman A: Experiences with the Kolff artificial kidney. *Am J Med* 7:15, 1949
36. De Leeuw NKM, Blaustein A: Studies of blood passed through an artificial kidney. *Blood* 4:653, 1949
37. Darmady EM: Dialysis of blood for the treatment of uraemia. *Proc R Soc Med* 41:410 and 418, 1948
38. Merrill JP: Dialysis in acute renal failure. In: *Replacement of Renal Function by Dialysis*, chapter 17, Edited by Drukker W, Parsons FM, Maher JF, Martinus Nijhoff, Medical Division, The Hague, Boston MA, London, 1st edition 1978, p 322
39. Bull GM, Joekes AM, Lowe KG: Conservative treatment of anuric uraemia. *Lancet* 2:229, 1949
40. Borst JGG: Protein katabolism in uraemia. Effects of protein-free diet, infections and blood transfusions. *Lancet* 1:824, 1948
41. Kolff WJ: Dialysis in treatment of uremia. *Arch Intern Med* 94:142, 1954
42. Alwall N: On the artificial kidney. I. Apparatus for dialysis of blood in vivo. *acta Med Scand* 128:317, 1947
43. Alwall N, Norviit L: On the artificial kidney. II. The effectivity of the apparatus. *Acta Med Scand (Suppl)*

196:250, 1947
44. Alwall N: *Therapeutic and Diagnostic Problems in Severe Renal Failure*, Copenhagen, Munksgaard; Stockholm, Svenska Bokförlaget; Oslo and Bergen, Universitetsforlaget, 1963 p 2
45. Alwall N, Bergsten BWB, Gedda PO, Norviit L, Steins AM: On the artificial kidney. IV. The technique in animal experiments. *Acta Med Scand* 132:392, 1949
46. Alwall N: Experiences with treatment of uremia by dialysis of the blood in vivo ('artificial kidney') *Twenty-third meeting of the Northern Surgical Association* held in Stockholm June 26–28, 1947. Copenhagen, Munksgaard, 1948, p 418 en 423
47. Alwall N, Norviit L, Steins AM: On the artificial kidney. VII. Clinical experiences of dialytic treatment of uremia. *Acta Med Scand* 132:587, 1949
48. Murray G, Delorme E, Thomas N: Artificial kidney. *JAMA* 137:1596, 1948
49. Von Garrelts B: *Twenty-third meeting of the Northern Surgical Association* held in Stockholm June 26–28, 1947, Copenhagen, Munksgaard, 1948, p 422
50. Von Garrelts B: A blood dialyzer for use in vivo. *Acta Med Scand* 155:87, 1956
51. Inouye WY, Engelberg J: A simplified artificial dialyzer and ultrafilter. *Surg Forum* 4:438, 1953
52. Kolff WJ: The artificial kidney – past and future. *Circulation* 15:285, 1957
53. Watschinger B, Kolff WJ: Further development of the artificial kidney of Inouye and Engelberg. *Trans Am Soc Artif Intern Organs* 1:37, 1955
54. Kolff WJ, Watschinger B: Further development of a coil kidney. *J Lab Clin Med* 47:969, 1956
55. Michielsen P: A single pass system with recirculation for the twin coil kidney. *Proc Eur Dial Transpl Assoc* 2:267, 1965
56. MacNeill AE, Doyle JE, Anthone R, Anthone S: Technic with a parallel flow straight tube blood dialyzer. *NY State J Med* 59:4137, 1959
57. Doyle JE, Anthone R, Anthone S, MacNeill AE: Treatment of renal failure with a parallel flow straight tubing blood dialyzer. *NY State J Med* 59:4149, 1959
58. Doyle JE: *Extracorporeal Hemodialysis Therapy in Blood Chemistry Disorders.* Am Lecture Series no 453, Springfield, IL, Charles C. Thomas, 1962, p 18
59. Skeggs LT Jr, Leonards JR: Studies on an artificial kidney. I. Preliminary results with a new type of continuous dialyzer. *Science* 108:212, 1948
60. Skeggs LT Jr, Leonards JR, Heisler CR: Artificial Kidney. II. Construction and operation of an improved continuous dialyzer. *Proc Soc Exp Biol Med* 72:539, 1949
61. Muercke RC: *Acute Renal Failure.* St Louis, The CV Mosby Company 1969, p 277
62. Maher JF, Schreiner GE, Waters TJ: Successful intermittent hemodialysis – longest reported maintenance of life in true oliguria (181 days). *Trans Am Soc Artif Intern Organs* 6:123, 1960
63. Giovannetti S, Bigalli A, Cioni L, Della Santa M, Ballestri P: Permanent vein cannulation for repeated hemodialysis. *Acta Med Scand* 173:1, 1963
64. Shaldon S, Rosen SM: Technique of refrigerated coil preservation haemodialysis with femoral venous catheterization. *Br Med J* 2:411, 1964
65. Quinton W, Dillard D, Scribner BH: Cannulation of blood vessels for prolonged hemodialysis. *Trans Am Soc Artif Intern Organs* 6:104, 1960
66. Sinclair ISR, Henderson MA, Simpson DC: Fluon arterio-venous shunt for repeated haemodialysis. *Lancet* 2:410, 1961
67. Quinton WE, Dillard D, Cole JJ, Scribner BH: Possible improvement in the technique of long-term cannulation of blood vessels. *Trans Am Soc Artif Intern Organs* 7:60, 1961
68. Sevitt L, Comty C, Rottka H, Shaldon S: The single break Silastic Teflon shunt. *Proc Eur Dial Transpl Assoc* 1:178, 1964
69. Shaldon S: *Proc Working Conf on Chron Dialysis*, Seattle (University of Washington), December 3–5, 1967, p 16
70. Ramirez O, Swartz C, Onesti G, Mailloux L, Brest AN: The winged in-line shunt. *Trans Am Soc Artif Intern Organs* 12:220, 1966
71. Buselmeier TJ, Kjellstrand CM, Ratazzi CC, Simmons RL, Najarian JS: A new subcutaneous prosthetic A–V shunt: advantageous over the standard Quinton-Scribner shunt and A–V fistula. *Proc Clin Dial Transpl Forum* 2:67, 1972
72. Wetzels E: *Hämodialyse und Peritonealdialyse* (Hemodialysis and Peritonealdialysis). Berlin, Heidelberg, New York, Springer-Verlag 1969, p 127 (in German)
73. Scribner BH, Caner JEZ, Buri R, Quinton WE: The technique of continuous hemodialysis. *Trans Am Soc Artif Intern Organs* 6:88, 1960
74. Kiil F, (Amundsen B): Development of a parallel flow artificial kidney in plastics. *Acta Chir Scand (Suppl)* 253:142, 1960
75. Kiil F, Glover JF Jr: Parallel flow plastic hemodialyzer as a membrane oxygenator. *Trans Am Soc Artif Intern Organs* 8:43, 1962
76. Scribner BH, Buri R, Caner JEZ, Hegstrom R, Burnell JM: The treatment of chronic uremia by means of intermittent dialysis: a preliminary report. *Trans Am Soc Artif Intern Organs* 6:114, 1960
77. Pendras JP, Cole JJ, Tu TH, Scribner BH: Improved technique of continuous flow hemodialysis. *Trans Am Soc Artif Intern Organs* 7:27, 1961
78. Cole JJ, Quinton WE, Williams C, Murray JS, Sherris JC: The pumpless low temperature hemodialysis system. *Trans Am Soc Artif Intern Organs* 8:209, 1962
79. Hegstrom RM, Murray JS, Pendras JP, Burnell JM, Scribner BH: Hemodialysis in the treatment of chronic uremia. *Trans AM Soc Artif Intern Organs* 7:136, 1961
80. Hegstrom RM, Murray JS, Pendras JP, Burnell JM, Scribner BH: Two years experience with periodical hemodialysis in the treatment of chronic uremia. *Trans Am Soc Artif Intern Organs* 8:266, 1962
81. Murray JS, Tu WH, Alberts JB, Burnell JM, Scribner BH: A community hemodialysis center for the treatment of chronic uremia. *Trans Am Soc Artif Intern Organs* 8:315, 1962
82. Brown HW, Maher JF, Lapierre L, Bledsoe FH, Schreiner GE: Clinical problems related to the prolonged artifial maintenance of life by hemodialysis in chronic renal failure. *Trans Am Soc Artif Intern Organs* 8:281, 1962
83. Gonzalez FM, Pabico RL, Walker Brown H, Maher JF, Schreiner GE: Further experience with the use of routine intermittent hemodialysis in chronic renal failure. *Trans Am Soc Artif Intern Organs* 9:11, 1963
84. Kolff WJ, Nakamoto S, Scudder JP: Experiences with long-term intermittent dialysis. *Trans Am Soc Artic Intern Organs* 8:292, 1962
85. Lindholm DD, Burnell JM, Murray JS: Experience in the treatment of chronic uremia in an outpatient community hemodialysis center. *Trans Am Soc Artif Intern Organs* 9:3, 1963
86. Sherris JC, Cole JJ, Scribner BH: Bacteriology of continuous flow hemodialysis. *Trans Am Soc Artif Intern Organs* 7:37, 1961

87. Fry DL, Hoover PL: Single pass dialysate flow for the Seattle pumpless hemodialysis system. *Trans Am Soc Artif Intern Organs* 10:98, 1964
88. Mion CM, Hegstrom RM, Boen ST, Scribner BH: Substitution of sodium acetate for bicarbonate in the bath fluid for hemodialysis. *Trans Am Soc Artif Intern Organs* 10:110, 1964
89. Mudge GH, Manning JA, Gilman A: Sodium acetate as a source of fixed base. *Proc Soc Exp Biol Med* 71:136, 1949
90. Grimsrud L, Cole JJ, Lehman GA, Babb AL, Scribner BH: A central system for the continuous preparation and distribution of hemodialysis fluid. *Trans Am Soc Artif Intern Organs* 10:107, 1964
91. Bower JD, Belle CH, Hench ME: Bactericidal properties of the concentrated artificial kidney bath solution. *Appl Microbiol* 14:45, 1966
92. Gutch GF, Swanson JR, Ogden DA: Failure of dialysis concentrate as a bactericidal agent. *Proc Clin Dial Transpl Forum* 4:234, 1974
93. Alberts C, Drukker W: Report on regular dialysis treatment in Europe. *Proc Eur Dial Transpl Assoc* 2:82, 1965
94. Drukker W, Schouten WAG, Alberts C: Report on regular dialysis treatment in Europe, IV, 1968. *Proc Eur Dial Transpl Assoc* 5:3, 1969
95. Shaldon S, Baillod RA, Comty C, Oakley J, Sevitt L: 18 Months experience with a nurse-patient operated chronic dialysis unit. *Proc Eur Dial Transpl Assoc* 1:233, 1964
96. Nosé Y: Discussion. *Trans Am Soc Artif Intern Organs* 11:15, 1965
97. Merrill JP, Schupak E, Cameron E, Hampers CL: Hemodialysis in the home. *JAMA* 190:466, 1964
98. Curtis FK, Cole JJ, Fellows HJ, Tyler LL, Scribner BH: Hemodialysis in the home. *Trans Am Soc Artif Intern Organs* 11:7, 1965
99. Baillod RA, Comty C, Ilahi M, Konotey-Ahulu FID, Sevitt L, Shaldon S: Overnight haemodialysis in the home. *Proc Eur Dial Transpl Assoc* 2:99, 1965
100. Hampers CL, Merrill JP, Cameron E: Hemodialysis in the home – a family affair. *Trans Am Soc Artif Intern Organs* 11:3, 1965
101. Scribner BH: Maintenance hemodialysis in perspective – 1969. *Proc 4th Congr Nephrol Stockholm* 3:110, edited by Alwall N, Berglund F, Josephson BS: Basel, München, New York, Karger 1970
102. Gurland HJ, Brunner FP, Chantler C, Jacobs C, Schärer K, Selwood NH, Spies G, Wing AJ: Combined report on regular dialysis and transplantation in Europe, VI. *Proc Eur Dial Transpl Assoc* 13:3, 1976
103. Brynger H, Brunner FP, Chantler C, Donckerwolcke RA, Jacobs C, Kramer P, Selwood NH, Wing AJ: Combined report on regular dialysis and transplantation in Europe, X, 1979, part I. *Proc Eur Dial Transpl Assoc* 17:3, 1980
104. Brescia MJ, Cimino JE, Appel K, Hurwich BJ: Chronic hemodialysis using venapuncture and a surgically created arteriovenous fistula. *N Engl J Med* 275:1089, 1966
105. Editorial (anonymous): Hemodialysis using an arteriovenous fistula. *N Engl J Med* 275:1134, 1966
106. Shaldon S: The use of the arteriovenous fistula in home haemodialysis. *Proc Eur Dia Transpl Assoc* 6:94
107. Gutch CF: Artificial kidneys: problems and approaches. *Annu Rev Biophys Bioeng* 4:405, 1975
108. Del Greco F, Ivanovich P, Krumlovsky FA (editors): Advances in dialysis. *Kidney Int* 18 (Suppl 10) 1980
109. Kolff WJ: The artificial kidney – past, present and future. *Trans Am Soc Artif Intern Organs* 1:1, 1955
110. Salisbury PF: History of The American Society for Artificial Internal Organs. *Trans Am Soc Artif Intern Organs* 6:II, 1960
111. The Book of Daniel 12:4. *The Holy Bible.* Cleveland, New York, World Publishing Company (year of original publication unknown) (cited in ref. 110)
112. Drukker W: Annual Business Meeting. *Proc Eur Dial Transpl Assoc* 2:346, 1965
113. Jacobs C, Broyer M, Brunner FP, Brynger H, Donckerwolcke RA, Kramer P, Selwood NH, Wing AJ, Blake PH: Combined report on regular dialysis and transplantation in Europe, XI, 1980. *Proc Eur Dial Transpl Assoc* 18:2, 1981
114. Edson H, Keen M, Gotch F: Comparative solute transport and therapeutic effectiveness of multiple point support and standard Kiil hemodialyzers. *Trans Am Soc Artif Intern Organs* 18:113, 1972
115. Von Hartitzsch B, Hoenich NA, Peterson RJ, Buselmeier TJ, Kerr DNS, Kjellstrand CM: Middle molecule clearance in current dialysers. *Proc Eur Dial Transpl Assoc* 10:522, 1973
116. Leonard EF, Bluemle LW Jr: The permeability concept as applied to dialysis. *Trans Am Soc Artif Intern Organs* 6:33, 1960
117. Bluemle LW Jr, Dickson JG Jr, Mitchell J, Podolnick MS: Permeability and hydrodynamic studies on the MacNeill-Collins dialyzer using conventional and modified membrane supports. *Trans Am Soc Artif Intern Organs* 6:38, 1960
118. Muldoon JF, Leonard EF: Measurement of dialyzing solution film permeability under idealized conditions. *Trans Am Soc Artif Intern Organs* 6:44, 1960
119. Hoeltzenbein J: Discussion. *Trans Am Soc Artif Intern Organs* 12:368, 1966
120. Drukker W, Jungerius NA, Alberts C: Report on regular dialysis treatment in Europe III. *Proc Eur Dial Transpl Assoc* 4:5, 1967
121. Anderson WW, Mann JB: Kiil versus coil dialysis – a comparative clinical study. In: *Hemodialysis, Principles and Practice.* Edited by Bailey GL, New York and London, Academic Press, 1972, p 373
122. Stewart RD, Lipps BJ, Baretta ED, Piering WR, Roth DA, Sargent JA: Short-term hemodialysis with the capillary kidney. *Trans Am Soc Artif Intern Organs* 14:121, 1968
123. Gotch F, Lipps BJ, Weaver J Jr, Brandes J, Rosin J, Sargent JA, Oja P: Chronic dialysis with the hollow fiber artificial kidney (HFAK). *Trans Am Soc Artif Intern Organs* 15:87, 1969
124. Alwall N: A new disposable artificial kidney: experimental and clinical experience. *Proc Eur Dial Transpl Assoc* 5:18, 1968
125. Scribner BH: Discussion. *Trans Am Soc Artif Intern Organs* 11:29, 1965
126. Babb AL, Popovich RP, Christopher TG, Scribner BH: The genesis of the square meter-hour hypothesis. *Trans Am Soc Artif Intern Organs* 17:81, 1971
127. Christopher TG, Cambi V, Harker LA, Hurst PE, Popovich RP, Babb AL, Scribner BH: A study of hemodialysis with lowered dialysate flow rate. *Trans Am Soc Artif Intern Organs* 17:92, 1971
128. Babb AL, Farrell PC, Uvelli DA, Scribner BH: Hemodialyzer evaluation by examination of solute molecular spectra. *Trans Am Soc Artif Intern Organs* 18:98, 1972
129. Milutinovic J, Halar EM, Harker LA, Babb AL, Scribner BH: Further experience with hemodialysis at 100 ml/min dialysate flow. *Proc Clin Dial Transpl Forum* 1:48, 1971
130. Ginn HE, Bugel HJ, James L, Hopkins P: Clinical experience with small surface area dialyzers (SSAD). *Proc Clin Dial Transpl Forum* 1:53, 1971

131. Rosenzweig J, Babb AL, Vizzo JF, Ginn HE: Large surface area hemodialysis. *Proc Clin Dial Transpl Forum* 1:56, 1971
132. Funck-Brentano JL: Experience with a new 'open membrane'. *Proc Clin Dial Transpl Forum* 1:80, 1971
133. Funck-Brentano JL, Sausse A, Man NK, Granger A, Rondon-Nucete M, Zingraff J, Jungers P: Une nouvelle méthode d'hémodialyse associant une membrane à haute perméabilité pour les moyennes molécules et un bain de dialyse en circuit fermé (A new method of haemodialysis with a membrane highly permeable for middle molecules and a closed dialysis fluid circuit). *Proc Eur Dial Transpl Assoc* 9:55, 1972 (in French)
134. Kjellstrand CM, Evans RI, Petersen RJ, Rust LW, Shideman J, Buselmeier TJ, Rozelle LT: Considerations of the middle molecule hypothesis. *Proc Clin Dial Transpl Forum* 2:127, 1972
135. Shaldon S, Florence P, Fontanier C, Polito C, Mion C: Comparison of two strategies for short dialysis using 1 m^2 and 2 m^2 surface area dialysers. *Proc Eur Dial Transpl Assoc* 12:596, 1975
136. Middle Molecules in Uremia and Other Diseases. Proceedings of the Symposium on Present Status and Future Orientation of Middle Molecules in Uremia and Other Diseases, Avignon, France, November 28-29, 1980. *Artif Organs* 4, Suppl 1981
137. Mirahmadi KS, Kay JH, Miller JH, Gorman JT, Rosen SM: Clinical evaluation of patients dialysed with double Gambro 4 hours, 3 times per week. *Proc Eur Dial Transpl Assoc* 11:121, 1974
138. Cambi V, Savazzi G, Arisi L, Bignardi L, Bruschi L, Rossi E, Migone L: Short dialysis schedules (SDS) - Finally ready to become routine? *Proc Eur Dial Transpl Assoc* 11:112, 1974
139. *Proceedings of the Conference on Natural and Synthetic Membranes.* Edited by Saravis C, Gershenkorn K, Brown ME. DHEW (NIH) publ 1967
140. Leonard EF, Colton CK, Craig LD, Gessler RM, Klein E, Lontz JF, Lyman DJ, Mason RG, Nossel HL: Evaluation of membranes for hemodialyzers. *Report of the Membrane Evaluation Study Group for the Artif Kidney-Chronic Uremia Program of NIAMDD* 1974, DHEW publ no (NIH) 74:605
141. Barbour BH, Bernstein M, Cantor PA, Fischer BS, Stone W Jr: Clinical use of NISR 440 polycarbonate membrane for hemodialysis. *Trans Am Soc Artif Intern Organs* 21:144, 1975
142. Langlois R, Kaye M: Two year clinical trial of polycarbonate membranes for hemodialysis. *Dial Transpl* 8:1111, 1979
143. Babb AL, Farrell PC, Strand MJ, Uvelli DA, Milutinovic J, Scribner BH: Residual renal function and chronic hemodialysis therapy. *Proc Clin Dial Transpl Forum* 2:142, 1972
144. Von Hartitzsch B: The middle molecule in present day hemodialysis. *Proc Clin Dial Transpl Forum* 2:149, 1972
145. Reiger J, Quellhorst E, Lowitz HD, Kong RG, Scheler F: Ultrafiltration for middle molecules in uraemia. *Proc Eur Dial Transpl Assoc* 11:158, 1974
146. Milutinovic J, Cutler RE, Hoover P, Meysen B, Scribner BH: Measurement of residual glomerular filtration rate in the patient receiving repetitive hemodialysis. *Kidney Int* 8:185, 1975
147. Gotch FA: Progress in hemodialysis. *Clin Nephr* 9:144, 1978
148. Babb AL, Strand MJ, Uvelli DA, Milutinovic J, Scribner BH: Quantitative describtion of dialysis treatment: a dialysis index. *Kidney Int 7 (Suppl 2)*:S23, 1975

149. Babb AL, Strand MJ, Uvelli DA, Scribner BH: The dialysis index. A pratical guide to dialysis treatment. *Dial Transpl* 6 (nr 9):9, 1977
150. Bergström J, Fürst P: Uremic middle molecules. *Clin Nephrol* 5:143, 1976
151. Dzúrik R, Adam J, Valončová E, Řezníček J, Zvara V: The effect of haemodialysis on blood peptide levels. *Proc Eur Dial Transpl Assoc* 8:167, 1971
152. Dzúrik R, Božek P, Řezníček J, Oborníková A: Blood level of middle molecular substances during uraemia and haemodialysis. *Proc Eur Dial Transpl Assoc* 10:263, 1973
153. Dall'Aglio P, Buzio C, Cambi V, Arisi L, Migone L: La rétention de moyennes molecules dans le sérum urémique (Retention of middle molecules in uraemic serum). *Proc Eur Dial Transpl Assoc* 9:409, 1972 (in French)
154. Migone L, Dall'Aglio P, Buzio C: Middle molecules in uremic serum, urine and dialysis fluid. *Clin Nephrol* 3:82, 1975
155. Funck-Brentano JL, Man NK, Sausse A: Effect of more porous dialysis membranes on neuropathic toxins. *Kidney Int 7 (Suppl 2)*:S52, 1975
156. Man NK, Ferlain B, Paris J, Werner G, Sausse A, Funck-Brentano JL: An approach to 'middle molecules' identification in artificial kidney dialysate, with reference to neuropathy prevention. *Trans Am Soc Artif Intern Organs* 19:320, 1973
157. Man NK, Granger A, Rondon-Nucete M, Zingraff J, Jungers P, Sausse A, Funck-Brentano JL: One year follow-up of short dialysis with a membrane highly permeable to middle molecules. *Proc Eur Dial Transpl Assoc* 10:236, 1973
158. Man NK, Cueuille G, Zingraff J, Drueke T, Jungers P, Sausse A, Billon JP, Funck-Brentano JL: Investigations on clinico-chemical correlations in uraemic polyneuritis. *Proc Eur Dial Transpl Assoc* 11:214, 1974
159. Bergström J, Gordon A, Fürst P, Ryhage R: A study of uremic toxicology. *Proc 7th Ann Contractors Conf Artif Kidney - Chronic Uremia Program of NIAMDD*, edited by Krueger KK, DHEW publ no (NIH) 75:248, 1974, p 19
160. Asaba H, Bergström J, Fürst P, Oulès R, Zimmerman L: Accumulation and excretion of middle molecules. *Proc Eur Dial Transpl Assoc* 13:481, 1976
161. Bergström J: Uraemic toxicity. *Proc Eur Dial Transpl Assoc* 12:579, 1975
162. Fürst P, Zimmerman L, Bergström J: Determination of endogenous middle molecules in normal and uremic body fluids. *Clin Nephrol* 5:178, 1976
163. Bergström J, Fürst P, Zimmerman L: Uremic middle molecules exist and are biologically active. *Clin Nephrol* 11:229, 1979
164. Zimmerman L, Baldesten A, Bergström J, Fürst P: Isotachophoretic separation of middle molecule peptides in uremic body fluids. *Clin Nephrol* 13:183, 1980
165. Higgins MR, Grace M, Bettcher KB, Silverberg DS, Dossetor JB: Blood access in hemodialysis. *Clin Nephrol* 6:473, 1976
166. Bell PRF, Calman KC: *Surgical Aspects of Haemodialysis.* Edinburgh and London, Churchill Livingstone, 1974
167. Foran RF, Shore E, Levin PM, Freiman RL: Vascular access for hemodialysis. In: *Clinical Aspects of Uremia and Dialysis*, edited by Massry SG, Sellers AL, Springfield IL, Charles C. Thomas, 1976, p 504
168. Ramirez O, Swartz C, Onesti G, Mailloux L, Brest AN: The winged in line shunt. *Trans Am Soc Artif Intern Organs* 12:220, 1966
169. Thomas GI: A large-vessel applique A-V shunt for hemodialysis. *Trans Am Soc Artif Intern Organs* 15:288, 1969

170. Thomas GI: The femoral shunt to-day. *Dial Transpl* 2 (nr 1):23, 1973
171. Buselmeier TJ, Kjellstrand CM, Simmons RL, Duncan DA, Von Hartitzsch B, Rattazzi LC, Leonard AS, Najarian JS: A totally new subcutaneous prosthetic arteriovenous shunt. *Trans Am Soc Artic Intern Organs* 19:25, 1973
172. Buselmeier TJ, Kjellstrand CM, Quinton WE, Von Hartitzsch B, Meyer RM, Shideman JR, Bosl BM, Toledo LH, Spanos PK, McCosh TM, Simmons RL, Najarian JS: The Buselmeier shunt. *Dial Transpl* 3 (nr 1):30, 1974
173. May J, Tiller D, Johnson J, Stewart J, Sheil AGR: Saphenous vein arteriovenous fistula in regular dialysis treatment. *N Engl J Med* 280:770, 1969
174. Chinitz JL, Yokoyama T, Bower R, Swartz C: Self-sealing prosthesis for arteriovenous fistula in man. *Trans Am Soc Artif Intern Organs* 18:452, 1972
175. Chinitz J, Bower R, Yokoyama T, Del Guercio E, Kim K, Swartz C: Further experience with a self-sealing prosthesis for A-V fistula. *Am Soc Artif Intern Organs (Abstracts)* 19th annual meeting 2:12, 1973
176. Richie RE, Johnson K, Walker PJ, Staab EV, Ginn HE: Use of bovine xenograft for problems in vascular access. *Am Soc Artif Intern Organs (Abstracts)* 19th annual meeting 2:54, 1973
177. VanderWerff BA, Rattazzi LC, Katzman HA, Schild AF: Three year experience with bovine graft arteriovenous (A-V) fistulas in 100 patients. *Trans Am Soc Artif Intern Organs* 21:296, 1975
178. Beemer RK, Hayes JF: Hemodialysis using a mandril grown graft. *Trans Am Soc Artif Intern Organs* 19:43, 1973
179. Flores L, Dunn I, Frumkin E, Forte R, Requena R, Ryan J, Knopf M, Kirschner J, Levowitz BS: Dacron arteriovenous shunts for vascular access in hemodialysis. *Trans Am Soc Artif Intern Organs* 19:33, 1973
180. Baker LD Jr, Johnson JM, Goldfarb D: Expanded polytetra-fluoroethylene (PTFE) subcutaneous arteriovenous conduit: an improved vascular access for chronic hemodialysis. *Trans Am Soc Artif Intern Organs* 22:382, 1976
181. Kaplan MS, Mirahmadi KS, Winer RL, Gorman JT, Dabirvaziri N, Rosen SM: Comparison of 'PTFE' and bovine grafts for blood access in dialysis patients. *Trans Am Soc Artif Intern Organs* 22:388, 1976
182. Buselmeier TJ, Rynasiewicz JJ, Sutherland DER, Howard KJ, David TD, Mauer SM, Simmons RL, Najarian JS, Kjellstrand CM: A prosthesis for blood access in patients with thrombosis of peripheral vasculature. *Dial Transpl* 6 (nr 8):48, 1977
183. Mindich BP, Silverman MJ, Elguezabal A, Levowitz BS: Umbilical cord vein fistula for vascular access in hemodialysis. *Trans Am Soc Artif Intern Organs* 21:273, 1975
184. Kester RC: Vascular access for the problem patient. In *Dialysis Review*, edited by Davison AM, Tunbridge Wells, Kent, UK, Pitman Medical Publishing Co Ltd, 1978, p 106
185. Blaney TL, Lindan O, Sparks RE: Adsorption: a step toward a wearable artificial kidney. *Trans Am Soc Artif Intern Organs* 12:7, 1966
186. Jützler GA, Keller HE, Klein J, Carius J, Floss K, Dijckmans J, Fürsattel L, Leppla W: Physico-chemical investigations in regeneration of dialysis fluid. *Proc Eur Dial Transpl Assoc* 3:265, 1966
187. Twiss EE, Paulssen MMP: Dialysis-system incorporating the use of activated charcoal. *Proc Eur Dial Transpl Assoc* 3:262, 1966
188. Van Leer E: *Hemodialyse met Koolstofadsorptie* (Haemodialysis with charcoal adsorption). MD Thesis 1970 Univ of Rotterdam, Drukkerij Bronder-Offset NV (in Dutch)
189. Gordon A, Greenbaum MA, Marantz LB, McArthur MJ, Maxwell MH: A sorbent-based low volume recirculating dialysate system. *Trans Am Soc Artif Intern Organs* 15:347, 1969
190. Gordon A, Gral T, DePalma JR, Greenbaum MA, Marantz LB, McArthur MJ, Maxwell MH: A sorbent-based low volume dialysate system: preliminary studies in human subjects. *Proc Eur Dial Transpl Assoc* 7:63, 1970
191. Gordon A, Better OS, Greenbaum MA, Marantz LB, Gral T, Maxwell MH: Clinical maintenance hemodialysis with a sorbent-based low volume dialysate regeneration system. *Trans Am Soc Artif Intern Organs* 17:253, 1971
192. Greenbaum MA, Gordon A: A regenerative dialysis supply system. *Dial Transpl* 1 (nr 1):18, 1972
193. Drukker W: Introduction to the Redy system. Two long-term patients. *Nieren- u Hochdruckkranckheiten 5, (Suppl)*: 3, 1976
194. Drukker W, Parsons FM, Gordon A: Practical application of dialysate regeneration: the Redy system. In: *Replacement of Renal Function by Dialysis*, chapter 14, edited by Drukker W, Parsons FM, Maher, JF. Martinus Nijhof, Medical Division, The Hague, Boston MA, London, 1st edn 1978, p 244
195. Briefel GR, Hutchisson JT, Galonsky RS, Hessert RL, Friedman EA: Compact travel hemodialysis system. *Proc Clin Dial Transpl Forum* 5:61, 1975
196. Jacobsen SC, Stephen RL, Bulloch EC, Luntz RD, Kolff WJ: A wearable artificial kidney: functional description of hardware and clinical results. *Proc Clin Dial Transpl Forum* 5:65, 1975
197. Stephen RL, Jacobsen SC, Atkin Thor E, Kolff WJ: Portable wearable artificial kidney (WAK) - initial evaluation. *Proc Eur Dial Transpl Assoc* 12:511, 1975
198. Delano B, Friedman EA: Regular dialysis treatment. The portable suitcase kidney. In: *Replacement of Renal Function by Dialysis*, chapter 22, edited by Drukker W, Parsons FM, Maher JF. Martinus Nijhoff, Medical Division, The Hague, Boston MA, London, 1st edn 1978, p 431
199. Kolff WJ: The future of dialysis. The WAK. In: *Replacement of Renal Function by Dialysis*, chapter 42, edited by Drukker W, Parsons FM, Maher JF. Martinus Nijhoff, Medical Division, The Hague, Boston MA, London, 1st edn 1978, p 708
200. Bergström J, Asaba H, Fürst P, Oulès R: Dialysis, ultrafiltration and blood pressure. *Proc Eur Dial Transpl Assoc* 13:293, 1976
201. Shaldon S: Discussion. *Proc Eur Dial Transpl Assoc* 13:300, 1976
202. Jones EO, Ward MK, Hoenich NA, Kerr DNS: Separation of dialysis and ultrafiltration - Does it really help? *Proc Eur Dial Transpl Assoc* 14:160, 1977
203. Ivanovich P, Huang C, Stefanovic N, Del Greco F: A useful adjunct to dialysis. *Proc Eur Dial Transplant Assoc* 14:605, 1977
204. Scribner BH: Substitution of bicarbonate for acetate in the dialysate for the care of a critically ill patient. *Dial Transpl* 6 (nr 3):26, 1977
205. Samar RE: Bicarbonate and acetate hemodialysis. *Contemp Dial*, August 1981, p 10
206. Tolchin DO: Acetate metabolism and high efficiency hemodialysis. *Int J Artif Organs* 2:1, 1979
207. Gotch FA, Sargent JA, Keen M, Lam M, Prowitt M: The solute kinetics of intermittent dialysis therapy. *Proc 11th Ann Contractors' Conf Artif Kidney Program of NIAMDD*, edited by Mackey BB. DHEW publication nr (NIH) 79-144, 1978, p 110
208. Muirhead EE, Reid AF: A resin artificial kidney. *J Lab*

Clin Med 33:841, 1948
209. Yatzidis H: A convenient haemoperfusion micro-apparatus over charcoal for the treatment of endogenous and exogenous intoxications, its use as an active artificial kidney. *Proc Eur Dial Transpl Assoc* 1:83, 1964
210. Chang TMS: Micro capsule artificial kidney in replacement of renal function: with emphasis on adsorbent hemoperfusion. In: *Replacement of Renal Function by Dialysis*, chapter 12, edited by Drukker W, Parsons FM, Maher JM. Martinus Nijhoff, The Hague, Boston MA, London, 1st edn, 1978, p 217
211. Yatzidis H, Oreopoulos D, Triantophyllidis D, Voudiclare S, Tsaparas N, Gavras C, Stravroulaki A: Treatment of severe barbiturate poisoning. *Lancet* 2:216, 1965
212. Editorial (anonymous): Haemoperfusion for acute intoxication with hypnotic drugs. *Lancet* 2:1116, 1979
213. Gelfland MC: Charcoal hemoperfusion in treatment of drug overdosage. *Dial Transpl* 6 (nr 8):8, 1977
214. Winchester JF, Apiliga MT, Mackay JM, Kennedy AC: Haemodialysis with charcoal haemoperfusion. *Proc Eur Dial Transplant Assoc* 12:526, 1975
215. Winchester JF, Apiliga MT, Kennedy AC: Short term evaluation of charcoal hemoperfusion combined with dialysis in uremic patients. *Kidney Int* 10 (Suppl 7):S315, 1976
216. Winchester JF: Symposium on sorbents in uremia: Part 4. Comparison of charcoal hemoperfusion with hemodialysis. *Dial Transpl* 6, (nr 9):46, 1977
217. Chang TMS: Haemoperfusion over micro-encapsulated adsorbent in a patient with hepatic coma. *Lancet* 2:1371, 1972
218. Williams R: Approaches to the development of artificial liver support. In: *Artificial Organs*, edited by Kennedy RM, Courtney JM, Gaylor JDS, Gilchrist T, London and Basingstoke, Macmillan Press, 1977, p 403
219. Henderson LW, Besarab A, Michaels A, Bluemle LW Jr: Blood purification by ultrafiltration and fluid replacement (diafiltration). *Trans Am Soc Artif Intern Organs* 12:216, 1967
220. Brull L: L'ultrafiltration in vivo (Ultrafiltration in vivo). *C R Soc Biol* (Paris) 99:1607, 1928 (in French)
221. Hamilton R, Ford C, Colton C, Cross R, Steinmuller S, Henderson L: Blood cleansing by diafiltration in uremic dog and man. *Trans Am Soc Artif Intern Organs* 17:259, 1971
222. Henderson LW, Livoti LG, Ford CA, Kelly AB, Lysaght MJ: Clinical experience with intermittent hemodiafiltration. *Trans Am Soc Artif Intern Organs* 19:119, 1973
223. Henderson LW, Colton CK, Ford C: Kinetics of hemodiafiltration. II Clinical characterization of a new blood cleansing modality. *J Lab Clin Med* 85:372, 1975
224. Quellhorst E, Rieger J, Doht B, Beckmann H, Jacob I, Kraft B, Mietzsch G, Scheler F: Treatment of chronic uraemia by an ultrafiltration kidney. First clinical experience. *Proc Eur Dial Transpl Assoc* 13:314, 1976
225. Henderson LW, Ford C, Bluemle LW, Bixler HJ: Uremic blood cleansing by diafiltration using a hollow fiber ultra filter. *Trans Am Soc Artif Intern Organs* 16:107, 1970
226. Baldamus CA, Schoeppe W, Koch KM: Comparison of haemodialysis (HD) and post dilution haemofiltration (HF) on an unselected dialysis population. *Proc Eur Dial Transpl Assoc* 15:228, 1978
227. Shaldon S, Beau MC, Claret G, Deschodt G. Oules R, Ramperez P, Mion H, Mion C: Haemofiltration with sorbent regeneration of ultrafiltrate: first clinical experience in end stage renal disease. *Proc Eur Dial Transpl Assoc* 15:220, 1978
228. Bergström J: Ultrafiltration without dialysis for removal of fluid and solutes in uremia. *Clin Nephrol* 9:156, 1978
229. Quellhorst E, Schuenemann B, Doht B: Treatment of severe hypertension in chronic renal insufficiency (CRI) by haemofiltration. *Proc Eur Dial Transpl Assoc* 14:129, 1977
230. Manis T, Friedman EA: Dialytic therapy for irreversible uremia. *N Engl J Med* 301:1321, 1979
231. Major RH: *A History of Medicine II*, Charles C. Thomas, Springfield, IL 1954, p 916
232. Peters DK, Rees AJ, Lockwood CM: Plasma exchange in glomerular and related auto-allergic diseases. *Proc Eur Dial Transpl Assoc* 14:409, 1977
233. Houwert DA, Kater L, Hené RJ, Struyvenberg A: Plasma exchange in immune complex disease. *Proc Eur Dial Transpl Assoc* 16:520, 1979
234. Agashi T, Kaneko I, Hasuo Y, Hayasaka Y, Sanaka T, Ota K, Amemiya H, Sugino N, Abe M, Ono T, Kowai S, Yamana T: Double filtration plasmapheresis. *Trans Am Soc Artif Intern Organs* 26:406, 1980
235. International symposium on plasma exchange, abstracts. *Nieren u Hochdruckkrankheiten* 9:136, 1980
236. Samtleben W, Blumenstein M, Gurland HJ: Membrane plasma separation: advantages and hazards. *Eur Dial Transpl Assoc Abstracts* XVIIth Congress, Prague, 1980, p 84
237. Sprenger K, Franz HE: Membrane plasma separation (MPS): procedural recommendations. *Proc Eur Dial Transpl Assoc* 17:353, 1980
238. Pineda AA, Taswell HF: Selective plasma component removal: alternatives to plasma exchange. *Artif Organs* 5:234, 1981
239. Bensinger WI: Plasma exchange and immunoadsorption for removal of antibodies prior to ABO incomptable bone marrow transplant. *Artif Organs* 5:254, 1981
240. Burgstaler EA, Pinedo AA: Immunoabsorption in an extracorporeal plasma perfusion system: in vitro studies. *Artif Organs* 5:259, 1981
241. Shinoda A, Kitada H, Suzuki S, Kurihara S, Sarto Y, Yuri T, Ishikawa I: Accessible plasma exchange using membrane filter – a successfully treated case of TTP with repeated plasma exchanges. *Artif Organs* 5:248, 1981
242. Lindner A, Charra B, Sherrard DJ, Scribner BH: Accelerated atherosclerosis in prolonged maintenance hemodialysis. *N Engl J Med* 290:697, 1974
243. Alberts C, Drukker W: Report on regular dialysis treatment in Europe. *Proc Eur Dial Transpl Assoc* 2:82, 1965
244. Gurland HJ, Brunner FP, Chantler C, Jacobs C, Schärer K, Selwood NH, Wing AJ: Combined report on regular dialysis and transplantation in Europe, VI, 1975. *Proc Eur Dial Transpl Assoc* 13:3, 1976
245. Bagdade JD, Porte D Jr, Bierman EL: Hypertriglyceridemia: a metabolic consequence of chronic renal failure. *N Engl J Med* 279:181, 1968
246. Bagdade JD, Shafrir E, Wilson DE: Mechanism(s) of hyperlipidemia in chronic uremia. *Trans Am Soc Artif Intern Organs* 22:42, 1976
247. Savdie E, Gibson JC, Crawford GA, Simons LA, Mahony JF: Impaired plasma triglyceride clearance as a feature of both uremic and posttransplant triglyceridemia. *Kidney Int* 18:774, 1980
248. Swamy AP, Cestero RVM, Campbell RG, Freeman RB: Long term effect of dialysate glucose on the lipid levels of maintenance hemodialysis patients. *Trans Am Soc Artif Intern Organs* 22:54, 1976
249. Gonzalez FM, Pearson JE, Garbus SB, Holbert RD: On the effects of acetate during hemodialysis. *Trans Am Soc*

Artif Intern Organs 20a:169, 1974
250. Boyle IT: Vitamin D and the kidney. *Proc Eur Dial Transpl Assoc* 12:113, 1975
251. Pappenheimer AM, Wilens SL: Enlargement of parathyroid glands in renal disease. *Am J Pathol* 11:73, 1935
252. Pappenheimer AM: Effect of reduction of kidney substance upon parathyroid glands and skeletal tissue. *J Exp Med* 64:965, 1936
253. Liu SH, Chu HI: Studies of calcium and phosphorus metabolism with special reference to pathogenesis and effects of dihydrotachysterol (AT10) and iron. *Medicine (Baltimore)* 22:103, 1943
254. Nicolaysen R: Studies upon the mode of action of vitamin D_3. III The influence of vitamin D on the absorption of calcium and phosphorus in the rat. *Biochem J* 31:122, 1937
255. Bauer GCH, Carlsson A, Lindquist B: Evaluation of accretion, resorption and exchange reactions in the skeleton. *Kungliga Fysiografiska, Sallskapet I Lund Forhandlinger* 25:3, 1955
256. Lund J, DeLuca HF: Biologically active metabolite of vitamin D_3 from bone, liver and bloodserum. *J Lipid Res* 7:739, 1966
257. Trummel GL, Raisz LG, Blunt JW: 25-Hydroxycholecalciferol: stimulation of bone resorption on tissue culture. *Science* 163:1450, 1969
258. DeLuca HF: The kidney as an endocrine organ for the production of 1,25-hydroxyvitamin D_3, a calcium-mobilizing hormone. *N Engl J Med* 298:359, 1973
259. Bhattacharyya MH, DeLuca HF: The regulation of rat calciferol 25-hydroxylase. *J Biol Chem* 248:2969, 1973
260. Fraser DR, Kodicek E: Unique biosynthesis by kidney of a biologically active vitamin D metabolite. *Nature* 228:764, 1970
261. Kodicek E: Recent advances in vitamin D metabolism. 1,25-dihydroxycholecalciferol, a kidney hormone controlling calciummetabolism. *Clinics in Endocrinology and Metabolism* 1 no 1 edited by McIntyre I, London, Philadelphia, Toronto, Saunders Comp Ltd, 1972, p 305
262. Holick MF, Schnoes HK, DeLuca HF: Identification of 1,25-dihydroxycholecalciferol; a form of vitamin D_3 metabolically active in the intestine. *Proc Natl Acad Sci USA* 68:803, 1971
263. Holick MF, Schnoes HK, DeLuka HF: Identification of 1,25-dihydroxycholecalciferol: a metabolite of vitamin D active in intestine. *Biochemistry* 10:2799, 1971
264. Reeve J: Therapeutic applications of vitamin D analogues. *Br Med J* 2:888, 1979
265. Velentzas C, Oreopoulos DG: 1,25-dihydroxyvitamin D_3 and osteomalacia: some unanswered questions. *Int J Artif Organs* 3:313, 1980
266. Ward MK, Feest TG, Ellis HA, Parkinson IS, Kerr DNS, Herrington J, Goode GL: Osteomalacic dialysis osteodystrophy: evidence for a water borne aetiological agent, probably aluminium. *Lancet* 1:84, 1978
267. Marsden SNE, Parkinson IS, Ward MK, Ellis HA, Kerr DNS: Evidence for aluminium accumulation in renal failure. *Proc Eur Dial Transpl Assoc* 16:588, 1979
268. Alfrey AC, Miskell JM, Burks J, Contiguglia SR, Rudolph H, Lewin E, Holmes JH: Syndrome of dispraxia and multifocal seizures associated with chronic hemodialysis. *Trans Am Soc Artif Intern Organs* 18:257, 1972
269. Spofforth J: Case of aluminium poisoning. *Lancet* 1:1301, 1921
270. Alfrey AC, LeGendre GR, Kaehny WD: The dialysis encephalopathy syndrome. Possible aluminium intoxication. *N Engl J Med* 294:184, 1976
271. Parkinson IS, Beckett A, Ward MK, Feest TG, Hoenich N, Strong A, Kerr DNS: Aluminium removal from water supplies. *Proc Eur Dial Transpl Assoc* 15:586, 1978
272. Flendrig JA, Kruis H, Das AH: Aluminium intoxication: the cause of dialysis dementia? *Proc Eur Dial Transpl Assoc* 13:355, 1976
273. Flendrig JA, Kruis H, Das AH: Aluminium and dialysis dementia. *Lancet* 1:1235, 1976
274. Elliott HL, Macdougall AI: Aluminium studies in dialysis encephalopathy. *Eur Dial Transpl Assoc* 15:157, 1978
275. Platts MM, Goode GC, Hislop JS: Composition of the domestic water supply and the incidence of fractures and encephalopathy in patients on home dialysis. *Br Med J* 2:657, 1977
276. Davison AM, Giles GR: The effect of transplantation on dialysis encephalopathy. *Proc Eur Dial Transpl Assoc* 16:407, 1979
277. Wing AJ, Brunner FP, Brynger H, Chantler C, Donckerwolcke RA, Gurland HJ, Jacobs C, Kramer P, Selwood H: Dialysis dementia in Europe (Report of the Registration Committee of the European Dialysis and Transplant Association). *Lancet* 2:190, 1980
278. Pierides AM, Edwards JWG, Cullum Jr UX, McCale JT, Ellis HA: Hemodialysis encephalopathy with osteomalacic fractures and muscle weakness. *Kidney Int* 18:115, 1980
279. Short AIK, Winney RJ, Robson JS: Reversible microcytic hypochromic anaemia in dialysis patients due to aluminium intoxication. *Proc Eur Dial Transpl Assoc* 17:226, 1980
280. Kaehny WD, Alfrey AC, Holman RE, Shorr WJ: Aluminium transfer during hemodialysis. *Kidney Int* 12:361, 1977
281. Gazek EM, Babb AL, Uvelli DA, Fry DL, Scribner BH: Dialysis dementia: the role of dialysate pH in altering the dialyzability of aluminium. *Trans Am Soc Artif Intern Organs* 25:409, 1979
282. Berlyne GM, Ben-Ari J, Pest D, Weinberger J, Stern M, Gilmore GR, Levine R: Hyperaluminaemia from aluminium resins in renal failure. *Lancet* 2:494, 1970
283. Berlyne GM: Aluminum toxicity in renal failure. *Int J Artif Organs* 3:60, 1980
284. Ulmer DD: Toxicity from aluminium antacids (Editorial). *N Engl J Med* 294:184, 1976
285. Graf H, Stumvoll HK, Meisinger V, Kovarik J, Wolf A, Pinggera WF: Aluminum removal by hemodialysis. *Kidney Int* 19:587, 1981
286. Dewberry FL, McKinney PD, Stone WJ: The dialysis dementia syndrome: report of fourteen cases and review of the literature. *asaio J* 3:102, 1981
287. Platts MM, Anastassiades E: Dialysis encephalopathy: precipitating factors and improvement in prognosis. *Clin Nephrol* 15:223, 1981
288. Levick SE: Dementia from aluminum pots? (Letter to the editor). *New Engl J Med* 303:164, 1980
289. Trapp GA, Cannon JB: Aluminum pots as a source of dietary aluminum (Letter to the editor). *New Engl J Med* 304:172, 1981
290. Koning JH: Aluminum pots as a source of dietary aluminum (Letter to the editor). *New Engl J Med* 304:172, 1981
291. Ackrill P, Ralston AJ, Day JP, Hodge KC: Successful removal of aluminium from patient with encephalopathy (Letter to the editor). *Lancet* 2:692, 1980
292. Platts MM: Dialysis encephalopathy (Letter to the editor). *Lancet* 2:1035, 1980
293. Adhemar JP, Laederich J, Jaudon MC, Masselot JP, Buisson C, Galli A, Kleinknecht D: Dialysis encephalopathy, diagnostic and prognostic value of clinical and EEG signs, and aluminium levels in serum and cerebrospinal fluid. *Proc Eur Dial Transpl Assoc* 17:234, 1980

294. Graf H, Stummvoll HK, Meisinger V: Dialysate aluminium concentration and aluminium transfer during haemodialysis. *Lancet* 1:46, 1982
295. Memorandum on the summary and conclusions of the International Workshop on the role of biological monitoring in the prevention of aluminium toxicity in man. 'Aluminium analysis in biological fluids'. (Luxembourg, 5-7 July, 1982). *CEC, Health and Safety Directorate*, JMO Building, Luxembourg 2920
296. Blumberg BS, Alter HJ, Visnich S: A 'new' antigen in leukaemia sera. *JAMA* 191:541, 1965
297. Blumberg BS: Australia antigen, hepatitis and leukaemia. *Tokyo J Med Sci* 76:1, 1968 (cited in ref 296)
298. Zuckerman AJ: *Hepatitis Associated Antigen and Viruses.* Amsterdam, London, North-Holland Publishing Co, 1972, p 12
299. Blumberg BS, Gerstley BJS, Hungerford DA, London WT, Sutnick AI: A serum antigen (Australia antigen) in Down's syndrome, leukaemia and hepatitis. *Ann Intern Med* 66:924, 1967
300. London WT, DiFiglia M, Sutnick AI, Blumberg BS: Hepatitis in hemodialysis unit: Australia antigen and host response. *N Engl J Med* 281:571, 1969
301. Drukker W, Alberts C, Odé A, Roozendaal KH, Wilmink J: Report on regular dialysis treatment in Europe, II, 1966. *Proc Eur Dial Transpl Assoc* 2:90, 1966
302. Sutnick AI, Millman I, London WT, Blumberg BS: The role of Australia antigen in viral hepatitis and other diseases. *Annu Rev Med* 23:161, 1972
303. Grob PJ, Bishof B, Naeff F: A cluster of hepatitis B transmitted by a physician. *Lancet* 2:1218, 1981
304. *Hepatitis and the Treatment of Chronic Renal Failure.* Report of the Advisory Group 1970-1972, chairman: Lord Rosenheim, Dept of Health and Social Security, Scottish Home and Health Dept, Welsh Office
305. *Advies inzake de Logistieke Consequenties van het Rapport van de Gezondheidsraad betreffende Maatregelen ter Profylaxe van Serumhepatitis.* (Recommendations concerning the logistic consequences from the report of the Dutch Health Council relating to the prophylaxis of serum hepatitis). Centrale Raad voor de Volksgezondheid, Rijswijk 1975 (in Dutch)
306. Le Bouvier GL: The heterogeneity of Australia antigen. *J Infect Dis* 123:671, 1971
307. Magnius LO, Espmark JA: New specificities in Australia antigen positive sera distinct from the Le Bouvier determinants. *J Immunol* 109:1017, 1972
308. Raimondo G, Smedile A, Gallo L, Babbo A, Ponzetto A, Rizetto M: Multicentre study of HBV-associated delta infection and liver disease in drug addicts. *Lancet* 1:249, 1982
309. Editorial (anonymous): Delta agent – a virus in disguise? *Lancet* 1:259, 1982
310. Leading article (anonymous): High-titre hepatitis B immune globulin. *Br Med J* 1:241, 1976
311. Robinson WS, Lutwick LI: The virus of hepatitis, type B (two parts). *N Engl J Med* 295:1168 and 1232, 1976
312. Kiernan TW, Ramgopal M: Viral hepatitis: progress and problems. *Med Clin North Am* 63:611, 1979
313. Feinstone SM, Kapikian AZ, Purcell RH, Alter HJ, Holland PV: Transfusion-associated hepatitis not due to viral hepatitis type A or B. *N Engl J Med* 292:767, 1975
314. Alter HJ, Holland PV, Morrow AG, Purcell RH, Feinstone SM, Moritsugu Y: Clinical and serological analysis of transfusion-associated hepatitis. *Lancet* 2:838, 1975
315. Alter HJ, Purcell RH, Holland PV, Popper H: Transmissible agent in non-A, non-B hepatitis. *Lancet* 1:460, 1978
316. Tabor E, Drucker JA, Hoofnagle JH, Apryl M, Gerety RJ, Sieff LB, Jackson DR, Barker LF, Pineda-Tamondong G: Transmission of non-A, non-B hepatitis from man to chimpanzee. *Lancet* 1:463, 1978
317. Vitviski L, Prince AM, Trepo C, Brotman B: Detection of virus-associated antigen in serum and liver of patients with non-A, non-B hepatitis. *Lancet* 2:1263, 1979
318. Galbraith RM, Dienstag JL, Purcell RH, Gower PH, Zuckerman AJ, Williams R: Non-A, non-B hepatitis associated with chronic liver disease in a haemodialysis unit. *Lancet* 1:951, 1979
319. Shirachi R, Shiraishi H, Tateda A, Kikuchi K, Ishida N: Hepatitis C antigen in non-A, non-B post transfusion hepatitis. *Lancet* 2:853, 1978
320. Wands JR, Kolff R, Isselbacker KJ: Acute viral hepatitis. In Harrison's *Principles of Internal Medicine*, 9th edn International Students Edition edited by Isselbacker KJ, Adams RD, Braunwald E, Petersdorf RG, Wilson JD, New York, McGraw-Hill Book Company, 1980, p 1466
321. Prince AM, Szmuness W, Mann MK: Hepatitis B immune globulin: Final report of a controlled, multicenter trial of efficacy in prevention of dialysis associated hepatitis. *J Infect Dis* 137:131, 1978
322. Zuckerman AJ: Why the world needs a hepatitis vaccine. *New Scientist* 88:167, 1980
323. Krugman S, Giles JP, Hammond J: Viral hepatitis, type B (MS-2 strain) studies on active immunization. *JAMA* 217:41, 1971
324. Purcell RH, Gerin JL: Hepatitis B subunit vaccine. A preliminary report of safety and efficacy tests in chimpanzees. *Am J Med Sci* 270:395, 1975
325. Maupas P, Goudeau A, Coursaget P, Drucker J, Bagros P: Hepatitis B vaccine: efficacy in high-risk settings, a two year study. *Intervirology* 10:196, 1978
326. Maupas P, Goudeau A, Coursaget P, Drucker J, Barin F, André M: Immunization against hepatitis B in man: a pilot study of two years duration. In *Viral Hepatitis*, edited by Vyas GN, Cohen SN, Schmidt R, Philadelphia, Franklin Institute Press, 1978, p 539
327. Crosnier J, Jungers P, Couroucé AM, Laplanche A, Benhamou E, Degos F, Lacour B, Prunet P, Cerisier Y, Guesry P: Randomised placebo-controlled trial of hepatitis B surface antigen vaccine in French haemodialysis units: I medical staff, II, haemodialysis patients. *Lancet* 1:455 and 797, 1981
328. Szmuness W, Stevens CE, Harley EJ, Zano EA, Oleszko WR, William DC, Sadovsky R, Morrison JM, Kellner A: Hepatitis B vaccine: demonstration of efficacy in a controlled clinical trial in a high-risk population in the United States. *New Engl J Med* 303:833, 1980
329. Dienstag JL: Toward control of hepatitis B (editorial). *New Engl J Med* 303:874, 1980
330. Szmuness W, Stevens CE, Oleszko WR, Goodman A: Passive-active immunisation against hepatitis B: immunogenicity studies in adult Americans. *Lancet* 1:575, 1981
331. Leading article (anonymous). *Br Med J* 281:1585, 1980
332. Blumberg BS, London WT: Hepatitis B virus and the prevention of primary hepatocellular carcinoma. *N Engl J Med* 304:782 1981 (Editorial)
333. Thölen VH, Stricker E, Feer H, Massini MA, Staub H: Über die Anwendung der künstlichen Niere bei Schizophrenie und Myasthenia gravis (The application of the artificial kidney in cases of schizophrenia and myasthenia gravis). *Dtsch Med Wochenschr* 85:1012, 1960 (in German)
334. Wagemaker H, Cade R: The use of hemodialysis in chronic schizophrenia. *Am J Psychiatry* 134:6, 1977

335. Cade R, Wagemaker H: Hemodialysis as treatment for chronic schizophrenia. *Abstr Am Soc Artif Intern Organs* 7:7, 1978
336. Wagemaker H, Cade R: The use of hemodialysis of fourteen chronic schizophrenics. *Abstr Am Soc Artif Intern Organs* 7:62, 1978
337. Palmour RM, Ervin FR, Wagemaker H, Cade R: Characterization of a peptide derived from the serum of psychiatric patients. *Abstr Ann Meeting Soc Neuroscience*, 1977
338. Kolff WJ: Dialysis of schizophrenics. Weird and novel applications of dialysis, hemofiltration, hemoperfusion and peritoneal dialysis: witchcraft? *Artif Organs* 2:277, 1978
339. Gurland HJ: Combination of hemodialysis and hemoperfusion used in conventional dialyser format in the treatment of uremia. *Proc 12th Ann Contractor's Conf Artif Kidney – Chronic Uremia Program of NIAMDD*, edited by Mackey BB, DHEW Publication nr (NIH) 81-1979, 1979 p 279
340. Twardowski ZJ: Abatement of psoriasis and repeated dialysis. *Ann Intern Med* 86:510, 1977
341. Buselmeier TJ, Dahl MV, Kjellstrand CM, Goltz RW: Dialysis therapy for psoriasis. *JAMA* 240:1270, 1978
342. Kramer P: Dialysis for psoriatic patients. *Proc 11th Ann Contractor's Conf Artif Kidney Program NIAMDD*, edited by Mackey BB, DHEW Publication nr (NIH 79-1442, 1978, p 217
343. Korz R, Klein H, Genth E: Myasthenia gravis und Lupus erythematosus Nephritis (myasthenia gravis and lupus erythematosus). *Dtsch Med Wochenschr* 103:1485, 1978 (in German)
344. Gurland HJ: Is blood purification suitable for an effective cure of psoriasis? *Paper presented at the 2nd symposium on chronic renal failure*, Prague, March 1979
345. Burton BT, Kirschman GH: Demographic analysis: end stage renal disease and its treatment in the United States. *Clin Nephrol* 11:47, 1979
346. Waterfall WK: Dialysis and transplantation. *Br Med J* 281:726, 1980
347. Relman AS, Rennie D: Treatment of end stage renal disease. Free but not equal (Editorial). *N Engl J Med* 303:996, 1980
348. Brunner FP, Brynger H, Chantler C, Donckerwolcke RA, Hathway RA, Jacobs C, Selwood NH, Wing AJ: Combined report on regular dialysis and transplantation in Europe, IX, 1978. *Proc Eur Dial Transpl Assoc* 16:2, 1979
349. Editorial (anonymous): Ethics and the nephrologist. *Lancet* 1:594, 1981
350. Gurland HJ, Wing AJ, Jacobs C, Brunner FP: Comparative review between dialysis and transplantation. Chapter 39 in *Replacement of Renal Function by Dialysis*, 1st edn, edited by Drukker W, Parsons FM, Maher JF, The Hague, Boston, London, Martinus Nijhoff, 1978, p 664
351. Evans RW, Blagg CR: Treatment of end-stage renal disease (Letter to the editor). *N Engl J Med* 304:357, 1981
352. Relman AS, Rennie D: Treatment of end-stage renla disease (Reply). *N Engl J Med* 304:357, 1981
353. Iglehart K: Funding the endstage renal-disease program. *N Engl J Med* 306:492, 1982
354. Parsons FM, Brunner FP, Burck HC, Gräser W, Gurland HJ, Härlen H, Schärer K, Spies GW: Statistical report. *Proc Eur Dial Transpl Assoc* 11:3, 1974
355. Manis Th, Friedman EA: Dialytic therapy for irreversible uremia I and II. *N Engl J Med* 301:1254 and 1321, 1979
356. Carmody M, Cattell WR, Cambi V, Koch KM, Baillod RA: Dialysis – petrified or progressive. *Proc Eur Dial Transpl Assoc* 11:537, 1974

3

PRINCIPLES AND BIOPHYSICS OF DIALYSIS

JOHN A. SARGENT and FRANK A. GOTCH

Introduction	53
Fundamentals of mass transport	54
Mechanisms of transport	54
The concentration driving force: concentration difference	56
Logarithmic mean concentration difference	56
Operational characteristics of the dialyzer	57
Ultrafiltration coefficient	57
Mass transport and solute flux	57
Consideration of flow rates	57
Dialysance and clearance	57
Measurement of dialysance and clearance	59
Effective blood water flow when ions traverse red cell membranes, e.g. bicarbonate	59
The interrelationship of operational constants, D, Q_B and Q_D and the overall mass transfer coefficient – membrane area product	59
The effective clearance of larger solutes with ultrafiltration	60
Transport determined by kinetic methods	60
The use of marker solutes	61
Mass balance principles applied to intermittent dialysis: solute kinetic modelling	61
Mass balance considerations as they apply to quantification of intermittent dialysis treatment	62
Formulation of a model: elements of the mass balance diagram	63
Writing the mass balance equation	64
Use of the mass balance equation	64
Solution of the mass balance equation	65
Mass balance as applied to various solute systems	65
Urea nitrogen mass balance	65
Consideration of steady state: chronic renal failure	66
Establishing a level of K_R	67
Urea nitrogen kinetics in the dialyzed patient	68

Use of mass balance equation solution	70
Modelling of the anticoagulant activity of heparin	70
Acid base control in dialysis patients	71
Acid generation from metabolic processes	71
Net acid generation as related to protein catabolism and intake	72
Acetate metabolism	72
Body base	74
Bicarbonate modelling	75
The body base model	75
Control of acid base: solution of the model	77
The effect of fluid retention and removal	77
Creatinine	78
Sodium	78
Sodium distribution volume	78
Calculation of ΔNa and ΔV over the dialysis cycle	79
Sodium-volume model	80
Clinical application of the sodium-volume model	82
Kinetic consideration of uremic toxins	83
The case with metabolic interactions	64
Appendix	86
Dialyzer transport measurements: the case with ultrafiltration	86
Average blood concentration during urine collection	87
Two pool analysis of "middle molecule" kinetics	87
Mathematical concepts and relational analysis	88
Independent and dependent variables and linear regressions	88
Therapeutic extension of clinical information through mathematical reduction of data	89
Nutritional management of acute dialysis	89
Summary	91
Nomenclature	91
References	92

INTRODUCTION

Intermittent dialysis therapy is used in chronic uremia to re-establish body water solute concentrations that cannot be achieved by the natural organ. In this sense, the dialyzer becomes an artificial kidney and it is through the transport of substances by this device that chemical and biophysical control consistent with continued survival is achieved. This chapter is organized as shown in Figure 1 and consists of two basic lines of development:

1. Consideration of the dialyzer and its operating principles,
2. Application of mass balance principles to various solute systems and the effect of dialyzer use on solute control during intermittent dialysis therapy.

Biophysical treatment of hemodialysis requires quantitative description of the interacting variables involved in this therapy; such a description, to be unambiguous, must use mathematical relationships. Certain fundamental relationships, because of their central role, have been developed in detail, such as clearance measurements and single pool solute kinetics. For solution techniques of equations and relationships that are mainly descriptive, such as double pool kinetics of larger molecules, the reader is either referred to the appendix or to specific texts on applied mathematics. The appendix section discusses independent and dependent variables, as well as the quantitative use of relational (linear) analysis. In most cases symbols are defined in the text. For reader convenience, however, a list of symbols used appears under Nomenclature on pages 91 and 92.

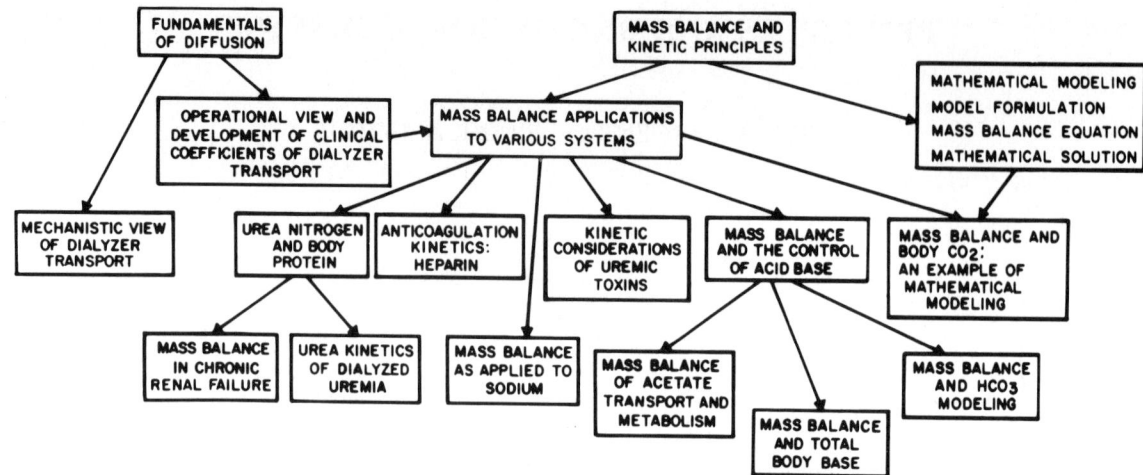

Figure 1. Diagrammatic outline of chapter organization.

In this chapter the dialyzer will be considered initially, starting with a brief discussion of the fundamentals of diffusion embodied in Fick's law. The pratical application of these concepts to dialyzer development or clinical use, however, requires the definition of several coefficients which are useful in either the design of dialyzers or their use in the clinic; these two aspects will be discussed in turn. The mechanistic view of transport is intended to describe what influences dialyzer properties; the discussion of the operational aspects of a dialyzer, which concerns itself with the development of relationships for dialysance and clearance, will be of value in the second part of the chapter when mass balance is considered with respect to the patient-dialyzer system.

The section which considers the mass balance of intermittent dialysis therapy begins with the fundamentals of conservation of matter and from them develops kinetic and steady state relationships that govern concentration control in dialyzed patients; these concepts are then applied to several solute systems.

FUNDAMENTALS OF MASS TRANSPORT

To remove a substance from the blood with a dialyzer, the species must move out of the blood across a membrane and into the dialysate by diffusion which is governed by Fick's Law:

$$J = -DA\frac{dc}{dx} = -DA\frac{\Delta c}{\Delta x} \quad [1]$$

This expression states that the flux, J, of a material over a short distance, dx, will be proportional to its concentration difference, dc, over this distance and the area of the diffusion front, A. The phenomenological constant of proportionality resulting in equality of the above statements is the *diffusivity,* **D**, which has units of cm²/sec and will be a unique property of the solute-solvent at a specific temperature. Finally, the sign convention is adopted that diffusion will be the positive direction; material moves from the region of higher to that of lower activity so that concentration will be decreasing (dc/dx < 0) in the direction of flux; mathematically, therefore, the right hand side of the equation must carry a negative sign.

Equation 1 is the fundamental relationship for undimensional diffusive movement of material and is the mass transfer analog to Fourier's Law which governs heat conduction. To be of practical use in the study of the operation of dialyzers, however, it is necessary to put equation 1 in less general form so that the mechanisms of transport of specific devices can be evaluated. This mechanistic approach is generally taken by engineers who desire to improve the operating characteristics and efficiency of a dialyzer. It can also be helpful to physicians in understanding the anticipated effects of different operational conditions on dialyzer performance. Typical changes in operational conditions would be dialyzer clotting, variable ultrafiltration, and non-standard flow rates. This approach also can give increased insight into what to expect from changes in the components of a dialyzer, such as the use of a different dialysis membrane.

MECHANISMS OF TRANSPORT

If the value of Δx in equation 1 is relatively constant in any one dialyzer design, the major variables that determine flux for the dialyzer will be concentration difference and area, **D** being a constant at any particular temperature for a specific chemical species. This being the case, equation 1 can be written as:

$$J = -K_o A \overline{\Delta C} \quad [2a]$$

Here $\overline{\Delta C}$ is an appropriately defined concentration difference. In equation 2a a new proportionality constant, the *overall mass transfer coefficient,* K_o, has appeared and is defined as:

$$K_o = \frac{\frac{J}{A}}{-\overline{\Delta C}} = \frac{\text{unit flux}}{\text{driving force}} \quad [2b]$$

K_o has units of cm/min and is independent of $\overline{\Delta C}$ in the concentration range experienced in dialysis. Comparison of equation 1 and 2a shows that K_o is proportional to the diffusivity of the solute being transfered and inversely proportional to the diffusion distances characteristic of the dialyzer; this transport coefficient can be calculated from basic transport values if blood and dialysate flows are known as will be shown below (1–3). If equation 2a is further rewritten, the flux per unit area can be described as:

$$\text{unit flux} = \frac{J}{A} = \frac{-\overline{\Delta C}}{1/K_o} = \frac{-\overline{\Delta C}}{R_o} \quad [2c]$$

If $1/K_o$ is viewed as a resistance to transport (R_o), equation 2c can be written as:

$$\frac{\text{Mass transfer}}{\text{per unit area}} = \frac{\text{Driving force}}{\text{Resistance to transfer}} \quad [3]$$

Equation 3 is a quantitative statement of a fundamental physical principle which applies throughout the physical sciences. It states that there will be a flux of material proportional to the driving force and that that flux will be opposed by (or is inversely proportional to) certain resistances. This is the same form as Ohm's law of electric current flow in the field of electricity, it is the same law that is applied to conductive heat flow, and it is in the same form as the relationship that is used to calculate peripherial resistance in circulation physiology (4).

Specifically, equation 3 shows that mass transfer is the result of the driving force relative to the resistance to transfer and is useful in that it demonstrates that flux per unit area can be improved only by increasing the driving force or decreasing the resistance. The overall resistance is an index of the difficulty in getting from the center of the blood stream to the center of the dialysate stream and is the sum of all the resistances of which it is composed (see Figure 2):

$$R_o = R_B + R_M + R_D \quad [4]$$

where R_B = blood side resistance
R_M = membrane resistance
R_D = dialysate side resistance

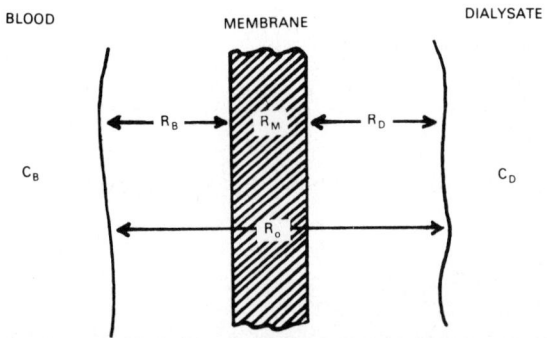

Figure 2. Schematic representation of resistances to transport in a dialyzer.

In this way, the diffusion path is divided into three segments representing the three fundamental elements of a dialyzer.

K_o was defined above as proportional to $D/\Delta x$ so that R_o, being proportional to $1/K_o$, is proportional to $\Delta x/D$. In the three segments described above, R will be:

$$R_B = \frac{\Delta x_B}{D_B}$$

$$R_M = \frac{\Delta X_M}{kD_M} = \frac{\Delta X_M}{D_{M^*}}$$

$$R_D = \frac{\Delta X_D}{D_D}$$

Where k is the solute distribution coefficient between the membrane material and the solution.

For any particular solute, the diffusivity in blood (D_B) and dialysate (D_D) of a given composition will be constant. Moreover, it should have the same value irrespective of the dialyzer, being a solution constant at operational temperatures. As a consequence, the R_B and R_D in a specific dialyzer will be governed by the Δx_B and Δx_D terms; these terms are the effective diffusion distances from the main stream to and from the membrane. To the extent that blood flows are swift and fluid channels are small, the value of Δx for both blood and dialysate will be small as will the values for R_B and R_D. The membrane resistance R_M still depends on Δx_M (the thickness of the membrane) but in addition, will be sensitive to the effective diffusivity in the membrane (D_{M^*}) which can vary considerably as a result of its chemical composition. In this context, a thin (small Δx_M) permeable (large D_{M^*}) membrane would have a small value for R_M. It should be noted, however, that the resistances are additive so that while a dialyzer with a highly permeable membrane will have low values for R_M, R_o may be high due to large values for R_B and R_D. Dialyzer efficiency can be best increased, therefore, by reducing the value of the largest resistance in equation 4. The relative values for the above resistances in four dialyzer-membrane combinations are shown in Table 1 and illustrate the importance of the various resistances in these dialyzers (5–7).

What becomes evident from Table 1 is that for urea, the predominant resistances to transport in the prototype parallel plate, Kiil dialyzer were R_B and R_D (i.e., in the fluid streams) whereas in the hollow fiber devices with narrow fluid paths, the major resistance is in the membrane. The overall resistance, however, is lower in the latter explaining why, in general, hollow fiber dialyzers have better urea transport. For large molecules all of these dialyzers, except the one with the noncellulosic membrane, have over two thirds of the resistance in the membrane.

The overall resistance, R_o (or overall mass transfer coefficient, K_o) can be readily calculated from the diffusive dialysance, D, and knowledge of blood and dialysate flow rates (see below for discussion of diffusive dialysance). Conversely, if R_o or K_o is known the expected

Table 1. Mass transfer resistances for various dialyzer-solute combinations.

Dialyzer and membrane	Membrane m^2	Solute	K_B^* ml/min	R_B^{**} ml/min	R_M min/cm	R_D^{**} min/cm	R_O min/cm	$\frac{R_B-R_D}{R_O}$	$\frac{R_M}{R_O}$	Ref.
Parallel ridge Kiil-Cuprophane	1.0	Urea	80	24	19	16	59	0.68	0.32	5
		Vitamin B_{12}	18	101	362	45	508	0.29	0.71	5
Parallel ridge Kiil-polycarbonate	1.0	Urea	110	24	14	16	54	0.74	0.26	6
		Vitamin B_{12}	37	101	90	45	236	0.62	0.38	6
Cordis-Dow Model 4 Hollow fiber regenerated cellulose	1.3	Urea	160	4	21	7	32	0.34	0.66	7
		Vitamin B_{12}	23	17	—	20	519	0.07	0.93	7
Cordis-Dow Model 5 Hollow fiber regenerated cellulose	2.5	Urea	185	5	21	9	35	0.40	0.60	7
		Vitamin B_{12}	40	21	—	25	536	0.09	0.91	7

* Clearances based on Q_B = 200 ml/min, Q_D 500 ml/min and 37 °C vitamin B_{12} *in vitro*
** The value of R_B and R_D have been established from

$$\frac{\text{R urea, follow fiber kidney}}{\text{R urea Kiil}} \text{ (R vitamin } B_{12}, \text{ Kiil)} = \text{R vitamin } B_{12}, \text{ hollow fiber kidney.}$$

diffusive dialysance under specific clinical conditions of flow can be calculated.

THE CONCENTRATION DRIVING FORCE: CONCENTRATION DIFFERENCE

Equation 2a states that with a specific dialyzer ($K_o A$ = a constant) the removal of solute will depend directly on the concentration difference, ΔC. It is important to develop this variable further so that it can be used in computations to follow.

Logarithmic mean concentration difference

There will be a linear change in concentrations of the blood and dialysate streams as solute is transfered from one to the other (see Figure 3). This figure is for counter-current flows and shows solute levels in the blood decreasing from its entry into the dialyzer at the right while concentrations in the dialysate are increasing from its entry into the dialyzer at the left. The concentration difference at any point in the dialyzer is represented by the difference between these two lines (see the intermediate line) and it is this concentration that will determine the local flux (see equation 2a). A similar figure can be constructed for co-current flow and the analytical results to be developed below will apply equally to this case. In Figure 3 the slope of the concentration difference line will be:

$$\text{slope} = \frac{d(\Delta C)}{dJ} = \frac{\Delta C_i - \Delta C_o}{J} \quad [5]$$

If equation 2a is differentiated and evaluated for the very small transport area, dA, then substituted into equation 5 for dJ:

$$\frac{d(\Delta C)}{-K_o \, dA \, \Delta C} = \frac{\Delta C_i - \Delta C_o}{J}$$

Rearrangement yields:

$$\frac{d(\Delta C)}{\Delta C} = \frac{-K_o(\Delta C_i - \Delta C_o) \, dA}{J}$$

And integration and solving the resulting expression for flux:

$$J = K_o A \left[\frac{\Delta C_i - \Delta C_o}{\text{Ln}(\Delta C_i / \Delta C_o)} \right] \quad [6]$$

The expression in parentheses in equation 6 is the logarithmic mean concentration difference which can be expanded as:

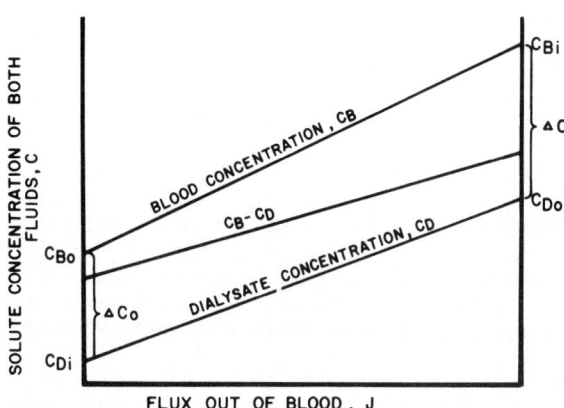

Figure 3. Graphical representation of blood and dialysate concentration as a function of flux between the two fluid streams.

$$C \text{ (Log-mean)} = \frac{(C_{Bi}-C_{Do})-(C_{Bo}-C_{Di})}{\text{Ln } (C_{Bi}-C_{Do})/(C_{Bo}-C_{Di})} \quad [7]$$

The log-mean concentration difference as represented in equation 7 is an operationally exact statement of the integrated concentration driving force in a dialyzer being operated in either counter-current or co-current mode. Equation 7, however, contains both inlet and outlet blood and dialysate concentrations which in the clinical operation of a dialyzer are tedious to obtain.

It is considerably more convenient to define a surrogate concentration driving force, $(C_{Bi}-C_{Di})$ in the clinical setting. This concentration difference can be shown to be directly proportional to the log-mean concentration difference and is clinically more reasonable than equation 7 because it uses undialyzed blood and inlet dialysis solution values as reference levels to evaluate and calculate dialyzer performance. This measurement of concentration difference also adapts well to system modelling because it is possible to determine fluxes from patient's systemic concentrations alone.

OPERATIONAL CHARACTERISTICS OF THE DIALYZER

During dialysis treatment the dialyzer is the point at which mass transfer takes place either *from* the patient (e.g. potassium and protein catabolites) or *to* the patient (e.g. calcium or acetate). There is also a transfer of water from the patient to the dialysate for volume control. The two mechanisms of transport are different and are effected by virtue of dissimilar driving forces: concentration differences for the various chemical constituents and a pressure difference in the case of water. To describe the operational characteristics of a dialyzer for clinical use, it is desirable to define operational coefficients which are the analog of K_o in equation 2b and which result in a linear proportionality relating flux and driving force. The two coefficients for dialyzer water and solute flux are the ultrafiltration coefficient and dialysance; clearance is a special case of dialysance as will be discussed below.

Ultrafiltration coefficient

Ultrafiltration coefficient $[K_{UF}(\text{ml/min/mm Hg})] =$

$$= \frac{\text{water flux}}{\text{transmembrane pressure}} = \frac{Q_F}{\overline{P}_B-\overline{P}_D} \quad [8]$$

The water flux is referred to as the ultrafiltration rate (Q_F ml/min) and the driving force is the difference in mean pressures from the blood side (P_B) to the dialysate side (P_D).

Mass transport and solute flux

Consideration of flow rates
A dialyzer is operated by manipulation of blood and dialysate flow rates. It is, therefore, appropriate to define the basis for these flows.

The dialysate and ultrafiltrate being homogeneous aqueous fluids, their flow rates are unambigious and represent those flows which would be calculated if a timed volumetric collection were done. Blood, in contrast, is a heterogeneous fluid which contains proteins and cellular elements. Its bulk flow rate will always exceed its water flow rate; indeed at times its non-cellular water flow rate (or plasma water) is a more relevant flow, as in the case of inulin transport; the non-cellular flow adjusted for cellular water participation is more appropriate when considering materials such as bicarbonate which readily enters cells but is in much lower cellular concentration due to Donnan effects [8–10]. Bulk blood flow, however, is routinely measured clinically and throughout the evolution of the dialysis field this quantity has been used.

In the development of the expressions to follow, Q_B will be used as the flow rate of the portion of the blood appropriate to the solute being discussed. Consequently, the quantity, $Q_B C_B$, will represent the mass of material in the flowing stream and Q_B will take its units from C_B (e.g. if C_B for bicarbonate is in millimoles per liter of blood water adjusted for red cell water and Donnan effects then Q_B will be in units of liters per minute of effective blood water flow). It should be recognized, however, that much dialysis literature and product information (such as dialyzer performance data) use the clinically measurable values of Q_B so that if other flow rates are desired they must be computed from the bulk flow and blood constants.

Dialysance and clearance
Consider the dialyzer under single pass conditions as shown in Figure 4. Once flows have stabilized, the system will be at steady state under which condition the mass balance will be:

$$Q_{Bi}C_{Bi}+Q_{Di}C_{Di} = (Q_{Bi}-Q_F)C_{Bo}+(Q_{Di}+Q_F)C_{Do}$$

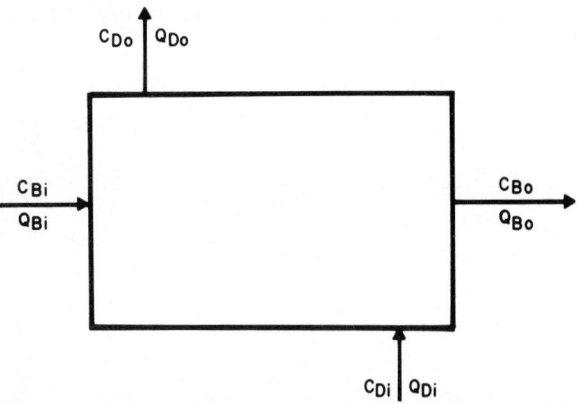

Figure 4. Schematic representation of flows and concentrations for a dialyzer operated with counter-current flows.

Rearrangement of this expression yields:

$$Q_{Bi}(C_{Bi} - C_{Bo}) + Q_F C_{Bo}$$
$$= Q_{Di}(C_{Do} - C_{Di}) + Q_F C_{Do} \quad [9]$$

The first term on each side of equation 9 can be viewed as the diffusive component of flux whereas the second term shows the deviation from the purely diffusive case when there is a convective component. Both sides of the equation are expressions of solute flux during the transit of the dialyzer: The left hand side represents the solute leaving the blood; the right hand side is the solute appearing in the dialysate.

We now define a term called *diffusive dialysance* (D) (11), which will be a constant for a dialyzer at any specific blood and dialysate flow *.

$$D = \frac{\text{Change in solute content of incoming blood}}{\text{Concentration driving force}}$$

$$D = \frac{Q_{Bi}(C_{Bi} - C_{Bo})}{\alpha C_{Bi} - C_{Di}} = \frac{Q_{Di}(C_{Do} - C_{Di})}{\alpha C_{Bi} - C_{Di}} \quad [10a]$$

Dialysance is the magnitude of flux to be expected per unit of concentration driving force. The next step in the mathematical development is to divide equation 9 by the concentration driving force from the blood to the dialysate. Using the inlet concentrations as discussed above the generalized inlet concentration driving force will be: $\alpha C_{Bi} - C_{Di}$. The term, α is a 'Donnan factor' defined as the ratio of cation concentrations in dialysate and blood at equilibrium and will be discussed further when sodium balance is considered:

$$\alpha = \frac{\text{Equilibrium cation concentration in dialysate}}{\text{Equilibrium cation concentration in plasma water}}$$

[11]

When non-charged solutes are being considered, $\alpha = 1$ and equation 10a becomes:

$$D = \frac{Q_{Bi}(C_{Bi} - C_{Bo})}{C_{Bi} - C_{Di}} = \frac{Q_{Di}(C_{Do} - C_{Di})}{C_{Bi} - C_{Di}} \quad [10b]$$

Dividing equation 9 by the concentration driving force, $C_{Bi} - C_{Di}$, yields:

$$\frac{Q_{Bi}(C_{Bi} - C_{Bo})}{C_{Bi} - C_{Di}} + \frac{Q_F C_{Bo}}{C_{Bi} - C_{Di}}$$
$$= \frac{Q_{Di}(C_{Do} - C_{Di})}{C_{Bi} - C_{Di}} + \frac{Q_F C_{Do}}{C_{Bi} - C_{Di}} \quad [12]$$

The left hand side of equation 12 becomes:

$$\frac{J}{C_{Bi} - C_{Di}} = D + \frac{Q_F C_{Bo}}{C_{Bi} - C_{Di}} = D' \quad [13]$$

---

* It should be noted that this is the special case of dialysance (which will appear later) and that in this unique case, ultrafiltration, Q_F, is zero.

Where D' is the total dialysance (11). The flux out of the blood compartment is then:

$$J = D(C_{Bi} - C_{Di}) + Q_F C_{Bo}$$

If $Q_F \ll Q_B$, equation 10b can be considered to represent the approximate relationship of blood inlet and outlet concentrations. In such a case, which is generally true during hemodialysis, equation 10 can be solved for C_{Bo}. If this rearrangement is substituted into the above expression:

$$J = D(C_{Bi} - C_{Di}) + Q_F \left[C_{Bi} - \frac{D}{Q_{Bi}}(C_{Bi} - C_{Di}) \right]$$

And expanding and rearranging:

$$J = \left[D\left(1 - \frac{Q_F}{Q_{Bi}}\right) + Q_F \right] C_{Bi} - D\left(1 - \frac{Q_F}{Q_{Bi}}\right) C_{Di} \quad [14]$$

Equation 14 when solved for D yields:

$$D = \frac{\dfrac{J}{C_{Bi} - C_{Di}} - \dfrac{Q_F C_{Bi}}{C_{Bi} - C_{Di}}}{1 - Q_F/Q_{Bi}} \quad [15]$$

The flux in equation 15 can either be measured by the amount of solute lost from the blood or the amount appearing in the dialysate. Equation 9 indicates that by using the left hand side as the value for J, an expression for dialysance based on the blood side results, D_b. Analogous steps and using the right hand side of equation 9 will result in D_d.

An important special case of these expressions is when $C_{Di} = 0$ which is the case with most single pass dialyzers and metabolic wastes. In this case, equation 10 becomes the definition of *diffusive clearance* K, which is the analog of the physiologic concept (12):

$$K = \frac{Q_{Bi}(C_{Bi} - C_{Bo})}{C_{Bi}} \quad [16]$$

and equations 14 and 13 become:

$$\frac{J}{C_{Bi}} = K + Q_F \frac{C_{Bo}}{C_{Bi}} = K' \quad [17a]$$

$$K = \frac{\dfrac{J}{C_{Bi}} - Q_F}{1 - \dfrac{Q_F}{Q_{Bi}}} \quad [17b]$$

Rearrangement of this expression, or alternatively, simplification of equation 13 when $C_{Di} = 0$ yields:

$$J = [K(1 - Q_F/Q_{Bi}) + Q_F] C_{Bi} = K' C_{Bi} \quad [18]$$

Here K' is the total clearance and is defined as the total flux divided by the inlet blood concentration. Equations 13 and 17 mathematically combine diffusive and convective components of transport into a single first order term D' or K'*.

Because they are defined as linear coefficients relating flux to the concentration driving force, they are very useful in the kinetic description of dialysis. It should be pointed out, however, that these terms are no longer a constant for a given set of blood and dialysate flows because of their dependence on the ultrafiltration rate, Q_F.

The appearance of a diffusive and a convective term in equations 13 and 17 should not be taken as identifying the mechanism of convective transport but as a description of the net contribution that ultrafiltration will make to flux and corresponding dialysance and clearance. It is seen in equations 13 and 17 that clearance and dialysance will increase in the presence of ultrafiltration to the extent of the actual concentration present in the outflow blood.

That these equations mathematically (as opposed to physically) describe net transport is illustrated by considering equation 13 for a cation such as K^+. In such a case, the cation will be retained as plasma is ultrafiltered due to Donnan effects and $C_{Bo} > C_{Bi}$. In fact it is possible to conceive of cases where the increased dialysance above the diffusive value, due to Q_F, may be greater than the ultrafiltration flux itself as a result of $C_{Bo}/(\alpha C_{Bi} - C_{Di}) > 1$.

An illustrative case would be if D (potassium) = 0.100 l/min, C_{Bi} = 4 mmol/l, C_{Di} = 2 mmol/l, and α = 0.95 (Gotch FA, Falkenhagen D, Sargent JA: Unpublished data); C_{Bo} will be approximately 3 mmol/l, and $C_{Bo}/(\alpha C_{Bi} - C_{Di}) = 1.67$, and there would be an increase of more than 3 ml/min in dialysance for each 2 ml/min of ultrafiltration.

Measurement of dialysance and clearance. In the context of equation 12 dialysance and clearance values should be identified for flux measured from blood and dialysate, and the selection of the location for sampling would appear to be based on the convenience of sampling and the analytical sensitivity of the assays used. While this is true *in vitro*, *in vivo* measurements are complicated by the complexity of blood. The unstated assumption of Figure 4 and equation 12 is that the flow rate, Q_B, is that of a homogenous fluid at concentration C_B. *In vivo* conditions are at variance with this assumption: 1) Blood is heterogenous because of suspended red cells which will result in transmural solute disequilibrium for large materials and rapid transits through the dialyzer, 2) Blood is composed of certain non-aqueous constitutents so that water flow (the distribution space for dissolved unbound solutes) equals the product of blood flow and the aqueous fraction.

In light of these difficulties, using dialysate values allows for direct measurement of fluxes without the complexities described above. It is prudent, however, to obtain both blood and dialysate side values as a check on methods and analyses. In general, dialysance and clearance measurements used throughout this chapter, will be specified in terms of the dialysate (K_D).

It should be noted that there are perferred methods of measuring the values in equation 9. Operationally Q_{Do} and C_{Do} can be determined from a timed aliquot of outflow dialysate and Q_B is determined from bubble time measurement (13) (see also chapters 5 and 11), C_{Bo} and C_{Do} should be obtained before C_{Bi} and C_{Di} so that sampling does not upset flow patterns. Q_F is determined from the product of ultrafiltration coefficient (K_{UF}) and the blood-dialysate pressure drop $(\overline{P}_B - \overline{P}_D)$ (see equation 8):

$$Q_F = K_{UF}(\overline{P}_B - \overline{P}_D) \quad [19]$$

Effective blood water flow when ions traverse red cell membranes, e.g. bicarbonate

The bicarbonate ion is a charged particle for which the red cell membrane is freely permeable (8). Hence, it is necessary to consider a modification of the general case of blood or plasma flow for this ion and those that distribute similarly. The Donnan ratio, red cell to plasma is

$$R_D = \frac{\text{anion concentration in red cell water}}{\text{anion concentration in plasma water}}$$

$$= 1/\alpha \text{ (red cell to plasma)}$$

An effective blood side water flow rate, Q_E, for bicarbonate can be calculated as:

$$Q_E = Q_B \left[F_P - \frac{Hct}{100}(F_P - F_R R_D) \right] \quad [20]$$

For values of: F_P = 0.94, F_R = 0.72, and R_D = 0.69 (10), equation 20 reduces to:

$$Q_E = Q_B \left(0.94 - 0.443 \frac{Hct}{100} \right) \quad [21]$$

The effective flow, Q_E, can then be used in place of Q_B in the forgoing expressions and those to be developed relating D, Q_D, and Q_B to $K_o A$.

The interrelationship of operational constants, D, Q_B, and Q_D and the overall mass transfer coefficient – membrane area product

It is useful to determine the relationship between the operational clinical constant, diffusive dialysance, and the overall mass transfer coefficient. Equation 6 shows that for a given dialyzer K_o will be a constant and flux will be determined solely by the magnitude of blood and dialysate concentrations; that is, the value of K_o will not change as flows or concentrations change. Inspection of equations 10 shows that this is not true for diffusive dialysance and that the value of this constant depends directly on the flow rate. It follows that under any particular flow conditions there should be a relationship between D and K_o (or $K_o A$) which would be useful in determining the value of the dialyzer constant K_o from a set of clinical chemistries. Conversely, it should be pos-

---

* These expressions are those generally used in defining clearance and dialysance and also appear in Chapters 5 and 12.

sible to determine what clinical performance a dialyzer should have when blood or dialysate flows change or when dialyzer membrane is compromised such as with clotting.

It is possible to develop the relation between K_oA and D by equating solute flux in a dialyzer using equation 14 (when $Q_F = 0$), the definition of D (see equation 10b), and equations 6 and 7. Such a combination and rearrangement yields:

$$D(C_{Bi} - C_{Di}) = K_oA \frac{(C_{Bi} - C_{Do}) - (C_{Bo} - C_{Di})}{\log \frac{C_{Bi} - C_{Do}}{C_{Bo} - C_{Di}}}$$

Manipulation of equation 10b yields the inlet and outlet concentration differences:

$$C_{Bi} - C_{Do} = (C_{Bi} - C_{Di})(1 - D/Q_D)$$

and

$$C_{Bo} - C_{Di} = (C_{Bi} - C_{Di})(1 - D/Q_B)$$

Substitution of these concentration terms into the equation above yields:

$$K_oA = \frac{Q_B}{1 - Q_B/Q_D} \log \frac{1 - D/Q_D}{1 - D/Q_B} \quad [22]$$

This is the expression describing K_oA and how this dialyzer constant can be computed from diffusive dialysance and clinical flows. This relationship can be rearranged to yield dialysance as a function of K_oA and flow rates:

$$D = \frac{e^{\frac{K_oA(1 - Q_B/Q_D)}{Q_B}} - 1}{\frac{e^{\frac{K_oA(1 - Q_B/Q_D)}{Q_B}}}{Q_B} - \frac{1}{Q_D}} \quad [23]$$

Equation 23 is extremely useful in predicting the dialysance (or clearance) of a particular solute under known flow conditions if the overall mass transfer coefficient – membrane area product is known. Quite often a family of dialyzers will have the same design and, therefore, similar transport resistances. In such cases, the clinical performance of other dialyzers of the same type can be estimated accurately by merely scaling the value of K_oA by the differing membrane areas in the various devices.

Equations 22 and 23 are for counter current flow. Similar expressions can be developed for co-current flow for K_oA:

$$K_oA = \frac{Q_B}{1 + Q_B/Q_D} \log \frac{Q_B}{Q_B - D(1 + Q_B/Q_D)} \quad [24]$$

and upon rearrangement for D:

$$D = Q_B \frac{1 - e^{-\frac{K_oA(1 + Q_B/Q_D)}{Q_B}}}{1 + Q_B/Q_D} \quad [25]$$

The effective clearance of larger solutes with ultrafiltration

It is generally recognized that convective transport (ultrafiltration) augments solute transport (14, 15). Equation 18 indicates that with smaller solutes and high clearance values (K), the effective clearance (K') will not be greatly influenced by ultrafiltration. This is not the case, however, with larger substances where K may be of the same order of magnitude as Q_F. The effect of ultrafiltration on mass transport of solutes of different size can be illustrated using urea and a hypothetical, large molecular weight, substance which is poorly removed by diffusive transport (see Table 2). The data in Table 2 confirm that ultrafiltration plays an extremely limited role in the case of a highly cleared solute like urea (adding only 2% at high rates of ultrafiltration) but can be a major means of transport with those materials whose diffusion transport is limited, being capable of augmenting clearance by as much as 45%.

Table 2. The effect of ultrafiltration on solute clearance for materials easily and poorly cleared by the dialyzer.

Solute	K_d $Q_F = 0$	$Q_F = 5$ ml/min K'_d	K'_d/K_d	$Q_F = 10$ ml/min K'_d	K'_d/K_d
Urea	150	151.25	1.01	152.5	1.02
Solute 'X'	20	24.5	1.23	29.0	1.45

Transport determined by kinetic methods

The measurement of dialyzer transport by single pass methods is straight forward and accurate as long as transport rates are high so that concentration differences are sizable. In this case, values for Q_{Do}, C_{Do}, Q_F and C_{Bi} when substituted into equation 17b will yield reliable K_D values. However, with a poorly diffusing solute where C_{Do} values may be small as will the drop in blood values, a closed loop method will yield more accurate results. With this procedure either the blood circuit or the dialysate circuit is recycled through a reservoir, and the rate of solute accumulation can be used to measure accurately the transport properties (see Figure 5). Consider the system's mass balance:

Accumulation in blood reservoir
= Flux in – flux out

There is no flux in and substitution of equation 14 into this expression yields:

$$\frac{d(VC_B)}{dt} = D\left(1 - \frac{Q_F}{Q_{Bi}}\right)C_{Di}$$

$$- \left[D\left(1 - \frac{Q_F}{Q_{Bi}}\right) + Q_F\right]C_B \quad [26]$$

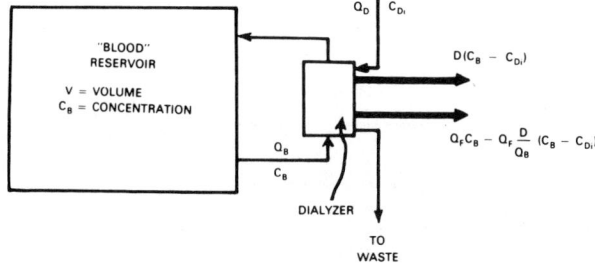

Figure 5. Schematic representation of recycle circuit for transport evaluation including flow rates and removal rates.

In Figure 5 where the blood loop is recycled, solute will be lost from the reservoir so that accumulation will be negative. Note that the second term of equation 26 is analogous to the one that appeared in equation 18 as the $K'C_{Bi}$ term (the product of the apparent clearance and blood inlet concentration) and accounts for the presence of convective transport.

The solution of this expression depends on the conditions of the measurement; when $Q_F = 0$, V is constant, the Q_F/Q_B terms drop out and the left hand side becomes $V(dc/dt)$ which is easily solvable and yields:

$$C_B = C_{Bo} \cdot e^{-Dt/V} + C_{Di}(1 - e^{-Dt/V}) \quad [27a]$$

Rearranging and solving for D:

$$D = \frac{V}{t} \text{Log} \frac{C_{Bo} - C_{Di}}{C_{Bt} - C_{Di}} \quad [27b]$$

Note that if the reservoir of Figure 5 is placed on the dialysate side, an equivalent expression to equation 26 results which when solved yields analogous solutions where the 'B' and 'D' sub-scripts are reversed.

If Q_F is not zero, then equation 26 must be solved and yields a more complicated expression which is the analog to equation 27a. (This case is solved in the Appendix.) Using the closed loop method for clearance determination, one of the streams is recycled through a reservoir and the reservoir concentration is sampled at two times, t minutes apart. The first concentration becomes C_{Bo} (or C_{Do}), the second C_{Bt} (or C_{Dt}). The dialysance can then be calculated from equation 27b. Another method using this recycle technique and equation 27a is to take serial reservoir samples and to plot the logarithm term as a function of time. The slope of the resulting straight line will then be D/V from which the value of D can be obtained.

This technique is most suitable for materials that are poorly transported by the dialyzer so that the reservoir concentration does not change rapidly. The model shown in Figure 5 assumes that all of the material in the system is in the reservoir which is well mixed. In actuality, a significant fraction of the recycle loop is represented by the dialyzer volume and tubing so that this assumption is not strictly true. If D is small and V is large, however, this non-ideality becomes negligible.

The use of marker solutes

It is common practice to describe a dialyzer or membrane by the transport properties of a series of marker substances such as those listed in Table 3 (16–20). These materials when used in controlled *in vitro* studies will yield transport as a function of molecular weight relationships that characterize the particular dialyzer. The difficulty with such characterizations is that *in vivo* performance cannot be predicted accurately from *in vitro* transport data because of the presence of proteins and the probability of their interaction with the membrane, the possibility of Donnan effects, and other phenomena unique to physiologic solutions. An added complication is that less than half of the listed materials (predominantly those of lower molecular weight) can be used *in vivo* so that the relationship between *in vitro* and *in vivo* values cannot be obtained easily. Finally, results of transport studies with higher molecular mass substances should be used circumspectly; membrane permeability depends on factors other than molecular mass such as molecular conformation (2, 16, 17) so that a substance of 1355 daltons (the mass of vitamin B_{12}) may have transport properties far different *in vivo* from those observed for vitamin B_{12} *in vitro*.

Table 3. Commonly used solute markers for transport studies.

Solute	Molecular weight	Reference
NaCl	58	2
Urea	60	2
Creatinine	113	2
Uric acid	168	2
Dextrose	180	2
Sucrose	342	2
Raffinose	594	2
Bromsulfophthalein (BSP)	838	16
Cyclohepta-amylose or β Schardinger or Cyclo-dextrin	1,152	2, 18
Vitamin B_{12}	1,355	2, 16
Bacitracin	1,411	2, 16
Inulin	5,200	2, 16
Cytochrom C	13,400	2, 16

MASS BALANCE PRINCIPLES APPLIED TO INTERMITTENT DIALYSIS: SOLUTE KINETIC MODELLING

Uremia results from the body's loss of control over its internal chemistry through the diminished capacity of the regulating organ, the kidney. The fundamental assumption of dialysis treatment is that some uremic abnormalities are a function of the concentration of ingested or metabolically produced toxic materials which are normally excreted by the natural kidney. The ability to keep the uremic patient alive by hemodialysis and peritoneal dialysis emphasizes that if some degree of chemical control can be restored, however imperfect, the results of uremia (particularily the predictable and imminent mortality) can be, in part, reversed. It is clear, therefore, that the passive transport of water, solutes and electolytes which is the sole capability of dialysis, is sufficient to control the imbalances which result from kidney failure.

In dialysis treatment a large number of materials, many of unknown composition (21-33) and toxicity are removed, all of them at unequel rates. In order to 'control' dialysis treatment, therefore, one might hope to select a key compound which would provide an index of treatment. To date there is no such compound although there have been numerous attemps to define one in order to develop an index of adequate treatment (5, 34-35). In reality, although control of toxic substances may be the goal of dialysis treatment, levels of a limited number of solutes, balance of fluid and electrolytes, and control of acid-base constitute the basis of current treatment adequacy on a day-to-day basis. It is with regard to the measurement and control of such substances that the concept of mass balance and solute kinetics can provide powerful tools and insights to guide treatment.

Dialysis was first mathematically modelled over three decades ago (11) and this approach has continued until the present time (34-47). Clinical dialysis, however, has not kept pace with these advances in the quantitative understanding and ability to describe and monitor treatment. The reasons for this vary. Not all physicians consider the task of clinical management of the dialysis patient as a completely quantifiable one, a view that is at least partially justified because of the multifactorial nature of most medical problems. In addition, much of the information required by some models is unavailable to the practicing physician in the time span required for his treatment decisions. These restrictions notwithstanding, the ability to describe quantitatively biochemical and physiologic processes and the abnormalities that exist in uremic patients makes the process of modelling an important one for greater understanding of the disease state and better management of subsequent therapy.

The mathematical modelling of dialysis therapy represents the structured application of the principles of conservation of matter to the patient undergoing dialysis. There are many advantages to this structured approach:
1. It enables one to describe a specific biochemical system and thereby monitor or investigate various physiologic processes, such as net rates of protein catabolism (48-50).
2. It enables one to prescribe the appropriate dialysis treatment to achieve a desired therapeutic goal, or to investigate the predictable results of altered treatment (39, 40, 51, 52).
3. It increases understanding of the controlling physiologic-biochemical mechanisms from the type of model required to describe the kinetics of a particular substance (10, 45, 53).
4. It allows determination of the controlling factors in any solute system through evaluation of the order of magnitude of various routes of input and output in a quantitatively defined system (10).

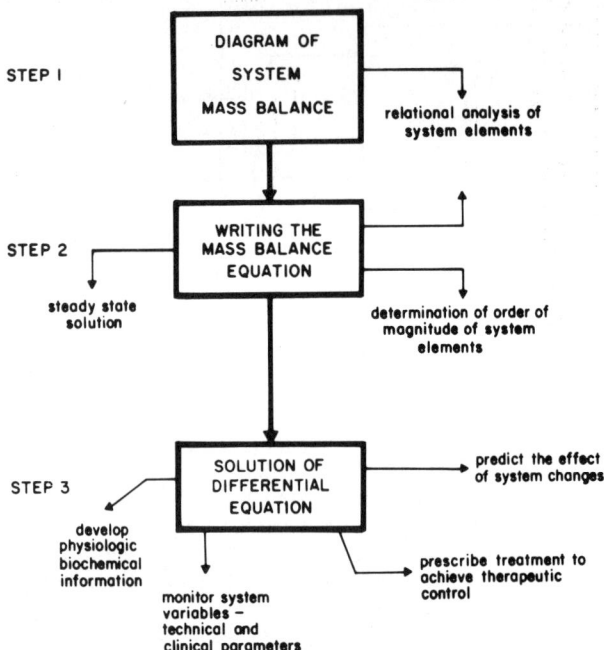

Figure 6. Diagram illustrating the steps in formulating and representing a mathematical model. Figure includes indications of uses of each stage of formulation.

5. It allows discrimination of the causes of clinical observations and problems such as hypotension caused by sodium flux or hypoxia (10, 45).

Mathematical modelling can be viewed as 'quantified intuition' in that it mathematically relates events that are known to take place. Two aspects of this should be stressed:
1. An individual who has a thorough basic understanding of the physiologic system being modelled is best able to construct and benefit from the model, i.e., the physician who deals with specific clinical problems.
2. Putting the qualitative relationship in a mathematical context increases its value and the usefulness of information by vastly extending its range of application and the value of analyzed data (see discussion of mathematical elements in the Appendix).

The basic steps of modelling are shown in Figure 6 and consist of: formulating the system description (step one) which usually involves a diagramatic representation of the system; writing the mass balance equation (step two) using the diagram; and solving it (step three). It should be noted that only step three requires any degree of advanced mathematical skills.

Mass balance considerations as they apply to quantification of intermittent dialysis treatment

The concept of conservation of matter or mass balance appears to be obvious; it is in the application of this law to a physical system, however, that it becomes an increasingly complex but an extremely powerful analytical and conceptual tool.

The law of conservation of mass can be restated in the word equation:

Accumulation (increase in system content) = input to system − output from system [28]

Equation 28 forms the basis for a substantial portion of this chapter in that most relationships to follow are either applications or solutions of it.

Formulation of a model: elements of the mass balance diagram

While the application of mass balance principles to a specific system would not appear to pose any great problem, in practice it is the most difficult aspect of modelling. The difficulty lies in the need to understand fully and isolate quantitatively the specific system being modelled. It should be stressed that once the model is formulated the mathematical description of the system is predetermined, so that a deliberate attempt to accurately and quantitatively represent the system will assure the validity of subsequent steps. It is helpful if the model is formulated by use of a structured diagram. Such a diagram consists of boxes for the system and arrows for inputs and outputs.

In the figures that follow, the model is shown as a box with arrows going into and out of it; these figures exemplify the two formal elements of this approach. The box describes the system content (generally in units of mass), such as the product of volume and concentration. Inputs add to the system content, and outputs decrease it. The manner (if any) that the inputs or outputs relate to the system content or concentration is indicated with respect to the appropriate arrows. In the case of a single box (the figures shown), the system is 'single pool' or one well-mixed compartment.

The system content is the total mass present at any instant. It can be contained in any physical space, such as the vascular space, the red blood cell, or the amount of dialysate recirculating through a dialyzer. The system content is the product of the compartment volume and the concentration in that space. Alternatively, it can be the total system mass (irrespective of its distribution space) or simply the effect of the total mass such as in the case of heparin (54).

The quantitative description of system inputs and outputs must be consistent with the description of system content. In general, there are two common types of input/outputs: those that depend on the amount of material present in the system (first-order processes) and those that are constant (zero-order processes). The clearance of a dialyzer (Kd) is a first-order process, because material is removed as a product of Kd and concentration (see Equation 18). In contrast, an effectively saturated metabolic process (such as acetate metabolism in most dialyzed patients) (53) is a constant output, or zero-order process.

The process of model formulation is best illustrated with an example.

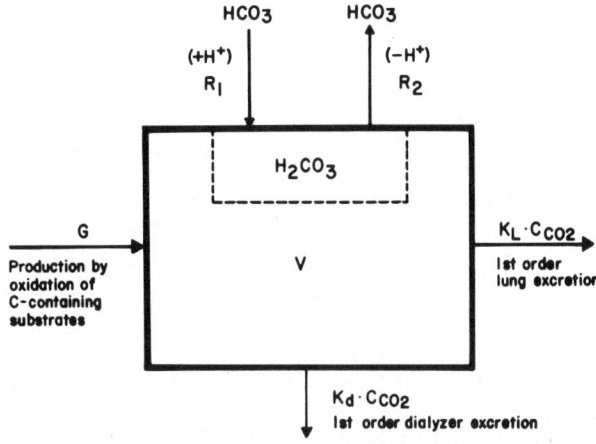

Figure 7. Model describing the CO_2 system in the dialyzed patient (Reprinted from Kidney International, with permission).

The transport of CO_2 in dialysis patients has attracted considerable attention (55–59) and represents a good illustration of modelling techniques. The first step is to define what is meant by the CO_2 system. One must decide what forms of CO_2 are to be included, (e.g. should bicarbonate be considered part of the system?) so that all elements of the model are consistent. For this analysis we will let the CO_2 system be the total dissolved CO_2 gas in body water and let it also include the hydrated form of CO_2 (carbonic acid), but not bicarbonate. We can then draw a box such as Figure 7, that will represent the total body content of CO_2 gas at any time shown as the product of body water and CO_2 concentration (10).

Once the system is identified it is necessary to define how CO_2 is added to, and leaves the system. There are two major means of CO_2 production. The first is the oxidative metabolism of carbon containing substrates which is the ultimate origin of all body CO_2. The other is the neutralization of acid (H^+) by body bicarbonate (see reaction R-2).

$$CO_2 + H_2O \rightleftarrows H_2CO_3 \rightleftarrows H^+ + HCO_3^- \quad [R1] [R2]$$

Carbon dioxide readily reacts with water to form carbonic acid, which will dissociate to yield H^+ and bicarbonate by reaction R1. This system of reactions is reversible and moves to the left by reaction R2, which represents the neutralization of acid (H^+) by bicarbonate to form H_2CO_3 and generation of CO_2. In fact, both of these reactions continue and to the extent that they are unbalanced there is net generation or consumption of CO_2.

There are two major means by which CO_2 is removed from the body water in the non-dialyzed patient. It is apparent that if reaction R1 predominates CO_2 is removed from the system. The other route of removal is by exhalation via the lungs which will be a first order process and which will depend on the CO_2 level of the system with the lungs representing a first order excretion route which can be viewed as a lung clearance, K_L. The amount of CO_2 removed by the lungs therefore is $K_L C$. In the patient not on dialysis this completely defines the system. In the dialyzed patient, however, the dialyzer will also have a CO_2 clearance (K_D) and flux by this route is $K_D C$.

It is important, at this point to re-emphasize the need for an unambigious, structured, and quantitative approach to the formulation of this model. The CO_2 system has been isolated and is the one being modelled. As such the transport of bicarbonate by the dialyzer is not relevant to the analysis; the flux of bicarbonate in the dialyzer will only affect the CO_2 through the balance of reactions R1 and R2 which have already been considered.

Note that the units of K_D and C must be consistent and their product equal the dialyzer flux of dissolved gaseous CO_2. Clearances will most conveniently be expressed in liters per minute because CO_2 concentrations are most commonly in units of grams or millimoles per liter. This is important, because many investigators have been impressed that the dialyzer totally 'clears' incoming blood of CO_2 having CO_2 clearances equalling or exceeding blood flow (10, 58, 59). The CO_2 content of incoming blood, however, when expressed in appropriate units is very low (about 1.1 mmol/l) so that the CO_2 removed by the dialyzer is very small (10, 45). Analysis of the system (which will be completed below) will show that a much more significant route of CO_2 removal during dialysis is reaction R2 which is promoted by bicarbonate loss and body re-alkalinization using acetate during treatment.

This completes the formulation of the CO_2 model. The CO_2 system itself is carbon dioxide, present as dissolved gas and its hydrated form (carbonic acid). It is generated by metabolic processes and the production of carbonic acid when acids are neutralized by combining with bicarbonate. It is removed by the reversal of this reaction (dissociation of H_2CO_3) and its first order removal (clearance) represented by the lungs (K_L) and the dialyzer (K_D).

Writing the mass balance equation

Once the system has been formulated the mass balance equation is written. This is basically a mechanical step of substituting terms into equation 28.

The accumulation, or change in system content, will be the rate of change of the system content with time (first derivative with respect to time of the system content: d(content)/dt). It should be noted that although this term gives the intimidating appearance of 'higher mathematics' it is merely a quantitative symbol of the time dependant change of system content (i e: accumulation). The only aspect that will change from one system to another is the representation of 'content'. In the current example, total disolved CO_2 'content' will be the product of total body water and CO_2 concentration (Not P_{CO_2}):

$$CO_2 \text{ content} = VC_{CO_2}$$

$$\text{Change system content} = \frac{d(VC_{CO_2})}{dt}$$

The input and output are taken directly from the system diagram (see Figure 7) and will be the algebraic sum of all the arrows in the diagram. The zero order terms will be constants and the first order terms will be the product of first order constants (clearances) and the concentration. Substitution of all of these terms in equation 28 yields:

$$\frac{(VC_{CO_2})}{dt} = G + R1 - R2 - K_L C_{CO_2} - K_D C_{CO_2} \quad [29]$$

Equation 29 is the mass balance equation for body CO_2 and, as has been stated, is a strictly mechanical reduction of the elements of the formulation, shown diagramed in Figure 7, to a mathematical form.

Use of the mass balance equation

One may be inclined to solve immediately the above expression to obtain the body CO_2 content as a function of time. For this substance this is not a very productive approach. The most useful mathematical relationship in this case, and a valuable one generally, is the mass balance equation itself.

It is instructive to consider all the terms in the specific equation to determine their relative magnitude and relation to one another. Common values for the terms listed are shown in Table 4.

Consider first the accumulation term on the left hand side of the equation 29. Computation of body CO_2 content using the values in Table 4 shows body CO_2 content is about 42 mmol. This is an interesting value from two stand points. First, it should be appreciated that the

Table 4. Typical values in a 70 kg patient undergoing acetate dialysis.

Inter dialytic	Intra dialytic	References
V = 40 l	40 l	—
C = 1.05 mmol/l (P_{CO_2} = 35 mm Hg)	1.05 mmol/l	10
G = 11 mmol/min	11 mmol/min	58,59
R_1 = —	0	—
R_2 = —	2.3 mol/min	10
K_L = 10.5 l/min	8.1 l/min	10,58
K_D = 0	0.20 l/min	10
ΔC = —	0.3 mmol (10 mm Hg)	—
$\frac{d(VC)}{dt}$ = —	0.05 mm/min	
$K_L C_{CO_2}$ = 11 mmol	8.5 mmol	—
$K_d C_{CO_2}$ = 0	0.21 mmol	—
R_2 = —	2.29 mmol	—

entire body content of CO_2 represents only 4 min of body CO_2 production. Stated differently, there is very little 'CO_2 storage' in the body. This is of enormous physiologic consequence, as is widely appreciated, in that ventilation can have a pronounced second to second effect on CO_2 levels which is extremely important in pH control through respiratory compensation in response to an acid/base insult. The second point is that a PCO_2 change of 10 mm Hg over a four hour dialysis represents an average rate of change in body CO_2 content of: $d(V_{CO_2})/dt = (40)(0.3)/240 = 0.05$ mmol/minute or less than 0.5% of the rate of body production. It becomes clear that the change in body CO_2 content represents a small difference between two very large numbers and that in fact the body is effectively in a steady state with respect to CO_2 content. Intuitively, it would be difficult to conclude otherwise.

The system being at steady state, all the terms on the right hand side of equation 29 must add to zero. Between dialyses equation 29 reduces to: $G = K_L C_{CO_2}$; the generated CO_2 is exhaled. During dialysis the situation is more complicated. The generation of CO_2 would be expected to remain relatively constant, which from the standpoint of energetics is reasonable. During acetate dialysis reaction R2 will predominate and R1 will equal zero. Bicarbonate loss, in itself, will not affect this model. Usually, however, the HCO_3^- lost in the dialyzer is almost quantitatively replaced by reaction R2. If plasma bicarbonate levels* are 18 mEq/l approximately 2.3 mEq/min will be lost and replaced by reaction R2.

Examination of the three routes of removal indicates that the effect of dialyzer CO_2 transport is vanishingly small (2%, see Table 4) and can be neglected with respect to its effect on PCO_2. This fact has not been widely appreciated (58, 59).

Rearrangement of equation 29 yields:

$$G - R2 - K_D C_{CO_2} = K_L C_{CO_2}$$

Solving for K_L

$$K_L = G/C_{CO_2} - R2/C_{CO_2} - K_D \quad [30]$$

The 'normal' steady state relationship (in the non-dialyzed patient) of G, $K_L(K_{Ln})$, and C_{CO_2} is:

$$K_{Ln} = G/C_{CO_2} \quad [31]$$

If equation 30 is divided by equation 31, the relative value of K_L will be

$$\frac{K_L}{K_{Ln}} = 1 - R2/G - K_D/K_{Ln} \quad [32]$$

Substituting values into this expression from Table 4 lung clearance would be expected to drop 77% from its normal value.

Adjustments of CO_2 levels to control pH is part of the feed back in the normal individual (8, 60) although this may be complicated by hypoxia particularly at low P_{CO_2} values. During dialysis P_{CO_2} remains relatively stable (57), and equation 32 indicates that this must reflect a reduction in K_L (which is directly related to respiratory rate) to approximately three quarters of non-dialysis values in order to adjust for extra-pulmonary CO_2 excretion. It is important, therefore, that the reduced ventilation predicted by equation 32 be explained when the observed dialysis hypoxia is considered (55–59).

Solution of the mass balance equation

Most kinetic models (and all those to be considered) are in the form of a first order linear differential equation for which solutions and solution techniques by classical methods of applied mathematics are well known (61, 62). The solutions describe the system concentration (or system content) as function of time. Essentially the expression can then be used to predict the effect of treatment changes on a particular solute being modelled and to monitor various system parameters. This aspect of modelling has been most extensively developed for urea as described below.

These are the key steps of modelling. It is well to emphasize again that the actual mathematical steps of writing the mass balance equation and solving it (steps two and three in Figure 6) are mechanical operations which totally depend upon the model formulation (step one). Consequently, the entire validity of the solutions depend on the correct and rigorous formulation of the model itself.

MASS BALANCE AS APPLIED TO VARIOUS SOLUTE SYSTEMS

Urea nitrogen mass balance

Urea is of interest because it is the major product of protein catabolism so it can be used as an index of the patient's catabolic status and, by extension, nutritional state. Furthermore, development of the uremic syndrome is dependent to a large extent on protein catabolism (63–67) for which urea* generation provides a quantitative measure (see equation A-16 in the Appendix).

Although urea is not considered highly toxic, its presence in high blood concentrations may result in increased morbidity in dialysis patients (68–71) (see also Chapter 19). It has been demonstrated in a large well controlled cooperative study that elevation of BUN in the presence of adequate protein intake results in increased rates of hospitalization (72, 73). In addition, there are nitrogenous compounds that are commonly found in the dialysis patient which may be stoichiome-

---

* For bicarbonate and hydrogen ion, concentrations are expressed as milliequivalents per liter, rather than as SI units (millimoles) unlike other sections of the book to facilitate mathematical consideration of ionic reactions and balances. For monovalent ions, the units are interchangeable quantitatively. This is not so for divalent ions.

* Because it is the nitrogen component of urea that is derived from protein, urea nitrogen is the expression used in quantitative considerations herein, but the solute itself is referred to as urea.

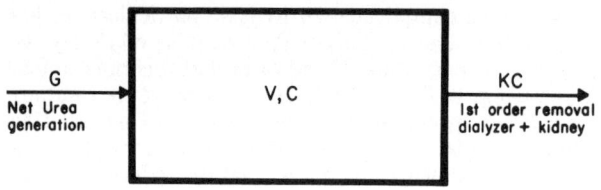

Figure 8. Model of urea nitrogen in the dialyzed patient (Reprinted from Kidney International, with permission).

trically related to the rate of protein catabolism and consequently, to the rate of urea production.

Urea distribution and metabolism can be described quantitatively as is shown in Figure 8. This figure considers urea to be distributed in a single pool (physically approximating total body water) (74) with one route of net entry (or generation) and one route of removal by first order processes.

Urea will enter the pool of body water as amino acids are oxidized (75, 76). As such its minute rate of net generation (absolute synthesis – absolute degradation) will not, in fact, be constant. The urea content of the body, however, is a thermodynamic property (its value being path independent) and will increase in a quasi-linear manner between dialyses. As a result the assumption that net urea generation is zero-order (constant) is considered to have practical validity.

Routes of removal are considered to be entirely first order (i.e. proportional to concentration) and accounted for solely by the residual kidney and the dialyzer. Urea diffuses into the gut where its nitrogen is converted into ammonia which is reabsorbed by the portal circulation (77–78). Because this path is internal to the model no net gut contribution to urea removal from total body water is considered.

The analysis of this model then proceeds by writing the mass balance relationship:

Accumulation = Input − Output

$$\frac{d(VC)}{dt} = G - (K_R + K_D)C \qquad [33]$$

Further expansion of equation 32 yields:

$$V\frac{dC}{dt} + C\frac{dV}{dt} = G - (K_R + K_D)C \qquad [34]$$

Consideration of steady state: chronic renal failure

Before considering the solution of equation 34 it is appropriate to contemplate the mass balance equation itself with respect to the special, but, more usual case of steady state when dC/dt and dV/dt are both negligible. These two quantities will always have some value, but when dialysis is not required there will be no net accumulation and these terms can be neglected. With respect to body solutes steady state is commonly called 'homeostasis' and in this physiological situation the left hand side of equation 34 is zero (steady state with respect to body protein and is usually called zero nitrogen or protein balance). Considering equation 34, steady state for the urea nitrogen system can be represented as:

$$G = K_R C \qquad [35a]$$

there are two other forms of this expression

$$K_R = G/C \qquad [35b]$$

and

$$C = G/K_R \qquad [35c]$$

Figure 9 interrelates the three parameters shown in equations 35. The figure itself shows the BUN as a function of time at two different levels of protein intake as renal function (urea clearance) declines. The Kr as a linear function of time is shown in a secondary K-time plot in the same figure. This figure also relates the net rate of urea nitrogen production resulting from a known quantity of protein catabolism. This relationship, which is discussed further in the Appendix, accurately relates the net amount of urea that will be generated for net protein catabolic rates (PCR) from 20 to 350 g/day in uremic and normal individuals (48, 76, 79, 80). The two forms of this relationship are (with G expressed in mg/min):

$$G = \frac{PCR - 0.294\,V}{9.35} \qquad [36a]$$

which when rearranged yields

$$PCR = 9.35\,G + 0.294\,V \qquad [36b]$$

Figure 9 represents a progression of steady states as renal function declines. In this figure there is no change in generation. As 70 g of protein is ingested and a like amount catabolized a net quantity of 6.23 mg/min of urea nitrogen or 13.4 mg/min of urea, i.e. 223 μmol/min is generated, both in the uremic patient with 10 ml/min of renal function, and in a normal individual. This same amount is excreted in both cases. The difference between the two is that because the flux is equal to the product of K_R and C (equation 35a) the BUN must be far higher in the uremic patient which is obviously the case.

There will be some BUN level above which every physician will consider clinical measures appropriate. For the following discussion 100 mg/dl (214 mg/dl of urea or 35.7 mmol/l) has been chosen as this level, to illustrate the use of steady state expressions shown in equation 35.

When K_R drops to 6 ml/min BUN will be slightly above 100 mg/dl (35.7 mmol/l of urea) (see equation 35c). At this point the clinical decision may be to start dialysis. As seen from the figure, however, a reduction in protein intake to 50 g/day would decrease the BUN to below 70 mg/dl (25 mmol/l of urea) and allow the patient to delay dialysis for an extended period. This has been the historic approach of the management of uremia (63, 81, 82). This, in fact is the spontaneous physiologic result of uremia and anorectic feed back. With an intake of 50 g/day (G = 4.09 mg/min) the BUN will reach 100 mg/dl (35.7 mmol/l of urea) when K_R is approximately 4 ml/min. Once again intake may be re-

3: *Principles and biophysics of dialysis*   67

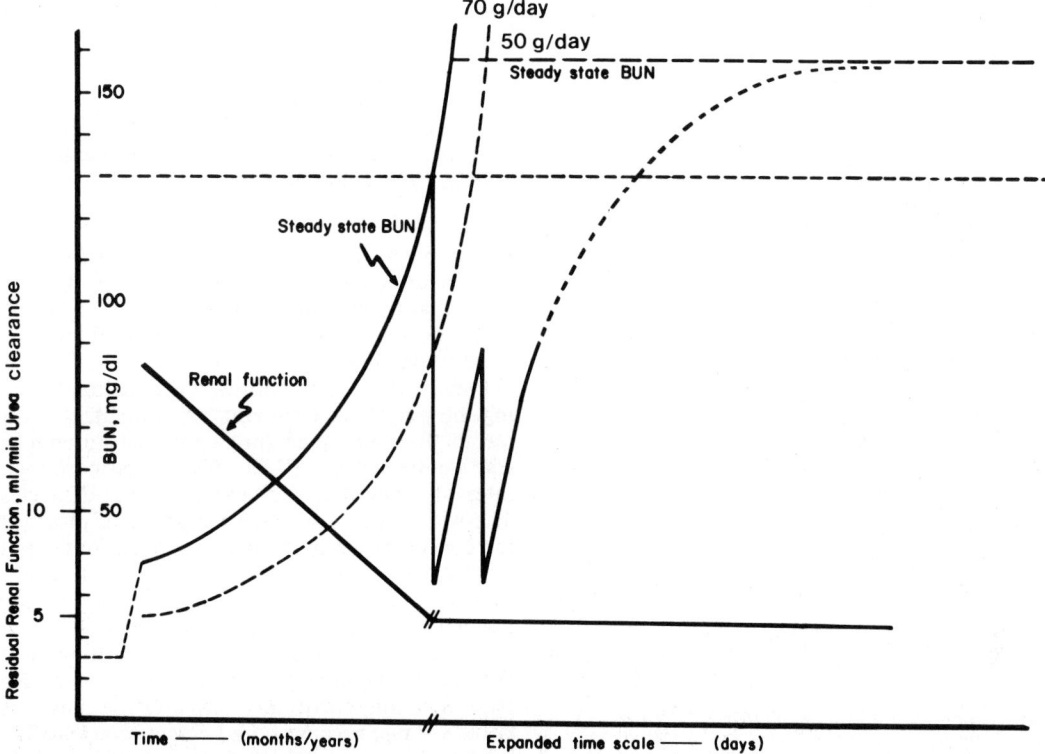

Figure 9. Blood urea nitrogen in a patient with chronic renal failure with decreasing renal function (see superimposed plot in bottom left of figure). Relationship is shown for two levels of protein intake (and net catabolism) up to the point where dialysis is instituted.
BUN mg/dl → mmol/l: multiply by 0.357.

duced. At some point, however, dialysis will be initiated to allow a tolerable intake with an acceptable BUN. It is important to realize, however, that a steady state concentration still exists. For an intake of 70 g/day with a K_R of 2 ml/min BUN would be 312 mg/dl (111.4 mmol/l of urea), for example. The patient undergoes dialysis to keep BUN below this level. But at the end of a dialysis BUN starts to increase towards this level and only the next dialysis interrupts it. The build up of BUN to a steady state value post dialysis is curvilinear because as BUN increases the residual kidney will remove more material and blunt the rate of increment (see right hand side of both equation 35a and Figure 9). It is also important to recognize that as long as there is some kidney function there is a steady state BUN, which will change as K_R does. In some cases K_R will improve slightly; in such cases a re-evaluation of intake and treatment is appropriate (83).

Establishing a level of K_R

The level of renal function is the major parameter to which all others must adjust. In the case of steady state its value is shown by equation 35b which can be expanded to yield:

$$K_R = \frac{G}{C} = \frac{\text{excretion rate}}{C} = \frac{V_{ur}C_{ur}}{T_{ur}} \frac{1}{C_B} \quad [37]$$

The right hand side of 37 is general for all solutes. It does not rely on the presence of steady state. In this case C_B will be the average blood value during the urine collection (see appendix for the mathematical determination of this quantity during dialysis). What is required is a urine collection of known volume, V_{ur}, and analysis of the solute concentration in that urine volume, C_{ur}, (urea nitrogen, creatinine, etc.) the duration of the collection, T_{ur}, and the average prevailing blood level of that solute C_B. In the case described above, typical values for a 1500 ml 24 h collection would be: C_{ur} – urea nitrogen = 600 mg/dl (= 214 mmol/l urea), creatinine = 92 mg/dl (8.1 mmol/l), which yield excretory rates (and generation for the steady state) of 9 g/day (6.25 mg/min) for urea nitrogen and 1380 mg/day (0.96 mg/min) for creatinine. For blood values of 104 mg/dl (= 37.1 mmol/l urea) (BUN) and 8 mg/dl (708 µmol/l) (creatinine), clearances will be K_R (BUN) = 6 ml/min; K_R creatinine = 12 ml/min.

This information is useful in a number of ways. The net rate of urea generation obtained from this urine collection can be used in equation 36b to compute net pro-

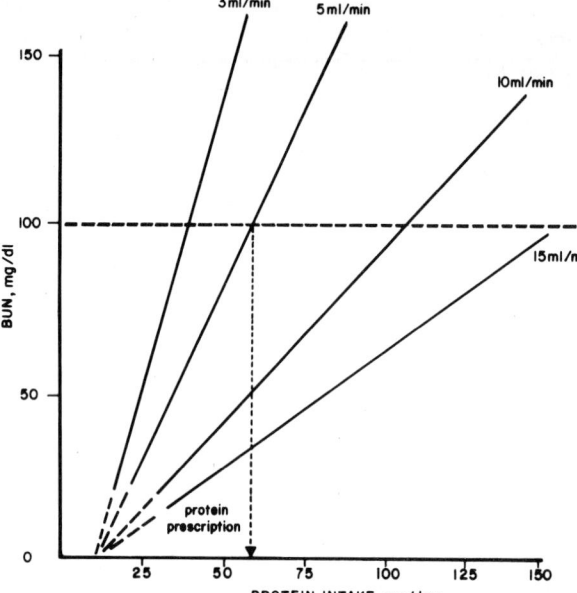

Figure 10. Blood urea nitrogen in the nutritionally stable adult chronic renal failure patient in relation to intake (and net catabolism)
BUN mg/dl → mmol/l: multiply by 0.357.

tein catabolism. Such data are useful in many disease states (not just uremia) for assessment of protein nutritional status and are readily available from urine collections analyzed for urea nitrogen. The rate of creatinine generation is useful as a nutritional parameter (84). Creatinine generation rate is also a convenient check on the accuracy of collection; its value is relatively stable because it is produced at a reasonably constant rate from muscle tissue. Consequently, variability of this parameter suggests inaccuracy in urine collection (either V_{ur} or T_{ur}) or analysis (C_{ur}).

The ratio of K_R urea to K_R creatinine is also a useful parameter because in chronic renal failure the ratio of these two basic clearances tends to remain relatively constant and can be used to estimate K_R urea from K_R creatinine values (85). Once K_R urea is known, it is possible using equation 35a and 36b both to determine the level of protein intake required to keep BUN below a desired value, and the actual protein intake when a patient presents with an elevated BUN (85).

This approach is shown graphically in figure 10 when BUN is plotted as a function of PCR for various levels of residual urea clearance and illustrates that if K_R is known in nutritionally stable (zero nitrogen balance) patients, PCR (intake) can be accurately prescribed and determined from BUN measurements. Once clearances have been measured, a great deal of information is available from routine blood values alone. From the initial clearance determinations levels of G (creatinine) and the ratio of K_R urea to K_R creatinine (K_R ratio) are known. Consequently, from subsequent values of BUN and plasma creatinine concentrations the following can be calculated:

K_R creatinine – from plasma creatinine concentration, G (creatinine) and equation 35b
K_R urea – from K_R creatinine and the K_R ratio
G urea – from K_R urea, BUN and equation 35a
PCR from equation 36b

It is apparent that with these data available from those two blood chemistries, reducing them to a ratio of BUN/plasma creatinine concentrations as has been suggested decreases their value as analytical and nutritional parameters (86).

Finally, it is worth considering equation 35c as showing the general determinants of both BUN and creatinine in the undialyzed (not necessarily uremic) patient. The solute levels will be directly proportional to net rates of generation and inversely related to clearances. The widespread use of the reciprocal of plasma creatinine concentration as an index of renal function (87) and the tendency to view elevated BUN levels as an indication of renal failure should be examined in the context of equation 35c. Plasma creatinine levels will reflect renal function only when creatinine generation is constant. When wasting occurs simultaneously with decreasing renal function, creatinine concentration may remain relatively stable because both G creatinine and Kr creatinine are decreasing at the same rate. Similarly, elevated BUN reflects the net rate of generation relative to clearance. Consequently, a high BUN may reflect a high rate of catabolism or intake (79) or reduced renal function or both. Appropriate clinical and nutritional management require, that the determinants of mass balance as represented by equation 35c be evaluated individually.

Urea nitrogen kinetics in the dialyzed patient
At the point in Figure 9 when dialysis is instituted solute concentration will oscillate at a point below steady state and the object of dialysis is to keep them within a tolerable range. Equation 34 must, therefore, be considered in its entirety.

When there is no significant change in the system volume the second term on the left of equation 34 can be dropped ($dV/dT = 0$) and:

$$V \frac{dC}{dt} = G - (K_R + K_D)C \quad [38a]$$

$$\frac{dC}{dt} = \frac{G}{V} - \frac{K_R + K_D}{V} C \quad [38b]$$

It should be pointed out that in the steady state analysis, concentration was insensitive to the system volume because there was no solute accumulation. Once dialysis is needed, however, body water serves as a container that stores solutes between treatments. Equation 38b describes this, and shows that V will play a significant role with respect to the rate of concentration increase, dC/dt, and by extension the corresponding treatment required.

The more general case, however, in the uremic patient is for V to change due to fluid retention between treatments and ultrafiltration during dialysis. In this case V, as a function of time, is represented as:

$$V = V_o + \beta t \quad [39a]$$

And

$$\frac{dV}{dt} = \beta \quad [39b]$$

Where β is the rate of weight gain. Combining equations 34, 39a, and 39b and letting $K = K_R + K_D$, yields:

$$\frac{dC}{G-(K+\beta)C} = \frac{dt}{V_o+\beta} \quad [40]$$

Solution of equations 38a and 40 by classical techniques (61, 62) yields analogous expressions for concentration as a function of time:

$$C = C_o e^{-\frac{Kt}{V}} + \frac{G}{K}[1-e^{-\frac{Kt}{V}}] \quad [41a]$$

$$C = C_o \left(\frac{V_o+\beta t}{V_o}\right)^{-\frac{K+\beta}{\beta}} + \frac{G}{K+\beta}\left[1 - \left(\frac{V_o+\beta t}{V_o}\right)^{-\frac{K+\beta}{\beta}}\right] \quad [41b]$$

Manipulations of expression 41a for the guidance of dialysis therapy have been discussed elsewhere (39). Analogous rearrangements of equation 41b provide for the same monitoring and guidance of treatment in the more general case in renal failure where volumes are changing due to expanding and contracting quantities of body water during different intervals of the therapy.

Equations 41 are used to predict the BUN concentration that will result from a specific set of therapy (t, K, and schedule) and patient (V_o, G, and β) parameters.

Although equation 41b is the more general solution of equation 34 examination of equation 41a can give some insight into the nature of these expressions. Reference to equation 35c shows that the coefficient of the second term on the right side of equation 41a is the steady state concentration if dialysis was performed indefinitely. Equation 41a can then be written as:

$$C = C_o e^{-\frac{Kt}{V}} + C_{SS}[1-e^{-\frac{Kt}{V}}] \quad [42]$$

The term, $e^{-Kt/V}$ is one that describes the rate of concentration decay in a first order system of volume V where material is being cleared at a rate K. It represents the reciprocal of $e^{+Kt/V}$ and therefore becomes small, approaching zero, as t becomes large. Also, by definition, any number, including e, raised to the power 0 will equal 1, so that when $t = 0$, equation 42 reduces to the trivial expression $C_B = C_{Bo}$ which is the case by definition at $t = 0$. Conversely, as t becomes large C_B approaches C_{Bss}.

If the patient is dialyzed for an infinite period of time, the exponential terms will approach zero, as mentioned above. The rate at which this happens depends on the relative values of (K_R+K_D) and V. If the numerator of the exponent (K_R+K_D) is large compared to V, then the exponent will disappear rapidly; if the converse is true,

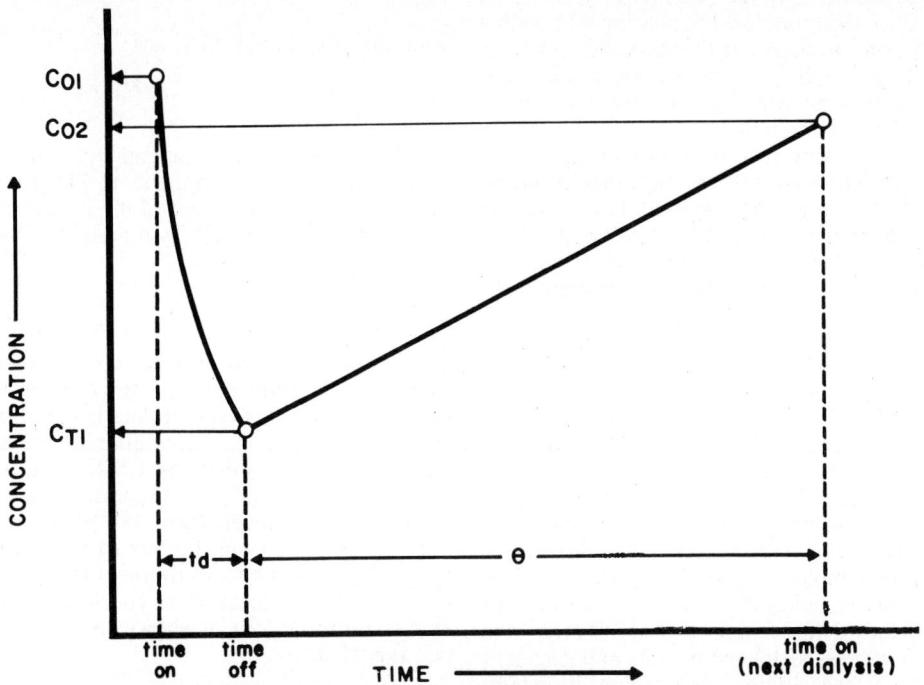

Figure 11. Blood urea nitrogen in the dialyzed patient during one dialysis cycle.

it will remain a significant factor for long intervals. When the exponential is no longer significant, equation 42 reduces to the steady state (i.e., when the concentration has ceased to change), the rate of material entering equals that leaving and there is no accumulation. Rarely is the patient actually dialyzed to steady state although it is important to note that even if long dialyses are used, the lowest possible concentration is that described by the ratio G/K.

A similar analysis of equation 41b will not lead to the same relationships. This is because the analysis that led to equation 41b is based on volume changing at a constant rate over time and at large values of t the inescapable, and impossible, result is that during very long treatments V could become negative (i.e.: $-Q_F t$ be larger than V_o, $-Q_F$ being β during dialysis – see equation 39a).

Use of mass balance equation solution

Equation 41b is used in two ways: to establish patient parameters (V and G) from clinical data (39) and to predict the effect of therapy changes and prescribe dialysis treatment to achieve clinical goals (39, 40, 51, 88, 89).

It is clear from equation 41b that desired BUN concentrations can be achieved by manipulation of K_D and T_D (the two direct therapy parameters). Dialysis frequency is also a treatment parameter which will determine the interval over which BUN is allowed to increase between treatments (89). The use of equation 41b for predictive and prescriptive computations, however, presupposes knowledge of the patient parameters V and G. Initially values for these parameters must be developed from clinical data for the specific patient for whom the model is to be used. If the patients level of renal function is known, examination of equation 41b shows that with BUN concentrations at the start and end of an interval as well as weight changes and treatment variables the only remaining undefined parameters in these expressions are patient volume, V_o, and urea nitrogen generation rate, G. Taking each of these constants separately, if one of them were known the other could be calculated directly from a single interval. It follows that both can be computed if the treatment parameters and BUN concentrations are known over two intervals, such as a dialysis and an inter-dialytic period (see Figure 11). The computations to obtain V and G as well as the predictive use of these solutions have been discussed elsewhere (39, 40, 45).

Modelling of the anticoagulant activity of heparin

Heparin is the anticoagulant universally used in dialysis treatment. The need to model this drug stems from the fact, which has generally been ignored in the pharmacology literature, that biological sensitivity and elimination of heparin varies widely (54). In the formulation of this model, a slightly different approach is followed. The characteristic of interest with heparin is its anticoagulant effect, measured as the clotting time prolongation (54), rather than concentration, that is the appropriate parameter to model. Clotting time prolongation relative to

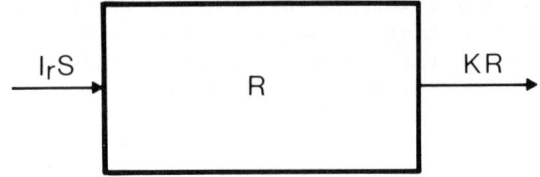

Figure 12. Model of heparin.

base line values which result from systemic heparin use, can be considered a direct measure of the system content (see Figure 12).

Input to the system after initial loading is a zero order infusion rate, Ir, with units of units/hour. A coefficient is required to convert the infusion rate to increased clotting time response, so input is IrS. In this term S is the sensitivity of the clotting system to added heparin. This response is found to be linear and insensitive to dose level for therapeutic quantities of this drug (54). Output is first order (90–92) and described as the product of the response and an elimination constant, KR. This completes the model formulation.

Mass balance is then written:

$$\frac{dR}{dt} = I_r S - KR \qquad [43]$$

At steady state the right side of equation 43 will equal zero and the steady state infusion rate necessary for the required response will be:

$$I_r = \frac{KR}{S} \qquad [44]$$

Solution of equation 43 yields:

$$R_t = R_o e^{-Kt} + \frac{I_r S}{K}(1 - e^{-Kt}) \qquad [45]$$

Both S and K are individual patient constants and must be determined for each patient. The sensitivity, S, is evaluated by measurement of the change in response to a step change in heparin as represented by bolus dose:

$$S = \frac{R - R_o}{dose} \qquad [46]$$

It is useful to be able to calculate the heparin elimination constant from serial clotting times for a dialysis patient because this type of data is commonly available in the clinical setting. Examination of equation 45 shows that K appears both in the $I_r S/K$ term as well as the exponent, and as such this expression cannot be directly solved for K although there will be a unique value for this metabolic constant for any specific value of R_t, R_o, I_r and S. A specific rearrangement of equation 45 which avoids the use of logarithms, common in analagous urea kinetic solutions (39), is shown in equation 47 (Trezek GJ unpublished):

$$K = \frac{I_r S (1 - e^{Kt})}{R_i - R_t e^{Kt}} \qquad [47]$$

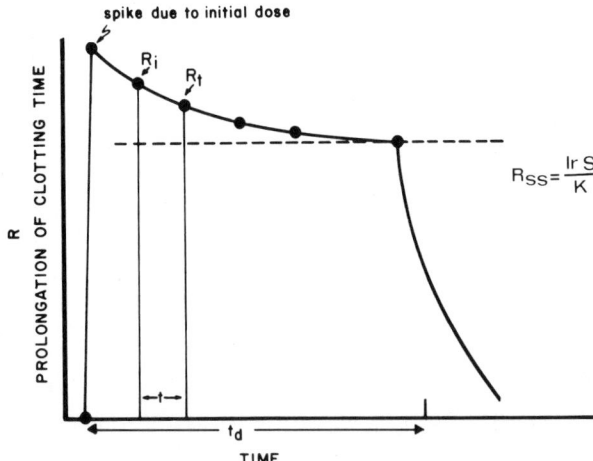

Figure 13. Clotting time prolongation in a dialysis patient with systemic heparinization consisting of a loading dose and a constant infusion thereafter.

Equation 47 is used when the infusion rate, I_r, is known and the sensitivity, S, has been calculated for clotting time response values after the start of dialysis as shown in Figure 13. Both R_i and R_t are measured by standard techniques (although some form of the whole blood partial thromboplastin time is preferred because of its speed and reproducibility). The computation requires that equation 47 be 'primed' with a 'starting' value of K. This value is then used to compute the right-hand-side of equation 47, which will yield a 'closer' value for K (the left-hand-side of the equation). This new K value is then used to recompute another value of K until this system of calculations converges on a unique value.

Acid base control in dialysis patients

Maintenance of body pH is a fundamental aspect of normal homeostasis ultimately controlled through net acid excretion by the kidneys. As with other solutes, impairment of renal function results in loss of homeostatic control over H^+. This upset must be considered as one of the most severe complications of renal failure, particularly because of the highly reactive nature of acids and bases and the narrow range of pH consistent with life (approximately 6.8 to 7.8 in man). The entire metabolic structure of the body relies on the maintenance of optimal pH; the clinical signs of lowered pH in acidosis are well known: hyperventilation due to respiratory compensation, K^+ elevation due to cellular neutralization of H^+, low bicarbonate from H^+ neutralization, and eventual bone deterioration from long term H^+ buffering. Perhaps one of the most critical aspects of this problem is that acid must be buffered immediately upon generation. Unlike other solutes where body water acts as a 'storage vessel' between treatments, it has a very low capacitance for H^+ and the bulk of H^+ storage must be accomplished by the body buffer system which then must be realkalinized during dialysis treatment.

Acid generation from metabolic processes

Metabolism of various substrates will have a net acid (H^+ producing) or basic (H^+ consuming) effect depending on their composition. Christensen (93, 94) pointed out that it is most convenient to consider the overall biochemical reaction (substrate to products) from the standpoint of a charge balance, and to add H^+ as a product or reactant to accomplish this overall adjustment of charge. In this manner acid producing reactions yield products that are more negative than their reactants and generate H^+. Conversely, reactions whose products have a higher electrical charge than the reactants, have consumed H^+ and have a basic effect. Consideration of NH_4Cl, which is a typical material to produce experimental acidosis, illustrates Christensen's point

$$NH_4Cl\,(+CO_2) \rightarrow urea + H_2O + Cl^- \quad [R3]$$

The complete catabolism of ammonium chloride will yield urea and water from the oxidation of nitrogen and hydrogen stranding the Cl^- in body water. The net effect is the same as adding equivalent amounts of HCl. To balance the reactions with respect to charge H^+ must be added to the right hand side of the reaction

$$2\,NH_4Cl\,(+CO_2) = urea + H_2O + 2\,Cl^- + 2\,H^+ \quad [R4]$$

Metabolism of an organic anion will have the reverse effect as can be illustrated with the acetate anion whose products are neutral CO_2 and water:

$$\text{Organic anion} + H^+ = H_2O + CO_2 \quad [R5a]$$
$$\text{acetate} + (H^+) = 2\,H_2O + 2\,CO_2 \quad [R5b]$$

Writing this expression in traditional biochemical form tends to confuse this point.

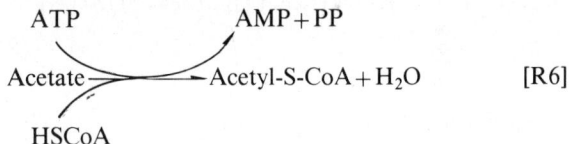

Chemical balance shows, however, that as written there is one more hydrogen in the products than in the reactants.

Reaction R5 and R6 illustrate that the popular concept that acetate produces bicarbonate is figurative at best (58, 59), the alkalanizing effet of acetate being through its consumption of H^+ as it is metabolized. Bicarbonate is produced by the unique reaction of carbonic acid dissociation (see reaction R1). The only connection between these two reactions is that one consumes hydrogen ion (acetate metabolism) whereas the other produces it (dissociation of carbonic acid).

This method of considering metabolic reactions would then predict that ingested citric acid, formic acid (even nitric acid) would have no net effect on body acid base status because these compounds are electrically neutral on ingestion and will produce only neutral products. Although pH will decrease transiently, metabolism of the anion (base equivalent) will eventually reverse the response.

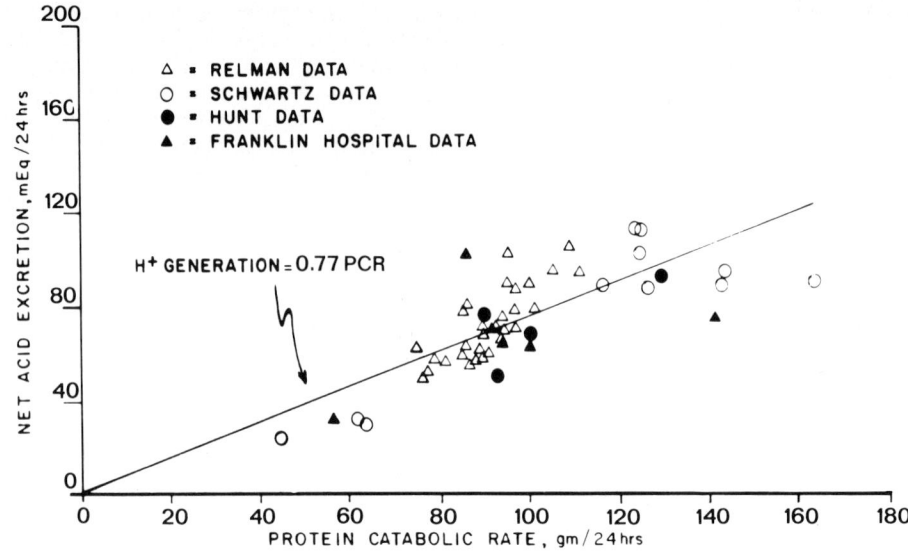

Figure 14. Hydrogen ion (acid) generation as a function of net rates of protein catabolism.

Net acid generation as related to protein catabolism and intake

Catabolism of protein would have a predictable acidic effect. This is because of the two sulfur containing amino acids – cystine and methionine – when metabolized will abandon their sulfur as a negatively charged sulfate ion.

$$H\text{-}\underset{H}{\overset{H}{C}}\text{-}S\text{-}\underset{H}{\overset{H}{C}}\text{-}\underset{H}{\overset{H}{C}}\text{-}\underset{\underset{H\ H\ H^+}{\diagup\,|\,\diagdown}}{\overset{}{C}}\text{-}COO^- \rightarrow H_2O + CO_2 + Urea + SO_4^= + (2\,H^+)$$

[R7]

(methionine)

In addition to its direct acidic effect, protein is a good index of general intake of various substances (47, 95). Analysis of metabolically and clinically controlled studies where both H and nitrogen balances were done (Figure 14) show that net rates of protein catabolism can be used to obtain good estimates of the net quantity of acid being produced (0.77 mEq/g of protein catabolized) (96–100).

Acetate metabolism

Appreciation of the alkalinizing effect of acetate metabolism, shown in reaction R5, lead Mion and coworkers in 1965 to substitute this anion for the more commonly used bicarbonate (101). This opened the way for the development of current dialysis proportioning systems (102). The disadvantages of using bicarbonate in dialysate solutions are its poor solubility, its instability, and the requirement of high concentrations of dissolved CO_2 to keep pH in the range where magnesium and calcium will remain soluble (103). The advantages of ace-

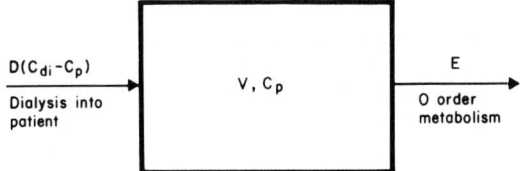

Figure 15. Model of acetate.

tate are its high solubility and perceived rapid rate of metabolism (104, 105).

Model formulation of acetate metabolism presents a major problem. Once again a single pool is sought (see Figure 15). Input to the system is uncomplicated being diffusive transport from dialysis fluid to blood in the dialyzer, as described in equation 14. The output from the system presents some difficulty, however. A typical acetate concentration profile during and immediately after dialysis is shown in Figure 16 and is the one that is commonly found in dialysis patients (52, 106). Examination of this figure reveals an asymmetry between the concentration build-up, which may take as long as 2 to 3 h during dialysis and the rapid reduction of acetate to low plasma levels in less than an hour after dialysis. These kinetics are not consistent with a first order metabolic process.

Many metabolic systems show non-linear behavior as described by Michaelis-Menten type kinetics and shown in Figure 17. The type of system shown indicates first order metabolism at low substrate levels (e.g.: a doubling of metabolic rate for a doubling of substrate); as substrate builds up, however, there is less of an increase in metabolic rate approaching saturation levels. If acetate metabolism were in the shaded region of the figure its conversion to acetyl CoA shown in reaction R6

3: *Principles and biophysics of dialysis* 73

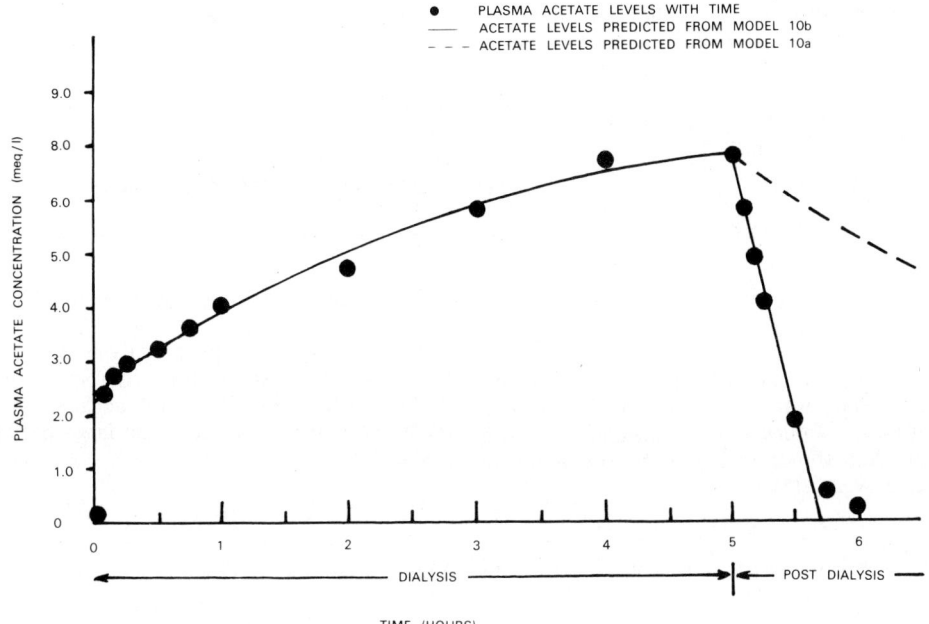

Figure 16. Plasma acetate concentrations with time in a typical dialysis patient during and shortly after a 5 hour treatment.

would show very little sensitivity to changing acetate levels and would be effectively constant (or zero order). When this output is used, the model in Figure 15 results. This yields the mass balance expression:

$$\frac{d(VC_P)}{dt} = D(C_{Di} - C_P) - E \quad [48]$$

whose solution is during dialysis:

$$C_P = C_{Po} e^{-Dt/V} + \frac{DC_{Di} - E}{D}(1 - e^{-Dt/v}) \quad [49]$$

and after dialysis:

$$C_P = C_{Pt} - \frac{E}{V}t \quad [50]$$

From Figure 16 it is clear that acetate metabolism slows when acetate concentration is below 2 mEq/l post dialysis. Reference to Figure 17 would indicate that below these acetate levels the metabolic reaction is below the shaded region and in the linear range (the reaction is now first order).

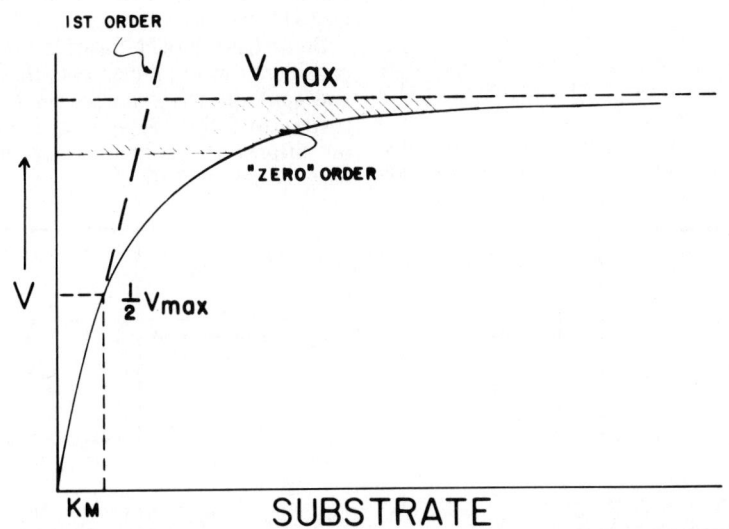

Figure 17. Velocity of a metabolic reaction (V, mEq/min) as a function of substrate levels (mEq/l) which would result from Michaelis-Menten kinetics.

It is seen that equation 49 is of the same form as equation 42 and that $(DC_{Di}-E)/D$ will be the steady state plasma level at large values of t (i.e. when $e^{-Dt/V}$ is very small). It is clear that if steady state concentrations are known or can be approximated and D is known then the value of E can be estimated from

$$E = D(C_{Di} - C_{P_{ss}}) \quad [51]$$

rearrangement of equation 48 allows another computation of E:

$$E = D\left(C_{Di} - \frac{C_B - C_{Bo} e^{-Dt/V}}{1 - e^{-Dt/V}}\right) \quad [52]$$

where V is assumed to be extracellular water and is taken as 1/3 of total body water (or V urea from the urea kinetic calculations). Values of E computed by both methods for the data shown in Figure 16 are shown in Table 5 and agree very closely.

Table 5. Acetate concentration in a patient dialyzed with 39 mmol/l in the dialysis fluid for 5 h. D acetate = 0.120 l/min.

Time: t-relative to the start of dialysis, 0-relative to its end (min)	Plasma concentration (mmol/l)	E (from equation 52)	E (from equation 51)
0	0	—	—
60	4.0	3.63	—
120	4.7	3.87	—
180	5.8	3.74	—
240	6.7	3.66	—
300	6.8	3.73	—
		3.73	3.74

Body base

Because of the critical nature of acid base control it is important to describe quantitatively the elements of H^+ and buffer base in the patient.

Acid-base kinetics are conceptually complex because of the labile nature of the solute, H^+, for which mass balance equations must be written. Although several hundred millimoles of H^+ may be generated and removed during a complete dialysis cycle, the free concentration in body water remains vanishingly small (0.000030 to 0.000045 mEq/l) because of instantaneous reactions between H^+ and the large buffer pool in the body.

$$H^+ + \text{buffer}^- = \text{buffer H} \quad [R8]$$

This can be more fully appreciated by refence to Table 6 which shows the various elements of H^+ balance in a 70 kg dialysis patient ingesting from 0.8 to 1.6 g protein/kg/day dialyzed with acetate dialysate using a CDAK-1.3 m² dialyzer.

Ironically, from a strict mass balance sense, the modeled species (H^+) can be ignored, because it is present in negligible quantities. In fact, H^+ balance is so treated, and the difference between H^+ production and elimination is taken as equal to the degree of buffer depletion (i.e.: reaction R8 goes to completion and $d(H^+)/dt = 0$). In the discussion to follow, the model is of the body content of basic equivalents, and their increase or decrease in content can be considerd as the negative of H^+ balance. In this manner hydrogen ion balance, can be considered as the negative of base balance; alkalinization of body buffer being 'negative H^+ balance', and acidification of body buffer being 'positive H^+ balance'.

Body base model formulation requires an in depth consideration of all elements that affect acid base status and consequently becomes quite complex. It is first necessary to define the system. However, consideration of the bicarbonate system is appropriate before the body base system is defined.

Table 6. Magnitude of elements in H^+ balances over one dialysis cycle.

Hydrogen generation (from dietary sources)	100–200 mEq
Bicarbonate loss during acetate dialysis	500 mEq
Acetate uptake	600–800 mEq
Organic acid production	0–200 mEq
Organic anion loss (net H^+ production)	0–100 mEq
Body H^+ content	0.0017 mEq

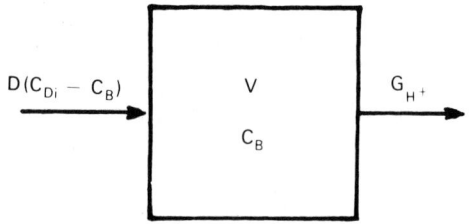

a. USING THE CONCEPT OF BICARBONATE SPACE

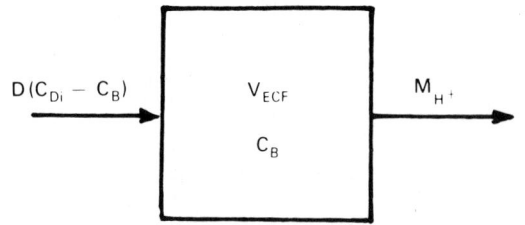

b. USING A FIXED VOLUME AND H^+ MOBILIZATION

Figure 18. Model of the bicarbonate system during bicarbonate dialysis showing two versions of the model: a) using apparent bicarbonate space, and b) using a fixed volume approximating extracellular volume and a mobilization constant.

Bicarbonate modelling
Bicarbonate is traditionally and superficially treated pharmokinetically as distributed in a single pool volume of 40% body weight (98, 99, 107 [see Figure 18]):

$$V \frac{dC_B}{dt} = D(C_{Di} - C_{Bi}) - g_{H^+} \quad [52a]$$

Solution of which yields:

$$C_B = C_{Bo} e^{-Dt/V} + \left(C_{Di} - \frac{g_{H^+}}{D}\right)(1 - e^{-Dt/V}) \quad [52b]$$

The volume of bicarbonate distribution, V, can be computed:

$$V = D t \, \text{Log} \, \frac{C_{Bo} - (C_{Di} - g_{H^+}/D)}{C_{Bt} - (C_{Di} - g_{H^+}/D)} \quad [52c]$$

From the change in plasma concentration under known dialysis conditions of D and C_{Di} during bicarbonate dialysis, V can be calculated (where g_{H^+}/D is considered negligible).

Values calculated using this equation occasionally show large and variable bicarbonate volumes (108). A similar variation of bicarbonate space depending on the level of acidosis has been reported (109). Re-evaluation of the model shows that the fault may lie with the use of traditional pharmacokinetic techniques. These methods are normally applied to a specific solute which occupies a unique physical volume. This may be modified in the case of protein binding because an additional capacity for the substance is present and V is correspondingly larger. Bicarbonate, however, because of its interrelation with H^+ and through it the other buffer systems, represents a highly labile material which may disappear from extracellular space either by diffusion into cells or by neutralization of H^+ released from other buffers (107).

It does not seem unreasonable to consider that during the interdialytic period, generated H^+ will progressively deplete buffer stores and that during dialysis the infused bicarbonate will have to restore these buffers. The extent of restoration may vary depending on the state of depletion which will reflect the magnitude of interdialytic H^+ generation. A constant term such as g_{H^+} must then be retained in the mass balance equation but its definition will differ as it will not be the generation of H^+ but the apparent movement of HCO_3^- out of extracellular space. The disappearance of bicarbonate from this space can be described in terms of m_{H^+} or 'hydrogen ion mobilization' which is intended to include diffusive movement of HCO_3^- out of the extracellular volume; the V term in the equation then becomes a constant which value is known or can be determined. Rearrangement of the mass balance equation shown in Figure 17 with the substitution of m_{H^+} for g_{H^+} yields:

$$V_{ecf} \frac{dC_B}{dt} = D(C_{Di} - C_B) - m_{H^+} \quad [53a]$$

$$m_{H^+} = D(C_{Di} - C_{Bo}) - \frac{(C_{Bt} - C_{Bo})}{1 - e^{-Dt/v}} D \quad [53b]$$

Equation 53b shows that m_{H^+} is the difference of two terms, the initial rate of diffusive flux into extracellular space, and a term that contains the rate of rise of bicarbonate in that space. The second term accounts for the fact that HCO_3^- content of extracellular space is increasing. The lack of equivalence of this increased content with the flux from the dialyzer is accounted for by basic equivalents that have moved into other anatomical areas. Consequently, using typical intradialytic values for C_{Di}, C_{Bo}, C_{Bt}, V, D, and t, the extent of titration of buffers can be calculated. Thus if $C_{Di} = 35$ mmol/l, $C_{Bo} = 20$ mmol/l, $C_{Bt} = 23$ mmol/l over a one-hour period and $V = 13$ l, $D = 0.100$ l/min, the bicarbonate is disappearing at a rate of 0.69 mmol/min during this interval. The average flux into the patient $D(C_{Di} - C_B)$ would be approximately 0.1 (35 − 21.5) or 1.35 mmol/min of which 49% would contribute to a rise in extracellular bicarbonate concentration. These illustrative data demonstrate an analytical technique that can estimate H^+ balance during the process of acid-base correction with dialysis treatment. The adoption of model b in Figure 18 should increase understanding of what is actually occuring in the body, whereas a 'distribution space' for bicarbonate tends to blur the fact that the kinetics of this substance are interrelated both to the movement of H^+ and the status of body buffers.

The body base model
The model shown in Figure 18 represents only the bicarbonate portion of the overall base content of the body. Figure 19 shows its incorporation into the overall model of body base equivalents. It is included as the bottom half of the inner box which is the bicarbonate portion of the buffer base equivalents, that are capable of interacting with other body buffers. The inner box represents the body base equivalents and is separated into three sections. Base equivalents in extracellular water are illustrated as including the HCO_3^-, just discussed, as well as the non-buffer materials in extracellular water (top right) such as lactate, acetate, and other organic anions (see reaction R5). The top left section of this box represents the non-extracellular buffers in basic form. The size of the space belies its extent which is actually greater than half of the total buffer base capacity of the body (107). Communication between these three compartments is indicated. As was discussed, addition of HCO_3^- to the extracellular pool will not quantitatively increase the extracellular bicarbonate content because there will be 'mobilization' of bicarbonate (or transfer of base equivalents) to other buffer systems. Similarly, when the buffers are acidified the buffer load will be distributed among bicarbonate and other buffer systems as shown by the H^+ accumulation term a_{H^+} which indicates that as the extracellular compartment sustains an acid load, base equivalents will move into that compartment to partially restore bicarbonate level (i.e. non extracellular buffers will neutralize some of the added H^+). In Figure 19 the outer box encloses the system but also contains internal sources capable of producing buffer base if alkalinized, such as carbonic acid, organic acids, and acidified non extracellular buffers.

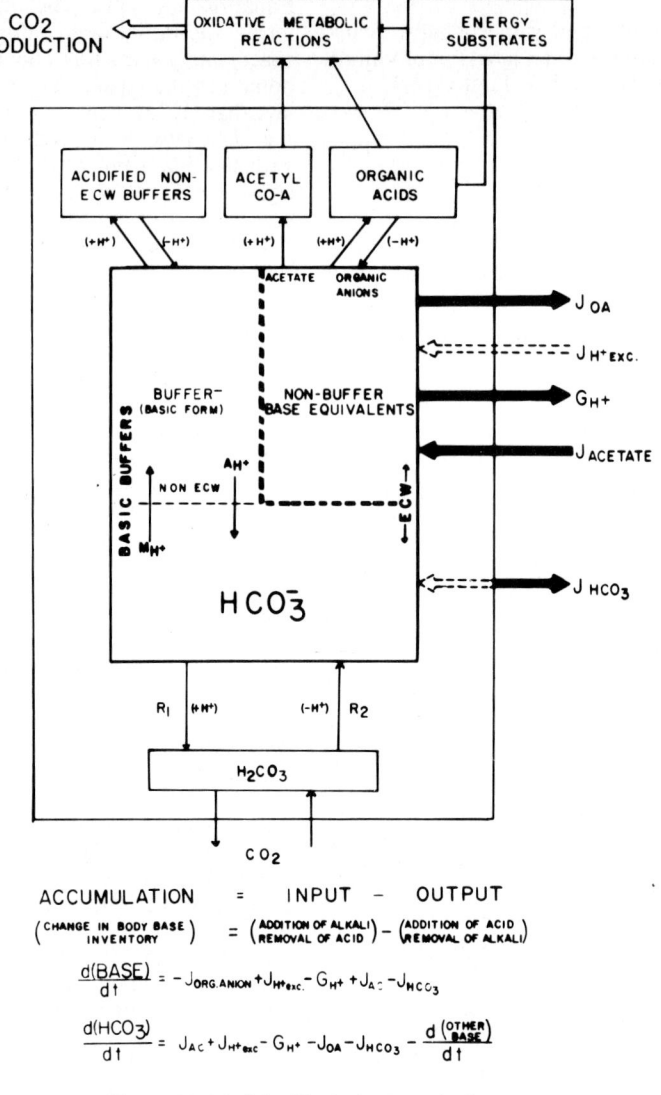

Figure 19. Model of body base equivalents.

Consider the example of lactic acid production by anaerobic metabolism:

glucose = lactate + (H⁺)   [R9]

Both lactate and H⁺ are added to the internal box of the figure. H⁺, however, will combine with a buffer base, HCO_3^- for example, and produce H_2CO_3, which may in turn be exhaled in its anhydrous form, CO_2. This series of reactions, however, will have no effect on the total base content because the decrease in HCO_3^- has been matched by the addition of lactate, a base equivalent (see reaction R5a).

It should be emphasized that carbon dioxide interaction with the body base system will have no net effect on the base content, for it is a neutral substance, although it can profoundly effect the system pH through its relation with the carbonic acid-bicarbonate system. The net excretion or retention of carbon dioxide, however, will not effect the body base content.

With reference to Figure 19 only the bold arrows represent net inputs and outputs for the system. All other arrows represent the transfer of neutral material which has no net effect on the overall acid base status.

Consider first the inputs to the system: The ways that the body buffer system content can increase. A total of three inputs are considered. Renal excretion of acids (J_{H^+} Exc), will effect a net increase because net removal of hydrogen ion will cause a net movement of base equivalents from one of the internal buffer systems (e.g.

alkalinization of non-extracellular buffers or dissociation of H_2CO_3 by reaction R1). Body base can be increased directly by flux of acetate into the patient (direct addition of base equivalents). Alternatively, bicarbonate (if used in the dialysis fluid) can be a pathway to increase base content of the system. Note that once in the system, the acetate to acetyl-CoA conversion will be coupled to one of the other internal systems alkalinizing a non-extracellular buffer or net dissociation of H_2CO_3. In this light it is apparent that non-stoichiometric appearance of bicarbonate during acetate metabolism (58, 59) should, in fact, be predicted because of the variety of substances capable of providing a hydrogen ion consumed in the acetate metabolic reaction.

Routes of output or ways in which base equivalent will be removed from the system will be: by removal of organic anions which are themselves base equivalents (e.g.: lactate); by acid generation g_{H^+}, or by bicarbonate loss during acetate dialysis. These outputs (and inputs) are totally general. If the diet is low in protein and high in alkaline material (sodium citric for example) g_{H^+} will be negative and there will be a net system increase. Also if bicarbonate is given by mouth, or some other unbalanced organic anion such as monosodium glutamate is ingested, this contribution can be dealt with by incorporating the flux of these substances in J_{HCO_3} or J_{OA} terms and appropriate adjustment of algebraic sign.

The writing of the mass balance equation yields

$$\frac{d(\text{Base})}{dt} = -J_{OA^-} + J_{H^+}\text{Exc} - g_{H^+} + J_{AC^-} - J_{HCO_3^-} \quad [54]$$

This expression is totally general and not restricted to dialysis or even uremia. Consider the stable individual, presumably in steady state ($d(\text{base})/dt = 0$):

$$J_{H^+}\text{Exc} = g_{H^+} + J_{OA} + J_{HCO_3^-} \quad [55]$$

Which indicates that H^+ excretion will balance H^+ generation plus the loss of organic anions and bicarbonate. Acid base upsets can also be described by Figure 19 and equations 54 and 55. Consider, for example, ketoacidosis in diabetes. When fat is a major energy substrate, there is generation and neutralization of organic acids represented by the dissociation of organic acids into the buffer pool. The immediate effect will be neutralization of H^+ by some other buffer, which the organic anion will replace as a body base equivalent, the body base content staying constant. The elevated levels or organic anions, however, will result in urinary excretion of these materials (J_{OA}). If, J_{H^+} exc, can increase to accommodate the buffer loss (see equation 55), there will be no net acidification of the system. If not there will be reduction in the base context (see equation 54).

If body base is separated into bicarbonate and other buffers, equation 54 can be rewritten and solved for the HCO_3^- terms:

$$\frac{d(HCO_3^-)}{dt} + J_{HCO_3^-}$$

$$= J_{AC} - g_{H^+} - J_{OA} - \frac{d(\text{other base})}{dt} \quad [56]$$

Equation 56 indicates that HCO_3^- removal from the system plus the increase in HCO_3^- content will equal the combination of the four terms on the right side. It should, once again, be noted that for acetate flux and metabolism to be equal to HCO_3^- mass balance as has been anticipated by some (58, 59) the algebraic sum of the last four terms must be zero an improbable result during such a metabolically disruptive event as dialysis. Consequently, the non-equivalence of acetate up-take and bicarbonate appearance described by others (58, 59) should not be surprising.

Control of acid base: solution of the model

The goal of acid base control during dialysis treatment is to minimize the depletion of body buffers between dialyses and the non-extracellular buffers (bone) in the long term, and to restore adequately the basic buffer forms during treatment.

As alluded to above, there is very little therapeutic control of interdialytic base depletion, which is primarily a result of acid forming foods in the diet and which appears in the foregoing relationships. In addition, intake of fluid, which will not have an overall effect on body buffers, causes movement of base equivalents into the extra-cellular compartment to supply buffer to this space as it expands (dilutional acidosis) (109). From these considerations it is clear that while Figure 19 represents a useful model it cannot yet be adequately formulated.

The system content as represented by the internal box in Figure 19 cannot be accurately specified. More information with the respect to the composition and interrelation of buffers as implied by the terms aH^+ and mH^+ is required. Because HCO_3^- is the measurable component of body buffer and the one to which output and input are related, knowledge of how HCO_3^- and other buffers interact is required. Also of interest in the location of the acetate alkalinization step and whether it has its effect directly on extracellular buffers or through non extracellular buffers. The dash lines shown in Figure 19 may have certain resistances associated with them so that the addition of HCO_3^- to the extracellular fluid may have a different effect than equivalent alkalinization using acetate and indications of this possibility have been observed (Gotch FA, unpublished). It is also possible that the alkalinizing effect of acetate may depend on transport of a co-ion, e.g. sodium, and therefore complete specification and the model will rely on another solute system which is changing during dialysis. For these reasons the model as described in Figure 19 must be considered as partially specified, for which the mass balance equation (equations 54, 55, and 56) are an accurate representation, but for which insufficient information is available for complete formulation for the purposes of guiding treatment.

The effect of fluid retention and removal

A few comments are appropriate with respect to the marginal ability to correct acid base during dialysis. The acidification of the system between treatments was discussed primarily with respect to protein and acid generation. In addition, as fluid is consumed and retained in body water some degree of dilutional acidosis occurs (i.e. base equivalents will move into extracellular fluid acidifying cell buffers in the process, to sustain extracellular buffer levels). Although this will not cause a change in total body base equivalents, non extracellular buffers will be depleted. The need to remove the retained fluid during dialysis, however, markedly blunts the ability to alkalinize the patient. Equation 14 shows that with Q_F of zero and 15 ml/min under the same bicarbonate conditions discussed above flux would be 1.35 mEq/min versus 0.91 mEq/min or a 33% drop when $Q_F = 15$ ml/min (900 ml/h).

Creatinine

Creatinine is traditionally grouped with urea as a major uremic catabolite, the concentration of which, should be controlled (112–114). That plasma creatinine concentration provides valuable nutritional information through its relationship to body muscle mass is well established (84). In this regard, it is probably more accurate to view creatinine or at least its production rate as an outcome measure of dialysis therapy rather than a control variable.

Plasma creatinine concentration is widely used in the predialysis patient as a rough inverse correlate to kidney function (87), although there is evidence that creatinine production drops in chronic uremia disproporionately to the decrease in lean body mass (115–117). Nevertheless, the relative constancy of creatinine production from the spontaneous and non-enzymatic dehydration of creatine phosphate has made it useful as an endogenous marker in progressive renal failure. Through its utility as a marker of renal function it has become associated with other catabolites and has assumed an importance that is unwarranted for its role as a metabolic product. It does not, like urea, represent the end product of a major metabolic pathway, although it is associated with the energy pathway in muscle tissue through its connection with the creatine – phosphocreatine system. It can be shown that creatinine follows single pool kinetics (113) although not as closely as urea does (114).

Sodium

There continues to be significant intradialytic morbidity associated with regular dialysis therapy. This morbidity during treatment is comprised of multiple symptoms including headache, nausea and vomiting, fatigue, hypotension and severe muscle cramps. The most frequent and objective symptoms are hypotension and muscle cramps which require medical intervention and occur in 15 to 40% of treatments in different centers.

Over the past 5 years, several studies have shown that increasing the dialysis fluid concentration of Na (C_{Di}) reduces morbidity during dialysis (118–120). This therapeutic maneuver has been empirically shown to be effective but has the potential risk of causing excessive body Na content and volume overload. Consequently a model would seem highly desirable for quantitative assessment of interdialytic Na and volume loading and intradialytic Na and volume removal.

Hemofiltration has been widely reported to reduce morbidity during treatment compared to hemodialysis (121–132). In view of the strong dependence of treatment morbidity during dialysis on dialysis fluid sodium concentration an evaluation of comparative hemofiltration morbidity should include assessment of Na flux in the compared therapies. This requires an analytic model to quantify Na flux in both hemodialysis and hemofiltration.

Sodium distribution volume

It has long been known that osmotic equilibrium exists throughout body water (111). Although there are multiple small anatomical subdivisions of total body water (V), (133), with respect to osmotic equilibrium it can be described as a two compartment system comprised of extracellular and intracellular water (V_E and V_C) as diagrammed in Figure 20. Osmotic equilibrium exists between compartments because of the extremely high hydraulic permeability of cell membranes; any change in the osmotically active solute content of V_C or V_E selectively results in rapid net water flux until the concentration of solute in both compartments is again equal.

Owing to the passive nature of water flux between V_E and V_C due only to the osmotic driving force, it follows that volume of each compartment will be determined by the relative contents of osmotically active solute in each compartment and the total amount of water distributed between the compartments. Although there are multiple solutes present in body water, the bulk of osmolality in V_E is contributed by sodium salts and in V_C it is contributed by potassium salts. The asymmetric distribution of Na and K is achieved by active transport mechanisms in cell membranes resulting in high transcellular concentration gradients for Na and K. It has been shown by isotope dilution studies that plasma Na (C_{Na}) over a wide concentration range is linearly dependent on the rapidly exchangeable body sodium and potassium content (Na_{Ex}, K_{Ex}) and total body water, V.

The relationship found was (19):

$$C_{Na} = \frac{Na_{Ex} + K_{Ex}}{V} \quad [57]$$

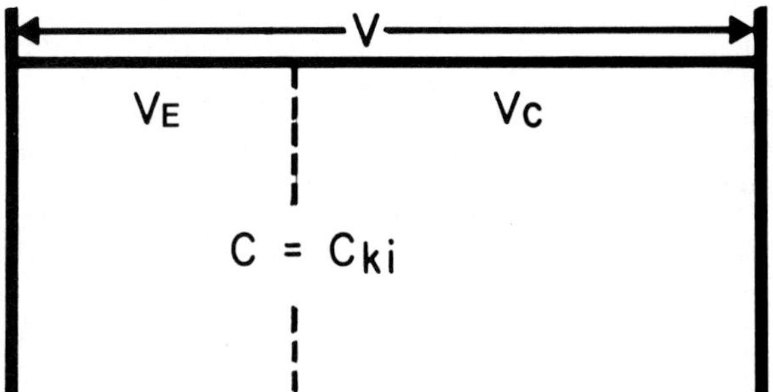

Figure 20. Two compartment distribution of osmotically active sodium and potassium in body water.

The rapidly exchangeable quantities, $Na_{Ex} + K_{Ex}$, were postulated to be measures of the osmotically active Na and K salts in V_E and V_C respectively. The relationship in equation 57 provided confirmation of this postulate and demonstrated that the effective osmotic driving force controlling body water distribution between V_E and V_C was determined by Na and K salts in the two compartments respectively. The sum of Na_{Ex} and K_{Ex} can be considered equal to the total osmotically active cation (C^+) in body water and equation 57 can then be written:

$$C_{Na} = \frac{C^+}{V} \qquad [58]$$

Equation 58 is a powerful physiologic statement showing that C^+ can readily be calculated from the product $C_{Na} V$. Serial change in C^+ can be computed from serial changes in C if V is either constant or undergoes a quantified change, ΔV. This can be illustrated as follows: Consider initial composition to be represented by C_{Na1}, V_1 and C_1^+; assume that C_{Na2} is measured after a known Δv and unknown change in C^+ due to changes in body water content of Na and K, ΔNa and ΔK. The serial composition relationships will be:

$$C_{Na1} = \frac{C_1^+}{V} \qquad [59a]$$

$$C_{Na2} = \frac{C_1^+ + \Delta Na + \Delta K}{V_1 + \Delta V} \qquad [59b]$$

The change in C^+, which is by definition $\Delta Na + \Delta K$, can be determined by subtraction of equation 59a from 59b:

$$(\Delta Na + \Delta K) = (C_{Na2} - C_{Na1}) V_1 + (C_{Na2})(\Delta V) \qquad [59c]$$

Assuming all quantities on the right hand side of equation 59c can be measured, the relationships in equation 59c provide a simple method to calculate ΔC^+ or $\Delta NA + \Delta K$.

The clinical material used to establish the relationships in equation 57 was comprised of a spectrum of patients with chronic illness with C_{Na} ranging from hyponatremic to modest hypernatremic levels (110). In the hyponatremia of chronic illness, depletion of cellular K^+ often was the major compositional change present causing H_2O to move out of cells diluting Na^+ in extracellular fluid.

In the dialysis patient there are regular small oscillations in body water K^+ content with interdialytic loading of excess K^+ followed after 2 or 3 days by dialytic removal of the excess. Thus, body K^+ content, in the absence of an associated severe K^+ depleting chronic illness, oscillates between mild excess and normal. Under these conditions it can be considered that the loaded and removed K^+ distribute fairly equally over total body water (13, 134) and will not contribute to the relationship between C_{Na}, ΔV and C^+ described by equation 59b even though a precise description of K^+ kinetics requires a 2 pool model (135, 136). Thus equation 59c can be rewritten as

$$\Delta Na = C_{Na2}(V_1 + \Delta V) - (C_1)(V_1) \qquad [60]$$

It is apparent from equation 60 that, although anatomically Na is confined to V_E, since its osmotic distribution is V, a single pool distribution volume equal to V can be used to model sodium. The magnitude of change in the Na^+ content of body water can be computed from equation 60 only if there are no unusual asymmetrically distributed solutes which are loaded or removed from body water during the dialysis cycle. The only two solutes which would satisfy these criteria are dextrose and mannitol, both of which can accumulate in V_E. Consequently in the diabetic patient with substantial changes in blood sugar during dialysis or in the mannitol treated patient, equation 60 would be invalid due to unaccounted changes in osmotically active solute in V_E resulting in net transcompartmental water flux independent of ΔNa.

Calculation of ΔNa and ΔV over the dialysis cycle
A flow diagram of body compositional relationships over the dialysis treatment cycle is shown in Figure 21. In order to calculate values for interdialytic dietary sodium loading and subsequent intradialytic sodium removal from serial values of C_{Na} it is necessary to determine V and ΔV. Total body water is coextensive with the urea distribution volume (74) so that the variable volume urea kinetic model described earlier can be used to determine V_t. Over short 2 to 3 day interdialytic intervals change in body weight is traditionally used as a measure of change in V (volume loading, V_L). Similarly, change in body weight from pre to post dialysis is used to measure the volume of fluid removal, V_R.

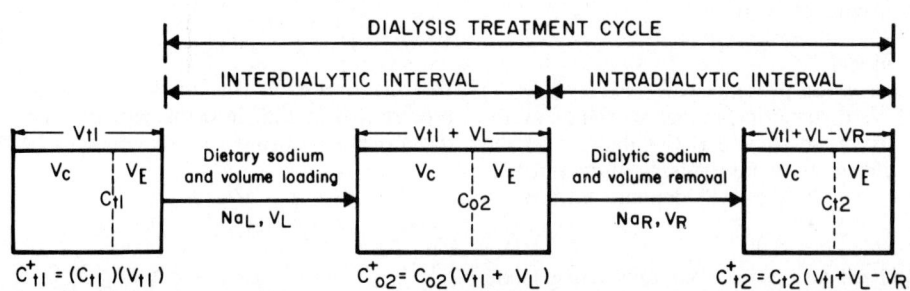

Figure 21. Flow diagram of interdialytic Na and volume loading and intradialytic Na and volume removal.

The magnitude of sodium removal is equal to $C_{o2}^+ - C_{t1}^+$ (see Figure 21) and described by:

$$\text{sodium loading} = C_{o2}(V_{t1} + V_L) - C_{t1})(V_{t1}) \quad [61]$$

The magnitude of sodium removal is equal to $C_{o2}^+ - C_{t2}^+$ and described by

$$\text{sodium removal} = C_{o2}(V_{t1} + V_L) - C_{t2}(V_{t1} + V_L - V_R) \quad [62]$$

Sodium balance $\Delta(VC_{Na})$ over the treatment cycle is by definition equal to sodium loading minus sodium removal and can be determined by subtracting equation 62 from 61 resulting in

$$\Delta CV = (C_{t2} - C_{t1})V_{t1} + C_{t2}(V_L - V_R) \quad [63]$$

Equations 61 to 63 provide a simple method to quantify Na loading, removal and balance over the treatment cycle from serial measured values of C_{Na} and use of urea kinetics to determine V_t and changes in weight to determine V_L and V_R.

The usual therapeutic goal for each treatment cycle is to achieve zero Na and V balance; that is, to exactly remove during dialysis the quantity of dietary sodium and water loaded since the previous dialysis. Inspection of equation 63 shows that to achieve this the end dialysis sodium concentration must always be returned to the same value ($C_{t2} = C_{t1}$) and the net fluid removed during dialysis must equal the interdialytic weight gain ($V_L = V_R$). The first term on the right side of equation 63 can be viewed as being controlled by the diffusive Na concentration gradient between blood and dialysate; the second term can be viewed as being controlled by the magnitude of ultrafiltration. Current state of the art of dialysis therapy provides reasonable assurance that $V_R = V_L$ by matching the ultrafiltration to the interdialytic weight gain but does not assure that $C_{t2} = C_{t1}$ since there is no attempt to individualize the diffusive Na gradient for each treatment. This would require measurement of C_{o2} and use of a model to individualize dialysis solution Na$^+$ concentration as will be discussed.

The relative impact on sodium balance resulting from mismatch of diffusive gradient and ultrafiltration can be shown by consideration of equation 63. Assume average values * of $V_t = 38.0$ l and $C_{t2} = 140$ mmol/l. For each mmol/l difference between C_{t2} and C_{t1} there will be a 38 mmol change in sodium balance and for each 0.1 l mismatch between V_L and V_R there will be a difference of 14 mmol. It is apparent that both diffusion and ultrafiltration must be individualized for each treatment if no change in sodium balance is to result.

Sodium-volume model
The preceding discussion provides the theoretical basis for a single pool Na distribution model as well as methods to compute change in Na and H$_2$O balance over the interdialytic and intradialytic intervals. Sodium and volume loading between dialyses will depend entirely on dietary Na and H$_2$O intake and can be quite variable. In order to reliably achieve zero Na balance over each dialysis cycle, it is necessary to target a constant end-dialysis Na concentration irrespective of predialysis concentration as shown by equation 63. A model is useful, therefore, to determine Na balance during dialysis as a function of combined diffusive and convective Na flux across the dialyzer.

The mathematical development of the flux expressions for charged as well as uncharged solutes, such as urea, starts from consideration of mass balance and concentration driving forces in the dialyzer (see equation 12a). As has been discussed in the case of Na$^+$, which is a positively charged solute, the effective diffusive gradient will not equal the inlet chemical concentration gradient because the Donnan effect of anionic plasma protein will result in asymmetric distribution of Na$^+$ across the membrane (137). The Donnan effect is most rigorously defined under equilibrium conditions as would prevail with a closed loop protein solution perfusate and an open loop aqueous dialysate. When such a system reaches equilibrium, the Donnan influence on the inlet Na concentration gradient can be defined by 'Donnan factor' α:

$$\alpha = \frac{C_{Di}}{C_{Pi}} \quad [64]$$

In this system at equilibrium net Na flux between perfusate and dialysate is zero so the effective diffusive driving force is zero although C_{Di} is less than C_{Pi} due to the Donnan effect. Rearrangement of equation 64, which describes the equilibrium Na concentration ratio across the membrane, can be viewed as the effective dialysis fluid concentration equivalent to plasma levels $C_{Di} = \alpha C_{Pi}$. Consequently, the Na concentration driving force, traditionally defined as $C_{Di} - C_{Pi}$, can be expressed as $C_{Di} - \alpha C_{Pi}$; the term α is a coefficient which can be applied to C_{Pi} to correct the chemical gradient for Donnan influence and defines the effective diffusive gradient.

Assuming that a similar relationship applies under non-equilibrium conditions when there is net Na flux, the development of the flux expression combines equations 11 and 14, i.e. incorporates the driving force, $(C_{Di} - \alpha C_{Pi})$:

$$J = D\left(1 - \frac{Q_F}{Q_E}\right)C_{Di} - \left[D\alpha\left(1 - \frac{Q_F}{Q_E}\right) + Q_F\right]C_{Pi} \quad [65]$$

In this expression (in contrast to equation 14) flux is represented as that into the patient. Body Na and H$_2$O mass balance during dialysis can now be described as

$$\frac{dVC}{dt} = D\left(1 - \frac{Q_F}{Q_E}\right)C_{Di} - \left[D\alpha\left(1 - \frac{Q_F}{Q_E}\right) + Q_F\right]C_{Pi} \quad [66]$$

---

* Sodium is considered here as an osmotically active solute, not as a reactant, thus concentrations are expressed as molar units (SI), not as equivalents (conventional).

Integration of equation 66 over an individual dialysis from beginning to end of the treatment (o to t) and solution for α, C_{Di} or C_t results in:

$$\alpha = C_{Di} \frac{1 - \left(\frac{V_t}{V_o}\right)^{D\alpha(1/Q_F - 1/Q_E)}}{C_t - C_o \left(\frac{V_t}{V_o}\right)^{D\alpha(1/Q_F - 1/Q_E)}} \quad [67a]$$

$$C_{Di} = \frac{\alpha \left[C_t - C_o \left(\frac{V_t}{V_o}\right)^{D\alpha(1/Q_F - 1/Q_E)} \right]}{1 - \left(\frac{V_t}{V_o}\right)^{D\alpha(1/Q_F - 1/Q_E)}} \quad [67b]$$

$$C_t = \frac{1}{\alpha}\left[C_{Di} - (C_{Di} - aC_o)\left(\frac{V_t}{V_o}\right)^{D\alpha(1/Q_F - 1/Q_E)} \right] \quad [67c]$$

The clinical application of equations 67b and 67c will be considered later. Equations 67 are transcendental in that they contain α in both the coefficients and exponents. As such it is not possible to separate α algebraically to obtain its value from dialysis data. A unique value for α, does exist, however, which can be computed from dialysis data by interactive solutions of equation 67a. Such a calculation requires that this equation be 'primed' with an α value, which is then used to compute the right side of equation 67a. This will yield a 'closer' value for α (the left side of the equation). This new value of α is then used to recompute another α value and this process continues until the system of calculation converges on a unique value. Values for α were calculated using these methods for *in vivo* hemodialysis as well as *in vitro* hemofiltration where α can be defined analogous to equation 64:

$$\alpha = C_F/C_{Pi} \quad [68]$$

In hemofiltration studies α values were determined from measurements of Na concentration in the inlet plasma stream and outlet ultrafiltrate stream (138). Since the magnitude of α would be expected to have an inverse relationship to the mean protein concentration in the blood compartment of these devices (C_{Pr}), the α values were analyzed as a function of C_{Pr}. These data, which are reported in detail elsewhere (138), are summarized in Figure 22 where it is apparent that α is a linear function of C_{Pr} for the combined data on *in vivo* hemodialysis, *in vivo* isolated ultrafiltration and *in vitro* hemofiltration over a wide range of C_{Pr}.

An *in vivo* Na flux expression for hemodialysis containing α as a function of C_{Pr} can now be developed. Since dialysis membranes are impermeable to protein, the mean total protein concentration can readily be derived from conservation of mass across the dialyzer in accordance with the following expression

$$C_{Pr} = 0.5\, C_{Pri}\left[1 + \frac{1}{1 - Q_F/Q_{Pi}} \right] \quad [69]$$

Combining equations 9 and 12 with the equation for regression of α on C_{Pri} in Figure 22 results in:

$$J = D\left(1 - \frac{Q_F}{Q_E}\right) C_{Di} - \left\{ D\left[1 - 0.0037\, C_{Pi}\left(1 + \frac{1}{1 - \frac{Q_F}{Q_E}}\right)\right]\left(1 - \frac{Q_F}{Q_E}\right) + Q_F \right\} C_{Pi} \quad [70]$$

A similar Na flux expression can also be developed for hemofiltration which is a much simpler system than hemodialysis with respect to Na flux. In hemofiltration, Na flux is physically separated into a purely convective ultrafiltrate stream, $(C_F)(Q_F)$, and a stream of substitution fluid, $(C_S)(Q_S)$, which is infused into either blood line of the hemofiltration circuit. The rate of substitution fluid infusion is matched to equal the ultrafiltration rate in the device (Q_F) minus the net rate of fluid removal (Q_f) prescribed for the treatment ($Q_S = Q_F - Q_f$). The Na flux expression is then:

$$J = (C_S)(Q_S) - (Q_S + Q_f)\, C_F \quad [71a]$$
$$J = C_S Q_S - (Q_S + Q_F)\, \alpha C_{Pi} \quad [71b]$$

The analogue of equation 69 for hemofiltration can similarly be developed from consideration of protein mass balance across the device:

$$\overline{C_{Pr}} = 0.5\, C_{Pri}\left(1 + \frac{1}{1 - FF}\right) \quad [72]$$

The Na flux expression for hemofiltration can now be developed by combining equations 68, 71 and 72 with the regression equation in Figure 22 resulting in

$$J = C_S Q_S - (Q_S + Q_F)\left[(1 - 0.0037\, C_{Pri})\left(1 + \frac{1}{1 - FF}\right) \right] C_{Pi} \quad [73]$$

If the sodium flux into the dialyzed patient (equation 65) and into the hemofiltration patient (equation 71b) are set equal and the dialysis fluid sodium concentration, C_{Di}, is determined for Na flux to equal that during hemofiltration, equation 74 results:

$$C_{Di} = \frac{Q_S}{D\left(1 - \frac{Q_F}{Q_E}\right)} C_S - \left[\frac{Q_S}{D\left(1 - \frac{Q_F}{Q_E}\right)} \alpha hf - \alpha hd + \frac{Q_S}{D\left(1 - \frac{Q_F}{Q_E}\right)}(\alpha hf - 1) \right] C_{Pi} \quad [74]$$

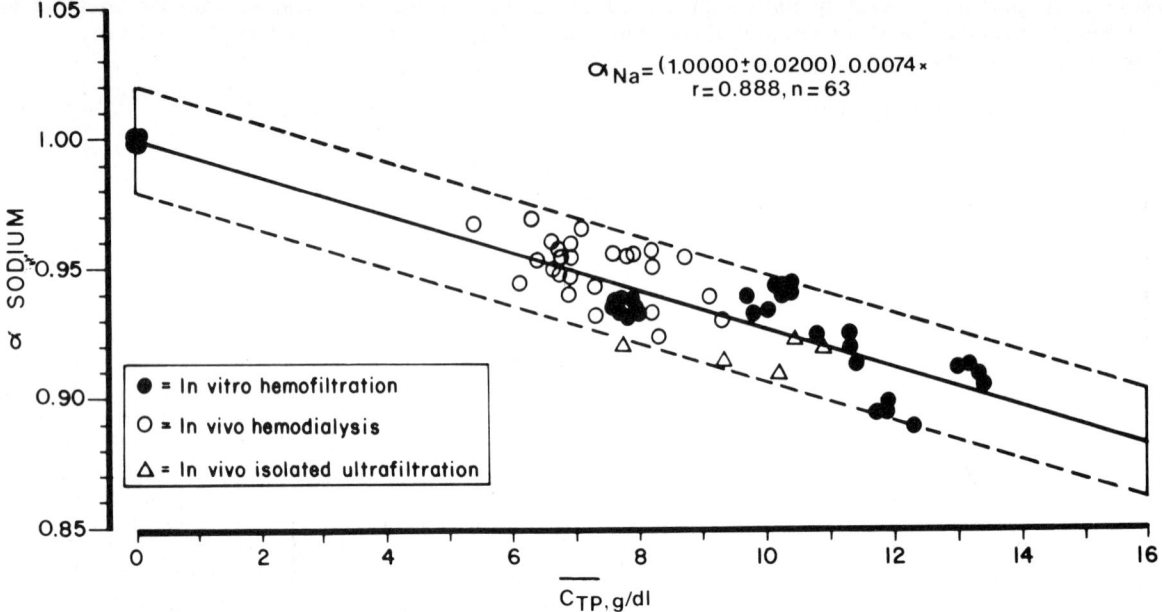

Figure 22. Overall regression of α for sodium on mean device total protein concentrations for hemodialysis and hemofiltration.

Therapeutically, Q_S and $D(1-Q_F/Q_E)$ can be considered equivalent. If $Q_S/D(1-Q_F/Q_E)$ is approximately 1 it can be seen from equation 74 that the coefficient of C_{Pi} will be negative (i.e.: $\alpha hf < \alpha hd$ and $\alpha hf < 1$). Consequently, dialysis fluid sodium concentration must be higher than the sodium level of replacement fluid for sodium flux to be equivalent.

Review of studies comparing morbidity in hemofiltration and hemodialysis (119-130) shows that in most instances $C_{Di} < C_S$, so that Na flux in hemodialysis can be predicted to exceed that in hemofiltration. Consequently, reduced morbidity in hemofiltration may be due wholly or in part to reduced net Na flux. Definitive evaluation of these two therapies will require studies designed with net Na flux equal in both treatments.

Clinical application of the sodium-volume model. Preliminary clinical results suggest that morbidity can be sharply reduced by modest adjustment of targeted C_t (138). The clinical sensitivity to relatively small changes in plasma Na concentration and body content of Na suggests that individualization of both Na and H_2O removal during dialysis is a promising method to control morbidity by assuring zero Na balance over each treatment cycle. This can be achieved by calculation of interdialytic Na and volume loading and use of the kinetic model to individualize C_{Di} for each dialysis to result in constant end dialysis plasma Na concentration in accordance with equation (67b).

Clinical implementation of sodium modelling for reduction of intradialytic morbidity requires a controllable removal of fluid and sodium to achieve the desired end dialysis weight and plasma sodium concentration. Functionally this requires that equation 67b be solved for the appropriate dialysate concentration. Consideration of equation 67b shows that the value of several parameters are required. Dialysance (D), the Donnan factor (α), and the effective flow rate (Q_E) can be considered constants for a specific dialyzer, flow rate, and plasma protein concentration. For a specific patient, a value of V_t can be determined using urea kinetics (see previous section). The patient's pre dialysis plasma sodium concentration and weight gain must be measured. The patient will also have a normally scheduled dialysis time. From the known value of V_t and weight gain, V_o can be easily determined. From the weight gain and the dialysis time, the rate of ultrafiltration can be computed. The only remaining parameter in equation 67b is the value of C_t, the desired end dialysis sodium concentration. This value must be set by the clinical staff for the specific patient. Once all of these values are known the required dialysis fluid sodium concentration can be properly computed.

The optimal targeted end dialysis plasma sodium concentration and body weight should be values that cause only minimal intradialytic morbidity without inducing hypertension mediated by sodium and water excess. Thus the C_t and V_t values targeted for individual patients would be those which facilitate achievement of therapeutic goals and C_t values and might range from 135 to 145 mmol/l over the total patient population. The clinical judgement based on individualized correlation of clinical signs and symptoms as well as defined C_t and V_t values will be required to arrive at the optimal prescribed therapy for each patient.

Kinetic consideration of uremic toxins

The concept of an uremic toxin is an old one. It is normal to consider that as other regulated substances accumulate in the absence of excretory capacity, so do certain substances that are systemic toxins. This concept is in part supported by the unresponsiveness of some lesions to the regulation of the commonly measured materials by dialysis. Toxic substances are generally presumed to be certain peptides which are excreted in the normal metabolic state, and this presumption has been supported by detection of various substances in normal urine (139) which are found in uremic plasma but are absent in uremic urine (26, 28). Peptide production can be pictured by the hypothetical scheme shown in Figure 23.

In this scheme are shown a protein and substance γ; the protein is initially cleaved to A and B, and these two peptide fragments subsequently break down into various intermediate peptide products until the final products G, H, I, and L result which are normally excreted in the urine. Substance γ is some other material that undergoes various metabolic steps which result in Z; Z may or may not be excreted by the kidney. It is only reasonable to presume in this scheme that the abnormal removal of these hypothetical catabolic products will cause disruptions, perhaps toxic in nature. There has been the feeling that one or more of such substances are toxins and that their accumulation results in various uremic lesions (15, 29, 34, 35, 140).

This concept was pursued in the early 1970s attempting to accelerate 'toxin' removal using different dialysis protocols (5, 141, 142) and more permeable dialysis membranes; in addition, certain quantifications and indices of therapy, partially based on these materials, were proposed (5, 34, 35). The rationale behind these studies was that the materials to be removed vary in size so that during dialysis they would be removed at different rates, the smaller ones being removed more rapidly than the larger ones (i.e. during dialysis the rates of elimination, V_{E1}, V_{E2}, V_{E3}, and V_{E4}, which might be similar in the natural organ, are different and depend on the size of the individual solute and the dialyzer characteristics). Consequently, the larger materials or 'middle molecules' (29, 140) would accumulate to a greater extent than the smaller catabolites and if toxic, would result in an aggravation of a given uremic lesion, the neurological system being one of the target areas (143).

In this regard, it has been suggested that the peritoneum is a far more permeable membrane than those used in hemodialyzers and that removal of 'middle molecules' is more efficient with peritoneal dialysis (5). Observation of patients undergoing this mode of therapy is said to support this hypothesis by the less frequent occurrence of neuropathy (144), a lesion thought to result from middle molecule accumulation (5, 18). More recent analysis of peritoneal dialysis brings this contention into question (145). Other analyses of patients undergoing peritoneal dialysis, however, suggests that there may be a lower rate of some catabolic reactions (protein catabolism and urea generation) than in hemodialysis patients (14); this would then result in a correspondingly lower level of several of the hypothetical catabolic substances discussed above but because this is caused by lower overall catabolic rates some level of under nutrition should be expected in such cases.

Nevertheless, the presence of several catabolic materials G, H, I, L in high concentration and the possible toxicity of one or more of these substances is certainly valid. The analysis becomes immediately more complex, however, due to the size of the materials involved and the heterogenicity of the body. Kinetic analysis of such solute systems requires multi-compartmental models so that the levels of these unknown catabolites which will result from different types of dialysis therapy can be estimated and the effects of different dialyzers and protocols can be evaluated.

The steps of model formulation are similar to those discussed above with the exception that it is now necessary to abandon the simplicity of a single well mixed system. Two basic models are shown in Figure 24 (a and b) the difference between the two being the site of solute generation. Figure 24a indicates that material is generated into the perfused pool which would be the case if the solute in question were produced in the liver so that it had to traverse the extracellular system to reach cells. Figure 24b represents the case where the material is produced in cells. In either case there is a resistance to

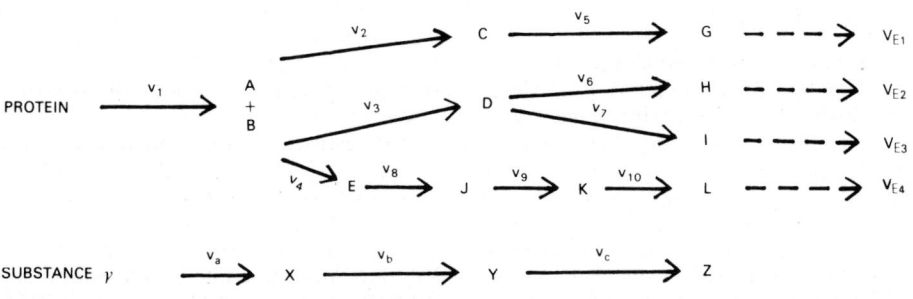

Figure 23. Hypothetical metabolic scheme involving catabolism of a protein and the biochemical pathways for some other substance γ.

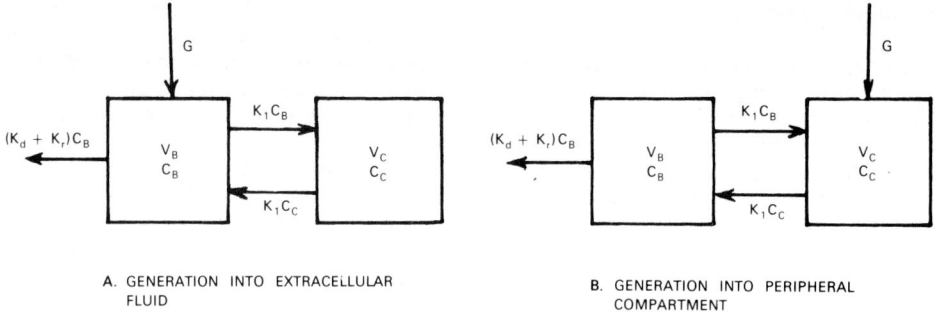

Figure 24. Two versions of a two compartment model for large molecular weight substances. Model A shows generation of material into the perfused (extracellular) compartment; model B shows generation into the perpherial (cellular) compartment.

movement between the two compartments. The transport constant in this case is the intercompartmental transport coefficient (K_i) which has units of flow.

These models have been discussed at length by others (41, 43) but it is instructive to consider briefly the basic differences between them. In 'case A' the peripheral pool acts as a capacitance, and the perfused compartment will go through large swings, the concentration being low immediately post dialysis and building up to levels higher than the peripheral compartment as the interdialytic period progresses. There will be solute movement alternately out of and into the peripheral pool during the dialysis cycle.

In contrast, 'case B' shows that the peripheral pool connects the site of generation and the site of excretion. As such the peripheral pool concentration will be elevated, because it is only through a high concentration difference that material can be transported into the perfused pool. Ironically, in 'case B' the uremic levels are closer to normal (relatively) because the same transport situation exists in health i.e., large concentration gradients are required for transport out of cells. This can perhaps be seen more clearly if steady state mass balance is examined in the two pools of model 24B:

$$G = K_1(C_{C_{ss}} - C_{B_{ss}}) \qquad [75a]$$
$$K_1(C_{C_{ss}} - C_{B_{ss}}) = K_R C_{B_{ss}} \qquad [75b]$$

Solution of these equations for the steady state concentration in pool C yields:

$$C_{C_{ss}} = \frac{G}{K_R}\left(1 + \frac{K_R}{K_1}\right) \qquad [76]$$

Equation 76 shows that for peripheral generation the concentration will approach G/K_R when K_1 becomes large but will be higher with decreasing values of K_1 (e.g., for $K_1 = 5$ ml/min and K_R (normal) of 125 ml/min, the K_R/K_1 term results in normal steady state concentrations in the peripheral pool 26 times G/K_R). Thus, a minimal toxic effect of decreased transport out of extracellular space with model 24b would be expected if the effector site was situated in pool C because of the high normal value in this pool.

In models such as Figure 24a and 24b mass balance expressions are written for each pool and the resulting differential equations are then solved simultaneously. Solutions for each of these cases are shown in the Appendix.

The case with metabolic interactions

The foregoing discussion of middle molecules in a multicompartmental setting is entirely hypothetical; such analyses point up the difficulties to be encountered when 'toxic' substances are not measured and their site of action is not known. In addition, the complexity of the kinetic system requiring knowledge of production rates and rates of transport between compartments coupled with the paucity of knowledge of these fundamental values makes this area of research a very demanding one.

Attempts to date to demonstrate a cause and effect relationship with respect to lowering levels of middle molecular weight toxins have been somewhat ambiguous (31, 146). There have been reports of improved blood pressure control (147) and decreased neuropathy (148) with similar high permeability protocols.

The 2 pool analysis of uremic toxins views the metabolic network shown in Figure 23 as a series of independent reactions that will depend on the removal rate alone for their level in the body. Reconsidering of this figure shows that while this approach may be attractive, it may be somewhat simplistic.

Consider the path for the protein to fragment B and the three pathways resulting in end products H, I, and L. If the clearances of L, H, and I are restricted, these substances will build up uniformly. However, if L is removed more rapidly than H and I, as would be the case during dialysis with urea (L) and large molecules, then the levels of H and I would be much higher relative to normal than the level of L would be; this interrelationship of catabolites has been the basis of the preceding discussion.

It is instructive, however, to consider the case where the paths are not independent. Let reaction V_4 be much faster than V_3 so that comparatively small amounts of H and I are formed with respect to L. At steady state, i.e., with the natural kidney still functioning, V_4, V_8, V_9, V_{10}, and V_{E4} will all be equal because none of the intermediates E, J, or K are accumulating. This will also be true of the chain of reactions resulting in H and I, i.e. $V_3 = V_6 + V_7 = V_{E2} + V_{E3}$. In this system, the complete blockage of pathways V_6 and V_7 will not significantly increase production of E because the predominant reaction is already in this direction. Reduction of V_4, however, would cause reaction V_{10}, V_9, V_8, and V_4 to slow which would increase B and the rates of reactions V_3 V_6 and V_7. If L is a common catabolite, such as urea, then its elevation in the steady state case would cause corresponding elevation of the levels of K, J, E, and B. Urea's immediate precursor arginine has, in fact, been shown to be higher than normal in uremic patients (149). In addition, if pathway V_3 existed, higher levels of D, H, and I would be expected. In fact, H and I would increase more than L even if they were cleared at the same rate because V_3 has been increased with respect to V_4. In the dialysis patient where V_{E2} and V_{E3} would possibly be less than V_{E4}, levels of H and I would be that much higher.

Up to this point, we have considered the ultimate products of these hypothetical biochemical reactions to be the potentially toxic materials. It is quite possible that intermediate substances C, D, E, J, or K might be metabolically active materials. As such, the elevated concentrations existing when the described pathways are blocked might reach toxic levels, or one of these materials (D, for example) might be an inhibitor for reaction V_6 in another metabolic pathway. This in turn might result in either toxic levels of X in the metabolic reaction series in which D does not itself participate, or the creation of some lesion because of the abnormally low levels of substance Z.

The above discussion has viewed the series of reactions with regard to what may occur at different steady state levels. In the dialysis patient, however, the levels of F, H, I and L will be continually changing, which will cause the levels of intermediates to change with lags appropriate to the kinetics of the individual reactions. This would then cause a system of metabolic perturbations to exist in the dialysis patient and would be a new syndrome not found in non-dialyzed patients and the perturbations themselves might cause toxic effects that would not be the result of any specific compound.

That the above discussion describes some catabolites is indicated by the kinetic behavior of various 'middle molecular' weight compounds (33) [see Figure 25]. Two 'typical' curves are shown in this figure and show markedly different behavior. Figure 25a shows classical double pool behavior (36) for compounds 7f and 7g of reference 33. The modest concentration rebound and short transient times indicate that there is only slight multipool behavior. The short rebound transient also indicates that K_i values are probably large relative to the dialyzer clearance so that re-equilibration takes place rapidly. The behavior shown by these materials is not much different than that of urea, creatinine, or uric acid (36, 112, 113).

Figure 25b shows a totally different and confusing concentration pattern, particularly post dialysis. It is clear from this curve (which is a composite of peptides 7a, 7b, and 7c of Asaba and coworkers [33]) that both models shown in Figure 24 are inadequate. What is most disturbing about these compounds is the rapid rise post treatment followed by a drop even below post dialysis levels. The model in Figure 25b should be viewed as a specific but hypothetical example of the general diagram shown in Figure 23 and constructed to represent a possible explanation of the concentration behavior of the peptide shown.

Consider that these peptides are metabolic intermediates and are ultimately catabolized to compound β.

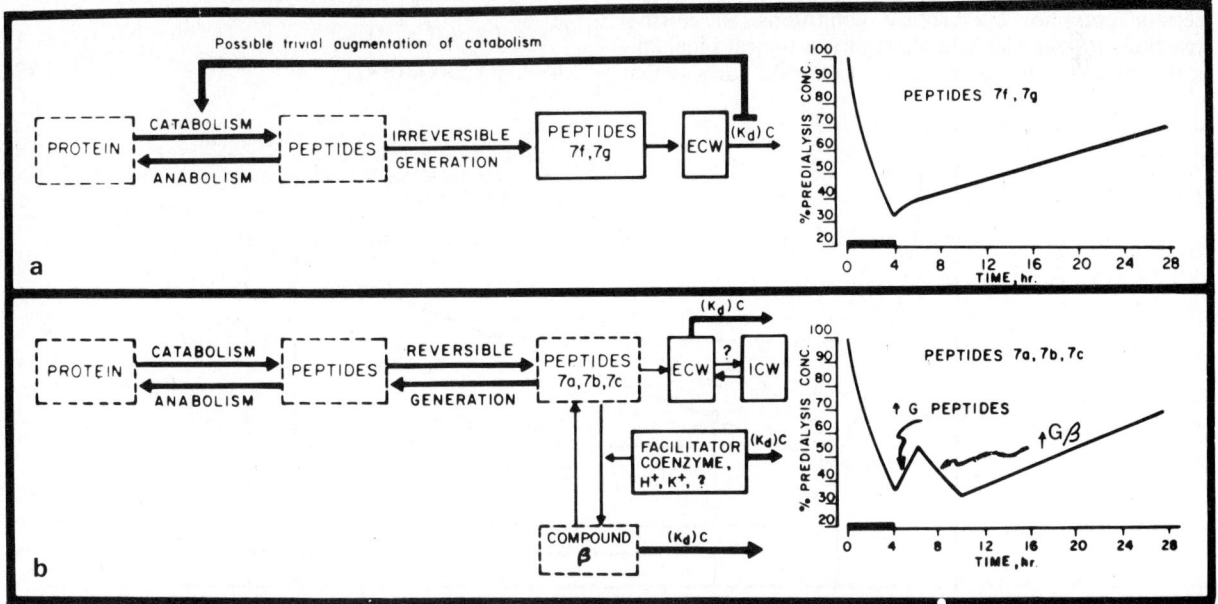

Figure 25. Concentration/time behavior of two types of peptides reported by Asaba et al [33] showing possible explanations for the kinetics of these materials. Reprinted by permission from Middle Molecules in Uremia and other diseases. Supplement to Volume 4, Artificial Organs, Copyright © 1981 by the International Society for Artificial Organs.

Both the peptides and β are dialyzable and will accumulate in the uremic patient after dialysis. Further, the metabolic reaction of the peptide to β requires a facilitator, co-enzyme, or cofactor (be it an electrolyte, optimal pH, etc.). Consider what, under these specific conditions, would happen as a result of dialysis. During dialysis all of these materials – the peptide, the facilitator, and β – decrease in concentration. Immediately at the end of treatment there is a marked increase in peptide levels both because of mass action and the increased production of this material from the precursor peptide. In addition, because the facilitator has been dialyzed to low concentrations, the degradation of 7a, b and c to β is temporarily blocked. The combination of increased production of these peptides into a 'dead-ended' system will result in a rapid rise in their concentration post dialysis.

The facilitator is gradually repleted post dialysis to the point where the catabolism of the peptide to β can proceeed and there is a rapid decrease of peptide levels as β (which was also removed during treatment) increases. Once this reaction scheme is back to 'normal' the concentration of the peptides gradually rises as levels of β increase, dependent on the reaction constant for the peptide/β reaction. Note also, that the final slope of peptide build-up is more gradual than that immediately post dialysis because the same amount of peptide generation is both accumulating and supplying substrate for the 'β reaction'.

This reaction scheme, while entirely hypothetical, is a possible explanation of curves such as the one shown in Figure 25b. Moreover, what this figure shows is not a traditional 'toxin' but a very labile compound which appears and is degraded by multiple pathways, and depends on the level of reactants and products for its kinetic behavior, and which may require co-factors and certain optimum biochemical conditions for normal reactions to take place. In short, it is a typical biochemical compound in a uremic setting. Curves such as that in Figure 25b serve to remind us that uremia, particularly dialyzed uremia, where homeostasis no longer exists, is a very disrupted metabolic state. And it is very likely that there is a high degree of 'toxicity' associated with such metabolic chaos.

APPENDIX

Dialyzer transport measurements: The case with ultrafiltration

The use of recycle methods of dialyzer transport measurement were described above for the case where there is no ultrafiltration. When ultrafiltration is present ($Q_F \neq 0$) a solution different from equations 26 result. Reconsider equation 25 with the left hand side expanded:

$$V \frac{dC_B}{dt} + C \frac{dV}{dt} = D \left(1 - \frac{Q_F}{Q_B}\right) C_{Di} - \left[D \left(1 - \frac{Q_F}{Q_B}\right) + Q_F\right] C_B \qquad [A1]$$

The size of the reservoir volume as a function of time will be:

$$V = V_o - Q_F t$$

and

$$\frac{dV}{dt} = -Q_F$$

Substitution of these relationships into equation A1 rearrangement and solution yield:

$$C_{Bt} = C_{Di} + (C_{Bo} - C_{Di}) \\ [(V_o - Q_F t)/V_o]^{(D/Q_F)(1 - Q_F/Q_B)} \qquad [A2]$$

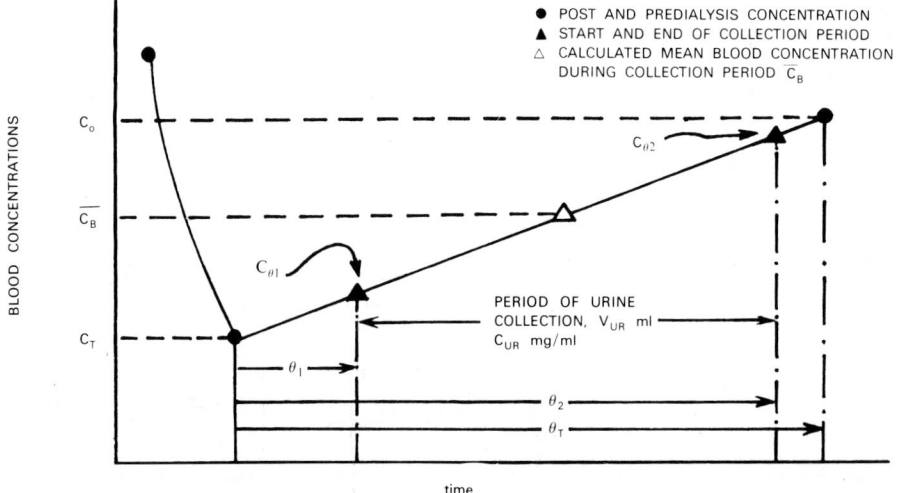

Figure A-1. Blood concentration and time values post dialysis required to calculate residual kidney clearance in the dialyzed patient.

Solving for D:

$$D = \frac{Q_F}{1 - Q_F/Q_B} \frac{\log \frac{(C_{Bt}-C_{Di})}{(C_{Bo}-C_{Di})}}{\log \frac{(V_o - Q_F t)}{V_o}} \quad [A3]$$

Appropriate reservoir sampling for equation variables will yield dialysance values (see text).

Average blood concentration during urine collection

Figure A1 shows that when concentration build up between dialysis is considered linear, it follows from the principle of similarity (150) that:

$$\frac{C_o - C_t}{\theta_t} = \frac{C_{o1} - C_t}{\theta_1} = \frac{C_{o2} - C_t}{\theta_2}$$

The value of starting and ending collection concentrations (C_{o1} and C_{o2}) will be:

$$C_{o1} = C_t + (C_o - C_t)\frac{\theta_1}{\theta_2}$$

and

$$C_{o2} = C_t + (C_o - C_t)\frac{\theta_2}{\theta_t}$$

The average collection concentration will be the average of C_{o1} and C_{o2} or:

$$\overline{C}_B = C_t + \frac{(C-G)(\theta_1 + \theta_2)}{2\theta_t} \quad [A4]$$

Two pool analysis of 'middle molecule' kinetics

The model in Figure 24 assumes distribution in two well mixed spaces: Compartment B, a perfused space and Compartment C, a non-perfused space. Between these two compartments there is transport by first order mechanism K_1. Two variations of the model are considered: (a) with generation into the perfused space and (b) with generation into the non-perfused space.

The removal of 'middle molecules' from the system is by first order elimination from compartment B by the dialyzer and natural organ if present.

MODEL A: This model represents the case where the solute is generated into the perfused space. This would be the mechanism of generation if such substances were synthesized in the liver during protein catabolism, for example. The defining equations for this model during all phases of dialysis are:

$$V_B \frac{dC_B}{dt} = G - K_1(C_B - C_C) - (K_R + K_D)C_B$$
$$\text{(Compartment B)} \quad [A5]$$

$$V_C \frac{dC_C}{dt} = K_1(C_B - C_C) \text{ (Compartment C)} \quad [A6]$$

The method of solution employed has been to put both equations A5 and A6 into Laplace transform space and alternately solve them simultaneously for the transformed concentration in each space. These expressions are then easily inverted by standard techniques to yield:

$$C_B = \left[\frac{C_{Co}K_1}{V_B} + \frac{C_{Bo}K_1}{V_C} + \frac{G}{V_B} - \frac{GK_1}{V_B V_C}\frac{1}{\beta} - C_{Bo}\beta\right]\frac{e^{-\beta t}}{\alpha - \beta} -$$
$$- \left[\frac{C_{Co}K_1}{V_B} + \frac{C_{Bo}K_1}{V_C} + \frac{G}{V_B} - \frac{GK_1}{V_B V_C}\frac{1}{\alpha} - C_{Bo}\alpha\right]\frac{e^{-\alpha t}}{\alpha - \beta} + \frac{GK_1}{V_B V_C \alpha \beta} \quad [A7]$$

$$C_C = \left[\frac{C_{Bo}K_1}{V_C} + \frac{C_{Co}(K_1 + K_R + K_D)}{V_B} - \frac{GK_1}{V_B V_C}\frac{1}{\beta} - C_{Co}\beta\right]\frac{e^{-\beta t}}{\alpha - \beta} -$$
$$- \left[\frac{C_{Bo}K_1}{V_C} + \frac{C_{Co}(K_1 + K_R + K_D)}{V_B} - \frac{GK_1}{V_B V_C}\frac{1}{\alpha} - C_{Co}\alpha\right]\frac{e^{-\alpha t}}{\alpha - \beta} + \frac{GK_1}{V_B V_C \alpha \beta} \quad [A8]$$

Where α and β are defined by:

$$\alpha \text{ and } \beta = \frac{1}{2}\left[\frac{K_1}{V_C} + \frac{K_1 + K_R + K_D}{V_B} \pm \right.$$
$$\left. \pm \sqrt{\left(\frac{K_1}{V_C} + \frac{K_1 + K_R + K_D}{V_B}\right)^2 - 4\frac{K_1(K_R + K_D)}{V_B V_C}}\right]$$

Off dialysis these equations still hold except in the case of the anephric patient; this special case can be approximated by letting K_R approach zero, i.e., by letting K_R have a very small value. C_{Bo} and C_{Do} will be the initial values for the particular interval being considered; pre-dialysis for the dialytic period, end dialysis values for the period between treatments.

MODEL B: This model represents the case where the solute is generated into the peripheral space in a manner similar to creatinine. The defining equations for this model during all phases of dialysis are:

$$V_B \frac{dC_B}{dt} = -K_1(C_B - C_C) - (K_R + K_D)C_B \quad [A9]$$

$$V_C \frac{dC_C}{dt} = G + K_1(C_B - C_C) \quad [A10]$$

The same solution method described above was used to solve equation A9 and A10 and results in:

$$C_B = \left[\frac{C_{Co}K_1}{V_B} + \frac{C_{Bo}K_1}{V_C} - \frac{GK_1}{V_B V_C}\frac{1}{\beta} - C_{Bo}\beta\right]\frac{e^{-\beta t}}{\alpha - \beta} -$$

$$- \left[\frac{C_{Co}K_1}{V_B} + \frac{C_{Bo}K_1}{V_C} - \frac{GK_1}{V_B V_C}\frac{1}{\alpha} - C_{Bo}\alpha\right]\frac{e^{-\alpha t}}{\alpha - \beta} + \frac{GK_1}{V_B V_C \alpha \beta} \quad [A11]$$

$$C_C = \left[\frac{C_{Bo}K_1}{V_C} + \frac{C_{Co}(K_1+K_R+K_D)}{V_B} + \frac{G}{V_B} - \frac{G(K_1+K_R+K_D)}{V_C V_B}\frac{1}{\beta} - C_{Co}\beta\right]\frac{e^{-\beta t}}{\alpha - \beta} -$$

$$- \left[\frac{C_{Bo}K_1}{V_C} + \frac{C_{Co}(K_1+K_R+K_D)}{V_B} + \frac{G}{V_B} - \frac{G(K_1+K_R+K_D)}{V_C V_B}\frac{1}{\alpha} - C_{Co}\alpha\right]\frac{e^{-\alpha t}}{\alpha - \beta} +$$

$$+ \frac{G(K_1+K_R+K_D)}{V_B V_C \alpha \beta} \quad [A12]$$

The value of α and β will be the same for the two models. Inspection of equations A11 and A12 shows that at steady state, i.e. $e^{-\alpha t}$ and $e^{-\beta t}$ equal zero, the concentration is represented by the constant term which is different for two compartments B and C. In the non-dialysis case, C_B will be less than C_C because the residual clearance, K_R appears in the numerator of the constant term for equation A12 but not in the corresponding one in equation A11. What is indicated is that in the normal patient where K_R may exceed 100 ml/min, there will be a profound intercompartmental concentration difference in the case of model B which was discussed previously.

Mathematical concepts and relational analysis

Independent and dependent variables and linear regressions

Medical science and clinical practice are characterized by, among other things, vast amounts of data and information both available and obtained for patients. It is important to consider such clinical data in a structured manner particularly if relationships between variables are to be investigated.

A broad distinction can be made between those parameters that cause other effects, or in terms of which other effects are measured (such as time) and the effects themselves. Those that are the cause or reference parameters are generally refered to as *independent variables* and their effects or results are *dependent variables*. Thus, as will be discussed below, when protein is catabolized, urea is generated. The protein being catabolized will cause the urea to be generated (not the other way around) so that the amount of protein being catabolized is considered to be the independent variable. The amount of urea produced is the dependent variable.

This independent/dependent variable relationship in many biological systems is linked. For example, protein catabolism will also produce acid (H^+), another dependent variable; the production of acid, however, will lower plasma bicarbonate concentration, which will neutralize the generated acid and in this context H^+ generation will be an independent variable and HCO_3 will be a dependent variable. Bicarbonate will be an independent variable in the buffer reactions which will cause respiratory changes (as quantified by the Henderson-Hasselbalch equation). These examples of related physiological variables illustrates that the examination of clinical data can be much more meaningful when the concept of independent and dependent variables is kept in mind.

This is clearly the case when relationships and correlations between variables are investigated using linear analysis. Analysis for linear correlations is an attempt to obtain a direct relationship between two variables. Most commonly when such a relationship is found the analysis is considered complete, when in fact it has only begun.

This is the starting point for in depth analysis because a non-trivial relationship between variables allows a fundamental property of that variable system to be described in an unequivocal mathematical form of a straight line. In addition, analysis of composite data will often reveal a fundamental relationship that is more accurate than any of the points that make it up. An example of this is the determination of bicarbonate dialysance values from the slope of a plot of $J = f(C_{Bi} - C_{Di})$ rather than by direct computation using equation 10 (10).

The relationship that results from a linear regression analysis is:

$$Y = aX + b \quad [A13]$$

The presence of an expression, in this exact form, on a linear regression plot, i.e. the use of x and y rather than the actual variables being related, however, belies a reluctance to take the next step. In addition, it should be noted that this general mathematical form indicates that the dependent variable should be plotted on the vertical axis (ordinate) as a function of the independent variable on the horizontal axis (abscissa) so that expression A13 shows that can be expected to happen to Y (a dependent variable) when X (an independent variable) changes.

Consider, for example, the data of Borah and colleagues (48, 49) relating net urea generation rate and net rates of protein catabolism (see Figure A2). The dependent variable will be the net urea generation because it is caused by protein catabolism and oxidation of amino acids; the net rate of protein catabolism will be the independent variable. The linear regression is shown in Figure A2 and results in the relationship:

$$G = 0.154\,PCR - 1.7$$
(not $Y = 0.154\,X - 1.7$) [A14]

This relationship can now be used in various ways. First, it can estimate the rate of urea generation at various levels of intake e.g., 60 g/day or 400 g/day protein intake such as the patient reported by Richards and Brown (79). Second, it is important to consider the equation constants, specifically the coefficient of PCR and the intercept.

The slope indicates that for each 10 g of protein catabolized, 1.54 g of urea nitrogen will be generated. This is 96% of the nitrogen content of protein and indicates that there may be some other non-urea products that will be generated in a linear manner when protein is catabolized. A slight dependence of creatinine generation on protein generation has been found (151) and there may be other trace catabolites whose net production increases as the net amount to protein catabolism does.

The intercept (-1.7) should also be considered. There are two intercepts that should be evaluated (when $G = 0$ and when $PCR = 0$). When $PCR = 0$, i.e. when there is no net catabolism, extrapolation of the relationship would indicate that there will be negative generation (or that urea will be consumed). Physically, this would mean that urea would be consumed to yield other nitrogen base materials that are produced and excreted at a fixed rate (see below). It appears that this conclusion is more a result of the mathematics than actual physiology, and would not be expected to actually occur under normal circumstances; the relationship will become discontinuous at some point before $G = 0$. In this context it is important to emphasize that one should be cautious in extrapolating relationships into domains outside the range of the data used. Extrapolation into ranges where discontinuity would be expected (very low levels of protein catabolism in the present case) should be attempted with caution. Evaluation of the PCR intercept (where $G = 0$) gives other information:

$$0 = 0.154\,PCR - 1.7$$
$$PCR = 1.7/0.154 = 11.04 \quad [A15]$$

The PCR intercept indicates that in the patients Borah and coworkers studied there is an obligatory rate of catabolism (i.e. not linearly related to PCR) of 11 g/day. This is in the form of creatinine production and nitrogen excretion in the stool. If, as is likely, this rate of obligatory nitrogen loss is a function of body size, then the Borah relationship can be generalized by adjusting this intercept value relative to body size by keeping the same slope, i.e., the same linear reaction of G to PCR. In this case, when the intercept is scaled by the volume of total body water (in Borah's patients 37.6 l), the relationship, when solved for PCR, becomes

$$PCR = 6.49\,G_u + 0.294\,V \quad [A16a]$$

or if G is in mg/min:

$$PCR = 9.35\,G_u + 0.294\,V. \quad [A16b]$$

Physically, this adaption to body size shifts the G/PCR line to the left (for smaller individuals) and to the right (for larger ones) with the slope remaining the same. Such a modification has been shown to be valid for estimation of PCR in pediatric patients (76, 152). Similarly, if obligatory or fixed losses are known to be different, i.e. as they would be in peritoneal dialysis, a similar shift in the relation of Figure A2 would be appropriate. Recent data on patients treated by continuous ambulatory peritoneal dialysis (CAPD) (see chapter 23) show such a shift, although the analysis did not follow the lines described above (80).

This example, while fundamental to the urea nitrogen discussion in this chapter, is meant to illustrate the logical progression and extensive use that can be made of linear relational analysis.

It is critical to add that when there is a linear relationship between variables, an extended evaluation of the elements of that relationship is important. If such analysis (examination of slopes and intercepts) does not result in useful information, it is likely that the key, or fundamental variables are not being related.

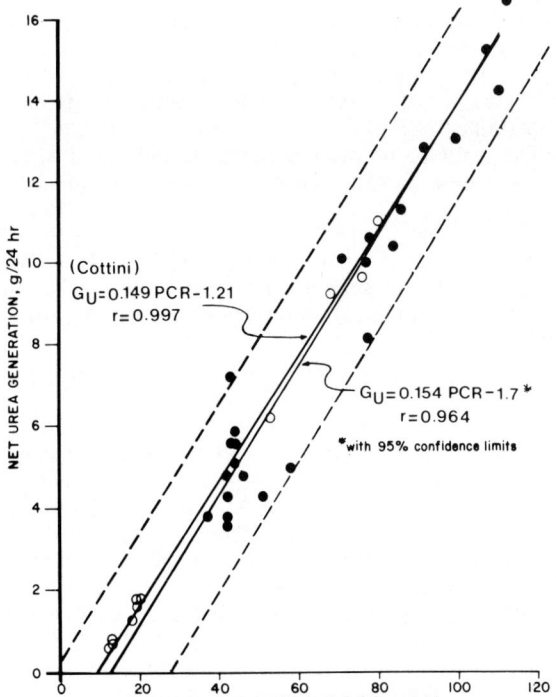

Figure A-2. Relationship between net protein catabolic rate and net urea nitrogen generation in uremic subjects. Data shown are those from two populations: Cottini et al (151) and Borah et al (48). Reprinted by permission, Dialysis and Transplantation 10(4):314, 1981.

Therapeutic extension of clinical information through mathematical reduction of data

Nutritional management of acute dialysis
Linear reduction of data reduces clinical information to

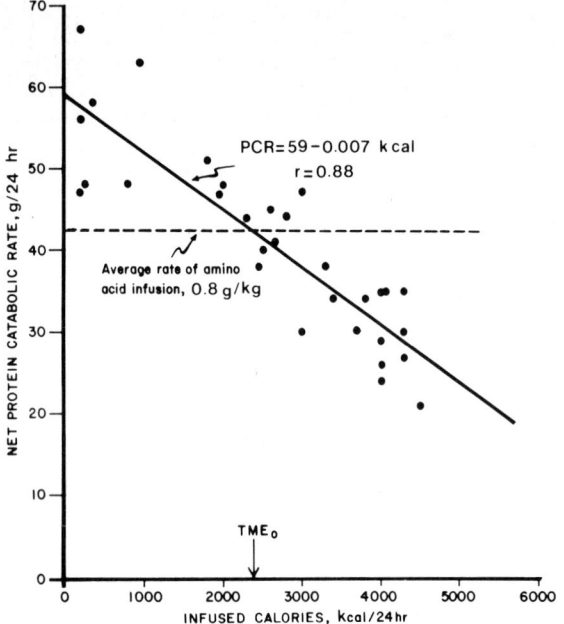

Figure A-3. Net protein catabolic rate as a function of dextrose calorie infusion in a 73 year old male with acute renal failure. PCR = 59−0.007 kcal (1 kcal = 4.2 kJ). Reprinted by permission, Dialysis and Transplantation 10(4):314, 1981.

quantitative form, increasing its therapeutic use as has been discussed above. It can also extend these collective data to broader areas of therapy and treatment decision. The relation of net rates of catabolism as a function of energy intake in the acute dialysis patient provides a pertinent example (49, 153, 154).

Often in the acute dialysis patient undergoing total parenteral nutrition, a relation will exist between the rate of energy input to the patient and the net rate of protein catabolism (see Figure A3 [153]). Such relationships have been found by many investigators (155–159); clinically observations are commonly made of negative nitrogen balance in patients with large energy demands that are not met, e.g. protein-calorie malnutrition.

This clinical 'understanding' of the interaction of net protein catabolism and energy intake, however, can be further extended and made into a powerful therapeutic tool if it is reduced to quantitative form. The relationship shown in Figure A3 is a PCR-Energy relationship for an acute dialysis patient receiving total parenteral nutrition (energy in the form of 70% dextrose monohydrate). In this figure energy is the independent variable because, as is shown, the change in the energy level is the factor influencing the net rate of protein catabolism. It should be noted that the metabolic interrelationships in the acute dialysis patient are clearly complex, but in terms of Figure A3 it is the change in energy that is shown to influence the PCR. For this particular patient during this specific illness the relation was:

$$PCR = 59 - 0.007 \text{ kcal} \quad [A17]$$

Equation A17 indicates that for each 1,000 kcal (4,200 kJ of additional dextrose energy given the PCR will be reduced by 7 g/day. When no exogenous dextrose is given the PCR will be 59 g/day. It should be stressed that Figure A3 is specific for the patient-illness for which it was determined. A different patient will have a different relation; the effect of dextrose input would be expected to be different for the same patient during another illness.

This expression which reduces the multiple PCR/energy observations to a mathematical relation can then be used to determine the probable effect of giving more or less energy in the form of dextrose, much the way that the G/PCR relation (see Figure A2) was used to determine the effect of increased catabolism on BUN or to determine the PCR from computed G values. The analysis, however, should not stop here.

In addition to the problems of catabolite accumulation in acute dialysis patients, there is the problem of volume control. As more protein and dextrose are administered there is an obligatory addition of water. This added volume load using an energy 'stock solution' with C_E kcal/ml 'energy concentration' and an amino acid stock solution of C_{AA} mg amino acids/ml, however, can be accurately estimated as:

$$V = \frac{PPI}{(1000 - E/C_E)C_{AA}} + V_A \quad [A18]$$

In this expression PPI is the 'effective parenteral protein intake' and V_A is the additional volume required to supply the desired electrolytes to the intraveneous solution. For 70% dextrose monohydrate C_E will be 2.38 kcal/ml; C_{AA} will be 0.085 g amino acids/ml for Freeamine *.

The amount of protein administered for a specific energy input, E, and volume of solution, V, will be:

$$PPI = (1000 - E/C_E) C_{AA} (V - V_A) \quad [A19]$$

For the degree of nitrogen balance PPI−PCR = dP/dt, equation A17 (in general form) and A19 can be combined (see graphical representation Figure A4) to yield:

$$dP/dt = (1000 - E/C_E) C_{AA} (V_F - V_A) - (PCR_0 - bE) \quad [A20]$$

In equation A20 PCR_0 is the PCR when no energy is given (the PCR intercept) and b is the slope of the PCR/E relation (see figure A4). Equation A20 presents the treatment/nutritional problem in unequivocal form. The three clinical factors that have to be considered, and their interrelations are shown:

1. dP/dt: The degree of protein balance (positive, negative, or zero)
2. E: The amount of energy to be administered.
3. V_F: The amount of fluid to be administered.

The choice of independent variable now rests with the physician. Volume may be controlling and dP/dt and E will then have to be adjusted to the need for control of

---

* Amino acid solution commercially available in the U.S.

3: Principles and biophysics of dialysis 91

fluid. Or the status of protein balance (dP/dt) may be the primary clinical consideration.

Summary

The essential point to be drawn from the foregoing development is that there is information contained in clinical data that remains untapped, even when such information is analyzed by elegant statistical techniques. The need is generally not for more data or more sophisticated analysis; it is for a more structured analysis of the information available.

The initial step, as in the process of modeling, is a conceptual one: which variables are controlling (the independent variables) and which ones respond (the dependent variables)? The independent-dependent variable statistical analysis will yield certain direct (or linear) relationships. The question must be asked: do they make sense? An important means to answer this question is by examination of the slope and intercept values of the specific linear relationship. If these show physically or physiologically impossible situations there is reason to re-examine the original data. If these basic parameters seem devoid of any physical meaning it is likely that a different presentation of the data will yield more important information.

Finally, once a linear relation has been discovered and found to be relevant it represents a precise analytical and clinical tool. The tool should be examined, 'fashioned', and used to predict clinical behavior and to estimate the magnitude of metabolic events. Such a tool, which represents the quantitative distillation of physiological properties and behavior in man, provides a unique means to use clinical information and an opportunity to greatly expand the domain of clinical investigation and medical understanding.

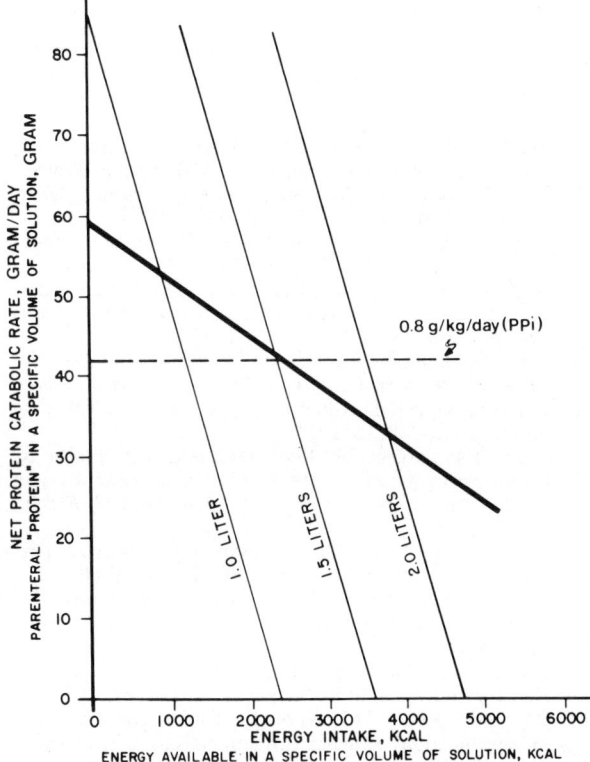

Figure A-4. The energy-catabolism-volume relationships in the acute renal failure patient. Isovolumic lines for total volumes of 1, 1.5, and 2 litres are shown superimposed on the PCR/energy relation of Figure A-3. The figure shows the nutrient constraints of parenteral fluid mixing as well as the therapeutic constraints of treating such a patient. Reprinted by permission, Dialysis and Transplantation 10(4): 314, 1981.

NOMENCLATURE

A   Area (cm^2); dA: differential area

α Donnan factor as defined by equation 11; αhd: α during hemodialysis; αhf: α during hemofiltration

a_{H^+} Addition of H$^+$ to extracellular water from intracellular water; this term is the reverse of m_{H^+} (mEq/min), also A_{H^+}

C   Concentration (mg/ml, mmol/l, mEq/l); C_{AA}: amino acid concentration in stock solution for parenteral nutrition; C_B: blood concentration; C_C: concentration in pool C in a two pool model; C_{CO_2}: concentration of gaseous CO$_2$; C_D: dialysate concentration; C_E: energy concentration of dextrose stock solution for parenteral nutrition; C_F: concentration in hemofiltrate; C_o: initial concentration – pre-dialysis; C_t: end-dialysis concentration; C_{ur}: urine concentration; C_{SS}, C_{Bss}, C_{Css}: steady state concentration; C_{o1}, C_{o2}: C_t for two sequential dialyses; C_{Bi}, C_{Di}: inlet concentrations; C_{Na}: sodium concentration; C_P: plasma concentrations, C_{Po}, C_{Pt}, and C_{Pss} represent initial, end dialysis, and steady state values; C_{Pr}: concentration of proteins in plasma; $\overline{C_B}$: mean concentration; ΔC: concentration difference in flux expressions; dc/dx: change of concentration with distance, indicates a concentration gradient; $\Delta c/\Delta x$: gradient over the fixed distance Δx; C(Log-mean): concentration driving force in a dialyzer as defined by equation 7; dC/dt: time rate of change in concentration

C$^+$ Total osmotically active cation: Na$_{Ex}$+K$_{Ex}$ (mmol)

D   Diffusive dialysance: (ml/min, l/min); D$'$: apparent dialysance as defined by equation 13

D   Diffusivity, (cm^2/sec); D_B: diffusivity in blood; D_D: diffusivity in dialysate; D_m: diffusivity in the membrane; D_{m^*}: effective diffusivity in the membrane

E   Zero order enzymatic conversion rate of acetate to acetyl-CoA (mmol/min); dextrose energy infused as part of parenteral nutrition (kcal, kJ)

F   Fraction; FF: filtration fraction in hemofiltration; F_P: water fraction in plasma; F_R: water fraction of the red cell

G   Generation rate (mg/min, mmol/min, mEq/min); in the case of urea: G = the net rate of urea nitrogen generation from net protein catabolism; g_{H^+}: rate of hydrogen ion production, also G_{H^+}

HCT   hematocrit (per cent)

I   Infusion rate of heparin: (units/hour)

J   Flux: mass/time, (mg/min, mmol/min, mEq/min); J_{Ac}: flux of acetate into a patient; $J_{H^+ \, Exc}$: flux of H$^+$ out of patient by renal excretion; J_{HCO_3}: flux of bicarbonate out of a patient; J_{OA}: flux of organic anions

K	Diffusive clearance or transport constant; K_o: overall mass transfer coefficient (cm/min); K: clearance (ml/min, l/min); K_B: clearance based on blood side flux; K_D: clearance based on dialysate side flux; K_L: lung clearance (of CO_2); K_{Ln}: normal lung clearance; K_R: residual renal clearance; K': apparent clearance as defined by equation 16a; K_i: intercompartmental transport coefficient in a two pool model; K_{UF}: ultrafiltration coefficient, (ml/min/mm Hg)
k	Solute distribution coefficient
K_{Ex}	Total exchangeable potassium: (mmol)
m_{H^+}	Mobilization of H^+ out of extracellular water into other buffers: (mEq/min) (see equation 52b), also M_{H^+}
Na_{Ex}	Total exchangeable sodium: (mmol)
P	Pressure: (mm Hg); P_B: blood side pressure; P_D: dialysate side pressure; $\bar{P}$: average pressure
P	Tissue protein content of the body (g); dP/dt: rate of change of tissue protein content with time, protein balance
PCR	Net rate of protein catabolism: (g/day); PCR_o: intercept value of PCR in equation A 17 and A 20; pcr: net rate of protein catabolism relative to normal body weight
PPI	Parenteral protein intake: (g/day)
Q	Flow rate (ml/min, l/min); Q_B: blood flow; Q_D: dialysate flow; Q_E: effective blood water flow rate as defined by equation 20, ultrafiltrate flow; Q_{Bi}, Q_{Di}: inlet flow rates to the dialyzer; Q_S: rate of addition of substitution fluid in hemofiltration
R	Mass transfer resistance (min/cm); R_B: mass transfer resistance in blood phase; R_D: mass transfer resistance in dialysate phase; R_M: mass transfer resistance in the membrane; R_o: overall mass transfer resistance
R	Response of body clotting mechanism to a heparin load; prolongation of clotting time (sec); R_i: R at the start of an interval; R_o: initial value of R, baseline value; R_t: R at the end of an interval
R_1, R_2	Rate of carbonic acid dissociation reaction; rate of bicarbonate neutralization reaction (mEq/min)
S	Sensitivity of an individual to heparin: response/unit (seconds clotting time prolongation/unit of heparin)
T(t)	Time (minutes); td: duration of dialysis; T_{ur}: length of a urine collection
V	Volume (ml, l); volume of distribution of specific species, volume of parenteral solutions given to a patient; V_A: volume of electrolytes added to parenteral solutions; V_B: volume of compartment b in a two pool model; V_C: volume of compartment c in a two compartment model; V_{Ecf}: volume of extra-cellular fluid; V_F: amount of fluid to be administered to the patient receiving total parenteral nutrition; V_L: inter-dialytic volume loading; V_R: intra-dialytic volume removal; V_D: initial volume; V_{ur}: volume of a urine collection; dV/dt: time rate of change in volume
X(x)	Distance (cm); dx: differential distance; Δx: diffusion distance; Δx_B: thickness of blood film; Δx_D: thickness of dialysate film; Δx_M: membrane thickness
α, β	Exponent in two pool analysis (min-1)
β	Rate of weight gain: (g/min, kg/day)
θ	Inter-dialytic interval (minutes); $\theta(\theta_t)$: total interval; θ_1: interval from the end of a dialysis to the start of a urine collection; θ_2: interval from the end of dialysis to the end of a urine collection

REFERENCES

1. Michaels AS: Operating parameters and performance criteria for hemodialyzers and other membrane-separation devices. *Trans Am Soc Artif Intern Organs* 12:387, 1966
2. Gotch FA, Autian J, Colton CK, Ginn HE, Lipps BJ, Lowrie EG: *The Evaluation of Hemodialyzers*, DHEW publ no (NIH) 72:103, 1971
3. Klein E, Autian J, Bower JD, Buffaloe G, Centella L, Colton CK, Darby TD, Farrell PC, Holland FF, Kennedy RS, Lipps B Jr, Mason R, Nolph KD, Villarroel F, Wathen RL: *Evaluation of Hemodialyzers and Dialysis Membranes* DHEW publ no (NIH) 77-1294, 1977
4. Guyton AC: *Textbook of Medical Physiology*, Philadelphia, WB Saunders Co, 6th edition, 1981, p 208
5. Babb AL, Popovich RP, Christopher TG, Scribner BH: The genesis of the square meter-hour hypothesis. *Trans Am Soc Artif Intern Organs* 17:81, 1971
6. Klein E: Membranes and materials evaluation. *Proc 7th Annu Contractors Conf Artif Kidney – Chronic Uremia Program* NIAMDD edited by Krueger KK, DHEW publ no (NIH) 75-248:85, 1974
7. Gotch FA, Sargent JA, Keen ML, Seid MA, Foster R: Comparative treatment time with Kiil, Gambro and Cordis-Dow kidneys. *Proc Clin Dial Transpl Forum*, 3:217, 1973
8. Comroe JH: *Physiology of Respiration*. Chicago, Year Book Medical Publishers, 2nd edition, 1975, p 60
9. Pitts RF: *Physiology of the Kidney and Body Fluids*, Chicago, Year Book Medical Publishers, Inc, 2nd edition, 1968, p 29
10. Sargent JA, Gotch FA: Bicarbonate and carbon dioxide transport during dialysis therapy. *asaio J* 2:61, 1979
11. Wolf AV, Remp DG, Kiley JE, Currie GD: Artificial kidney function: Kinetics of hemodialysis. *J Clin Invest* 30:1062, 1951
12. Smith HW: *The Kidney: Structure and Function in Health and Disease*. New York, Oxford University Press, 1951, p 39
13. Gotch FA: Hemodialysis: Technical and kinetic considerations. Chapter 41 in *The Kidney*, edited by Brenner BM, Rector FC Jr, Philadelphia, WB Saunders Company, 1976, p 1672
14. Nolph KD, Nothum RJ, Maher JF: Effects of ultrafiltration on dialysance in commercially available coils. *Kidney Int* 2:293, 1972
15. Nolph KD, Nothum RJ, Maher JF: Ultrafiltration: A mechanism for removal of intermediate molecular weight substances in coil dialyzers. *Kidney Int* 6:55, 1974
16. Farrell PC, Babb AL: Estimation of the permeability of cellulosic membranes from solute dimensions and diffusivities. *J Biomed Mater Res* 7:25, 1973
17. Bottomley S, Parsons FM, Broughton PMG: The dialysis of non-electrolytes through regenerated cellulose (Cuprophane). I. The effect of molecular size: *J Appl Polym Sci* 16:2115, 1972
18. Babb AL, Farrell PC, Uvelli DA, Scribner BH: Hemodialyzer evaluation by examination of solute molecular spectra. *Trans Am Soc Artif Intern Organs* 18:98, 1972
19. Popovich RP, Hlavinka DJ, Bomar JB, Moncrief JW, Dechard JF: The consequences of physiological resistances on metabolic removal from the patient – artificial kidney system. *Trans Am Soc Artif Intern Organs* 21:108, 1975
20. French D: The Schardinger dextrins. *Adv Carbohydrate Chem* 12:189, 1957
21. Schreiner GE: The search for the uremic toxin(s). *Kidney Int* 7 (suppl 3):S270, 1975
22. Horowitz HI: Uremic toxins and platelet function. *Arch Intern Med* 127:823, 1970
23. Cohen BD: Guanidinosuccinic acid in uremia. *Arch Intern Med* 126:846, 1970

24. Giovannetti S, Biagini M, Cioni L: Evidence that methyl guanidine is retained in chronic renal failure. *Experientia* 24:341, 1968
25. Schmidt EG, McElvian NS, Bowen JJ: Plasma amino acids and the ether soluble phenols in uremia. *Am J Clin Path* 20:253, 1950
26. Gordon A, Bergström J, Fürst P, Zimmerman L: Separation and characterization of uremic metabolites in biologic fluids: A screening approach to the definition of uremic toxins. *Kidney Int* 7 (suppl 2):S45, 1975
27. Giovanetti S, Barsotti G: Dialysis of methylguanidine. *Kidney Int* 6:177, 1974
28. Fürst P, Bergström J, Gordon A, Johnsson E, Zimmerman L: Separation of peptides of 'middle' molecular weight from biological fluids of patients with uremia. *Kidney Int* 7 (Suppl 3):S272, 1975
29. Funck-Brentano J, Man NK, Sausse A, Zingraff J, Boudet J, Becker A, Cueille GF: Characterization of a 1100–1300 MW uremic neurotoxin. *Trans Am Soc Artif Intern Organs* 22:163, 1976
30. Bergström J, Fürst P: Uremic toxins. *Kidney Int* 12 (Suppl 8):S-9, 1978
31. Berström J, Fürst P, Zimmerman L: Uremic middle molecules exist and are biologically active. *Clin Nephrol* 11:229, 1979
32. Asaba H, Bergström J, Fürst P, Oulès R, Zimmerman L: Accumulation and excretion of middle molecules. *Proc Eur Dial Transpl Assoc*, 13:481, 1976
33. Asaba H, Fürst P, Oulès R, Ward M, Yahiel V, Zimmerman L, Bergström J: The effect of hemodialysis on endogenous middle molecules in uremic patients. *Clin. Nephrol* 11:257, 1979
34. Babb AL, Strand MJ, Uvelli DA, Milutinovic J, Scribner BH: Quantitative description of dialysis treatment: A dialysis index. *Kidney Int* 7 (Suppl 2):S23, 1975
35. Babb AL, Strand MJ, Uvelli DA, Scribner BH: The dialysis index: A practical guide to dialysis treatment. *Dial Transpl* 6(6):9, 1977
36. Bell RL, Curtis FK, Babb AL: Analog simulation of the patient-artificial kidney system. *Trans Am Soc Artif Intern Organs* 11:183, 1965
37. King PH, Baker WR, Ginn HE, Frost AB: Computer optimization of hemodialysis. *Trans Am Soc Artif Intern Organs* 14:389, 1968
38. Dedrick RL: Pharmacodynamic considerations for chronic hemodialysis. *Kidney Int* 7 (Suppl 2):S-7, 1975
39. Sargent JA, Gotch FA: The analysis of concentration dependence of uremic lesions in clinical studies. *Kidney Int* 7 (Suppl 2):S35, 1975
40. Gotch FA, Sargent JA, Keen ML, Lee M: Individualized quantified dialysis therapy of uremia. *Proc Clin Dial Transpl Forum* 4:27, 1974
41. Popovich RP, Hlavinka DJ, Bomar JB, Moncrief JW, Dechard JF: The consequences of physiological resistances on metabolite removal from the patient–artificial kidney system. *Trans Am Soc Artif Intern Organs* 21:108, 1975
42. Gotch FA, Farrell, PC, Sargent JA: Theoretical considerations of molecular transport in dialysis and sorbent therapy for uremia. *J Dial* 1:105, 1976
43. Frost TH, Kerr DNS: Kinetics of hemodialysis: A theoretical study of the removal of solutes in chronic renal failure compared to normal health. *Kidney Int* 12:41, 1977
44. Sargent JA: Kinetic modeling in the guidance of dialysis therapy. *Dial Transpl* 8:1101, 1979
45. Sargent JA, Gotch FA: Mathematical modelling of dialysis therapy. *Kidney Int* 18 (Suppl 10):S-2, 1980
46. Sargent JA: Which mathematical model to guide clinical dialysis? Chapter 41 in *Uremia – Pathobiology of Patients Treated For 10 Years Or More: Third Capri Conference on Uremia,* edited by Giordano C, Friedman EA, Milan, Wichtig Editore, 1980, p 209
47. Sargent JA, Lowrie EG: Which mathematical model to study uremic toxicity? *Clin Nephrol* 17:303, 1982
48. Borah MF, Schoenfeld PY, Gotch FA, Sargent JA, Wolfson M, Humphreys MH: Nitrogen balance during intermittent dialysis therapy of uremia. *Kidney Int* 14:491, 1978
49. Sargent JA, Gotch FA, Borah M, Piercy L, Spinozzi N, Schoenfeld P, Humphreys M: Urea kinetics: A guide to nutritional management of renal failure. *Am J Clin Nutr* 31:1696, 1978
50. Cogan MG, Sargent JA, Yarbrough S, Vincenti F, Amend W: Prevention of prednisone-induced negative nitrogen balance. *Ann Intern Med* 95:158, 1981
51. Gotch FA, Sargent JA, Keen ML, Lam M, Prowitt M, Grady M: Clinical results of intermittent dialysis therapy (IDT) guided by ongoing kinetic analysis or urea metabolism. *Trans Am Soc Artif Intern Organs* 22:175, 1976
52. Sargent JA: Urea Kinetics: A quantitative guide to nutrition and treatment in renal disease. *Dial Transpl* 10:275, 1981
53. Sargent JA: *The Role of Acetate in Acid Base Corrections during Hemodialysis Treatment,* PhD Thesis, University of California, Berkeley, 1976
54. Gotch FA, Keen ML: Precise control of minimal heparinization for high bleeding risk hemodialysis. *Trans Am Soc Artif Intern Organs* 23:168, 1977
55. Sherlock JE, Yoon Y, Ledwith JW, Letteri JM: Respiratory gas exchange during hemodialysis. *Proc Clin Dial Transpl Forum* 2:171, 1972
56. Sherlock JE, Ledwith JW, Letteri JM: Hypoventilation and hypoxemia during hemodialysis: reflex response to removal of CO_2 across the dialyzer. *Trans Am Soc Artif Intern Organs* 23:406, 1977
57. Aurigemma NM, Feldman NT, Gottlieb M, Ingram RH, Lazarus JM, Lowrie EG: Arterial oxygenation during hemodialysis. *N Engl J Med* 297:871, 1977
58. Tolchin N, Rogers JL, Hayashi J, Lewis EJ: Metabolic consequences of high mass-transfer hemodialysis. *Kidney Int* 11:366, 1977
59. Tolchin N, Roberts JL, Lewis EJ: Respiratory gas exchange by high efficiency hemodialysis. *Nephron* 21:137, 1978
60. Guyton AC: *Textbook of Medical Physiology,* Philadelphia PA, WB Saunders, 6th edition, 1981, p 518
61. Kreyszig E: *Advanced Engineering Mathematics.* New York, John Wiley and Sons, 1972, p 24, 147
62. Sokolnikoff IS, Redheffer RM: *Mathematics of Physics and Modern Engineering.* New York NY, McGraw Hill, 1958, p 23, 756
63. Giovanetti S, Maggiore Q: A low nitrogen diet with proteins of high biological value for severe chronic uraemia. *Lancet* 1:1000, 1964
64. Shaw AB, Bazzard FJ, Booth EM, Nilwarangkur S, Berlyne GM: The treatment of chronic renal failure by modified Giovanetti diet. *Q J Med* 34:237, 1965
65. Kerr DNR, Robson A, Elliott RW, Ashcroft R: Diet in chronic renal failure. *Proc R Soc Med* 60:115, 1967
66. Franklin SS, Gordon A, Kleeman CR, Maxwell MH: Use of a balanced low-protein diet in chronic renal failure. *JAMA* 202:477, 1967
67. Kopple JD, Sorensen MK, Coburn JW, Gordon A, Rubini ME: Controlled comparison of 20 g and 40 g protein diets in the treatment of chronic uremia. *Am J Clin Nutr* 21:553, 1968

68. Hewlett AW, Gilbert QO, Wickett AD: The toxic effetcs of urea on normal individuals. *Arch. Intern Med* 18:636, 1916
69. Grollman EF, Grollman A: Toxicity of urea and its role in the pathogenesis of uremia. *J Clin Invest* 38:749, 1959
70. Cohen BD, Handelsman DG, Narayan PB: Toxicity arising from the urea cycle. *Kidney Int* 7 (Suppl 3): S285, 1975
71. Johnson WJ, Hagge WW, Wagoner RD, Dinapoli RP, Rosevear JW: Toxicity arising from urea. *Kidney* Int 7 (Suppl 3):S288, 1975
72. Lowrie EG, Laird NM, Parker TF, Sargent JA: Effect of the hemodialysis prescription on patient morbidity. *N Engl J Med* 305:1176, 1981
73. Luke RG: Uremia and the BUN. *N Engl J Med* 305:1213, 1981
74. Steffenson KA: Some determinations of the total body water in man by means of intravenous injections of urea. *Acta Physiol Scand* 13:282, 1947
75. Lehninger AL: *Biochemistry,* New York NY, Worth Publishers, 1970, p 433
76. Sargent JA, Gotch FA: Is urea generation adaptive? *Controv Nephrol* 1:451, 1979
77. Walser M, Bodenlos LJ: Urea metabolism in man. *J Clin Invest* 38:1617, 1959
78. Wolpert E, Phillips SF, Summerskill WHJ: Transport or urea and ammonia production in the human colon. *Lancet* 2:1387, 1971
79. Richards P, Brown CL: Urea metabolism in an azotemic woman with normal renal function. *Lancet* 2:207, 1975
80. Blumenkrantz MJ, Kopple JD, Moran JK, Grodstein GP, Coburn JW: Nitrogen and urea metabolism during continuous ambulatory peritoneal dialysis. *Kidney Int* 20:78, 1981
81. Berlyne GM, Shaw AB, Nilwarangkur S: Dietary treatment of chronic renal failure. Experience with a modified Giovanetti diet. *Nephron* 2:129, 1965
82. Walser M: The conservative management of the uremic patient. Chapter 39 in *The Kidney,* edited by Brenner BM, Rector FC Jr, Philadelphia PA, WB Saunders Co, 1976, p 1613
83. Bennett N: Urea kinetics: A dietitian's clinical tool in the nutritional management of patients with end stage renal disease. *Dial Transpl* 10:332, 1981
84. Forbes G, Bruining GJ: Urinary creatinine excretion and lean body mass. *Am J Clin Nutr* 29:1359, 1976
85. Sargent JA, Gotch FA: Mass balance: A quantitative guide to clinical nutritional therapy I: The predialysis renal disease patient. *J Am Dietetic Assoc* 75: 547, 1979
86. Kopple JD, Coburn JW: Evaluation of chronic uremia. Importance of serum urea nitrogen, serum creatinine, and their ratio. *JAMA* 227: 41, 1974
87. Rutherford WE, Blondin J, Miller JP, Greenwalt AS, Vavra JD: Chronic progressive renal disease: Rate of change of serum creatinine concentration. *Kidney Int* 11:62, 1977
88. Cestero RVM, Thunberg B, Jain VK: Diagnostic value of modelled therapy: nutritio.al status and technical problems of treatment. *Dial Transpl* 10:302, 1981
89. Acchiardo SR, Moore LW: Urea kinetics: the possibility of selectively-reduced treatment frequency. *Dial Transpl* 10:295, 1981
90. Olsson P, Lagergen H, Er S: The elimination from plasma of intravenous heparin. *Acta Med Scand* 173:619, 1963
91. Eiber HB, Danishefsky I, Borelli JJ: Studies with radioactive heparin in humans. *Angiology* 2:40, 1960
92. Estes JW: The kinetics of heparin. *Ann N Y Acad Sci* 179:187, 1971
93. Christensen HN: General concepts of neutrality regulation. *Am J Surg* 103:286, 1962
94. Christensen HN: *Diagnostic Biochemistry: Quantitative Distributions of Body Constituents and Their Physiological Interpretation.* New York, NY, Oxford University Press, 1959, p 122
95. Isaksson B: Urinary nitrogen output as a validity test in dietary surveys. *Am J Clin Nutr* 33:4, 1980
96. Gotch F, Sargent J: Measurement of H^+ balance (H^+b) during acetate and bicarbonate dialysis (AD, BD) therapy. *Abstracts Am Soc Nephrol* 12:117A, 1979
97. Relman AS, Schwartz WB: The effects of DOCA on electrolyte balance in normal man and its relation to sodium chloride intake. *Yale J Biol Med* 24:540, 1952
98. Schwartz WB, Jenson RL, Relman SA: The disposition of acid administered to sodium – depleted subjects: the renal response and the role of the whole body buffers. *J Clin Invest* 33:587, 1954
99. Schwartz WB, Orning KJ, Porter R: The internal distribution of hydrogen ions with varying degrees of metabolic acidosis. *J Clin Invest* 36:373, 1957
100. Hunt JH: The influence of dietary sulfur on the urinary output of acid in man. *Clin Sci* 5:119, 1956
101. Mion CM, Hegstrom RM, Boen ST, Scribner BH: Substitution of sodium acetate for sodium bicarbonate in the bath fluid for hemodialysis. *Trans Am Soc Artif Intern Organs* 10:110, 1964
102. Grimsrud L, Cole JJ, Lehman GA, Babb AL, Scribner BH: A central system for the continuous preparation and distribution of hemodialysis fluid. *Trans Am Soc Artif Intern Organs,* 10:107, 1964
103. Sargent JA, Gotch FA, Lam MA, Prowitt M, Keen, ML: Technical aspects of on line proportioning of bicarbonate dialysate, *Proc Clin Dial Transpl Forum* 7:109, 1977
104. Krebs HA: The biochemical lesions in ketosis. *Arch Intern Med* 107:119, 1961
105. Lundquist F: Production and utilization of free acetate in man. *Nature* 193:579, 1962
106. Kaiser BA, Potter DE, Bryant RE, Vreman HJ, Weiner MW: Acid-base changes and acetate metabolism during routine and high-efficiency hemodialysis in children. *Kidney Int* 19:70, 1981
107. Swan RC, Pitts RF: Neutralization of infused acid by nephrectomized dogs. *J Clin Invest* 34:205, 1955
108. Gotch FA, Borah MF, Keen ML, Lam MA, Prowitt M, Sargent JA: The solute kinetics of intermittent dialysis therapy. *Third Annual Report to Artificial Kidney – Chronic Uremia Program* NIAMDD 1977, p 48 (unpublished)
109. Garella S, Dana CL, Chazan JA: Severity of metabolic acidosis as a determinant of bicarbonate requirements. *N Engl J Med* 289:121, 1973
110. Edelman IS, Leibman J, O'Meara MP, Birkenfeld LW: Interrelations between serum sodium concentration, serum osmolarity and total exchangeable sodium, total exchangeable potassium and total body water. *J Clin Invest* 37:1236, 1958
111. Maffly RH: The body fluids: volume, composition, and physical chemistry. In *The Kidney,* edited by Brenner BM, Rector FC Jr, Philadelphia PA, WB Saunders Company, 1976, p 65
112. Dombec DH, Klein E, Wendt RP: Evaluation of two pool model for predicting serum creatinine levels during intra and interdialytic periods. *Trans Am Soc Artif Intern Organs* 21:117, 1975
113. Sanfelippo ML, Hall DA, Walker WE, Swenson RS: Quantitative evaluation of hemodialysis therapy using a

simple mathematical model and a programmable pocket calculator. *Trans Am Soc Artif Intern Organs*, 21:125, 1975
114. Katz MA, Hull AR: Transcellular creatinine disequilibrium and its significance in hemodialysis. *Nephron* 12:171, 1974
115. Jones JD, Burnett PC: Implication of creatinine and gut flora in the uremic syndrome: Induction of 'creatininase' in colon contents of the rat by dietary creatinine. *Clin Chem* 18:280, 1972
116. Jones JD, Burnett PC: Creatinine metabolism in humans with decreased renal function: creatinine deficit. *Clin Chem* 20:1204, 1974
117. Mitch WE, Walser M: A proposed mechanism for reduced creatinine excretion in severe chronic renal failure. *Nephron* 21:248, 1978
118. Wehle B, Asaba H, Castenfors J, Fürst P, Grahn A, Gunnarson B, Shaldon S, Bergström J: The influence of dialysis fluid composition on the blood pressure response during diaysis. *Clin Nephrol* 10:62, 1978
119. Ogden DA: A double crossover comparison of high and low sodium dialysis. *Proc Clin Dial Transpl Forum* 8:157, 1978
120. Van Stone JC, Cook J: Decreased postdialysis fatigue with increased dialysate sodium concentration. *Proc Clin Dial Transpl Forum* 8:152, 1978
121. Quellhorst E, Reiger J, Doht B, Beckman H, Jacob I, Kraft B, Mietzsch G, Scheler F: Treatment of chronic uraemia by an ultrafiltration kidney – first clinical experience. *Proc Eur Dial Transpl Assoc* 13:314, 1976.
122. Maekawa M, Kishimoto T, Ohyama T, Tanaka H: Present status of hemofiltration and hemodiafiltration in Japan. *Artif Organs* 4:85, 1980.
123. Kakagwa S: Multifactorial evaluation of hemofiltration therapy in comparison with conventional hemodialysis. *Artif Organs* 4:94, 1980
124. Streicher E, Schneider H: Clinical experience in hemofiltration. *Int J Artif Organs* 3:221, 1980
125. Schneider H, Streicher D, Hachmann H, Chmiel H, von Mylius U: Clinical experience with haemofiltration. *Proc Eur Dial Transpl Assoc* 14:136, 1977
126. Baldamus CA, Knobloch M, Schoeppe W, Koch KM: Hemodialysis/hemofiltration. A report of a controlled cross-over study. *Int J Artif Organs* 3:211, 1980
127. Shaldon S, Beau MC, Claret G, Deschodt G, Oulès R, Ramperez P, Mion H, Mion C: Haemofiltration with sorbent regeneration of ultrafiltrate: first clinical experience in end stage renal disease. *Proc Eur Dial Transpl Assoc* 15:220, 1978
128. Shaldon S, Deschodt G, Beau MC, Claret G, Mion H, Mion C: Vascular stability during high flux haemofiltration (HF). *Proc Eur Dial Transpl Assoc* 16:695, 1979
129. Shaldon S, Beau MC, Deschodt G, Ramperez P, Mion C: Vascular stability during haemofiltration. *Trans Am Soc Artif Intern Organs* 26:391, 1980
130. Baldamus CA, Ernst W, Fassbinder W, Koch KM: Differing haemodynamic stability due to differing sympathetic response: comparison of ultrafiltration, haemodialysis and haemofiltration. *Proc Eur Dial Transpl Assoc* 17:205, 1980
131. Shaldon S, Beau MC, Deschodt G, Flavier JL, Gullberg CA, Ramperez P, Mion C: Two years clinical experience with short hour high efficiency haemofiltration (HF). *Abstracts Clin Dial Transpl Forum*, p 52, 1980
132. Quellhorst E, Schuenemann B, Hildebrand U, Falda Z: Response of the vascular system to different modifications of haemofiltration and haemodialysis. *Proc Eur Dial Transpl Assoc* 17:197, 1980

133. Edelman IS, Leibman J: Anatomy of body water and electrolytes. *Am J Med* 27:256, 1959
134. Flear CTG, Bhattacharya SS, Sung CM: Solute and water exchanges between cells and extracellular fluids in health and disturbances after trauma. *J Parenteral Enteral Nutr* 4:98, 1980
135. Feig PU, Shook A, Sterns RH: Effect of potassium removal during hemodialysis on the plasma potassium concentration. *Nephron* 27:25, 1981
136. Feig PU, Pring M, Guzzo J, Singer I: Disposition of intravenous potassium in anuric man: A kinetic analysis. *Kidney Int* 15:651, 1979
137. Donnan FG: The theory of membrane equilibria. *Chem Review* 1:73, 1924
138. Gotch FA, Lam MA, Prowitt M, Keen ML: Preliminary clinical results with sodium-volume modeling of hemodialysis therapy. *Proc Clin Dial Transpl Forum* 10:12, 1980
139. Burzynski SR: Biologically active peptides in human urine: I. Isolation of a group of medium size peptides. *Physiol Chem Physics* 5:437, 1973
140. Scribner BH, Babb AL: Evidence for toxins of middle molecular weight. *Kidney Int* 7 (Suppl 3):349, 1975
141. Shinaberger JH, Miller JH, Rosenblatt MG, Gardner PW, Carpenter GW, Martin FE: Clinical studies of 'low flow' dialysis with membranes highly permeable to middle weight molecules. *Trans Am Soc Artif Intern Organs* 18:82, 1972
142. Rattazzi T, Wathen R, Comty C, Raij L, Leonard A, Shapiro F: The comparison of low flow (Q_D 200) to regular flow (Q_D 500) dialysis. *Trans Am Soc Artif Organs* 20:402, 1974
143. Ginn HE, Teschan PE, Walker PJ, Bourne JR, Macalyne F, Ward JW, McLain LW, Johnson HB, Hamel B: Neurotoxicity in uremia. *Kidney Int* 7 (Suppl 3):S357, 1975
144. Tenckhoff H, Curtis FK: Experience with maintenance peritoneal dialysis in the home. *Trans Am Soc Artif Intern Organs* 16:90, 1970
145. Gotch FA: A quantitative evaluation of small and middle molecule toxicity in therapy of uremia. *Dial Transpl* 9:183, 1980
146. Gotch FA, Sargent JA: Modelling of middle molecules in clinical studies. Symposium on present status and future orientation of middle molecules in uremia and other diseases. *Artif Organs* 4:133, 1980
147. Henderson LW, Stone RA, Ford CA, Lysaght MJ: Blood pressure control with hemodiafiltration. *Proc 10th Annu Contractons' Conf Artif Kidney – Chronic Uremia Program* NIAMDD DHEW Publication No. (NIH) 77:1442, 1977, p 110
148. Funck-Brentano JL, Man NK, Sausse A, Cueille G, Zingraff J, Drueke T, Jungers P, Billon JP: Neuropathy and 'middle' molecule toxins. *Kidney Int* 7 (Suppl 3):S352, 1975
149. Gulyassy PRF, Peters JH, Lin SC, Ryan PM: Hemodialysis and plasma amino acid composition in chronic renal failure. *Am J Clin Nutr* 21:565, 1968
150. Bartsch HJ: *Handbook of Mathematical Formulas*. Translated by Liebscher H, New York NY, Academic Press, 1974, p 139
151. Cottini ERP, Gallina DK, Dominguez JE: Urea excretion in adult humans with varying degrees of kidney malfunction fed milk, egg or an amino acid mixture: Assessment of nitrogen balance. *J Nutr* 103:11, 1973
152. Bleiler RE, Schedl HP: Creatinine excretion: variability in relationship to diet and body size. *J Lab Clin Med* 59:945, 1962

153. Harmon WE, Spinozzi N, Meyer A, Grupe WE: Use of protein catabolic rate to monitor pediatric hemodialysis. *Dial Transpl* 10:324, 1981
154. Sargent JA, Gotch FA: Nutrition and treatment of the acutely ill patient using urea kinetics. *Dial Transpl* 10:314, 1981
155. Sargent JA: Urea mass balance: Nutrition and treatment of the acutely ill patient. *Nutritional Support Services* 2 (No. 2):33, 1982
156. Cuthbertson DP: The metabolic response to injury and its nutritional implications: retrospect and prospect. *J Parenter Enter Nutr* 3:1078, 1979
157. Long JM, Wilmore DW, Mason AD: Effect of carbohydrate and fat intake on nitrogen excretion during total intravenous feeding. Ann Surg, 185:417, 1977
158. Clowes GHA Jr, O'Donnell TF Jr, Blackburn GL, Maki TN: Energy metabolism and proteolysis in traumatized and septic man. *Surg Clin North Am* 56:1169, 1976
159. Clowes GHA Jr, O'Donnell TF Jr, Ryan NT: Energy metabolism in sepsis: treatment based on different patterns in shock and high output stage. *Ann Surg* 179:684, 1974
160. Wolfe BM, Culebras JM, Sim AJW, Ball MR, Moore FD: Substrate interaction in intravenous feeding: comparative effects of carbohydrate and fat on amino acid utilization in fasting man. *Ann Surg* 186:518, 1977

4

MEMBRANES

DONALD J. LYMAN

Introduction	97
Cellulosic membranes	98
New membranes for artificial kidney use	99
Non-cellulosic membranes	99
Crosslinked water-soluble polymers	99
Poly-N-vinylpyrrolidone membranes	99
Polyvinyl alcohol membranes	99
Precipitated polyelectrolyte membranes	99
Polypeptide membranes	100
Poly α-aminoacid membranes	100
Collagen membranes	100
Block copolymer membranes	100
Copolyether-ester membranes	100
Copolyether-urethane membranes	101

Copolyether-carbonate membranes	101
Modifications of non-water swellable films	102
Radiation grafted membranes	102
Nucleopore membranes	102
Nylon/epoxy membranes	102
Polyacrylonitrile membranes	102
Membranes based on cellulose	102
Cellulose-acetate membranes	102
Ultra-thin membranes	103
Sorbent membranes	103
Membranes currently under clinical trials	103
Membrane sterilization and leachables	104
References	104

INTRODUCTION

A membrane may be defined as an imperfect barrier between two fluids, thus implying that fluid mass is transported unevenly with the result that mixtures may be separated (1–3). In the most general sense, this definition would encompass the more common polymer membranes, the bilayer membranes believed to be surrounding living cells, liquid membranes, metal, glass and fabric ultrafilters, as well as vapor gaps (i.e. no material at all). A variety of processes can also be used to facilitate separation and can influence the type of membrane used.

These membrane processes can be grouped into nine major categories: membrane permeation, dialysis, osmosis, reverse osmosis, membrane filtration, electrodialysis, electrodecantation, thermo-osmosis, and electron osmosis. Of primary importance to our discussion are the polymer membranes interposed between blood and a dialyzing fluid so as to effect exchange between these fluids, usually by the processes of dialysis and ultrafiltration.

The processes of dialysis and ultrafiltration have been investigated for over a century since the pioneering work of Graham and Fick in the 1850's (4, 5) (see also Chapter 2). Most of the studies in this period involved cellulosic membranes, initially the collodion or cellulose nitrate derivatives and later cellulose itself as a regenerated material. These membranes are essentially devoid of any charge or adsorption property. Transport through these membranes appears to be primarily due to passage of solute through 'micro holes' or pores in the membrane. In other words, the membrane acts as a microporous barrier or sieve, with the driving force for solute transport being a concentration gradient between the two separate fluids. Most theories of membrane diffusion are based on data obtained from cellulosic membranes. It was not until the middle of the 1930's with the expansion of the polymer industry that other polymeric materials, such as ion-exchange resins, were used as membranes for industrial applications.

The first blood dialyzers, developed by Abel, Rowntree and Turner, used tubular membranes prepared from cellulose nitrate (6). Problems in fabrication leading to poor reproducibility in properties contributed, along with other factors, to the slow acceptance of this device (7). It was not until the availability of a more consistently uniform regenerated cellulose membrane (cellulose tubes developed for sausage casings) that the stage was set for the successful clinical utilization of blood dialysis. In 1943, Kolff reported on the use of his rotating drum artificial kidney device to assist acute kidney failure patients, using tubular membranes of cellulose (8).

During the next 15 years, a variety of devices was explored as blood dialyzers, but the membrane remained essentially the same. That is, regenerated cellulose in tubular, then later in sheet form. Variations in the properties of these membranes reflected the differences in both the method and the reproducibility of preparation. It was not until after the successful pioneering efforts of Scribner and colleagues in 1960 in utilizing intermittent hemodialysis for endstage chronic kidney failure patients (9) that the question of new membranes, designed specially for artificial kidney devices, was examined. The success of the cellulose membrane in saving the life of the terminal renal failure patient, plus the lack of basic knowledge of what a membrane should accomplish in terms of separation (and conservation) of solutes from blood, made the search for a replacement membrane more difficult. Indeed, it is possible that we do not want a general purpose membrane (in which terms cellophane may be more ideal) but a series of membranes tailored to do a specific job, so that in combination they may more accurately perform the removal-retention functions shown by the natural kidney. Much of the effort in this area to develop new membranes came from the support of the Artificial Kidney – Chronic Uremia program of the National Institute of Arthritis Metabolism and Digestive Diseases in the USA (10–22), though earlier support from other sources, such as the John Hartford Foundation, initiated the quest.

A number of new, synthetic polymer membranes have been prepared and partially characterized. Many of these membranes appear to possess new and unusual separation properties. However, the lack of basic clinical knowledge on what needs to be accomplished by the membrane has prevented any judgment to be made on which might be the best membrane(s) for hemodialysis.

In the following sections, the general methods of polymer synthesis and membrane fabrication are discussed, along with selected data on solute dialysis to indicate the similarities and differences between various membranes.

CELLULOSIC MEMBRANES

The cellulose membranes that have been the basis for most hemodialysis treatments have been prepared by a regeneration process. Cellulose is a polysaccharide which does not melt below its decomposition temperature and dissolves only upon chemical reaction. Two major processes are used to form these regenerated cellulose membranes. The first involves solution of purified cellulose in sodium hydroxide, followed by an aging process to lower molecular weight oxidatively. Carbon disulfide is then added to convert this material to the cellulose xanthate. This gelatinous solution, called viscose, is then dissolved in excess sodium hydroxide and extruded in the form of a sheet into an acid bath to effect the regeneration of the cellulose and to coagulate the polymer into a membrane:

$$(R)\text{-OH} \xrightarrow{\text{NaOH}} (R)\text{-ONa} \xrightarrow{CS_2} (R)\text{-OCSNa} \xrightarrow{H^+} (R)\text{-OH}$$
$$\overset{\overset{\displaystyle S}{\displaystyle \|}}{}$$

Films made by this process are called cellophane or Visking tubing. The Cuprophan membrane (also called Cuprophane) is a regenerated cellulose prepared by a second process which involves the solubilization of cellulose in an ammonia solution of cupric oxide. This cuprammonium-cellulose complex is extruded into an acid bath to yield the regenerated cellulosic film:

$$(R)\text{-OH} \xrightarrow[\text{NH}_4\text{OH}]{\text{CuO}} (R)\text{-OCu(NH}_4)_4(\text{OH})_2 \xrightarrow{H^+} (R)\text{-OH}$$

Structural differences in the film do occur as a result of the method of film formation and result in slight differences in dialysis and ultrafiltration properties. These are due to differences in the microstructure or morphology of the membranes and result in somewhat higher diffusion rates to be observed for the Cuprophan membranes. However, variations in a production run of either film often cause greater differences in dialysis and ultrafiltration properties than those observed between the two types. In addition, differences in dialysis and ultrafiltration can also result from unsuitable storage conditions. For example, to preserve permeability and ultrafiltration properties, Cuprophan should be stored at 20 to 25 °C and a relative humidity between 35 and 40% if unpacked (the original packing Cuprophan may be stored at any temperature and humidity). However, the material should be gradually brought to room temperature to avoid condensation of water vapor on the membrane surface. More recently, the Artificial Kidney-Chronic Uremia program of NIAMDD has sponsored research to define the manufacturing and processing parameters necessary to yield optimum and reproducible regenerated cellulose membranes (11–13, 23).

The work of many investigators, especially that of Craig (24), has shown that a wide range of membrane porosity can be obtained by mechanical stretching of wet membranes. If the stretching is done in a biaxial manner, for example, by subjecting a cellulose tubing to hydrostatic pressure, the pores are enlarged and the resulting membrane allows ready passage of solutes that were barely able to diffuse before. If the stretching is done in a linear manner, for example, by the longitudinal stretching of a film, solutes which formerly diffused through the unstretched film at a reasonable rate, now barely pass through the membrane. Stretching of the film in a linear manner can be visualized as changing the shape of the holes in the membrane from a circular to an elliptical shape, thereby reducing the effective diameter of the passage. Since transfer is due primarily to passage of solute through micropores, the permeability is directly related to the molecular volume (which often is approximated by the molecular weight) of the diffusing solute and the size of the pore. Thus, Craig, showed that the half-time rates of transfer for ribonuclease were 6.6 h for the unstretched membrane, 0.9 h for the biaxially stretched membrane, and 17.5 h for the linearly stretched membrane. While this technique offers an interesting method of changing the size of the holes and thereby the size of the molecules that will pass through the membrane, this change can only be made within certain limits without adversely affecting the integrity of the film.

Larger pores have been obtained by swelling and annealing of films at elevated temperatures, by forming networks in the films by extracting compounds which had been dispersed in the original film, or by chemical reactions with the membrane material (24–27, Lyman DJ unpublished work). An example of this latter method, in which cellulose membranes were treated with aqueous $ZnCl_2$ solutions, has given membranes which were reported to be permeable to solutes having molecular weights as high as 134 000 (dimer of serum albumin) (24). In a similar manner, the porosity of the cellulose film can be decreased by suitable chemical reactions. For example controlled acetylation of the membrane with acetic anhydride-pyridine mixtures has been very effective in producing membranes with reduced pore sizes (24).

However, since the primary action of the cellulose membrane is that of a sieve, there is little selectivity in the separation of molecules which are closely related in size except when their size is approximately that of the pore. When this occurs, there is the possibility that forces acting between the solute and the surface of the pore channel come into play and influence the rate of transfer. If the pores are enlarged to obtain improved rate for transfer of large molecules, a loss of selectivity of smaller molecules results. All commercial cellulosic film materials appear to be similar to cellophane in this respect.

NEW MEMBRANES FOR ARTIFICIAL KIDNEY USE

The establishment of the Artificial Kidney-Chronic Uremia program of NIAMD in 1966, was the major driving force in the search for new synthetic polymers for dialysis membranes. The limitations inherent in the current regenerated cellulose membranes led investigators to search for new membranes that might more directly imitate the function of the natural kidney in its overall efficiency and in its selectivity for solute removal. These studies have ranged from the synthesis of homogeneous membranes to the preparation of membranes having heterogeneous and asymmetric structures, and have led to the development of many interesting membrane systems, test dialyzers and new theories of diffusion. However, new developments in membrane research depend upon (a), basic knowledge on what must be removed (or retained) for the best patient maintenance and (b), research combined with actual clinical trials and (c), financing.

In the following sections, the synthesis and fabrication of many of the new membrane materials which came out of this early search for improved artificial kidney membranes are briefly described. Selected membrane properties are also reported to indicate the differences between various membranes. The dialysis properties were often measured using a variety of diffusion cells and techniques; for example, the simple Relative Cell (28), the Rotating Dialysis Cell (29), the Thin Film Dialysis Cell (30), the Babb-Grimsrud Miniature Artificial Kidney Cell (31), the modified Katchalsky Cell (32), and the Leonard-Bluemle Cell (33). Each of these cells is useful for measuring diffusion though the variables controlled in each cell are different. More recently, in the USA a Membrane Evaluation Study Group has recommended more standardized procedures for assessing membranes (34, 35).

Non-cellulosic membranes

Crosslinked water-soluble polymers
Water-soluble polymers can be made into a water-insoluble gel structure by interconnecting the polymer chains into a three-dimensional network structure. This crosslinking may be achieved in a variety of ways; for example, by reaction of –OH or –NH groups in the polymer with formaldehyde, glutaraldehyde, or a di-isocyanate; by incorporating a divinyl monomer into the polymerization of a water soluble vinyl monomer; by the formation of a polymeric salt from mixtures of a polycation and polyanion. Since the crosslinking renders the material intractable, the membrane must be formed prior to or during the crosslinking step. In general, the rate of dialysis is inversely related to the degree of cross-linking of the membrane whereas the mechanical strength is directly related to the degree of crosslinking.

Poly-N-vinylpyrrolidone membranes. These membranes were of interest since the polyvinylpyrrolidones (PVP) are compatible with blood. The membranes were prepared by mixing a solution of PVP in N,N-dimethylformamide and pyridine with 5 to 20% by weight methylene bis(4-phenyl isocyanate) (MDI). Films were cast at once since gelation occurs within minutes. These films were highly swollen in water and one film crosslinked with 10% MDI had a half-time rate of urea transfer three times as fast as gel cellophane (36). A major disadvantage appeared to be the poor wet strength of the membrane.

Polyvinyl alcohol membranes. In the early 1960's polyvinylalcohol (PVA) membranes were investigated as dialysis membranes by Shaldon. These membranes, obtained commercially from Japan, were prepared by crosslinking PVA films containing about 10% glytaraldehyde by the action of aqueous HCl. Shaldon's *in vitro* and *in vivo* data indicated diffusion properties two to three times slower for urea, creatinine, uric acid and dextrose than that shown for Cuprophan (unpublished observations, personal communication of Dr Shaldon (University of Nîmes, France) to the author, 1965).

Other membranes prepared from water-soluble polymers include those from polyoxyethylene glycol crosslinked with MDI and polyoxypropylene triol, polyhydroxyethyl methacrylate crosslinked via ethylene dimethacrylate (the HEMA hydrogels). In general, when sufficient mechanical strength was obtained, the dialyzing properties of these membranes (for urea) were slower than of cellophane.

Precipitated polyelectrolyte membranes. A new type of membrane composed of a precipitated gel resulting from the interaction of a polystyrene sulfonic acid and a polyvinylbenzyltrimethyl ammonium hydroxide was developed by the Amicon Corp., Cambridge, MA, USA:

These Dia-Flo membranes have been widely studied for hemodiafiltration (37, 38). These membranes show higher clearances of intermediate molecular weight solutes and higher ultrafiltration than does Cuprophan. One possible problem with these membranes, which might be correctable by modification of the composition, is the adherence of a layer of protein to the membrane surface due to a concentration polarization (37).

Polypeptide membranes

A variety of polypeptide membranes have been investigated, ranging from naturally occurring materials which have been crosslinked (i.e. solubilized collagen and albumin) to synthetic co-polypeptides which can be made cationic, anionic or non-ionic by proper choice of aminoacids and/or post-treatments.

Poly α-aminoacid membranes. A variety of homopolymers, random and block copolymers based on methyl-L-glutamate have been synthesized and characterized (11–19, 39). The aminoacid polymers are synthesized via their N-carboxy-anhydrides (see formule A below).

especially for higher molecular weight solutes, compared to Cuprophan (15) (Table 1).

Collagen membranes. Collagen is uniquely suited for preparing membranes since it can be easily isolated and purified, solubilized and cast into films, then crosslinked to give an insoluble hydrogel. The collagen used in these dialysis experiments was from calf skin, which had been treated to isolate the soluble collagen fraction. Membranes were then solvent cast from acetic acid onto polyethylene and air dried. The films were then washed with ammonium hydroxide, followed by acetone-water mixtures, then crosslinked by UV irradiation or by heating at 110 °C (40).

The collagen membranes can be made with a wide variety of permeability properties by varying the degree of crosslinking and by chemically blocking the positively and negatively charged amino acid side groups. In general, the membranes having good strength properties, dialyzed low molecular weight solutes similar to Cuprophan, but showed improved dialysis rates for solutes with a greater molecular mass than 500 daltons (41, 42).

A) $H_2N-CH-COOH \xrightarrow{COCl_2}$ ... $\xrightarrow{H_2O}$ $\{NH-CH-CO\}_n$

Co-monomers that have been used in the polymerization include L-lysine, L-leucine, DL-methionine and DL-leucine. By proper choice of comonomer, followed by removal of any blocking agent, one can obtain anionic, cationic, or neutral polymers. Films are usually solvent cast from ethylene dichloride and tetrachloroethylene. In some instances, inclusion of a water soluble additive, such as polyoxyethylene glycol, in the film forming step improves porosity.

Of particular interest was the membrane prepared from polymethyl glutamate. *In vitro* tests seemed to indicate that this material had good compatibility, good mechanical properties and improved dialysis properties,

Table 1. Polymethyl glutamate membrane resistance for various solutes, min/cm.

Solute	Polymethyl glutamate-6000	Cuprophan
Urea	21.5	18.4
Creatinine	32.5	32.8
Uric Acid	38.0	39.1
Sucrose	49.9	67.1
Raffinose	67	112
Vitamin B-12	73	205
Bacitracin	101	450

Block copolymer membranes

A variety of block copolymers ranging from the typical ABA type to the multiple block $(AB)_n$ type have been explored as membrane materials. These latter multiple block copolymers represent the first attempts at molecular tailoring of membranes to achieve selectivity in diffusion based on both solute size and chemical structure. These types of copolymers are based on combining a water soluble chain segment or block to impart water swelling and selectivity to the membrane and a hydrophobic block to impart mechanical strength.

Copolyether-ester membranes: The first of these multiple block copolymers to be studied were based on polyoxethylene glycol and polyethylene terephthalate (28) and were prepared by melt polymerization:

$$2\ CH_3OC-\bigcirc-COCH_3 + HOCH_2CH_2OH + HO(CH_2CH_2O)_mH \xrightarrow{\Delta}$$

$$\left[\left(C-\bigcirc-C-OCH_2CH_2\right)_n \left(OC-\bigcirc-CO(CH_2CH_2O)_m\right)\right]_x$$

They could be dissolved in solvents like dichloromethane and solution cast into clear tough films. Compar-

Table 2. Relative half-time escape rates/min for a copolyester membrane containing 30% polyethylene glycol, 1540 daltons.

Solute	Copolyester membrane	Cuprophan
Urea	58	68
Creatinine	117	123
Uric Acid	217	320
Dextrose	268	223
Raffinose	930	450
Bacitracin	568	720
Insulin	26% in 30 hours	None

Table 3. Relative half-time escape rates/min for four copolyether-urethane membranes *.

Solute	I	II	III	IV
Urea	122	153	164	115
Creatinine	214	364	309	360
Dextrose	390	820	665	1080

* Contains 70 mole % of: I. cis/trans 1,4-cyclohexanediol; II. trans 1,4-cyclohexanediol; III. 1,5-pentanediol; IV. α,α'-dihydroxy-p-xylene.

ison of dialysis rates through one of these membranes showed faster dialysis of certain solutes as compared to Cuprophan (Table 2).

Apparently, these differences are based on both solubility and viscosity effects between the solute-water-polyoxyethylene segments. However, the lack of long-term hydrolytic stability of these membranes would limit their uses. Replacement of the ester linkage by the more hydrolytically stable carbonate linkage has shown promise in improving membrane stability.

Copolyether-urethane membranes. These copolymers were prepared by a two-step solution polymerization method (43) (see formula A below).

Films could be solvent cast from N,N-dimethyl formamide solutions of the copolymers in a 75°C forced draft oven. Striking variations in solute transport were observed as the chemical structure of the hydrophobic block was changed (Table 3). Preliminary studies indicate that differences in domain-matrix phase separation, influencing solute solubility and solute-water-membrane viscosity are principal factors in these diffusion differences (44).

Copolyether-carbonate membranes. The substitution of a carbonate linkage $-Ar-O-\overset{\overset{O}{\|}}{C}-O-Ar-$, in place of the ester linkage, $-Ar-\overset{\overset{O}{\|}}{C}-OCH_2-$, gave membranes with improved hydrolytic stability (13–19). These block polymers can be prepared by adding a Bisphenol-A capped polyoxyethylene glycol to the normal polycarbonate synthesis (see formule B below).

Table 4. Membrane clearance, ml/min of copolyether-polycarbonate membrane.

Solute	Polycarbonate membrane	Cuprophan
Urea	120.0	124.0
Creatinine	92.0	86.0
Sucrose	67.0	60.0
Vitamin B-12	43.0	22.0
Inulin	7.0	4.4

The optimum mechanical and dialysis properties were obtained with copolymers containing 25% polyethylene glycol of 6000 daltons. Membranes can be solvent cast from chloroform and either air dried or using methanol for gelation of the membrane; or alternatively by using a water miscible solvent and water for the membrane gelation step. This membrane showed ultra-filtrating properties 2 to 5 times that of Cuprophan and much better middle molecule permeability than Cuprophan (18, 45, [see Table 4]). In addition, this membrane can be easily heat sealed, thus allowing the formation of membrane envelopes.

Modifications of non-water swellable films
The ready availability of commercial hydrophobic film materials have led many investigators to investigate methods of treating these films so as to develop possible dialysis membranes. The use of high energy radiation to make holes in films or to graft water-soluble monomers onto films are notable examples of these methods. Another method is to introduce extractable additives into the hydrophobic film. Examples of these are discussed below.

Radiation grafted membranes. A number of investigators have explored the use of radiation grafting of water-soluble monomers onto non-water soluble films. This represents an attempt to modify inexpensive preformed films by radiation grafting processes. Typically water soluble monomers which have been used include vinyl alcohol (via the acetate, followed by hydrolysis), N-vinylpyrrolidine, acrylamide, acrylic acid and N-vinyl pyridine; typical films used as substrates include polyethylene, polypropylene, poly(4-methylpentene-1), polytetrafluoroethylene etc.

In general, better dialysis properties were obtained at high degrees of grafting, at which point the strength properties of the membranes decrease rapidly. However, the N-vinylpyrrolidone grafted poly(4-methylpentene-1) films did show adequate strength with dialysis properties similar to Cuprophan (46).

Nucleopore membranes. These membranes were prepared by a two-step process called 'track-etch'. The first step consists of bombarding a dielectric film, such as poly-bisphenol-A-carbonate, with massive energetic nuclear (^{235}U fission) fragments. These produce narrow trails, or 'tracks', of radiation damage as they pass through the film. The second step is the etching of the film with NaOH which selectively dissolves the damaged material. This leaves straight-through cylindrical pores of quite uniform diameter, in contrast to pores in other films that are of variable diameter and quite tortuous in path.

Nylon/epoxy membranes. The incorporation of a water miscible solvent into the casting solution of a hydrophobic polymer can result in a membrane having sufficient water passage (even though it is essentially non-swellable), to act as a good dialysis membrane. Of note is the work (47) on nylon/epoxy membranes which were prepared from a solution of Dupont Elvamide 8061 in methanol-trichloroethylene to which had been added 10 to 25% Epon 828 and 130% of dimethyl sulfoxide. The films were air dried, then extracted with water. The addition of the dimethyl sulfoxide is the key to the improved dialysis performance. The epoxy appears to add stability to the storage of the wet membrane. A membrane containing 25% epoxy had adequate strength at a 0.7 mm film thickness, and showed the following improvements over Cuprophan permeability: urea 35%, creatinine 45%, uric acid 30% and NaCl 20%.

Polyacrylonitrile membranes (see also Chapter 14). Two industrial groups (Monsanto (48) and Rhône-Poulenc (49)) have used copolymerization of acrylonitrile (with methylvinyl pyridine and sodium methallyl sulfonate) coupled with a fabrication process to achieve a workable hemodialysis membrane from a normally hydrophobic polymer. Both types of these polyacrylonitrile membranes have shown increased ultrafiltration with similar or slightly better dialysis properties than Cuprophan, especially in the middle molecular weight range (49) (see Table 5).

Membranes based on cellulose

The initial success with cellophane and Cuprophan membranes has led researchers to investigate the use of reverse osmosis membrane technologies developed in water desalination programs. These membranes were usually based on cellulose acetate and prepared from polymer solutions containing swelling agents and other additives (50). By controlling the additives and the film casting conditions, anisotropic membranes can be formed possessing a very thin, essentially dense skin on one surface, with the remainder of the membrane being a highly porous structure that serves as a support.

Cellulose acetate membranes
The membranes prepared for artificial kidney uses were usually cast from 60/40 acetone-formamide mixtures (by

Table 5. Polyacrylonitrile membrane permeability, cm/min 10^3.

Solute	Polyacrylonitrile (R-P)	Cuprophan
Urea	95.2	66.6
Creatinine	55.5	33.3
Dextrose	45.4	22.2
Sucrose	31.2	11.7
Inulin	4.1	0.4

Table 6. Permeabilities (cm/min 10³) of membranes based on cellulose.

Solute	Cellulose acetate	Cuprophan
Urea	22.5	20.7
Creatinine	28.5	24.4
Vitamin B-12	9.1	1.9
Inulin	1.6	0.1

Table 7. Membrane clearance, ml/min of ultra-thin cellulose membrane.

Solute	Ultra-thin membrane	Cuprophan
Urea	48	37
Creatinine	35	29
Uric Acid	34	22
Vitamin B-12	9	8

weight) (13–18, 21). They showed permeability properties 2 to 8 times better (especially for higher molecular weight solutes) and ultrafiltration rates 2 to 20 times faster than Cuprophan. Annealing the high flux membrane in hot water (85°C for 10 min) reduces water and solute permeabilities to more optimum levels (Table 6). This technology could also be adapted to the fabrication of hollow fibers. Permeability properties can be further modified by partially hydrolyzing the acetate group (i.e. partially regenerating the cellulose).

Ultra-thin membranes

Other workers (13–19) investigated the use of ultra-thin membranes (0.15 to 1.5 μ), similar to the skin formed in the anisotropic desalination membranes described above, but without the coarse backing membrane. These were prepared by casting a solution of nitrocellulose onto water (51). Evaporation and diffusion of solvent into the water leads to an ultra-thin membrane which was then converted to cellulose by treatment with alcoholic ammonium hydroxide. Similar films could be made from cellulose acetate (17). The film was then attached to a sheer nylon tricot support backing. These ultra-thin membranes have shown 100% increases in permeabilities to solutes such as sucrose and 25% increase in permeability to solutes such as vitamin B-12. The ultrafiltration was three times that of Cuprophan PT 150. More typical data are given in Table 7.

Sorbent membranes

The application of sorbents in extracorporeal circulation has shown promise of treatment of drug intoxication, as well as assisting in the removal of more conventional solutes in the traditional artificial kidney. Of interest recently, has been sorption-dialysis techniques where a membrane is used to prevent direct interaction of the sorbent with blood (22, 52). The Enka sorbent membranes, utilizing a Cuprophan membrane with a backing of a carbon sorbent in a cellulose matrix (available in hollow fiber, tubing, or sheet form), are currently being evaluated (52).

MEMBRANES CURRENTLY UNDER CLINICAL TRIALS

Some of the membranes described in the previous section have undergone preliminary clinical trials. Their selection appeared to be based on (a), the ease of scaled-up synthesis and membrane fabrication and (b), improved *in vitro* solute diffusion and (or) ultrafiltration characteristics as compared to the standard Cuprophan membrane. These include the polypeptide membrane based on polymethyl glutamate (Gulf South Research Institute, USA), the block copolyether-carbonate (National Institute for Scientific Research, USA), the polyacrylonitrile (Rhône-Poulenc, France), the Dia-Flo precipitated polymer complex (Amicon, USA), the cellulose acetate (Celanese, USA) and regenerated ultrathin cellulose (North Star Research Institute, USA) membranes (14–22, 35, 51), and regenerated cellulose hollow fibers (Cordis Dow, USA) and anisotropic polysulfone hollow fibers (Amicon Corp., USA) (35). Selected membrane permeability data are shown in Table 8 for some of these membranes. While patient well-being (i.e. less nausea, improvement of neuropathy, etc.) seem to be obtained with all of these membranes, with the non-cellulosic material the hematocrits also improved. However, the *in vivo* dialysis data of small molecules did not show the results one would expect from *in vitro* data.

Table 8. Selected membrane permeability data *.

Solute	Molecular weight	Cuprophan	Celanese 3×	Rhône-Poulenc RP-AN-69	NISR M-37-36-29	Amicon PMD Hollow fiber	Cordis Dow Hollow fiber
Urea	60	11.5	9.22	15.5	17.7	8.21	6.67
Creatinine	113	5.82	4.74	9.38	9.22	5.59	3.65
Dextrose (anhydrous)	180	3.75	2.86	6.88	5.59	3.97	2.28
Sucrose	342	1.76	2.68	4.87	4.42	3.21	1.22
Raffinose	504	1.62	1.44	4.09	2.98	–	–
Vitmin B-12	1355	0.59	0.84	2.66	1.80	1.46	0.26
Inulin	5200	0.12	0.25	0.88	0.30	0.28	0.04
Ultrafiltration rate × 10⁵ (ml/cm²-sec-atm)	–	5.05	11.1	63.9	7.94	45.3	2.58

* A Kaufman-Leonard stirred batch dialyzer cell (33) was used. (Data are from [21] and [35]).

For example, the copolyether-carbonate membrane showed *in vivo* dialysance coefficients similar to Cuprophan for small solutes (53). However, for solutes greater than 1000 molecular weight, the copolyether-carbonate membrane was somewhat more efficient in removal. Part of this may be due to the fact that dialyzer design can influence membrane permeabilities. Also, preliminary data in our laboratory has indicated that for membranes in which transport is influenced by membrane-solute interactions, dialysis rates of a single solute can be different when it is mixed with other solutes.

MEMBRANE STERILIZATION AND LEACHABLES

The toxicologic potential of a polymer material must be assessed when it is brought in contact with the blood. A variety of screening tests including the Pyrogen test, the Hemolysis test, the Tissue culture-Agar Overlay test, the Tissue culture ICG test, the Intradermal test in Rabbits, Systemic Toxicity test in mice and the Isolated Heart test (in rabbits) have been applied to this question (18, 19, 34, 35). Most polymers described in the previous sections can be controlled so that during manufacture toxic materials (reaction products or additives) are not retained in the membranes. However, in regard to this aspect it should be ascertained that only high quality membranes (and tubing) are supplied.

A greater problem is that of residual chemicals (formaldehyde, ethylene oxide, etc.) from sterilization procedures. The various polymers have different tendencies toward retention of these chemicals and as a result, they are not always completely removed by standard washing or degassing procedures. Any chemicals not removed can later be infused into the patient's blood. Studies have shown that gas chromatographic analysis is not always sufficient to detect residual formaldehyde; a better technique appears to be the acetyl-acetone test (54).

REFERENCES

1. Tuwiner SB: *Diffusion and Membrane Technology.* New York, Reinhold Publishing Corp, 1962
2. Friedlander HZ, Rickles RN: Membrane technology. Part II: Theory and development. *Anal Chem* 37:27A, 1965
3. Kesting RE: *Synthetic Polymer Membranes.* New York, McGraw-Hill Book Co, 1971
4. Graham T: The Bakerian Lecture – On Osmotic Force. *Phil Trans Roy Soc London* 144:177, 1854
5. Fick A: Ueber Diffusion. *Ann Physik Chem* 94:59, 1855
6. Abel JJ, Rowntree LG, Turner BB: On the removal of diffusable substances from the circulating blood of living animals by dialysis. *J Pharmacol Exp Ther* 5:275, 1913–14
7. Doyle JE: *Extracorporeal Hemodialysis Therapy in Blood Chemistry Disorders.* Springfield, IL, Charles C Thomas Publishers, 1962, p 11
8. Kolff WJ, Berk HTJ, ter Welle M, Van Der Ley AJW, Van Dijk EC, Van Noordwijk J: De kunstmatige nier; een dialysator met groot oppervlak. (The artificial kidney, a dialyzer with a large surface area). *Geneesk Gids* 21:409, 1943 (in Dutch)
9. Hegstrom RM, Murray JS, Pendras JP, Burnell JM, Scribner BH: Hemodialysis in the treatment of chronic uremia. *Trans Am Soc Artif Intern Organs* 7:136, 1961
10. *Proc Conf on Hemodialysis NIAMD and NHI,* edited by Connally NTJ, Publ Health Service publ no 1349, 1964
11. *Proc 1st Annu Contractors' Conf Artif Kidney Program of NIAMD,* edited by Lieberman RA, NIH Publ no 101, 1968
12. *Proc 2nd Annu Contractors' Conf Artif Kidney Program of NIAMD,* edited by Krueger KK, DHEW publ (NIH) 1969
13. *Proc 3rd Annu Contractors' Conf Artif Kidney Program of NIAMD,* edited by Krueger KK, DHEW publ (NIH), 1970
14. *Proc 4th Annu Contractors' Conf Artif Kidney Program of NIAMD,* edited by Krueger KK, DHEW publ (NIH), 1971
15. *Proc 5th Annu Contractors' Conf Artif Kidney Program of NIAMD,* edited by Krueger KK, DHEW publ no (NIH) 72-278, 1972
16. *Proc 6th Annu Contractors' Conf Artif Kidney Program of NIAMDD,* edited by Krueger KK, DHEW publ no (NIH) 74-248, 1973
17. *Proc 7th Annu Contractors' Conf Artif Kidney Program of NIAMDD,* edited by Krueger KK, DHEW publ no (NIH) 75-248, 1974
18. *Proc 8th Annu Contractors' Conf Artif Kidney Program of NIAMDD,* edited by Mackey BB, DHEW publ no (NIH) 76-248, 1975
19. *Proc 9th Annu Contractors' Conf Artif Kidney Program of NIAMDD,* edited by Mackey BB, DHEW publ no (NIH) 77-1167, 1976
20. *Proc 10th Annu Contractors' Conf Artif Kidney Program of NIAMDD,* edited by Mackey BB, DHEW publ no (NIH) 77-1442, 1977
21. *Proc 11th Annu Contractors' Conf Artif Kidney Program of NIAMDD,* edited by Mackey BB, DHEW publ no (NIH) 79-1442, 1978
22. *Proc 12th Annu Contractors' Conf Artif Kidney Program of NIAMDD,* edited by Mackey BB, DHEW publ no (NIH) 81-1979, 1979
23. Meltzer TH, Gutfreund K, Kulshrestha VK, Stake AM: Optimized cellulose membranes for artificial kidney dialysis applications. *Trans Am Soc Artif Intern Organs* 14:12, 1968
24. Craig LC, Konigsberg W: Dialysis studies. III. Modification of pore size and shape in cellophane membranes. *J Phys Chem* 65:116, 1961
25. Biget AM: A procedure for rapid dialysis. *C R Acad Sci (D) (Paris)* 224:827, 1947
26. Immergut EH, Rollin S, Salkind A, Mark H: Membranes for osmotic pressure measurements. *J Polymer Sci* 12:439, 1954
27. Michaels AS, Baddour RF, Bixler HJ, Chov CV: Conditioned polyethylene as a permselective membrane. *Ind Eng Chem Process Design Develop* 1:14, 1962
28. Lyman DJ, Loo BH, Crawford RW: New synthetic membranes for dialysis. I. A copolyether-ester membrane system. *Biochemistry* 3:985, 1964
29. Laug OB, Stokesbery DP: *The Development of Standard Test Methods for Hemodialysis Membranes.* Nat Bureau of Stand, Report no 9872, Nat Tech Inform Serv (PB 179669), Springfield, VA
30. Craig LC: *Advances in Analytical Chemistry and Instru-*

mentation. Vol 4 edited by Reilly CN, New York, NY, Interscience Publishers, 1965, p 35
31. Babb AL, Maurer CJ, Fry DL, Popovich RP, McKee RE: The determination of membrane permeabilities and solute diffusivities with applications to hemodialysis. *Chem Eng Prog Symp Ser* 64:59, 1968
32. Fritzinger BK, Brauman SK, Lyman DJ: Membrane characteristics, permeability parameters, and frictional coefficients for Cuprophane. *J Biomed Mater Res* 5:3, 1971
33. Kaufmann TG, Lenard EF: Mechanism of interfacial mass transfer in membrane transport. *Am Inst Chem Eng* 14:421, 1968
34. *Evaluation of Membranes for Hemodialyzers*. Report from the Membrane Evaluation Study Group for the Artif Kidney Chronic Uremia Program of NIAMDD, DHEW publ no (NIH) 74-605, 1974
35. *Evaluation of Hemodialysis and Dialysis Membranes*. Report of the Study Group for the Artificial Kidney-Chronic Uremia Program, DHEW publ no (NIH) 77-1294, 1977
36. Markle RA, Falb RD, Leininger RI: Improved membranes for artificial kidney dialysis. *Rub and Plasts Age* 45:800, 1964
37. Bixler HJ, Nelsen LM, Bluemle LW Jr: The development of a diafiltration system for blood purification. *Trans Am Soc Artif Intern Organs* 14:99, 1968
38. Silverstein ME, Ford CA, Lysaght MJ, Henderson LW: Response to rapid removal of intermediate molecular weight solutes in uremic man. *Trans Am Soc Artif Intern Organs* 20:614, 1974
39. Bamford CH, Elliott A, Hanby WE: *Synthetic Polypeptides*, New York NY, Academic Press, 1956
40. Nishihara T, Rubin AL, Stenzel KH: Biologically derived collagen membranes. *Trans Amer Soc Artif Intern Organs* 13:243, 1967
41. Rubin AL, Riggio RR, Nachman RL, Schwartz GH, Miyata T, Stenzel KH: Collagen materials in dialysis and implantation. *Trans Am Soc Artif Intern Organs* 14:169, 1968
42. Stenzel KH, Rubin AL, Yamayoshi W, Miyata T, Suzuki T, Sohde T, Nishizawa M: Optimization of collagen dialysis membranes. *Trans Am Soc Artif Intern Organs* 17:293, 1971
43. Lyman DJ, Loo BH: New synthetic membranes for dialysis. IV. A copolyether-urethane membrane system. *J Biomed Mater Res* 1:17, 1967
44. Thakore YB, Shieh DF, Lyman DJ: Chemical and morphological effects on solute diffusion through block copolymer membranes, in *Ultrafiltration, Membranes and Applications* edited by Cooper AR, Polymer Science and Technology, New York, NY, Plenum Press, vol 13. 1980, p 45
45. Pitts T, Mackey M, Barbour GL: In vitro permeability studies of peritoneal, Cuprophan, and polycarbonate membranes. *Trans Am Soc Artif Intern Organs* 24:150, 1978
46. Ishigaki I, Lyman DJ: Preparation and properties of N-vinylpyrrolidone grafted polymer by radiation-induced graft polymerization. *J Membrane Sci* 1:301, 1976
47. Luttinger M, Cooper CW, Leininger RI: Preparation of novel hemodialysis membranes. *Trans Am Soc Artif Intern Organs* 14:5, 1968
48. Salyer IO, Ball GL, Beemsterboer GL: The Monsanto polyacrylonitrile hollow fiber artificial kidney, in *Membrane Processes in Industry and Biomedicine* edited by Bier M, Chapter 3, New York NY, Plenum Press, 1971
49. Man NK, Terlain B, Paris J, Werner G, Sausse A, Funck-Brentano JL: An approach to middle molecular identification in artificial kidney dialysis, with reference to neuropathy prevention. *Trans Am Soc Artif Intern Organs* 19:320, 1973
50. Loeb S, Sourirajan S: Sea Water Demineralization by means of an osmotic membrane, in: *Adv Chem Series 38*, edited by Gould RF, ACS Press, 1963, p 117
51. Kjellstrand CM, Petersen RJ, Evans RL, Shideman JR, Santiago EA, Buselmeier TJ, Rozelle LT: In vitro studies of a new ultrathin membrane for hemodialysis. *Trans Am Soc Artif Intern Organs* 18:106, 1972
52. Malchesky PS, Piatkiewicz W, Varnes WG, Onderen L, Nose Y: Sorbent membranes: device designs, evaluation and potential applications. *Artif Organs* 2:367, 1978
53. Bianchi R, Bionda A, Carmassi F, Palla R, Donadio C, Galli M, Chiellini E, Molea N, Mariani G: Evaluation of new membranes for hemodialysis: preliminary studies with a polycarbonate membrane. *J Dial* 3:383, 1979
54. Nash T: Colorimetric estimation of formaldehyde by means of the Hantzsch reaction. *Biochem J* 55:416, 1953

5
DIALYSERS

NICHOLAS A. HOENICH and DAVID N.S. KERR

Introduction	106
The history of dialyser design – a brief survey	107
Haemodialysers in current clinical use	107
Non-disposable flat plate designs	108
Disposable flat plate dialysers	109
Coil dialysers	111
Hollow fibre dialysers	114
Large surface area haemodialysers	116
Dialysers using high permeability membranes	118
Dialysers utilising sorbent materials	118
Paediatric dialysers	119
Dialyser performance measurement	120
Blood flow	120
Clearance and dialysance	122
Factors influencing clearance	125
Ultrafiltration	125
Red cell effects	125
Temperature	125
Flow rate	125
Dialysate degassing	125
Membrane characteristics	126
Clearance of middle molecules	126
Factors influencing clearance of middle molecules	126
Ultrafiltration	126
Flow rate	127
Membrane characteristics	127
Ultrafiltration rate	127
Factors influencing ultrafiltration rate	129
Membrane characteristics	129
Plasma protein concentration	129
Thermo-osmotic effects	129
Blood compartment volume and compliance	129
Flow resistance	130
Resistance to blood flow	130
Resistance to dialysate flow	130
Flow distribution	131
Blood-membrane interactions	131
Thrombogenecity	131
Damage to blood components	131
Haemodialysis leucopenia	131
Haemodialysis complement activation	132
Damage to platelets by membranes	132
Blood loss in haemodialysers	132
Haemodialyser washout characteristics	134
Elution of toxic substances from the dialyser	134
Bacterial contamination	135
Cost	135
Choosing a dialyser	135
Future trends in haemodialyser design	135
Nomenclature	137
References	137

INTRODUCTION

During the early years of treatment of renal failure by haemodialysis, there were rapid technical developments in dialyser design. Early models of dialysers, notably disposable types, were inefficient and often varied considerably in their performance.

These problems stimulated extensive work which resulted in a large variety of disposable dialysers of varying configurations offering improved and predictable performance characteristics. The growth has persisted to date, as shown by data from the European Dialysis and Transplant Association (EDTA) registry surveys (Table 1).

Before undertaking a survey of existing haemodialysers, the requirements of an ideal haemodialyser need to be considered and these are shown in Table 2. A number of these requirements are interrelated while others are mutually exclusive. The extent to which currently used designs conform to these ideals may vary considerably

Table 1. Numbers of different types of dialysers manufactured 1976 to 1980.

		Disposable		
Year	Non disposable	Flat plate	Coil	Hollow fibre
1976	13	13	27	4
1977	7	21	37	15
1978	7	30	38	20
1979	6	32	40	33
1980	8	54	40	73

Table 2. Requirements of an ideal haemodialyser.

High clearance of small and middle molecular weight solutes
Negligible loss of vital solutes across the semipermeable membrane
Adequate range of ultrafiltration
Low residual blood volume and good washback characteristics
High reliability
Non toxic construction
Low cost
Re-use potential

as each design represents a compromise between conflicting demands.

The choice of dialyser, therefore, becomes a compromise. On one hand, it may be desirable to select a dialyser whose performance characteristics are 'tailored' to the needs of the patient. On the other hand, fiscal or other considerations may prevent such a choice being made. It is, therefore, fortunate that patients with chronic renal failure are tolerant of a wide range of treatment produced by a variety of different dialyser designs since it may not be possible to select the 'best' dialyser for each patient.

The history of dialyser design – a brief survey

A brief review of the major developments of haemodialyser design is given here. A more detailed survey of the development of the basic design is presented in Chapter 2, while other historical reviews have been published by Hoeltzenbein (1) and Dittrich and colleagues (2).

The artificial kidney or haemodialyser dates from 1913 when Abel, Rowntree and Turner (3) demonstrated the feasibility of removing metabolites from animals by passing their blood through nitrocellulose tubes bathed in saline. The therapeutic potential of this technique was realised and applied by Haas in 1923 (4) but further application and use was prevented by technical difficulties.

The commercial production of heparin and the availability of cellulose tubing permitted the clinical application of this technique in 1937 by Thalhimer (5) but it was not until the development of the rotating kidney by Kolff and Berk (6) that haemodialysis became an accepted procedure. This first successful dialyser was of an intricate design comprising a coiled cellophane tube on a revolving drum which was originally made from aluminium strips and subsequently from wooden laths. Almost half of the drum was immersed in a bath containing dialysis fluid. As the drum rotated it carried a film of fluid with it from the bath so that solute exchange occurred across the membrane whether in or out of the bath. Paradoxically, this design, while once dominating the scene, like Neanderthal man, disappeared without leaving any progeny. A number of factors contributed to its disappearance. A rotating coupling was required between the blood tubing and the blood lines which, together with other non-disposable components, gave rise to frequent pyrogen reactions. The membrane was unsupported on the outer side and considerable skill was required to balance the inflow and outflow so that the extracorporeal volume did not oscillate too widely. Even with an experienced operator the extracorporeal volume could not be kept below 1 litre which necessitated blood priming, while the low pressure in the system made fluid removal difficult and possible only by means of a high dextrose concentration in the dialysis fluid.

Alwall (7), working independently in Sweden, developed an alternative design which, while more complex to operate and less efficient than Kolff's design, was the first machine suitable for fluid removal using hydrostat-

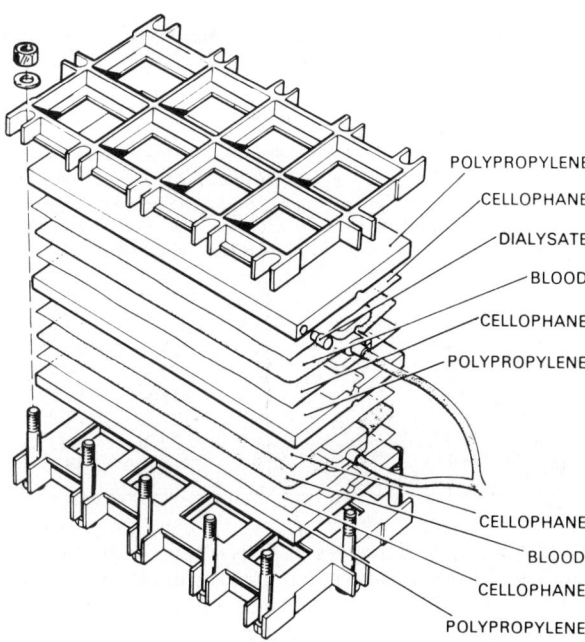

Figure 1. The Kiil non-disposable haemodialyser (Not to scale).

ic pressure. This design was the evolutionary father of modern coil dialysers.

The first flat plate design was described by Skeggs and Leonards (8) who used sheets of cellulose membrane supported on corrugated rubber pads to separate the blood and dialysate which flowed in opposite directions. In subsequent designs, two sheets of membrane were used between which the blood flowed. This latter design was subsequently adapted by Kiil (9) who initially manufactured his dialyser from Araldit, an epoxy resin compound, later from polypropylene (Figure 1). This basic design, modified by Scribner and colleagues (10, 11), remained in extensive use for the treatment of chronic renal failure until the late 1960's.

While the design described by Abel, Rowntree and Turner may be considered as the first hollow fibre dialyser, the forerunner of current hollow fibres was the experimental design described by Stewart and colleagues (12). It comprised a perspex outer jacket which incorporated dialysate connectors encasing a bundle of hollow fibres potted at the ends in polyurethane.

HAEMODIALYSERS IN CURRENT CLINICAL USE

Up to 1968, four fifths of European dialyses were undertaken using either the non-disposable flat plate (Kiil) or the disposable twin coil dialyser (13). The early 1970's saw the introduction of disposable flat plate designs. More recently, the solution of problems associated with large scale production together with the wider availability of hollow fibres resulted in an increased use of hollow fibre designs (Table 3).

Table 3. Use of haemodialysers in Europe showing percentage of patients reported as using a certain dialyser most frequently in the year.

Year	Haemodialyser type			
	Non disposable flat plate	Disposable		
		Flat plate	Coil	Hollow fibre
1973	25.9	29.7	38.2	4.5
1974	20.4	33.5	37.7	7.5
1975	13.7	40.2	35.4	10.4
1976	11.0	42.2	35.8	10.4
1977	8.7	43.2	31.4	14.6
1978	6.4	46.0	27.7	19.8
1979	4.7	44.7	22.3	28.3
1980	3.1	45.7	16.6	34.6

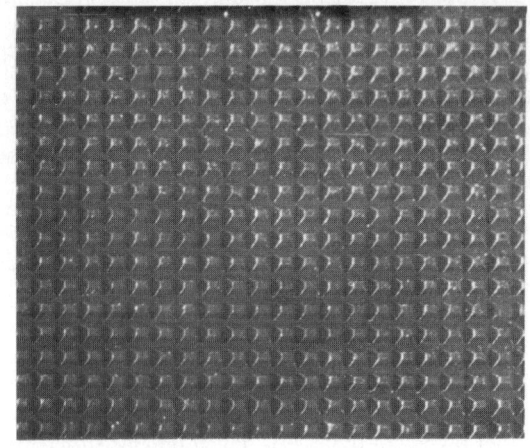

Figure 2. Multipoint structure used in Meltec haemodialysers.

These four major types of dialyser constitute the categories of haemodialysers in current clinical use. Each of these categories may be further sub-divided into standard (Table 4), large surface area (Table 5) and paediatric designs (Table 6).

Non-disposable flat plate designs

The earlier Kiil type dialysers produced by a number of manufacturers throughout the world, have largely been replaced by multi-point variants. The superiority of multiple cone supports was demonstrated by Bluemle and colleagues in 1960 (14), but such designs were not adopted on a large scale until the 1970's when the pyramid support, obtained by cross cutting the longitudinal grooves and creating an array of close packed flat topped pyramids (Figure 2) was introduced by the Western Gear Company in the USA (15) and by Meltec in the United Kingdom (16). This modification resulted in a substantial improvement in clearance of small and middle molecules due to the reduction of obstructed membrane surface and improved mixing of the dialysate during its passage through the dialyser. Meltec has developed a recent further modification (Meltec M3 Micropoint) in which the depth of the cross cut has been reduced and the blood manifold modified (17).

Non-disposable flat plate haemodialysers have a number of disadvantages. They are somewhat bulky with heavy boards which some patients find difficult to handle. They have a leak rate which is inversely proportional to the skill of the person building the dialyser and they are prone to cause pyrogenic reactions. The dialysate pathway is readily colonised by bacteria and power-

Table 4. Physical characteristics of standard haemodialysers.

Dialyser type	Name	Manufacturer	Surface area m^2	Membrane type	Membrane thickness micron
Non disposable flat plate	M3 Micropoint	Meltec Ltd. UK	1.03	Cuprophan	11
	Multipoint	Meltec Ltd. UK	1.03	Cuprophan	11
Disposable flat plate	GLP	Ab Gambro, Sweden	1.0	Cuprophan	11 [a]
	BL 500 Bravo	Bellco SpA, Italy	1.1	Cuprophan	16
	EXP 400	Extracorporeal SA Belgium	1.15	Cellulose	20
	MTL 104	Secon GmbH, Germany	1.20	Cellulose-hydrate	20
Disposable coil	EX 25	Extracorporeal SA Belgium	1.0	Cuprophan	18
	ALT 100	Bentley/Sorin, Italy	1.0	Cuprophan	18
	Vita 2HP [b]	Bellco SpA, Italy	1.2	Cuprophan	18
Disposable hollow fibre	CDAK 3500	Cordis, USA	0.9	Cellulate	40/210 [c]
	Triex 1	Extracorporeal, USA	1.0	Cuprophan	11/200
	CF 1200	Travenol, USA	1.2	Cuprophan	16/215
	MTS	MTS, Germany	1.3	Cuprophan	11/200
	HF 130	Cobe Labs. USA	1.3	Cuprophan	19/300

[a] Available with other thickness Cuprophan.
[b] Single pass coil.
[c] Internal diameter.

Table 5. Physical characteristics of large surface area haemodialysers.

Dialyser type	Name	Manufacturer	Surface area m²	Membrane type	Membrane thickness micron
Non disposable flat plate	Multipoint	Meltec Ltd, UK	1.53	Cuprophan	11
Disposable flat plate	GLP	Ab Gambro, Sweden	1.36	Cuprophan	11
	RP 514	Rhone Poulenc, France	1.35	Cuprophan	11
	PPD	Cobe Labs, USA	1.6	Cuprophan	11
Disposable coil	ALT 140	Bentley/Sorin, Italy	1.39	Cuprophan	18
	EX 29	Extracorporeal SA, Belgium	1.4	Cuprophan	18
	EX 55 [a]	Extracorporeal SA, Belgium	1.4	Cuprophan	18
Disposable hollow fibre	CDAK 4000	Cordis, USA	1.4	Cellulate	40/210 [b]
	HF 150	Cobe Labs, USA	1.5	Cuprophan	16/300
	AM 20	Asahi Medical, Japan	1.6	Cuprammonium rayon	15/200
	Triex 3	Extracorporeal, USA	1.6	Cuprophan	11/200
	GF 180M	Gambro GmbH, Germany	1.8	Cuprophan	11/200

[a] Single pass coil.
[b] Internal diameter.

Table 6. Performance characteristics of haemodialysers suitable for paediatric use.

Dialyser type	Name	Manufacturer	Surface area	Clearance (ml/min) Urea	Clearance (ml/min) Creat	Blood compartment volume (ml) [a]	Ultra filtration coefficient ml/hr/mmHg	Ref. [d]
Non disposable flat plate	Multipoint	Meltec Ltd UK	0.6	116	90	102	1.68 [b]	—
		Meltec Ltd UK	0.77	131	103	110	2.58	—
Disposable flat plate	Mini Minor	Ab Gambro, Sweden	0.28	61	42	20	0.5 [c]	181
	Minor	Ab Gambro, Sweden	0.51	100	73	33	1.7 [c]	181
	EXP 200	Extracorporeal SA, Belgium	0.85	106	83	88	2.34	—
Disposable coil	EX 20	Extracorporeal, USA	0.3	—	57	84	1.36	—
	EX 21	Extracorporeal, USA	0.7	—	87	158	2.76	—
	ALT 77	Bentley/Sorin, Italy	0.77	110	89	204 [b]	2.76	—
Disposable hollow fibre	CDAK	Cordis, USA	0.6	118	90	53	0.84	—
	Triex L	Extracorporeal, USA	0.86	141	106	79	2.61	—

[a] At transmembrane pressure of 100 mmHg.
[b] At transmembrane pressure of 150 mmHg.
[c] In vivo.
[d] Where no reference is quoted in this and subsequent tables, the data are those obtained at Newcastle upon Tyne.

ful antiseptics such as a solution of 2% formaldehyde (5% formalin) are required for sterilisation. Formaldehyde is toxic, has an unpleasant smell, may give rise to allergic skin reactions, irritates the respiratory tract and is difficult to eliminate totally from the dialyser (18). It is probably the cause of anti-N antibodies in the blood of patients who use non-disposable or re-use disposable dialysers (19-21) (see also Chapter 11 and 15).

On the other hand, such dialysers have a low resistance to blood flow, offer a wide range of ultrafiltration, are efficient in their clearance of both small and middle size toxins and in countries where labour costs are low, they are comparatively inexpensive to use.

Although several designs are in clinical use their popularity has declined over the past five years in favour of the more compact and convenient disposable types. The Meltec Multipoint is still widely used in the United Kingdom and in consequence, it has been included in our tables of comparative performance, together with its more recent Micropoint version.

Disposable flat plate dialysers

Early disposable flat plate designs were a compromise between the previously described non-disposable flat plate dialysers and the current disposable designs. Such dialysers consisted of a disposable membrane insert with a solid clamping frame (22). The first truly disposable haemodialyser was the Gambro-Alwall (23, 24). In con-

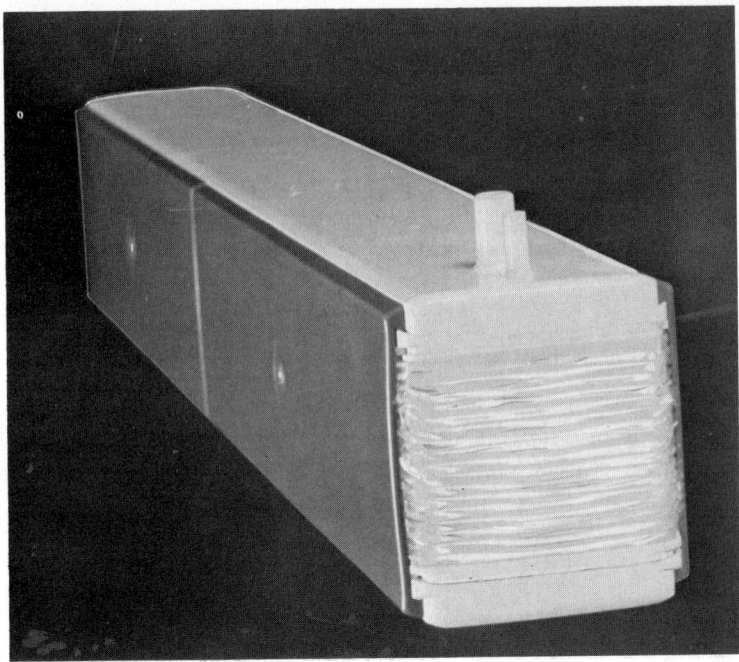

Figure 3. Multiple layer configuration in a disposable haemodialyser offering a range of surface areas based upon a single basic design.

trast to current designs it was bulky, suffered from a poor flow distribution through the multiple layers and had a high residual blood volume. It was succeeded by more successful designs, and current models are smaller and more compact than their predecessors. Since they are pre-sterilised they are more convenient than their non-disposable counterparts; the reduction in size for current designs has been achieved by the use of multi-layer design (Figure 3). Such designs require high precision during manufacture to ensure an even distribution of the blood and dialysis fluid through the multiple layers. These exacting requirements have meant that early disposable flat plate designs were inferior to their non-disposable counterparts. Improvements and advances in manufacturing techniques have meant that the earlier inferiority of this category of dialysers has been largely eliminated and current performance characteristics are comparable with those of non-disposable dialysers (25).

The early disposable flat plate dialysers used moulded plastic plates for the support of the membrane. The trend towards thinner fluid films in the search for improved performance (26) has resulted not only in the reduction of the support size (27) but also their replacement by alternate forms of support structure such as non-woven polypropylene mesh. The use of this mesh not only eliminated the use of expensive moulded supports, but also further reduced the size of the dialyser (Figure 4). Its use, however, may adversely influence the performance in the presence of inadequately degassed dialysis fluid due to the adherence of air bubbles to the mesh structure causing a reduction in the effective surface area of the dialyser (28).

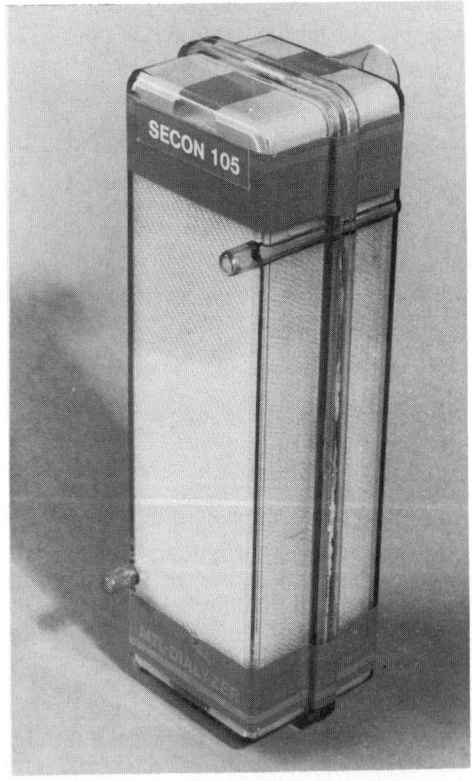

Figure 4. Miniature multilayer flat plate disposable haemodialyser in which the moulded membrane support plate has been replaced by a non-woven polypropylene mesh.

5: Dialysers 111

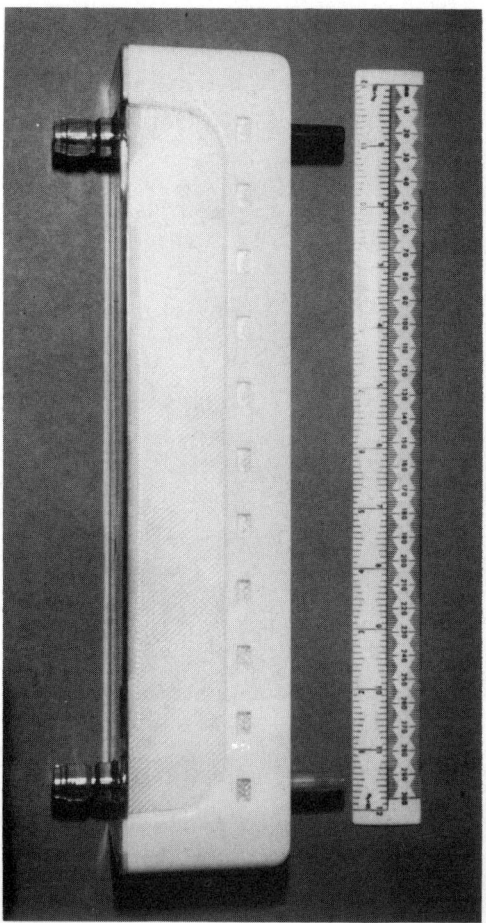

Figure 5. The Extracorporeal EX-P400 multilayer disposable haemodialyser.

Disposable flat plate dialysers retain the advantages of non-disposable dialysers, i.e. low flow resistance, high efficiency and a wide range of ultrafiltration. They overcome many of the objections to their non-disposable counterparts. Being fully disposable and pre-sterilised, they avoid the use of formaldehyde and are rarely associated with pyrogen reactions.

A number of different designs are available from the major haemodialyser manufacturers (Figures 5 and 6), and, as shown in Table 3, their use accounts for nearly half of European dialyses.

Coil dialysers

The first disposable coil utilised a tubular membrane supported by a fibre glass mesh, wound around a solid central core (Figure 7). This original design had a high blood compartment volume and compliance due to the poor support given by the mesh and required priming by blood prior to use. Performance was poor and unpredictable because of the escape of fluid around the coil in its holding can, a defect which was soon overcome by enclosing the coil in an inflatable plastic cuff (29).

A subsequent modification of this design was the replacement of the fibre glass mesh by a new mesh support of the type described by Hoeltzenbein (30) (see Chapter 2) and today, virtually all coils use some modification of this mesh as the support structure.

Current designs are developments of these early models. The tubular membrane is wider and shorter than in the earlier designs. The inflatable cuff has been replaced by a solid perspex outer casing (Figure 8) while in some models, the traditional folding of the membrane at the join with the blood inlet and outlet tubing has been replaced by distribution manifolds. The use of this manifold is beneficial not only in ensuring the even flow distribution through the membrane, but also in eliminating the trapping of blood in the folds. In one design (Bellco Vita 2) the Hoeltzenbein mesh has been replaced by an extruded multipoint support sheet bearing a series of truncated pyramids.

Coil dialysers originally used a high dialysate flow rate (25–30 l/min) obtained by recirculation of the dialysate, using a high speed pump, through the supporting struc-

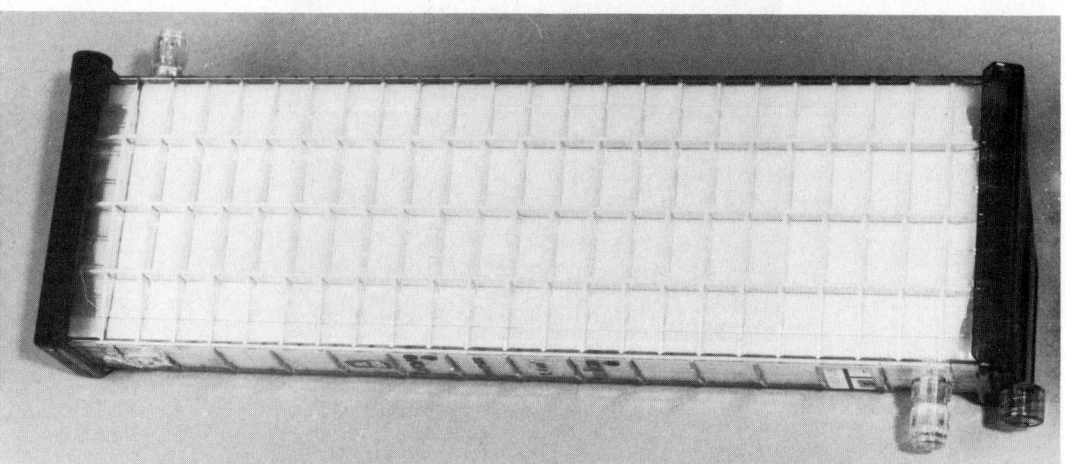

Figure 6. The Bellco Bravo 1.4 m² multilayer disposable haemodialyser.

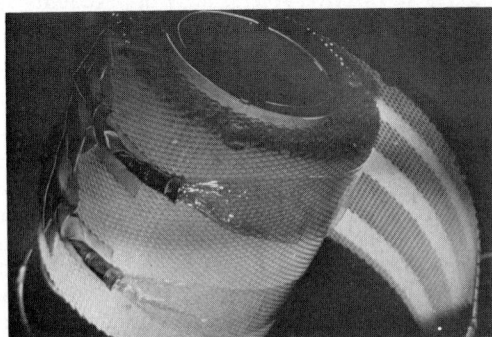
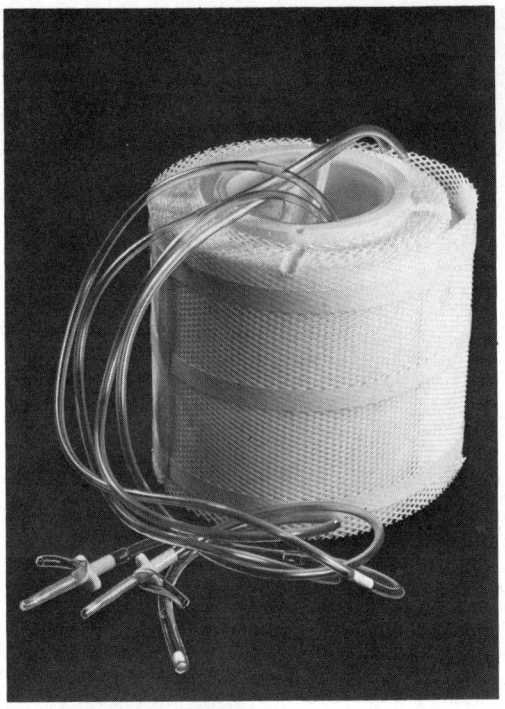
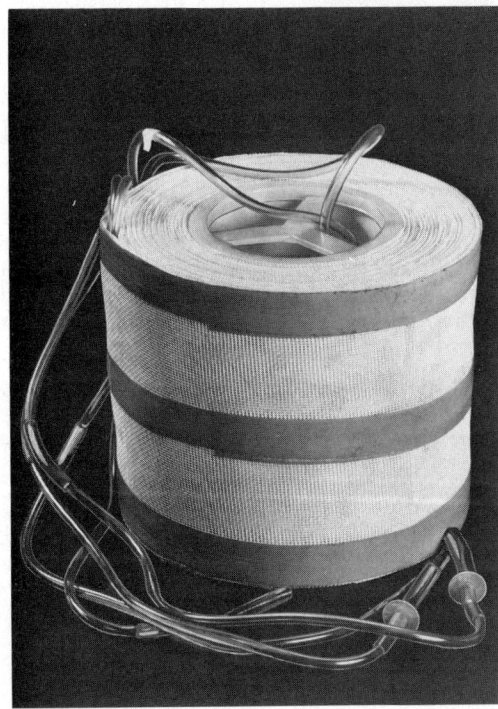

Figure 7. Early coil haemodialysers.

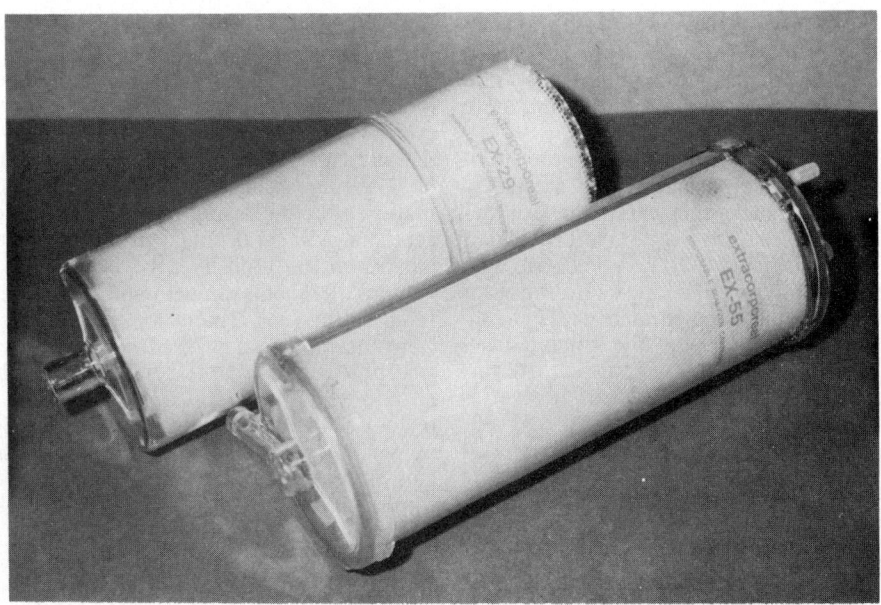

Figure 8. The Extracorporeal EX series of coil haemodialysers designed for both recirculating and single pass dialysate supply systems.

ture over the outside of the membrane at right angles to the direction of blood flow. This high flow rate limited the use of these dialysers to recirculating or recirculating single-pass (RSP) systems. To enable the dialysers to be used with conventional single pass dialysate systems, fully encased coils have been developed (Figure 9); this permits their use with a dialysate flow rate of 500 ml/min but at the expense of some reduction in clearance.

Coil dialysers have a high blood flow resistance which is an inevitable consequence of their construction. This resistance generates high pressure in the blood pathway which varies from patient to patient due to the influence of the patient's haematocrit on blood viscosity. Conse-

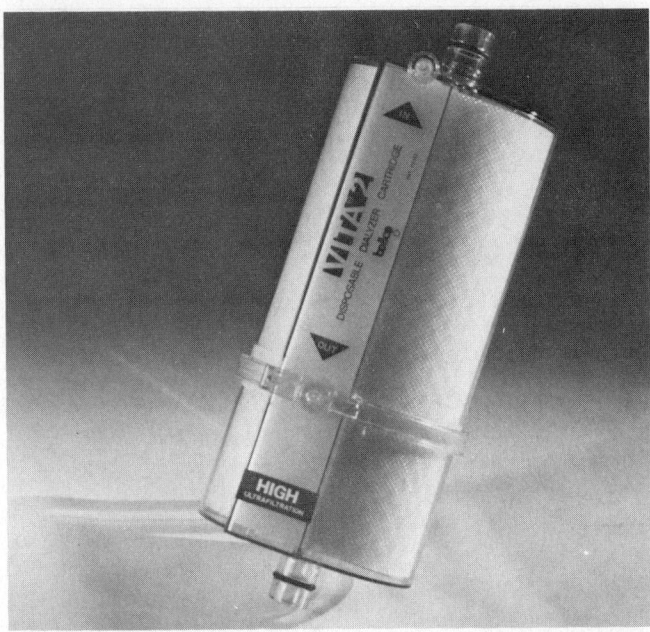

Figure 9. The Bellco Vita 2 enclosed coil haemodialyser.

quently such dialysers have a high ultrafiltration rate which, in addition, is difficult to predict. The blood compartment volume of coil dialysers is higher than that of flat plate and hollow fibre dialysers and they are more compliant.

Coil dialysers have a number of advantages to compensate for their high internal resistance and obligatory ultrafiltration. They are inexpensive compared to other disposable dialysers, are easy to use and prepare, and may be used with less sophisticated dialysate supply systems than single pass dialysers. The high ultrafiltration can be an advantage for the overhydrated patient.

When used in recirculation systems, the solute removal characteristics of such dialysers is expressed in terms of dialysance (see page 122) since their clearance varies according to the type of recirculating system used. Allowance for this fact must be made when comparing coil dialysers with other types which do not utilise dialysis fluid recirculation. Fully encased coils which are an adaption of the recirculating models use the lower dialysis fluid flow rates of single pass systems and, in consequence, have a lower dialysance than the corresponding models used in recirculation, but this reduction is compensated by the use of fresh dialysate in single pass so that the average effectiveness is comparable.

Major manufacturers of coil dialysers include Travenol (Ultraflo series), Extracorporeal (EX series) and Bentley/Sorin (ALT series). There are also licence built copies of these and other designs available in some countries. Coil dialysers were widely used in the late 1960's (13); their use in Europe is declining in comparison with other disposable dialysers (Table 3) but total consumption is still rising.

Hollow fibre dialysers

The forerunner of currently used hollow fibre dialysers (HFAK's) was the experimental design produced by the Dow Chemical Company which used cellulose hollow fibres manufactured for desalination purposes. This early design retained the basic characteristics of Abel, Rowntree and Turner's design and comprised a perspex outer jacket incorporating dialysate connectors and containing a bundle of hollow fibres, potted at the ends in polyurethane. It was subsequently manufactured by Cordis Dow in a range of sizes ($1.3-2.5 \, m^2$) and used formalin as the sterilising agent. This, while clinically acceptable, was far from ideal and more recent variants have been sterilised by ethylene oxide.

Until 1975, the regenerated cellulose fibres manufactured as the replacement for the earlier cellulose fibres, were the only source of raw material used in the construction of hollow fibre devices. These fibres had a lower permeability than Cuprophan (also called Cuprophane) and consequently required a high transmembrane pressure to produce sufficient ultrafiltration for clinical requirements. They necessitated the use of unconventional proportioning machines generating high transmembrane pressure or larger than usual surface area to overcome this limitation.

In 1975, Enka AG complemented their production range of haemodialysis membranes with a range of hollow fibres manufactured by the cuprammonium process. The availability of this alternative source of fibres, manufactured in a wider range of wall thickness and hydraulic permeability than the original regenerated cellulose acetate has led a large number of manufacturers to extend their range of dialysers and include hollow fibre designs. More recently Asahi Medical has introduced a series of HFAK dialysers using fibres manufactured from cuprammonium rayon. The original Cordis hollow fibres have been replaced by Cellulate, a cellulose acetate membrane with higher permeability to water and middle molecules giving comparable performance to cuprammonium fibres. Recent developments include the introduction of polymethyl-methacrylate (31) polyacrylonitrile (32) and polysulphone hollow fibres (33) with higher permeabilities designed specifically for ultrafiltration and haemofiltration but which can be employed for

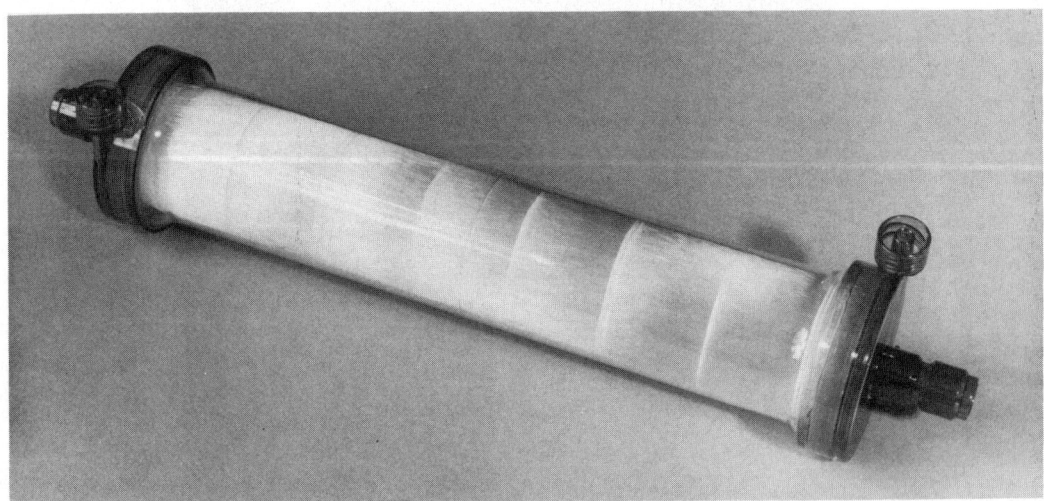

Figure 10. The Braun Dia-cap hollow fibre haemodialyser.

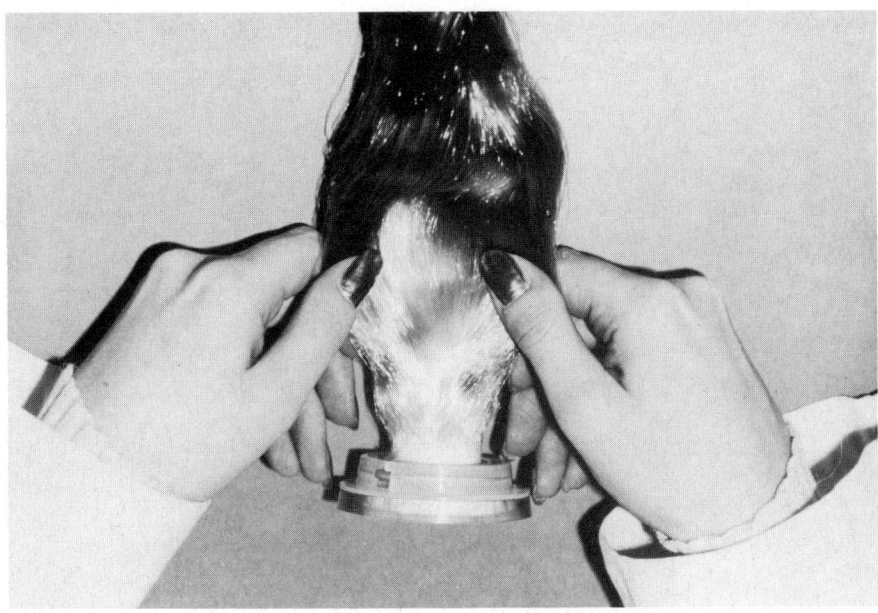

Figure 11. Flow maldistribution observed in the dialysate pathway of a hollow fibre haemodialyser.

haemodialysis with an apparatus that creates zero transmembrane pressure (see Chapters 4 and 14).

Many of these designs have been copies of the classical design described by Stewart and colleagues (12) in which the dialysate flows on the outside of the fibres which are arranged in a bundle while blood flows in a countercurrent direction through the fibres whose internal diameter is 200–300 micron (Figure 10). Although this design is theoretically the most efficient, in contrast with flat plate designs, a decrease in efficiency may be present as a consequence of flow maldistribution or channelling in the dialysate pathway (Figure 11). In order to minimise this channelling, a number of novel fibre configurations have been developed. Nakagawa and colleagues (34) arranged the fibres in a rectangular block designed to direct dialysate back and forth through the bundle. This arrangement has been incorporated in a number of commercial designs (Figure 12). Lee and Taylor (35) developed a triple bundle configuration used in the Extracorporeal Triex series of dialysers in which the dialysate flow paths of each bundle are inter-connected in series while the blood compartments are connected in parallel (Figure 13).

Cobe Laboratories in their HFAK designs use a baffled cross flow system to improve the flow configuration (Figure 14) while the development of secondary flow patterns was envisaged in the Sorin Spiraflo series in which the fibres are spirally wound around a central core, this concept also being used by several other manufacturers.

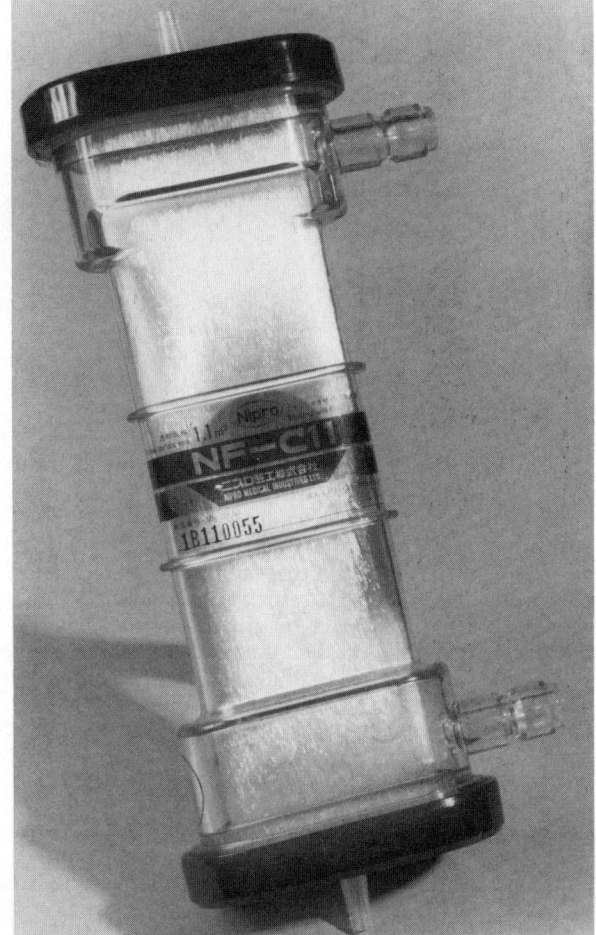

Figure 12. Rectangular block arrangement of fibres designed to minimise flow maldistribution in the dialysate pathway (Nipro, NF-CII).

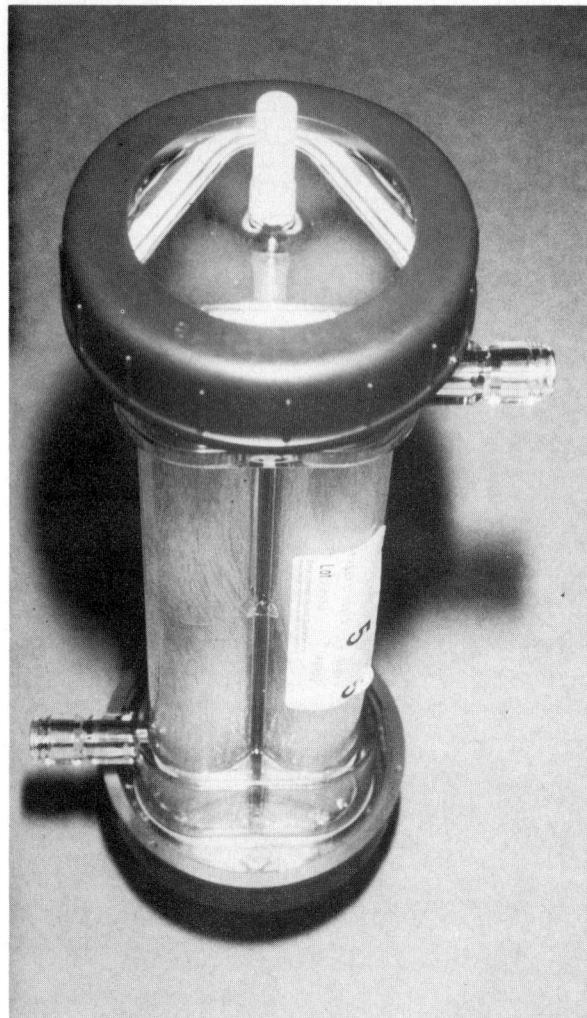 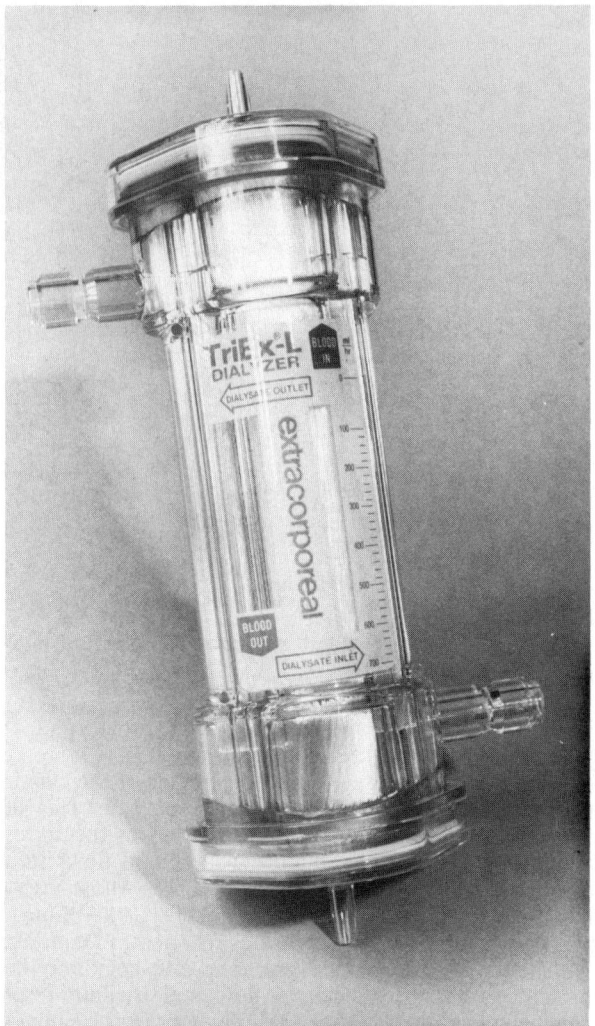

Figure 13a and 13b. The extracorporeal Triex 2 (1.3 m^2) and Triex L (paediatric) hollow fibre haemodialysers.

Early models of hollow fibre dialysers suffered from thrombogenecity in the header manifold, distortion of fibres by the potting process and an irregular blood flow distribution (36). Many of these problems have been solved by improvements in the manufacturing technology, but, in those designs in which blood enters the dialyser via a manifold and is distributed by the shape of the manifold and the pressure gradient, blood may stagnate at the bundle edge resulting in clotting of the peripheral fibres. Sigdell (37) described an optimised design of the inlet and outlet manifold in which the blood enters the header manifold tangentially to the orientation of the fibres (Figure 15). This creates a circular and turbulent flow pattern in the manifold eliminating stagnation areas. This optimised design has been adopted by the MTS series of hollow fibre dialysers which are produced under licence by Erika (HPF series) for the United States' market.

Large surface area haemodialysers

Several of the early dialysers such as the rotating drum and the Skeggs-Leonards Kidney had large surface areas – up to 3 to 4 m^2, but with the abandonment of blood priming of dialysers the membrane area contracted to about 1 m^2.

The development of haemodialysers took, however, a radical turn in 1971 when the Seattle group formulated the first theory of toxicity of larger molecules, the 'square meter/hour hypothesis' (38). In 1972 this hypothesis was revised and renamed the 'middle molecule hypothesis' (39). The basis of this hypothesis (see Chapters 2, 3 and 19) was that some features of uraemia were caused by middle molecules in the range of 300–2000 molecular weight, the clearance of which was much more dependent upon the effective membrane surface area and membrane permeability than upon the

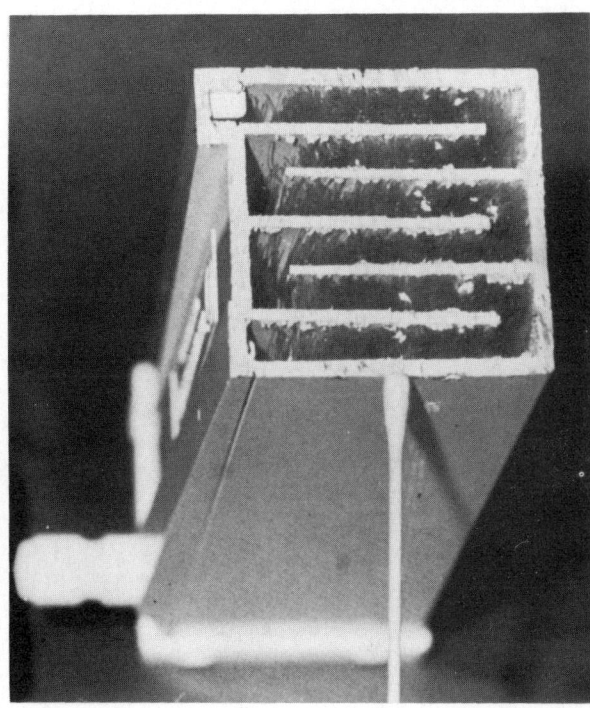

Figure 14. Baffled cross flow arrangement of fibres used in the Cobe HF haemodialyser to minimise flow maldistribution in the dialysate pathway.

thickness of the drag film on the blood and dialysate sides of the membrane. This hypothesis led to the extensive development of large surface area dialysers which were based on well proven standard dialysers and whose design features were similar to their smaller surface area counterparts. The increase in surface area for flat plate designs was achieved by the addition of extra blood layers (Figure 3). The addition of these extra blood compartments can result in flow maldistribution which, in turn, reduces the increase in performance due to reduction in the effective surface area of the dialyser. Minimisation of this problem may be achieved by alteration of the internal geometry of the dialyser. For coil dialysers, the commonest way of increasing the surface area was to increase the length of the membrane tubing. An increase in the width of the tubing would have been preferable but was prevented by difficulties in producing wider membrane tubing. This increase in the surface area results in a further increase in the blood volume of such dialysers and a tighter winding tension during manufacture may be applied to minimise such increases. This tighter winding increases the flow resistance in the blood pathway which, in turn, increases the basal ultrafiltration rate, while overwinding may result in partial nonperfusion of the blood pathway during practical use.

For hollow fibre dialysers, either the number of fibres or the fibre length could be increased. In contrast to plate designs, the dialysate pathway of hollow fibre dialysers is not so well defined geometrically since the fibres do not completely fill the pathway and may not be straight as a result of cross winding on the bobbins during manufacture, giving rise to maldistribution or channelling, and a consequent lowering of performance.

Consequently, large surface area dialysers offer higher solute removal rates notably for middle molecules and a higher ultrafiltration than their smaller surface area counterparts, but the improvement offered may not be quite in proportion to the increase in surface area (40). Despite this, they have been used to operate short dialysis schedules in which the reduction in treatment time has exceeded that dictated by performance considerations.

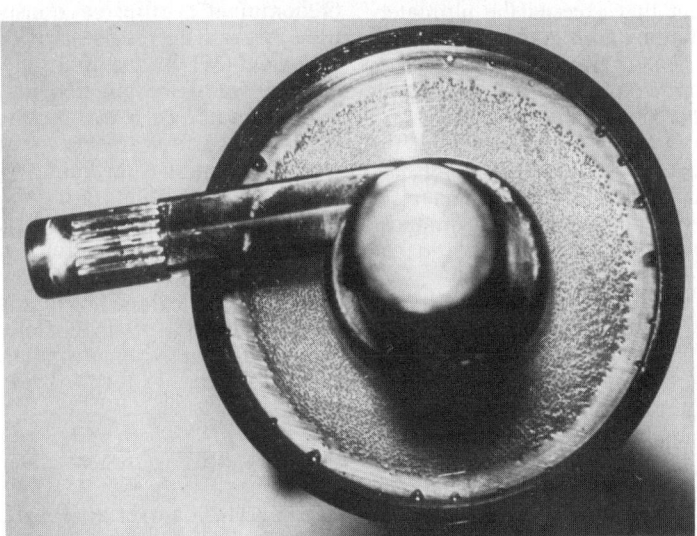

Figure 15. Optimised blood manifold used in hollow fibre haemodialysers designed to eliminate the clotting of peripheral fibres (Erika, HTS series).

Dialysers using high permeability membranes

The success of cellulose based membranes in clinical practice coupled with the lack of knowledge concerning the precise requirement for solute removal have hindered the development of new haemodialysis membranes. The advent of the middle molecule hypothesis resulted in the development of alternative methods of treatment of chronic renal failure such as haemofiltration (41-44), controlled sequential ultrafiltration (45-48) and simultaneous dialysis and haemofiltration (49-51) which required membranes that were more permeable than the classical dialysis membranes and has resulted not only in the production of non-cellulosic membranes such as polymethylmethacrylate (PMMA [31]) and polyacrylonitrile (AN 69 or PA membrane [52, 53]) but also in the production of modified cellulosic membranes (Cuprophan-HDF) making them suitable for use with the above techniques (see also Chapters 4 and 14).

High permeability membranes may be used in conventional haemodialysis systems but since the improved middle molecular clearance in these membranes is associated with a high hydraulic permeability compared to conventional membranes, their use may only be safely undertaken using modified dialysis systems which permit control of ultrafiltration during clinical use. Alternatively, single needle dialysis may be performed using a double head pump system which enables the ultrafiltration characteristics of such membranes to be controlled with comparative ease (54). In general, however, such membranes are used in haemofiltration, isolated ultrafiltration or simultaneous dialysis and haemofiltration rather than conventional haemodialysis.

Haemofiltration imitates the glomerular filtration process of the human kidney and is a process whereby the uraemic blood is cleansed by a combination of ultrafiltration (convective solute removal) and dilution in which a sterile pyrogen-free diluting fluid replaces the fluid loss from the patient that exceeds the ultimately required fluid loss. The diluting fluid may be introduced upstream of the device (pre-dilution) or downstream (post-dilution). The use of such devices (Figure 16) requires special equipment capable of automating the task of balancing the flow rates of the ultrafiltrate and the diluting fluid. Requirements of devices suitable for haemofiltration are shown in Table 7 (See also Chapters 11 and 13). Current devices (Table 8) utilise asymmetric porous membranes whose molecular cut off is determined by the pore size. The filtrate produced as a result of hydrostatic pressure in the blood compartment or a vacuum on the filtrate side contains all molecules whose molecular size is below the cut off value of the membrane. In contrast with conventional dialysis which is predominantly diffusive transport and in which the transport rate decreases sharply with increasing molecular weight (39), in haemofiltration all metabolites which are well below the cutoff point cross the membrane at the same rate. To overcome the disadvantage of lower small molecular clearance with this technique compared with conventional haemodialysis, simultaneous haemodialysis and haemofiltration provides an alternative technique which may be undertaken with haemodialysers using high flux membranes such as the Rhône-Poulenc RP-6 (Figure 17). Such devices thereby offer both an improved clearance of middle molecules and an enhanced clearance of small molecules by diffusion compared with pure haemofiltration (see also Chapters 12 and 13).

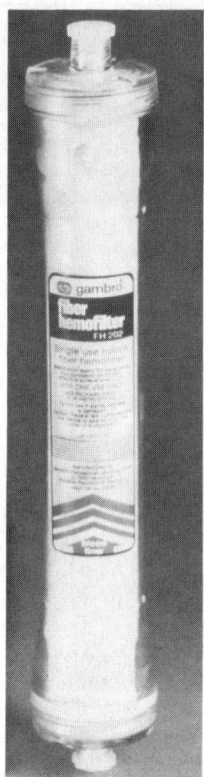

Figure 16. The Gambro fibre haemofilter FH102.

Table 7. Comparison of haemodialysis (HD) and haemofiltration (HF).

	HD	HF
Driving force	Concentration gradient	Pressure
Primary flux	Solutes	Solvent
Separation mechanism	Diffusion	Sieving Coefficient
Membrane requirements	Low resistance to diffusion	Low resistance to pressure

Dialysers utilising sorbent materials

Haemoperfusion over activated charcoal has been widely used in treating drug intoxications (see Chapter 16). However, in uraemia it has been used only as an adjunct to other methods, such as haemodialysis which can remove water and additional substances (55, 56).

Table 8. Characteristics of devices with high permeability membranes.

Application	Name	Manufacturer	Surface area	Membrane type	Ultrafiltration ml/hr/mmHg	Ref.
Haemodialysis/ sequential dialysis	Lundia Ultraflux	Ab Gambro, Sweden	2.25	Cuprophan HDF	29	181
Haemofiltration	Filtryzer Bl	Toray Industries, Japan	1.15	Polymethylmethacrylate hollow fibres 40[a]/240[b]	11	182
	RP6	Rhône Poulenc, France	1.03	Polyacrylonitrile sheet 40[b]	30	—
Haemofiltration	Diafilter 20	Amicon	0.2	Polysulphone hollow fibres 31[a]	30–40	183
	Diafilter 30	Amicon	0.5	Polysulphone hollow fibres 31[a]	60–75	183
	SM 40002	Sartorius	0.3	Triacetate sheet-120[a]	13	184

[a] (Wall) thickness (micron).
[b] Internal diameter (micron).

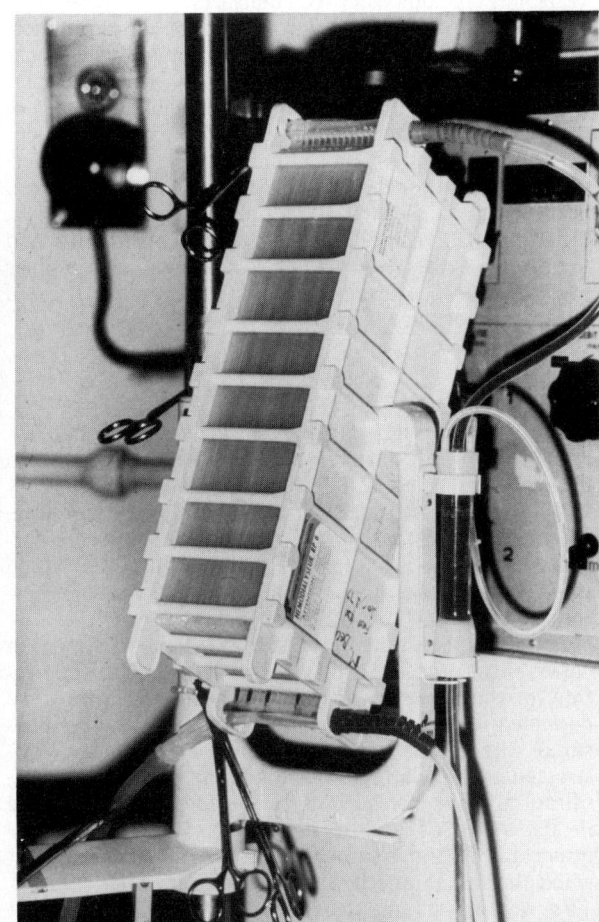

Figure 17. The Rhône Poulenc RP6 multilayer haemodialyser utilising polyacrylonitrile membrane.

As an alternative, sorbent membranes were developed in 1976 by Enka AG. These membranes contain two layers, one mainly of activated charcoal bonded by a small amount of cellulose and the second a thin layer of Cuprophan, that serves as the blood interface (57). This membrane is available in flat sheet, tubular and hollow fibre form, is well suited for use in conventional haemodialysers, and offers the possibility of combining dialysis and haemoperfusion in a single device. A number of dialysers incorporating these membranes have been produced (58, 59). They have not been used extensively in the treatment of uraemia but have been employed for the treatment of psoriasis (60), schizophrenia (60, 61) and hepatic failure (62).

Paediatric dialysers

Children with renal failure face numerous problems which are unique to their age group. Although the techniques of dialysis in children and adults are comparable, adaptations of the equipment and dialysis schedules to meet the paediatric needs are necessary (63, 64).

The choice of dialyser in the treatment of children is largely governed by the extracorporeal blood volume which at no time should be greater than 10% of the child's total blood volume (65).

Examples of dialysers suitable for the treatment of children are shown in Table 6. Of these dialysers, hollow fibre configurations offer the greater flexibility since they have a low blood compartment volume. Multi-layer flat plate configurations, on the other hand, allow a number of blood compartments to be selectively clamped to meet the needs of the paediatric patient.

In addition to adjusting the blood compartment volume to the clinical needs, careful attention should also be paid to the selection of the blood lines in ensuring

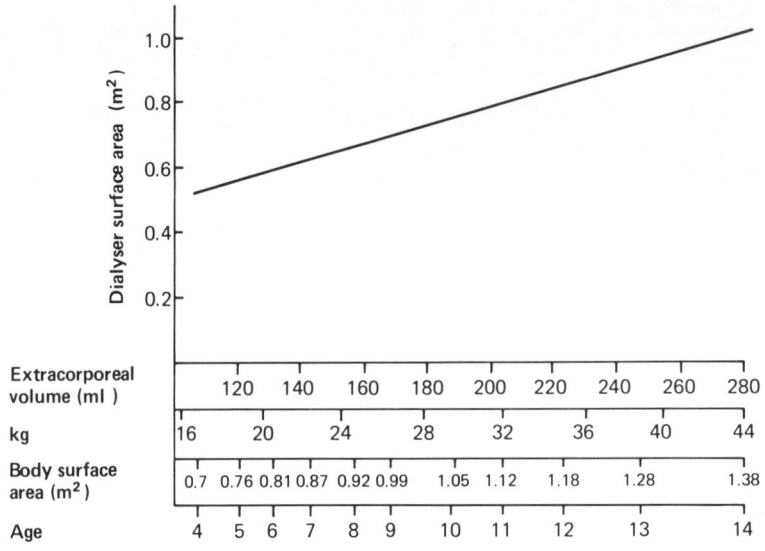

Figure 18. Nomogram for selection of paediatric haemodialyser.

that their contribution to the total extracorporeal volume is such that it remains within the limit discussed above.

For adults who are treated with a variety of haemodialysers ranging from 1 to 2.5 m² the mean ratio between body surface area and dialyser surface area is 0.75. This ratio should ideally be the same for children and, in consequence, a nomogram may be used in the selection of the appropriate dialyser (Figure 18). Using this nomogram, it may be seen that the most appropriate dialyser for a 10 year old child would be one with a surface area of 0.7 m² while the total extracorporeal volume should be approximately 190 ml or less.

The metabolic rate of children is greater than that of adults. Consequently children accumulate nitrogenous waste products, electrolytes and water at a greater rate than adults and, therefore, need more dialysis in relation to their body weight than an adult. Ideally dialysis in children should be performed more frequently than for adults. Since this is often impractical either longer or higher efficiency dialyses are necessary. However, it must be remembered that the rate of removal of fluid and small metabolites must also be matched to the size of the patient.

Excessively high solute removal can cause disequilibrium and convulsions (63, 64) while excessively fast removal of fluid causes shock.

Control of disequilibrium may be accomplished by the use of high dialysate dextrose concentration or mannitol infusion during dialysis (66, 67), but the use of these techniques is potentially more hazardous than for adults and therefore best avoided. (For comprehensive information on paediatric dialysis the reader is refered to Chapter 25).

DIALYSER PERFORMANCE MEASUREMENT

The choice of haemodialysers has grown in the past five years and the choice between dialysers has become more difficult. In this section, we shall describe the parameters which are of importance to the clinician and which enable him to make a rational comparison of rival designs. It is not the intention to provide an extensive review of dialyser performances which may be obtained from published surveys (68–71) or from our own studies undertaken on behalf of the Department of Health and Social Security in the United Kingdom (72), but to highlight differences between dialysers of similar construction and to introduce the reader to the fundamental principles involved in measuring performance characteristics of clinical importance.

Blood flow

Blood flow through the dialyser influences both clearance and ultrafiltration rate, the latter particularly in designs which have a high blood pathway resistance.

The accurate measurement of blood flow is, therefore, of critical importance in all studies of dialyser performance (see also Chapter 11). Despite this, it is often neglected by investigators studying haemodialyser performance.

In vitro measurement of simulated blood flow can easily be accomplished by a timed collection at the outflow of the dialyser. The measured flow rate must be corrected for the ultrafiltration rate which may be measured directly or calculated from a previously constructed graph relating transmembrane pressure to ultrafiltration. This correction is of considerable importance in the study of middle molecular clearance but less important in the clearance of small molecules except when the membrane permeability is very high.

In vivo measurement of blood flow is more difficult since variations in the occlusion and dimension of the pump segment may be present. One popular method is to calibrate the blood pump *in vitro* and assume that the same dial setting generates a comparable blood flow *in vivo*. There are several pitfalls in this method. Two important sources of error – incomplete occlusion of the blood pump segment and variation in blood flow with varying pressure downstream of the pump – can be avoided by choice of blood pump and punctilious attention to detail. Blood pump segments vary a little in diameter from sample to sample and, since the blood flow is proportional to the square of this diameter, small variations cause appreciable errors. If circuits are bought from a single reliable supplier this error can be ignored for clinical purposes but in research studies, the pump should be recalibrated at the end of each *in vivo* study. All roller pumps respond to a low inflow pressure by producing a decreased flow at a given dial setting and the fall off begins before most circuits collapse upstream of the pump (H Tanboga and N Hoenich, unpublished observations 1977).

This source of error can be avoided by monitoring pressure in the arterial blood line upstream of the pump or by incorporating with that line a thin-walled collapsible sac ('mouse') that detects a fall in pressure more readily than the thicker walled tubing (see Chapter 11).

Inexpensive in-line disposable flow meters (Figure 19) have been produced. Such systems are unable to provide a sufficient degree of accuracy at low blood flow rates, while at clinical flow rates, the accuracy of the reading may be vitiated by the presence of froth in the measuring chamber.

In vivo blood flow rates may be also measured by electro-magnetic or ultrasonic flow meters. Such systems, apart from their cost, have a number of disadvantages. Electro-magnetic flow meters use probes which are incorporated into the blood lines necessitating autoclaving between uses which shortens the life of the probe. Clip on probes used with ultrasonic flow meters are sensitive to changes in the blood tube dimensions and rely upon the attainment of an accoustic contact between the blood tubing and the probe which cannot be checked after the experiment. The accuracy of ultrasonic and electro-magnetic flow meters ranges between ± 5 and $\pm 15\%$ (73).

The most widely used mode of *in vivo* blood flow measurement has been the bubble transit measurement in which the passage of a small air bubble is measured between two fixed marks. This method has been used in our *in vivo* studies and the factors affecting the transit time have been studied. An accuracy of $\pm 3\%$ over the clinical range of blood flow rates can be achieved with routine use of this technique.

In order to achieve this level of accuracy, the following requirements are essential:

(1) An adequate length of race track (200 cm). This race track length ensures that the transit time lies between 8 and 30 sec. when using 5 mm internal diameter tubing over the clinical range of blood flows.
(2) The race track should be kept horizontal to avoid errors introduced by the lower density of air compared with blood.
(3) The length of the race track should be measured prior to commencement of dialysis to minimise

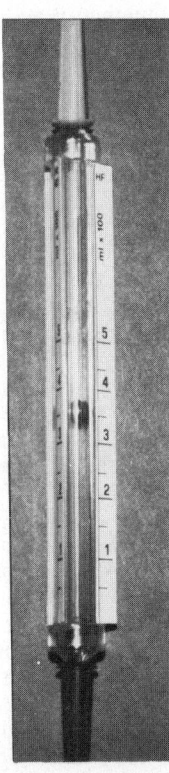

Figure 19. In line disposable blood flow meter.

stretching. Commercial PVC tubing is sufficiently constant to give an accuracy of $\pm 3\%$ provided it is not stretched when the track is measured.
(4) The blood line should be calibrated with bank blood whose haematocrit is of the same range as the patient's, since the bubble speed is influenced by fluid viscosity. *In vitro* studies have shown that the variation introduced by the haematocrit range 27 to 40% is 5% (74).
(5) A single air bubble (0.5 ml) has to be injected and transit time has to be measured in triplicate by a stopwatch measuring to 0.1 sec. If the air bubble fragments, the observation is discarded.
(6) The diameter of the circuit tubing should be sufficiently constant. Variation in this diameter has the same effect on calculated blood flow as variation in the blood pump insert with the method discussed above. We have found that commercial circuits supplied in the UK by two manufacturers are sufficiently constant that recalibration is not necessary at each experiment. However, it is a wise precaution to recheck calibration from time to time during a series of experiments.

Measurement of bubble transit time involves inserting a needle repeatedly into the injection site. Inexperienced staff run a considerable risk of impaling a finger on the far side of the tubing, unless the bloodline is provided with a semicircular plastic cover. Careful instruction in the technique is therefore necessary and in our view it should not be used with patients who are $HB_s Ag$ positive.

The bubble transit method is suitable for conventional two-needle haemodialysis. Single needle systems, apart from those using double lumen catheters or needles, generate an intermittent flow rate due to the alternating occlusion (from 0.2 to 2 sec.) of the arterial and venous blood lines; thus the techniques described above cannot be used. Furthermore, in mechanical single needle systems the blood flow rates in different parts of the extracorporeal circuit differ with high transient blood flows occurring during the in-flow and out-flow phases of the cycle. However in the extracorporeal circuit between the dialyser venous outlet and the venous bubble chamber blood flow is largely independent of the cyclic variations introduced by the blood pump which are damped out by the dialyser so that blood flow can be measured with the bubble transit method in that section. We have used two alternative techniques. In our early studies, we maintained the 200 cm race track in the arterial blood line, but instead of making the bubble transit measurements in triplicate, we measured the transit time for ten bubbles. This has the same effect as lengthening the race track but avoids the problems of increased extracorporeal volume and washback volume at the end of dialysis. In more recent studies, we have used a 400 cm race track in the venous segment of the extracorporeal circuit placed between the blood outlet of the dialyser and the venous bubble trap and measured the transit time of five bubbles. This produces an error comparable with that for two needle measurement provided the flow interruption in switching from the arterial to the venous phase does not exceed 1 second.

Clearance and dialysance

In analogy to the clearance concept of the human kidney the overall solute transport characteristics of a dialyser may be expressed in terms of clearance or dialysance. Of these, the clearance is preferred by the clinician, since it describes the haemodialyser as part of the circulatory system. Dialysance is used by engineers in the comparison of the overall solute removal at a given blood flow for different dialyser designs.

The clearance of the dialyser may be expressed in terms of concentration gradients and flow rates such that

$$K_B = \frac{(C_{Bi} - C_{Bo})Q_{Bi}}{C_{Bi}} + \frac{Q_f C_{Bo}}{C_{Bi}}$$

for the blood side of the dialyser and

$$K_D = \frac{(C_{Do} - C_{Di})Q_{Di}}{C_{Bi}} + \frac{Q_f C_{Do}}{C_{Bi}}$$

for the dialysis fluid side of the dialyser.

Dialysance may also be expressed in a similar format such that

$$D_B = \frac{(C_{Bi} - C_{Bo})Q_{Bi}}{(C_{Bi} - C_{Di})} + \frac{Q_f C_{Bo}}{(C_{Bi} - C_{Di})}$$

for the blood side of the dialyser and

$$D_D = \frac{(C_{Do} - C_{Di})Q_{Di}}{(C_{Bi} - C_{Di})} + \frac{Q_f C_{Do}}{(C_{Bi} - C_{Di})}$$

for the dialysis fluid side of the dialyser.

Under conditions of zero ultrafiltration ($Q_f = 0$) these expressions reduce to the commonly used relationships shown below:

$$K_B = \frac{(C_{Bi} - C_{Bo})Q_B}{C_{Bi}}$$

$$K_D = \frac{(C_{Do} - C_{Di})Q_D}{C_{Bi}}$$

$$D_B = \frac{(C_{Bi} - C_{Bo})Q_B}{C_{Bi} - C_{Di}}$$

and

$$D_D = \frac{(C_{Do} - C_{Di})Q_D}{(C_{Bi} - C_{Di})}$$

The relationship between clearance and dialysance is given by

$$K_B = \frac{(C_{Bi} - C_{Di})D_B}{C_{Bi}}$$

and the two terms are equivalent only when $C_{Di} = 0$, as in single pass dialysis.

In all other cases clearance is less than dialysance; therefore, if dialysers are compared in terms of their dialysance, when their construction demands different dialysate supply systems, an erroneous impression of their relative efficiency will be created. For instance, in the case of coil dialysers used with rapid recirculation of dialysate, the dialysance is higher than that for dialysers used in single pass systems. However, in the former, the dialysance is equal to the clearance only in the initial minutes of dialysis and decreases throughout dialysis as the solute accumulates in the tank, whereas for single pass dialysis, it remains equal throughout dialysis. It would be possible to compare dialysers fairly in terms of 'mean clearance', but practically this is not feasible since the answer depends upon the size of patient, duration of dialysis, recirculation volume and the dialyser.

There are a number of special cases in which the relationship described above between dialysance and clearance is more complex. The first of these is when a coil dialyser is used with recirculating single pass dialysate flow (RSP) in which a small volume of dialysate (5 to 10 l) is recirculated through the dialyser at a flow rate corresponding to that which would be used in pure recirculation. Simultaneously, fresh dialysate at a slower rate is added. For such systems an expression relating clearance to dialysance has been devised by von Hartitzsch et al. (75), viz:

$$K_B = \frac{D_B}{1 + \dfrac{D_B}{Q_D}}$$

permitting a comparison of coil dialysers with parallel plate and hollow fibre types. This relationship does not hold during the first hour of dialysis during which time there may be rapidly changing solute concentration in the recirculating reservoir.

A second case in which the clearance is modified is in single needle systems where partial blood recirculation through the dialyser may be experienced. The degree of recirculation in such systems is a function of the system, the fistula blood flow and the needle used (76, 77). Under these conditions the modified relationship derived by Gotch (74) and given by

$$K_R = \frac{K(1-R')}{1-R'\left(1-\frac{K}{Q_B}\right)} \text{ is applicable.}$$

Certain modifications to the widely used formula defining clearance are necessary when dealing with haemofiltration because using this technique, solute is cleared from the blood by physical removal of plasma water and in consequence, greater attention must be paid to the solute distribution, compared with haemodialysis. The relationships for the calculation of whole blood clearance for specified operating conditions have been described in detail by Colton et al. (78) and Henderson et al. (79) and are as follows:

$$K_B = Q_B \frac{(1-H)}{(1-H+H_k)} \times$$
$$\times \left\{ 1 - \left[\frac{(1-\emptyset)(1-H) + \frac{Q_D}{Q_B}\left(1-\frac{Q_f}{Q_D}\right)}{(1-\emptyset)(1-H) + \frac{Q_D}{Q_B}} \right]^s \right\}$$

for pre-dilution

$$K_B = Q_B \frac{(1-H)}{(1-H+H_k)} \times$$
$$\times \left\{ 1 - \left[\frac{(1-\emptyset)\left(1-H+\frac{Q_f}{Q_B}\right)}{(1-\emptyset)(1-H)} \right]^s \right\}$$

for post-dilution.

In the case of sequential dialysis and ultrafiltration during the ultrafiltration phase, whole blood clearance is defined as

$$K_B = \frac{Q_f C_f}{C_{Bi}}$$

Table 9. Relationship of dialysance to total mass transfer resistance.

Flow Geometry	Dialysance (D)	Total mass transfer resistance (R_T)
Co-Parallel	$Q_B \left[\dfrac{1-\left[\exp -J\left(1+\frac{Q_B}{Q_D}\right)\right]}{1+\frac{Q_B}{Q_D}} \right]$	$\dfrac{S(Q_B+Q_D)}{Q_B Q_D \ln\left[\dfrac{1}{1-\frac{D}{Q_B}-\frac{D}{Q_D}}\right]}$
Contra-Parallel	$Q_B \left[\dfrac{1-\left[\exp -J\left(1-\frac{Q_B}{Q_D}\right)\right]}{1-\frac{Q_B}{Q_D}\exp\left[-J\left(1-\frac{Q_B}{Q_D}\right)\right]} \right]$	$\dfrac{S(Q_B-Q_D)}{Q_B Q_D \ln\left[\dfrac{1-\frac{D}{Q_B}}{1-\frac{D}{Q_D}}\right]}$
Cross-Flow *	$\dfrac{Q_B}{2}\left[\left[\dfrac{1-\exp\left[-J\left(1+\frac{Q_B}{Q_D}\right)\right]}{1+\frac{Q_B}{Q_D}}\right] + \left[\dfrac{1-\exp\left[-J\left(1-\frac{Q_B}{Q_D}\right)\right]}{1-\frac{Q_B}{Q_D}\exp\left[-J\left(1-\frac{Q_B}{Q_D}\right)\right]}\right]\right]$	$\dfrac{S}{2Q_B Q_D}\left[\dfrac{Q_B+Q_D}{\ln\left[\dfrac{1}{1-\frac{D}{Q_B}-\frac{D}{Q_D}}\right]} + \dfrac{Q_B-Q_D}{\ln\left[\dfrac{1-\frac{D}{Q_B}}{1-\frac{D}{Q_D}}\right]}\right]$

Where $J = \dfrac{S}{R_T Q_B}$

---

* Approximate equation only. For exact equations refer to Kays and London, Compact Heat Exchangers, 2nd ed., New York, McGraw Hill, 1964.

See Appendix for key to symbols.

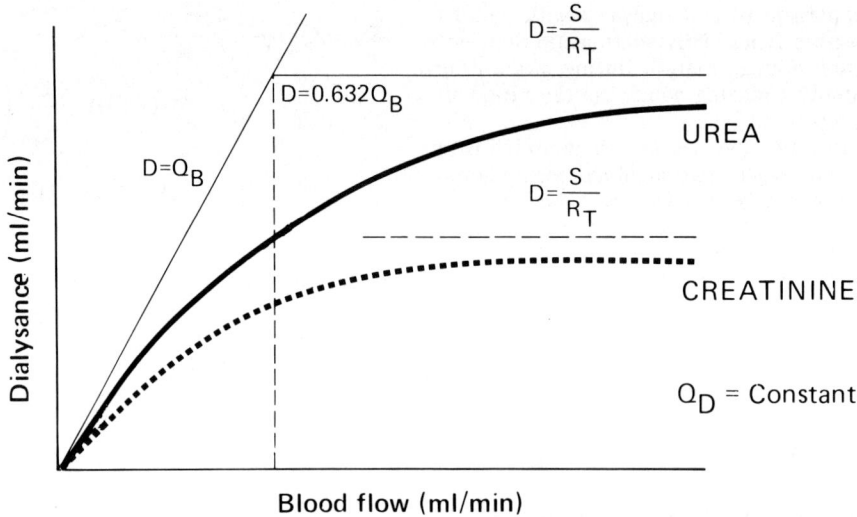

Figure 20. The relationship of dialysance to blood flow: applicable to any haemodialyser. The curves are limited by the two constraints shown whose interception is given by 0.632 Q_B.

If the effects of the exclusion volume of the hydrated proteins and the exclusion of larger molecular weight solutes from the erythrocytes are neglected this relationship may be simplified to

$$K_B = Q_f \dot{S}$$

Measurement of clearance is normally sufficient for clinical comparison purposes. The engineer sees the haemodialyser as a mass exchanger and therefore he wishes to gain insight into the physical phenomena occurring in the dialyser in order that he may analyse or improve the design; mass transfer coefficient or resistance provides a more fundamental approach.

In the absence of significant ultrafiltration, relationships between mass transfer resistance and dialysance have been derived and may be used to analyse the phenomena occurring in a haemodialyser in any of the clinically used flow configurations (Table 9).

For conventional haemodialysers, dialysance is related to blood flow and governed by the constraints shown in Figure 20. The shape of the relationship is the same for all modern dialysers and consequently the data on any new design can be fitted by computer to a curve of standard shape (75). In addition, the error of this estimate may also be established. A typical analysis obtained by this technique for the Meltec Multipoint dialyser is shown in Figure 21. The bars above and below

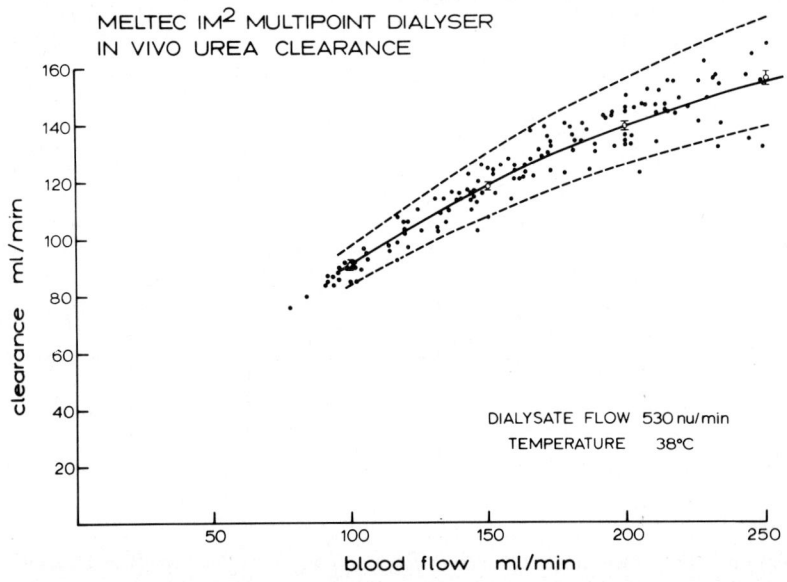

Figure 21. Experimental data obtained for the Meltec haemodialyser showing the 95% confidence and probability limits.

Table 10. Standard haemodialysers studied at Newcastle upon Type. *In vivo* small molecule clearance at a blood flow of 200 ml/min. Dialysate flow 530 ml/min. Temperature 38 °C.

	ml/minute			
	Urea clearance	Range	Creatinine clearance	Range
M3 Micropoint	147±1.1	141–156	118±0.7	111–123
Multipoint	143±1.0	113–155	119±0.7	114–127
GLP	133±4.0	118–154	109±3.0	95–128
BL 500 Bravo	139±1.9	130–149	114±3.3	97–139
EXP 400	147±3.2	133–161	114±1.9	102–127
MTL 104	139±2.9	127–154	111±3.7	96–132
EX 25	118±0.7	111–124	99±1.0	94–105
ALT 100	122±1.0	115–130	102±1.5	92–114
Vita 2 HP	122±2.2	114–129	98±1.0	93–105
CDAK 3500	125±2.4	114–141	104±1.6	96–114
Triex 1	145±3.1	130–164	122±2.3	110–137
CF 1200	152±3.4	135–172	125±3.1	109–147
MTS	172±1.5	159–192	147±3.3	130–169
HF 130	141±1.9	130–156	118±2.1	105–133

Table 11. Large surface area haemodialysers studied at Newcastle upon Tyne. *In vivo* small molecule clearance characteristics at a blood flow of 200 ml/min. Dialysate flow 530 ml/min. Temperature 38 °C.

	ml/minute			
	Urea clearance	Range	Creatinine clearance	Range
Multipoint	168±1.6	160–177	149±5.0	129–176
GLP	152±2.3	137–169	132±2.6	116–149
RP 514	137±1.0	130–147	111±1.9	103–122
PPD	139±2.9	125–159	121±2.2	110–133
ALT 140	125±3.2	109–150	114±1.3	105–122
EX 29	132±0.8	127–135	113±1.7	109–118
EX 55	132±2.6	120–143	104±1.6	96–114
CDAK 4000	156±1.6	147–168	128±1.6	118–141
HF 150	147±2.2	137–159	127±2.4	115–141
AM 20	173±1.5	161–182	154±4.8	140–175
Triex 3	167±1.4	150–175	147±2.2	132–167

the line at standard blood flow rates indicate the 95% confidence limits of the estimate while the probability limits of the data are represented by the dashed lines. In such analyses, the confidence limits may be made as narrow as desired by increasing the number of observations. Increasing the number of observations does not influence the probability limit of the observations since this represents the variability in observations caused by the experimental technique and the dialyser variability. Provided gross inaccuracies from a single dialyser are excluded, this parameter may be used as a measure of consistency. Therefore, in Tables 10 and 11 the mean clearance at a blood flow rate of 200 ml/min is presented with 95% confidence limits for comparison and the 95% probability range of data to indicate dialyser variability

for our *in vivo* studies carried out on patients whose mean haematocrit was 25% (range 19–40%).

Factors influencing clearance

Ultrafiltration

The effects of ultrafiltration on small molecule clearance, as has been shown by Kramer (80), are in the order of 3% provided the ultrafiltration rate is less than 5 ml/min. The effects of ultrafiltration on the clearance of coil, hollow fibre and parallel plate dialysers have been studied extensively by Nolph and colleagues (81–83). In all dialysers total clearance rises when transmembrane pressure is raised to increase ultrafiltration. In coil and flat plate dialysers, there is a decrease in diffusive clearance due to expansion of the blood pathway and increased draping of the membrane over supports, but this is more than offset by the contribution of increased ultrafiltration. Hollow fibre dialysers are non-compliant and have no membrane supports so there is no fall in diffusive clearance with increasing transmembrane pressure, simply an unopposed increase due to ultrafiltration.

Red cell effects

In vivo studies involve a complex heterogenous solution in which the solute diffusion rates are reduced due to the movement of solutes around or through the formed elements (84). Furthermore, there may be significant binding of some solutes in the blood (85–87) causing higher *in vitro* results than *in vivo*. These effects have been studied by Grossman, Kopp and Frey (88) who showed that the difference between *in vitro* and *in vivo* clearance for urea, is of the order of 3% for the haematocrit range 20 to 30% over the clinical range of blood flows.

Temperature

The importance of measurement of solute transport characteristics at a constant temperature was established by Fritz (89) and today, the majority of studies are undertaken at a constant temperature (37±1 °C).

Flow rate

The relationship between solute removal and blood flow rate is shown in Figure 20. The relationship between solute removal and dialysate flow is similar. A modest improvement in small molecule removal can be achieved by raising the dialysate flow rate above the conventional 500 ml/min but this technique is not widely employed due to the extra cost incurred.

Dialysate degassing

Adequate degassing of dialysate has become an important factor influencing solute removal by dialysers (see also Chapters 7 and 11). In the presence of poorly degassed dialysate, loss of surface area from masking of the membrane by air bubbles or flow channelling from air locking of the flow passages may occur (Figure 22), resulting in decreased solute clearance with duration of dialysis (28).

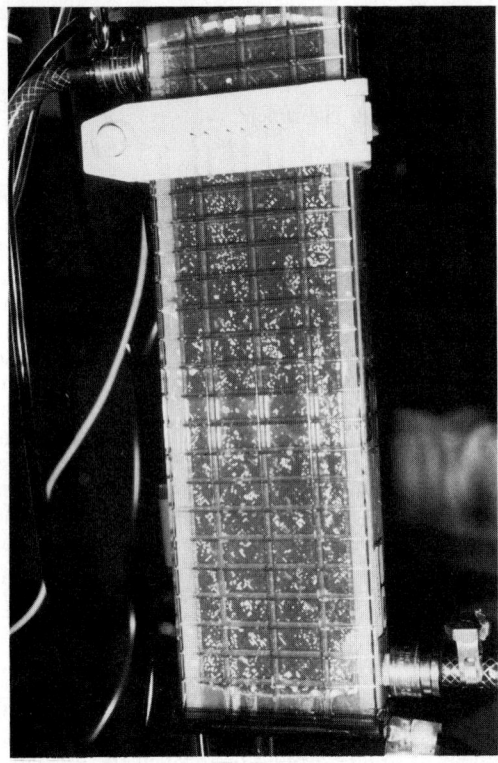

Figure 22. Accumulation of air in the dialysate pathway as a consequence of poorly degassed dialysis fluid.

Membrane characteristics
The membrane permeability of the widely used cellulosic based membranes decreases with increased molecular size, and consequently, the membrane becomes the principal barrier to diffusion for middle and large weight solutes in contrast to low molecular weight solutes for which the principal barrier to diffusion lies in the fluid films surrounding the membrane.

Membrane thickness has a reduced effect on small molecule clearance compared with large molecules (90).

Table 12. Compounds suitable for *in vitro* clearance studies.

Compound	Molecular mass daltons	
Sodium chloride	58	
Urea	60	
Creatinine	113	Small molecules
Uric Acid	168	
Dextrose	180	
Sucrose	342	
EDTA	380	
Raffinose	504	Middle molecules
Vitamin B_{12}	1355	
Inulin	5200	
Cytochrome C	13400	
Haemoglobin	68000	Large molecules
Albumin	69000	

Table 13. Standard haemodialysers. In vitro middle molecule clearances at a blood flow of 200 ml/min. Dialysate flow 530 ml/min. Temperature 38 °C.

	^{3}H Vitamin B_{12} (1355 daltons) (ml/min)	Ultrafiltration * (ml/min)
M3 Micropoint	45.3±4.8	3.0
Multipoint	33.7±1.1	2.1
GLP	25.9±2.0	5.2
BL 500 Bravo	33.6±5.7	5.0
EXP 400	39.9±3.0	6.5
MTL 104	41.9±4.4	7.8
EX 25	—	—
ALT 100	38.7±2.7	5.5
Vita 2 HP	36.1±2.6	6.6
CDAK 3500	33.2±2.1	6.2
Triex 1	29.2±3.8	3.9
AM 10	29.9±3.2	3.3
CF 1200	—	—
MTS	39.4±3.5	5.0
HF 130	27.8±2.3	2.6

Mean ± SD shown
* Ultrafiltration rate at the time of the experiment. Vitamin B_{12} clearances shown are corrected for ultrafiltration rates at the time of the experiment.

Quoted membrane thickness refers to dry thickness; the membrane swells considerably on contact with dialysis fluid (91). This swelling, however, does not affect small molecule clearance directly but may contribute to the maldistribution of flow in multilayer dialysers (92).

Clearance of middle molecules

Prior to 1968, publications dealing with haemodialyser performance included only information relating to the clearance of small molecular weight solutes.

More recently, it has been postulated that some complications of intermittent dialysis treatment are due to the inadequate removal of compounds in the range of 500 to 2000 daltons (38, 39). While this hypothesis is not universally accepted the study of this characteristic of haemodialysers has been recommended (93). It is carried out with substances which have no claim to be uraemic toxins and which may not appear in human plasma (Table 12). Measurements of middle molecule clearance characteristics have been undertaken on dialysers shown in Tables 13 and 14.

Factors influencing clearance of middle molecules

Ultrafiltration
For low molecular weight solutes the rate of diffusion across the membrane overshadows the contribution from convective mass transfer. As molecular weight increases solute permeability of haemodialysis membranes decreases and for solutes greater than 300 daltons the

Table 14. Large surface area haemodialysers. In vitro middle molecule clearances at a blood flow of 200 ml/min.

	^3H Vitamin B_{12} (1355 daltons) (ml/min)	Ultrafiltration [a] (ml/min)
Multipoint	41.9±3.1	4.2
GLP	35.6±4.4	6.0
RP 514	44.4±8.6	3.7
PPD	—	—
ALT 140	40.7±5.0 [b]	8.1
EX 29	—	—
EX 55	32 ±3.1	7.7
CDAK 4000	43.6±7.9	5.4
HF 150	35.9±7.9	3.7
AM 20	42.2±5.5	5.9
Triex 3	40.9±4.3 [b]	4.1
GF 180M [c]	58	5.7

[a] Ultrafiltration rate at the time of the experiment. Vitamin B_{12} clearances shown are corrected for ultrafiltration rates.
[b] Unlabelled Vitamin B_{12}.
[c] Reference 181.
Mean ± SD shown.

contribution from ultrafiltration to solute transport becomes significant and a correction for ultrafiltration effects becomes necessary. Studies shown in Tables 13 and 14 were undertaken under basal ultrafiltration conditions and the results obtained corrected for ultrafiltration effects (80).

Flow rate
The removal of middle and large molecules is much less dependent on dialysate flow and low flow rates (100 to 200 ml/min) have been used as a technique for selective removal of middle molecules (94, 95). The excellent condition of patients on this treatment regimen has been quoted as supporting evidence for the middle molecule hypothesis. Although these observations have not been challenged, low flow rates of dialysate have not been widely employed and a flow rate of 500 ml/min remains the standard.

Membrane characteristics
The membrane is the principal barrier to diffusion for large and middle molecule substances.

Studies have shown that thick membranes selectively retard higher molecular weight solutes (90, 96). Early Cordis-Dow dialysers used cellulose acetate fibres in their construction, the thickness of which was three times that of Cuprophan fibres. This factor accounted for the low middle molecule clearance characteristics of these dialysers in relation to their surface area. Improvements in membrane technology have made it possible to improve membrane permeability, yet retain a comparatively high membrane thickness. This concept is demonstrated by the new generation of cellulose membranes produced by the Cordis-Dow Corporation (Cellulate) for conventional haemodialysers. It is also widely used in the membranes specifically developed for haemofiltration (Table 8).

Ultrafiltration rate

Fluid removal during haemodialysis has two components: one due to the hydrostatic transmembrane pressure gradient ($Q_{f(h)}$) and the other due to the osmotic transmembrane pressure gradient ($Q_{f(osm)}$) such that

$$Q_f = Q_{f(h)} + Q_{f(osm)}$$

The rate of fluid removal due to hydrostatic pressure is a function of the haemodialyser fluid dynamic conditions, surface area and membrane hydraulic permeability such that

$$Q_{f(h)} = L_h A \Delta P_{M(h)}$$

Fluid losses due to osmotic gradients are much more difficult to measure. The osmotic gradient across the membrane is the algebraic sum of the osmotic gradients for each of the molecular species present on either side of the membrane. Since the overall molarity of the dialysis fluid is close to that of the blood, the influence of this factor is small. Solutes such as dextrose may be added to the dialysate to enhance fluid removal; this exerts a powerful osmotic force drawing fluid from the patient. With modern dialysers which provide an adequate range of ultrafiltration, such techniques are presently rarely used. A special case of an osmotic pressure gradient is that due to the proteins in plasma; since the membrane is impermeable to protein and the dialysate is protein-free, these molecules exert their full osmotic force which is referred to as the plasma oncotic pressure or colloid osmotic pressure. At normal plasma protein concentrations, this pressure is about 25 mm Hg and under these conditions, the relationship between fluid loss and hydrostatic pressure is modified to

$$Q_f = L_h A (\Delta P_{M(h)} - \Delta P_{osm})$$

The mean hydrostatic pressure in a dialyser is given by

$$\Delta P_{M(h)} = \frac{(P_{Bi} + P_{Bo})}{2} - \frac{(P_{Di} + P_{Do})}{2}$$

This pressure may not be measured readily in clinical practice and a series of formulae showing the relationship between measured pressure and ultrafiltration rate may be established (Figure 23).

Transmembrane pressure calculations in coil haemodialysers have neglected the influence of dialysis fluid inlet pressure due to the difficulty in measurement of this pressure. Furthermore, it was assumed that the transmembrane pressure is equal to:

$$\frac{(P_{Bi} + P_{Bo})}{2}$$

This simple formula, however, assumes that the coil dialyser has a stable flow path section, and a linear fall in pressure along the blood pathway. Gagneaux and

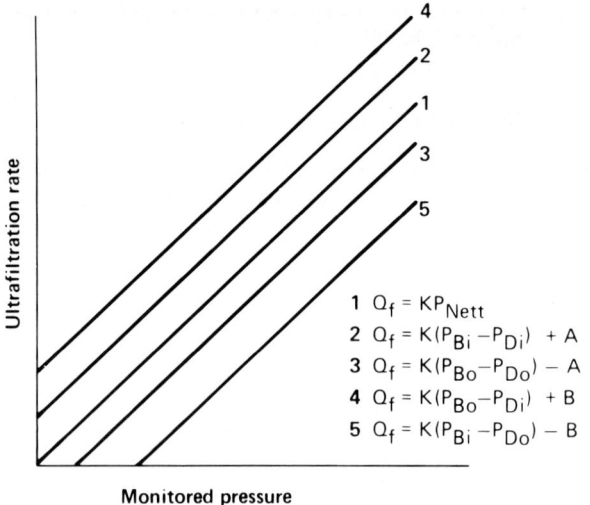

Figure 23. Ultrafiltration rate of a haemodialyser as a function of monitored pressure where K is a constant dependent upon membrane permeability and A B are intercepts on the axes.

Lowrie (97) have indicated that these assumptions significantly underestimate the transmembrane pressure and have suggested that a more appropriate relationship is given by

$$P_{nett} = \frac{4 (P_B^5 \text{ in} - P_B^5 \text{ out})}{5 (P_B^4 \text{ in} - P_B^4 \text{ out})}$$

In practice, the relationship between the ultrafiltration rate and transmembrane pressure may most readily be studied *in vitro* under conditions of balanced osmolarity using the same fluid on both sides of the membrane. Under these conditions, a very satisfactory straight line relating the two parameters may be obtained. If the appropriate correction for plasma osmotic pressures is made, then it is possible to predict the *in vivo* ultrafiltration based on *in vitro* measurements.

These relationships, however, are only of limited value clinically, since the pressure may not be measured at all parts of the circuit. However, as Figure 23 shows, the slopes of the lines are identical. This slope, which is a function of the membrane hydraulic permeability and the haemodialyser surface area, is defined as the ultrafiltration coefficient, whose units are ml/hr/mm Hg. *In vitro* and *in vivo* ultrafiltration coefficients measured with the aid of an electronic weighing system are shown in Tables 15 and 16; ideally, these two values should be comparable. In general, the ultrafiltration coefficients measured *in vivo* are lower than those obtained *in vitro* even after correction for the colloid osmotic pressure of plasma proteins. This reduction may be a consequence of the coating of the membrane surface by proteins and other blood components (platelets, lipids, red cells, white cells, fibrin).

Provided transmembrane pressure (TMP) is measured directly ultrafiltration *in vivo* rarely exceeds ultrafiltration *in vitro* at the same TMP. The rare occasions when this happens are probably explained by inter-dialyser variability.

However, if ultrafiltration *in vitro* is related to *calculated* TMP (based on direct measurement of blood and dialysate outlet pressures and predicted pressure drops across the dialyser) results are much more variable. The assumed pressure drop across the dialyser may be affected by poor degassing of the dialysis fluid, thrombus formation, channelling in the blood compartment or the variable relationship between haematocrit and viscosity. The difficulty in predicting *in vivo* ultrafiltration from *in vitro* results has been responsible for many episodes of hypotension during dialysis; these should be avoidable in the future as more proportionating units incorporate direct ultrafiltration monitors or measurement of true TMP.

Table 15. Standard haemodialysers. Ultrafiltration coefficients (ml/hr/mm Hg). Blood flow 200 ml/min. Dialysate flow 530 ml/min. Temperature 38 °C.

	In vitro	In vivo
M3 Micropoint	4.26	—
Multipoint	3.48	3.12
GLP	3.67	5.87
BL 500 Bravo	3.30	2.79
EXP 400	3.90	2.35
MTL 104	5.64	3.96
EX 25	2.20	—
ALT 100	3.44	—
Vita 2 HP	3.89	4.86
CDAK 3500	5.85	4.73
Triex 1	3.37	3.58
AM 10	3.17	3.09
CF 1200	2.74	4.98
MTS	5.10	5.25
HF 130	3.09	2.84

Table 16. Large surface area haemodialysers. Ultrafiltration coefficients (ml/hr/mm Hg). Blood flow 200 ml/min. Dialysate flow 530 ml/min. Temperature 38 °C.

	In vitro	In vivo
Multipoint (1.5 m²)	4.91	—
GLP	6.47	5.96
RP 514	3.71	4.86
PPD	4.77	—
ALT 140	3.70	—
EX 29	4.34	—
EX 55	4.76	—
CDAK 4000	4.48	4.72
HF 150	4.06	3.86
AM 20	4.59	4.15
Triex 3	5.35	4.46
GF 180M [a]	5.70	5.10

[a] Reference 181.

Blood compartment volume and compliance

The blood compartment volume of a dialyser is an important parameter for both the clinician and the engineer. In clinical practice it contributes to the extracorporeal circuit volume. In engineering terms, the blood compartment volume is expressed in terms of blood film thickness which is an important factor in governing the dialyser's small molecule clearance.

The blood compartment of early dialysers was so large that priming with donor blood was essential. Since the 1960's there has been a steady reduction in the blood compartment volume of dialysers and in many cases the volume of the blood lines exceeds that of the dialyser.

The dialyser is normally primed at low transmembrane pressure and the static blood compartment volume is established at this pressure. As transmembrane pressure is increased, the blood compartment volume increases – this increase is a function of the membrane characteristics such as thickness and grain orientation and the shape of the membrane supports. The value of the blood compartment volume may also be expressed in terms of blood path geometry. For hollow fibres it is given by:

$$\frac{\pi \& L N}{4}$$

and for flat plate or coil dialysers by:

$$\dot{L} W h_B N$$

It is difficult to establish limits on the priming volume and compliance of dialysers. Ideally, the priming volume should be as low as possible but the 100 ml achieved in many modern dialysers presents no problem to most adult patients and further reduction is not a

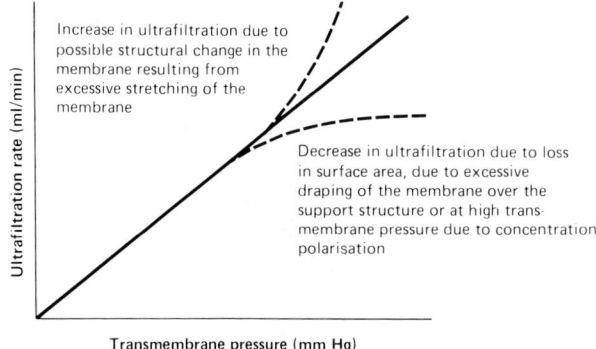

Figure 24. Causes of variation in ultrafiltration during clinical use.

Factors influencing ultrafiltration rate

Membrane characteristics

With increasing transmembrane pressure, changes in the membrane structure may occur, causing either an increase or decrease in ultrafiltration (Figure 24). Decrease of ultrafiltration may occur due to excessive stretching of the membrane resulting in draping of the membrane over the support structure while an increase in ultrafiltration may be a result of structural changes resulting in an increased membrane permeability.

Shrinkage of membranes due to variation in storage conditions and humidity may also occur causing alteration of membrane permeability (W. Bandel [Enka AG, Wuppertal, FRG], personal communication to the authors). Variability of membrane permeability due to interbatch variations of the membranes used have been described in the literature (98). Such variations while present, are not true interbatch variations but reflect the day to day fluctuations which may be present in large scale production, since membranes used in haemodialysers are produced not in batches but on a continuous basis.

Plasma protein concentration

The influence of plasma protein concentration on ultrafiltration rates used in conventional haemodialysis is small. When the ultrafiltration rate becomes sufficiently high (e.g., 50 ml/min or more) the ultrafiltration is no longer linearly dependent upon the transmembrane pressure but begins to flatten out, due to the build up of a concentrated layer of protein at the membrane surface (99, 100).

Thermo-osmotic effects

Osmotic effects are created by temperature differences between the blood and dialysate (101) and a linear relationship exists between temperature and ultrafiltration rate over the range of temperatures seen in clinical practice (102).

Table 17. Standard haemodialysers. Blood compartment volume (ml).

	Transmembrane pressure (mmHg)	
	100	200
M3 Micropoint	151	+16
Multipoint	125	+15
GLP	85	+19
BL 500 Bravo	90	+12
EXP 400	98	+20
MTL 104	51	+ 8
EX 25	166	+78
ALT 100	240	+72
Vita 2 HP	238	+23 [b]
CDAK 3500	75	—
Triex 1	98 [a]	—
AM 10	99 [a]	—
CF 1200	114	—
MTS	95	—
HF 130	200 [a]	—

[a] Includes hydraulic uptake of the fibres.
[b] For 50 mm increase in TMP.

Table 18. Large surface area haemodialysers. Blood-compartment volume (ml).

	Transmembrane pressure (mmHg)	
	100	200
Multipoint	166	27
GLP	203	+19
RP 514	177	+11
PPD	119	+17
ALT 140	354	—
EX 29	230	+72
EX 55	274	+24 [b]
CDAK 4000	93	—
HF 150	171	—
AM 20	140 [a]	—
Triex 3	116	—
GF 180M	140 [c]	—

[a] Includes hydraulic uptake of the fibres.
[b] For 50 mm increase in TMP.
[c] Reference 181.

clinically important goal. Compliance over the clinical range of pressures should be minimal or zero; this ideal, however, is difficult to achieve except in hollow fibre dialysers.

Measurement of blood compartment volume and compliance is most readily carried out *in vitro*. It can be combined with the measurement of ultrafiltration using a solution to which the membrane is permeable, however, for highly permeable membranes and dialysers a non-permeable fluid such as corn oil may be preferable. In Tables 17 and 18 the blood compartment volume and compliance is shown for selected clinically used dialysers.

Flow resistance

Resistance to blood flow

The resistance to flow in the blood compartment is governed by the pathway geometry; for flat plate dialysers with a large width to height ratio the relationship is given by

$$\Delta P_B = \frac{0.009\ \mu \dot{L} Q_B}{Wh^3 N} \text{ mm Hg}$$

while in circular tubes (hollow fibre dialysers) the pressure drop is given by

$$\Delta P_B = \frac{0.096\ \mu \dot{L} Q_B}{\pi N d^4} \text{ mm Hg}$$

Both these relationships are linear and highly dependent upon the blood pathway geometry and the blood viscosity which depends upon the haematocrit. Deviations in linearity may occur from dimensional instabilities introduced by manufacture or membrane deformation.

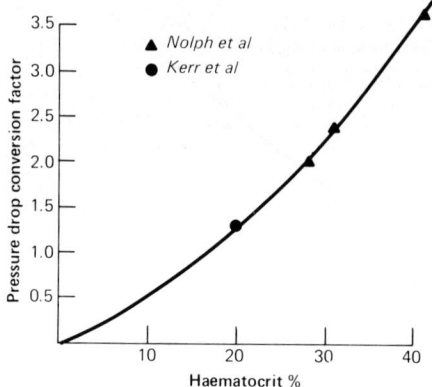

Figure 25. Conversion factor for blood compartment pressure drop from aqueous solution measurement to blood of varying haematocrit.

Blood flow resistance can be measured *in vitro* using blood or an aqueous solution or *in vivo*. It is most commonly measured *in vitro* using an aqueous solution. To estimate the *in vivo* pressure drop a conversion factor may be used if direct measurement is unavailable. To establish this conversion factor we have measured the pressure drop directly using blood with a haematocrit of 20%, and combined the results with those obtained by Nolph and colleagues (102) for haematocrit values of 26, 31 and 41% (Figure 25). Care should be exercised in the use of this conversion factor since there is a considerable scatter in the relationship between haematocrit and blood viscosity.

Resistance to dialysate flow

The equations governing the pressure drop in the dialysate pathway with flow rate are comparable with those

Table 19. Standard haemodialysers. Flow resistance (mm Hg).

	Blood compartment	Dialysate compartment
	At saline flow of 200 ml/min	At dialysate flow of 530 ml/min
M3 Micropoint	29	18
Multipoint	35	26
GLP	13	15
BL 500 Bravo	62	24
EXP 400	36	4
MTL 104	11	40
EX 25	39	—
ALT 100	216	—
Vita 2 HP	90	4
CDAK 3500	11	6
Triex 1	8	49
CF 1200	10	13
MTS	20	18
HF 130	9	65

To estimate the flow resistance for blood with a haematocrit of 25% multiply the figures shown by 1.8.

Table 20. Large surface area haemodialysers. Flow resistance (mm Hg).

	Blood compartment	Dialysate compartment
	At saline flow of 200 ml/min	At dialysate flow of 530 ml/min
Multipoint	49	15
GLP	16	6
RP 154	15	19
PPD	31	6
ALT 140	203	—
EX 29	202	—
EX 55	95	3
CDAK 4000	11	11
HF 150	8	14
AM 20	12	14
Triex 3	7	77
GF 180M	20	10

To estimate the flow resistance for blood with a haematocrit of 25% multiply the figures shown by 1.8.

established for the blood pathway. As the majority of conventional haemodialysers are operated in conjunction with a negative pressure in the dialysate pathway excessive pressure drops in that pathway may limit the use of the device to certain delivery systems, while significant variations in this parameter in disposable dialysers or successive reassembly of reusable dialysers can lead to an unpredictability of both solute and water removal.

Blood and dialysate flow resistances for selected haemodialysers are shown in Tables 19 and 20.

Flow distribution

The uniformity of flow distribution in both the blood and dialysate compartments is important since variations not only influence the solute transport characteristics of the device, but may also result in flow stagnation in the blood pathway leading to increased thrombus formation and consequent blood loss.

Flow non-idealities may occur in both the blood and dialysate pathways due to random dimensional variations in the path geometry during manufacture or systematic defects in the design of a particular dialyser. The influence of these effects may be demonstrated by the injection of a non-dialysable dye into the dialyser. Elimination or reduction of these flow non-idealities is the aim of every manufacturer but only a moderate degree of success has been achieved in this area (see Figure 11).

Blood-membrane interactions

Thrombogenicity

Clotting within the dialyser was a serious problem with some past models (103, 104) but improvements in dialyser design have tended to reduce thrombus formation. Nevertheless, thrombus formation can occur in spite of adequate anticoagulation. The underlying mechanisms for this are complex, multifactorial and poorly understood.

Clotting within the dialyser may be a function of the fluid dynamic conditions within the device. Recent studies have shown that the convective and diffusive phenomena occurring near the membrane surface also play an important part in determining the extent of thrombus formation (105, 106). It is also a function of the patient's blood, the dose, administration and half life of heparin. Patients vary considerably in their heparin requirements (107, 108) (see also chapter 9).

Precise heparin administration during routine haemodialysis is possible by the application of a technique described by Gotch and Keen (109) and elaborated by others (110, 111) enabling heparin requirements to be tailored to each patient's needs and thereby reducing thrombus formation (see also chapter 10).

An additional potential hazard associated with haemodialyser thrombogenecity is the formation of microthrombi and subsequent release into the patient's circulation of microemboli (112).

Damage to blood components

During dialysis, platelets, white cells and red cells are deposited on the membrane (104, 113–115). Damage to platelets is shown by a fall in platelet count, loss of mature platelets from the circulation (114, 116) and the release of serotonin (116). Lindsay and colleagues (104) in their studies, also demonstrated a correlation between platelet damage and clot formation in the dialyser.

Destruction and damage of red cells occur in blood flowing through tubing (118, 119). The influence of shear rates on red cells has been studied by Blackshear (120) who concluded that under laminar blood flow conditions, the damage to red cells is not significant. This is confirmed by the near normal red cell survival in haemodialysis patients in whom blood loss has been minimised (121). Some damage, however, may arise from the blood pump (122) and until this can be eliminated, the contribution due to the dialyser may be difficult to assess.

Haemodialysis leucopenia

In the early phase of haemodialysis (0 to 45 minutes) there is a fall in circulating leucocytes (neutrophils, macrophages and probably eosinophils) which is reversed by the end of the first hour of dialysis (Figure 26). The studies of Toren and colleagues (123) and Craddock et al. (124–126) showed that the cause of this phenomenon is sequestration of leucocytes in the lungs.

All authors agree that the type of membrane used has an influence on the extent of this leucopenia. Cellulose membranes produce a profound leucopenia; the newer synthetic alternatives such as polymethylmethacrylate, polycarbonate and cellulose acetate produce an intermediate leucopenia; the PA (PAN69) and polysulphone membranes cause little leucopenia (127–129).

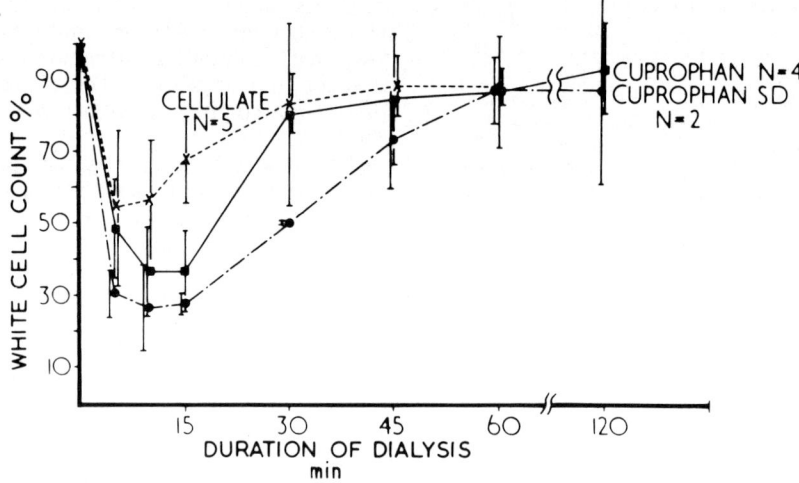

Figure 26. Variation of white cell count with duration of dialysis for cellulose and modified cellulose membranes.

Consequently, it might be assumed that a study of dialysis leucopenia would have become a routine part of dialyser evaluation many years ago. In practice, this has not happened because, until recently, it was assumed that this was a harmless laboratory aberration with no influence on the patient's condition. In 1977, Craddock and his colleagues (124–126) suggested that sequestration of leucocytes in the lungs was responsible for the hypoxia which characteristically develops during haemodialysis with acetate containing dialysis fluid. Although interpretation of the facts has been disputed by several authors (130–133) there is now some pressure from licencing bodies to include a study of dialysis leucopenia in the evaluation of new membranes. In the absence of any clear-cut evidence that leucopenia is of importance in causing symptoms during haemodialysis, and in the light of the 20 year survival of some patients who have been subjected to this phenomenon more than 150 times a year, we remain unconvinced that it should be taken into account in the selection of dialysers or dialysis membranes.

Haemodialysis complement activation
In 1977, Craddock and colleagues (124–126) formulated a hypothesis that contact between membrane and plasma, which is essential for the production of dialysis leucopenia, resulted in activation of complement and demonstrated that the incubation of plasma with a cellulose membrane activates complement through an alternative pathway and releases a substance which produces leucopenia similar to that seen in haemodialysis. Subsequent studies by the same group (124, 134) showed that activation of complement fraction C5 (C5a) induced granulocyte aggregation. The influence of membrane type on complement activation has been studied by Aljama and colleagues (135), Jacob et al. (128) and Jones and coworkers (136).

The conflicting results obtained by these authors and Craddock and his colleagues probably reflect the different methods used to assess complement activation. Most authors measured the levels of complement fractions in the serum which may not be the best index of complement activation, particularly as the immunological assays employed in some cases react with breakdown products of the original fraction.

Complement activation by membranes, like leucopenia which has been attributed to it, remains at the moment an interesting laboratory phenomenon without definite clinical implications. Should it be shown in the future to have clinical importance, complement activation will have to be incorporated in the evaluation of dialysers and membranes; at the moment, there is not sufficient published information to compare dialysers and membranes meaningfully in respect of this characteristic.

Damage to platelets by membranes
So far, the testing of this phenomenon has not been sufficiently standardised to make it possible to compare dialysers in respect of their effects on platelets, but it is likely to become a part of dialyser evaluation in the future.

Blood loss in haemodialysers

The total blood loss in patients receiving regular dialysis treatment for chronic renal failure may be as high as 5 l/annum (137). This blood loss is a consequence of a number of factors such as sampling for biochemical control and bleeding from fistula sites. Blood loss into the dialyser and blood lines remains also an important component of this overall loss and its measurement and optimisation is an important parameter.

The blood loss in a dialyser may be due to a number of causes such as the accidental rupture of the membrane, clotting episodes during dialysis and blood loss at the termination of dialysis.

Large amounts of blood may be lost as a consequence of membrane leak or rupture. A high leak rate is a serious disadvantage since it not only has a deleterious effect on patient and staff morale but may also contribute significantly to the patient's anaemia. Current haemodialysers are tested during manufacture and in consequence, have low leak rates but this has not always been the case (138). The leak rate for non-disposable dialysers depends upon the skill and care of the persons building them. Improvements in manufacturing technology of both the dialyser and the membrane have made significant contributions to the reduction of this problem and leak rates for current dialysers are difficult to assess since multiple centre studies extending over several thousand dialyses would be required even for dialysers with an (unacceptable) leak rate of 5% or higher. When leaks occur, they are presently more likely to be related to the shipment, storage and handling prior to and during use.

All currently used haemodialysers are sufficiently thrombogenic to require the administration of an anticoagulant for successful operation. The formation of thrombus in the dialyser is a consequence of the patient's thrombus generating potential, the surface properties of the material in contact with the blood such as surface charge, surface roughness, the geometry of the flow path and the local fluid dynamic and mass transfer conditions (139–141).

The reduction of thrombus formation has been explored by giving antiplatelet drugs along with heparin (142) and by the attachment of heparin molecules to the membrane surface (143–145). More recently, prostaglandins with and without anticoagulants have been used to reduce thrombus formation in haemodialysers (146).

At the termination of dialysis, the contents of the extracorporeal circuit are returned to the patient by the use of a rinseback technique involving either normal saline, isotonic dextrose or air to displace the circuit contents. A considerable amount of blood may remain at the termination of this procedure. This residue is made up of two distinct components.

First, the fluid blood component, which is related to the design of the dialyser, the volume of rinseback solution, the technique of washback (147, 148) and the heparinisation during dialysis. The second component is the clotted residue formed, despite adequate heparinisation, which is trapped and cannot be removed by increasing the volume of washback or altering the technique, short of disrupting the clot.

Measurement of these two components differs: fluid blood retained in the extracorporeal circuit is measured by haemoglobinometry, whereby the haemoglobin concentration of the patient's arterial blood is compared with that of the extracorporeal circuit at the termination of dialysis. A number of methods for this purpose are available (148, 150, 151). In our own studies after the washback, one litre of ammoniated water (0.04% NH_3) is circulated through the dialyser under minimal ultrafiltration conditions. Once thorough mixing has been achieved the haemoglobin content of the patient's blood and the ammoniated water is measured using a technique described by Cripps (152). The blood retained is calculated from a simple formula (75) which incorporates an estimate of the extracorporeal circuit based upon previous measurements or estimated by draining the contents of the circuit into a measuring cyclinder; while both these methods are subject to inaccuracies their influence on the final result is small.

The accuracy of fluid residual blood measurements was questioned by Lindsay and colleagues (149) but we have found the procedure used by us accurate and reproducible when compared with other techniques (T. White and M. Scott, Department of Medical Physics and Clinical Biochemistry, Royal Victoria Infirmary, Newcastle Upon Tyne, unpublished observations, 1974).

Clotted blood residue may be assessed visually but is most readily measured by the labelling of the patient's red cells with a radioactive tracer and comparing the tracer concentration in the dialyser with a sample of the patient's blood taken prior to the termination of dialysis and diluting it in a geometry of similar dimensions as

Table 21. Standard haemodialysers. Residual blood loss (ml).

	Fluid blood		Clotted blood		Saline rinse volume (ml)	Rinse volume circuit volume [a]
	Mean	Range	Mean	Range		
M3 Micropoint	5.3	2.2–10.9	—	—	600	1.64
GLP	2.1	0.4–3.7	—	—	600	1.73
BL 500 Bravo	1.0	0.0–2.3	—	—	600	2.14
EXP 400	3.7	2.4–7.0	1.7	1.3–2.1	600	1.91
MTL 104	4.3	0.3–7.9	—	—	400	1.47
EX 25	8.1	0.4–20.1	4.5	3.9–4.9	800	1.90
ALT 100	5.6	0.2–19.1	—	—	800	1.71
Vita 2HP	2.0	0.3–3.9	3.8	0.7–7.0	800	0.60
CDAK 3500	1.9	0.3–12.8	—	—	600	1.83
Triex 1	1.2	0.1–2.4	0.9	0.4–1.4	600	1.72
CF 1200	1.7	0.9–2.3	—	—	600	1.52
MTS	1.5	0.2–3.0	—	—	600	2.15
HF 130	2.3	0.4–8.5	—	—	600	1.70

[a] Circuit volume = volume of dialyser + blood lines.

Table 22. Large surface area haemodialysers. Residual blood loss (ml).

	Fluid blood		Clotted blood		Saline rinse volume (ml)	Rinse volume / circuit volume[a]
	Mean	Range	Mean	Range		
Multipoint	4.3	1.8–8.0	–	–	800	2.52
GLP	3.3	1.5–5.5	–	–	600	1.76
RP 514	3.9	1.7–8.9	–	–	800	1.87
PPD	8.9	2.8–17.1	–	–	600	1.69
ALT 140	8.9	2.2–24.5	–	–	800	1.86
EX 29	6.0	1.9–26.2	7.7	4.8–10.6	800	2.11
EX 55	4.2	1.0–15.3	–	–	800	1.74
CDAK 4000	2.0	0.6–4.0	–	–	600	1.74
HF 150	3.9	2.0–5.8	–	–	600	1.48
AM 20	1.7	0.9–2.8	–	–	600	1.59
Triex 3	2.1	0.5–8.7	–	–	600	1.63
GF 180M	–	–	–	–	–	–

[a] Circuit volume = volume of dialyser + blood lines.

the dialyser and counting it in a bulk sample or whole body counter. The two most commonly used tracer substances are ^{51}Cr and ^{59}Fe. Of the two, ^{51}Cr is preferable since it may be used immediately with relative ease whereas some two weeks must be allowed for the incorporation of ^{59}Fe into the red cells. The radiation dose from these studies is small – a single dose of 50 µCi of ^{51}Cr permits measurements of residual blood volume of about six consecutively used dialysers. Unfortunately, the dose cannot be repeated too many times since the procedure is not for the benefit of the patients and in consequence, we restrict our patients to a maximum of two labellings. This limits the number of measurements possible and accounts for the scanty literature on this subject.

Comparison between different dialysers' residual blood loss characteristics are given in Tables 21 and 22. These results show a wide scatter but the mean loss from this source is small in comparison with loss from other sources.

Haemodialyser washout characteristics

The residual blood loss characteristics of haemodialysers are generally established after a standard saline rinseback – in our unit 600 ml. The introduction and availability of large surface area dialysers, miniature dialysers and the growing trend towards the reduction of treatment time has resulted in the desirability of minimising fluid given to the patient at the end of dialysis without incurring unacceptable blood losses. This requirement has led to the need to determine the washout characteristics of a dialyser to permit optimisation of washback volume and minimisation of fluid blood loss. A non invasive technique to enable this to be undertaken has been developed using ^{51}Cr labelled red cells (153). Using this technique, blood recovery curves for the haemodialyser may be established and related to the ratio of washback volume/circuit volume (Figure 27). This method is suitable for both in vitro and in vivo measurements but the need to expose the patient to radiation

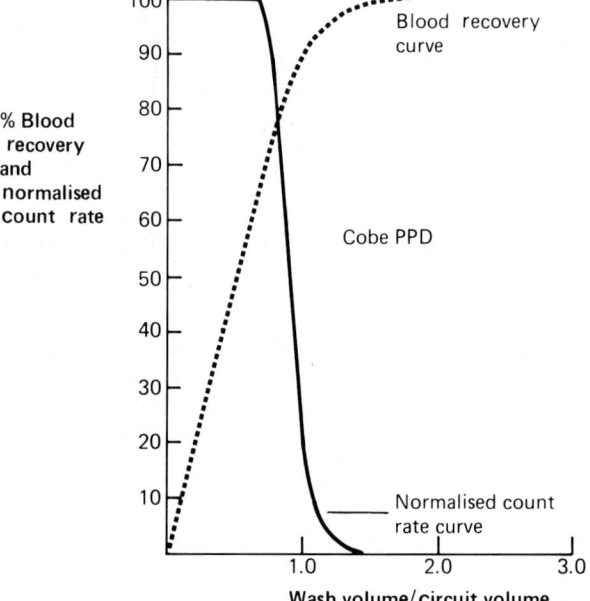

Figure 27. Normalised count rate curve and its derived blood recovery curve.

limits the clinical use of this technique. Furthermore, extrapolation of *in vitro* data to *in vivo* where the membrane may be distorted or clotted can lead to the introduction of errors. The visual observation of the colour of the blood-saline mixture at the venous bubble trap may well prove a more acceptable and sufficiently accurate clinical guide to dialyser washout effectiveness (154, 155).

Elution of toxic substances from the dialyser

Materials used in the construction of dialysers are considered 'non-toxic' in the sense that they conform to toxicity standards drawn up for quite different applications. There are no internationally accepted standards for purity and little attention has been paid to this aspect in dialyser evaluation.

Haemodialysis membranes contain some zinc and copper which may be released during dialysis (156, 157) and interactions have been reported between the sterilising agent and membrane (158) and other materials used in the construction of the dialyser (159) while allergic reactions in dialysis patients have been attributed to residual ethylene oxide (160).

Occasional allergic and anaphylactic reactions have been observed with Cuprophan hollow fibre dialysers possibly due to the inadequate removal of the isopropyl myristate from the membrane or due to the organic solvents (methanol and freon) used in the removal of the myristate (161).

Plasticisers and other compounds may leach out of the blood lines and bags used in intravenous infusion (162-165). Recently a foreign body reaction to silicone was identified in the spleen of a haemodialysis patient with decreasing haemoglobin levels and pancytopenia. The patient was dialysed 20 to 24 h per week during 4 years. Silicone rubber tubing and pumps inserts were used (166, 167).

The repeated exposure of regular dialysis patients to these hazards renders them vulnerable but hard evidence of harm is scant although eluates from the tubing sets and dialysers have been shown to produce cardiac arrythmias (159).

Bacterial contamination

Pyrogen reactions were common in the early days of haemodialysis when many were due to the reuse of components in direct contact with the blood which were autoclaved between use. Many problems described in the literature relate to non-disposable dialysers where the blood-contacting surfaces are subject to considerable handling (168). They are not a problem of great magnitude with disposable dialysers. Although bacterial contamination may occur during manufacture, it appears to be a rare cause of pyrogen reactions; with a few exceptions (169) single use disposable dialysers are free of this complication.

In vitro studies have shown that bacteria and endotoxins are too large to cross the haemodialysis membrane (170). However, scanning electron microscopy has confirmed the presence of bacteria on both sides of the membrane (169). Nevertheless the cause of outbreaks of pyrogen reactions often remains a mystery. They are attributed to bacterial growth in the dialysate (171, 172) or to water contamination by pyrogens (173). Certainly, endotoxin enters the blood stream of some patients and stimulates the formation of antibodies (174, 175), but there is no convincing evidence that the origin of these endotoxins is the dialysis fluid and consequently, any reaction that occurs during haemodialysis should first be blamed on the blood compartment, not the dialysis fluid.

Cost

The haemodialyser constitutes the most expensive disposable component of the extracorporeal circuit. In general, hollow fibre dialysers and designs using high permeability membranes are more expensive than flat plate and coil dialysers. Previous surveys of haemodialyser performance included cost (75). A recent survey of European dialysis centres showed that cost is no longer an important parameter in the choice of dialyser in most countries (176).

The cost of dialysers can vary substantially from country to country or even from centre to centre and depends, in part, on the quantities purchased. The recent market trend has been towards the reduction in price of disposable dialysers in the presence of increasing costs of labour, production and transport, reflecting destocking by manufacturers.

CHOOSING A DIALYSER

The choice of a dialyser for a patient receiving regular dialysis treatment is a complex decision involving not only the basic performance parameters of the device and cost, but also the clinician's philosophy of treatment. For many years, a single size dialyser was used for patients ranging from 40 to over 80 kg. The market now is large enough to allow the sale of dialysers in different sizes and ultrafiltration characteristics to allow some individualisation of therapy and a greater effort has to be made by clinicians to find the right haemodialyser for each patient. Furthermore, the ability to model mathematically the processes involved in the biochemical control of the patient will make it possible to achieve a desired therapeutic goal and to assess the results of altered treatment, leading to the better management of the haemodialysis patient (177, 178).

FUTURE TRENDS IN HAEMODIALYSER DESIGN

The relationship between dialyser design parameters and the basic performance characteristics are shown in Table 24. The narrow choice of materials available for dialyser designers has limited the possibility of radical changes in design trends. Of the design parameters shown, only four – surface area, geometry of the blood and dialysate pathway and membrane thickness – have received attention from the designers. Current flat plate designs use an improved membrane support geometry permitting better control of blood film thickness. This not only limits the dialyser's blood compartment volume, but also influences the clearance of small molecules and accounts for much of the improvements demonstrated by the current generation of designs.

Dialysate pathway geometry in the flat plate design is well defined, but is far from optimal in the case of hollow fibre designs. Mathematical analysis by Sigdell (37) and Lee and Taylor (35) have indicated ways of improv-

Table 23. Optimisation of haemodialyser design. Influence of design variables on clinical parameters.

Design variable	Clinical parameters					
	Clearance					
	Small molecules	Large molecules	Ultrafiltration	Blood flow resistance	Blood compartment	Blood loss
Surface area	+	+	+	−	+	+
Blood path geometry	+ +	+	−	+	+	+ +
Dialysate path geometry	+ +	+	−	−	+	−
Membrane thickness	+	+	+	+	+	−
Membrane permeability	+	+ +	+ +	−	−	−
Membrane strength	+	+	+	+ +	+ +	−

+ + Positive influence.
+   Marginal influence.
−   No effect.

ing fluid dynamic characteristics and application of these design concepts will doubless lead to further improvements.

Further improvements of performance may be achieved by the elimination of the blood and dialysis fluid film boundary layers which for small molecules are the principal barriers to diffusion. Elimination of these boundary layers for a flat plate design has been achieved in a 'vortex mixing' dialyser developed by Bellhouse and Abel and colleagues (179, 180) which uses pulsatile reversing blood and dialysis fluid flows generated by rolling diaphragm and piston pumps in the blood and dialysate circuits (Figure 29).

Preliminary results using this design with a surface area of $0.32 \, m^2$ show that it achieves ultrafiltration rates and clearances of small and middle molecules comparable with those of conventional m^2 dialysers (personal communication to authors, 1981).

Some further improvements in the consistency of performance are likely, due to better quality control of dialysers during manufacture. But major advances in performance may be expected only as a result of introduction of new membranes. At the time of writing, cellulosic membranes (Cuprophan, cellulose acetate) remain the most widely used membranes. Modified cellulose membranes offer an increased permeability to middle molecules and an increased ultrafiltration as do non-cellulosic membranes (polyacrylonitrile, polymethylmethacrylate); their use to date has been largely limited to the newer, alternative techniques of treatment of terminal renal failure such as haemofiltration. Further developments in membrane technology can be anticipated re-

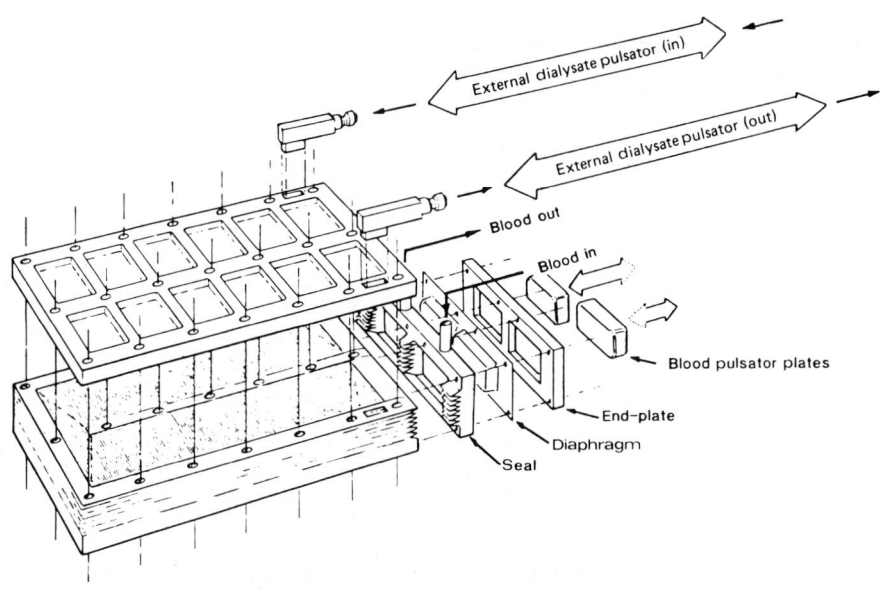

Figure 28. The 'Oxford' vortex mixing haemodialyser.

sulting in more selective membranes, and future radical developments in haemodialyser design will depend on the identification of uraemic toxins. With their positive identification, the designers of haemodialysers will be able to concentrate upon designs which selectively remove uraemic toxins while retaining essential compounds such as amino acids and water soluble vitamins.

NOMENCLATURE

A	Cross sectional area
C	Concentration
D	Dialysance
H	Haematocrit
K	Clearance
L_h	Membrane hydraulic permeability
L	Length
N	Integer
P	Pressure
Q	Volumetric flow rate
R	Mass transfer resistance
R'	Recirculation
S	Surface area
S	Sieving coefficient
W	Blood path width
Ø	Volume fraction of hydrated proteins
π	Constant
d	Fibre internal diameter
h	Blood pathway height
k	Equilibrium solute distribution between red cells and plasma
s	Integer
μ	Viscosity

Subscripts

B	Blood
Bi	Blood inlet
Bo	Blood outlet
D	Dialysate
Di	Dialysis fluid inlet
Do	Dialysate outlet
f	Flux
h	Hydraulic
M	Membrane
Osm	Osmotic
R	Recirculation
T	Total

REFERENCES

1. Hoeltzenbein J: *Die künstliche Niere* (The artificial kidney) Stuttgart, Ferdinand Enke Verlag 1969, p 270 (in German)
2. Dittrich P, Gurland HJ, Kessel M, Massini M-A, Wetzels E: *Hämodialyse und Peritonealdialyse* (Haemodialysis and peritoneal dialysis) Berlin, Heidelberg, New York, Springer-Verlag 1969, p 477 (in German)
3. Abel JJ, Rowntree LG, Turner BB: On the removal of diffusible substances from the circulating blood of living animals by dialysis. *J Pharmacol Exp Ther* 5:275, 1913-1914
4. Haas G: Dialysieren des stromenden Blutes am Lebenden (Dialysis of the circulating blood in vivo). *Klin Wochenschr* 2:1888, 1923 (in German)
5. Thalhimer W: Experimental exchange transfusion for reducing azotemia. Use of artificial kidney for this purpose. *Proc Soc Exp Biol Med* 37:641, 1937
6. Kolff WJ, Berk HTJ, ter Welle M, van der Ley AJW, van Dijk EC, van Noordwijk, J: De kunstmatige nier; een dialysator met groot oppervlak (The artificial kidney; a dialyser with a large surface area). *Geneesk Gids* 21: 409, 1943 (in Dutch)
7. Alwall N: On the artificial kidney. I. Apparatus for dialysis of the blood in vivo. *Acta Med Scand* 128:317, 1947
8. Skeggs LT Jr, Leonards JR: Studies on an artificial kidney: I. Preliminary results with a new type of continuous dialyzer. *Science* 108:212, 1948
9. Kiil F, (Amundsen B): Development of a parallel flow artificial kidney in plastics. *Acta Chir Scand (Suppl)* 253:142, 1960
10. Scribner BH, Caner JE, Buri R, Quinton WE: The technique of continuous hemodialysis. *Trans Am Soc Artif Intern Organs* 6:88, 1960
11. Pendras JP, Cole JJ, Tu WH, Scribner BH: Improved technique of continuous flow hemodialysis. *Trans Am Soc Artif Intern Organs* 7:27, 1961
12. Stewart RD, Cerny JC, Mahon HI: The capillary 'Kidney'. Preliminary report. *Univ Michigan Med Centre J* 30:116, 1964
13. Drukker W, Haagsma-Schouten WAG, Alberts Chr, Spoek MG: Report on regular dialysis treatment in Europe V, 1969, *Proc Eur Dial Transpl Assoc* 6:99, 1969
14. Bluemle LW, Dickson JG, Mitchell J, Podolnick MS: Permeability and hydrodynamic studies on the MacNeil Collins dialyzer using conventional and modified membrane supports. *Trans Am Soc Artif Intern Organs* 6:38, 1960
15. Edson H, Keen M, Gotch F: Comparative solute transport and therapeutic effectiveness of multiple point support and standard Kiil hemodialyzers. *Trans Am Soc Artif Intern Organs* 18:113, 1972
16. von Hartitzsch B, Hoenich NA: Meltec Multipoint haemodialyser *Br Med J* 1:237, 1972
17. Hoenich NA, Johnston S, Laing C, Evans C, Kerr DNS: The Meltec Micropoint M3 haemodialyser *Report No 92 to Department of Health and Social Security* London, UK 1980
18. Lewis KJ, Dewar PJ, Ward MK, Kerr DNS: Formation of anti-N-like antibodies in dialysis patients: effect of different methods of dialyzer rinsing to remove formaldehyde. *Clin Nephrol* 15:39, 1981
19. Shaldon S, Chevallet M, Maraoui M, Mion C: Dialysis associated auto-antibodies. *Proc Eur Dial Transpl Assoc* 13:339, 1976
20. Fassbinder W, Pilar J, Scheuermann E, Koch M: Formaldehyde and the occurrence of anti-N-like cold agglutinins in RDT patients. *Proc Eur Dial Transpl Assoc* 13:333, 1976
21. Fassbinder W, Seidl S, Koch KM: The role of formaldehyde in the formation of haemodialysis-associated anti-N-like antibodies. *Vox Sang* 35:41, 1978
22. McDonald HP, Merrill JP: A disposable parallel flow unit for the MacNeill-Collins artificial kidney – Description and evaluation. *Trans Am Soc Artif Intern Organs* 6:7, 1960
23. Malchesky PS, Mrava GL, Nosé Y: A totally disposable presterilized dialyzer. *Arch Intern Med* 127:278, 1971
24. Alwall N: A new disposable artificial kidney: experimen-

tal and clinical experience. *Proc Eur Dial Transpl Assoc* 5:18, 1968
25. Hoenich NA, Kerr DNS: A comparative evaluation of three high efficiency disposable dialyzers. *Clin Nephrol* 3:211, 1975
26. Frost TH: Artificial kidney machines: thin films or else? *Engineering in Medicine* 2:82, 1973
27. Hoenich NA, Frost TH: Influence of design and operating variables on conventional haemodialysis. In *Renal Dialysis,* edited by Whelpton D, London, Sector Publishing Ltd, 1974 p 85
28. Hoenich NA, White T, Luno J, Liano F, Kerr DNS: Disposable dialysers – current trends and experiences. In *Technical Aspects of Renal Dialysis,* edited by Frost TH, Tunbridge Wells, Pitman Medical, 1977, p 38
29. Elliott W, Kerr DNS, Horn DB, Pearson DT: In-vitro performance of the twin-coil artificial kidney with suggested improvements. *Lancet* 1:248, 1961
30. Hoeltzenbein J: Efficient and inexpensive, no-prime, no blood-loss haemodialysis system. *Proc Eur Dial Transpl Assoc* 5:316, 1969
31. Ota K, Okazawa T, Kumagaya E, Agishi T, Sugino N, Mitani N, Fujii Y, Kinura M, Nagao Y, Tsukamoto H, Tanzawa H, Sakai Y: Polymethylmethacrylate capillary kidney highly permeable to middle molecules. *Proc Eur Dial Transpl Assoc* 12:559, 1975
32. Anonymous: Asahi Hemofilter PAN-15 *Manufacturer's Literature,* Tokyo, Japan Asahi Medical Co Ltd, no date
33. Lysaght MJ, Ford CA, Colton CK, Stone RA, Henderson LW: Mass transfer in clinical blood ultrafiltration devices – a review. In *Technical Aspects of Renal Dialysis,* edited by Frost TH, Tunbridge Wells Pitman Medical, 1977, p 81
34. Nakagawa S, Koshikawa S, Ishida Y, Uematsu M, Ishibashi K: Development of flat type hollow fibre dialyser (NF-01): achievement of better performance than cylinder type with same membrane area. In: *Technical Aspects of Renal Dialysis* edited by Frost TH, Tunbridge Wells, Pitman Medical, 1977, p 29
35. Lee KH, Taylor JA: Multi-chambered dialyzers and their efficiencies. *Artif Organs* 3:137, 1979
36. Agishi T, Ota K, Nosé Y: Is hollow fibre occlusion due to maldistribution of blood? *Proc Eur Dial Transpl Assoc* 12:519, 1975
37. Sigdell JE: *A mathematical theory for the capillary artificial kidney.* Stuttgart, Hippokrates Verlag, 1974
38. Babb AL, Popovich RP, Christopher TG, Scribner BH: The genesis of the square meter-hour hypothesis. *Trans Am Soc Artif Intern Organs* 17:81, 1971
39. Babb AL, Farrell PC, Uvelli DA, Scribner BH: Hemodialyzer evaluation by examination of solute molecular spectra. *Trans Am Soc Artif Intern Organs* 18:98, 1972
40. Hoenich NA, Conceicao S, Ward MK, White T, Kerr DNS: Large surface area dialysers. A question of performance. *Proc Eur Soc Artif Organs* 3:78, 1976
41. Reiger J, Quellhorst E, Lowitz HD, Kong RG, Scheler F: Ultrafiltration for middle molecules in uraemia. *Proc Eur Dial Transpl Assoc* 11:158, 1974
42. Quellhorst E, Reiger J, Dcht B, Beckmann H, Jacob I, Kraft B, Mietzsch G, Scheler F: Treatment of chronic uraemia by an ultrafiltration kidney – first clinical experience. *Proc Eur Dial Transpl Assoc* 13:314, 1976
43. Quellhorst E, Doht B, Schuenemann B: Hemofiltration: treatment of renal failure by ultrafiltration and substitution. *J Dial* 1:529, 1977
44. Smeby LC, Jørstad S, Widerøe T-E: Design analyses of a new selective filtration system for removal of uremic toxins. *Clin Nephrol* 13:125, 1980
45. Ivanovich P: Sequential ultrafiltration-hemodialysis. 18 months' experience. *Dial Transpl* 7:1077, 1978
46. Lynggaard F: One year's experience with sequential filtration/hemodialysis. *Dial Transpl* 7:1106, 1978
47. Rowland S: Isolated ultrafiltration and sequential dialysis with a new dialysis fluid module. *Dial Transpl* 9:1080, 1980
48. Bergström J: Ultrafiltration without dialysis for removal of fluid and solutes in uremia. *Clin Nephrol* 9:156, 1978
49. Jones EO, Ward MK, Hoenich NA, Kerr DNS: Separation of dialysis and ultrafiltration – does it really help? *Proc Eur Dial Transpl Assoc* 14:160, 1977
50. Leber HW, Wizemann V, Goubeaud G, Rawer P, Schutterle G: Hemodiafiltration: A new alternative to hemofiltration and conventional hemodialysis. *Artif Organs* 2:150, 1978
51. Jørstad S, Smeby LC, Widerøe T-E, Berg KJ: Removal of uremic toxins and regeneration of hemofiltrate by a selective dual hemofiltration artificial kidney (SEDUFARK) system. *Clin Nephrol* 13:85, 1980
52. Man N-K, Terlain B, Paris J, Werner G, Sausse A, Funck-Brentano JL: An approach to 'middle molecules' identification in artificial kidney dialysate with reference to neuropathy prevention. *Trans Am Soc Artif Intern Organs* 19:320, 1973
53. Lyman DJ: Membranes. In *Replacement of Renal Function by Dialysis,* edited by Drukker W, The Hague, Parsons FM, Maher JF, The Hague, Boston, London, Martinus Nijhoff 1978 p 69
54. Hilderson J, Ringoir S, van Waeleghem JP, van Egmond J, van Haelst JP, Schelstraete K: Short dialysis with a polyacrylonitrilmembrane (RP6) without the use of a closed recirculating dialyzate delivery system. *Clin Nephrol* 4:18, 1975
55. Winchester JF, Apiliga MT, Kennedy AC: Short-term evaluation of charcoal hemoperfusion combined with dialysis in uremic patients. *Kidney Int* 10 (Suppl 7), S315, 1976
56. Odaka M, Tabata Y, Kobayashi H, Nomura Y, Soma M, Hirasawa H, Sato H, Suenaga E, Nabeta K: Three-hour maintenance dialysis combining direct haemoperfusion and haemodialysis. *Proc Eur Dial Transpl Assoc* 13:257, 1976
57. Anonymous: Cuprophan. *Technical Information Bulletin* No 12, 1. Wuppertal, Germany, Enka AG, 1977
58. Gurland HJ, Castro LA, Samtleben W, Fernandez JC: Combination of hemodialysis and hemoperfusion in a single unit for treatment of uremia. *Clin Nephrol* 11:167, 1979
59. Denti E, Walker JM, Brancaccio D, Tessore V: Evaluation of novel sorbent systems for joint hemodialysis and hemoperfusion. *Medical Instrumentation* 11:212, 1977
60. Gurland HJ, Fernandez JC, Samtleben W, Castro LA: Sorbent membranes: used in conventional dialyser format in vitro and clinical evaluation *Symposium on Hemoperfusion, Dialysate and Diafiltrate Purification.* Munich, DBR, Gemeinschaftsfachausschuss Medizinische Verfahrenstechnik, Abs 48, 1978
61. Stephen RL, Velick SF, Grosser B: Dialysis/hemofiltration in schizophrenia – review. *Symposium on Hemoperfusion, Dialysate and Diafiltrate Purification.* Munich, DBR; Gemeinschaftsfachausschuss Medizinische Verfahrenstechnik. Abs 92, 1978
62. Al Mardini H, Hoenich N, Bartlett K, Record CO: Comparative value of different dialysis membranes, including a carbon-coated membrane for removal of noxious substances in hepatic coma. *Int J Artif Organs* 2:290, 1979

63. Broyer M, Loirat C, Kleinknecht C: Technical aspects and results of regular hemodialysis in children. *Acta Paediatr Scand* 61:677, 1972
64. Grushkin CM, Korsch B, Fine RN: Hemodialysis in small children. *JAMA* 221:869, 1972
65. Shideman JR, Meyer RM, Streifel AJ, Lynch RE, Mauer SM, Kjellstrand CM: The evaluation and applications of hemodialyzers for pediatric patients. *J Dial* 2:217, 1978
66. Gutman RA, Hickman RO, Chatrian GE, Scribner BH: Failure of high dialysis-fluid glucose to prevent the disequilibrium syndrome. *Lancet* 1:295, 1967
67. Hagstam KE, Lindergard B, Tibbling G: Mannitol infusion in regular haemodialysis treatment for chronic renal insufficiency. *Scand J Urol Nephrol* 3:257, 1969
68. Hone PWE, Randerson D, Farrell PC: Performance characteristics of disposable hemodialyzers. *Dial Transpl* 8:689, 1979
69. Cvejich L, Finnigan M, Brown P, Lindsay RM: Which hollow fiber dialyzer? *Dial Transpl* 7:990, 1978
70. Finnigan M, Cvejich L, Vandierendonck R, Lindsay RM: Which parallel plate dialyzer? *Dial Transpl* 8:882, 1979
71. Hone PWE, Ward RA, Mahony JF, Farrell PC: Hemodialyzer performance: an assessment of currently available units. *J Dial* 1:285, 1977
72. Hoenich NA, Kerr DNS: *Dialyser evaluation reports to Department of Health and Social Security,* different dates. (Available on request from authors)
73. Lunt MJ, Powell RJ, Cattell WR: Evaluation of an ultrasonic doppler flowmeter for measurement of extracorporeal blood flow during renal dialysis. In *Technical Aspects of Renal Dialysis,* edited by Frost TH, Tunbridge Wells, Pitman Medical, 1977, p 210
74. Gotch FA: Hemodialysis: technical and kinetic considerations. In *The Kidney,* edited by Brenner BM, Rector FC Jr, Philadelphia, London, Toronto, Sydney, WB Saunders Company, 1976, p 1672
75. von Hartitzsch B, Hoenich NA, Samson P, Erickson J, Ashcroft RA, Kerr DNS: A clinical evaluation of the new dialysers. *Kidney Int* 3:35, 1973
76. Piron M, Becaus I, Lameire N, Bleyn J, Ringoir S: An in vitro study of recirculation in single needle dialysis with the double headpump. In *Technical Aspects of Renal Dialysis,* edited by Frost TH, Tunbridge Wells, Pitman Medical, 1977, p 169
77. Ogden DA, Cohen IM: Blood recirculation during hemodialysis with a coaxial counterflow single needle blood access catheter. *Trans Am Soc Artif Intern Organs* 25:325, 1979
78. Colton CK, Henderson LW, Ford CA, Lysaght MJ: Kinetics of hemodiafiltration. I. In vitro transport characteristics of a hollow-fiber blood ultrafilter. *J Lab Clin Med* 85:355, 1975
79. Henderson LW, Colton CK, Ford CA: Kinetics of hemodiafiltration. II. Clinical characterization of a new blood cleansing modality. *J Lab Clin Med* 85:372, 1975
80. Kramer P, Tonnis HJ, Eichelberg B, Kattermann R, Scheler F: Distortion of dialysance by ultrafiltration, and its correction by means of a simple method. *Proc Eur Dial Transpl Assoc* 8:460, 1971
81. Nolph KD, Nothum RJ, Maher JF: Effects of ultrafiltration on dialysance in commercially available coils. *Kidney Int* 2:293, 1972
82. Nolph KD, Hopkins C, Van Stone J: Effects of ultrafiltration on solute clearances in parallel plate dialyzers. *Clin Nephrol* 8:453, 1977
83. Nolph KD, Twardowski ZJ, Hopkins CA, Rubin J, Van Stone JC: Effects of ultrafiltration on solute clearances in Cuprophan and cellulose hollow fiber dialyzers: in vitro and clinical studies. *J Lab Clin Med* 91:998, 1978
84. Colton CK, Smith KA, Merrill EW, Reece JM: Diffusion of organic solutes in stagnant plasma and red cell suspensions. *Chemical Engineering Progress Symposium Series* 66:85, 1970
85. Farrell PC, Ward RA, Hone PW: Uric acid: binding levels of urate ions in normal and uraemic plasma, and in human serum albumin. *Biochem Pharmacol* 24:1885, 1975
86. Farrell PC, Grib NL, Fry DL, Popovich RP, Broviac JW, Babb AL: A comparison of in vitro and in vivo solute-protein binding interactions in normal and uremic subjects. *Trans Am Soc Artif Intern Organs* 18:268, 1972
87. Skalsky M, Schindhelm K, Farrell PC: Creatinine transfer between red cells and plasma: a comparison between normal and uremic subjects. *Nephron* 22:514, 1978
88. Grossman NDF, Kopp KF, Frey J: Transport of urea by erythrocytes during haemodialysis. *Proc Eur Dial Transpl Assoc* 4:250, 1967
89. Fritz KW: Comparable dialysance measurement. *Proc Eur Dial Transpl Assoc* 1:59, 1964
90. Hoenich NA, von Hartitzsch B, Samson PJ, Erickson J, Reed B, Kerr DNS: Comparative performance characteristics of different thickness Cuprophane membrane. *Proc Eur Dial Transpl Assoc* 9:594, 1972
91. Leonard EF, Colton CK, Craig LD, Gessler RM, Klein E, Lontz JF, Lyman DJ, Mason RG, Nossel HL: Evaluation of membranes for hemodialyzers. *Report of the Membrane Evaluation Study Group for the Artificial Kidney-Chronic Uremia Program of NIAMDD* DHEW Publication No (NIH) 74-605, 1974
92. Muir WM: Editorial Review. *Proc Eur Dial Transpl Assoc* 8:359, 1971
93. Klein E, Autian J, Bower JD, Buffaloe G, Centella LJ, Colton CK, Darby TD, Farrell PC, Holland FF, Kennedy RS, Lipps B Jr, Mason R, Nolph KD, Villarroel F, Wathen RL: Evaluation of hemodialyzers and dialysis membranes. *Report of a Study Group for the Artificial Kidney-Chronic Uremia Program of NIAMDD* DHEW Publication No (NIH) 77-1294, 1977
94. Christopher TG, Cambi V, Harker LA, Hurst PE, Popovich RP, Babb AL, Scribner BH: A study of hemodialysis with lowered dialysate flow rate. *Trans Am Soc Artif Intern Organs* 17:92, 1971
95. Shinaberger JH, Miller JH, Rosenblatt MG, Gardner PW, Carpenter GW, Martin FE: Clinical studies of 'low flow' dialysis with membranes highly permeable to middle weight molecules. *Trans Am Soc Artif Intern Organs* 18:82, 1972
96. Klein E, Holland FF, Donnaud A, Lebeouf A, Eberle K: Diffusive and hydraulic permeabilities of commercially available cellulosic hemodialysis films and hollow fibers. *J Membrane Science* 2:349, 1977
97. Gagneux SA, Lowrie EG: Mean transmembrane pressure within coil hemodialyzers. *Dial Transpl* 5 (nr 5):61, 1976
98. Frost TH, Jolly D, Kerr DNS: Effect of membrane grain orientation on in vitro performance of a Kiil dialyzer. *Kidney Int* 3:186, 1973
99. Blatt WF, David A, Michaels AS. Nelsen L: Solute polarization and cake formation in membrane ultrafiltration: causes, consequences and control techniques. In *Membrane Science and Technology,* edited by Flinn FE, New York, Plenum, 1970, p 47 (Cited in ref 100)
100. Jaffrin MY, Vantarg G, Granger A: A concentration polarization model of hemofiltration with highly permeable membranes. *asaio J* 2:73, 1979
101. Grossmann DF, Kopp KF: Thermo-osmotic effect and ultrafiltration in the artificial kidney. Experience with the 'coil kidney'. *Proc Eur Dial Transpl Assoc* 3:299, 1966

102. Nolph KD, Fox M, Maher JF: Factors affecting the ultrafiltration rate from standard dialysis coils. *Trans Am Soc Artif Intern Organs* 16:487, 1970
103. Gotch FA, Sargent JA, Teisinger CL, Jones PO, Lipps BJ: The hollow fibre artificial kidney (Cordis Dow) 1968-71. *Proc Eur Dial Transpl Assoc* 8:568, 1971
104. Lindsay RM, Prentice CRM, Davidson JF, Burton JA, McNicol GP: Haemostatic changes during dialysis associated with thrombus formation on dialysis membranes. *Br Med J* 4:454, 1972
105. Blackshear PL Jr, Forstrom RJ: Fluid dynamics of blood cells and applications to hemodialysis. *Proc 10th Annual Contractors' Conference, Artificial Kidney Program of NIAMDD*, edited by Mackey BB, DHEW Publication No (NIH) 77-1442, 1977, p 58
106. Blackshear PL Jr, Forstrom RJ: Fluid dynamics of blood cells and applications to hemodialysis. *Proc 8th Annual Contractors' Conference, Artificial Kidney Program of NIAMDD*, edited by Mackey BB, DHEW Publication No (NIH) 75-248, 1975, p 59
107. Tourkantonis A: Heparin concentration during haemodialysis with heparinisation by automatic infusion pump. *Proc Eur Dial Transpl Assoc* 2:257, 1965
108. Lindsay RM: Variable heparin requirements during hemodialysis. Why? *asaio J* 3:81, 1980
109. Gotch FA, Keen ML: Precise control of minimal heparinization for high bleeding risk hemodialysis. *Trans Am Soc Artif Intern Organs* 23:168, 1977
110. Flicker W, Russell LW, Farrell PC: Precise anticoagulation-reagents and artifacts. *Dial Transpl* 9:1042, 1980
111. Ward RA: Precise anticoagulation for hemodialysis: importance of whole blood coagulation time test reagent. *Dial Transpl* 8:606, 1979
112. Bischel MD, Scoles BG, Mohler JG: Evidence for pulmonary microembolization during hemodialysis. *Chest* 67:335, 1975
113. Gotch FA: Solute transport and ultrafiltration in hemodialysis. In *Clinical Aspects of Uremia and Dialysis*, edited by Massry SG, Sellers AL, Springfield IL, Charles C. Thomas, 1976, p 639
114. Buscarini L, Bassi F: Leucocyte loss in haemodialysis. *Acta Haematol (Basel)* 48:278, 1972
115. Marshall JW, Ahearn DJ, Nothum RJ, Esterly J, Nolph KD, Maher JF. Adherence of blood components to dialyzer membranes; morphological studies. *Nephron* 12:157, 1974
116. Papadimitriou M, Baker LRI, Seitanidis B, Sevitt LH, Kulatilake AE: White blood count in patients on regular haemodialysis. *Br Med J* 4:67, 1969
117. Lawson LJ, Crawford N, Dawson Edwards P, Blainey JD: Platelet destruction and serotonin release during haemodialysis. *Proc Eur Dial Transpl Assoc* 2:63, 1965
118. Indeglia RA, Shea MA, Forstrom R, Bernstein EF: Influence of mechanical factors on erythrocyte sublethal damage. *Trans Am Soc Artif Intern Organs* 14:264, 1968
119. Blackshear PL Jr, Dorman FD, Steinbach JH: Some mechanical effects that influence hemolysis. *Trans Am Soc Artif Intern Organs* 11:112, 1965
120. Blackshear PL Jr, Patankar SV: Fluid dynamics of blood cells and applications to hemodialysis. *Proc 11th Annual Contractors' Conference, Artificial Kidney Program of NIAMDD*, edited by Mackey BB, DHEW Publication No (NIH) 79-1442, 1978, p 97
121. von Hartitzsch B, Carr D, Kjellstrand CM, Kerr DNS: Normal red cell survival in well dialyzed patients. *Trans Am Soc Artif Intern Organs* 19:471, 1973
122. Veitch P, Hawkins F, Frost TH, Jolly D, Kerr DNS: Factors affecting haemolysis in extracorporeal dialysis circuits. In: *Technical Aspects of Renal Dialysis*, edited by Frost TH, Tunbridge Wells, Pitman Medical, 1977, p 218
123. Toren M, Goffinet JA, Kaplow LS: Pulmonary bed sequestration of neutrophils during hemodialysis. *Blood* 36:337, 1970
124. Craddock PR, Hammerschmidt D, White JG, Dalmasso AP, Jacob HS: Complement (C5a)-induced granulocyte aggregation in vitro. *J Clin Invest* 60:260, 1977
125. Craddock PR, Fehr J, Brigham KL, Kronenberg RS, Jacob HS: Complement and leukocyte-mediated pulmonary dysfunction in hemodialysis. *N Engl J Med* 296:769, 1977
126. Craddock PR, Fehr J. Dalmasso AP, Brigham KL, Jacob HS: Hemodialysis leukopenia. Pulmonary vascular leukostasis resulting from complement activation by dialyzer cellophane membranes. *J Clin Invest* 59:879, 1977
127. Hakin RM, Lowrie EG: Effect of dialyzer reuse on leukopenia, hypoxemia and total hemolytic complement system. *Trans Am Soc Artif Intern Organs* 26:159, 1980
128. Jacob AI, Gavellas G, Zarco R, Perez G, Bourgoignie JJ: Leukopenia, hypoxia, and complement function with different hemodialysis membranes. *Kidney Int* 18:505, 1980
129. Shin J, Matsuo M, Shinko S, Fujita Y, Inoue S, Sakai R, Nishioka M: A study on hemodialysis leukopenia using various dialyzers. *J Dial* 4:51, 1980
130. Dumler F, Levin NW: Leukopenia and hypoxemia. Unrelated effects of hemodialysis. *Arch Intern Med* 139:1103, 1979
131. Aurigemma NM, Feldman NT, Gottlieb M, Ingram RH Jr, Lazarus JM, Lowrie EG: Arterial oxygenation during hemodialysis. *N Engl J Med* 297:871, 1977
132. Aurigemma NM, Feldman NT, Gottlieb M, Ingram RH Jr, Lazarus JM, Lowrie EG: Pulmonary dysfunction in hemodialysis. *N Engl J Med* 298:283, 1978
133. Sherlock JE, Ledwith JW, Letteri JM: Hypoxemia during dialysis. *N Engl J Med* 297:558, 1977
134. Hammerschmidt DE, Weaver LJ, Hudson LD, Craddock PR, Jacob HS: Association of complement activation and elevated plasma-C5a with adult respiratory distress syndrome. *Lancet* 1:947, 1980
135. Aljama P, Bird PAE, Ward MK, Feest TG, Walker W, Tanboga H, Sussman M, Kerr DNS: Haemodialysis-induced leucopenia and activation of complement: Effects of different membranes. *Proc Eur Dial Transpl Assoc* 15:144, 1978
136. Jones RG, Broadfield JB, Parsons V: Arterial hypoxemia during hemodialysis for acute renal failure in mechanically ventilated patients: observations and mechanisms. *Clin Nephrol* 14:18, 1980
137. Longnecker RE, Goffinet JA, Hendler ED: Blood loss during maintenance hemodialysis. *Trans Am Soc Artif Intern Organs* 20:135, 1974
138. Stewart WK, Fleming LW: The rupture problem with haemodialysers. *Br J Hosp Med (Equip Suppl)* May 1974, p 47
139. Butruille YA, Leonard EF, Litwak RS: Platelet-platelet interactions and non-adhesive encounters on biomaterials. *Trans Am Soc Artif Intern Organs* 21:609, 1975
140. Schultz JS, Lindenauer SM, Penner JA, Barenberg S: Determinants of thrombus formation on surfaces. *Trans Am Soc Artif Intern Organs* 26:279, 1980
141. Petschek H, Adamis D, Kantrowitz AR: Stagnation flow thrombus formation. *Trans Am Soc Artif Intern Organs* 14:256, 1968
142. Dawson A, Lawinski C, Weston M, Parsons V: Sulphin-

pyrazone as a method of keeping dialysis membranes clean. In *Technical Aspects of Renal Dialysis,* edited by Frost TH, Tunbridge Wells, Pitman Medical, 1977, p 133
143. Grode GA, Anderson SJ, Grotta HM, Falb RD: Non-thrombogenic materials via a simple coating process. *Trans Am Soc Artif Intern Organs* 15:1, 1969
144. Gott VL, Whiffen JD, Dutton RC: Heparin bonding on colloidal graphite surfaces. *Science* 142:1297, 1963
145. Schmer G, Teng LNL, Vizzo JE, Graefe U, Milutinovich J, Cole JJ, Scribner BH: Clinical use of a totally heparin grafted hemodialysis system in uremic patients. *Trans Am Soc Artif Intern Organs* 23:177, 1977
146. Woods HF, Weston MJ, Bunting S: Haemodialysis without heparin. *Proc Eur Dial Transpl Assoc* 15:122, 1978
147. Evans DB, Clarkson EM, Curtis JR: Blood loss using the modified two-layer Kiil dialyser. *Br Med J* 4:651, 1967
148. Lindsay RM, Burton JA, Edward N, Dargie HJ, Prentice CRM, Kennedy AC: Dialyzer blood loss. *Clin Nephrol* 1:29, 1973
149. Lindsay RM, Burton JA, King P, Davidson JF, Boddy K, Kennedy AC: The measurement of dialyzer blood loss. *Clin Nephrol* 1:24, 1973
150. Miller JH, Shinaberger JH, Gardner PW: Comparison of new hemodialyzers: 1974-1975. *Dial Transpl* 4(nob):40, 1975
151. Gorgels J, Tan BH: An evaluation of the performance of current dialyzers in routine use and in vitro. *Dial Transpl* 5(nob):68, 1976
152. Cripps CM: Rapid method for the estimation of plasma haemoglobin levels. *J Clin Pathol* 21:110, 1968
153. Clayton CB, Hoenich NA, Keir MJ. The measurement of dialyser washout characteristics. In: *Technical Aspects of Renal Dialysis,* edited by Frost TH, Tunbridge Wells Pitman Medical 1977, p 65
154. Easterling RE, Schulz M, Knepley W: Comparison of the hollow fiber artificial kidney with the coil dialyzers. *Proc Clin Dial Transpl Forum* 1:25, 1971
155. Easterling RE: Comparison of the EX03 dialyzer cartridge and the high performance Ultra-flo II (UFII) coil dialyzer with the Gambro-Lundia plate dialyzer (GL). *Proc Clin Dial Transpl Forum* 2:48, 1972
156. Zazgornik J, Schmidt P: Effects of zinc-containing dialysis membranes on zinc metabolism in patients on RDT. *Proc Eur Dial Transpl Assoc* 9:548, 1972
157. Barbour BH, Bischel M, Abrams DE: Copper accumulation in patients undergoing chronic hemodialysis. The role of Cuprophan. *Nephron* 8:455, 1971
158. Gutch CF, Eskelson CD, Ziegler E, Ogden DA: 2-Chloroethanol as a toxic residue in dialysis supplies sterilized with ethylene oxide. *Dial Transpl* 5(nr 4):21, 1976
159. Autian J, Lawrence WH, Dillingham EO, Beyer SA, Bigelow CL, Kleiman A: Detection of toxicity of extracted constituents from dialyzers and components *Proc 10th Annual Contractors' Conference, Artificial Kidney Program of NIAMDD* edited by Mackey BB, DHEW publication No (NIH) 77-1442, 1977, p 71
160. Poothullil J, Shimizu A, Day RP, Dolovich J: Anaphylaxis from the product(s) of ethylene oxide gas. *Ann Intern Med* 82:58, 1975
161. Keshaviah P, Luehmann D, Shapiro F, Comty CM: Investigation of the risks and hazards associated with hemodialysis devices. *FDA Medical Device Standards Publication, Technical Report,* DHEW publication, contr no 223-78-5046. June 1980
162. Jaeger RJ, Rubin RJ: Extraction, localization, and metabolism of Di-2-ethylhexyl phthalate from PVC plastic medical devices *Environ Health Perspect* Jan 1973, p 95
163. Ono K, Ikeda T, Fukumitsu T, Tatsukawa R, Wakimoto T: Migration of plasticiser from haemodialysis blood tubing. *Proc Eur Dial Transpl Assoc* 12:571, 1975
164. Neergaard J, Nielsen B, Faurby V, Christensen DH, Nielsen OF: On the exudation of plasticizers from PVC haemodialysis tubings. *Nephron* 14:263, 1975
165. Lewis LM, Flechtner TW, Kerkay J, Pearson KH, Nakamoto S: Bis(2-ethylhexyl) phthalate concentrations in the serum of hemodialysis patients. *Clin Chem* 24:741, 1978
166. Bommer J, Ritz E, Waldherr R: Silicone induced splenomegaly. Treatment of pancytopenia by splenectomy in a patient on hemodialysis. *N Engl J Med* 305:1077, 1981
167. Albisser AM, Jackman WS, Lougheed WD: Avoiding silicone cell inclusions from peristaltic pumps. *Lancet* 1:563, 1982
168. Curtis JR, Wing AJ, Coleman JC: Bacillus cereus bacteraemia. A complication of intermittent haemodialysis. *Lancet* 1:136, 1967
169. Jans H, Bretlau P, Nielsen B: Bacteriological contamination of dialyzers. *Nephron* 20:10, 1978
170. Bernick JJ, Port FK, Favero MS, Brown DG. Bacterial and endotoxin permeability of hemodialysis membranes. *Kidney Int (Abstract)* 14:670, 1978
171. Johnson WJ, Zabransky RJ, Mueller GJ, Wagoner RD, Maher FT: Modifications in the assembly and sterilization of the Kiil dialyzer and Quinton-Scribner tank. *Mayo Clin Proc* 40:462, 1965
172. Favero MS, Petersen NJ, Boyer KM, Carson LA, Bond WW: Microbial contamination of renal dialysis systems and associated health risks. *Trans Am Soc Artif Intern Organs* 20:175, 1974
173. Blagg CR, Tenckhoff H: Microbial contamination of water used for hemodialysis. *Nephron* 15:81, 1975
174. Bernick JJ, Port FK, Favero MS, Brown DG: Bacterial and endotoxin permeability of hemodialysis membranes. *Kidney Int* 16:491, 1979
175. Raij L, Shapiro FL, Michael AF: Endotoxemia in febrile reactions during hemodialysis. *Kidney Int* 4:57, 1973
176. Taber S: EDTNA Transplantation report *Proc Eur Dial Transpl Nurses Assoc* 34:1979
177. Parnell S, Sawyer RF, Meister MJ, Levin NW: Individualized dialysis prescription based on urea kinetic modeling. *Dial Transpl* 10:288, 1981
178. Sargent JA, Gotch FA: Mathematic modeling of dialysis therapy. *Kidney Int* 18:(Suppl 10)S2, 1980
179. Bellhouse BJ, Haworth WS, Jeffree MA, Bellhouse EL: A practical vortex-mixing haemodialyser. *Proc Eur Soc Artif Organs* 7:112, 1980
180. Abel K, Jeffree MA, Bellhouse BJ, Bellhouse EL, Haworth WS: A practical secondary-flow haemodialyzer. *Trans Am Soc Artif Intern Organs* 27:639, 1981
181. Anonymous: Gambro Lundia Mini Minor 13.5 µ. *Manufacturer's Technical Information* – Ab Gambro, Lund, Sweden
182. Anonymous: Filtryzer Typ B-11.15 m² *Manufacturer's Technical Information* – Hoechst (Toray Industries Inc 2, Niholbaghi-Muro Machi 2 Chrome Chuo-Ku, Tokyo, Japan)
183. Anonymous: *Clinical Ultrafilters. Manufacturer's Technical Information* – Amicon Corporation, (25 Hartwell Avenue, Lexington, MA, 02173, USA)
184. Schneider H, Streicher E: Technical aspects of hemofiltration. *Dial Transpl* 8: 371, 1979

6
PRETREATMENT AND PREPARATION OF CITY WATER FOR HEMODIALYSIS

CHRISTINA M. COMTY and FRED L. SHAPIRO

Introduction	142
Hazards of contaminants to dialyzed patients	142
Proposed standards of water quality for hemodialysis systems	144
Methods of water treatment – their uses and their hazards	145
Water softening	145
Deionization	145
Reverse osmosis	145
Filters	146
Monitoring of water quality	146
References	147

INTRODUCTION

In the early years of chronic hemodialysis, water used for dialysis was rarely treated. Because average patient survival was short, there was a general unawareness of acute or chronic complications from exposure to tap water contaminants. Since the late 1960's, however, nephrologists have become increasingly aware of both acute and chronic problems resulting from exposure to untreated water. Contaminants present in both tap water and concentrate used for dialysate preparation, may enter the patient's blood stream across the dialyzer membrane in large amounts because of the large volume of fluid to which the patient is exposed during treatment (140 to 240 l). Trace amounts of contaminants expecically the metals, present in dialysate may result in considerable accumulation as a result of protein binding after entry into the blood stream (1). Such accumulation is worsened as a result of a longer biological half-life because of the absence of urinary excretion. There is evidence that pediatric patients may be more susceptible to trace metal-induced complications than adults.

Regulation of the maximum limits of contaminants permitted in U.S. drinking water are specified in the National Interim on Primary Drinking Water Regulations, drafted under the auspices of the environmental protection agency (EPA) and became effective in 1977 (2, 3). These regulations (Table 1) replaced the Public Health Service drinking water standards of 1962. These regulations only apply to community water supplies and are based on an average daily intake of two liters of drinking water. As these contaminants are known to be hazardous in drinking water, they are likely to be hazardous to dialysis patients. Nevertheless, other metals are not recognized as hazardous in drinking water, but have been found to cause problems in dialyzed patients. Water standards in other countries also don't recognize the unique exposure to potential toxins that dialysis patients regularly encounter.

Table 1. National interim primary drinking water standards. Maximal concentrations allowed for contaminants in drinking water sources.

Contaminant	Concentration mg/l	SI (µmol/l)
Arsenic	0.05	1.5
Barium	1.0	7.3
Cadmium	0.01	0.1
Chromium	0.05	1.0
Lead	0.05	0.2
Mercury	0.002	0.01
Nitrate	10.0	161.3
Selenium	0.01	0.1
Silver	0.05	0.5
Chlorinated hydrocarbons (Pesticides)		
Endrin	0.002	—
Lindane	0.004	—
Methoxchlor	0.100	—
Toxaphane	0.005	—
Chlorophenoxys (Herbicides)	0.010	—
Combined α particle activity	5 pCi/l [a]	—
β Particle and photon radioactivity from man-made nuclides	4 mrem/year [b]	

[a] Pico curies per liter.
[b] Rem is a biologically effective dose of radiation exposure.

HAZARDS OF CONTAMINANTS TO DIALYZED PATIENTS

The contaminants that have been implicated as causing toxic effects in dialysis patients are listed in Table 2. *Alum* (Aluminum sulfate) has been used since the days of Pliny (77 A.D.) as a coagulant for purifying drinking water. A syndrome of progressive dementia and neurological deterioration which is frequently fatal has been ascribed to high levels of brain aluminum resulting from

Table 2. Water contaminants and their toxic effect on dialysis patients.

Contaminant	Lowest concentration associated with symptoms mg/l	SI (µmol/l)	Toxicity	References	Method of removal
Aluminum	0.06	2.2	Encephalopathy (dialysis dementia)	4–9	RO, DI
			Renal bone disease (vitamin D resistant osteomalacia)	10, 11	
			Proximal myopathy		
Calcium	88	2,200	Hard water syndrome	12–14	Softener, RO
Magnesium	88	3,667	Hard water syndrome	12–14	DI
Chloramines	0.25	5	Heinz body hemolytic anemia	15–17	Carbon filter
Copper	0.49	8	Nausea, chills, fever, liver damage, severe hemolysis	18–20	RO, DI
Fluoride	1.0	53	Bone disease	21–24	RO, DI
Nitrates	2.0	32	Methemoglobinemia	25	RO, DI
Sodium	300	13,043	Hypernatremia, hypertension, pulmonary edema, seizures	27, 28	RO, DI
Sulfate	200	2,083	Nausea, vomiting	29	RO, DI
Zinc	0.20	3	Hemolytic anemia, nausea, vomiting	30, 31	RO, DI
Iron	2.0	36	Damage to equipment	32	Iron filter
Manganese	2.0	36	Damage to equipment	32	Iron filter

RO = Reverse osmosis; DI = Deionizer.

elevated aluminum levels in community dialysate water supplies (4–9). Aluminum has also been implicated as being an etiological factor in the development of some types of renal bone disease and proximal myopathy (10, 11). Although there is evidence to suggest that chronic therapy with aluminum-containing phosphate binders in the dialysis patient may result in an increase in the body burden of aluminum, the amount of aluminum ingested is relatively small compared to the enormous load of aluminum these patients may acquire from water. (See also chapter 42)

Hardness of water is due to the presence of calcium and magnesium, and is a common problem in municipal water supplies. If calcium and magnesium concentrations in the dialysate solution (because of the use of hard water for preparation) are in excess of normal plasma diffusible calcium and magnesium levels, the 'hard water syndrome' consisting of hypercalcemia and hypermagnesemia may occur (12–14). This is a syndrome of nausea, vomiting, muscle weakness, skin flushing and hyper- or hypotension and is a constant hazard to the dialysis patient. On technical grounds it is preferable to maintain a constant dialysate calcium and magnesium level by mixing fixed proportions of softened water with either solid salts or concentrated salt solutions to prepare dialysis fluid.

Chlorination of water is a widely accepted method of reducing bacterial contamination and in many areas this is achieved by the addition of chloramines (condensation products of chlorine and ammonia). Chloramines denature hemoglobins both by direct oxidation and by inhibition of the hexose monophosphate shunt. Chloramines have been implicated as the agents responsible for an acute hemolytic anemia in dialysis patients, characterized by the presence of Heinz bodies. This hemolytic anemia is especially severe in patients with a hexose monophosphate shunt deficiency (15–17).

Copper may be present in water from natural sources and high copper concentrations are a potential hazard in certain municipal areas obtaining their water supply from shallow surface water which is periodically treated with copper sulfate to kill algea. Other reported sources of copper in the dialysate are leaching from copper tubing in dialysis equipment itself, or using an exhausted deionizer with copper tubing present in the equipment (18–20). However, the commonest source for copper is from plumbing. Copper intoxication causes acute symptoms of nausea, chills and headache with liver damage and often fatal hemolysis.

Fluoridation of water supplies for the prevention of dental caries is widely practiced in many areas of the world, the recommended level being 1 mg/l (53 µmol/l). However the fluoride concentration of drinking water is highly variable depending on the annual maximum air temperature and in some areas a concentration of up to 1.7 mg/l (89 µmol/l) is accepted. In addition very high natural fluoride levels of above 2 mg/l (105 µmol/l) are observed in certain geographic locations. The role of fluoride in the pathogenesis of bone disease in the chronic dialysis patient is controversial (21–24). Nevertheless because of the accumulation of fluoride in bone there is suggestive evidence that the use of fluoridated water for dialysate may be harmful on a long term basis. Significant quantities of fluoride probably do not pass across the dialyzer membrane when the dialysate concentration is less than 0.1 mg/l (5 µmol/l).

Nitrates present in tap water are indicative of either bacterial contamination (despite sterile cultures), or the use of fertilizers in agriculture areas. A nitrate concentration up to 10 mg/l (161 µmol/l) is permitted in drinking water, but high nitrate levels can cause problems in infants fed dried milk formula mixed with tap water. In the patient treated by hemodialysis nitrate concentrations above 10 mg/l (161 µmol/l) can cause severe methemoglobinemia with hypotension and nausea. A safe dialysis concentration is probably less than 2 mg/l (32 µmol/l) (25).

Sodium concentration may be high in some parts of the world where the water is brackish or frankly salty (26). Likewise when water is very hard the sodium concentration may be very high if a water softener is used as removal of calcium and magnesium occurs in exchange for sodium. High concentrations of naturally occurring potassium may also be encountered, usually in association with sodium and other minerals. Further treatment of water may be required unless adjustments in the sodium content of the concentrate can be made. Excessively high levels of sodium in the dialysis fluid cause hypernatremia with hypertension and pulmonary edema, confusion, vomiting, tachycardia and shortness of breath. If the sodium concentration is sufficiently high seizures, coma and death may occur (27, 28).

Drinking water with a high *sulfate* content has a cathartic effect when the concentrations are greater than 250 mg/l (2.6 mmol/l). Sulfate concentrations above 200 mg/l (2.1 mmol/l) increase the amounts of lead dissolved from lead pipes. A clinical syndrome of nausea, vomiting, and metabolic acidosis has been observed in patients dialyzed against high concentrations of sulfate (29). There is no other information in the literature concerning the effect of sulfate in the uremic patient, although sulfate is an end product of protein metabolism.

A syndrome consisting of hemolytic anemia associated with nausea, vomiting and fever has been described as a result of excessively high dialysate *zinc* levels. This has resulted from the use of galvanized iron in the water supply namely in water storage tanks, in softeners and piping (30, 31).

Iron transfer to the patient during dialysis is probably small (32). However excessive iron in the water supply damages both water treatment and dialysate supply equipment. A concentration of less than 2 mg/l (36 µmol/l) can be handled by a water softener very adequately and does not appear to impair the efficiency of the softener.

Other trace elements such as cadmium, tin, arsenic, lead, strontium and manganese may be present in municipal water supplies in quantities that are insufficient to interfere with the drinking water quality. Nevertheless accumulation of these elements in tissues of dialyzed patients has been documented for strontium, manganese, tin and cadmium (33). In some areas the *pH* of the treated water may be excessively low (less than 6.7 pH units).

This has reportedly caused excessive clotting of dialyzers and subsequently reduction of dialyzer performance and increased blood loss. Itching, nausea, vomiting and acidosis have been described. In combination with copper containing pipes and fittings water of low pH can cause symptoms of acute copper intoxication.

A fresh water louse, Asellus aquaticus, lives and breeds in water mains, but does not produce human disease. During the breeding season, the males die after copulation, and they may give the water an unpleasant odor and taste. To overcome this problem water supplies are frequently treated with *pyrethrins*. The residual pyrethrins concentration is approximately 0.001 mg/l (±3 nmol/l).

The toxicity of pyrethrins is not accurately known but a fatal dose by intravenous injection is thought to be about 2.5 mg/kg (71 µmol/kg). This would require dialysis with about 20,000 liters over a 24 hour period before an average 70 kg man had been exposed to a presumed fatal dose. Dialysis has been performed with pyrethrin treated water and no untoward effects have been noted.

Pyrogenic reactions are a frequent problem in dialysis units, an incidence of between 5 and 6% being reported (34–36). These pyrogenic reactions may be due to microbial contamination of the municipal water supply. They are often due to multiplication of microorganisms during dialysate preparation and delivery, particularily if stagnant and dead spaces exist such that the colony count may increase several fold over that found in the supply water.

Although municipal water supplies are extensively treated to remove *particulate matter,* suspended particles may still be present in many water supplies. Suspended particles greater than 5 µm are highly undesirable because they may plug tubing and orifices and require removal by a 5 µm sediment filter. Smaller particulate matter may be present in certain water supplies where treatment in the supply plant has been incomplete and may cause deterioration of reverse osmosis equipment and deionizers. Reusable or disposable filters down to 0.02 µm are available for their removal.

PROPOSED STANDARDS OF WATER QUALITY FOR HEMODIALYSIS SYSTEMS

Various standardizing organizations including the Association for the Advancement of Medical Instrumentation (AAMI), have proposed water standards for hemodialysis systems (37). The AAMI standards for water used for hemodialysis are considered to be the most comprehensive and are shown in Table 3. Significant omissions in such standards, including those of AAMI, are maximum contaminant levels for organic and radioactive contaminants. Additionally, proposed limits for some trace metals, while appropriate for drinking water standards, are considered excessively high for dialysis purposes. It is estimated that there are at least 30,000 chemicals in use in the U.S.A. and approximately 1,000 new chemicals are developed each year. Many of these are dialyzable and are potentially toxic and find their way into drinking water supplies through municipal and industrial pollution. This has been observed in Louisiana where chloroform and carbon tetrachloride, two known carcinogens have been found in the plasma of residents of New Orleans attributed to the contamination of the drinking water in that area (38).

Table 3. Standards proposed by the Association for the advancement of medical instrumentation for hemodialysis water [a].

Contaminant	Maximum allowable level mg/l	SI (µmol/l)
Calcium	10	250
Magnesium	4	167
Sodium	70 [b]	3043
Potassium	8	205
Fluoride	0.2	11
Chlorine	0.5	7
Chloramines	0.1	2
Nitrate (N)	2.0	32
Sulfate	100.0	1,042
Copper	0.1	1.6
Barium	0.1	0.7
Zinc	0.1	1.5
Arsenic	0.05	0.7
Chromium	0.05	1.0
Lead	0.05	0.24
Silver	0.05	0.46
Cadmium	0.01	0.09
Selenium	0.01	0.13
Aluminum	0.01	0.37
Mercury	0.002	0.01
Microbial load	Total viable counts shall not exceed 100/ml	

[a] To be used if water is not purified by a deionizer.
[b] 230 mg/l (10 mmol/l) for water used to prepare dialysis fluid in sorbent regeneration systems.

METHODS OF WATER TREATMENT – THEIR USES AND THEIR HAZARDS

Water softening

Water softening is a well known method of removing calcium and magnesium ions present in water in exchange for sodium ions as shown in the following equations:

$$CA^*(HCO_3)_2 + Na_2R \rightarrow Ca^*R + NaHCO_3$$

carbonate hardness   soluble nonhardness

$$Ca^*SO_4 + Na_2R \rightarrow Ca^*R + Na_2SO_4$$
$$Ca^*Cl_2 + Na_2R \rightarrow Ca^*R + 2NaCl$$

(* also for magnesium. R represents the anionic component of the ion exchanger).

The sodium load introduced by the softener is related to the hardness of the feed water and can be calculated from the equation Na(mmol/l) = total hardness as $CaCO_3$(mg/l) ÷ 50. Water softeners vary in capacity. The capacity required can be calculated from the number of liters required to perform a single dialysis and multiplying this by the hardness of the water in mg/l which will give the capacity of the softener required in mg. If reverse osmosis is also to be used the volume of the water to be softened will be considerably higher. This must be taken into account when estimating the capacity of softener required. When exhausted, the ion exchanger is regenerated with sodium chloride (brine). Other ions such as iron and manganese are also removed from the feed water during the softening process, but are only removed from the softener to a slight degree during the regeneration cycle. Resins handling high concentrations of these elements may lose their efficiency because of contamination.

Certain hazards have been described in relation to the use of water softeners for hemodialysis. These include bacterial contamination of the softener, and inadequate regeneration because of insufficient water pressure, which will result in the 'hard water syndrome' (39). Finally there is a very high risk of hypernatremia if the water softener is not equipped with an automatic valve to bypass the dialysis equipment during the regeneration cycle or a monitor to detect excessive sodium concentrations (27). Inadequate rinsing of brine from exchange tanks after regeneration can also result in the same type of hazard.

Deionization

Deionizers like water softeners, work on the ion exchange principle but differ in that they remove both anions and cations replacing them with hydrogen and hydroxide ions which combine to form water. There are basically two types of resins, cationic and anionic, and deionizers may be dual-bed or mixed-bed in type. The dual-type of deionizer consists of two tanks, one containing the cationic resin and the other the anionic resin. These systems do not produce as good a quality of water as a mixed-bed system but are less expensive. In the mixed-bed deionizer unit both cation and anion resins are mixed together in the same tank and can produce extremely pure water with resistances greater than 1 Mohm/cm (10^6 ohm/cm).

A deionizer is costly to operate if the feed water contains high concentrations of total dissolved solids and is highly dangerous if used when exhausted. Deionizers are subject to bacterial contamination or organic fouling because of the porous structure of the resins. Although the deionizer removes chloramines it should not be used for this purpose unless water has been pretreated with a carbon filter to remove organic nitrogen and avoid the danger of formation of the highly carcinogenic nitrosamines (40). Deionizers are often used to 'polish' reverse osmosis water when other treatment alone is not adequate for the removal of certain ions such as nitrates and fluorides. In many instances the cost of water treatment can be considerably reduced by pretreatment of water by softening and reverse osmosis prior to passage through the deionizer (29).

Reverse osmosis

Since 1968, reverse osmosis has been advocated as the method of choice for the preparation of dialysis water (41). When two solutions of different ionic concentration are separated by a semipermeable membrane solvent of the solution flows from the less concentrated to the more concentrated side, a process known as osmosis. Osmotic pressure is defined as the hydrostatic pressure required on the side of the concentrated solution to prevent such a flow. Hydrostatic pressures greater than the osmotic pressure cause a reversal of solvent flow, the solvent moving from the concentrated to the more dilute solution, a process that is called reverse osmosis. Reverse osmosis is based on molecular weight seiving and also on ionic exchange.

Cellulose acetate membranes have been extensively used for reverse osmosis equipment, and are generally used as 1) spirally wound cartridges or 2) as hollow fiber modules. The hollow fiber modules are very compact but very susceptible to plugging and leaks from ruptured fibers. The cellulose acetate membrane is damaged by excessive hardness, iron, manganese and free chlorine in the water. A pH of 8 or over deacetylates the membrane. The membrane is also very sensitive to bacterial attack which may cause digestion.

Reverse osmosis removes between 85 and 95% of dissolved solutes present in feed water. Some solutes are very efficiently removed, e.g. sulfates, while others, especially dissolved gases are not efficiently removed. The quality of pure water is dependent on pump size and on the membrane surface area. The quality and quantity of the water produced falls when the water is cold and warming of feed water may be required in very cold climatic conditions.

For good results reverse osmosis should be used only after pretreatment of feed water by removing hardness, particulate matter and dissolved free gases. The 5 to 15% of solutes remaining in water treated by reverse osmosis may be in excess of the maximum safety concentrations for dialysate preparation (e.g. fluorides and nitrates), and further treatment with a deionizer may be required.

Filters

Filters used for the treatment of dialysate water are one of two types: 1) sediment filters and 2) adsorptive filters. *Sediment filters* remove particulate matter from the water supply, the 5 µm filter being used in many centers to remove large particles, and the 1 µm filter only for the final filtration of water for dialyzer reuse and for preparing formaldehyde solution. Some water supplies may contain undesirable amounts of smaller particulate matter including sediments of sand, organic material and vegetable matter, so that further filtration in the dialysis unit may be required to protect equipment. Disposable filters of down to 0.45 µm are available but may be costly to use. A reusable 0.02 µm filter is commercially available (Continental Water Conditioning Corporation, PO Box 26428, El Paso TX, USA) and is highly effective for the pretreatment of poor quality water. The risks of use of a sediment filter are those of pyrogenic reactions, sepsis and bacteremia due to microbiotic growth on the filter media, and can be alleviated by proper disinfection or replacement and periodic culturing. Problems associated with the use of sediment filters include inadequate filtration due to seal leaks and sloughing of filter media itself into the water.

Carbon filters are *adsorptive filters* and consist of activated carbon housed in a pressure canister through which the water flows. Free chlorine, chloramine, organic materials, endotoxins and pyrogens are adsorbed onto the particle filter. The carbon filter is essential for the treatment of city water containing chlorine or chloramine. Frequent replacement or servicing is required, however, if the chlorine content is high. The carbon filter can also be a source of bacterial contamination and should be serviced or replaced frequently. In addition to bacterial contamination, carbon filters can occasionally slough off small particles of the carbon media referred to as 'fines' which tend to plug orifices of equipment down stream the filter. The inclusion of a 3 to 5 µm sediment filter after the carbon filter is an effective method of removing carbon fines and preventing damage to the equipment. Carbon filters should be tested for adequate removal of chlorine or chloramine, using test kits.

Oxidizing filters to remove iron and manganese are probably unnecessary since municipal water supply would already have been pretreated for removal of these contaminants. Small amounts of residual iron and manganese (less than 2 mg/l [about 36 µmol/l]) can be removed safely by the water softener.

MONITORING OF WATER QUALITY

The efficiency of softening equipment should be checked periodically, the frequency depending to some extent on the degree of hardness of the feed water and the softener's capacity. Daily testing using a commercially available test kit is performed by most centers. (Test kits are available from Hach Chemical Company, P.O. Box 907, Ames, Iowa 50010, USA and Ecodyne Company, Lindsey Division, P.O. Box 3420, St. Paul, Minnesota 55165, USA.)

In multipatient hospital systems automatic hardness monitoring at 10 to 30 min intervals by means of a Testomat apparatus (Heyl KG, 32 Hildesheim, P.O. Box 305, West Germany) is a most efficient and inexpensive method of preventing the hard water syndrome.

It is desirable to monitor the efficiency of removal of chloramines. A commercially available test kit is now available utilizing a modified orthotolidine reagent. This reagent is very stable and a positive test is indicated by the rapid development of an intensely yellow color with minimal fading. The test detects as little as 0.1 mg/l (1.4 µmol/l) of total chlorine. As mentioned in the previous section where formaldehyde is used for a sterilization of certain parts of the water treatment system some sensitive method of detecting residual formaldehyde should be used (see chapter 15).

Monitoring of the water purification by deionizers is a relatively simple process in which water quality (ionic content) is determined by continuous reading electrical 'specific' resistance meters. The higher the resistance, the better the quality of water. When the resistance falls to a predetermined level (below 300,000 ohms/cm^2) the exhausted unit must be exchanged for a fresh unit.

Monitoring of water treated by reverse osmosis is also

accomplished by specific electrical resistance equipment. Use of a dual probe to monitor both feed and purified water determines whether or not alteration in water quality is due to changes in equipment or changes in feed water (29). Meters are equipped with internally set alarms which are activated when the quality of the feed water or the treated water deteriorates.

REFERENCES

1. NIH Report: *Trace Metal Protein Binding*, Gulf South Research Institute, 1979
2. National Academy of Sciences National Research Council, Committee on Safe Drinking Water: *Drinking Water and Health*. National Academy of Sciences, Washington, DC, 1977
3. Environmental Protection Agency, Office of Water Supply: *National Interim Primary Drinking Water Regulations* US Government Printing Office, Washington, DC, 1978
4. Alfrey AC, Mishell M, Burks SR, Contiguglia P, Rudolph H, Lewin E, Holmes JH: Syndrome of dyspraxia and multifocal seizures associated with chronic hemodialysis. *Trans Am Soc Artif Intern Organs* 18:257, 1972
5. Alfrey AC: Dialysis encephalopathy syndrome. *Annu Rev Med* 29:93, 1978
6. Platts MM, Morehead PJ, Grech P: Dialysis dementia. *Lancet* 2:159, 1973
7. Cartier F, Allain P, Gary J, Chatel F, Menault F, Pecker S: Progressive myoclonic encephalopathy in dialysis patients. *Nouv Presse Méd* 7:97, 1978
8. Kaehny WD, Alfrey AC, Holman RE, Shorr WJ: Aluminum transfer during hemodialysis. *Kidney Int* 12:361, 1977
9. McDermitt JR, Smith AI, Ward MK, Parkinson IS, Kerr DNS: Brain-aluminum concentration in dialysis encephalopathy. *Lancet* 1:901, 1978
10. Platts MM, Goode GC, Hislop JS: Composition of the domestic water supply and the incidence of fractures and encephalopathy in patients on home dialysis. *Br Med J* 2:657, 1977
11. Ward MK, Ellis HA, Feest TG, Parkinson IS, Kerr DNS, Herrington J, Goode GL: Osteomalacic dialysis osteodystrophy: evidence for a water-borne aetiological agent, probably aluminum. *Lancet* 1:841, 1978
12. Freeman RM, Lawton RL, Chamberlain MA: Hard-water syndrome. *N Engl J Med* 276:1113, 1967
13. Evans DB, Slapak ML: Pancreatitis in the hard water syndrome. *Br Med J* 3:748, 1975
14. Drukker W: The hard water syndrome. A potential hazard during hemodialysis *Proc Eur Dial Transpl Assoc* 5:284, 1968
15. Yawata Y, Kjellstrand C, Buselmeier T, Howe R, Jacob H: Hemolysis in dialyzed patients: tap water-induced red blood cell metabolic deficiency. *Trans Am Soc Artif Intern Organs* 18:301, 1972
16. Botella J, Traver JA, Sanz-Guajardo D, Torres MT, Sanjuan I, Zabala P: Chloramines, an aggravating factor in the anaemia of patients on regular dialysis treatment. *Proc Eur Dial Transpl Assoc* 14:192, 1977
17. Yawata Y, Howe R, Jacob HS: Abnormal red cell metabolism causing hemolysis in uremia. A defect potentiated by tap water hemodialysis. *Ann Intern Med* 79:362, 1973
18. Ivanovich P, Manzler A, Drake R: Acute hemolysis following hemodialysis. *Trans Am Soc Artif Intern Organs* 15:316, 1969
19. Manzler AD, Schreiner AW: Copper-induced acute hemolytic anemia. A new complication of hemodialysis. *Ann Intern Med* 73:409, 1970
20. Matter BJ, Pederson J, Psimenos G, Lindeman RD: Lethal copper intoxication in hemodialysis. *Trans Am Soc Artif Intern Organs* 15:309, 1969
21. Siddiqui JY, Simpson SW, Ellis HE, Kerr DNS, Appleton DR, Robinson BH, Hawkins JB, Robertson PW, Taves DR: Fluoride and bone disease in patients on regular haemodialysis. *Proc Eur Dial Transpl Assoc* 8:149, 1971
22. Lough J, Noonan R, Gagnon R, Kaye M: Effects of fluoride on bone in chronic renal failure. *Arch Pathol* 99:484, 1975
23. Jowsey J, Johnson WJ, Taves DR, Kelly PJ: Effects of dialysate calcium and fluoride on bone disease during regular hemodialysis. *J Lab Clin Med* 79:204, 1972
24. Posen GA, Gray DG, Jaworski ZF, Couture R, Rashid A: Comparison of renal osteodystrophy in patients dialyzed with deionized and non-deionized water. *Trans Am Soc Artif Intern Organs* 18:405, 1972
25. Carlson DJ, Shapiro FL: Methemoglobinemia from well water nitrates: A complication of home dialysis. *Ann Intern Med* 73:757, 1970
26. Steinkamp RC, Young CL, Nyhus D, Greenberg AE: Sodium content of community water supplies in California. *Calif Med* 109:126, 1968
27. Nickey WA, Chinitz VL, Kim KE, Onesti G, Swartz C: Hypernatremia from water softener malfunction during home dialysis. *JAMA* 214:915, 1970
28. Robson M: Dialysate sodium concentration, hypertension, and pulmonary edema in hemodialysis patients. *Dial Transpl* 7:678, 1978
29. Comty C, Luehmann D, Wathen R, Shapiro F: Prescription water for chronic hemodialysis. *Trans Am Soc Artif Intern Organs* 20:189, 1974
30. Gallery EDM, Blomfield J, Dixon SR: Acute zinc toxicity in haemodialysis. *Br Med J* 4:331, 1972
31. Petrie JJB, Row PG: Dialysis anaemia caused by subacute zinc toxicity. *Lancet* 1:1178, 1977
32. Lawson DH, Boddy K, King PC, Linton AL, Will G: Iron metabolism in patients with chronic renal failure on regular dialysis treatment. *Clin Sci Mol Med* 41:345, 1971
33. Alfrey AC, LeGendre GR, Kaehny WD: The dialysis encephalopathy syndrome: possible aluminum intoxication. *N Eng J Med* 294:184, 1976
34. Biagini M, Rindi P, Rizzo G, Giovannetti S: Removal of pyrogens from dialysate of artificial kidney. *Proc Eur Dial Transpl Assoc* 7:467, 1970
35. Raij L, Shapiro FL, Michael AF: Endotoxemia in febrile reactions during hemodialysis. *Kidney Int* 4:57, 1973
36. Robinson PJA, Rosen SM: Pyrexial reactions during haemodialysis. *Br Med J* 1:528, 1971
37. *Hemodialysis systems standard (proposal)*. Association for the Advancement of Medical Instrumentation, Arlington, VA, 1978
38. Bowty B, Carlisle D, Laseter JL, Storer J: Halogenated hydrocarbons in New Orleans drinking water and blood plasma. *Science* 187:75, 1975
39. Stamm JM, Engelhard WE, Parsons JE: Microbiological study of water-softener resins. *Appl Microbiol* 18:376, 1969
40. Simenhoff M, Dunn S, Smiley J: Nitrosodimethylamine (NDMA) in dialysate water and blood of chronic dialysis patients (CDP). *Abstracts Am Soc Nephrol* 13:52A, 1980
41. Madsen RF, Nielsen B, Olsen OJ, Raaschou F: Reverse osmosis as a method of preparing dialysis water. *Nephron* 7:545, 1970

7

THE COMPOSITION OF DIALYSIS FLUID

FRANK M. PARSONS and WILLIAM K. STEWART

Historical	148
Individual concentrations of electrolytes and dextrose	149
Sodium	149
Current usage	149
Relationship to disequilibrium and osmolal changes	150
Reduction of osmolal change	151
Limitations of higher sodium dialysis	151
Limitations of methods reducing osmolal change	152
Future trends	152
Potassium	152
Acute renal failure	152
Chronic renal failure	153
Calcium	153
Magnesium	155
Hard-water syndrome	157
Acetate	157
Chloride	158
Dextrose	159
Fluoride	160
Contaminants and other substances	161
Constituting the dialysis fluid	161
Tank systems	161
Proportioning systems	162
De-aeration of dialysis fluid	163
Acknowledgements	164
References	164

HISTORICAL

Kolff (1) described most of the problems that have been encountered subsequently in formulating a suitable dialysis fluid. After many trials, and in the absence of modern analytical techniques, he advocated the following composition:

Sodium	126.5 mmol/l
Potassium	5.4 mmol/l
Calcium (in tap water)	1.0 mmol/l
Magnesium not stated	
Bicarbonate	23.9 mmol/l
Chloride	109.0 mmol/l
Dextrose *	1.36 g/dl (76 mmol/l)
(or for dehydration)	2.72 g/dl (151 mmol/l)

The major problem was the high pH of the solution because of the bicarbonate which affected the solubility of calcium. Kolff attempted to correct pH by bubbling CO_2 into the dialysis fluid but technically this proved too difficult. Once he even used NaH_2PO_4. He finally added no calcium to the tap water (which contained 1.0 mmol/l) and gave calcium gluconate intravenously post-dialysis. To avoid haemolysis, dextrose monohydrate was added to the dialysis fluid to 'strengthen' erythrocytes. Alwall (2), using a closed container for dialysis fluid and dialyser, was able to bubble CO_2 into the dialysis fluid to reduce pH to acceptable levels, thereby preventing precipitation of calcium, but NaH_2PO_4 still had its advocates (3).

Skeggs and Leonards (4) used both CO_2 and phosphate to control pH but the composition to be favoured subsequently was (in mmol/l) Na 140; K 4.0; Mg 0.5; Ca 1.25; HCO_3 26.8; Cl 120.7 and dextrose 182 mg/dl with CO_2 added to correct the pH to 7.4 (5); concentrations of calcium and magnesium were thus about equal to the ionic values found in plasma. For dialysers immersed in a fixed volume of dialysate it was essential to replenish the dialysis fluid every 2 h in order to achieve higher clearances (6). Initially calcium was only added to the dialysis fluid after its pH had been corrected with CO_2 during which time the two units of citrated blood, used to prime the dialyser and hence unsaturated with calcium ions, had entered the circulation. The severe symptoms produced were prevented by adding calcium to the dialysis fluid after pH had been corrected and dialysing the citrated blood, to which heparin had been added, before it entered the circulation (7).

The concentration of the principal electrolytes in extracellular fluid is given in Table 1 (8). In theory the composition of dialysis fluid should probably be similar to that of interstitial fluid with suitable correction for

Table 1. Composition of extracellular fluid (8).

	Serum mmol/l	Serum water mmol/l	Interstitial fluid mmol/l
Sodium	142	152.7	145
Potassium	4	4.3	4
Calcium	2.5	1.5	1.5
Magnesium	0.8	0.5	0.5
Chloride	101	108.5	114
Bicarbonate	27	29.3	31

---

* In most countries it is necessary to specify whether dextrose anhydrous (180.2 daltons) or dextrose monohydrate (198.2 daltons) has been prescribed. In this chapter dextrose concentrations have been expressed, whenever possible, as dextrose anhydrous.

Table 2. Early composition of dialysis fluid for intermittent dialysis.

		Reference
Sodium	130 to 135 mmol/l	(10)
Potassium	0 to 1.5 mmol/l as needed	(9)
Calcium	1.25 mmol/l	(9)
Magnesium	0.5 mmol/l	(9)
Chloride	100.5 mmol/l	(9)
Bicarbonate or equivalent	35 mmol/l	(11)
Dextrose	1818 mg/dl (101 mmol/l)	(10)

the small protein fraction. In practice considerable variation has been advocated in both cation and anion concentrations (*vide infra*). The most common composition of dialysis fluid used in the early 1960's is given in Table 2. Later, the content of dextrose was reduced to 182 mg/dl (10.1 mmol/l) once ultrafiltration by hydrostatic pressure had been shown to be superior to the hyperosmolar method of achieving dehydration (9).

The importance of the concentration of each electrolyte and dextrose will be examined in detail.

INDIVIDUAL CONCENTRATIONS OF ELECTROLYTES AND DEXTROSE

Sodium

In dialysis fluid, as in extracellular fluid, sodium is the major determinant of osmolality. The early 1970's saw enquiries into the hitherto unquestioned usage of dialysis fluid with a low sodium concentration relative to those of plasma and plasma water (Table 2) (12–14). The use of sodium in dialysis fluid as low as 115 mmol/l (information courtesy of Macarthy's Laboratories Ltd.) and as high as 155 mmol/l (15, 16) has been described, but until the middle of the last decade most United Kingdom and continental European dialysis centres used a sodium concentration of less than 135 mmol/l with a mean level of 130 mmol/l (17). The use of a low sodium concentration was justified by the assumption that the kidney is unable to excrete sodium so that sodium accumulation with consequent hypertension, thirst and fluid overload tends to develop. With a gradient of about 20 mmol/l between dialysis fluid sodium at 130 mmol/l and plasma water sodium at 150 mmol/l (18), the rate of removal of sodium from the patient is determined by the concentration difference across the dialysis membrane. Extraction of water in these early haemodialysers was effected by osmotically-induced ultrafiltration, osmolality of dialysis fluid being increased by using unphysiologically high concentrations of dextrose (1.5 g/dl) which more than out-weighed the osmotic reduction in dialysis fluid due to low sodium concentrations.

Current haemodialysers are more satisfactory than earlier models and rupture of membranes is uncommon. Consequently such dialysers are capable of withstanding perfusion with blood at comparatively high hydrostatic pressures generated by roller pumps. With these physical changes in dialyser characteristics, ultrafiltration nowadays can be effected by hydrostatic pressure difference across the dialysis membrane. Ultrafiltration is capable of inducing net convective shifts of water, sodium and solutes from plasma to dialysate even in the absence of those concentration gradients necessary for passive diffusion induced transfers. In consequence there has been a movement upwards in transmembrane pressures and in dialysis fluid sodium concentrations, accompanied by a need for increased ultrafiltration (17, 19). The ultrafiltration of 2 kg of plasma water will remove concomitantly about 260 mmol of sodium (as well as other solutes), an amount approximately equal to that ingested by the average patient during 3 days. Thus it is practicable to remove accumulated dietary sodium by hydrostatic ultrafiltration alone (20) and the original justification for a sodium concentration gradient across the dialyser has gone.

Dialysis centres imposing severe restrictions of salt and water intake on their patients may avoid the need for much ultrafiltration. Such centres continue to emphasise the need for minimal interdialytic weight gain by the patient and prefer the use of hyponatric dialysis fluid, possibly because its use appears to minimise thirst and spontaneous water intake in the patients. However, there have always been some patients who, despite adequate dialysis and removal of sodium with a concentration of sodium in dialysis fluid at 130 mmol/l, remained hypertensive (21, 22).

Current usage

Figure 1 illustrates the current pattern of usage of dialysis fluids of various sodium strengths in the United Kingdom. Half of the dialysis fluid concentrates supplied are for a sodium concentration of 130 mmol/l with the rest mainly between 132 and 137 mmol/l and a small proportion at 139 to 140 mmol/l. One dialysis centre only is supplied with a concentrate to give a final sodium concentration of 145 mmol/l.

It should be recognised, however, that concentrate supplied is not always a reliable indicator of the final dialysis fluid concentrations as used. Some dialysis units underdilute the concentrate, or use water-softening devices which may increase the final sodium concentration by up to 6 mmol/l. Based on data available to the major supplier of concentrate solutions in the United Kingdom the most likely concentrations used are shown in Figure 2. This diagram of the estimated usage, and, therefore, probable actual usage, takes on a different pattern from that of the concentrate supplied. Thus the number of litres used of dialysis fluid containing 136 to 137 mmol/l sodium exceed other concentrations, although a considerable proportion of users still apparently prefer concentrations as low as 130 mmol/l. The relative proportions as percentages (Figure 2) show that an estimated 28% of dialysis centres still use 130 mmol/l sodium in dialysis fluid, 51% use between 135 and 137 mmol/l and 12.5% use a concentration greater than 139 mmol/l of sodium.

The 1980 figures show a clear trend upwards in the

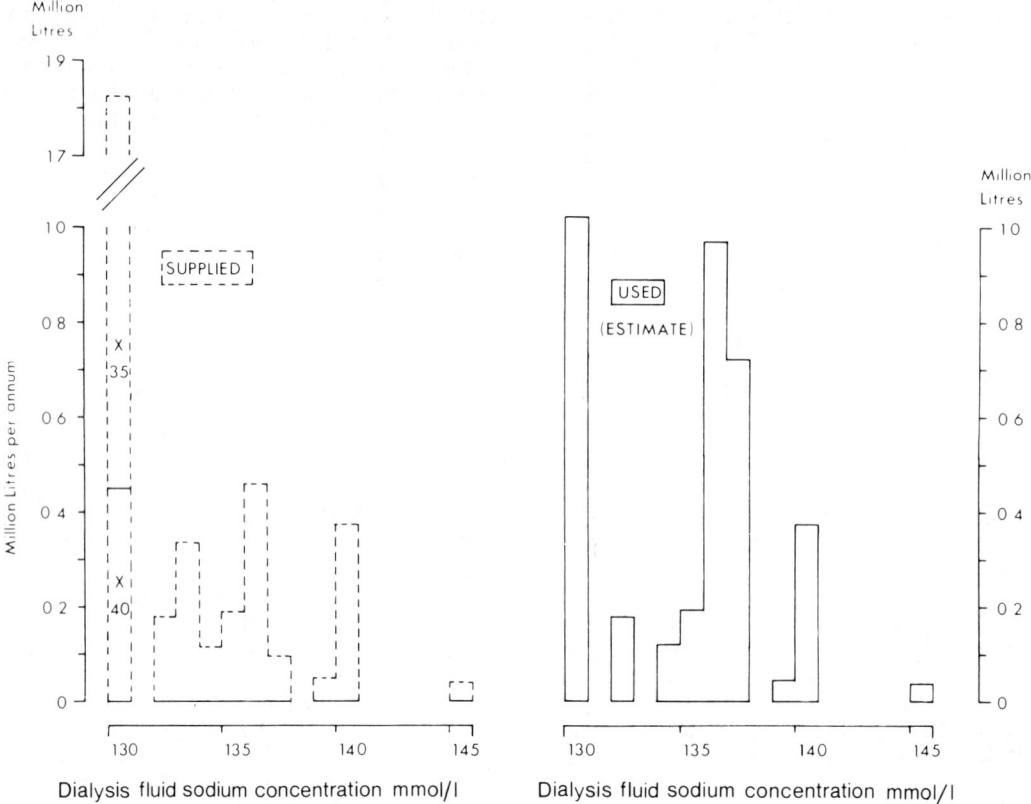

Figure 1. Sodium concentrations of supplied dialysis fluid (left) and estimated concentrations of dialysis fluid as used (right) in the United Kingdom at 1980.

sodium concentration used compared with 1974 (17). The change is particularly noticeable compared with the figures for 1967, when 80% of European dialysis centres were using sodium concentrations of 130 mmol/l (23). This has dropped to 28% for United Kingdom centres in 1980 (Figure 2). The average sodium concentration used has now become 134.7 mmol/l, whereas between 1970 and 1974 it was between 128.4 and 130.6 mmol/l (17). In 1974, 13.4% of solutions had a sodium concentration greater than 135 mmol/l, whereas the equivalent percentage for 1980 was 58.4% (17).

Boquin and colleagues in 1977 (24) surveyed the concentration of sodium in the dialysis fluid obtained from concentrate supplied by the three main manufacturers in the United States (covering 75% of the market) and found that 35% had a sodium concentration of 130 to 133 mmol/l, 61% had 134 to 136 mmol/l, but only 4% were in the 137 to 140 mmol/l range.

Relationship to disequilibrium and osmolal changes
The role of sodium in dialysis fluid is best comprehended in the light of recent work on dialysis disequili-

Figure 2. Concentrate supplied and used in the United Kingdom, expressed as a percentage to show the relative proportions at each sodium concentration.

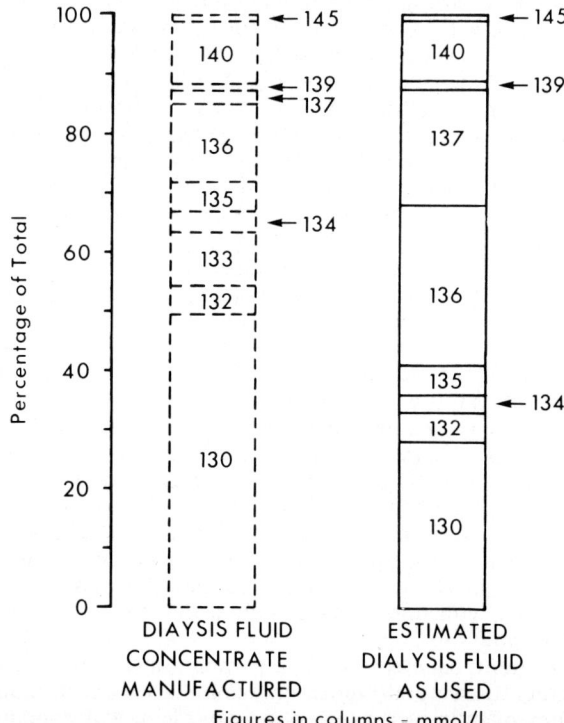

brium syndrome. This has been largely equated with dialysis-induced change in extracellular fluid osmolality and resultant movements of water between body compartments. Every dialysis treatment necessarily induces a drop in plasma osmolality except for ultrafiltration alone.

During dialysis with a sodium concentration in dialysis fluid of 130 mmol/l or less, the blood returning to the patient will be hyponatraemic. Consequently the plasma sodium concentration will decrease progressively. This reduction in extracellular sodium concentration, as well as the lowering of plasma urea concentration, will produce a situation where the intracellular fluid is relatively hyperosmolar and there will be a consequent movement of water from the extracellular space to the intracellular space. In the case of hyponatric dialysis the decrease in extracellular osmolality is of the order of 30 mOsm/kg plasma water, from about 310 mOsm/kg plasma water pre-dialysis to 280 mOsm/kg plasma water post-dialysis. Clinically these osmolality-related changes are expressed mainly by nausea and vomiting, muscle cramps, hypotension and headaches (25, 26). Cerebral overhydration is also thought to play a part in this syndrome (27).

It has to be recognised that maintenance dialysis treatment cannot be undertaken without the extraction of osmotically-active substances from the patient. The therapeutic aim must be to minimise both the extent and rate of osmolal changes. The concentrations of sodium in dialysis fluid should be chosen with these desiderata in mind. Sodium concentration is the variable which can most easily be manipulated so as to reduce the extent of osmolal change in dialysis fluid. It follows that no single sodium concentration is ideal.

The concentration selected will vary according to the haemodialysis technique employed, particularly to the extent of ultrafiltration used and the temporal inter-relation between ultrafiltration and dialysis.

Reduction of osmolal change
The use of increased sodium concentration in dialysis fluid has been part of a general trend evoked by awareness of the need to minimise changes in the osmolality of body fluids during the dialysis period. Other ways of achieving this end have been described, such as sequential dialysis, i.e., ultrafiltration followed by dialysis to separate solute diffusion from fluid removal (28–33), infusions of mannitol to counteract the reduction in plasma osmolality as urea is dialysed out of the extracellular fluid (34–36), high concentrations of dextrose in dialysis fluids (35, 37, 38), glycerol in dialysis fluid (39), and hypertonic saline infusions (40). Other investigators have advocated the use of haemofiltration (diafiltration or haemodiafiltration) in which infusions of replacement fluids are given either before or after the ultrafiltration process (41–46), and have claimed a reduction in the symptoms of disequilibrium which so often accompany low sodium dialysis. Cambi and colleagues (47) have recommended ultrashort dialysis (2 h) with recirculation of 20 to 40 l dialysate in a closed system, using sodium concentrations of 132 mmol/l or 140 mmol/l.

Coincidental with the observations that higher rates of ultrafiltration could be tolerated as long as sodium concentrations in dialysis fluid were higher (14, 16, 24, 48–50), Bergström and his co-workers (31) recommended the temporal separation of the ultrafiltration process from the dialysis process, so that urea and other small solute diffusion did not occur concurrently with fluid removal, thus reducing osmolar decreases in the critical first hours of ultrafiltration. It is of interest that in these reports the dialysis which followed ultrafiltration was carried out with sodium concentrations of 145 mmol/l and the dialysis was tolerated better than when the sodium concentration was only 133 mmol/l (28, 30). Reduction in blood volume has been shown to be less during dialysis with 145 mmol/l of sodium in dialysis fluid compared with 130 mmol/l (51). Liebau and colleagues (15) recommended increasing the sodium concentration of dialysis fluid to as high as 155 mmol/l in order to allow gradual removal of excess fluid and better control of blood pressure in patients whose hypertension was 'uncontrollable' when lower concentrations were used. Locatelli and colleagues (16) also showed that sodium concentrations in dialysis fluid as high as 155 mmol/l enabled toleration of high ultrafiltration rates (3 l/h) at the same time as dialysis.

The advent of shorter-duration dialysis (around 12 h weekly) with larger surface area dialysers capable of high ultrafiltration rates has brought about an appreciation of the limits of tolerance in some patients to the dialysis process, and the critical role of plasma sodium concentrations and changes therein. Schuenemann and colleagues (52) have pointed out that the body is more sensitive to concentration changes than to volume changes. It used to be thought that the reduction in plasma volume was responsible for much dialysis-related upset but it has gradually become apparent that it is the diffusion-produced changes in plasma concentrations and consequent reduction in osmolality, that seem to mediate the trouble (16, 26, 35). There is no doubt that higher sodium concentrations can minimise osmotic shifts (53, 54).

Limitations of higher sodium dialysis
Some authors, however, have found that the higher sodium concentrations, although reducing disequilibrium, have given rise to problems of thirst and unacceptable inter-dialysis weight-gains (55, 56), and Redaelli and colleagues (57) have shown that truly isonatric dialysis, with sodium concentrations the same as the patient's plasma water, actually gives rise to hypernatraemia. The movement of water from extracellular to intracellular space is probably responsible for an increase of around 3 mmol/l in plasma water sodium concentrations during dialysis with isonatric dialysis fluid. Locatelli and colleagues (58) have pointed out that any sodium concentration in dialysis fluid (e.g. 140 mmol/l) is not 'high' or 'low' in itself, but should be related to the individual patient's plasma water sodium. A sodium in dialysis fluid of 140 mmol/l could be high for a hypoproteinaemic hyponatraemic patient, and low for a sodium overloaded patient. Redaelli and colleagues (57) recommend matching sodium concentration in dialysis fluid to the individual patient to counteract ultrafiltration-produced increases in plasma water sodium, which in prac-

tical terms means a sodium concentration in dialysis fluid several mmol/l lower than the patient's plasma water sodium. In their experience this turned out to be, on average, a sodium concentration of 142 mmol/l (termed by them 'adequate' sodium in dialysis fluid). It has been suggested that raised intracellular sodium concentrations are responsible for the increased thirst and weight gains seen in diabetic dialysed patients (58, 59). In the past individual matching of dialysis fluid concentration to patient needs has not proved practical in most dialysis units, though it has much to recommend it. With the advent of variable dilution proportioning machines, however, this may well prove the ideal approach for the future.

Limitations of methods reducing osmolal change
The contribution to osmolal change from diffusion of other plasma components like creatinine and phosphate is minimal relative to urea and sodium in molar terms. Other methods aimed at reducing plasma osmolality changes to the unavoidable minimum necessitated by urea diffusion tend to have various disadvantages. Mannitol, being possibly toxic in prolonged usage, is seldom used (39, 60). The use of glycerol has been criticised by Van Stone and colleagues (61) who consider sodium or dextrose to be more physiological. Haemofiltration has its advocates (33, 45) but tends to be expensive and may have clinical disadvantages such as causing increased parathormone (PTH) levels (62).

Future trends
At this time sodium could be the tool of choice, and current proportionating machines allow easy manipulation of sodium concentration. The future trend may well be to vary sodium in dialysis fluid throughout an individual dialysis, such as described by Dumler and colleagues (63), Maeda and colleagues (64) and Chen and co-workers (65). This approach avoids the loss of valuable dialysis diffusion and extraction time, which occurs using ultrafiltration and dialysis sequentially, a factor especially important in the face of the trend towards shorter dialysis times. Locatelli and colleagues (66) believe that the use of higher dialysis fluid sodium concentration is better than sequential ultrafiltration and dialysis in all but the fluid-overloaded patient. Some disadvantageous side-effects have been reported with high ultrafiltration, even without dialysis (67). Maeda and colleagues (64) gradually lowered the sodium concentration from 140 to 150 mmol/l to 133 to 140 mmol/l in dialysis fluid throughout a dialysis period, but also used haemodiafiltration, with replacement fluid at a sodium concentration of 140 mmol/l injected after the dialyser, and found that patients with cellular overhydration responded well to this treatment. Chen and colleagues (65) found that an extra litre of fluid could be removed with a continuously decreasing sodium concentration in dialysis fluid from 150 to 133 mmol/l compared with standard dialysis at 130 mmol/l before arterial blood pressure was affected. Dumler and colleagues (63) dialysed patients against a sodium concentration of 150 mmol/l for 3 h and then at 130 mmol/l for 1 h and found fewer symptoms of disequilibrium compared to using sodium concentrations of 140 mmol/l throughout a dialysis. These two groups counteracted the osmolality fall of urea removal by allowing sodium influx during the first hours of dialysis and then removing sodium during the later period of dialysis, a revolutionary new approach which may prove useful in those refractory patients who have excessive thirst and weight gain when treated with a higher sodium concentration in dialysis fluid, and hypotension and cramps when treated with a lower sodium concentration.

Potassium

Potassium homeostasis is considerably affected in renal failure. This may be particularly so in patients with acute renal failure and there is thus a need for some degree of flexibility in the potassium concentration used in dialysis fluid. In this section the dialysis solution suitable for acute renal failure and that for chronic renal failure will be discussed separately.

Acute renal failure
Control of hyperkalaemia during the phase of renal insufficiency is important, being particularly difficult in patients with a severe metabolic response * when the initial rise in the level of potassium in the plasma frequently exceeds other biochemical markers of uraemia. If internal bleeding has been an additional complication the rapid release of potassium from lysis of red blood cells leads to an increased hazard. In the early days of haemodialysis, using fixed volume tanks for preparing dialysis fluid, hyperkalaemia was most readily corrected by withholding potassium from the dialysis fluid (68) for the first 30 to 60 min of dialysis (provided the patient was not receiving digitalis or similar drugs). When release of potassium was excessive (i.e. from large haematomas) a deliberate attempt to produce a partial depletion of total body potassium (TBK) using a zero or relatively low potassium concentration in dialysis fluid for a longer period of time delays the recurrence of hyperkalaemia. In other situations, such as prolonged diarrhoea and vomiting, the development of hypokalaemia can be prevented by adding additional potassium to the dialysis fluid.

Using the more modern flow-to-waste proportioning systems control of plasma potassium in acute renal failure is more difficult; ideally a range of concentrate solutions should be available to provide a dialysis fluid of potassium content capable of being varied from 1 to 4 mmol/l so that patients with either hyperkalaemia or hypokalaemia can be treated successfully. Alternatively we have found that a known volume of an accurately prepared solution of concentrated KCl added to a container filled to a calibrated mark with concentrate is satisfactory. Preferably the potassium concentration in

---

* Severe metabolic response was the original terminology (69); subsequently it was renamed 'hypercatabolic' which is an unfortunate term, for the disturbance is more likely to be due to a reduction in protein synthesis rather than an increase in catabolism (70).

the dialysis fluid passing into the dialyser should be checked by flame photometry or a potassium measuring electrode system before dialysis is commenced.

Chronic renal failure

For potassium and magnesium there are ranges of plasma values which are not associated with adverse clinical symptoms. This is fortuitous, for total body accumulation is inevitable between dialyses when the patient is eating normal food. There is considerable flexibility automatically included in a dialysis system, because the quantity of each cation removed, assuming a constant concentration in the dialysis fluid, increases as the plasma value rises, and, conversely, decreases as that in the plasma falls. There may also be a 'reverse dialysis' of potassium against a concentration gradient between blood and dialysis fluid in potassium depleted subjects (71). Thus small changes in daily dietary intake are permissible. The concentration of potassium used in the dialysis fluid must depend on dietary intake, type of dialyser used and the duration and frequency of dialysis (72, 73) so that there is no single ideal value applicable to all clinical conditions. Intracellular potassium is also dependent on the acid-base balance so that the relative levels of sodium, chloride and acetate (hence bicarbonate) in dialysis fluid are also important determinants of potassium balance. Unfortunately all those factors which affect potassium balance in patients treated by regular dialysis have not been stated in the majority of reported investigations so that it becomes difficult, if not impossible, to make an accurate assessment (74).

The plasma concentration of potassium is not a reliable guide to total body content though most would agree that persistently low values, particularly before dialysis, are suggestive of a total body deficit. Red cell concentrations (71, 75) may give some indication of TBK. As a result investigations to ascertain the optimum concentration of potassium in dialysis fluid have been mainly directed towards measurement of either TBK or potassium content of muscle obtained by biopsy. Exchangeable potassium values using ^{42}K or ^{43}K (76, 77) underestimate TBK in renal failure, even though 64 hours had been allowed in some instances for equilibration to occur, so that investigations using exchangeable isotopic techniques will not be reviewed here. Using ^{40}K techniques (71, 76, 78–81) several investigators found no evidence of potassium depletion, presumably because potassium intake was adequate, whilst the frequency of dialysis and the potassium concentration in the dialysis fluid were suitable for the type of dialyser used, even though dissimilar dialysis techniques were employed. Full details of all the factors involved in potassium metabolism were, however, not recorded. But when the potassium intake was low or the level in the dialysis fluid was less than 1.5 mmol/l (or both) (73, 80) then TBK was below normal. Some caution is necessary in the interpretation of the data. For instance an attempt was made to correct the acidosis resulting from the use of one of the dialysis fluids shown to give normal values of TBK (79) by elevating the acetate in the dialysis fluid by 5 mmol/l at the expense of chloride (82). Profound symptomatic hypokalaemia developed in all patients which was corrected by temporarily raising the potassium concentration in dialysis fluid to 5 mmol/l. As no other changes had been introduced presumably potassium had moved intracellularly in response to correction of a metabolic acidosis. Thus TBK, as measured by ^{40}K, is not necessarily an infallible guide to the state of potassium balance but it is a non-invasive investigation allowing measurements to be made repeatedly over an indefinite period of time. It must also be remembered that some reduction in TBK should be expected because most patients with renal failure have a reduced red cell mass (73).

The other main method used for estimating potassium content of the body has been obtained by analysis of muscle biopsies (74, 77, 83–85). Intracellular potassium appears to be low in chronic renal failure but returns to normal after institution of dialysis (77) provided dialysis fluid potassium is not too low (74). Whether this improvement in potassium content after starting intermittent dialysis is due to improved dietary intake, decreased intracellular water or correction of acidosis is not clear.

On the available evidence a free dietary intake of 60 to 80 mmol potassium per day with a thrice weekly dialysis schedule, each dialysis lasting 6 to 8 h, seems to give a reasonable potassium balance when the dialysis fluid contains about 1.5 mmol/l. There will inevitably be some minor asymptomatic hyperkalaemia before dialysis and hypokalaemia immediately after dialysis. When current shorter dialysis times with a larger dialyser (1.5 m^2) were used (86) potassium balance seemed to remain unaltered. If the concentration of potassium in the dialysis fluid is greater than 1.5 mmol/l or dialysis is undertaken only twice per week some dietary restriction of potassium is probably required for hyperkalaemia is still a major cause of death in patients treated by regular dialysis (87).

If dietary intake is temporarily reduced (i.e. during intercurrent illness) then oral supplementation of potassium (or an increased level in the dialysis fluid) may be necessary. However, prolonged fasting, particularly preoperatively, may give rise to hyperkalaemia, which can be overcome by oral or intravenous dextrose. Should the time interval between dialysis be temporarily lengthened (e.g. in case of difficulties with vascular access) plasma potassium must be measured frequently and any tendency for the development of hyperkalaemia corrected by using an orally administered cation-exchange resin, preferably in the calcium phase (88).

Calcium

Since 1964, acetate (11) has replaced bicarbonate in dialysis fluid. This change solved the problem of preparing dialysis fluid 'concentrates' with calcium retained in stable solution. Earlier attempts to supply bicarbonate-containing concentrate were unsatisfactory because calcium precipitates in an alkaline medium. Currently, calcium in dialysis fluid is determined by the calcium content of the commercial concentrate chosen (a range is available) and the dilution characteristics of the proportioning system employed. Account must always be taken of the calcium content of the water supply used to dilute the concentrate for this may add up to 1 or 1.5 mmol/l (4 to 6 mg/dl) of calcium. When the mains water content exceeds 0.25 to 0.3 mmol/l of calcium (1 to 1.2 mg/dl), water softeners, deionisation or reverse osmosis devices become mandatory since seasonal or other variations in water calcium content could effect unacceptably large changes. For occasional use it is possible to increase calcium in dialysis fluid by adding a known amount of calcium chloride dihydrate in solution to a known quantity of concentrate in a container and mixing well.

Calcium concentration in dialysis fluid in the earliest years of intermittent dialysis was 1.25 to 1.3 mmol/l (5.0 to 5.2 mg/dl) (9, 23). Later the diffusible fraction of calcium in the plasma of patients with renal failure was reported to be higher than in normal subjects, values ranging from 57.6 to 64.3% (89-91) of the total plasma calcium value, so that the minimum amount of calcium in dialysis fluid to achieve a zero or slightly positive balance to the patients was found to be about 1.5 to 1.55 mmol/l (6 to 6.2 mg/dl) (90, 91), although the exact concentration will vary from patient to patient (92). Early studies on mineralisation of bone indicated that calcium was lost from the skeleton when calcium fell below 1.5 mmol/l (6 mg/dl) in dialysis fluid (93-96). Increasing the concentration to 1.75 mmol/l (7 mg/dl) (96) prevented a fall in the metacarpal bone index and a further increase to 2.0 mmol/l (8 mg/dl) resulted in an increase in total body calcium in patients with osteomalacia (97). Discussion on adequacy of calcium concentration in dialysis fluid has been focused on the range 1.5 to 2.0 mmol/l (6 to 8 mg/dl).

Some modes of treatment technique, such as ultrafiltration and haemofiltration, lead to loss of calcium from plasma to dialysate. During ultrafiltration, for example, diffusible calcium will be removed together with water and sodium. In conventional dialysis the interdialytic fluid accumulation with calcium is removed by ultrafiltration plus the additional volume of plasma water with calcium which is removed to make space for the calcium-free saline used to 'wash-back' the blood from the dialyser. If this combined volume is two litres (a conservative estimate) then about 3 mmol (120 mg) of calcium will be removed per dialysis or 9 mmol (360 mg) per week if the patient receives three dialyses per week. There could also be an additional deficit if calcium-free saline solutions are used to prime the dialyser. Such saline fluids do not attain the same concentration of calcium present in the dialysis fluid because of the low dialysance of calcium (7). To this 'loss' by dialysis must be added the net calcium balance occurring in the gastrointestinal tract which may be negative by as much as 5 mmol (200 mg) daily (90, 98) or 35 mmol (1400 mg) per week. Thus the combined loss of calcium from the body stores, by dialysis and via the gastrointestinal tract, could be as high as 45 mmol (1800 mg) per week. Even higher rates of loss, determined by neutron activation balance techniques, have been reported (97). This hidden negative calcium balance could be corrected by either transferring calcium from dialysis fluid to plasma (reverse dialysis) or improving dietary absorption.

Manipulation of calcium concentration in dialysis fluid can be used readily to augment the delivery of calcium to the patient during haemodialysis. The calcium concentration in dialysis fluid and the concomitant levels of plasma inorganic phosphate have been shown to be the two major influences controlling the flux of calcium across the dialyser during haemodialysis (99).

The quantity of calcium transferred to the patient during haemodialysis has been estimated relative to the concentration present in the dialysis fluid. With a calcium concentration of 1.25 to 1.5 mmol/l (5 to 6 mg/dl) in dialysis fluid only around 2.8 mmol (112 mg) is transferred to the patient during a six hour dialysis, insufficient to correct the deficit of 3 mmol (120 mg) lost as a consequence of ultrafiltration alone. Any accompanying negative calcium balance in the gastrointestinal tract will add to the loss of total body calcium. In contrast, by raising the calcium concentration in dialysis fluid to 1.75 to 2.0 mmol/l (7 to 8 mg/dl) the rate of calcium transferred to the patient rises five fold (100) so that on a weekly schedule of three, six hour dialyses, some 43.2 mmol (1728 mg) could be transferred to the patient weekly. This 'reverse dialysis' of calcium seems a practicable method of correcting potential calcium deficits when using a single-pass system, provided a dialysis fluid of accurately controlled composition is fed continuously to the dialyser. In recirculating dialysis fluid systems 'reverse dialysis' of calcium is more difficult to control as the concentration of calcium in the dialysis fluid will tend to fall progressively throughout each treatment.

During the last decade the traditional level of 1.25 to 1.5 mmol/l (5 to 6 mg/dl) calcium in dialysis fluid has been increased by some (101, 102) in the hope of normalising overall calcium balance (103) and perhaps obviating hyperparathyroidism and osteodystrophy (104). Levels as high as 2.0 mmol/l (8 mg/dl) of calcium in dialysis fluid have been recommended (99). Overt post-dialytic hypercalaemia has been reported as uncommon when using 1.75 mmol/l (7 mg/dl) of calcium in dialysis fluid (105), yet nausea and vomiting may be provoked during dialysis with 1.63 mmol/l (6.52 mg/dl) of calcium (90).

Even transient dialysis-related hypercalcaemia readily provokes unpleasant nausea, vomiting and hypertension (106) and should be avoided. Moreover, covert soft tissue calcification is widespread in dialysed patients, and of obscure causation (107). A positive calcium balance and (or) an intermittent rapid influx of extraneous calcium cannot be assumed to be entirely beneficial, indeed it may be harmful.

Despite the trend to higher calcium concentration in dialysis fluid some advocate (108), and many continue to use, traditional lower and possibly safer levels between 1.5 to 1.6 mmol/l (6 to 6.4 mg/dl). Effective treatment with active vitamin D sterols may be hindered by high calcium concentrations in dialysis fluid through the ready emergence of hypercalcaemia (109) and lower concentrations (1.4 to 1.5 mmol/l) (5.6 to 6 mg/dl) may be preferable (110).

Higher calcium concentrations in dialysis fluids, equal to or greater than 1.75 mmol/l (7 mg/dl), do suppress PTH secretion, measured by N-terminal-type assays in some short-term studies (111) but not in others (112). Any effect on calcium metabolism produced by intermittent dialysis on parathyroid function or bone status is not necessarily persistent and may be less potent than the contrasting effect produced by pharmacologic doses of vitamin D_3 metabolites (113). Anomalous results have been reported with acute studies when high calcium concentrations in dialysis fluid appeared to decrease plasma C-terminal PTH actively while N-terminal PTH increased (114).

Measurable changes in body calcium content can be monitored during the course of maintenance haemodialysis by using photon densitometry (81), balance technique (97) and *in vivo* neutron activation methods (102). In one study a dialysis fluid with a calcium concentration of 1.63 mmol/l (6.52 mg/dl) was shown to correlate with unchanged (18 patients) or increased (6 patients) total body calcium over two years whereas 1.25 mmol/l (5 mg/dl) resulted in a uniformly negative balance (102). However, even protracted zero overall balance for calcium cannot be assumed to imply normal bone structure or a normal distribution of calcium between osseous and soft tissue.

A rational alternative approach to the associated problems of calcium deficit, hyperparathyroidism and osteodystrophy, utilises the active forms of vitamin D or synthetic analogues which primarily increase absorption of dietary calcium (115–119).

The currently popular urge to increase calcium concentrations in dialysis fluid should be tempered by realisation that the effect of active vitamin D metabolites and analogues such as 1,25-dihydroxyvitamin D_3 $(1.25(OH)_2D_3)$ or 1α hydroxyvitamin D_3 $(1\alpha(OH)D_3)$ is additional to any effect of high calcium in dialysis fluid on bone and body calcium content (109, 120). Some investigators, without altering conventional calcium concentrations in dialysis fluids, have employed these active forms of vitamin D, in well-controlled studies with evident improvement in plasma calcium and PTH (N-terminal) levels (121–123) and even bone structure in the longer term studies (124–127). Although the therapeutic or prophylactic use of the active forms of vitamin D can also induce hypercalcaemia (125, 127, 128) the effect of these sterols on the intestinal absorption of calcium is inherently more constant, controllable and physiological than the use of high calcium concentrations in dialysis fluids which in effect is only an intermittent intravenous infusion of that element. Unlike high calcium in dialysis fluids, these sterols more reliably suppress parathyroid overactivity (129, 130) but long established parathyroid hyperplasia only regresses slowly (131).

Utilisation of high calcium concentrations in dialysis fluids may be complementary with and advantageous relative to the active forms of vitamin D in the early post operative management of maintenance dialysis patients who required parathyroidectomy. Hypocalcaemia in such patients can be remedied using high calcium concentrations in dialysis fluids but careful selection of concentrations and biochemical control is essential if gross interdialytic hypercalcaemia is to be avoided.

Thus, there are now available two approaches to the correction of negative calcium balance in patients being treated by intermittent dialysis, one using dialysis to 'reverse dialyse' calcium into patients, the other using $1,25(OH)_2D_3$ or $1\alpha(OH)D_3$. The first of these, using an increased calcium concentration in the dialysis fluid, presents some administrative difficulties in preparing appropriate concentrates and ensuring that only the correct one is used for individual patients. Furthermore it will have little effect in suppressing parathyroid overactivity. The second, using active forms of vitamin D, certainly increases absorption of dietary calcium and this absorption can seemingly balance any tendency to calcium loss even when a low calcium concentration in dialysis fluid (1.375 mmol/l) (5.5 mg/dl) is used (120). The major problems in the use of vitamin D metabolites is their potential toxic action in producing hypercalcaemia, although the existing calcium concentration is usually re-established soon after discontinuing the drug (131). The major toxic manifestations include metastatic calcification, manifested by radiologically identifiable soft tissue calcification, pruritus and corneal calcification. The degree of toxicity is also dependent on the plasma phosphate concentration (see also Chapter 35).

Control of disordered calcium metabolism in patients being treated by intermittent dialysis is fraught with multiple difficulties. The effect of concomitant aluminium accumulation, and possibly fluoride retention, on calcium metabolism in bone has not been fully assessed and it may be that modification of existing views will become necessary. As a policy the concentration of calcium in dialysis fluid should be just high enough to avoid the development of a negative calcium balance across the dialyser. It is recognised that this will not restore bone to normal. If symptoms of osteodystrophy arise (or a myopathy of vitamin D deficiency develops) then treatment with $1,25(OH)_2D_3$ or $1\alpha(OH)D_3$ is probably necessary (124, 127). This will alter the previously established overall calcium balance as absorption of dietary calcium will be improved. There is no failure to receptors of $1,25(OH)_2D_3$ in the gut although there may be a lack of response in the receptors in bone (132). There is also evidence of the value of vitamin D therapy in the prophylaxis of hypocalcaemia and bone disorder of predominantly osteitis fibrosa type in dialysed patients.

All workers agree that frequent monitoring of plasma calcium and phosphate is essential whenever $1,25(OH)_2D_3$ or $1\alpha(OH)D_3$ is given, particularly as acute attacks of hypercalcaemia can develop spontaneously (131).

Magnesium

Magnesium, the neglected cation, is predominantly intracellular, but the physiological plasma concentration is stabilised within the range 0.70 to 1.10 mmol/l (1.7 to 2.7 mg/dl), approximately 25% being protein-bound, and the rest diffusible (0.52 to 0.82 mmol/l), mostly in the ionised form (133). Absorption of dietary magnesium in renal failure appears to be normal (134) and is

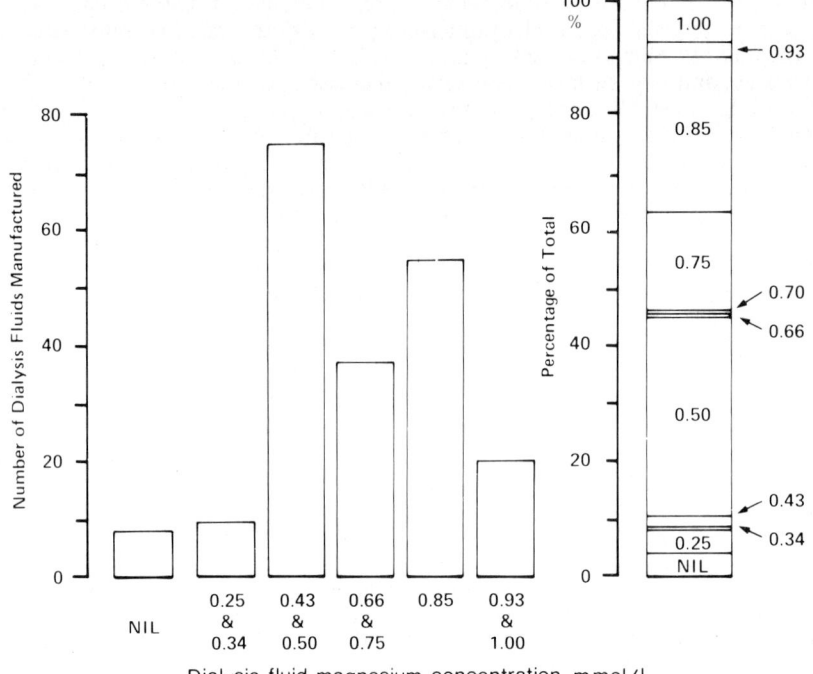

Figure 3. Magnesium concentrations of supplied dialysis fluids in the United Kingdom at 1980.

unaltered by changes in vitamin D metabolism (135). In particular magnesium absorption continues unaltered despite the development of hypermagnesaemia or tissue excess (133) so that in renal failure care must be taken to avoid magnesium containing drugs or a high magnesium intake (136).

The kidney is the main regulator of extracellular magnesium concentration. As renal failure progresses with reduced glomerular filtration, hypermagnesaemia is inevitable if dietary intake is normal. Magnesium excess has been associated with cardiac abnormalities (at plasma concentrations approaching 5 mmol/l, 12.3 mg/dl) and with effects on the nervous system, such as loss of deep tendon reflexes, at plasma concentrations above 3 mmol/l (7.4 mg/dl) (133). Magnesium deficiency also affects the nervous system, causing neuromuscular disturbances and tremor.

The relationships between magnesium, PTH and bone metabolism, both in the presence and absence of renal failure, are complex and require further elucidation. Investigations have been beset by problems of PTH assay and have often been inconsistent (137). Much of the immunologically reactive part of PTH is not biologically reactive and assays measuring the C and N terminals of the molecule, respectively, can give differing results. However, most studies have indicated that acute hypermagnesaemia tends to reduce PTH production (133, 138) whereas hypomagnesaemia has been variously associated with lower (139), higher (140) and unchanged PTH levels (141). In chronic renal failure, the effect of magnesium is subservient to the overriding effect of calcium on PTH production, hypocalcaemia being a far more potent stimulus than varying magnesium concentrations (133).

Haemodialysis using a 1.0 m² dialyser for 6 h will remove around 10.3 mmol (250 mg) from a patient when the plasma magnesium is normal at the start of dialysis and the dialysis fluid contains no magnesium (142). Therefore, using a thrice weekly dialysis schedule some 30.9 mmol (750 mg) of magnesium can be removed which approximates to the quantity of magnesium absorbed from a normal diet per week. Thus, in patients on dialysis, plasma concentrations of magnesium are dependent on the concentration in the dialysis fluid, the dietary intake and the dialysance of magnesium (143). The amount of magnesium removed at each dialysis will vary with the extent of the increase in the pre-dialysis plasma magnesium concentration (134).

A survey of dialysis fluid concentrates for the United Kingdom market in 1980 indicated a magnesium concentration in dialysis fluid ranging from nil to 1.0 mmol/l, with 80% of fluids between 0.50 and 0.80 mmol/l (Figure 3), nearly 50% being equal to or greater than the normal minimal plasma diffusible concentration. In the early days of maintenance haemodialysis a magnesium in dialysis fluid of 0.5 to 0.7 mmol/l was common so the current practice has not changed markedly over two decades. Low magnesium concentrations in dialysis fluids (0.0 to 0.2 mmol/l) have been advocated (144–146). Such fluids result in normal to high normal pre-dialysis plasma magnesium concentrations, decreasing to mildly low concentrations post-dialysis which return to normal a few hours later. Thus plasma magnesium can be made to fluctuate across the normal range. Similar effects can be demonstrated for potassium when the potassium concentration in dialysis fluids is varied. For both magnesium and potassium the plasma concentration of each can move over a wide range without any overt clinical change.

Lowering magnesium in dialysis fluid to 0.0 to 0.2 mmol/l (0.5 mg/dl) has resulted in improved nerve conduction velocities (146), more normal erythrocyte magnesium concentrations (145), less pruritus (147) and improvements of renal osteodystrophy (148), though some of these claims have been disputed (149, 150). Although increases in plasma PTH levels have been reported during low magnesium dialysis (151, 152) recent more prolonged studies (153) have indicated no significant changes in plasma PTH levels during variations in dialysis fluid magnesium concentrations which significantly affected plasma magnesium. Although magnesium concentrations above 0.25 mmol/l (0.6 mg/dl) in dialysis fluids have been recommended to inhibit hyperparathyroidism (152), the evidence for magnesium influences on parathyroid activity in dialysed patients remains conflicting. Whilst hypermagnesaemia can suppress PTH production, hypomagnesaemia can both inhibit PTH release from the gland and increase end organ resistance (154) – effects of possible benificial value in chronic renal failure, where progressive parathyroid overactivity is common due to calcium disturbances.

It is accepted that magnesium retention, rather than deficiency, is the main problem in renal failure and excess magnesium may be a factor in both renal bone disease (155) and soft tissue calcification (137, 156). Erythrocyte and tissue magnesium concentrations appear to remain high even with the long term use of low magnesium dialysis fluid (145, 150). Although the overt effects of acutely high plasma magnesium concentrations are seldom seen in patients on intermittent dialysis, the avoidance of even moderate hypermagnesaemia would seem a desirable goal. The majority of dialysis units, however, accept moderate hypermagnesaemia as a matter of course, with pre-dialysis values in the 1.5 to 2.0 mmol/l (3.7 to 4.9 mg/dl) range using a dialysis fluid magnesium concentration of around 0.7 mmol/l (1.7 mg/dl). Concentrations in dialysis fluid above 0.25 mmol/l (0.6 mg/dl) continue to be recommended (150–152). Few, however, have continued to dialyse for long periods at magnesium concentrations greater than 1.0 mmol/l (2.45 mg/dl).

The future trend in dialysis fluid magnesium concentrations will probably be downwards, to a possible mean between 0.2 (0.5 mg/dl) and 0.3 mmol/l (0.7 mg/dl) which, on present evidence, would appear to be the most acceptable level. As dialysis times become shorter, magnesium retention may be increased, and it would seem sensible to lower magnesium in dialysis fluids accordingly, in order to keep plasma magnesium as near normal as possible. On the other hand if dietary intake of magnesium decreases for any reason then it would be wise to monitor plasma magnesium concentrations and supplement by oral, parenteral or higher dialysis fluid concentrations if sub-normal pre-dialysis values are found.

Hard water syndrome (see also Chapter 6)

Failure of a plant used for pretreatment of hard water can mean that the final concentration of calcium and magnesium can be excessively high. Discontinuation of the use of a base exchanger (water softener), without informing the dialysis centre, elevated the calcium content of dialysis fluid from 1.5 to 3.6 mmol/l (6 to 14.4 mg/dl) and the magnesium from 0.5 to 1.5 mmol/l (1.2 to 3.7 mg/dl) (157). In another instance failure of the electrical timers controlling regeneration of a base exchanger (158) caused an elevation of the calcium concentration in dialysis fluid from 1.5 mmol/l to 3.0 to 3.3 mmol/l (6 mg/dl to 12 to 13.4 mg/dl) and magnesium from 0.75 mmol/l to 1.45 to 1.5 mmol/l (1.8 to 3.6 to 3.7 mg/dl). In both reports the clinical symptoms occurring with the elevated calcium and magnesium concentrations were similar. There was a marked rise in blood pressure 3 to 6 h after commencing treatment accompanied by sweating and abnormal sensation of warmth. Nausea, progressing to vomiting, developed and there was profound lethargy and weakness. Because both calcium and magnesium concentrations were elevated in each report it was impossible to ascribe a symptom to the elevation of one element, although hypertension was more likely to be caused by the hypercalcaemia.

Acetate

Acetate was first used in dialysis fluid to replace the chlorides of potassium, calcium and magnesium as they are less deliquescent salts (6). In the first description of 'refrigerated' intermittent dialysis (10) sodium acetate was added to dialysis fluid to overcome 'bubbling' in the venous return blood-line. In 1964 the Seattle physicians (11) replaced all bicarbonate with acetate, considered by some the second major advance in intermittent dialysis after the introduction of the Scribner shunt (159). The use of acetate was most successful but it is surprising that only in relatively recent years has its metabolism been studied in patients with renal failure. Acetate has some bacteriostatic and bactericidal properties (160).

In normal subjects acetate appears in the plasma during the metabolism of ethanol (161) being formed in the liver and metabolised to carbon dioxide and water in the peripheral tissues (162). The maximum amount of acetate that can be metabolised is about 300 mmol/h, furnishing some 62.5 kcals/h (263 kJ/h) (163). The dialysance of acetate in pure solution was determined in 1964 (11) as 55 to 65 ml/min using a simulated blood flow of 150 ml/min and a dialysing surface area of 0.9 m². The amount of acetate gaining access to the circulation during a normal haemodialysis was estimated at about 90 mmol/h. The ideal concentration of acetate in dialysis fluid (11) was determined as 35 mmol/l and values close to this concentration are used at the present time.

This earlier work has now to be reassessed as efficiency of dialysis has improved. Present day dialysers are

trose in dialysis fluid has not yet been fully determined. It could, perhaps, be argued on first principles that the concentration of dextrose present in dialysis fluid should not cause a major disturbance of normal blood values (about 5 mmol/l).

Several authors have investigated the effect of dextrose concentrations in dialysis fluid on fat metabolism. Lipaemia and 'glucose' intolerance is a common finding in chronic renal failure and not surprisingly this has been linked with the mortality and morbidity from cardiovascular complications. There is an increased incidence of hypertriglyceridaemia and relatively low incidence of hypercholesterolaemia in the chronic maintenance haemodialysis population (200). The hypertriglyceridaemia and hypercholesterolaemia tended to fall when the dextrose concentration in dialysis fluid was reduced from 455 mg/dl (25.3 mmol/l) to zero over a six month period (200). On the other hand a decrease in triglycerides during dialysis has been reported when dialysis fluid contained 400 mg/dl (22.2 mmol/l) of dextrose (201), triglycerides rising when the fluid contained no dextrose. When the dextrose concentration was 182 mg/dl (10.1 mmol/l) it was concluded that this did not contribute to hypertriglyceridaemia (192). However, there does seem to be a gradual fall in triglyceride and cholesterol concentrations with increasing duration of dialysis (200, 201).

Unfortunately a number of studies of triglyceride concentrations in dialysed patients have been undertaken at widely different dextrose concentrations in dialysis fluid, ranging 0 to 455 mg/dl (0 to 25.3 mmol/l), which were not considered as a material variable. Even so it would seem that dextrose in modest amounts (182 mg/dl or 10.1 mmol/l) is unlikely to contribute to the incidence of hypertriglyceridaemia (see also Chapter 29).

The effect of omitting dextrose on gluconeogenesis is probably of importance. Blood pyruvate (192, 202) fell and acetoacetate and β-hydroxybutyrate were markedly increased (192) during dextrose-free dialysis in the fasting state. In the presence of dextrose there was little change in all three substances, the modest rise in acetoacetate and β-hydroxybutyrate probably occurring as a result of an influx of acetate. Using dextrose-free dialysis fluid there was up to 60% reduction in whole blood alanine concentration (202) (a precursor of pyruvate), so it was concluded that gluconeogenesis was profound, glycogenolysis being inadequate to maintain blood sugar concentration (199). However, dextrose in dialysis fluid did not prevent the increased protein catabolic rate observed during dialysis, so this increase is apparently not the result of gluconeogenesis but due to some other metabolic event (199).

In summary it would appear that dextrose in modest amounts (up to 182 mg/dl or 10.1 mmol/l) is safe but its absence is probably not deleterious. Despite the findings that modest amounts of dextrose may be beneficial, on specialised investigation, many nephrologists use dextrose-free dialysis fluids which seem to cause few, if any, clinical abnormalities.

Fluoride

Fluoride is frequently added to tap water to achieve a final concentration of 1.0 mg/l (0.05 mmol/l or 1.0 ppm) (203) giving an intake from tap water of 1.4 to 1.8 mg/day in normal subjects to which must be added the fluoride content of food of 0.5 to 1.5 mg/day (26–78 µmol/day). This is 0.5 mg/day higher (204) if fluoridated water is used in food processing and preparation. The main route for excretion of fluoride is through the kidney but some is deposited in apatite mineral in bone. The normal plasma concentration of fluoride is about 0.02 to 0.032 µg/ml (appr. 1.0 to 1.7 µmol/l) (205, 206) and some increase is found in patients with renal failure (reaching 0.094 µg/ml (appr. 5 µmol/l)) when the serum creatinine exceeds 265 µmol/l (205). The highest recorded values, reaching about 10 times normal, have been found in patients dialysed against dialysis fluid constituted with fluoridated tap water (205–208) showing a progressive increase with time on dialysis (209). This rise takes place because excess fluoride cannot be eliminated in renal failure and the patient may gain 10 to 30 mg (0.53 to 1.59 mmol) fluoride per dialysis (208, 210, 211). An equilibrium in the plasma concentration occurs about 4 to 6 h after the start of dialysis (207, 211) then falls between dialyses (205) presumably as fluoride moves into bone where it accumulates (212) and may contribute to the increased osteoid seen in bone biopsies of dialysis patients.

The high incidence of osteodystrophy in patients treated by regular dialysis has led to the speculation that excessive fluoride retention could play a role. Unfortunately the evidence is conflicting and no controlled long term trial with fluoride in the dialysis fluid as the only variable has been undertaken (213). This is probably because other advances have been occurring in understanding the aetiology of osteodystrophy (such as accumulation of aluminium, see Chapters 35 and 42). Some studies present evidence that fluoride does contribute to the development of bone disease (207, 214, 215) but other investigators found inconclusive evidence or no clear-cut demonstrable effect (205, 207–209, 211, 216, 217). It may be that fluoride retention is beneficial (212) making bone more resistant to PTH induced resorption. Faced with such conflicting reports some may prefer to deionise tap water before use (215) in the hope that the severity and incidence of bone disease will be lessened or, very simply, to adjust the constancy of the internal environment to as near normal as possible (213); others consider that it is still premature to state that fluoridated tap water leads to damaging accumulation in bone (217).

If a deioniser is used it must be correctly maintained (218) otherwise excessive quantities of fluoride may be eluted before saturation for divalent ions is recognised as the apparatus becomes exhausted (see also Chapter 6).

CONTAMINANTS AND OTHER SUBSTANCES

Harmful chemicals present in tap water must be removed before the water enters a dialysis system (see also Chapter 6). At all times vigilance is required as frequently water authorities add substances at irregular intervals to raw water to make it potable. Aquatic animals growing in town mains water frequently require energetic methods, in the form of chemical agents, to suppress multiplication. In the case of turbidity from earthy or algal sources water authorities commonly add aluminium sulphate (alum) or ferrous sulphate to remove discolouration. The residuum of such additives are usually considered quite harmless when ingested in normal quantities but may cause problems in conventional dialysis systems which use hundreds of litres of tap water per week. Rarely, unexpected material such as zinc or copper may, inadvertently, be introduced to water supplies near to the point of delivery, especially in home dialysis installations in rural areas. Most authorities maintain high standards of purification in water supplied to domestic establishments (particular attention being paid to bacterial contamination) but these standards vary throughout the world and it is advisable for each dialysis centre to make appropriate enquiries for there may be potential hazards peculiar to certain areas. For example water may contain nitrates originating from fertilisers in agricultural areas.

Many dialysis centres are now pre-treating mains water with reverse osmosis (R.O.) plants. These process the water supply usually using an activated charcoal bed and base-exchanger (water softener) prior to forcing the water at high pump-generated pressure through a semipermeable membrane. This special membrane, in addition to providing a sterile product, rejects a very high percentage of inorganic ions (Table 3) and organic substances greater than 200 daltons. It is to be noted that R.O. units work on a percentage rejection basis and not to any given absolute value in the product water so that it is essential for all dialysis centres to analyse the product at regular intervals. This is important for the composition of town mains water commonly varies on a seasonal basis. Such measurement also gives warning of a partial breakdown of an R.O. unit. Table 3 shows that fluoride has a relatively low rejection ratio (and, though not shown, a similar value is found for bicarbonate).

Table 3. Average rejection rates of a reverse osmosis unit.

Substance	% Rejection
Calcium	96–98
Magnesium	96–98
Sodium	85–95
Potassium	85–95
Aluminium	98–99
Sulphate	95–98
Chloride	85–95
Nitrate	60–85
Fluoride	86–95

The rejection of fluoride (and bicarbonate) is affected by the pH of the feed water, being greater than 95% at pH 8.0 but only 85% at pH 6.3 (Hendryck Y, personal communication). In unfavourable situations it may be necessary to treat further the product water from an R.O. unit by adding a deioniser. Highly purified water is 'corrosive' and must not be allowed to come into contact with ordinary metals. It is commonly stored or transported in inert plastic containers or tubing.

The accepted standard for maximum allowable impurity for inorganic constituents in the water supply to dialysis machines, currently advocated by the Association for the Advancement of Medical Instrumentation (AAMI), Haemodialysis Systems Standard Committee, U.S.A., is recorded in Table 3 of Chapter 6. As yet there are no special regulations regarding the purity of chemicals used in the manufacture of concentrate (with the exception of a higher grade of purity required for hydrated $MgCl_2$ used in dialysis fluid [219]). In one dialysis fluid tested, the aluminium concentration was 10 µg/l (JP Day, P Ackrill, personal communication) when the commercial concentrate was appropriately diluted with aluminium-free distilled water. More work on the purity of concentrate solution seems indicated.

Although dialysis removes certain essential substances, such as water soluble vitamins and amino acids, these are not added to dialysis fluid on account of expense and can usually be replaced by an adequate diet and some supplements.

CONSTITUTING THE DIALYSIS FLUID

Tank systems

Once the concentration of electrolytes (and dextrose if required) in the dialysis fluid has been chosen the exact quantities of a mixture of chloride and acetate (or bicarbonate) salts can be decided. It is important to take into account the composition of the water supply and pretreat if necessary. In the early days of dialysis each salt, of pharmaceutical grade, was weighed out individually and stored in separate sealed containers prior to adding to a known volume of water in a tank. Frequently the water added to the tank was obtained from a thermostatically controlled mixer tap connected to a hot and cold water supply to give the required temperature. Proper mixing of the fluid was usually achieved by using either manually operated or electrically driven paddles. A more satisfactory mixing procedure was to introduce a stream of filtered air into the bottom of the tank. If bicarbonate was used in place of acetate it was customary to replace the air with a mixture of 10% CO_2 and 90% O_2 and add the salts of calcium and magnesium after the pH had fallen to 7.4, thereafter the flow of gas into the mixture was reduced to maintain this pH.

The disadvantages of a tank supply would include physical size, limited capacity, the labour intensive procedure, problems associated with unequal mixing and infection. The bacteriology problem led to the development of 'refrigerated recirculation dialysis' (220). Cool-

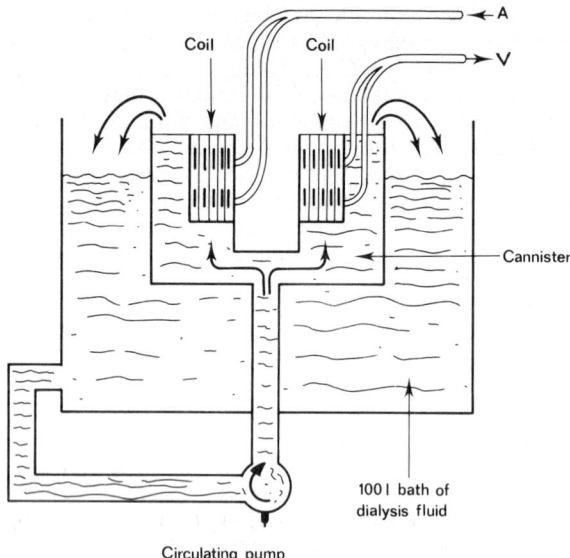

Figure 4. Diagram of the Kolff-Twin Coil dialyser.

ing reduced the bacterial count but great care was necessary in undertaking adequate sterilising of the tank between dialyses, using chemical agents. Frequently the chemical composition of the dialysis fluid was not checked but electric conductivity could be used or the chloride content measured by adapting the Schales and Schales method (221) using disposable syringes, the final titration being done with a hypodermic needle attached to a 1.0 ml syringe graduated in hundredths. Neither procedure satisfactorily guarded against the accidental omission of one or more chemicals, particularly salts of potassium, calcium and magnesium. Advantages of the tank system would include a low initial capital cost, its simplicity and the ability to vary the composition of dialysis fluid with relative ease.

In the single patient systems developed during the 1940's and 1950's the tank contained about 100 l of dialysis fluid, a fresh solution being used every 2 h. When a coil dialyser was used (222) the dialysate was recirculated through the coil, which was held in a rigid container situated above the level of the main 100 l tank, at about 20 to 30 l/min (Figure 4 and in Chapter 2 Figure 23b). Later this system was modified so that fresh dialysis fluid was fed at 500 ml/min into a small tank of about 6 l capacity, containing the dialyser, through which the dialysate recirculated at 10 to 15 l/min, before being discarded to drain, the so-called 'Recirculating Single Pass (RSP)' system. When intermittent dialysis for chronic renal failure was established in the 1960's tanks of 500 to 1,000 l, made of plastic or stainless steel, were used to store the dialysis fluid. Either one tank was reserved for each patient or several were connected together to provide a supply to several dialysis stations. The dialysis fluid was delivered to the dialyser either by positive pressure from a small header tank situated up-

stream of the dialyser or sucked through by an efflux pump situated downstream of the dialyser.

Proportioning systems

In 1964 three developments revolutionised the preparation of dialysis fluid; firstly, replacement of bicarbonate with acetate (11) so that calcium and magnesium were not precipitated, secondly, the development of a concentrate containing the relative proportion of electrolytes in solution which had to be diluted 35 times with tap water (pre-treated if necessary) and thirdly, development of mechanical proportioning systems (223) continuously blending concentrate with tap water (pre-treated if necessary) in the correct proportions. These systems and the necessary monitoring devices required to ensure safety to the patient are described in Chapters 2 and 11. Complete analysis of all electrolytes (except acetate) and dextrose (if used) in every batch of concentrate manufactured is essential to make sure that each ingredient has been added in the correct amount.

Because the optimum concentrations of electrolytes in dialysis fluid has not been decided there has been no single composition of concentrate advocated. Indeed, the commercial manufacturers of concentrate in the United Kingdom have been requested over the past years to provide more than 156 different compositions varying from 30 to 40 times concentration although 35 times was the most frequently employed.

With the introduction of methods capable of providing a continuous supply of dialysis fluid the needs for undertaking 'refrigerated' intermittent dialysis ceased because the bacterial content of the fluid fell to acceptable levels and the concentrate remained 'sterile' for long periods of time (9). This allowed dialysis to be undertaken at body temperature, the spent dialysis fluid going straight to drain (9), the so-called 'flow-to-waste' system. The efficiency of dialysis was thus increased.

If the recent disquiet directed towards the use of acetate rather than bicarbonate, described previously, is confirmed then considerable modification to our current method of undertaking dialysis will be necessary, particularly for seriously ill patients with acute renal failure. These patients frequently have a severe metabolic response so that acetate intolerance is likely to occur, even if its metabolic degradation rate is unimpaired, when a dialyser with a surface area in excess of 1.5 m^2 is used. Thus, the problem of retaining divalent ions in solution in dialysis fluids containing bicarbonate will return. The original dialysis machines developed in the 1940's and 1950's were satisfactory for they used bicarbonate, pH being corrected by CO_2, and ultrafiltration was achieved by elevating the pressure of blood in the dialyser, the dialysis fluid being kept at normal atmospheric pressure. One method of continuous blending tap water with concentrate containing bicarbonate has been suggested (224). Two concentrate solutions were pumped separately into the pumped water stream. The first contained NaCl and $NaHCO_3$ whilst the second contained the chlorides of sodium, potassium, calcium and magnesium plus sufficient HCl or acetic acid to produce a suitable pH and PCO_2 on mixing. By using NaCl in both concentrates the detection of incorrect flow rates of the two concentrates and water was readily detectable by a conductivity device. Another system available commercially uses a similar principle of acidification but the first concentrate contains only $NaHCO_3$, all the NaCl, acid and other chlorides being added to the second concentrate. In these bicarbonate systems the tap water, usually pre-treated with an R.O. unit, should be de-aerated and warmed to body temperature before receiving the two concentrates. Considerable care must be exercised to avoid an excess of acid as this will cause degassing problems if an excess of CO_2 is produced and, if HCl is used, also cause a metabolic acidosis from hyperchloraemia. Most machines now available commercially using these principles are able to dispense either acetate or bicarbonate containing dialysis fluid according to requirement.

De-aeration of dialysis fluid

The solubility of air in water decreases as the temperature rises (Table 4). As town mains water is invariably pressurised the volume of air in solution at a given temperature may be higher than that quoted, particularly if the temperature of the water rises during distribution or air is injected into the supply pipes for cleansing purposes. When cold water is warmed to 37 °C the dissolved air is not released instantaneously, passing through a 'supersaturated phase', so that PO_2 values may be significantly elevated above those found under normal atmospheric pressure (225). Equilibration eventually occurs after about 4 h but takes place more rapidly if the water is agitated. This means that some device is required to remove excess air when cold town mains water is warmed to 37 °C. In earlier types of single patient proportioning machines the dialysis fluid was first warmed to 37 °C and then entered the headertank which contained sharp pointed ceramic beads or polypropylene mesh screens to speed the process of de-aeration. Even so the time taken for the dialysis fluid to traverse the headertank was inadequate to allow equilibration to occur, so that the PO_2 in the dialysis fluid entering the dialyser was at least 200 mm Hg (225). This meant that conductivity devices were frequently coated with air resulting in false low alarms. In addition the excessive partial pressure of air was 'dialysed' through the membrane to enter the blood where the mean 'arterial' PO_2 rose from 89 mm Hg to 116 mm Hg in the blood returning to the patient. Frequently, and particularly in winter months when the cold tap water contained more dissolved air (see Table 4), this resulted in air coming out of solution in the dialyser and return blood lines. This could adversely interfere with the performance of the dialyser (225) and also increase fibrin deposition in some types of hollow fibre dialysers (226) (see also Chapter 5). The released air accumulated in the bubble trap, where frothing also occurred, thus displacing the blood in the bubble trap and air embolus was a very real danger. The problem of air coming out of solution in the blood stream when coil dialysers were used was less when dialysis fluid was recirculated at atmospheric pressure from a static tank (thereby allowing more time for air to come out of solution), dehydration being achieved by elevating the blood pressure which, incidentally, allows a small additional quantity of air to be carried in solution.

In many modern dialysers ultrafiltration is achieved by applying a negative pressure to the dialysis fluid. If the pressure of the dialysis fluid is reduced to −200 mm Hg then the maximum solubility of air in water at 37 °C is decreased by about 4 ml/l (Table 4). This means that simple de-gassing procedures undertaken at normal atmospheric pressure will not usually prevent air coming out of solution in the blood circuit, particularly during the winter months. Two methods have been developed to remove excess air from the town mains water on warming to 37 °C.

(a) Negative pressure. Creation of a negative pressure (Figure 5) by means of an electric pump sucking the dialysis fluid through a constricting nozzle was originally developed for a tank supply system operating at the temperature of town mains (227). The flow rate through the de-aerer at such temperatures should be about twice that passing through the dialyser, the pressure in the vacuum chamber being at approximately −600 mm Hg (226). The system is more efficient at 37 °C when the flow rate through the vacuum chamber can be reduced to that passing through the dialyser. The

Table 4. Approximate solubility of air in water at varying temperatures and pressures.

Temperature of town mains °C	Saturated air content at 760 mm Hg ml/l	Quantity to be removed on heating to 37 °C at 760 mm Hg ml/l	Additional quantity of air to be removed at 37 °C if pressure reduced to 560 mm Hg (i.e.: −200 mm Hg)
5	25.5	11.5	
10	23.0	9.0	
15	20.5	6.5	
20	18.5	4.5	4.0 ml/l
25	17.0	3.0	
30	15.5	1.5	
35	14.5	0.5	
37	14.0	—	

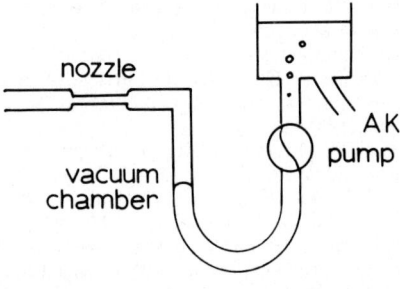

Figure 5. De-aeration using negative pressure.

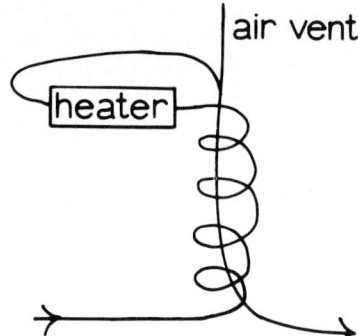

Figure 6. De-aeration using a heat-exchanger.

device is most conveniently attached to a headertank as a recirculating system. One reason for the efficiency of the method is the profound agitation produced as the fluid, at a negative pressure, passes through the pump.

Further improvement has been obtained by incorporating plastic mesh screens in the vacuum chamber but this was abandoned as the mesh tended to trap particulate matter and was also difficult to 'sterilise'.

(b) Heat exchanger. Heating incoming town mains to 68° to 70°C with subsequent cooling to normal dialysis fluid temperatures in a heat exchanger (Figure 6) is an efficient method of driving air out of solution. At equilibration the solubility of air in water at 70°C and 760 mm Hg is 8.0 ml/l (228). This is less than the solubility of air in water at 37°C and −200 mm Hg (Table 4). Heating town mains to 70°C is equivalent to 'pasteurisation' so that most pathogenic non-spore types of bacteria will be killed.

According to present practice sufficient air should be removed from town mains so that the PO_2 of dialysis fluid at 37°C is less than 150 mm Hg, provided the negative pressure applied to dialysis fluid in the dialyser is not too great (225). If air still tends to come out of solution further treatment with an additional negative pressure device will usually cure the fault.

ACKNOWLEDGEMENTS

Figure 5 is reproduced from the Proceedings of the European Dialysis and Transplant Association Volume V, 1968 by kind permission of the Editors and Excerpta Medica Foundation.

Table 3 was kindly provided by Culligan, High Wycombe, U.K.

We thank Macarthy's Laboratories, Romford, U.K. for details of the composition of concentrates supplied to dialysis centres in U.K.

We also thank J.P. Day and P. Ackrill, Withington Hospital, Manchester, U.K. and Y. Hendryk, Culligan, Brussels, Belgium for their personal communications.

REFERENCES

1. Kolff WJ: *New ways of treating uraemia*, London, J & A Churchill, 1947
2. Alwall N: On the artificial kidney. I. Apparatus for dialysis of the blood *in vivo*. *Acta Med Scand* 128:317, 1947
3. Murray G, Delorme E, Thomas N: Artificial kidney. *JAMA* 137:1596, 1948
4. Skeggs LT Jr, Leonards JR: Studies on an artificial kidney: I. Preliminary results with a new type of continuous dialyzer. *Science* 108:212, 1948
5. Murphy WP, Swan RC, Walter CW, Weller JM, Merrill JP: Use of an artificial kidney. III Current procedures in clinical hemodialysis. *J Lab Clin Med* 40:436, 1952
6. Wolf AV, Remp DG, Kiley JE, Currie GD: Artificial kidney function: kinetics of hemodialysis. *J Clin Invest* 30:1062, 1951
7. Parsons FM, McCracken BH: The use and function of the artificial kidney. *Br J Urol* 30:463, 1958
8. Diem K, Lentner C (Editors): *Documenta Geigy Scientific Tables* 7th Ed. Basle, J.R. Geigy, 1970 p 523
9. Cole JJ, Fritzen JR, Vizzo JE, van Paasschen WH, Grimsrud L: One year's experience with a central dialysate supply system in a hospital. *Trans Am Soc Artif Intern Organs* 11:22, 1965
10. Scribner BH, Hegstrom RM, Buri R: Treatment of chronic uremia by means of hemodialysis: a progress report. In *Proc 1st Int Congr Nephrol*, Basel, New York, S. Karger, 1961, p 616
11. Mion CM, Hegstrom RM, Boen ST, Scribner BH: Substitution of sodium acetate for sodium bicarbonate in the bath fluid for hemodialysis. *Trans Am Soc Artif Intern Organs* 10:110, 1964
12. Stewart WK, Fleming LW, Manuel MA: Benefits obtained by the use of high sodium dialysate during maintenance haemodialysis. *Proc Eur Dial Transpl Assoc* 9:111, 1972
13. Port FK, Johnson WJ, Klass DW: Prevention of dialysis disequilibrium syndrome by use of high sodium concentration in the dialysate. *Kidney Int* 3:327, 1973
14. Stewart WK, Fleming LW: Blood pressure control during maintenance haemodialysis with isonatric (high sodium) dialysate. *Postgrad Med J* 50:260, 1974
15. Liebau H, Eisenbach GM, Mariss P, Hilfenhaus M: Role of sodium and water in hypertensive patients on maintenance hemodialysis. *Contrib Nephrol* 8:126, 1977
16. Locatelli F, Costanzo R, Di Filippo S, Pedrini L, Marai P, Pozzi C, Ponti R, Sforzini S, Redaelli B: Ultrafiltration and high sodium concentration dialysis: pathophysiological correlation. *Proc Eur Dial Transpl Assoc* 15:253, 1978
17. Stewart WK, Fleming LW, McLean S: Is hyponatric dialysis appropriate? a survey of dialysate sodium concentration in the United Kingdom. *Dial Transpl* 6 (nr 7):9, 1977
18. Moriarty MV, Parsons FM: Hypernatraemia during peritoneal dialysis. *Proc Eur Dial Transpl Assoc* 3:359, 1966
19. Redaelli B, Sforzini S, Limido D, Mimmo R, Di Filippo G, D'Amico P, Palumbo A: La concentrazione del Na nel liquido di dialisi nel trattamento emodialitico. Considerazioni teoriche e risultati clinici a breve termine. (The concentration of sodium in the dialysis fluid for haemodialysis treatment. Theoretical considerations and short term clinical results) *Minerva Nefrol* 23:301, 1976 (In Italian)
20. Nolph KD, Hopkins CA, New D, Antwiler GD, Popovich RP: Differences in solute sieving with osmotic vs. hydro-

static ultrafiltration. *Trans Amer Soc Artif Int Organs* 22:618, 1976
21. Wilkinson R, Scott DF, Uldall PR, Kerr DNS, Swinney J, Robson V: Plasma renin and exchangeable sodium in the hypertension of chronic renal failure. *Q J Med* 39:377, 1970
22. Haruyama T, Shitomi K, Kaneda H, Takeuchi M, Murata T: Development of malignant hypertension as a result of negative sodium balance. *Nippon Jinzo Gakkai Shi* 19:441, 1977
23. Drukker W, Jungerius NA, Alberts C: Report on regular dialysis treatment in Europe III, 1967. *Proc Eur Dial Transpl Assoc* 4:3, 1967
24. Boquin E, Parnell S, Grondin G, Wollard C, Leonard D, Michaels R, Levin NW: Crossover study of the effect of different dialysate sodium concentrations in large surface area short-term dialysis. *Proc Clin Dial Transpl Forum* 7:48, 1977
25. Arieff AI, Massry SG: Dialysis disequilibrium. In: *Clinical Aspects of Uremia and Dialysis*. Edited by Massry SG, Sellers AL. Springfield IL, CC Thomas 1976
26. Gordon A, Maxwell MH: Water, electrolyte, and acid-base disorders associated with acute and chronic dialysis. In: *Clinical Disorders of Fluid and Electrolyte Metabolism*, 3rd edn. Edited by Maxwell MH, Kleeman CR. New York, McGraw-Hill, 1980, p 827
27. Kennedy AC, Linton AL, Luke RG, Renfrew S: Electroencephalographic changes during haemodialysis. *Lancet* 1:408, 1963
28. Asaba H, Bergström J, Fürst P, Lindh K, Mion C, Oulès R, Shaldon S: Sequential ultrafiltration and diffusion as alternative to conventional hemodialysis. *Proc Clin Dial Transpl Forum* 6:129, 1976
29. Bergström J, Asaba H, Fürst P, Oulès R: Dialysis, ultrafiltration, and blood pressure. *Proc Eur Dial Transpl Assoc* 13:293, 1976
30. Wehle B, Asaba H, Castenfors J, Fürst O, Grahn A, Gunnarsson B, Shaldon S, Bergström J: The influence of dialysis fluid composition on the blood pressure response during dialysis. *Clin Nephrol* 10:62, 1978
31. Bergström J: Ultrafiltration without dialysis for removal of fluid and solutes in uremia. *Clin Nephrol* 9:156, 1978
32. Wehle B, Asaba H, Castenfors J, Fürst P, Gunnarsson B, Shaldon S, Bergström J: Hemodynamic changes during sequential ultrafiltration and dialysis. *Kidney Int* 15:411, 1979
33. Hampl H, Paeprer H, Unger V, Kessel MW: Hemodynamics during hemodialysis, sequential ultrafiltration and hemofiltration. *J Dial* 3:51, 1979
34. Hagstam KE, Lindergård B, Tibbling G: Mannitol infusion in regular haemodialysis treatment for chronic renal insufficiency. *Scand J Urol Nephrol* 3:257, 1969
35. Rodrigo F, Shideman J, McHugh R, Buselmeier T, Kjellstrand C: Osmolality changes during hemodialysis: natural history, clinical correlations, and influence of dialysate glucose and intravenous mannitol. *Ann Intern Med* 86:554, 1977
36. Henrich WL, Woodard TD, Blachley JD, Gomez-Sanchez C, Pettinger W, Cronin RE: Role of osmolality in blood pressure stability after dialysis and ultrafiltration. *Kidney Int* 18:480, 1980
37. Drukker W, Alberts C, Jungerius NA: Dialysate glucose concentration and plasma osmolality during haemodialysis in acute renal failure. *Proc Eur Dial Transpl Assoc* 2:7, 1965
38. Leski M, Niethammer T, Wyss T: Glucose-enriched dialysate and tolerance to maintenance hemodialysis. *Nephron* 24:271, 1979

39. Arieff AI, Lazarowitz VC, Guisado R: Experimental dialysis disequilibrium syndrome: prevention with glycerol. *Kidney Int* 14:270, 1978
40. Jenkins PG, Dreher WH: Dialysis-induced muscle cramps: treatment with hypertonic saline and theory as to etiology. *Trans Amer Soc Artif Intern Organs* 21:479, 1975
41. Quelhorst E, Rieger J, Doht B, Beckmann H, Jacob I, Kraft B, Mietzsch G, Scheler F: Treatment of chronic uraemia by an ultrafiltration kidney – first clinical experience. *Proc Eur Dial Transpl Assoc* 13:314, 1976
42. Kohnle W, Heimsch E, Schmidt-Wiederkehr P, Franz HE: Acid base status during treatment of chronic uremia with diafiltration. *J Dial* 1:419, 1977
43. Schünemann B, Girndt J, Quellhorst E: Hemofiltration as a treatment for 'dialysis-resistant' hypertension and hypotensive hyperhydration. *J Dial* 1:575, 1977
44. Stiller S, Mann H, Gürich W: Theoretical aspects of various ultrafiltration methods in artificial kidney therapy. *Artif Organs* 2:137, 1978
45. Henderson LW: Pre vs. post dilution hemofiltration. *Clin Nephrol* 11:120, 1979
46. Kishimoto T, Yamagami S, Tanaka H, Ohyama T, Yamamoto T, Yamakawa M, Nishino M, Yoshimoto S, Maekawa M: Superiority of hemofiltration to hemodialysis for treatment of chronic renal failure: comparative studies between hemofiltration and hemodialysis on dialysis disequilibrium syndrome. *Artif Organs* 4:86, 1980.
47. Cambi V, Arisi L, Bignardi L, Garini G, Rossi E, Savazzi G, Migone L: Critical appraisal of hemofiltration and ultra-filtration. The development of ultra-short dialysis: preliminary results. *J Dial* 2:143, 1978
48. Levin NW, Grondin G: Dialysate sodium concentration. *Int J Artif Organs* 1:255, 1978
49. Levine T, Falk B, Henriquez M, Raja RM, Kramer MS, Rosenbaum JL: Effects of varying dialysate sodium using large surface area dialyzers. *Trans Am Soc Artif Intern Organs* 24:139, 1978
50. Man NK, Pils P, Di Guilio D, Zingraff J, Drueke T, Jungers P, Funck-Brentano J-L: Tolerance to high ultrafiltration rates during closed batch hemodialysis. *Artif Organs* 2:154, 1978
51. Funck-Brentano J-L: Ultrafiltration and diffusion techniques with the polyacrylonitrile membrane dialyzer. *Proc Renal Physicians Assoc* 2:9, 1978
52. Schuenemann B, Borghardt J, Falda Z, Jacob I, Kramer P, Kraft B Quellhorst E: Reactions of blood pressure and body spaces to hemofiltration treatment. *Trans Am Soc Artif Intern Organs* 24:687, 1978
53. Garini G, Savazzi GM, Arisi L, Bignardi L, David S, Rossi E, Cambi V: Attuali orientanenti sulla composizione del bagno di dialisi (Current orientation on the composition of the dialysis bath fluid). *Minerva Nefrol* 26:599, 1979 (In Italian)
54. Aizawa Y, Hirasawa Y, Shibata A: A fall of plasma osmolality created at dialyzer and its possible effect on circulating blood volume. *Clin Nephrol* 12:269, 1979
55. Wilkinson R, Barber SG, Robson V: Cramps, thirst and hypertension in hemodialysis patients – the influence of dialysate sodium concentration. *Clin Nephrol* 7, 101, 1977
56. Robson M, Oren A, Ravid M: Dialysate sodium concentration, hypertension and pulmonary edema in hemodialysis patients. *Dial Transpl* 7:678, 1978
57. Redaelli B, Sforzini S, Bondoldi G, Dadone C, Di Filippo S, Filoramo F, Limido D, Mimmo R, Pincella G, Vigano MR: Hemodialysis with 'adequate' sodium concentration in dialysate. *Int J Artif Organs* 2:133, 1979
58. Locatelli F, Costanzo R, Di Filippo S: High sodium

dialysate. *Int J Artif Organs* 2:171, 1979
59. Jones R, Poston L, Hinestroso H, Parsons V, Williams R: Weight gain between dialyses in diabetics: possible significance of raised intracellular sodium content. *Br Med J* 280:153, 1980
60. Swamy AP, Cestero RVM: Mannitol and maintenance hemodialysis. *Artif Organs* 3:116, 1979
61. Van Stone JC, Meyer R, Murrin C, Cook J: Hemodialysis with glycerol dialysate. *Trans Am Soc Artif Intern Organs* 25:354, 1979
62. Streicher E, Schneider H, Knödler U, Müller H, Spohr U, Schmidt-Gayk H: Chronic hemofiltration treatment. *Artif Organs* 4:48, 1980
63. Dumler F, Grondin G, Levin NW: Sequential high/low sodium hemodialysis: an alternative to ultrafiltration. *Trans Am Soc Artif Intern Organs* 25:351, 1979
64. Maeda K, Saito A, Kawaguchi S, Asada A, Niwa T, Ohta K, Kobayashi K: Hemodiafiltration with sodium concentration-controlled dialysate. *Artif Organs* 4:121, 1980
65. Chen W-T, Ing TS, Daugirdas JT, Humayun HM, Brescia DJ, Gandhi VC, Hano JE, Kheirbek AO: Hydrostatic ultrafiltration during hemodialysis using decreasing sodium dialysate. *Artif Organs* 4:187, 1980
66. Locatelli F, Costanzo R, De Filippo S, Pedrini L, Marai P, Pozzi C, Ponti R, Sforzini S, Redaelli B: Controlled sequential ultrafiltration dialysis, iso-osmotic dialysis, isonatric dialysis: pathophysiological and clinical evaluations. *Dial Transpl* 8:622, 1979
67. Lynggaard F, Nielsen B: Rapid fluid extraction with the Gambro Ultradiffuser. *Artif Organs* 2:134, 1978
68. Merrill JP: *The Treatment of Renal Failure*. New York, Grune and Stratton Inc 1955, p 185
69. Parsons FM, McCracken BH: The artificial kidney. *Br J Urol* 29:424, 1957
70. O'Keefe SJD, Sender PM, James WPT: 'Catabolic' loss of body nitrogen in response to surgery. *Lancet* 2:1035, 1974
71. Johny KV, Lawrence JR, O'Halloran MW, Wellby ML, Worthley BW: Studies on total body, serum and erythrocyte potassium in patients on maintenance haemodialysis. The value of erythrocyte potassium as a measure of body potassium. *Nephron* 7:230, 1970.
72. Seedat YK: Total body potassium and chronic renal failure. *Br Med J* 2:405, 1972
73. Oh MS, Levison SP, Carroll HJ: Content and distribution of water and electrolytes in maintenance hemodialysis. *Nephron* 14:421, 1975
74. Butkus DE, Alfrey AC, Miller NL: Tissue potassium in chronic dialysis patients. *Nephron* 13:314, 1974
75. Hagemann I, Schilling E, Krocker B, Precht K, Buchali K, Kruse I, Pietsch R, Eichhorst E, Seewald R: Untersuchungen des Elektrolytgehaltes in Erythrozyten im chronischen Hämodialyse-Programm bei Anwendung unterschiedlicher Spüllösungen. (The electrolyte content in erythrocytes in the long term dialysis programme during use of different irrigating solutions) *Z Urol Nephrol* 66:255, 1974 (In German)
76. Boddy K, King PC, Lindsay RM, Briggs JD, Winchester JF, Kennedy AC: Total body potassium in non-dialysed and dialysed patients with chronic renal failure. *Br Med J* 1:771, 1972
77. Bilbrey GL, Carter NW, White MG, Schilling JF, Knochel JP, Borroto J: Potassium deficiency in chronic renal failure. *Kidney Int* 4:423, 1973
78. Blainey JD, Hilton DD: The composition of the body in renal failure. *Ann R Coll Surg Engl* 47:45, 1970
79. Morgan AG, Burkinshaw L, Robinson PJA, Rosen SM: Potassium balance and acid-base changes in patients undergoing regular haemodialysis therapy. *Br Med J* 1:779, 1970
80. Delwaide PA, Rorive G: Etude du potassium total chez des patients en insuffisance renale chronique. Influence de la dialyse. (Study of total body potassium in patients with chronic renal failure. Effect of dialysis) *Nephron* 8:173, 1971 (in French)
81. Cohn SH, Cinque TJ, Dombrowski CS, Letteri JM: Determination of body composition by neutron activation analysis in patient with renal failure. *J Lab Clin Med* 79:978, 1972
82. Atkinson PJ, Hancock DA, Acharya VN, Parsons FM, Proctor EA, Reed GW: Changes in skeletal mineral in patients on prolonged maintenance dialysis. *Br Med J* 4:519, 1973
83. Bittar EE, Watt MF, Pateras VR, Parrish AE: The pH of muscle in Laennec's cirrhosis and uraemia. *Clin Sci* 23:265, 1962
84. Graham JA, Lawson DH, Linton AL: Muscle biopsy water and electrolyte contents in chronic renal failure. *Clin Sci* 38:583, 1970
85. Maschio G, Bazzato G, Bertaglia E, Sardini D, Mioni G, D'Angelo A, Marzo A: Intracellular pH and electrolyte content of skeletal muscle in patients with chronic renal acidosis. *Nephron* 7:481, 1970
86. Martin AM, Oduro-Dominah A, Gibbins JK, Devapal D, Mitchell DC: Regular short haemodialysis in end-stage renal failure. *Br Med J* 3:758, 1975
87. Brynger H, Brunner FP, Chantler C, Donckerwolcke RA, Jacobs C, Kramer P, Selwood NH, Wing AJ. Combined report on regular dialysis and transplantation in Europe, X, 1979. *Proc Eur Dial Transpl Assoc* 17:4, 1980
88. Berlyne GM, Janabi K, Shaw AB, Hocken AG: Treatment of hyperkalaemia with a calcium-resin. *Lancet* 1:169, 1966
89. Ogden DA, Holmes JH: Changes in total and ultrafilterable plasma calcium and magnesium during hemodialysis. *Trans Am Soc Artif Intern Organs* 12:200, 1966
90. Wing AJ: Optimum calcium concentration of dialysis fluid for maintenance haemodialysis. *Br Med J* 4:145, 1968
91. Wilmink JM: Some aspects of problems of calcium in maintenance dialysis. *Folia Med Neerl* 12:117, 1969
92. Soyannwo MAO, Oreopoulos DG, Mustafo G, McGeown MG: Studies on dialysate calcium requirements on maintenance haemodialysis: with observations on phosphate and magnesium. *Proc Eur Dial Transpl Assoc* 5:288, 1969
93. Sokol A, Gral T, Edelbaum DN, Rosen V, Rubini ME: Correlation of autopsy findings and clinical experience in chronically dialyzed patients. *Trans Am Soc Artif Intern Organs* 13:51, 1967
94. van Amstel WJ, Spijkerman MG, De Graeff J: Regulation of plasma calcium in patients on chronic haemodialysis. *Folia Med Neerl* 12:118, 1969
95. Fournier AE, Johnson WJ, Taves DR, Beabout JW, Arnaud CD, Goldsmith RS: Etiology of hyperparathyroidism and bone disease during chronic hemodialysis. I. Association of bone disease with potentially etiologic factors. *J Clin Invest* 50, 592, 1971
96. Bone JM, Davison AM, Robson JS: Role of dialysate calcium concentration in osteoporosis in patients on haemodialysis. *Lancet* 1:1047, 1972
97. Denney JD, Sherrard DJ, Nelp WB, Chesnut CH, Baylink DJ, Murano RI, Hinn G: Total body calcium and long-term calcium balance in chronic renal disease. *J Lab Clin Med* 82:226, 1973
98. Kaye M, Mangel R, Neubauer E: Studies in calcium

metabolism in patients on chronic haemodialysis. *Proc Eur Dial Transpl Assoc* 3:17, 1966
99. Goldsmith RS, Furszyfer J, Johnson WJ, Beeler GW Jr, Taylor WF: Calcium flux during hemodialysis. *Nephron* 20:132, 1978
100. Goldsmith RS, Furszyfer J, Johnson WJ, Fournier AE, Arnaud CD: Control of secondary hyperparathyriodism during long-term hemodialysis. *Am J Med* 50:692, 1971
101. Suzuki M, Hirasawa Y: Azotemic renal osteodystrophy; clinical features and bone pathology. *Endocrinol Jpn* 26 (Suppl):85, 1979
102. Asad SN, Ellis KJ, Cohn SH, Letteri JM: Changes in total body calcium on prolonged maintenance hemodialysis with high and low dialysate calcium. *Nephron* 23:223, 1979
103. Ritz E: Azotemic osteodystrophy – indications for intervention. *Prog Biochem Pharmacol* 17:251, 1980
104. Regan RJ, Peacock M, Rosen SM, Robinson PJ, Horsman A: Effect of dialysate calcium concentration on bone disease in patients on hemodialysis. *Kidney Int* 10:246, 1976
105. Johnson WJ: Persistent severe hypercalcemia during maintenance hemodialysis. *Ann Intern Med* 93:272, 1980
106. Zawada ET Jr, Bennett EP, Stinson JB, Ramirez G: Serum calcium in blood pressure regulation during hemodialysis. *Arch Intern Med* 141:657, 1981
107. Kuzela DC, Huffer WE, Conger JD, Winter SD, Hammond WS: Soft tissue calcification in chronic dialysis patients. *Am J Pathol* 86:403, 1977
108. Conceicao S, Hoenich NA, Ward MK, White T, Aljama P, Dewar J, Kerr DNS: Ionised calcium during haemodialysis. *Proc Eur Dial Transpl Assoc* 14:229, 1977
109. Winney RJ, Bone JM, Anderson TJ, Robson JS: Treatment of renal osteodystrophy with 1 alpha-hydroxycholecalciferol (1 alpha-OH-D$_3$) in conjunction with a high dialysate calcium. *Calcif Tissue Res* 22 (Suppl):94, 1977
110. Smith MA, Winney RJ, Strong JA, Tothill P: Long-term effect of dialysate calcium and 1 α-hydroxycholecalciferol on bone calcium content in hemodialysis patients as measured by neutron activation analysis of the forearm. *Nephron* 28:213, 1981
111. Goldsmith RS, Furszyfer J, Johnson WJ, Fournier AE, Sizemore GW, Arnaud CD: Etiology of hyperparathyroidism and bone disease during chronic hemodialysis III. Evaluation of parathyroid suppressibility. *J Clin Invest* 52:173, 1973
112. Drueke T, Bordier PJ, Man NK, Jungers P, Marie P: Effects of high dialysate calcium concentration on bone remodelling, serum biochemistry, and parathyroid hormone in patients with renal osteodystrophy. *Kidney Int* 11:267, 1977
113. Bouillon R, Verberckmoes R, de Moor P: Influence of dialysate calcium concentration and vitamin D on serum parathyroid hormone during repetitive dialysis. *Kidney Int* 7:422, 1975
114. McIntosh CHS, Fuchs C, Dorn D, Quellhorst E, Henning HV, Hesch RD, Scheler F: Effect of dialysate calcium concentration on plasma parathyroid hormone during hemodialysis. *Nephron* 19:88, 1977
115. Chalmers TM, Hunter JO, Davie MW, Szaz KF, Pelc B, Kodicek E: 1-Alpha-hydroxycholecalciferol as a substitute for the kidney hormone 1,25-dihydroxycholecalciferol in chronic renal failure. *Lancet* 2:696, 1973
116. Brickman AS, Coburn JW, Massry SG, Norman AW: 1,25-Dihydroxyvitamin D$_3$ in normal man and patients with renal failure. *Ann Intern Med* 80:161, 1974
117. Peacock M, Gallagher JC, Nordin BEC: Action of 1 α-hydroxy-vitamin D$_3$ on calcium absorption and bone resorption in man. *Lancet* 1:385, 1974
118. Catto GRD, MacLeod M, Pelc B, Kodicek E: 1 α-Hydroxycholecalciferol: a treatment for renal bone disease. *Br Med J* 1:12, 1975
119. Pierides AM, Ward MK, Alvarez-Ude F, Ellis HA, Peart KM, Simpson W, Kerr DNS, Norman A: Long term therapy with 1,25(OH)$_2$D$_3$ in dialysis bone disease. *Proc Eur Dial Transpl Assoc* 12:237, 1975
120. Winney RJ, Tothill P, Robson JS, Abbot SR, Lidgard GP, Cameron EHD, Smith MA, Macpherson JN, Strong JA: The effect of dialysate calcium concentration and 1 α-hydroxyvitamin D$_3$ on skeletal calcium loss and hyperparathyroidism in haemodialysis patients. *Clin Endocrinol (Oxf)* (Suppl):151s, 1977
121. Nielsen HE, Melsen F, Christensen MS, Hansen HE, Rødbro P, Johannsen A: 1 α-Hydroxycholecalciferol treatment of long-term hemodialyzed patients. Effects on mineral metabolism, bone mineral content and bone morphometry. *Clin Nephrol* 8:429, 1977
122. Lamperi S, Vagge R: Effects of 1-alpha OH D$_3$ therapy in uremic patients in conservative or dialytic treatment. *Int J Artif Organs* 2:243, 1979
123. Fischer JA, Binswanger U: 1,25-Dihydroxycholecalciferol in dialysed patients with clinically asymptomatic renal osteodystrophy. A controlled study. *Contrib Nephrol* 18:82, 1980
124. Goldstein DA, Malluche HH, Massry SG: Management of renal osteodystrophy with 1,25(OH)$_2$D$_3$. 1. Effect on clinical, radiographic and biochemical parameters. *Miner Electrolyte Metab* 2:35, 1979
125. Kanis JA, Cundy T, Earnshaw M, Henderson RG, Heynen G, Naik R, Russell RGG, Smith R, Woods CG: Treatment of renal bone disease with 1 α-hydroxylated derivatives of vitamin D$_3$. *Q J Med* 48:289, 1979
126. Berl T, Berns AS, Huffer WE, Alfrey AC, Arnaud CD, Schrier RR: Controlled trial of the effects of 1,25 dihydroxycholecalciferol in patients treated with regular dialysis. *Contrib Nephrol* 18:72, 1980
127. Moorthy AV, Harrington AR, Mazess RB, Simpson DP: Long-term therapy of uremic osteodystrophy in adults with calcitriol. *Clin Nephrol* 16:93, 1981
128. Baker LR, Muir JW, Cattell WR, Tucker KA, Sharman VL, Goodwin FJ, Marsh FP, Hately W, Morgan AG, de Saintonge DM: Use of 1,25(OH)$_2$-vitamin D$_3$ in prevention of renal osteodystrophy: preliminary observations. *Contrib Nephrol* 18:147, 1980
129. Care AD, Bates RFL, Pickard DW, Peacock M, Tomlinson S, O'Riordan JLH, Mawer EB, Taylor CA, Deluca HF, Norman AW: The effects of vitamin D metabolites and their analogues on the secretion of parathyroid hormone. *Calcif Tissue Res* 21 (Suppl): 142, 1976
130. Norman AW, Okamura WH, Friedlander EJ, Henry HL, Johnson RL, Mitra MN, Proscal DA, Wecksler W: Current concepts of the chemical conformation, metabolism, and interaction of the steroid, vitamin D, with the endocrine system for calcium homeostasis. *Calcif Tissue Res* 21 (Suppl):153, 1976
131. Madsen S: Calcium and phosphate metabolism in chronic renal failure, with particular reference to the effect of 1 α-hydroxy-vitamin D$_3$. *Acta Med Scand Suppl 638*:1, 1980
132. Peacock M, Heyburn PJ, Aaron JE, Taylor GA, Brown WB, Speed R. Osteomalacia: treated with 1 α hydroxy- or 1,25 dihydroxy-vitamin D. In *Vitamin D: Basic Research and its Clinical application.* Edited by Norman AW, Shaefer K, Herrath DV, Grigoleit HG, Coburn JW,

DeLuca HF, Mawer EB, Suda T, Berlin, New York, De Gruyter, 1979, p 1177
133. Massry SG: The clinical pathophysiology of magnesium. Contrib Nephrol 14:64, 1978
134. Schmidt P, Kotzaurek R, Zazgornik J, Hysek H: Magnesium metabolism in patients on regular dialysis treatment. Clin Sci 41:131, 1971
135. Kanis JA, Smith R, Walton RJ, Bartlett M: Magnesium intoxication during 1-α-hydroxycholecalciferol treatment. Br Med J 2:878, 1976
136. Paymaster NJ: Magnesium metabolism: a brief review. Ann R Coll Surg Engl 58:309, 1976
137. Brautbar N, Kleeman CR: Disordered divalent ion metabolism in kidney disease: comments on pathogenesis and treatment. Adv Nephrol 8:179, 1979
138. Buckle RM, Care AD, Cooper CW, Gitelman HJ: The influence of plasma magnesium concentration on parathyroid hormone secretion. J Endocrinol 42:529, 1968
139. Anast CS, Mohs JM, Kaplan SL, Burns TW: Evidence for parathyroid failure in magnesium deficiency. Science 177:606, 1972
140. Connor TB, Toskes P, Mahaffey J, Martin LG, Williams JB, Walser M: Parathyroid function during chronic magnesium deficiency. Johns Hopkins Med J 131:100, 1972
141. Levi J, Massry SG, Coburn JW, Llach F, Kleeman CR: Hypocalcemia in magnesium-depleted dogs: evidence for reduced responsiveness to parathyroid hormone and relative failure of parathyroid gland function. Metabolism 23:323, 1974
142. Parsons FM, Young GA: Regression of malignant tumors in potassium and magnesium depletion. In Magnesium in Health and Disease. Edited by Cantin M, Seelig MS. New York, SP Medical and Scientific books, 1980, p 233
143. Heierli C, Hill AVL: The relationship between the magnesium concentration in the dialysis fluid used and in the plasma and erythrocytes of patients with chronic renal failure being treated by regular haemodialysis. Clin Sci 43:779, 1972
144. Johny KV, Lawrence JR, O'Halloran MW, Wellby ML: Effect of haemodialysis on erythrocyte and plasma potassium, magnesium, sodium and calcium. Nephron 8:81, 1971
145. Stewart WK, Fleming LW: The effect of dialysate magnesium on plasma and erythrocyte magnesium and potassium concentrations during maintenance haemodialysis. Nephron 10:222, 1973
146. Fleming LW, Lenman JAR, Stewart WK: Effect of magnesium on nerve conduction velocity during regular dialysis treatment. J Neurol Neurosurg Psychiatry 35:342, 1972
147. Graf H, Kovarik J, Stummvoll HK, Wolf A: Disappearance of uraemic pruritus after lowering dialysate magnesium concentration. Br Med J 2:1478, 1979
148. Burnell JM, Teubner E: Effects of decreasing dialysate magnesium in patients with chronic renal failure. Proc Clin Dial Transpl Forum 5:191, 1976
149. Hollinrake K, Thomas PK, Wills MR, Baillod RA: Observations on plasma magnesium levels in patients with uremic neuropathy under treatment by periodic hemodialysis. Neurology 20:939, 1970
150. Catto GRD, Reid IW, MacLeod M: The effect of low magnesium dialysate on plasma, ultrafiltrable, erythrocyte and bone magnesium concentrations from patients on maintenance haemodialysis. Nephron 13:372, 1974
151. Pletka P, Bernstein DS, Hampers CL, Merrill JP, Sherwood LM: Effects of magnesium on parathyroid hormone secretion during chronic haemodialysis. Lancet 2:462, 1971

152. Parsons V, Papapoulos SE, Weston MJ, Tomlinson S, O'Riordan JLH: The long term effect of lowering dialysate magnesium on circulating parathyroid hormone in patients on regular haemodialysis therapy. Acta Endocrinol (Copenh) 93:455, 1980
153. Gonella M, Bonaguidi F, Buzzigoli G, Bartolini V, Mariani G: On the effect of magnesium on the PTH secretion in uremic patients on maintenance hemodialysis. Nephron 27:40, 1981
154. Anast CS, Winnacker JL, Forte LR, Burns TW: Impaired release of parathyroid hormone in magnesium deficiency. J Clin Endocrinol Metab 42:707, 1976
155. Alfrey AC, Miller NL: Bone magnesium pools in uremia J Clin Invest 52:3019, 1973
156. Posner AS, Betts F, Blumenthal NC: Role of ATP and Mg in the stabilization of biological and synthetic amorphous calcium phosphates. Calcif Tissue Res 22 (Suppl):208, 1977
157. Freeman RM, Lawton RL: The hard-water syndrome. Med Instrum 8:201, 1974
158. Drukker W: The hard water syndrome: a potential hazard during regular dialysis treatment. Proc Eur Dial Transpl Assoc 5:284, 1968
159. Quinton W, Dillard D, Scribner BH: Cannulation of blood vessels for prolonged hemodialysis. Trans Am Soc Artif Intern Organs 6:104, 1960
160. Borchardt KA, Richardson JA: Human plasma and the antibacterial effect of peritoneal dialysis solutions. Br Med J 1:205, 1971
161. Lundquist F: The concentration of acetate in blood during alcohol metabolism in man. Acta Physiol Scand 50 (Suppl 175):97, 1960
162. Lundquist F, Tygstrup N, Winkler K, Mellemgaard K, Munck-Petersen S: Ethanol metabolism and production of free acetate in the human liver. J Clin Invest 41:955, 1962
163. Lundquist F: Production and utilization of free acetate in man. Nature 193:579, 1962
164. Rorke SJ, Shippey W, Davidson WD: Acetate delivery to hemodialysis patients. Kidney Int (Abstracts) 8:433, 1975
165. Novello A, Kelsch RC, Easterling RE: Acetate intolerance during hemodialysis. Clin Nephrol 5:29, 1976
166. Tolchin N, Roberts JL, Hayashi J, Lewis EJ: Metabolic consequences of high mass-transfer hemodialysis. Kidney Int 11:366, 1977
167. Lewis EJ, Tolchin N, Roberts JL: High mass-transfer hemodialysis and acetate metabolism. Proc Renal Physicians Assoc 1:10, 1977
168. Port FK, Wright DL, Easterling RE: Acetate intolerance. Proc Renal Physicians Assoc 1:17, 1977
169. Graefe U, Milutinovich J, Follette WC, Vizzo JE, Babb AL, Scribner BH: Less dialysis-induced morbidity and vascular instability with bicarbonate in dialysate. Ann Intern Med 88:332, 1978
170. Viljoen M, Gold CH: Danger of haemodialysis using acetate dialysate in combination with a large surface dialyser. S Afr Med J 56:170, 1979
171. Kaiser BA, Potter DE, Bryant RE, Vreman HJ, Weiner MW: Acid-base changes and acetate metabolism during routine and high-efficiency hemodialysis in children. Kidney Int 19:70, 1981
172. Van Stone JC, Cook J: The effect of bicarbonate dialysate in stable chronic hemodialysis patients. Dial Transpl 8:703, 1979
173. Kveim M, Nesbakken R: Utilization of exogenous acetate during hemodialysis. Trans Am Artif Intern Organs 21:138, 1975

174. Kirkendol PL, Pearson JE, Holbert RD, Bower JD: Some cardiovascular (C-V) effects of sodium acetate. *Pharmacologist (Abstracts)* 17:218, 1975
175. Kirkendol PL, Devia CJ, Bower JD, Holbert RD: A comparison of the cardiovascular effects of sodium acetate, sodium bicarbonate and other potential sources of fixed base in hemodialysis solutions. *Trans Am Soc Artif Intern Organs* 23:399, 1977
176. Aizawa Y, Ohmori T, Imai K, Nara K, Matsuoka M, Hirasawa Y: Depressant action of acetate upon the human cardiovascular system. *Clin Nephrol* 8:477, 1977
177. Frohlich ED: Vascular effects of the Krebs intermediate metabolites. *Am J Physiol* 208:149, 1965
178. Nissenson AR: Prevention of dialysis-induced hypoxemia by bicarbonate dialysis. *Trans Am Soc Artif Intern Organs* 26:339, 1980
179. Raja R, Kramer M, Rosenbaum JL, Bollisay C, Krug M: Dialysis hypoxemia with varying dialyzers and dialysate – role of acetate in etiology. *Abstracts Am Soc Artif Intern Organs* 9:60, 1980
180. Dolan MJ, Whipp EJ, Davidson WD, Weitzman RE, Wasserman K: Hypopnea associated with acetate hemodialysis: carbon dioxide-flow-dependant ventilation. *N Engl J Med* 305:72, 1981
181. Toren M, Goffinet JA, Kaplow LS: Pulmonary bed sequestration of neutrophils during hemodialysis. *Blood* 36:337, 1970
182. Bischel MD, Scoles BG, Mohler JG: Evidence for pulmonary microembolization during hemodialysis. *Chest* 67:335, 1975
183. Craddock PR, Fehr J, Brigham KL, Kronenberg RS, Jacob HS: Complement and leucocyte-mediated pulmonary dysfunction in hemodialysis. *N Engl J Med* 296:769, 1977
184. Gonzalez FM, Pearson JE, Garbus SE, Holbert RD: On the effects of acetate during hemodialysis. *Trans Am Soc Artif Intern Organs* 20:169, 1974
185. Rorke SJ, Davidson WD, Guo SS, Morin RJ: Metabolic fate of ^{14}C-Acetate during dialysis. *Proc Eur Dial Transpl Assoc* 13:394, 1976
186. Cattran DC, Steiner G, Fenton SSA, Wilson DR: Hypertriglyceridemia in uremia and the use of triglyceride turnover to define pathogenesis. *Trans Am Soc Artif Intern Organs* 20:148, 1974
187. Ibels LS, Reardon MF, Nestel PJ: Plasma post-heparin lipolytic activity and triglyceride clearance in uremic and hemodialysis patients and renal allograft recipients. *J Lab Clin Med* 87:648, 1976
188. Gotch FA, Sargent JA, Keen M, Lam M, Prowitt MH: The solute kinetics of intermittent dialysis therapy. *Proc 11th Annu Contractor's Conf Artif Kidney Program of NIAMDD*. Edited by Mackey BB, DHEW publ no (NIH) 79.1442, 1978, p 110
189. Gotch FA, Boah MF, Keen ML, Lam MA, Prowitt MH, Sargent JA: The Solute Kinetics of intermittent dialysis therapy. *Third Annu Report to Artif Kidney Chronic Uremia Program NIAMDD* 1977, p 51 (unpublished)
190. Scribner BH: Indications for bicarbonate-containing dialysate in the care of the critically ill patient. *Proc Renal Phys Assoc* 1:25, 1977
191. Bjaeldager PAL, Christiansen E, Jensen HA, Paulev PK: Improved effect of hemodialysis on acidemic patients from an acetate concentration of 38 mmol/l. *Nephron* 27:142, 1981
192. Wathen R, Keshaviah P, Hommeyer P, Cadwell K, Comty C: Role of dialysate glucose in preventing gluconeogenesis during hemodialysis. *Trans Am Soc Artif Intern Organs* 23:393, 1977
193. Wathen RL, Keshaviah P, Hommeyer P, Cadwell K, Comty CM: The metabolic effects of hemodialysis with and without glucose in the dialysate. *Am J Clin Nutr* 31:1870, 1978
194. Young GA, Parsons FM: Amino nitrogen loss during haemodialysis, its dietary significance and replacement. *Clin Sci* 31:299, 1966
195. Ginn HE, Frost A, Lacey WW: Nitrogen balance in hemodialysis patients. *Am J Clin Nutr* 21:385, 1968
196. Kopple JD, Swendseid ME, Shinaberger JH, Umezawa CY: The free and bound amino acids removed by hemodialysis. *Trans Am Soc Artif Intern Organs* 19:309, 1973
197. Rubenfeld S, Garber AJ, Impact of hemodialysis on the abnormal glucose and alanine kinetics of chronic azotemia. *Metabolism* 28:934, 1979
198. Alwall N, Hagstam KE, Lindergard B, Lindholm T: A clinical trial with a glucose-free dialysate. *Proc Eur Dial Transpl Assoc* 7:55, 1970
199. Ward RA, Shirlow MJ, Hayes JM, Chapman GV, Farrell PC: Protein catabolism during hemodialysis. *Am J Clin Nutr* 32:2443, 1979
200. Swamy AP, Cestero RVM, Campbell RG, Freeman RB: Long-term effect of dialysate glucose on the lipid levels of maintenance hemodialysis patients. *Trans Am Soc Artif Intern Organs* 22:54, 1976
201. Hubner W, Sieberth HG, Diemer A, Finke K, Prange E: Effects of regular haemodialysis with glucose and glucose free dialysate on hyperlipaemia. *Proc Eur Dial Transpl Assoc* 8:174, 1971
202. Ganda OP, Aoki TT, Soeldner JS, Morrison RS, Cahill GF Jr: Hormone-fuel concentrations in anephric subjects. *J Clin Invest* 57:1403, 1976
203. Diem K, Lentner C (Editors): *Documenta Geigy Scientific Tables 7th Ed*, Basle, JR Geigy, 1970, p 497
204. Marier JR, Rose D: The fluoride content of some foods and beverages – a brief survey using a modified Zr SPADNS method. *J Food Sci* 31:941, 1966
205. Siddiqui JY, Simpson W, Ellis HE, Kerr DNS: Serum fluoride in chronic renal failure. *Proc Eur Dial Transpl Assoc* 7:110, 1970
206. Nielsen E, Solomon N, Goodwin NJ, Siddhivarn N, Galonsky R, Taves D, Friedman EA: Fluoride metabolism in uremia. *Trans Am Soc Artif Intern Organs* 19:450, 1973
207. Taves DR, Freeman RB, Kamm DE, Ramos CP, Scribner BH: Hemodialysis with fluoridated dialysate. *Trans Am Soc Artif Intern Organs* 14:412, 1968
208. Siddiqui JY, Simpson SW, Ellis HE, Kerr DNS, Appleton DR, Robinson BH, Hawkins JB, Robertson PW, Taves DR: Fluoride and bone disease in patients on regular haemodialysis. *Proc Eur Dial Transpl Assoc* 8:149, 1971
209. Oreopoulos DG, Taves DR, Rabinovich S, Meema HE, Murray T, Fenton SS, deVeber GA: Fluoride and dialysis osteodystrophy: results of a double-blind study. *Trans Am Soc Artif Intern Organs* 20:203, 1974
210. Taves DR, Terry R, Smith FA, Gardner DE: Use of fluoridated water in long-term hemodialysis. *Arch Intern Med* 115:167, 1965
211. Prosser DI, Parsons V, Davies C, Goode GC: The movement of fluoride across the cuprophane membrane of the Kiil dialyser. *Proc Eur Dial Transpl Assoc* 7:103, 1970
212. Parsons V, Davies C, Ogg CS, Siddiqui JY, Goode GC: The ionic composition of bone from patients with chronic renal failure and on RDT, with special reference to fluoride and aluminium. *Proc Eur Dial Transpl Assoc* 8:139, 1971
213. Rao TKS, Friedman EA: Fluoride and bone disease in

uremia, *Kidney Int* 7:125, 1975
214. Cordy PE, Gagnon R, Taves DR, Kaye M: Bone disease in hemodialysis patients with particular reference to the effect of fluoride. *Trans Am Soc Artif Intern Organs* 20:197, 1974
215. Rashid A, Posen GA, Gray D, Jaworski ZF: Bone disease in patients dialyzed with untreated water. *Med Instrum* 8:204, 1974
216. Kim D, del Greco F, Hefferen JJ, Levin NW: Bone fluoride in patients with uremia maintained by chronic hemodialysis. *Trans Am Soc Artif Intern Organs* 16:474, 1970
217. Parsons V: Fluoridated drinking-water and renal dialysis. *Lancet* 1:813, 1974
218. Johnson WJ, Taves DR: Exposure to excessive fluoride during hemodialysis. *Kidney Int* 5:451, 1974
219. *British Pharmacopoeia*, London, Her Majesty's Stationery Office 1980, Volume 1, p 264
220. Pendras JP, Cole JJ, Tu WH, Scribner BH: Improved technique of continuous flow hemodialysis. *Trans Am Soc Artif Intern Organs* 7:27, 1961
221. Schales O, Schales SS: A simple and accurate method for the determination of chloride in biological fluids. *J Biol Chem* 140:879, 1941
222. Watschinger B, Kolff WJ: Further development of the artificial kidney of Innouye and Engelberg. *Trans Am Soc Artif Intern Organs* 1:37, 1955
223. Grimsrud L, Cole JJ, Lehman GA, Babb AL, Scribner BH: A central system for the continuous preparation and distribution of hemodialysis fluid. *Trans Am Soc Artif Intern Organs* 10:107, 1964
224. Sargent JA, Gotch FA: On line proportioning of bicarbonate dialysate for acid-base correction during intermittent dialysis treatment. *Abstracts Am Soc Artif Intern Organs* 6:75, 1977
225. Von Hartitzsch B, Hoenich NA, Johnson J, Brewis RAL, Kerr DNS: The problem of de-aeration – cause, consequence, cure. *Proc Eur Dial Transpl Assoc* 9:605, 1972
226. Drukker W, v d Werff B, Meinsma K: De-aeration of dialysis fluid. *Dial Transpl* 3 (nr 3):33, 1974
227. Parsons FM, Meffan P: De-airing of dialysis fluid. *Proc Eur Dial Transpl Assoc* 5:314, 1968
228. Winkler LW: Die Löslichkeit der Gase in Wasser. (The solubility of gases in water). *Ber Dtsch Chem Ges* 34:1408, 1901 (in German)

8
ANGIOACCESS

KHALID M. H. BUTT

Introduction	171	Aneurysms and pseudoaneurysms	178
Strategies for angioaccess	171	Congestive heart failure	179
Percutaneous venous access	172	Graft arteriovenous fistula	179
External prosthetic devices	173	Materials	179
Technical considerations	173	Technical considerations	179
Complications	174	Complications	180
Thrombosis	174	Infections	181
Infections, bleeding and dislodgement	175	Thrombosis	181
Erosion of the skin	175	Pseudoaneurysm or pulsating hematoma	181
Restrictions of activities and psychological problems	175	Aneurysm	181
Progressive exhaustion of the vessels	175	Ischemia and arterial steal syndrome	181
Ischemia and gangrene	175	Venous hypertension and stasis	181
Congestive heart failure	175	Cardiac failure	181
Internal arteriovenous fistula	176	Lymphoceles	182
Technical considerations	176	Angioaccess for children	182
Complications	177	New approaches	183
Thrombosis	177	Hybrid devices	183
Infection	177	Shuntless access	183
Venous hypertension	177	Conclusions	183
Ischemia and arterial steal syndrome	177	References	183

INTRODUCTION

The hardware of hemodialysis, the sophisticated electronic gadgetry and the membranes with acceptable clearances, would be of no avail to a patient with end-stage renal disease for whom access to circulation could not be satisfactorily achieved. Angioaccess for a patient on maintenance hemodialysis continues to be his Achilles' heel (1). Although in 1975, it was predicted that 18% of the patients with end-stage renal disease would die prematurely because hemodialysis would become impossible for lack of access to circulation (2), I believe that today's sophisticated access techniques should interdict death ascribable to this cause (3). Proper planning and selection of appropriate technique, depending on vasculature and associated pathology, will go a long way in decreasing the angioaccess related morbidity, which for most hemodialysis patients accounts for the majority of hospital days.

STRATEGIES FOR ANGIOACCESS

Strategic planning for angioaccess is all important (4). In an ideal situation, where patients are being followed closely by a nephrologist as they progressively lose their kidney function, an internal arteriovenous fistula in the non-dominant forearm, approximately three months in advance of the necessity for hemodialysis, would constitute the best approach. After several weeks of maturation, the angioaccess thus developed may continue to serve uneventfully for many years, possible a lifetime. Periodic determinations should allow fairly accurate prediction of the time when the endogenous creatinine clearance will fall to about 5 ml/min, necessitating the institution of regular dialytic therapy.

If the patient has no patent superficial forearm veins due to multiple previous cutdowns or episodes of thrombophlebitis, as is commonly seen in heroin addicts, then a primary graft arteriovenous fistula may be placed approximately two to three weeks prior to the initiation of hemodialysis. For massively obese patients, where placement of needles even in adequately arterialized forearm veins is virtually impossible, and in severely cachectic patients, mostly in the elderly age group, where an arterialized superficial forearm vein may be easily accessible but repeated hematomas due to lack of elastic support predictably abbreviate the life of the access, a primary graft arteriovenous fistula also may be a preferable approach (5).

In patients developing acute post-traumatic or post-surgical reversible renal failure, an external prosthetic shunt (Scribner's) placed in the non-dominant forearm may provide the most appropriate access, permitting daily dialysis if necessary and almost always lasting for the duration of the therapy. When a patient in uremic coma appears in an emergency room, or one with renal failure presents with pulmonary edema where no time can be lost before starting dialysis therapy, a percutaneous access to the veins and a veno-venous dialysis is generally the most expeditious and effective approach.

For patients who present at the threshold of need for dialysis, permitting little time to plan and develop an angioaccess, several options may be considered:

1. If particularly large and thick-walled superficial forearm veins are available, a direct arteriovenous fistula can be constructed in the non-dominant forearm, and with extreme care, used almost immediately. When it is estimated that the veins are not of large caliber and several weeks of maturation may be necessary, then a simultaneous external prosthetic shunt may be placed in the *dominant* forearm and used for the initial period of therapy. Lower extremity vessels near the ankle (posterior or anterior tibial artery and saphenous vein) can also be profitably used in such circumstances.

2. If such a patient has marginal cardiac reserve, and a combination of an arteriovenous fistula and an external shunt is likely to tip the balance and cause cardiac decompensation, it is wise to perform veno-venous dialysis by percutaneous approach to the femoral or subclavian veins, or alternatively to tide the patient over the period of maturation of the internal arteriovenous fistula by peritoneal dialysis.

3. In the event that indications for a primary graft arteriovenous fistula are present, it should be implanted in the non-dominant forearm and allowed to heal for approximately two weeks prior to needle puncture. In dire circumstances, however, a graft arteriovenous fistula can indeed be used for dialysis access almost immediately after implantation.

4. One of the clever strategies recently utilized (6) is the placement of an external prosthetic shunt in the non-dominant upper extremity and nursing it meticulously to avoid any complications, thereby encouraging the appropriate arterialization changes in the vein. After an interval of a few weeks with antibiotic treatment, the shunt can be removed, and, proximal to the site of original cannulation, the artery and vein can be anastomosed to form an end-to-end arteriovenous fistula, with immediate availability of this access following surgery.

PERCUTANEOUS VENOUS ACCESS

Shaldon and coworkers (7, 8) in 1963, described a method of placing two catheters in the femoral veins, utilizing Seldinger's technique. Many workers have used this access repetitively for weeks to months with relatively low morbidity (9, 10). Under aseptic conditions and with local anesthesia, a needle with a plastic sheath is inserted into the femoral vein. The needle is withdrawn when the tip of the plastic cannula is in the lumen of the vein, as indicated by free efflux of blood. A guidewire is now passed through the plastic cannula and advanced up the vein. The cannula is removed leaving the guidewire in place, and a Shaldon catheter is now threaded onto the guidewire and passed up into the vein. The guidewire can now be removed. Another Shaldon catheter is placed in the contralateral femoral vein. One catheter is passed up to the lower inferior vena cava,

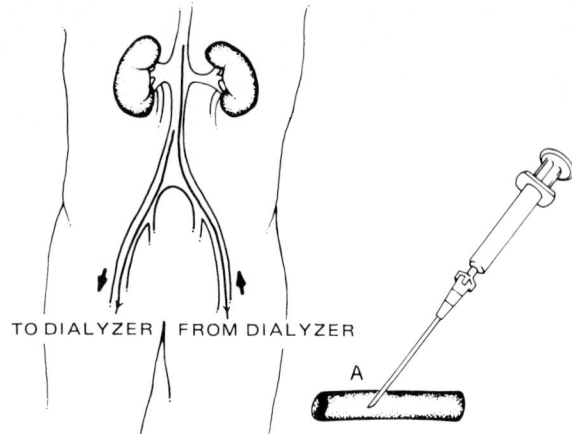

SHALDON CATHETERS IN PLACE

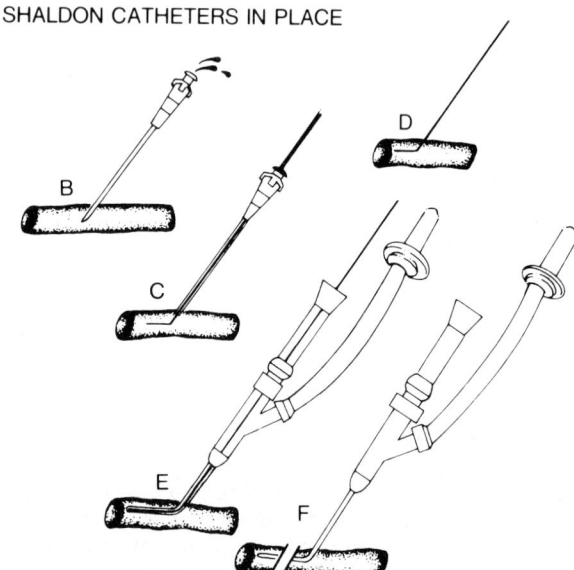

PERCUTANEOUS VEIN ACCESS

Figure 1. In a step-wise manner, this figure depicts the Seldinger technique of replacing a needle in the blood vessel with a catheter.
(A) A needle with an attached syringe is advanced into the lumen of the femoral vein; (B) The syringe is removed; (C) The guidewire is passed through the lumen of the needle into the blood vessel and advanced; (D) The needle is now removed, leaving the guidewire in place; (E) A catheter is now threaded over the guidewire and advanced into the lumen of the blood vessel; (F) The guidewire is now removed and the catheter is flushed with heparinized saline solution.
As depicted in the accompanying diagram, one of the catheters is advanced into the inferior vena cava for return of the blood and the other catheter is left either in the iliac vein or the beginning of the inferior vena cava for pull.

while the other is placed in the iliac vein; the latter used for 'pull' while the former is used for the 'return' of blood to the patient (Figure 1).

A single catheter can be used with a single needle device (see Chapter 11) to allow intermittent pull and return of blood, with some diminution of the efficiency of dialysis. Alternatively, blood can be drawn from the femoral venous catheter, and after a pass through the extra-corporeal circuit, can be returned into one of the superficial veins of the upper extremity.

Percutaneous venous access to the femoral vein is a safe procedure, with local hematomas as the only frequent complication. Occasionally, the guidewire or the catheter may perforate the vein, leading to retroperitoneal hematoma. Usually not very significant, such a hematoma may become life threatening if the catheter is used for 'return' and inadvertently large quantities of blood are pumped into the extraperitoneal space.

In the event of inadvertent puncture of the femoral artery, the initial plastic cannula can be left in the artery and an arteriovenous circuit set up. At the time of removal of the cannula from the artery care must be taken to achieve good hemostasis before releasing digital pressure. In rare circumstances, an arteriovenous fistula has resulted from repeated punctures of the groin (11). The only such case in my personal experience was repaired easily at surgery.

The disadvantage of percutaneous femoral access is the necessity for an experienced physician to perform the procedure practically every time the dialysis has to be done. In hospitalized, bed-ridden patients however, a catheter can be left in-situ with intermittent instillation of heparin for short periods of time. In patients with known thrombophlebitis or when thrombosis of the femoral and iliac veins is strongly suspected, attempts to install Shaldon catheters are theoretically hazardous, and may be associated with pulmonary embolism. In a large experience of over 2000 percutaneous femoral vein catherizations in Downstate Medical Center, no infection, thrombosis of the iliofemoral venous system, pulmonary embolism, vascular compromise of the lower limb, or death attributable to this procedure has been observed (10). In addition to providing a most expeditious access, this technique has the further merit of sparing the access surgeon the acute anxiety of inserting an urgent external prosthetic shunt before dialysis.

Erben, in 1967 (12), applied the technique of percutaneous venous access to the subclavian vein, and a considerable experience has recently been detailed by Uldall (13-15). A catheter can be passed into the subclavian vein after having been drawn through a subcutaneous tunnel, stabilized by sterile transparent adhesive dressings, and left in place for days to weeks. The patency is maintained by intermittent injections of heparin into the catheter, generally twice a day. Patients are ambulatory, comfortable and may indeed leave the hospital. In the event of malfunction, the guidewire can be replaced, the catheter withdrawn, and a new one inserted.

Because of the risk of pneumothorax, hemopneumothorax or hemomediastinum, it is important that experienced, well trained physicians should carefully place the subclavian catheter, with the patient in the Trendelenberg position to avoid air embolism. The catheter must not be used for dialysis until the position of this radio-opaque device has been ascertained with a chest radiograph. Episodes of bacteremia and local infection, because of the device transgressing the skin before entering the vessel, continue to be matters of concern, as is the case with all external prosthetic devices.

EXTERNAL PROSTHETIC DEVICES

The epochal demonstration in 1960, by Scribner and colleagues (16), that an indwelling Teflon shunt can be used repetitively for gaining access to the circulation, made it possible to maintain patients with end-stage renal failure with hemodialysis. Shortly thereafter the rigid all Teflon cannula was replaced by a composite device made of a Teflon tip and a Silastic tubing (see also chapter 2). This extended the cannula life considerably, but the majority of the problems common with all prosthetic devices still defy solutions.

Most commonly, the vessels in the distal forearm (the radial artery and cephalic vein or ulnar artery and basilic vein) are cannulated through a single longitudinal incision. However, any pair of vessels in reasonable juxtaposition can be cannulated to provide a shunt.

Technical considerations

An appropriate pair of blood vessels are selected and the correct size cannula tip is chosen. Generally the largest cannula tip that will just fit the lumen of the given vessel is used. Extreme caution has to be exercised not to strip the intima, particularly in the arteries. For safe cannulation a technique of passing the Fogarty embolectomy catheter through the lumen of the cannula, and advancing the tip of the cannula while pressing it against the semi-inflated balloon in the arteriotomy is useful (Figure 2). The recurved cannula devices initially employed were advantageous in that the distal joint was allowed free mobility, but they were more prone to thrombosis and difficult to thrombectomize. Straight cannulas, with wings to provide stability (17), placed proximally enough to allow freedom of the distal joint, are the devices of choice today.

Avoiding the problems of cannulation is the Allen-Brown modification (18), with a skirt of Dacron instead of a Teflon stip. This device necessitates careful microvascular anastomosis.

A Buselmeier shunt ([19], see Figure 29, chapter 2), a short subcutaneous U tube, with two nipples the only parts projecting beyond the skin, is a device that is extremely stable and has no chance of being accidently dislodged, but is technically difficult to implant and has not gained extensive popularity. Instead of using Teflon tips with this Silastic tubing, an Allen-Brown type of modification, using a Dacron skirt, has recently been utilized with some advantage.

Thomas, in 1969 (20), described a composite device for use in the groin (Figure 3). A Dacron face plate of appliqué is sutured to the femoral vessels, and Silastic tubing is brought through the skin and joined on the outside to construct the shunt. This device provides a large flow and has a good patency record, with about 50% lasting for up to two years. The remaining 50%,

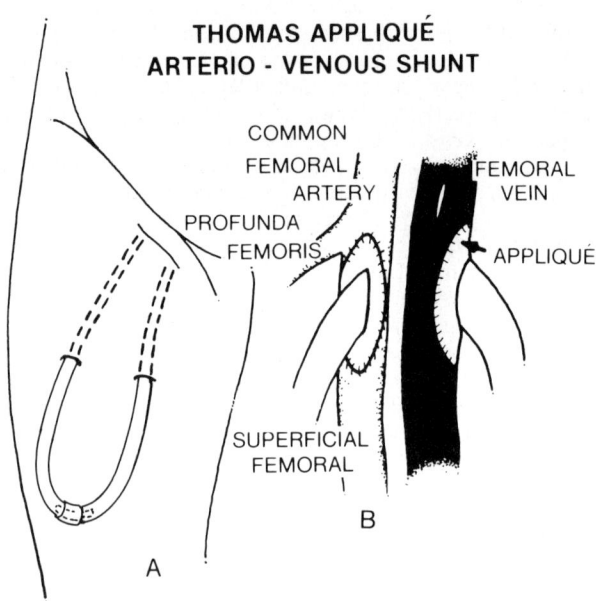

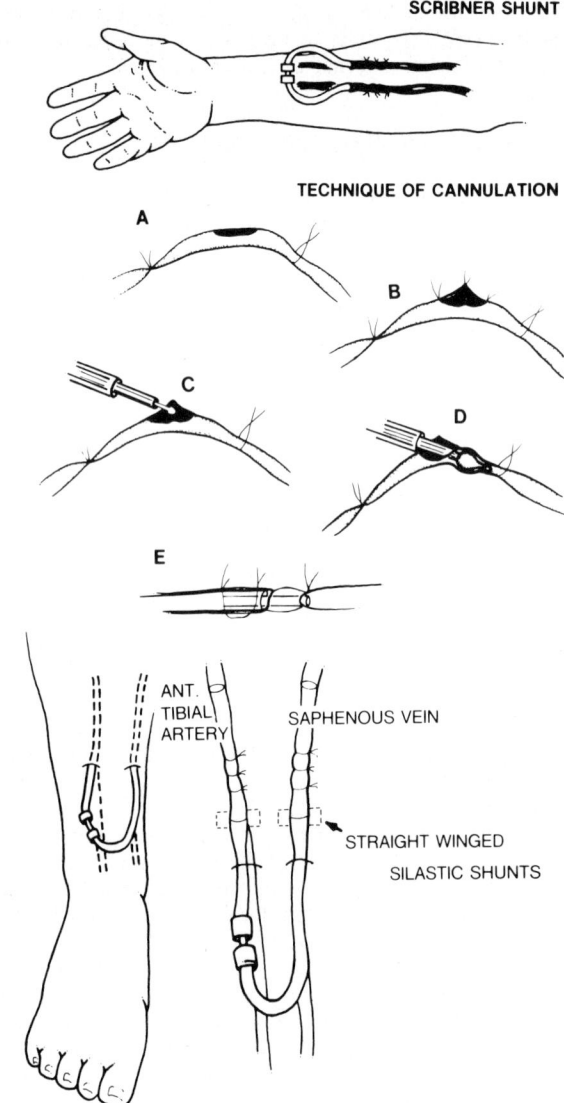

Figure 3. (A) External shunt in the thigh; (B) Details of the suturing of the faceplates (appliqué) of the Thomas shunt to the femoral artery and femoral vein.

Figure 2.
Top. Scribner shunt with cannulation of the radial artery and cephalic vein in the distal third of the forearm, with straight Silastic catheters cut to appropriate length to clear the wrist joint.
Center. The safest technique for cannulation of the blood vessel is depicted in a step-wise diagram. (A) Mobilization of the blood vessel with a distal ligature and a proximal loop around the vessel, with a longitudinal incision in the vessel; (B) Fine sutures placed in the vessel wall to facilitate cannulation; (C) A special technique of cannulation with a Fogarty balloon catheter passed through the cannula into the incision in the vessel; (D) A Fogarty catheter balloon is inflated in the incision in the vessel and the tip of the cannula is abutting against it as the entire assembly is advanced in the lumen of the vessel, avoiding injury to the intimal layer from the edge of the catheter tip; (E) With the catheter now in place inside the vessel, appropriate ligatures have been applied and the Fogarty catheter has been withdrawn.
Bottom. Cannulation of the ankle vessels, anterior tibal artery and saphenous vein, with straight winged Silastic shunts is depicted.

however, become infected which may lead to a limb-threatening or life-threatening hemorrhage. The high morbidity of the Thomas shunt (21, 22) and the availability of alternative techniques, leaves no continued justification for its use.

Complications

Thrombosis
Early post-implantation thrombosis may be a technical problem of non-alignment of the cannula with the vessel, or of stripping of the intima. If the flow of a small air bubble from the arterial to the venous side is slower than instantaneous, requiring two, three or more heartbeats, an early failure can almost certainly be predicted. Such problems should be corrected before the patient comes off the operating table.

After weeks of use, a progressive slowing of the blood flow through the shunt is generally due to intimal hyperplasia, most often in the vein. In the past, this always necessitated dissection of the more proximal vein and recannulation, but currently the availability of the transluminal angioplasty catheter has made it possible to restore the lumen of the cannulated vein without the need for surgery.

Forceful flushing of the venous cannula can lead to small pulmonary emboli, which are not clinically significant except when they are infected and lead to the formation of pulmonary abscesses. Forceful flushing of the arterial cannula in the upper extremity, particularly with large volumes of heparinized saline, may cause embolic complications in the cerebral vasculature (23, 24) and should always be avoided.

A number of mechanical devices for restoring the patency of external prosthetic cannulae have been devised; probably the safest is the Fogarty balloon catheter, and even that has to be used carefully so as not to dislodge the entire cannula assembly. Of the fibrinolytic agents for the dissolution of thrombi, the commonly used streptokinase has been associated with an unacceptably high incidence of side effects. Urokinase, theoretically the ideal agent, has limited availability and is prohibitively costly.

Anti-platelet agents and vitamin K antagonists have been used to decrease the frequency of thrombosis of the external prosthetic shunts in prospective studies (25). In the experience of several groups, including our own, the anti-platelet agents (26) dipyridamole (Persantine) and aspirin, have been found to be useful in conserving the patency of all modes of angioaccess. The use of vitamin K antagonists (27) has been associated with serious complications, including intracranial hemorrhage.

Infection, bleeding and dislodgement
External prosthetic devices invariably become infected since the body surface is colonized by microbes and the device provides a convenient route for these organisms to invade the tissues. More than 90% of these infections are of staphylococcal origin, and the remainder of gram negative enteric organisms, particularly in immunosuppressed patients. At the earliest sign of redness, tenderness or purulent discharge along the cannula, a staphylocidal, semi-synthetic, beta lactamase resistant penicillin should be started, and for the patient allergic to penicillin, vancomycin or clindamycin should be substituted. So common are cannula infections that some workers have recommended an ongoing antibiotic prophylaxis with intermittent vancomycin injections (28).

Infection leads to necrosis and dissolution of the vessel wall. Initially a pulsating hematoma may form, with intermittent leakage of blood along the track of the cannula. If the cannula is completely loose and becomes dislodged, there may be severe, at times exsanguinating, hemorrhage. The patient should be surgically treated at the time of the formation of the pseudoaneurysm or the initial minor leaks of blood. The only possible corrective measure is to remove the cannula, ligate the blood vessel, and find an alternative site.

An external prosthetic shunt has provided some patients with a potent instrument for suicide. Disconnecting the arterial and venous cannulae leads to a painless blood loss of 250 to 400 ml/min, causing rapid exsanguination. In addition to properly taping the cannulae at the junction, the entire area should be carefully bandaged for maximal protection. The parents of children with external prosthetic shunts should be carefully trained to control bleeding in the event of accidental dislodgement during play.

Erosion of the skin
This complication is infrequently seen, and can be completely avoided by providing a good padding of subcutaneous tissue over the Silastic cannula. In addition, utilizing a single incision instead of two parallel ones, helps to avoid devascularization of the skin. Straight cannulae are less bulky than the recurved ones, and therefore cause less stretching of the skin and less chance of ulceration. Early and aggressive control of infection is of paramount importance in preventing skin necrosis.

Restriction of activities and psychological problems
An external prosthetic device causes severe restrictions of the activities of the patient, particularly swimming, bathing, etc. Although some patients have been able to maintain these shunts for years, their anxiety has led to their holding the extremity in a protective posture, causing stiffening of the joints. Constant preoccupation with the protection of the life-line can indeed produce severe psychological stress.

Progressive exhaustion of the vessels
Prior to the advent of the internal arteriovenous fistula many patients needed repeated cannulations of their extremity vessels, often at short intervals, leading to exhaustion of their sites for access. A small subset of patients, having undergone multiple cannulations, now require particularly ingenious techniques for providing vascular access.

Ischemia and gangrene
Cannulation of the vessels in the distal extremity usually causes no serious consequence with regard to viability of the tissues perfused by the given artery. Ligation and cannulation of the main artery of the limb (brachial in the upper arm and femoral in the thigh) may indeed lead to severe ischemia of the distal extremity, even so it may be absolutely necessary in small children. To avoid the ischemic problem, an arterio-arterial external prosthesis was devised by Lawton (29). The superficial femoral artery is cannulated proximally and distally, and ligated in-between. Such a device can only be used for a short period of time, and when not needed any longer has to be removed with reconstruction of the arterial trunk. When it is necessary to approach the main limb vessel, it may be prudent to take a segment of autogenous vein and anastomose it to the main artery to construct a new branch. This may then be cannulated with continuing prograde flow of blood down the distal extremity. We have used this technique for femoral artery cannulation in infants with acute renal failure.

Rarely ischemia of the hand or foot may lead to gangrenous changes of the digits. In some referred cases we have been able to remove the shunts from the wrist, and reconstruct the radial artery with a segment of reversed cephalic vein, restoring circulation and avoiding amputation of the digits.

Congestive heart failure
Arteriovenous shunts using external prosthetic devices usually have limited blood flow, not amounting to much more than 500 ml/min. A high flow Thomas appliqué shunt, however, may cause cardiac failure in marginally compensated patients.

INTERNAL ARTERIOVENOUS FISTULA

In 1966, Brescia and colleagues described the technique of arterializing the superficial forearm veins (30) by side-to-side anastomosis of the radial artery and cephalic vein. An internal arteriovenous fistula, either of the classical or a modified type, is undoubtedly the ideal angioaccess for maintenance hemodialysis today (Figure 4).

Technical considerations

Examination of the forearm veins should be carried out very carefully by applying a sphygmomanometer cuff on the upper arm, and inflating it to a pressure of 40 mm Hg. Evaluation of the arteries should be carried out by palpation of the pulses and determination of the arterial pressure using an ultrasound probe. An assessment of the collateral circulation is made by performing the Allen test. Clenching the first while compressing both the radial and the ulnar arteries causes blanching of the skin of the palm. Releasing one vessel at a time while observing the speed and extent of the return of color to the palm will provide an index of collateral blood flow. In patients who have had multiple angioaccess procedures an angiographic survey, including bilateral brachial arteriograms and upper extremity venograms, is of great value (31).

Ideally the cephalic vein is anastomosed to the radial artery in the distal third of the forearm, with the connection made slightly larger than twice the diameter of the radial artery. The length of the anastomosis is commonly from 8 to 10 mm. An unhurried surgical procedure, avoiding vessel wall hematomas by careful ligation of the small branches while skeletonizing the vessels, and meticulous suturing with fine monofilament material, is rewarded with a nearly 100% initial success rate of fistulization. In the experience of most groups, if adequate time for maturation is allowed before use of the access, an 85 to 90% functional rate is achieved for two to three years (10).

The basilic vein on the postero-medial aspect of the forearm generally escapes the trauma of needle punctures, and may be of adequate size to be connected to the ulnar artery to form an internal arteriovenous fistula. If anatomically cumbersome to approach, the basilic vein can be translocated in a tunnel across the front of the forearm and anastomosed to the radial artery.

When the vessels in the distal third of the forearm are either obliterated or of inadequate size, a fistula may be located in the middle or the proximal third of the fore-

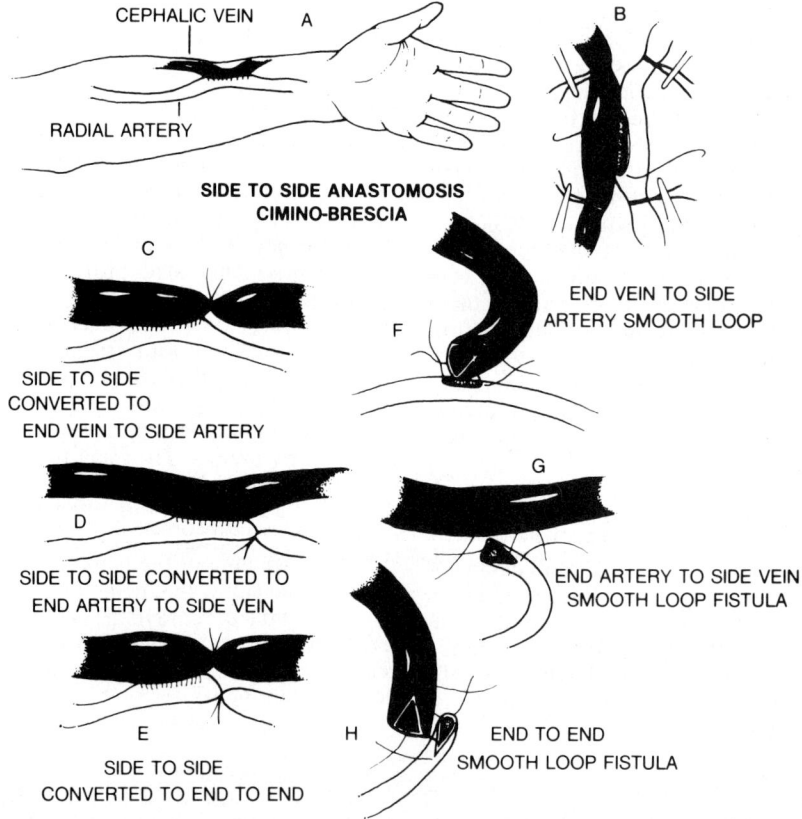

Figure 4. (A) Classical side-to-side cephalic vein-radial artery fistula; (B) Proximal and distal controls of the artery and vein in juxta-position and a double arm vascular suture for the construction of the anastomosis. Figures 4 C, D, E, F, G and H depict the various modifications of the classical Cimino-Brescia fistula.

arm. If the forearm veins are not usable at all, the cephalic vein above the elbow, or the basilic vein, either superficialized on the medial aspect of the arm or translocated in a curvilinear tunnel along the anterior aspect of the arm, can be connected to the brachial artery. The latter technique in particular has shown excellent patency, as high as 95% at five years in the experience of Dagher et al. (32). When anastomosing a vein to the brachial artery the anastomotic stoma must be smaller than the diameter of the brachial artery in order to avoid ischemia of the distal extremity.

A direct internal arteriovenous fistula in the lower extremity is to be avoided because of the propensity to develop varicosities of the venous system. In the thigh however, a superficialized greater saphenous vein can be anastomosed to the superficial femoral artery and provide an excellent access. The ischemic problems in the lower extremity are even more devastating than those of the upper extremity.

Bleeding from the open arteriotomy provides a good gauge of the inflow through the fistula. The ease with which large quantities of heparinized saline can be injected through an 8F* umbilical artery catheter threaded up the vein through the venotomy affords an assessment of the venous runoff. In the event that the vein is narrow in some areas, a small (3F or 4F) Fogarty embolectomy catheter can be passed up the vein and withdrawn with the balloon slightly inflated to produce a dilation.

Complications

Thrombosis

A common complication of external prosthetic devices, thrombosis in the established internal arteriovenous fistula is an uncommon event. A long standing arteriovenous fistula with aneurysmal dilations of the arterialized vein at the sites of needle punctures may develop mural thrombi. Sometimes these thrombi get dislodged from the aneurysm and obstruct a more proximal normal caliber vein. A simple thrombectomy can be performed, and the patient maintained on anticoagulants for a period of time. Rarely it may be necessary to excise the aneurysm partially or completely, and repair the vein.

Turbulence of the arteriovenous flow at the site of anastomosis because of angulation may, in part, be responsible for thrombotic complications. A variety of techniques have been devised to position the vessels in a 'smooth loop' (33) to allow a more streamlined flow (Figure 4). Another technique to reduce turbulence is to take the two tributaries of the cephalic vein, transect them, slit them to construct a 'venous bell', and construct an end vein-side artery fistula (34).

Stenosis of the arteriovenous fistula site developing after months to years can be diagnosed by angiography, either by injection into the main artery of the limb or into the arterialized vein, and refluxing the dye through the arteriovenous communication back into the artery (35). This stenotic lesion may progress to total occlusion. Remedial surgery involves an arteriovenous anastomosis of the same two vessels just proximal to the original site of the fistula. In some hypercoagulable states (e.g. polycystic kidney disease), long term use of heparin and/or anti-platelet agents may be necessary to insure the continued patency of the internal arteriovenous fistula.

Infection

Primary infection at the site of arteriovenous fistula is a rarity as opposed to the external prosthetic devices, where it is a rule. In our experience of more than 1,000 direct internal arteriovenous fistulae, primary suture line infection has been seen only twice; once in a diabetic patient where the sutures were removed prematurely and the vessels exposed with subsequent development of infection at the anastomosis, and another time in a malnourished patient with Crohn's Disease and amyloidosis, who was also on steroids at the time the arteriovenous fistula was constructed. He developed redness in the wound, and sought no surgical advice, and several weeks later started to have purulent drainage with subsequent dehiscence of the anastomotic line.

The incidence of infection in established internal arteriovenous fistulae is estimated to be one per hundred patient years of experience, whereas with external devices, it may be 60 to 100 time higher (36).

Venous hypertension

Occasionally, with predominant arterial flow going in a distal direction in the veins, increased venous pressure leads to edema and cyanosis of the extremity. When this occurs in connection with the radial artery-cephalic vein fistula in the distal forearm, the brunt of the pathology involves the thumb, which may be exceedingly sore ('sore thumb syndrome') (37), may manifest varicose veins, ulcerations, eczematoid changes, and seeping of serosanguinous fluid from the nail bed. The proximal venous channels are either stenotic or occluded, and the distal veins, with incompetent valves, provide the only egress for the arterial inflow (Figure 5). Swelling of tissues at the wrist may cause the carpal tunnel syndrome (38).

Angiography with sequential radiographs defines the pathophysiology and suggests the corrective measures. Distal venous flow has to be interrupted while providing a better proximal run-off channel. The latter can be accomplished either by correcting the stenotic areas in the vein, or finding a new vein and anastomosing it to the previously arterialized cephalic vein. Occasionally it may be necessary to completely close off the arteriovenous fistula and construct an alternative angioaccess.

Ischemia and arterial steal syndrome

Shunting of the arterial blood into the venous channels may cause ischemia of the distal extremity. This is further compounded by a reversal of the blood flow in the segment of the artery distal to the site of the arteriovenous communication (arterial steal) (39, 40). If the radial

---

* F = French; 1 F = 0.3 mm.

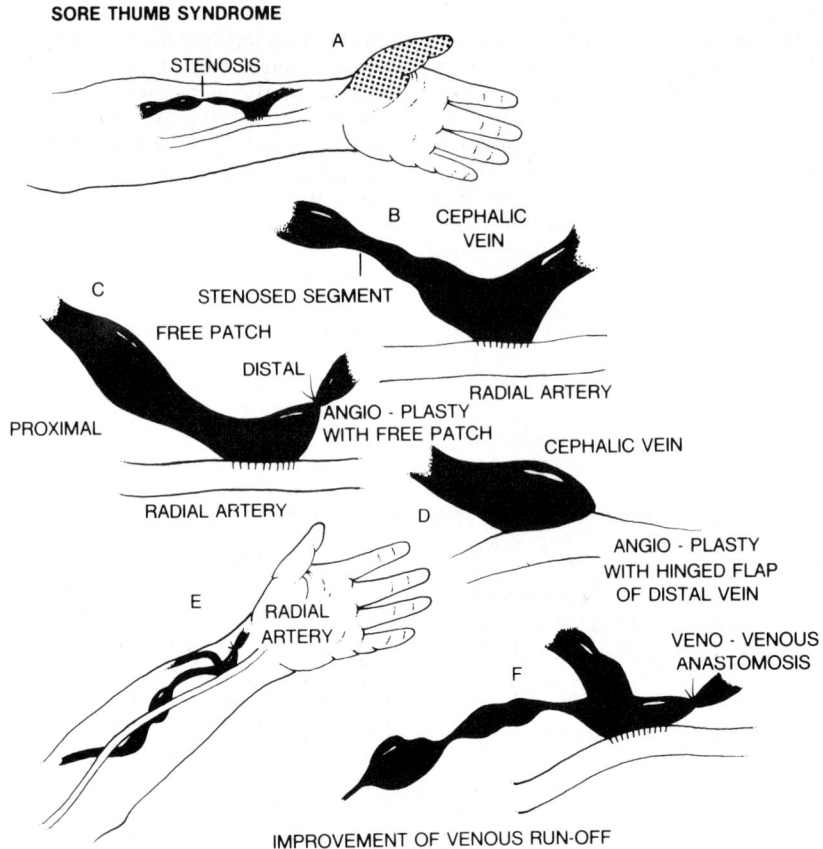

Figure 5. (A) Pathologic hemodynamics of 'sore-thumb' syndrome with stenosis of the proximal vein and predominant arteriovenous flow into the distal cephalic vein, with swollen cyanotic thumb; (B) The magnified sketch of the pathologic anatomy; (C) A free patch of vein used to enlarge the stenotic segment, with ligation of the cephalic vein distal to the arteriovenous anastomosis; (D) A flap of segment of cephalic vein distal to the arteriovenous anastomosis being turned over and used to enlarge the stenotic segment, simultaneously converting the fistula to an end vein-side artery variety; (E) Anastomosis of a patent vein to the previously arterialized vein to provide a better run-off and ligature of the cephalic vein distal to the arteriovenous fistula; (F) Enlarged representation of the technique of improving the venous runoff by employing a veno-venous anastomosis.

artery-cephalic vein connection is a large one, and resistance in the venous run-off is particularly low, a painful cold hand, mostly in the area of the radial supply (thumb, index and middle fingers), may progress to ischemic ulcerations or gangrene if corrective measures are not taken in time. In end vein-side artery fistulae approximately one-third of the arterial inflow into the vein is retrograde from the distal artery. Digital compression of the distal artery to interrupt the retrograde flow of blood may show improvement in the circulatory status of the hand and suggest a simple therapy of ligating the artery distal to the arteriovenous fistula with continuing function of the access for hemodialysis.

As mentioned previously, the ischemic complications of the distal extremity may be particularly pronounced when the major proximal arterial trunks are shunted into large sized veins, notably cephalic and basilic veins at, or about, the level of the elbow. The simple remedy of a ligature on the artery distal to the arteriovenous communication may not suffice, and to protect the viability of the distal limb, complete disconnection of the arteriovenous fistula may be absolutely necessary.

Aneurysm and pseudoaneurysm
Multiple punctures at the same site may eventually weaken the wall of the arterialized vein and cause an aneurysmal dilatation. In most circumstances these aneurysms do not cause any clinical problems. Occasionally mural thrombi as noted earlier, may lead to complete occlusion of the arteriovenous fistula. Very rarely a threatened rupture, as indicated by adherent, ulcerated skin, may necessitate resection of the aneurysm. Pseudoaneurysm, an exceedingly uncommon complication due to a low mean pressure in the arterialized vein, may occasionally become manifest when a puncture has been made in the vicinity of the arteriovenous anastomosis. In proximal fistulae a pseudoaneurysm, or pulsating hematoma, may occur as a result of

inadvertant puncture of the arterial trunk. Surgical correction may be necessary to prevent progressive enlargement and rupture.

Congestive heart failure

Most studies indicate an approximate 10% increase in the cardiac output (41, 42) with a direct arteriovenous fistula in the upper extremity. Flow rates through arteriovenous fistulae have been estimated from 300 to 500 ml/min. Occasionally as much as 1000 ml of blood may flow through an arteriovenous fistula that has been in place for a long time and has led to massive dilatation of both the feeding artery and the draining veins. In marginally compensated patients cardiac failure may develop. Surgical correction can be achieved by converting the fistula into an end-to-end variety and, while constantly measuring the flow through the veins with electromagnetic probes, progressively tightening a Teflon tape which has been wrapped around the artery to reduce the flow to approximately 300 ml/min (37). Empirically, this has been determined to be the lowest possible flow for adequate hemodialysis.

GRAFT ARTERIOVENOUS FISTULA

There is unanimity of opinion that a classical or modified direct arteriovenous fistula in the non-dominant forearm is the ideal angioaccess for maintenance hemodialysis. There are groups of patients, however, for whom the next best alternative, that of interposing a graft between an artery and a vein, may have to be utilized (Table 1). Indications for a graft arteriovenous fistula have been given in the discussion of strategies of angioaccess.

Table 1. Materials for graft arteriovenous fistulae.

A. Autologous grafts
  1. Saphenous vein
B. Allogeneic grafts
  1. Saphenous vein
      Cadaver donor
      Living donor (stripped varicose veins)
  2. Femoral artery
      Cadaver donor
  3. Umbilical vein (placental)
C. Prosthetic grafts
  1. Biologic
      Modified bovine carotid artery
  2. Synthetic
      Dacron
      Velour
      Mandril
      Teflon (expanded polytetrafluoroethylene)
  3. Composite
  4. Dacron reinforced
      Modified bovine carotid artery
      Umbilical vein

Materials

Although the 'gold standard' of reconstructive vascular surgery, the autogenous vein graft, served well in the initial era of graft arteriovenous angioaccess surgery (43, 44), today, with the possible exception of a patient with particular predilection for infection, autogenous saphenous vein is not the ideal graft material (45, 46). The major disadvantages of using autogenous saphenous vein for construction of graft arteriovenous fistulae are: 1) the additional surgery required in the thigh for harvesting of the vein, 2) availability only in a certain proportion of patients, and 3) difficulty in passing the thrombectomy (Fogarty) catheter through the valves in the event of early post-operative thrombosis. Approximately 50% of these grafts may be expected to be patent at one year.

Although in the experience of one group (47), allogeneic saphenous vein used as a straight graft arteriovenous fistula in the upper arm served extremely well, the limited availability and possible allogeneic sensitization make this and cadaver femoral artery (48) undesirable graft materials. There is extensive experience with the use of modified bovine carotid artery (Artegraft, Johnson & Johnson), and it does indeed have many distinct advantages (5, 49). The modified umbilical vein grafts (50), even with Dacron mesh reinforcement, and the mandril grafts have particular propensity to form aneurysms and pseudo-aneurysms with large bore needle punctures. In addition, the latter imposes a waiting period for tissue ingrowth into the Dacron mesh between the initial implantation and later anastomosis to the artery and vein.

The majority of access surgeons today favor the use of expanded polytetrafluoroethylene grafts (PTFE) for the construction of arteriovenous fistulae. These grafts share many of the virtues of the bovine heterograft and have some additional advantages: somewhat reduced incidence of junctional stenosis and almost no chance of hemorrhage during localized perigraft infections.

Technical considerations

The basic principles of reconstructive vascular surgery apply to the construction of the graft arteriovenous fistulae, namely a good arterial inflow, and appropriately long, wide lumen, smooth graft without kinks or twists, and a wide open venous run-off. These three prerequisites insure initial success in establishing arteriovenous flow. In my opinion, the ideal site for the implantation of the graft is the forearm. In the majority of patients the distal forearm vessels have been judged inadequate, and therefore a straight graft, starting from an artery in the distal forearm and draining into a vein at the antecubital fossa or in the upper arm, is generally not feasible. In my own experience a loop graft, starting from the antecubital fossa from one of the two divisions of the brachial artery (radial or ulnar), curving in a gentle wide loop and ending in a large vein (generally above the elbow and crossing the joint on the medial aspect), is the commonest configuration for the graft arteriovenous fis-

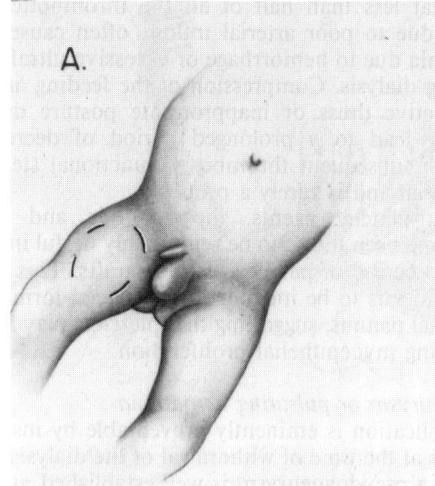
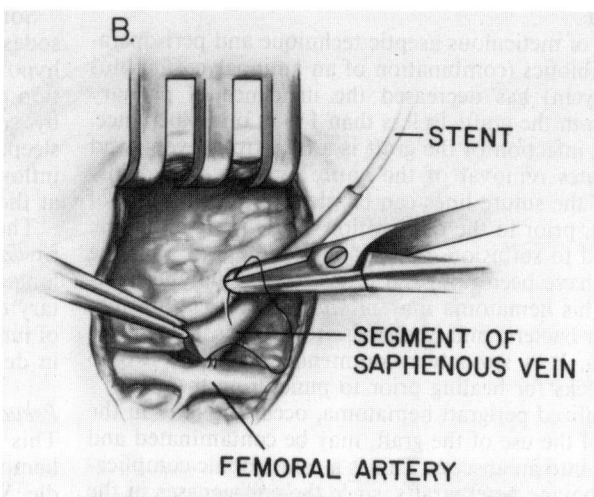
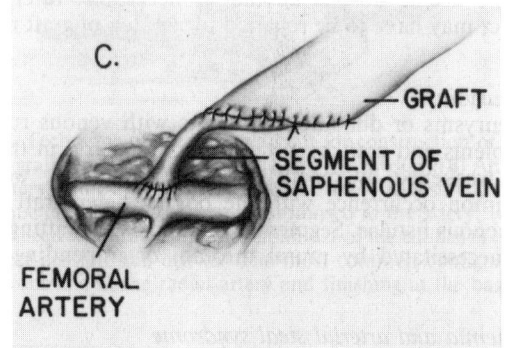
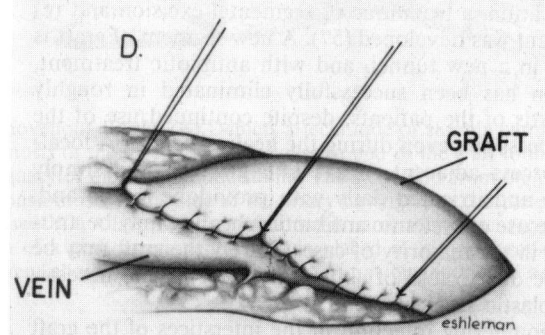

Figure 7. Technique of a composite graft arteriovenous fistula in an infant. (A) Position of incisions in the thigh; (B) Anastomosis of a small segment of saphenous vein to the superficial femoral artery. A stent is used passing from the vein through the anastomotic site into the femoral artery; (C) The other end of the segment of saphenous vein is spatulated and is anastomosed to a 6 mm PTFE graft; (D) A large venous anastomosis to the upper part of the saphenous vein at the sapheno-femoral junction.

or femoral) to a big vein (axillary or sapheno-femoral) may have as much as 4 l of blood flowing through it per minute (59–61). This can double the cardiac output and easily cause congestive heart failure, particularly in diabetic patients and the aged who are usually candidates for graft arteriovenous fistulae. After angiographic assessment, operative correction of this problem can be done by either placing a constricting Teflon tape around the graft at the arterial end, or narrowing the artery-graft anastomotic stoma with sutures. Using the electromagnetic probe during this procedure to assess the flow through the graft is almost imperative (37).

Lymphoceles
Transected and unligated lymphatic channels around the veins may lead to collection of fluid in the vicinity of the graft. This rare complication, more commonly seen in the groin, is treated by repeated aspirations which, however, may lead to disastrous infections.

ANGIOACCESS FOR CHILDREN

Technological progress has furnished small dialyzers, small volume tubings and equipment to monitor small fluctuations in weight, but angioaccess in 'small people' (62, 63) is no small problem. Extraordinary surgical skill, coupled with meticulous technique and enhanced by magnifying optical equipment are absolute prerequisites for success. The care of angioaccess in children is plagued by frequent trauma during play, and increased likelihood of microbial contamination (excreta and dirt). The caliber of the peripheral vessels imposes limitations as to the choice of available access sites, which of necessity has to be either the upper limbs or the thigh.

The preferred access for infants weighing 5 kg or less in an external prosthetic shunt located either in the upper arm or the thigh. To avoid damaging the main artery a segment of autogenous saphenous vein is used to construct a branch of the artery, which is then cannulated. A venous cannula can be inserted directly into the corresponding vein.

Techniques applicable to adults may be used for children 15 kg and above. The theoretical fear of overgrowth of the limb with an internal arteriovenous fistula has not materialized. Placement of needles is simplified by using local anesthesia injected by an air gun.

A graft arteriovenous fistula may be constructed using a 6 mm expanded PTFE prosthesis. As in the case of external prosthetic shunts, a segment of autogenous saphenous vein should be used to create an arterial branch (Figures 7A-D).

NEW APPROACHES

Hybrid devices

A combination of an internal graft arteriovenous fistula with an external access, which has the lure of sparing the pain of needle punctures, has been developed by two groups, one in Minneapolis (64) and the other in Los Angeles (65). Implantable either in the upper arm or in the thigh, these hybrid devices have side-arms which present on the skin surface, and can be attached to the extracorporeal circuit.

These innovations, in my opinion, have all the disadvantages of the external prosthetic devices, most prominently infection. A 25% infection rate, in the published experience of one of the above groups is totally unacceptable and makes continued use of this device difficult to justify.

Shuntless access

In some cases where no other technique was applicable, Bittinger et al. (66) utilized a technique of superficializing the femoral artery permitting the placement of two needles, the proximal one for 'pull' and the distal one for 'return'. The 'arterial jump graft' (67), a prosthesis placed between the common femoral and popliteal arteries, even in the face of arteriosclerotic occlusion of the superficial femoral artery, may provide an alternative avenue for blood access.

These shuntless techniques have the advantage of eliminating the hemodynamic problems of ischemia and arterial steal, venous hypertension and limb swelling, and increased cardiac load and decompensation. At the same time, they have two major disadvantages: transmission of the relatively high arterial pressure to the dialyzing membrane leading to excessive filtration, and painful sensations in the distal extremity whenever saline, heparin or any other drugs are injected into the return line of the extracorporeal circuit.

CONCLUSIONS

Angioaccess is the most important determinant for the continued well-being of patients with end-stage renal disease who are supported on hemodialysis. Although the problems of establishing and maintaining a reliable access continue to challenge the ingenuity and resourcefullness of vascular surgeons, from the therapeutic armamentarium today, one can be selected to suit the needs of almost every patient. Even patients with systemic vasculopathies (diabetes mellitus (68), lupus erythematosus, etc.) may now be enrolled in dialysis programs without the incessant fear of loss of their 'life-line'.

Repeated thrombosis, inevitable infection, limitations on activity, and threat of dislodgement dictate that external prosthetic shunts be used only sparingly today. Percutaneous venous access is an excellent stop-gap measure. A direct internal arteriovenous fistula, whenever applicable, is the procedure of choice and provides the best possible blood access. Alternatively, an interposed graft (bovine heterograft or expanded polytetrafluoroethylene) may be employed.

REFERENCES

1. Kjellstrand CM: The Achilles' heel of the hemodialysis patient. *Arch Intern Med* 138:1063, 1978
2. Bryan FA: Seventh Annual Progress Report: Oct. 1, 1974-Oct. 1, 1975 *Report No. AK-7-7-1387,* Research Triangle Institute, Triangle Park, NC. *The National Dialysis Registry-Artificial Kidney-Chronic Uremia Program,* Bethesda, MD, National Institute of Health, 1975
3. Butt KMH: Blood access. *Clin Nephrol* 9:138, 1978
4. Butt KMH, Kountz SL, Friedman EA: Angioaccess for hemodialysis, which, when, why? *Clin Nephrol* 3:207, 1975
5. Butt KMH, Rao TKS, Maki T, Mashimo S, Manis T, Delano BG, Kountz SL, Friedman EA: Bovine heterograft as a preferential hemodialysis access. *Trans Am Soc Artif Intern Organs* 20B:339, 1974
6. Simonian SJ, Stuart FP, Hill JL, Mahajan SK: Conversion of Scribner Shunt to an arteriovenous fistula for chronic dialysis. *Surgery* 8:44, 1977
7. Shaldon S, Rae AI, Rosen SM, Silva H, Oakley J: Refrigerated femoral venous-venous haemodialysis with coil preservation for rehabilitation of terminal uraemic patients. *Br Med J* 1:1716, 1963
8. Shaldon S, Silva H, Pomeroy J, Rae AI, Rosen SM: Percutaneous femoral venous catheterization and reusable dialysers in the treatment of acute renal failure. *Trans Am Soc Artif Intern Organs* 10:133, 1964
9. Kjellstrand CM, Merino GE, Mauer SM, Casali R, Buselmeier TJ: Complications of percutaneous femoral vein catherization for hemodialysis. *Clin Nephrol* 4:37, 1975
10. Friedman EA, Butt KMH, Pascua LJ, Hardy MA, Lawton RL, Uldall PR: Panel conference: Vascular access update. *Trans Am Soc Artif Intern Organs* 25:526, 1979
11. Shapiro WB, Faubert PF, Chou SY, Porush JG: Arteriovenous fistula as a complication of percutaneous femoral vein catherization for hemodialysis. *J Dial* 1:757, 1977
12. Erben J, Kvasnicka J, Bastecky J, Vortel V: Experience with routine use of subclavian vein cannulation in a haemodialysis. *Proc Eur Dial Transpl Assoc* 6:59, 1969
13. Uldall PR, Dyck RF, Woods F, Merchant N, Martin GS, Cardella CT, Sutton D, DeVeber GA: A subclavian cannula for temporary vascular access for hemodialysis or plasmapheresis. *Dial Transpl* 8:963, 1979

14. Uldall PR, Woods F, Merchant N, Bird M, Crichton E: Two years experience with the subclavian cannula for temporary vascular access for hemodialysis and plasmapheresis. *Proc Clin Dial Transpl Forum* 9:32, 1979
15. Uldall PR, Woods F, Merchant N, Crichton E, Carter H: A double-lumen subclavian cannula (DLSC) for temporary hemodialysis access. *Trans Am Soc Artif Intern Organs* 26:93, 1980
16. Quinton W, Dillard D, Scribner BH: Cannulation of blood vessels for prolonged hemodialysis. *Trans Am Soc Artif Intern Organs* 6:104, 1960
17. Ramirez O, Swartz C, Onesti G, Mailloux L, Brest AN: The winged in-line shunt. *Trans Am Soc Artif Intern Organs* 12:220, 1966
18. Rajagopalan PR, Fitts CT: Use of Allen-Brown shunt between profunda femoris artery and long saphenous vein for hemodialysis access. *Am Surg* 44:226, 1978
19. Buselmeier TJ, Simmons RL, Najarian JS, Duncan DA, Von Hartitsch B, Kjellstrand CM: The clinical application of a new prosthetic arteriovenous shunt. *Nephron* 12:22, 1973
20. Thomas GI: A large-vessel applique A-V shunt for hemodialysis. *Trans Am Soc Artif Intern Organs* 15:288, 1969
21. Morgan AP, Knight DC, Tilney NL, Lazarus JM: Femoral triangle sepsis in dialysis patients; frequency, management and outcome. *Ann Surg* 191:460, 1980
22. May J, Johnson JR, Evans R, Sheil AGR: Experience with large vessel applique (Thomas) shunts for haemodialysis. *Med J Aust* 2:1163, 1970
23. Gaan D, Mallick NP, Brewis RAL, Seedat YK, Mahoney MP: Cerebral damage from declotting Scribner shunts. *Lancet* 2:77, 1969
24. Clyne DH, Epstein J, Sloman G, Andrews JT, Hare WSC, Morris PJ, Marshall VC, Kincaid-Smith P: Retrograde cerebral emboli during procedures to clear arterial thrombi from haemodialysis shunts. *Med J Aust* 1:359, 1970
25. Kaegi A, Pineo GF, Shimizu A, Trivedi H, Hirsh J, Gent M: Arteriovenous shunt thrombosis prevention by sulfinpyrazone. *N Engl J Med* 290:304, 1974
26. Salzman EW: Influence of antiplatelet drugs on platelet-surface interactions. *Adv Exp Med Biol* 102:265, 1978
27. Wing AJ, Curtis JR, de Wardener HE: Reduction of clotting in Scribner shunts by long term anticoagulation. *Br Med J* 3:143, 1967
28. Morris AJ, Bilinsky RT: Prevention of staphylococcal shunt infections by continuous vancomycin prophylaxis. *Am J Med Sci* 262:87, 1971
29. Lawton RL, Sharzer LS: Vascular access for patients on maintenance dialysis. *Surg Gynecol Obstet* 135:279, 1972
30. Brescia MJ, Cimino JE, Appel K, Hurwich BJ: Chronic hemodialysis using venipuncture and a surgically created arteriovenous fistula. *N Engl J Med* 275:1089, 1966
31. Thomas ML, Rappaport AS, Wing AJ: Arteriography and phlebography of the limbs in planning shunt and fistula operations in patients with chronic renal failure. *Am J Roentgenol Radium Ther Nucl Med* 12:551, 1974
32. Dagher FJ, Gelber R, Reed W: Basilic vein to brachial artery, arteriovenous fistula for long term hemodialysis; a five year followup. *Proc Clin Dial Transpl Forum* 10:126, 1980
33. Karmody AM, Lempert N: 'Smooth loop' arteriovenous fistulas for hemodialysis. *Surgery* 75:238, 1974
34. Ehrenfeld WK, Grausz H, Wylie EJ: Subcutaneous arteriovenous fistulas for hemodialysis. *Am J Surg* 124:200, 1972
35. Anderson CB, Gilula LA, Sicard GA, Etheradge EE: Venous angiography of subcutaneous hemodialysis fistulas. *Arch Surg* 114:1320, 1979
36. Ralston AJ, Harlow GR, Jones DM, Davis P: Infections of Scribner and Brescia arteriovenous shunts. *Br Med J* 3:408, 1971
37. Butt KMH, Friedman EA, Kountz SL: Angioaccess. *Curr Probl Surg* 8:9, 1976
38. Bosanac PR, Bilder B, Grunberg RW, Banach SF, Kintzel JE, Stephens HW: Post-permanent access neuropathy. *Trans Am Soc Artif Intern Organs* 23:162, 1977
39. Bussell JA, Abbott JA, Lim RC: A radial steal syndrome with arteriovenous fistula for hemodialysis. Studies in seven patients. *Ann Intern Med* 75:387, 1971
40. Lawton L: Steal, stasis, swelling and stenosis. *Int J Artif Organs* 2:9, 1979
41. Johnson G Jr, Blythe WB: Hemodynamic effects of arteriovenous shunts used for hemodialysis. *Ann Surg* 171:715, 1970
42. Von Bibra H, Castro L, Autenrieth G, McLeod A, Gurland HJ: The effects of arteriovenous shunts on cardiac function in renal dialysis patients – an echocardiographic evaluation. *Clin Nephrol* 9:205, 1978
43. Girardet RE, Hackett RE, Goodwin NJ, Friedman EA: Thirteen months experience with the saphenous vein graft arteriovenous fistula for maintenance hemodialysis. *Trans Am Soc Artif Intern Organs* 16:285, 1970
44. Calman KC, Quin RO, Paton AM, Briggs JD, Bill PRF: Autogenous saphenous vein loop for hemodialysis. *Br J Surg* 60:383, 1973
45. May J, Harris J, Fletcher J: Long-term results of saphenous vein graft arteriovenous fistulas. *Am J Surg* 140:387, 1980
46. Haimov M, Burrows L, Schanzer H, Neff M, Baez A, Kwun K, Slifkin R: Experience with arterial substitutes in the construction of vascular access for hemodialysis. *J Cardiovasc Surg (Torino)* 21:149, 1980
47. Piccone VA Jr, Sika J, Ahmed N, LeVeen HH, DiScala V: Preserved saphenous vein allografts for vascular access. *Surg Gynecol Obstet* 147:385, 1978
48. Abu-dalu J, Urca I, Zonder HB, Rosenfeld JB: Hemodialysis treatment by means of a cadaver arterial allograft. *Arch Surg* 105:798, 1972
49. Chinitz JL, Yokoyama T, Bower R, Swartz C: Self-sealing prosthesis for arteriovenous fistula in man. *Trans Am Soc Artif Intern Organs* 18:452, 1972
50. Kester RC: Early results with human umbilical cord vein allografts for haemodialysis. *Br J Surg* 65:609, 1978
51. Kester RC: Arteriovenous grafts for vascular access in haemodialysis. *Br J Surg* 66:23, 1979
52. Tellis VA, Kohlberg WI, Bhat DJ, Driscoll B, Veith FJ: Expanded polytetrafluoroethylene graft fistula for chronic hemodialysis. *Ann Surg* 189:101, 1979
53. Gross GF, Hayes JF: PTFE graft arteriovenous fistulae for hemodialysis access. *Am Surg* 45:748, 1979
54. Merickel JH, Anderson RC, Knutson R, Lipschultz ML, Hitchcock CR: Bovine carotid artery shunts in vascular access surgery. Complications in the chronic hemodialysis patient. *Arch Surg* 109:245, 1974
55. Rosenthal JJ, Spigelman A, Gaspar MR, Movius HJ: Problems with bovine heterografts for hemodialysis. Recognition, correction and prevention. *Am J Surg* 130:182, 1975
56. Corry RJ, Patel NP, West JC: Surgical management of complications of vascular access for hemodialysis. *Surg Gynecol Obstet* 151:49, 1980
57. Butt KMH: Bovine heterograft for arteriovenous fistulas. In *Vascular Grafts,* edited by Sawyer PN, Kaplitt MJ, New York, Appleton-Century-Crofts, 1978, p 278
58. Rosenberg N, Lord GH: Prestenotic turbulence in arteries as the cause of mural thrombosis and embolism. *J Cardiovasc Surg,* Spec. Suppl 6:271, 1965
59. van der Werf BA: In discussion of van der Werf BA, Rat-

tazzi LC, Katzman HA, Schild AF: Three year experience with bovine graft arteriovenous (A-V) fistulas in 100 patients. *Trans Am Soc Artif Intern Organs* 21:299, 1975
60. van der Werf BA, Kumar SS, Pennell P, Gottleib S: Cardiac failure from bovine graft arteriovenous fistulas; diagnosis and management. *Trans Am Soc Artif Intern Organs* 24:474, 1978
61. Kaye M, D'Avirro M, Baird C, McCloskey B, Oscar G: Hemodynamic data on polytetrafluoroethylene (PTFE) grafts. *Trans Am Soc Artif Intern Organs* 25:328, 1979
62. Buselmeier TJ, Kjellstrand CM: A-V shunts and fistulae in neonates, infants and children. *Proc Eur Dial Transpl Assoc* 10:511, 1973
63. Arbus GS, DeMaria JE, Galiwango J, Irwin MA, Churchill BM: The first 10 years of the dialysis-transplantation program at The Hospital for Sick Children, Toronto. 1: Predialysis and dialysis. *Can Med Assoc J* 122:655, 1980
64. Collins AJ, Shapiro FL, Keshaviah P, Ilstrup K, Andersen R, O'Brien T, Martinez FJ, Cosentino LC: Blood access without skin puncture. *Trans Am Soc Artif Intern Organs* 27:308, 1981
65. Golding AL, Nissenson AR, Raible D: Carbon transcutaneous access device (CTAD). *Proc Clin Dial Transpl Forum* 9:242, 1979
66. Bittinger WO, Strauch M, Huber W, von Henning GE, Twittenhoff WD, Ewald R, Wittenmeier KW, Schworzbeck A, Stegaru B: Sixteen month experience with the subcutaneous fixed superficial femoral artery for chronic hemodialysis. *Proc Eur Dial Transpl Assoc* 7:408, 1970
67. Butt, KMH, Kountz SL: A new vascular access for hemodialysis, the arterial jump graft. *Surgery* 79:476, 1976
68. Butt KMH, Ortega MG, Shirani KZ, Hong JH, Adamsons RJ, Manis T, Friedman EA: Angioaccess in uremic diabetics. In *Diabetic Renal-Retinal Syndrome,* edited by Friedman EA, L'Esprance FA Jr, New York, Grune & Stratton Inc, 1980, p 209

9
EXTRACORPOREAL THROMBOGENESIS: MECHANISMS AND PREVENTION

REGINALD G. MASON[*], HANSON Y. K. CHUANG and S. FAZAL MOHAMMAD

Introduction	186
Interactions of blood components with artificial surfaces	187
Adsorption of plasma proteins to artificial surfaces	187
Adhesion of platelets to artificial surfaces	188
Adhesion of leukocytes to artificial surfaces	189
Adhesion of erythrocytes to artificial surfaces	190
Blood soluble and cellular components that adhere to hemodialysis membranes in clinical applications	190
The influences of blood flow rate and different geometries on deposition of blood soluble and cellular components on artificial surfaces	191
Approaches to the prevention of thrombosis during hemodialysis	191
Effects of soluble antithrombotic and antiplatelet agents	191
Modifications of surfaces of biomaterials that contact blood	192
Heparinization of surfaces	192
Other modifications of surfaces	193
Surface passivation with adsorbed plasma protein	194
Endothelialization of materials	194
Final comments	194
References	194

INTRODUCTION

The exposure of blood to artificial surfaces either extracorporeally or intracorporeally initiates a number of diverse reactions (1–4). Immediately following the exposure of most artificial surfaces to blood, various plasma proteins begin to adsorb to those surfaces. The interaction of plasma proteins with artificial surfaces can initiate the activation of the intrinsic and extrinsic blood coagulation, the kinin, the complement, and the fibrinolytic systems. Ultimately, thrombin may be formed, and this enzyme may adhere to artificial surfaces in an active state. While various proteins are adsorbing to an artificial surface and establishing an equilibrium state, blood cells begin to adhere to the adsorbed protein layer. Erythrocytes seem to adhere poorly to such a surface, but platelets and leukocytes, especially neutrophils, are attracted to the adsorbed protein layer, frequently in large numbers. Adhesion of leukocytes to the artificial surface may lead to activation of the extrinsic blood coagulation system through the exposure of tissue factor on the plasma membranes of the adherent cells.

Exposure of blood to an artificial surface may lead only to protein adsorption followed by adhesion of a few blood cells, or the reaction may be more intense. The series of events outlined above may culminate ultimately in the formation of a white mural thrombus composed of fibrin, platelets, leukocytes, and a few erythrocytes. Numerous diverse factors influence formation of mural thrombi and many of these are poorly understood even now. The chemical and physical nature of the artificial surface itself appears to play an important role not only in protein adsorption, but also in the subsequent adhesion of platelets and leukocytes. Rheologic factors are important also, since turbulence enhances thrombus formation, while laminar flow decreases the possibility of thrombosis. Stasis or vortical flow, even when confined to relatively small areas, can serve as powerful initiators of thrombosis. The activity states of the various blood components themselves appear to play poorly understood roles in thrombus formation. Normally the blood coagulation sequences are maintained in a fine state of balance by the interaction of activating mechanisms with numerous inactivating or neutralizing mechanisms (5, 6). Increased production of activated coagulation factors through contact of blood with artificial surfaces and adherent cells coupled with the possible loss of inactivating factors due to their adsorption to these surfaces or by denaturation can enhance thrombus formation. Similarly, alterations in the state of reactivity of platelets and leukocytes brought about by their contact with, or proximity to, artificial surfaces or by shear stress-induced changes may enable these activated cells to enhance their contributions toward the thrombotic process.

Formation of a mural thrombus, whether it be simply a single layer of adherent leukocytes and platelets, or whether it be a true fibrin thrombus that contains erythrocytes, platelets, and leukocytes, can be associated with the formation of emboli. If these emboli are small, they frequently cause no problems for the host, but if they are large or if their numbers are sufficiently great, they can obstruct blood vessels distal to the point of embolus origin and produce tissue damage. Certain pharmaceuticals, apart from the anticoagulants heparin and warfarin, can inhibit formation of thrombi by their actions on platelets and leukocytes.

The various effects of artificial surfaces in activation of blood coagulation and enhancement of thrombus formation have made necessary the use of anticoagulants in

---

[*] Deceased in October 1981.

patients undergoing hemodialysis. Heparin is the most commonly used anticoagulant today, although the coumarin derivatives are possible alternatives. Heparin has been used not only as a soluble anticoagulant but also to coat artificial surfaces in efforts to improve their blood compatibility. The slow leaching of heparin from such a coated surface into blood appears to diminish thrombus formation. Alternatively, heparin can be covalently bonded to a surface with resultant diminution in formation of thrombi by processes that are poorly understood. More recently, use of so-called antiplatelet agents, such as aspirin, dipyridamole, sulfinpyrazone, and PGI_2, has led in some clinical applications to improved compatibility of blood with artificial surfaces.

INTERACTIONS OF BLOOD COMPONENTS WITH ARTIFICIAL SURFACES

The importance of the interactions of blood soluble and cellular components with artificial surfaces is obvious in the use of any extracorporeal or intracorporeal device that interfaces with blood. The comments that will be made below concerning the various mechanisms whereby interaction of blood soluble and cellular components with surfaces may lead to thrombus formation will emphasize events that can take place during hemodialysis. However, the same comments will apply in most instances to events that take place when blood contacts other artificial organs and devices such as cannulas, catheters, vascular shunts, blood conduit tubing, blood oxygenators, artificial heart valves, artificial blood vessels, ventricular assist devices, and artificial hearts.

In the discussions that follow, the authors have been selective in their references to the literature, have referred wherever possible to review articles and have attempted to monitor both the United States and European literature where it concerns thrombosis and hemodialysis.

Adsorption of plasma proteins to artificial surfaces

The adsorption of plasma proteins to artificial surfaces has been studied for many years. Soon after hemodialysis for chronic renal failure was introduced into clinical medicine, concern was voiced about denaturation of plasma proteins exposed to surfaces in various dialyzers and in other extracorporeal devices (7). Concern for the effects of denatured plasma proteins persists, and recently probable denaturation of plasma protein was shown to influence platelet function adversely (8).

Interest in the mechanisms of activation of the intrinsic blood coagulation system led to numerous studies of the interaction of certain blood coagulation factors with artificial surfaces. Activation of the intrinsic blood coagulation system by exposure of blood to artificial surfaces has been shown to be due to adsorption of certain of the procoagulants to these surfaces, and work in this area continues with exciting advances in our understanding of the earlier reactions reported only recently (9–15). The studies of Vroman and coworkers (16–19) deserve special comment, since these investigators have studied for years the interaction of certain of the procoagulants and fibrinogen at the blood-artificial surface interface. Vroman and his associates have devised a number of unique methods for studying the interaction of proteins with artificial surfaces and have used several ingenious techniques for visualizing these reactions. These investigators have shown that a number of plasma proteins including albumin, globulins, and fibrinogen interact with artificial surfaces in a highly complex manner. This has been confirmed by others (20, 21) who used similar techniques. Oja and coworkers (22) used a different approach and studied the removal from plasma of specific blood coagulation factors following exposure of the plasma to artificial surfaces.

Lyman and Brash (23–26) have studied the interactions of plasma proteins with a large number of artificial surfaces, particularly hydrophobic polymer surfaces, and they published a review on protein adsorption to artificial surfaces. The importance of flow effects in studies of plasma protein adsorption to surfaces has been given emphasis by their work and that of others (27–29) as has the effects of erythrocytes. These and other investigators (30, 31) have shown that in the early stages of blood-material interaction adsorbed plasma protein frequently exists in a state of equilibrium with nonadsorbed protein. This equilibrium is influenced both by the specific surfaces tested and by the presence and amounts of different species of proteins in solution. It is now generally agreed that unless protein concentration is low, protein molecules are adsorbed to most artificial surfaces to form a monolayer with relatively little distortion of the various species of molecules present. Adsorption of molecular species that take part in activation of the intrinsic blood coagulation system (9–14, 16) and certain other protein species may represent important exceptions to this statement.

Thrombin adsorption to artificial surfaces presents a unique problem in the study of blood compatibility. Thrombin is adsorbed firmly to many artificial surfaces, and in most cases it is adsorbed in an enzymatically active form. Waugh and coworkers (32, 33) were early leaders in studies of this type. Recently, Chuang and coworkers (34, 35) have added new insights in the area of thrombin interactions with artificial surfaces. Further thought and investigation should be given to the phenomenon of thrombin adsorbed to artificial surfaces and its role in the formation of mural thrombi. Artificial surfaces exposed to blood may serve as foci for adsorption and concentration of active thrombin molecules. Indeed, platelets bind thrombin (36, 37) and platelets adherent to an artificial surface could serve as points for concentration of thrombin. It is evident that thrombin forms even in well heparinized blood that is exposed to various artificial surfaces extracorporeally. These artificial surfaces may then act to adsorb out the activated thrombin molecules and concentrate them, so that they can serve to enhance the activation of the blood coagulation system further.

Recently, *ex vivo* studies of protein adsorption involving use of different types of flow chambers and various flow conditions have been reported (38–40). In some of this work purified, radiolabeled plasma proteins have been used. Results from these studies generally support earlier investigations conducted with different techniques in that protein adsorption has been shown to occur rapidly. Of more interest are findings showing that protein species adsorbed initially apparently are replaced later by different protein species. These recent studies are of particular importance, because they have been conducted with blood that is returned to living experimental animals permitting the organism to react to surface-exposed blood in various ways. Equally exciting are recent reports of changes in supposedly 'immobile' polymer surface groups brought about by contact of the polymer with water that render the surface less reactive with proteins. The latter studies are expansions of the pioneer work of Merrill (3).

In summary, many workers have documented the fact that various proteins from plasma interact in a complex manner with artificial surfaces (1-4, 41-45). The consequences of these interactions are numerous and diverse, but our understanding of these complex interactions is still in its infancy. In a more optimistic vein, it must be noted that several investigators have reported the formation of a 'passivating' or blood-compatible protein layer on certain artificial surfaces exposed to blood for prolonged periods of time; these studies deserve further attention (46).

Adhesion of platelets to artificial surfaces

Reactions of platelets with adsorbed plasma proteins have received attention from a number of different investigators. Lyman and coworkers (23-25) found that proteins adsorbed to hydrophobic polymers were not denatured. However, platelets adhered to these plasma proteins, and this platelet adhesion appeared in their studies to be related to the critical surface tension of the supporting artificial surface (23, 25, 47). In most test systems, albumin adsorbed to artificial surfaces has little effect on the subsequent adherence of platelets to such surfaces, but a fibrinogen coating of a surface enhances platelet adherence, while a gamma globulin coating enhances adhesion and stimulates the platelet release reaction (48). A number of other workers have reported that fibrinogen adsorbed to glass and other surfaces enhances platelet adhesion (49-52). This effect can be demonstrated at extremely low concentrations of fibrinogen (51). In interpreting experiments of this type, it must be realized that in the absence of protein, platelets adhere avidly to bare or uncoated artificial surfaces (53, 54). A number of investigators have (47, 50, 53-56) shown that exposure of the mixed proteins of plasma to artificial surfaces appreciably decreases the subsequent reactions of platelets with these surfaces. Purified albumin was found to be a useful coating on artificial surfaces when inhibition of platelet adhesion was desired.

Others also have investigated the roles of a variety of plasma proteins in platelet adhesion to artificial surfaces (48, 50, 53, 54). Fibrinogen was found to enhance platelet adhesion, while as noted above, the presence of plasma decreased the adhesion of cells to artificial surfaces. Recently, several different naturally occurring components of plasma has been shown to inhibit markedly the adhesion of platelets to artificial surfaces (57-59).

The surface energies of artificial surfaces that have acquired coatings of plasma proteins were found to be remarkably similar regardless of the composition of the material (60-63). This finding may explain why so many different types of artificial surfaces react similarly when placed in contact with blood. However, surface energy alone does not determine the degree of compatibility with blood. Other factors must be influential also.

The role of the carbohydrate content of proteins in influencing platelet adhesion to artificial surfaces was studied by Lee and Kim (64). These workers found that platelet adhesion to adsorbed proteins paralleled the saccharide content of these proteins. These findings may explain why albumin, a protein that contains no carbohydrate, produces less platelet adhesion than do fibrinogen, fibronectin (65), or gamma globulin, each of which contain sugar moieties.

Treatment of heparinized surfaces with fibrinogen solutions, platelet-free plasma, or serum does not protect against subsequent platelet adhesion, whereas incubation of the heparinized surface with albumin reduces adhesion of platelets to that surface (43, 45, 66, 67). Hence, heparinization of a surface in itself does not prevent subsequent protein adsorption but may influence the types and amounts of protein adsorbed.

It is now generally recognized that the adsorption of plasma proteins to artificial surfaces plays important roles in the generation of thrombi as well as in prevention of thrombus formation (41-43, 68-72). Despite this, our knowledge of the composition of thrombus-generating surface coatings and of passive or protective coatings is remarkably scanty. This lack of knowledge is due largely to our lack of techniques for detecting and quantitating the various components of the adsorbed protein layers that form on surfaces of extracorporeal devices conducting blood. Not only must we come to understand the mechanisms whereby adsorbed protein layers attract platelets, but we must also develop protein or other adsorbed or bound layers that will discourage or prevent platelet and leukocyte adhesion. In all of this work the important effects of rheologic factors must be borne in mind (73-78).

Recently, new insights have been gained concerning the increasingly complex ways in which platelet adhesion to protein-coated artificial surfaces can enhance thrombus formation. In some, but by no means all, cases adhesion stimulates platelets to undergo a complex series of reactions that enhance the platelet aggregation and blood coagulation reactions. Activated platelets change shape to produce pseudopods that appear to enhance the spreading of these cells on a surface. Shape change frequently is followed by the release reaction (79-81), generation and release of thromboxane A_2 (TXA_2), production of platelet activating factor (PAF) (82, 83), and platelet factor 3 (PF3) activity (84, 85); binding of fibrinogen (86-88), Factor Va

(89, 90), and Factor Xa (91, 92) to specific 'receptors' on the outer surface of the platelet plasma membrane, and generation of Factor XIa on the plasma membrane surface (93, 94). Release of serotonin, ADP, TXA_2, and PAF leads to aggregation of nearby platelets that bind to already adherent platelets. Release of platelet factor 4 (PF4) (95, 96) can result in neutralization of heparin by this basic platelet protein. Binding of fibrinogen to platelets is essential for ADP-induced aggregation. Production of PF3 activity enhances the blood coagulation cascade and may be related to the binding of activated Factors V and X on the platelet surface. Activation of factor XI and binding of Factors Va and Xa by platelets markedly enhances blood coagulation sequences in the neighborhood of adherent and aggregated platelets with the ultimate formation of thrombin, an enzyme that also binds to platelets (97, 98) and converts fibrinogen to fibrin. Fibrin stabilizes adherent platelet aggregates. Thus, appropriate stimuli, admittedly incompletely understood at present, arising from adsorbed plasma proteins or from artificial surfaces themselves trigger a variety of changes in platelets that can lead to their adhesion and aggregation and to their active enhancement of blood coagulation processes as well as to alterations in their function (99–101).

Adhesion of leukocytes to artificial surfaces

Adhesion of leukocytes to artificial surfaces has been less well studied than has the adhesion of platelets, although research in this area has accelerated during the past few years. It was realized early that hemodialysis was associated with a precipitous but short lasting fall in the peripheral leukocyte count (102, 103) (see Chapters 5 and 32). This fall in leukocytes was followed by a gradual rise to normal or even supranormal levels (104). Various studies have shown that the initial fall in leukocytes is due only in small part to adhesion of these cells to artificial surfaces that contact blood. The major part of the leukopenia that develops soon after hemodialysis is initiated appears due to sequestration of leukocytes within the patient's vascular system (104). The role of activated complement components, particularly C5a desarg, in dialysis-associated leukopenia has received considerable attention (105–108). Another active area of research involves studies of alteration of leukocyte function secondary to exposure of blood to artificial surfaces.

The consequences of the adhesion of leukocytes to artificial surfaces are several, including potential immunologic consequences (see Figure 1). On the other hand, several studies suggest that adhesion of leukocytes to artificial surfaces is associated with the exposure of tissue factor activity in or on the leukocyte plasma membrane to blood (109–111). Adherent leukocytes also may release certain factors stored in cytoplasmic granules or generated within these cells that can influence blood coagulation (112–115) as well as platelet aggregation. In the latter case, it has been shown that stimulated leukocytes can release PAF (116) and TXA_2 (117, 118). Morphologic studies indicate that adherent leukocytes may

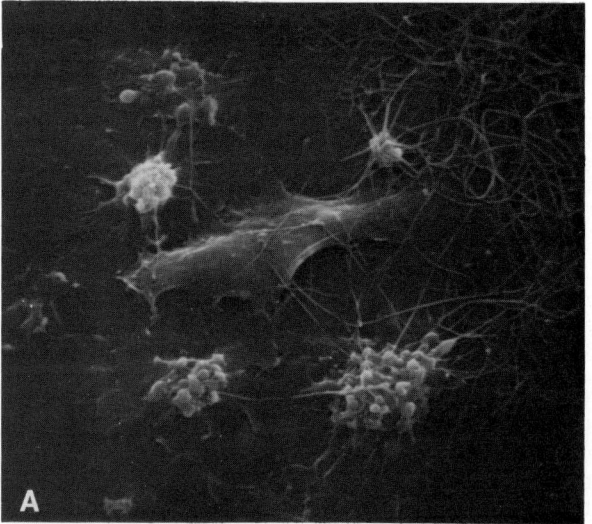

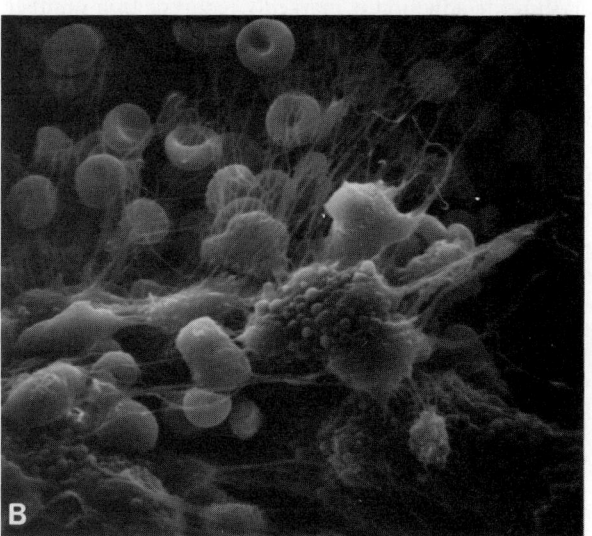

Figure 1. Thrombotic deposits present on different areas of the same hemodialysis membrane. (A) This view shows several platelet aggregates interconnected and intimately associated with fibrin fibers of varying size; (B) This view shows leukocytes, erythrocytes, and at least one platelet aggregate enmeshed in a fibrin network.

attract platelets that subsequently adhere to them (119–124). These interactions of leukocytes and platelets deserve further investigation.

Adherent leukocytes may serve as scavengers that remove adherent platelets and fibrin. This role has not yet been clarified fully, but there are numerous reports in the literature indicating that neutrophils and macrophages can phagocytose adherent platelets, fibrin, or denatured protein.

Despite the presence of numerous adherent platelets and leukocytes (123–127), the efficiency of reused dialysis membranes does not seem to be noticeably impaired (128, 129), although not all investigators agree (130) (see also Chapter 15). This raises the question of whether adhesion of leukocytes and platelets to hemodialysis membranes has any significance, unless it leads to the formation of mural thrombi or emboli or produces changes in blood that alter certain functions of circulating platelets or leukocytes.

Adhesion of erythrocytes to artificial surfaces

Although erythrocytes have been shown to adhere to artificial surfaces *in vitro* (131), morphologic studies of hemodialysis membranes following their clinical use indicate that relatively few erythrocytes adhere firmly to these surfaces (127, 130, 131). Adherent platelets and leukocytes far outnumber adherent erythrocytes in these studies unless a fibrin clot is present to entrap the red cells (see Figure 1). As with platelets and leukocytes, erythrocytes will adhere to artificial surfaces avidly in the absence of protein (131), but when protein is present, erythrocyte adhesion is markedly reduced. In a number of *in vitro* studies, erythrocytes have been shown to adhere to artificial surfaces by a small area of their plasma membrane (132). Such adherent erythrocytes can be deformed by shear stresses, and the main part of the cell may be torn away from the adherent portion. It has been shown that flow conditions are important in determining the approach of erythrocytes to hemodialysis membranes and other artificial surfaces (133, 134). Also important in attraction of erythrocytes and other blood cells to a dialysis membrane is the force produced by passage of fluid through the membrane itself (135, 136).

The interaction of erythrocytes with artificial surfaces including hemodialysis membranes can lead to enhancement of blood coagulation through several mechanisms. First, if erythrocytes are disrupted during their adhesion on an artificial surface, thromboplastic substances may appear on the surface of the cell or can be released from the injured cells (44, 45). These thromboplastic substances can enhance the function of the intrinsic blood coagulation system. If erythrocytes are damaged or disrupted, they release a number of substances including ADP that enhance the adhesion of circulating platelets to those platelets already adherent to the hemodialysis membrane or other artificial surfaces, and this can lead to formation of a mural white thrombus (44, 45).

BLOOD SOLUBLE AND CELLULAR COMPONENTS THAT ADHERE TO HEMODIALYSIS MEMBRANES IN CLINICAL APPLICATIONS

During hemodialysis, the blood that is exposed to dialysis membranes is heparinized. The degree to which plasma proteins are adsorbed to hemodialysis membranes and the degree to which platelets and leukocytes adhere to this adsorbed protein layer vary from patient to patient. This may depend on the effective level of heparin present in the blood of the patients. The dose of heparin that must be used to achieve a certain degree of inhibition of blood coagulation also varies from one patient to another for reasons that are not understood completely (137). Heparin carries a considerable negative charge, and this permits these anticoagulant molecules to interact with certain artificial surfaces, numerous different plasma proteins, and with platelets and leukocytes. The amount of heparin present appears to be highly important in determining the interaction of soluble and cellular components of the blood with hemodialysis membranes (66). As stated above, PF4 (95, 96) release from stimulated platelets will neutralize the anticoagulant activities of heparin, so that increased platelet adhesion can lead to the need for larger doses of heparin. Certain basic proteins released from stimulated leukocytes also can neutralize heparin.

In certain hemodialysis patients, increased numbers of thromboembolic complications occur during hemodialysis compared to the experiences of other patients. These thromboembolic prone individuals may require increased amounts of heparin for prevention of thromboembolism. The reasons for this are not well understood. Hemodialysis patients have been shown to have circulating platelets that are altered in certain of their functional properties (99, 100). Perhaps altered rheologic states within dialyzers have injured or activated the platelets. Certain other aspects of the blood coagulation and fibrinolytic systems also may be altered in these patients (138). The inclusion of certain antithrombotic or antiplatelet drugs in the patient's therapeutic regimen may decrease the propensity to thromboembolism. Finally, heparinization of surfaces in the *ex vivo* blood circuit including membrane surfaces may decrease interactions of blood with these surfaces and may permit dialysis to be performed with little or no anticoagulant added to the blood.

Recent evidence indicates that heparin may lower plasma prostaglandin I_2 (PGI$_2$) levels (139). PGI$_2$ is a potent antiplatelet agent and inhibits platelet adhesion, aggregation, and the release reaction. Thus heparin, a two edged sword, may enhance reactions of platelets with artificial surfaces while inhibiting blood coagulation.

Undesirable reactions of blood with artificial surfaces continue to be some of the most challenging problems encountered in the use of hemodialyzers. These blood-artificial surface interactions appear to be major obstacles in the way of successful use of artificial organs that contact blood. In other chapters in this book, the necessity of using heparin or other anticoagulants as a means of overcoming the thrombogenicity of artificial surfaces is discussed. Further, the interactions between artificial surfaces and plasma proteins on one hand and the cellular elements of blood on the other have been discussed earlier in this chapter.

A variety of surface physical and rheologic factors appear also to play important roles when blood comes in contact with a foreign surface. Exposure of blood to an artificial surface may result in rapid contact activation of certain of the blood coagulation factors in addition to alterations of platelets and leukocytes. In addition, rheologic conditions such as turbulence, pressure fluctuations, and shear stresses generated at the interface between the artificial surface and flowing blood appear to influence thrombus formation to a large degree. Further, the electrokinetic surface charge of an artificial surface determines to some extent the degree of thrombus formation.

THE INFLUENCE OF BLOOD FLOW RATE AND DIFFERENT GEOMETRIES ON DEPOSITION OF BLOOD SOLUBLE AND CELLULAR COMPONENTS ON ARTIFICIAL SURFACES

Blood and plasma both exhibit non-newtonian behavior particularly under low rates of shear (140–143). It has been demonstrated that due to inward migration of cells in the laminar flow circulation mode, erythrocytes tend to circulate away from the vessel or container wall leaving a cell-free marginal zone of plasma (144, 145). Goldsmith (145) demonstrated that this cell-free marginal zone of plasma shrinks when circulating cell concentrations increase as occurs at the surface of a dialysis membrane. Erythrocyte interactions and collisions give rise to sideways or radial movements, and cells including platelets and leukocytes are occasionally pushed against the chamber wall by these forces. This behavior of erythrocytes under conditions of flow can compel collisions of platelets with the container wall (146). At high rates of shear (1500 dynes/cm^2), erythrocytes undergo morphologic alterations; further increases in shear rates result in leakage of potassium and hemoglobin, while even further increases ultimately can cause lysis of the cells (144, 147–150). Leakage of various substances, particularly ADP, from erythrocytes under high shear stresses can induce the aggregation of platelets. Moreover, it has been shown that circulating platelets are even more sensitive to shear stress than are erythrocytes. Brown et al. (73, 151) observed that a shear stress of only 50 dynes/cm^2 resulted in liberation of adenine nucleotides and serotonin from intact platelets, whereas a shear stress of 100 dynes/cm^2 caused lysis of these cells in a rotational viscometer. These observations clearly suggest a marked susceptibility of platelets to shear stress. Even slight damage to platelets can induce the release reaction which in turn will induce further changes in nearby circulating platelets leading to formation of mural thrombi or circulating aggregates. The amount of mural thrombus formed and the size of circulating platelet or leukocyte aggregates are factors that can influence flow conditions markedly.

In addition to increased chances of interaction between a container wall and the cellular components of blood in an area of disturbed flow, alterations in the pattern of adsorption of soluble plasmatic components to the container wall can occur also. This altered deposition of soluble components onto the surrounding container walls can influence greatly the attractiveness of the wall for cellular components, especially in areas of persistently distorted flow. Increased adsorptive deposition of various plasma proteins on container walls in an area of turbulent or vortical flow and an associated increase in adherence of platelets have been demonstrated experimentally. Copley (152, 153) has suggested that in addition to fibrin deposition and aggregation of cellular elements of blood, a time dependent progressive adsorption of certain other plasma proteins also contributes to thrombogenesis. If this indeed is true, this latter process could be enhanced due to the newly generated electrokinetic status of a particular artificial surface. Such a surface thus would become thrombogenic only after a certain period of time had elapsed even under laminar flow conditions.

It is obvious that thrombogeneity of artificial surfaces is a result of the interplay of a variety of factors. This complexity makes the task of elucidating the various mechanisms involved in thrombus formation difficult. Most certainly, rheologic factors and the chemical and physical nature of the particular artificial surface in contact with flowing blood all play important roles.

APPROACHES TO THE PREVENTION OF THROMBOSIS DURING HEMODIALYSIS

Practical approaches to prevention of thrombosis during hemodialysis include use of improved dialysis membranes, various modifications of surfaces of biomaterials, endothelizations of blood contacting surfaces, and use of soluble antithrombotic and antiplatelet agents. Membrane selection and improvement of membranes have been discussed fully in Chapter 4. Several new or improved membranes currently under clinical trial should provide, in the near future, surfaces that will be more compatible with blood than those presently available. Various modifications of blood contacting surfaces will be discussed below.

Effects of soluble antithrombotic or antiplatelet agents

Two undesirable but commonly observed events that frequently follow the extracorporeal circulation of blood are deposition of fibrin and adherence of platelets and leukocytes to the blood-contacting artificial surface. While anticoagulants such as heparin are effective in preventing the formation of fibrin, they generally have little inhibitory effect on platelet adherence at the concentrations commonly used clinically. Therefore, even with clinically adequate levels of a circulating anticoagulant such as heparin, the ability of platelets to adhere to artificial surfaces and the possibility of formation of platelet aggregates due to altered flow conditions remain relatively unchanged or may even be enhanced. It may be important in this context to note a recently published observation that suggests that heparin, at low concentration, can stimulate platelet aggregation, the platelet release reaction, and TXA$_2$ production in the presence of subthreshold concentrations of a variety of aggregating agents (154, 155). It may be difficult to avoid excessive shear stresses completely during extracorporeal circulation. Platelets and possibly other blood cells subjected to shear stresses could release small concentrations of substances such as ADP, serotonin, PAF, and TXA$_2$; such substances then could produce a substantial degree of platelet aggregation in the presence of heparin. Indeed, heparin enhances TXA_2 production in the presence of serotonin, ADP or thrombin (155).

One approach to overcoming injurious alteration of blood cells with subsequent enhancement of platelet aggregation has been the use of antiplatelet or antithrombotic drugs. Dipyridamole appears to be one of the agents of choice (156). Aspirin also has been shown to decrease the adhesion of platelets to hemodialysis membranes (157, 158) as has RA-233, an analogue of dipyridamole. However, in another study, Mielke et al. (159) found aspirin ineffective in extracorporeal circulation in oxygenators, while dipyridamole used under similar conditions was a markedly effective inhibitor of platelet stimulation. Recently, Gurewich and Lipinski (160) found suloctodil, a vascular antispasmodic, to be the most effective antithrombotic agent in a 3 drug trial in animal models of thrombosis. In the same study, dipyridamole was shown to be more effective than aspirin. Dipyridamole also inhibits fibrin deposition in experimental animal models of thrombosis (161). The drug has been shown to reduce effectively the thromboembolic complications associated with the use of prosthetic heart valves (162, 163). Sulfinpyrazone, another antiplatelet agent, also has been found effective in inhibiting thrombus formation when given to patients with prosthetic heart valves (164). Suggestions have been made in several publications that prostaglandin E_1 (PGE_1) (165, 166) and PGI_2, a potent platelet aggregation inhibitor synthesized predominantly by endothelial cells in vivo, might be important in preventing platelet aggregation. The possibility of using PGI_2 alone or in the presence of heparin in extracorporeal circulation of blood has been investigated in several laboratories with promising results. Coppe et al. (167) observed that PGI_2 prevented loss of platelets during extracorporeal circulation. Weston et al. (168) and Bunting and associates (169) found that PGI_2 prevents thrombocytopenia, adhesion of platelets to dialyzer surfaces, and microembolization. They also observed that in the presence of PGI_2 it was possible to perform dialysis without the presence of anticoagulants. These reports point to the possibility of using PGI_2 routinely in extracorporeal circulation in the future; hypotension is a significant side effect of PGI_2 use, however.

It has been observed that when the use of any one antiplatelet agent fails to prevent thrombosis, the use of a combination of two different agents often proves effective (170). Well designed extensive trials are in progress to test the effectiveness of a variety of antiplatelet agents in human subjects in which blood is exposed to artificial surfaces (156). Results obtained from such trials will be useful in establishing the relative efficacies of antiplatelet drugs in prevention of thromboembolism during hemodialysis. It should be pointed out, that though much attention has been focused on the clinical use of oxygenators or artificial heart valves, thromboembolic problems associated with the use of any artificial devices that contact blood are generally a clinically significant problem. Thus, an agent found to be effective in prevention of mural thrombosis on surfaces of any one type of artificial organ may well prove useful in preventing thromboembolic complications in hemodialyzers.

Although a number of antiplatelet agents are presently known, the effects of only a few of these drugs have been studied carefully in patients undergoing hemodialysis. Several symposia proceedings and reviews have appeared recently reporting the effectiveness of a number of antiplatelet drugs in prevention of thromboembolism (156, 171–173). In many cases, these antiplatelet agents have been evaluated critically.

Modifications of surfaces of biomaterials that contact blood

Heparinization of surfaces

Heparinized surfaces were developed by Gott and associates in the early 1960s, when artificial prosthetic valves were beginning to be used increasingly in open heart surgery (174). In their original method, an ionic binding of the negatively charged sulfate groups of the heparin molecule with a quarternary ammonium salt on a graphite polymer surface took place. This graphite-benzalkonium-heparin (GBH) surface showed remarkably good blood compatibility compared to surfaces such as glass, polycarbonate, or silicone. Unfortunately, it was found later that this GBH procedure could not be applied to flexible materials such as cellophane or polyvinyl chloride. In addition, desorption of heparin from the surface was found to occur rapidly.

Investigators at Batelle Laboratories (175) improved the GBH technique using chloromethylation of a polystyrene surface followed by quarternization with dimethyl aniline. Heparin can be attached to such a treated surface by ionic binding. Several polymer surfaces such as polyethylene, polyvinyl chloride, cellophane, and silicone rubber have been heparinized successfully by this technique. More recently, numerous other methods have been introduced for quarternization of polymer surfaces with subsequent binding of heparin by ionic forces. Yen and Rembaum (176) used a polyurethane containing pendant amino groups and quarternized these by treatment with hydrochloric acid. Merker et al. (177) introduced as a heparin binder a quarternized 3-amino-propyltriethoxysilane on the silica filler present in commercially available silicone rubber. Heparin milled into a silicone rubber (Hepacone) during fabrication was used by Hufnagel et al. (178). Grode and associates (179) succeeded in quarternizing a number of different polymers by use of an oil soluble quarternary ammonium salt, tridodecylmethylammonium chloride (TDMAC). A heating and cooling technique was used by Langeren and coworkers (180) to induce penetration of a cationic surfactant into polymer surfaces; heparin then could bind to the deeply deposited cationic sites. Chawla and Chang (181) used a radiation grafting method to achieve the binding of heparin to a cellulose membrane. An inorganic heparin complex system was used by Dyck (182) to prepare several 'nonthrombogenic' polymer surfaces. Martin et al. (183) have shown that quarternary ammonium salts of polymers containing tertiary amino groups such as ANDMAEMA (acrylonitrile-dimethylaminoethyl methacrylate) could be formed by treatment of the polymer surface with acid at 50 °C. Lindsay and associates (67) modified this procedure by further treatment of these membranes with ethylene oxide after heparin was bonded. A hydrophilic polymer surface that also binds heparin ionically was developed by Idezuki et al. (184). Cross-linking of TDMAC (185) or cationic bonded heparin (180) with 1% glutaraldehyde has been used successfully to reduce the desorption of heparin. Unfortunately, the surface-bonded heparin achieved by ionic exchange reactions has been shown to be unstable. Desorption and dissociation of heparin from polymer surfaces can occur under both *in vivo* and *in vitro* conditions unless heparin is bonded covalently to the substrate.

Attempts have been made to bond heparin covalently to polymer surfaces, since there are carboxylic groups, amino groups, and hydroxyl groups available on the heparin molecule. Leininger and his associates (186) have modified their previous efforts by developing a one step heparin-TDMAC complex for heparin binding. Halpern and Shibakawa (187) have shown that polystyrene can be converted into isocyanato-polystyrene, and that heparin can be coupled to this modified polystyrene by a formamide bond. A polymer with crosslinked heparin was prepared by Merrill et al. (188). In addition, these workers were able to attach heparin molecules to cellulose membranes with ethylene amine (189). Schmer (190, 191) has shown that amino groups of heparin can be attached to either substituted or unsubstituted agarose by cyanogen bromide activation as in peptide synthesis. Hoffman and coworkers (192) have shown that heparin and protein molecules can be bound covalently to radiation grafted hydrogels using an approach similar to that of Schmer. Surfaces with covalently bonded heparin have shown great improvement over surfaces with ionically bonded heparin with respect to decreased *in vitro* or *in vivo* leaching of the bound heparin. However, these surfaces still do not appear ideal, since complete prevention of thrombus formation has not been achieved to date (193).

Major problems in the early development of heparin-bonded surfaces for clinical usage were the slow leaching of heparin as well as leaching of toxic agents used in grafting and quarternizing polymer surfaces. The use of covalently bonded, heparinized surfaces has come close to solving the problem of desorption of heparin following exposure of heparinized surfaces to blood. However, in some cases these surfaces were found to be less effective in prevention of thrombosis than were ionically heparinized surfaces. This is most probably due to the fact that harsher conditions are required to attach heparin to polymers covalently than in the case with ionic attachments. These harsh conditions likely resulted in increased physical damage to the surface. Such changes as craze, roughness, and opacification were observed (194), but this is to be expected. In addition, the heterogeneity of heparin preparations used for virtually all studies may have contributed to some of the adverse effects. For example, it was shown that several commercial preparations of heparin could contain as many as 21 different components with molecular sizes ranging from 3,000 to 39,000. Only heparin of polymer size greater than 7,000 (66% of the total) has been shown to have anticoagulant activities (195). Recently, multiple functional domains of the heparin molecule have been shown by Oosta et al. (196). The conditions used to attach heparin to surfaces will undoubtedly cause denaturation and fragmentation of heparin molecules before, during, or after bonding. Another obvious disadvantage in grafting heparin to dialysis surfaces has been the resultant impairment of diffusion in these membranes. Further, radioautography of ^{35}S-heparin-coated surfaces has shown clearly that the surface concentration of heparin was nonhomogeneous for the several polymers tested. This nonuniformity of heparin distribution may permit the formation of small thrombi at specific loci deficient in bound heparin (197). Difficulties in sterilization of heparinized surfaces also have been encountered in clinical applications.

In order to develop a heparin-bonded surface that is highly thromboresistant, it is essential to understand the mechanisms by which such surfaces may interact with blood. Unfortunately, these mechanisms have not been elucidated clearly to date. An attractive hypothesis states that a microatmosphere of heparin is created at the polymer surface (194). Hence, according to this hypothesis a heparinized surface is simply serving as a heparin reservoir during contact with blood. However, recent progress in covalently bonding heparin seems to refute this hypothesis, since these new surfaces have been shown to be thromboresistant under conditions in which there is little or no evidence for desorption of heparin. Recent findings suggest that plasma proteins adsorbed to heparinized surfaces may play important roles in the interaction of these surfaces with other soluble plasma components and with blood cells. Heparinized surfaces are known not to activate Hageman factor (factor XII) (188). The patterns of radioactively labeled plasma proteins adsorbed to heparin bonded surfaces and to nonheparinized parent polymer surfaces are surprisingly similar (198). Preincubation of heparinized surfaces with albumin solutions resulted in some inhibition of platelet adhesion (198, 199), an effect found also with the same surfaces that had not been coated with heparin. Recently, heparin 'cofactors' have been eluted from heparinized surfaces and one of these has been identified as antithrombin III, an agent known to inhibit thrombin function (200, 201). However, it is highly likely that as yet unidentified proteins adsorb on heparin-bonded surface in minute quantities. These unidentified proteins may be responsible for the antithrombogenicity of heparinized surfaces. Highly sensitive techniques, such as radioimmunoassays, have been used (202, 203) to identify and quantitate plasma proteins adsorbed on artificial surfaces. These techniques may be applied also to identify and quantitate plasma protein(s) adsorbed to heparinized surfaces.

Other modifications of surfaces
The use of prostaglandin derivatives known to inhibit platelet functions to coat materials may be another approach to enhancing the blood compatibility of artificial surfaces. PGI_2 has been shown to be effective in reduc-

ing thrombogenesis (204), especially when it is used in combination with heparin (205). However, the short half life of PGI_2 in aqueous solutions (about 3.5 min) and the difficulty of conjugating PGI_2 to surfaces without reducing its potency make the use of surface-bound PGI_2 as a nonthrombogenic surface unattractive. The presence of heparin decreases the effect of PGI_2 on platelets (139). Grode et al. (206) have shown that artificial surfaces with covalently bound PGE_1 were effective in inhibition of platelet adherence. A controlled release of PGE_1 from polymer matrices has been designed and tested by McRea and Kim (207). PGE_1 was incorporated into Biomer and polyvinyl chloride during casting and was released at a slow rate from the polymer into the soluble phase. This system will not only protect the potency of PGE_1 but will permit the antithrombogenic effect to last for an extended period of time. Such a system may be applicable also to labile agents such as PGI_2. On the other hand, pharmacologists have searched vigorously in the past few years for analogues of PGI_2 that possess greater stability and are of equal or better potency. Several analogues are available at this time (208–211). However, the biological activities of those analogues, especially when used *in vivo* or *ex vivo* in humans have not been studied fully.

Surface passivation with adsorbed plasma protein
Passivation of hemodialysis or other materials with blood or blood components has attracted some attention in the past, since no artificial surfaces have been found to be totally unattractive to plasma proteins. Surfaces precoated with albumin (26, 212), gelatin (213), or whole blood (214) have been used with varying degrees of success. The use of platelet adhesion inhibitor (57, 85) and lipoprotein (58) as a precoating to discourage platelet interaction with artificial surface may be feasible also. The major task of 'passivation' is the immobilization of the precoated substances. Although formalin or glutaraldehyde seem to be highly effective in stabilizing precoated surfaces (213, 214), the leaching of those chemicals into blood is undesirable, since both are toxic. Furthermore, the passivated surface may not have a long effective lifespan, since new proteins or blood cellular components may be adsorbed to these stabilized coatings.

Reuse of a hemodialyzer by the same patient has been shown to produce a lesser degree thrombosis than use of a new device (see Chapter 15). The efficacy of dialysis with reused hemodialyzers surprisingly was found not to be diminished appreciably. Furthermore, with dialyzer reuse the cost reductions are substantial initially. However, because of the temporal limitations of dialyzer reuse with the same patient, the high risks of contamination with bacteria during flushing and storage, and the threat that toxic or immunologically active substances may leach from the sterilized dialyzer, this practice is not recommended generally by manufacturers.

Endothelialization of materials
A radically different approach to increase the blood compatibility of materials is to cover the material surface with a viable layer of endothelial cells (215). However, this approach remains academic because of the numerous problems concerning the growing of endothelial cells on artificial surfaces. Further, in clinical applications the endothelial cells must be obtained initially from the same patient who will use the cell-coated device. Whether an endothelial monolayer present on a hemodialysis membrane will decrease the efficiency of dialysis is unknown at present. Other cell types, such as fetal fibroblasts, have been used with some success in work with nonhuman mammals.

FINAL COMMENTS

Obviously much remains to be learned of the interactions of blood with artificial surfaces. The eventual goal of many workers in the artificial organs field is to design surfaces that are so highly compatible with blood as to permit use of artificial organs including hemodialyzers without the use of anticoagulant and antithrombotic agents. The pathway for attainment of this goal has not yet been clearly delineated. To date the ultimate answer does not appear to be in heparinization of surfaces. Perhaps the use of antithrombotic agents will decrease thromboembolism in patients who use artificial organs that contact blood, but this is not likely to be the final answer either. Efforts to produce polymer or metal surfaces that in themselves are highly compatible with blood have met with failure for the most part. This failure is largely due to our lack of knowledge of the mechanisms by which artificial surfaces activate blood coagulation system and permit adhesion and alteration of platelets and leukocytes. When these reactions are better understood, it may then be possible to devise means of inhibiting these activating mechanisms. The clinician, while impatient with the slow progress of the basic scientist in this area, must appreciate the magnitude of the problem. We must all await with patience the performance of the numerous and diverse studies now under way and hope that they will lead in the near future to a basic understanding of blood-artificial surface interactions and suggest methods for controlling these.

REFERENCES

1. Forbes CD, Prentice CRM: Thrombus formation and artificial surfaces. *Br Med Bull* 34:201, 1978
2. Lindsay RM, Mason RG, Kim SW, Andrade JD, Hakim RM: Blood surface interactions – report of ASAIO panel conference. *Trans Am Soc Artif Intern Organs* 26:603, 1980
3. Merrill EW: Properties of material affecting the behavior of blood at their surface. *Ann NY Acad Sci* 283:6, 1977
4. Andrade JD, Coleman DL, Van Wagener R: Perspectives and future developments in the field of blood-materials

interactions. In: *Interactions of the Blood with Natural and Artificial Surfaces,* edited by Salzman E, New York Marcel Dekker, 1981, p 201
5. Jackson CM, Nemerson Y: Blood coagulation. *Annu Rev Biochem* 49:765, 1980
6. Nemerson Y, Furie B: Zymogens and cofactors of blood coagulation. *CRC Crit Rev Biochem* 9:45, 1980
7. Lee WH Jr, Krumhaar D, Fonkalsrud EW, Scheide OA, Maloney JV Jr: Denaturation of plasma proteins as a cause of morbidity and death after intracardiac operations. *Surgery* 56:29, 1961
8. Wallace HW, Liquoir EM, Stein TP, Brooks H: Denatured plasma and platelet function. *Trans Am Soc Artif Intern Organs* 21:450, 1975
9. Nossel HL: Activation of factors XII and XI in thrombogenesis. *Bull NY Acad Med* 48:281, 1972
10. Cochrane CG, Revak SD, Wuepper KD: Activation of Hageman factor in solid and fluid phases. *J Exp Med* 138:1564, 1973
11. Schiffman S, Lee P: Partial purification and characterization of contact activation cofactor. *J Clin Invest* 56:1082, 1975
12. Griffin JH, Cochrane CG: Mechanisms for the involvement of high molecular weight kininogen in surface-dependent reactions of Hageman factor. *Proc Natl Acad Sci USA* 73:2554, 1976
13. Cochrane CG, Wiggins RC, Revak SD: Activation of the contact system on a surface. In *Hemostasis, Prostaglandins, and Renal Disease,* edited by Remuzzi G, Mecca G, de Gaetano G, New York, Raven Press, 1980, p 125
14. Silverberg M, Dunn JT, Garen L, Kaplan AP: Autoactivation of human Hageman factor. *J Biol Chem* 255:7281, 1980
15. Mannhalter C, Schiffman S: Surface adsorption of factor XI. Association of adsorption sites with the heavy chain of activated factor XI. *Thromb Haemost* 43:124, 1980
16. Vroman L, Adams AL: Possible involvement of fibrinogen and proteolysis in surface activation. *Thromb Diath Haemorrh* 18:510, 1967
17. Vroman L, Adams AL, Klings M: Interactions among human blood proteins at interfaces. *Fed Proc* 30:1494, 1971
18. Vroman L: What factors determine thrombogenicity? *Bull NY Acad Med* 48:302, 1972
19. Vroman L, Adams AL, Fischer GC, Munoz PC: Interaction of high molecular weight kininogen, factor XII, and fibrinogen in plasma at interfaces, *Blood* 55:156, 1980
20. Morrissey BW, Stromberg RR: The conformation of adsorbed blood proteins by infrared bound fraction measurements. *J Colloid Interface Sci* 46:152, 1976
21. Morrissey BW, Smith LE, Stromberg RR, Fenstermaker CA: Ellipsometric investigation of the effect of potential on blood protein conformation and adsorbance. *J Colloid Interface Sci* 56:557, 1976
22. Oja PD, Holmes GW: Specific coagulation factor adsorption as related to functional groups on surfaces. *J Biomed Mater Res* 3:165, 1969
23. Lyman DJ, Brash JL, Chikin SW, Klein KG, Carini M: The effect of chemical structure and surface properties of synthetic polymers on the coagulation of blood. II. Protein and platelet interaction on polymer surfaces. *Trans Am Soc Artif Intern Organs* 14:250, 1968
24. Brash H, Lyman DJ: Adsorption of plasma proteins in solution to uncharged, hydrophobic polymer surfaces. *J Biomed Mater Res* 3:175, 1969
25. Lyman DJ, Klein KG, Brash JL, Fritzinger BK: The interaction of platelets with polymer surfaces. I. Uncharged hydrophobic polymer surfaces. *Thromb Diath Haemorrh* 23:120, 1970
26. Brash JL, Lyman DJ: Adsorption of proteins and lipids to nonbiological surfaces. In *The Chemistry of Biosurfaces,* edited by Hair ML, New York, Marcel Dekker, 1971, vol 1, p 177
27. Friedman LI, Liem H, Grabowski EF, Leonard EF, McCord CW: Inconsequentiality of surface properties for initial platelet adhesion. *Trans Am Soc Artif Intern Organs* 16:63, 1970
28. Turitto VT, Leonard EF: Platelet adhesion to a spinning surface. *Trans Am Soc Artif Intern Organs* 18:348, 1972
29. Eberhart RC, Lynch ME, Bilge FH, Arts HA: Effects of fluid shear and temperature on protein adsorption on Teflon surfaces. *Trans Am Soc Artif Intern Organs* 26:185, 1980
30. Lee RG, Kim SW: Adsorption of proteins onto hydrophobic polymer surfaces: adsorption isotherms and kinetics. *J Biomed Mater Res* 8:251, 1974
31. Lee RG, Adamson C, Kim SW, Lyman DJ: Determination of the surface energy of proteinated polymer surfaces. *Thromb Res* 3:87, 1973
32. Waugh DF, Baughman DJ: Thrombin adsorption and possible relations to thrombus formation. *J Biomed Mater Res* 3:145, 1969
33. Waugh DF, Lippe JA, Freund Y: Interaction of bovine thrombin and plasma albumin with low-energy surfaces. *J Biomed Mat Res* 12:599, 1978
34. Chuang HYK, Sharma NC, Mohammad SF, Mason RG: Adsorption of thrombin onto artificial surfaces and its detection by an immunoradiometric assay. *Artif Organs* 3 (Suppl):226, 1979
35. Chuang HYK, Mohammad SF, Sharma NC, Mason RG: Interaction of human α-thrombin with artificial surfaces and reactivity of adsorbed α-thrombin. *J Biomed Mater Res* 14:467, 1980
36. Shuman MA, Tollefsen DM, Majerus PW: The binding of human and bovine thrombin to human platelets. *Blood* 47:43, 1976
37. Mohammad SF, Whitworth C, Chuang HYK, Lundblad RL, Mason RG: Multiple active forms of thrombin-binding to platelets and effects on platelet function. *Proc Natl Acad Sci USA* 73:1660, 1976
38. Didisheim P, Stropp JQ, Borowick JH, Grabowski AF: Species differences in platelet adhesion to biomaterials: investigation by a new two-stage technique. *asaio J* 2:124, 1979
39. Schultz JS, Lindenauer SM, Penner JA, Barenberg S: Determinants of thrombus formation on surfaces. *Trans Am Soc Artif Intern Organs* 26:279, 1980
40. Hanson SR, Harker LA, Ratner BD, Hoffman AS: In vivo evaluation of artificial surfaces with a nonhuman primate model of arterial thrombosis. *J Lab Clin Med* 95:289, 1980
41. Scarborough DE, Mason RG, Dalldorf EG, Brinkhous KM: Morphologic manifestations of blood-solid interfacial reactions. *Lab Invest* 20:164, 1969
42. Salzman EW: Role of platelets in blood-surface interactions. *Fed Proc* 30:1503, 1971
43. Salzman EW: Nonthrombogenic surfaces: critical review. *Blood* 38:509, 1971
44. Scarborough DE: The pathogenesis of thrombosis in artificial organs and vessels. *Curr Top Pathol* 54:95, 1971
45. Salzman EW: Surface effects in hemostasis and thrombosis. In *The Chemistry of Biosurfaces,* edited by Hair ML, New York, Marcel Dekker, 1972, vol 2, p 489
46. Baier RE, DePalma VA, Furuse A, Gott VL, Lucas T, Sawyer PN, Srinivasan S, Stanczweski B: Thrombo-resistance of glass cleaned by glow discharge treatment in argon. Abstracts *Am Soc Artif Intern Organs* 2:3, 1973
47. Lyman DJ, Klein KG, Brash JJ, Fritzinger BK, Andrade

JD, Bonomo FS: Platelet interaction with protein-coated surfaces: an approach to thrombo-resistant surfaces. In *Platelet Adhesion and Aggregation in Thrombosis: Countermeasures*, edited by Mammem EF, Anderson GF, Barnhard MI, Stuttgart FRG, FK Schattauer Verlag, 1970, p 109
48. Evans G, Mustard JF: Platelet-surface reaction and thrombosis. *Surgery* 64:273, 1968
49. Zucker MB, Vroman L: Platelet adhesion induced by fibrinogen adsorbed onto glass. *Proc Soc Exp Biol Med* 131:318, 1969
50. Packham MA, Evans G, Glynn MF, Mustard JF: The effect of plasma proteins on the interaction of platelets with glass surfaces. *J Lab Clin Med* 73:686, 1969
51. Mason RG, Read MS, Brinkhous KM: Effect of fibrinogen concentration on platelet adhesion to glass. *Proc Soc Exp Biol Med* 137:680, 1971
52. Mason RG, Shermer RW, Zucker WH: Effects of certain purified plasma proteins on the compatibility of glass with blood. *Am J Pathol* 73:183, 1973
53. George JN: Direct assessment of platelet adhesion to glass: a study of the forces of interaction and the effects of plasma and serum factors, platelet function, and modification of the glass surface. *Blood* 40:862, 1972
54. Mohammad SF, Hardison MD, Glenn CH, Morton BD, Bolan JC, Mason RG: Adhesion of human blood platelets to glass and polymer surfaces. I. Studies with platelets in plasma. *Haemostasis* 3:257, 1974
55. Andrade JD, Kunitomo K, Van Wagenen R, Kastigir B, Gough D, Kolff WJ: Coated adsorbents for direct blood perfusion: hema/activated carbon. *Trans Am Soc Artif Intern Organs* 17:222, 1971
56. Andrade JD: Interfacial phenomena and biomaterials. *Med Instrum* 7:110, 1973
57. Mohammad SF, Hardison MD, Chuang HYK, Mason RG: Adhesion of human blood platelets to glass and polymer surfaces. II. Demonstration of the presence of a natural platelet adhesion inhibitor in plasma and serum. *Haemostasis* 5:96, 1976
58. Sharma NC, Mohammad SF, Chuang HYK, Mason RG: Inhibition of platelet adhesion to glass by certain human plasma and serum proteins. *asio J* 3:43, 1980
59. Sharma NC, Mohammad SF, Chuang HYK, Mason RG: Isolation and some of the physiochemical and immunologic properties of a platelet adhesion inhibitor from human serum. *Thromb Res* 17:683, 1980
60. Leininger RI, Mirkovitch V, Beck RE, Andrus PG, Kolff WJ: The zeta potentials of some selected solids in respect to plasma and plasma fractions. *Trans Am Soc Artif Intern Organs* 10:239, 1964
61. Baier RE, Gott VL, Feruse A: Surface chemical evaluation of thromboresistant materials before and after venous implantation. *Trans Am Soc Artif Intern Organs* 16:50, 1970
62. Lee RG, Adamson C, Kim SW: Competitive adsorption of plasma proteins onto polymer surfaces. *Thromb Res* 4:485, 1974
63. Kaelble DH, Moacanin J: A surface energy analysis of bioadhesion. *Polymer* 18:475, 1977
64. Lee RG, Kim SW: The role of carbohydrate in platelet adhesion to foreign surfaces. *J Biomed Mater Res* 8:393, 1974
65. Barber TA, Lambrecht LK, Mosher DL, Cooper SL: Influence of serum proteins on thrombosis and leukocyte adherence on polymer surfaces. *Scan Electron Microsc* 3:881, 1979
66. Salzman EW, Merrill EW, Binder A, Wolf CFW, Ashford TP, Austen WG: Protein-platelet interaction on heparinized surfaces. *J Biomed Mater Res* 3:69, 1969
67. Lindsay RM, Rourke J, Reid B, Friesen M, Linton AL, Courtney J, Gilchrist, T: Platelets, foreign surfaces, and heparin. *Trans Am Soc Artif Intern Organs* 22:292, 1976
68. Mason RG: The interaction of blood hemostatic elements with artificial surfaces. *Prog Hemost Thromb* 1:141, 1972
69. Berger S, Salzman EW, Merrill EW, Wong PSL: The reaction of platelets with prosthetic surfaces. In *Platelets: Production, Function, Transfusion and Storage*, edited by Baldini MG, Ebbe S, New York, Grune and Stratton, 1974, p 299
70. Berger S, Salzman EW: Thromboembolic complications of prosthetic devices. *Prog Hemost Thromb* 2:273, 1974
71. Mason RG, Mohammad SF, Chuang HYK, Richardson PD: The adhesion of platelets to subendothelium, collagen and artificial surfaces. *Semin Thromb Hemostas* 3:98, 1976
72. Weathersby PK, Horbett TA, Hoffman AS: A new method for analysis of the adsorbed plasma protein layer on biomaterial surfaces. *Trans Am Soc Artif Intern Organs* 22:242, 1976
73. Brown CH III, Lemuth RF, Hellums JD, Leverett LB, Alfrey CP: Response of human platelets to shear stress. *Trans Am Soc Artif Intern Organs* 21:35, 1975
74. Brown CH III, Leverett LB, Lewis SW, Alfrey CP Jr, Hellums JD: Morphological, biochemical, and functional changes in human platelets subjected to shear stress. *J Lab Clin Med* 86:462, 1975
75. Johnston GG, Marzec U, Bernstein EF: Effects of surface injury and shear stress on platelet aggregation and serotonin release. *Trans Am Soc Artif Intern Organs* 21:413, 1975
76. Roohk HV, Pick J, Hill R, Hung E, Bartlett RH: Kinetics of fibrinogen and platelet adherence to biomaterials. *Trans Am Soc Artif Intern Organs* 22:1, 1976
77. Hung TC, Hochmuth RM, Joist JH, Sutera SP: Shear-induced aggregation and lysis of platelets. *Trans Am Soc Artif Intern Organs* 22:285, 1976
78. Butruille YA. Leonard EF. Litwak RS: Platelet-platelet interactions and non-adhesive encounters on biomaterials. *Trans Am Soc Artif Intern Organs* 21:609, 1975
79. Whicher JS, Uniyal S, Brash JL: Platelet-foreign surface interactions: the release reaction from singly adherent platelets and adherent platelet aggregates. *Trans Am Soc Artif Intern Organs* 26:268, 1980
80. Clagett GP, Russo M, Hufnagle H, Collins GJ Jr, Rich NM: Platelet serotonin changes in dogs with prosthetic aortic grafts. *J Surg Res* 28:223, 1980
81. Malmgren R, Larsson R, Olsson P, Radegran K: Serotonin uptake and release by platelets adhering to polyethylene. *Haemostasis* 8:400, 1979
82. Chignard M, LeCouedic JP, Tence M, Vargaftig BB, Benveniste J: The role of platelet-activating factor in platelet aggregation. *Nature* 279:799, 1979
83. Chap H, Mauco G, Simon MF, Benveniste J, Douste-Blazy L: Biosynthetic labelling of platelet activating factor from radioactive acetate by stimulated platelets. *Nature* 289:312, 1981
84. Sharma NC, Mohammad SF, Chuang HYK, Mason RG: Isolation and physiochemical and immunologic characterization of human platelet factor 3. *Thromb Res* 16:673, 1979
85. Sharma NC, Mohammad SF, Chuang HYK, Mason RG: Characterization of a platelet adhesion inhibitor from human serum and plasma as a complex of albumin with immunoglobulin G. *Fed Proc* 40:810, 1981
86. Mustard JF, Packham MA, Kinlough-Rathbone RL, Perry DW, Regoeezi E: Fibrinogen and ADP-induced platelet

aggregation. *Blood* 52:453, 1978
87. Marguerie GA, Plow EF, Edgington TS: Human platelets possess an inducible and saturable receptor specific for fibrinogen. *J Biol Chem* 254:5357, 1979
88. Tomikawa M, Iwamoto M, Soderman S, Blomback R: Effect of fibrinogen on ADP-induced platelet aggregation. *Thromb Res* 19:841, 1980
89. Osterud B, Rapaport SI, Lavine KL: Factor V activity of platelets: evidence for an activated factor V molecule and for a platelet activator. *Blood* 49:819, 1977
90. Vicic WJ, Lages B, Weiss HJ: Release of human platelet factor V activity is induced by both collagen and ADP and is inhibited by aspirin. *Blood* 56:448, 1980
91. Miletich JP, Jackson CM, Majerus PW: Interaction of coagulation factor Xa with human platelets. *Proc Natl Acad Sci USA* 74:4033, 1977
92. Miletich JP, Jackson CM, Majerus PW: Properties of the factor Xa binding site on human platelets. *J Biol Chem* 253:6908, 1978
93. Lipcomb MS, Walsh PN: Human platelets and factor XI. Localization in platelet membranes of factor XI like activity and its functional distinction from plasma factor XI. *J Clin Invest* 63:1006, 1977
94. Walsh PN, Griffin JH: Contributions of human platelets to the proteolytic activation of blood coagulation factors XII and XI. *Blood* 57:106, 1981
95. Kaplan KL, Owen J: Plasma levels of β-thromboglobulin and platelet factor 4 as indices of platelet activation in vivo. *Blood* 57:199, 1981
96. Kaplan KL, Owen J: Radioimmunoassay of platelet factor 4, in *Methods in Enzymology*, edited by Vunakis HV, Langone JJ, New York, Academic Press, 70, 1981, p 226
97. McGregor JL, Clemetson KJ, James E, Luscher EF, Dechavanne M: Characterization of human blood platelet membrane proteins and glycoproteins by their isoelectric point (pI) and apparent molecular weight using two-dimensional electrophoresis and surface-labelling techniques. *Biochim Biophys Acta* 599:473, 1980
98. Ganguly P, Fossett NG: Inhibition of thrombin-induced platelet aggregation by a derivative of wheat germ agglutinin. Evidence for a physiologic receptor of thrombin in human platelets. *Blood* 57:343, 1981
99. Hennessy VL Jr, Hicks RE, Niewiarowski S, Edmunds LH Jr, Coleman RW: Function of human platelets during extracorporeal circulation. *Am J Physiol* 232:4622, 1977
100. Clagett GP, Russo M, Hufnagle H: Platelet changes after placement of aortic prostheses in dogs. *J Lab Clin Med* 97:345, 1981
101. Harker LA, Malpass TW, Branson HE, Hessel EA II, Slichter SJ: Mechanism of abnormal bleeding in patients undergoing cardiopulmonary bypass: acquired transient platelet dysfunction associated with selective–granule release. *Blood* 56:824, 1980
102. Kaplow JS, Goffinet JA: Profound neutropenia during the early phase of hemodialysis. *JAMA* 203:1335, 1968
103. Toren M, Goffinet JA, Kaplow LS: Pulmonary bed sequestration of neutrophils during hemodialysis. *Blood* 36:337, 1970
104. Jensen DP, Brubaker LH, Nolph KD, Johnson CA, Nothum RJ: Hemodialysis coil-induced transient neutropenia and overshoot neutrophilia in normal man. *Blood* 41:399, 1973
105. O'Flaherty J, Craddock PR, Jacob US: Altered granulocyte adhesiveness (GA) during in vivo complement (C) activation. *Blood* 48:987, 1976
106. Wauters JP, Lambert PH: Hemodialysis induced leukopenia: role of cellophane membrane and complement activation. *Kidney Int* (Abstract) 12:77, 1977
107. Aljama P, Bird PAE, Ward MK, Feest TG, Walker W, Tanboga H, Sussman M, Kerr DNS: Haemodialysis-induced leukopenia and activation of complement: effects of different membranes. *Proc Eur Dial Transpl Assoc* 15:144, 1978
108. Skubitz KM, Craddock PR: Reversal of hemodialysis granulocytopenia and pulmonary leukostasis. *J Clin Invest* 67:1383, 1981
109. Zacharski LR, McIntyre OR: Membrane-mediated synthesis of tissue factor (thromboplastin) in cultured fibroblasts. *Blood* 41:679, 1973
110. Garg SK, Niemetz J: Tissue factor activity of normal and leukemic cells. *Blood* 42:729, 1973
111. Rickles FR, Hardin JA, Pitlick FA, Hoger LW, Conrad ME: Tissue factor activity in lymphocyte cultures from normal individuals and patients with hemophilia A. *J Clin Invest* 52:1427, 1973
112. Rapaport SI, Hjost PF: The blood clotting properties of rabbit peritoneal leukocytes in vitro. *Thromb Diath Haemorrh* 17:222, 1967
113. Kociba GJ, Griesemer RA: Disseminated intravascular coagulation induced with leukocyte procoagulant. *Am J Path* 69:407, 1972
114. Saba HI, Herion JC, Walker RJ, Roberts HR: Effect of lysosomal cationic proteins from polymorphonuclear leukocytes upon the fibrinogen and fibrinolysis system. *Thromb Res* 7:543, 1975
115. Niemetz J, Muhlfelder T, Chievego ME, Troy B: Procoagulant activity of leukocytes. *Ann NY Acad Sci* 283:208, 1977
116. Camussi G, Mencia-Huerta JM, Benveniste J: Release of platelet activating factor and histamine. I. Effect of immune complexes, complement and neutrophils on human and rabbit mastocytes and basophils. *Immunology* 33:523, 1977
117. Morley J, Bray MA, Jones RW, Nugtenen DH, Van Dorp DA: Prostaglandin and thromboxane production by human and guinea-pig macrophages and leukocytes. *Prostaglandins* 17:729, 1979
118. Beckman RS: Prostaglandin production by human blood monocytes and mouse peritoneal macrophages: synthesis dependent on in vivo culture conditions. *Protaglandins* 21:9, 1981
119. Dutton RC, Webber AJ, Johnson SA, Baier RE: Microstructure of initial thrombus formation on foreign materials. *J Biomed Mater Res* 3:13, 1969
120. Baier RE. Dutton RC: Initial events in interactions of blood with a foreign surface. *J Biomed Mater Res* 3:191, 1969
121. Ahearn DJ, Marshall JW, Nothum RJ, Esterly JA, Nolph KD, Maher JF: Morphologic studies of dialysis membranes–adherence of blood components to air rinsed coils. *Trans Am Soc Artif Intern Organs* 19:435, 1973
122. Mason RG, Wolf RH, Zucker WH, Shinoda BA: Dynamics of thrombus formation upon an artificial surface in vivo: effects of antithrombotic agents. *Am J Path* 82:187, 1978
123. Mason RG, Zucker WH, Bilinsky RT, Shinoda BA, Mohammad SF: Blood components deposited on used and reused dialysis membranes. *Biomater Med Devices Artif Organs* 4:333, 1976
124. Lindsay RM, Prentice CRM, Burton JA, Ferguson D, Kennedy AC: The role of the platelet-dialysis membrane interaction in thrombus formation and blood loss during hemodialysis. *Trans Am Soc Artif Intern Organs* 19:487, 1973
125. Bjornson J, Kierulf P, Eika C, Godal HC: Fibrin deposits in the Kiil dialyzer. *Scand J Haematol* 11:379, 1973
126. Marshall JW, Ahearn DJ, Nothum RJ, Esterly J, Nolph

KD, Maher JF: Adherence of blood components to dialyzer membranes. Morphological studies. *Nephron* 12:157, 1974
127. Schwartz GH, Stenzel RH, Kohno I, Ast D, Miyata T, Rubin AL: Deposition of blood cells on collagen and Cuprophane membranes. *J Biomed Mater Res* 9:453, 1975
128. Bilinsky RT, Morris AJ: Hemodialysis coil reuse. *JAMA* 218:1806, 1971
129. Siemsen AW, Lumeng J, Wong EGC, Wong LMF, Ching A, Ennio JA, McGowan RF: Clinical laboratory evaluation of coil reuse. *Trans Am Soc Artif Intern Organs* 20:585, 1974
130. Kramer P, Matthaei D, Go JG, Winckler K, Schieler F: Effect of blood factor deposits in reused dialysers on the dialysance of middle weight molecules. *Proc Eur Dial Transpl Assoc* 9:278, 1972
131. George JN, Weed RI, Reed CF: Adhesion of human erythrocytes to glass: the nature of the interaction and the effect of serum and plasma. *J Cell Physiol* 77:51, 1971
132. Hochmuth RM, Mohandas N, Spaeth EE, Williamson JR, Blackshear PL Jr, Johnson DW: Surface adhesion, deformation and detachment at low shear of red cells and white cells. *Trans Am Soc Artif Intern Organs* 18:325, 1972
133. Goldsmith HL: The flow of model particles and blood cells and its relation to thrombogenesis. *Prog Hemostas Thromb* 1:97, 1972
134. Goldsmith HL: The effects of flow and fluid mechanical stress on red cells and platelets. *Trans Am Soc Artif Intern Organs* 20:21, 1974
135. Bartett K, Forstrom R, Blackshear PL Jr: Blood platelet deposition onto filtering surfaces – effect of concentration polarization. Abstracts *Am Soc Artif Intern Organs* 5:7, 1976
136. Forstrom RJ, Bartlett K, Blackshear PL Jr, Wood T: Formed element deposition onto filtering walls. *Trans Am Soc Artif Intern Organs* 21:602, 1975
137. Wessler S, Gitel S: Control of heparin therapy. *Prog Hemost Thromb* 3:311, 1976
138. Lindsay RM, Prentice CRM, Davidson JF, Burton JA, McNicol GP: Haemostatic changes during dialysis associated with thrombus formation on dialysis membranes. *Br Med J* 2:454, 1972
139. Saba HI, Saba SR, Blackburn CA, Hartman RC, Mason RG: Heparin neutralization of PGI_2: effects upon platelets. *Science* 205:499, 1979
140. Charm S, Kurland GS: Viscometry of human blood for shear rates of 0–100,000 sec^{-1}. *Nature* 206:617, 1965
141. Copley AL, Scott-Blair GW: Hemorheological method for the study of blood systems and of processes in blood coagulation. In *Flow Properties of Blood*, edited by Copley AL, Stainsby G, London, Pergamon Press, 1960, p 412
142. Rand PW, Lacombe E, Hunt HE, Austin WH: Viscosity of normal human blood under normothermic and hypothermic conditions. *J Appl Physiol* 19:117, 1964
143. Peric B: Viscosity of the blood at low shear rates. *Isr J Exp Med* 11:139, 1963
144. Blackshear PL Jr, Forstrom RJ, Dorman FD, Voss GO: Effect of flow on cells near walls. *Fed Proc* 30:1600, 1971
145. Goldsmith HL: Red cell motions and wall interactions in tube flow. *Fed Proc* 30:1578, 1971
146. Grabowski EF, Friedman LI, Leonard EF: Effects of shear rates on the diffusion and adhesion of blood platelets to a foreign surface. *Indust Eng Chem Fundam* 11:224, 1972
147. Nevaril CG, Lynch EC, Alfrey CP Jr, Hellums JD: Erythrocyte damage and destruction induced by shear stress. *J Lab Clin Med* 71:784, 1968
148. Bernstein EF: Certain aspects of blood interfacial phenomena – red blood cells. *Fed Proc* 30:1510, 1971
149. MacCallum RN, O'Bannon W, Hellums JD, Alfrey CP, Lynch EC: Viscometric instruments for studies on red blood cell damage. In *Rheology of Biological Systems*, edited by Gabelnick HL, Litt M, Springfield, IL, Charles C. Thomas, 1973, p 70
150. Solen KA, Whiffen JD, Lightfoot EN: The effect of shear, specific surface and air interface on the developments of blood emboli and hemolysis. *J Biomed Mater Res* 12:381, 1978
151. Brown CH III, Lemuth RF, Hellums JD, Leverett LB, Alfrey CP: Response of human platelets to shear stress. *Trans Am Soc Artif Intern Organs* 21:35, 1973
152. Copley AL: Hemorheological aspects of the endothelium-plasma interface. *Microvasc Res* 8:192, 1974
153. Copley AL: Non-newtonian behavior of surface layers of human plasma protein systems and a new concept of the initiation of thrombosis. *Biorheology* 10:541, 1971
154. Anderson WH, Mohammad SF, Chuang HYK, Mason RG: Heparin potentiates synthesis of thromboxane A_2 in human platelets. *Adv Prostaglandin Thromboxane Res* 6:287, 1980
155. Mohammad SF, Anderson WH, Smith JB, Chuang HYK, Mason RG: Effects of heparin on platelet aggregation, release reaction and thromboxane A_2 production. *Am J Pathol*, 104:132, 1981
156. Harker LA, Hirsch J, Gent M, Genton E: Critical evaluation of platelet inhibiting drugs in thrombotic disease. *Prog Hematol* 9:229, 1975
157. Stewart JH, Farrell PC, Dixon M: Reduction of platelet and fibrin deposition in haemodialysers by aspirin administration. *Aust NZ J Med* 5:117, 1975
158. Lindsay RM, Prentice CRM, Ferguson D, Burton JA, McNicol GP: Reduction of thrombus formation on dialyser membranes by aspirin and RA 233. *Lancet* 2:1287, 1972
159. Mielke CH, deLeval M, Hill JD, Macur MF, Gerbode F: Drug influence on platelet loss during extracorporeal circulation. *J Thorac Cardiovas Surg* 66:845, 1973
160. Gurewich V, Lipinski B: Evaluation of antithrombotic properties of 'Suloctodil' in comparison with aspirin and dipyridamole. *Thromb Res* 9:101, 1976
161. Gurewich V, Lipinski B, Wetmore R: Inhibition of intravascular fibrin deposition by dipyridamole in experimental animals. *Blood* 45:569, 1975
162. Harker LA, Slichter SJ: Studies of platelets and fibrinogen kinetics in patients with prosthetic heart valves. *N Engl J Med* 293:1302, 1970
163. Arrants JE, Hairston P, Lee WH Jr: Use of dipyridamole in preventing thromboembolism following valve replacement. *Chest* 58:275, 1970
164. Welly HS, Genton E: Altered platelet function in patients with prosthetic mitral valves – effect of sulfinpyrazone therapy. *Circulation* 42:967, 1970
165. Addonizio VP, Macarak EJ, Niewiarowski S, Colman RW, Edmunds LH: Preservation of human platelets with PGE_1 during in vitro cardiopulmonary bypass. *Trans Am Soc Artif Intern Organs* 23:639, 1977
166. Addonizio VP, Strauss JF, Macavak EJ, Colman RW, Edmunds LH: Preservation of platelet number and function with PGE_1 during total cardiopulmonary bypass in rhesus monkeys. *Surgery* 83:619, 1978
167. Coppe D, Wonders T, Snider M, Salzman EW: Preservation of platelet number and function during extracorporeal membrane oxygenation by regional infusion of prostacyclin. In *Prostacyclin*, edited by Vane JR, Bergstrom S, New York, Raven Press, 1979, p 385
168. Weston, MJ, Woods HF, Ash G, Bunting S, Moncada S, Vane JR: Prostacyclin as an alternative to heparin in

dogs. In *Prostacyclin,* edited by Vane JR, Bergstrom S, New York, Raven Press, 1979, p 349
169. Bunting S, Moncada S, Vane J, Woods HF, Weston MJ: Prostacyclin improves hemocompatibility during charcoal hemoperfusion. In *Prostacyclin,* edited by Vane JR, Bergstrom S, New York Raven Press, 1979, p 361
170. Harker LA: In vivo evaluation of antithrombin therapy in man. *Thromb Diath Haemorrh* 60 (suppl):481, 1974
171. Didisheim P, Shimomoto T, Yamazaki H: Platelets, thrombosis and inhibitors. *Thromb Diath Haemorrh* 60 (suppl), 1974
172. Mason RG, Sargi K, Brinkhous KM: Antithrombotic agents – their effects on platelets and methods for their evaluation. In *Cardiovascular Drugs,* edited by McMahon FG, New York, Futura, 1974, p 183
173. Hirsh J, Cade JF, Gallus AS, Schonbaum E: *Platelet, Drugs and Thrombosis.* New York, Basel, Karger S, 1975
174. Gott VL: Wall-bound heparin – historical background and current clinical applications. *Adv Exp Med Biol* 52:351, 1974
175. Leininger RI, Cooper CW, Epstein MM, Falb RD, Grode GA: Nonthrombogenic plastic surfaces. *Science* 152:1625, 1966
176. Yen SPS, Rembaum A: Complexes of heparin with elastomeric positive polyelectrolytes. *J Biomed Mater Res* 1:83, 1971
177. Merker RI, Elyash LJ, Mayhew SH, Wany JYC: The heparinization of silicone rubber using aminoorganosilane coupling agents. *Artificial Heart Program Conference,* edited by Hagyeli RJ, National Heart Institute, Washington DC, 1969, p 29
178. Hufnagel CA, Conrad PW, Gillespie JF, Pifarre R, Ilano A, Yokoyama T: Comparative study of cardiac and vascular implants in relation to thrombosis. *Surgery* 61:11, 1967
179. Grode GA, Anderson SJ, Crotte HM, Falb RD: Nonthrombogenic materials via a simple coating process. *Trans Am Soc Artif Intern Organs* 15:1, 1969
180. Lagergren HR, Eriksson JC: Plastics with a stable surface monolayer of cross-linked heparin – preparation and evaluation. *Trans Am Soc Artif Intern Organs* 17:10, 1971
181. Chawla AS, Chang TMS: Nonthrombogenic surface by radiation grafting of heparin – preparation, *in vitro* and *in vivo* studies. *Biomater Med Devices Artif Organs* 2:157, 1974
182. Dyck MF: Inorganic heparin complexes for the preparation of nonthrombogenic surfaces. *J Biomed Mater Res* 6:115, 1972
183. Martin RE, Shuey HF, Saltonstall GW Jr: Improved membranes for hemodialysis. *J Macromol Sci Chem A* 4:635, 1970
184. Idezuki Y, Watanabe H, Hagiwara M, Kanasugi K, Mori Y, Nagaoka S, Hagio M, Yamamoto K, Tanjawa H: Mechanism of antithrombogenicity of a new heparinized hydrophilic polymer: Chronic in vivo studies and clinical application. *Trans Am Soc Artif Intern Organs* 21:436, 1975
185. Eberle JW, Manton JR, Meals CR, Whitley DE, Rea WJ: Cross-linked heparin binding of a membrane oxygenator system. *J Biomed Mater Res* 7:145, 1973
186. Leininger RI, Crowley JP, Falb RD, Grode GA: Three year's experience in vivo and in vitro with surfaces and devices treated by the heparin complex method. *Trans Am Soc Artif Intern Organs* 18:312, 1972
187. Halpern BD, Shibakawa R: Heparin covalently bonded to polymer surface. *Adv Chem Ser* 87:197, 1968
188. Merrill EW, Salzman EW, Wong PSL, Ashford TP, Brown AH, Austen WG: Polyvinyl alcohol-heparin hydrogel 'G'. *J Appl Physiol* 29:723, 1970
189. Merrill EW, Salzman EW, Lipps BJ Jr, Gilliland ER, Austen WG, Joison E: Antithrombogenic cellulose membranes for blood dialysis. *Trans Am Soc Artif Intern Organs* 12:139, 1966
190. Schmer G: The biological activity of covalently immobilized heparin. *Trans Am Soc Artif Intern Organs* 18:321, 1972
191. Schmer G, Teng LNL, Cole JJ, Vizzo JE, Francisco MM, Scribner BH: Successful use of a totally heparin grafted hemodialysis system in sheep. *Trans Am Soc Artif Intern Organs* 22:654, 1976
192. Hoffman AS, Schmer G, Harris C, Kraft WG: Covalent binding of biomolecules to radiation-grafted hydrogel on inert polymer surfaces. *Trans Am Soc Artif Intern Organs* 18:10, 1972
193. Lansson R, Eriksson JC, Lagesgren H, Olsson P: Platelet and plasma coagulation compatibility of heparinized and sulphated surface. *Thromb Res* 15:157, 1979
194. Falb RD, Leininger RI, Grode G, Crowley J: Surface-bound heparin. *Adv Exp Med Biol* 52:365, 1974
195. Nader HG, McDuffe NM, Diettich CP: Heparin fractionation by electrofocusing. Presence of 21 components of different molecular weights. *Biochem Biophys Res Commun* 57:488, 1974
196. Oosta GM, Gardner WT, Beeler DL, Rosenberg RD: Multiple functional domains of the heparin molecule. *Proc Natl Acad Sci USA,* 78:829, 1981
197. Stewart GP, Wilkow MA: Mechanism of failure of biocompatible-treated surfaces. *J Biomed Mater Res* 10:413, 1976
198. Falb RD, Takahashi MT, Grode GA, Leininger RI: Studies on the stability and protein adsorption characteristics of heparinized polymer surfaces by radioisotopic labeling techniques. *J Biomed Mater Res* 1:239, 1967
199. Coleman DL, Atwood AI, Andrade JD: Platelet retention by albuminated glass and polystyrene beads. *J Bioengineering* 1:33, 1976
200. Gentry PW, Alexander B: Specific coagulation factor adsorption to insoluble heparin. *Biochem Biophys Res Commun* 50:500, 1973
201. Thaler E, Schmer G: A simple 2-step isolation procedure for human antithrombin II/III and its biological activity after insolubilization to agarose. *Trans Am Soc Artif Intern Organs* 20:516, 1974
202. Chuang HYK, Crowther PE, Mohammad SF, Mason RG: Identification and quantitation of plasma proteins adsorbed to artificial surfaces by use of ^{125}I-labeled specific antibodies. *Fed Proc* 37:444, 1978
203. Chuang HYK, Mohammad SF, Sharma NC, Mason RG: Radioimmunoassays of human fibrinogen and α-thrombin adsorbed to artificial surfaces. *Fed Proc* 40:806, 1981
204. Woods HF, Ash G, Weston MH, Bunting S, Moncada S, Vane JR: Prostacyclin can replace heparin in haemodialysis in dogs. *Lancet* 2:1075, 1978
205. Turney JH, Woods HF, Weston MJ: The use of prostacyclin in extracorporeal circuits. In *Hemostasis, Prostaglandins, and Renal Disease,* edited by Remuzzi G, Mecca G, Gaetano G, New York, Raven Press, 1981, p 353
206. Grode GA, Putman J, Crowley, Leininger RI, Falb RD: Surface-immobilized prostaglandin as a platelet protective agent. *Trans Am Soc Artif Intern Organs* 20:38, 1974
207. McRea JC, Kim SW: Characterization of controlled release of prostaglandin from polymer matrices for thrombus prevention. *Trans Am Soc Artif Intern Organs* 24:746, 1978
208. Van Drup DA, Van Evert WC, Van der Wolf L: 20-methylprostacyclin, a powerful unnatural platelet aggrega-

tion inhibitor. *Prostaglandins* 16:953, 1978
209. Dembinska-Kiec A, Rucker W, Schomhofer PS, Gandolf C: Prostacyclin analogs: antiaggregatory potency and enhancement of cAMP levels in human platelet rich plasma. *Thromb Haemost* 42:1340, 1979
210. Whittle BJR, Moncada S, Whiting F, Vane JR: Carbacyclin – a potent stable prostacyclin analogue for the inhibition of platelet aggregation. *Prostaglandins* 19:605, 1980
211. Malmstem C, Claesson HE: Inhibition of platelet aggregation and elevation of cyclic-AMP levels in platelets by 13, 14-dehydro PGI_2 methyl ester. *Prostaglandins Med* 4:453, 1980
212. Imai Y, Tajima K, Nosé Y: Biolized materials for cardiovascular prosthesis. *Trans Am Soc Artif Intern Organs* 17:6, 1971
213. Havasaki H, Kivaly R, Murabayashi S, Pepoy M, Fields A, Kambic H, Hillegass D, Nose Y: Cross-linked gelatin as a blood contacting surface. *Proc 2nd Meeting of ISAO,* 1979, p 203
214. Kambic H, Barenburg S, Havasaki H, Gibbons D, Kiraly R, Nose Y: Glutaraldehyde-protein complexes as blood compatible coatings. *Trans Am Soc Artif Intern Organs* 24:426, 1978
215. Mansfield PB, Wechezak AR, Sauvage LR: Preventing thrombus on artificial vascular surfaces: true endothelial cell linings. *Trans Am Soc Artif Intern Organs* 21:264, 1975

10

PRACTICAL USE OF ANTICOAGULANTS

ROBERT M. LINDSAY

Introduction	201
A summary of the hemostatic system	201
Platelets and platelet function	204
The basic platelet reaction	204
Induction	205
Transmission	205
Execution – the four stages	205
Coagulation tests and their use	206
Test of procoagulants	206
The partial thromboplastin time	206
The prothrombin time	206
The thrombin time	206
Reptilase time	206
Fibrinopeptide A	206
Fibrinogen	206
Fibrin-fibrinogen degradation products	206
Tests for monitoring dialysis anticoagulation	207
Whole blood clotting time	207
Whole blood activated clotting time	207
Whole blood activated partial thromboplastin time	207
Tests of platelet function	207
Peripheral smear evaluation and platelet count	207
Bleeding time	207
Platelet aggregometry	208
Platelet factor 4 and betathromboglobulin estimation	208
Anticoagulants	208
Heparin	208
Coumarin or indanedione anticoagulant drugs	209
Fibrinolytic agents	209
The conceptual basis for fibrinolytic therapy	210
Streptokinase	210
Urokinase	210
EACA and antiplasmins	210
The Sherry hypothesis	211
Ancrod	211
Antiplatelet agents	211
Inhibitors of induction	211
Inhibitors of early transmission	211
Inhibitors of late transmission	212
Inhibitors of execution	212
Antiplatelet agents: effect on vessel wall prostacyclin production	212
Ideal dose and therapeutic combinations of antiplatelet agents	212
Acetylsalicylic acid (aspirin)	212
Dipyridamole and its combination with aspirin	212
Sulfinpyrazone	213
Drug side effects	213
Aspirin	213
Dipyridamole	213
Sulfinpyrazone	213
The bleeding tendency of uremia	213
Hemodialysis: the problems of thrombosis and anticoagulation	214
Practical use of anticoagulants	215
Hemodialysis anticoagulation	215
Systemic heparin anticoagulation for the majority of hemodialysis patients	215
Heparinization procedures for the at-risk hemodialysis patient	215
Minimal heparinization	215
Regional heparinization	216
Protamine at the termination of dialysis	216
Dialysis by prostacyclin infusion	216
Dialysis using ancrod	216
Anticoagulant use with blood access devices	216
Prophylaxis for shunts	216
Anticoagulants in the treatment of thrombosed shunts and grafts	217
Future developments	217
Appendix	218
References	219

INTRODUCTION

To use anticoagulants optimally during dialysis it is necessary to understand hemostasis, how to evaluate it and how therapeutic agents interfere with it. Knowledge of the hemostatic defects found in uremia and the influence of dialysis upon these is necessary, as is an understanding of foreign surface induced coagulation. This chapter presents such information before providing a practical guide to anticoagulant use.

SUMMARY OF THE HEMOSTATIC SYSTEM

(This section is not referenced; further details may be obtained from any major coagulation text)

Vascular injury induces a rapid, localized, controlled hemostatic response. Endothelial disruption exposes blood to underlying collagen, basement membrane, and microfibrils. Platelets immediately adhere to these substances and secrete substances found in intracellular granules, while the contents of cell membranes, cytoplasm, and mitochondria are retained. This secretory process is called the 'release reaction' and the substances released include adenine nucleotides, serotonin, platelet factor 4 (heparin-neutralizing factor), acid hydrolases, permeases, calcium, and fibrinogen. After adhesion to the damaged surface, the platelets produce arachidonic acid metabolites, in particular, prostaglandin G_2 and thromboxane A_2, which, along with adenosine diphosphate (ADP) and serotonin from storage granules,

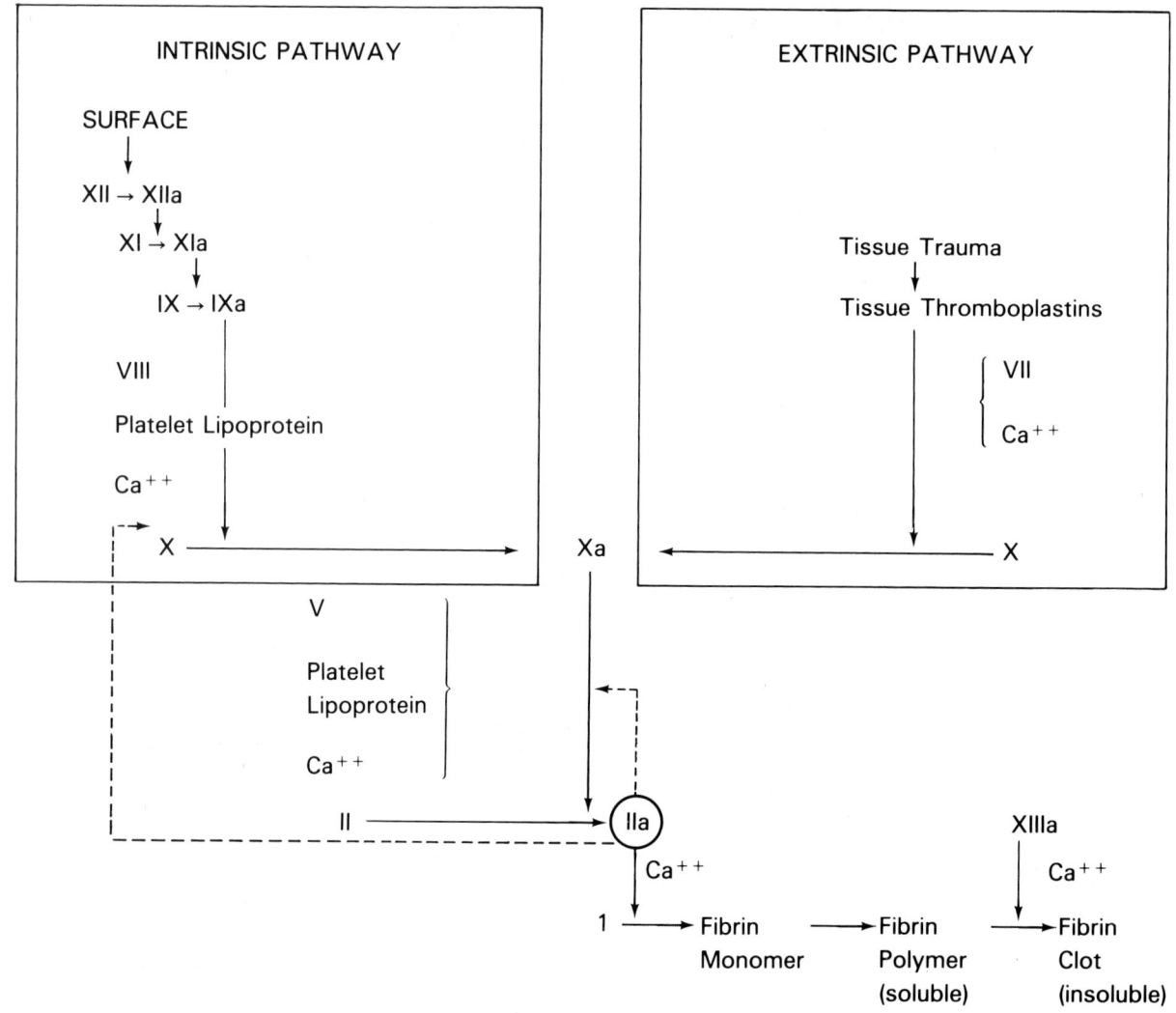

Figure 1. The classical view of the intrinsic and extrinsic coagulation pathways; they converge at the activation of Factor X. Activated factors are indicated by 'a' e.g. Xa. The dotted lines show that Factor IIa (thrombin) enhances the activation of Xa and itself.

stimulate further platelet aggregation, amplifying the release reaction. A 'white thrombus', or platelet plug, thus forms as the initial hemostatic event. The loosely packed platelet-collagen aggregate must consolidate to arrest bleeding permanently. As the platelet plug is forming, the tissue damage causes the release of 'tissue factor' which activates the extrinsic pathway of the coagulation cascade by interacting with factor VII. The factor VII-tissue factor complex can then convert factor X to factor Xa, rapidly generating small amounts of thrombin (factor IIa), which in turn amplifies platelet aggregation and release. Thrombin further augments the coagulation scheme by activating factors V and VIII.

The disrupted vascular surface also activates Hageman factor (factor XII), a part of the intrinsic coagulation pathway (see Figure 1), and it stimulates the fibrinolytic system (Figure 2) and other pathways such as kinin and complement. The inter-relationship between the intrinsic and extrinsic coagulation pathways are shown in Figure 1 and Table 1 lists the plasma procoagulants found in man with their plasma concentration and biologic half-life.

The hemostatic process is completed as the platelet-fibrin mass is consolidated and retracted into the wound by a mechanism that probably depends on the contractile properties of platelets. This retraction plus the local vasoconstriction mediated by serotonin and thromboxane A_2 from platelets permanently arrests bleeding.

The potentially autoamplified system outlined in Figure 1, would suggest that each time a wound occurs there would be generalized coagulation and permanently occluded vessels. This does not happen, however, because of 1) antagonism of the activated procoagulants by circulating inhibitors and 2) activation of the fibrinolytic system. The most important inhibitor antagonizes the serine protease procoagulants: Factors XIIa, XIa, Xa,

Table 1. Plasma procoagulants.

	Factor	Biological half-life (hours)	Plasma concentration (μg/ml)
I	Fibrinogen	95 to 120	2,500 to 3,500
II	Prothrombin	65 to 90	150
V	Proaccelerin	15 to 24	10
VII	Proconvertin	4 to 6	0.5
VIII	Antihemophilic factor	10 to 12	15
IX	Christmas factor	18 to 30	3
X	Stuart-Prower factor	40 to 60	15
XI	Thromboplastin antecedent	45 to 60	5
XII	Hageman factor	50 to 70	5
XIII	Fibrin-stabilizing factor	70 to 120	20

and IIa (thrombin). It may also inhibit VIIa. This inhibitor, called antithrombin III or heparin co-factor, is an alpha II globulin of molecular weight 63,000 and is normally present in human plasma. It forms an undissociable complex with the various proteases; for thrombin the complex is composed of one molecule of antithrombin III and one molecule of the protease. Its action is markedly enhanced by heparin.

Both contact activation and tissue damage trigger the fibrinolytic system which resembles the coagulation process in that both have intrinsic and extrinsic schemes (Figure 2). An activator of fibrinolysis, plasminogen activator, is released from the walls of peripheral veins. Circulating plasminogen is in equilibrium with that in clots, so when the concentration in the clot falls, plasminogen is converted to plasmin which then dissolves the clot to restore vessel patency. Plasmin is a proteolytic enzyme which, if uncontrolled, will attack fibrinogen, factor VIII, factor V, complement and pro-insulin in addition to lysing fibrin. Plasmin antagonists, antiplasmins, found in plasma, prevent uncontrollable hyperplasminemia. The fibrinolytic agents urokinase and streptokinase have been used to treat pulmonary embolism and other thrombo-embolic conditions. These agents (Figure 2) cause hyperplasminemia and the risk of severe hemorrhage.

These interactions are most relevant to the formation and degradation of fibrin-rich red thrombi which form in veins during stasis. White thrombi consist mostly of aggregated platelets and are formed in higher flow conditions where there is turbulence; they may be found on damaged arterial endothelium and foreign surfaces such as dialyzers and shunts.

There are important interactions between the components of the hemostatic system. For example, activated platelets vastly enhance the rate of interaction between factor Xa and factor II on the platelet membrane. Factor Xa in solution is readily neutralized by anti-thrombin

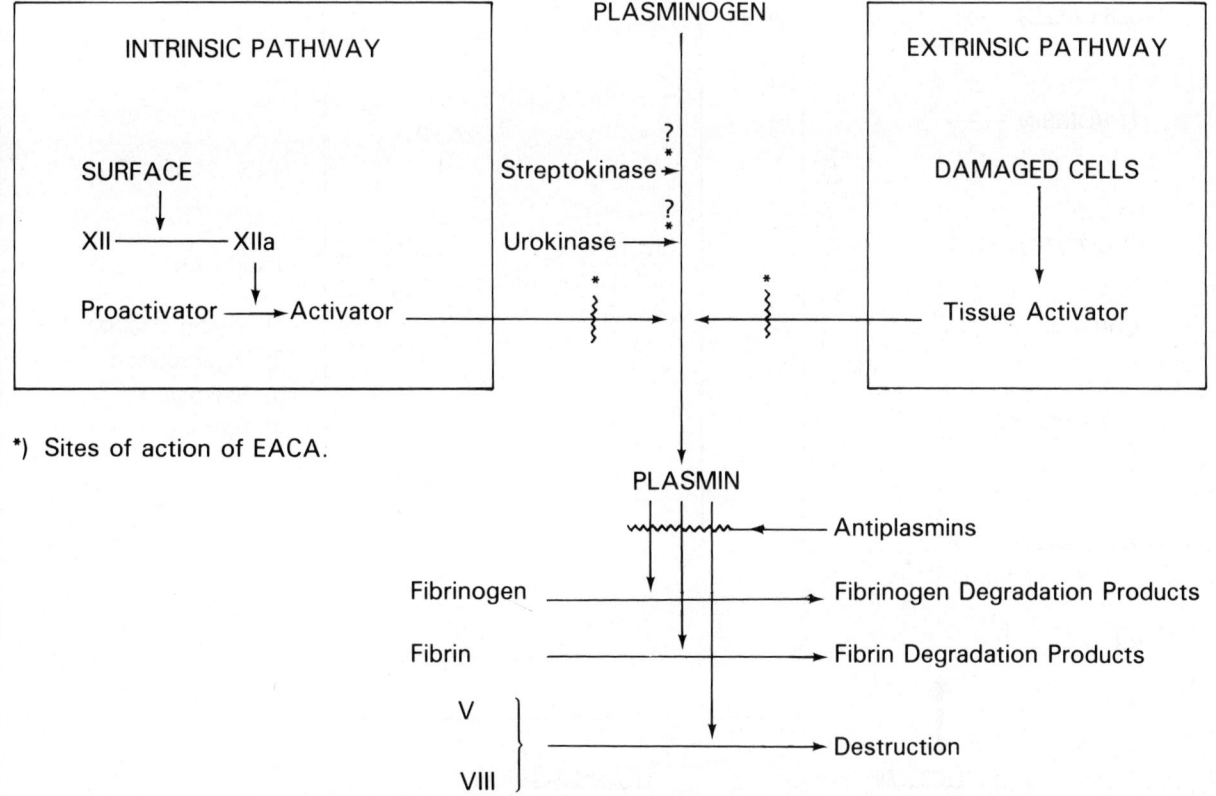

*) Sites of action of EACA.

Figure 2. The fibrinolytic system (EACA = epsilon-aminocaproic acid).

III, whereas Xa bound to the platelet membrane is not inactivated by that inhibitor nor by the heparin-antithrombin complex. These findings help to explain why hemostasis is localized. Because the reactions occur on surfaces, particularly on platelet membranes in damaged vessel walls, the hemostatic process is localized to the wound area; the rate of reaction at the appropriate site is markedly enhanced, but spread of the processes beyond the wound site is limited.

All the plasma procoagulants except factor VIII are synthesized in the liver; at least a proportion of factor VIII is synthesized by endothelial cells. Factors II, VII, IX, and X are vitamin K-dependent.

PLATELETS AND PLATELET FUNCTION
(This section is not referenced; further details may be obtained from any major coagulation text)

Platelets are derived from megakaryocytes which are produced by pluripotent myeloid stem cells. They have anucleate bodies approximately 2 μm in diameter and a circulating life span of about 10 days. With the renewal rate, or 'turnover' of approximately $35,000 \pm 1,200/\mu l$ of blood per day, the steady circulating platelet count averages $200,000/mm^3$ ($200 \times 10^9/l$). About 1/3 of the platelets are in a splenic pool that may freely exchange with the circulation. When necessary, platelet production can increase seven to eightfold. There is no marrow pool of platelets awaiting release. Increasing requirements for platelets must be met by augmented synthesis. Megakaryocyte maturation time does not shorten, but megakaryocyte volume may increase with platelet need. During equilibrium, platelet turnover (production rate) equals the disappearance rate. Platelets can disappear from the circulation through senescence, immunologic destruction or platelet consumption (non-immune platelet destruction including coagulation) in physiological or pathological states associated with platelet activity. Any platelet destructive process is usually associated with increased thrombocytopoiesis. When platelet production increases to keep pace with destruction, the levels of circulating platelets remain normal; if not, thrombocytopenia occurs. Excessive destruction accelerates platelet turnover and the average age of circulating platelets decreases. Platelets recently formed by the bone marrow are generally larger and have a greater functional metabolic capacity.

The basic platelet reaction

Platelets can be activated by many substances. These can be divided into three categories: proteolytic en-

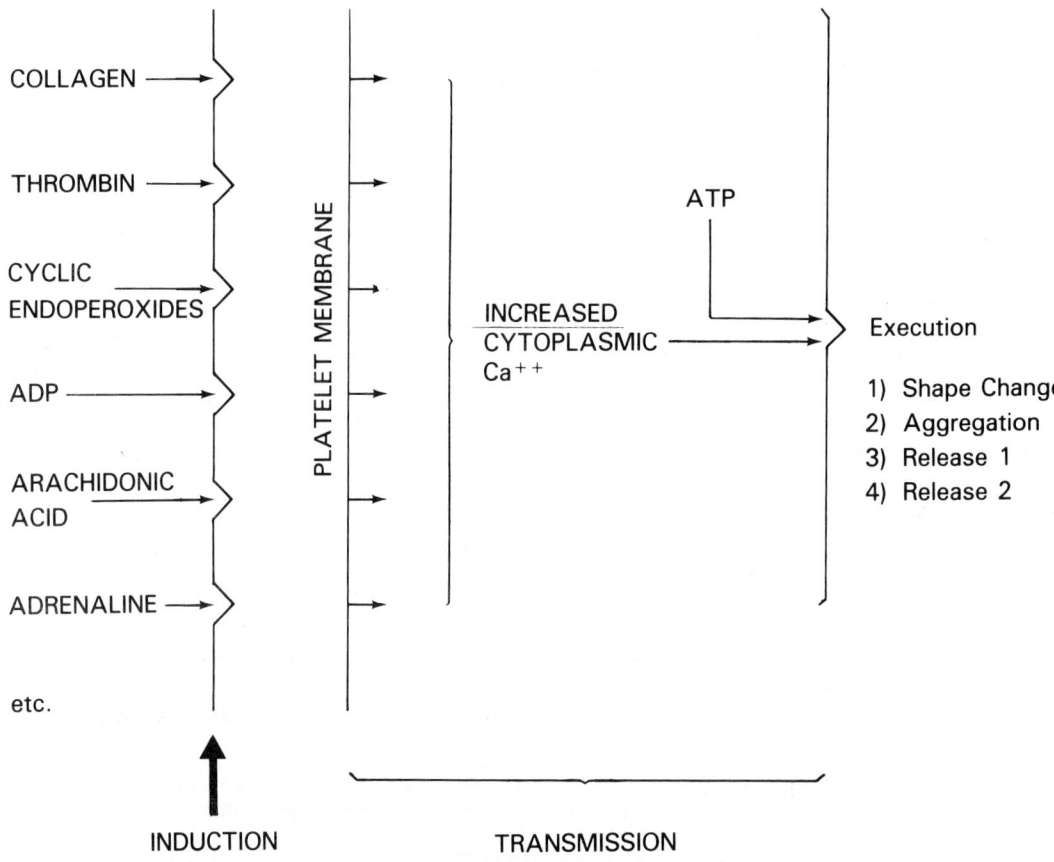

Figure 3. The basic platelet reaction (BPR).

zymes, such as thrombin or trypsin; large molecules, such as collagen fibers, aggregated IgG and insoluble immune complexes; and small molecules, such as ADP, serotonin, arachidonic acid, and epinephrine. The uniformity of the platelet response implies that every type of stimulation leads either to the same membrane alteration or always activates the same 'second messenger' system. This speculation has led to a unifying hypothesis for platelet responses to 'aggregating' agents, called the 'basic platelet reaction' (BPR).

The mature platelet has unique morphologic features that subserve platelet function. When platelets combine with aggregating agents under physiological conditions they rapidly lose their disc shape and become irregular spheres with multiple pseudopods. Surface contour changes are accompanied by movement of cytoplasmic granules toward the cell center, where they are closely encircled by the centrally displaced circumferential band of microtubules and microfilaments. This is the so-called 'shape change' reaction. During shape change, the individual cells become adhesive and begin to aggregate. Shape change-aggregation may induce fusion of the cytoplasmic granules within the plasma membrane and secretion of the granule contents via a canalicular system. The 'basic platelet reaction' is subdivided into three stages: induction, transmission, and execution (Figure 3), and can be summarized as follows.

Induction
The inducer interacts with the outer surface of the platelet membrane, possibly with a specific receptor for a given inducer.

Transmission
Induction causes a membrane response leading to the appearance of a transmitter in the cytoplasm, likely ionized calcium, which stimulates an ATP dependent (contraction) process. The more transmitter liberated the farther the contraction process proceeds and the more ATP is required.

Execution – The four stages
Stage 1 – Shape change and centralization of cytoplasmic granules
Stage 2 – Platelet aggregation
Stage 3 – Dense granule secretion or Release I (ADP, ATP, serotonin, calcium)
Stage 4 – Alpha granule release or Release II (acid hydrolases, potassium, fibrinogen, platelet specific proteins e.g., beta thromboglobulin, platelet factor 4)

Each of these platelet responses will be executed only when the basic platelet reaction has reached the corresponding stage and the proper internal and external conditions exist. At Stage 3 the platelets secrete ADP and serotonin, both of which induce the basic platelet reaction and thus strengthen the extracellular stimulus. At, or immediately before, Stage 3 arachidonic acid is liberated from the platelet membrane and converted to short-lived endoperoxides and thromboxane A_2 which are also potent inducers of the basic platelet reaction. This positive feedback greatly augments the overall stimulus. Figure 3 depicts the basic platelet reaction and a simplified version of the arachidonic pathway is indicated in Figure 4, which also shows that cyclic AMP

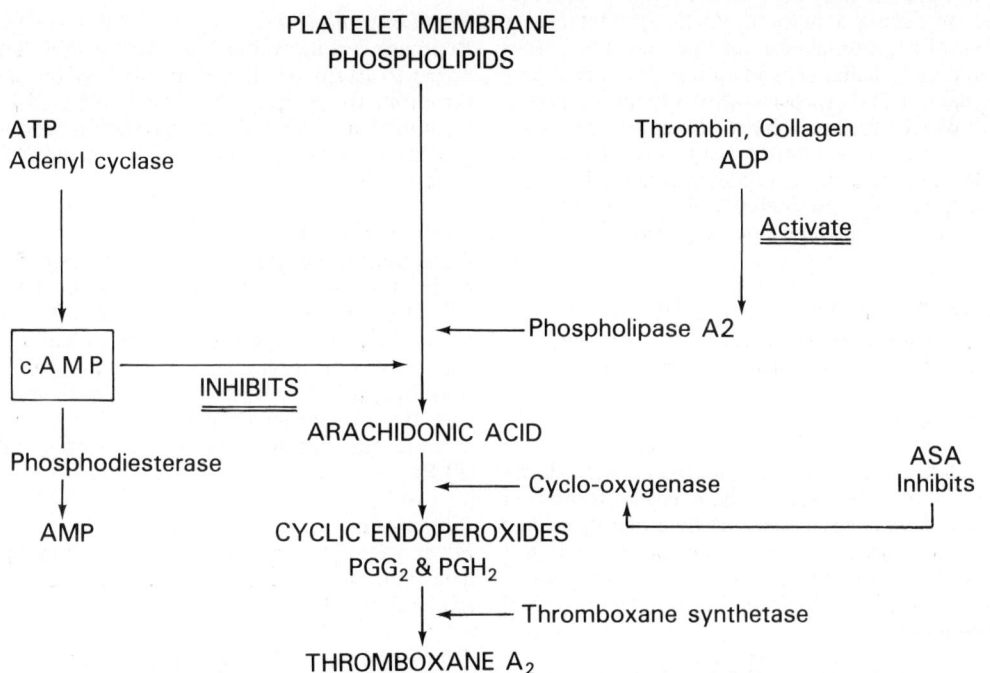

Figure 4. A simplified version of platelet cyclic endoperoxide and thromboxane A_2 production.

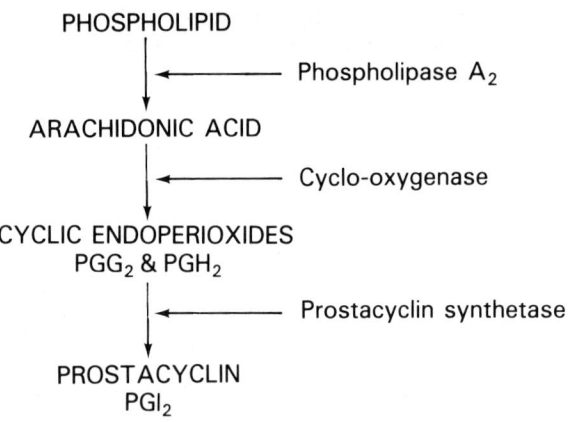

Figure 5. A simplified version of vessel wall prostaglandin generation.

(cAMP) blocks the production of arachidonate from platelet phospholipids. Therefore, circumstances that elevate cAMP levels such as increased adenyl cyclase activity and decreased phosphodiesterase activity will inhibit the platelet release reaction.

Clot retraction is mediated by thrombosenin which is platelet actomyosin. Platelets also help to maintain the integrity of small vessels: with thrombocytopenia red blood cells seem to leak through vessel walls. Platelets serve a key role in hemostasis by providing specific surface features for the intrinsic and extrinsic systems of coagulation. Platelets may also be involved in atherosclerosis by producing a myointimal factor that causes proliferation of subintimal smooth muscle cells. Vascular tissue and endothelial cells in culture produce a unique prostaglandin PGI_2 (prostacyclin) which is a potent inhibitor of platelet release thereby preventing thrombus formation. Remarkably similar pathways produce in platelets thromboxane A_2, a potent platelet release inducing agent, and in endothelial cells, prostacyclin, a powerful inhibitor of platelet release (Figure 5).

COAGULATION TESTS AND THEIR USE.
(This section is not referenced; further details may be obtained from any major coagulation text)

Tests of procoagulants

A few coagulation tests can evaluate procoagulant function (Figure 1). All are based on the eventual formation of fibrin strands that can be detected by either optical or electrical devices. In each case prolongation of a test time may represent an abnormally low factor concentration, the presence of a biologically inactive factor or factors, or inhibitors.

The partial thromboplastin time (PTT)
The PTT tests the intrinsic coagulation system (Figure 1). Kaolin, which provides a foreign surface, is added to whole plasma 6 min prior to the test to achieve maximal surface activation of factors XII and XI. Cephalin, a platelet lipid surrogate, is then added to the plasma and the time required to produce fibrin is recorded. Normal PTT values vary in different laboratories, but generally are 25 to 40 sec. This broad normal range makes it impractical to express the PTT as percent of normal. Because the normal prothrombin time is 10 sec and the time required to form a clot on optimal addition of thrombin to plasma is 6 sec, much of the PTT precedes factor X activation (Figure 1). The PTT is, therefore, most sensitive to abnormalties and deficiencies in the procoagulant sequence proximal to factor X.

The prothrombin time (PT)
The PT tests the extrinsic system. Tissue factor is added to whole plasma and the resulting fibrin can be measured in 9 to 10 sec. The PT can detect deficiencies in factors I, II, V, VII, and X. Antagonists of the extrinsic coagulation system, including heparin-antithrombin III complex, or fibrin degradation products, can prolong the PT.

The thrombin time (TT)
The TT evaluates the conversion of fibrinogen to fibrin. When optimal amounts of thrombin are added to plasma, fibrin appears in 5 to 6 sec. Because thrombin is such a powerful enzyme it can overwhelm inhibitors *in vitro*. However, if dilutions of thrombin are added to plasma until the normal TT becomes about 16 sec, inhibitors of fibrinogen-fibrin conversion such as fibrin degradation products or heparin-antithrombin III complex, can prolong the TT.

Reptilase time (RT)
Reptilase is a thrombin-like enzyme that converts fibrinogen to fibrin but is not affected by the heparin-antithrombin III complex. RT is also affected less than the thrombin time is by fibrin degradation products. Thus, a prolonged thrombin time with a normal RT suggests a heparin effect.

Fibrinopeptide A
A radioimmunoassay for fibrinopeptide A can assess recent thrombin generation or action. Thrombin acts primarily on fibrinogen by splitting off two molecules each of the fibrinopeptides A and B leaving one molecule of fibrin monomer. The radioimmunoassay for fibrinopeptide A will probably displace attempts to measure the circulating monomer by the ethanol gelation test or the plasma protamine paracoagulation test (PPP).

Fibrinogen
Fibrinogen is present in amounts that can be chemically measured and the results are usually reported quantitatively as mg/dl or as g/l.

Fibrin-fibrinogen degradation products
The fibrinolytic system is activated by the same factors that initiate coagulation (Figures 1 and 2). Plasmin at-

tacks both fibrinogen and fibrin producing degradation products (FDP's) that can be detected by various techniques, mainly immunological. A high titer of FDP's implies extensive hyperplasminemia, e.g., in disseminated intravascular coagulation but can also occur with extensive injuries or inflammatory disease.

These tests can be performed by the nephrology team and are sufficient for preliminary investigation of the renal patient with a coagulation abnormality. More specific assays of the coagulation and fibrinolytic systems should remain within the realm of the hematologist whose help may be required.

Tests for monitoring dialysis anticoagulation

Whole blood clotting time
The test is carried out in new glass test tubes measuring 3″ by 3/8″ (76 mm by 9.5 mm). Venous blood is collected in a plastic or siliconized glass syringe by clean venipuncture using a 19 to 21 gauge needle. One milliliter of blood is placed directly in each of four tubes at 37 °C and the tubes are tilted in turn at 30 sec intervals until each tube can be inverted without spilling blood. A stop watch is started once the blood is placed in the tubes and the clotting time is recorded from this time until the blood solidifies. The clotting time of each tube is recorded separately and the average of the four tests is reported. The clotting time of normal blood usually lies between 3 and 6 min.

Dialysis heparinization used to be monitored by whole blood clotting times and with systemic use of heparin, clotting times of around 15 to 20 min were usual. The obvious difficulty with this technique is that rapid adjustments in heparin dose cannot be made due to the prolonged clotting time. Whole blood activated clotting time improves such monitoring.

Whole blood activated clotting time (WBACT)
This test differs from the whole blood clotting time in that an activator of surface contact factors is added (Kaolin, earth, or ground glass) to speed up the initial stages of the coagulation cascade. Thus, a normal WBACT ranges from 90 to 140 sec. During dialysis when 'ideal' amounts of heparin are given (i.e., sufficient to prevent thrombus formation on artificial surfaces without causing bleeding) the WBACT lies between 200 and 240 sec. This time is short enough to adjust heparin dosage rapidly, if necessary. To carry out a WBACT the following are required:
1) Dry heat block calibrated to 37 °C ± 0.5°
2) Automatic pipette to deliver 0.2 ml
3) Stop watch
4) 12 mm × 75 mm glass test tubes
5) Tuberculin syringes with 21 gauge needles
6) Reagent (which will vary according to the manufacturer).

Set up:
1) Preheat test tubes in the heat block for 30 min.
2) Dispense 0.2 ml of reagent in test tubes.
3) Allow 10 min for reagents to warm.

Test procedure:
1) With tuberculin needle and syringe withdraw 0.4 ml sample of blood.
2) Remove needle from syringe and immediately dispense blood into warm test tube with reagent.
3) Start stop watch.
4) Gently swirl the mixture, return to heat block.
5) At 35 sec withdraw tube with tilt so that blood spreads along one half of its length.
6) Return tube to heat block.
7) Repeat steps 6 and 7 exactly every 5 sec.
8) The WBACT is when blood gels or turns into a solid clot.

Some companies manufacture a device which will perform the WBACT and electrically rotate the glass tube and record electronically the clotting time. Such a device which has been found useful by the author is the Hemochron System (International Technidyne Corporation, New Jersey, USA).

Whole blood activated partial thromboplastin time (WBAPTT)
This test can also monitor dialysis heparinization and is based on the same principle as the WBACT except that the activator contains a platelet lipid surrogate as well as a foreign surface. An example of such a reagent is Thrombofax (Ortho-diagnostics) which was until recently widely used in dialysis units but unfortunately is now difficult to obtain. The procedure for the WBAPTT is identical to that for the WBACT, but the clotting times are somewhat shorter.

TESTS OF PLATELETS AND PLATELET FUNCTION

(This section is not referenced; further details may be obtained from any major coagulation test)

Peripheral smear evaluation and platelet count

Examination of a peripheral blood smear quickly provides definitive information. On a well-stained normal smear there will be 8 to 12 platelets per high power (× 1000) magnification field, which corresponds to a normal platelet count ranging from 150,000 to 300,000/mm^3 (150 to 300 × 10^9/l).

Bleeding time

A carefully performed template bleeding time or use of a device such as the Simplate (Warner-Lambert Co, Morris Plains, NJ, USA) which makes a standard small skin incision, can give useful information about the platelet count, platelet function or both. The bleeding time is usually normal when platelet counts exceed 100,000/mm^3 (100 × 10^9/l) and is prolonged in an inverse linear fashion when counts are lower. If the bleeding time is prolonged despite adequate numbers of platelets, then platelet function is impaired. The bleeding time is the most clinically useful test of platelet function.

Platelet aggregometry

A platelet aggregometer is a simple device that records light transmission through a suspension of platelets. When platelets aggregate, light passes through the suspension more readily. To test aggregation a scale for each sample is set up from 0% (using platelet rich plasma) to 100% (platelet free plasma). Platelet rich plasma is placed in a cuvette and gently stirred and to this, concentrations of an appropriate aggregating agent, such as ADP, collagen or thrombin are added. As platelets aggregate, the rate of increase of light transmission can be measured and recorded on a scale thereby estimating the velocity of platelet aggregation (percent/minute).

Platelet factor 4 (PF4) and betathromboglobulin (BTG) estimation

PF4 and BTG are platelet specific proteins which are released from the alpha granules as part of the basic platelet release reaction. These proteins can be measured by radioimmunoassay and elevated levels indicate recent platelet activity.

ANTICOAGULANTS

Heparin

Heparin is present in most tissues but exists in highest concentration in the liver and the lungs. It is water soluble and may be precipitated by alcohol, acetone and acid. Heparin is usually prepared by extraction from animal tissue in water, alkali or potassium thiocyanate and purified by repeated precipitations with alcohol or acetone. From chemical analysis of the purest preparations, Jorpes (1) found that it was composed almost entirely of hexuronic acid, hexosamine, and ash. The ash contained 7 to 8% sulfur and the anticoagulant activity was proportional to the sulfur content. Heparin carries a strong electronegative charge; in a 2% solution the specific conductance is 85×10^{-4} mhos. Commercial heparins consist of a polydisperse mixture of polysaccharides of variable molecular weights (approximately 10,000) and other properties (2). Furthermore, heparin can be separated into fractions with active and inactive anticoagulant properties (3). Because heparins are variable, a suitable chemical assay is impossible. Therefore, standardization of a sample of heparin is based on comparison in vitro with a known standard in a non-specific assay of anticoagulant activity. The USP unit of heparin is the quantity that will prevent 1.0 ml of citrated sheep plasma from clotting for 1 hour after the addition of 0.2 ml of 1:100 $CaCl_2$ solution. Heparin Sodium USP must contain at least 120 USP units/mg and is available in sterile water for intravenous injection in concentrations of 250 to 40,000 USP units/ml (4).

The anticoagulant effect of heparin occurs because it acts on the intrinsic coagulation pathway (Figure 1), accelerating the rate at which antithrombin III neutralizes the proteolytic enzymes in the hemostatic cascade mechanism (5-8). In doing so it acts as a catalyst, increasing the rate of the protease inhibitor reaction without itself being consumed. Therefore, a major role of heparin is to accelerate the normal capacity of antithrombin III to neutralize the proteolytic activities of Xa, thrombin, XIa, IXa, and plasmin. The neutralization of Xa and thrombin requires less heparin than is needed to inhibit completely the other proteases. Before coagulation begins, the effect of heparin on Xa may be physiologically more important than the neutralization of thrombin since antithrombin III inhibition of one unit of Xa prevents the potential production of more than 15 units of thrombin (9). Conversely, after intravascular coagulation has occurred the principal function of antithrombin III will be to neutralize thrombin. This explains why the amount of heparin required to prevent thrombosis is less than is needed after thrombosis has developed.

Two mechanisms for heparin's potentiating effect on antithrombin III activity have been suggested. The first proposes that heparin binds to antithrombin III causing a confirmational change in the inhibitor that increases its reactivity towards its substrates (10). The second hypothesis suggests that heparin binds both to antithrombin III and to the substrates (11, 12). Both mechanisms may be involved.

There are two general types of assays of the action of heparin on coagulation: those determining the effect on clotting in general and those measuring the rate of specific clotting protease inactivation. Present experience suggests that neither type can, in the individual patient, predict with assurance antithrombotic efficacy or protect from hemorrhage.

As noted earlier, less heparin is required for thrombosis prophylaxis than to prevent extension of thrombosis after intravascular coagulation has occurred. When overt thrombosis is extensive, more heparin may be required than when intravascular coagulation is minimal. On this basis, heparin therapy can be divided into three categories: *low dose* (10,000 to 20,000 units/day), *medium dose* (20,000 to 60,000 units/day), and *large dose* (60,000 to 100,000 units/day). Low-dose heparin, usually given subcutaneously, reduces significantly the incidence of postoperative pulmonary emboli, does not produce significant bleeding and requires no monitoring (13). Medium dose heparin, given by constant intravenous infusion, is probably effective and safe for established venous thromboembolism. Monitoring is not essential but can give early warning of impending hemorrhage (13). Large dose heparin for florid thromboembolism is apparently safe if limited to under 48 h, but thereafter the risk of hemorrhage is high (13). The dosages of heparin required to conduct hemodialysis safely are given subsequently.

There have been conflicting reports of the action of heparin on platelet function. As early as 1938 Best (14) showed that heparin did not prevent 'white thrombus' formation in cellophane arteriovenous shunts in rabbits but did so in other species. A fall in platelet count has been noted after the injection of heparin into patients (15, 16) although other studies have not confirmed this observation (17–19). When blood is passed through glass bead columns, decreased (20), increased (21, 22) and unchanged (23) retention of platelets have been reported in the presence of heparin. These disparities may reflect variation in techniques for measuring platelet retention. Thompson and his colleagues (19) clearly demonstrated that heparin in final concentrations of 3 to 4 units/ml, in vitro or in plasma from volunteers given the drug, caused both increased retention of platelets within a test cell lined by cuprophan dialysis membranes (24) and also potentiation of platelet aggregation by ADP and adrenaline. Neither different heparin brands nor batch variations influenced these effects. Furthermore, Lindsay and colleagues (25) showed that commercial heparin in concentrations used during hemodialysis increases the retention of platelets on foreign surfaces such as those in the dialyzer circuit.

Coumarin or indanedione anticoagulant drugs

These agents produce the anticoagulant effect after 36 to 48 h by inhibiting the synthesis and hence reducing the plasma concentration of prothrombin and factors needed in its conversion, i.e., factors VII, IX and X (see Figure 1). The delay of the anticoagulation effect is likely to be due to persistent plasma concentrations of factors that were synthesized prior to the drug administration. The diminished concentration of these factors can be readily reflected by appropriate tests in circulating blood. Blockade of coagulation factor synthesis at the site of action of vitamin K_1 is attributed to interchange of physiological vitamin K with the coumarin or indanedione molecule.

When a high initial dose of one of these drugs is given, synthesis is completely blocked and the rate of decrease of plasma concentration of each of the factors depends on its biological half life (see Table 1). The rate of decay is also influenced by metabolic aspects in the particular patient; for example, in hypothyroidism catabolism is decreased so there is a slower disappearance rate, whereas the reverse holds true in hyperthyroidism and in febrile states (26). Ordinarily, total disappearance of the four factors is effected when the short acting coumarin derivatives are given in doses many times larger than the maintenance dose. The initial loading dose of the longer acting indanedione drugs is intentionally relatively small, so it does not block synthesis completely. When a constant maintenance dose has been established a stable depression of the production rate is achieved and the residual concentration of factor II (prothrombin) tends to be higher than that of factors VII, IX, and X.

It has been postulated that vitamin K may act at one or more of the four following sites: 1) completion of the structural gene components of the operon to form messenger RNA, 2) formation of peptide chains on the polyribosomes, 3) release of the completed peptide chains from the polyribosomes and formation of the complete vitamin K dependent factors from a polypeptide precursor or 4) transport of the foreign clotting factor across the cell membrane from intracellular to extracellular compartments (27).

The 4-hydroxycoumarin derivatives include: phenprocoumon, warfarin sodium, cyclocoumarol, dicumarol and ethyl biscoumacetate. The indanedione derivatives are from indan-1:3-dione and include the drugs phenindione, diphenadione, and chlorphenylindanedione. Serious and sometimes fatal sensitivity reactions to the indanedione drugs can occur whilst the coumarin drugs appear to be almost free from this problem. Sensitivity reactions have usually been reported with phenindione and may occur at any time from a few days to 6 weeks after starting the drug, most often at 3 to 4 weeks. The serious sensitivity phenomena include skin rashes, pyrexia, diarrhea, neutropenia, thrombocytopenia, hepatitis, and nephropathy. For this reason, these drugs are now rarely used and most renal units prefer warfarin or dicumarol. The dose of dicumarol for the initiation of therapy is 10 to 15 mg (30 to 45 µmol)/day until therapeutic prolongation of the prothrombin time occurs. Once the PT lies between 1½ and 2½ times the control value, a lower maintenance dosage is found and individually adjusted by the PT.

Certain drugs potentiate the action of oral anticoagulants. Salicylates produce the same disturbance of blood coagulation as that produced by coumarin and there may therefore be a summation of effect. Drugs or other agents such as alcohol, which may cause liver damage and hence decrease the synthesis of the vitamin K dependent factors, can also potentiate the coumarin effect. Other agents, for example, phenothiazines, may induce cholestasis diminishing absorption of vitamin K. Phenylbutazone causes a striking increase in sensitivity to the coumarin drugs (28); other drugs similarly incriminated include thyroxine, clofibrate, norethandrolone, methandrostenolone and sulfinpyrazone (29). Broad spectrum antibiotics which suppress the normal bacterial flora of intestines and reduce the production of vitamin K may also increase anticoagulant activity. Drugs that decrease the prothrombin time response, i.e., inhibit coumarin action, include barbiturates, ethchlorvynol, glutethimide, rifampin and griseofulvin. An interesting observation (unpublished) has been made in patients with very heavy proteinuria; the drug is lost in urine bound to protein. Thus, a higher dosage of coumarin may be required in severely nephrotic individuals.

FIBRINOLYTIC AGENTS

The fibrinolytic system (Figure 2) can be activated by factors present in the blood or extrinsically by a tissue activator provided by damaged cells in the blood vessel wall. Streptokinase and urokinase can be used therapeutically to enhance fibrinolysis; urokinase activates plasminogen directly and specifically, streptokinase, on the other hand, converts a normally inert proactivator to activator. Epsilon aminocaprioc acid (EACA) acts to block fibrinolysis by interfering with the action of the plasminogen activators.

The conceptual basis for fibrinolytic therapy

Under suitable circumstances it may be possible to deliver a fibrinolytic enzyme to a preformed thrombus *in vivo* and by markedly accelerating physiological fibrinolytic processes restore vascular patency before deleterious effects occur. Thus, fibrinolytic therapy is theoretically more attractive than anticoagulant therapy in which, at best, further fibrin formation is prevented and restoration of vascular patency depends on the relatively slow physiological fibrinolytic processes. It should be noted that the pre-formed thrombus consists mainly of fibrin and platelets. Perfusion with streptokinase in an artificial circulation of thrombi prepared *in vitro* in a Chandler's tube suggests that complete lysis of the fibrin, but not of the platelet component is possible, although large platelet masses can be broken down into smaller aggregates (30). This effect may be locally beneficial but theoretically could cause problems in certain circulations e.g. the cerebral.

Streptokinase

Streptokinase, the first activator of the fibrinolytic system to become available for investigation is commercially available in some countries. It is a protein with the electrophorectic mobility of human β-globulin and its molecular weight is about 43,000 (31). It is produced from many forms of streptococci from which it acquires its name, but plasminogen activator activity can be produced by many organisms including E coli, staphylococci, pseudomonas, and clostridia. There is very marked species variability in the response to streptokinase; human plasminogen is more readily activated than rabbit, canine or bovine plasminogens.

Streptokinase, like other streptococcal proteins, can be antigenic in man, and antibodies are detected in the normal population in varying amounts. Because it is rapidly bound by antibody, enough streptokinase must be given to bind antibody and any other non-specific inhibitors before the fibrinolytic enzyme system is affected. Thus, the effect on lysis times *in vitro* is dose dependent. The optimum concentration of streptokinase is considered to be 1000 to 2000 units/ml of plasma (32). When streptokinase is discontinued, fibrinolytic activity declines to pre-infusion levels within an hour. However, a coagulation defect persists for up to 24 h because of the digestion of coagulation factors such as fibrinogen, factors V, and VIII (see Figure 2) and, perhaps, some inhibition of platelet aggregation (30). Streptokinase can be given intravenously or by intra-arterial infusion. The loading dose can be an individually calculated antibody neutralizing dose or a standard initial dose of 1,250,000 units which will neutralize inhibitors in 97% of the population. Thereafter, a maintenance dose of around 100,000 units/h is infused (33).

After a course of streptokinase, and particularly when plasminogen has been substantially depleted, conventional anticoagulants should be given as soon as streptokinase is discontinued to prevent re-thrombosis with unlysable fibrin during the relatively long period of plasminogen regeneration (24 h). McNicol and Douglas (33) recommend the intravenous infusion of heparin (1,500 units/h) for 24 h after streptokinase and concurrent oral anticoagulant therapy for at least 7 days.

Streptokinase has toxicity, inherent in its effect as an activator of plasminogen; there is a risk of bleeding. The main non-hemorrhagic complication is pyrexia, which does not appear to be prevented by hydrocortisone. Allergic reactions include bronchospasm, tachycardia, and hypotension; some of these respond to antihistamines and to hydrocortisone.

Urokinase

It has been known since 1885 that urine had proteolytic activity. Specific fibrinolytic activity was noted by Macfarlane and Pilling (34), and shown by Williams (35) to be due to a plasminogen activator in urine; the name urokinase was suggested by Sobel and colleagues (36).

Urokinase is a colorless protein of molecular weight 54,000 that is highly stable over a wide pH and temperature range. It is, itself, a proteolytic enzyme which activates plasminogen according to first order kinetics likely by splitting lysine and/or arginine bonds. It seems likely that urokinase is elaborated by the kidneys. Urokinase appears to be non-antigenic and less toxic than streptokinase. Although a serum inhibitor is present, its levels are much more constant than with streptokinase so it is easier to use a fixed priming dose and a uniform maintenance dose on a body weight basis (33). Moreover, in *in vitro* systems containing both fibrinogen and fibrin, urokinase as compared with streptokinase, produces relatively more fibrinolysis and less break down of fibrinogen so anticoagulant effects are less likely (37). Urokinase does have the disadvantages of very high cost and potential thromboplastic or coagulative activity. In this latter regard, Prentice et al (38) studies a highly purified preparation of urokinase (Hoffmann-La Roche Inc, Nutley, NJ, USA) which *in vitro* had a 'zero coagulative assay' (39) of about 1,000 units/ml. Infused in patients in an initial dose of 3,600 units/kg body weight over 10 min followed by 3,600 units/kg/body weight/h it reduced the recalcification time in glass and plastic, decreased the PTT, and increased factor VIII concentration and platelet adhesiveness. Fibrinolysis predominated so much *in vivo*, however, that probably the coagulative effects are irrelevant (33). Nevertheless, it would be desirable to have a urokinase preparation free of such effects or a dosage schedule designed to minimize them.

EACA and antiplasmins

A variety of aliphatic amino compounds including lysine and ornithine competitively inhibit plasminogen activation (40). The most important of these is epsilon-aminocaproic acid (aminocaproic acid – EACA) (41). Aprotinin (Transylol, Boehringer, Ingelheim Ltd) is a polypeptide of molecular weight about 6,500 which is commercially prepared from bovine, lung is also a potent competitive inhibitor of plasminogen activation (42).

Plasma and serum exert a substantial inhibitory action on plasmin. Part of this is due to alpha-2-macroglobulin which reacts quickly as a competitive inhibitor of plasmin, one molecule of alpha-2-macroglobulin inhibiting two molecules of plasmin (43).

The Sherry hypothesis

A fibrinolytic system that does not necessarily cause hemorrhage has been attributed to the 'Sherry hypothesis' which is a postulated explanation of why the relatively non-specific proteolytic enzyme, plasmin, is largely restricted *in vivo* to a single highly specific action, namely, that of digestion of fibrin. Alternative explanations have been suggested, however.

According to this hypothesis, plasminogen in the plasma represents the soluble phase and in the clot, the gel phase (44). The results of plasminogen activation in the two phases differ strikingly. Plasminogen activation in the soluble phase, provided that it is not unduly rapid, produces no effect on susceptible substrates in the plasma because plasma antiplasmin rapidly inhibits plasmin as it is formed (see Figure 2). On the other hand, plasminogen activation in the clot or gel phase, where the effect of inhibitors on absorbed activator and plasminogen is weaker than in the plasma, produces a different result. In this circumstance, because of the intimate spatial relationship of plasminogen and fibrin, plasminogen activation produces fibrinolysis or thrombolysis. Lytic activity is, therefore, viewed as a function of clot plasminogen content and the main function of plasma plasminogen is to endow any intravascular fibrin which may form with the means to mediate its subsequent lysis when activator is either adsorbed upon it during its formation or subsequently diffuses into it from the plasma. Both plasminogen and activator are known to have a strong affinity for formed fibrin.

ANCROD

Ancrod is the approved name for 'Arvin' (Twyford Laboratories Ltd, United Kingdom) a purified fraction of the venom of the Malayan pit-viper. *In vivo* it anticoagulates by converting plasma fibrinogen to an unstable form of fibrin which is rapidly removed from the circulation without producing clinical evidence of vascular occlusion. Ancrod appears to be relatively free from serious side and toxic effects and control of therapy is easily achieved.

Crude venom and ancrod have been found to be almost identical in their actions in the blood coagulation mechanism. The coagulant fraction constitutes 5 to 10% of whole venom. One unit of ancrod (2 µg) has approximately equivalent coagulant activity to one NIH unit of thrombin when tested on a fibrinogen substrate at 37°C.

The thrombin-like action of ancrod on fibrinogen has been established; it will convert fibrinogen to fibrin directly in the absence of other coagulation factors. The actions of thrombin and ancrod on fibrinogen are not, however, identical since fibrinopeptide B is not released from fibrinogen by ancrod and the fibrin stabilization factor (factor XIII) is not activated. Thus, the fibrin formed by ancrod is unstable and rapidly removed from the circulation. Ancrod does not affect other blood coagulation factors nor does it have any significant action on platelets. Furthermore, it does not appear to activate the fibrinolytic enzyme system directly (45).

Ancrod is available in 1.0 ml sterile ampoules, each containing 67 units, which should be stored at 4°C. The initial dose of ancrod should be given by slow intravenous infusion over 2 to 12 h. Adequate hypofibrinogenemia can be achieved by 1 to 3 units/kg body weight without risk of dangerous intravascular coagulation. Thereafter, a maintenance dose of 1 to 2 units/kg body weight intravenously every 12 h will usually keep plasma fibrinogen levels below 60 mg/dl (46).

ANTIPLATELET AGENTS

A large number of agents (drugs and related chemicals) can inhibit platelet reactions *in vitro*. Many such agents suppress platelet function at concentrations that cannot be used in humans because of toxicity or pharmacokinetic considerations. This section reviews only those drugs that have been observed in humans to inhibit platelet function in hemostasis or to alter thromboembolic processes through an ascribed antiplatelet action.

If we consider the inhibition of platelet function in terms of the 'basic platelet reaction' (Figure 3), then inhibitors can be divided into four main categories:
1) substances that inhibit induction
2) substances that inhibit early transmission
3) substances that inhibit late transmission
4) substances that inhibit execution

It will be seen that many platelet suppressant drugs inhibit more than one of these reactions.

Inhibitors of induction

Both ATP and AMP derivatives are competitive inhibitors of *in vitro* ADP-induced induction (46, 47), but are not useful *in vivo* due to rapid inactivation (48) or to undesirable side effects (47, 49). Prescribable drugs, such as amitriptyline, imiprimine, penicillin G, pyrimidopyrimidine compounds, lidocaine, and the non-steroidal anti-inflammatory agents, affect the adhesion of platelets to collagen and thus inhibit induction (50–52).

Inhibitors of early transmission

Substances that activate adenyl cyclase or inhibit cyclic AMP (cAMP) phosphodiesterase cause a rise in the cytoplasmic level of cAMP. This is accompanied by inhibition of the basic platelet reaction in such a way that when the cAMP concentrations increase gradually, first granular secretion, then aggregation, and finally shape change are inhibited (53). PGE$_1$, PGD$_2$ (54) and PGI$_2$ (prostacyclin) (55) are potent stimulators of adenyl cyclase. Typical inhibitors of cAMP phosphodiesterase are papaverine (56), pyrimidopyrimidine compounds (e.g., dipyridamole, RA233 [57]) and the methylxanthines (theophylline, caffeine, and aminophylline [58]). Adenyl cyclase activators and phosphodiesterase inhibitors work synergistically and are much more effective when used in combination.

Inhibitors of late transmission

In response to the appearance of calcium in the cytoplasm, platelets contract provided that a critical threshold level of metabolic ATP is also present (see Figure 3). Inhibitors of contraction such as colchicine or vinblastine (59) interfere with this process, but only in high concentrations. A metabolic poison such as 2-deoxyglucose will lower metabolic ATP concentration (60) and inhibit platelet activation. Neither class of drug is specific for platelets, so they are unsuitable for use *in vivo*.

Inhibitors of execution

As indicated previously, this stage of the basic platelet reaction is associated with the conversion of arachidonic acid to short-lived cyclic endoperoxides and thromboxane A$_2$. This prostaglandin synthesis in the platelet can be blocked by inhibiting the enzyme cyclo-oxygenase (Figure 4). Acetylsalicylic acid covalently alters this enzyme (61) and produces an irreversible inhibition which lasts the life time of the platelet. Most other non-steroidal anti-inflammatory drugs are cyclo-oxygenase inhibitors as well but none of these drugs are covalently linked to the enzyme and, thus, the inhibition produced is short-lived and reversible (62). Examples of this type of agent are indomethacin, sulfinpyrazone, naproxen, sodium meclofenamate, and phenylbutazone.

Antiplatelet agents: effect on vessel wall prostacyclin production

Understanding of the use of platelet inhibitor drugs in thrombosis has to take into account the natural contribution of the vessel wall to the inhibition of thrombosis. The vessel wall may inhibit the process of thrombosis in at least two ways. One of these is in the release of plasminogen activator which can cause the localized formation of plasmin to lyse fibrin. The second mechanism is associated with formation of a prostaglandin metabolite which was initially discovered by Moncada and colleagues (55) and was subsequently named prostacyclin (63). This compound seems to be the main prostaglandin metabolite in vascular tissue, being most highly concentrated on the endothelium, and progressively decreasing in activity towards the adventitial surface (64, 65). Prostacyclin is a potent systemic vasodilator (66) and the most potent inhibitor of platelet aggregation yet discovered (55). It has been shown to inhibit platelet adherence to damaged vessel walls (67–69) and to possess antithrombotic properties (69, 70). As indicated above prostacyclin could be defined as an inhibitor of early transmission by activating platelet membrane adenyl cyclase which in turn increases platelet cyclic AMP.

Presumably, similar to the synthesis of the prostaglandin, thromboxane A$_2$, by the platelet, the vessel wall synthesizes prostacyclin from its own precursors (see Figure 5); arachadonic acid is converted into cyclic endoperoxides by the cyclo-oxygenase enzyme and such endoperoxides are subsequently converted into prostacyclin by a prostacyclin synthetase enzyme. It appears, therefore, that the generation of prostacyclin is a physiologic mechanism that protects the vessel wall from platelet deposition and an imbalance between the formation of prostacyclin and thromboxane A$_2$ may be one of the mechanisms leading to thrombosis. If this is the case, one might expect that drugs used to inhibit platelet activation might also inhibit prostacyclin formation and hence, nullify the desired effect of preventing thrombosis in natural vessels.

Ideal dose and therapeutic combinations of antiplatelet agents

Recent evidence indicates that the prescribed dose of each of the platelet inhibitor drugs may be crucial in determining the final therapeutic outcome of the patient. A summary of this evidence has recently been made and is outlined below (71).

Acetylsalicylic acid (aspirin)
A very low dosage of aspirin (160 to 325 mg/day [0.9 to 1.8 mmol]) is sufficient in most patients to have an antithrombotic effect inhibiting platelet cyclo-oxygenase without affecting vessel wall prostacyclin synthesis.

An intermediate dosage of aspirin (0.5 to 1.5 g/day, [2.8 to 8.3 mmol]) may be potentially beneficial to some patients whereas to others the antithrombotic effect may be partially abolished by the inhibition of prostacyclin synthesis.

Larger doses of aspirin (more than 1.5 g/day, [8.3 mmol]) may be potentially beneficial in a few patients and it appears that only very high dosages (perhaps more than 10 g/day, [55.6 mmol]) might promote thrombosis.

Dipyridamole and its combination with aspirin
Most of the information regarding the ideal potential anti thrombotic dose of dipyridamole has been obtained by platelet survival studies (72). The decreased platelet survival found in patients with prosthetic heart valves could be lenthened by high dosage dipyridamole therapy (100 mg [198 µmol] qid). A similar correction could be produced by the combination of intermediate dosages of dipyridamole (100 mg/day) and aspirin (1 g/day [5.6 mmol]) (73). Moncada and Korbut (74) examined various intravenous doses of both drugs singly and in combination in the rabbit and observed that maximal inhibition of platelet aggregation in flowing blood was obtained by combining intermediate dosages of dipyri-

damole (3 mg/kg [6 µmol/kg]) and aspirin (10 mg/kg, [5.6 µmol/kg]). Such a combination has therapeutic attraction because each drug affects platelet metabolism at a different level and, therefore, might be expected to increase the probability of therapeutic effectiveness.

Sulfinpyrazone
The available evidence suggests that 400 mg (1.1 mmol) of sulfinpyrazone per day has virtually no effect on platelets whereas 800 mg/day (2.1 mmol) is highly effective and that this latter dosage has only a minimal effect on prostacyclin formation so it is unlikely to promote thrombus formation.

Drug side effects

The most commonly used platelet inhibitor drugs (aspirin, dipyridamole, and sulfinpyrazone) are potent pharmacological agents with known side effects. This factor is important because if they are used as anti-thrombotic agents they usually are given for prolonged periods. Table 2 summarizes the most important side effects when compared with placebo; the data have been compiled by Fuster and Chesebro (71) from recent prospective studies.

Table 2. Side effects of antiplatelet agents.

Side effect	Percentage of patients using		
	Aspirin	Sulf-inpyrazone	Dipyridamole
Gastrointestinal upset	18	? (Negligible)	12
Bleeding	7	3	4
Headache	4	? (low)	9
Skin rash	2	?	3

Aspirin
The taking of 1.0 g (5.6 mmol) of aspirin per day will cause gastrointestinal side effects in about 20% of patients and 7% will have a bleeding complication, most often of the gastroduodenal tract that will necessitate medical attention. Plasma uric acid levels can increase in patients with good renal function and clinical gout can be precipitated. This latter complication is not relevant to the dialysis population. Allergy, particularly in the form of skin rashes, is uncommon.

Dipyridamole
Gastrointestinal symptoms such as epigastric discomfort and nausea occur in approximately 10% of patients. These symptoms, however, tend to subside after a few days of medication particularly if the drug is given with meals. In contrast with aspirin when dipyridamole is given alone or in combination with anticoagulants it does not seem to increase the incidence of gastritis, gastroduodenal ulcer, or the tendency to bleed. Because dipyridamole is a vasodilator headaches occur in almost 10% of patients but they become a major problem only rarely.

Sulfinpyrazone
Side effects caused by sulfinpyrazone seem to be less pronounced than those noted with aspirin or dipyridamole. In particular, there are fewer gastrointestinal side effects. As noted above sulfinpyrazone increases the sensitivity to oral coumarin anticoagulants and prolongs the prothrombin time. Thus, modification of coumadin dosage is highly likely when the two drugs are used together. The drug is, of course, a potent uricosuric agent. In the non dialysis population the possibility of precipitation of uric acid stones must be considered. Sulfinpyrazone also increases the sensitivity of sulfonylurea hypoglycemic agents and, if prescribed, attention should be given to the blood glucose level.

THE BLEEDING TENDENCY OF UREMIA

A bleeding tendency is common in uremia; this has been known since 1907 (75). While deficiencies in factors V and VII occur in some uremic patients (76), platelet abnormalities form the major coagulation defects in such patients and these may be both quantitative and qualitative. These abnormalities, which have been reviewed by Rabiner (77) often result in a prolonged bleeding time (78, 79). However, whether the uremic individual has a prolonged bleeding time, thrombocytopenia, or qualitative platelet abnormalities either alone or in combination, platelet life span appears to be normal (78) even when the patient is maintained on dialysis (80). When arteriovenous shunts are used for vascular access, however, platelet survival is shortened (72).

Improvement in both the qualitative and quantitative platelet abnormalities can be induced by dialysis therapy. This was first noted over 10 years ago by several groups (78, 81–83), who concluded that the thrombocytopathy of uremia was due to dialyzable factors that suppressed megakaryocytes and hence decreased platelet production and, in addition, acted as circulating toxins impairing the platelet release reaction. More recent studies have confirmed this and have shown that efficient hemodialysis or peritoneal dialysis can return platelet function to normal in spite of the trauma of the extracorporeal circuit (84–88). It appears, however, that the uremic platelet defect is not entirely explained by dialyzable toxins and that there may be non dialyzable plasma factors as well. There may be decreased concentrations of factor VIII-Von Willebrand activity which are not corrected by dialysis (89) and there is a non dialyzable heat labile factor in the plasma of uremic individuals capable of inhibiting production of platelet cyclo-oxygenase and at the same time stimulating endothelial prostacyclin production (90). Both effects, of course, will lead to defective platelet adhesion-aggregation.

The platelet defect and its ability to be improved by dialysis may influence the interaction between blood foreign surfaces and anticoagulants that occurs during hemodialysis. This interaction will now be discussed in some detail.

HEMODIALYSIS: THE PROBLEMS OF THROMBOSIS AND ANTICOAGULATION

When blood flows over a foreign surface, protein adsorption occurs immediately (91). Frequently, this is followed by platelet adhesion (92) and activation of the intrinsic coagulation pathway (93). The last two phenomena occur more or less independantly (94), but in the latter stages of blood clotting on a foreign surface there is a mutual interaction between the coagulation process and the platelet reaction. When prothrombin is converted to thrombin the platelet release reaction will be stimulated leading to enhanced platelet-adhesion-aggregation. On the other hand, during the platelet release reaction which follows platelet foreign surface contact, platelet factor III is released and augments the classical coagulation pathway. The end result is, of course, thrombus formation. The situation may also be enhanced by adherence of leukocytes since Niemetz and his colleagues (95) have demonstrated that leukocytes obtained from the used membranes of an artificial kidney have enhanced procoagulant activity. The relative importance of white cell adhesion in the final common pathway (i.e. thrombus formation) is not fully determined. There is recent interest, however, in alternative pathway complement activation occurring when blood comes in contact with the cellulose based membranes used in the artificial kidney and it is known that this is associated with a transient leukopenia and leukocyte aggregation (96). Further studies have suggested that C_{5a} production in the complement cascade is the factor which causes both neutropenia and leukocyte aggregation (97). It is highly possible, therefore, that C_{5a} induced leukocyte aggregation is associated with the release of leukocyte thromboxane A_2 which, in turn, may lead to *in vivo* platelet aggregation and destruction by those platelets on the foreign surface. Studies of this possible interaction are indicated.

The role of the platelet in surface induced thrombus formation appears to be well-defined. To prevent thrombosis taking place during hemodialysis, heparin is used. But, it has been pointed out that heparin has no inhibitory effect on the platelet foreign surface interaction. Indeed, it has been shown that in concentrations used during hemodialysis it actually enhances ADP induced platelet aggregation (19) and the retention of platelets on a foreign surface (25). Thus, heparin cannot be considered as an ideal anticoagulant for extracorporeal use. Thrombus formation can take place upon the membranes of the artificial kidney in spite of adequate heparinization and this may be associated with the fall in platelet count over the course of dialysis and with demonstrable rentention of platelets by that membrane surface (98). The hypothesis that platelet retention by that membrane is an important step in the reaction which subsequently leads to thrombus formation has been proven by a double blind trial involving antiplatelet agents (99). Furthermore, the substitution of a dialysis membrane with low platelet retaining properties into a dialyzer known to have enhanced *in vivo* thrombus formation also reduced the amount of thrombus formed during the dialysis procedure (100). Thus, the nature of the dialysis membrane and the geometry to which that membrane conforms are important (101).

From the heparin anticoagulation point of view the patient walks a tight rope between under anticoagulation with the resulting problems of blood clotting, and over heparinization with bleeding from cannulation sites and other miscellaneous areas such as the gut and uterus. Because of these problems more precise control of heparin anticoagulation has been recommended using a series of WBACTs (or WBAPTTs) to delineate a 'heparin profile' for the patient. From this profile an indication of the heparin loading dose required and the rate of constant infusion necessary during dialysis can be calculated (102). Details of the mathematical modelling approach to heparin therapy are given in Chapter 3. There is no doubt that with a given patient, over a short period of time, the 'heparin profile' works and trouble free dialysis anticoagulation can be achieved. However, in spite of this technique, variability in heparin requirements has been noted in dialysis patients. It appears that heparinization cannot be uniformly judged on a body weight basis and that a given patient may require different heparin dosages from time to time. It may be that currently available commercial heparin has variable potency. On the other hand, it may equally be possible that some of the variability rests with the uremic patient and his dialysis treatment; for example, efficient hemodialysis can improve platelet function in spite of extracorporeal trauma. Thus, it can be anticipated that platelet function in a given patient will be different at the commencement of renal replacement therapy from that found after 6 months of adequate dialysis. Accordingly, the patient's propensity to have platelet retention by relatively non biocompatible materials will change with improvement of uremia by dialysis treatment. Furthermore, the platelet dialysis membrane interaction is implicated in thrombus formation during hemodialysis. Platelet retention by foreign surfaces in this situation is followed by the release of platelet constituents including platelet factor 4 (PF4) which is released in parallel with serotonin (103). PF4 appears to be a substance in the molecular weight range of 7,000 to 9,000 which has heparin neutralizing activity (HNA) (104). Any demonstrable HNA in plasma is believed to be a function of PF4 released by platelets and its level, if raised, is likely to affect recent or continuing platelet activity as might be found in arterial thrombosis (105). HNA levels have been found to be increased in the plasma of patients with end-stage renal disease treated by hemodialysis but were not raised in non-dialyzed patients with severe chronic renal failure or patients treated by peritoneal dialysis nor in patients with normal renal function who have been exposed to the extracorporeal circulation of the heart lung bypass, 48–72 h before testing (106). It was postulated, therefore, that the trauma of extracorporeal circulation causes platelets to release PF4 which is not cleared by dialysis but is by the human kidney. The elevation of plasma HNA, so caused, must have therapeutic implications for heparin dosage schedules during hemodialysis. For example, a 70 kg man with end-stage renal failure and a hematocrit of 20% is likely to have a plasma volume of about 4,000 ml and at a plasma HNA level of 0.140 units/ml has the immediate ability to neutralize 560 units of heparin. A continuous infusion of 7,000 units of heparin over 3 h will run at 40 units/min, a common dialysis procedure. There is, therefore, the potential for complete neutralization of heparin over the first 14 min of infusion. During this period, the platelet foreign surface interaction will generate further HNA release and prolong the period of serious underdosage. If a continuous heparin infusion is contemplated it may be advisable to start this at least 15 min before dialysis commences or to use an adequate systemic loading dose. It has already been confirmed that there is a correlation between an elevated plasma HNA level and the necessity to give greater than normal heparin dosages during hemodialysis (106).

There has been interest recently in the use of prostacyclin (PGI_2) for dialysis anticoagulation. Woods and his colleagues (107) demonstrated that the dialysis of dogs could be carried out without heparin if a constant infusion of prostacyclin (2 μg/min; equivalent to 60 to 100 ng/kg/min) was used. These investigators subsequently demonstrated that this agent can be used safely for human dialysis and that an infusion rate of 9 ng/kg/min has significant heparin sparing effects (108). They proposed that the sparing of heparin consumption and the enhancement of its biological activity by prostacyclin are due to the prevention of release of platelet antiheparin activity (PF4). In a more recent study it was shown that prostacyclin could be used as a sole anticoagulant in 10 patients on long-term dialysis and in one patient undergoing dialysis for acute renal failure who had bled on three occasions when heparin was used. The authors administered prostacyclin intravenously for 10 min before starting dialysis and via the arterial line during the procedure adjusting the dosage to avoid induced hypotension. Each patient underwent 240 min of dialysis and received an average of only 423 ng of prostacyclin/kg of body weight. No clinically important changes in the intrinsic clotting system were noted and there was no evidence of hemorrhage or thrombosis within the dialyzers. It was concluded, therefore, that prostacyclin could replace heparin safely as a sole antithrombotic agent during hemodialysis and that this agent might be advantageous if ordinary anticoagulation is contraindicated (109). Whether or not widespread use of prostacyclin for dialysis will occur will depend upon the frequency of undesirable clinical side effects such as drug induced hypotension and, of course, on its availability and cost.

PRACTICAL USE OF ANTICOAGULANTS

With this background a practical guide to the use of the various anticoagulant agents for dialysis patients can be given. This will be presented separately as it relates to hemodialysis anticoagulation and to the prevention of clotting in blood access devices.

Hemodialysis anticoagulation

Systemic heparin anticoagulation for the majority of hemodialysis patients
It will be clear from the data presented that heparin is not an ideal anticoagulant for hemodialysis and yet is the only one generally available. Thrombus formation may take place during hemodialysis in spite of apparently adequate heparinization and the platelet foreign surface interaction is of major importance in its occurrence. The ability of platelets to release their contents is likely to be enhanced by the improvement in the uremic syndrome resulting from adequate dialysis and will be stimulated by the materials used in the hemodialysis circuit which are of poor biocompatability. It is likely, therefore, that variations in heparin dosage for hemodialysis are common within the dialysis population and these cannot necessarily be judged by body weight. Taking all this into account, the following have been suggested as guidelines for the better monitoring of heparin anticoagulation for the patient on maintenance dialysis (110):

1) The patient should have heparin requirements assessed during a series of WBACT's (or WBAPTT's as described by Gotch and Keen [102]) during the first three hemodialyses the patient receives. From the information, so obtained, an indication of the heparin loading dose and the rate of constant infusion required during dialysis will be ascertained. (Details of the methodology and calculations are provided as an appendix to this chapter.)

2) When the patient is established on a regular hemodialysis schedule the heparin/WBACT profile should be assessed on a monthly basis.

3) Should any untoward clotting or hemorrhagic tendencies be noted, emergency reassessment of the heparin/WBACT profile should be made.

4) If it appears that untoward clotting episodes are occurring in spite of apparently good heparinization techniques then ideally, the patient's platelet function should be examined with particular reference to the release of PF4 and assessment of plasma HNA levels. If enhanced platelet activity and elevated plasma HNA levels are found, it is reasonable to treat the patient with an anti-platelet agent such as acetylsalicylic acid in low dose. If such investigations are not available then empirically the antiplatelet agent should be tried.

Heparinization procedures for the at risk hemodialysis patient
Frequently a hemodialysis has to be performed on an acute or chronic uremic patient with an intercurrent hemorrhagic problem (such as gastrointestinal bleeding or menorrhagia) or a situation exists when over heparinization might be dangerous, as in the patient with pericarditis or in association with recent surgery. In such situations minimal heparinization or 'regional heparinization' with neutralization of circulating heparin by protamine sulphate has been employed.

Minimal heparinization. A technique of 'minimal heparinization' has been evaluated (Hood SA, Holmes L, and Lindsay RM, unpublished) which is suitable for such a high risk situation and appears to obviate successfully the need for the regional technique. The basis of the minimal heparinization technique is to reduce the total heparin dosage given to the dialysis patient by 50%. The dialyzer and lines are primed with saline in the usual way and 1,000 units of heparin are added to the system 2 min prior to the termination of (re)circulation. The patient then receives an initial bolus of heparin into the venous return cannula and after the commencement of dialysis, heparin is given at a constant infusion which is terminated 30 min before the planned termination of dialysis. The amounts of heparin given as initial bolus and at a constant infusion are 50% of those known to be ideal according to the standard systemic heparinization schedule. The heparin dosage can be safely reduced to a mean of 2,750 units/4 h of dialysis without inducing significant thrombus formation and whilst maintaining a blood loss in the dialyzers and lines of less than 5 ml. Further reductions in heparin are possible but then the dialyzer blood loss increases and the risk of clotting the venous return system is greater. The investigators also felt there might be some advantage in using dialyzers with cellulose acetate membranes as opposed to Cuprophan membranes when utilizing such a technique. Throughout the course of each dialysis it is important to conduct serial WBACTs at hourly intervals and these should be maintained at around 200 sec throughout the course of dialysis. Close monitoring of WBACT in each individual patient can allow fine adjustments, if necessary, in the rate of heparin infusion.

Regional heparinization. A constant heparin infusion with a solution of 200 units of heparin/ml in 0.9% saline is infused into the inlet line of the dialyzer. Simultaneously, a constant infusion of a solution of 2 mg of protamine sulfate/ml in 0.9% saline is infused into the outlet line before the blood returns to the patient. At the beginning of dialysis a minimal loading dose of heparin is given i.e., 50% of that normally required, if known, or empirically 500 units plus that in the priming solution. At the commencement of dialysis both infusion pumps are started; separate pumps being employed so that the rate of heparin or protamine can be increased or decreased. The objective is to keep the patient's WBACT between 80 to 100 sec and the extracorporeal circuit of the artificial kidney at the therapeutic level, namely, 200 to 250 sec. The good dialysis nurse becomes very adept at adjusting the infusions of heparin and protamine sulfate to regulate the desired clotting times.

A 'heparin rebound' phenomenon may occur after regional heparinization. Even with a normal WBACT at the end of dialysis a rebound state of anticoagulation may occur from 2 to 4 h after the cessation of dialysis and persist for up to 10 h, possibly causing hemorrhage. It is believed that this heparin rebound is caused by the heparin-protamine complex being broken down in the reticuloendothelial system and the anticoagulant re-entering the circulation.

In view of this rebound and the fact that protamine sulfate in large doses also has an anticoagulant action, large amounts of protamine should be avoided. In other words, the secret of good regional heparinization is to decrease the heparin infusion thereby decreasing the WBACT rather than increase the protamine.

Protamine at the termination of dialysis. However dialysis anticoagulation has been carried out in a high risk situation, should the patient's WBACT be prolonged and if it is felt that there is a significant risk of bleeding, then the intravenous administration of protamine can be given to the patient to neutralize any remaining heparin. Should it be necessary to neutralize heparin urgently, one has to accept that the potency of batches both of heparin and protamine sulfate vary, but the usually accepted dose of protamine sulfate is 1 to 1.5 mg per 100 units of heparin. By personal experience, the author considers that generally only 50% of the recommended protamine dosage should be given and no more than 50 mg in any 10 min period.

Should time permit, it is possible to have a heparin:protamine titration test carried out. Here a known volume (10 ml) of blood is taken from the patient immediately post-dialysis and protamine is added by titration until a WBACT (or other test such as a thrombin time) is returned to normal. By estimating the patient's blood volume, the exact amount of protamine required to neutralize circulating heparin can be calculated. Again, this author would suggest that only half the recommended protamine dosage should be given and then protamine titration checked once more.

Dialysis with prostacyclin infusion
The use of prostacyclin would seem very appropriate for the high risk group and its use could increase rapidly in the next few years. In many countries, certainly in North America, the drug is only available for experimental use at this time. When available, the dosage regimes previously suggested would be appropriate.

Dialysis using ancrod
Ancrod with its unique effect on fibrinogen has been used in place of heparin as an anticoagulant during dialysis and was observed to reduce the formation of fibrin on the membranes of the Kiil dialyzer (111). However, it would be impractical to use this drug routinely for dialysis as its administration is more complex than heparinization and, as it is not easily neutralized, the patient would have a hypofibrinogenemic clotting defect for sometime after dialysis which might lead to excessive blood loss from arteriovenous fistula cannulation sites.

Anticoagulant use with blood access devices

Prophylaxis for shunts
We have to consider how best to maintain patency of devices, such as Teflon-Silastic arteriovenous shunts and foreign material grafts, which may be implanted subcutaneously to be used as blood conduits. It has been shown that both sulfinpyrazone (112) and acetylsalicylic acid (113) will prolong shunt life without causing significant morbidity. Anticoagulation with coumadin, on the other hand, will also prolong shunt life (114) but increased hemorrhagic complications will be encountered.

As far as the dose of the antiplatelet agent that is required to keep the Teflon-Silastic arteriovenous shunt patent, one can theorize that this device will not endothelialize and, therefore, it is not necessary to be concerned about suppressing prostacyclin generation. Most centers prescribe aspirin in the intermediate dosage range i.e., 650 mg (3.6 mmol)/day but theoretically, the low dose (160 to 325 mg [0.9 to 1.8 mmol]/day) is probably sufficient. Sulfinpyrazone is usually given in the dosage range of 200 mg (525 µmol), 3 or 4 times a day. In view of the fact that aspirin irreversibly inhibits the cyclo-oxygenase system in the platelet, it might be thought that the drug could be given once or twice a week and still have the desired effect. It must be remembered, however, that if platelet survival is approximately 10 days (likely to be even less in a patient with an A-V shunt) then 10% of a platelet population will be renewed each day by new non-affected platelets. For this reason, aspirin should be given daily. The efficacy of dipyridamole either alone or in combination with aspirin on patency should be studied. As mentioned previously, however, there is a theoretical advantage of combining the two drugs, so it would be perfectly reasonable to prescribe a low to intermediate dosage of aspirin in combination with dipyridamole 100 mg (198 µmol)/day.

There does not appear to be any prospective study which has clearly demonstrated the value of antiplatelet agents in maintaining patency of foreign material grafts. There is no doubt that platelet foreign surface interaction takes place with their use. Clagett and his colleagues (115) have demonstrated shortened platelet survival after the placement of Dacron aortic prostheses in dogs. Harker et al (116) have also demonstrated that the decreased platelet survival associated with prosthetic arterial grafts will return towards normal within 9 months in humans and within 6 weeks in baboons. In the baboon it was shown that normalization of platelet survival correlated with the degree of graft endothelialization. Both aspirin and dipyridamole can prevent platelet aggregation and adherence to such vascular grafts in animal studies (117). In the author's own unit the actuarial survival curve of PTFE (Gortex) (polytetrafluoroethylene) grafts (see Chapter 8) was assessed within the hemodialysis population and it was found that 50% of the grafts are lost within the first 10 months. Thereafter, the survival curve improves dramatically. It would appear, therefore, that this might be the time when graft endothelialization takes place. If an antiplatelet agent is to be used, therefore, it would seem that the dosage of the drug is not important in the early stages, but after 10 months when endothelialization has taken place one might have to consider the potential effects on decreasing prostacyclin production. Prospective trials of antiplatelet agents in various dosages with the use of such grafts is indicated.

A policy that has been adopted by many units, including the author's, which appears to be satisfactory is that antiplatelet agents are prescribed to the patient with a previous history of blood access thrombosis or after his first clotting episode. They are, however, not prescribed routinely. Coumadin anticoagulation is only employed after further thrombotic episodes in spite of the use of antiplatelet agents.

Anticoagulants in the treatment of thrombosed shunts and grafts
When a Teflon-Silastic shunt clots, it can often be declotted mechanically either by irrigation with heparinized saline and the dextrous use of suction by syringe (see also Chapter 8). If one is fortunate and restores a flow through the shunt, there is a clear indication for the commencement of either antiplatelet agents or a coumadin type of anticoagulant. If the declotting procedures are not successful, surgical help is needed and replacement of the clotted tip or tips is necessary. In the past many units attempted lytic therapy and infused streptokinase (118, 119) or urokinase (120-122) to declot such shunts. None of these authors gave detailed follow up regarding the long term patency achieved by such methods and most nephrologists would now agree that the success rate of lytic therapy in this area is poor. There are no reports to suggest that lytic therapy has a place in the management of thrombosed fistulae or prosthetic grafts and the management of such problems rests with early surgical intervention.

FUTURE DEVELOPMENTS

In the future we will undoubtedly see improvements in the biocompatability of surfaces used in the artificial kidney and in other artificial organ systems. Considerable research work is currently being done in the field of pharmacological manipulations of surfaces bringing about the controlled release of bioactive agents such as heparin and prostaglandins which will significantly reduce the surface thrombosis without upsetting the coagulation status of the patient. This topic has been reviewed recently (125 and Chapter 9).

In addition, there is considerable research at the present time into the understanding of the anticoagulant, antithrombotic, and hemorrhagic effects of heparin; these three effects are not necessarily directly related to each other. Stemming from this research is the development of heparinoids which have been shown in experimental animals to be as effective in preventing thrombosis but at the same time induce less hemorrhage than heparin. It is almost certain, therefore, that in the not too distant future such heparinoids will be available and which may be ideal for hemodialysis anticoagulation.

APPENDIX

1) To use the WBACT to calculate heparin dosage for dialysis in a given patient.

   Procedure:

Action	Comments
1. Use non-heparinized saline in priming the dialyzer.	1. This allows accurate assessment of heparin received by the patient.
2. Do a baseline whole blood activated clotting time (WBACT) (#1).	2. This is unheparinized blood.
3. Administer loading dose of 1,500 to 2,000 units of heparin to the patient.	3. Systemic heparinization is recommended before the extracorporeal circuit is attached to the patient.
4. Follow with 10 ml of normal saline.	4. To ensure that entire loading dose of heparin enters the patient's circulation.
5. Allow 3 to 5 min to pass.	5. To ensure optimal patient response.
6. Do a WBACT (#2)	6. —
7. Initiate dialysis.	7. Do *not* begin heparin pump at this time.
8. Calculate patient response to heparin.	8. Response = WBACT #2 - WBACT #1
9. Calculate patient sensitivity to heparin.	9. Sensitivity = $\dfrac{\text{response}}{\text{heparin dose}}$
10. Do a WBACT (#3) *exactly* 30 min. after bolus dose of heparin was given.	10. This will allow calculation of patient's elimination rate of heparin (K)*
11. Begin the heparin pump at the desired dosage.	11. Give bolus as well if WBACT is below 200 sec.
12. Do a WBACT on a 1/2 hourly basis.	12. Hourly infusion rate = $\dfrac{(\text{desired WBACT} - \text{WBACT \#1})(K)}{\text{sensitivity}}$
13. Stop heparin prior to termination of dialysis according to calculations.	13. Time (hours) = $1/K \, \text{Log}_e \left[\dfrac{\text{desired WBACT} - \text{WBACT \#1}}{\text{lowest WBACT before take-off} - \text{WBACT \#1}} \right]$
14. Do a final WBACT just prior to finishing dialysis.	

2) To use the WBACT to monitor a given dialysis.

   Procedure:

Action	Comments
1. Do a baseline WBACT.	1. —
2. Administer loading dose of 1,500 to 2,000 units of heparin to the patient.	2. Systemic heparinization is recommended. Loading dose of 1,500 units is based on average patient sensitivity of 0.06 sec/unit, thereby elevating WBACT to 230 to 260 sec, i.e., peaking above the ideal range.
3. Follow with 10 ml normal saline.	3. To ensure that loading dose enters patient for optimal patient response.

* K (elimination rate in hours) = $\text{Log}_e \left[\dfrac{\text{Response}}{\text{WBACT \#3} - \text{WBACT \#1}} \right] \times \dfrac{1}{\text{Time (hours)}}$

  = $2 \times \text{Log}_e \left[\dfrac{\text{Response}}{\text{WBACT \#3} - \text{WBACT \#1}} \right]$ (for 30 min test period.)

The data will give an ideal hourly infusion rate for heparin (see 12 above) and an ideal loading dose can also be calculated as follows:

Loading dose = $\dfrac{\text{Desired WBACT} - \text{WBACT \#1}}{\text{Sensitivity}}$

4. Allow 3 min to pass.
5. Do a WBACT 3 min after venous line is attached.
6. Give bolus dose as necessary.

7. Do a WBACT 30 to 60 min later.
8. Adjust infusion rate if necessary.

9. Do WBACT test at hourly intervals.
10. Stop heparin infusion 1/2 hour before termination of dialysis.
11. Do a WBACT test.

12. Do a final WBACT 30 min after discontinuing infusion – just before taking the patient off.

4. Follow usual procedures.
5. This will give patient's response to heparinized saline in dialyzer.
6. For every 10 sec WBACT is below 200 sec give 250 units.
7. To check constant infusion rate.
8. For every 10 sec WBACT is above or below 220 sec, change heparin infusion rate by 250 units. NOTE: If WBACT is below 200 sec, give bolus dose of heparin.
9. To check infusion rate.
10. —
11. A WBACT value at this time is most desirable to help determine the exact time for discontinuing the heparin infusion for subsequent dialysis.
12. For every 20 sec WBACT is above 200 sec stop heparin pump 15 min earlier next dialysis. For every 20 sec WBACT is below 200 sec, leave heparin pump on 15 min longer.

The clotting times can be graphed as shown in Figure 6.

Note the WBACT times given in this appendix are those found in the author's unit using the Hemochron (International Technidyne Corp., New Jersey) system. Times found in other units may vary according to the reagent and system used; each unit must set up its own standards.

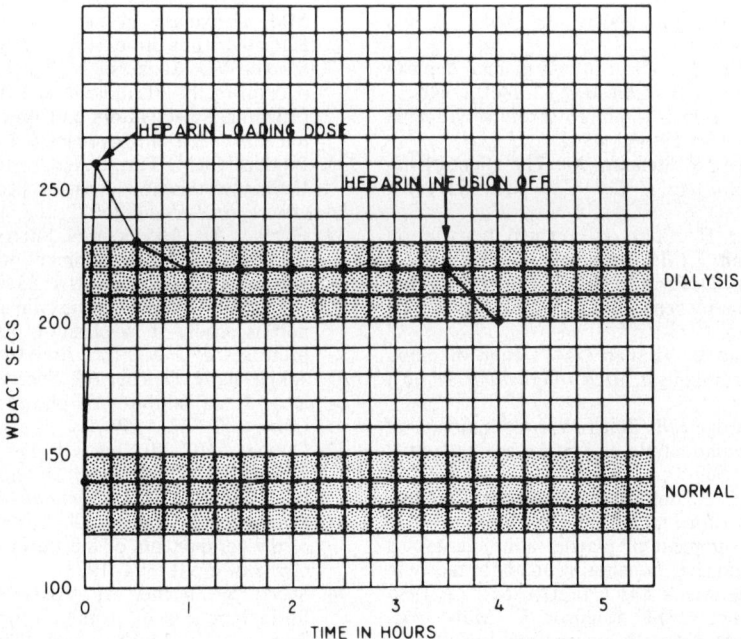

Figure 6. A typical heparin/WBACT profile for a 4 h hemodialysis. The ideal loading dose of heparin should cause a slight overshoot of desired dialysis WBACT range. If it does not, it is slightly more difficult to achieve a steady heparin infusion rate.

REFERENCES

1. Jorpes JE: *Heparin In The Treatment of Thrombosis. An Account of its Chemistry, Physiology and Application in Medicine*, London, Oxford University Press, 1946
2. Cifonelli JA, King J: Structural studies on heparins with unusually high N-acetylglucosine contents. *Biochim Biophys Acta* 320:331, 1973
3. Rosenberg RD, Lam LH: Heparinized surface – a comment. *Ann NY Acad Sci* 283:404, 1977
4. O'Reilly RA: Anticoagulant, antithrombotic and thrombolytic drugs. In: *The Pharmacological Basis of Thera-*

peutics, edited by Gilman AG, Goodman LS, Gilman A, 6th edn, New York, NY, MacMillan Publishing Co, 1980, p 1351
5. Brinkhous KM, Smith HP, Warner ED, Seegers WH: The inhibition of blood clotting: an unidentified substance which acts in conjunction with heparin to prevent a conversion of prothrombin into thrombin. *Am J Physiol* 125:683, 1939
6. Seegers WH, Cole ER, Harmison CR, Monkhous FC: Neutralization of autoprothrombin-C activity with antithrombin. *Can J Biochem* 42:359, 1964
7. Damus PS, Hicks M, Rosenberg RD: Anticoagulant action of heparin. *Nature* 246:355, 1973
8. Rosenberg JS, McKenna P, Rosenberg RD: Inhibition of human factor IXa by human antithrombin. *J Biol Chem* 250:8883, 1975
9. Yin ET, Wessler S, Stoll PJ: Biological properties of the naturally occurring plasma inhibitor to activated factor X. *J Biol Chem* 246:3703, 1971
10. Rosenberg R, Damus PS: The purification and mechanism of action of human antithrombin-heparin co-factor. *J Biol Chem* 248:6490, 1973
11. Gitel S: Evidence of catalytic role of heparin in anticoagulation reactions. In: *Heparin: Structure, Function, and Clinical Implications*, edited by Bradshaw RA, Wessler S, New York, NY, Plenum Press, 1975, p 243
12. Wilson-Gentry P, Alexander B: Specific coagulation factor adsorption to insoluble heparin. *Biochem Biophys Res Commun* 50:500, 1973
13. Wessler S, Gitel S: Control of heparin therapy. *Prog Hemost Thromb* 3:311, 1976
14. Best CH: Heparin and thrombosis. *Br Med J* 2:977, 1938
15. Fidlar BA, Jaques LB: The effect of commercial heparin on the platelet count. *J Lab Clin Med* 33:1410, 1948
16. Gollub S, Ulin AW: Heparin-induced thrombocytopenia in man. *J Lab Clin Med* 59:430, 1962
17. Quick AJ, Shanberge JN, Stefanini M: The effect of heparin on platelets *in vivo*. *J Lab Clin Med* 33:1424, 1948
18. Davey MG, Lander H: Effect of injected heparin on platelet levels in man. *J Clin Pathol* 21:55, 1968
19. Thomson C, Forbes CD, Prentice CRM: The potentiation of platelet aggregation by heparin *in vitro* and *in vivo*. *Clin Sci Mol Med* 45:485, 1973
20. Moolten SE, Vroman L, Vroman GMS: Role of blood platelets in thromboembolism. *Arch Intern Med* 84:667, 1949
21. O'Brien JR, Shoobridge SM, Finch WJ: Comparison of the effect of heparin and citrate on platelet aggregation. *J Clin Pathol* 22:28, 1969
22. Bowie EJW, Owen CA, Thompson JH: A test of platelet adhesiveness. *Mayo Clin Proc* 44:306, 1969
23. Salzman EW: Measurement of platelet adhesiveness: a simple *in vitro* technique demonstrating an abnormality in Von Willebrand's disease. *J Lab Clin Med* 62:724, 1963
24. Lindsay RM, Prentice CRM, Ferguson D, Muir WM, McNicol GP: A method for the measurement of platelet adhesiveness by use of dialysis membranes in a test-cell. *Br J Haematol* 24:377, 1973
25. Lindsay RM, Rourke JTB, Reid BD, Linton AL, Gilchrist T, Courtney J, Edwards RO: The role of heparin on platelet retention by acrylonitrile co-polymer dialysis membranes. *J Lab Clin Med* 89:4, 1977
26. Loeliger EA: General considerations on coumarin induced hypocoagulability and its control. In: *Human Blood Coagulation* edited by Hemker HC, Loeliger EA, Veltkamp JJ, Leyden, Leyden University Press, 1969, p 283
27. Douglas AS, McNicol GP: Anticoagulant therapy. In: *Human Blood Coagulation Haemostasis and Thrombosis* edited by Biggs R, 2nd edn, Oxford, London, Edinburgh, and Melbourne, Blackwell Scientific Publications, 1976, p 571
28. Aggeler PN, O'Reilly RA, Leong L, Kowitz PE: Potentiation of anticoagulant effect of warfarin by phenylbutazone. *N Engl J Med* 276:496, 1967
29. O'Reilly RA, Aggeler PN: Determinants of the response to oral anticoagulant drugs in man. *Pharmacol Rev* 22:35, 1970
30. McNicol GP, Bain WH, Walker F, Rifkand BM, Douglas AS: Thrombolysis studied in an artificial circulation; thrombi prepared in vitro in a Chandler's tube. *Lancet* 1:838, 1965
31. Blatt WF, Segal H, Grey JL: Purification of streptokinase and human plasmin and their interaction. *Thromb Diath Haemorrh* 11:393, 1964
32. Konttinen Y: Some observations on the effect of thrombin on the antifibrinolytic aspect of streptokinase. *Scand J Clin Lab Invest* 14:568, 1962
33. McNicol JP, Douglas AS: Thrombolytic therapy and fibrinolytic inhibitors. In: *Human Blood Coagulation, Haemostasis and Thrombosis* edited by Biggs R, 2nd edn, Oxford, London, Edinburgh, and Melbourne, Blackwell Scientific Publications 1976, p 436
34. Macfarlane RG, Pilling J: Fibrinolytic activity of normal urine. *Nature* 159:779, 1947
35. Williams JRB: The fibrinolytic activity of urine. *Br J Exp Pathol* 32:530, 1951
36. Sobel GW, Mohler SR, Jones NW, Dowdy AB, Guest MM: Urokinase: an activator of plasma profibrinolysin extracted from urine. *Am J Physiol* 171:768, 1952
37. Sawyer WD, Alkjaersig N, Fletcher AP, Sherry S: A comparison of the fibrinolytic and fibrinogenolytic effects of plasminogen activators and proteolytic enzymes in plasma. *Thromb Diath Haemorrh* 5:149, 1960
38. Prentice CRM, Turpie AGG, McNicol GP, Douglas AS: Urokinase therapy: dosage schedules and coagulant side effects. *Br J Haematol* 22:567, 1972
39. Fletcher AP, Alkjaersig N, Sherry S, Genton E, Hirsch J, Bachman F: The development of urokinase as a thrombolytic agent. *J Lab Clin Med* 65:713, 1965
40. Mullertz S: Effect of carboxylic and amino acids on fibrinolysis produced by plasmin, plasminogen activator and proteases. *Proc Soc Exp Biol Med* 85:326, 1954
41. Alkjaersig N, Fletcher AP, Sherry S: Epsilon-aminocaproic acid: an inhibitor of plasminogen activation. *J Biol Chem* 234:832, 1959
42. Dubber AHC, McNicol GP, Douglas AS: *In vitro* and *in vivo* studies with Trasylol, an anticoagulant and a fibrinolytic inhibitor. *Br J Haematol* 14:31, 1968
43. Schreiber AD, Kaplen AP, Austen KF: Plasma inhibitors of the components of the fibrinolytic pathway in man. *J Clin Invest* 52:1394, 1973
44. Sherry S, Fletcher AP, Alkjaersig N: Fibrinolysis and fibrinolytic activity in man. *Physiol Rev* 39:343, 1959
45. Turpie AGG, McNicol GP, Douglas AS: Ancrod ('Arvin') a new anticoagulant. In *Human Blood Coagulation, Haemostasis and Thrombosis* edited by Biggs R, 2nd edn, Oxford, London, Edinburg, and Melbourne, Blackwell Scientific Publications, 1976, p 476
46. Macfarlane DE, Mills DCB: The effects of ATP on platelets: evidence against the central role of released ADP in primary aggregation. *Blood* 46:309, 1975
47. Michal F, Maguire MH, Gough G: 2-methylthyo-adenosine 5-phosphate: a specific inhibitor of aggregation. *Nature* 222:1073, 1969
48. Holmsen H, Holmsen I, Bernhardsen A: Microdetermi-

nation of ADP and ATP in plasma with the firefly luciferase system. *Ann Biochem* 17:456, 1966
49. Angus JA, Cobbin LB, Einstein R, Maguire MH: Cardiovascular actions of substituted adenosine analogues. *Br J Pharmacol* 41:592, 1971
50. Mohammad SF, Mason RG: Inhibition of human platelet collagen adhesion reaction by amitriptyline and imiprimine. *Proc Soc Exp Biol Med* 145:1106, 1971
51. Cazenave JP, Packham MA, Guiccione MA, Mustard JF: The effects of penicillin G on platelet aggregation, release and adherence to collagen. *Proc Soc Exp Biol Med* 142:159, 1973
52. Cazenave JP, Packham MA, Guiccione MA, Mustard JF: Inhibition of platelet adherence to collagen-coated surface by non steroidal anti-inflammatory drugs, pyrimido--pyrimidine and tricyclate compounds and lidocaine. *J Lab Clin Med* 83:797, 1974
53. Holmsen H: Classification and possible mechanisms of action of some drugs that inhibit platelet aggregation. *Ser Haematol* 8:50, 1976
54. Mills DCB, Macfarlane DE: Stimulation of human platelet adenyl-cyclase by prostaglandin D2. *Thromb Res* 5:401, 1974
55. Moncade S, Gryglewski R, Bunting S, Vane JR: An enzyme isolated from arteries transforms prostaglandin endoperoxides to an unstable substance that inhibits platelet aggregation. *Nature* 263:663, 1976
56. Markwardt F, Hoffman A: Effects of papaverine on cyclic AMP phosphodiesterase of human platelets. *Biochem Pharmacol* 19:2519, 1970
57. Rozenberg MC, Walker CM: The effect of pyrimidine compounds on the potentiation of adenosine inhibition of aggregation, on adenosine phosphorilation and phosphodiesterase activity on blood platelets. *Br J Haematol* 24:409, 1973
58. Mills DCB, Smith JB: The influence of platelet aggregation of drugs that effect the accumulation of adenosine 3-5 cyclic monophosphate in platelets. *Biochem J* 121:185, 1971
59. Sneddon JM: The effect of mitosis inhibitors of blood platelet tubules and aggregation. *J Physiol* (Lond) 214:145, 1971
60. Holmsen H, Cetkowsky CA, Day HJ: The effects of antimycin and 2-deoxyglucose on adenine nucleotides in human platelets: role of metabolic ATP in aggregation, secondary aggregation, and shape change of platelets. *Biochem J* 144:385, 1974
61. Roth GJ, Majerus PW: The mechanism of the effect of aspirin on human platelets I. Acetylation of a particulate fraction protein. *J Clin Invest* 56:624, 1975
62. Ali M, McDonald JWD: Reversible and irreversible inhibition of platelet cyclo-oxygenase and serotonin release by non-steroidal anti-inflammatory drugs. *Thromb Res* 13:1057, 1978
63. Johnson RA, Morton DR, Kinner JH, Gorman RR, McGuire JC, Sun FF, Whitaker N, Bunting S, Salman J, Moncada S, Vane JR: The chemical structure of prostaglandin x (prostacyclin). *Prostaglandins* 12:915, 1976
64. Moncada S, Herman AG, Higgs EA, Vane JR: Differential formation of prostacyclin (PGx or PGI$_2$) by layers of the arterial wall: An explanation for the anti-thrombotic properties of vascular endothelium. *Thromb Res* 11:323, 1977
65. MacIntyre DE, Pearson JD, Gordon JL: Localization and stimulation of prostacyclin production in vascular cells. *Nature* 271:549, 1978
66. Armstrong JN, Lattimer N, Moncada S, Vane JR: Comparison of the vasodepressor effects of prostacyclin and 6-oxyl-prostaglandin F$_1$ alpha with those of prostaglandin E$_2$ in rats and rabbits. *Br J Pharmacol* 62:125, 1978
67. Cazenave JP, Degana E, Kinlough-Rathbone RL, Richardson M, Packham MA, Mustard JF: Prostaglandins I$_2$ and E$_1$ reduce rabbit and human platelet adherence without inhibing serotonin release from adherent platelets. *Thromb Res* 15:273, 1979
68. Higgs EA, Moncada AS, Vane JR, Caen JP, Michel H, Tobelen G: Effect of prostacyclin (PGI$_2$) and platelet adhesion to rabbit arterial subendothelium. *Prostaglandins* 16:17, 1978
69. Weiss HJ, Turitto VT: Prostacyclin (prostaglandin I$_2$, PGI$_2$) inhibits platelet adhesion and thrombus formation on subendothelium. *Blood* 53:244, 1979
70. Higgs EA, Higgs GA, Moncada S, Vane JR: Prostaglandin (PGI$_2$) inhibits the formation of platelet thrombi in arterioles and venules of the hamster cheek pouch. *Br J Pharmacol* 63:535, 1978
71. Fuster V, Chesebro JH: Series on pharmacology in practice. 10. Anti thrombotic therapy: role of platelet-inhibitor drugs. 11. Pharmacological effects of platelet-inhibitor drugs. *Mayo Clin Proc* 56:185, 1981
72. Harker LA, Slichter S: Platelet and fibrinogen consumption in man. *N Engl J Med* 287:999, 1972
73. Harker LA: *In vivo* evaluation of antithrombotic therapy in man. *Thromb Diath Haemorrh (suppl 60)*:481, 1974
74. Moncada S, Korbut R: Dipyridamole and other phosphodiesterase inhibitors act as antithrombotic agents by potentiating endogenous prostacyclin. *Lancet* 1:1286, 1978
75. Riesman D: Hemorrhages in the course of Bright's disease with a nephrotic origin. *Am J Med Sci* 134:709, 1907
76. Donner L, Neuwirtova: The hemostatic defect of acute and chronic uraemia. *Thromb Diath Haemorrh* 5:319, 1960
77. Rabiner SF: Uremic bleeding. *Proc Hemost Thromb* 1:233, 1972
78. Castaldi PA, Rosenberg MC, Stewart JH: The bleeding disorder of uraemia. *Lancet* 2:66, 1966
79. Salzman EW, Neri LL: Adhesiveness of blood platelets in uremia. *Thromb Diath Haemorrh* 15:84, 1966
80. George CRP, Slichter SJ, Quadracci LJ, Striker GE, Harker LA: A kinetic evaluation of hemostasis in renal disease. *N Engl J Med* 291:1111, 1974
81. Stewart JH, Castaldi PA: Uraemic bleeding: A reversible platelet defect corrected by dialysis. *Q J Med* 36:409, 1967
82. Rabiner SF, Hrodek O: Platelet factor 3 in normal subjects and patients with renal failure. *J Clin Invest* 47:901, 1968
83. Joist JH, Pechan J, Schikowski U, Hubner G, Gross R: Studies on the nature and etiology of uremic thrombocytopathy. *Verh Dtsch Ges Inn Med* 75:476, 1969
84. Lindsay RM, Moorthy AV, Koens F, Linton AL: Platelet function in dialyzed and non-dialyzed patients with chronic renal failure. *Clin Nephrol* 4:52, 1975
85. Lindsay RM, Friesen M, Koens F, Linton AL, Oreopoulos D, DeVeber G: Platelet function in patients on long term peritoneal dialysis. *Clin Nephrol* 6:335, 1976
86. Lindsay RM, Friesen M, Aronstam A, Andrus F, Clark WF, Linton AL: Improvement of platelet function by increased frequency of hemodialysis. *Clin Nephrol* 10:67, 1978
87. Nenci GG, Berrettini M, Agnelli G, Parise P, Buincristiani U, Ballatori E: Effect of peritoneal dialysis, haemodialysis and kidney transplantation on blood platelet function. I. Platelet aggregation by ADP and epinephrine. *Nephron* 23:287, 1979
88. Jorgenson KA, Ingeberg S: Platelets and platelet function

in patients with chronic uremia on maintenance hemodialysis. *Nephron* 23:233, 1979
89. Kazatchkine M, Sultan Y, Caen JP, Bariety J: Bleeding in renal failure: a possible cause. *Br Med J* 2:612, 1976
90. Remuzzi G, Livio M, Cavenaghi AE, Marchesi D, Mecca G, Donati MB, de Gaetano G: Unbalanced prostaglandin synthesis and plasma factors in uraemic bleeding a hypothesis. *Thromb Res* 13:531, 1978
91. Brash JL, Lyman DJ: Adsorption of proteins and lipids to non-biological surfaces. In: *The Chemistry of Biosurfaces*, edited by Hair ML, New York, NY, Marcel Dekker Inc., 1971, p 177
92. Salzman EW: Role of platelets in blood-surface interactions. *Fed Proc* 30:1503, 1971
93. Vroman L, Adams AL, Klings M: Interactions among human blood proteins at interfaces. *Fed Prod* 30:1494, 1971
94. Feijen J: Thrombogenesis caused by blood foreign surface interaction. In: *Artificial Organs: Proceedings of a seminar on the clinical applications of membrane oxygenators and sorbent-based systems*, edited by Kenedi RM, Courtney JM, Gaylor JDS, Gilchrist T, London, Basingstoke, MacMillan Press Ltd, 1977, p 235
95. Niemetz J, Muhlfelder T, Chierego ME, Troy B: Procoagulant activity of leukocytes. *Ann NY Acad Sci* 283:208, 1977
96. Craddock PR, Fehr J, Brigham KL, Kronenberg RS, Jacob HS: Complement and leukocyte-mediated pulmonary dysfunction in hemodialysis. *N Engl J Med* 296:769, 1977
97. Jacob HS, Craddock PR, Hammerschmidt DE, Moldow CF: Complement-induced granulocyte aggregation: an unsuspected mechanism of disease. *N Engl J Med* 302:89, 1980
98. Lindsay RM, Prentice CRM, Davidson JF, Burton JA, McNicol GP: Haemostatic changes during dialysis associated with the thrombus formation on dialysis membranes. *Br Med J* 4:454, 1972
99. Lindsay RM, Ferguson D, Prentice CRM, Burton JA, McNicol GP: Reduction of thrombus formation on dialyzer membranes by aspirin and RA233. *Lancet* 2:1287, 1972
100. Lindsay RM, Rourke J, Reid B, Friesen M, Linton AL, Courtney J, Gilchrist T: Platelets, foreign surfaces and heparin. *Trans Am Soc Artif Intern Organs* 22:292, 1976
101. Wilkinson R, Lindsay RM, Burton JA: The membrane support system and thrombus formation on dialysis membranes. *Proc Eur Dial Transpl Assoc* 10:306, 1973
102. Gotch FA, Keen ML: Precise control of minimal heparinization for high bleeding risk hemodialysis. *Trans Am Soc Artif Intern Organs* 23:168, 1977
103. Harada K, Zucker MB: Simultaneous development of PF4 activity and release of ^{14}C-serotonin. *Thromb Diath Haemorrh* 25:41, 1971
104. Rucinski B, Niewiarowski S, James P, Walz DA, Brudzynski AZ: Antiheparin proteins secreted by human platelets. Purification, characterization and radioimmunoassay. *Blood* 53:47, 1979
105. O'Brien JR: Antithrombin III and heparin clotting times in atherosclerosis and thrombosis. *Thromb Diath Haemorrh* 32:116, 1974
106. Aronstam A, Dennis B, Friesen MJ, Clark WF, Linton AL, Lindsay RM: Heparin neutralizing activity in patients with renal disease on maintenance haemodialysis. *Thromb Haemorrh* 35:695, 1978
107. Woods HF, Ash G, Weston MJ, Bunting S, Moncada S, Vane JR: Prostacyclin can replace heparin in haemodialysis in dogs. *Lancet* 2:1075, 1978
108. Turney JH, Fewell MR, Williams LC, Parsons V, Weston MJ: Platelet protection and heparin sparing with prostacyclin regular dialysis therapy. *Lancet* 2:219, 1980
109. Zusman RM, Rubin RH, Cato AE, Cocchetto DM, Crow JW, Tolkoff-Rubin N: Haemodialysis using prostacyclin instead of heparin as the sole antithrombotic agent. *N Engl J Med* 304:934, 1981
110. Lindsay RM: Variable heparin requirements during hemodialysis-Why? *Am Soc Artif Intern Organs* 3:81, 1980
111. Hall GH, Holman HM, Webster ADB: Anticoagulation by ancrod for haemodialysis. *Br Med J* 4:591, 1970
112. Kaedi A, Pinio GF, Shimizu A, Drivedi H, Hirsch J, Gent M: Arteriovenous shunt thrombosis: Prevention by sulfinpyrazone. *N Engl J Med* 290:304, 1974
113. Harter HR, Burch JW, Majerus PW, Stanford N, Delmez JA, Anderson CB, Weerts CA: Prevention of thrombosis in patients on hemodialysis by low dose aspirin. *N Engl J Med* 301:577, 1979
114. Wing AJ, Curtis JR, de Wardener HE: Reduction of clotting in Scribner shunts by long-term anticoagulation. *Br Med J* 3:143, 1976
115. Clagett GP, Russo M, Hugnagel H: Platelet changes after placement of aortic prostheses in dogs. I. Biochemical and functional alterations. *J Lab Clin Med* 97:345, 1981
116. Harker LA, Slichter S, Sauvage LR: Platelet consumption by arterial prostheses: The effects of endothelialization and pharmacologic inhibition of platelet function. *Ann Surg* 186:594, 1977
117. Oblath RW, Buckley FO, Green RM, Schwartz SI, De Weese JA: Prevention of platelet aggregation and adherence to prosthetic vascular grafts by aspirin and dipyridamole. *Surgery* 84:37, 1978
118. Cluney GJA, Martin AM, Nolan B: Intermittent haemodialysis: insertion and care of the Silastic Teflon cannula. *Br Med J* 3:88, 1967
119. Anderson DC, Martin AN, Cluney JGA, Stewart WK, Robson AS: The use of streptokinase in the declotting of arteriovenous shunts. *Proc Eur Dial Transpl Assoc* 4:55, 1967
120. Watt DL, Dun BP, Livingston WR, MacDougall AI, MacKay RKS, Obineche EN, Rennie JB: The use of urokinase in declotting arteriovenous shunts. *Proc Eur Dial Trans Assoc* 6:88, 1969
121. McIntosh CS, Petrie JC, MacLeod N: Maintenance of Silastic-Teflon shunts for haemodialysis. *Brit Med J* 4:717, 1969
122. Cluney GJA, Hartley L: Treatment of clotting in external-arteriovenous shunts with a fibrinolytic enzymes. *Med J Aust* 2:463, 1969
123. Lindsay RM, Mason R, Kim SW, Andrade JD, Hawkin RM: Blood surface interactions. *Trans Am Soc Artif Intern Organs* 26:603, 1980

11

HAEMODIALYSIS MONITORS AND MONITORING

PRAKASH R. KESHAVIAH and STANLEY SHALDON

Introduction	223
The extracorporeal blood circuit	225
Flow monitoring	225
Flow output of a blood pump	225
Bubble transit time	226
Electromagnetic flow devices	226
Ultrasonic flow meters	226
Bubble trap flow indicator	226
Pressure monitoring	226
Mechanical manometers	227
Electronic manometers	228
Enclosed pressure sack or pillow pressure monitor	228
Air leak monitors	229
Visible light photocell	229
Infra red photocell	230
Capacitance devices	230
Ultrasonic devices	230
Blood line clamp	230
Infusion pumps for anticoagulation	230
The dialysis fluid circuit	230
Conductivity monitoring	232
Temperature monitoring	232
Pressure monitoring	233
Flow monitoring	234
Blood leak monitoring	234
Dialysis fluid deaeration	235
Disinfection of the dialysis fluid delivery system	235
Electrical safety	236
Overview of system safety	236
Special monitoring schemes	237
Single needle systems	237
Sequential ultrafiltration and diffusion	238
Patient monitoring	239
References	240

INTRODUCTION

The world-wide acceptance of haemodialysis as a long term means of achieving survival for patients with end stage renal failure may have obscured the inherent danger of this technique to the patient. The technique evolved rapidly from the intensive care unit with continuous nursing and medical observation of the patients in 1960 (1), to the patient's own home, where unattended overnight haemodialysis was first performed in 1964 with a passive flow system and without the use of a blood pump (2). The universal preference for the arteriovenous (A-V) fistula (3) and its implied use of a blood pump, the use of more efficient dialysers (4) together with the requirement that the patient accepts more responsibility for his own treatment (5), have placed an even greater emphasis on the need for adequate equipment and monitoring.

It is difficult to estimate the true incidence and severity of technical mishaps in haemodialysis from a review of the scientific literature. This may, in part, be due to the reluctance of dialysis centres to publish their unfortunate accidents. It may also be a consequence of a major secondary complication obscuring the primary origin of the complication. For example, infections are still a principal cause of death among dialysis patients, accounting for 20% of all patient mortality (6). It is likely that many of these infections are related to primarily technical faults as opposed to reduced immune response of uraemic patients. A comprehensive survey of the risks and hazards associated with haemodialysis equipment has been published recently (7). The reader is also referred to Chapter 31 of this book for a survey of the acute complications associated with haemodialysis.

In striving for safety in haemodialysis, one must recognise that safety is a relative rather than an absolute concept. The addition of safety features should be considered in terms of added cost, complexity, increased maintenance and most importantly, overall effectiveness of treatment. Equipment should be designed around the 'fail-safe' concept defined by Grimsrud (8) as follows:

'In the event of an excursion of the variables outside their control limits, or a breakdown of the monitoring or control equipment itself, the system will automatically return to a safe configuration'.

Safe configuration refers to patient isolation, and hence protection from the malfunction and its effects but does not usually include rectification of the cause of an alarm. Such rectification is usually dependent on appropriate human action. It is, therefore, important to note that safety depends not only on an equipment design, but also on a properly trained operator. It is not possible to substitute one for the other.

Several national and international agencies are in the process of formulating standards for haemodialysis equipment (9–12). A comparative assessment and critical review of these standards may be found in the survey of the risks and hazards associated with haemodialysis equipment cited above (7). This survey also includes a definition of minimum system design from the viewpoint of monitoring and recommendations related to equipment performance.

This chapter will focus on the monitoring of the extracorporeal blood circuit and the dialysate circuit. Equipment used in these circuits will be described and the parameters that need to be measured and monitored will be defined. Principles of measurement and the accuracy and resolution requirements of these monitors will also be defined. In addition to the monitoring requirements of the blood and dialysis fluid circuits, special dialysis schemes such as single needle dialysis and sequential ultrafiltration and diffusion will be discussed. Monitoring of the patient during dialysis will also be considered briefly.

Before proceeding to a detailed discussion of individual monitors, certain requirements that are common to all monitors and constitute an approach to the ideal monitoring system will be enumerated:

1. The location and sensitivity of monitors should detect changes in the variable monitored before the changes can affect the patient.
2. Functional testing of alarms should be easily accomplished without special tools so that testing may be incorporated into the dialysis procedure. It should also be possible to test and calibrate each monitor independently using external standards.
3. The minimum sensitivity and maximum spread of alarm limits should be internally set with operator adjustments being possible only within this range. Operator adjustments should not result in the alarm being disabled.
4. Fail-safe design and system stability may be compromised with interdependence of monitors and their circuitry. This may also be true if control and monitoring functions have common sensors and circuitry. It is therefore desirable to have control and monitoring functions independent of each other and individual monitors independent of each other. Further, the monitor should be critically sensitive to only one variable.
6. Audible and visual alarms should be provided. A muting switch, if provided, should affect *only* the audible alarm and for a limited time duration (e.g. 90 to 120 seconds). It should be impossible to resume dialysis as long as the alarm condition exists or with the monitors inactivated. Visual alarms should be designed for clarity and readability at a distance of 2 m. Audible alarms should be rated at no less than 70 decibels ('A' scale) at 3 m.
7. In an alarm condition, patient protection should occur as a consequence of passive mechanisms inherent to system design rather than specific reactive mechanisms.
8. When there is isolated loss of power, the affected monitor displays should indicate either the high or low range rather than the central normal range to prevent the operator from assuming normal operation. Loss of power to the overall system should be indicated by an alarm (audible and visual) and patient protection schemes should be automatically activated.
9. The hydraulic and electrical components within a piece of equipment should be separated, the electrical circuits being adequately isolated from liquid leaks.

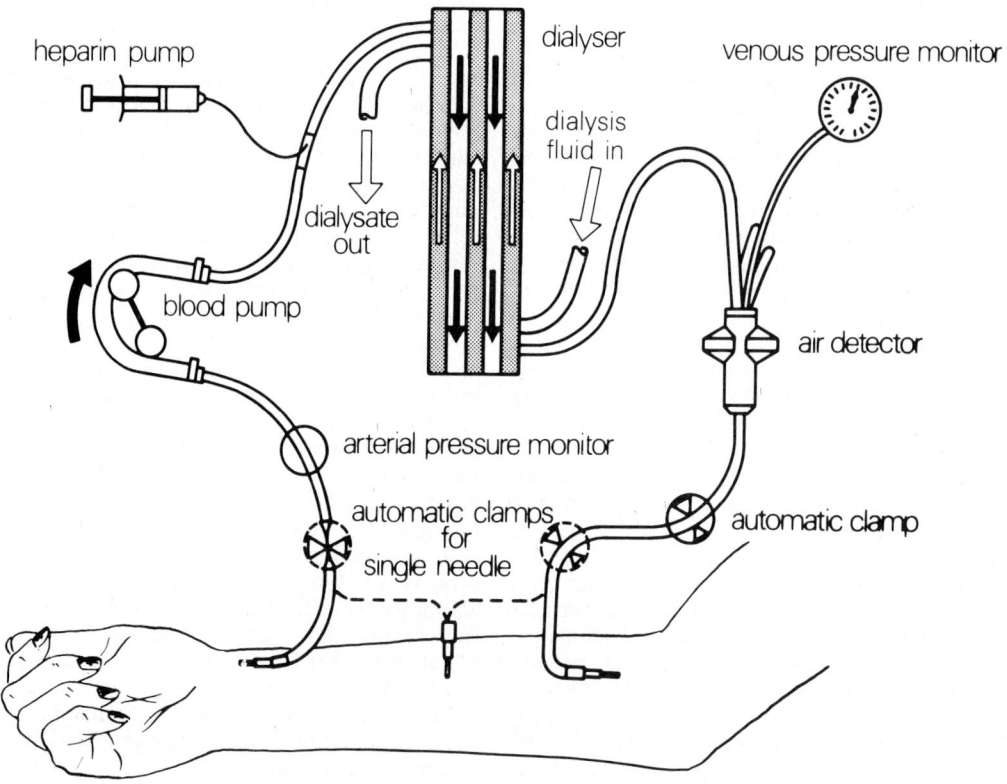

Figure 1. Typical haemodialysis blood circuit.

The outside of the equipment should be shielded from liquid spills.

THE EXTRACORPOREAL BLOOD CIRCUIT

A typical haemodialysis blood circuit is illustrated in Figure 1. With the use of the A-V fistula, blood is pumped from the patient via his access site through the dialyser and back to the patient. The segment of the circuit from the patient to the dialyser is commonly referred to as the arterial segment and that from the dialyser back to the patient as the venous segment. The sites at which pressures in the blood circuit are usually measured are between the patient's access and the blood pump and at the venous air trap located downstream of the dialyser. Sometimes pressures are also monitored at an arterial air trap between the blood pump and the dialyser. The air detector is usually located on the venous air trap with the clamp that is activated by the air detector being positioned just below the air trap. Heparin, for anticoagulation, is typically infused downstream of the blood pump. Patient isolation from alarm conditions in the blood circuit is usually effected by stopping the blood pump and clamping the venous blood tubing.

Flow monitoring

The flow rate at which the blood compartment of the dialyser is perfused is an important parameter as it influences the efficiency of solute transport across the dialyser membrane. Small solutes such as urea and creatinine are said to be flow limited, as the clearances of these solutes are influenced to a greater extent by the blood and dialysis fluid flow rates than by the diffusive resistance of the dialyser membrane. On the other hand, large solutes such as Vitamin B_{12} (which is often used as a test substance and has a molecular weight of 1357) are membrane limited, their clearance being mainly influenced by the diffusive resistance of the membrane and to a much smaller extent by blood and dialysis fluid flow rates. Dialyser clearances of small solutes increase as blood and dialysis fluid flow rates are increased but at a diminishing rate, a relative clearance plateau being reached beyond a certain blood or dialysis fluid flow rate.

In the early days of haemodialysis, cannulae were used for blood access, thereby allowing passive perfusion of the blood circuit by the patient's systemic blood pressure. The predominant use of the A-V fistula nowadays, necessitates the use of a blood pump for perfusion of the blood circuit, because of the large pressure drops in the fistula needles.

Blood pumps used in haemodialysis may be freestanding or an integral part of the dialysis fluid delivery system. The type of blood pump most commonly used is the peristaltic roller pump. A compressible segment of the 'arterial' blood tubing is inserted into a curved roller track in the blood pump and the rotation of the rollers compresses the tubing, forcing blood out of the pump segment. After passage of the roller, the tubing resumes its original shape and blood is drawn in to refill the pump segment.

The roller pumps used in haemodialysis have between one and three rollers on the pump head, two rollers being most common. Increasing the number of rollers on the pump head increases the frequency of pulsation but decreases the pulse amplitude (pulse pressure). The occlusion of the pump segment between the roller track and the rollers is usually adjustable. Inadequate occlusion results in back flow, foaming and possibly haemolysis. Over occlusion can lead to tubing damage, and hence blood leaks, as well as increased haemolysis. In many blood pumps, spring loaded rollers are used to achieve optimal occlusion, correcting for small variations in tubing diameter, wall thickness and elastic modulus.

Blood pumps are usually designed to accommodate a range of tubing sizes as well as single/dual pump segments. In pumps that incorporate a direct display of blood flow rate, provisions are made to correlate choice of tubing size and number of segments to flow rate, either through the use of multiple scales on the display or through use of selector switches. Blood pumps are usually provided with a tool for manual operation in the event of a power failure.

Haemolysis is a problem of considerable magnitude in blood pumps used for cardiopulmonary bypass because of the high blood flow rates. In haemodialysis, however, the flow rates are much lower and studies indicate that immediate and delayed haemolysis in the extracorporeal circuit are too small to be of consequence (13, 14). It has also been shown that, in well-dialysed patients, red cell survival approaches normal, suggesting that there is no delayed haemolysis due to sublethal damage in the extracorporeal circulation (15).

In some blood pumps there are inadequate provisions for protecting the operator from the rotating parts of the pump. Either there is no safety cover or there are rotating parts that protrude through the safety cover. Some pumps have a mechanical or electrical safety shut-off feature in high torque situations. This not only protects the pumps from damage but also provides for operator safety.

It is highly desirable to have the electrical components of blood pumps shielded from liquid spills. In the absence of such shielding, a saline spill may not only damage the pump circuit but could also result in dangerous current leakage. High current leakage may also be observed in older pumps that have been subjected to salt corrosion. The use of a low voltage DC motor reduces the electrical hazard associated with a blood pump.

Flow output of the blood pump

The flow output of a blood pump is the product of pump speed and stroke volume. If stroke volume is constant, flow output is directly proportional to pump speed. Many blood pumps have a meter that supposedly indicates the speed of operation and hence the flow rate. The displayed parameter is not really pump speed but armature voltage, pump speed being proportional to armature voltage. Under normal inlet voltage conditions this is valid. However, inlet voltages do fluctuate by at least ±10%, if not more. Therefore, the same meter indication could result in varying pump speeds, depending on the voltage. There are pumps that have a true tachometer display, and this is more desirable than an armature voltage indicator. If stroke volume varies, accurate measurement of pump speed will not guarantee accurate flow rates. Stroke volume variations, arising from variations in the internal diameter of the pump segment, may result in flow rate errors as large as ±20%. With extreme inlet suction pressures (subatmospheric pressures), there is incomplete refilling of the pump segment resulting in a reduced stroke volume. The stroke volume is also reduced by retrograde flow when the pump outlet pressure exceeds the occlusive pressure setting of the rollers. In both situations, the actual flow rate is less than that indicated by pump speed.

A blood pump that displays armature voltage may be calibrated using banked blood or a fluid that has a viscosity similar to blood. The calibration is however valid only if the pressures at the pump inlet and outlet simulate those in clinical use. As the pressures in clinical use vary considerably, the calibration may be inaccurate because of the changes in stroke volume associated with different inlet and outlet pressures.

Bubble transit time
A method that is widely used clinically for measuring the blood flow rate is the 'bubble transit time' method. In this method an air bubble is injected into the arterial segment of the blood circuit and the transit time of the bubble across a certain length of tubing is measured. A suitable calibration is used to convert the transit time to a flow rate. Blood tubing for haemodialysis usually incorporates a 50 cm 'race track'. The race track is merely a segment of blood tubing with two markings spaced at the required distance to allow convenient measurement of the bubble transit time. There are several factors that contribute to inaccuracies with this method. The race track should be horizontal during the measurement and this is often neglected in clinical use. The bubble size has a significant influence on the accuracy of the method. Small bubbles that travel along the axis of flow result in an overestimation of the actual flow rate because the velocity profile across the tube cross-section is parabolic, the centre line velocity being twice the mean velocity. The method is more accurate when the bubble fills the entire tubing cross-section. Variations in the internal diameter of the blood tubing and hence the volume of the race track are another source of error. Inaccuracies in the time measurement also add to the error of the method. At a typical blood flow rate of 200 ml/min, a race track length of 50 cm, and an internal diameter of 0.48 cm (3/16''), the bubble transit time is as small as 2.5 sec. To improve the accuracy of the method, race track lengths as large as 2 m have been used but if this increases the length of blood tubing used, the extracorporeal volume may be larger than desired. The risk of hepatitis transmission through an accidental needle stab exists with this method. The risk is minimised if there is a protective guard on the underside of the injection site. Aerosol transmission of virus particles from puncturing a tube under positive pressures does, however, exist. The risk of accidental needle stabs and aerosol transmission can be eliminated with an infusion 'T' for injecting the bubble. In spite of these criticisms, under ideal conditions of measurement, a good correlation can be established between the bubble transit time and the blood flow rate (see Chapter 5 for further details of the 'bubble transit time' method).

Electromagnetic flow devices
These have been employed in haemodialysis; the electromagnetic method is an invasive technique which requires that the electrodes are in direct contact with blood. Although the method is very accurate the need to clean and sterilise the blood contaminated transducers together with the risk of transmission of hepatitis have largely precluded its clinical use.

Ultrasonic flow meters
Ultrasonic flow meters employ the principle that the passage of a blood cell will reflect part of the transmitted ultrasonic wave and cause a frequency change which can be detected by the 'Doppler shift' which is directly proportional to the particle speed. This value in cm/min multiplied by the inner cross-section of the blood tubing in cm^2 yield a flow rate in ml/min. The calibration of the inner diameter of the tubing is critical. In addition, the sonic contact between transducer and tubing must be adequate and requires the use of a silicone gel to improve the sonic transport. It is possible to monitor the electrical read out of blood flow with a high/low alarm contact system. In spite of the theoretical advantages, the expense and unreliability of current ultrasonic meters have prevented their use as a routine clinical monitor.

Bubble trap flow indicator
A visual flow indicator has been incorporated into the disposable bubble trap which has been modified into two chambers separated by a disc containing a central hole through which the blood flows. A small tube allows free communication of air between the top of each chamber. As a result the height of the column of blood in the upper chamber is related to flow-rate. An appropriate scale is fixed to the upper chamber graduated from 100 to 400 ml/min.

Pressure monitoring

Pressures in the blood circuit are monitored for two reasons. Firstly monitors can detect disconnection of tubing as well as obstructions caused by clots, kinks or clamps. Secondly pressures are also measured to aid in controlling fluid removal from the patient. In haemodialysis, fluid removal is achieved by applying a hydrostatic pressure differential across the dialyser membrane, fluid being forced through membrane pores. This process is called ultrafiltration and the applied pressure differential is referred to as the transmembrane pressure (TMP). The TMP may be generated by applying positive (above-atmospheric) blood compartment pressures, ne-

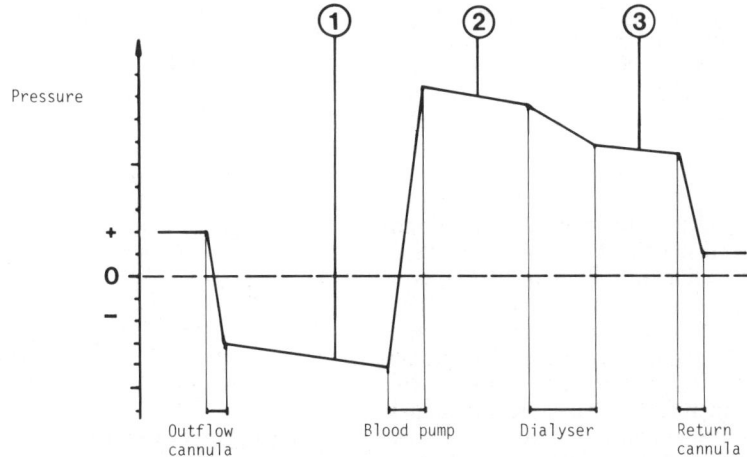

Figure 2. Pressure profile in the blood circuit. Pressure ① is negative before the pump and pressures ② and ③ are positive after it.

gative dialysis fluid compartment pressures, or both. The blood compartment pressure used in calculating the TMP is estimated by averaging the pressures at the inlet and outlet of the dialyser. In routine clinical practice, as the pressure drop across the blood compartment is small (except in coil dialysers), the pressure in the venous air trap is used as a reasonable approximation of the blood compartment pressure. The indirect control of the ultrafiltration rate by controlling the TMP reflects current state of the art. Some of the newer dialysis fluid delivery systems are capable of directly controlling the rate of ultrafiltration, the TMP then becoming a dependent parameter rather than an independent controlling parameter.

The pressure profile in the blood circuit is depicted in Figure 2. Pressures that exceed atmospheric pressure are considered positive and those below atmospheric are negative. As seen in the figure, pressures upstream of the blood pump may be negative while those downstream of the pump are positive. It is the energy supplied by the pump that raises pressure. Pressure monitoring is desirable at the locations indicated in Figure 2 for the following reasons:

The pressure before the blood pump (① - Figure 2) is negative due to the resistance of the access site needle and tubing set. It is desirable to have as little negative pressure as possible for a given blood flow rate to avoid suction of the vessel wall into the lumen of the needle and to minimise the risk of air entry at bad joints. The length and internal bore of the fistula needle can increase the resistance by 100% if 38 mm by 1.5 mm needles are used instead of 15 mm by 2.0 mm needles (16).

The pressure between the blood pump (② - Figure 2) and the dialyser is always positive. As indicated earlier, its measurement permits a calculation of the TMP when used in conjunction with the venous pressure. The 'venous' pressure, that is the pressure after the dialyser (③ - Figure 2), is measured in the air trap downstream of the dialyser. Increase in resistance between the air trap and the return access site will cause a rise in pressure which may rupture the dialyser membrane. In addition, any alarm which stops the blood pump will cause the pressure at this point to drop and will usually result in a low pressure alarm. Reductions in blood flow as well as any disruption of the tubing between the bubble trap and the venous needle will cause a drop in pressure as well, and activate a low pressure alarm.

Blood circuit pressure monitors and alarms are usually incorporated into the dialysis fluid delivery system. There are three types of pressure monitors commonly in use.

Mechanical manometers
Mechanical manometers have mechanical, optical, or electronic contacts and depend upon a change in pressure causing a movement within bellows or Bourdon tubes which, by means of amplifying levers and gears, is then registered by a pointer. The pointer position is related to a graduated pressure scale. The mechanical alarm contacts are essentially make or break contacts which depend upon a junction between the moving pointer and the fixed alarm contact. In selecting a mechanical contact from the fail safe point of view it is essential that the circuit be broken by the alarm situation. It is also important that the voltage and current passing through the contact be sufficient to make the circuit. This will depend upon the surface area and the material used. Low resistance gold plating is frequently used as it is resistant to oxidation which would cause an increase in resistance. DC circuits (12 to 24 V) are commonly employed, with high resistance components to safeguard against possible increase in resistance by oxidation of contacts. This type of alarm monitor with a range of -250 to $+400$ mm Hg is the oldest and perhaps the least reliable of pressure monitors.

Mechanical manometers with optical or electronic contacts are more reliable theoretically. The contact between the moving pointer and the fixed alarm setting depends upon the fact that the pointer interrupts a light beam to a photosensitive cell. With electronic contacts the pointer changes the frequency of an oscillator circuit and thereby triggers an alarm. Although these methods involve more components and are more expensive, the mechanical moving parts are reduced resulting in greater reliability.

Electronic manometers
A pressure transducer picks up the pressure signal and converts it to an electrical signal. This is then amplified and the value is displayed either on a meter or as a digital read-out graded in millimetres of mercury. The alarm settings in the electronic system are preset and usually not adjustable on the display panel. Alterations are made by the use of trim potentiometers inside the monitor. It is difficult therefore to visualise the actual alarm settings under these conditions. However, using an adjustable graduated dial indicator with a fixed pressure range between high and low alarm points which can be set to the pressure determined by the pointer on the meter, a compromise situation is obtained. An alternative to this is the use of the electronic signal to record the pressure, with adjustable visible alarm contacts operated either by an optical device or by changing the frequency within an oscillator. The advantage of this system is a more reliable measurement of pressure with visible adjustable alarm settings.

Enclosed pressure sack or pillow monitor
The enclosed pressure sack or pillow pressure monitor (Figure 3), is a device, usually situated between the patient and the blood pump, that offers a crude method of detecting excessive negative pressure. The sack maintains the pressure when full and holds a microswitch in the make position; when the sack collapses the microswitch breaks and causes an alarm. The sack and the microswitch may be calibrated to alarm at a minimum given negative pressure which will depend upon the thinness of the wall of the sack and the spring force of the microswitch. Even with such calibration, the pillow monitor is susceptible to frequent false alarms. It cannot be used in single needle dialysis.

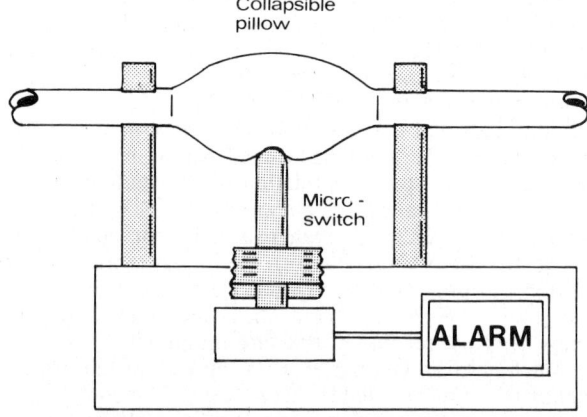

Figure 3. Collapsible 'pillow' pressure monitor.

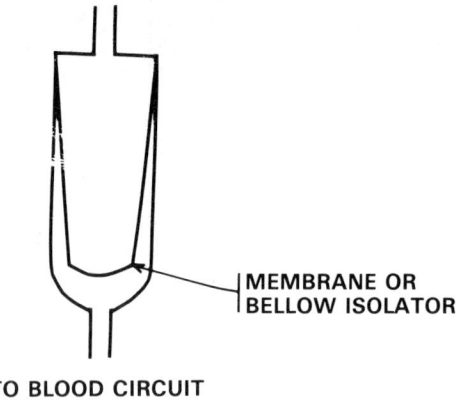

Figure 4. Blood pressure monitor isolator.

With all manometers and pressure transducers it is desirable that there is some form of isolation between the blood and the actual monitoring device. The development of isolators was necessitated originally because of the risk of transmission of hepatitis. Subsequently, protection of the monitor from blood contamination and the difficulty in cleaning it, resulted in a rapid adoption of some form of disposable elastic non-permeable membrane or bellows used as a pressure monitor isolator (Figure 4). The alternative type of pressure isolator, in the form of a pore filter which closes on contact with liquids, is excellent for protecting the monitor but has a major disadvantage. After closure, no further pressure change can be recorded; thus unless the filter is changed, the monitor is rendered inoperative.

Pressure monitors should have an accuracy of ± 10 mm Hg at pressures less than 50 mm Hg and $\pm 10\%$ of the indicated pressure at pressures greater than 50 mm Hg. The tolerance of ± 10 mm Hg is necessary to detect blood line separations occuring when blood circuit pressures are low. The tolerance of $\pm 10\%$ of the indicated pressure at pressures greater than 50 mm Hg is based on considerations of ultrafiltration control and prediction. The accuracy of the alarms should be ± 10 mm Hg relative to the indicated alarm setting.

Blood circuit pressure alarms, when activated, should shut the blood pump off and activate audible and visual signals of the alarm condition. When the cause of the alarm has been corrected, there should be a manual obligation to restart the blood pump. The maximum spread of pressure alarm limits should be internally set, with operator adjustments being possible only within this range. For detection of disconnections, it would be desirable to restrict the low limit setting to pressures that are above atmospheric. If the low limit were set in the subatmospheric range, disconnections may remain undetected. This requirement may create a problem in priming the circuit before the initiation of dialysis. It is common practice to spread the alarm limits beyond the safety range during the priming procedure. A possible solution to this problem would be to incorporate a time delay of up to 60 seconds inactivating the low alarm thereby enabling the pump to prime the circuit. It is undesirable to be able to by-pass the low alarm setting.

Air leak monitors

When haemodialysis is performed without a blood pump, the whole blood circuit is under positive pressure and air embolism consequent to air entry into the blood circuit is extremely unlikely. However, with the predominant use of the A-V fistula pump circuit nowadays, the risk of air embolism has increased enormously as negative pressures are developed between the arterial fistula needle and the blood pump. The incidence of major air embolism has been reported as 1 per 2000 haemodialyses (17). Foam-emboli with micro-bubbles of air mixed with blood are more common than pure air emboli and the mortality is around 25% of all reported cases. The causes of air entry include dislodgement of the outflow needle, leaks around any connection between the outflow needle and the blood pump, air entry from an intravenous infusion system inserted before the blood pump, with an empty glass fluid container and air entry from the heparin infusion system also placed before the blood pump. Reduction in the incidence of these accidents can be achieved by eliminating all connections and needle punctures before the blood pump and by infusion of heparin and saline downstream of the blood pump. Efficient degassing of the dialysis fluid will also reduce micro-bubble transport across the dialyser membrane. However, despite minimising these risks, air detectors remain essential. They are recommended for all haemodialysis blood circuits where subatmosphere pressure can be generated.

The ideal air detector will respond to the presence of foam or air and not to saline. It should not require by-passing in order to prime the blood circuit. It should register an audible and visible alarm, fulfil the basic requirements of fail safe monitoring, be powered independently of the blood pump (not from the pump's electrical supply) and in an alarm situation must stop the blood pump. Because of the high compliance of many disposable dialysers, stopping the blood pump will not prevent an air embolism, however, as the passive expulsion of air from an air-filled dialyzer under pressure will still reach the patient in most cases. Therefore, a solenoid clamping device which occludes the venous tube below the bubble trap is also essential (see Figure 1). The air detector devices are usually placed around the venous bubble trap (Figure 5A), but some models are situated on the venous tubing itself below the bubble trap (Figure 5B). Many different physical principles have been employed in current air detectors.

Visible light photocell

The earliest air detectors consisted of a light source which triggered a photocell situated on the opposite side of the bubble trap; the cell did not react if blood

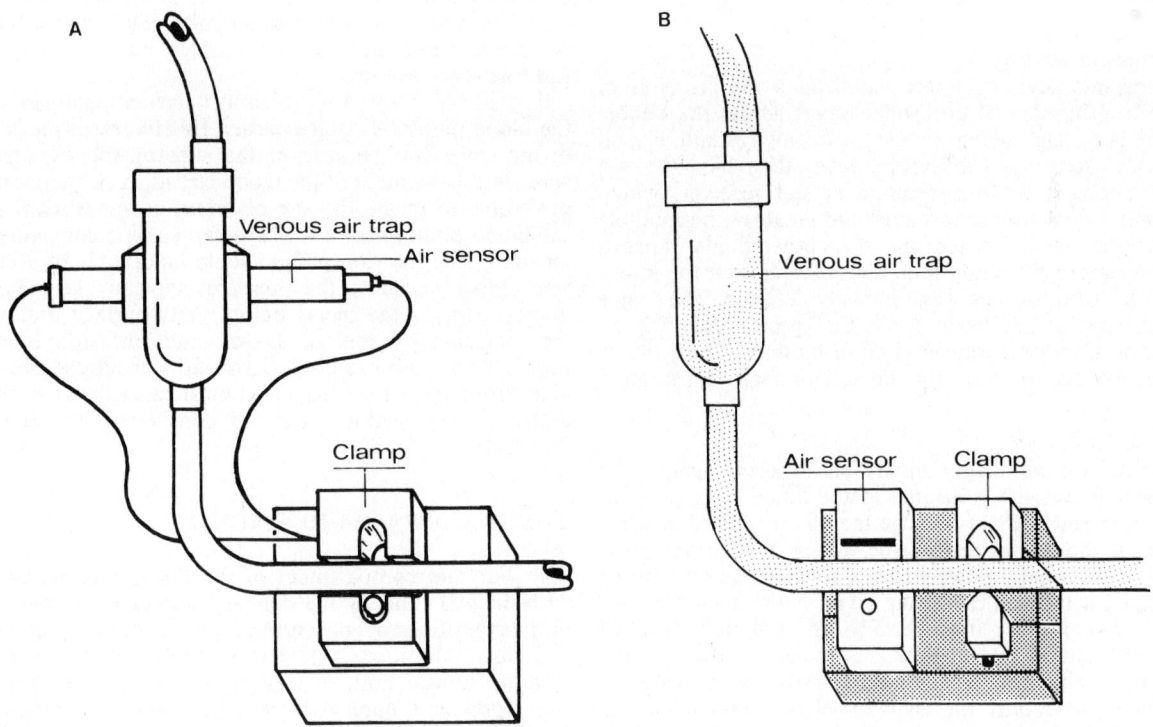

Figure 5. A. Air detector with sensor positioned on venous air trap and clamp on venous blood return line; B. Air detector with sensor and clamp positioned on venous blood return line.

obstructed the light path. These devices were insensitive to foam and could not react if the light path was obstructed by fibrin deposits on the inner wall of the bubble trap. In addition, ambient light could reach the photocell and cause false alarms.

Infrared photocell
Infrared light photocell devices have increased the sensitivity to air but are still not foolproof against obstruction to the passage of the infrared waves, or sensitive enough to be 100% reliable against foam without causing multiple false alarms.

Capacitance devices
Capacitance devices (18) are based upon the principle of change in the frequency of an oscillator circuit, which will vary with the presence of air or fluid within the range of the circuit, and with the thickness of the bubble trap wall, or an admixture of the two. By using two or more capacitor plates to surround the bubble trap sensitive to different frequencies, changes in oscillation can predict the presence of air, foam, saline or blood in the bubble trap. Theoretically this device could fulfill all the requirements of the ideal detector. This device has proven too difficult to use, however, because of volume changes within the bubble trap associated with alterations in the venous pressure, variations in wall thickness of the bubble trap and alterations in the blood viscosity according to individual haemotocrit levels. It must be calibrated for each patient and the sensitivity adjusted accordingly. In addition, it is not 100% reliable for foam.

Ultrasonic devices
Ultrasonic devices (19) are based upon the principle of the transmission of ultrasonic waves across the bubble trap. A voltage source to a transmitting ceramic crystal causes vibrations; ultrasonic waves then pass through the bubble trap to a ceramic crystal receiver, which vibrates on sensing the waves and creates a measurable electrical signal. Because blood or other fluids transmit sound more efficiently than air, a decrease in the intensity of the ultrasonic wave is easily detected. The major advantage of this technique is the specific damping effect on ultrasonic transmission of bubbles. Thus, this is probably the most reliable device for foam detection.

Bloodline clamp
The ideal blood clamp should be occlusive against the maximal pressure generated in the blood circuit (up to 800 mm Hg) and not damage the blood tubing. In addition, it should not restrict the tubing in the open position. It is usually powered by a solenoid valve with or without a mechanical spring lever working on the 'anvil' principle. For it to be fail-safe, it should close on 'break' and be held open in the 'make' position. In the event of electrical power failure, however, it becomes difficult to return the dialyser blood content to the patient. For this reason some clamps are designed to function in the reverse sequence, which is basically undesirable.

The volume of air required to cause clinical symptoms is uncertain. It has been reported that as little as 5 ml of air can be fatal (20), but it is generally accepted that volumes necessary to cause death range from 65 to 125 ml of rapidly injected air (21). Ward and co-workers (17) in analysing their experience with air embolism suggest that humans are probably sensitive to less than 1.0 ml/kg/min of air. In the haemodialysis setting, air entering the patient may range from a massive bolus of air to a short stream of microbubbles. Von Hartitzsch and Medlock (22) report symptoms of nausea and vomiting attributed to a continuous stream of microbubbles which were 1 to 1.5 mm in diameter. Others report that no symptoms have occurred as a consequence of microbubble embolisation (23). It is, therefore, difficult to specify minimum sensitivity of air detection until further research has established susceptibility limits for air occurring as large boluses, as large visible bubbles and as microbubbles or foam. If the air detector is extremely sensitive, it becomes subject to numerous false alarms and runs the risk of being inactivated by dialysis personnel or the patient.

Infusion pumps for anticoagulation

Infusion pumps are used to infuse heparin, and sometimes protamine, into the blood circuit to control anticoagulation of blood. There are two types of infusion pumps used in haemodialysis, syringe pumps and peristaltic pumps. Syringe pumps are more commonly used. Infusion pumps may have fixed rates of infusion or variable rates ranging from 0.5 to 6.0 ml/h. They may either be free-standing units or incorporated into the dialysis fluid delivery system.

The site of infusion is sometimes located upstream of the blood pump. As stated earlier, this increases the risk of air embolism because of the subatmospheric pressures in this segment of the blood circuit. It is, therefore, preferable to locate the site of infusion downstream of the blood pump, the venous air trap being a convenient location. The infusion pump should be capable of accurate delivery against the pressures typically generated downstream of the blood pump. With syringe pumps, the inclusion of 'end of stroke' and 'infusion interrupted' (e.g. power failure) alarms are considered desirable. However, with adequate clinical surveillance of the dialysis, these features are not considered absolutely essential.

THE DIALYSIS FLUID CIRCUIT

The dialysate compartment of the dialyser is perfused with dialysis fluid by the delivery system under appropriate conditions of concentration, temperature, pressure and flow. Monitors and alarms incorporated into the system monitor and, in some systems, control hydrostatic pressures applied across the dialyser membrane for fluid removal. They also safeguard against dialyser blood leaks and sudden changes of pressure in the blood circuit associated with disconnections and obstructions.

In some delivery systems, the blood pump, heparin infusion pump and air detector are built into the system with provisions for appropriate connections to, and positioning of, the blood tubing. The advantages of such an integrated system include a less cluttered treatment area, simplified operations and elimination of human errors in interconnecting free-standing devices.

Dialysis fluid delivery systems may be single pass, recirculating single pass or recirculating systems. Each type may be further divided into single patient or multiple patient (central) systems. In the single pass system, dialysis fluid is delivered to the dialyser and, after a single pass, is pumped out to the drain. In the recirculating single pass system, dialysis fluid is recirculated in the dialysate circuit with fresh dialysis fluid being continuously introduced into the circuit, displacing dialysate in the circuit and causing it to overflow to the drain. In the recirculating system, a large volume of dialysis fluid is recirculated in the dialysate circuit with no provisions for supplying fresh dialysis fluid or overflow from the recirculating dialysate. At the treatment's beginning, the closed loop is filled with fresh dialysis fluid; at the treatment's end, the spent dialysate is drained from the closed loop.

Dialysis fluid may be prepared as a batch process (manual or automated) or may be continuously proportioned (on-line). In single pass systems, dialysis fluid is generally prepared on-line by proportioning pretreated water, and concentrate. Recirculating systems are usually batch systems. Recirculating single pass systems may be either batch or proportioning systems.

The composition of dialysis fluid and its preparation in recirculating and recirculating single pass systems are discussed in Chapter 7 and the clinical problems associated with incorrect formulation are discussed in Chapter 31 of this book. This chapter will deal primarily with the single pass system, the system most commonly used today.

The introduction of dialysis fluid concentrate and the principle of fluid proportioning in 1964 revolutionised haemodialysis. It eliminated the need for manual production of large quantities of dialysis fluid used in batch systems, reduced the bacteriological problem and opened the way for single pass dialysis at 37 °C. The basic single pass dialysis fluid circuit used with either a central supply system and bedside monitors or an individual patient unit is illustrated in Figure 6. The continuous production of dialysis fluid is achieved with a proportioning device, mixing water and concentrate. Water is pretreated, heated and deaerated before being mixed with concentrate. The quality of the resulting dialysis fluid is assured by conductivity and temperature monitoring. If the quality of the fluid is outside prescribed limits, it by-passes the dialyser. Normally dialysis fluid perfuses the dialyser under conditions of controlled flow and pressure. The presence of red cells in dialysate, in case of a membrane rupture, is detected by a blood leak monitor situated after the dialyser. The dialysate pressure is monitored by a pressure monitor and the dialysate then passes to drain via an effluent pump which creates the flow and pressure requirements of the circuit.

The dialysis fluid delivery system consists of the proportioning device, conductivity monitoring, temperature regulation and monitoring, blood leak detection, dialysis fluid pressure and flow regulation and monitoring. In addition to these functions the delivery system also deaerates the dialysis fluid, interfaces with the air in blood detector and blood pump and incorporates a disinfection scheme using chemicals or hot water. Typically, blood circuit pressure monitors and alarm circuitry

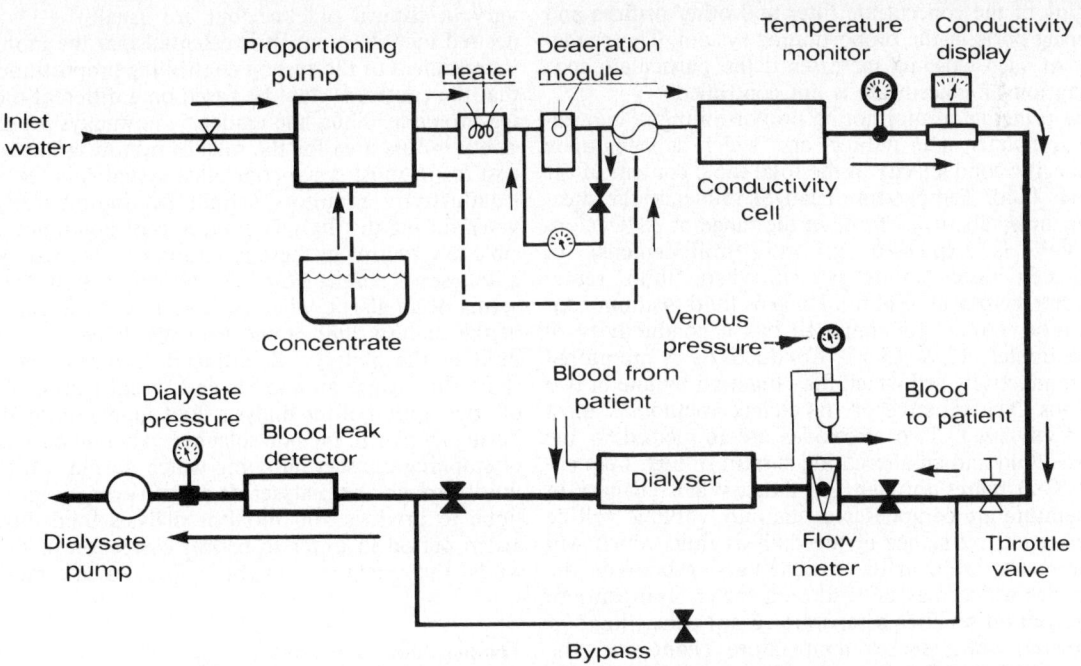

Figure 6. Schematic presentation of single pass dialysis fluid circuit.

are incorporated into the dialysis fluid delivery system.

Conductivity monitoring

In proportioning systems, treated water and concentrate are mixed in the desired ratio, electrical conductivity being the parameter commonly used to monitor appropriate proportioning. The porportioning ratio may be fixed, adjustable to a desired value or continuously variable with a servo-control system based on continuous, internal conductivity monitoring.

Proportioning pumps may be motor or water driven pumps. Motor driven pumps may be of the piston, plunger or membrane type and are usually bulky and noisy but have functioned well for over 10 years with very few problems. Water driven pumps are driven by water pressure and are generally quieter and smaller than motor driven pumps. Servo-control systems may have a peristaltic pump whose speed is servo-controlled or a venturi orifice whose opening is servo-controlled. Though separate sensors are usually used for monitoring and for control of the produced fluid, the two conductivity cells are often identical in design and the possibility of simultaneous failures exists. Further, crystallisation of concentrate in a venturi orifice can cause problems. The advantages of the servo-controlled system are that it permits miniaturisation and lower costs.

Fatalities associated with improper proportioning of dialysis fluid have been reported (24–26). Often human error and negligence were contributing factors. Easily accessible by-pass switches or a re-zeroing feature constitute poor design practice and increase the potential for human errors. Improper proportioning can result from clogging of the concentrate filter and other orifices and metering ports in the proportioning system. The probability of such clogging increases if the particulate contamination of concentrate is not controlled.

The principle of monitoring proportioning of concentrate and water is an indirect one, which depends upon the specific conductivity of the total ionic content of the dialysis fluid. Temperature changes influence the measurement by about 1.7%/°C in the range of 38°C. Conductivity is expressed in mS (milliSiemens) or mmhos/cm (milii 'mhos' per cm where 'mho' represents the reciprocal of ohm). Dialysis fluid (sodium concentration 130 to 150 mmol/L) has a conductivity of approximately 13 to 15 mS. Conductivity is monitored in a conductivity cell which may function by one of two methods. The resistive or impedance method is most commonly used. Two electrodes are immersed in the dialysis fluid and an alternating current of high frequency (1 Khz) pulses through the fluid. When changes in temperature are compensated, the only variable will be the electrical resistance of the dialysis fluid which will cause an alteration in the current passing between the electrodes which may be read on a meter. Temperature compensation requires a separate circuit consisting of a thermistor which senses temperature changes in the range of 34 to 41 °C and corrects the conductivity output signal accordingly. The alternative method is inductive where two electro-magnetic coils replace electrodes and the alteration in the current passing through them represents changes in the conductivity of the dialysis fluid. Temperature compensation is again necessary. It is always mandatory, when calibrating a new conductivity cell or changing the concentrate formula, to correlate a given conductivity reading to a direct measurement of the sodium content in the dialysis fluid by flame photometry, as the conductivity also varies with the ratios of chloride to acetate or bicarbonate and the presence or absence of dextrose.

Problems arising with conductivity measurement are usually due to coating of the electrodes with deposits from the dialysis fluid or with air bubbles from inadequate deaeration of the fluid. These artefacts increase the resistance resulting in a false low conductivity measurement. Design of the cell to prevent gas accumulation is important. It should have a small fluid channel pathway, and the electrodes should be made of an anticorrosive and non-toxic material. The induction coil method has the advantage that air bubbles have a smaller effect upon current changes. Design of the conductivity monitoring system is extremely important for the safety of the haemodialysis procedure. It must follow the fail-safe basis described in the beginning of this chapter. The meter design is usually of the continuous scale type where its range should not exceed the physiological limits of safety, i.e. the equivalent of 120 to 160 mmol/l sodium (approximately 12 to 16 mS). If, however, the meter is of the zero type, the percentage deviation from a precalibrated known conductivity set at zero should not exceed $\pm 10\%$. Both types should detect 1% changes easily. The alarm setpoints should not be movable beyond the safe limits of the physiological range of conductivity. The acceptable limits of the alarm setpoints vary in clinical practice, but are usually $\pm 3\%$ of the desired measurement. It is essential that the monitor be independent of the system controlling proportioning and that the control system be based on a different monitoring principle. Thus, the tendency, nowadays, to sacrifice safety in this area for the sake of minimisation and low cost (as in most servo-controlled systems) is regrettable. Conductivity monitors should be automatically activated during the dialysis mode and it should not be possible to circumvent these monitors or their alarms when a dialyser is connected to the delivery system. The triggering of an alarm, when there is an error in the quality of the dialysis fluid, must stop the delivery of dialysis fluid to the dialyser, diverting it to drain, and at the same time cause an audible and visual alarm. Methods of interruption of the dialysis fluid supply to the dialyser during an alarm, include solenoid valve by-pass systems or stopping the suction pump which normally draws the fluid through the dialyser. It is, however, usual to continue to produce and monitor dialysis fluid during an alarm period in order to permit correction of the error whilst the machine is in the by-pass or safe modality.

Temperature monitoring

Early designs of delivery systems used cold dialysis fluid

to retard bacterial growth in the recirculation reservoir with heat exchangers provided for rewarming the blood. Modern delivery systems utilise a thermostatically controlled heater to warm the incoming water which is then mixed with concentrate at room temperature, the temperature sensor being located downstream of the point of mixing. The temperature of the dialysis fluid is maintained within the range of 36 °C to 42 °C. Though red cell haemolysis may result only at temperatures greater than 45 °C, protein denaturation can take place at temperatures above 42 °C (27).

Overheated dialysis fluid can cause haemolysis and even death (28, 29). One report (29) indicates that exposure of blood to temperatures between 47 °C and 51 °C caused a form of chronic haemolysis rather than sudden, massive haemolysis. Underheated dialysis fluid causes patient discomfort from chilling but does not usually cause damage to the formed elements in blood. It has, however, been reported that low temperature dialysis fluid can activate an anti-N-like cold agglutinin precipitating extracorporeal coagulation (30).

Heat exchangers and (or) immersion heating elements are used to generate the required temperature. They should be constructed from passivated stainless steel and never from copper or aluminium, because of the risk of copper or aluminium intoxication. To reduce the risk of corrosion, it is preferable that water alone is in contact with the heating element and that dilution of the concentrate occurs after the heating of the water. With a single pass (500 ml/min) delivery system, 1.5 kW is sufficient to raise cold water to the dialysing temperature. If hot water disinfection is required, a reduction in flow to 200–300 ml/min will permit the 1.5 kW heating source to raise the water temperature to 85 °C. The 1.5 kW energy requirement enables the machine to draw its electrical supply from a standard domestic wall socket in most countries.

The heating system control may employ a mechanical thermostat with large temperature swings between the on and off settings or a precise closed loop proportioning band with continuous adjustment of the heating element current compensating for temperature fluctuations detected by the sensor. The advantage of the latter system is that the lag time between a temperature deviation and its correction is much shorter, so that the volume of the fluid dead space, necessary to damp out temperature fluctuations, can be reduced considerably. The thermostat system usually requires a reservoir of at least one litre to produce a constant temperature. This is undesirable as it constitutes a source of bacterial growth during dialysis and presents problems of cleaning and adequate sterilisation, which tend to be time consuming because of the large volume.

The accuracy of temperature control and monitoring should be ± 1 °C. The monitor should have at least a high alarm limit with audible and visual alarms. The accuracy of the monitor and high alarm set point should be such that dialysis fluid temperature does not exceed 42 °C, inclusive of monitor and alarm set point errors. Temperature monitors and alarms should be independent of temperature controls and adjustments should be possible only within the physiological range of 36 °C to 42 °C. It should not be possible to circumvent the monitor or its alarm when a dialyser is connected to the delivery system. If hot water disinfection is used, means, such as a shunt-interlock system, should be provided to prevent dialysis during the disinfection cycle.

Pressure monitoring

As indicated earlier, the determination of transmembrane pressure for fluid removal requires a measurement of the pressure in the dialysate compartment of the dialyser. Single pass proportioning systems are sometimes referred to as negative pressure systems because they provide the capability for generating negative dialysis fluid pressures for facilitating fluid removal. The negative pressure may be generated either by locating a constricting valve upstream of the dialyser and the dialysate pump downstream of the dialyser or by using two pumps, one on either side of the dialyser, the downstream pump being operated at a faster flow setting than the upstream one. Dialysate pumps should be self-priming and capable of pumping air during the priming of the dialysis fluid circuit.

As with the blood compartment pressure, the dialysate compartment pressure can be estimated by averaging the inlet and outlet dialysate pressures. However, as the dialysate compartment pressure drop is usually small, in most delivery systems only one of the two pressures is measured for calculating the TMP.

Dialysis fluid pressures are measured with mechanical or electronic manometers which are similar to those used for blood circuit pressures. If the manometer is located on a 'T' fitting rather than in a 'flow through' configuration, stagnant areas inaccessible to sterilant exist and there is the potential for bacterial contamination and proliferation.

Dialysis fluid pressure monitors usually include high and low limit alarms with visual and audible indications of the alarm condition.

Some dialysis fluid delivery systems display the TMP. The TMP is usually based on one blood compartment and one dialysate compartment pressure and is, therefore, an approximation of the true TMP. Some systems also provide servo-control of the TMP, thus maintaining a constant TMP even with changing blood compartment pressures.

Dialysis fluid pressure monitors should have a measurement range of -400 to $+200$ mm Hg and be accurate to ± 20 mm Hg or $\pm 10\%$ of the indicated reading, whichever is greater. The same limits on accuracy apply to the TMP display for systems that display this parameter rather than the dialysis fluid pressure. Alarms which are adjustable should not allow settings outside the monitor's scaled range. The alarm setting accuracy should be ± 10 mm Hg or $\pm 10\%$ of the setting whichever is greater.

If positive dialysis fluid pressures are achievable, safeguards should be provided to prevent dialysate compartment pressures from exceeding blood compartment pressures. This is necessary because if a membrane leak develops, not only will the leak go undetected because of the pressure gradient from dialysis fluid to blood, but contamination of the blood circuit with non-sterile dialysis fluid will also result.

Many new dialysis fluid delivery systems have provisions for controlling the ultrafiltration rate directly without relying on control of the TMP. In such systems, measurement of the dialysis fluid pressure may be unnecessary other than to provide alarm limits to prevent membrane rupture or to prevent dialysate compartment pressures exceeding blood compartment pressures.

Flow monitoring

As with blood flow rates, dialyser clearances of small solutes increase as the dialysis fluid flow rate is increased but at a diminishing rate until a relative clearance plateau is reached. The dialysis fluid flow rate is therefore one of the determinants of solute transport across the dialyser membrane. Typically, the dialysis fluid flow rate is 500 ml/min for single pass systems. At this level of dialysis fluid flow, dialyser clearances are less sensitive to changes in dialysis fluid flow rate than to changes in the blood flow rate.

In some single pass delivery systems, the proportioning pumps deliver dialysis fluid to a storage vessel from which the dialyser is perfused by a separate pump. In other systems, the proportioning pump also functions as the dialysis fluid delivery pump. Not all delivery systems display the flow rate and few systems incorporate alarms for out of range flow rates. In some systems, the dialysis fluid flow rate is internally set and operator adjustment of flow rates is not easily accomplished. These features are all related to the non-critical nature of the flow rate in terms of patients safety. In systems that display dialysis fluid flow rate, a calibrated flow meter is usually provided situated either before or after the dialyser. An accuracy of ±10% of indicated flow is considered quite adequate.

Blood leak monitoring

Delivery systems incorporate a sensor, usually of the photo-optical type, that can detect the presence of blood in dialysate. Some sensors use the visible light spectrum, while others use the blue light of the spectrum for improved sensitivity. In the event of a blood leak, there are audible and visual indications of the alarm condition and power to the blood pump is interrupted. In addition, in some systems, the flow of dialysis fluid bypasses the dialyser. The threshold of blood leak detection is adjustable in some systems, so that, with a minor blood leak, the threshold can be increased and dialysis continued.

As the osmolality of dialysis fluid is not very different from that of blood, the red cells entering dialysate, in the event of a membrane leak, are not haemolysed. Blood leak detection is, therefore, accomplished by measuring the change in optical transmission caused by the scattering of light by haemoglobin-containing red cells. Some manufacturers use haemoglobin standards for calibrating blood leak sensors. This may lead to inaccuracies of calibration, because with a membrane leak the haemoglobin is within the red cell membrane rather than in solution.

The blood leak sensor usually has a 'flow-through' configuration (Figure 7). Some sensor designs are susceptible to false alarms produced by trapping of air bubbles in the optical path. The incidence of this artefact can be minimised by efficient deaeration of dialysis fluid and by appropriate design of the sensor. For example, if the light path is situated at the bottom of the sensor cuvette and the fluid enters and leaves at the top, buoyancy of the air bubbles will help keep the air bubbles out of the optical path. The sensitivity of blood leak detection may be diminished if the windows of the cuvette become coated with deposits from the dialysate. The cuvette should, therefore, be easily accessible for regular cleaning and it should be possible to introduce a control filter to check the sensitivity of the sensor and intactness of the electrical monitoring circuits.

In some delivery systems, the blood leak is not quantitated, and instead, a relative index of the magnitude of the leak is provided. This makes estimation of the actual blood loss difficult especially if haemoglobin standards have been used for calibration. For quantitation of the detector in units of ml blood/l of dialysate, a detection threshold of 0.25 ml blood/l dialysate for nonadjustable

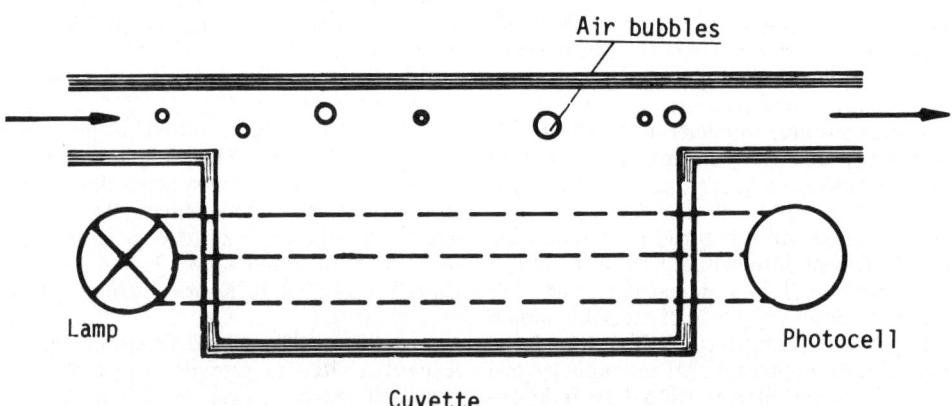

Figure 7. Bloodleak sensor with a flow-through configuration.

detectors and a maximum threshold of 0.35 ml blood/l of dialysate for adjustable detectors are recommended. Such a calibration can be achieved using a blood standard having the characteristics of uraemic blood which has a lower haematocrit than normal. Having initially calibrated the detector with a blood standard, subsequent testing of the detector can be done by more convenient methods such as the interposition of an optical filter.

Dialysis fluid deaeration

The feed water to the delivery system usually has a considerable amount of dissolved air, especially during the cold winter months (see also Chapter 7). Dialysis fluid prepared from this water has a tendency to 'degas' under conditions of negative pressure and heating to operating temperature. The gas that comes out of solution may result in flow maldistribution in the dialyser's dialysis fluid compartment by 'air-locking' or obstructing flow passages. Membrane masking by air bubbles may also result. As a consequence, the dialyser's solute clearances may be reduced. In addition, dialysis fluid compartment pressure drops could increase, making TMP estimation, and hence ultrafiltration prediction, unreliable. Observations in the literature indicate that, when dialysis fluid has a high concentration of dissolved air, air may cross the dialyser membrane into blood and contribute to foaming in the venous air trap (31, 32). Foaming is undesirable because of the potential for air embolism as well as microembolism from small clots formed at the blood-air interface.

Deaeration of dialysis fluid in delivery systems is usually achieved by first heating incoming water to physiologic temperatures, and then subjecting it to extreme negative pressures (300–600 mm Hg) and venting air released from solution. The negative pressures are usually achieved by a constricting valve upstream from a pump that recirculates water in a closed loop which contains an air trap and vent (Figure 6). Some systems use elevated temperatures rather than negative pressure for deaeration. The incoming water is heated to temperatures around 85 °C to facilitate deaeration. In such systems, a heat exchanger is used to cool the deaerated stream by heat transfer to the incoming water. Some delivery systems do not have good deaeration capabilities and merely incorporate a filter that provides nucleation sites for air bubble formation. These small bubbles are then coalesced into larger ones which are vented. This scheme does not accomplish effective removal of dissolved air.

Von Hartitzsch and colleagues (31) suggested limiting the PO_2 of dialysis fluid entering the dialyser to no more than 150 mm Hg. Drukker and coworkers (32), based on more recent experience, have indicated that problems related to air in dialysis fluid are non-existent at PO_2 values under 130 mm Hg. Inlet water temperatures and pressures greatly influence the amount of air which comes out of solution. Therefore, rather than rely on dialysis fluid PO_2 values, the efficacy of deaeration should be quantitated. An example of such quantitation would be to assume a standard inlet water condition (e.g. 4 °C at 760 mm Hg) and to then choose the lowest clinically relevant negative pressure (e.g. −500 mm Hg at 37 °C) at which no air comes out of solution. The volume of air at inlet conditions less the saturation volume at the chosen negative pressure at 37 °C is denoted as 100% removal and the actual removal expressed as a percentage of this total removal.

Disinfection of the dialysis fluid delivery system

The input water to the dialysis machine is usually contaminated with common water bacteria unless it has been adequately pretreated. Water softeners and deionizers can contribute to bacterial proliferation because of the inherent 'dead spaces' within these devices. Dialysis fluid at 37 °C, especially if it contains dextrose, supports bacterial growth. Delivery systems, therefore, require periodic disinfection to prevent excessive bacterial contamination of dialysis fluid. Disinfection may be achieved either with hot water at 90° to 95 °C or with chemicals such as formaldehyde or sodium hypochlorite.

Delivery systems usually have a mode switch that initiates the disinfection, cool-down (for hot water sterilisation) and rinse cycles. The disinfection cycle should not only allow adequate contact time, but also expose all parts of the flow circuit to the disinfectant. In systems designed to introduce disinfectant in the concentrate line the dialysis fluid-contacting, but not the water-containing parts of the flow circuit, are disinfected. With hot water disinfection, cooling may be achieved by rinsing the whole circuit with cool dialysis fluid, thereby accomplishing cool down and rinse-out of the water simultaneously. Hot water disinfection may cause caramelisation of residual dextrose and lead to flow obstructions and coating of blood leak detector lenses. In some delivery systems the disinfection, cool-down (for hot water disinfection) and rinse phases are automatically sequenced with adequate time for each phase.

An important requirement of a delivery system is that it prevents the operator from dialysing a patient during the disinfection, cool or rinse cycles. Once the disinfection cycle is initiated, it should be impossible for the dialysis mode to be selected until the cycle has been completed. This can be achieved by means of a shunt interlock switch. The shunt connector activates a microswitch that prevents initiation of dialysis. Further, the temperature and conductivity monitors are overridden during this phase. An additional safeguard would be to have no power to the blood pump during this phase. Further, in systems that proportion the disinfectant, some means should be provided that will necessitate replacing the disinfectant with concentrate before selecting the dialyse mode. This is especially important for central systems.

In systems that have dead ends, 'T-joints' and areas of reduced flow, inadequate disinfection may result with consequent contamination of the dialysis fluid by bacteria and pyrogens. The problem is magnified because these systems are also susceptible to bacterial proliferation. Such system designs may also lead to inadequate rinse-out of disinfectant and potential toxic reactions.

The connection of the drain line of the delivery system to the drain receptacle should be such as to prevent back-siphoning and contamination due to retrograde growth of drain pipe organisms. An air gap at the drain connection is one means of achieving this.

Formaldehyde is a very effective disinfectant and is widely used in dialysis for disinfecting delivery systems as well as for disinfecting dialysers for multiple use. Formaldehyde is, however, an unpleasant toxic substance and there is, hence, the risk of patient and staff exposure to formaldehyde from spills, splashes and fumes. Inhalation of formaldehyde has been associated with asthmatic reactions (33) and contact dermatitis due to formaldehyde in clothing textiles has been reported (34). Inadequate rinsing of formaldehyde could result in formaldehyde crossing over into the blood circuit across the dialyser membrane. Toxic symptoms produced by formaldehyde include transitory burning sensation in the vascular region, an uneasy feeling with a smothering sensation, a drop in blood pressure and a strange taste in the mouth (35). Chronic toxicity of formaldehyde is not well documented but neurological and retinal disturbances, metabolic acidosis and haemolysis have been speculated (36). Formaldehyde may also be a potent inactivator of heparin (35) and thereby contribute to clotting and resultant blood loss. There is considerable circumstantial evidence (37–41) linking the use of formaldehyde to the formation of anti-N-like antibodies especially in the context of dialyser disinfection with formaldehyde. The clinical significance of this relatively rare antibody is not well known but it has been implicated in renal allograft failure (42) and a shortened red cell life span (43). It has been demonstrated recently (43, 44) that the formaldehyde-induced alteration of red cell membranes is dose-dependent and that the formation of anti-N-like antibodies can be prevented by reducing the residual formaldehyde concentration below 10 µg/ml (see also Chapter 15).

Clinitest tablets, which are widely used for formaldehyde detection, have been shown to be incapable of detecting concentrations under 15 µg/ml (35). The Hantzsch test has been proposed as a more sensitive screening test for residual formaldehyde (35).

Hypochlorite has also been used for disinfecting dialysis fluid delivery systems. A major disadvantage of hypochlorite is its corrosive effect on metals. It is also considered to be a less effective disinfectant than formaldehyde.

Electrical safety

The potential for electric shock in dialysis patients exists because of the current transmission capability of a circuit which includes extracorporeal blood, the dialyser membrane, and dialysis fluid. If the equipment is appropriately grounded, this hazard does not exist. However, with restrictions on equipment current leakage, the seriousness of the hazard can be minimised when equipment grounding is absent or inappropriate.

Lefferson and Goss (45) have described circumstances in which an electric current may flow through this circuit. These include broken ground wires and dialysis machinery and other appliances not being at the same ground potential. These authors illustrate methods of reducing the hazards from a broken ground wire by reducing the amount of current leakage using isolation transformers or high impedance leakage current paths. Reducing the hazard of dialysis machinery and other appliances not at the same ground potential is described as a particular risk for home dialysis patients, hospitals generally having equipotential ground systems.

Deller (46) has shown recently that the typical total impedance of the combination of dialysis fluid, blood lines, blood, and dialyser is about 400 kiloohms. Because of this, dialysis patients have little danger of electric shock during normal conditions of no ground or insulation failures. However, when direct contact is made with the device, the protective impedance of the blood and dialysis fluid circuit is by-passed and the potential for electric shock exists. Frize and colleagues (47), recently described the results of an experiment in which a dog was connected to a current source and ground via the cephalic vein in the left foreleg and muscles or the right rear leg. Current at 60 Hz was applied to a level of 85 milliamperes, root mean square (RMS). No pump (heart) failure or fibrillation occurred.

Proposed limits for dialysis machines range from 100 to 500 microamperes. The American Association for the Advancement of Medical Instrumentation (AAMI) and the American National Standards Institute, Inc (ANSI) have determined that risk current limits for dialysis machines should be set at 100 microamperes, RMS (48). We believe that this limit implies a large margin of safety.

Other electrical hazards of dialysis equipment exist in addition to those described as leakage currents or grounds at unequal potential. Electrical components of dialysis devices operate in an environment in which liquid spills are common. The spills occur as a result of frequent intravenous fluid administration, priming of extracorporeal circuits with saline, connection of dialysis fluid supply hoses to dialysers, and maintenance of hydraulic components within dialysis fluid supply devices. External switches and plugs or receptacles are especially susceptible to spills. Such spills cause violent short circuits to develop, with fire and destruction of circuitry being a common result.

Overview of system safety

Some manufacturers allow the user to choose the specific configuration of monitors desired. A basic system is offered, and other system monitors are optional. Although such flexibility is sometimes desirable, it may allow patient safety to be compromised in favour of low equipment cost. Relative to patient safety, a minimum system can be proposed. The minimum system should have the following monitors:

1. Temperature monitor with at least a high limit alarm.

2. Conductivity monitor with high and low limit alarms.
3. At least one manometric device with high and low limit alarms for blood circuit pressure monitoring.
4. Blood leak detector with a quantifiable level of detection.
5. Provisions for interfacing with an air detector, if not included as part of the system.
6. At least one dialysate pressure monitor with high and low limit alarms (for delivery systems that rely on dialysate pressure control for fluid removal).

The recommendations made earlier for each type of monitor also apply to the minimum system.

The integrated systems approach is a recent innovation. When free standing devices such as the air detector, blood pump and infusion pump are used in conjunction with the dialysis fluid delivery system, suitable interfacing should be provided so that the addition of accessories does not compromise the integrity of monitoring and alarms.

As indicated earlier, functional testing of monitors and alarms should be easily accomplished without the need for special tools so that such testing may be incorporated into the dialysis procedure. Such testing should not be limited to a check of the electronic monitoring and alarm circuitry but should include the sensors. It should be possible to test and calibrate each monitor independently using external standards.

SPECIAL MONITORING SCHEMES

Single needle systems

The need for the single needle technique arose on the basis that two needles were more difficult to insert than one and that one puncture gave a longer fistula life (49). The latter hypothesis has not been proven, although 7% (50) of fistula dialyses are presently performed with single needle systems. However, the technique works poorly where it is most needed, namely in patients with poor vascular access, particularly where there is a low blood flow through the A-V fistula. The disadvantages of this technique are multiple. There is an increase in mechanical devices, reduction in blood flow, and an ever present risk of recirculation and inefficient dialysis. In addition, the dialyser must be compliant or a compliant chamber used for optimal results. This may result in an increase in the extracorporeal blood volume.

The basic principle involves alternating the direction of blood flow through a single access needle joined to a Y-junction which connects the two ends of the classical blood circuit (Figure 1). The alteration of direction of flow can be achieved in different ways. One system (Figure 8) uses two clamps, one situated on the arterial and the other on the venous line as close to the Y-junction as possible. When the arterial clamp is opened, the pump draws blood out against the closed venous clamp and

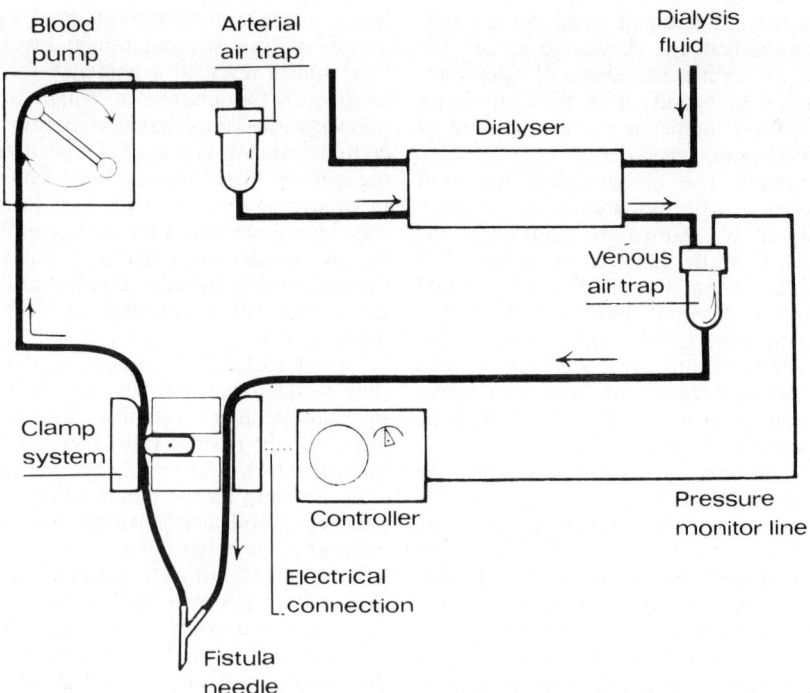

Figure 8. One type of single needle system with continuous blood pump operation and alternate activation of arterial and venous clamps.

the situation is reversed when the venous clamp is opened and the arterial clamp is closed. Pressure monitoring of the venous bubble trap with high/low-alarm contacts can be made to operate the clamps, i.e. the high pressure contact opens the venous clamp and closes the arterial clamp and vice versa. Under these conditions of pressure/pressure regulation, the blood pump never stops and this is contrary to all basic pressure monitoring considerations. An alternative is the timed opening and closing of the clamps with pressure monitoring still controlling the blood pump. Time-time systems may be hazardous because of the relative independence of the stroke volumes for the two phases with the possibility of a mismatch. The continuous operation of the blood pump even when the arterial clamp is closed leads to extreme subatmospheric pressures between the patient's access and the blood pump. This can lead to foaming from 'degassing' of blood with the potential for clotting in the dialyser. Also the effective blood flow is reduced because of the incomplete filling of the pump segment. Further, upon the opening of the arterial clamp, the sudden exposure of the patient's access to an extreme subatmospheric pressure can be detrimental. The generation of extreme subatmospheric pressures also increases the potential for air embolism.

In another type of single needle system, there is intermittent operation of the blood pump with a single venous clamp. When the blood pump is on, the venous clamp is closed and blood is drawn out of the patient into the extracorporeal circuit. The venous air trap pressure increases as a consequence and at a pre-set high pressure limit, the pump is shut off and the clamp opened, blood being returned to the patient. This causes a fall in venous air trap pressure and when the low pre-set pressure limit is reached, the clamp closes and the pump is turned on to begin a new cycle of operation. This system is simpler to operate than the two clamp system but is a relatively inefficient system because of the intermittent blood pump operation.

In yet another system, two blood pumps are used which operate sequentially, one situated before and the other after the dialyser. No clamps are required as the occlusive pumps also serve the function of clamps. The objection to this system is that an unmonitored pressure can build up between the 'venous' blood pump and the patient's vascular access with the risk of haematoma formation and damage to the fistula. Newer versions of this system include a second pressure monitor to prevent this problem. In addition, two sites of sub-atmospheric pressure are developed in the blood circuit.

Single needle systems are more complex from the view point of operation and safety monitoring. The efficiency of solute transport is compromised by recirculation. It is difficult to measure the 'true' blood flow with most single needle systems. The beneficial effect on fistula longevity with one instead of two punctures for each dialysis has not been established. The use of single needle dialysis as a last resort in the face of fistula problems is ill-advised when fistula perfusion is poor because of increased recirculation and, hence, less effective treatment. When fistula perfusion is adequate but only a short segment of fistula is available, as in paediatric dialysis, however, single needle dialysis may permit satisfactory use of the fistula. In acute renal failure, the use of percutaneous catheterisation (51) of a major vein (femoral or subclavian) with a single needle system reduces the 'indwelling cathether risk' (see also Chapter 8). Double lumen, single needles are beginning to find wider application in haemodialysis and some of the early problems with the double lumen concept are being eliminated. With a well-designed double lumen needle, the benefits of a single venipuncture may be utilised without the use of special, more complex equipment.

Sequential ultrafiltration and diffusion

Sequential ultrafiltration and diffusion is a fairly recent mode of therapy that requires the divorcing and sequencing of fluid and solute removal, these two processes being simultaneous during conventional haemodialysis. Isolated ultrafiltration, i.e. fluid removal without simultaneous solute removal by diffusion, may precede or follow the phase of pure diffusive solute removal. The observation that isolated ultrafiltration did not produce symptomatic hypotension was first reported in 1972 (52), and later confirmed in 1975 (53). However, the demonstration that ultrafiltration alone was well tolerated but not when combined with diffusion, as in classical acetate dialysis in susceptible patients, was first reported in 1976 (54). The potential benefit of separating diffusion and ultrafiltration sequentially during one treatment session was also first described in 1976 with the Rhône-Poulenc high flux dialyser (RP6) when the patient lost 4 kg during 1 h without change in pulse or blood pressure and then tolerated 3 h of asymptomatic acetate dialysis without weight loss (55). However, further studies revealed a tendency for the blood pressure to drop in the absence of weight loss (56). Subsequent investigations of the haemodynamic changes indicated a compensatory increase of the peripheral resistance during isolated ultrafiltration, but a failure of the peripheral resistance to rise during classical acetate dialysis (57–59). This observation has been confirmed and shown to be associated with a rise in circulating catecholamines during isolated ultrafiltration but not during acetate haemodialysis with ultrafiltration (60). This phenomenon is unexplained.

During isolated ultrafiltration, dialysis fluid does not flow through the dialyser but the required hydrostatic pressure gradient is established across the dialyser membrane for the desired rate of fluid removal. This can be accomplished in several ways. The simplest is to use a venous clamp on the blood tubing to generate adequate positive blood compartment pressures, the dialysate compartment being open to the atmosphere. With this scheme, the ultrafiltrate can be collected readily and the rate of fluid removal easily determined. The generation of high blood compartment pressures does, however, increase the possibility of tubing disconnections and membrane ruptures as in coil dialysis. Monitoring of the pressure in the blood compartment is therefore essential, especially as it is difficult to regulate the blood compartment pressure precisely with most venous clamps. Also,

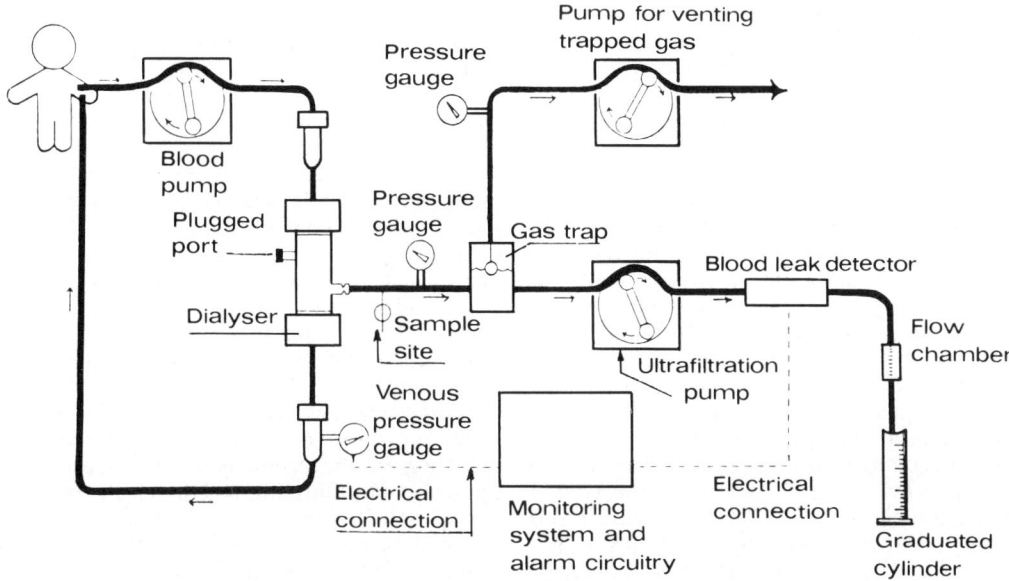

Figure 9. A hardware scheme for isolated ultrafiltration.

some form of blood leak detection should be used, to prevent excessive blood loss in the ultrafiltrate should membrane rupture occur. Isolated ultrafiltration can also be performed using negative pressures in the dialysate compartment. The negative pressure may be generated either by a suction pump, or a vacuum source or by using a conventional dialysis fluid delivery system that can generate negative pressures in the dialysate compartment during the by-pass mode of operation. With the negative pressure schemes, it may be more difficult to measure the rate of ultrafiltration than with the positive pressure scheme but it is easier to control the negative pressure generated. If a suction pump is used, the rate of ultrafiltration can be controlled by controlling the speed of the pump. The difficulty, however, lies in the fact that the ultrafiltrate has a tendency to 'degas' under subatmospheric pressures, resulting in a mixture of fluid and gas being pumped. To avoid this, a gas trap with provisions for venting the gas under conditions of negative pressure is required (Figure 9). If a vacuum source is used, a graduated collection vessel can be used for measuring the rate of ultrafiltration. With the dialysis fluid by-pass scheme, the ultrafiltrate mixes with dialysis fluid and is, therefore, not accessible for direct measurement of flow rate unless special provisions for diverting the ultrafiltrate flow through a flow meter are included. In all of the schemes discussed, monitoring of patient weight can be also used to assess the rate of fluid removal. The negative pressure schemes should also incorporate some form of blood leak detection. It is desirable to locate the blood leak detector as close to the dialyser as possible, to prevent delays between the incidence of the membrane rupture and the activation of the blood leak alarm.

PATIENT MONITORING

One of the most difficult parameters to measure in the dialysis patient is the dry body weight (see also Chapter 12). Indeed, it is possible that the true dry weight is never known, as measurements of total body water and the extracellular space have to be related to a standard derived from a normal population (61). The observation that most dialysis patients have an appreciable diuresis and weight loss following successful transplantation suggests that these patients were overhydrated. Because of the ever-present risk of overhydration and associated volume hypertension, the monitoring of body weight and blood pressure before and after each dialysis has become a traditional ritual. The aim is to control the blood pressure by ultrafiltration (inducing weight loss) and avoid hypertension or orthostatic hypotension. To succeed, the patient must cooperate and restrict salt and water intake to avoid large swings in body weight. On a thrice weekly dialysis schedule, weight gains in excess of 2.5% of the estimated dry body weight in the longest interdialytic period are often associated with predialysis hypertension or postdialysis fatigue and hypotension after ultrafiltration. The majority of cooperative patients, however, are capable of maintaining a reasonable blood pressure with this regimen.

The monitoring of the patient's blood pressure and heart rate during dialysis is also traditional, the frequency of the observation depending upon the unit and staff availability. Measurement of weight loss during a dialysis is rarely required today, as with most modern dialysers, the ultrafiltration rate is predictable based on the estimation of the TMP. With certain recirculating systems, the actual increase in dialysate volume due to ultrafiltration can be measured directly. With isolated ultrafiltration, direct collection and measurement of the volume of ultrafiltrate obviates the need for weight measurement during dialysis.

Long term monitoring of body weight is a difficult problem for the dialysis physician. In the absence of overt clinical signs of dehydration or overhydration, the blood pressure is often used as an index of correct hydration. However, this rule may prove fallacious and much clinical experience may be necessary to adjust the individual body weight according to circumstances. In the early months of treatment following initial progressive weight loss with blood pressure control, the patient should gain weight at the rate of 0.5 to 1.0 kg per month if he is receiving an adequate protein and calorie intake and was malnourished initially (61). True weight gains of 5 kg are not unusual during the first year of treatment. After this, it is uncommon to see significant weight gain in stable adult patients. It is difficult to judge this type of weight gain and a tendency to ultrafilter the patient into shock to prove whether the weight gain is dry weight gain or not, is a bad practice. In the absence of overt oedema, it is better to allow progressive weight gain if the blood pressure does not exceed normal limits and to ask the patient if he feels better keeping the extra weight. With patients over the age of 60 years, a mild systolic hypertension is often better tolerated than the rigorous prescription of a dry body weight designed to produce a normal blood pressure. However, some patients feel bloated when they are too heavy and will insist upon a lower weight. The monitoring of the haematocrit may be useful in judging changes in body weight. Weight gain associated with water retention dilutes the red cell mass and may be associated with an unexplained progressive reduction of the haematocrit. Conversely, unexpected rises in the haematocrit may suggest the presence of dehydration. A frequent problem among dialysis patients is wasting with maintenance of actual body weight. This can lead to a state of hypertension without apparent weight gain or to signs of overt overhydration. The cause of such wasting is usually malnutrition due to an inadequate diet or any catabolic process, particularly infection. The clue to recognising it is often a rise in blood pressure without weight gain associated with a reduction in the haematocrit. The treatment is more aggressive ultrafiltration together with the correction of the causative factor. The continuous monitoring of blood pressure and weight are the fundamentals by which the dry body weight of the dialysis patient is judged. It is often difficult for the patient to monitor this correctly for himself and a regular review of blood pressure and body weight is necessary for all dialysis patients.

REFERENCES

1. Scribner BH, Buri R, Caner JEZ, Hegstrom R, Burnell JM: The treatment of chronic uremia by means of intermittent hemodialysis. A preliminary report. *Trans Am Soc Artif Intern Organs* 6:114, 1960
2. Shaldon S: Experience to date with home hemodialysis. *Proc Working Conf on Chronic Dialysis,* University of Washington, Seattle, WA, 1964, p 66
3. Brescia MJ, Cimino JE, Appel K, Hurwich BJ: Chronic hemodialysis using venipuncture and surgically created arterio-venous fistula. *N Engl J Med* 275:1089, 1966
4. Cambi V, Savazzi G, Arisi L, Bignardi L, Bruschi G, Rossi E, Migone L: Short dialysis schedules (SDS) – Finally ready to become a routine? *Proc Eur Dial Transpl Assoc* 11:112, 1974
5. Shaldon S: Independence in maintenance haemodialysis. *Lancet* 1:520, 1968
6. Gurland HJ, Brunner FP, v Dehn H, Härlen H, Parsons FM, Schärer K: Combined report on regular dialysis and transplantation in Europe, III, 1972. *Proc Eur Dial Transpl Assoc* 10:XVII, 1973
7. Keshaviah P, Luehmann D, Shapiro FL, Comty CM: *Investigation of the risks and hazards associated with hemodialysis devices.* Technical Report, a FDA Medical Device Standards Publication, U.S. Department of Health, Education and Welfare, 1980
8. Grimsrud HJ, Cole JJ, Eschbach JW, Babb AL, Schribner BH: Safety aspects of hemodialysis. *Trans Am Soc Artif Intern Organs* 20:770, 1974
9. Association for the Advancement of Medical Instrumentation: *Hemodialysis Systems Standard* (proposed), Arlington VA, 1978.
10. Canadian Standards Association: *Fluid Supply Systems and Accessories for Hemodialysis,* Draft CSA standard Z364.2, Rexdale, Ont, Canada, 1978.
11. British Standards Panel, LEL/103/2/12, Draft British Standard: *Single Patient Continuous Flow Type Supply and Monitoring Machines for Haemodialysis,* London, England, 1975.
12. (Japanese) Ministry of Health and Welfare. *Standards of Artificial Kidneys for Dialysis* (draft), Tokyo, Japan, 1979. Translated by C-D Medical Systems Ltd, Cordis Dow Corp Company, Miami FA
13. Bernstein EF, Indeglia RA, Shea MA, Varco RL: Sublethal damage to the red blood cell from pumping. *Circulation* (Suppl) 1:226, 1967
14. Hyde SE III, Sadler JH: Red blood cell destruction in hemodialysis. *Trans Am Soc Artif Intern Organs* 15:50, 1969
15. Von Hartitzsch B, Carr D, Kjellstrand CM, Kerr DNS: Normal red cell survival in well dialyzed patients. *Trans Am Soc Artif Intern Organs* 19:471, 1973
16. Shaldon S, Ahmed R, Oag D, Crockett R, Opperman F, Koch KM: The use of the A-V fistula in overnight home haemodialysis in children. *Proc Eur Dial Transpl Assoc* 8:65, 1971
17. Ward MK, Shadforth M, Hill AVL, Kerr DNS: Air embolism during haemodialysis. *Br Med J* 2:74, 1971
18. Beullens T, Beelen R, Van Ypersele de Strihou C: Devices for air detection during dialysis. *Proc Eur Dial Transpl Assoc* 8:412, 1971
19. Nishi RY: Ultrasonic detection of bubbles with doppler flow transducers. *Ultrasonics* 10:173, 1972
20. Blagg CR: Acute complications associated with hemodialysis. In *Replacement of Renal Function by Dialysis,* edited by Drukker W, Parsons FM, Maher JF, 1st edn, the Hague, Boston, London, Martinus Nijhoff 1978, p 486
21. Weseley SA: Air embolism during hemodialysis. *Dial Transpl* 2:14, 1972
22. Von Hartitzsch B, Medlock R: New devices to prevent air foam emboli. *Dial Transpl* 8:515, 1979

23. De Palma JR, Shinaberger JH, Abukurah AR: Air embolism hazards in maintenance hemodialysis. *Trans Am Soc Artif Intern Organs* (Abstract), 1976, p 20
24. Said R, Quintanilla A, Levin N, Ivanovich P: Acute hemolysis due to profound hypo-osmolality. A complication of hemodialysis. *J Dial* 1:447, 1977
25. Linder A, Moskovtchenko JF, Traeger J: Accidental mass hypernatremia during hemodialysis. *Nephron* 9:99, 1972
26. Bluemle LW Jr: Current status of chronic hemodialysis. *Am J Med* 44:749, 1968
27. Kachmar JF, Grant GH: Proteins and amino acids. In: *Fundamentals of Clinical Chemistry,* edited by Norbert W. Tietz, Philadelphia, London, Toronto, Sydney, W.B. Saunders Company 1976, p 264
28. Fortner RW, Nowakowski A, Carter CB, King LH, Knepshield JH: Death due to overheated dialysate during dialysis. *Ann Intern Med* 73:443, 1970
29. Berkes SL, Kahn SI, Chazan JA, Garella S: Prolonged hemolysis from overheated dialysate. *Ann Intern Med* 83:363, 1975
30. Harrison PB, Jansson K, Kronenberg H, Mahony JF, Tiller D: Cold agglutinin formation in patients undergoing haemodialysis. A possible relationship to dialyser re-use. *Aust NZ J Med* 5:195, 1975
31. Von Hartitzsch B, Hoenich NA, Johnson J, Brewis RAL, Kerr DNS: The problem of de-aeration – cause, consequence, cure. *Proc Eur Dial Transpl Assoc* 9:605, 1972
32. Drukker W, van der Werff B, Meinsma K: Deaeration of dialysis fluid. *Dial Transpl* 3:33, 1974
33. Hendrick DJ, Lane DJ: Formaline asthma in hospital staff. *Br Med J* 1:607, 1975
34. O'Quinn SE, Kennedy CB: Contact dermatitis due to formaldehyde in clothing textiles. *JAMA* 194:123, 1965
35. Ogden DA, Myers LE, Eskelson CD, Ziegler EJ: Iatrogenic administration of formaldehyde to hemodialysis patients. *Proc Dial Transpl Forum* 3:141, 1973
36. Reveillaud RJ, Deschamps A, Aubert Ph: Risks of i.v. administration of formaldehyde to hemodialyzed patients. *Kidney Int* 11:292, 1977
37. Howell D, Perkins HA: Anti-N-like antibodies in the sera of patients undergoing chronic hemodialysis. *Vox Sang* 23:291, 1972
38. White WL, Miller GE, Kaehny WD: Formaldehyde in the pathogenesis of hemodialysis-related anti-N antibodies. *Transfusion* 17:443, 1977
39. Crosson JT, Moulds J, Comty CM, Polesky F: A clinical study of anti-N_{DP} in the sera of patients in a large repetitive hemodialysis program. *Kidney Int* 10:463, 1976
40. Shaldon S, Chevallet M, Maraoui M, Mion C: Dialysis associated auto-antibodies. *Proc Eur Dial Transpl Assoc* 13:339, 1976
41. Fassbinder W, Pilar J, Scheuermann E, Koch M: Formaldehyde and the occurrence of anti-N-like cold agglutinins in RDT patients. *Proc Eur Dial Transpl Assoc* 13:333, 1976
42. Belzer FO, Kountz SL, Perkins HA: Red cell cold autoagglutinins as a cause of failure of renal allotransplantation. *Transplantation* 11:422, 1971
43. Koch KM, Frei U, Fassbinder W: Hemolysis and anemia in anti-N like antibody positive hemodialysis patients. *Trans Am Soc Artif Intern Organs* 24:709, 1978
44. Lewis KJ, Dewar PJ, Ward MK, Kerr DNS: Formation of anti-N-like antibodies in dialysis patients: Effect of different methods of dialyzer rinsing to remove formaldehyde. *Clin Nephrol* 15:39, 1981
45. Lefferson P, Goss J: Risk current vs leakage current. *Dial Transpl* 2:42, 1973
46. Deller AG: Electrical safety in dialysis. *J Med Eng Technol* 3:186, 1979
47. Frize M, Scott J, Durie N, Park G: Fibrillation caused by leakage from dialysis machines – What is the danger? *Med Biol Eng Comput* 16:124, 1978
48. Association for the Advancement of Medical Instrumentation. *Safe Current Limits for Electromedical Apparatus,* American National, Standard Arlington, VA, 1978.
49. Kopp KF, Gutch CF, Kolff WJ: Single needle dialysis. *Trans Am Soc Artif Intern Organs* 18:75, 1972
50. Gurland HJ, Brunner FP, Chantler C, Jacobs C, Schärer K, Selwood NH, Spies G, Wing AJ: Combined report on regular dialysis and transplantation in Europe, VI, 1976. *Proc Eur Dial Transpl Assoc* 13:3, 1976
51. Shaldon S, Chiandusse L, Higgs B: Haemodialysis by percutaneous catheterisation of the femoral artery and vein with regional heparinisation. *Lancet* 2:857, 1961
52. Kobayashi K, Shibata M, Kato K, Kato S, Nakamura S, Kurachi K, Yasuda B, Ohta K, Maeda K, Imai T, Kawaguchi S, Shimizu K, Yamazaki T, Maji T, and Nomura T: Studies on the development of a new method of controlling the amount and contents of body fluids (extracorporeal ultrafiltration method: ECUM) and the application of this method for patients receiving long term hemodialysis. *Jap J Nephrol* 14:1, 1972
53. Ing TS, Ashbach DL, Kanter A, Oyama HJ, Armbruster KFW, Merkel FK: Fluid removal and negative-pressure hydrostatic ultrafiltration using a partial vacuum. *Nephron* 14:451, 1975
54. Bergström J, Asaba H, Fürst P, Oulès R: Dialysis ultrafiltration and blood pressure. *Proc Eur Dial Transpl Assoc* 13:293, 1976
55. Shaldon S: Sequential ultrafiltration and dialysis. *Proc Eur Dial Transpl Assoc* 13:300, 1976
56. Asaba H, Bergström J, Fürst P, Lindh K, Mion C, Oulès R, Shaldon S: Sequential ultrafiltration and diffusion as alternative to conventional haemodialysis. *Proc Clin Dial Transpl Forum* 6:129, 1976
57. Hampl H, Paeprer H, Unger V, Kessel M: Hemodynamic studies during hemodialysis in comparison to sequential ultrafiltration and hemofiltration. *J Dial* 3:51, 1979
58. Wehle B, Asaba H, Castenfors J, Fürst P, Gunnarson B, Shaldon S, Bergström J: Hemodynamic changes during sequential ultrafiltration and dialysis. *Kidney Int* 15:411, 1979
59. Keshaviah P, Ilstrup K, Constantini E, Berkseth R, Shapiro F: The influence of ultrafiltration (UF) and diffusion (D) on cardiovascular parameters. *Trans Am Soc Artif Intern Organs* 26:328, 1980
60. Koch KM, Ernst W, Baldamus CA, Brecht HM, Georges J, Fassbinder W: Sympathetic activity and hemodynamics in hemodialysis ultrafiltration and hemofiltration. *Kidney Int* Abstract) 16:891, 1979
61. Comty CM: Factors influencing body composition in terminal uraemics treated by regular haemodialysis. *Proc Eur Dial Transpl Assoc* 4:216, 1967

12

BIOPHYSICS OF ULTRAFILTRATION AND HEMOFILTRATION

LEE W. HENDERSON

Introduction	242	Membrane toxicity	252
Theoretical background	242	Peritoneal dialysis	252
Hemodialysis	242	Solute transport by ultrafiltration during dialysis	252
Peritoneal dialysis	246	Hemodialysis	252
Sieving coefficient measurement	248	Peritoneal dialysis	254
Hemodialysis	248	Impact of convection on diffusion	254
Peritoneal dialysis	249	Hemofiltration (Convective solute transport without hemodialysis)	256
Clinical application of ultrafiltration	249	Theoretical aspects	256
Hemodialysis	249	Factors affecting ultrafiltration flow rate	257
Dialysis induced symptomatic hypotension	250	*Membrane sieving*	259
Vascular volume depletion	250	*Clearance*	259
Physiochemical toxicity	251	References	262
Autonomic neuropathy	251		

INTRODUCTION

Removal of excess body water is an important function of both the artificial kidney and peritoneal dialysis. Recently, solute removal in conjunction with ultrafiltration has been exploited as an alternative to diffusion as a means for cleansing uremic blood. This chapter deals with the practical and theoretical aspects of ultrafiltration and convective mass transfer across the artificial kidney and peritoneal dialysis membranes.

THEORETICAL BACKGROUND

Hemodialysis

When a concentration gradient exists across a semipermeable membrane, both solute and water tend with time to move in a direction to discharge that gradient. Solute and water move in opposite directions across the membrane to achieve equilibrium. The gradient may be expressed in terms emphasizing the solute (e.g., number of mg/dl of solute on side A, minus number of mg/dl of solute on side B) or in terms emphasizing the water (e.g., number of milliosmoles on side A, minus number of milliosmoles on side B). Osmolality is generally considered as the number of solute particles per kilogram of water. Alternatively, it may be considered as a measure of the number of water molecules per kilogram of solution i.e., the 'concentration of water'. There are two ways in which a concentration gradient for water may be achieved: osmotically and hydrostatically. For artificial kidney membranes both osmotic and hydrostatic (hydraulic) force may be used to achieve the concentration gradient necessary to cause ultrafiltration, i.e., the separation of plasma water from macromolecular constituents such as protein and cellular elements. For reasons that will become apparent hydrostatic force is the more effective.

An equation that relates ultrafiltration rate to these forces is frequently written

$$J_f = \frac{Q_f}{A} = L_p(\Delta P + \Delta \pi) \quad [1]$$

Ultrafiltration rate per unit area of membrane = (permeability of membrane to water) × (hydrostatic force + osmotic force) where

J_f = the volume flux rate per unit membrane area across the membrane for water (ml/min/cm^2),[1]

L_p = the permeability of the membrane for water, i.e., the volumetric flow rate of water per unit area of membrane per unit pressure gradient (ml/min·cm^2·mm Hg),

Q_f = flow rate of ultrafiltrate (ml/min),

A = area of the membrane (cm^2),

ΔP = the hydraulic pressure gradient from blood path to dialysis fluid path (mm Hg),

$\Delta \pi$ = the osmotic pressure gradient from blood path to dialysis fluid path (mm Hg);

$\Delta \pi$ is frequently expressed as mOsm/l and may be converted to mm Hg using 1.0 mOsm $\cong$ 19 mm Hg.

The hydrostatic and osmotic forces are summed in this equation, since with hemodialysis there is a deliberate, usually hydrostatic, gradient favoring water movement

---

[1] Since milliliters equal cubic centimeters, cm^3/min/cm^2 can be reduced to cm/min.

from blood to dialysate. When isotonic dialysis fluid is used, the osmotic pressure provided by the plasma proteins favors water movement from the dialysis solution to blood and the contribution of $\Delta\pi$ to J_f is negative. The two forces $\Delta\pi$ and ΔP may be examined conceptually for an artificial kidney membrane with the aid of Figures 1 and 2. Consider Figure 1 showing two perfectly mixed solutions (blood and dialysis fluid) separated by a membrane which contains homogeneously distributed water filled pores (drawn in cross section as right circular cylinders). Further, the membrane is perfectly semipermeable with respect to blood proteins and formed elements. That is, no cells or protein traverse the pores because the pores have too small a diameter to accomodate these comparatively large molecules and blood cells. Figure 1 shows the events at the pore when an osmotically active solute such as glucose (as anhydrous d-glucose, mass = 180 daltons) is present in high concentration (280 mg/dl = 15,6 mmol/l) on the dialysis fluid side of the membrane (side B). As noted, the concentration of water may be considered to be inversely related to the concentration of solute. That is, for a given volume of solution the greater number of dissolved solute particles (molecules, ions) the fewer number of water molecules can be present. The osmolality of the plasma is 300 mOsm/l and that of the dialysis fluid which contains an identical concentration of electrolytes to that found in the plasma water, but with 180 mg/dl more of glucose is 310 mOsm/l. Figure 1 depicts the instant after these two solutions appear on each side of the membrane. Further, there is no difference in hydrostatic pressure across the membrane (consider the membrane 'floppy', such that no hydrostatic pressure gradient can be sustained). At this instant, there is a concentration gradient for water across the pores from A to B. The magnitude of this pressure gradient is 10 mOsm/l or 190 mm Hg (1.0 mOsm/l = 19 mm Hg). Water moves very swiftly to discharge such concentration gradients. Water rarely if ever moves by single molecule diffusion [2], but rather by 'bulk' or 'plug' flow in which movement of 'blocks' of water occur much as you would consider the movement of pure water in a pipe when an inlet to outlet pressure gradient is applied. It is apparent that in subsequent instances this rather straight forward conceptualization becomes much more complicated. To cite some of the events, glucose is small enough to move by diffusion down its concentration gradient from B to A reducing the osmotic driving force; further, the water arriving on side B dilutes the glucose concentration adjacent to the membrane lengthening the diffusion path over which the concentration gradients apply and slowing their discharge. Further, protein, a macromolecular structure present in solution on the blood side (A), cannot cross the membrane and will exert an osmotic effect (oncotic pressure) favoring water reabsorption from the dialysis bath. Finally, the distribution of charges on the solute particles and the requirement for electroneutrality across the membrane will modulate the movement of electrolytes in response to their concentration gradient. Before moving to a somewhat more rigorous description, it can be helpful to consider a comparable conceptualization for the circumstance in which a hydraulic (hydrostatic) pressure gradient exists. Figure 2 depicts a rigid membrane with blood on side A

---

[2] The distribution of tritiated water in a beaker can occur by single molecule diffusion.

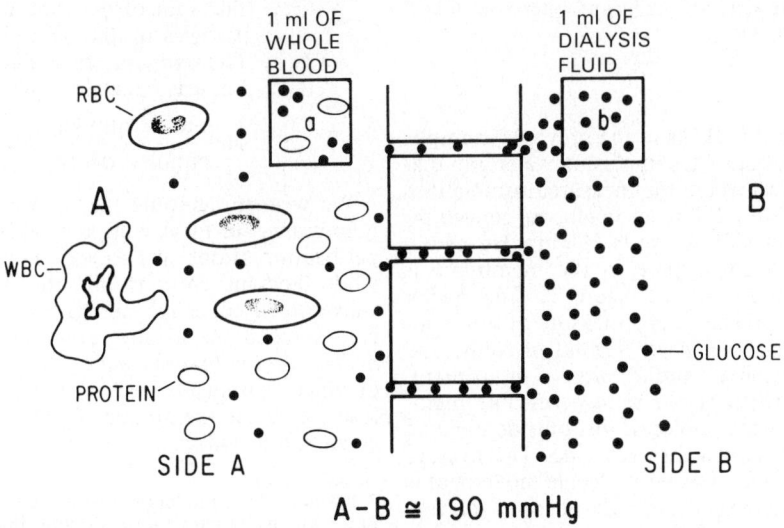

Figure 1. Diagrammatic sketch of a semipermeable membrane dividing whole blood (side A) and dialysis fluid (side B). Glucose (anhydrous) is present on side B at 280 mg/dl (15,6 mmol/l). The pores in the membrane are too small to allow passage of cell elements and protein. An osmolar gradient from A to B of approximately 190 mm hg (5890–5700 mm Hg) is diagrammatically shown in 1 ml control volumes a and b where the amount of water per milliliter of solution is greater in a than b (see text for further discussion).

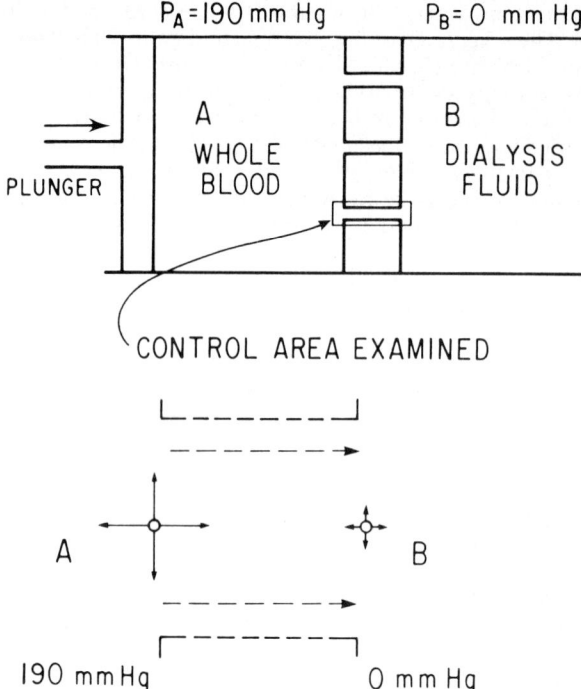

Figure 2. Diagrammatic sketch of a rigid membrane dividing whole blood (side A) and dialysis fluid with osmolality equal to that of whole blood (side B). A piston on side A provides 190 mm Hg pressure on the whole blood. A single pore in the membrane is depicted below. An average water molecule just outside each end of the pore is depicted as an open circle (○). Vectors for the random motion of these water molecules are given. The length of the vector depicts the number of water molecules moving in the direction indicated. It is apparent that there is an imbalance in the vectors within the pore such that more water molecules are moving into the pore from side A than from side B with a resultant net flux of water from A to B down the length of the pore.

and dialysis fluid on side B. As in the previous example, the composition of electrolytes in plasma water and dialysis fluid are identical as are the measured osmolalities and this time there is no difference in glucose concentration. The plunger on side A exerts 190 mm Hg of hydrostatic pressure. A single pore in the membrane is depicted in the lower part of Figure 2. The higher hydrostatic pressure on side A is a measure of the greater number of bombardments per second of solute and solvent particles on a given surface area of the container, one surface of which is our semi-permeable membrane. An 'average' water molecule just outside the pore in the membrane is shown for each side. The average magnitude and direction of water molecule movement is given by the vector arrows. In the bulk phase of solution outside the pore such motion is random and is schematically shown in Figure 2 as four arrows of equal length reflecting the sums of all intermediate vectors for each quadrant. The greater number of bombardments of the end of the pore on side A as opposed to side B means that there is a net movement of water from A to B down the pore. It should be noted that solute particles that are small enough not to be hindered by the pore, (the pore diameter being substantially larger than the hydrated radius of the solute), will move with the water as a result of the frictional forces between water and the solute particle. This convecting of solutes along with water through a membrane in response to a pressure gradient (osmotic or hydrostatic) is termed 'solvent drag'. When the membrane exerts no restraining force (sieving effect) on the solute, i.e., the solution does not change in concentration as it traverses the membrane, then the terms 'bulk', 'plug' or 'Possilian' flow describe the events. In the present example, of course, protein and cell elements are blocked from crossing the membranes by pore size and the solute concentration of plasma water does change as the ultrafiltrate is formed.

Let us return now to equation 1, and a more formal description of the above events. In general, the hydraulic pressure gradient of equation 1 (ΔP) may be taken as the average blood path pressure (P_B) minus the average dialysate path pressure (P_D). These values are readily measured in most artificial kidney monitors. The osmotic pressure gradient is somewhat more complicated to compute. Van't Hoff's Law of Osmotic Pressure adequately describes the osmotic pressure difference between two solutions (e.g., blood and dialysis fluid) *in the absence of a membrane:*

$$P_B - P_D = \Delta\pi = RT\left[\sum_{j=1}^{m} C_j^B - \sum_{j=1}^{n} C_j^D\right] \quad [2]$$

where B and D identify the two solutions and

$\sum_{j=1}^{m} C_j^B$ = The sum $(1+2+3\ldots m)$ of the concentrations [3] of all solute particles in blood (B)

$\sum_{j=1}^{n} C_j^D$ = The sum of the concentrations of all solute particles in dialysis fluid (D)

T = The temperature in degrees Kelvin

R = The gas constant = 0.0623 when units of $\dfrac{\text{liter} \times \text{mm Hg}}{\text{mmol} \times \text{degree}}$ are used

We wish to compute the $\Delta\pi$ across a semipermeable membrane. An ideal semipermeable membrane permits permeation of one species, e.g. water, with no resistance while blocking entry to all other species, e.g. protein. Currently used cellulosic dialysis membranes may be considered to be ideally semipermeable for water and protein. In the dialysis setting, however, there are a host of other osmotically active solutes, most of which diffuse across the membrane. To assess the contribution a given solute makes to the over-all transmembrane os-

---

[3] Partially or completely dissociated electrolytes contribute more solute particles to the solution than their molar concentration would identify. For example, NaCl at concentrations used in dialysis fluid, dissociates almost completely into its constituent ions, providing nearly double the number of osmotically active particles that would be expected from consideration of the molality and Avogadro's number.

motic pressure gradient, it is necessary to know how readily it permeates the membrane, as compared with water in response to an applied hydraulic pressure gradient. This may be expressed as

$$\frac{N}{Q_f} = C_w(1-\varepsilon) \qquad [3]$$

where
N = the net flux rate of solute movement across the membrane (moles/min);
Q_f = the net flux rate of water movement across the membrane (ml/min);
C_w = the average concentration (molality) of solute in the bulk phase or retentate, in this instance the concentration of the solute in the plasma water (mmol/ml);
ε = a property of the membrane termed the 'rejection coefficient' and is a measure of the degree to which the membrane restrains movement of the solute.

If the membrane pore is much larger than both the water molecule and the solute particle, both will traverse the membrane without hindrance, and the ultrafiltrate's concentration (C_f)

$$C_f = \frac{N}{Q_f} \qquad [4]$$

is unchanged from the retentate, i.e., the concentration of the solution does not change as it crosses the membrane. In this instance

$$C_f = C_w$$

and by equation 3,

$\varepsilon = 0$ = rejection coefficient.

For protein, which is completely rejected by the membrane, however,

$\varepsilon = 1$

The rejection coefficient, therefore, will have values that range from zero to 1, depending on the degree of stearic hindrance presented by the membrane to the hydrated solute particle. At times, it is more convenient to refer to the sieving coefficient (S) of a membrane for a given solute:

$$\varepsilon = 1 - S \qquad [5]$$

$$S = \frac{C_f}{C_w} \qquad [6]$$

The Van't Hoff equation applied *across the membrane* may be written using Staverman's reflection coefficient (σ), which may be considered the measure of a membrane's 'semipermeability' for a given solute and as such is closely related to, but different from the rejection coefficient (ε) [4]

$$\Delta\pi = RT\sigma_j \left[\sum_{j=1}^m C_j^B - \sum_{j=1}^n C_j^D \right] \qquad [7]$$

or, converting concentration terms for each side of the membrane into osmolar gradients we have the more useful

$$\Delta\pi = \sum_{j=1}^n (\Delta\pi_j \sigma_j) \qquad [8]$$

$$= (\Delta\pi_1 \sigma_1) + (\Delta\pi_2 \sigma_2) + \ldots \text{etc.} \qquad [9]$$

Equation 2 may now be written more precisely as

$$Q_f = AL_p \left(\Delta P + \sum_{j=1}^n \Delta\pi_1 \sigma_1 \right) \qquad [10]$$

The concentration of the ultrafiltrate C_f under carefully controlled conditions is not only dependent on σ, but, as has been shown by Spiegler and Kadem (1), varies with the volume flow rate J_f (ml/min/cm^2) of ultrafiltrate.

$$C_f = \frac{J_s}{J_f} = (1-\varepsilon)C_w \qquad [11]$$

where J_s, is the solute flux rate (mol/min/cm^2).
ε then may be related to σ using the Spiegler equation (2):

$$\varepsilon = \sigma \frac{\varepsilon^\beta - 1}{\varepsilon^\beta - \sigma} \qquad [12]$$

where $\beta = J_f(1-\sigma)/P_m$ and P_m = the permeability of the membrane for the solute considered (cm/min)

when J_f is very large ε approaches σ

when J_f is very small ε approaches $\frac{J_f \sigma}{P_m}$

The ultrafiltration rate in the human glomerulus and capillary beds such as that in the splanchnic circulation, interestingly, are dominated by considerations of oncotic pressure. The importance of oncotic pressure lies not in its magnitude, which is small in absolute terms (1 to 1.5 mOsm/l or 19 to 28 mm Hg), but rather in the fact that it is nearly equal to the hydraulic pressure gradient across the capillary wall. By contrast, in the artificial kidney, under usual operating conditions (where ΔP ranges from 20 to 250 mm Hg) hydraulic pressure (ΔP)

---

[4] ε is readily measured during clinical application or on the bench whereas σ is not. There is a considerable body of theoretical information for both synthetic and biological membranes available for σ that will not be included in this chapter. However, an understanding of ε and an appreciation of how ε and σ differ will provide a satisfactory theoretical background with which the forces at work when ultrafiltration occurs can be understood. A useful way to conceptualize σ is as the ratio of the flow of water relative to solute (J_d) over the total volume flow of water (J_v) that results from the hydrostatic pressure gradient alone, i.e. $\sigma = J_d/J_v$ with $\Delta C_s = 0$. If the membrane does not distinguish between solute and water as they move through, then there will be no relative flow, i.e. $J_d = 0$ and $\sigma = 0$ and the ultrafiltered solution does not change concentration as it crosses the membrane. Should the membrane, however, totally restrain the solute, then $J_d = J_v$; $\sigma = 1$ and the ultrafiltrate is totally free of the solute.

almost invariably exceeds oncotic pressure. Small solutes, other than protein, present in dialysis fluid or in uremic plasma (e.g., glucose, urea) contribute substantially to the osmolality of the solution (25 to 100 mOsm/l or 475 to 1900 mm Hg), but because of their low reflection coefficient with cellophane result in comparatively little water flux across the membrane.

Peritoneal dialysis

A detailed description of the peritoneal membrane appears in chapter 22. The present analysis will consider the peritoneal membrane as the domain that separates the bulk phase of plasma water from the bulk phase of well-mixed dialysis fluid. Such a description then comprises both the anatomical structures such as the vascular endothelium, mesothelium etc., and in addition, all of their attendant unstirred layers. Unlike hemodialysis ultrafiltration across the peritoneal membrane is accomplished almost exclusively by osmotic force.

The peritoneal membrane is not perfectly semipermeable (i.e. is somewhat leaky) for the solutes to be considered, making our task of quantitating the driving force for ultrafiltration more complicated. Glucose moves across the peritoneal membrane at a rate consonant with its rather small size (180 daltons). Even protein molecules such as albumin (60,000 daltons) traverse the peritoneal membrane to some small extent.

As noted for the artificial kidney the peritoneal membrane is not ideally semipermeable and the correction factor (σ) for each solute concentration gradient ($\Delta\pi$) must be applied to adjust that gradient for the degree of the membrane's 'semipermeability' for that solute. Analogous to equation 10 for artificial membranes these concepts could be set down as follows:

$$Q_f = AL_p (\Delta\pi_1 \sigma_1 \text{ and } \Delta\pi_2 \sigma_2 + \ldots \text{etc.}) \quad [13]$$

where: $\Delta\pi_1 \sigma_1$ would equal the osmotic driving gradient for sodium $\Delta\pi_2 \sigma_2$ would equal that for potassium, etc., until each of the solutes present on each side of the membrane was represented. This equation was previously written for the artificial kidney (eq. 10) with a term to express the hydrostatic driving force resulting from the blood to bath (ΔP). Because the peritoneal space under normal circumstances is free of significant quantities of fluid, we may reasonably assume that the hydrostatic and oncotic forces at play across the capillary membrane from arteriolar to venular end are in balance with lymphatic run off. In order to effect net accumulation of ultrafiltrate in the peritoneal space, these forces must be unbalanced by the osmotic force contributed by the presence of glucose in the dialysis fluid. For a two liter exchange added to the peritoneal space, the hydrostatic force contributed would result either from the elastic recoil of the abdominal wall and/or the hydrostatic head of pressure generated by the 'column' of water above the dependent portion of the peritoneal membrane. As such it would be expected to be small and in a direction favoring net uptake across the peritoneal membrane from 'bath to blood'. To be precise, this force must be added as a component of ΔP. Lastly,

in considering this simplification there is the unlikely possibility that hypertonic dialysis fluid by some mechanism may alter the afferent/efferent resistances of the peritoneal capillary bed in such a manner as to enhance the hydrostatic pressure gradient thereby causing ultrafiltration. Solutes that were nearly equal or equal in concentration on both sides of the membrane would, of course, contribute little or no driving force for ultrafiltration. Solutes such as glucose, urea and protein, for example, which by therapeutic intent or biological circumstance will have significant concentration gradients across the membrane, may contribute significant osmotic driving force.

To understand just how much, or even relatively how much force for ultrafiltration across the peritoneal membrane would be contributed, for example, when glucose is contrasted with protein or urea, requires further exploration of the term σ and an appreciation that the larger a solute is in terms of its molecular size the less likely it is to be present in biologic solutions at a concentration that contributes much to the total osmolality.

Albumin, for example, has a reasonable high σ. That is to say albumin moves through the membrane with difficulty. It is commonly present in the plasma at a concentration of 3.5 g/dl. Taking an average molecular

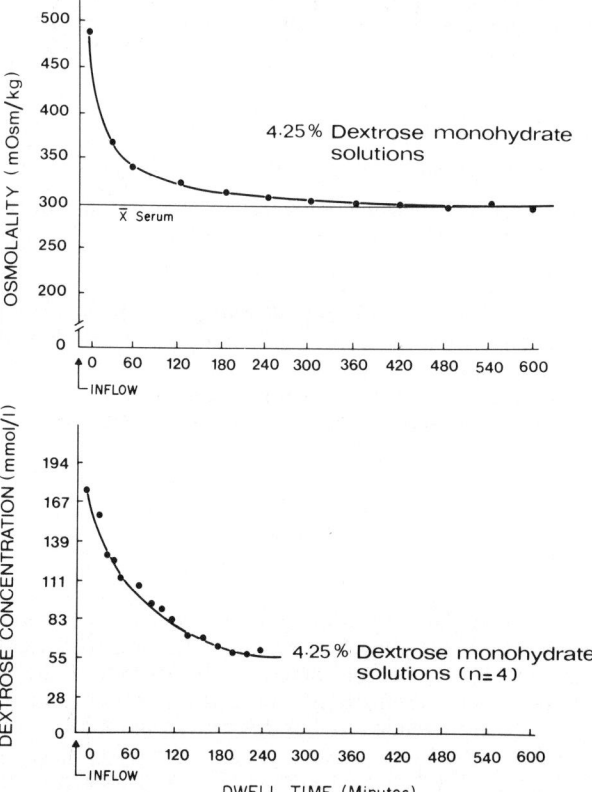

Figure 3. Change in d-glucose concentration and osmolality of a solution containing 4.25% dextrose monohydrate plotted vs. dwell time.

weight of 60,000 and assuming $\sigma = 1$, the osmolar contribution of albumin to resisting movement of plasma water into the peritoneal space is only

$$\frac{35 \text{ g/kg H}_2\text{O}}{60,000} = 0.0006 \text{ Osm/kg H}_2\text{O}$$
$$= 0.6 \text{ mOsm/kg H}_2\text{O} = 11 \text{ mm Hg}$$

Dextrose monohydrate on the other hand at a concentration of 1.5 or 4.25 g/dl in the dialysis fluid (1.36 or 3.86 g/dl of dextrose anhydrous) and 100 mg/dl in plasma would contribute a maximum potential osmolar driving gradient for ultrafiltration of either 70 mOsm (1330 mm Hg) or 209 mOsm (3987 mm Hg) [5]. This maximum is never manifest, however, because of the relatively low σ for dextrose across the peritoneal membrane. Furthermore, with time, the concentration gradient deteriorates (Figure 3). There are at least two components to this discharge of the gradient. The first is diffusion of dextrose into the plasma and the second is convective water movement countercurrent to the dextrose. Clinically, the net movement of water is obtained

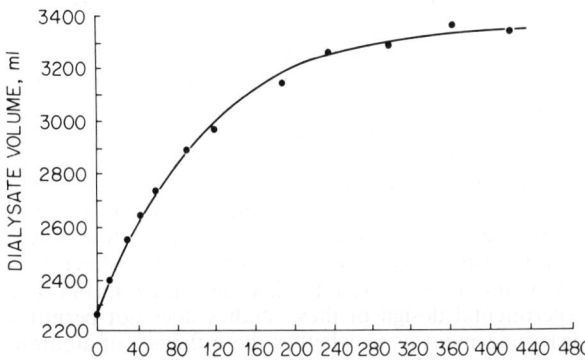

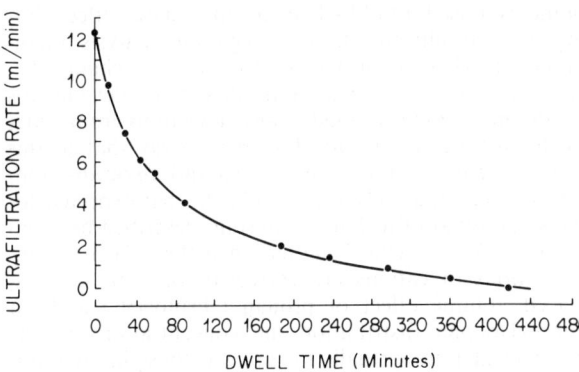

Figure 4. Dialysate volume and the rate of ultrafiltration are plotted vs. dwell time for a solution containing 4,25% dextrose monohydrate.

---

[5] Dextrose (d-glucose) is added to dialysis solution to provide an osmolar gradient for ultrafiltration. Expressed as d-glucose . H$_2$O (dextrose monohydrate, 198 daltons), the concentrations are 1.5 g/dl or 4.25 g/dl, whereas the concentrations of dextrose anhydrous are 1.36 or 3.86 g/dl.

Table 1. Comparison of membrane sieving coefficients.

			Sieving coefficients		
Solute	Daltons	Mol diam Å	Cuprophan	AN69 [a]	XM50 [b]
Urea	60	5.1	1.00	1.00	0.99 ± 0.01
Sucrose	342	9.2	0.79	0.98	1.02 ± 0.02
B$_{12}$	1355	14.6	0.63	0.94	—
Inulin	5200	22.9	0.31	0.78	0.96 ± 0.05

[a] AN69 = polyacrilonitrile membrane distributed in sheet plate dialyser format by Rhône Poulenc Corporation, France.
[b] XM50 = An experimental polysulfone membrane produced by the Amicon Corporation, USA.

as the difference between inflow and outflow volumes. As such, it represents an average value. Figure 4 shows the relationship of water flow rate and dialysate volume with time for a solution containing 4.25% dextrose monohydrate (3) while Figure 3 relates the osmolar gradient and the dextrose concentration with time. To determine the osmotic force contributed by urea (u), with a molecular weight of 60, consider the following circumstance: for a plasma urea concentration of 300 mg/dl (50 mmol/l) (BUN of 140 mg/dl) it offers a 50 mOsm (950 mm Hg) maximum potential osmolar driving gradient for water movement. Clinical wisdom identifies that 'isotonic' (1.5% dextrose containing) dialysis solutions used in patients with a blood urea nitrogen concentration of 150 ± 20 mg/dl (about 54 mmol/l of blood urea) usually results in little or no net removal of excess total body water. In this circumstance then for average values of π for a 60 min exchange time then $\sigma_u \pi_u \simeq \sigma_g \pi_g$ where starting values for $\pi_u = 950$ and $\pi_g = 1482 \therefore \sigma_u < \sigma_g$ and $\frac{\sigma_u}{\sigma_g}$ = about 0.6. With cellulose membranes for laboratory use (i.e. not Cuprophan) studied *in vitro* (4), the values obtained are $\sigma_u = 0.024$ and $\sigma_g = 0.20$, i.e. $\frac{\sigma_u}{\sigma_g}$ = about 0.1 suggesting that this synthetic membrane is a good deal 'tighter' than peritoneal membrane. A similar conclusion for Cuprophan was arrived at by another line of reasoning (5). At present, there is very limited information about σ for the peritoneal membrane and the various solutes that are present in the peritoneal dialysis system (i.e. soluble constituents of uremic plasma water and dialysis fluid) (6). Direct measurement of the peritoneal membrane characteristic σ for a given solute is not presently possible. Even indirect or relative measurements such as described above are not easy and are subject to criticism. As with hemodialysis what is usually measured clinically is the sieving coefficient(s) (eq. 6) or rejection coefficient (ε) as described in equations 5 and 6. Table 1 lists these values for several relevant solutes (6–9). In order to gain insight into the relationship of the rejection coefficient and Staverman's reflection coefficient for the peritoneal membrane where direct measurements are difficult to

(2) the ultrafiltration rate of the artificial kidney to be used.

The concept of 'dry' weight of a hemodialysis patient is widely accepted and usually defined as the body weight below which hypotension and/or symptoms such as muscle cramps particularly in the legs occur. Should the patient be upright, signs and symptoms of postural hypotension may be manifest. The patient's 'dry' weight is only established after several weeks of conscious effort by the hemodialysis staff to achieve an asymptomatic minimum weight level. Implied in this definition is the absence of clinically demonstrable fluid accumulation in tissues or body cavities unexplained by local derangements, e.g. thrombophlebitis, or pericarditis. Once established, this value is the basis for the judgement of excesses of total body water requiring removal. This empirical concept is clinically exceedingly useful. Table 3 gives total body water (tritiated water space) in liters and as a percent of body weight in 16 stable end stage renal failure patients on hemodialysis treatment for at least six months. Whole blood volume (I^{131}-Albumin + ^{51}Cr-RBC) in liters and as a fraction of total body weight is given for the same group. The measurements were made post treatment and all were considered to be at 'dry' weight. The values given do not differ from those of normal subjects (Henderson LW, San Felippo ML, Barg AP, O'Connor DT: Unpublished observations).

The ultrafiltration rate of the membrane package used is usually offered by the manufacturer as a graph of the rate of fluid loss vs. transmembrane pressure. Reasonable prediction of fluid loss per treatment time can be made from these graphs. For unencased coils the pressure gradient may be clearly estimated by averaging the inflow and outflow pressures of the blood path. Most dialysis fluid delivery systems do not provide an inflow pressure. Estimates of the transmembrane pressure from outflow pressure measurements alone modified by experience with a given piece of equipment are, however, quite satisfactory clinically. As Nolph, Fox and Maher (17) have identified, encased coils through which dialysis fluid is pumped have a significant back pressure which reduces the transmembrane pressure as estimated from blood path pressure measurement alone. Experience with the coil/fluid delivery system combination and/or information from the manufacturer is then required to predict fluid loss accurately with time. With coil dialyzers there is a significant obligatory fluid loss due to the comparatively high resistance to flow through the blood path. Encased coils show a somewhat lower obligatory fluid loss due to the lower intrinsic transmembrane pressure (17). Membrane packages using hollow fiber or sheet/plate format in general do not have an obligatory ultrafiltration rate as the blood path resistance to flow is low. In these units dialysis fluid is often pulled through the dialyzer rather than pushed and a hydrostatic pressure for ultrafiltration is achieved by the dialysis fluid pump pulling against a partially occluded (by an adjustable clamp) inflow line or the blood pump pumping against a partially occluded blood return line or both. Resistance to flow in the unclamped dialysate path is sufficiently low so that at satisfactory flow rates (200 to 500 ml/min) little, if any, obligatory ultrafiltration occurs.

New fluid delivery equipment for hemodialysis is now available that will provide direct measurement of the flow rate of ultrafiltrate as a difference in flow rates of dialysis fluid entering and leaving the membrane package. In addition the total volume of ultrafiltrate generated at any point in the treatment may be displayed. Lastly, this information will provide the ability to program fluid loss for a given treatment to achieve any pattern desired, e.g. linear loss.

Dialysis induced symptomatic hypotension

Symptomatic hypotension is common during hemodialysis treatments, but a distinct rarity with peritoneal dialysis. A clinical pattern of dizziness, malaise, nausea, and cramps accompanied by a fall in blood pressure, requiring some therapeutic intervention occurs in approximately 25% of hemodialysis treatments. The common perception is that this syndrome is the result of the rate and volume of removal of excess body water.

Vascular volume depletion

'Dry weight', as defined above, is that weight at the end of a dialysis treatment below which the patient, more often than not, will become symptomatic and go into shock. Clinical wisdom relates symptomatic hypotension not only to the *amount* of ultrafiltrate removed during hemodialysis treatment (net negative fluid balance) but also to the *rate* of removal. Shear et al. (18-20), demonstrated the rather constant rate of reabsorption of fluid from the peritoneal space. We may reasonably extrapolate from the capillaries of the splanchnic bed to those throughout the body and argue that each patient has a finite rate of recruitment of fluid from the extravascular into the vascular space and that if removal of plasma water by the artificial kidney exceeds that rate for long enough, hypovolemic shock with its attendant symptoms will occur. The logic of shock occurring when ultrafiltration sufficiently depletes the vascular volume is undeniable but overly simplistic in the setting of maintenance dialysis for chronic uremia. It should be recognized that vascular volume may be partitioned into intrathoracic and peripheral 'compartments'. To date, no studies address changes in these compartments with artificial kidney treatment. In addition, Bergström and associates (21, 22), Schuenemann and coworkers (23), Rouby et al (24), and Rodrigo et al. (25) recently have called attention to the importance of osmolar changes

Table 3. Total body water and whole blood volume in 16 stable maintenance dialysis patients at 'dry' weight.

	$\bar{X}$[a]	SEM[a]
Total body water (liters)	43.17	1.1
Total body water/kg body wt (%)	59.81	1.6
Whole blood volume (ml)	4480	283
Whole blood volume/kg body wt (%)	5.92	0.37

[a] $\bar{X}$ = mean, SEM = standard error of the mean.

occurring during dialysis therapy. When 1 to 3 l of plasma water are removed over a 4 h period, plasma proteins are concentrated, providing an enhanced oncotic force to recruit extravascular fluid into the vascular space. This force, when quantitated in terms of milliosmoles per liter, would seem to be trivial at best, as it would provide less than 0.5 mOsm (that is, < 10 mm Hg) driving gradient for capillary water reabsorption. This is quite sufficient, however, to unbalance the Starling forces of the microcirculation in favor of reabsorption of extravascular fluid. With the abrupt reduction of the plasma water concentration of such small solutes as urea and creatinine during dialysis and the lag in their equilibration across biologic membranes, an additional osmotic driving gradient for cell uptake of water occurs, leaving the vascular space to be refilled from the already diminished interstitial space (24, 26). For a given ultrafiltration rate, the magnitude of this volume depletion would clearly be a direct function of the rate of fall in plasma urea concentration with dialysis. 'High efficiency' dialyzers, especially when used in the clinical setting of a high plasma urea nitrogen concentration, would then put the patient at greater risk for symptomatic hypotension than would less efficient (smaller area) dialyzers or peritoneal dialysis, where the urea clearance rate is less (27–31) [7]. Further, dialyzers with large surface areas offer the potential for shorter treatment periods, and hence, the fluid removal required to maintain the patient 'dry' must be accomplished in this shorter treatment time, accentuating the problem of symptomatic hypotension.

From this pathophysiologic schema, we may then examine the observation that when ultrafiltration is conducted separately in time from diffusional solute loss, symptomatic hypotension is less frequent. By separating ultrafiltration from diffusional urea removal, we may speculate that only a single force depletes the vascular volume (ultrafiltration) and that this is partially offset by the enhanced oncotic force recruiting extravascular volume.

Note that all empirical therapies offered for symptomatic hypotension (hypertonic mannitol, isotonic and hypertonic saline and plasminate [8]) provide an extracellular solute particle with osmotic or oncotic capability to recruit vascular volume.

The data obtained on cardiac output and peripheral vascular resistance of uremic patients undergoing hemodialysis bear comment. The studies in humans by Wehle et al. (32), Hampl and coworkers (33), and Chen and associates (34) used either invasive or noninvasive techniques to assess these autonomic nervous system compensatory mechanisms. Compensatory peripheral vasoconstriction with fluid removal was better maintained with both sequential ultrafiltration and dialysis (32) and hemofiltration (33) than it was for hemodialysis (simultaneous dialysis and ultrafiltration). Nevertheless, the underlying cause for the differences noted remains obscure. The functional 'lesion' identified may result from an acute vasculopathy or autonomic neuropathy mediated by an osmotic fluid shift with failure of the afferent and efferent resistances of the microvasculature to constrict appropriately when the vascular volume is depleted.

Physiochemical toxicity
The work of Graefe et al. (30) and Novello and coworkers (35) in humans and that of Keshaviah et al. (26) and Kirkendol and colleagues (36) in animals suggest that acetate may cause symptomatic hypotension in certain instances. The rate at which acetate may be metabolically disposed of, varies among patients. Symptomatic hypotension occurs in those where the rate of acetate uptake from the dialysis fluid exceeds its rate of metabolism and the plasma level of acetate increases considerably. Kishimoto et al. (37), correlated the serum acetate concentration with symptomatic hypotension in a series of 27 patients treated with acetate dialysis fluid. Hypotension occurred when serum acetate was about 5 mmol/l. High efficiency dialysis predisposes toward higher plasma acetate concentrations. The mechanism for the acetate's reaction remains unclear; that is, is it cardiotoxic, or is the toxicity primarily microcirculatory with venular pooling secondarily compromising cardiac output, or both?

Autonomic neuropathy
Classical compensatory cardiovascular mechanisms protect us from changes in vascular volume. Carotid, aortic, and cardiopulmonary baroreceptors sense a depletion in arterial vascular volume. A compensatory increase in both cardiac output and peripheral vascular resistance occurs in an effort to hold blood pressure stable. Sympathetic nervous system insufficiency occurs in some patients with end stage renal failure (38–44). Lilley, Golden, and Stone (43) suggest a defect in the afferent limb of the baroreceptor reflex arc in a subset of uremic patients. Typical clinical findings in this group were hypertension, lability of blood pressure with symptomatic hypotension when fluid was removed during hemodialysis, and a significantly higher plasma dopamine-β-hydroxylase (DBH) activity. Total peripheral resistance in such patients is high when corrected for the low hematocrit typically present with chronic uremia (45, 46). Patients with baroreceptor reflex dysfunction show findings similar to animals in which surgical section of the afferent nerve from the baroreceptors has been performed, i.e., hypertension, high peripheral resistance resulting from unopposed sympathetic nervous system activity, and lability of blood pressure in response to sodium and volume loading (47–50). Present thinking (51) indicates that a resetting of the level of the 'servo point', around which the reflex modulates changes in blood pressure, occurs at a higher level in nonuremic patients with hypertension. Studies to determine the reflex resetting and altered sensitivity in patients with renal failure and hypertension are few (40–44). They indicate, primarily, a reduction in sensitivity of the mechanisms involving baroreceptor pulse interval

---

[7] Dialyzers with a greater than 1.0 m² of membrane area and with a urea clearance of 150 ml/min or higher at 200 ml/min blood flow rate are considered to be high efficiency dialyzers when compared with more standard equipment where urea clearances of 120 ml/min are common.

[8] Plasminate is a reconstituted plasma protein solution.

regulation. In addition, although data from Kersh and coworkers (42) suggest a normal end-organ responsiveness to catecholamines, Romoff and colleagues (52) have data to suggest end-organ unresponsiveness.

DBH is a presynaptic enzyme that catalyzes the synthesis of norepinephrine. DBH is not rapidly degraded biochemically or eliminated, unlike norepinephrine so it has a substantially longer half life (48, 53, 54). Plasma DBH reflects the longer-term (day to day) level of activity of the sympathetic nervous system more closely than does plasma norepinephrine. Increased plasma DBH, therefore, also reflects excess sympathetic nervous system traffic.

Hemofiltration has been noted to result in a lower incidence of symptomatic hypotension (55–57). While the membranes most frequently used for this technique are more biocompatible than cellulosic membranes it is not clear whether this factor or the less efficient rate of removal of osmotically important solutes is the reason for this lower incidence.

Membrane toxicity

Exposure of blood to cellulosic membranes clearly triggers surface sensitive proteins discharging the complement cascade. This, in turn, relates temporally to the pulmonary sequestration of leukocytes early in the course of cellulosic hemodialysis (58–63). This leukocyte sequestration may underlie the fall in arterial partial pressure of oxygen (PAO_2) noted with hemodialysis (62, 63). The dissociation between leukocyte sequestration and the reduction in PAO_2 casts doubt, however, on this as the etiologic mechanism (64). The Amicon XM-50 membrane does not cause changes in such leukocyte functions as random mobility, phagocytosing ability, or response to a chemotactic stimulus, unlike the Dow regenerated cellulose acetate membrane (61). The closely related XP-50 membrane from Amicon, now commonly being used for hemofiltration, also does not cause hemodialysis leukopenia (Henderson LW, unpublished observations), nor does the AN-69 polyacrilonitrile (PA) membrane from Rhône Poulenc, although the latter does activate complement (65). To date, no prospective studies have been reported to test the hypothesis that cellulosic membrane toxicity may be responsible for some of the symptomatic hypotension noted during hemodialysis.

It is apparent that symptomatic hypotension is multifactorial in etiology and that volume and rate of removal of excess body water are only two of the causative factors.

Peritoneal dialysis

Ultrafiltration across the peritoneal membrane must be accomplished osmotically. Glucose, sorbitol, mannitol and other osmotically active solutes have been used to create the pressure gradient. Commercially available dialysis solutions most often offer a 1.5 g/dl and 4.25 g/dl glucose solution. The measured osmolality of the 1.5 g/dl solution is 350 mOsm/l a figure well above that for a normal plasma, but quite comparable to that of the patient with renal failure when the blood urea nitrogen concentration is 150 to 200 mg/dl (blood urea 54 to 72 mmol/l). The 4.25 g/dl dextrose monohydrate solution, however, is considerably more hypertonic than even uremic plasma and a two liter exchange will induce about 300 to 500 ml of ultrafiltrate per exchange. There is considerable variability among patients with regard to the negative fluid balance due to ultrafiltration. An explanation may well be that the membrane involved is biological and subject to differences between patients as well as changes with time in the same patient. With a duration of each exchange of 30 to 70 min an ultrafiltration rate of 7 to 16 ml/min is achieved, which contrasts with rates of 0 to 35 ml/min that may be easily obtained with a standard Cuprophan dialysis membrane. As peritoneal dialysis is usually conducted over at least 12 h and not uncommonly in acute renal failure for 24 to 48 h compared to 4 to 6 h for extracorporeal hemodialysis many clinicians prefer peritoneal dialysis when large volumes (over 5.0 l) of body water must be removed. The slower removal rate permitted by the longer treatment time, means fewer symptoms related to depletion of vascular volume, since the rate of movement of fluid entering the vascular compartment from interstitial and possibly intracellular sources is sufficient to compensate for the fluid removal. The rate of mobilization of extravascular fluid is specific to the individual. Fluid sequestered in body cavities such as the pleura or the pericardium usually is recruited very slowly and may take weeks or months of repeated efforts to remove, even in the absence of any identifiable cause for local fluid accumulation like active pleuritis or pericarditis.

SOLUTE TRANSPORT BY ULTRAFILTRATION DURING DIALYSIS

Hemodialysis

While the concept of solute rejection by the membrane is important, in order to understand why $\Delta\pi\sigma$ contributes comparatively little to the transmembrane pressure when fluid is removed from a patient during dialysis, it is vital to the understanding of convective mass transfer. From equation 2 it is apparent that the membrane property (ε) dictates the respective velocities of solute (N) and solvent (Q_f) movement across the membrane. No concentration gradient is necessary for solute transport by convection. While transport by diffusion is always size-dependent (i.e. small solutes are transported faster than large ones), convective mass transfer is not necessarily dependent on particle size. The respective contributions of convection and diffusion in conventional dialyzers has been ignored until recently (66–68), largely because of the comparatively low hydraulic permeability of Cuprophan. The advent of more water-permeable ('high flux') membranes, however, has directed interest to this area. At present there is comparatively little information on sieving coefficients for uremic solutes across cellulosic dialysis membranes. In Table 1 Cuprophan is compared with high flux polyacrilonitrile (PA) and polysulfone (XM-50) membranes for sieving coefficients (67, 68).

An expression for combined diffusive and convective clearance (and dialysance) may be derived from equations for clearance (and dialysance) and from consideration of mass balance across a dialyzer in which ultrafiltration is occurring:

$$Q_{Bi}C_{Bi} = Q_{Bo}C_{Bo} + Q_f C_f$$

$$\text{Clearance} = \frac{Q_{Bo}(C_{Bi} - C_{Bo})}{C_{Bi}} + Q_f \quad [17]$$

$$= \frac{Q_{Di}(C_{Do} - C_{Di})}{C_{Bi}} + \frac{Q_f C_{Do}}{C_{Bi}} \quad [18]$$

$$\text{Dialysance} = \frac{Q_{Bo}(C_{Bi} - C_{Bo}) + Q_f C_{Bi}}{C_{Bi} - C_{Di}}$$

$$= \frac{Q_{Di}(C_{Do} - C_{Di}) + Q_f C_{Do}}{C_{Bi} - C_{Di}} \quad [19]$$

These equations provide a clinically statisfactory means for describing mass transfer when both solute transport processes are ongoing. Two points of importance should be noted. *First*, equations relating dialysance and membrane mass transfer resistances are not valid in the presence of ultrafiltration. Hence, values obtained from equations 18 and 19 should not be used to calculate the overall mass transfer resistance of a membrane/solute pair. The hydraulic permeability of Cuprophan is low so that the transmembrane pressure gradients, resulting from the blood path resistance to flow, which is intrinsic to many clinical dialyzers, results in low enough ultrafiltration rates to permit use of these equations. If high flux membranes are used and transmembrane pressure is regulated by adjustment of pressure on the dialysis fluid side of the membrane to block net ultrafiltration, these equations again will be in error. In this situation, convective flux will continue at the inflow end of the blood path where a blood-to-dialysate pressure gradient exists. At the outflow end the pressure gradient is reversed, and, owing to the comparatively high flow rate for dialysis fluid ($Q_D \gg Q_B$), the solute concentration of the dialysis fluid re-entering the blood path is lower than the ultrafiltrate formed at the inflow end ('Starling flow'). Calculated mass transfer resistances for poorly diffusing solutes are then artifactually low. *Second*, while equations 18 and 19 are useful in deriving expected chemical benefits from treatment, they offer little insight into the interaction between convection and diffusion when both are operating in a given dialyzer (as noted in the section on ultrafiltration, σ changes with J_f).

Villarroel and colleagues (2) have developed a simplified form of the Spiegler and Kadem equation (1) that describes solute transport as the sum of a convective and diffusive term:

$$J_s = P_m \Delta C + \overline{C}(1 - \sigma) J_v \quad [20]$$

where J_v is volume flux and

$$\overline{C} = C_B - Z(C_B - C_D) \quad [21]$$

and (the factor)

$$Z = \frac{1}{\beta} - \frac{1}{e^\beta - 1} \quad [22]$$

Beta is given by

$$\beta = (1 - \sigma)\frac{J_v}{P_m} \quad [23]$$

If $0 < \beta < 3$ then $\frac{1}{3} < Z < \frac{1}{2}$

If $\beta > 3$ then $Z = \frac{1}{\beta}$ and

$$J_s = C_B(1 - \sigma)J_v \quad [24]$$

These relationships point up the fact that as ultrafiltration rate, *in vitro*, increases, the overall contribution to net solute transport made by diffusion decreases to zero, an observation already made by Nolph and associates (12, 66). The studies of Villarroel and colleagues (2) demonstrated that for dialysis membranes tested *in vitro*, equation 16 shows a reasonable degree of agreement (within 5%) with the results obtained with the more rigorous and complex Spiegler equation. As can be predicted, the impact of convective mass transport is most impressive on solutes that diffuse poorly through the membrane. Figure 5 plots clearance by diffusion (curve A) and clearance by convection (curve B) against log molecular weight. It is apparent that for

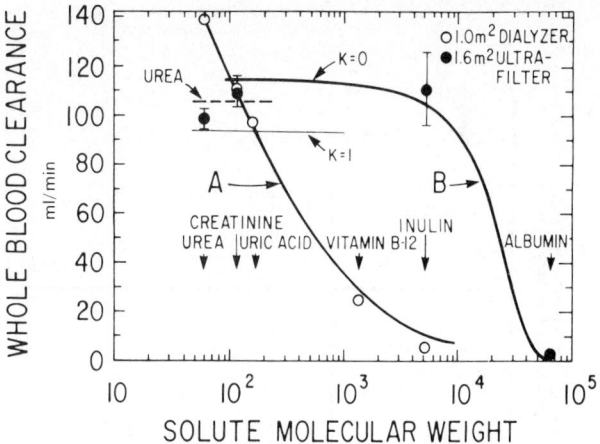

Figure 5. Whole blood clearance is plotted against the log of solute molecular weight. Curve A shows the solute clearance pattern for a 1.0 m² dialyzer operated with no ultrafiltration where solute transport is by diffusion. Curve B shows such a pattern for a 1.6 m² ultrafilter where solute transport is by convection. Normal human kidneys display a clearance pattern very similar to curve B. Small solutes (<200 molecular weight) are better cleared by diffusion. K ranges from 0 to 1 and describes the distribution of solute between plasma and the red blood cell (see text on hemofiltration for further discussion of K).

'conventional' uremic solutes (less than 200 daltons) curve A shows a higher clearance than curve B (68, 69).

Peritoneal dialysis

The ability of solutes to move across the peritoneal membrane in the absence of a driving concentration gradient was demonstrated in 1966 for urea (69). Important to the understanding of the mechanism for movement of solutes into the dialysis fluid is the role that the membrane plays in restraining or modulating such movement. The concept of membrane sieving or rejection as explored above, is central to an understanding of how solute movement occurs. Solute mass transfer and its quantitation has been dealt with in some detail elsewhere (see Chapter 3). Therefore, these comments are restricted to convective mass transfer across the peritoneal membrane and the impact that this may have on simultaneously occurring diffusive mass transfer. The usual calculation of peritoneal clearance using the conventional relationship

clearance =

$$\frac{\text{average mass removed per minute in the dialysate}}{\text{plasma concentration}}$$

will provide an average rate of plasma clearance that will not distinguish the comparative contributions of convection and diffusion, but which is perfectly satisfactory for clinical judgements relating to the rate of solute removal. Table 2 offers sieving coefficient values for urea, inulin, glucose, sodium, potassium and chloride.

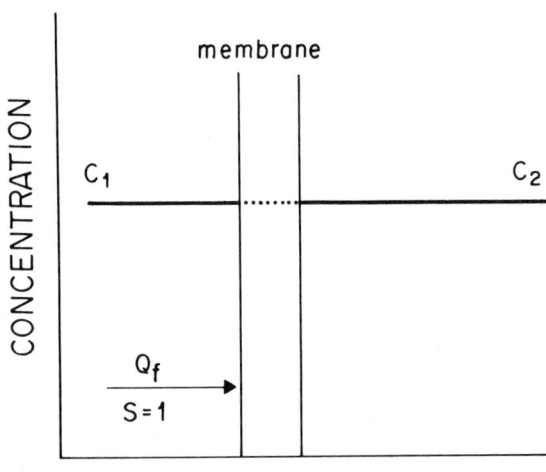

Figure 6. Concentration profile for a solute with sieving coefficient (S) = 1 during ultrafiltration across a membrane. The dialysis fluid has been made up to contain a concentration of the solute (C_2) that is equal to that in plasma water (C_1).

Take the case of an uncharged solute of small molecular weight for which S = 1. Let us assume for the moment that urea fulfills these criteria. Figure 6 depicts this concentration profile across a membrane separating blood and dialysis fluid. The concentration for urea has been adjusted to be equal in plasma water and dialysis fluid and, for the present, we will assume the sieving coefficient to be 1.0. The concentration profile is drawn for the conditions existing a few moments after the onset of ultrafiltration and is linear. That is, there is no change in the concentration of the ultrafiltered plasma water as it crosses the membrane and its attendant 'unstirred' layers. In this circumstance the average convective clearance of urea will be the product of the sieving coefficient and the ultrafiltration rate.

$$S_u = \frac{\overline{C}_{f_u}}{\overline{C}_{w_u}} \qquad [25]$$

$$S_u \overline{Q}_f = \frac{\overline{C}_{f_u}}{\overline{C}_{w_u}} \overline{Q}_f = \text{Average clearance of urea from plasma water by convection} \qquad [26]$$

$$= \frac{\text{Mass removed by ultrafiltration/exchange time}}{\text{Plasma water concentration}}$$

$\overline{Q}_f$ would usually be obtained as the volume difference (Inflow volume − Outflow volume) divided by the exchange time.

It is apparent that the average convective clearance for a solute with S = 1 is equal to the ultrafiltration rate.

The measurement of the ultrafiltration rate as usually performed clinically provides an average value. The glucose generated osmotic gradient deteriorates exponentially with time. The convective clearance described then is also an average value for the plasma cleared over the time interval of the exchange rather than an instantaneous value.

In the usual clinical situation where one may wish to quantitate the convective clearance for a solute such as urea there is *no* urea present in the dialysis fluid. Diffusion and convection then occur simultaneously during the exchange.

Impact of convection on diffusion

While there are theoretical treatments for the comparative contributions of diffusion and convection to overall clearance rate for the peritoneal (69–71) and hemodialysis membrane (2, 72), there are only a limited number of *in vivo* experiments to substantiate the respective contributions of these forces to net mass transfer (6, 12). Reasoning from this work and from analogy with synthetic membranes *in vitro* a qualitative appreciation of the interaction between these two modes of solute transport may be developed. Figure 7 differs from Figure 6 in that there is no ultrafiltration occurring and the circumstance is presented where there is no urea present in the dialysis fluid. Figure 7 depicts the concentration profile when

12: Biophysics of ultrafiltration and hemofiltration 255

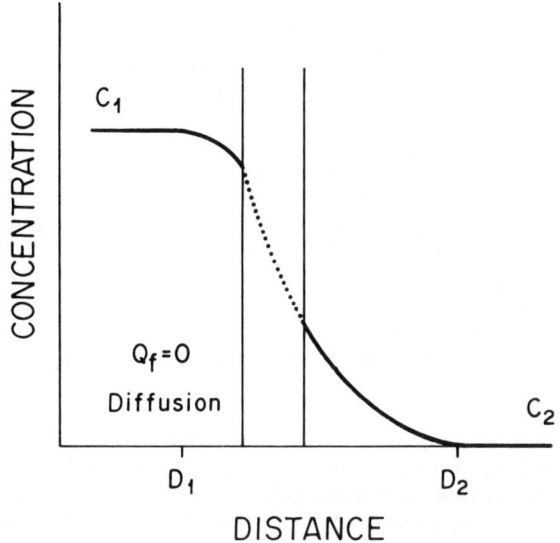

Figure 7. Concentration profile for a solute that diffuses across a membrane in the absence of any ultrafiltration. The 'steepness' of the driving gradient for diffusion is depicted by the difference in concentrations between the bulk phase of the plasma water (C_1) and that of the dialysis fluid (C_2) acting over the distance D_1 to D_2, i.e. $\frac{C_1 - C_2}{D_1 - D_2}$

diffusion alone occurs. The fall in concentration from bulk phase plasma to the surface of the membrane represents the 'blood side' unstirred layer that is partially depleted of solute by diffusion across the membrane into the dialysis fluid. Similarly, the 'dialysate side' unstirred layer is depicted as a continuing reduction in concentration with distance in the dialysis fluid before achieving the dialysate bulk phase concentration (which at the start will be zero). With peritoneal dialysis there is comparatively little mixing of unstirred layers of dialysate when compared with hemodialysis. One may then expect this component of resistance to transport for peritoneal dialysis to be significant. Imposing a transmembrane driving force for ultrafiltration on the conditions shown in Figure 7 results in the changes shown in Figure 8. The reduction to zero (or toward zero for a more diffusively permeable solute) of the blood side fluid film will enhance diffusion by shortening the length of the path over which the gradient for diffusion is acting (D_1 to D_2) between bulk phase blood and bulk phase dialysate. In addition the drop in concentration within the membrane has been obliterated, also shortening the path over which the concentration gradient is exercised. Finally, there is a shift of the dialysate side film away from the membrane. In the event that mechanical mixing may be somewhat better away from the membrane, there will be some enhancement of diffusion. Alternatively, if mechanical mixing is less good the diffusion path may be lengthened and diffusive transport reduced (12). This formulation assumes no mechanical changes such as increased membrane blinding on support structures or stretching of the membrane to alter permeability characteristics.

Figure 9 shows the circumstance for a larger uncharged solute where there is significant membrane restraint ($S < 1$). The solute is convected to the membrane surface where the concentration builds up ('concentration polarization' or 'solute polarization') (67, 68, 73,

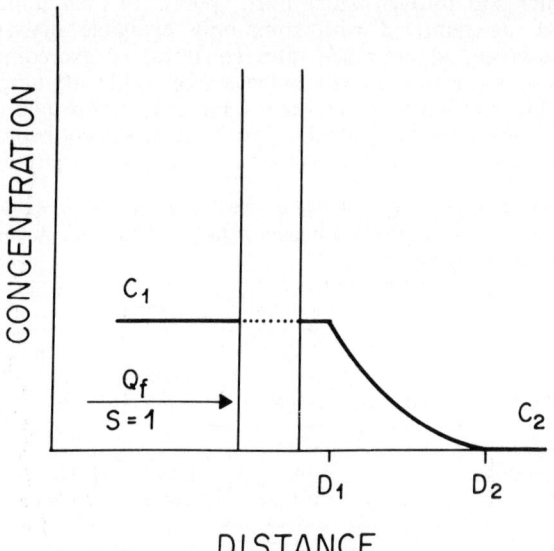

Figure 8. Concentration profile for a solute with $S = 1$ moments after ultrafiltration has begun. Note the steeper driving gradient for diffusion created by the obliteration of the unstirred layer on the blood side, i.e. D_1 to D_2 for diffusion (Figure 7) is larger than that depicted here.

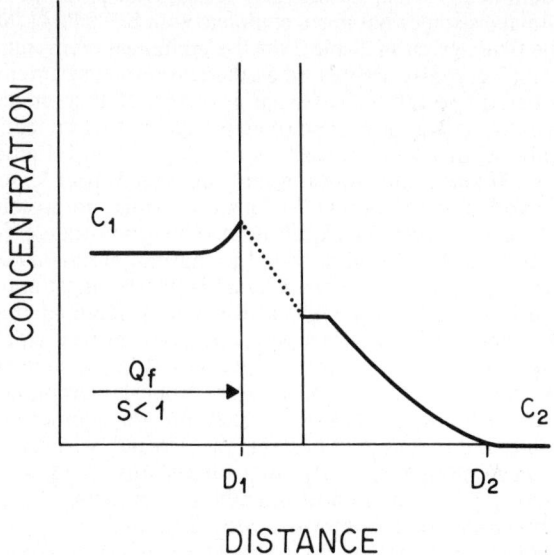

Figure 9. Concentration profile for a solute that is partially restrained by the membrane ($S<1$) moments after the onset of ultrafiltration. The concentration gradient is made steeper by the buildup of solute on the membrane (C_1) and acts over a shorter distance than was the case for simple diffusion (as in Figure 7).

74). The concentration within the membrane falls with distance and the dialysate side film is displaced in a manner analogous to the situation in Figure 8. Again the overall effect is to steepen the concentration gradient enhancing the diffusive component of transport. Precise quantitation of this enhancement for the solutes routinely dealt with in uremic plasma, is not presently possible for the peritoneal membrane and may not be in view because of data, that indicate that exposure to hypertonic solutions not only increase membrane permeability, but membrane area (increase in number of capillary loops perfused?) as well (7).

Finally, in considering the impact of convection on diffusion it should be apparent that solute size is important. For larger solutes with poor diffusive permeability for the membrane (referred to now without its attendant fluid films), convective mass transport, if the sieving coefficient for that solute is high enough, can contribute the major portion of the total mass transported. As a corollary, the fraction of overall mass transfer resistance to diffusion contributed by unstirred fluid films becomes less as the solute considered becomes larger due to the membrane dominating the serial resistance to transport (75).

Albumin, the smallest of the traditional plasma proteins and plasma protein in general, bears some special comment with respect to peritoneal dialysis. The presence of protein in the initiating exchange (i.e. the 'ascites' present) and its subsequent decline over the next few exchanges to a steady state level points up the fact that under usual circumstances there is a loss of protein from the plasma into the peritoneal space. The capillary membrane is the likely source. Albumin is the predominant protein. Table 2 lists a sieving coefficient (S) for albumin of < 0.02. Glomerular restraint of albumin in animals is somewhat more complete with $S \simeq 0.003$ (76). The figure given in Table 2 for the peritoneal membrane is not rigorously arrived at, as there are no experiments to determine this value so far reported. Rather, it derives from data for protein (precipitable by trichloracetic acid) loss in a series of isotonic exchanges $(1.3 \pm 0.1$ gms, $n = 13)$ taken after washout and subtracted from losses in hypertonic solution $(1.7 \pm 2$ gms) to which no protein had been added to block diffusion. The ultrafiltrate concentration of 0.06 g/dl divided by a normal plasma albumin of 3.5 g/dl = 0.02. This figure is purely an estimate as diffusive loss is not blocked and it is assumed that only albumin is convected when, in point of fact, small amounts of globulin are also present. It is of interest, however, that this estimate of 'peritoneal membrane' restraint in man approaches that for the glomerular membrane in animals. Further, the presence of protein in spent peritoneal dialysate is frequently cited as a point for the peritoneal membrane as being 'very permeable' when contrasted with hemodialysis or hemofiltration membranes. It should be noted, however, that more than 98% of the protein is held back by this 'very permeable' membrane even under the stress of hypertonic solutions. For perspective, Cuprophan PT-150 has a transmittance (T_r) value $(T_r \simeq S)$ for egg albumin (44,000 daltons, 46.6 Å) of 0.002 and the more permeable Rhône-Poulenc AN 69 (PA) dialysis membrane has a value of 0.04 (72). In light of its slow diffusivity, it seems likely that the predominant mechanism for protein loss across the peritoneal membrane is convective even in the presence of isotonic dialysis solutions. The presence of dialysis fluid would, of course, 'trap' by massive dilution, protein lost from the capillary that normally would, under steady state circumstances, be either returned to the vascular space via the lymphatics or less likely be convected back across the venular end of the capillary bed.

HEMOFILTRATION
(Convective solute transport without hemodialysis) [9]

At present hemofiltration has moved from an experimental technique to clinical application. More efficient clearance of intermediate molecular weight solutes with hemofiltration compared with conventional hemodialysis suggests that this technique will become more widespread in the near future.

Theoretical aspects

Several indirect lines of reasoning and more recently the identification of uremic solutes of comparatively large size (> 500 daltons) using molecular separation methods based on size, prompted the development of a convective cleansing method of the blood (hemofiltration) to remove these poorly diffusing solutes (77–79). Solute removal by hemodialysis as a diffusion based process in size discriminatory, i.e. small molecules such as the conventionally recognized uremic solutes, (urea [60 daltons], creatinine [113], uric acid [168]) diffuse rapidly in water and through water filled 'pores' in membranes and are removed with commonly available dialysis equipment at clearance rates equal to, or exceeding, those for intact human kidneys (see Table 4). Large solute molecules on the other hand that diffuse poorly are cleared badly by hemodialysis. The process of hemofiltration in which whole blood is diluted with a physio-

Table 4. Comparison of whole blood clearance patterns for 1.6 m² hemofiltration, the human kidney and for 1 m² hollow fiber hemodialysis.

Solute	Daltons	Clearance (ml/min)		
		1.6 m² Hemo-filtration	Human kidney	1.0 m² Hemo-dialysis
Inulin	5200	117	218	6
Creatinine	113	108	218	110
Urea	60	101	136	139

---

[9] The process of convective solute removal from uremic whole blood has been called hemofiltration, hemodiafiltration or hemoultrafiltration. The term hemofiltration has been adopted by workers in the field at the 1977 Gstaad Meeting in Switzerland.

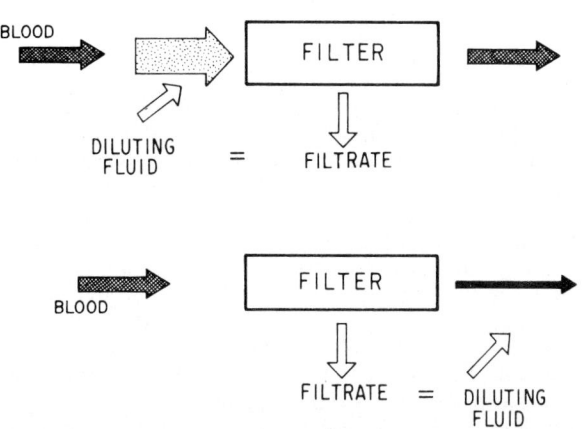

Figure 10. Diagram of hemofiltration showing two modes of replacing ultrafiltrate to the blood path.

Table 5. Diluting fluid composition [a].

	mmol/l		mmol/l
Sodium	133 (132-140)	Chloride	105 (100-110)
Potassium	2 (0-4.0)	Acetate	37 (35-40)
Calcium	1.75 (1.25-2.0) [b]	—	—
Magnesium	0.75 [b]	—	—
Dextrose anhydr 0-5.6 mmol/l [b]			

[a] Common values given, with range in brackets.
[b] Conversions:
  Calcium   3.5 (2.5-4.0) mEq/l
  Magnesium 1.5 mEq/l
  Dextrose   0-100 mg/dl

logic solution of electrolytes either before or after it is ultrafiltered across a membrane to remove convectively undesirable solutes, is diagrammatically shown in Figure 10. Blood is introduced into the membrane package and a transmembrane pressure gradient is accomplished either by creating a negative pressure in the casing outside of the membrane and (or) positively pressurizing the blood path by partially clamping the blood outflow line while pumping blood into the inflow port. The membrane used is selected for its high hydraulic permeability and retentivity characteristics. The latter should mimic those of the human glomerular basement membrane.

The ultrafiltrate formed should contain little or no macrosolutes (protein) and no cellular elements. All other microsolutes, e.g. electrolytes, urea, creatinine, uric acid, glucose, phosphate, sulfate etc. should be present in the ultrafiltrate in the same concentration as they appear in plasma water. Intermediate molecular weight solutes (500 up to 10,000 daltons) identified (but not characterized) as present in abnormal concentrations in uremic plasma will be removed convectively along with the microsolutes. Depending on the size of the pores in the membrane and the solute particles, a certain percentage of these intermediate molecular weight solutes will be retained. Figure 5 shows the clearance pattern for an Amicon XM-50 ultrafilter. It is apparent that like the human kidney, inulin with a molecular weight of 5200 is cleared at the same rate (approximately 100 ml/min) as creatinine (113 daltons) at the operating conditions of this 1.6 m² device.

It is obvious that replacement of water, desirable electrolytes and glucose, simulating 'tubular reabsorption' will be required to maintain a satisfactory blood volume and composition. Table 5 gives the composition of a typical replacement solution. Diluting fluid may be introduced before (predilution) or after (postdilution) the ultrafilter (see Figure 10 [see also next chapter]).

At present there are at least seven membrane modules specifically made in Europe and Japan to perform hemofiltration. The expectation is for even more membranes to become available in the next few years. Table 6 is a partial list of those for which some performance data has been generated. It should be noted that, for some membranes, restraint of larger solutes such as inulin is strongly affected by the presence or absence of plasma proteins in the 'blood' used as test solution. There appears to be no significant difference between use of out dated bank blood and in vivo animal or human studies (80, 81).

Table 6. Inulin sieving coefficients for hemofiltration membranes at common clinical operating parameters.

	Inulin sieving coefficient	
Membrane	Saline	Whole blood
Amicon XP-50	0.97±0.04	0.29±0.08
Asahi PAN-15	0.94±0.09	0.13±0.05
Daicel-Hemofresh	—	0.83±0.06
Sartorius Hemofilter	—	0.59±0.10
Rhône Poulenc RP-6	0.84±0.01	0.79±0.05

Factors affecting ultrafiltration flow rate

Solute mass transfer rate across the membrane is governed by the rate of ultrafiltration and the sieving coefficient of the membrane. Equation 1 gives the general form of the relationship of forces governing the ultrafiltrate flux (J_f) across membranes that have a relatively low hydraulic permeability. A more useful equation for membranes having a high hydraulic permeability (e.g. polyacrilonitrile, polysulfone) and used to ultrafilter protein containing solutions such as plasma or blood is needed. Figure 11 shows the results of an experiment in which a sheet of high flux membrane is placed in a stirred cell and transmembrane pressure is induced. Saline flux is linearly related to transmembrane pressure. When protein is present, however, the flux rate shows a linear relationship early but eventually reaches a plateau at

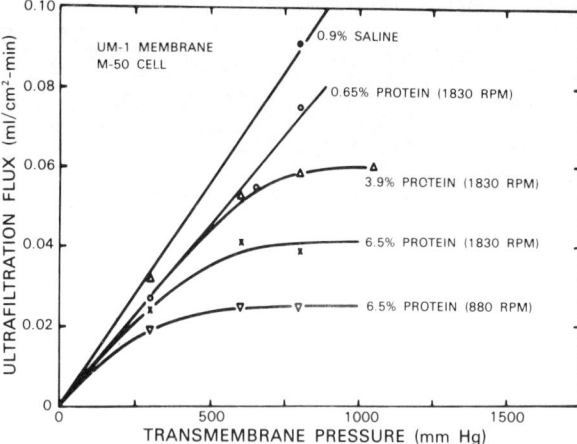

Figure 11. Ultrafiltration flux rate is plotted against transmembrane pressure. Data were collected in a stirred cell with sheet ultrafiltration membrane. The influence of changes in protein concentration can be seen. For saline (0% protein) the response is linear. Increasing protein concentration in the bulk solution decreases the plateau value for the flux rate of water. Increasing stirrer speeds reduce the thickness of the polarized layer of protein on the membrane and increases the flux rate for water at any given protein concentration. (RPM = stirrerspeed, revolutions per minute, see text).

which time further increases in transmembrane pressure result in no further increase in flux rate. An increase in protein concentration of the solution being filtered results in a lower plateau of water flux but increasing stirrer speed elevates the level of this plateau. Experiments such as these have permitted a reasonable description of the events at the membrane level (67, 68, 74, 82). Figure 12 is a diagrammatic representation of such events. During the ultrafiltration of blood, protein containing solution moves to the membrane surface where water and the microsolutes continue to move unimpeded across the discriminating surface. Protein, however, is sieved out and remains behind (concentration polarization). The thickness of this polarized protein layer is determined by the amount of protein delivered to the surface (protein concentration in the bulk phase of plasma times the flow rate for water through the membrane) and the amount diffusing back from the surface (back flux). Factors that influence the back flux are the concentration gradient and the shear forces that 'stir' the protein layer. In the stirred cell with sheet membrane used to generate the data for Figure 11 increasing stirrer speed decreases the thickness of the polarized protein layer and increases the water flux rate. In a hollow fiber unit increasing flow rate down the fiber reduces the thickness of this layer. Previous work with hollow fiber ultrafilters and whole blood permitted several useful correlations relating variables of protein concentration in the bulk phase of plasma (C_p), (67, 68, 74, 82, 83) the slope of the velocity profile for whole blood at the fiber wall, that is the shear rate (γ_w) and the fiber length from the inlet (x):

$$J_f = 1.28 \times 10^{-3} \left(\frac{\gamma_w}{x}\right)^{1/2} \ln\left(\frac{28.7}{C_p}\right) \qquad [27]$$

One may take from this relationship that for a hollow fiber unit the water flux rate falls with increase of plasma protein concentration, that the faster the end to end flow rate down the fiber the higher the flux, but the longer the fiber the lower the flux rate.

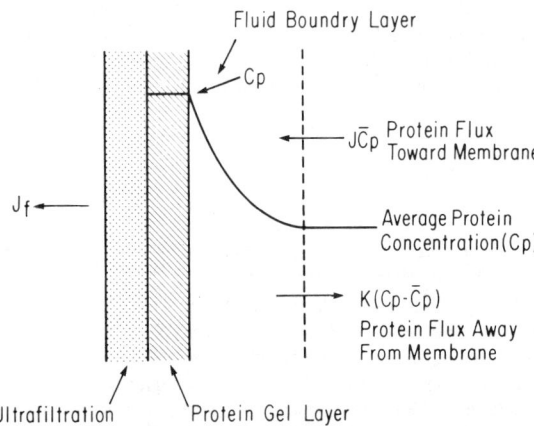

Figure 12. Diagram of the events at the membrane during ultrafiltration of a protein containing solution. Protein is moved to the membrane surface (polarized) in conjunction with the water traversing the membrane. It is moved away from the membrane by diffusion and shear forces generated by flow over the membrane. Thickness of the protein layer at steady state represents the net balance of these two processes. The concentration profile for protein is shown.

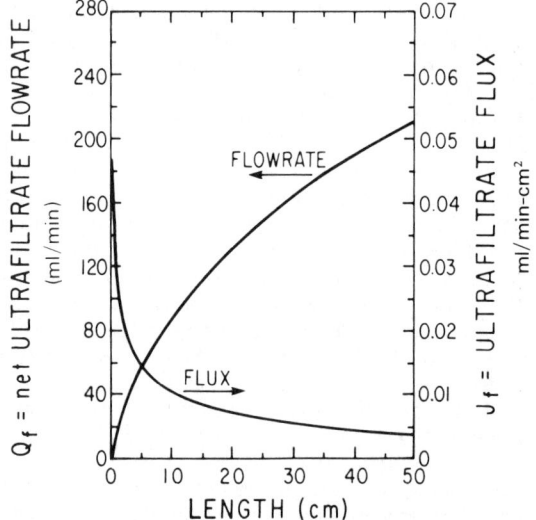

Figure 13. Net ultrafiltrate flow rate and ultrafiltrate flux are plotted against distance from the fiber inlet, for a 4000 fiber unit with fiber internal diameter of 200 μm operated in the predilution mode ($Q_B = Q_f = 200$ ml/min). With a 20 cm length, a 1.0 m² total transport area is present.

Another useful formulation relates net ultrafiltration flow rate (Q_f) to the membrane area of the device (A), the diameter of the fiber (d) and the blood flow rate entering the device:

$$Q_f \alpha (A/d)^{2/3} (Q_{Bi})^{1/3} \qquad [28]$$

This points up that Q_f is independent of fiber length so long as (A/d) is held constant. It might be incorrectly assumed from equation 24 that for a given total membrane area J_f could be increased by shortening the length of the fibers and increasing their numbers holding total surface area constant. However this is not true; if a given blood flow is directed into a greater number of fibers the shear rate in each fiber will fall and J_f will decrease as a result. Figure 13 depicts the differences in net flow of ultrafiltrate (Q_f) and ultrafiltrate flux (J_f) and their dependence on fiber length, i.e. (A/d) increasing.

Membrane sieving

The other factor governing solute clearance is the membrane sieving coefficient. Conceptually this may be considered a pore filled membrane with water moving through the pores. Solutes that are small in size in comparison with the pore diameter pass with the water and are not held back (sieved out). For such solutes, the concentration of the solute does not change as it traverses the pores in the membrane. i.e. the concentration of a solute in the ultrafiltrate (C_f) is the same as in the plasma water (C_w) and their ratio, the sieving coefficient (S), is 1.0:

$$S = \frac{C_f}{C_w} = 1 \qquad [29]$$

Equation 29 is valid locally anywhere along the fiber, but C_f and C_w vary with length. Operationally, we have access to the inflow and outflow blood of the ultrafilter as well as to the ultrafiltrate. S can be measured using the average of inflow and outflow plasma water concentration as an approximation of C_w for solutes with S < 1, i.e.

$$S = \frac{2 C_f}{C_{wi} + C_{wo}} = 1 \qquad [30]$$

This approximation has been shown to be reasonably accurate (better than 1%) for flow conditions reported with hollow fiber hemofiltration (67, 68).

For solutes large enough to impinge on the pore, the membrane will hold back a part or all of that solute as the ultrafiltrate is formed. The concentration of the solute changes as the ultrafiltrate is formed. As noted for dialysis membranes the sieving coefficient then may range from 0 (for macromolecules such as protein) to 1 for microsolutes unimpeded by the membrane. To characterize an ultrafiltration membrane, it would be necessary to know its hydraulic permeability (J_f) and the correlation between sieving coefficient and molecular size. It should be noted that change of charge on the solute molecule as noted for biological filtration membranes may play a role in establishing its degree of sieving by a given membrane (84). Charges on the membrane surface or within the pore may expedite or retard the solutes passage. In addition, the polarized layer of protein that accumulates on the ultrafiltration membrane may in fact become the discriminating layer that determines the presence or absence of sieving. The data from Table 6 show that inulin sieving for some membranes is strongly dependent on the presence of protein.

Solute concentration in plasma water (C_w) is related to the measured concentration of that solute (in the absence of protein binding) by the relationship:

$$\frac{C_p}{C_w} = 1 - \phi \qquad [31]$$

where ϕ (the volume fraction of plasma proteins- the 'protocrit') may be calculated as the product of 0.0107 and the total concentration of plasma proteins in g/dl (16). Whole blood concentration (C_B) is related to plasma concentration as

$$\frac{C_B}{C_p} = 1 - H + HK \qquad [32]$$

where H is the hematocrit, expressed as a decimal, and K is the distribution coefficient between red cells and plasma. For a solute entirely excluded from the red cell such as inulin, K = 0 whereas if there is no difference in concentration across the red cell membrane then K = 1. The high hemoglobin concentration precludes K ever reaching 1.0 for passively distributed solutes. Typical K values (67, 68) for some solutes are

Inulin = 0.00

Urea = 0.86

Creatinine = 0.73

Clearance

We may now express clearance for a solute in terms of flow rates and the sieving coefficient for that solute. By definition clearance is the mass of solute removed divided by the concentration of that solute in the whole blood or plasma. The mass removed in the ultrafiltrate ($C_f Q_f$) is easily determined.

$$\text{Plasma clearance} = \frac{C_f Q_f}{C_w} \qquad [33]$$

For certain solutes where a significant plasma blank may be present, e.g. for inulin, a form of the clearance equation may be useful if balanced operation pertains (i.e. the flow rates for diluting fluid and ultrafiltrate are equal).

$$\text{Whole blood clearance} = Q_B \left(\frac{C_{pi} - C_{po}}{C_{pi}} \right) \qquad [34]$$

Concentration corrections for K and H cancel out of the fraction as do the blank values. In predilution mode, C_{pi} should be sampled before dilution. In post dilution mode, C_{po} should be sampled after dilution.

Measurements of solute concentration and flow on the blood side of the membrane make it possible to compute a mass balance:

rance is subject to inaccuracy, because the precise space of distribution and rate of intracellular contribution to the plasma water is not known for most solutes of interest. It should be noted that, if plasma clearance is reported, the mass balance errors that may be calculated by using plasma flow rates and concentrations taken pre- and post-addition of diluting fluid will reflect not only the errors in measuring blood flow rate and those of the analysis used to determine solute concentration, but also those caused by the movement of intracellular solutes into the plasma water. Studies on urea movement out of the cell in response to the concentration gradient established by 50% dilution of whole blood in predilution mode hemofiltration indicate swift equilibration between red cell and plasma water (87).

As information on the kinetics of solute distribution grows, it will be possible to report clearances in terms of the rate at which a particular solute's space of distribution is cleared. It is important to note the potential limitations imposed on hemofiltration techniques by the kinetics of solute movement from the intracellular to the vascular space.

REFERENCES

1. Spiegler KS, Kadem O: Transport coefficients and salt rejection in uncharged hyperfiltration membranes. *Desalination* 1:311, 1966
2. Villarroel F, Klein E, Holland F: Solute flux in hemodialysis and hemofiltration membranes. *Trans Am Soc Artif Intern Organs* 23:225, 1977
3. Rubin J, Nolph KD, Popovich RP, Moncrief JW, Prowant B: Drainage volume during continuous ambulatory peritoneal dialysis. *asaio J* 2:54, 1979
4. Durbin RP: Osmotic flow of water across permeable cellulose membranes. *J Gen Physiol* 44:315, 1960
5. Henderson LW: The problem of peritoneal membrane area and permeability. *Kidney Int* 3:409, 1973
6. Pyle WK, Moncrief JW, Popovich RP: Peritoneal transport evaluation in CAPD. In: *CAPD Update; Continuous Ambulatory Peritoneal Dialysis* edited by Moncrief JW, Popovich RP, New York, Masson Publ USA Inc, 1981, p. 35
7. Henderson LW, Nolph KD: Altered permeability of the peritoneal membrane after using hypertonic peritoneal dialysis fluid. *J Clin Invest* 48:922, 1969
8. Nolph KD, Hano JE, Teschan PE: Peritoneal sodium transport during hypertonic peritoneal dialysis. *Ann Intern Med* 70:931, 1969
9. Brown ST, Ahearn DJ, Nolph KD: Potassium removal with peritoneal dialysis. *Kidney Int* 4:67, 1973
10. Landis EM, Pappenheimer JR: Exchange of substances through the capillary walls. *Handbook of Physiology* Section 2, Circulation, edited by Hamilton WF, vol 2, Washington DC, American Society of Physiology, 1963, p 961
11. Rosenbaum RW, Hruska KA, Anderson C, Robson AM, Slatopolsky E, Klahr S: Inulin: an inadequate marker of glomerular filtration rate in kidney donors and transplant recipients? *Kidney Int* 16:999, 1979
12. Husted FC, Nolph KD, Vitale FC, Maher JF: Detrimental effects of ultrafiltration on diffusion in coils. *J Lab Clin Med* 87:435, 1976
13. Henderson LW: Redy or not. *asaio J* 2:49, 1979
14. Nolph KD, Stolz ML, Carter CB, Fox M, Maher JF: Factors affecting the composition of ultrafiltrate from hemodialysis coils. *Trans Am Soc Artif Intern Organs* 16:495, 1970
15. Donnan FG: Theory of membrane equilibria. *Chem Reviews* 1:73, 1924-25
16. Colton CK, Smith KA, Merrill EW, Friedman S: Diffusion of urea in flowing blood. *Am Inst Chem Engineering J* 17:800, 1971
17. Nolph KD, Fox M, Maher JF: Factors affecting the ultrafiltration rate from standard dialysis coils. *Trans Am Soc Artif Intern Organs* 16:487, 1970
18. Shear L, Swartz C, Shinaberger JA, Barry KG: Kinetics of peritoneal fluid absorption in adult man. *N Engl J Med* 272:123, 1965
19. Shear L, Castellott JJ, Barry KG: Peritoneal fluid absorption: I. Effect of dehydration on kinetics. *J Lab Clin Med* 66:232, 1965
20. Shear L, Castellott JJ, Shinaberger JA, Poole L, Barry KG: Enhancement of peritoneal fluid absorption by dehydration, mercaptomerin and vasopressin. *J Pharmacol Exp Ther* 154:289, 1966
21. Bergström J, Asaba H, Fürst P, Oulès R: Dialysis ultrafiltration and blood pressure. *Proc Eur Dial Transpl Assoc* 13:293, 1976
22. Bergström J: Ultrafiltration without dialysis for removal of fluid and solutes in uremia. *Clin Nephrol* 9:156, 1978
23. Scheunemann B, Borghardt J, Falda Z, Jacob I, Kramer P, Kraft B, Quellhorst E: Reactions of blood pressure and body spaces to hemofiltration treatment. *Trans Am Soc Artif Intern Organs* 14:687, 1978
24. Rouby JJ, Rotembourg J, Durande JP, Bassett JY, Legrain M: Importance of the plasma refilling rate in the genesis of hypovolaemic hypotension during regular dialysis and controlled sequential ultrafiltration-haemodialysis. *Proc Eur Dial Transpl Assoc* 15:239, 1978
25. Rodrigo F, Shideman J, McHugh R, Buselmeier T, Kjellstrand C: Osmolality changes during hemodialysis. *Ann Intern Med* 86:554, 1977
26. Keshaviah P, Berkseth RO, Shapiro FL, Davidman M: Mechanisms and control of fluid removal by ultrafiltration. *Proc 12th Annu Contractor's Conf Artif Kidney-Chronic Uremia Program* NIAMDD edited by Mackey BB, DHEW publ no (NIH 81-1979) 1981 p 166
27. Kennedy AC, Linton AL, Eaton JC: Urea levels in cerebrospinal fluid after haemodialysis. *Lancet* 1:410, 1962
28. Sitprija V, Holmes JH: Preliminary observations on the change in intracranial pressure and intraocular pressure during hemodialysis. *Trans Am Soc Artif Intern Organs* 8:300, 1962
29. Wakin KG: The pathophysiology of the dialysis disequilibrium syndrome *Mayo Clin Proc* 44:406, 1969
30. Graefe U, Milutinovich J, Follette WC, Vizzo JE, Babb AL, Scribner BH: Less dialysis-induced morbidity and vascular instability with bicarbonate in dialysate. *Ann Intern Med* 88:332, 1978
31. Rosenzweig J, Babb AL, Vizzo JE, Scribner BH, Ginn HE: Large surface area hemodialysis. *Proc Clin Dial Transpl Forum* 1:56, 1971
32. Wehle B, Asaba H, Castenfors J, Fürst P, Gunnarson B, Shaldon S, Bergström J: Hemodynamic changes during sequential ultrafiltration and dialysis. *Kidney Int* 15:411, 1979
33. Hampl H, Paeprer H, Unger V, Kessel M: Hemodynamic

studies during hemodialysis in comparison to sequential ultrafiltration and hemofiltration. *J Dial* 3:51, 1979
34. Chen WT, Chaignon M, Tarazi R, Bravo EL, Nakamoto S: Hemodynamics of post dialysis hypotension. *Abstracts Am Soc Nephrol* 10:41, 1977
35. Novella A, Kelsch R, Easterling R: Acetate intolerance during hemodialysis. *Clin Nephrol* 5:28, 1976
36. Kirkendol PL, Devia CJ, Bower JD, Holbert RD: A comparison of the cardiovascular effects of sodium acetate, sodium bicarbonate and other potential sources of fixed base in hemodialysate solutions. *Trans Am Soc Artif Intern Organs* 23:399, 1977
37. Kishimoto T, Tanaka H, Yamakawa M, Mizutani Y, Yamamoto T, Hirata S, Horiuchi N, Maekawa M: Morbidity, instability and serum acetate level during hemodialysis. *Abstracts Artif Organs* 3:22, 1979
38. Goss JE, Alfrey AC, Vogel JHK, Holmes JH: Hemodynamic changes during hemodialysis. *Trans Am Soc Artif Intern Organs* 13:68, 1967
39. Kim KE, Neff M, Cohen B, Somerstein M, Chinitz J, Onesti G, Swartz C: Blood volumes changes and hypotension during hemodialysis. *Trans Am Soc Artif Intern Organs* 16:508, 1970
40. Pickering TG, Gribbon B, Oliver DO: Narrow reflex sensitivity in patients on long-term hemodialysis. *Clin Sci* 43:645, 1972
41. Lazarus JM, Hampers CL, Lowrie EG, Merrill JP: Baroreceptor activity in normotensive and hypertensive uremic patients. *Circulation* 47:1015, 1973
42. Kersh ES, Kronfield JS, Unger A, Popper RW, Cantor S, Cohn K: Autonomic insufficiency in uremia as a cause of hemodialysis induced hypotension. *N Engl J Med* 290:650, 1974
43. Lilley JJ, Golden J, Stone RA: Adrenergic regulation of blood pressure in chronic renal failure. *J Clin Invest* 57:1190, 1976
44. McGrath BP, Tiller DJ, Bune A, Chalmers JP, Korner PI, Uther JB: Autonomic blockade and the Valsalva maneuver in patients on maintenance hemodialysis: A hemodynamic study. *Kidney int* 12:294, 1977
45. Kim KE, Onesti G, Schwartz AB, Chinitz JL, Swartz C: Hemodynamics of hypertension in chronic end stage renal disease. *Circulation* 46:456, 1972
46. Neff MS, Kim KW, Persoff M, Onesti G, Swartz C: Hemodynamics of uremic anemia. *Circulation* 43:876, 1971
47. Liedtke AJ, Urschel CW, Kirk ES: Total systemic autoregulation in the dog and inhibition by baroreceptor reflexes. *Circ Res* 32:673, 1973
48. DeQuattro V, Nagatsu T, Maronde R, Alexander N: Catecholamine synthesis in rabbits with neurogenic hypertension. *Circ Res* 24:545, 1969
49. Mancia G, Donald DE: Demonstration that the atria, ventricles and lungs are each responsible for atonic inhibition of the vasomotor center in the dog. *Circ Res* 36:310, 1975
50. Dobbs WA: Relative importance of nervous and intrinsic mechanical factors in cardiovascular control system (Ph D dissertation), Jackson Mississippi, University of Mississippi 1970, cited by Young DB: Neurocontrol of fluid volumes: Volume receptors in autonomic control, in chapter 18, *Circulatory Physiology II: Dynamics and Control of the Body Fluids*, edited by Guyton AC, Taylor AE, Granger HJ, Philadelphia, PA, WB Saunders Co, 1975, p 262
51. Editorial (anonymous): Baroreceptors and high blood pressure. *Lancet* 1:1279, 1979
52. Romoff MS, Campese VM, Lane K, Massry SG: Mechanism of autonomic dysfunction in uremia: evidence for reduced end organ response to norepinephrine *Kidney Int* 14:731, 1978

53. Rush RA, Geffen LB: Radioimmunoassay and clearance of circulatory dopamine-β-hydroxylase. *Circ Res* 31:444, 1972
54. Molinoff PB, Brimijoin S, Weinshilboum R, Axelrod J: Neurally-mediated increase in dopamine-β-hydroxylase activity. *Proc Natl Acad Sci USA* 66:453, 1970
55. Quellhorst EA, Schuenemann B: A controlled study to compare hemodialysis and hemofiltration treatment in patients with chronic renal failure. *Proc 12th Annu Contractor's Conf Artif Kidney-Chronic Uremia Program* NIAMDD edited by Mackey BB, DHEW Publ No (NIH 81-1979) 1981, p 173
56. Bosch JP, Glabman S, von Albertini B, Geronemus R, Kahn T, Goldstein MH, Kupfer S: Comparison of hemofiltration and ultrafiltration plus hemodialysis to conventional hemodialysis. *Prox 12th Annu Contractor's Conf Artif Kidney-Chronic Uremia Program* NIAMDD edited by Mackey BB, DHEW Publ No (NIH 81-1979) 1981, p 184
57. Henderson LW: Symptomatic hypotension during hemodialysis. *Kidney Int* 17:571, 1980
58. Kaplow LS, Goffinet JA: Profound neutropenia during the early phase of hemodialysis. *JAMA* 203:1135, 1968
59. Gral T, Schroth P, DePalma JR, Gordon A: Leukocyte dynamics with three types of hemodialyzers. *Trans Am Soc Artif Intern Organs* 15:45, 1969
60. Brubaker LH, Nolph KD: Mechanisms of recovery from neutropenia induced by hemodialysis. *Blood* 38:623, 1971
61. Henderson LW, Miller ME, Hamilton RW, Norman ME: Dialysis leukopenia polymorph, random mobility and the control of peripheral white cell levels – a preliminary observation. *J Lab Clin Med* 85:191, 1975
62. Craddock PR, Fehr J, Brigham KL, Kronenberg RS, Jacob HS: Complement and leukocyte mediated pulmonary dysfunction in hemodialysis. *N Engl J Med* 296:769, 1977
63. Craddock PR, Fehr J, Dalmasso AP, Brigham KL, Jacob HS: Hemodialysis leukopenia. *J Clin Lab Invest* 59:879, 1977
64. Aurigemma NM, Feldman NT, Gottliev M, Ingram RH Jr, Lazarus JM, Lowrie EG: Arterial oxygenation during hemodialysis. *N Engl J Med* 297:871, 1977
65. Alijama P, Bird PAE. Ward MK, Feest TG, Walker W, Tanboga H, Sussman M, Kerr DNS: Hemodialysis-induced leukopenia and activation of complement: Effects of different membranes. *Kidney Int* 14:103, 1978
66. Nolph KD, Hopkins CA. Van Stone JC: Decreases in small solute clearances with ultrafiltration in parallel plate dialysers. *Abstracts Am Soc Artif Intern Organs* 6:63, 1977
67. Henderson LW, Colton CK, Ford C: Kinetics of hemodiafiltration. II. Clinical characterization of a new blood cleansing modality. *J Lab Clin Med* 85:372, 1975
68. Colton CK, Henderson LW, Ford CA, Lysaght MJ: Kinetics of hemodiafiltration. I. In vitro transport characteristics of a hollow fiber blood ultrafilter. *J Lab Clin Med* 85:355, 1975
69. Henderson LW: Peritoneal ultrafiltration dialysis: enhanced urea transfer using hypertonic peritoneal dialysis fluid. *J Clin Invest* 45:950, 1966
70. Babb AL, Johansen PJ, Strand MJ, Tenckhoff H, Scribner BH: Bidirectional permeability of the human peritoneum to middle molecules. *Proc Eur Dial Transpl Assoc* 10:247, 1973
71. Randerson DH, Farrell PC: Mass transfer properties of the human peritoneum. *asaio J* 3:140, 1980
72. Green DM, Antwiler GD, Moncrief JW, Decherd JF, Popovich RP: Measurement of the transmittance coefficient spectrum of Cuprophan and RP 69 membranes: Applications to middle molecule removal via ultrafiltration. *Trans Am Soc Artif Intern Organs* 22:627, 1976

73. Andreoli TE, Schafer JA, Troutman SL: Coupling of solute and solvent flows in porous lipid bilayer membranes. *J Gen Physiol* 57:479, 1971
74. Blatt WF, Dravid A, Michaels AS, Nelson L: Solute polarization and cake formation in membrane ultrafiltration: Causes, consequences and control techniques. *Membrane Science and Technology,* edited by Flinn JE, New York, Plenum Corporation, 1970, p 47
75. Colton CK: Permeability and transport studies in batch and flow dialyzers with application to hemodialysis. *Ph D Thesis,* Massachusetts Institute of Technology, Cambridge, MA, 1969
76. Carone FA, Banks DB, Post RS: Micropuncture study of albumin excretion in the normal rat. *Am J Physiol* 55:19A, 1969
77. Henderson LW: Middle molecules re-examined. *Nephron* 22:146, 1978
78. Bergström J, Fürst P, Zimmerman L: Uremic middle molecules exist and are biologically active. *Clin Nephrol* 11:229, 1979
79. Gutman RA, Huang AT, Bouknight NS: Inhibitor of marrow thymidine incorporation from sera of patients with uremia. *Kidney Int* 18:715, 1980
80. Henderson LW, Beans E, Prestidge H, Forc CA, Colton C, Frigon R: Evaluation of hemofiltration membranes. *Kidney Int* 16:779, 1979
81. Ramenofsky L, Lai F, Schroeder P, Hosokawa S, Kato Y, Henderson L: Comparison of hemofiltration (HF) membrane performance: Sieving coefficients (SC): *Abstracts Am Soc Artif Intern Organs* 10:55, 1981
82. Okazaki M, Yoshida F: Ultrafiltration of blood: Effect of hematocrit on ultrafiltration rate. *Ann Biomed Eng* 4:138, 1976
83. Lysaght MJ, Ford CA, Colton CK, Stone RA, Henderson LW: Mass transfer in clinical blood ultrafiltration devices – a review. Chapter 9 in *Technical Aspects of Renal Dialysis,* edited by Frost TH, Tunbridge Wells, UK, Pitman Medical Publishing Co Ltd 1978, p 81
84. Chang RLS, Deen WM, Robertson CR, Brenner BM: Permselectivity of the glomerular capillary wall: III Restricted transport of polyanions. *Kidney Int* 8:212, 1975
85. Murdaugh V, Doyle EM: Effecti of hemoglobin on erythrocyte urea concentration. *J Lab Clin Med* 57:579, 1961
86. Nolph KD, Bass OE, Maher JF: Acute effects of hemodialysis on removal of intracellular solutes. *Trans Am Soc Artif Intern Organs* 20:622, 1974
87. Henderson LW, Sanfelippo ML: Extracorporeal access to intracellular solutes of whole blood. *Kidney Int* 14:676, 1978

13

ULTRAFILTRATION AND HAEMOFILTRATION PRACTICAL APPLICATIONS

EDUARD A. QUELLHORST

Principles of ultrafiltration and haemofiltration	265	Influence on calcium and phosphate metabolism	270
Definitions	265	Influence on lipid metabolism	271
Technical aspects of haemofiltration	265	Influence on polyneuropathy	271
Membranes	265	Influence on subjective symptoms	271
Dilution site	260	Haemofiltration in acute renal failure and for exogenous	
Monitoring systems	267	intoxications	271
Diluting fluid	267	Spontaneous arterio-venous ultrafiltration	272
Clinical aspects of haemofiltration	267	Sequential ultrafiltration/dialysis	272
Indications	267	Haemodiafiltration	272
Elimination of uraemic toxins	267	Acknowledgment	272
Influence on the cardiovascular system	268	References	272
Influence on hormone levels	270		

PRINCIPLES OF ULTRAFILTRATION AND HAEMOFILTRATION

The concept of removing water and solutes from the human body by filtration, thus imitating the function of the natural kidney was originally proposed in 1907 (1), but it did not become a practical reality until 1947, when the first artificial kidney, to be based on the principle of ultrafiltration was described (2). Using this very simple apparatus the investigators achieved a filtrate flow of 1.2 l/h. In 1967 Henderson and coworkers (3) published a new method of blood purification, in which considerable amounts of ultrafiltrate, extracted from the human blood by a hydrostatic gradient across highly permeable membranes, were replaced by a solution resembling as closely as possible the composition of the extracellular fluid. The first favourable results obtained with this new method, initially called 'diafiltration', were reported by American (3) and German (4, 5, 6) investigators. As suggested by Burton (5) in 1976 at the first symposium on this new technique of blood purification in Braunlage (W. Germany) the name 'diafiltration' was replaced by 'haemofiltration'.

Definitions

Although the terms haemofiltration, diafiltration and haemodiafiltration (6) have been used as synonyms for some years, the terminology has recently been standardised and each term now has a somewhat different meaning. During *ultrafiltration* fluid and solutes are removed by convective transport through semi-permeable membranes. In *haemofiltration* the ultrafiltrate flow is augmented by using high flux membranes requiring the substitution of fluid before or after the haemofilter (pre- or post dilution).

In *haemodiafiltration* or *diafiltration*, haemofiltration and haemodialysis are performed simultaneously. Finally, *sequential ultrafiltration/haemodialysis* signifies a process in which a period of pure ultrafiltration precedes or follows a period of haemodialysis in the course of the same treatment session (7).

TECHNICAL ASPECTS OF HAEMOFILTRATION

Membranes

For clinical use of haemofiltration, special, highly permeable membranes had to be developed. Cellophane and cuprophane membranes were suitable for haemodialysis, but the possibility of controlling the hydrostatic pressure during haemofiltration made the use of 'asymmetric', highly permeable membranes (8) possible. The main characteristics of membranes and filters commonly used for haemofiltration are compared with those of the glomerulus in Table 1. Haemofiltration membranes differ in chemical structure from those fabricated for haemodialysis and the question arises as to whether some of the favourable results of haemofiltration should be attributed to the replacement of cellulosic membranes by the special membranes designed for haemofiltration rather than to the method itself.

The molecular cutoff of haemofiltration membranes is considerably higher than that of haemodialysis membranes and approaches the cutoff diameter of the natural kidney (see Table 1). Whereas the tubules of the natural kidney employ various mechanisms for the conservation of substances of vital importance, the filtrate in haemofiltration systems, in contrast is discarded and replaced by a simple modified Ringer-lactate solution. The development of depletion syndromes with haemofiltration was therefore to be expected, but so far none have been

Table 1. Characteristics of different haemofiltration membranes and filters in comparison to the natural kidney.

Membrane	Type of filter	Surface area m^2	Cutoff($\pm$) daltons	Filtrate flow (post-dilution) ml/min/mm Hg/cm$^2 \times 10^5$
—	Natural kidney	± 3.0	50 000	8.3
Triacetate	Flat membrane (Haemofilter Sartorius)	0.3	20 000	7.5
Polysulfone	Capillary filter (Amicon)	0.6	50 000	3.6
Polyamide	Capillary filter (Berghof)	1.0	15 000	2.8
Polyacrylonitrile	Flat membrane (Rhône Poulenc RP 6)	1.0	40 000	1.9

observed even though many patients have been treated for more than ten years.

Dilution site

In the first publication concerning clinical application of haemofiltration Henderson (3) recommended the addition of replacement fluid *before the filter (pre-dilution)*. This mode of dilution however requires about 30% more substitution fluid than re-infusion *after the filter (post-dilution)*. Therefore many, in particular European groups (9–11) prefer the post-dilution mode. With infusion of the substitution fluid before the filter, the filtrate flow can be increased considerably and independently of the blood flow. The concentration of solutes removed is lower in the pre-dilution mode than in post-dilution haemofiltration, but there is virtually no practical difference between the two modes of treatment with the exception of substances with a molecular weight of about 5000 and more, which are more efficiently removed with the pre-dilution technique (12). However, the increased elimination of solutes of such high molecular weight does not ordinarily justify the use of the required additional amounts of dilution fluid.

Other technical modifications have been developed such as combined pre- and post-dilution modes and filtrate regeneration. Compared with post-dilution haemofiltration these techniques can achieve a considerably higher filtrate flow with re-infusion either before or after

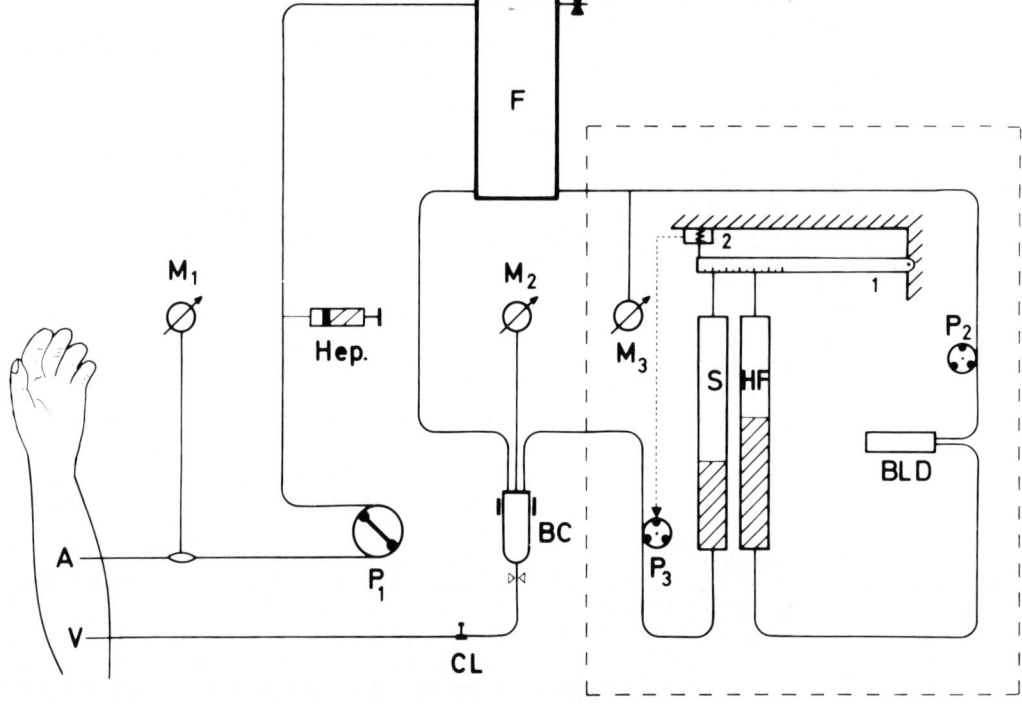

Figure 1. Diagram of a post-dilution haemofiltration monitoring system. A = artery, V = vein, M$_1$–M$_3$ = pressure gauges, P$_1$ = blood pump, P$_2$ = filtrate pump, P$_3$ = substitution fluid pump, F = filter, Hep = heparin pump, BC = bubble trap, BLD = blood leak detector, HF = filtrate, S = substitution fluid, 1 = beam for the suspension of canisters, 2 = load cell.

the filter, without necessarily sacrificing the advantage of smaller amounts of replacement fluid (13). The same objective was attained by other authors (14) who increased the surface area of the haemofilters.

Haemofiltration monitoring systems

Depending on the method of treatment, 20 to 40 l of body fluid has to be filtered from the blood and to be replaced by almost identical quantities of a modified Ringer-lactate solution in the course of one treatment session lasting 3 to 6 h (see also the previous Chapter). This large fluid exchange requires a very accurate balancing and monitoring system (Figure 1). From clinical experience it became clear that this monitoring system should fulfil two conditions: the fluid volume, by which the body weight of the patient has to be reduced, should be removed at a constant rate during the whole haemofiltration procedure and fluid replacement has also to be given at a continuous and constant rate rather than abruptly or intermittently. In order to avoid deleterious side effects of unbalance, the necessary precautions have to be made by the use of programmable monitoring systems. Figure 1 presents a gravimetric balancing system used in different haemofiltration devices, which are now commercially available.

Diluting fluid

During the course of one haemofiltration session (with the post-dilution technique) at least 20 l of extracellular fluid, removed by ultrafiltration, have to be replaced by a fluid with a composition as close as possible to the composition of normal extracellular fluid. In contrast to haemodialysis the electrolyte balance in haemofiltration depends primarily on the composition and volume of the replacement fluid. For example: a negative fluid balance of about 2 litres induces a negative sodium balance of somewhat less than 300 mmol per treatment. The close correlation between fluid and electrolyte balance in haemofiltration was originally demonstrated by Fuchs et al. (15), who showed that calcium and fluid balance in an individual patient were equilibrated when the calcium concentration in the diluting fluid was 1.9 mmol/l (7.6 mg/dl) and fluid removal was 3.9 kg per treatment. Fluid loss exceeding this amount caused a negative calcium balance while less ultrafiltration resulted in a positive calcium balance. Such a correlation also applies to other electrolytes and has to be considered when large fluid volumes must be removed by haemofiltration.

Since the first publication on haemofiltration as a practical method for treatment of patients with uraemia, opinions diverged about the optimal composition of the diluting fluid. Numerous recommendations have been made. Recommended sodium concentrations have varied between 135 and 160 mmol/l, potassium concentrations from 0 to 4 mmol/l and calcium concentrations from 1.0 to 2.0 mmol/l (4 to 8 mg/dl). Most investigators prefer bicarbonate as the buffer anion, but there is no clinical indication that acetate is superior to lactate or vice versa. Most investigators, however, prefer bicarbonate as the buffer anion.

In spite of the fact, that a considerable amount of various substances (e.g. amino acids) is lost by haemofiltration, there is no need to add amino acids or dextrose to the substitution fluid. Some investigators, however, have contrary views and recommend the addition of dextrose to stabilise the extracellular osmotic pressure.

Whereas the effectivity of haemodialysis concerning the elimination of 'middle' molecules is mainly time-dependent, the effect of haemofiltration depends on the volume of fluid filtered. There is a consensus of opinion among all investigators, that the fluid volume exchanged during each treatment with the post-dilution technique should be approximately 20 l or more.

Baldamus et al. (16) have proposed a formula to predict the efficiency of the removal of low molecular weight substances, e.g. for urea:

$$V^{1/2} = 0.47 \times BW - 3.03,$$

where $V^{1/2}$ = volume of fluid necessary to reduce serum levels to 50% and BW = body weight.

As the production of large amounts of sterile diluting fluid is one of the most expensive components of haemofiltration, efforts have been made to regenerate filtrate by the use of sorbents (17, 18) or oxidation (19) and to re-infuse the filtrate into the blood. The on-line production of diluting fluid by proportioning concentrate and processed tap-water (pretreated with reverse osmosis) has been proposed (20). But, so far, not one of these methods has obtained practical application on a large scale.

CLINICAL ASPECTS OF HAEMOFILTRATION

Indications

Long-term haemofiltration treatment of patients with terminal chronic renal failure started in 1974. With increasing experience the new method became increasingly popular. Many patients now have been on regular haemofiltration treatment for more than 8 years. In 1980, 893 patients out of a European dialysis population numbering 48 408, were treated regularly by haemofiltration. According to the registry of the European Dialysis and Transplant Association the majority of them were treated for 12 to 13 hours weekly, but 17% were treated for only 4 to 5 hours per week (21). In addition an increasing number of patients with acute renal failure, due to a variety of causes, have been treated by haemofiltration. Other applications reported in the literature are glycoside and diuretic resistant cardiac failure with pulmonary oedema (22), exogenous intoxications and hepatic coma (23, 24).

Elimination of uraemic toxins

As had to be expected the removal of low molecular

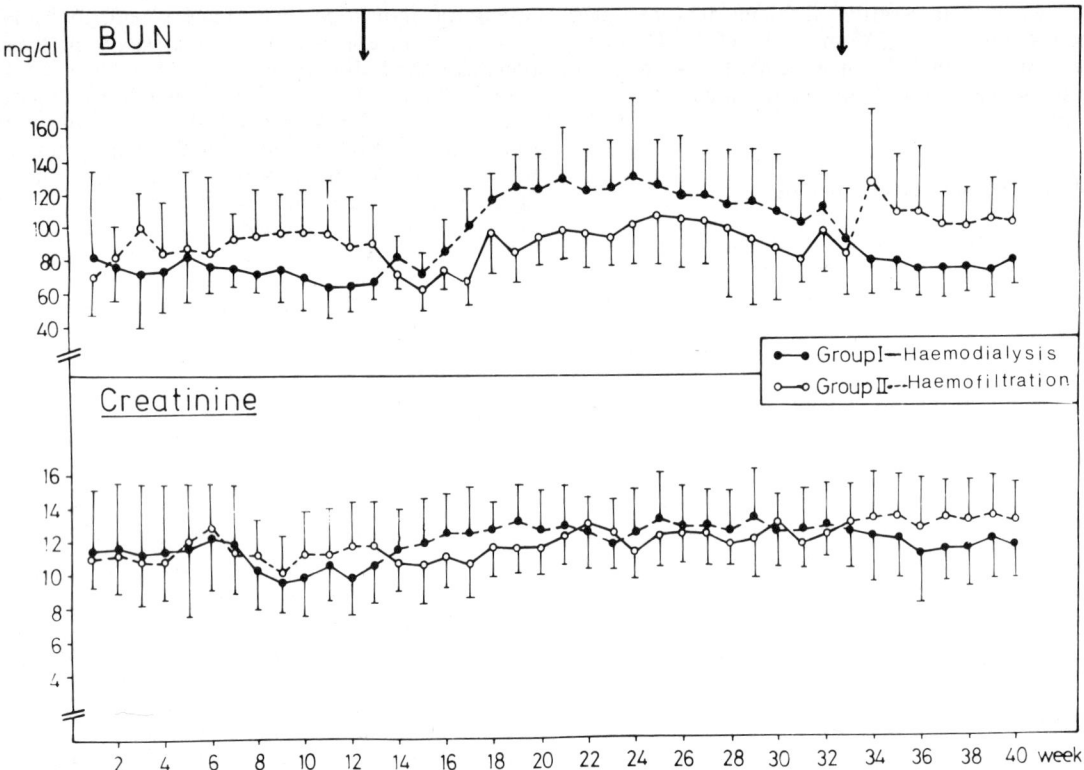

Figure 2. Blood urea nitrogen (BUN) and creatinine levels ($\bar{X} \pm SD$) in two groups of 30 patients each during regular haemodialysis and haemofiltration treatment. Arrows indicate changes of the methods of treatment. The interrupted line indicates haemofiltration and the solid line haemodialysis.
(BUN mg/dl → mmol/l: multiply by 0.714.
BUN mg/dl → blood urea mmol/l: multiply by 0.357.
Creatinine mg/dl → µmol/l: multiply by 88.4).

weight substances (urea, creatinine) with post-dilution haemofiltration is less effective than with haemodialysis. The haemofiltration clearance rates of small solutes, however, are considerably higher than with intermittent peritoneal dialysis. When patients are transferred from haemodialysis to haemofiltration treatment, a slight increase of plasma creatinine and urea concentrations occurs (Figure 2). But with protein intake remaining unchanged, there is no further increase once plasma levels have stabilised. This may be partly explained by a decrease in the urea generation rate in haemofiltration as observed by Baldamus et al. (25), but this does not explain the stabilisation of plasma creatinine levels. Signs or symptoms of uraemic complications (e.g. pericarditis, pleuritis or progressing neuropathy) in patients undergoing regular haemofiltration treatment have not been reported so far.

In contrast to haemodialysis and intermittent peritoneal dialysis, haemofiltration is considerably more effective in removing substances of higher molecular weight. But no clinical symptoms have been unequivocally related to the accumulation of middle molecular substances in renal failure. Thus, the significance of a more effective removal of these middle molecules requires further evaluation.

Influence on the cardiovascular system

Patients with hypotension and fluid overload or those with hypertension are difficult to treat with regular haemodialysis and constitute high risk groups. In addition symptomatic hypotension occurs in as many as 25% of haemodialysis treatments (26). Hypotensive episodes resulting from ultrafiltration during conventional haemodialysis can be deleterious, in particular in older patients with restricted cardiovascular reserve and cardiovascular complications.

From a recent report compiled by the French Diaphane Dialysis Registry (27) the annual death rate of approximately 2500 chronic dialysis patients appeared to be 12 times higher than the death rate of the French population in general, adjusted for sex and age. During the same period death rates from cardiovascular complications and from strokes were respectively 19 and 20 times higher among dialysis patients than the national

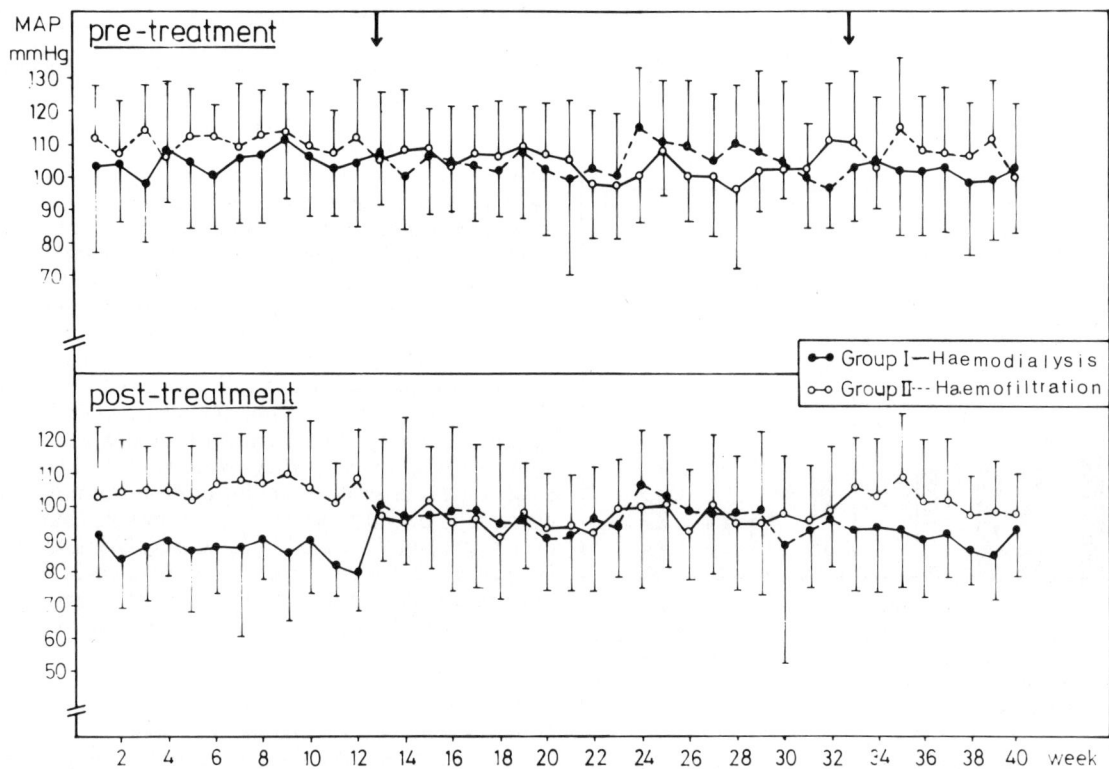

Figure 3. Pre- and post-treatment mean arterial pressure (MAP) in two groups of 30 patients each. The mean fluid removal per treatment was kept constant in both groups ($\bar{X} \pm SD$). (See also legend Figure 2).

death rates in France from these two causes. This high incidence of cardiovascular complications in chronic dialysis patients suggests that treatment modalities, which are less likely to provoke symptomatic hypotension, should be preferred.

Bergström et al. (28) observed that fluid removal achieved by pure ultrafiltration (without simultaneous dialysis) causes less hypotension and is better tolerated than fluid removal during conventional dialysis. These observations were also noted later in patients treated by haemofiltration (14, 16). These findings have been confirmed by the results obtained from a comparative study of two groups each of 30 patients. Both groups were alternately treated with haemofiltration and haemodialysis each time for periods of three months, according to an A-B-A or B-A-B sequence (A = haemodialysis, B = haemofiltration). Mean pre-treatment arterial blood pressure readings did not differ in the two groups. Post-treatment blood pressures were however significantly higher during haemofiltration treatment (Figure 3). The number of hypotensive episodes with collapse reactions during and after treatment with haemofiltration was only one tenth of the number of collapse reactions observed with haemodialysis.

Although a definite explanation for the different reactions of the cardiovascular system cannot be given as yet, some observations pertaining to the pathogenesis should be mentioned. Under similar conditions of fluid removal, total peripheral resistance remained unchanged or increased slightly during haemofiltration, but decreased during haemodialysis (29–32). The vascular system apparently reacts in a more physiological way to fluid removal by haemofiltration than to combined ultrafiltration and haemodialysis. It was also demonstrated that serum-catecholamine levels remained stable during haemofiltration, but decreased considerably during haemodialysis (31, 32). In spite of removal of more body fluid with haemofiltration, the extracellular volume is obviously reduced to a lesser degree by haemofiltration than by haemodialysis (33), which may be explained by a more substantial fluid shift from the intracellular to the extracellular space (Figure 4 [see also Chapter 12]). Evidence for this 'refilling phenomenon' was presented for ultrafiltration by Rouby et al. (34) and was confirmed by observations from Sausse and co-workers (35), who calculated the extracellular volume on the basis of the sodium free water clearance.

Hypertensive patients in the haemodialysis population can be divided into two groups. In one (large) group hypertension is predominantly volume dependent. In this group blood pressure can be lowered by fluid removal. In a small group of patients (about 5 to 10% of the dialysis population) hypertension is volume independent and cannot be corrected by ultrafiltration. In

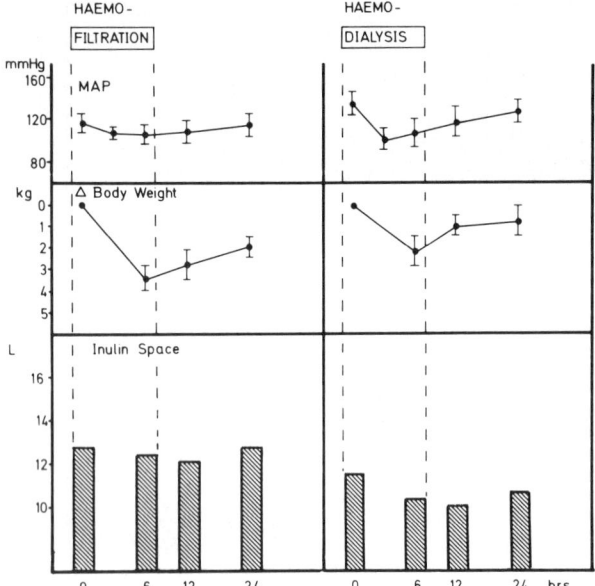

Figure 4. Changes of inulin space, body weight and mean arterial pressure (MAP) in 4 patients undergoing post-dilution haemofiltration and, after restitution of their initial body weight, haemodialysis treatment.

the former group plasma renin activity is usually normal or only slightly elevated. The latter group usually shows very high plasma renin levels and blood pressure can be reduced or normalised by Saralasin infusion. Both groups of hypertensive patients may profit from haemofiltration; volume dependent hypertension can be favourably influenced by this method which, in contrast to haemodialysis, allows a linear fluid removal without cardiovascular collapse. Because of the minimal number of hypotensive episodes saline infusions are usually unnecessary: which facilitates correction of hypertension. But also volume-independent, dialysis and antihypertensive drug resistant hypertension may also react favourably during haemofiltration treatment. In one study (36) blood pressure could be normalised in 13 patients who were transferred from haemodialysis to haemofiltration because of dialysis resistant severe hypertension. Ten patients had a very high plasma renin activity at the start of haemofiltration treatment, which could be normalised in all patients except one, during an 8 month course of treatment. Similar results were obtained by Henderson et al. (37), but another group of investigators (16) observed no differences between haemofiltration and haemodialysis in the control of blood pressure. It has to be emphasised however, that blood pressure values in these patients at the start of the treatment were considerably lower than in the patients of the other two studies. Irrespective of the different results, haemofiltration should be tried before bilateral nephrectomy is considered in cases of severe dialysis resistant hypertension.

Influence on hormone levels

A considerable loss of vital substances and the development of depletion syndromes during haemofiltration treatment was expected because of the high porosity of asymmetric membranes with a molecular cutoff ranging from 15 000 to 50 000 daltons. Because most hormones have molecular weights in the range of the 'middle molecules' haemofiltration associated endocrine changes were anticipated. The effect of a single haemofiltration treatment on serum levels of different hormones has been investigated by Kramer and coworkers (38) who showed that plasma testosterone, cortisone, gastrin and thyroid stimulating hormone levels did not change, but human growth hormone levels decreased. Concentrations in the filtrate were low for testosterone and immeasurable for cortisone, growth hormone and thyroid stimulating hormone, perhaps because of the high molecular weights or protein binding of these hormones. The decrease of growth hormone concentrations could however be explained by food intake during haemofiltration. Gastrin levels which are generally elevated in uraemia did not decrease; insulin and gastric inhibitory peptide levels increased. The plasma activity of somatomedin B was very low at the start of treatment and remained unaltered during haemofiltration. In contrast to these findings Schneider and associates (39) observed a decrease of thyroid stimulating hormone levels in the course of a haemofiltration procedure and suggested loss of this hormone in the filtrate. In long term studies, T_3, T_4 and TSH levels decreased continuously during a haemofiltration period of 5 to 20 months. Serum TSH decreased markedly during five hours of haemofiltration treatment, possibly because of loss in the filtrate. Nevertheless peripheral euthyroidism was maintained because of a normal and stable T_4/TBG ratio. Long term studies however, are required for detection of hypothyroidism during regular haemofiltration treatment. No definite data on parathormone activity during long-term haemofiltration are currently available. No influence (15) as well as a decrease (40) in parathormone activity have been reported. The lack of a consensus may be explained by differences in calcium balance and variable determinations of parathormone and its metabolites.

Influence on serum calcium and phosphate

In spite of a more or less strong correlation between fluid and electrolyte equilibrium in haemofiltration in contrast to haemodialysis there is no evidence for a specific influence of this mode of treatment on serum calcium levels. A decrease in serum phosphate, allowing a decrease of oral phosphate binders (e.g. aluminum hydroxide) has been reported previously (5, 41) but was later questioned (16). In a controlled study it appeared that phosphate binders could be reduced but not omitted during regular haemofiltration treatment. This, however, cannot be explained by improved elimination of phosphate in the filtrate and further investigations are indicated to clarify this controversy.

Influence on lipid metabolism

Shortly after the introduction of haemofiltration as a method of treatment for end-stage renal disease a favourable effect on plasma triglyceride levels was reported (5, 42). Patients with severe hypertriglyceridaemia during long-term haemodialysis treatment showed a dramatic improvement after changing to haemofiltration. This effect however, might be attributed to the application of a diluting fluid containing lactate instead of acetate and not to haemofiltration treatment per se (11), or to a change in dextrose balance. Plasma cholesterol levels, which may be more important for the development of vascular complications in haemodialysis patients, were not affected by haemofiltration.

Effect on polyneuropathy

A rapid improvement of uraemic neuropathy in chronic haemodialysis patients was obtained by Funck-Brentano et al. (43) by replacing the Cuprophan membrane by the polyacrylonitrile membrane which is highly permeable, allowing much better removal of substances with a molecular mass of 1000 to 1300 daltons. Similar favourable results were obtained when the same membrane was used for haemofiltration (44). With improved dialysis techniques clinical signs and symptoms of uraemic neuropathy or even a reduction of motor nerve conduction velocity (measured on the peroneal nerve) have become very rare. Sensory nerve conduction velocity and vibratory perception threshold, which are more sensitive parameters for early detection of uraemic neuropathy, were found to be abnormal in about 30% of an adequately treated haemodialysis population. In a controlled study improvement was noted by changing from haemodialysis treatment to haemofiltration. The number of patients with an increasing vibratory perception threshold and a decreasing sensory nerve conduction velocity was decreased reversibly when haemofiltration was employed.

Influence on subjective symptoms

Subjective symptoms of a disequilibrium syndrome (headaches, nausea, vomiting, muscle cramps) frequently occur during haemodialysis or peritoneal dialysis treatment, in particular when azotaemia is severe, dialysis is rapid or when large amounts of fluid have to be removed by ultrafiltration. These symptoms mostly occur during hypotensive episodes, but they are also observed without impairment of the circulation. In Table 2 the incidence of muscle cramps, nausea and headaches is presented in 1000 haemodialysis and peritoneal dialysis sessions and during haemofiltration in relation to the removal of fluid (in percentage of initial body weight). Clearly the percentage of these side reactions correlates closely with the ultrafiltration rate in haemodialysis and peritoneal dialysis, but remains low during haemofiltration.

Table 2. Occurrence of muscle cramps, nausea and/or headache (% of treatment procedures) in relation to the reduction of body weight (% of pre-treatment body weight) in 1,000 procedures each of haemodialysis (HD), peritoneal dialysis (PD) and haemofiltration (HF).

Reduction of (body weight (%))	Muscle cramps			Nausea/headache		
	HD	PD	HF	HD	PD	HF
1	2	3	2	6	8	7
2	4	3	3	10	9	10
3	21	5	4	25	21	9
4	26	12	5	33	22	10
5	40	19	4	33	19	10
6	49	21	9	50	34	9
7	48	23	9	49	36	9

HAEMOFILTRATION IN ACUTE RENAL FAILURE AND EXOGENOUS INTOXICATIONS

For patients with acute renal failure removal of large amounts of fluids is often indicated. This can be performed by haemofiltration without the risk of adverse circulatory reactions, which is particularly important for acute renal failure patients. In addition haemofiltration requires only 20 to 30 l of (sterile) diluting fluid in contrast with haemodialysis, which uses approximately 150 l of (not absolutely sterile) dialysis fluid per treatment of five hours. This obviously requires a proportioning system, an adequate supply of (pretreated) water and a drain, which are not always available in intensive care units.

Haemofiltration is, therefore, usually easier to perform in the intensive care setting where acute renal failure patients are commonly admitted. In addition no dialysis fluid (which may not be sterile) comes in contact with the filter. Moreover the haemofilter and supply lines for the substitution fluid are all disposable. Sterility is, therefore, more easily maintained during haemofiltration. This is obviously of special importance for patients with acute renal failure who are particularly susceptible to infection.

Because of less effective removal of small molecular substances, however, post-dilution haemofiltration should not be applied in cases of 'hypercatabolic' acute renal failure. In these cases haemodialysis, which removes small molecules such as urea and creatinine more efficiently, has to be preferred in order to avoid undesirable and potentially dangerous accumulation of urea.

Shortly after its introduction, haemofiltration was used for treatment of exogenous intoxications. A number of drugs are re-absorbed from the glomerular filtrate by the tubular system of the human kidney and many others are eliminated slowly by metabolism, suggesting that such treatment would augment removal appreciably. It was indeed demonstrated that some barbiturate derivatives are more efficiently removed by haemofiltration than by haemo- or peritoneal dialysis (45). But haemoperfusion has proved to be even more efficient and easier to perform.

SPONTANEOUS ARTERIO-VENOUS HAEMOFILTRATION

In 1974 Silverstein and coworkers (46) reported connecting an ultrafilter in series with a dialyser and could thereby remove large amounts of fluid from patients without disrupting the electrolyte- and acid-base balance. This mode of treatment has also been suggested for treatment of pulmonary oedema and peripheral oedema resistant to conventional therapy. A modification of this method, called *spontaneous arterio-venous haemofiltration* was described in 1977 by Kramer et al. (47). These investigators removed ultrafiltrate with a capillary haemofilter without using a blood pump. The arterio-venous pressure difference appeared to be sufficient for an adequate blood flow through the haemofilter and a satisfactory production of filtrate. In practice, catheters are introduced into a femoral artery and a femoral vein using the Seldinger technique. The capillary haemofilter is inserted in between. With a blood flow of 100 ml/min, 200 to 600 ml/h of filtrate is obtained, allowing a rapid removal of oedema. This method is particularly suitable for treatment of pulmonary oedema and is also useful for anuric and oliguric patients who have to be treated with high caloric parenteral feeding, which inevitably causes a fluid overload. The fluid excess can be removed intermittently by pumpless arterio-venous haemofiltration.

SEQUENTIAL ULTRAFILTRATION/DIALYSIS

Bergström and coworkers (28) reported in 1976 that substantial amounts of fluid could be removed from patients by ultrafiltration without causing a fall in blood pressure, when carried out before or after dialysis. Apparently sequential ultrafiltration/dialysis was much better tolerated haemodynamically, than was conventional dialysis (in which both procedures are carried out simultaneously). In practice approximately 4 hours of pure dialysis (removal of solutes by diffusion) with zero transmembrane pressure is carried out before or after performing one or two hours of pure ultrafiltration (removal of fluid and solutes by convection [see also chapters 3 and 12]). In contrast with haemofiltration usually no automatic monitoring of the amount of ultrafiltrate removed is carried out during this procedure. This makes careful clinical observation during the ultrafiltration period mandatory, in order to prevent too rapid and too drastic a reduction of body fluid volume. Currently however several dialysis machines are provided with special facilities for sequential ultrafiltration and dialysis and automatic monitoring of the amount of ultrafiltrate removed.

With this technique not only is adequate fluid removal much better tolerated (without a fall in blood pressure), but also a better removal of small molecular substances is obtained than with haemofiltration alone. Bergström and co-workers (28) concluded that ultrafiltration is far better tolerated if a significant decrease of plasma osmolality was avoided during ultrafiltration.

HAEMODIAFILTRATION

In haemodiafiltration conventional haemodialysis and haemofiltration are performed simultaneously, using highly permeable membranes and applying substantial transmembrane pressure differences during treatment. This offers a combination of the advantages of haemodialysis (high clearance of small molecular substances) and those of haemofiltration (fluid removal without circulatory impairment [48]). However a rather complex monitoring system is necessary to regulate both haemofiltration and haemodialysis in a single unit. The introduction of a new type of filter for haemofiltration, which allows a high ultrafiltrate flow (120–150 ml/min) could make the differences between haemodialysis and haemofiltration negligible as far as the elimination of small molecular substances are concerned. This may make a technically complex monitoring device for the haemodiafiltration unnecessary in the near future.

ACKNOWLEDGEMENT

This study was supported by a grant from the Chronic Uremia Program NIAMDD, NIH Bethesda, MD (under contract NO1-AM-8-2229).

REFERENCES

1. Bechhold H: Ultrafiltration. *Biochem Z* 6:379, 1907 (in German)
2. Malinow MR, Korzon W: An experimental method for obtaining an ultrafiltrate of the blood. *J Lab Clin Med* 32:461, 1947
3. Henderson LW, Besarab A, Michaels A, Bluemle LW: Blood purification by ultrafiltration and fluid replacement (Diafiltration). *Trans Am Soc Artif Intern Organs* 12:216, 1967
4. Quellhorst E, Plashues E: Ultrafiltration: Elimination harnpflichtiger Substanzen mit Hilfe neuartiger Membrane (Removal of waste materials with the aid of new membranes). In *Aktuelle Probleme der Dialyseverfahren und der Niereninsuffizienz*, edited by v. Dittrich P und Skrabal F, Friedberg Hessen, Bindernagel Verlag 1977, p 216 (in German)
5. Quellhorst E, Doht B, Schuenemann B: Haemofiltration: Treatment of renal failure by ultrafiltration and substitution. *J Dial* 1:529, 1977
6. Streicher E, Schneider H, v. Mulius U, Mahler B: Haemodiafiltration mit asymmetrischen Kapillarmembranen (Haemodiafiltration with asymmetric capillary mem-

branes). *Nieren- und Hochdruckkrankh* 5:191, 1976 (in German)
7. Robinson BHB, Hawkins JB: Preface *Proc Europ Dial Transpl Assoc* 15:IX, 1978
8. Loeb S, Sourirajan S: Sea water demineralization by means of an osmotic membrane. *Adv Chem Ser* 38:117, 1962
9. Man NK, Funck-Brentano JL: Haemofiltration, an alternative method for the treatment of end stage renal failure. *Adv Nephrol* 7:293, 1977
10. Scheler F: Haemofiltration. In: *Haemofiltration*, edited by Scheler F, Henning HV, Muenchen, Dustri-Verlag 1977, p 1
11. Schneider H, Streicher E, Hachmann H, Chmiel H, v. Mylius U: Clinical experience with haemofiltration. *Proc Eur Dial Transpl Assoc* 14:136, 1977
12. Streicher E, Schneider H: Asymmetric polyamide hollow-fiber filters in the haemofiltration system. *J Dial* 1:727, 1977
13. Bosch JP, Glabman S, v. Albertini B, Geronemus R, Kahn T, Goldstein MH, Kupfer S: Comparison of haemofiltration and ultrafiltration plus hemodialysis to conventional hemodialysis. *Proc 12th Annu Contractor's Conf Artif Kidney-Chronic Uremia Programm NIAMDD* edited by Mackey BB, DHEW publ No (NIH) 81-1979, 1979, p 184
14. Ramperez P, Flavier JL, Deschodt G, Beau MC, Issantier R, Mion C, Shaldon S: Preliminary experience with short hour high-efficiency haemofiltration (HF) at home. *Eur Dial Transpl Assoc* (Abstracts) 1980, p 79
15. Fuchs C, Dorn D, Henning HV, Matthaei D, McIntosh C, Kramer P, Ritter D, Schuenemann B, Scheler F: Calcium-Phosphat-Stoffwechsel und Haemofiltration (Calcium-phosphate metabolism and haemofiltration). *Klin Wochenschr* 56:1163, 1978 (in German)
16. Baldamus CA, Schoeppe W, Koch KM: Comparison of haemodialysis (HD) and post dilution haemofiltration (HF) on an unselected dialysis population. *Proc Eur Dial Transpl Assoc* 15:228, 1978
17. Shaldon S, Beau MC, Claret G, Deschodt G, Oulès R, Ramperez P, Mion H, Mion C: Haemofiltration with sorbent regeneration of ultrafiltrate: First clinical experience in end stage renal failure. *Proc Eur Dial Transpl Assoc* 15:220, 1978
18. Henderson LW, Parker HR, Schroeder JP, Frigon R, Sanfelippo ML: Continuous low flow hemofiltration with sorbent regeneration of ultrafiltrate. *Trans Am Soc Artif Intern Organs* 24:178, 1978
19. Quellhorst E, Schuenemann B, Borghardt J: Haemofiltration: Current clinical applications and revolution of techniques. *Renal Physicians Assoc Proc* 2:1, 1978
20. Henderson LW, Beans E: Successful production of pyrogen-free electrolyte solution by ultrafiltration. *Kidney Int* 14:522, 1978
21. Jacobs C, Broyer M, Brunner FP, Brynger H, Donckerwolcke RA, Kramer P, Selwood NH, Wing AJ, Blake PH: Combined Report on Regular Dialysis and Transplantation in Europe, XI, 1980. *Proc Eur Dial Transpl Assoc* 18:3, 1981
22. Quellhorst E, Schuenemann B, Doht B: Haemofiltration – a new method for the treatment of chronic renal insufficiency. In: *Technical Aspects of Renal Dialysis*, edited by Frost TH, Tunbridge Wells, Pitman Medical Publishing Co Ltd, 1978, p 96
23. Machesky PS, Ouchi K, Piatkiewicz W, Nosé Y: Membrane plasma filtration systems with multiple reactors for hepatic support. *Artif Organs* 2:265, 1978
24. Denis J, Opolon P, Delorme ML, Granger A, Darnis F: Long term extra-corporeal assistance by continuous haemofiltration during fulminant hepatic failure. *Gastroenterol Clin Biol* 3:337, 1979
25. Baldamus CA, Knobloch M, Rosak C, Koch KM: Die Kompensation der metabolischen Azidose und die Harnstoff-Stickstoff-Generationsrate unter Haemodialyse und unter Haemofiltration (Compensation of metabolic acidosis and the urea nitrogen generation with haemodialysis and haemofiltration). *Mitt Arbeitsgem Klin Nephrol* 8:118, 1979 (in German)
26. Henderson LW: Symptomatic hypotension during hemodialysis. *Kidney Int* 17:571, 1980
27. Degoulet P, Reach J, Aime F, Rioux P, Jacobs C, Legrain M: Risk factors in chronic haemodialysis. *Proc Eur Dial Transpl Assoc* 17:149, 1980
28. Bergström H, Asaba H, Fürst P, Oulès R: Dialysis, ultrafiltration and blood pressure. *Proc Eur Dial Transpl Assoc* 13:293, 1976
29. Hampl H, Paeprer H, Unger V, Kessel MW: Hemodynamics during hemodialysis, sequential ultrafiltration and hemofiltration. *J Dial* 3:51, 1979
30. Shaldon S, Deschodt G, Beau MC, Claret G, Mion H, Mion C: Vascular stability during high flux haemofiltration (HF). *Proc Eur Dial Transpl Assoc* 16:695, 1979
31. Baldamus CA, Ernst W, Fassbinder W, Koch KM: Differing haemodynamic stability due to differing sympathetic response: comparison of ultrafiltration, haemodialysis and haemofiltration. *Proc Eur Dial Transpl Assoc* 17:205, 1980
32. Quellhorst E, Schuenemann B, Falda Z: Response of the vascular system to different modifications of haemofiltration and haemodialysis. *Proc Eur Dial Transpl Assoc* 17:197, 1980
33. Schuenemann B, Borghardt J, Falda Z, Jacob I, Kramer P, Kraft B, Quellhorst E: Reactions of blood pressure and body spaces to hemofiltration treatment. *Trans Am Soc Artif Intern Organs* 24:687, 1978
34. Rouby JJ, Rottembourg J, Durande JP, Basset JY, Legrain M: Importance of the refilling rate in the genesis of hypovolaemic hypotension during regular dialysis and controlled sequential ultrafiltration-haemodialysis. *Proc Eur Dial Transpl Assoc* 15:239, 1972
35. Sausse A, Man NK, Di Gulio S, Zingraff J, Drueke T, Jungers P, Funck-Brentano JL: Evidence for Na-free water clearance during haemodialysis. *Proc Eur Soc Artif Organs* 5:186, 1978
36. Quellhorst E, Schuenemann B, Doht B: Treatment of severe hypertension in chronic renal failure by haemofiltration. *Proc Eur Dial Transpl Assoc* 14:129, 1977
37. Henderson LW, Ford CA, Lysaght MJ, Grosman RA, Silverstein ME: Preliminary observations on blood pressure response with maintenance diafiltration. *Kidney Int* 7 (Suppl 3):S-413, 1975
38. Kramer P, Matthaei D, Arnold R, Ebert R, Köbberling D, McIntosh C, Schwinn E, Scheler F, Ludwig H, Reichel J, Spitella G: Changes of plasma concentration and elimination of various hormones by haemofiltration. *Proc Eur Dial Transpl Assoc* 14:144, 1977
39. Schneider H, Streicher E: Thyroid function in long term haemofiltration. *Proc Eur Dial Transpl Assoc* 15:187, 1978
40. Schaefer K, Offermann G, Asmus G, v. Herrath D: Das Verhalten von Calcium, Phosphat und Parathormon unter chronischer Hämofiltration (Calcium, phosphate and parathyroid hormone changes during chronic haemofiltration). *Nieren- und Hochdruckkrankh* 7:40, 1978 (in German)
41. Fuchs C, Doht B, Dorn D, McIntosh C, Ritter D, Scheler F: Parathyroid hormone, calcium and phosphate balance in hemofiltration. *J Dial* 1:631, 1977
42. Henning HV, Balusek E: Lipid metabolism in uremia: effect of regular hemofiltration and hemodialysis treatment *J Dial* 1:595, 1977

43. Funck-Brentano JL, Man NK, Sausse A: Effect of more porous membranes on neuropathic toxins. *Kidney Int* 7, (Suppl 2):S52, 1975
44. Beckmann H, Ossenkop Ch, Quellhorst E: Changes in peripheral nerve function with long-term hemofiltration treatment. *J Dial* 1:585, 1977
45. Quellhorst E, Scheler F: Die Behandlung von Vergiftungen mittels Ultrafiltrations- Peritonealdialyse (Treatment of intoxications with peritoneal dialysis with ultrafiltration). In: *Vergiftungen*, edited by Frey R, Halmagyi M, Lang K, Oettel P, Berlin, Heidelberg, New York, Springer Verlag, 1970, p 24, (in German)
46. Silverstein ME, Ford CA, Lysaght MJ, Henderson LW: Treatment of severe fluid overload. *New Engl J Med* 291:747, 1974
47. Kramer P, Wigger W, Rieger J, Matthaei D, Scheler F: Arteriovenous hemofiltration. A new and simple method for treatment of overhydrated patients resistant to diuretics. *Klin Wochenschr* 55:1121, 1977
48. Leber HW, Wizemann V, Goubeaud G, Rawer P, Schütterle G: Simultaneous hemofiltration/hemodialysis: An effective alternative to hemofiltration and conventional hemodialysis in the treatment of uremic patients. *Clin Nephrol* 9:150, 1978

14

THE POLYACRYLONITRILE MEMBRANE; USE IN DIALYSIS WITH THE RHODIAL SYSTEM. USE IN HAEMOFILTRATION

JEAN-LOUIS FUNCK-BRENTANO and NGUYEN-KHOA MAN

The polyacrylonitrile membrane	275
Physical properties	275
Permeability for solutes	276
Permeability for water	276
Thrombogenicity	276
The RP 6 dialyser	276
Characteristics and performance	276
Clearance of solutes	276
Ultrafiltration	277
Reuse	277
The dialysate recirculating system	278
Description and practical application	278
Control of ultrafiltration	279
The middle molecule hypothesis and the RP 6 dialyser	279
Short dialysis	279
Middle molecules and polyneuropathy	279
The RP 6 dialyser with PA membrane as a haemofilter	281
Haemofiltration with the PA membrane: mass transfer characteristics	281
The haemofiltration system	281
Ultrafiltration parameters of the PA membrane	282
Comparison of haemodialysis and haemofiltration *in vitro* clearances	283
Clinical results with haemofiltration	283
References	285

THE POLYACRYLONITRILE (PA) MEMBRANE

The polyacrylonitrile (PA, AN69) membrane is a synthetic membrane which is highly permeable for middle molecules and water, consisting of an acrylonitrile sodium methallylsulphonate copolymer, with a wet thickness of 30 μm. There is no dense layer on the surface as in cellulosic membranes (1); when used for dialysis, its resistance to solute transfer is, therefore, low. (For additional information see also Chapter 4).

Physical properties

Pressure and stretching at breaking point are 0.9 kg/cm and 80%, respectively, in a longitudinal direction and 0.3 kg/cm and 200%, respectively, in a transverse direction. Thus, the PA membrane is more elastic and less anisotropic than cellulosic membranes. Because of its resistance to oxidising agents, sterilisation with hypochlorite is possible. The material has no toxic properties when tested under either acute or chronic conditions. The PA membrane is impermeable to bovine albumin

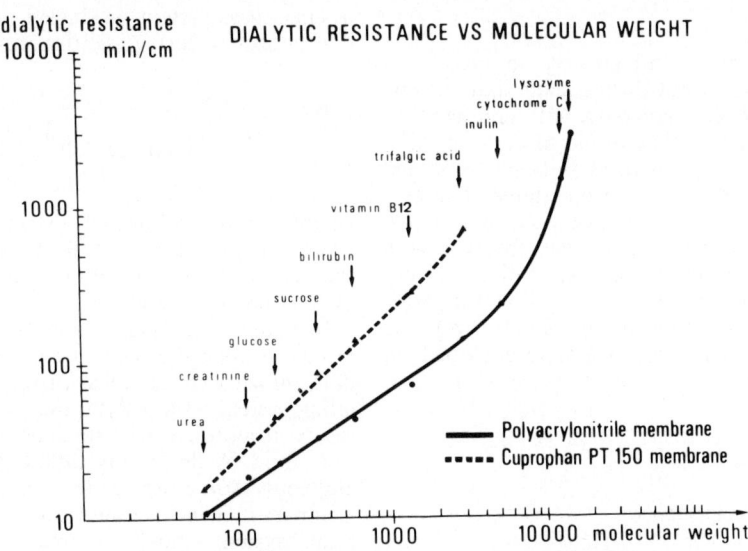

Figure 1. Membrane resistance of Cuprophan PT 150 and polyacrylonitrile membrane for solutes with different molecular weights.

(60,000 daltons). Its permeability limit is in the range of 40,000 daltons.

Permeability for solutes

The dialytic resistance of the membrane (R_M) to solutes of different molecular weights is shown in Figure 1. The R_M for vitamin B_{12} is 3.8 times less than that of Cuprophan PT 150. With solutes of higher molecular weight the ratio increases exponentially.

Permeability for water

The permeability of the PA membrane for water is high compared with conventional dialysis membranes, being in the order of 36.5 to 45.6 ml/min/m²/100 mm Hg, about 10 times greater than that of Cuprophane (Figure 2).

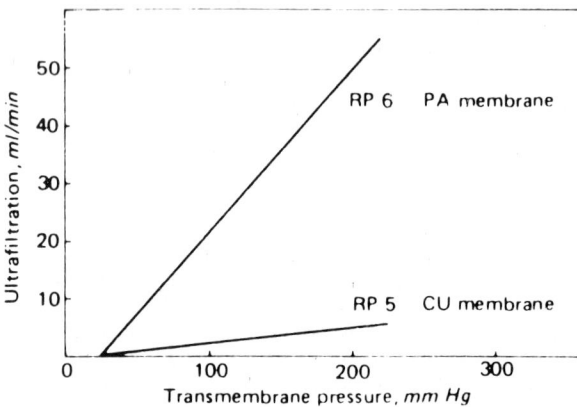

Figure 2. Ultrafiltration rate of RP 6 dialyser with PA membrane and RP5 dialyser with Cuprophane (CU) membrane.

Thrombogenicity

Blood coagulation studies and changes in blood cell counts have been carried out during acute and chronic dialysis. Induced platelet aggregation with collagen was unchanged whereas it was slightly increased with ADP 0.5 γ/ml. Platelet adhesiveness to glass beads remained low and fibrinogen and factor V were stable. The erythrocyte and platelet counts remained unchanged. An early and transient fall in leucocytes was observed with both PA and cellulosic membranes. After dialysis, very few cells were found on the PA membrane and identification of proteins interacting at the blood/membrane interface indicated that Clq and C4 were adsorbed on the PA membrane (2).

THE RP 6 DIALYSER

Characteristics and performance

The RP 6 dialyser is a disposable parallel grooved plate artificial kidney with 16 blood compartments, sterilised by gamma ray, and with a dialysing surface area of 1.03 m². The pressure drops are 15 mm Hg for the blood compartment and 30 mm Hg for the dialysis fluid compartment at a blood flow of 200 ml/min and a dialysis fluid flow of 1000 ml/min. The priming volume of the blood compartment is 150±20 ml at 70 mm Hg transmembrane pressure. At the conclusion of dialysis, blood is returned to the patient by gravity with a final rinse of 250 ml of normal saline. Blood loss in the dialyser is approximately 3 to 5 ml.

Clearance of solutes

The clearances of different solutes were determined at a blood flow rate of 200 ml/min and a dialysis fluid flow rate of 500 ml/min and are shown in Table 1. In a recir-

Table 1. RP 6 dialyser (with PA membrane), *in vitro** solute clearances.

Solute	MW	Clearance ml/min
Urea	60	150
Creatinine	113	125
Uric acid	168	110
Vit B_{12}	1,355	68
Inulin	5,200	34
Myoglobin	17,800	19

* Q_B = 200 ml/min
Q_D = 500 ml/min

culating dialysis system, the clearances of all solutes decrease with time although their dialysance remains constant (Figure 3). This dialysance can be calculated using the formulae of Wolf and Graetz (3, 4). For comparison with single pass systems we developed the concept of equivalent clearance K_E which is the clearance of a single pass system producing the same fall in plasma concentration during identical time intervals:

$$K_E = \frac{v}{t_d} \ln\left(\frac{v+q}{v+q \exp -\left[\frac{V t_d (v+q)}{vq}\right]}\right)$$

where v is the volume of distribution in the patient in litres, q is the volume of the dialysis fluid in litres, V is the dialysance in litres/week, t_d is the total dialysis time in fractions of a week.

In Figure 4 dialysance and equivalent clearances are plotted against molecular weight for seven solutes. The data shown were obtained *in vitro* using a dual recirculating system with a RP 6 dialyser, a 30 l 'body water' reservoir representing a standard patient and 50 l of dialysis fluid. A decreasing difference between dialysance and equivalent clearance for increasing molecular weight is apparent. This phenomenon indicates that the recirculating system tends to correct the relatively excessive permeability of the membrane for small molecules, simulating more closely normal renal function.

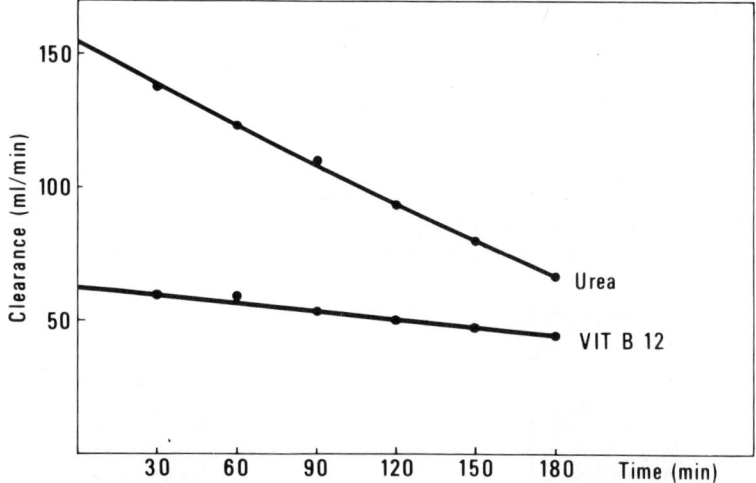

Figure 3. Decrease of equivalent clearances of urea and vitamin B_{12}, with the closed tank system (*in vitro*).

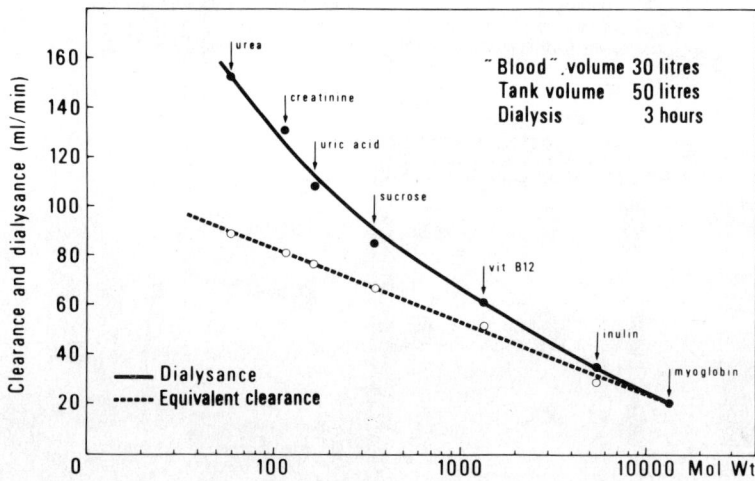

Figure 4. Dialysance and equivalent clearance vs. MW with RP 6 dialyser and closed tank system (*in vitro*).

Ultrafiltration

As the permeability of the PA membrane to water is about 10 times that of Cuprophane, the pressure gradient which is needed to achieve the same transfer of water is approximately 10 times less. A special single batch, closed circuit recirculating dialysis fluid delivery system – the Rhodial System – has been devised for use with the RP 6 dialyser, allowing accurately controlled ultrafiltration by a volumetric pump (see below).

Reuse of the RP 6 dialyser (see also Chapter 15)

Because of the resistance of the PA membrane to oxidising agents, sodium hypochlorite solution can be used both as a cleansing and a sterilising agent.

The recommended procedure for reuse of the RP 6 dialyser is as follows: (a) After returning the blood from the dialyser to the patient, the dialysis fluid compartment is drained. (b) The blood circuit is rinsed with 5,0 l of 1.0% sodium hypochlorite solution (water used to make this 1% solution must be filtered to 1 μm). This takes about 15 min. The deposits of fibrin and blood, either dissolved or loosened by the action of hypochlorite, are washed out of the dialyser. (c) The unit is stored at room temperature after the dialysate compartment and blood circuit have been filled with hypochlorite solution. (d) Prior to reuse the unit is drained by gravity. The dialysate compartment is rinsed with tap water at a flow rate of 1,0 l/min for 15 min. Some of the water penetrates in the blood compartment, partially removing hypochlorite. The blood circuit is then further rinsed with 1,0 l of normal saline and the efflux is tested for residual hypochlorite, using Clinistix, the sensivity of this test being approximately 1 part to 1000. This procedure allows the reuse of the dialyser and blood tubing for at least three successive dialyses. No untoward reactions have occurred and no decrease in dialyser performance has been observed.

THE DIALYSATE RECIRCULATING SYSTEM

Description and practical application

The dialysis fluid delivery system to be used with the RP 6 dialyser (Figure 5) consists of an airtight tank system with a 75 l capacity, designed for recirculation of the dialysis fluid and for presetting the ultrafiltration rate (see diagram presented in Figure 6). The tank is filled with softened or deionised water and the appropriate volume of dialysis concentrate is added. In a separate reservoir 2,0 l of dialysis fluid are available for rinsing the dialyser circuit. The dialysis fluid is heated to the appropriate temperature (37° to 39°C) by an external heater. A centrifugal pump ensures dialysate circulation at a flow rate of 1,0 l/min. At the end of dialysis the

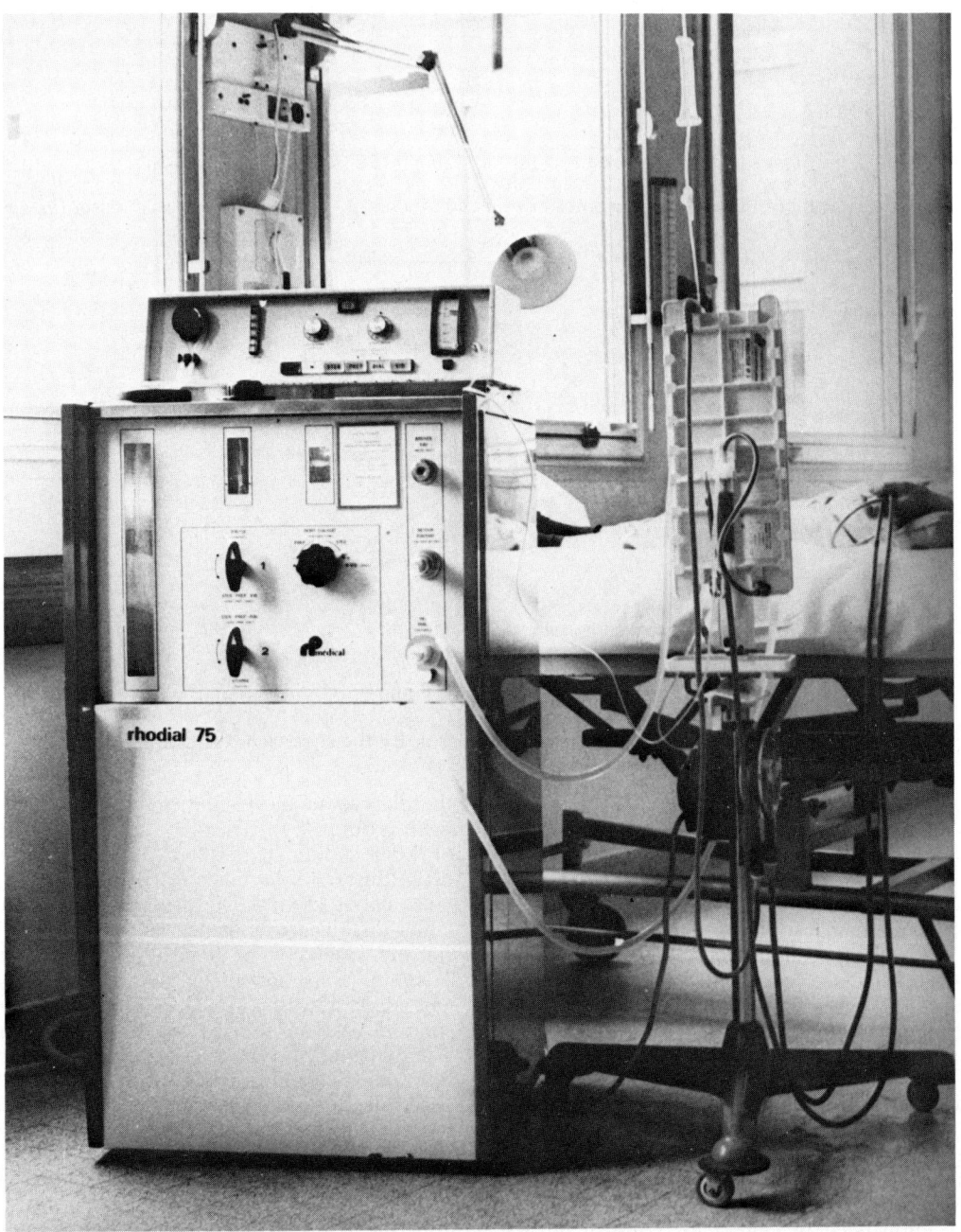

Figure 5. The 75 l airtight tank system with dialysate recirculation.

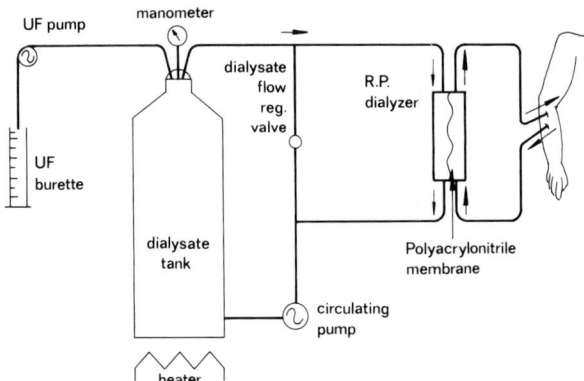

Figure 6. Diagram of the recirculating system showing the dialysate recirculation and the ultrafiltrate pump (UF) and burette, to be used with the RP6 dialyser.

used dialysate is drained and a sample may be collected for analysis and for calculation of the total solute removal. The solute content of the dialysis fluid at the end of dialysis reflects the plasma predialysis concentration level, the mass transfer and input and output balance. In addition the sample can be used for research investigations, such as identification of yet unknown substances removed during dialysis (5). Sterilisation of the tank can be achieved by either circulation of internally generated steam, or with chemical disinfectants.

Control of ultrafiltration

The amount of ultrafiltration and the flow of ultrafiltrate are regulated by a volumetric pump (Figure 6). Since the rigidity of the tank and tubing allows no variation in volume, the fluid removed from the system by the volumetric pump is necessarily replaced by an equal volume of ultrafiltrate, transferred through the membrane from the patient's plasma. Contrary to traditional forms of ultrafiltration the pressure across the membrane is entirely controlled by the preset ultrafiltration rate. The outflow from the volumetric pump is collected in a burette and permits accurate measurement of the total amount of ultrafiltrate.

THE MIDDLE MOLECULE HYPOTHESIS AND THE RP 6 DIALYSER

It is well known that patients treated with regular peritoneal dialysis have a low incidence of uraemic neuropathy despite relatively high blood urea and creatinine concentrations. It is equally well known that prevention of neuropathy in regular dialysis patients depends on the total amount of dialytic treatment given per week. This led Babb and coworkers (6, 7) to formulate the so called 'middle molecule' hypothesis (see also Chapters 2 and 19). These investigators suggested that uraemic polyneuropathy was due to the retention of certain solutes of relatively high molecular weight during haemodialysis

treatment, their passage through the Cuprophane membrane being constrained because of the relatively high membrane resistance for these metabolites. Removal by peritoneal dialysis, however, was supposed to be much better because of the higher permeability of the peritoneal membrane for these middle weight solutes, which explained the low incidence of polyneuropathy in patients treated with regular peritoneal dialysis.

Short dialysis

According to the middle molecule hypothesis reduction in the total number of dialysis hours/week required a better transfer of middle molecules than is obtained with the $1 m^2$ Cuprophane membrane commonly used in artificial kidneys. The higher permeability of the PA membrane for middle molecules opened the opportunity of shortening dialysis time. Because of transfer of middle molecules across the PA membrane is twice that of Cuprophane, it seemed possible to cut total dialysis time/week into half.

This was confirmed in four stable dialysis patients, who were initially treated with a dialyser with a $0.9 m^2$ Cuprophane membrane. Their condition was adequate according to the criteria of DePalma et al (8). Three patients had no residual kidney function at all, one had a residual creatinine clearance of 1.8 ml/min. The total dialysis time per week was halved and the $0.9 m^2$ Cuprophane dialyser was replaced by the RP 6 dialyser with a $1.03 m^2$ PA membrane. After one year of treatment all four patients were in an excellent condition, notwithstanding an increase of predialysis plasma concentrations of urea and creatinine of about 50%. Plasma uric acid and haemoglobin levels did not change significantly (9).

Mean nerve conduction velocity remained unchanged during the entire period of short dialysis.

It should be mentioned, however, that dialysis time can also be shortened with other membranes which are highly permeable to middle molecules and/or by increasing the active surface area of conventional cellulosic membranes, e.g. of the hollow fibre dialyser configuration, which has the advantage of a marked reduction of the surface/volume ratio (10).

Middle molecules and polyneuropathy

The high permeability of the PA membrane in combination with a closed circuit tank system made further investigations possible.

In an attempt to identify a number of middle molecules which could be responsible for the development of polyneuropathy, the first dialysate of patients with a severe peripheral neuropathy was analysed and compared with the dialysate of control patients without neuropathy (11). Gel chromatography of samples was performed on Sephadex G 15 and absorption was measured at 254 nm. We arbitrarily chose a spectrum of middle molecules between 300 and 1,500 daltons. Chromatographic analysis of the first dialysate from patients with severe neuropathy showed a middle molecule content, higher than found in the control (Figure 7).

For a tentative identification the solutes which may cause uraemic neuropathy, high performance gel chromatography was carried out with plasma ultrafiltrate from uraemic patients with and without neuropathy (12a). Amongst the peaks within the middle molecule range, peak b showed an appreciably higher absorbance than in uraemic patients without neuropathy (Figure 8).

Ion exchange chromatography of peak b showed a striking increase of fraction b4 (Figure 9).

This fraction contains two sub-peaks: one detected at 206 nm (b_{4-1}), the other detected at 254 nm (b_{4-2}). Only the sub-peak b_{4-2} apparently correlates with neuropathy in uraemic patients (28).

The b_{4-2} purified from urines of healthy subjects and from uraemic hemofiltrate were shown to be identical.

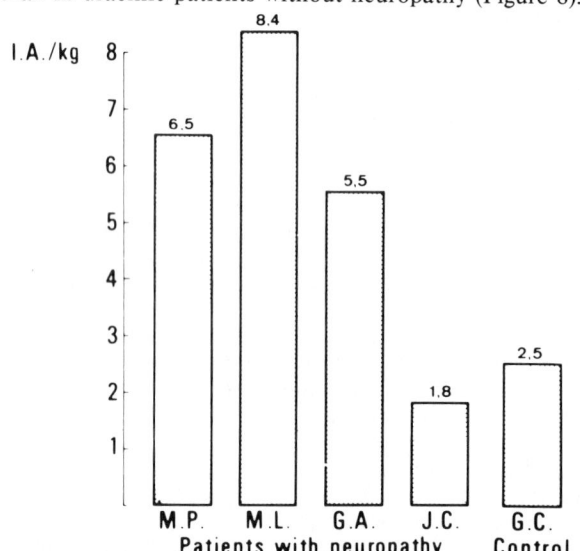

Figure 7. Middle molecule integrated absorbance (IA) of first PA dialysates.

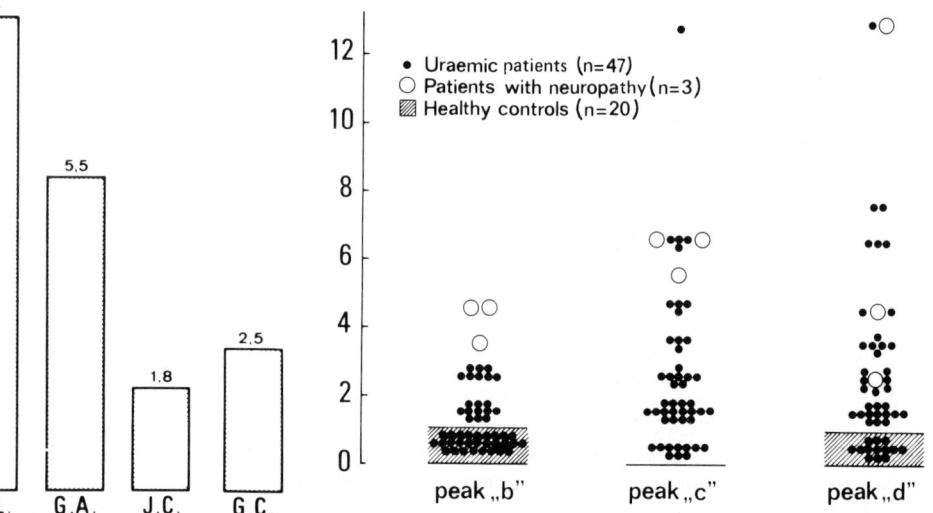

Figure 8. Integrated absorbance of peaks b, c and d in uraemic patients (●) and uraemic patients with polyneuropathy (○). Hatched areas represent normal range.

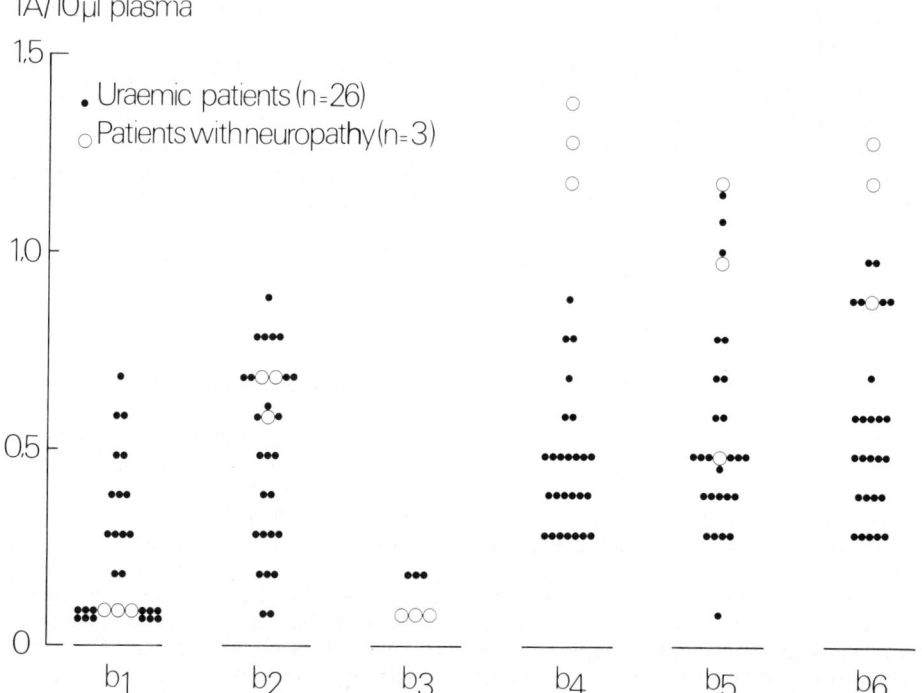

Figure 9. Integrated absorbance of subpeaks b_1 to b_6 in uraemic patients (●) and in uraemic patients with neuropathy (○).

This purified solute was used to determine b_{4-2} concentrations in biological fluids. In healthy subjects, the b_{4-2} plasma concentration was below 1 mg/l and the 24-h urinary excretion was about 35 mg. Regular dialysis treated patients had a mean b_{4-2} plasma concentration of about 4 mg/l ranging from 10 to 20 mg/l in polyneuropathic patients. Mass spectrometry showed that this solute is a glucuronic acid conjugate with a MW of 568 (12b).

In the frog sural nerve test, described elsewhere (13), fraction b appeared to be neurotoxic. Fractions c and d did not have neurotoxic properties.

Evidently the RP 6 dialyser with the PA membrane offers interesting opportunities of investigating plasma chromatographic patterns in uraemic patients with the techniques developed by Bergström and associates (14, 15).

A possible relationship between middle molecules and uraemic polyneuropathy was clinically investigated in four patients with severe neuropathy, attributed to inadequate dialysis. They were transferred to treatment with the RP 6 dialyser and the PA membrane after being dialysed for periods of 8 to 38 months, twice weekly, 6 or 10 h with a 1 m² Cuprophane dialyser. All were able to walk without help within 3 months. Motor nerve conduction velocity of the peroneal nerve was not measurable at the onset of treatment with the PA membrane, but reappeared in one patient after 12 months. In all patients the cubital motor nerve conduction velocity increased simultaneously with the improvement of the clinical neurological condition (5, 9, 16). The dramatic and rapid improvement was comparable with the initial phase of recovery ('the rapid improvement phase') observed after successful renal transplantation (see Chapter 37).

THE RP 6 DIALYSER WITH PA MEMBRANE AS A HAEMOFILTER (see also chapters 12 and 13)

Haemofiltration has in recent years moved from an investigational procedure to clinical application as an alternative method for treatment of uraemia (17).

Solute removal by convection is comparable to glomerular filtration: intermediate molecular weight solutes (the so called middle molecules) are more efficiently removed than with conventional haemodialysis.

Development and clinical application of haemofiltration have been hampered for a long time by a lack of suitable membranes with high hydrodynamic permeability, adequate rejection characteristics, good biocompatability and sufficient mechanical strength to endure high transmembrane pressures (18–22).

Quellhorst and co-workers (1976 [23]) used the RP 6 dialyser with the highly permeable PA membrane as a haemofilter with promising results.

Haemofiltration with the PA membrane: mass transfer characteristics

Haemofiltration is, as mentioned above, a predominantly convective solute transfer procedure, limited by the membrane transmittance or sieving coefficient.

Table 2 shows transmittance data of Cuprophane 150 PM and PA membranes as presented by Green and co-workers (24) compared with sieving coefficients of the glomerular basement membrane (GBM), for different solutes, derived from Pitts (25).

Table 2. Transmittance coefficients for artificial membranes (Cuprophane 150 PM and PA) and for the glomerular basement membrane (GBM).

Solute	MW	CU 150 PM	PA	GBM
Urea	60	1.000	1.000	1.00
Creatinine	113	0.891	0.985	1.00
Vitamin B_{12}	1,355	0.629	0.940	1.00
Inulin	5,200	0.309	0.776	0.98
Ovalbumin	44,000	0.002	0.044	0.22
Haemoglobin	64,500	–	0.009	–

The transmittance (T_r) of the PA membrane for vitamin B_{12} (1,355 daltons) and of the glomerular basement membrane are similar (0.94 and 1.00). The vitamin B_{12} transmittance of Cuprophane 150 is less (0.62).

The transmittance coefficients for inulin (5,000 daltons) of the PA and GBM are comparable – the T_r of the PA membrane being only slightly less (0.77 versus 0.98), T_r for inulin of Cuprophane 150 PM being only 0.30.

Clearances of 1,000 to 5,000 molecular weight solutes by haemofiltration with the PA membrane will be apparently of the same order of magnitude as by the glomerulus.

The haemofiltration system

The characteristics of the PA membrane make the RP 6 dialyser suitable for haemofiltration purposes. A flow diagram of a haemofiltration system is presented in Figure 10.

Ultrafiltrate is removed from the blood passing the haemofilter and a nearly equal volume of substitution fluid is administered to the blood prior its return to the patient (so called post dilution substitution). The composition of the substitution fluid as commonly used is shown in Table 3.

Table 3. Composition of the substitution fluid.

Na	140 mmol/l	Cl	105 mmol/l
K	0 mmol/l	Acetate	40 mmol/l
Ca	1.75 mmol/l		
Mg	0.75 mmol/l		

Ca mmol/l → mg/dl: multiply by 4
Mg mmol/l → mg/dl: multiply by 2.4

The amount of substitution fluid injected in the venous bubble trap is equal to the amount of ultrafiltrate minus the required loss of body weight. This is accomplished by using a weighing balance which holds the

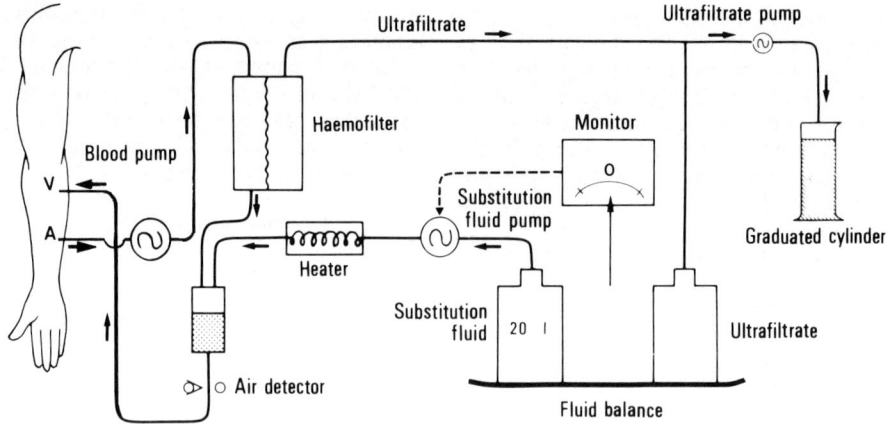

Figure 10. Flow diagram of a haemofiltration system including monitoring of fluid balance and air leak monitors.

ultrafiltrate reservoir on one side and the reservoir with sterile substitution fluid on the other. A volumetric pump, responding to an electronic feed back signal from the weighing balance, injects the required amount of substitution fluid. Another volumetric pump monitors the weight loss of the patient by collecting a predetermined volume of ultrafiltrate in a graduated cylinder.

Ultrafiltration parameters of the PA membrane

Ultrafiltrate flow rates (Q_{UF}) plotted as a function of the transmembrane pressure (TMP) both for water and blood (at different flow rates) are presented in Figure 11. There is a linear correlation between the ultrafiltration of pure water and TMP. The ultrafiltrate flow rates of blood plotted as a function of the TMP, however, are different and it should be mentioned that the ultrafiltrate flow of anaemic blood (haematocrit 30%) is always less than of the 'undiluted' blood and approaches a plateau with high transmembrane pressures.

As shown in Figure 11 Q_{UF} at 300 mm Hg is approximately 70 ml/min at a Q_B of 200 ml/min and 95 ml/min at a Q_B of 400 ml/min, which is about 30% of the flow rates of the blood and 50% of the values obtained with water.

This phenomenon has to be explained by the formation of a stagnant protein layer (called 'cake') at the blood/membrane interface. This layer, consisting of a concentrated protein solution, reduces ultrafiltration as a result of increased colloid osmotic pressure at the membrane surface and by an increase of the hydrodynamic resistance of the membrane (26).

Obviously it is of no advantage to increase TMP beyond 300 mm Hg. A further increase produces a minimal increase of Q_{UF}, because of membrane polarisation. In addition it increases the risk of membrane rupture.

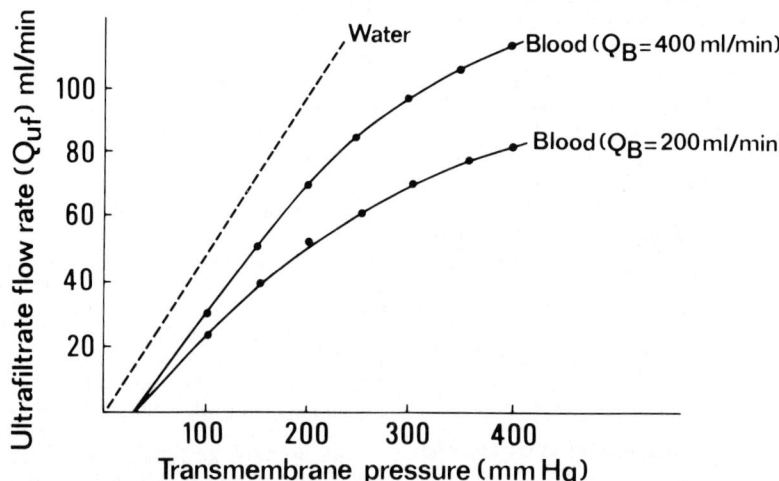

Figure 11. Ultrafiltrate flow rate as a function of transmembrane pressures for various blood flow rates.

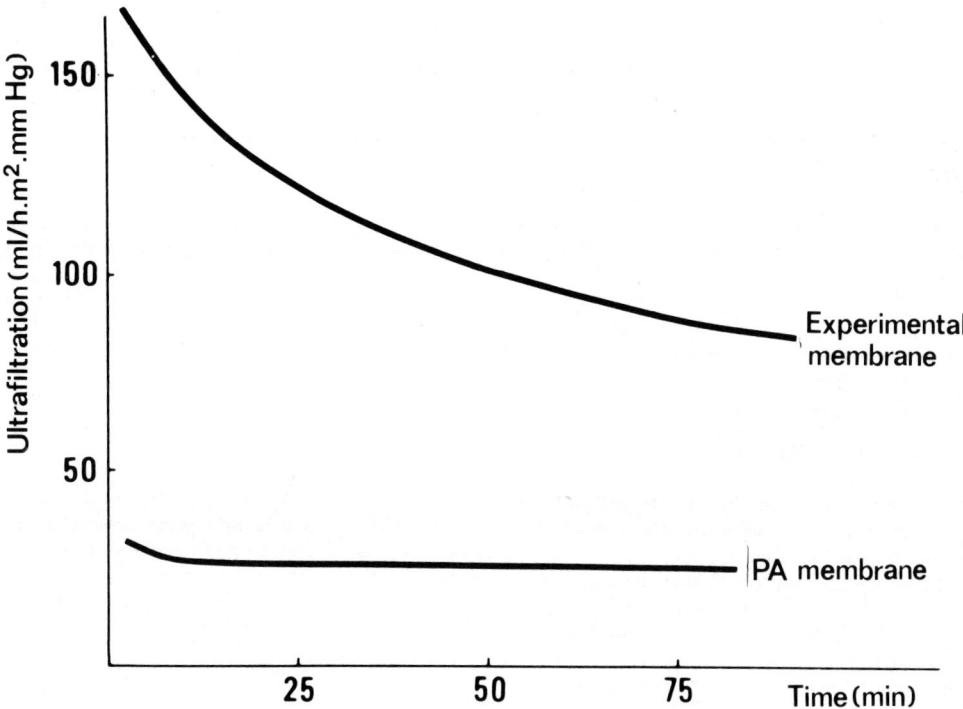

Figure 12. Evolution of ultrafiltration slopes as a function of time for an experimental ultrafiltration membrane and for the polyacrylonitrile PA membrane.

In Figure 12 the good biocompatibility properties of the PA membrane are compared with an experimental ultrafiltration membrane: when Q_{UF} was maintained at very low values (2 ml/min), no polarisation occurred with the PA membrane, whereas the Q_{UF} with the experimental membrane decreased markedly with time (2).

Comparison of haemodialysis and haemofiltration *in vitro* clearances

Haemofiltration clearances of various solutes with a RP 6 haemofilter (provided with the PA membrane) at a Q_{UF} of 70 ml/min are presented in Table 4 and are compared with haemodialysis clearances with a RP 5 dialyser with Cuprophan membrane and a RP 6 with the PA membrane.

Urea clearances with haemofiltration are 50% less than with haemodialysis, either with the RP 5 of the RP 6 dialyser. Haemofiltration clearances of vitamin B_{12} (1,355 daltons) are equal to haemodialysis with the RP 6 dialyser provided with the PA membrane. But haemofiltration clearances of higher molecular weight solutes (1,000–20,000) are more than 2 to 7 times higher than those obtained with haemodialysis with the same RP 6.

Quellhorst and co-workers (22) and Henderson et al. (27) reported similar results.

Table 4. In vitro clearances (ml/min) with haemodialysis and haemofiltration.

Solute	MW	Haemodialysis [a] RP 5 Cuprophan	RP 6 PA	Haemofiltration [b] RP 6 PA
Urea	60	125	135	70
Vitamin B_{12}	1,355	21	60	65.8
Inulin	5,200	2	23	54.4
Myoglobin	17,800	—	3	22.4

[a] Haemodialysis: Q_B 200 ml/min Q_D 500 ml/min.
[b] Haemofiltration: Q_{UF} 70 ml/min.

Clinical results obtained with haemofiltration

Haemofiltration was first introduced for clinical application by Henderson and associates in 1975 (2). The original haemofilter was a device with a polysulfone membrane (XM 50 produced by Amicon Corporation in the USA) in a format of 12,000 hollow fibers. The hydrodynamic permeability of this membrane was 1.75 ml/min/cm^2/mm Hg/10^4.

Quellhorst and co-workers in West-Germany and Funck-Brentano and associates in the Necker unit in Paris used the RP 6 dialyser as an ultrafilter for clinical application.

Haemofiltration treatment appeared to be well tolerated; fluid removal dit not evoke hypotensive episodes or muscle cramps. Removal of urea, creatinine and uric

Table 5. Removal of urea, creatinine, uric acid and phosphate (g/dialysis).

	Body weight	Urea	Creatinine	Uric acid	Phosphate
Haemodialysis 1 m² PA, 5 hrs (n = 10)	57.7±2.10	28.1±2.16	2.22±0.209	0.839±0.053	0.678±0.059
Plasma concentrations before dialysis		33 ±1.5 mmol/l	1560±84 µmol/l	0.49±0.025 mmol/l	3.6±0.3 mmol/l
Haemofiltration 1 m² PA, 5 hrs (n = 8)	53.7 kg±4.79	29.5±4.25	1.76±0.213	0.952±0.112	0.679±0.122
Plasma concentrations before haemofiltration		36 ±4.9 mmol/l	1137±97 µmol/l	0.52 ±0.059 mmol/l	2.9 ±0.4 mmol/l

Urea mmol/l → mg/dl: multiply by 6
Creatinine µmol/l → mg/dl: multiply by 0.0113
Uric acid mmol/l → mg/dl: multiply by 16.8
Phosphate mmol/l → mg/dl: multiply by 1.8

acid by haemofiltration was approximately similar to the removal by haemodialysis with comparable pretreatment blood concentrations (Table 5).

The amount of phosphate removed with haemofiltration was also similar to the amount removed by haemodialysis (Figure 13). Half of the total amount is apparently removed during the first 2 hours of treatment. Afterwards a plateau is reached. That suggests that a steady state occurs and that the phosphate moved from intra to extra-cellular fluid as fast as it was removed by the haemofilter.

Table 6 shows the removal of middle molecules (b_{4-2}) [28] by 5 hours haemodialysis and 5 hours haemofiltration. Obviously removal by haemofiltration is more effective: regarding the removal of middle molecules haemofiltration operates in a similar fashion as the natural kidney.

Table 6. Plasma concentration and removal of middle molecular weight (b_{4-2}) solutes in healthy subjects and in uraemic patients on haemodialysis and haemofiltration.

	Plasma concentration (mg/l)	Removal
Healthy subjects (n = 24)	≤1	urinary excretion 38±3 mg/24 h
Uraemic patients Haemodialysis (n = 18)	4.0±0.7	by machine 57±9 mg/session
Haemofiltration (n = 17)	3.5±0.6	61±5 mg/session

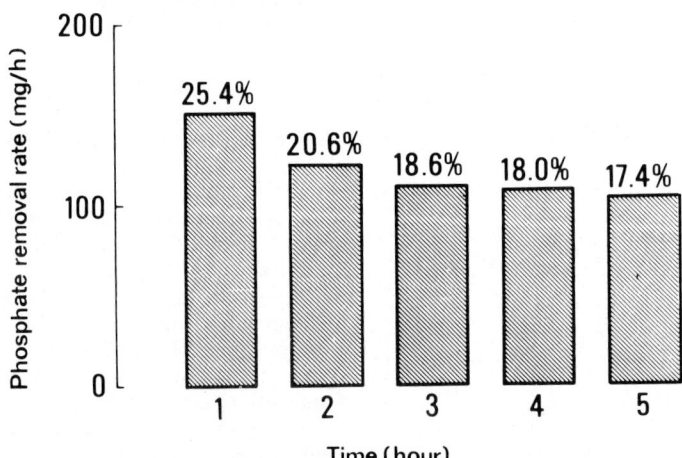

Figure 13. Phosphate removal rate during 5 hour haemofiltration (mean value of 5 sessions). Percentages of total removal are shown.

REFERENCES

1. Rickles RN: *Membranes, Technology and Economics,* Park Ridge, NJ, Noyes Development Corporation 1967, p 11
2. Vroman L, Kling M: Identification of proteins interacting at blood/artificial kidney material interfaces: relation to platelets and white blood cells. *Proc 8th Annu Contractors' Conf Artif Kidney – Chronic Uremia Program of NIAMDD* edited by Mackey BB, DHEW publ No (NIH) 76–248, 1975, p 69
3. Wolf AV, Remp DG, Kiley JE, Currie GD: Artificial kidney function: kinetics of hemodialysis. *J Clin Invest* 30:1062, 1951
4. Wolf AV: The artificial kidney. *Science* 115:193, 1952
5. Man NK, Terlain B, Paris J, Werner G, Sausse A, Funck-Bretano JL: An approach for 'Middle Molecule' identification in artificial kidney dialysate with reference to neuropathy prevention. *Trans Am Soc Artif Intern Organs* 19:320, 1973
6. Babb AL, Farrel PC, Uvelli DA, Scribner BH: Hemodialyzer evaluation by examination of solute molecular weight spectra *Trans Am Soc Artif Intern Organs* 18:98, 1972
7. Babb AL, Popovich RP, Christopher TG, Scribner BH: The genesis of the square meter-hour hypothesis. *Trans Am Soc Artif Intern Organs* 17:81, 1971
8. De Palma JR, Abukurah A, Rubini ME: 'Adequacy' of haemodialysis *Proc Eur Dial Transpl Assoc* 9:265, 1972
9. Man NK, Granger A, Rondon-Nucete M, Zingraff J, Jungers P, Sausse A, Funck-Brentano JL: One year follow-up of short dialysis with a membrane highly permeable to middle molecules. *Proc Eur Dial Transpl Assoc* 10:236, 1973
10. Gotch F, Sargent J, Keen M, Holmes G, Teisinger C: Development and long term clinical evaluation of thromboresistant hollow fiber kidney (HFK). *Trans Am Soc Artif Intern Organs* 18:135, 1972
11. Funck-Brentano JL, Man NK, Sausse A: Effect of more porous dialysis membrane on neuropathic toxins. *Kidney Int* 7:52, 1974
12a. Funck-Brentano JL, Man NK, Sausse A, Zingraff J, Boudet J, Becker A, Cueille GF: Characterization of a 1100–1300 MW uremic neutoxin. *Trans Am Soc Artif Intern Organs* 22:163, 1976
12b. Cueille G, Man NK, Sausse A, Farges JP, Funck-Brentano JL: Further characterization of a neurotoxic uremic middle molecule. *Proc 8th Int Congr Nephrol Athens,* edited by Zurukzoglu W, Papadimitriou M, Pyrposopoulos M, Sion M, Zamboulis C, Basel, Karger 1981, p 606
13. Boudet J, Cueille GF, Benoist JM, Man NK, Funck-Brentano JL: In vitro frog sural nerve test: a monitor for detecting neurotoxin solutes. *Artif Organs* 4 (Suppl):94, 1980
14. Fürst P, Bergström J, Gordon A, Johnsson E, Zimmerman L: Separation of peptides of 'middle' molecular weight from biological fluids of patients with uremia. *Kidney Int* 7 (Suppl no 3), S272, 1975
15. Funck-Brentano JL, Man NK, Sausse A, Cueille G, Zingraff J, Drueke T, Jungers P, Billon JP: Neuropathy and 'middle' molecules toxins. *Kidney Int* 7, (Suppl no 3): S352, 1975
16. Funck-Brentano JL, Man NK: The polyacrylonitrile membrane and the Rhodial system: their practical application. In *Replacement of Renal Function by Dialysis,* edited by Drukker W, Parsons FM, Maher JF, 1st edition, The Hague, Boston, London, Martinus Nijhoff 1978, p 125
17. Man NK, Funck-Brentano JL: Hemofiltration, an alternative method for treatment of end-stage renal failure. *Adv Nephrol* 7:293, 1978
18. Bixler HJ, Nelsen LM, Bluemle LW Jr: The development of a diafiltration system for blood purification. *Trans Am Soc Artif Intern Organs* 14:99, 1968
19. Dorson WJ, Pizziconi VB, Woorhees ME, Calkins JM, Christianson JD, Cotter DJ, Fargotstein R, Markovitz M, Monty DE Jr, Tomisaka DM: Initial trials of a molecular separation artificial kidney. *Trans Am Soc Artif Intern Organs* 19:109, 1973
20. Hamilton R, Ford C and Colton C, Cross R, Steinmuller S, Henderson LW: Blood cleansing by diafiltration in uremic dog and man. *Trans Am Soc Artif Intern Organs* 17:259, 1971
21. Henderson LW, Besarab A, Michaels A, Bluemle LW Jr: Blood purification by ultrafiltration and fluid replacement (diafiltration). *Trans Am Soc Artif Intern Organs* 13:216, 1967
22. Quellhorst E, Fernandez E, Scheler F: Treatment of uraemia using an ultrafiltration-filtration system. *Proc Eur Dial Transpl Assoc* 9:584, 1972
23. Quellhorst E, Rieger J, Doht B, Beckmann H, Jacob I, Kraft B, Mietzsch C, Scheler F: Treatment of chronic uraemia by an ultrafiltration kidney. First clinical experience *Proc Eur Dial Transpl Assoc* 13:314, 1976
24. Green DM, Antwiller GD, Moncrief JW, Decherd JF, Popovich RP: Measurement of the transmittance coefficient spectrum of Cuprophan and RP-69 membranes: Application to middle molecule removal via ultrafiltration, *Trans Am Soc Artif Intern organs* 22:627, 1976
25. Pitts RF: *Physiology of the Kidney and Body Fluids* (3d ed) Chicago IL, Year Book Medical Publishers Inc 1974
26. Colton CK, Henderson LW, Ford CA, Lysaght MJ: Kinetics of hemodiafiltration. I: In vitro transport characteristics of a hollow-fiber blood ultrafilter. *J Lab Clin Med* 85:355, 1975
27. Henderson LW, Colton CK, Ford CA: Kinetics of hemodiafiltration. II: Clinical characterization of a new blood cleansing modality. *J Lab Clin Med* 85:372, 1975
28. Man NK, Cueille G, Zingraff J, Boudet J, Sausse A, Funck-Brentano JL: Uremic neurotoxin in the middle molecular weight range. *Artif Organs* 4:116, 1980

15
MULTIPLE USE OF HEMODIALYZERS

NORMAN DEANE and JAMES A. BEMIS

History and rationale	286
Components of reuse processing techniques	287
Storage of the dialyzer	288
Rinsing	288
Cleaning	289
Sterilization	292
Preparation for subsequent use	295
Reuse of tubing	295
Functional studies of reused dialyzers	295
Patient experience	296
Survival	296
Morbidity	297
Biocompatibility	297
Acceptance	298
Complications	298
Pyrogenic	298
Infectious	299
Immunologic	299
Technical	299
Some practical aspects of a reuse program	300
The reprocessing area	300
Equipment	300
Control of components	300
Process controls	300
Labeling control	300
Records	307
Environmental protection	307
Appendices	307
A. Storage procedure for hollow fiber dialyzers	307
B. Preparation for use of stored hollow fiber dialyzers	307
C. Process and quality control in a dialyzer multiple use program: organization and personnel	307
References	302

HISTORY AND RATIONALE

Repeated hemodialysis treatment for chronic failure was initiated by Belding Scribner and colleagues (1) in 1960. The earliest procedures included several aspects that were shortly employed for multiple use of dialyzers. Scribner selected the Kiil dialyzer (2) which he modified into a 2-layer flat membrane dialyzer. As seen in the expanded diagram of the Kiil dialyzer (Figure 1), two sheets of membrane enclose a blood port positioned between grooved boards at each end of the dialyzer (3) (see also chapters 2 and 5). The large plastic boards must be scrubbed and washed to prepare for dialysis. The dialyzer is then 'built' by creating a tight alignment between the boards, membranes and blood ports. A torque wrench, used on the stabilizing nuts and bolts, firmly balanced the pressure of the boards and maintained the boards and membranes in exact position. Blood flows between the membranes as dialysis fluid flows countercurrently between the membranes and the boards. Scribner and coworkers rinsed the blood and dialysate compartments with water and sterilized both compartments with formalin, since they were not sterile when assembled. The dialyzer remained filled with formalin until the time for dialysis when it was flushed with saline to remove the formalin. The steps in this process are comparable to those now employed for multiple use of dialyzers.

Following the initial reports of repeated hemodialysis for chronic renal failure from the Seattle group (1, 4), other nephrologists also initiated chronic treatment programs (5). Disposable coil dialyzers were readily available in many facilities (6), so repetitive hemodialysis was begun in many centers with coil dialyzers despite their large blood compartment volumes (300 to 600 ml) as compared to those of the 2-layered Kiil dialyzer. To avoid circulatory instability, blood was needed to prime the coil before each dialysis. After dialysis, the blood left in the coil was discarded.

To avoid such waste a technique was developed in which, at the end of dialysis, blood was removed from the coil under sterile conditions into a blood donor collection bag and stored at the blood bank until the patient's next treatment. This type of blood 'donation' differed logistically and administratively from approved blood banking procedures. In 1964 Shaldon and colleagues (7), to avoid excessive blood handling, devised a method by which the coil, with its contained blood, was refrigerated at the end of dialysis. The coil dialyzer and blood were then used for the next dialysis. This was the first dialyzer reuse. The main problem with this technique was the occasional development of pyrogenic reactions when the blood and coil were reused. The method became outmoded as coil and other dialyzers with smaller blood compartments became available.

In 1967 Pollard and co-workers (8) described a technique for reusing the Kiil dialyzer which employed cleaning with sodium hypochlorite, rinsing and sterilization with formalin. Blood handling was avoided since the blood within the dialyzer could be returned at the end of treatment, leaving the dialyzer filled with sterile saline.

Stimuli for the development of reuse of the Kiil dialyzer were the desire to reduce the time and effort

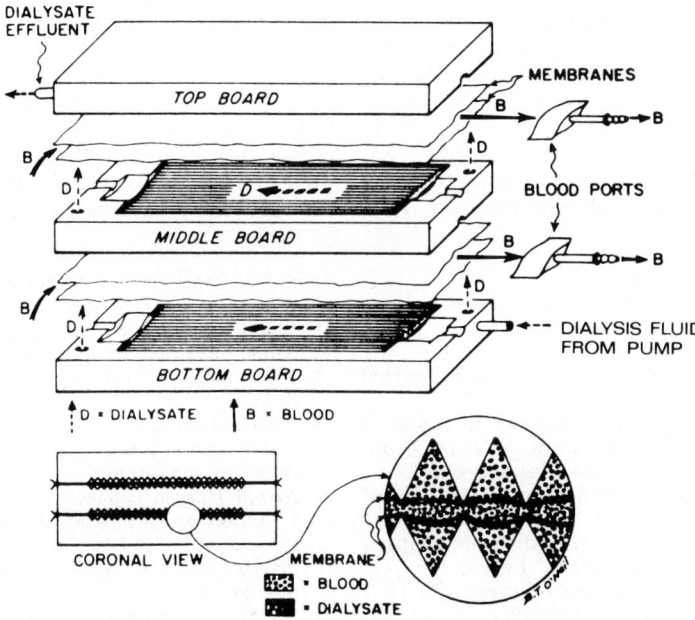

Figure 1. Structure and components of the Kiil parallel flow boards. (Not to scale). Reproduced from Myers (3, [with permission]).

required to assemble the equipment and to conserve materials, so reducing cost. Since the sterilization was the same for initial and repeated use and the rinsing and cleaning processes posed no obvious hazards, the safety of the procedure was anticipated and subsequently demonstrated.

Employing variations of the techniques of Shaldon and of Scribner, multiple use of dialyzers has continued since 1967. It is widely employed throughout the world. Data are available from Europe (9–11), Australia and New Zealand (12), Hawaii and the South Pacific (13, 14) and the United States (15).

Continued multiple use of dialyzers does seem appropriate in view of the favorable results for mortality, morbidity, complications, dialyzer function, biocompatibility and the implications for cost containment. As with any medical treatment, the process has evolved and developed with continued familiarity and control. Figure 2 summarizes factors influencing the evolution of reuse procedures since 1962. Further optimization and standardization of multiple use techniques is required for continued development of the method.

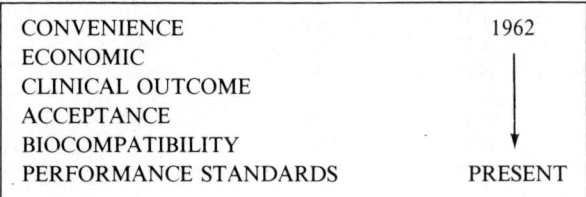

Figure 2. Factors influencing evolution of dialyzer reuse procedures.

COMPONENTS OF REUSE PROCESSING TECHNIQUES

The processing of a dialyzer for subsequent use at the end of a treatment consists of two main phases: 1) the dialyzer is stored for later use; 2) the dialyzer is prepared for use when the next treatment is due. In published procedures the details of the methods used for these two phases vary considerably, often with insufficient definition of the exact technical conditions to permit validation or replication. This chapter analyzes the components of these techniques and presents the results of certain studies that help define the parameters and conditions for optimization of multiple use techniques. Although tubing, when re-used, is reprocessed along with the dialyzer, this subject is treated separately below.

Storage of dialyzers

Storage of the dialyzer involves the following processes:
1) rinsing to effect maximum removal of blood,
2) cleaning to remove residual blood components,
3) sterilization of the blood and dialysate compartments.

Rinsing

The rinsing process begins after the blood has been returned to the patient by displacement with saline. The dialyzer usually is then transported to a separate area where the appropriate connections are made for rinsing blood and dialysate compartments. This should be accomplished within 10 min, if possible. Conditions for rinsing various dialyzers have included an air rinse technique (8) and fluid rinses employing tap water (16, 17), saline (18, 19), reverse osmosis water (20), deionized water (21), and heparinized water (22, 23) or heparized saline (24). Water temperature, flow rate, pressure (continuous or pulsatile), use of reverse flushing and, for hollow fiber dialyzers, reverse ultrafiltration are variables in the rinsing procedure. The published literature does not provide sufficient data or definition to identify the essential factors in adequate rinsing techniques.

To establish whether special steps in the rinsing procedure would result in more effective reprocessing, a comparison of a simple rinsing process with unidirectional water flush of blood and dialysate compartments ('simple case') was made with that of an involved pro-

Table 1. Simple case rinse procedure.

1. Blood rinse-back with sterile saline.
2. Saline-filled dialyzer to storage room within 5 min.
3. Place dialyzer in rack with arterial side (red headers) down.
4. Attach room temperature RO water line to arterial side of blood compartment and flush for 2 min at 25 psi [a] with 3.5 to 4.0 l/min, tap headers to remove pockets of air.
5. After 2 min, disconnect RO water line from blood side of dialyzer.
6. Connect RO water to dialysate side, rinse dialysate compartment one minute; flow 3.5 to 4.0 l/min.
7. Wash both compartments of the dialyzer through with 2.0% formaldehyde and leave this agent in the dialyzer.

[a] 25 psi = 1,7 atm.

Table 2. Complex case rinse procedure.

1. Blood rinse-back with sterile saline.
2. Saline-filled dialyzer to storage room within 5 min.
3. Place dialyzer in rack with arterial side (red header) down.
4. Attach dialysate line to arterial side of blood compartment and flush for 5 min at 500 ml/min with warmed (37°C) dialysate; tap headers to remove pockets of air.
5. Attach Hansen connectors to both dialysate ports. Run 37°C RO water through the dialysate compartment with the inlet at the dialysate port nearest the arterial end of the dialyzer. Flush at 5 psi [a], 500 m/min, for 5 min and tap to remove air.
6. Once air is removed, clamp inflow and outflow dialysate compartment lines. Continue dialysate flow through the blood compartment.
7. Immediately after clamping both dialysate lines, release the clamp on the inflow line and abruptly increase the pressure in the dialysate compartment to 25 psi [b]. Discontinue flow through the blood compartment by clamping the inflow line to the blood compartment.
8. Release the pressure in the dialysate compartment after 5 min and flush the blood compartment with 37°C dialysate for one minute.
9. Repeat steps 7 and 8 six times. The direction of flushing of the blood compartment is reversed after three releases of pressure. Tap headers occasionally.
10. After six releases, flush 37°C RO water through the dialysate compartment and 37°C dialysate through the blood compartment for 5 min.
11. Wash both compartments of the dialyzer through with 2.0% formaldehyde and leave this agent in the dialyzer.

[a] 5 psi = 0,34 atm.
[b] 25 psi = 1.7 atm.

Table 3. Summary of experimental rinse procedures.

	Rinse procedure	
Variable	Simple case	Complex case
Solution		
Blood side	RO water	Dialysate
Dialysate side	RO water	RO water
Temperature	20–25 °C	37 °C
Time	short	long
Flow	fast	slow
Pressure pulsing	no	yes
Reverse UF	no	yes
Reverse flushing	no	yes

Table 4. Comparison of properties of Travenol 1200 dialyzers processed after one use by simple and complex rinsing procedures [a].

	Mean [b] ± 2 S.D.			P-value		
Property	Simple (S) (N = 9)	Complex (C) (N = 9)	New (N) (N = 8)	S vs C	S vs N	C vs N
Cell Vol, ml [b]	107 ± 5	104 ± 7	110 ± 4	NS [d]	0.015	0.0005
C_{urea}, ml/min	156 ± 16	165 ± 9	164 ± 10	0.02	0.04	NS
C_{creat}, ml/min	125 ± 23	136 ± 8	131 ± 11	0.02	NS	NS
C_{inulin}, ml/min	3.3 ± 1.8	3.3 ± 3.0	3.8 ± 1.4	NS	NS	NS
Q_F, [c]						
100 mm Hg	4.9 ± 0.6	4.8 ± 0.6	4.8 ± 0.6	NS	NS	NS
200 mm Hg	11.0 ± 1.8	10.4 ± 1.5	9.8 ± 3.2	NS	NS	NS

[a] From Ketteringham et al. (26 [with permission]).
[b] 'Cell volume' represents the total intraluminal volume of the fibers in the dialyzer plus the volume in the headers.
[c] Q_B = 200 ml/min; Q_D = 500 ml/min, Q_F = ultrafiltration, ml/min.
[d] Not significant by Wilcoxon Matched-pairs Signed Rank Test.

Table 5. Comparison of properties of once used and new Travenol 1200 dialyzers rinsed by the standard Manhattan Kidney Center procedure [a].

Property	Mean ± 2 S.D.		P-value
	Once used	New	
FBV, ml [b]	104±6	110±6	0.0001
C_{urea}, ml/min	166±6	164±10	NS
C_{creat}, ml/min	135±7	131±11	NS
C_{inulin}, ml/min	3.7±1.0	3.8±1.4	NS
Q_F, ml/min [c]			
100 mm Hg	5.2±0.6	4.8±1.2	NS
200 mm Hg	10.7±1.8	9.8±3.2	NS

[a] From Ketteringham et al. (26 [with permission]).
[b] Total intraluminal volume of the hollow fibers is called the 'fiber bundle volume' (FBV).
[c] Q_B = 200 ml/min; Q_D = 500 ml/min; Q_F = ultrafiltration ml/min.

cess utilizing altered direction of water flow, pressure pulsing and reverse ultrafiltration ('complex case'), using pairs of once-used hollow fiber dialyzers from the same patients (20, 25). The rinsing procedures are described in Tables 1 and 2 and compared in Table 3. The results of rinsing studies on Travenol 1200 hollow fiber dialyzers (26) are summarized in Table 4.

These data suggest enhanced urea and creatinine clearances with the complex case rinsing procedure but no change in inulin clearance or ultrafiltration. These slight differences in clearances with the more involved rinsing procedures must be balanced against the extra time required. A standard rinsing procedure intermediate between these two techniques has been used extensively at the Manhattan Kidney Center (See Appendix A), and found to be satisfactory (Table 5).

Cleaning

In the cleaning process a chemical agent is used to remove any blood remaining in the dialyzer after the rinse process. Cleaning precedes sterilization of the dialyzer. Because cell volume of hollow fiber dialyzers may be well maintained by rinsing alone, multiple use techniques may be entirely satisfactory without cleaning agents. To determine their usefulness, a variety of cleaning agents has been studied employing used hollow fiber dialyzers with unacceptably low cell volumes as an index of cleaning efficiency. A similar parameter is not available for coil dialyzers or plate dialyzers.

Sodium hypochlorite, first used by Pollard and colleagues (8) for cleaning Kiil dialyzers, has been widely used for cleaning coil dialyzers (20, 27) and flat plate dialyzers (20, 28, 29) but until recently (30) has not been used for hollow fiber dialyzers (20, 31–33). Because other cleaning agents have been used infrequently, the impact of various cleaning agents on decreased cell volume has been evaluated by perfusing the dialyzer with the test substance for 5 to 20 min at 200 to 250 ml/min or at 100 ml/min. At 5 min intervals cell volume was measured. The test substance, if ineffective in the short-term study, was also allowed to remain in the dialyzer blood compartment for up to 48 h. Cell volume was measured after 3 h and 24 h. All test substances were evaluated on three different dialyzers demonstrating a range of cell volumes. Because household bleach (5.25% sodium hypochlorite) was an effective regenerative cleaning agent for hollow fiber dialyzers, it was used as a standard to which the others (listed in Table 8) were compared. Undiluted bleach (5.25% sodium hypochlorite) was as effective at 25 °C as at 37 °C and increased cell volume regardless of how often the dialyzer had been previously used. Perfusing the blood compartment with undiluted bleach at room temperature for 7 min at 250 ml/min conveniently and effectively cleansed these hollow fiber dialyzers.

Figure 3 shows the kinetics of cleaning Travenol 1200 dialyzers with 5.25%, 0.525% and 0.21% sodium hypochlorite, when the blood compartment is perfused at 250 ml/min. With each concentration cell volume increased to 90 to 100 ml, even when the initial volume before bleach treatment was as low as 26 ml. (The mean cell volume of several new Travenol 1200 dialyzers was 115 ml.) At a flow rate of 250 ml/min the half-time for cleaning these dialyzers was about one minute when per-

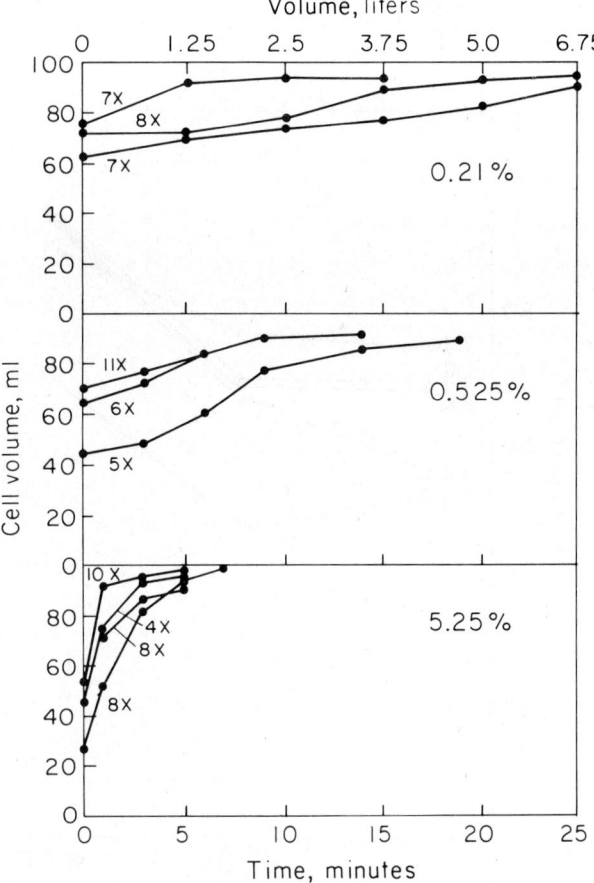

Figure 3. Effect of different concentrations of sodium hypochlorite on cell volume of reused dialyzers (see text).

fusing the blood compartment with 5.25%, 6 min with 0.525% and 20 min with 0.21% sodium hypochlorite.

Bleach was equally effective as a cleaning agent of used Cordis-Dow 3500 hollow fiber dialyzers. Neither dialyzer can be left for a long time, however, with undiluted bleach in the blood compartment. Within 20 to 30 min, bleach interacts exothermically with these dialyzers, which soon become porous and leak.

As shown in Figure 4 the cell volume of only one of five dialyzers increased after perfusion with undiluted hydrogen peroxide (H_2O_2) (3%) for periods ranging from 5 to 20 min. After rinsing the H_2O_2 from the blood compartment each dialyzer was flushed with undiluted bleach for 7 min which increased the cell volume substantially. Thus, H_2O_2 does not clean the Travenol 1200 dialyzer blood compartment effectively. Dialyzers treated for 20 min with H_2O_2 leaked badly after bleach treatment.

Seven detergents, chosen to represent the possible charge states of detergents (cationic, anionic, non-ionic and zwitterionic) were evaluated (Table 6). An eighth detergent, a commercial mixture of anionic and non-ionic detergents and containing solubilizers and a complexing agent produced extensive foam, did not improve cell volume in preliminary experiments and was not investigated further. Each detergent was evaluated both by perfusing the blood compartment of three multiply

Table 6. Cleaning agents for evaluation in used dialyzers.

Sodium hypochlorite
Hydrogen peroxide
Detergents
    Cationic
    Anionic
    Zwitterionic
    Nonionic
Enzymes
    Trypsin
    Chymotrypsin
    Elastase
    Plasmin
EDTA [a]

[a] Ethylene diamine tetra-acetic acid.

used Travenol 1200 dialyzers with low cell volumes for up to 20 min as well as by incubation for 18 to 48 h intervals.

Figures 5 and 6 show the effects observed with two of the cationic detergents. Cetylpyridinium chloride (Figure 5) and the mixed alkyltetramethylammonium bromide (Figure 6) increased cell volume about 15% in three out of five dialyzers incubated overnight with these detergents. The third cationic detergent benzylammonium chloride (Totil), produced increases in cell volume of at most 5% during overnight incubation. In contrast, a

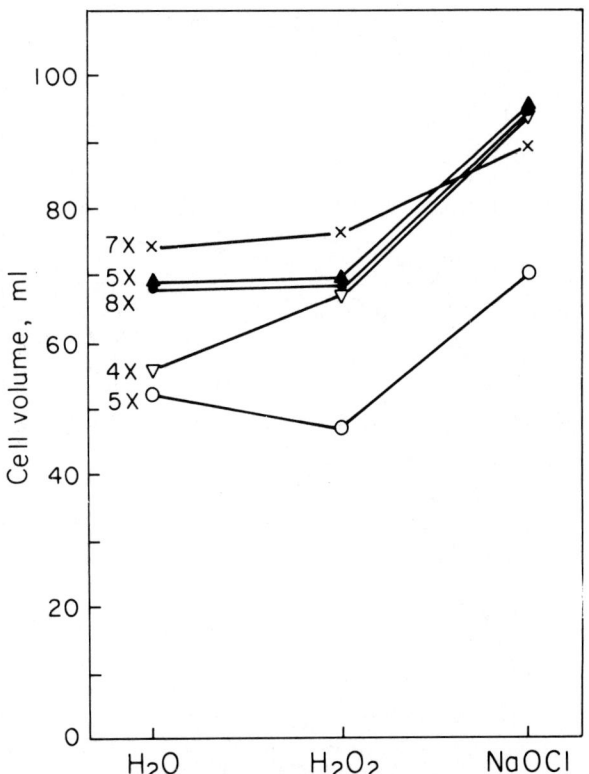

Figure 4. Effect of hydrogen peroxide treatment on cell volume of reused dialyzers. (see text).

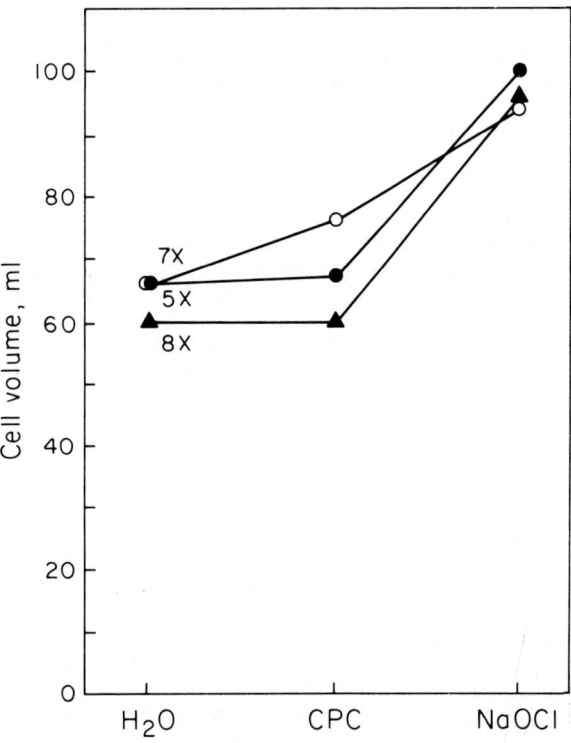

Figure 5. Effect of 1% cetylpyridinium chloride (CPG) treatment on cell volume of reused dialyzers.

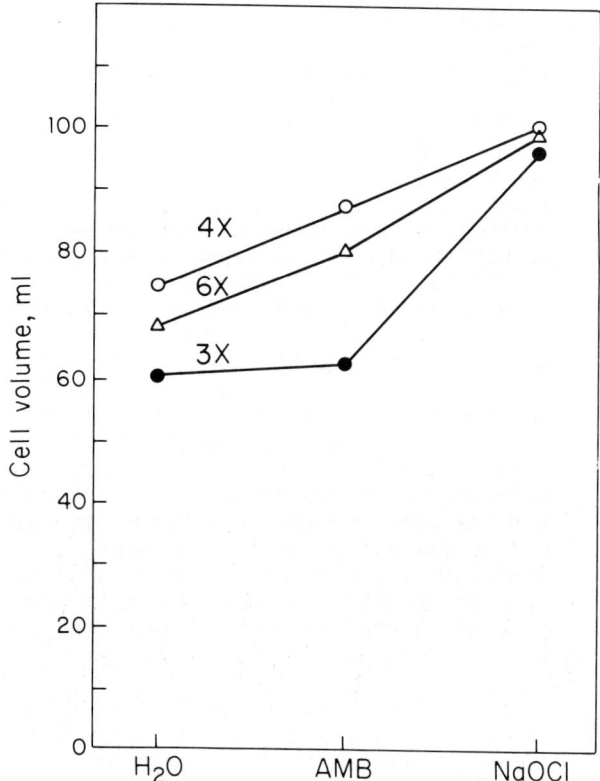

Figure 6. Effect of 1% mixed alkyltetramethylammonium bromide (AMB) on cell volume of multiply used dialyzers.

7 min treatment with bleach substantially increased the cell volume of these dialyzers.

The anionic detergents sodium dodecyl sulphate and -cholate increased the cell volume only about 5% in half of the dialyzers, as did the non-ionic detergent Triton X-100 and the zwitterionic detergent Zwittergent. Again, with each dialyzer a 7 min treatment with bleach caused large increases in cell volume. The proteolytic enzymes trypsin, α-chymotrypsin and plasmin were also ineffective cleaners of hollow fiber dialyzers despite incubation from 3 to 48 h. Elastase, on the other hand, modestly increased cell volume (Figure 7). With one dialyzer cell volume increased about 10% after 4 h, while with the other cell volume increased 10% and 20% after 48 h incubation. With bleach, however, a substantial further increase of the cell volume of these dialyzers was obtained.

With the calcium chelator, EDTA, a 20 h incubation in the Travenol 1200 dialyzers did not increase the cell volume of two out of three dialyzers tested. The cell

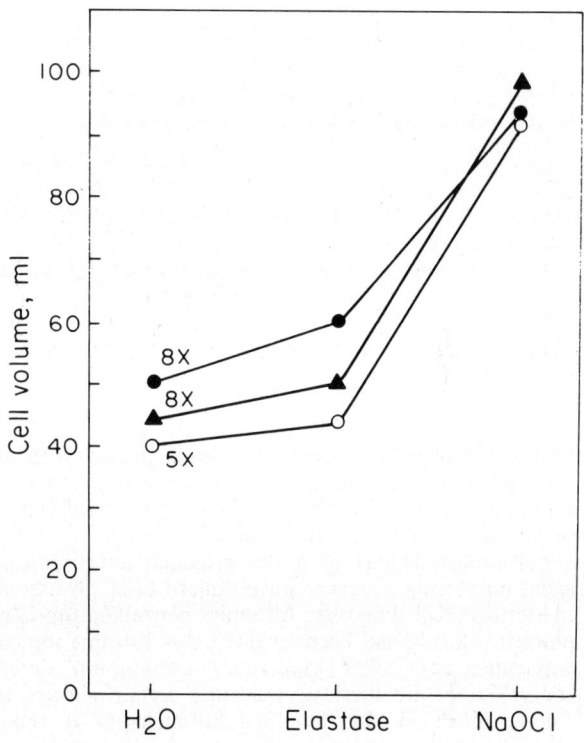

Figure 7. Effect of 0.1 mg/ml elastase treatment on cell volume of reused dialyzers.

Table 7. Clearances and ultrafiltration rates for multiple-used Travenol 1200 HF dialyzers after standard rinse + bleach after last rinse [a].

	No uses	Cell vol.[b] after/before bleaching (ml)	Clearance (ml/min)				Ultrafiltration ml		Bleach
			Urea	Creatinine	Inulin	B_{12}	100 mm TMP^a	200 mm TMP	
n = 7	6±3	97±4 70±16	167±4	135±1	4.0	29±4	5.5±8	11.9±1.5	5.25% NaOCl 37°C
n = 9	7±2	93±4 54±12	168±6	134±5	4.3±5	26±3	5.6±0.5	12.2±0.7	5.25% NaOCl 25°C
n = 2	8±1	97±4 62±6	164±6	133±2	3.3	22±3	5.2±0.2	11.2±0.8	0.21% NaOCl
n = 2	6±1	93±1 48±14	166	131	4.6	25±4	5.5	11.7±0.9	0.53% NaOCl
n = 1	7	96 74	159	132	9.0	20	6.0	12.5	5.25% NaOCl+H_2O_2

[a] Modified from Ketteringham et al. (26 [with permission]).
[b] Cell volume: see legend Table 4.
[c] TMP = transmembrane pressure.

Table 8. Functional comparison of used Travenol 1200 dialyzers treated with NaOCl and new dialyzers [a].

Property	New (N = 8) Mean ± 2 S.D.	NaOCl-treated (N = 16) Mean ± 2 S.D.	P-value
FBV, ml [b]	110 ± 6	95 ± 8	0.0001
C_{urea}, ml/min	164 ± 10	167 ± 10	NS
C_{creat}, ml/min	131 ± 11	134 ± 7	NS
C_{B12}, ml/min	—	27 ± 8	—
C_{inulin}, ml/min	3.8 ± 1.4	4.7 ± 0.8	NS
Q_F, ml/min			
100 mm Hg	4.8 ± 1.2	5.6 ± 1.2	0.02
200 mm Hg	9.8 ± 3.2	12.1 ± 2.2	0.0007

[a] From Ketteringham et al. (26 [with permission]).
[b] FBV = fiber bundle volume (see legend Table 5).

volume of the third increased 20% after 10 min, but then stabilized.

Thus, sodium hypochlorite was the only agent that effectively cleaned hollow fiber dialyzers. As shown in Tables 7 and 8, function of dialyzers treated with sodium hypochlorite is essentially normalized with this treatment (26).

Sterilization

Filling the blood and dialysate compartments with an appropriate concentration of the selected antimicrobial agent and leaving this agent in the dialyzer until subsequent use is the final step in dialyzer storage.

Formaldehyde has been the principal antimicrobial agent for storing dialyzers since Pollard et al. (8) used it to sterilize Kiil dialyzers. Although benzalkonium (Zephiran) chloride had been tried (23, 34–36), this topical antiseptic, and other quaternary ammonium detergents (37–41) are ineffective against certain species of *Pseudomonas* (35, 36, 42, 43). Outbreaks of *P. cepacia* (35) and *P. aeruginosa* (36) septicemia have occurred in dialysis patients when dialyzers were stored with this agent.

Although 27% saline has controlled bacterial contamination (18, 44) Gutch et al. (45) demonstrated that this concentration of salt is not entirely adequate for this purpose. Wielgosz et al. (46) reported using 5% acetic acid but experience is too limited to judge its effectiveness. Glutaraldehyde and an iodophor are being employed in the United Kingdom, while peracetic acid (Acetoper) has had limited use in the Federal Republic of Germany. Published reports of the technique and the microbiologic effects are too limited with these agents to permit evaluation. Activated chlorine dioxide also has been used to disinfect dialyzers but the published data indicate inadequacy.

Process controls to determine that bacteriologic control has been accomplished in a reprocessing procedure should meet the following criteria:
1. A minimum of 20 samples obtained by the technique of membrane filtration from dialyzers reprocessed by a standard procedure should all have negative cultures.
2. Appropriate bacteriologic studies of the total dialysis system should include cultures of incoming supply water, treated water prior to distribution to individual patient stations on prior mixing with concentrate, and the effluent dialysate prior to discard. Adequate disinfection of the total dialysis system is essential whether or not reprocessing of dialyzers occurs in the facility. Microbial contamination of water used to prepare dialysis fluids and the dialysate should meet or exceed proposed guidelines (47–50). For water the bacterial count should be less than 100/ml and for dialysis fluid less than 1,000/ml.

With single-pass systems, dialysate samples should be collected at the point where the fluid leaves the dialyzer. In recirculating systems, samples should be collected at the periphery of the recirculation cannister containing the coil dialyzer. Samples should be collected at least bimonthly and whenever pyrogenic and/or septicemic complications are suspected.
3. The log kill of the sterilant should be defined by standard bacteriologic techniques *in vitro* and by dialyzer inoculation studies. The conditions used in the total dialysis system should be well within the safety margin of the documented log kill capability of the concentration of the sterilant employed.

Sterility implies total absence of viable organisms in a solution or an apparatus. Sterilants are agents to achieve sterility, but this condition must be defined in terms of testing procedures and a particular set of conditions.

The United States Pharmacopeia guidelines for sterility testing (51) are used by manufacturers of new dialyzers. These guidelines are not rigorous enough for all prevailing considerations, however. Therefore, testing procedures and conditions must be specified. Sterility is a condition achieved in a statistical and legal sense and defined by using specified concentrations of sterilants under carefully described conditions.

The effectiveness of a sterilant is evaluated in terms of particular microbiologic organisms, the number of these organisms, the concentration of the sterilant, the duration of exposure of the organisms to the sterilant and the culture technique by which the action of the sterilant is tested. Clearly, a sterilant effective under one set of conditions may have its concentration reduced to an ineffective level under other conditions. Alternatively, the number of bacteria to which the sterilant is exposed may exceed the number which that concentration of the sterilant can eradicate. Bacteria vary in their individual susceptibility to sterilants and a given sterilant concentration may be effective against one organism but not against others. Inadequate exposure time of the bacteria to the sterilant can fail to kill the organisms. Further, the technique by which the action of the sterilant is assayed is of critical importance in investigation. An appropriately rigorous assay requires use of a large volume of fluid, whenever possible, with filtration of fluid by a membrane of an appropriate diameter by the standard membrane filtration technique (51).

Sterilant action against test organisms is defined in terms of a log kill function. Thus, an agent with a 5-log

Table 9. Lowest concentration of each antimicrobial required to give a 6-log kill of each indicator organism in 5 h [a].

Antimicrobial	Indicator organism			
	C. albicans	E. coli	P. Aeruginosa	Staph. aureus
Formaldehyde	0.1%	—	0.05%	—
Glutaraldehyde	—	0.05%	0.05%	0.05%
Betadine	0.8%	0.8%	0.8%	0.8%
Acetoper	0.2%	0.2%	0.2%	0.2%

[a] From Ketteringham et al. (26 [with permission]).

kill function against 10^5 bacteria/ml would reduce the number of bacterial or colony-forming units (CFU) to 10^0/ml, or 1 organism/ml. The reduction would be $10^5 \rightarrow 10^0$ (i.e. $100,000 \rightarrow 1$) = 99,999/ml. An agent with a 2-log kill function would reduce the number of bacteria from 10^5/ml to 10^3/ml. In this case the reduction would be $10^5 \rightarrow 10^3$ (i.e. $100,000 \rightarrow 1,000$) = 99,000/ml.

Sterility of a particular constellation of organisms which pose risk is achieved, when the log-kill property of the antimicrobial agent is known. Sterility is documented by defining conditions and demonstrating that they have been met in a specified number of samples.

The minimum concentrations of a sterilant required to achieve *in vitro* a 6-log kill in 5 h and in 24 h with a number of test organisms (*C. albicans, E. coli, P. aeruginosa* and *staph aureus* [25, 26]) are shown in Tables 9 and 10. The minimum concentrations required were: formaldehyde 0.1%; glutaraldehyde 0.1%; Betadine 0.8% and Acetoper 0.2%. The minimum concentration of formaldehyde achieving 6-log kill of the test organisms is much lower than the 1.5 to 4.0% concentrations ordinarily employed in multiple use techniques.

Betadine, a topical antiseptic, was chosen only because it served as a convenient source of active iodine. The iodine-organic complex would dissociate when diluted and presumably remain effective even after considerable dilution.

Gram-negative bacteria can multiply rapidly in many hospital-associated fluids including distilled, deionized, reverse osmosis and softened water (52–56). These bacteria can proliferate excessively in dialysate and cause

Table 10. Lowest concentration of two antimicrobials required to give a 6-log kill of each indicator organism in 24 h [a].

Antimicrobial	Indicator organism		
	C. albicans	E. coli	S. aureus
Formaldehyde	—	0.05%	0.1%
Glutaraldehyde	0.1%	—	—

[a] From Ketteringham et al. (26 [with permission]).

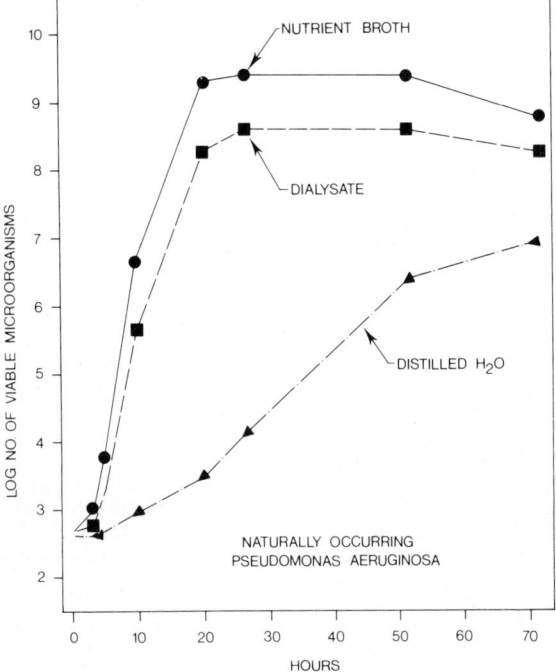

Figure 8. Comparative growth of *Ps aeruginosa* in distilled water, nutrient broth and dialysis fluid. From Favero et al. (53 [with permission]).

pyrogenic reactions, sepsis or both. Favero et al. (53) demonstrated the growth of these organisms in water and the effect of dialysis fluid in enhancing this growth curve (Figure 8). Factors influencing the microbial contamination and the variety of gram-negative bacteria detected in hemodialysis systems are summarized in Tables 11 and 12.

The number of the gram-negative water bacteria in post-hemodialyzer dialysate correlates with the incidence of pyrogenic reactions in the dialysis patients (Table 13). Virtually all such gram-negative bacteria contain lipopolysaccharide materials (endotoxin). Endotoxin has a molecular weight of approximately one million and cannot pass through the intact dialyzer membranes (57, 58) which have molecular weight limits in the range of 10^4. Bernick and coworkers (59, 60) confirmed that endotoxin does not cross the intact dialyzer membrane. Alterations can occur in the dialyzer membrane that permit passage of bacterial endotoxin, however. Therefore, water employed for reprocessing of dialyzers should be free of detectable endotoxin.

In addition to the gram-negative bacteria, some non-tuberculosis mycobacteria grow quite rapidly in distilled water and are more resistant to disinfectants than the gram-negative bacteria (61). The most resistant of these strains as judged from acute studies employing 8% formaldehyde (61) at 25 °C is the TM-7 strain of *M. chelonei* (Figure 9). In view of the unique nature and resistance of this organism to antimicrobials, we evaluated

Table 11. Factors influencing microbial contamination in hemodialysis systems [a].

		Comments
I.	Water supply	
	A. Source	
	Ground water	Can be a source of endotoxin and bacteria
	Treated surface water	
	B. Treatment	
	1. None	Not recommended
	2. Filtration	
	Prefilter	Unless properly disinfected can act as bacterial reservoir
	Absolute	
	Carbon	
	3. Ion exchange	
	Softening	Not recommended: both softeners and deionizers can be significant bacterial reservoirs and do not remove endotoxins
	Deionizing	
	4. Reverse osmosis	Highly efficient; removes bacteria and endotoxins: can be colonized downstream from membrane if not properly disinfected
II.	Water and dialysis fluid distribution systems	
	A. Distribution pipes	
	Size	Oversized diameter and length increase bacterial reservoir for both treated water and centrally prepared dialysate
	Construction	Rough joints, dead-ends and unused branches can act as bacterial reservoirs
	Elevation	Outlet taps at highest elevation to prevent loss of disinfectant
III.	Dialysis machines	
	A. Single pass	Disinfectant should have contact with all parts of the machine
	B. Recirculating-single pass or recirculating (batch)	Recirculating pumps and machine design allow for massive contamination levels if not properly disinfected. Overnight formaldehyde treatment is recommended

[a] From Favero et al. (53 [with permission]).

Table 12. Types of Gram-negative water bacteria detected in dialysis systems [a].

Pseudomonas	Achromobacter
Falvobacterium	Aeromonas
Acinetobacter	Serratia
Alcaligenes	Moraxella
Erwinia	

[a] From Favero et al. (53 [with permission]).

Table 13. Relationship between levels of Gram-negative water bacteria in post membrane dialysate and attack rates of pyrogenic reactions among dialysis patients during an outbreak [a].

Log 10 No/ml	No dialyses	Pyrogenic reactions	Attack rates
1–100	25	1 [b]	4%
100–10,000	31	4	13%
10,000+	21	5	24%

[a] From Favero et al. (53 [with permission]).
[b] Questionable laboratory data with sample taken during this reaction.

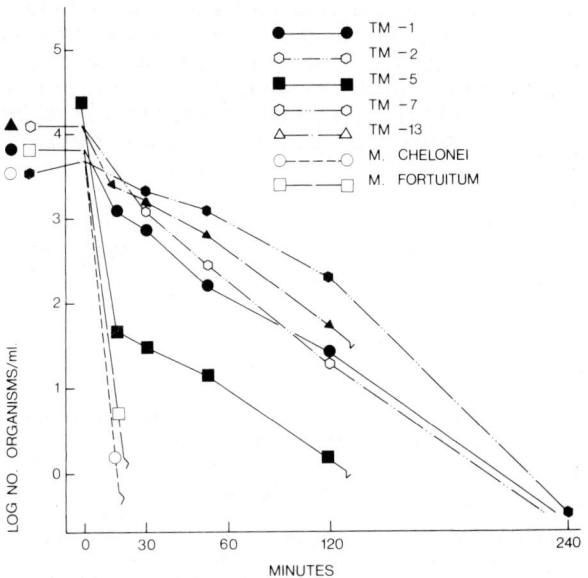

Figure 9. Comparative resistance of mycobacterial organisms in distilled water to 8% formaldehyde at 25 C. From Carson et al. (61 [with permission]).

Table 14. Growth curve of *M chelonei*-like organisms in varying concentrations of formaldehyde.

	HCHO Conc	Concentration (CFU/ml)	log kill
Initial	0%	1.9×10^6	—
After 24 hours:	0%	2.2×10^6	0
	2.0%	5.0×10^2	4
	4.0%	8.5×10^1	5
	6.0%	3×10^0	6
	8.0%	no growth	6

the log kill function of formaldehyde after 24 h exposure at concentrations ranging from 2 to 8% (Table 14).

Formaldehyde has been the principal antimicrobial agent used during the 15 year experience with multiple use of dialyzers. No infectious complications have resulted from multiple use techniques when appropriate concentrations of formaldehyde were employed with well defined techniques. The *in vitro* effectiveness of formaldehyde in minimum concentrations against the more common bacteria and in greater concentrations against the relatively resistant organisms presented herein support the value of formaldehyde for sterilization with multiple use techniques.

Preparation for subsequent use

Dialyzers must be flushed to remove the stored antimicrobial agent prior to their next use. Procedures have been described for flushing the Kiil dialyzer (8), disposable parallel plate dialyzers (62, 63), coil dialyzers (18, 23, 31, 34, 35) and hollow fiber dialyzers (31, 64, 65). Preparation for use involves rinsing with 1 to 5 l of sterile water and/or 1 to 3 l of sterile saline with or without added heparin. Water or dialysis fluid is used to flush the dialysate compartment. The Clinitest tablet method has been used to screen for residual formaldehyde (when water or dialysis fluid without dextrose is used to flush). A Clinitest reaction upon initiating the flushing procedure confirms the presence of formaldehyde in the hemodialyzer and it is essential to demonstrate a negative Clinitest reaction after flushing.

When standard preparation techniques for reuse are employed (Appendix B) the flushing procedure will reduce the concentration of formaldehyde in the initial effluent which would enter the patient (25) to less than 2 µg/ml. This reduction in concentration is documented by the negative Clinitest reaction.

Few studies have described methods to optimize the flushing of the antimicrobial agent from the dialyzer. Ogden and associates (66) used the more sensitive Hantzsch reaction with (acetyl-acetone and ammonium salts) (67) to determine residual formaldehyde concentrations in Kiil, Gambro and Cordis-Dow hollow fiber dialyzers. An increase of formaldehyde concentrations in the effluent after blood lines were clamped and then released demonstrated the reversible binding of formaldehyde to the dialyzer membrane. Release of formaldehyde from the membrane occurs because of a concentration gradient between the membrane and the blood compartment. Formaldehyde in the blood compartment is dialyzed into the dialysate compartment from which it is removed by the flushing. Recently Lewis and coworkers (68) emphasized the importance of formaldehyde removal in the dialysate effluent by a dialysis fluid rinse of extended duration.

In addition, particulate matter must be removed from the effluent of the stored dialyzer. Particulate matter consists of extraneous, mobile, undissolved substances, other than gas bubbles (51), in a solution. There should be not more than 50 particles/ml > 10.0 µm and no more than 5 particles/ml > 25.0 µm in effective linear dimension (51).

Particulate matter collected onto membrane filters is quantified by light microscopy at 100× magnification (51). This method is currently used to assess particulates in the effluent from new and used dialyzers (25). Gravimetric determination of particulates by membrane filtration also has been attempted (26).

Reuse of tubing

Reuse of dialyzer tubing, reported many times (8, 13, 20, 24, 28, 29, 32, 62, 64, 69–77), has been incidental to dialyzer reuse in terms of technique, and there has been little description of procedures or difficulties, if any, associated with reuse of tubing. A separate standardized procedure is not available since the conditions of rinsing, cleaning and sterilization will be those used for the dialyzer. Where fibrin or other proteinaceous material is noted in the mesh of the bubble trap, methods wherein the bubble trap is filled with bleach solution, allowed to stand, then flushed, should be defined.

FUNCTIONAL STUDIES OF REUSED DIALYZERS

There are numerous reports of clearance and ultrafiltration studies on dialyzers which have been reused a variable number of times. They document the evolution of the multiple use techniques but fail to provide a consistent body of interpretable data.

Table 15. Relationship of clearance to physical characteristics of reused plate and coil dialyzers.

Membrane area	Membrane permeability	Clearance
NC	NC	NC
NC	↓	↓
NC	↑	↑
↓	NC	↓
↓	↑	NC

NC = no change.

Table 16. Clearances and ultrafiltration rates for multiply-used Travenol 1200 HF dialyzers [a] after standard rinse.

Dialyzer	No Uses	Cell volume	Clearance (ml/min)				Ultrafiltration ml/min	
			Urea	Creatinine	Inulin	Vitamin B_{12}	100 mm TMP [b]	200 mm TMP
Used n = 16	6±3	76±15	148±15	111±18	3.1±0.9	19±5	4.7±0.6	10.4±1.0
New n = 8	0	110±2	164±5	131±6	3.8±0.7	—	4.8±0.6	9.8±1.6

[a] Modified from Ketteringham et al. (26 [with permission]).
[b] TMP = transmembrane pressure.

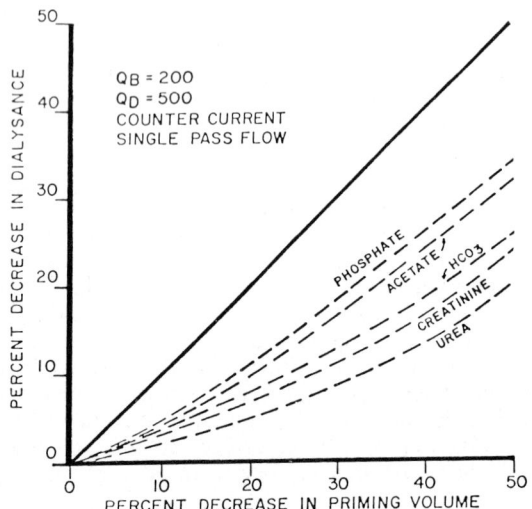

Figure 10. Relationship between dialysance and priming volume for C-Dak 1.8 hollow fiber dialyzer. From Gotch (71 [with permission]).

Table 17. Annual mortality in dialysis centers [a].

Study	Patients (number)		Mortality (%)		P
	reusing	not reusing	reusing	not reusing	
Five European countries (EDTA Registry, 1976)	591	3491	6.8	8.8	0.057
Five European Countries (EDTA Registry, 1977)					
Ages 35-44	175	749	1.2	8.8	0.0001
Ages 45-54	242	1021	5.0	5.3	0.40
United Kingdom	98	130	6.5	15.6	0.022

[a] From Lowrie and Hakim (72 [with permission]).

Interpretation of a change in clearance or ultrafiltration rate of a multiple used dialyzer is difficult to evaluate unless there is a concomitant ability to measure the (functional) surface area of the dialyzer. For example, reduction of clearance in a parallel plate dialyzer may be due to a lower functional surface area of the dialyzer or to a decrease in the membrane permeability or both. Alterations of clearances and ultrafiltration rates cannot be interpreted in the light of these permutations when techniques for multiple use vary widely or are insufficiently defined.

Because membrane surface area correlates with cell volume of hollow fiber dialyzers, changes in clearance and ultrafiltration rates can be related to membrane area or permeability with this dialyzer, unlike the coil and flat plate dialyzers as illustrated in Table 15. Gotch (78) showed that changes in clearances of hollow fiber dialyzers are somewhat less than predicted from a linear relationship to changes in fiber bundle volume (Figure 10).

For multiple used Travenol 1200 HF dialyzers using our standard rinse technique (Appendix A), clearances of small solutes and ultrafiltration rates correlate and are satisfactorily maintained (Table 16).

PATIENT EXPERIENCE

Multiple use dialyzer experiences should be compared with those obtained from initial dialyzer use techniques in terms of patient survival, morbidity, and evidence of biocompatibility.

Survival

Patient survival data on reused dialyzers were collected by the Registry of the European Dialysis and Transplant Associaton (EDTA) in 1976 and 1977. The data from eight European countries (9-11) (Table 17) indicate that patients treated with reused dialyzers fare as well or better than those treated with single use dialyzers (79).

Morbidity

With Ogden's description (80) of the 'new-dialyzer syndrome', a constellation of symptoms has been identified with increasing frequency in recent years. This reaction to treatment with a new dialyzer is characterized by back or chest pain, respiratory distress, malaise and sometimes chills or fever. Reactions may be mild but occasionally are severe enough to require replacement of the dialyzer and use of analgesics, antihistamine or epinephrine.

A double-blind study using new or used hollow fiber dialyzers contained in an opaque box documented the incidence of back pain to be 19.5% for new dialyzers versus 6.5% for reprocessed dialyzers (81). As Figure 11 demonstrates, the back pain was also more severe with new than with reused dialyzers. Similarly, the incidence of chest pain was 11% for new versus 2.5% for reprocessed dialyzers and severe reactions were more frequent with new than with reused dialyzers (Figure 12).

Kant and Pollak (82) also compared the incidence of symptoms and hospitalization rates at similar intervals in separate dialysis facilities practicing single use and reuse. There were no significant differences in the number of days of hospitalization for problems unrelated to dialysis but days of hospitalization for dialysis-related complications were almost twice as many with single use as with multiple use (Table 18).

Biocompatibility

After the first pass of a patient's blood through a dialyzer with cellophane or Cuprophan membranes, white blood count and serum complement decrease (83, 84)

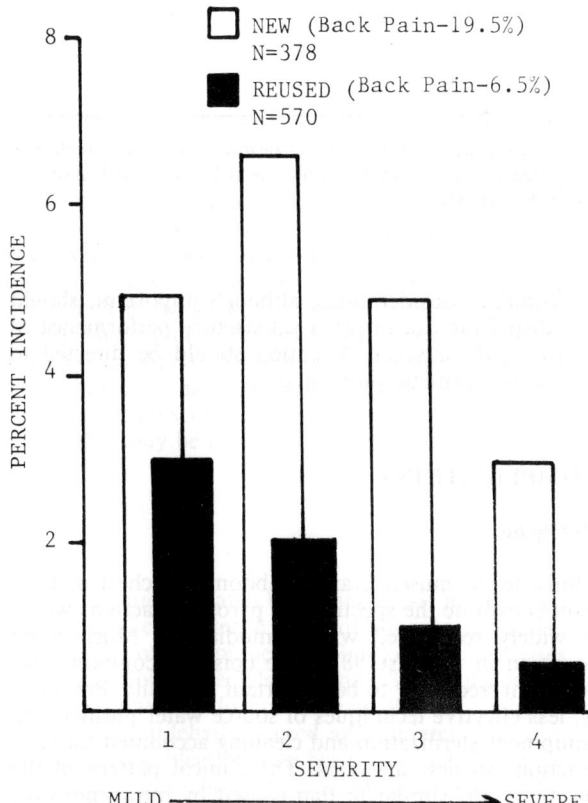

Figure 11. The incidence of back pain in patients treated with new dialyzers is significantly greater than with reused dialyzers (p = 0.0005). From Bok et al. (74 [with permission]).

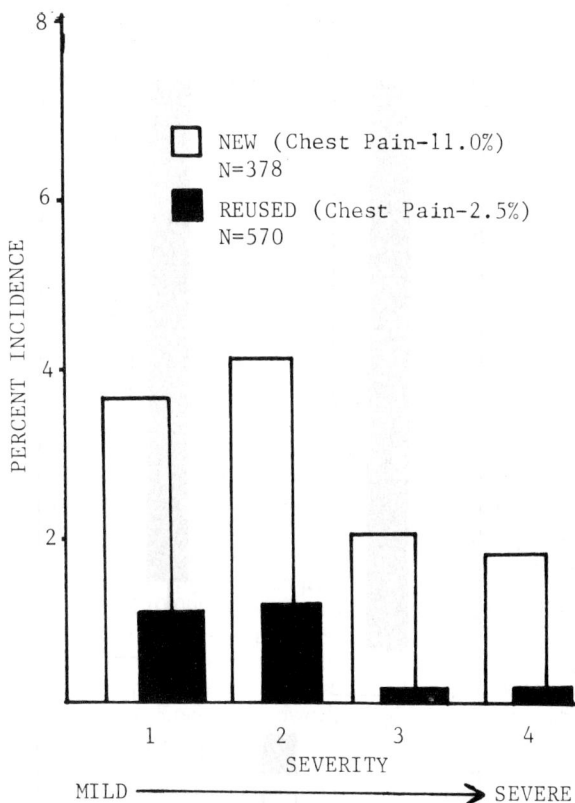

Figure 12. The incidence of chest pain is significantly greater in patients treated with new dialyzers than with reused dialyzers (p = 0.013). From Bok et al. (74 [with permission]).

Table 18. Frequency of hospitalization of ESRD patients [a].

	Single use (320 Pt months)	Multiple use unit (334 Pt months)	P-Value
Days of hospitalization/month, not related to dialysis	0.43	0.48	0.3
Days of hospitalization/month, related to dialysis	0.90	0.48	<0.001

[a] From Kant and Pollak (75 [with permission]).

SOME PRACTICAL ASPECTS OF A REUSE PROGRAM

The reprocessing area

The area employed for reprocessing must be isolated from other functions. Temperature and humidity in the reprocessing area should be reasonably controlled. There should be no passage for other personnel in the area.

Total enclosure is desirable with provision for venting excess gas without allowing it to enter the work place. When total enclosure is not possible, processes should be designed and operated to limit occupational exposure by contact or inhalation of any gas, liquid, splash or mist.[1]

The installation should be adequately ventilated to insure that formaldehyde concentrations in the workroom will not exceed the recommended limit. A hood should be installed with an open face velocity of 150 ft^3/min (about 43 m^3/min).[2]

Equipment

The equipment should have controls to establish pressures and flow of water and sterilant at appropriate times during reprocessing. The equipment should insure the production of processed water (RO) for thorough rinsing of dialyzers as specified in the techniques. A schedule of preventive maintenance of reprocessing equipment, including periodic sterilization of tubing systems and reservoirs, if present, should be documented.

Control of components

All water used for reprocessing dialyzers, including that used for preparing antimicrobial and cleaning solutions, should be reverse osmosis water. (Deionized water has also been reported to be satisfactory for reprocessing of dialyzers [DA Ogden, personal communication, April 1981])

Periodically this water should be analyzed for endotoxin by the Limulus Amebocyte Lysate (LAL) test and for sterility by a membrane filtration culture technique. Water quality should meet draft standards of the American Association of Medical Instrumentation (AAMI) and should be monitored as recommended.

The concentration of any solution employed for cleaning of dialyzers should be specified and conditions of exposure of the dialyzer specifically defined. Concentrations of the cleaning solution and its concentration in the effluent from the dialyzer should be measured periodically.

The concentrated formaldehyde (37%) should be diluted in a well ventilated hood with reverse osmosis endotoxin-free water. Where possible, flushing of equipment or dialyzers with formaldehyde should be done by a suction or gravity flow technique.

Fluid used for flushing should meet the draft standards for hemodialysis systems of the AAMI. Endotoxin should be measured periodically in effluents from randomly selected initial use and reprocessed dialyzers.

Process controls

The process must be described in a clear and detailed fashion. Copies of this description should be available in the work place where reprocessing of hemodialyzers is accomplished. This process description or immediately related material should identify the quality control requirements for the process.

A system should be in place for device evaluation with documentation. For hollow fiber dialyzers, this would include visual inspection and measurement of cell volume at each reprocessing. Measurements of cell volume should be checked against a dialyzer of known volume and there should be periodic checks of cell volume of in-use dialyzers to verify the technique. Should the manufacturer change the membrane or when a different species of dialyzer is used, clearances and ultrafiltration rates should be measured to verify that multiple use does not adversely influence function and that the relationship between fiber bundle volume and clearance is maintained.

Dialyzers should be tested for the presence of antimicrobial agents before preparation for use. Clinitest tablets may be used to assess process control after the preparation for use procedure. Weekly, or once per 200 hemodialyses, a sensitive test for formaldehyde, such as the Schiff's reagent or Hantzsch test (67), should confirm the efficacy of rinse-out of formaldehyde from randomly selected dialyzers. If different dialyzers are being reprocessed in a dialysis unit, it should be verified that procedures for reprocessing each dialyzer, if different, are standardized. The bacteriology of water and dialysis fluid should be tested at least monthly in the facility. A regular schedule of functional evaluation of reprocessed dialyzers should be maintained, although the schedule will be influenced by the total activity of the hemodialysis unit.

Labeling control

A system for reprocessed hemodialyzers should be implemented which assures specific, readily visable labeling of each patient's hemodialyzer and the date of each use. This record should be reviewed by a nurse each time the dialyzer is used.

---

[1] National Institute for Occupational Safety and Health (NIOSH), Criteria for a Recommended Standard: Occupational Exposure to Formalhyde, Dec 1976. Superintendent of Documents, U.S. Government Printing Office, Washington, D.C.
[2] American Conference of Governmental Industrial Hygienists (ACGIH), Laboratory Hood Data, January 1978.

Records

Daily records of reprocessing activity should be kept in an accurate and systematic manner. Daily and weekly summaries should indicate the number of dialyzers used during each interval. The number of uses for each dialyzer, the average number of uses, details of unusual findings in the reprocessing activity and the basis of rejection of dialyzers should be indicated.

Environmental protection

Records of water quality, air quality, microbiologic environment, and staff medical records should be maintained in an organized and accurate fashion.

ACKNOWLEDGMENT

This study was supported in part by NIAMDD, contract No. 1-AM-9-2214.

APPENDICES

Appendix A. Storage procedure for hollow fiber dialyzers

1. Return blood to the patient by rinsing-back with sterile saline.
2. Take the saline-filled dialyzer to the storage room within 10 min.
3. Place the dialyzer in a support rack with the arterial side down.
4. Attach the reverse osmosis (RO) water line to the arterial side of the blood compartment; flush the blood side for 5 min at 20 psi[3] at 3 to 4 l/min.
5. After 5 min disconnect the RO line from the arterial side of the blood compartment.
6. Attach lines with Hansen connectors to both dialysate ports. Attach the line nearest the arterial side to the RO water outlet and flush the dialysate compartment. Once all air is displaced, clamp the outflow of the dialysate compartment creating pressure to a predetermined value[4] and maintaining it for at least an hour.
7. Fifteen minutes into step 6, slowly release the clamp on the dialysate outflow. Return to step 4, flushing the blood compartment for 2 min at 20 psi at 3 to 4 l/min.
8. Repeat step 7 three more times during the procedure, alternating the direction of flushing. The first and third flushes are with the arterial line connected to the RO water outlet, while the second is with the venous line connected to the RO water outlet. During each 2 min rinse of the blood side, clamp the outflow tubing three times and release.
9. After completing step 8, measure cell volume.
10. Fill both the blood and dialysate compartments with 2.0% formaldehyde solution. Tie off tubing on blood side and place caps on dialysate ports.
11. Record date of use, cell volume and operator's initials, noting that formaldehyde was added.

Appendix B. Preparation for use of stored hollow fiber dialyzers

1. Inspect the dialyzer carefully and test to insure presence of formaldehyde in blood compartment by observing a strongly positive reaction with Clinitest tablet.
2. Check the dialyzer and double check documenting that the dialyzer chosen belongs to the patient to be treated.
3. Place dialyzer in holder with arterial side up. Place the date and operator's initials on the preparation label.
4. Connect dialysate lines and blood lines and flush dialysate compartment with dialysate for a minimum of 10 min at 500 ml/min. Retain this flow rate throughout steps 5 to 8.
5. At the end of the 10 min flush of the dialysate compartment, flush 1000 ml heparinized saline (2000 units of heparin/1000 ml saline) through the blood compartment. The blood pump is set to deliver the saline at a flow rate of 125 ml/min. The venous side is clamped intermittently to allow all the air to be purged from the dialyzer.
6. After the 1000 ml heparin-saline flush, clamp the blood side and allow the dialysate to flow for an additional minimum of 10 min.
7. After 10 min invert the dialyzer so that arterial side is down with the saline connected and flush 700 ml of heparinized saline (2000 units heparin/1000 ml saline) through the dialyzer, clamping the venous side intermittently to allow all of the air to be purged from the dialyzer. The flow rate of saline is kept at 125 ml/min.
8. After the 700 ml flush, and with dialysate still flowing, obtain a sample of saline from the venous side for Clinitest determination of formaldehyde. If the test shows a deep blue, the dialyzer is ready for use. If the test shows any color but deep blue, flush another 1000 ml of saline through the dialyzer and test again.
9. Allow the dialysate to continue flowing at 500 ml/min until the patient is connected.
10. A process control should be conducted weekly with 5 dialyzers (minimum) to insure that residual formaldehyde is less than 10 μg/ml (0.33 μmol/ml) when Schiff's reagent is used.

---

[3] 20 psi = 1.36 atm.
[4] The appropriate pressure must be established in the dialysate compartment for each hemodialyzer reprocessed. The dialysate compartment pressure for the Travenol 1211 can be 25 psi (1.7 atm).

Appendix C. Process and quality control in a dialyzer multiple use program: organization and personnel

The personnel who are involved in a hemodialyzer multiple use program (Fig. C-1) have operational and quality assurance responsibilities.

The operational staff perform the dialyzer reprocessing techniques. Technical aides are trained in the reprocessing procedures, while the supervisory staff monitors the performance of these aides periodically. They verify the accuracy of labels, records and techniques. They conduct intermittant checks on the quality of performance of reprocessing procedures.

The quality assurance personnel have the responsibility for implementing procedures necessary for process and quality control. Quality assurance personnel cannot have responsibility for performing reprocessing techniques or be responsible to the supervisor who monitors the reprocessing procedures.

Both categories of personnel report to the medical director or administrator of the unit. The qualifications of staff performing these roles should be described in writing. The training procedures should be explicit and check lists are necessary to verify the accomplishment of various steps in the training process. Policy should be defined for appropriate attire, as well as the measures to achieve environmental protection and maximum sanitary control in the reprocessing area.

In several countries in Europe, where hepatitis B in dialysis units apparently is a greater risk than it is in the USA, a strict code of practice and measures for the control of cross infection have been instituted.

According to these measures, dialyzers used in HB_sAg positive patients should not be reused, except possibly in the home dialysis setting.

In addition HB_sAg positive members of staff should not work in dialysis units and should be barred from work in reprocessing areas (98–100).

Routine screening for HB_sAg among staff in dialysis units is therefore recommended.

These restrictions may become redundant when immunization against hepatitis B for staff and patients in dialysis (and renal) units is effectuated (101).

Nasal carriage of staphylococci should not prohibit personnel from reprocessing dialyzers, but aseptic technique must be rigorous under these circumstances.

A schedule of documentation of the periodic review by supervisory operational personnel and quality assurance of staff should be maintained.

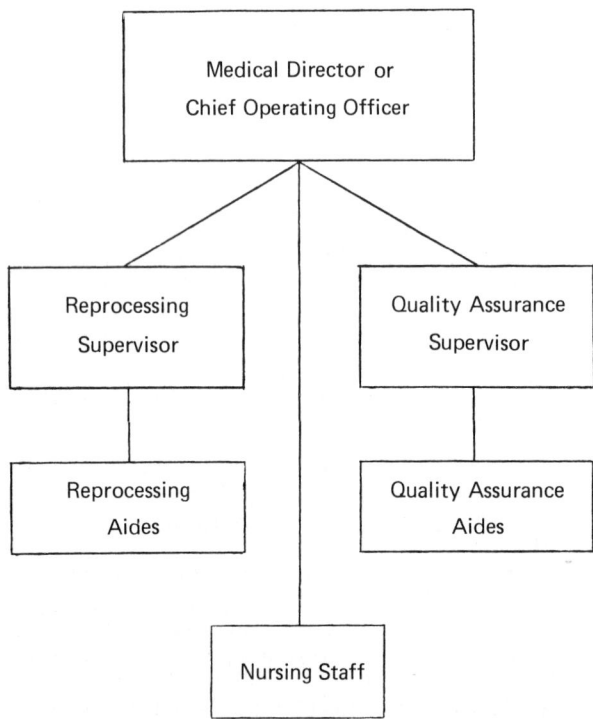

Figure C-1. Organizational structure of hemodialysis multiple use facility.

REFERENCES

1. Scribner BH, Buri R, Caner JEZ, Hegstrom R, Burnell JM: The treatment of chronic uremia by means of intermittent dialysis: a preliminary report. *Trans Am Soc Artif Intern Organs* 6:114, 1960
2. Kiil F, Amundsen B: Development of a parallel flow artificial kidney in plastics. *Acta Chir Scand (Suppl)* 253:142, 1960
3. Myers CH: Parallel flow hemodialyzer systems. In *Hemodialysis: Principles and Practice,* edited by Bailey GL, New York and London, Academic Press, 1972, p 324
4. Pendras JP, Cole JJ, Tu WH, Scribner BH: Improved technique of continuous flow hemodialysis. *Trans Am Soc Artif Intern Organs* 7:27, 1961
5. Brown HW, Maher JF, Lapierre L, Bledsoe FH, Schreiner GE: Clinical problems related to the prolonged artificial maintenance of life by hemodialysis in chronic renal failure. *Trans Am Soc Artif Intern Organs* 8:281, 1962
6. Merrill, JP, Schupak E, Cameron E, Hampers CL: Hemodialysis in the home. *JAMA* 190:468, 1964
7. Shaldon SH, Silva H, Rosen SM: Technique of refrigerated coil preservation haemodialysis with femoral venous catheterization. *Br Med J* 2:411, 1964
8. Pollard TL, Barnett BMS, Eschbach JW, Scribner BH: A technique for storage and multiple reuse of the Kiil dialyzer and blood tubing. *Trans Am Soc Artif Intern Organs* 13:24, 1967
9. Jacobs C, Brunner FP, Chantler C, Donckerwolcke RA, Gurland HJ, Hathway RA, Selwood NH, Wing AJ: Combined report on regular dialysis and transplantation in Europe VII, 1976 *Proc Eur Dial Transpl Assoc* 14:2, 1977
10. Wing AJ, Brunner FP, Brynger H, Chantler C, Donckerwolcke RA, Gurland HJ, Hathway RA, Jacobs C: Combined report on regular dialysis and transplantation in Europe, VIII, 1977. *Proc Eur Dial Transpl Assoc* 15:3, 1978
11. Wing AJ, Brunner FP, Brynger H, Chantler C, Donckerwolcke RA, Gurland HJ, Jacobs C, Selwood NH: Mortal-

ity and morbidity of reusing dialysers. *Br Med J* 2:853, 1978
12. Disney APS, Correll R: Report of the Australia and New Zealand combined dialysis and transplant registry. *Med J Aust* 1:117, 1981
13. Siemsen AW, Ennis J, McGowan R, Wong EGC, Wong LMF: Limited-care hemodialysis. *Trans Am Soc Artif Intern Organs* 18:70 1972
14. Siemsen AW, Study of reuse of cuprophan and cellophane coils. *Annual Progress Report, NIH Contract* 72-2217, 1973 (unpublished)
15. Deane N, Blagg CR, Bower J, De Palma JR, Gutch C, Kanter A, Ogden DA, Sadler J, Siemsen A, Teehan B, Sosin A: A survey of dialyzer reuse practice in the United States. *Dial Transpl* 7:1128, 1978
16. De Palma JR, Pecker EA, Maxwell MH: A new automatic coil dialyzer system for daily dialysis. *Proc Eur Dial Transpl Assoc* 6:26, 1969
17. Lazarus JM, Friedrich RA. Merrill JP: Hollow fiber kidney reuse. *Dial Transpl* 2, (no) 1:14, 1973
18. Bilinsky RT, Morris AJ: Hemodialysis coil reuse: A safe and economical new method. *JAMA* 218:1806, 1971
19. Gotch F, Sargent J, Keen M, Holmes G, Teisinger C: Development and long term clinical evaluation of a thromboresistant hollow fiber kidney (HFK). *Trans Am Soc Artif Intern Organs* 18:135, 1972
20. Miller JH, Shinaberger JH, Gardner PW, Mirahmadi K: Comparison of new dialyzers 1974–1975. *Dial Transpl* 4, (no 6):40, 1975
21. Juncos LI, Marbuy CT, Cade R, Mahoney JJ, Bucci CM, Ayers A: Reusing the follow-fiber dialyzer. *Dial Transpl* 6, (no 12):32, 1977
22. Ben-Ari J, Berlyne GM: Excessive ultrafiltration due to intracoil fibrin deposition as a complication of coil reuse. *Nephron* 9:189, 1972
23. Gottloib L, Servadio C: The routine reutilization of 'disposable' coils for hemodialysis. *Isr J Med Sci* 8:79, 1972
24. Bell RP, Figueroa JE: Haemodialysis cost reduction by artificial kidney storage: a simple, effective technique for re-use of coil kidneys. *Br Med J* 1:788, 1970
25. Deane N, Bemis JA: Multiple use of hemodialyzers. *Final Report, NIAMDD Contract* No 1-AM-9-2214, 1981 (unpublished)
26. Ketteringham JM, Broome MG, Johnston FL, Sturgeon ML, Wood AM: The in-vitro evaluation of certain issues related to the multiple use of hemodialyzers. *Subcontract report to National Nephrology Foundation, NIAMDD Contract* No 1-AM-9-2214, 1981
27. Siemsen AW, Lumeng J, Wong ECG, Wong LMF, Ching A, Ennis JA, McGowen RF: Clinical and laboratory evaluation of coil use. *Trans Am Soc Artif Intern Organs* 20:589, 1974
28. Mirahmadi KS, Kaye JH, Kastagir BK, Miller JH, Imparto B, Williams T, Gorman JT: Clinical evaluations of patients dialyzed with two Gambros four hours, three times per week. *Proc Clin Dial Transpl Forum* 3:247, 1973
29. Teehan BP, Smith LJ, Hartigan MF, Griesemer GA, Gilgore GS, Sigler MH: Functional and morphological changes in reused Gambro-Lundia Nova dialyzers. *Proc Clin Dial Transpl Forum* 5:51, 1975
30. Lanning JT, Winterich C, Zuanaich N: Multiple use of hollow fiber dialyzers in a free-standing center. *Dial Transpl* 9:36, 1980
31. Smith LJ: Large surface area dialysis. *Nurs Clin North Am* 10:481, 1975
32. Hirsch K, Grist G, Crouch T: A reuse method for the Cordis-Dow artificial kidney. *Dial Transpl* 5, no 2:76, 1976
33. Hardy DW, Higgins MR, McFarlane DF, Hughes RV: An automated cleaning device for dialyzers; machine design and technology. *Clin Nephrol* 5:275, 1976
34. Johnson CE, Octaviano GN, Beirne GJ, Haynie GD, Burns RO: Cleaning, storage and repeated use of twin coil dialyzing units. *JAMA* 207:2087, 1969
35. Wagnild JP, McDonald P, Craig WA, Johnson C, Hanley M, Wamn SJ, Ramgopal V, Beirne GJ: Pseudomonas aeruginosa bacteremia in a dialysis unit, II. Relationship to reuse of coils. *Am J Med* 62:672, 1977
36. Kuehnel E, Lundh H: Outbreak of Pseudomonas cepacia bacteremia related to contaminated reused coils. *Dial Transpl* 5:44, 1978
37. Mitchell RG, Hayward AC: Postoperative urinary tract infections caused by contaminated irrigating fluid. *Lancet* 1:793, 1966
38. Burdon DW, Whitby JL: Contamination of hospital disinfectants with Pseudomonas species. *Br Med J* 2:153 1967
39. Cragg J, Andrews AV: Bacterial contamination of disinfectants. *Br Med J* 3:57, 1969
40. Bassett DJC, Stockes KJ, Thomas WRG: Wound infection with Pseudomonas multivorans, a water-borne contaminant of disinfection solutions. *Lancet* 1:1188, 1970
41. Speller DC, Stephans ME, Viant AC: Hospital infections by Pseudomonas cepacia. *Lancet* 1:798, 1971
42. Plotkin AA, Austrian R: Bacteremia caused by Pseudomonas sp. following the use of material stored in solutions of cationic surface-active agents. *Am J Med Sci* 235:621, 1958
43. Phillips I: Pseudomonas cepacia septicemia in an intensive care unit. *Lancet* 1:375, 1971
44. Mason RG, Zucker WH, Bilinsky RT, Shinoda BA, Sharp DE, Mohammad SF: Blood components deposited on used and reused dialysis membranes. *Biomater Med Devices Artif Organs* 4:333, 1976
45. Gutch CF, Swanson JR, Ogden DA: Failure of dialysis concentrate as a bactericidal agent. *Proc Clin Dial Transpl Forum* 4:234, 1974
46. Wielgosz A, Rutkoswki B, Maritius A: Utilization of acetic acid solution for resterilization of dialyzers. *Abstracts Eur Dial Transpl Assoc* 1979, p 103
47. Favero MS, Petersen NJ: Microbiologic guidelines for hemodialysis systems. *Dial Transpl* 6, (no 11):34, 1977
48. ASAIO-AAMI Standard, 1977 (not published)
49. Health Care Financing Administration, U.S. Dept of HEW. Bureau of Health Standards and Quality Letter No. 10 *End Stage Renal Disease Program – Guidelines for Testing of HBsAg and Dialysis Fluids,* March 1, 1978
50. Association for the Advancement of Medical Instrumentation, HS-D, 11/80: *Standards for Hemodialysis Systems* (Draft) (not published)
51. *The United States Pharmacopeia, Twentieth Revision,* July 1, 1980. United States Pharmacopeial Convention, Inc Rockville, MD 20852
52. Favero MS, Carson LA, Bond WA, Petersen NJ: Factors that influence microbial contamination of fluids associated with hemodialysis machines. *Appl Microbiol* 28:822, 1974
53. Favero MS, Petersen NJ, Carson LA et al.: Gram-negative water bacteria in hemodialysis systems. *Health Lab Sci* 12:321, 1975
54. Katz D, Laney H, Linquist JA and Persike EC: Formaldehyde disinfection to eliminate bacterial contamination of deionizers. *Dial Transpl* 5, (no 3):42, 1976
55. Dawids SG, Vejlsgaard R: Bacteriological and clinical evaluation of different dialysate delivery systems. *Acta Med Scand* 199:151, 1976

56. Petersen NJ, Boyer KM, Carson LA, Favero MS: Pyrogenic reactions from inadequate disinfection of a dialysis fluid distribution system. *Dial Transpl* 7 (no 1):52, 1978
57. *Hemodialysis Manual,* DHEW (HSM), Publ No 72-7002. Washington DC, US Government Printing Office, 1971
58. Work F: Production, chemistry and properties of bacterial pyrogens and endotoxins. In *Pyrogens and Fever,* Edited by Wolstenholme GEW, Birch J, Edinburgh, Churchill Publ Co, 1971, p 23
59. Bernick JJ, Port FK, Favero MS, Brown DG: Bacterial and endotoxin permeability of hemodialysis membranes. *Kidney Int* 16:491, 1979
60. Bernick JJ, Port FK: Endotoxin does not permeate the intact cellophane dialyzer membrane. *Chronic Renal Disease Conference NIAMDD,* January 1980, p 30
61. Carson LA, Petersen NJ, Favero MS, Aguero SM: Growth characteristics of atypical mycobacteria in water and their comparative resistance to disinfectants. *Appl Environ Microbiol* 36:839, 1978
62. Miach PJ, Evans SM, Wilcox AA, Dewborn JK: Reuse of a disposable dialyzer for home dialysis. *Med J Aust* 1:146, 1976
63. Vercellone A, Piccoli G, Aloatti S, Segoloni GP, Stratta P, Triolo G, Canavese C and Grott G: Reuse of dialyzers. *Dial Transpl* 7:350, 1978
64. Eschbach JW, Vizzo JE: Evaluation of Dow hollow fiber artificial kidney. *Proc 5th Annual Contractor's Conference (Artificial Kidney Program, NIAMDD)* edited by Krueger KK, DHEW Publ No (NIH) 72-248, p 17
65. Kaehny WD, Miller GE, White WL: Relationship between dialyzer reuse and the presence of anti-N-like antibodies in chronic hemodialysis patients. *Kidney Int* 12:56, 1977
66. Ogden DA, Myers LE, Eskelson CD, Ziegler EJ: Iatrogenic administration of formaldehyde to hemodialysis patients. *Proc Clin Dial Transplant Forum* 3:141, 1973
67. Nash T: The colorimetric estimation of formaldehyde by means of the Hantzsch reaction. *Biochem J* 55:416, 1953
68. Lewis KJ, Dewar PJ, Ward MK, Kerr DNS: Formation of anti-N-like antibodies in dialysis patients: effect of different methods of dialyser rinsing to remove formaldehyde. *Clin Nephrol* 15:39, 1981
69. Fawcett KC, Mangles MD: Reuse of the Gambro Lundia 17-layer dialyzer. *Dial Transpl* 3, (no 1):38, 1974
70. Ahmad R, Goldsmith HJ: Automated dialyser rinsing machine. *Dial Transpl* 4, (no 5):29, 1975
71. Cane T: The Cordis-Dow artificial kidney. *Dial Transpl* 4, (no 2):59, 1975
72. Harrison PB, Jansson K, Kronenberg H, Mahony JF, Tiller D: Cold agglutinin formation in patients undergoing haemodialysis. A possible relationship to dialyzer reuse. *Aus NZ J Med* 5:195, 1975
73. Snyder D, Louis BM, Gorfien P, Mordujovich J: Clinical experience with long-term brief, daily haemodialysis. *Proc Eur Dial Transpl Assoc* 11:128, 1977
74. Crockett E: Development of successful and economic re-use of disposable dialysers and lines without complication. *Abstracts Eur Dial Transpl Nurs Assoc* 1979, p 114
75. Keggie J, Powell J, Beare J, Nicholls M, Greenaway H, Pavitt L: The advantages of re-using the dialyser and the blood lines *Abstracts Eur Dial Transpl Nurs Assoc* 1979, p 116
76. Hill K, Clinkard S: Elimination of formalin and the re-use of dialysers. *Abstracts Eur Dial Transpl Nurs Assoc* 1979, p 116
77. Ahmad R, Hussler J: Reusing dialysers. *Br Med J* 1:123, 1979
78. Gotch FA: Mass transport in reused dialyzers. *Proc Clin Dial Transpl Forum* 10:81, 1980
79. Lowrie EG, Hakim RM: The effect on patient health of using reprocessed artificial kidneys. *Proc Clin Dial Transpl Forum* 10:86, 1980
80. Ogden DA: New dialyzer syndrome. *N Engl J Med* 302:1262, 1980
81. Bok DV, Pascual L, Herberger C, Sawyer R, Levin NW: Effect of multiple use of dialyzers on intradialytic symptoms. *Proc Clin Dial Transpl Forum,* 10:92, 1980
82. Kant KS, Pollak VE: Dialyzer reuse: safety and efficacy. Chronic Renal Disease Conference NIAMDD, January 1980 (Abstract), p 33
83. Kaplow LS, Goffinet JA: Profound neutropenia during the early phase of hemodialysis. *JAMA* 203:1135, 1968
84. Gral T, Schrotl P, De Palma JR, Gordon A: Leukocyte dynamics with three types of hemodialyzers. *Trans Am Soc Artif Int Organs,* 15:45, 1969
85. Savdi E, Bruce L, Vincent PC: Modified neutropenic response to reused dialyzers in patients with chronic renal failure. *Clin Nephrol* 8:422, 1977
86. Hakim R, Fox K, Lowrie EG: Biocompatibility of cellulosic and non-cellulosic hemodialyzer membranes. Chronic Renal Disease Conference NIAMDD January, 1980 (Abstract), p 32
87. Hakim RM, Lowrie EG: Effect of dialyzer reuse on leukopenia, hypoxemia and total hemolytic complement system. *Trans Am Soc Artif Int Organs* 26:159, 1980
88. Robinson PJA, Rosen SM: Pyrexial reactions during haemodialysis. *Br Med J* 1:528, 1971
89. Bennett IL, Cluff LE: Bacterial pyrogens. *Pharmacol Rev* 9:427, 1957
90. Petersen NJ, Carson LA, Favero MS: Bacterial endotoxin in new and reused hemodialyzers: a potential cause of endotoxemia. *Trans Am Soc Artif Intern Organs* 27:155, 1981
91. Keshaviah P: Investigation of the risks and hazards associated with hemodialysis devices. *FDA, DHEW contract* 223-78-5046, 1980, p 350 (Can be obtained at Bureau of Medical Devices (HFK-310) FDA, 8750 Georgia Ave, Silver Spring MD 20910)
92. Favero MS, Deane N, Leger RT, Sosin AE: Effect of multiple use of dialyzers on hepatitis B incidence in patients and staff. *JAMA* 245:166, 1981
93. Belzer FO, Kountz SL, Perkins HA: Red cell cold autoagglutinins as a cause of failure of renal allotransplantation. *Transplantation* 11:422, 1971
94. Howell D, Perkins HA: Anti-N-like antibodies in the sera of patients undergoing chronic hemodialysis. *Vox Sang* 23:291, 1972
95. Fassbinder W, Pilar J, Scheuermann E, Koch KM: Formaldehyde and the occurrence of anti-N-like cold agglutinins in RDT patients. *Proc Eur Dial Transpl Assoc* 13:333, 1976
96. Shaldon S, Chevallet M, Maraoui M, Mion C: Dialysis associated auto-antibodies. *Proc Eur Dial Transp Assoc* 13:339, 1976
97. Koch KM, Frei U, Fassbinder W: Hemolysis and anemia in anti-N-like antibody positive hemodialysis patients. *Trans Am Soc Artif Intern Organs* 24:709, 1978
98. Report of the Advisory Group 1970-1972. *Hepatitis and the Treatment of Chronic Renal Failure (Rosenheim Report).* London, Department of Health and Social Security (DHSS) 1972
99. Grob PJ, Bischof B, Naeff F: Cluster of hepatitis B transmitted by a physician. *Lancet* 2:1218, 1981
100. Letter to Regional and Area Medical Officers with appendix. London, DHSS, December 1981
101. Zuckerman AJ: Priorities for immunisation against hepatitis B, *Br Med J* 1:686, 1982

16
HEMOPERFUSION

JAMES F. WINCHESTER

Introduction	305
Principles of hemoperfusion	306
Sorbents	306
Solute spectrum adsorbed and effects of coating sorbents	307
Side effects of hemoperfusion	307
Hemoperfusion in uremia	308
Historical background	308
Short-term clinical studies	310
Long-term clinical studies	311
Comparison of devices	313
Potential clinical benefits and present role in treatment of end-stage renal disease	313
Hemoperfusion in drug intoxication	314
Clinical and laboratory studies	314
Indications for hemoperfusion	316
Hemoperfusion in hepatic encephalopathy	316
Clinical and laboratory studies	316
Indications for hemoperfusion	318
Other uses of sorbent hemoperfusion	318
Schizophrenia	318
Psoriasis	318
Anti-cancer drug removal	318
Immunoadsorption	318
Future developments	319
Acknowledgments	319
References	319

INTRODUCTION

Classically, the treatment of chronic uremia has focused on reducing the generation of nitrogenous end products of protein breakdown or their removal by dialysis techniques. The treatment of many thousands of patients with chronic uremia has demonstrated that diet and dialysis are feasible treatments, although these methods do not correct all the metabolic consequences of renal failure and many features of uremia continue unabated. To

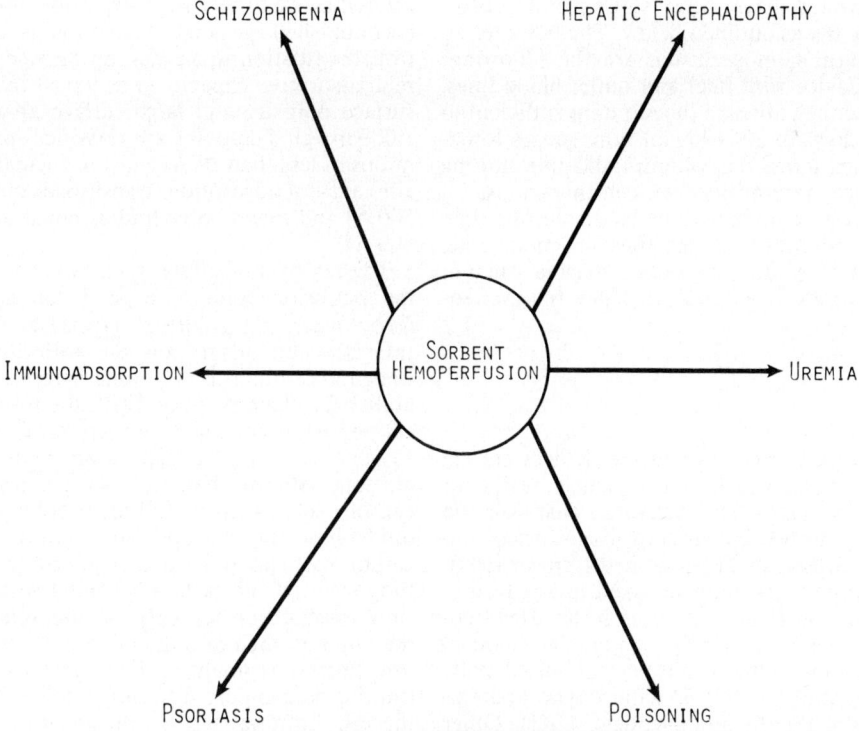

Figure 1. Uses of sorbent hemoperfusion.

increase the efficiency or otherwise improve dialysis techniques, attention has been directed over the last two decades to the properties of sorbents. Oral use of sorbents such as oxy-starch and charcoal (see chapter 18), has been of considerable interest, but as yet remains of unproven value as the only treatment of severe uremia. On the other hand, sorbent regeneration of dialysate (see chapter 17), is now accepted in the clinical management of uremia.

This chapter is concerned with direct contact of blood with sorbents within cartridges (columns), primarily reviewing the potential use of hemoperfusion in uremia, but also discussing the application of hemoperfusion in drug intoxication, hepatic encephalopathy, and other interesting areas (Figure 1).

PRINCIPLES OF HEMOPERFUSION

The term, hemoperfusion, implies the direct contact of blood from the patient or animal with a sorbent system. Most clinically available sorbent systems employ plastic housings incorporating particulate sorbent materials within them, through which blood percolates in a laminar flow throughout the system. The sorbent system must be of sufficient biocompatibility to allow direct blood contact without allowing appreciable destruction of blood elements to occur. To overcome the problem of incompatibility of early hemoperfusion systems (1, 2), Chang (3) introduced a microencapsulation process by which the sorbent particles were coated with a polymer membrane, such as albumin-collodion. Many other encapsulation polymers have been subsequently introduced for clinical use as outlined below. The basic requirements for clinical hemoperfusion are the following: hemoperfusion device with inlet and outlet blood lines, vascular access to the patient, a blood pump sufficient to maintain blood flows of 200–300 ml/min, gauges to detect pressure drops across the column indicating clotting within the device, intermittent or continuous use of heparin sufficient to maintain whole blood clotting time greater than 30 minutes, and facilities for monitoring safety (platelet and white cell counts, plasma calcium and glucose concentrations) and efficiency (plasma solute or drug levels).

Sorbents

Typical sorbents used in hemoperfusion devices are the activated carbons (charcoals), ion-exchange resins or non-ionic macroporous resins. Activated charcoals are available in many forms, but principally consist of uncoated granular carbons in the loose-bed form or fixed-bed form (whereby the particles are fixed to a polyethylene backing and wound in a spiral as in the Hemodetoxifier [Becton-Dickinson, USA]) or granular charcoal coated with albumin cellulose nitrate (collodion) polymer (Chang's research model) or with acrylic hydrogel polymer (Hemocol [Smith and Nephew, UK]). Other devices containing charcoals are prepared from extruded charcoal coated with cellulose acetate (Ab Gambro, Sweden), or with methacrylic hydrogel (Tecnologie Biomediche, Italy). Other columns contain spherical charcoals derived from pyrolized macroporous resins (uncoated with polymer: XE-336 [Extracorporeal Medical Specialties Inc, USA]) or spherical charcoals derived from petroleum and coated with albumin-collodion solutions (Hemosorba [Asahi Medical Inc, Japan]). Two other cartridges contain cellulose/collodion coated petroleum based spherical charcoal (Teijin Co, Ltd, Japan) or pitch-based polyhema coated spherical charcoal (Kuraray Co, Japan).

Ion-exchange resins have been used in various studies, but are not yet available for clinical use; they include the amberlite series, Zerolit 225 and the Zeolite series. The non-ionic resins consist of macroporous crosslinked polystyrene amberlite series such as XAD-2, and XAD-4 which has been clinically available for several years (XR-004 cartridge, [Extracorporeal Medical Specialties Inc., USA]). The latter contains 650 g (wet weight) of washed, heat sterilized, pyrogen free XAD-4.

The devices used in clinical studies commonly contain 100 to 300 g of activated charcoal in the uncoated form or coated with polymer membranes ranging in thickness from 0.05 to 0.5 µm. The details of each sorbent device are given below in the section on clinical studies of hemoperfusion in uremia.

Activated carbons are prepared from biological substances (coconut shells, peach pits, sawdust, coal, peat, molasses, etc.) or from nonbiological substances (petroleum or pitch). Although the physical properties of activated carbon are more influenced by the activation process, the choice of starting material produces such characteristics as fine pore distribution, for example, with coconut shell carbons. Activation is induced by controlled oxidation in air, carbon dioxide or steam. Maximal adsorptive capacity is achieved by inducing a high surface porosity and large surface area (approximately 1,000 m^2/g). The pores are classified into micropores (a radius of less than 20 Å) which principally determine the efficiency of adsorption, transitional pores (radius 20 to 500 Å) and macropores (radius equal to or greater than 500 Å).

The removal of solutes such as toxic compounds from the perfusion solution depends on complex physical forces where the solute is trapped at the liquidsorbent interface and adsorption fits with the Freundlich or Langmuir isotherms (4). Some carbons also possess the ability for chemisorption (with the formation of chemical bonds) or chemical conversion of some compounds. In general, non-polar solutes are better adsorbed from aqueous solution than are polar solutes. With activated carbon, solutes must diffuse externally through the liquid phase (plasma and from within red cells) to the carbon particles and are then subject to several rate limiting steps. If the carbon is coated with polymer, diffusion must occur through the membrane, through the macropores, then into the micropores where the adsorption process is finalized. For uncoated carbon, the rate limiting step is pore diffusion, while with coated carbon the rate limiting step is diffusion through the polymer coating. For medical use in hemoperfusion devices, activated carbons must possess the following qualities: freedom from 'microparticulate fines', easy washability, resistance to attrition within devices, high adsorptive capacity, smooth surface morphology, low microparticle generation, minimal elution of toxic ions, high blood compatibility, and easy sterilization, low toxicity and low pyrogenicity. All these qualities determine the manufacturers' choice of charcoal for the inclusion within clinical hemoperfusion cartridges and such properties have been reviewed recently by Denti and Walker (5).

Ion exchange resins possess the ability to exchange one ion for another, the same quantity of charge being removed and replaced by another, to maintain electrical neutrality. Some of the materials used for ion exchange also function as adsorbents, but presently no system has been developed for continuous hemoperfusion because of the prohibitive side effects of removal of biologically important ions such as calcium and magnesium, although the removal of such compounds can be minimized by pretreating the ion exchange resin with appropriate electrolyte solutions.

Chemical adsorbents (chemisorbents) depend on the formation of chemical bonds between the solute and the adsorbent, and although not yet clinically accepted, it has been demonstrated in man that oral polyaldehydes (oxy-starch and oxy-cellulose) are able to remove urea and ammonia from the gastrointestinal tract under physiologic circumstances.

The *macroporous resins* are non-ionic, gel type resins which are formed in beads by an agglomerate of microspheres that are cross-linked to a high degree, thereby producing less swelling of the beads in physiologic solutions. The macroporous resins have a high ability to adsorb organic solutes on the surfaces of the microspheres, which possess surface areas of 300 to 500 m²/g. Uncharged macroporous resins (e.g. XAD-4) are similar to activated charcoal, however, they adsorb solutes with less energetic forces and consequently, the adsorption is more reversible than with organic sorbents such as activated carbon. The elution of organic solutes (such as barbiturates, methaqualone, glutethimide, etc.) from XAD-4 is more readily obtained with the use of methanol or ethanol than can ever be achieved using similar elution techniques with activated carbon.

Solute spectrum adsorbed and effects of coating of sorbents

The solute spectrum adsorbed, particularly with activated charcoal and with special regard to uremic solutes, is shown in Table 1. Removal by activated carbon of solutes ranging in molecular mass from 60 to 21,500 daltons has been demonstrated *in vitro* and *in vivo*. As mentioned above, diffusion of solutes into the microporous structure of coated carbon depends on the polymer membrane thickness and for substances of low molecular mass (creatinine [113 daltons], uric acid [168 daltons], hippuran [363 daltons], vitamin B_{12} [1,355 daltons]) a thin cellulose coating reduces the adsorption

Table 1. Putative uremic toxins removed by sorbents (molecular weight range 60 to 21,500).

Adrenocorticotrophin	(Myoinositol) *
(Aldosterone) *	Non-protein nitrogen
Amino acids *	Nor-epinephrine
Calcium *	Organic acids *
25,OH-cholecalciferol *	Oxalate *
Creatinine *	Parathyroid hormone *
Cyclic AMP	Phenols *
Epinephrine	(Phosphate) *
Folic acid **	Polyamino acids
Gastrin *	(Renin) *
Glucagon	Ribonuclease
Glucose *	Serotonin
(Growth hormone) *	Thyroxine *
Guanidines *	Trace metals; As, Co, Cr, Se
Indoles *	Triglycerides *
Insulin *	Triiodothyronine *
L-Dopamine	(Urea) *
(Magnesium) *	Uric acid *
Middle molecule peaks *	Vitamin B_{12} **

* Studied during hemoperfusion in uremic patients.
** Unpublished.
(Incompletely removed.)

only slightly. At higher molecular weights (greater than 3,500), however, substantial reduction of adsorption occurs with polymer coating (6). Nevertheless, it is this capacity to adsorb molecules of the 'middle molecular weight' size (300 to 1,500) that has stimulated interest in activated charcoal hemoperfusion in uremia. Adsorption of molecules larger than most middle molecular mass solutes (>1,500 daltons) is limited by the pore structure of the specific semi-permeable membrane coating. It must be borne in mind, however, that adsorption of biologically important small solutes also occurs. This is most noticeable clinically with adsorption of glucose, calcium, amino acids, and middle molecules, all of which exhibit finite saturation rates for adsorption. It has been recently appreciated that 25-hydroxycholecalciferol and other hormones (7, 8) have been removed by charcoal hemoperfusion *in vivo*, and important trace metals such as arsenic, cobalt, chromium, and selenium are also removed *in vitro* with perfusion of protein solutions through activated charcoal devices (9). No experience with long term effects of such removal is available, but the observations do attest to the wide spectrum adsorbent capacity of activated carbon.

Side effects of hemoperfusion

Particle embolization was a feature of the early poorly washed hemoperfusion devices and this has been essentially improved by selecting charcoal resistant to attrition and using polymer coating techniques, various methods for fixing carbon to a fixed bed structure, and washing procedures applied on a commercial scale, each of which reduce particulate matter to acceptable infusion fluid limits (required by Federal or other agencies).

emic toxins as reported earlier by Yatzidis (1), but also could remove polyamino acids (36) and medium molecular weight substances (36, 37). In addition, Chang and co-workers (36, 37) demonstrated both *in vitro* and *in vivo* that plasma creatinine and urate clearances with hemoperfusion alone in man were greater than with conventional hemodialysis. These reports noted, however, that urea could not be adsorbed in the quantities thought necessary for the treatment of uremia. Stimulated by Yatzidis' work in Greece and Chang's work in Canada, many others throughout the world have become involved in the development and use of charcoal hemoperfusion devices in experimental uremia and also in the treatment of uremic man. These studies are outlined in detail in Table 2.

Short-term clinical studies

Some of the sorbent devices used in the treatment of clinical uremia are shown in Figure 2. Table 2 shows that in short term studies (repetitive or non-repetitive studies over a period of time less than three months) there is a wide variability, in terms of solute clearance and response to hemoperfusion, depending on the clinical device used. It is apparent, however, that creatinine and uric acid are cleared efficiently by charcoal hemoperfusion alone in contrast with urea which is much better removed by standard hemodialysis. The addition of charcoal hemoperfusion to dialysis increases the total clearance rates of creatinine, urate and middle molecules. While there is some question as to the total quantity of middle molecules removed by hemoperfusion (38), middle molecular weight substances removal is greater than with hemodialysis. Moreover, hemoperfusion in conjunction with hemodialysis can augment middle molecular weight substances clearances. Figure 3 shows middle molecular weight substances removal, assayed by a simple chromatographic technique, before and after hemoperfusion alone in a uremic patient. Middle molecule removal approaches 144 ml/min at blood flow rates of 300 ml/min as reported by Chang (39), while Oulès et al. (38), examining specific subpeaks of middle molecular weight substances reported that extraction of peaks 7a-d was initially 60 to 70% of blood flow rates, but decreased to 10 to 30% during the course of a 2 to 3 hour hemoperfusion. Rosenbaum et al. (40) obtained with XE-336 hemoperfusion a middle molecular weight substance removal of 273 ml/min at blood flow rates of 300 ml/min in uremic animals.

Critical analysis of the total solute removed during hemoperfusion has been reported by Winchester et al. (7). Figure 4 shows that total solute removal with a 2 hour hemoperfusion alone or combined with hemodialysis for standard markers of uremia such as creatinine and urate is substantially less than achieved during a 5 hour standard hemodialysis. Subsequent analysis by Gelfand and Winchester (41), has shown that small molecular weight substances (urea, urate, guanidines, and

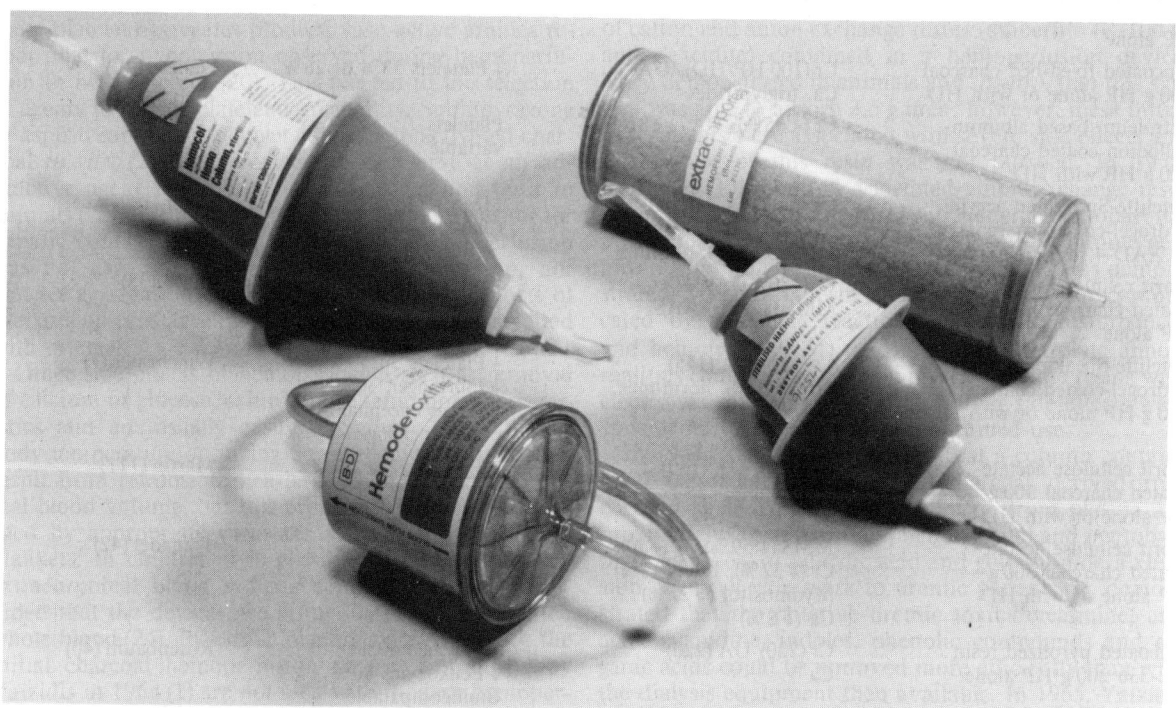

Figure 2. Selected hemoperfusion devices. Acrylic hydrogel coated charcoal hemoperfusion devices (300 g and 100 g columns, center; XAD-4 resin hemoperfusion device, right. Fixed bed uncoated charcoal hemoperfusion device, left. For details see text.

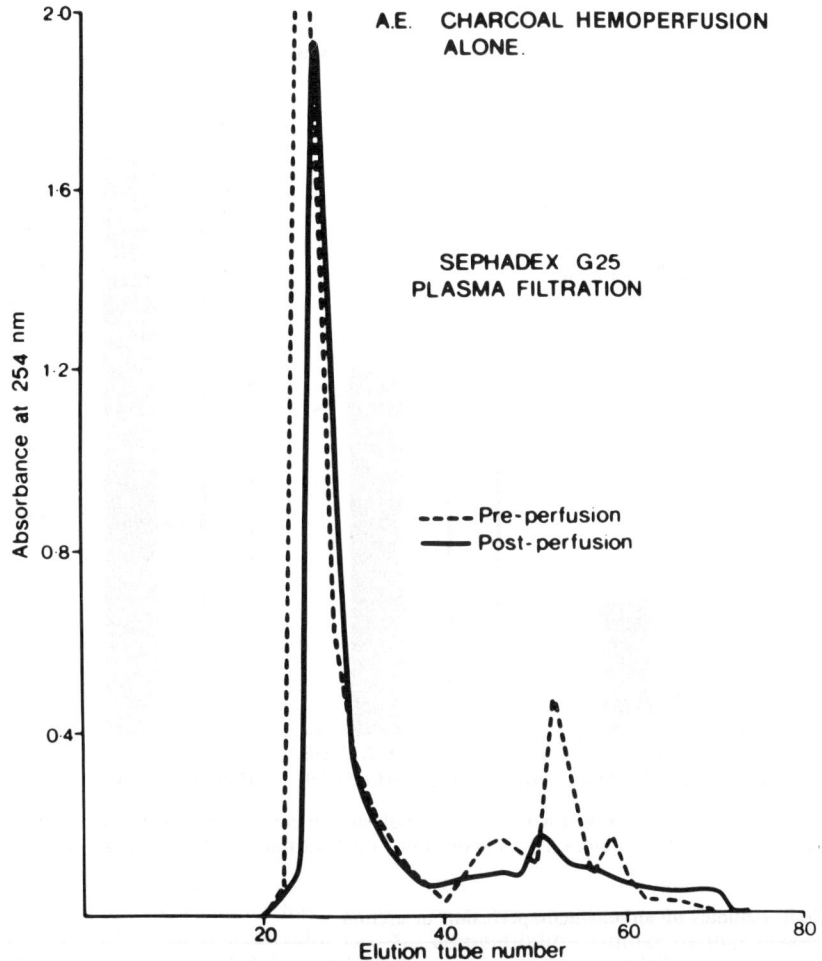

Figure 3. Reduction of 'middle molecular weight' substances with 2 hours coated charcoal hemoperfusion.

phenols) with the exception of creatinine are not removed by hemoperfusion alone with any substantially greater efficiency than by hemodialysis. Creatinine and urate clearances *in vitro* are close to blood flow rates, but these values are reduced *in vivo* due to the competitive adsorption of the other compounds. Significant quantities of organic acids, indoles and myoinositol (42) are also removed by hemoperfusion *in vivo* and *in vitro*.

The structure of amino acids determines their adsorption to activated carbon. Amino acids with aromatic groups are more efficiently adsorbed than branched-chain amino acids (43). In studies of uremia, amino acids not only are removed by charcoal hemoperfusion (7, 28) but are also released from charcoal or other body pools after initial adsorption (38).

Winchester et al. (7) have observed appreciable alterations in plasma insulin, plasma growth hormone, plasma total thyroxine and total triiodothyronine concentrations during hemoperfusion in uremic patients, not substantially different from that occurring during hemodialysis.

The latter observations have recently been confirmed by Stefoni et al. (28). Other hormones and metabolites removed during *in vitro* or *in vivo* hemoperfusion are listed in Table 1.

Most short term studies have not reported any clinical improvement with the use of charcoal hemoperfusion in uremia, although the initial observation of Yatzidis and coworkers (1), suggested that improvement in pericarditis, gastrointestinal symptoms and lethargy occurred. Martin and associates (44) and Odaka et al. (45), also reported that pericarditis appeared to resolve faster when patients are treated with short term charcoal hemoperfusion, than when treated with hemodialysis.

Long-term clinical studies

It has become appreciated that charcoal hemoperfusion alone is insufficient for the control of symptoms or removal of water in uremic subjects (Table 3). For suf-

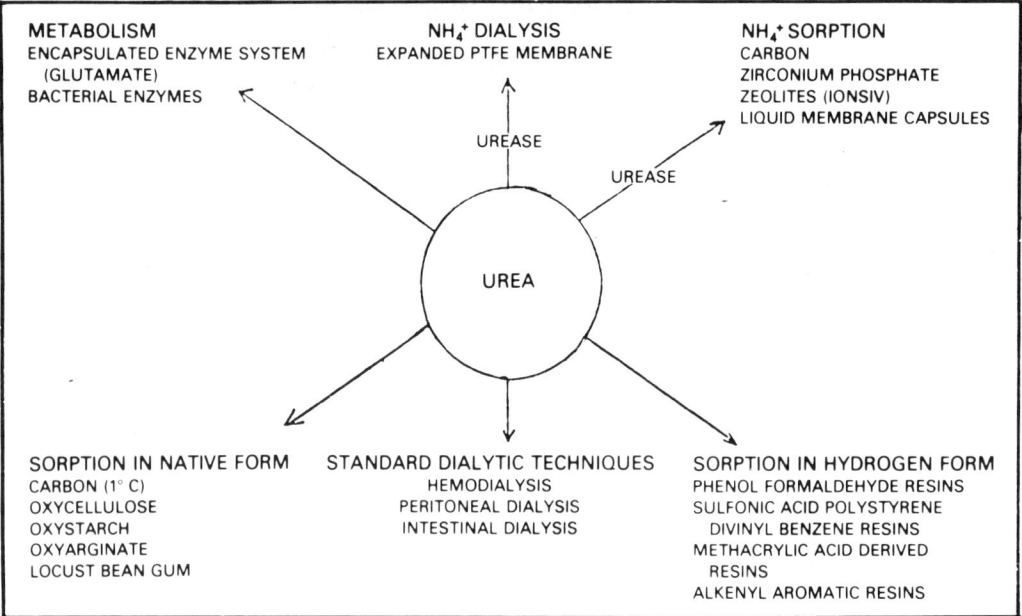

Figure 6. Methods for urea removal currently under study (reprinted from Winchester et al. (114), with permission of the copyright holder).

HEMOPERFUSION AND DRUG INTOXICATION

Since World War II, acute self poisoning with drugs in major industrialized societies has reached almost epidemic proportions. It has been pointed out that 10 to 11.3% of all medical emergencies presenting at hospitals in the United Kingdom result from acute self-poisoning with a distinct female preponderance, reaching 50% of all female medical admissions in certain areas. In the United Kingdom, approximately 120,000 patients were admitted to hospitals in 1973 with a diagnosis of poisoning by medicinal or non-medicinal agents, and the latest epidemiological statistics for England and Wales show that in 1977 there were over 4,000 deaths from poisoning; similar statistics for the United States in 1977 show that there were 6,681 deaths from poisoning, while the number of patients discharged from non-Federal short-stay hospitals with a diagnosis of poisoning, totaled 145,000 (25). While intensive supportive management without the use of central stimulants has reduced the mortality from acute sedative drug overdosage from 25% in 1945 to less than 1% in 1966 (50), it has been appreciated that if serious cases of sedative self-poisoning are considered (Grade III or Grade IV coma [51]) the overall mortality ranges from 8.3% to 34% (52).

In very severely poisoned patients recourse has often been made, under the guidelines proposed by Maher and Schreiner (53), to the use of dialytic techniques for removing drugs. Because of its simplicity and efficiency, attention in the last decade has also been directed to the use of sorbent hemoperfusion in the treatment of severely drug intoxicated patients. This subject has been reviewed in depth by Winchester and coworkers (52, 54) in 1977 and 1978. While hemodialysis is a most effective method for removing highly diffusible substances, it has become clear that hemoperfusion is more efficient with regard to certain other poisons. Lipid soluble drugs and protein bound drugs which are inefficiently removed by hemodialysis can be removed more rapidly by hemoperfusion. Drugs such as salicylate and barbiturates can also be more effectively removed by hemoperfusion *in vitro* and *in vivo* than by hemodialysis under the same conditions of blood flow rate and plasma drug concentrations.

Clinical and laboratory studies

Table 4 shows the drugs removed by various hemoperfusion devices *in vitro* and *in vivo*. The studies quoted deal principally with activated charcoal preparations, rarely with ion exchange resins, and non-ionic macroporous resins. Table 5 shows that for similar conditions of blood flow rate and drug concentrations the extraction ratio for certain drugs (inlet concentration – outlet concentration divided by inlet concentration) is most efficient with the macroporous, non-ionic resin XAD-4. In terms of spectrum of activity, however, although XAD-4 can remove lipid soluble drugs particularly well, activated charcoal is more non-specific and can be used in a wide variety of clinical poisonings.

Using pharmacokinetic modeling, Winchester et al. (55), first demonstrated that drug elimination could be substantially enhanced with hemoperfusion and since

Table 4. Drugs removed by sorbent hemoperfusion.

Barbiturates *
  Amobarbital
  Butabarbital
  Heptabarbital
  Hexobarbital
  Pentobarbital
  Quinalbital
  Secobarbital
  Thiopental
  Vinalbital

Nonbarbiturate hypnotics,
Sedatives, tranquilizers
  Bromisovalum
  Carbamazeline
  Carbromal *
  Chlorpromazine *
  Chloral hydrate *
  (Diazepam) *
  Ethchlorvynol *
  Glutethimide *
  Meprobamate *
  Methaqualone *
  Methyprylon *
  Phenytoin
  Promazine
  Promethazine

Antidepressants
  Amitriptyline *
  Clomipramine
  Desipramine
  Nortriptyline *

Plant/animal toxins,
Herbicides/insecticides
  Amanita phalloides *
  Amanitin
  Chlorinated insecti-
    cides
  Demeton-S-methyl
    sulfoxide *
  Dimethoate *
  Methyl-parathion *
  Nitrostigmine
  Paraoxon *
  Parathion *
  Paraquat *
  Phenol *
  Phalloidin
  Polychlorinated biphenyls

Solvents/gases
  Carbon tetrachloride *
  Ethylene-oxide

Cardiovascular agents
  Digoxin *
  β-Methyl-digoxin *
  Digitoxin *
  Methylproscillarin
  N-Acetylprocainamide
  Procainamide

Alcohols
  (Ethyl-alcohol)
  (Methyl-alcohol)

Analgesics
  Acetyl salicylic acid *
  Methyl salicylate *
  Acetaminophen */paracetamol *
  Phenylbutazone *

Antimicrobials/anticancer agents
  Adriamycin *
  Ampicillin
  Cephalothin *
  Chloramphenicol *
  Chloroquine *
  Clindamycin
  Erythromycin
  Gentamicin *
  Isoniazid
  Methotrexate *
  Penicillin *

Miscellaneous
  Caffeine
  Camphor
  Phencyclidine *
  Phenformin
  Theophylline *

* Studied in vivo. ( ) = Ineffective removal.

Table 5. Plasma drug extraction ratios *.

	Standard hemodialysis	Coated or uncoated charcoal hemoperfusion	XAD-4 or XAD-2 resin hemoperfusion
Acetaminophen	0.4	0.5	0.7
Amobarbital	0.26	0.3	0.9
Carbromal	0.31	0.55	1.0
Digoxin	0.15	0.27	0.46
Ethchlorvynol	0.32	0.7	1.0
Glutethimide	0.16	0.65	0.8
Paraquat	0.5	0.6	0.9 **
Phenobarbital	0.27	0.5	0.85
Salicylates	0.5	0.5	—
Theophylline	0.49	0.7	0.8
Tricyclic drugs	0.35	0.35	0.8

* At similar conditions of blood flow rate (200-300 ml/min) and plasma drug concentrations (derived from literature).
** Ion exchange resin.

that time several animal and clinical studies have confirmed that for specific drugs elimination rates can be substantially increased during the hemoperfusion periods (56–59).

Adverse reactions are observed during hemoperfusion in poisoning similar to those seen in treatment of uremia, although these are less troublesome in view of the fact that rarely is it necessary to proceed with repetitive hemoperfusion except in the case of glutethimide and ethchlorvynol, or poisoning by other drugs which possess slow intercompartmental transfer rates and large volumes of distribution (52). Thrombocytopenia developing during hemoperfusion in poisoning cases usually recovers within 24 to 48 h, and very rarely is associated with hemostatic problems (52).

Several authors oppose the use of hemoperfusion in poisoning (60, 61), arguing that conservative management alone is almost invariably associated with a favorable clinical outcome. It must, however, be pointed out that the geographic and other variations in poisoning are such (62) that consideration must be given to hemoperfusion or dialysis in severe cases with specific toxic agents. In general, patients that are poisoned with agents that cause metabolic abnormalities such as acidosis, should not be treated by hemoperfusion. Hemodialysis is still recommended as the treatment of choice for severely poisoned patients with ethanol poisoning (sorbent devices saturate rapidly with ethanol), methanol (because of formaldehyde and formic acid formation and profound acidosis) ethylene glycol (acidosis and oxalate formation) and salicylate (acidosis and the risk of bleeding from the effects on platelets). It must be pointed out, however, that there are several controversial areas where the indications for hemoperfusion remain, as yet, unproven. Acetaminophen (paracetamol) poisoning is best treated by administering sulfhydryl compounds, such as n-acetyl cysteine within 14 h of ingestion (63). The only controlled clinical trial of hemoperfusion in acetaminophen poisoning started within the first 14 h of ingestion was not associated with a favorable clinical outcome (64). Our recent observations, however, suggest that in the treatment of patients who present later than 14 h after ingestion hemoperfusion may be associated with a lesser rise in hepatic enzyme (SGOT, SGPT) concentrations, than occurs with conservative management alone (65). The value of hemoperfusion in acetaminophen poisoning remains, nevertheless, unproven.

Clinical benefit of hemoperfusion for amitriptyline poisoning has been reported using either activated charcoal (66) or resin hemoperfusion (67). Others have not supported this contention (68). Tricyclic drugs have large volumes of distribution and intoxication occurs at low plasma concentrations. Hemoperfusion for tricyclic drug poisoning has been singularly unimpressive (unpublished personal observation). Although a 60% (activated charcoal) to 90% (XAD-4 resin) extraction of nortriptyline occurred during hemoperfusion, no substantial alteration in arterial plasma drug concentrations occurred during four hemoperfusions each lasting 4 h in a patient who subsequently died of severe tricyclic poisoning.

Several studies attest to the beneficial effects of hemoperfusion in digitalis poisoning in animals (69–71) and man (72–73), showing increased drug elimination rates and reduction in plasma digitalis concentrations; but other clinical studies of hemoperfusion in digoxin poisoning have reported somewhat disappointing results (74–76).

Although initially disappointing results were obtained with hemoperfusion in paraquat poisoning (77), it has recently been appreciated that repetitive (almost continuous) activated charcoal hemoperfusion treatment, can prevent pulmonary fibrosis, and induce a favorable clinical outcome (78).

Indications for hemoperfusion

Patients should only be considered for sorbent hemoperfusion if, in addition to fulfilling clinical criteria outlined below, they also have been poisoned with adsorbable drugs such as those outlined in Table 4. It must be stressed that the more important criteria are clinical, as listed below:
1. Severe clinical intoxication leading to progressive deterioration despite intensive supportive management.
2. Severe intoxication with depression of mid-brain function leading to hypoventilation, hypothermia, or hypotension.
3. The development of complications of coma such as pneumonia or septicemia or the presence of underlying conditions predisposing to such complications (e.g., chronic obstructive pulmonary disease).
4. Impairment of the normal drug elimination pathway because of hepatic, cardiac, or renal insufficiency.

In addition to these criteria, hemoperfusion should be considered in the management of patients with the following drugs concentrations:
phenobarbital > 430 µmol/l (100 µg/ml)
short and intermediate acting barbiturates
> 200 µmol/l (50 µg/ml)
glutethimide and methaqualone
> 160 µmol/l (40 µg/ml)
salicylates > 5 mmol/l (800 µg/ml)
ethchlorvynol > 1 mmol/l (150 µg/ml)
meprobamate > 460 µmol/l (100 µg/ml)
trichloroethanol > 335 µmol/l (50 µg/ml)
paraquat > 0.5 µmol/l (0.1 µg/ml)

It is unknown, however, at which concentration toxicity is exerted with diquat and amanita phalloides poisoning. If two or more drugs are present on toxicological screening, hemoperfusion may even be considered at lower individual plasma drug concentrations. As mentioned above, it is probably more correct to use hemodialysis for severe drug intoxication with ethanol, methanol, ethylene glycol and salicylates in view of the rapid correction of both the drug intoxication and the associated metabolic abnormalities.

HEMOPERFUSION IN HEPATIC ENCEPHALOPATHY

Clinical and laboratory studies

The pathogenesis of hepatic encephalopathy, like that of uremia, is poorly understood and consequently therapy directed at removing specific toxins has been limited. In 1972, Chang (79) reported improvement in consciousness in a 50 year old woman treated with charcoal hemoperfusion. This report stimulated the application of charcoal hemoperfusion in the management of fulminant hepatic encephalopathy in the most severe grade of

Table 6. Effect of charcoal hemoperfusion on stage IV fulminant hepatic encephalopathy.

References	No of patients	Recovery of consciousness	Survival	Biochemical changes
Gazzard et al. 1974 (80)	31	48%	39%	↓ Amino acids
Chang et al., 1976 (107)	6	66%	16%	— —
Yamazaki et al., 1977 (113)	13	69%	38.5%	— —
Silk and Williams, 1978 (112)	71	—	23.9%	— —
Gelfand et al., 1978 (85)	10	90%	40%	↑ Amino acid B/A ratio ** ↓ CSF cAMP
Odaka et al., 1978 (49)	10*	70%	30%	↓ Amino acids
Agishi et al., 1980 (47)	18	70%	22%	— —
Gimson et al., 1980 (23)	12	Not reported	Not reported	— —

* Includes 5 patients in stage III coma.
** B/A ratio = Branched chain/aromatic (see text).

coma (stage IV). Initial studies of large series of patients in London by Williams and coworkers (80) were highly encouraging but subsequent studies by the same group have not been confirmatory and attention was for some time directed to the use of hemodialysis with the polyacrylonitrile membrane (82, 83). Studies reporting the use of charcoal hemoperfusion in fulminant hepatic encephalopathy are shown in Table 6. In comparison to conservative therapy alone, which is associated with a 13–17% survival, in some series a substantially greater survival was achieved. Berk (84) however, has pointed out that survival with charcoal hemoperfusion may not be statistically significantly different from that achieved with conservative management. The focus on survival, however, does not emphasize that in most series a large number of patients recover consciousness at some point during the hemoperfusion treatment schedule. Attention should now be directed to instituting hemoperfusion at a much earlier stage of hepatic encephalopathy (prior to stage IV, when irreversible changes, most likely cerebral edema with brain-stem herniation, may have already occurred).

The substances which may be relevant to the development of hepatic encephalopathy and that are removed by sorbent hemoperfusion are shown in Table 7. Gazzard et al. (80), demonstrated that the aromatic amino acids, particularly methionine, were reduced with charcoal hemoperfusion, while Gelfand et al. (85) demonstrated in plasma and also in cerebrospinal fluid that the ratio of branched chain amino acids to aromatic amino acids was appreciably increased after hemoperfusion. (The ratio of branched chain to aromatic amino acids holds an inverse correlation with the degree of hepatic coma.)

Unquestionably, coagulation abnormalities associated with or induced by charcoal hemoperfusion in hepatic encephalopathy, are more common than observed in the treatment of other conditions, and it is our routine practice to administer infusions of platelets and fresh frozen plasma following hemoperfusion (85). Recent work, however, suggests that the antiplatelet-aggregating agent, prostacyclin, may improve the biocompatibility of hemoperfusion for hepatic encephalopathy (23).

Certainly, charcoal hemoperfusion as a definitive treatment for hepatic encephalopathy has fallen short of its goals for several reasons. Controlled clinical trials of hemoperfusion are, at present, logistically impossible, while optimal timing and frequency of hemoperfusion have not been determined. It has been suggested by Berk (84), on the basis of kinetic modeling, that hepatic toxins move in a slowly equilibrating pool and for optimal results detoxification procedures should be performed every 12 h. Chang et al. (86), have shown that in animals, hemoperfusion may improve the prognosis if applied at an earlier coma staging (stage III). Recently

Table 7. Substances relevant to hepatic coma removed by sorbent hemoperfusion.

Amino acids * – aromatic > branched	Fatty acids – oleic, hexanoic, octanoic, N-valeric
(Ammonia) *	(Glucose) *
Bile acids *	Mercaptan
Bilirubin *	Middle molecules
(Calcium) *	Norepinephrine
Coagulation factors *	Octopamine
(Cyclic AMP) *	Phenols *
Dopamine	(Protein bound molecules)
Epinephrine	

* Studied in vivo.
( ) Ineffectively removed.

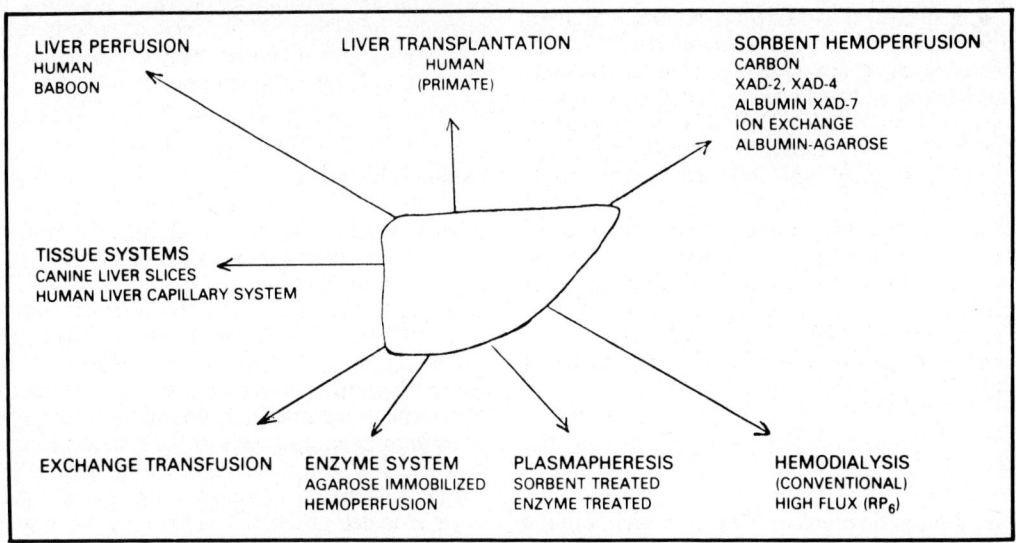

Figure 7. Current investigative methods used in conjunction with standard therapy for the treatment of hepatic coma (reprinted from Winchester et al. (114), with permission of the copyright holder).

clinical hemoperfusion studies have supported this contention (115). Other limitations underline the fact that charcoal hemoperfusion does not supply nutritive or reparative properties associated with normal hepatic function and that it is not yet possible to design a specific sorbent for removing the hepatic failure 'toxin'. Like uremia, hepatic encephalopathy is more likely of multi-factorial origin and, at present, the design of a specific sorbent cannot be undertaken, although it is felt that toxins responsible for hepatic encephalopathy are probably tightly protein bound and consequently poorly removed by adsorption. New techniques for the treatment of hepatic encephalopathy, including the design of systems for removing protein bound toxins are shown in Figure 7.

Indications for hemoperfusion

At present, it is impossible to give definitive criteria for the adoption of charcoal hemoperfusion in fulminant hepatic encephalopathy, since survival from this disorder depends on many factors such as the etiology of the liver disease, age and sex, and clear results will only emerge from a large, well-conducted controlled clinical trial. However, until alternative approaches are better defined, hemoperfusion should be used in carefully selected patients, at an earlier stage of coma and perhaps more frequently than has been the position so far, since hemoperfusion probably represents the most effective available treatment for acute fulminant hepatic failure at the present time.

OTHER USES OF SORBENT HEMOPERFUSION

Schizophrenia

In 1977 Wagemaker and Cade (87) reported dramatic improvement of five of six schizophrenic patients treated with regular (once weekly) hemodialysis; later they observed similar beneficial results in an additional series of patients (in 16 out of 23). They attributed the therapeutic effect to removal of leucine-endorphin by dialysis (88), although this was not confirmed by others (89).

Several clinical investigators were stimulated to apply other treatment techniques such as hemoperfusion and hemofiltration in the treatment of this serious psychiatric disorder (90–94). The variable clinical results have not proved clinical efficacy of such treatment.

This somewhat controversial therapy is discussed in chapter 49.

Psoriasis

In a similar fashion favorable results have been found in patients with severe psoriasis treated with peritoneal dialysis (95) and hemodialysis (96). Others, however, have observed psoriasis developing during regular dialysis (97) and have noted negative results with hemodialysis treatment (98).

Patients with psoriasis have also been treated with hemoperfusion and hemofiltration (99, 100). The treatment of psoriasis with hemodialysis and related techniques is also discussed by Gurland and his co-authors in chapter 49.

Anti-cancer drug removal

Since the use of anti-cancer drugs may be limited by the presence of hepatic or renal dysfunction, the full benefits of such drugs as adriamycin or methotrexate may be curtailed in patients with diseases of these systems. Several authors have attempted to remove anti-cancer drugs from patients with inadvertent excessive dosage of these drugs, while it has been our own theory that exposure of patients to a high therapeutic drug load with subsequent rapid removal might obviate the known tissue toxicity of high dose anti-cancer drug therapy (59, 101). Although initial reports of uncoated charcoal hemoperfusion in removal of methotrexate were encouraging, subsequent reports of XAD-4 resin or uncoated charcoal hemoperfusion and hemodialysis or peritoneal dialysis have been somewhat disappointing (101). Methotrexate removal is more efficiently achieved with the use of uncoated charcoal hemoperfusion, than with XAD-4 resin hemoperfusion or with hemodialysis or peritoneal dialysis. But, although substantial methotrexate clearance is initially achieved, the charcoal columns rapidly saturate and become inactive. Therefore there is no substantial change in drug elimination kinetics (101). It is unlikely, consequently, that tissue concentrations of methotrexate can be substantially reduced. Further work in this area is needed. Similarly, although substantial removal of the anthracycline antibiotic and anti-cancer drug, adriamycin, can be achieved with charcoal hemoperfusion and substantial increases in drug elimination rates can be achieved (59), further work is required before any statement can be made on the reduction of tissue levels of this drug with hemoperfusion.

Immunoadsorption

One of the most exciting possibilities for hemoperfusion involves the specific adsorption of immune proteins on antigen or antibody coated carrier particles. This technique has been introduced by Terman and co-workers (102), who have shown that it is possible to remove antibodies to such proteins or polypeptides as bovine serum albumin, deoxyribonucleic acid and antiglomerular basement membrane antibody from blood percolated through these immunoadsorbent systems. Recently, Terman and his coworkers, have shown that DNA-collodion coated charcoal removed significant quantities of single stranded anti-DNA antibodies and immune complexes from the circulating blood of a patient with systemic lupus erythematosus. In addition to the reduction of immune reactants in blood, subendothelial glomerular deposits were also very much reduced on comparison of pre- and post treatement renal biopsy specimens (103). Certainly, immunoadsorption for the treatment of lupus erythematosus appears to be a promising approach.

Recent work from Terman's lab has shown that this technique may also benefit hyperacute renal xenograft rejection in animals (104). In a dog model with spontaneous breast cancer, passage of blood over a column containing staphylococcal A protein was associated with regression and complete disappearance of the breast cancer lesions (105). Studies of this technique in human breast cancer are underway and the results are awaited with considerable interest.

FUTURE DEVELOPMENTS

It is the feeling of most workers in the field of artificial organs that the future development of treatment of uremia will involve the hybridization of sorbent technology in conjunction with dialysis/hemofiltration techniques. At present, the problem of the identification of specific uremic toxins is a major barrier to development in this field. Current interest in this complex area centers around the removal of middle molecules and recent attention has also been directed toward the removal of urea, which has been the classic 'marker' of uremia. In this respect, several approaches to extracorporeal removal of urea have been made which involve enzyme degradation of urea and development of specific sorbents such as the Ionsiv series and cation exchange resins. Such techniques are shown in Figure 6. Urea sorbents which combine the necessary properties of effectiveness and biocompatibility along with control of pH and electrolyte abnormalities are certainly a feasible prospect for the treatment of uremia. At present, however, no sorbents have been developed which have all of these desirable properties. But it is likely that a 'wearable' kidney which combines the properties outlined above should be a feasible prospect over the next few years.

It certainly would appear that hemoperfusion has a definitive role in the management of acute drug intoxication, a less definitive role in the management of uremia, and a questionable role in the management of hepatic encephalopathy. A most exciting prospect is the development of the specific extracorporeal immunoadsorbent columns which not only offer the prospect of treatment of severe refractory immune mediated diseases but theoretically may allow examination of the role of specific antibodies in the mediation of such diseases.

ACKNOWLEDGEMENTS

The author thanks Mrs Patti Werr and Mrs Donna Sullivan for secretarial assistance in preparing the manuscript.

REFERENCES

1. Yatzidis H: A convenient haemoperfusion micro-apparatus over charcoal for the treatment of endogenous and exogenous intoxications. Its use as an artificial kidney. *Proc Eur Dial Transpl Assoc* 1:83, 1964
2. Dunea G, Kolff WJ: Clinical experience with the Yatzidis charcoal artificial kidney. *Trans Am Soc Artif Intern Organs* 11:178, 1965
3. Chang TMS: Semipermeable aqueous microcapsules (artificial cells): with emphasis on experiments in an extracorporeal shunt system. *Trans Am Soc Artif Intern Organs* 12:13, 1966
4. Asher WJ: Introduction to sorbents. In: *Sorbents and Their Clinical Applications,* edited by Giordano C, New York, Academic Press, Inc 1980, p 3
5. Denti E, Walker JM: Activated carbon: properties, selection and evaluation. In: *Sorbents and Their Clinical Applications,* edited by Giordano C, New York, Academic Press Inc, 1980, p 101
6. Denti E, Luboz MP, Tessore V: Adsorption characteristics of cellulose acetate coated charcoals. *J Biomed Mater Res* 9:143, 1975
7. Winchester JF, Ratcliffe JG, Carlyle E, Kennedy AC: Solute, amino acid, and hormone changes with coated charcoal hemoperfusion in uremia. *Kidney Int* 14:74, 1978
8. Kokot F, Pietrek J, Seredynski M: Influence of haemoperfusion on plasma levels of hormones and β-methyldigoxin. *Proc Eur Dial Transpl Assoc* 15:604, 1978
9. Cornelis R, Ringoir S, Mees L, Hoste J: Behavior of trace metals during hemoperfusion. *Mineral Electrol Metab* 4:123, 1980
10. Hagstam KE, Larsson LE, Thysell H: Experimental studies on charcoal haemoperfusion in phenobarbital intoxication and uraemia, including histopathologic findings. *Acta Med Scand* 180:593, 1966
11. Winchester JF: Hemoperfusion in uremia. In: *Sorbents and Their Clinical Applications,* edited by Giordano C, New York, Academic Press, Inc., 1980, p 387
12. Chang, TMS. Microcapsule artificial kidney in replacement of renal function. With emphasis on adsorbent hemoperfusion. In: *Replacement of Renal Function by Dialysis,* First Edition, edited by Drukker W, Parsons FM, Maher JF, The Hague, Boston, London, Martinus Nijhoff Publishers, 1978, p 217
13. Odaka M, Tabata Y, Kobayashi H, Nomura Y, Soma M, Hirasawa H, Sato H, Suenaga E, Nabeta K: Three hour maintenance haemodialysis combining direct haemoperfusion and haemodialysis. *Proc Eur Dial Transpl Assoc* 13:257, 1976
14. Ota K, Ohta T, Kobayashi M, Yoshida S, Kaneko I, Agishi T, Sugihara M: Petroleum based activated charcoal for direct haemoperfusion. *Proc Eur Dial Transpl Assoc* 13:250, 1976
15. Stefoni S, Feliciangeli G, Coli L, Bonomini V: Evaluation of a new coated charcoal for hemoperfusion in uremia. *Int J Artif Organs* 2:320, 1979
16. Craddock PR, Fehr J, Brigham KL, Kronenberg R, Jacob

HS: Complement and leukocyte-mediated pulmonary dysfunction in hemodialysis. *N Engl J Med* 296:769, 1977
17. Gurland HJ, Fernandez JC, Samtleben W, Castro LA: Sorbent membranes used in a conventional dialyzer format: In vitro and clinical evaluation *Artif Organs* 2:372, 1978
18. Davis TA, Cowsar DR, Harrison SD, Tanquary AC: Artificial carbon fibers for hemoperfusion. *Trans Am Soc Artif Intern Organs* 20:353, 1974
19. Malchesky PS, Varnes WG, Nokoff R, Nose Y: The charcoal capillary haemoperfusion system. *Proc Eur Dial Transpl Assoc* 13:242, 1976
20. Weston MJ, Langley PG, Rubin MH, Hanid MA, Mellon P, Williams R: Platelet function in fulminant hepatic failure and effect of charcoal haemoperfusion. *Gut* 18:897, 1977
21. Winchester JF, Forbes CD, Courtney JM, Reavey M, Prentice CRM: Effect of sulphinpyrazone and aspirin on platelet adhesion to activated charcoal and dialysis membranes in vitro. *Thromb Res* 11:443, 1977
22. Bunting S, Moncada S, Vane JR, Woods HF, Weston MJ: Prostacyclin improves hemocompatibility during charcoal haemoperfusion. In: *Prostacyclin,* edited by Vane JR, Bergström S, New York, Raven Press, 1979, p 361
23. Gimson AES, Langley PG, Hughes RD, Canalese J, Mellon PG, Williams R, Woods HF, Weston MJ: Prostacyclin to prevent platelet activation during charcoal haemoperfusion in fulminant hepatic failure. *Lancet* 1:173, 1980
24. Mauer S, Chavers BM, Kjellstrand CM: Treatment of an infant with severe chloramphenicol intoxication, using charcoal-column hemoperfusion. *J Pediatr* 96:136, 1980
25. Winchester JF: *Evaluation of Sorbent Haemoperfusion in Poisoning and Uraemia.* MD Thesis, University of Glasgow, Scotland, 1980
26. Lindsay RM, Prentice CRM, Davidson JF, Burton JA, McNicol GP: Haemostatic changes during dialysis associated with thrombus formation on dialysis membranes. *Br Med J* 4:454, 1972
27. Chang TMS, Chirito E, Barre B, Cole C, Hewish M: Clinical performance-characteristics of a new combined system for simultaneous hemoperfusion-hemodialysis-ultrafiltration in series. *Trans Am Soc Artif Intern Organs* 21:502, 1975
28. Stefoni S, Coli L, Feliciangeli G, Baldrati L, Bonomini V: Regular hemoperfusion in regular dialysis treatment. A long-term study. *Int J Artif Organs* 3:348, 1980
29. Muirhead EE, Reid AF: Resin artificial kidney. *J Lab Clin Med* 33:841, 1948
30. Schreiner GE: The role of hemodialysis (artificial kidney) in acute poisoning. *Arch Intern Med* 102:896, 1958
31. Rosenbaum JL, Onesti G, Heider C: The removal of cation from dogs with an ion-exchange column. *JAMA* 180:762, 1962
32. Kissack AS, Gliedman L, Karlson KE: Studies with ion exchange resins. *Trans Am Soc Artif Intern Organs* 8:219, 1962
33. Nealon TF Jr, Ching N: An extracorporeal device to lower blood ammonia levels in hepatic coma. *Trans Am Soc Artif Intern Organs* 8:226, 1962
34. Yatzidis H, Voudiclari S, Oreopoulos D, Tsaparas N, Triantaphyllidis D, Gavras C, Stavroulaki A: Treatment of severe barbiturate poisoning. *Lancet* 2:216, 1965
35. Chang TMS, Gonda A, Dirks JH, Malave N: Clinical evaluation of chronic intermittent and short term hemoperfusion in patients with chronic renal failure using semipermeable microcapsules (artificial cells) formed from membrane coated activated charcoal. *Trans Am Soc Artif Intern Organs* 17:246, 1971
36. Chang TMS, Migchelsen M: Characterization of possible 'toxic' metabolites in uremia and hepatic coma based on the clearance spectrum for larger molecules by the ACAC microcapsule artificial kidney. *Trans Am Soc Artif Intern Organs* 19:314, 1973
37. Chang TMS, Migchelsen M, Coffey JF, Stark R: Serum middle molecule levels in uremia during long term intermittent hemoperfusion with the ACAC (coated charcoal) microcapsule artificial kidney. *Trans Am Soc Artif Intern Organs* 20:364, 1974
38. Oulès R, Asaba H, Neuhauser M, Yahiel V, Gunnarsson B, Bergström J, Fürst P: Removal of uremic small and middle molecules and free amino acids by carbon hemoperfusion. *Trans Am Soc Artif Intern Organs* 23:583, 1977
39. Chang TMS: Assessments of clinical trials of charcoal hemoperfusion in uremic patients. *Clin Nephrol* 11:111, 1979
40. Rosenbaum JL, Kramer MS, Raja R, Henriquez M: Hemoperfusion in uremia: Effect of time, solute competition and biocompatibility on column adsorption. In: *Hemoperfusion, Kidney and Liver Support and Detoxification,* edited by Sideman S, Chang TMS, Washington DC, Hemisphere Publishing Corp, 1980, p 245
41. Gelfand MC, Winchester JF: Hemoperfusion results in uremia. *Clin Nephrol* 11:107, 1979
42. Trznadel K, Walasek L, Kidawa Z, Lutz W: Comparative studies on the effect of hemoperfusion and hemodialysis on the elimination of some uremic toxins. *Clin Nephrol* 10:229, 1978
43. Weber WJ, Morris JC: Kinetics of adsorption on carbon from solutions. *Proc Am Soc Civil Eng* 89:31, 1963
44. Martin AM, Gibbins JK, Kimmitt J, Rennie F: Hemodialysis and hemoperfusion in the treatment of uremic pericarditis. A study of 13 cases. *Dial Transpl* 8:135, 1979
45. Odaka M, Hirasaw H, Kobayashi H, Ohkawa M, Soeda K, Tabata Y, Soma M, Sato H: Clinical and fundamental studies of cellulose coated bead-shaped charcoal haemoperfusion in chronic renal failure. In: *Hemoperfusion, Kidney and Liver Support and Detoxification,* edited by Sideman S, Chang TMS, Washington DC, Hemisphere Publishing Corp, 1980, p 45
46. Otsubo O, Kuzuhara K, Simada Y, Yamauchi Y, Takahashi I, Yamada Y, Otsubo K, Inou T: Treatment of uraemic peripheral neuritis by direct haemoperfusion with activated charcoal. *Proc Eur Dial Transpl Assoc* 16:731, 1979
47. Agishi T, Yamashita N, Ota K: Clinical results of direct charcoal hemoperfusion for endogenous and exogenous intoxication. In: *Hemoperfusion, Kidney and Liver Support and Detoxification,* edited by Sideman S, Chang TMS, Washington DC, Hemisphere Publishing Corp, 1980, p 255
48. Siemsen AW, Dunea G, Mamdani BH, Guruprakash G: Charcoal hemoperfusion for chronic renal failure. *Nephron* 22:386, 1978
49. Odaka M, Tabata Y, Kobayashi H, Nomura Y, Soma A, Hirasawa A, Sato H: Clinical experience of bead-shaped charcoal hemoperfusion in chronic renal failure and fulminant hepatic failure. In: *Artificial Kidney, Artificial Liver and Artificial Cells,* edited by Chang TMS, New York, Plenum Press, 1978, p 79
50. Lawson AA, Mitchell I: Patients with acute poisoning seen in a general medical unit (1960-1971). *Br Med J* 4:153, 1972

51. Reed CE, Driggs MF, Foote CC: Acute barbiturate intoxication: A study of 300 cases based on a physiologic system of classification of the severity of the intoxication. *Ann Intern Med* 37:290, 1952
52. Winchester JF, Gelfand MC, Tilstone WJ: Hemoperfusion in drug intoxication – Clinical and laboratory aspects. *Drug Metab Rev* 8:69, 1978
53. Maher JF, Schreiner GE: The dialysis of poisons and drugs. *Trans Am Soc Artif Intern Organs* 13:369, 1967
54. Winchester JF, Gelfand MC, Knepshield JH, Schreiner GE: Dialysis and hemoperfusion of poisons and drugs – Update. *Trans Am Soc Artif Intern Organs* 23:762, 1977
55. Winchester JF, Tilstone WJ, Edwards RO, Gilchrist T, Kennedy AC: Hemoperfusion for enhanced drug elimination – A kinetic analysis in paracetamol poisoning. *Trans Am Soc Artif Intern Organs* 20:358, 1974
56. Gibson TP, Lucas SV, Nelson HA, Atkinson AJ, Okita GT, Ivanovich P: Hemoperfusion removal of digoxin from dogs. *J Lab Clin Med* 91:673, 1978
57. Zmuda MJ: Resin hemoperfusion in dogs intoxicated with ethchlorvynol (Placidy ®), *Kidney Int* 17:303, 1980
58. Ehlers SM, Zaske DE, Sawchuk RJ: Massive theophylline overdose. Rapid elimination by charcoal hemoperfusion. *JAMA* 240:474, 1978
59. Winchester JF, Rahman A, Tilstone WJ, Kessler A, Mortensen L, Schreiner GE, Schein PS: Sorbent removal of adriamycin in vitro and in vivo. *Cancer Treat Rep* 63:1787, 1979
60. Lorch JA, Garella S: Hemoperfusion to treat intoxications. *Ann Intern Med* 91:301, 1979
61. Farrell PC: Commentary: Acute drug intoxication and extracorporeal intervention. *asaio J* 3:39, 1980
62. Maher JF: In discussion on hemoperfusion for poisoning – Is it really necessary? *Controversies in Nephrology*, Volume 2, edited by Schreiner GE, Winchester JF, Washington, Georgetown Nephrology Press, 1980, p 228
63. Rumack BH, Peterson RG: Acetaminophen overdose: Incidence, diagnosis, and management in 416 patients. *Pediatrics* 62:898, 1978
64. Gazzard BG, Willson RA, Weston MJ, Thompson R, Williams R: Charcoal haemoperfusion for paracetamol overdose. *Br J Clin Pharmacol* 1:271, 1974
65. Winchester JF, Gelfand MC, Helliwell M, Vale JA, Goulding R, Schreiner GE: Extracorporeal treatment of salicylate or acetaminophen poisoning – Is there a role? *Arch Intern Med* 141:370, 1981
66. Diaz-Buxo JA, Farmer CD, Chandler JT: Hemoperfusion in the treatment of amitriptyline poisoning. *Trans Am Soc Artif Intern Organs* 24:699, 1978
67. Trafford JAP, Jones RH, Evans R, Sharp P, Sharpstone P, Cook J: Haemoperfusion with R-004 amberlite resin for treating acute poisoning. *Br Med J* 2:1453, 1977
68. Crome P, Braithwaite RA, Widdop B, Medd RK: Haemoperfusion in clinical and experimental tricyclic antidepressant poisoning. In: *Hemoperfusion, Kidney and Liver Support and Detoxification*, edited by Sideman S, Chang TMS, Washington DC, Hemisphere Publishing Corp, 1980, p 301
69. Carvallo A, Ramirez B, Honig H, Knepshield J, Schreiner GE, Gelfand MC: Treatment of digitalis intoxication by charcoal hemoperfusion. *Trans Am Soc Artif Intern Organs* 22:718, 1976
70. Gibson TP, Atkinson AJ: Effect of changes in intercompartmental rate constants on drug removal during hemoperfusion. *J Pharm Sci* 67:1178, 1978
71. Shah G, Nelson HA, Atkinson AJ, Okita GT, Ivanovich P. Gibson TP: Effect of hemoperfusion on the pharmacokinetics of digitoxin in dogs. *J Lab Clin Med* 93:370, 1979
72. Marbury T, Mahoney J, Juncos L, Conti R, Cade R: Advanced digoxin toxicity in renal failure – Treatment with charcoal hemoperfusion. *South Med J* 72:279, 1979
73. Tobin M, Cerra F, Steinbach J, Mookerjee B: Hemoperfusion in digitalis intoxication: A comparative study of coated versus uncoated charcoal. *Trans Am Soc Artif Intern Organs* 23:730, 1977
74. Warren SE, Fanestil DF: Digoxin overdose: Limitations of hemoperfusion-hemodialysis treatment. *JAMA* 242:2100, 1979
75. Freed CR, Gerber JG, Gal J, Rumack BH, Nies AS: Hemoperfusion in drug overdose. *JAMA* 241:1575, 1979
76. Slattery JR, Koup JR: Hemoperfusion in the management of digoxin toxicity. Is it warranted? *Clin Pharmacokinet* 4:395, 1979
77. Gelfand MC, Winchester JF, Knepshield JH, Hanson KM, Cohan SL, Strauch BS, Geoly KL, Kennedy AC, Schreiner GE: Treatment of severe drug overdosage with charcoal hemoperfusion. *Trans Am Soc Artif Intern Organs* 23:599, 1977
78. Okonek S, Baldamus CA, Hofman A, Schuster CJ, Bechstein PB, Zoller B: Two survivors of severe paraquat intoxication by 'continuous hemoperfusion'. *Klin Wochenschr* 57:957, 1979
79. Chang TMS: Haemoperfusion over microencapsulated adsorbent in a patient with hepatic coma. *Lancet* 2:1371, 1972
80. Gazzard BG, Portmann BA, Weston MJ, Langley PG, Murray-Lyon IM, Dunlop EH, Flax H, Mellon PJ, Record CO, Ward MB, Williams R: Charcoal haemoperfusion in the treatment of fulminant hepatic failure. *Lancet* 1:1301, 1974
81. Silk DBA, Williams R: Sorbents in hepatic failure. In: *Sorbents and Their Clinical Applications*, edited by Giordano C, New York, Academic Press, Inc, 1980, p 415
82. Opolon P, Rapin JR, Huguet C, Granger A, Delorme ML, Boschat M, Sausse A: Hepatic failure coma treated by polyacrylonitrile membrane hemodialysis. *Trans Am Soc Artif Intern Organs* 22:701, 1976
83. Silk DBA, Trewby PN, Chase RA, Mellon PJ, Hanid MA, Davies M, Langley PG, Wheeler PG, Williams R: Treatment of fulminant hepatic failure by polyacrylonitrile membrane haemodialysis. *Lancet* 2:1, 1977
84. Berk PD: A computer simulation study relating to the treatment of fulminant hepatic failure by hemoperfusion. *Proc Soc Exp Biol Med* 155:535, 1977
85. Gelfand MC, Winchester JF, Knepshield JH, Cohan SL, Schreiner GE: Reversal of hepatic coma by coated charcoal hemoperfusion: Clinical and biochemical observations. *asaio J* 1:37, 1978
86. Chang TMS, Lister C, Chirito E, O'Keefe P, Resurreccion E: Effects of hemoperfusion rate and time of initiation of ACAC charcoal hemoperfusion on the survival of fulminant hepatic failure rats. *Trans Am Soc Artif Intern Organs* 24:243, 1978
87. Wagemaker H, Cade R: The use of hemodialysis in chronic schizophrenia. *Am J Psych* 134:684, 1977
88. Cade R, Wagemaker H: Hemodialysis as a treatment for chronic schizophrenia. (Abstr) *Am Soc Artif Intern Organs* 7:1, 1978
89. Kolff WJ: Dialysis of schizophrenics. Weird and novel applications of dialysis, hemofiltration, hemoperfusion, and peritoneal dialysis: Witchcraft? *Artif Organs* 2:277, 1978

90. Gurland HJ: Chronic schizophrenia. *The S. Neaman Workshop on Hemoperfusion: Devices and Clinical Applications,* edited by Sideman S, Chang TMS, Haifa, Publication No. 01/108/80, Technion-Israel Institute of Technology, 1980, p 123
91. Chang TMS: Hemoperfusion in chronic schizophrenia. *Int J Artif Organs* 1:253, 1978
92. Kinney MJ: Hemoperfusion for chronic schizophrenia: Preliminary psychiatric results (Cited in Gurland, ref. 90)
93. Nedopil N, Dieterle D, Gurland HJ: Blood purification treatment of schizophrenia. *Int J Artif Organs* 3:76, 1980
94. Schulz SC, VanKammen DP, Balow JE, Flye MW, Bunney WE: Dialysis in schizophrenia: A double blind evaluation. *Science* 211:1066, 1981
95. Twardowski ZJ, Nolph KD, Rubin J, Anderson PC: Peritoneal dialysis for psoriasis. *Ann Intern Med* 88:349, 1978
96. McEvoy J, Kelly AMT: Psoriatic clearance during hemodialysis. *Ulster Med J* 45:76, 1976
97. Breathnach SM, Boon NA, Black MM, Jones NF, Wing AJ: Psoriasis developing during dialysis. *Br Med J* 1:236, 1979
98. Nissensson AB, Rapaport M, Gordon A, Narins RG: Controlled study demonstrates that psoriasis is not improved by hemodialysis. *Kidney Int* 14:682, 1978
99. Maeda K, Saito A, Kawaguchi S, Niwa T, Sezaki R, Kobayashi K, Asada H, Yamamoto Y, Ohta K: Psoriasis treatment with direct hemoperfusion. In: *Hemoperfusion, Kidney and Liver Support and Detoxification.* Edited by Sideman S, Chang TMS, Washington, DC, Hemisphere Publishing Corp, 1980, p 349
100. Tagami H, Ofuji S: Leukotactic properties of soluble substances in psoriasis scale. *Br J Dermatol* 95:1, 1978
101. Winchester JF, Rahman A, Bregman H, Mortensen LM, Gelfand MC, Schein PS, Schreiner GE: Role of hemoperfusion in anticancer drug removal. In: *Hemoperfusion, Kidney and Liver Support and Detoxification,* edited by Sideman S, Chang TMS, Washington DC, Hemisphere Publishing Corp, 1980, p 369
102. Terman DS: Extracorporeal immunoadsorbents for extraction of circulating immune reactants. In: *Sorbents and Their Clinical Applications,* edited by Giordano C, New York, Academic Press, Inc 1980, p 470
103. Terman DS, Buffaloe G, Mattioli C, Cook G, Tillquist R, Sullivan M, Ayus JC: Extracorporeal immunoadsorption: Initial experience in human systemic lupus erythematosus. *Lancet* 2:824, 1979
104. Terman DS, Garcia-Rinaldi R, McCalman R, Crumb CC, Mattioli C, Cook G, Poser, R: Modification of hyperacute renal xenograft rejection after extracorporeal immunoadsorption of heterospecific antibody. *Int J Artif Organs* 2:35, 1979
105. Terman DS, Yamamoto T, Mattioli M, Cook G, Tillquist R, Henry J, Poser R, Daskal Y: Extensive necrosis of spontaneous canine mammary adenocarcinoma after extracorporeal perfusion over staphylococcus aureus Cowans I. *J Immunol* 124: 795, 1980
106. Yatzidis H, Oreopoulos D: Early clinical trials with sorbents. *Kidney Int* 10 (Suppl 7):S215, 1976
107. Chang TMS: Hemoperfusion alone and in series with ultrafiltration or dialysis for uremia, poisoning and liver failure. *Kidney Int* 10 (Suppl 7):S305, 1976
108. Yatzidis H, Yulis G, Digenis P: Hemocarboperfusion-hemodialysis treatment in terminal renal failure. *Kidney Int* 10 (Suppl 7):S312, 1976
109. Leber XE, Neuhauser M, Goubeaud G: Chronic uraemia: haemodialysis or haemoperfusion? In: *Artificial Organs,* edited by Kenedi RM, Courtney JM, Gaylor JDS, Gilchrist T, London and Basingstoke, MacMillan Press, Ltd, 1977, p 220
110. Dunea G, Rizvi ZH, Mamdani BH, Anicama HJ, Mahurkar SD: Charcoal hemoperfusion and combination dialysis-hemoperfusion in chronic renal failure. *(Abstr) Am Soc Artif Intern Organs* 5:22, 1975
111. Martin AM, Gibbins JK, Oduro M, Herbert R: Clinical experience with cellulose coated carbon hemoperfusion. In: *Artificial Liver, Artificial Kidney, and Artificial Cells,* edited by Chang TMS, Plenum Press, New York, 1978, p 143
112. Silk DBA, Williams R: Experiences in the treatment of fulminant hepatic failure by conservative therapy, charcoal haemoperfusion and polyacrylonitrile haemodialysis. *Int J Artif Organs* 1:29, 1978
113. Yamazaki Z, Fujimori Y, Sanjo K, Kojima Y, Sugiura M, Wada T, Inoue N, Sakai T, Oda T, Kominami N, Fujisaki U, Kataoka K: New artificial liver support system (Plasma perfusion detoxification) for hepatic coma. *Artif Organs* 1:148, 1977
114. Winchester JF, Gelfand MC, Knepshield JH, Schreiner GE: Realities in evaluating the clinical uses of sorbent hemoperfusion. *Int J Artif Organs* 2:310, 1979
115. Gimson AES, Braude S, Melion PJ, Canalese J, Williams R: Earlier charcoal haemoperfusion in fulminant hepatic failure. *Lancet* 2:681, 1982

17

DIALYSATE REGENERATION

ANTONY J. WING, FRANK M. PARSONS and WILLIAM DRUKKER

Introduction	323
Previous attempts to regenerate dialysate	323
Practical application of dialysate regeneration	326
The Redy-Sorb system	326
The regeneration cartridge	326
Practical application and guidelines for use of the Redy system	330
Urea removal; available cartridges	331
Low dialysate flow rate through the circuit	331
Kinetics of pH and CO_2	331
Sodium kinetics	333
Calcium, magnesium and potassium kinetics	334
Acetate kinetics and correction of metabolic acidosis	334
The Redy system in patients with normal or low plasma urea concentrations	335
Long-term treatment with the Redy system	335
Toxicology of the Redy system	336
Acknowledgments	338
New model Redy 2000	338
References	339

INTRODUCTION

Conventional haemodialysis performed 6 h, thrice weekly, requires some 600 l of water for preparation of dialysis fluid per week. The usual equipment requires water and drainage connections and is, in practice, immobile.

In many areas there may be inadequate plumbing or a natural shortage of water; in other parts of the world water may become increasingly scarce either on a temporary, periodic or permanent basis. In addition mains water has to be pre-treated, often with complicated equipment, which is expensive and requires adequate professional maintenance (see chapter 6).

Several attempts have been made to treat spent dialysate by activated carbon for reuse, in order to reduce the required water volumes (1–5).

It was shown, that activated carbon is an effective adsorbent for many urinary nitrogenous waste products urea being an important exception. Although 100 g of activated carbon is sufficient to adsorb the quantities of creatinine, uric acid and phenols produced daily, some 10 to 20 kg would be required to adsorb the daily production of urea (2). Although the toxic potential of urea, per se, is questionable (see chapter 19), it is a traditional marker of the uraemic state and increases the osmolality of the body fluids. It should obviously be removed in the treatment of uraemia.

Urea is, however, an unreactive molecule, which is difficult to adsorb, in particular from dialysis fluid, where the electrolyte concentration, the dextrose content, pH and temperature cannot be manipulated readily outside narrowly restricted limits. In addition, activated carbon has virtually no affinity for mono- and divalent ions and therefore cannot correct abnormalities of sodium, potassium, phosphate, chloride, calcium or magnesium.

This chapter reviews various attempts to develop efficient regeneration of dialysis fluid and describes the only system that is practical and available commercially and rather widely used.

PREVIOUS ATTEMPTS TO REGENERATE DIALYSATE

Several attempts have been made to purify a small volume of dialysate fit for reuse, making a dialysis system with a small volume of recirculating dialysis fluid possible.

In Japan Maeda and coworkers (6) in 1971 constructed a portable artificial kidney system, utilising 30 l of dialysate which were regenerated by recirculation through a column containing 500 g of activated charcoal and a second column containing 200 g of alumina. These two substances were selected on the basis of their adsorption rates for creatinine, uric acid and inorganic phosphate. In addition appreciable amounts of methylguanidine and guanidino acetic acid were adsorbed. The adsorbents were tested for the release of potentially toxic trace metals, including aluminium, by atomic absorption spectophotometry and it was concluded that the system was safe. *In vitro* experiments demonstrated satisfactory adsorption of creatinine and uric acid by the activated carbon and of phosphate by the alumina column. It should be mentioned, however, that the investigators did not use the sensitive flameless atomic absorption spectrophometric technique, as later described by Fuchs and coworkers (7), which is required for accurate aluminium determinations in biological fluids.

The Japanese investigators used their 30 l system for at least 46 months in a number of patients in a comparative study with a single pass system, which required 210 l of dialysis fluid. Six hundred dialyses were performed and on average plasma concentrations were reduced by 59% for creatinine, 67% for uric acid and 58%

for phosphate. A possible rise of the blood urea was, however, a matter of concern. Surprisingly in an anuric patient, being dialysed 7 hours thrice weekly with the new system during 14 months, a fall of the blood urea concentration was observed after an initial rise. The patient was eventually fully rehabilitated.

In 1974 the same investigators (8) reported favourable results in an additional group of patients. At that time, according to the authors, almost all home dialysis patients in Japan were using their system.

Subsequently the authors changed to a 10 l system, increasing the acetate concentration to 50 mmol/l, which normalised post-dialysis bicarbonate concentration. Equally good results were obtained; pre-dialysis levels of blood urea initially increased but gradually decreased after 6 weeks, stabilising at approximately 420 mg/dl (70 mmol/l). The authors explained this phenomenon by postulating the incorporation of urea into plasma and tissue proteins.

Nevertheless no further papers on this system have been published in the current literature and we do not know of any application of this system outside Japan.

Italian investigators (9) prepared a sorbent cartridge with a bottom layer of granulated oxidised starch for removal of urea and a layer with aluminium silicate which removed phosphate and substantial amounts of calcium and magnesium. Therefore, a cation exchange resin layer was inserted in between. This layer served a dual purpose: by exchanging cations, calcium replenishment and potassium removal were obtained. Remaining organic metabolites such as creatinine and uric acid were removed by a top layer containing activated carbon. A number of animal experiments were performed with encouraging results in 1974 but the system had not yet been used in patients. No further reports have been published in the literature.

In England dialysate regeneration was reviewed and studied at the Atomic Weapons Research Establishment at Aldermaston by Bultitude and Gower (10). They tried to regenerate the dialysis fluid by circulating through a 4 kg (dry weight) activated charcoal pack. A 30 l batch of a somewhat modified dialysis fluid was used, containing (in mmol/l) sodium 132, potassium 1.3, calcium 1.5, magnesium 0.5, acetate 43 and chloride 94 (without dextrose).

Up to 2.5 l of body water (including solutes) could be removed from the patient by ultrafiltration by means of a negative pressure pump situated down stream of the dialyser as is used in a conventional flow-to-waste system. The 30 l of dialysis fluid was chosen partly to correct electrolyte imbalance as equilibration would occur with the plasma water across the dialyser and partly to equilibrate urea in a similar manner. A very limited clinical trial was undertaken by one of the authors (FMP). Certainly during dialysis, equilibration between plasma water and dialysis fluid occurred, but unexplained hypocalcaemia developed and it seemed that with this type of regeneration system, further work on calcium kinetics was required.

The wearable artificial kidney, developed by Stephens and Kolff and coworkers (11, 12) in the mid 70's, is a somewhat miniaturised haemodialysis system, using a 20 l dialysate batch with (partial) regeneration through a 250 g activated charcoal column, which gives the patient the opportunity of greater mobility by disconnecting himself from the 20 l reservoir for brief periods of time (up to 15 minutes).

Basically these designs shared one, crucial problem: the efficient removal of urea, which so far was unsolved.

Kolff (13, 14) suggested the insertion of an additional dialyser, provided with an asymmetric, positively charged cellulose acetate, anion exchange membrane, attached to a secondary recirculation circuit incorporating a column containing urease and an ion exchange resin. This secondary urea removal system, originated at the Weizmann Institute of Science in Israel, allowed urea to diffuse through the (secondary) membrane, but electrolytes did not diffuse through the charged membrane. Urea was converted by urease into ammonium ions and bicarbonate. The ammonium ions were removed by a cation exchange resin inserted into the secondary circuit. The exchange resin was a zeolite with a high affinity for ammonium ions, which exchanged ammonium for sodium. Neither ammonium nor sodium could diffuse back through the positively charged secondary membrane into the primary dialysis circuit. Insertion of an activated carbon column in the secondary circuit also removed creatinine, uric acid and other organic substances.

The same group of investigators later (1979) designed a somewhat simplified system, omitting the secondary circuit with the second dialyser (15).

This system (Figure 1) incorporated a urease column which hydrolysed urea to ammonium carbonate, and a cation exchange resin (a selective zeolite) which exchanged ammonium ions for sodium. Another cation resin exchanged sodium ions for protons, and, finally, an activated carbon column adsorbed organic waste substances like creatinine, uric acid and others. Sensors were incorporated to monitor pH, calcium and potassium ions and these regulated the bypass flow through the cation resins, to maintain pH between narrow limits.

Another method of removing ammonia generated by urease has recently been presented by Pişkin and coworkers (16). The dialysis fluid, after passing through a

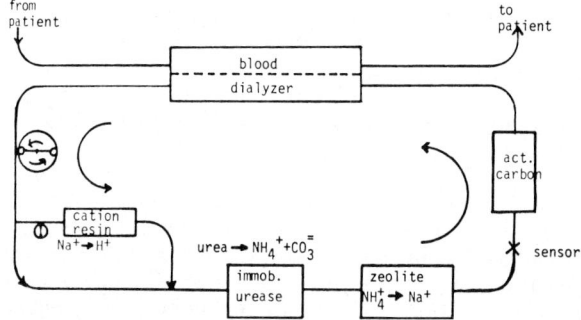

Figure 1. Dialysate regeneration system designed by Kolff and coworkers, incorporating a urease column, an exchange resin (selective zeolite) and an activated carbon column (see text). (From Kolff et al. [14] with permission).

urease column, entered a packed bed gas desorption column, a powerful air stream flowing countercurrently through the degassing column.

Several other ways of removing urea have been suggested. They are either derived from animal physiology or from waste-disposal processes (13, 17). One concept, originated by Harmsen and Kolff (18), dates back to 1947. Bacterial cultures were grown inside a cellophane membrane or tube, nutrients coming from the dialysate outside the membrane. It was hoped that microbial enzymes would convert urea into small amino acids, which would dialyse back into the dialysate, finally reaching the patient. Several years later it was demonstrated that decomposition of urea can be achieved by soil bacteria (19) and also by a certain bacterial strain from the rumen of cattle (13). However less desirable bacterial products could also be formed and reach the patient.

Malchesky and Nosé (17) studied the removal of nitrogenous waste products in batch reactors, using human urine as substrate, and initially selected bacteria from activated sludge provided by a local sewage treatment plant. They obtained encouraging results for their cultures removed substantial amounts of urea, creatinine and uric acid from the substrates.

Although the goal of these investigators was to use these 'biological reactors' as renal substitutes (20) their systems could also be used for dialysate regeneration. This was investigated by Ackerman and coworkers (21), who used an immobilised strain of gram positive (presumably non-pyrogenic) bacteria in a bioreactor. The selected bacteria were capable of converting urea to nitrogenous gases with a minimal production of ammonia. They recirculated the dialysis fluid through the bioreactor and used a bacterial filter and a powerful ultraviolet light disinfector to control bacterial contamination (Figure 2).

So far these investigators like others have not bridged the gap from laboratory investigations to clinical application. Their *in vitro* results, however, were promising.

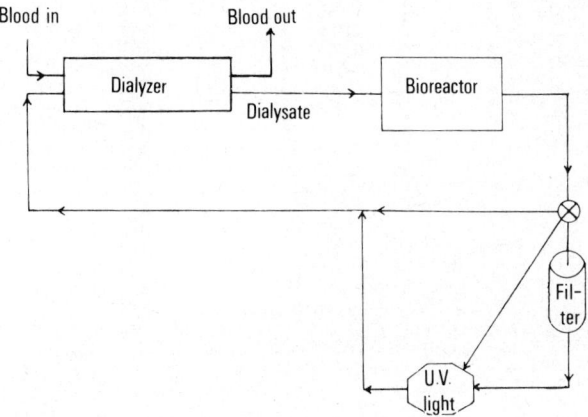

Figure 2. Regeneration of dialysate by bacteria in a 'bioreactor'. In the recirculation circuit a bacterial filter and a UV disinfector are incorporated. (From Ackerman et al. [21], with permission).

Another, ingenious approach dates back to the mid 1960's, when Tuwiner (22) reported on the application of electrochemical degradation of organic compounds in urine with the aim of producing potable water for manned space vehicles.

When a direct electric current is passed through a solution containing NaCl, chlorine is produced at the anode and sodium hydroxide and hydrogen at the cathode. The chlorine and sodium hydroxide react to produce sodium hypochlorite, a strong oxidant. It appeared possible to oxidise organic compounds in urine by electrolysis (23, 24). Two French investigators, Bizot and Sausse (25) applied this principle to used dialysate and presented evidence that urea, creatinine and uric acid could be oxidised to nitrogen, water and carbon dioxide.

This work was pursued by Fels (24) in Canada, who showed that the decomposition rate of urea is a strong function of both voltage and current and that for every mole of urea degraded one mole of carbon dioxide, one mole of nitrogen and two moles of hydrogen were produced.

Similar experimental work, using electro-oxidation to regenerate haemofiltrate, is presently underway in the Federal Republic of Germany (26, 27).

In summary, several groups around the world have tried to develop an efficient system for dialysate regeneration that would eliminate the large quantities of pretreated water, thereby reducing the cost of dialysis treatment, while retaining reliability and safety. So far these efforts have not resulted in systems suitable for clinical application with the single exception of the Japanese system described by Maeda (6, 8).

To understand the development of the only practical and commercially available dialysate regeneration system we have to recall another approach which also originated from manned space flight technology.

In the mid 1960's the aerospace industry in Southern California began to seek diversification by applying aerospace research technology to biomedical engineering, more specifically to dialysis associated engineering. In the absence of a suitable adsorbent, the problem of urea removal could only be solved in an indirect way. An experimental system was designed, using enzymatic hydrolysis of urea by urease, zirconium phosphate (ZiP) being selected to bind the produced ammonium.

ZiP acts partially as a molecular sieve, but primarily as a cation exchange resin, having a high affinity for ammonium ions exchanging them for H^+ ions and sodium ions, even in the presence of relatively high concentrations of sodium ions. Hydrated zirconium oxide was added to bind phosphate.

A sorbent system consisting of urease, zirconium phosphate, hydrous zirconium oxide and activated carbon was subjected to animal testing (28, 29). Initially utilising a total dialysate volume of 1 l, anephric dogs were dialysed with this sorbent dialysate regeneration system, resulting in survivals for as long as 37 days without evidence of uraemic or other toxicity. Subsequently two human subjects were dialysed successfully for periods of 9 and 10 months (30, 31).

It was concluded that sorbent regeneration of dialysate

provided a realistic approach to a portable dialysis system, independent of a fixed water supply and drain and without the need for pre-treatment of water (32).

PRACTICAL APPLICATION OF DIALYSATE REGENERATION

The Redy-Sorb system

The system, originally named Redy, which was derived from REcirculating DialYsis system[1] (Figure 3), incorporates a dialysate reservoir containing 5.5 l of dialysis fluid (Figure 4), which is continuously recirculated at a flow rate of 200 ml/min through a disposable five layer cartridge, which regenerates the dialysate.[2]

The apparatus is provided with the usual monitors of temperature and electrical conductivity of the dialysate and a gauge for continuously measuring the volume of ultrafiltrate. Alarm systems include a low pressure alarm for the recirculation circuit, a blood leak detector and an additional safety device, which activates the acoustic alarm in case of failure of the calcium-magnesium acetate infusion pump in delivering the predetermined amount of infusate per minute. A flow diagram of the system is presented in Figure 5.

The regeneration cartridge

The cartridge basically accomplishes three functions:
1. enzymatic decomposition of urea
2. ion exchange
3. adsorption.

The original cartridge, which had only four layers, was later modified by adding an extra bottom or *first layer* acting as a scavenger proximal to the urease. This layer consists of activated carbon and hydrated zirconium oxide and prevents inactivation of the urease from trace metal contaminants (especially copper) and oxidising agents such as chlorine, chloramine, sodium hypochlorite and others, which might be present after disinfecting and rinsing the system or in the water used for preparation of dialysis fluid (see Figures 6, 7a, 7b, 8, 9a and 9b).

The *second layer* contains urease, which catalyses the conversion of urea into ammonia and carbamic acid, which, is converted into ammonium ions and bicarbon-

---

[1] The name Redy was changed to Sorb System for unknown (commercial) reasons. The name Redy is better known, so will be used in this chapter.
[2] The amount of dialysis fluid has been increased recently to 6 l.

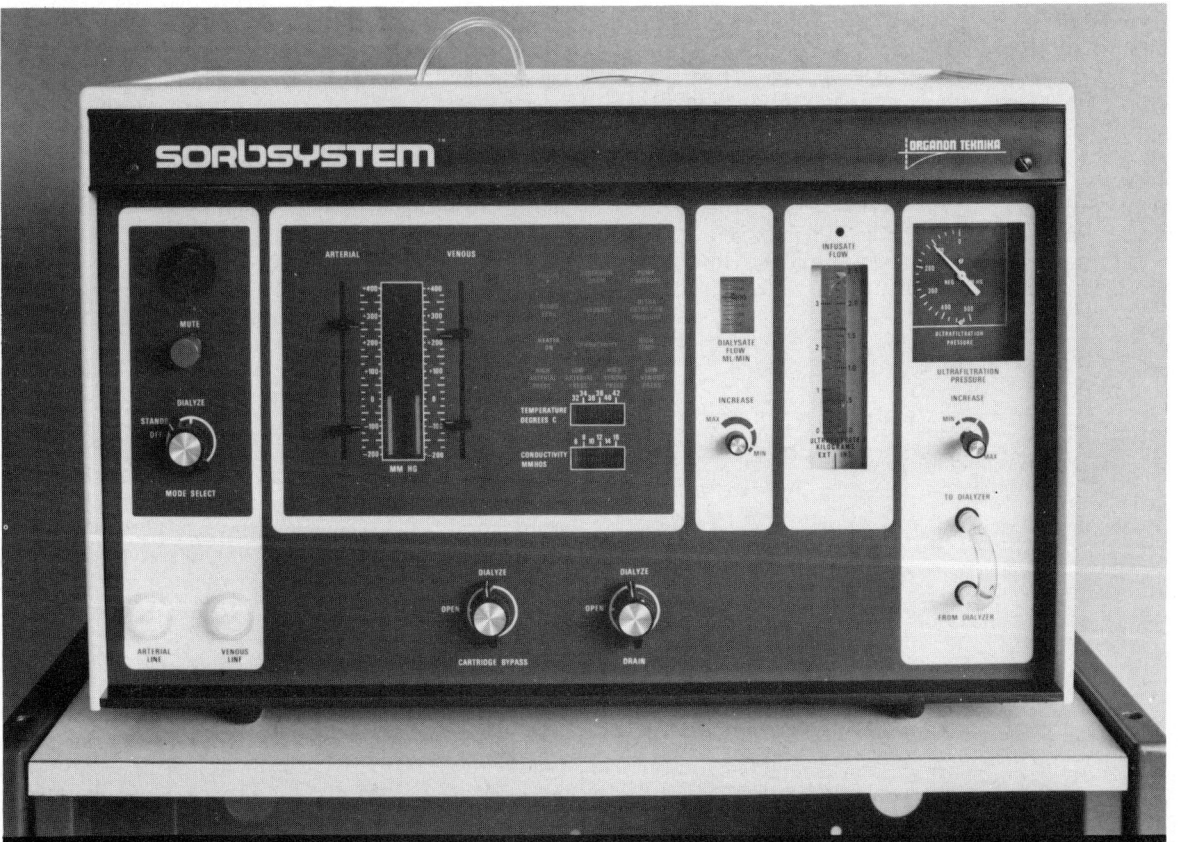

Figure 3. Front view of the Redy (= Sorb System) unit.

17: *Dialysate regeneration*   327

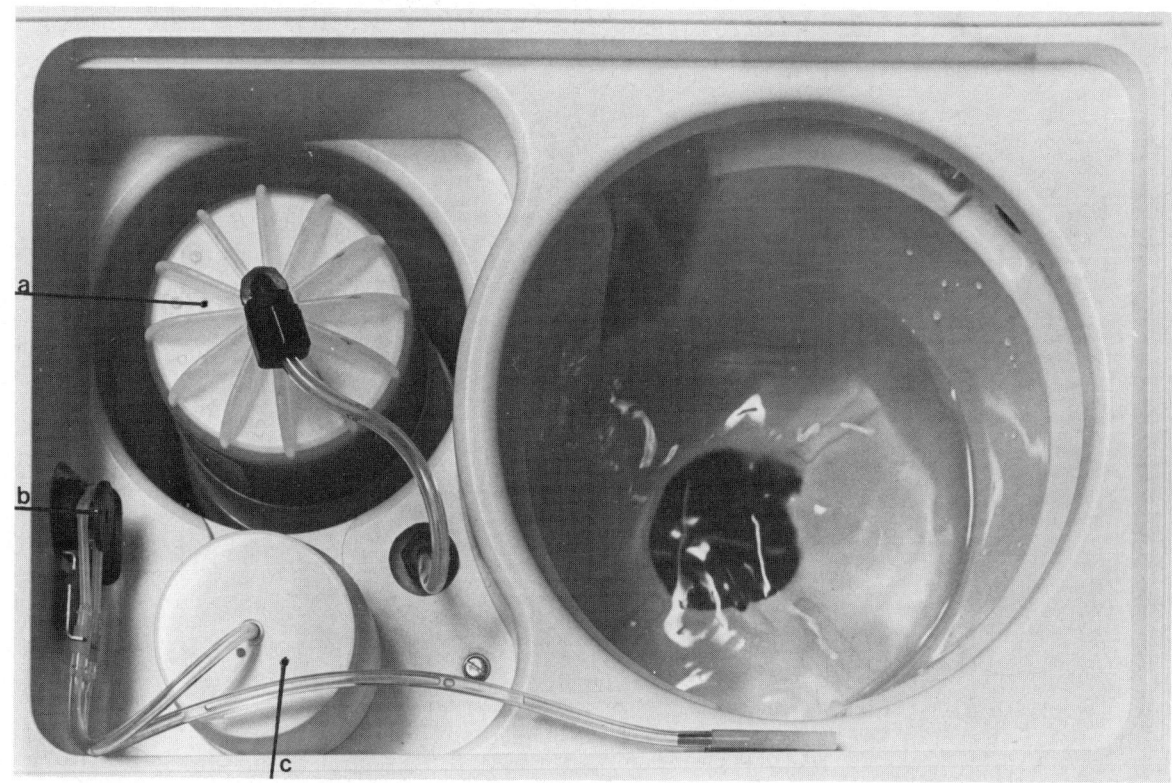

Figure 4. Redy (= Sorb System) unit, top view. (a) Regeneration cartridge; (b) Infusate pump; (c) Calcium and magnesium infusate reservoir.

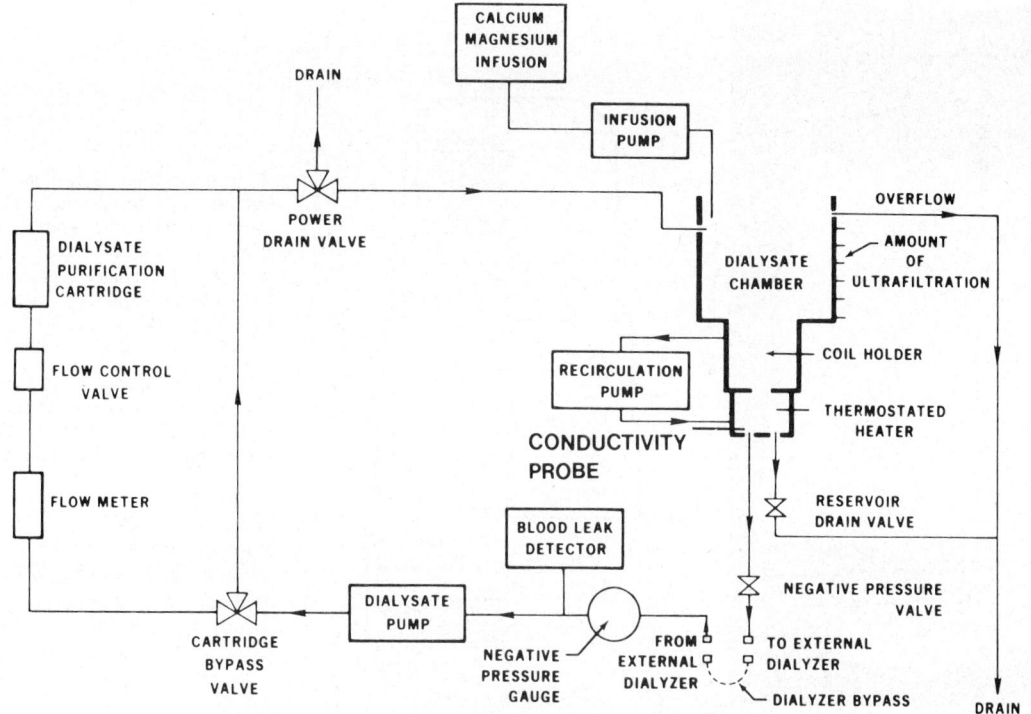

Figure 5. Flow diagram of the Redy system (see text).

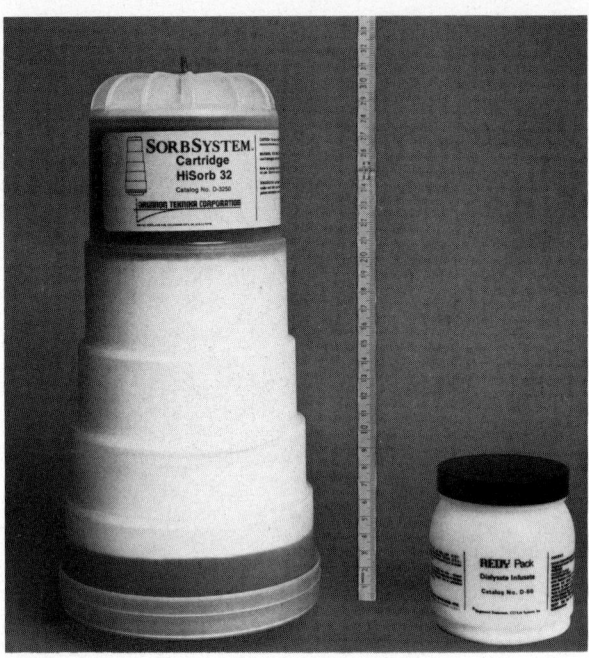

Figure 6. D 32 regeneration cartridge (old model) with infusate reservoir, containing calcium and magnesium acetate (and sometimes potassium acetate, see text).

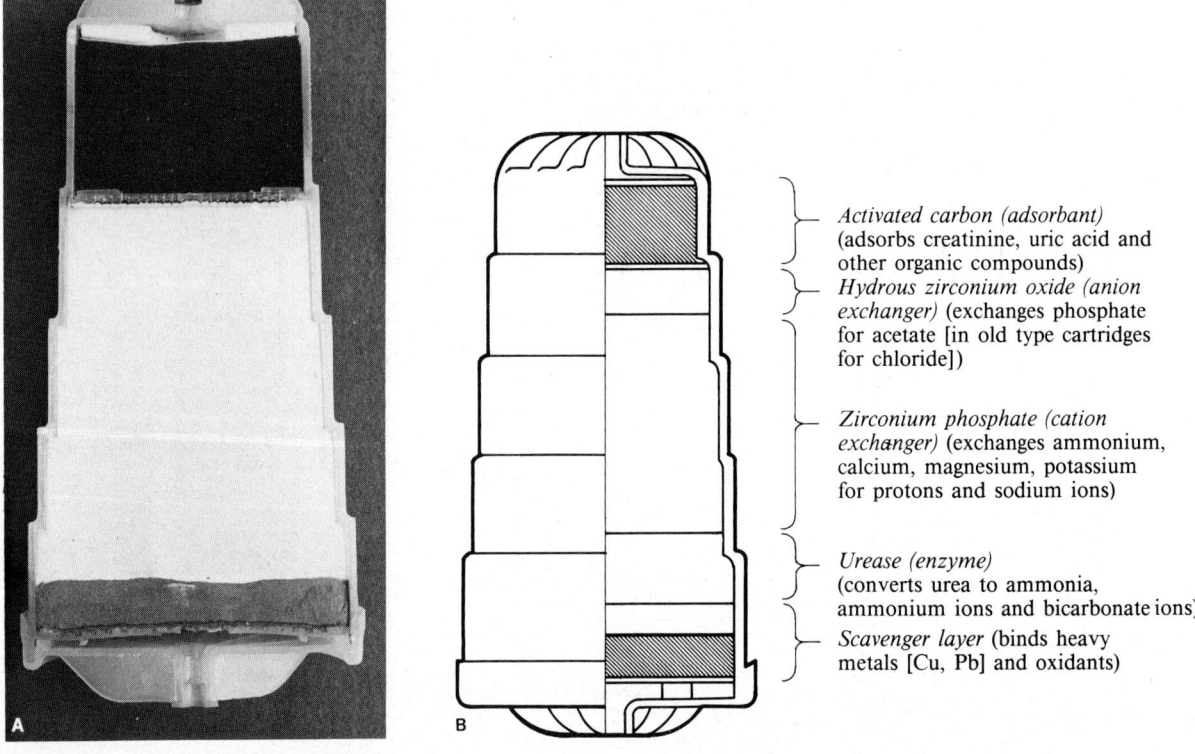

Figure 7. A. Old model regeneration cartridge, longitudinal section; B. Operation of the sorbent cartridge (see text).

17: Dialysate regeneration 329

ate ions (33–36 [see Figure 10]). Ammonia, in watery solution, will also be converted into ammonium ions:

$$NH_3 + H_2O \rightarrow NH_4^+ + OH^-.$$

The net result of urea splitting may be written as:

$$NH_2\text{-}CO\text{-}NH_2 + 3H_2O \rightarrow 2NH_4 + HCO_3^- + OH^-.$$

In addition bicarbonate lost from the patient across the dialyser membrane enters the dialysis fluid. The fluid recirculates through the cartridge which is supplied by the manufacturers at a pH of 6 (36). The bicarbonate both generated by the conversion of urea and originating from the patient enters the *third layer* of the cartridge, consisting of zirconium phosphate and reacts with protons delivered by the ZiP:

$$ZiPH + NaHCO_3 \rightarrow ZiPNa + H_2O + \overset{\nearrow}{CO_2}.$$

The stability of the bicarbonate in the dialysis fluid depends on the pH. When pH of this fluid drops below 7 (see Figure 12) bicarbonate will also decompose into water and carbon dioxide.

Ammonium ions also enter the zirconium phosphate layer which acts as a cation exchanger loaded with hydrogen ions and sodium ions, in a ratio of 1:8 (35, 36). The ammonium ions are, along with calcium, magnesium and potassium ions, exchanged for hydrogen and sodium ions (28–30, 35, 36 [Figure 11]). The released hydrogen ions will be buffered partially by the bicarbonate but this does not prevent an initial drop of dialysate

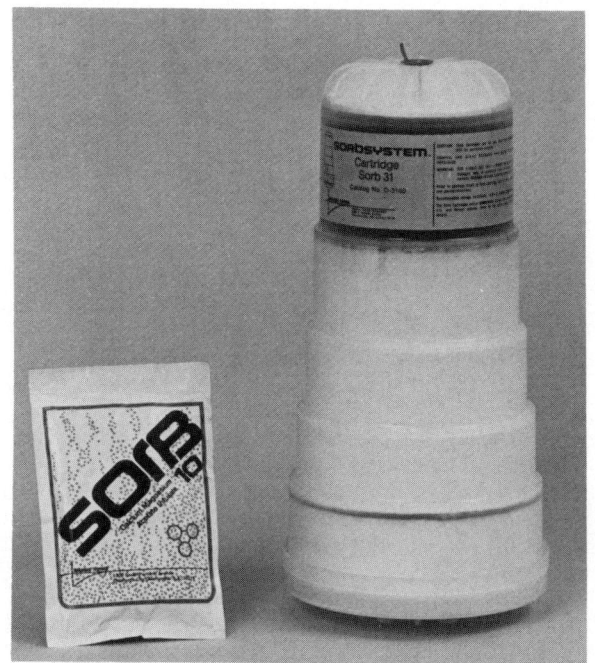

Figure 8. New Model (D 31) regeneration cartridge containing reduced amount of aluminium oxide, with package containing calcium and magnesium acetate (for infusate).

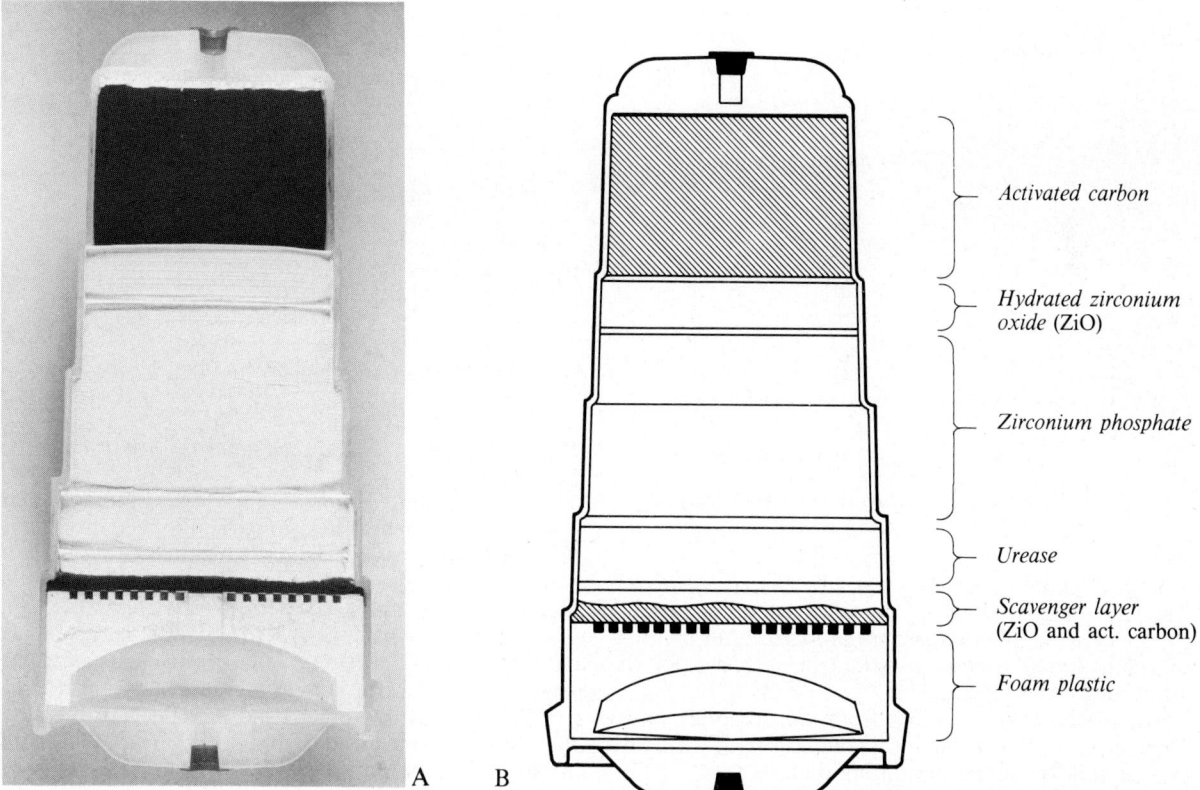

Figure 9. A. New model cartridge, longitudinal section; B. Diagram of new model cartridge showing different layers.

$$\text{H}_2\text{N-CO-NH}_2 + 2\,\text{H}_2\text{O} \xrightarrow{\text{urease}} \text{NH}_4^+ + \text{NH}_2\text{COO}^- + \text{H}_2\text{O}$$
$$\text{urea} \qquad\qquad\qquad\qquad\qquad \text{carbamic acid}$$

$$\rightleftarrows 2\,\text{NH}_4^+ + \text{CO}_3^{--}$$
$$\rightleftarrows \text{NH}_4^+ + \text{NH}_3 + \text{HCO}_3^-$$

Figure 10. Conversion of urea into ammonium ions, ammonia, bicarbonate and water by urease. (From Reithel FJ in Boyer PD: The Enzymes, 3rd edition, 1971, [33] with permission).

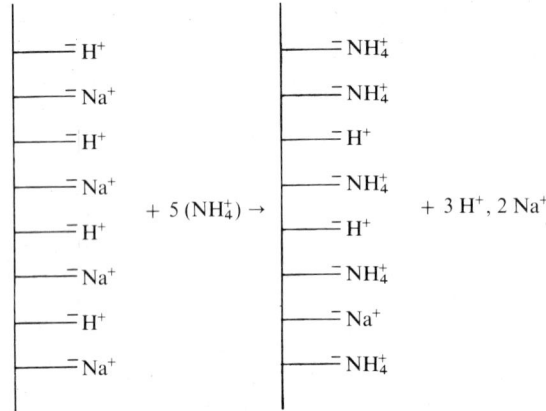

Figure 11. Exchange of NH_4^+ for H^+ and Na^+ in the zirconium phosphate layer. (From Van Doorn and Thomas [29], modified, with permission).

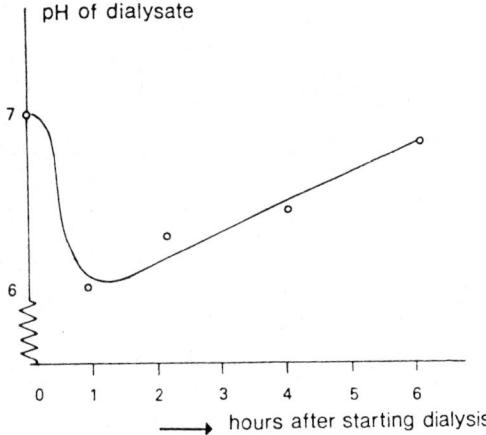

Figure 12. Dialysate pH during the course of dialysis.

pH (see Figure 12), which is partially caused by the release of hydrogen ions from the third layer and partially through release of anions from the *fourth layer* (consisting of hydrated zirconium oxide) in exchange for the adsorption of phosphate.

The release of sodium ions from the zirconium phosphate layer is responsible for a gradual rise of the dialysate sodium concentration during dialysis.

Because of complete removal of calcium, magnesium and potassium ions from the dialysis fluid by the cartridge, calcium and magnesium ions (and in some cases potassium ions) have to be added continuously to the dialysate. The desired calcium and magnesium concentrations are achieved by continuously infusing a solution of calcium and magnesium acetate (and in some cases also potassium acetate) from a small container, utilising a small Holter-type metering pump (Figures 4, 5 and 6) into the main dialysate reservoir.

The *fourth layer* of the cartridge consists of hydrous zirconium oxide (ZiO), which acts as an anion exchange resin. In the earliest (D 11) cartridge it was loaded with chloride, as in the later D 41 and D 42 cartridges. However, (for reasons to be discussed below) cartridges are now marketed with zirconium oxide in the acetate form (type D 31 and D 32) which exchange phosphate for acetate (in the old cartridges [D 11, D 41 and D 42], which are taken off the market, phosphate was exchanged for chloride). The cartridge does not remove sulphate from the dialysate to any appreciable degree. Sulphate bypasses the cartridge and accumulates in the dialysis fluid. Plasma sulphate levels in patients treated with the Redy system are therefore higher than in patients treated with single pass dialysis (37, 38).

Finally the *fifth layer*, consisting of activated carbon, adsorbs creatinine, uric acid, phenols, indican and other nitrogenous waste substances. It also adsorbs amino acids and a limited quantity of dextrose (7.5–15 g) (Van Doorn AWJ, 1979, unpublished observations). The cartridge, however, becomes quickly saturated with dextrose after which the system equilibrates with the blood sugar of the patient (39 [see Table 1]).

Table 1. Dextrose. Initially a small amount of dextrose is adsorbed by the cartridge. Patient's blood sugar values remain within normal limits.

	Patient mmol/l	Reservoir (dialysate) mmol/l	Cartridge effluent mmol/l
Start	5.4	4.2	3.5
4 h	4.1	6.6	6.6
8 h	6.6	6.6	6.4

(SI → conventional units: multiply by 18 (= mg/dl).

Practical application and guidelines for use of the Redy system

The practical application of this low volume sorbent regeneration system differs in several aspects from conventional single pass or recirculating dialysis systems. In conventional dialysis the concentration of solutes in the dialysis fluid is the one chemical variable which the operator must consider. In Redy dialysis he also must pay attention to the effects of the regeneration cartridge, which extracts waste substances and adds electrolytes continuously. On the other hand the effects of the variable composition of the dialysis fluid are mitigated by the small volume of dialysis fluid as compared with the total body water (see below) and the low dialysate flow rate (36).

Urea removal; available cartridges. The ability to remove urea is basically limited by the capacity of the zirconium phosphate layer of the cartridge to exchange ammonium ions.

Different types of cartridges are available: the D 31 has an average capacity for 20 g urea nitrogen, that is approx. 43 g (approx. 716 mmol) of urea. In muscular patients or (and) after high protein intake or during a hypercatabolic state, when the urea generation rate and the pre-dialysis plasma urea concentration are particularly high, the binding capacity of this cartridge may be exceeded, resulting in free ammonia entering the effluent from the cartridge. When the critical ammonia level of 2 mg/dl (1.11 mmol/l) in the dialysis fluid is exceeded, a syndrome of acute ammonia intoxication may occur, characterised by (rapidly reversible) symptoms of headaches, nausea and vomiting. Ammonia test paper is available, which permits rapid screening of dialysate ammonia levels, whenever an ammonia 'breakthrough' is anticipated or suspected.

A special high capacity cartridge (type D 32) has been introduced with an average capacity of 28 g urea nitrogen, that is 60 g (1000 mmol) of urea.

Most patients can be treated by thrice weekly dialysis using D 31 cartridges per week, provided that their protein intake is not excessive, and does not exceed 60 g per day.

Should intercurrent infections develop protein catabolism will be increased and either the higher capacity cartridge (D 32) should be used or conventional dialysis should be employed.

Some larger patients require routinely more capacity for urea than provided by the D 31 cartridges and a weekly routine of two D 31 cartridges with one D 32 after the week-end interval has proved satisfactory.

Because there is a linking of the sodium/hydrogen balance to the load of ammonium ions presented to the ZiP layer, which in turn depends on the amount of urea removed from the patient, the selection of the correct type of cartridge for the individual patient is also important (36, *vide infra*).

Low dialysate flow rate through the circuit. For adequate regeneration of the dialysate by the cartridge the dialysate flow rate through the system, including the dialyser, had to be limited to 200 ml/min (in contrast with the standard flow rate of 500 ml/min through the dialyser in conventional single pass systems). Thus the 5.5 l volume circulates through the dialyser cartridge circuit about twice every hour. In addition the amount of cations (Ca^{++}, Mg^{++} and K^+) bound by the cartridge (in exchange for sodium ions and protons) would proportionally increase with a higher dialysate flow rate, not only requiring a higher calcium and magnesium infusate flow, but also resulting in a decrease of the ammonium binding capacity and release of an undesirable additional amount of sodium and hydrogen ions.

The effect of low dialysate flow has been studied by Babb and associates (40–42): the clearances of low molecular weight (readily dialysable) solutes are reduced. Clearances of less dialysable middle molecules are not (or much less) affected. Small molecule clearances (urea, creatinine) using the Redy system are some 15–20% less than with standard dialysis systems. This, however, does not influence post-dialysis plasma concentrations of urea and creatinine.

In contrast with conventional single pass dialysate delivery systems both the dialysate pH and the sodium concentration in the rinsing fluid vary during the course of dialysis, as has been mentioned earlier.

Kinetics of pH and CO_2. The ammonium ions produced in the urease layer are exchanged in the ZiP layer for hydrogen ions and sodium ions, which are released into the dialysis fluid. In addition, acetate ions (with the old D 11, D 41 and 42 chloride ions) are released from the hydrated ZiO layer in exchange for phosphate. Obviously both a drop of pH and a progressive increase in sodium concentration in the dialysis fluid occur during dialysis (Figure 12, Table 2). The drop in pH, however, is partially buffered by bicarbonate and has no significant effect on the acid-base balance of the blood passing the dialyser. Any hydrogen ions passing through the membrane into the patient's blood will be immediately buffered.

Table 2. An increase in dialysate and plasma sodium concentration occurs during dialysis; blood pressure remains stable.

		Blood pressure, Plasma Na, dialysate Na pre- and postdialysis					
		Blood pressure supine mm Hg		Plasma Na mmol/l		Dialysate Na mmol/l	
Pat	Sex	pre-	post-	pre-	post-	pre-	post-
1. Lo	m	120/80	105/60	139	145	138	149
2. Ze	f	125/78	120/70	140	141	—	—
3. Ru	f	130/80	125/75	139	143	—	—
4. Sm	f	125/78	120/70	140	142	135	144
5. Wa	f	120/70	110/60	140	143	132	147

But as the pH of the dialysate drops below 7 during recirculation through the cartridge, a further conversion of the bicarbonate will occur, producing CO_2 and H_2O. Gaseous carbon dioxide escapes from the top of the cartridge (Figure 13), entering the dialysis fluid. The dialysate becomes supersaturated with carbon dioxide (the excess escaping in the air), generating a very high PCO_2 in the dialysate (200 mm Hg at 120 min [43, 44]). Consequently total CO_2 of the blood passing through the dialyser increases. Simultaneously there is a loss of bicarbonate (see below).

The blood leaving the dialyser in a Redy system is hypercapnic and presents the phenomenon of combined 'respiratory' and 'metabolic' acidosis and has a very low pH (36, 45–47).

In conventional dialysis systems using acetate in place of bicarbonate, the blood leaving the dialyser also has a low bicarbonate concentration, but a normal pH, because of a simultaneous loss of carbon dioxide to the dialysate (which is going to drain).

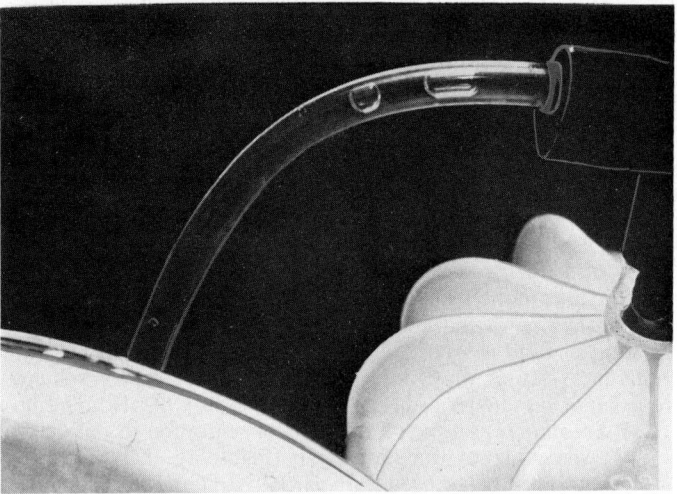

Figure 13. Carbon dioxide produced by conversion of bicarbonate escaping from the top of the cartridge.

The blood leaving the dialyser in a Redy system rapidly mixes with the patient's blood-pool and any excess of CO_2 is immediately lost in the expired air. Therefore this interesting phenomenon seems to have little if any clinical significance (36, 47). However, adverse effects may occur when the extracorporeal circuit is maintained by connecting venous and arterial blood lines (after disconnecting the patient for temporary interruption of dialysis with continuing extracorporeal recirculation of the blood, while correcting positions of fistula needles). This is sometimes done while the dialysate flow is continued. When the recirculated hypercapnic blood from the dialyser reaches the patient's respiratory centre after reconnection and reestablishing dialysis, rather unpleasant side effects occur, like hyperventilation with facial flushing, oppression and acute headaches.

The excess of CO_2 in the dialysis fluid of the Redy system requires degassing of the bath fluid (43, 47): the CO_2 (and also nitrogen from dissolved air) will escape from the blood when negative pressure on the dialysate is applied. This causes foaming of the blood which leaves the dialyser and could adversely interfere with mass transfer and also increase fibrin deposition in hollow fibre dialysers. These effects can be minimised by degassing of the dialysis fluid (47; see also chapter 7).

If an external dialyser is used (partial) degassing may be achieved by replacing the standard pump in the recirculation circuit by a small high power (Micro Giant) pump and inserting an adjustable constriction in the circuit (Figure 14), thus creating a negative pressure area (47, 48). To prevent temperature instability a simple stirrer has to be added in the reservoir (Figure 14). So far, this modification has not been incorporated by the manufacturers. Alternatively, it seems possible to

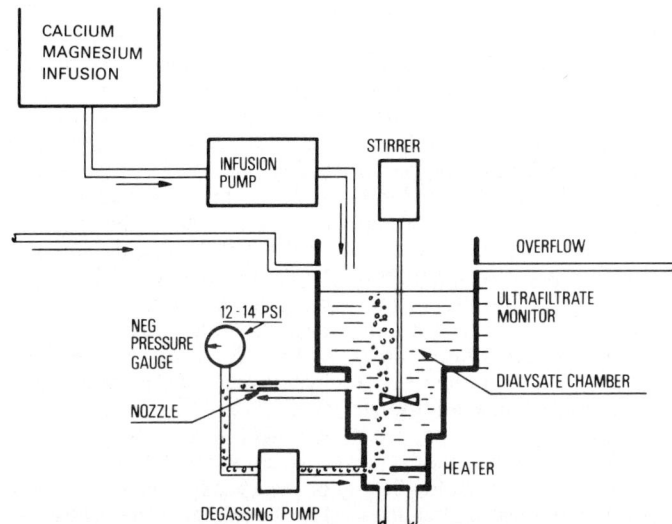

Figure 14. Partial flow diagram of the Redy system (see also Figure 5) with degassing of the dialysate by negative pressure (only possible with an external dialyser). (12-15 PSI = approx. 0.82-0.95 atmosphere.)

insert a device with a degassing membrane for removal of carbon dioxide and nitrogen (44).

Sodium kinetics. Ammonium ions produced by the enzymatic conversion of urea are exchanged in the ZiP layer for hydrogen ions and sodium ions. Therefore an increase of dialysate sodium occurs during dialysis. The increase depends on the amount of urea removed from the patient. Removal of 18.7 g of urea nitrogen or 40 g of urea (668 mmol) releases from the cartridge some 70 to 140 mmol sodium, so that the sodium concentration in the 5.5 l of dialysate rises 13 to 25 mmol/l. In addition, some 50 mmol of Na are liberated from the cartridge during the first passage of the dialysis fluid (49) and this amount will be even greater if hard water is used to make up the priming dialysis fluid. Furthermore, the initial recirculation of the dialysis fluid through the dialyser, which is usually primed with normal saline (155 mmol/l sodium), increases dialysate sodium 8 mmol/l. Finally potassium, calcium and magnesium ions are also bound by the cartridge in the ZiP layer in exchange for hydrogen and sodium ions. This increases total dialysate sodium by approximately 10 mmol/h. Thus, during a 6 h dialysis a total sodium increment of 200 to 250 mmol occurs. This increases dialysate sodium concentration approximately 35 to 45 mmol/l. It is therefore recommended that the dialysate sodium concentration should be 105 to 110 mmol/l prior to insertion of the cartridge. Thus a negative sodium concentration gradient exists between dialysate and patient during the first hours of dialysis, sodium being transferred from the patient to the dialysis fluid. Thereafter following a brief period of equilibrium with zero transfer, sodium transfer occurs in the opposite direction (from dialysate to the patient) counteracted of course by convective sodium loss from the patient during ultrafiltration. It should be kept in mind that an unsuitable large urea load (in excess of that for which the cartridge was designed) causes an additional increase of sodium ions released by the cartridge with a further rise of dialysate sodium. The selection of a suitable cartridge is therefore of importance.

Recently the relationship between urea removal and sodium release has been expressed in a somewhat complicated equation (Schilb and coworkers [50]), allowing a calculation of the sodium increase, using predialysis plasma urea concentration and dialysis time as parameters.

The sodium kinetics of the Redy system have raised some concern about the management of hypertension, in particular in the early period of clinical trials when pre-dialysis sodium concentrations of 132 to 138 mmol/l were used (see Table 2).

Several clinical investigators have now confirmed that in practice there is no difference in hypertension control with the Redy system and with conventional dialysis systems (47, 49, 51). During Redy dialysis diffusion of sodium clearly varies with the concentration gradient and is therefore a dynamic variable; but the effects are mitigated by the small volume of dialysis fluid and the low dialysate flow. The ratio between the 5.5 l total volume in the Redy system and the sodium space of the patient is approximately 1 to 2.5, contrasting with a ratio of approximately 10 to 1 in conventional single pass dialysis.

An increase in dialysate sodium concentration of 5 to 7 mmol/l results in an increase of only 1 mmol/l in the patient's plasma during a Redy dialysis (Roberts M and Pecker EA, Organon Teknika Corp., unpublished data). A hypernatric bath late in treatment may add some 50 to 100 mmol sodium to the patient (36). This is counteracted by a convective sodium loss of about 135 mmol with each litre of ultrafiltrate removed.

Clearly net sodium balance is much more importantly influenced by convective sodium transfer from the patient, due to ultrafiltration than by diffusive factors and the 'metabolism' of the cartridge.

Summarising, dialysate sodium concentration in the Redy system is a variable (rising) parameter. Obviously the initial sodium concentration depends on the composition of the dialysis fluid placed in the reservoir.

The degree and tempo of the rise in sodium concentration depend on the following factors:

1. The equilibration time between commencing the flow of the dialysis fluid through the cartridge and the start of dialysis.
2. The amount of urea extracted from the patient (in turn depending on pre-dialysis plasma urea concentration, the clearance rate of the dialyser and the 'urea' capacity of the cartridge).
3. Duration of dialysis, which will determine the amount of sodium released by the cartridge in exchange for ammonium ions (derived from urea) and calcium, magnesium and potassium ions removed from circulating dialysate.
4. The accuracies of both the flow meter and infusion pump. Both are not entirely satisfactory, which can result in variations of the rate of cation exchange in the cartridge, which in turn will affect sodium release.

Clearly anion release (with the present cartridges: acetate) will vary between different patients, depending on the amount of anions (predominantly phosphate) exchanged.

Fortunately in practice the majority of the above conditions is remarkably constant in the individual stable chronic dialysis patient; the major factors affecting the final dialysate composition are the initial concentrations in the dialysis fluid, timing of the commencement of dialysis, the duration of dialysis and the amount of urea, removed from the patient.

Thus each dialysis unit should ascertain these variables and adjust the initial dialysis fluid composition accordingly. As a guide it would not be unreasonable to use an initial dialysis fluid of the following composition:

Sodium: 95–110 mmol/l
Potassium: 0–1 mmol/l
Calcium: 1.5–1.75 mmol/l
Magnesium: 0.5–0.85 mmol/l
Chloride: 65–75 mmol/l
Acetate: 35–45 mmol/l
Dextrose monohydrate: 0–10.1 mmol/l (0–200 mg/dl).

Moreover the correct cartridge 'size' with normal or 'high' urea capacity should be selected.

As explained earlier because of the 1 to 2.5 relationship of the dialysate volume as compared with the patient's sodium space and also because of the low dialysate flow (36) the impact of the dialysis fluid on the patient's body fluid composition is much less than in conventional 500 ml/min single pass dialysis. Nevertheless pre- and post-dialysis plasma and dialysate analyses should be undertaken in patients not yet stabilised on treatment with the Redy system.

An adult patient can commence dialysis after a 15 min equilibration following insertion of the cartridge, when the sodium in the dialysis fluid is usually 115 to 120 mmol/l. A small or paediatric patient should not commence dialysis until the sodium concentration reaches 125 mmol/l. The conductivity meter can be used to judge the moment to start dialysis.

If hard water is used for preparation of dialysis fluid, the calcium in the initial fluid placed in the reservoir should be either omitted or much reduced.

Calcium, magnesium and potassium kinetics. Calcium, magnesium and potassium ions are completely removed by the cartridge from the dialysis fluid. Therefore calcium and magnesium have to be added continuously. The manufacturer supplies calcium and magnesium as acetate salts in the appropriate amounts as dry powder with each cartridge (see Figures 6 and 8). This is dissolved in water to the graduated 300 ml mark in a suitable container. This solution is infused into the dialysate at a rate of 18 mmol calcium plus 6 mmol magnesium (and 48 mmol of acetate) per hour with the calibrated infusion pump (see Figures 4 and 5).

Attention should be paid to maintaining the correct dialysate flow rate of 200 ml/min for which the infusate pump has been calibrated, in order to maintain the correct calcium and magnesium concentrations of 1.5 mmol/l (6 mg/dl) and 0.5 mmol/l (1.2 mg/dl) respectively. Obviously, it is possible to alter the calcium and magnesium concentrations in the dialysate by varying the concentration in the infusate.

As previously explained, potassium is also completely removed from the dialysis fluid and, if potassium free dialysate is undesirable for a particular patient, potassium acetate should also be added via the infusate system. For this purpose commercially prepared packages are available containing the correct amount of potassium acetate to increase dialysate potassium concentration in increments of 1 mmol/l.

Acetate kinetics and correction of metabolic acidosis. In conventional dialysis correction of acidosis occurs by metabolic conversion of acetate into bicarbonate (52). Several clinical investigators noted incomplete correction of metabolic acidosis in patients treated with the Redy system with a cartridge containing chloride loaded ZiO (43, 46, 47, 53). This was particularly obvious in so called 'short dialysis', when large (2 m^2) surface area dialysers were used (46). Various explanations have been presented (47).

In the Redy system with the original (presently obsolete) D 11 regeneration cartridge utilising the chloride form of hydrous zirconium oxide the total amount of acetate available to the patient was small: with an initial sodium concentration of 105 to 110 mmol/l and an acetate concentration of 26 to 29 mmol/l the total quantity of acetate in the 5.5 l of dialysis fluid was 140 to 160 mmol/l. However, the chloride loaded D 11 cartridge adsorbed 50 mmol acetate, which was exchanged for chloride ions, leaving approximately 100 mmol of acetate. The infusion of the acetate salts of calcium and magnesium (and sometimes potassium) adds an additional 290 mmol of acetate in 6 hours. This makes a total of only 390 mmol available to the patient, which is clearly insufficient for correction of acidosis.

In contrast, in a single 6 h haemodialysis with a standard single pass system 180 l dialysis fluid with 35 mmol/l acetate traverse the dialyser, confronting the patient with a total of 6300 mmol of acetate, which is a considerable load. Obviously the amount of acetate actually transferred into the patient by reverse dialysis is less and depends on the clearance for acetate of the dialyser, the duration of dialysis, the concentration of acetate in the dialysate and the rate of disappearance of the acetate from the patient's blood. This, in turn, depends on the rate with which an individual patient metabolises acetate. It has been suggested that the excess of acetate in standard single pass haemodialysis may cause dialysis associated problems and side effects, such as vascular instability with hypotension and post-dialysis hangover (see chapter 7). It may therefore be advantageous in providing less acetate during conventional dialysis, in particular to patients who are 'slow metabolisers' of acetate (54). Presently clinicians are inclined to replace acetate by bicarbonate either in selected patients or as a routine (55, 56). On the other hand the persistent metabolic acidosis as observed with the previous 'chloride loaded' cartridges D 11, D 41 and D 42 was considered as less desirable by several clinical investigators, even while the clinical significance was unknown. It could worsen or accelerate renal bone disease (57) and could have an adverse effect on haemoglobin synthesis, but it might also be a minor blemish without much significance.

Nevertheless several measures for improved correction of metabolic acidosis with the Redy system have been suggested (47).

Van Doorn and Thomas (35) showed that with the old D 11 cartridge an increase of the initial acetate concentration in the dialysis fluid from 40 to 60 mmol/l corrected the metabolic acidosis satisfactorily. However this also raised the sodium concentration by 20 mmol/l, which was less desirable (see above).

An elegant and simple solution was offered by the cartridge experts by introducing the D 31 and D 32 cartridges, containing hydrous zirconium oxide loaded with acetate instead of chloride. This provides the patient with an additional 100 mmol acetate, because the initial loss of 50 mmol into the cartridge is eliminated and an extra 50 mmol acetate is released from the acetate loaded cartridge in exchange for phosphate. Thus a total of 490 mmol of acetate is made available during a 6 hour Redy dialysis. Since the cartridge also produces bicarbonate and the bicarbonate loss from the patient across the dialyser membrane is considerably less than in single pass dialysis, the pre-dialysis plasma bicarbonate values achieved with the D 31 and D 32 'acetate loaded' cartridges seem to be comparable to those achieved with standard single pass dialysis techniques (49).

The Redy system in patients with normal or low plasma urea concentrations. As discussed earlier an unexpectedly low urea load or a cartridge with an unsuitable high urea binding capacity may cause persistence or aggravation of metabolic acidosis. Unless adequate quantities of urea enter the cartridge dialysate sodium is adsorbed by the cartridge and severe hyponatraemia and acidosis may develop, the concentration of chloride in the dialysate remaining unaltered. Obviously the Redy system should not be used with the standard cartridges (containing urease) in patients with normal or only marginally raised plasma urea (e.g. in cases of drug overdose).

For (haemoperfusion) treatment of patients who have taken an overdose of a dialysable poison that is adsorbed by charcoal, a special sorbent cartridge (type D 13) is available, containing activated carbon only. (This system is, however, not as efficient as a standard haemoperfusion system, without a dialyser.)

Long-term treatment with the Redy system. The Redy system was commercially introduced in 1972. Until recently, only a few reports have been published on the results of long-term treatment, in particular compared with treatment with conventional dialysis systems (47, 49, 58–60). Apart from incomplete correction of metabolic acidosis in the earlier years with the 'chloride loaded' cartridges no major differences in clinical status, blood chemistries and blood pressure have been noted compared to patients treated with standard single pass dialysis techniques.

Irrespective of brief and rapidly reversible episodes of acute ammonia intoxication in the early clinical trials, until recently no specific adverse reactions or complications had been reported.

Lately Whalen and associates (61) in a comparative study found elevated serum alkaline phosphatase values in 12 out of 19 patients after being treated with the Redy system for 12 months or longer, with peak values after 2 years. All patients responded to therapy with dihydrotachysterol and the authors concluded that their findings indicated early renal osteodystrophy; which might have eventually caused symptoms and radiographic abnormalities when the patients had been left untreated with a vitamin D metabolite for a longer period of time.

The investigators suggested that as the sorbent cartridge does not remove sulphate (38) elevated plasma concentrations of sulphate (twice as high as in single pass dialysis patients) could have played a role in bone metabolism.

Recently several cases of aluminium intoxication in patients treated with the Redy system have been reported, both from the USA and France (62–64). This toxicologic aspect will be discussed later.

Since 1974 the Redy system has been used in a integrated programme at St Thomas' Hospital, London, UK. Nineteen patients treated by one of the authors (AJW) have used the Redy system for home dialysis, two of these patients having been treated for 7 years; eight were treated for shorter periods (5–36 months) while awaiting transplantation. Total patient experience amounted to 43 patient-years. At any one time between six and ten of the St Thomas' haemodialysis population (up to 10% of the total) were using the Redy system in the home.

Reasons for choice of the Redy system have mostly arisen from the disadvantages of using a conventional single pass system, requiring formal installation for regular dialysis at home (65). The use of a portable system solved the delay and problems of adapting or extending the house or even rehousing the family (66).

Some factors influencing the choice of the system have now altered: continuous ambulatory peritoneal dialysis (CAPD) has become an alternative temporary therapy for patients awaiting transplantation (see also chapters 23 and 24).

Cost of treatment with the Redy system was higher than with conventional systems, because of the cost of cartridges, but this was balanced by savings made on home adaptations and by reducing time on hospital haemodialysis. (The extra cost of Redy home dialysis for 2 years has proved equivalent to the price of one of the more expensive home conversions or the cost difference between 6 months hospital dialysis as opposed to 6 months conventional home dialysis [66]).

For safety purposes the original Redy monitor has been modified by the introduction of a conductivity monitor to ensure that the correct quantity of priming concentrate was added. The presence of the conductivity meter proved instructive during dialysis, monitoring the progressive rise in conductivity as sodium was released by the cartridge (66).

The conductivity monitor is presently incorporated into the standard commercial machine.

The greatest advantage is the mobility of the equipment as dialysis can be performed without being in the immediate vicinity of either a water tap or/and a drain.

The system makes travelling for holiday (Figure 15) and business purposes possible. It has been used for dialysis in hotels, in a caravan, on camping sites and even in a sailing boat (60), and while sunbathing on the beach. If necessary the Redy can be operated from a small electric power generator driven by an petrol engine.

Airlines have agreed to accept the monitor without freight charge and in many countries the required rather bulky disposables can be obtained through the manufacturers' local representatives.

The mobility of the Redy system has also proved extremely useful when emergencies interrupted the function of St Thomas' renal unit, on one occasion by a prolonged disruption in electric supply, on another when fire in the hospital rendered the unit temporarily uninhabitable.

The Redy system represents the St Thomas' unit's standby for evacuation if the low lying part of London,

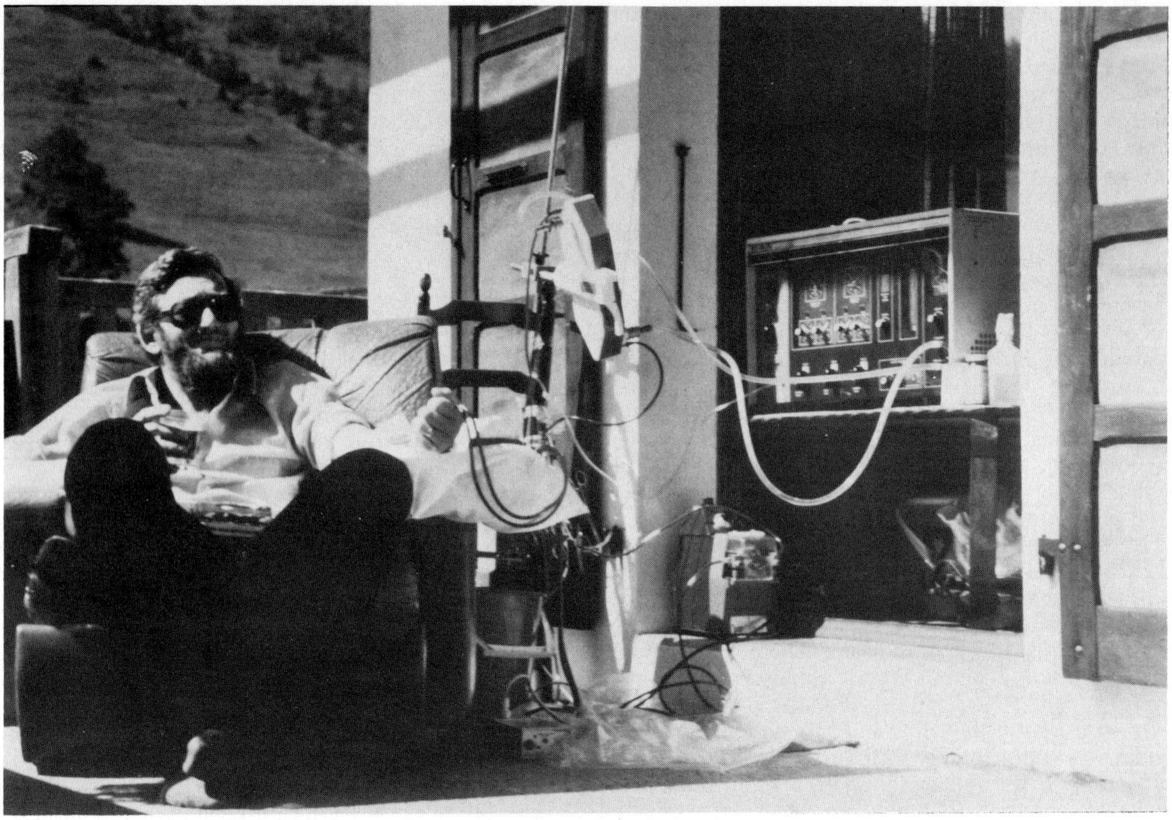

Figure 15. A London patient travelling with the Redy: holiday in France.

in which St. Thomas' Hospital is situated, should be flooded by the river Thames.

Toxicology of the Redy system

Toxicology studies have been performed by Møller et al. (67). Their primary concern was a potential toxicity of zirconium, which according to these authors is an essential human trace metal. Using emission spectrochemical analysis they found in a series of Redy dialysate samples, values far below normal serum values. Other trace elements analysed (copper, silicon, aluminium) gave similar results. Only boron levels appeared to be three times normal, which the investigators explained either by high boron plasma levels in uraemic patients or by release from the cartridge. Boron seems to be toxic to man, but the Danish investigators concluded that the Redy system carried no obvious toxicological risk.

Møller and coworkers, using formaldehyde as a sterilising agent found however 'alarmingly high' formaldehyde concentrations, even after an extra (third) rinse of the system, when the Clinitest check (which is notoriously insensitive) was negative. This, however, is obviously not a specific Redy problem: many dialysis systems presently in use are disinfected with formaldehyde (see also chapters 11 and 15 for formaldehyde toxicity), and may present a similar problem.

It should be emphasised that Møller and his colleagues (67) did study the early release of aluminium from the cartridge (see following pages) but their flame emission analysis had a sensitivity limit of 100 µg/l (3.7 µmol/l) and was obviously far too insensitive for measuring aluminium concentrations in dialysate and biological fluids, which require a minimal sensitivity of 5 µg/l (0.18 µmol/l). It is now appreciated that flameless spectophotometric analysis, using a high temperature graphite furnace, is required to detect low concentrations of aluminium [3] (7).

It is not generally known, that the Redy cartridge in addition to the active reactants, described previously, contained a substantial amount of aluminium oxide (Al_2O_3), which so far was considered as an inert (non-reactive) and non-toxic substance. It is used as filling material and as a binding vehicle for the urease in the second layer of the cartridge. In addition, activated carbon is commonly contaminated with substantial amounts of aluminium oxide (AJW Van Doorn, Organon Teknika, Turnhout, Belgium, unpublished data, 1980). Release of aluminium from the cartridge with substantial contamination of the recirculating dialysis fluid seems a potential hazard of the system. Aluminium contaminated dialysis fluid is considered as the principal cause of aluminium intoxication in chronic dialysis pa-

---

[3] Inductively Coupled Plasma (ICP) emission spectrometry seems to be a promising new analytical technique (74).

tients, but conflicting opinions concerning dialysibility of aluminium have been recorded in the literature (67–73).

Aluminium kinetics in the dialysis setting have been studied in detail by a Seattle group of investigators (75).

It was demonstrated that both solubility and dialysibility of aluminium ions are strongly pH dependent. Aluminium solubility and (reverse)clearances were negligible at pH values ranging from 6.5 to 7.6, but increased dramatically at pH below 6.5 and above 7.6.

Initial dialysis fluid pH in the Redy system obviously depends on the pH of the water used for preparation; during dialysis pH decreases for reasons explained earlier (see Figure 12). Obviously the risk of aluminium release from the cartridge and transfer of this element into the patient is small as long as dialysate pH fluctuates between 6.5 and 7.6 (74).

On the other hand aluminium ions are eagerly adsorbed in the ZiP layer of the cartridge (and are exchanged for sodium ions and protons). Aluminium released from the bottom layer will be bound in the zirconium layer, however aluminium released from the top layer (the activated carbon) enters the dialysis fluid, but will be removed by the cartridge during recirculation.

Recently Pierides and Frohnert (62) reported six patients with end stage renal failure who were dialysed for periods of 18 to 34 months on the Redy system and who developed aluminium associated osteomalacia with pathological fractures. Five of them subsequently developed dialysis dementia and four died (bone aluminium was measured in three patients and was very high [135 to 360 ppm = 5 to 13 mmol/kg]).

This is the first report on aluminium intoxication in patients dialysed with the Redy system. No details are given by Pierides and Frohnert on the administration of oral aluminium containing phosphate binders and on previous dialysis treatment with other systems. Perfusion studies of Redy D 31 cartridges with aluminium free water indicated a variable but often considerable release of aluminium. Most of it was released during the first hour, but some cartridges showed a prolonged release, lasting throughout the 4 h experiments. In most cartridges aluminium concentration in the perfusate decreased during continued recirculation and in half of the cartridges aluminium levels of less than 50 µg/l (50 ppb, approximately 1.9 µmol/l) (62) were obtained after recirculating the dialysate for 90 to 120 min. Some cartridges, however, needed 4 h of recirculation until the 50 µg/l level was obtained. It was demonstrated that the aluminium present in the perfusate readily diffused through the membrane of a Cordis Dow dialyser, with one exception. The discrepancies could be explained by different pH values of the dialysis fluid in these experiments: no pH values were reported. In addition aluminium levels of 50 µg/l are no longer considered as safe: recently the upper limit has been set to 10–15 µg/l (0.37 µmol-0.56 µmol/l) in Europe (74) and to 10 µg/l (0.37 µmol/l) in the USA (see also chapter 42).

It should be mentioned that Van Doorn (personal communication) obtained in similar experiments both *in vitro* and *in vivo* very low dialysate aluminium values

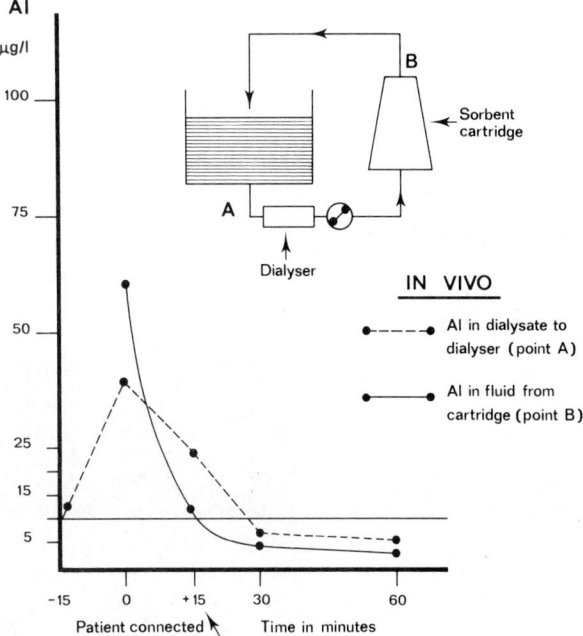

Figure 16. Aluminium concentrations in Redy dialysate during actual dialysis. (From Van Doorn AWJ, 1981, unpublished data. With permission). (µg/l → µmol/l divide by 27)

(<10 µg = <0.37 µmol/l), even after 30 minutes of recirculation (Figure 16). Both Pierides and coworkers and Van Doorn used the sensitive flameless absorption photometric analysis technique.

The unloading of aluminium into the patient increases considerably when bicarbonate rinsed cartridges or dialysis fluid containing bicarbonate instead of acetate are used. Mion and associates (63) observed three cases of fracturing osteomalacia with very high bone aluminium values after treatment with regular haemofiltration for 15 to 20 months, the haemofiltrate, being regenerated by passage via a bicarbonate rinsed Redy cartridge and being reinfused in the patient. Bicarbonate dialysis with the Redy system should be definitely discouraged until aluminium is totally eliminated from the regeneration cartridge (63, 64).

Recently the aluminium oxide content of the cartridge has been substantially reduced. All aluminium above the ZiP layer has been removed, and the aluminium contamination of the activated carbon in the top layer seems also to be reduced. In addition aluminium released from this layer presumably will be bound in the 'scavenger' layer and in the ZiP layer during recirculation. The urease layer also still contains aluminium oxide, acting as binding agent.

The geometry of this improved D 31 cartridge (coded D 3160) is somewhat different from the previous model (see Figures 8, 9a and 9b). Similarly the older D 32 cartridge will be replaced by an improved model from which the aluminium oxide also has been largely removed.

According to preliminary reports from the manufac-

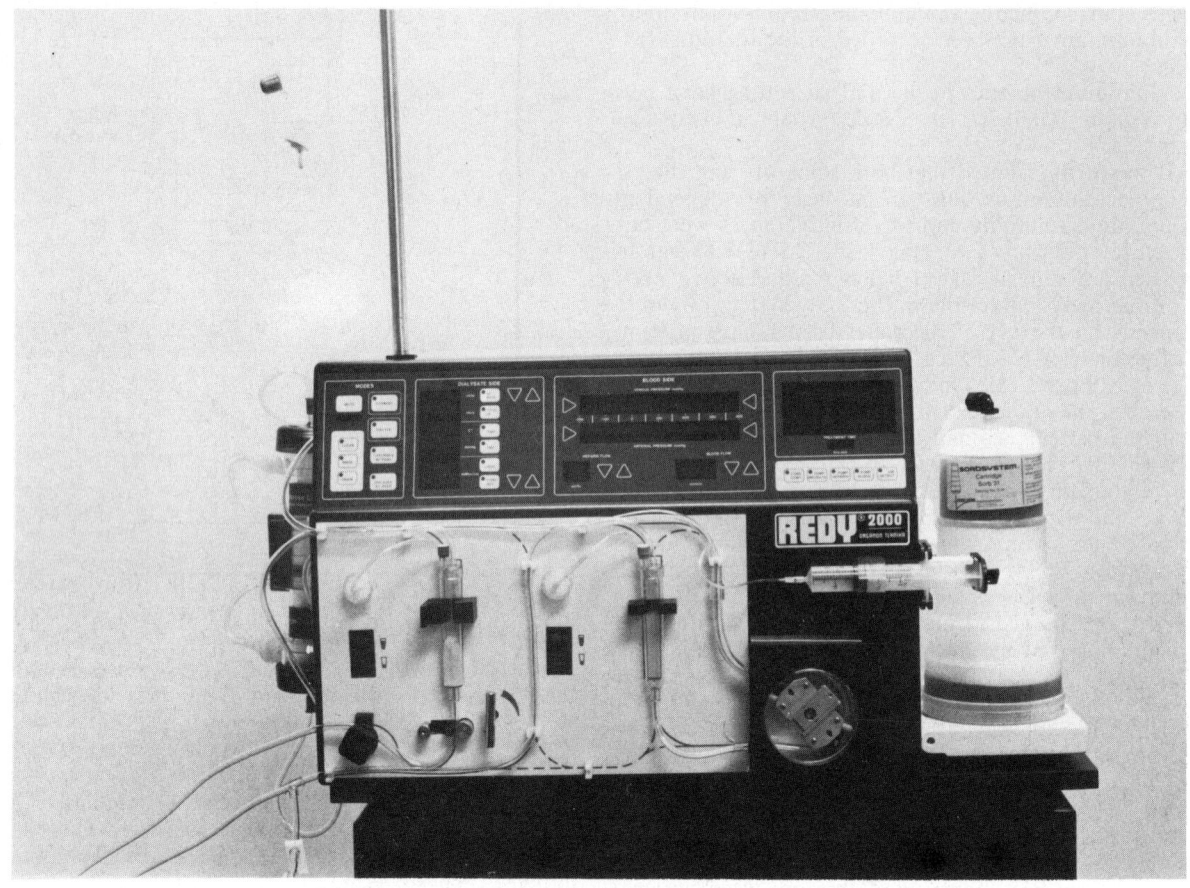

Figure 17. A new and more compact model (Redy 2000) will be marketed soon. The sorbent cartridge is at the outside of the dialysis fluid reservoir. (Picture by courtesy of Messrs Organon Teknika).

turers soluble aluminium *in vitro* with the new D 3160 cartridge never rises above 10 ppb ([= 10 µg/l = 0.37 µmol/l], see also chapters 6 and 7). *In vivo* similar low aluminium values were obtained. Sometimes an increase of aluminium output occurred at the end of dialysis, which raised the aluminium level to about 10 µg/l (0.37 µmol/l). This was explained by aluminium release from the patient. A recent report confirms that the new cartridge will reduce the aluminium concentration of the bath fluid to less than 10 µg/l (0.37 µg/l) in the first ½ h of (*in vivo*) dialysis, maintaining a level of 5 µg/l ± 1 (0.185 µmol/l ± 0.037) throughout a 4 h dialysis (76). The new cartridges will be marketed in due course.

For the time being a pre-dialysis rinsing period of the cartridge with (acetate containing) dialysate of 60 min is recommended and fresh dialysate should be prepared before the patient is connected to the dialyser.

Finally, in long-term treatment checking of pH of the dialysate during the course of dialysis may be a good additional safety measure.

With the new 'low' aluminium cartridges these safety measures may be superfluous and can perhaps be omitted. However, a serious warning has been sounded and physicians who use this system must be alert to this newly recognised potential complication.

New model Redy 2000

A new model, reduced in size and weight and provided with improved electronics and monitoring systems has been constructed (Figure 17). This model (Redy 2000) will be marketed soon.

ACKNOWLEDGMENTS

The authors are indebted to A.W.J. Van Doorn Ph.D. and M. Roberts Ph.D., both from Organon Teknika Corp., for their critical comments on this chapter as published in the first edition of this book and their views on the physical chemistry of the cartridge. However, the opinions expressed by the authors in different sections of this chapter do not necessarily reflect their conceptions.

The authors also gratefully acknowledge the courtesy of the directors of Organon Teknika Corporation, Turnhout, Belgium, who made the photographs available of the new Redy-Sorb system model of the D 32 cartridge (Figures 3, 4 and 6) and of the new 'low' aluminium cartridge (Figures 8 and 9a) giving permission for publication.

They also wish to thank the Organon Teknika scientific staff for providing the authors with preliminary data on the new 'low aluminium' cartridge.

REFERENCES

1. Blaney TL, Lindan O, Sparks RE: Adsorption: a step forwards to a wearable artificial kidney. *Trans Am Soc Artif Intern Organs* 12:7, 1966
2. Jutzler GA, Keller HE, Klein J, Carius J, Floss K, Dijckmans J, Fürsattel L, Leppla W: Physico-chemical investigations in regeneration of the dialysis fluid. *Proc Eur Dial Transpl Assoc* 3:265, 1966
3. Twiss EE, Paulssen MMP: Dialysis-system incorporating the use of activated carbon. *Proc Eur Dial Transpl Assoc* 3:262, 1966
4. Van Leer E: *Hemodialyse met koolstof adsorptie.* (Haemodialysis with carbon adsorption). MD Thesis 1970 University of Rotterdam, the Netherlands. Rotterdam, Bronder-Offset N.V., 1970 (in Dutch)
5. Kolobow T, Dedrick RL: Dialysate capacity augmentation with activated carbon slurry. *Proc Eur Dial Transpl Assoc* 3:375, 1966
6. Maeda K, Kawaguchi S, Manji T, Kobayashi K, Ohta K, Saito A, Shimoji T, Yui T, Hori M: Portable artificial kidney system with adsorbents. *Proc Eur Dial Transpl Assoc* 10:298, 1973
7. Fuchs C, Brasche M, Paschev K, Nordbeck H, Quellhorst E: Aluminium-Bestimmung in Serum mit flammenloser Atomabsorption. (Determination of aluminium in serum with flameless atomic absorption). *Clin Chim Acta* 52:71, 1974 (in German)
8. Maeda K, Kawaguchi S, Shimizu K, Manji T, Kobayashi K, Ohta K, Saito A, Amano I, Yoshiyama N, Nakagawa S, Koshikawa S: Ten-litre dialysate supply system with adsorbents. *Proc Eur Dial Transpl Assoc* 11:180, 1974
9. Petrella E, Orlandini GC, Bigi L: Regeneration of dialysis fluid. *Proc Eur Dial Transpl Assoc* 11:173, 1974
10. Bultitude FW, Gower RP: Sorption based haemodialysis system. In *Renal Dialysis,* edited by Whelpton D, London, UK, Sector Publishing Ltd., 1974, p 74 (distributed in the U.S. and Canada by JB Lippincott Company)
11. Stephens RL, Jacobsen SC, Atkin Thor E, Kolff WJ: Portable/wearable artificial kidney (WAK) – initial evaluation. *Proc Eur Dial Transpl Assoc* 12:511, 1975
12. Kolff WJ: The future of dialysis. In Replacement of *Renal Function by Dialysis,* edited by Drukker W, Parson FM, Maher JF, 1st edn, The Hague, Boston, London, Martinus Nijhoff, 1978, p 702
13. Kolff WJ: Longitudinal perspectives on sorbents in uremia. *Kidney Int* 10 (Suppl 7):S211, 1976
14. Kolff WJ, Walker JM, Gregonis D, Klein E: A membrane system to remove urea from the dialyzing fluid of the artificial kidney. *Proc 11th Annu Contractors' Conf Artif Kidney Program* NIAMDD, edited by Mackey BB, DHEW publ no (NIH) 79-1442, 1978, p 162
15. Kolff WJ, Gregonis D, Wisniewski S, Klein E, Wendt R: A membrane system to remove urea from dialysate. *Proc 12th Annu Contractors' Conf Artif Kidney Program NIAMDD,* edited by Mackey BB, DHEW publ no (NIH) 81-1979, 1981, p 215
16. Pişkin E, Evren V, Azdural AR, Chang TMS: Design of a packed bed gas desorption column for the removal of urea as ammonia. *Artif Organs* 5 (Abstracts):56, 1981
17. Malchesky PS, Nosé Y: Biological reactors for renal support. *Trans Am Soc Artif Intern Organs* 23:726, 1977
18. Harmsen GW, Kolff WJ: Cultivation of micro organism with the aid of cellophane membranes. *Science* 105:582, 1947
19. Setälä K, Heinonen H, Schreck-Pulona I: Uraemic waste recovery II: in vitro studies. *Proc Eur Dial Transpl Assoc* 9:514, 1972
20. Malchesky PS, Nosé Y: Biological reactors as renal substitutes. *Artif Organs* 3:8, 1979
21. Ackerman RA, Crosby SC, Morefield EF, Stevenson RS: Dialysate delivery and regenerative system. *Trans Am Soc Artif Intern Organs* 25:398, 1979
22. Tuwiner SB: Research, design and development of an improved water reclamation system for manned space vehicles. *RAI Research Corp Report 364 for NASA Contract NASA-4373* (cited in reference 24)
23. Fels M: Electrochemical degradation of waste metabolites in dialysate solution. In *Technical Aspects of Renal Dialysis,* edited by Frost TH, Tunbridge Wells, UK, Pitman Medical Publishing Company 1978, p 226
24. Fels M: Recycle of dialysate from the artificial kidney by electrochemical degradation of waste metabolites: small-scale laboratory investigation. *Med Biol Eng Comput* 16:25, 1978
25. Bizot J, Sausse A, German patent no 2261220. French patent application no 7144868 (cited in reference 23)
26. Quellhorst E, Schuenemann B: Regeneration of hemofiltrate by using charcoal-coated membranes and electro-oxidation. *Int J Artif Org* 4:265, 1981
27. Köster K, Wendt H, Gallus J, Krisam G, Lehmann HD: Regeneration of hemofiltrate by anodic oxidation of urea. *Int J Artif Org* 4:264, 1981
28. Gordon A, Greenbaum MA, Marantz LB, McArthur MJ, Maxwell MH: A sorbent-based low volume dialysate system. *Trans Am Soc Artif Intern Organs* 15:347, 1969
29. Gordon A, Popovitzer M, Greenbaum MA, Marantz LB, McArthur MJ, DePalma JR, Maxwell MH: Zirconium phosphate – a potentially useful adsorbent in the treatment of chronic uraemia. *Proc Eur Dial Transpl Assoc* 5:86, 1969
30. Gordon A, Gral T, DePalma Jr, Greenbaum MA, Marantz LB, McArthur MJ, Maxwell MH: A sorbent-based low volume dialysate system: preliminary studies in human subjects. *Proc Eur Dial Transpl Assoc* 7:63, 1970
31. Gordon A, Better OS, Greenbaum MA, Marantz LB, Gral T, Maxwell MH: Clinical maintenance hemodialysis with a sorbent-based, low volume dialysate regeneration system. *Trans Am Soc Artif Intern Organs* 17:253, 1971
32. Greenbaum MA, Gordon A: A regenerative dialysis supply system. *Dial Transpl* 1 (no 1):18, 1972
33. Reithel FJ: Ureases. In *The Enzymes,* edited by Boyer PD, volume IV: Hydrolysis, 3rd edn, New York and London, Academic Press, 1971, p 1
34. Better OS, Gordon A, Greenbaum MA, Marantz LB, Maxwell MH: Acid-base balance in patients on sorbent hemodialysis. Role of bicarbonate generation in dialysate. *Am Soc Nephrol (Abstracts)* 4:8, 1970
35. Van Doorn AWJ, Thomas HCL: The working of the cartridge, with special regard to bicarbonate and acetate aspects. *Nieren- u Hochdruckkrankheiten (Suppl 1)* 5:9, 1976
36. Henderson LW: Redy or not. *asaio J* 2:49, 1979
37. Van Doorn AWJ, Drukker W, Thomas HCL, Verdickt L: Regeneration dialysis; handling of sulfate by the cartridge. *Eur Dial Transpl Assoc* (Abstracts) 5:177, 1976
38. Freeman RM, Richards CJ: Studies on sulfate in end-stage renal disease. *Kidney Int* 15:167, 1979
39. Lewin AJ, Gordon A, Greenbaum MA, Maxwell MH: Sorbent based regenerative delivery system for use in peritoneal dialysis. *Proc Clin Dial Transpl Forum* 3:126, 1973

40. Babb AL, Popovich RP, Christopher TG, Scribner BH: The genesis of the square meter-hour hypothesis. *Trans Am Soc Artif Intern Organs* 17:81, 1971
41. Christopher TG, Cambi V, Harker LA, Hurst PE, Popovich RP, Babb AL, Scribner BH: A study of hemodialysis with lowered dialysate flow. *Trans Am Soc Artif Intern Organs* 17:92, 1971
42. Eberhard K, Thomae U, Von Frowein G, Kuhlmann H: Anwendung der Adsorptionsmethode zur Regeneration von Spüllösungen in der Hämodialysebehandlung (Redy System). (Application of the adsorption method to regeneration of rinsing fluids used in haemodialysis (Redy System). *Med Klin* 70:323, 1975 (in German)
43. Farrell PC, Hone PW, Ward RA, Abernethy PE, Mahony JF: Development of a sorbent-based wearable artificial kidney. *Second Australasian Conference on Heat and Mass Transfer.* The University of Sidney, 1977 (February) p 207
44. Shaldon S: Early clinical trial of hemofiltrate recycling via sorbents. *Proc 12th Annu Contractors' Conf Artif Kidney Program NIAMDD,* edited by Mackey BB, DHEW publ no (NIH) 81-1979, 1981, p 265
45. Rohmer D, Nassri M, Sherlock J, Letteri J, Ledwith J: A comparison of the respiratory dynamics during hemodialysis using acetate and bicarbonate dialysate in a sorbent regenerative system. *Trans Am Soc Artif Intern Organs* 27:176, 1981
46. Farrell PC, Mahony JF, Jones BV, Mathew TH, Dawborn JK, Disney AP: Clinical evaluation of a dialysate regeneration system for maintenance haemodialysis. *Aust NZ J Med* 6:292, 1976
47. Drukker W: Introduction to the Redy System. Two long-term patients. *Nieren- u Hochdruckkrankheiten (Suppl 1)* 5:5, 1976
48. Drukker W, Van Der Werff B, Meinsma K: De-aeration of dialysis fluid. *Dial Transpl* 3 (no 3):33, 1974
49. Roberts M, Pecker EA, Lewin AJ, Gordon A, Maxwell MH: Clinical experience with adsorptive recirculation dialysis. *Dial Transpl* 6 (no 5):16, 1977
50. Schilb Th, Shapiro W, Porush J: Sodium kinetics of the Redy sorbent cartridge (RSC) when used to recycle ultrafiltrate (UF). *Artif Organs (Abstracts)* 5:61, 1981
51. Bisson P: Redy System for home haemodialysis. *Nieren- u Hochdruckkrankheiten (Suppl 1)* 5:9, 1976
52. Mudge CH, Manning JA, Gilman A: Sodium acetate as a source of fixed base. *Proc Soc Exp Biol Med* 71:136, 1949
53. Hampl H, Kessel M, Horn G: Short duration dialysis employing the Redy System with special consideration of buffer capacity. *Nieren- u Hochdruckkrankheiten (Suppl 1)* 5:34, 1976
54. Novello A, Kelsch RC, Easterling RE: Acetate intolerance during hemodialysis. *Clin Nephrol* 5:29, 1976
55. Scribner BH: Substitution of bicarbonate for acetate in the dialysate for the care of a critically ill patient. *Dial Transpl* 6 (no 3):26, 1977
56. Kirkendol PL, Devia CJ, Bower JD, Holbert RD: A comparison of the cardiovascular effects of sodium acetate, sodium bicarbonate and other potential sources of fixed base in hemodialysate solutions. *Trans Am Soc Artif Intern Organs* 23:399, 1977
57. Boyle IT: Vitamin D and the kidney. *Proc Eur Dial Transpl Assoc* 12:113, 1975
58. Lewin AJ, Greenbaum MA, Gordon A, Maxwell MH: Current status of the clinical application of the Redy ® dialysate delivery system. *Proc Clin Dial Transpl Forum* 2:52, 1972
59. Mansell MA, Wing AJ: Long term experience of home dialysis with sorbent regeneration of dialysate. *Proc Eur Dial Transpl Assoc* 13:275, 1977
60. Drukker W, Parsons FM, Gordon A: Practical application of dialysate regeneration: the Redy system. In *Replacement of Renal Function by Dialysis,* edited by Drukker W, Parson FM, Maher JF. The Hague, Boston, London, Martinus Nijhoff Publishers, 1st ed, 1978, p 255
61. Whalen JE, Freeman RM, Richards CJ: Elevated serum alkaline phosphatase in patients receiving sorbent cartridge hemodialysis. *asaio J* 4:9, 1981
62. Pierides AM, Frohnert PP: Aluminum related dialysis osteomalacia and dementia, after prolonged use of the Redy cartridge. *Trans Am Soc Arti Intern Organs* 27:629, 1981
63. Mion C, Branger B, Issautier R, Ellis HA, Rodier M, Shaldon S: Dialysis fracturing osteomalacia without hyperparathyroidism in patients treated with HCO_3 rinsed Redy cartridge. *Trans Am Soc Artif Intern Organs* 27:634, 1981
64. Branger B, Ramperez P, Marigliano N, Mion H, Shaldon S, Mion C: Aluminium transfer in bicarbonate dialysis using a sorbent regenerative system: an in vitro study. *Proc Eur Dial Transpl Assoc* 17:213, 1980
65. Wing AJ: Discussion in *Proc Eur Dial Transpl Assoc* 11:550, 1975
66. Wing AJ, Mansell MA: Home dialysis with the Redy system – socio-economic and biochemical observations. *Nieren- u Hochdruckkrankheiten (Suppl 1)* 5:21, 1976
67. Møller BB, Bahnsen M, Solgaard P, Sørensen E: Toxicological problems with the Redy ® system. *Scand J Urol Nephrol (Suppl)* 30:23, 1976
68. Pierides AM, Edwards WG, Cullum UX, McCall JT, Ellis HA: Hemodialysis encephalopathy with osteomalacic fractures and muscle weakness. *Kidney Int* 18:115, 1980
69. Whittier FC, Hurwitz A, Scott JA: Aluminum toxicity in uremia, a preliminary report. *Abstracts Am Soc Artif Intern Organs* 2:72, 1973
70. Knepshield JH, Schreiner GE, Lowenthal DT, Gelfland MC: Dialysis of poisons and drugs – annual review. *Trans Am Soc Artif Intern Organs* 19:609, 1973
71. Alfrey AC, LeGendre GR, Kaehny WD: The dialysis encepalopathy syndrome: possible aluminum intoxication. *N Engl J Med* 294:184, 1976
72. Alfrey AC, Kaehny WD: Letter to the editor. *N Engl J Med* 294:1131, 1976
73. Kaehny WD, Alfrey AC, Holman RE, Shorr WJ: Aluminum transfer during hemodialysis. *Kidney Int* 12:361, 1977
74. Savory J, Berlin A: *Memorandum on the summary and conclusions of the International Workshop on the role of biological monitoring in the prevention of aluminium toxicity in man (aluminium analysis in biological fluids),* Luxembourg, 1982. Commission of the European Communities Directorate-General of Employment, Social Affairs and Education, Luxembourg, 1982
75. Gacek EM, Babb AL, Uvelli DA, Fry DL, Scribner BH: Dialysis dementia: the role of dialysate pH in altering the dialyzability of aluminum. *Trans Am Soc Artif Intern Organs* 25:409 1979
76. Odell RA, Yang J, George CR, Farrell PC: Aluminum kinetics during sorbent (Redy) dialysis. *Contemp Dial* 3, nr 7:57, 1982

18

ORAL SORBENTS IN UREMIA

ELI A. FRIEDMAN

Introduction	341
Sorbents; definition	341
Gastrointestinal perfusion	342
Diarrhea therapy	343
Ingestible sorbents	343
Charcoal	344
Oxidized starch and oxidized cellulose	344
Locust bean gum	347
Liquid membrane capsules	347
Other applications of sorbents	348
Antacids	348
Hyperkalemia	348
Lipid reduction	348
Conclusion	351
References	351

INTRODUCTION

In late 1981, more than 56,000 Americans were being kept alive, despite irreversible uremia, by maintenance peritoneal or hemodialysis, at an annual governmental expenditure exceeding 1.2 billion dollars. Dialytic therapy, as now practiced, and renal transplantation, from a living or cadaveric donor, extend useful life for years, for most patients. Because of its extraordinary cost, however, approximately three out of four people around the world will have no chance of receiving contemporary uremia therapy should their kidneys fail (1). Extreme variation in availability and quality of health care between industrialized and 'third world' nations, is no where better illustrated than in the statistics of uremia therapy. Whereas Japan, for example, sustained 251 uremic patients per million population in 1981, Egypt could afford to treat only one per million, and China and India treat less than one per million people (2). Nigeria, at the bottom of the list, with a population of 70 million, has no uremia therapy at all. Texts on modern management of renal insufficiency, therefore, are pertinent, for the time being, to only a minority of a rapidly growing world population. Health planners in developed countries stressed by the advancing expense of uremia therapy, are exploring shortened, more efficient hemodialyses, employing reused dialyzers and the benefits of continuous ambulatory peritoneal dialysis, to contain costs. By contrast, third world nations must await still cheaper alternatives before affording uremia therapy as a competitive priority and before diverting funds now committed to coping with malaria, trachoma, and malnutrition. One rational, though elusive approach to reducing the price of dialysis is an extension of the interdialytic interval, perhaps avoiding the need for dialysis, by repeated or continuous extraction of nitrogenous and other solutes from intestinal fluids. Investigational strategies designed to exploit the gut as a substitute nephron, include administration of oral sorbents and intestinal perfusion ('intestinal dialysis').

SORBENTS; DEFINITION

Sorbent systems for solute extraction in uremic patients have been devised utilizing three contact methods between sorbent and solute (sorbate): 1) The sorbent may be kept on the opposite side of a synthetic membrane to reduce the volume of dialysate during hemodialysis, or may be used to regenerate a small volume of hemofiltrate, which is reinfused during hemofiltration (3). 2) The sorbent may be placed in direct contact with a body fluid, usually blood (hemoperfusion) after which the treated fluid is either intermittently or continuously returned to the patient (4). 3) The sorbent can be instilled within an organ or body cavity of the patient, with sorbent and body fluid on opposite sides of a membrane. Experiments thus far have used both the peritoneal and gastrointestinal membranes, but any accessible membrane, including the alveolar membrane (5), might be employed.

The term sorbents includes absorbents, adsorbents, ion exchange materials and complexing agents. Asher (16) reviewed the theoretical basis underlying various possible interactions between sorbent and sorbate. An *absorbent* usually refers to a liquid that incorporates an absorbate into solution by physical forces. The absorbent liquid must be immiscible with the treated aqueous liquid. *Adsorbents* hold sorbed (adsorbed) materials on a gas-liquid, liquid-liquid, or solid-liquid interface. Solid sorbents have most often been ingested in the form of highly porous granules with internal surface areas as high as 1000 m^2 per gram of adsorbent. It is often not possible to classify adsorbents absolutely as developing either exclusively physical or chemical binding to sorbed substances. Both reactions may occur simultaneously. Carbon, the most extensively studied adsorbent, binds multiple materials which vary in affinity, depending on the source of the carbon (bone, coal, coconut shell, petroleum) and its physical form (particle size, texture, chemical form of surface oxygen).

Ion *exchange materials* substitute ions from the exchange substance for those in solution. Included in this category of sorbents are zeolite crystals, gel structure resins, and macroporous resins. Sorbents acting as *complexing agents,* the last category to be considered, are molecules or ions (termed ligands) that coordinate a metal in more than one position of a molecule. Coordination is effected by sharing two or more ligand electron groups. Should the resulting complex be insoluble in the solvent used, the sorbing substance is termed a chelating agent. If soluble, it is termed a sequestering agent. To illustrate a common use of complexing agents, blood is routinely anticoagulated by sequestering calcium ion with citrate ion.

Clinically valuable mixtures of sorbents might be formulated to accomplish several objectives by different mechanisms. Thus, an oral dose of dialdehyde starch which binds urea chemically, could be added to charcoal to adsorb creatinine physically, along with an aliquot of an ion exchange resin to sorb phosphate. This mixture extracts three solutes known to exist in high concentrations in the uremic patient.

GASTROINTESTINAL PERFUSION

Sparks (7) reviewed the literature pertaining to the employment of gastrointestinal perfusion (intestinal dialysis) as a uremia therapy. Intestinal perfusion was first discussed by Claude Bernard in 1847 (8) and reassessed by Auguste in 1929 (9). Pendleton and West (10) in 1932, designed studies in the dog to ascertain whether urea would pass from blood to the small bowel lumen. Infusing solutions through a rubber tube inserted into the duodenum, and recovering drainage from the ileum at the ileo-cecal junction, they found that 'when normal saline solution was placed in the small bowel its urea content rapidly rose to that of blood'. Within 15 min, the concentration of urea in the bowel was 'slightly in excess' of blood urea concentration. When this experiment was repeated in four anephric dogs infused with urea to produce blood levels as high as 265 mg/dl (44 mmol/l) at two hours, urea levels in the bowel reached 153 mg/dl (25.5 mmol/l) in 15 min and 299 mg/dl (50 mmol/l) at two hours. No discussion of the clinical applicability of these results was offered though derivative applications have included intestinal dialysis, peritoneal dialysis and oral sorbent trials.

A negative, but well conducted and pertinent study was reported in 1933, by Hessel, Pekelis, and Meltzer (11). They prepared total external jejunal fistulae in nephrectomized dogs who were stimulated with cholagogues and histamine, but did not live longer than anephric controls. Similar negative results were reported in 1946, by Seligman, Frank, and Fine (12), who also termed their efforts at aspirations of the intubated duodenum in a uremic patient 'futile'. Enthusiastic, though often poorly controlled reports of the benefits of perfusing some or all of the intestine of uremic patients, have been published since. Vermooten and Hare (13), for instance, stated, in 1948, that gastric lavage when performed continuously, will extract so much urea '... that as a result, an unconscious uremic patient will be transformed overnight into a bright, normal and conscious individual'. All of seven uremic patients with prostatism in this study improved within 24 h of beginning gastric lavage. The authors could not extend these results to three cases of chronic nephritis, who became worse, even though as much 'as a gram or more of urea was removed in 24 h by continuous gastric lavage'. Quantitation of the urea clearance obtainable by lavage of the stomach, was provided by Maluf's report (14 [1950]) of a 27 year old man with chronic glomerulonephritis, who had gastric intubation, and was lavaged with 11.5 l of a 2.0% solution of Na_2SO_4 over 4.5 h achieving a urea clearance of 2.7 ml/min. Intestinal irrigation in the same patient, at the rate of 22.2 ml/min, resulted in a urea clearance of 19.1 ml/min though neither type of lavage caused an appreciable fall in serum creatinine concentration which was 9.7 mg/dl (858 µmol/l) at the start, and 9.6 mg/dl (850 µmol/l) at the conclusion, of a 24 h lavage. Gastric aspiration or lavage, is too inefficient in solute extraction to affect the course of chronic uremia. Improvement, sometimes truly dramatic, which has been described consequent to gastric lavage, is most likely attributable to correction of uremic acidosis, by removal of hydrochloric acid in gastric secretions.

The first unequivocal evidence of the clinical usefulness of intestinal dialysis was reported by Kolff in 1947 (15). By means of a double ended ileostomy, Kolff perfused the isolated intestinal loop of a 57 year old uremic man with a warmed rinsing fluid extracting 0.48 g (8 mmol) of urea/h (5 g [83 mmol] in 10 h) with obvious clinical improvement. Kolff's anticipatory vision can be appreciated from the fact that he arranged for this patient to be dialyzed at home by his wife for two months before he died, effecting the first successful home dialysis 20 years before hemodialysis was introduced into the home in Seattle, Boston and London.

Twiss and Kolff (16) subsequently treated a 36 year old uremic man by dialysis of an isolated 2.5 m loop of midintestine for 8 to 10 h daily for 16 consecutive days at a flow of 500 to 2100 ml/h. During treatment of this patient, it was appreciated that his hypertension was 'sodium responsive' and not of renal origin, an insight later to be confirmed in hemodialyzed patients. An average of 8.6 g/day (1433 mmol/day) of urea was removed, but creatinine was extracted at only 6.8%, and uric acid at only 4.8% of the rate of urea. Life was clearly prolonged in this patient, who was totally anuric (left aplastic kidney and right nephrectomy for hydronephrosis), for 9 of the 16 days of intestinal perfusion.

Schloerb (17) performed elegant studies of perfusion of an isolated jejunal segment in uremic patients. He concluded in 1958, (two years before Scribner and colleagues [18] devised the external arterio-venous shunt, and initiated long term hemodialysis), that 'intestinal dialysis is probably the only method that affords the possibility of repeated dialysis over a long period'. Schloerb (19) studied an 18 year old man with chronic nephritis who had an isolated loop of the proximal half of his intestine lavaged a total of 74 times; 24 of the perfusions were performed at home. Employing six hour perfusions, at a rate of 2 l/h, it was found that the passage of substances across the intestinal mucosa was dependent on flow rate, osmolality of perfusate, concentration gradient between blood and perfusate, and temperature of the perfusate. A flow rate of 2 l/h optimized nitrogen extraction at 0.92 g/h or 5.5 g in 6 h, removing urea nitrogen at a rate of 0.8 g/h (28.6 mmol of urea) or 4.8 g (171 mmol of urea) per 6 h perfusion period. Mean urea clearance was 13.4 ml/min, which was 17.9% of calculated normal renal clearance. As was previously noted by Maluf (14), intestinal perfusion in Schloerb's study failed to extract significant amounts of either creatinine or uric acid. Perhaps the most important aspect of Schloerb's investigations was the effect of omitting perfusion for five days during which plasma urea concentration rose from 86 to 129 mg/dl (14.3 to 21.5 mmol/l), and the patient deteriorated, developing nausea, vomiting and irritability, all of which subsided after the next perfusion.

According to Spark's (20) calculations, in which solute clearances in all reported human trials of intestinal dialysis were 'adjusted' to a 630 cm intestinal length, and a perfusate flow rate of 2000 ml/h, the average clearances were: urea, 31.4 ± 14.4 ml/min; creatinine, 14.1 ± 10.1 ml/min; uric acid, 18.3 ± 10.4 ml/min; phosphate 3.9 ± 2.7 ml/min.

Evidence that gastrointestinal perfusion extends life in uremic animals is limited. Nephrectomized dogs lavaged via a 50 to 100 cm Thira-Vella intestinal fistula at a rate of 26 to 66 ml/min, for 2.3 to 10.5 h/day, did not have their survival extended significantly (21). Although blood urea levels were reduced, and as much as 14 mg [0.5 mmol of urea] of urea nitrogen were removed per 2.5 cm of intestine, per hour of irrigation (1.4 g (50 mmol of urea) per perfusion), six treated dogs lived a mean of 81 h, only 8 h longer than controls. To assess the ultimate place of intestinal dialysis, it is helpful to consider Spark's computation of the mean flux into the bowel of four solutes viz. urea, creatinine, uric acid, and phosphorus, based on 53 patients reported in the literature (20). The calculated quantities of each solute available within the intestinal lumen each 24 h were: urea 71 g (1183 mmol), creatinine 2.9 g (25.7 mmol), uric acid 2.5 g (15 mmol) and phosphate 2.0 g (21 mmol). As a minimum goal for effective substitution of renal function, Sparks suggested that the extraction of 6 g (100 mmol) urea, 0.5 g (4.4 mmol) creatinine, 0.5 g (3 mmol) uric acid and 1.2 g (12.6 mmol) phosphate would be necessary. These quantities are much less than the amount contained in luminal fluids, and thus, might be extractable during gastrointestinal perfusion (22-25).

Consequent to Scribner's introduction of maintenance hemodialysis, interest in gastrointestinal perfusion for renal insufficiency fell off sharply. In a review through 1962, Clark, Templeton, and McCurdy (26) found 16 cases in the literature, of which only five patients lived for as long as three months. In a discouraging study of five patients, this group had only one survivor for more than three months and suggested that intestinal dialysis be reserved for patients whose urine output exceeds 1500 ml/day and who are free of widespread vascular disease. Based on a study of six patients 'subjected' to intestinal perfusion for 6 to 26 weeks, Pateras et al (27), reached a similar conclusion. While 'water, electrolyte, and acid base balance were easily controlled, intestinal dialysis was found inadequate in correcting the uremic syndrome on a long term basis'.

Diarrhea therapy

More recently, however, Young and co-workers (28) stimulated by their inability, because of cost, to offer uremia therapy in Taipei (Taiwan), explored the use of gut perfusion in renal insufficiency. These workers devised what they termed diarrhea therapy, in which the large volumes of oral fluid replacement given in cholera (29) were reformulated as a warmed mannitol-saline solution. Diarrhea therapy consists of a treatment session costing 3 dollars, and lasting 3 h, in which a uremic patient drinks 7 l of the solution at the rate of 200 ml every 5 min. The solution contains in each liter: mannitol 180 mmol; sodium 60 mmol; potassium 4 mmol; calcium 1 mmol; chloride 46 mmol; and bicarbonate 20 mmol. Diarrhea, first semiformed, and then liquid begins within 45 min and ends within 25 min of completion of drinking. Gastro-intestinal tract clearance over eight months, in a uremic patient with a residual mean creatinine clearance of 3.4 ml/min (0.7 ml/min in the eighth month), were: 29.0 ± 2.6 ml/min for urea, and 6.4 ± 0.9 ml/min for creatinine. Diarrhea therapy was subsequently initiated in 17 patients thrice weekly, including the performance of 3 h sessions at home, so long as the patient's residual renal function exceeded 1.0 ml/min. The mean duration of home diarrhea therapy was 6.8 ± 4 months (range of 1.3 to 16 months). The patients improved; they experienced increased appetite, while itching and weakness decreased, and body weight, blood pressure, and hematocrit remained constant. In the author's impression, diarrhea therapy is inexpensive, simple, can be performed at home, and most importantly, will maintain uremic patients for as long as 16 months.

For the 75% of the world's population for whom conventional dialytic therapy is out of the question due to its high cost, a choice between diarrhea and death is a realistic proposal. A well constructed field trial, accomplishable at modest cost, is appropriate. If the results are confirmative, diarrhea therapy holds great potential for life prolongation in uremic citizens of poor countries.

INGESTIBLE SORBENTS

History's first oral sorbent, described in Dioscorides' Materia Medica in 40 B.C. is *terra sigillata,* the sacred earth initially found, and still mined on the Greek island of Lemnos. According to Pliny's writing in 100 A.D., *terra sigillata* is effective '... against complaints of the spleen and kidneys, copious menstruation, also against poisons and wounds caused by serpents'. Several ancient Egyptian *papyri* detail the benefits of charcoal, given orally, for chemical or disease induced intoxications.

Charcoal

Yatzidis (30) introduced charcoal hemoperfusion for the treatment of uremia at the first meeting of the European Dialysis and Transplant Association in 1964. The technique and current status of hemoperfusion is discussed by Winchester in the preceding chapter. Charcoal hemoperfusion as presently practiced, is inadequate as a sole treatment for uremia.

Yatzidis also explored the use of charcoal given by mouth, to remove retained nitrogenous solutes from the intestinal tract. In preliminary *in vitro* studies of gastric fluid, bile and intestinal fluid, Yatzidis found that concentrations of 'uremic substances' were elevated in proportion to their serum levels. Intestinal fluid, contains urea, for example, at 92% of its serum level while the creatinine concentration in gastric fluid was 33% that of serum drawn simultaneously from the same uremic patient.

Charcoal has great adsorption capacity for many organic molecules, including drugs and metabolic wastes of low water solubility (31, 32). Davis (33) determined the adsorptive capacity of activated charcoal *in vitro*, from solutions containing 5 mg/dl of different solutes. Each gram of carbon under the conditions tested will bind 0.24 mg (4 µmol) of urea, 19 mg (168 µmol) of creatinine, 90 mg (536 µmol) of uric acid, 140 mg (539 µmol) of secobarbital, 230 mg (927 µmol) of pentobarbital and 290 mg (1.16 mmol) of methaqualone. Other investigators have confirmed the broad sorbing properties of charcoal in buffered solutions. Sparks and co-workers (34) however, found that the actual binding of creatinine by charcoal was much lower in small intestinal fluid than in buffered saline.

Based on this encouraging result, Yatzidis and Oreopoulos (35) next initiated a clinical trial and treated 12 patients in chronic renal failure with 20 to 50 g of powdered charcoal per day, combined with a 40 g protein diet. Control periods of eight weeks were alternated with eight weeks of charcoal treatment. The 16 week control-treatment cycle was then repeated. Significant reductions were observed in the serum concentration of guanidines, uric acid, and phenols. There were, however, no decreases in the serum levels of creatinine, urea, organic acids, electrolytes, sulfate, or phosphate. Patients recounted marked subjective improvement in uremic signs and symptoms, including anorexia and vomiting. It was concluded, that oral charcoal in the doses given, might be a helpful adjunct to dialytic therapy, but extracted insufficient nitrogen to substitute for regular hemodialysis. Yatzidis's patients, it should be stipulated, had a relatively high residual renal function (creatinine clearances ranging from 10 to 15 ml/min, [personal communication to the author]) precluding direct comparison with the usual hemodialysis patient. From our own later trials in uremic patients and healthy volunteers, we can confirm the acceptability and lack of toxicity of activated charcoal ingested in a divided daily dose of 35 g, for as long as eight weeks. We were also unable to substantiate its efficacy as a nitrogen extracting ingestible sorbent.

In daily doses of 50 g of powdered activated charcoal, Denti et al (36) found that healthy volunteers suffered nausea, vomiting and constipation of sufficient severity to interrupt further trial. A further negative note on the potential oral use of charcoal was sounded by Maxwell and co-workers (37), who administered 'various forms of carbon in doses up to 90 g daily' to uremic dogs without evidence of 'significant effect on the lowering of any of the metabolites associated with the uremic state'. The severity of azotemia was only mild in Maxwell's dogs; a greater sorbing effect of nitrogenous metabolites might have occurred at higher blood and intestinal fluid concentrations. Encapsulation of activated charcoal within a cellulose acetate butyrate membrane did not improve its efficacy as a sorbent, as judged by feeding 40 g to a uremic dog, who showed no discernible reduction in serum creatinine concentration (38). Oral charcoal, in contrast to charcoal in hemoperfusion devices, must thus be regarded as an ineffective nitrogen binding sorbent (Figure 1). It is intriguing to appreciate that the mechanism proffered to explain the inefficacy of charcoal as an intraintestinal nitrogen sorbent, which is the coating of adsorption pores with lipids in gut fluids, may provide a rationale for charcoal's use as a hypolipidemic agent.

Oxidized starch and oxidized cellulose

Following the disappointment over the failure of ingested charcoal to prove active as a nitrogen binder, interest in oral sorbents for treating uremia lay dormant

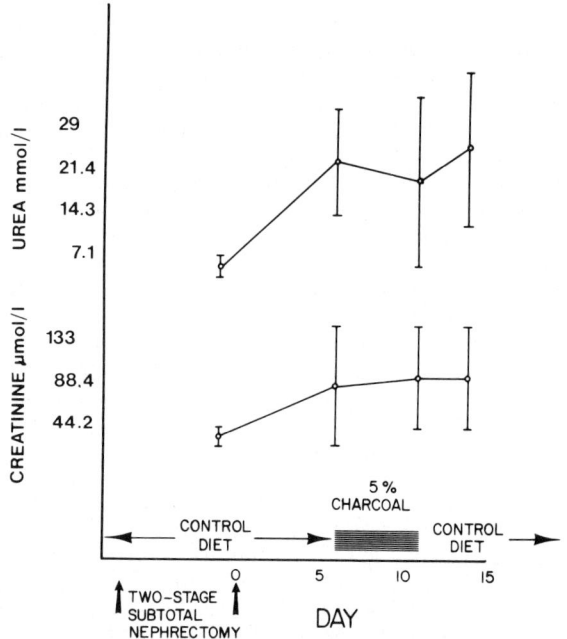

Figure 1. Oral charcoal fed to azotemic rats is an ineffective nitrogen binding sorbent. In this study the animals showed no response in terms of BUN or serum creatinine concentrations to a 5% charcoal diet.
(Blood urea mmol/l → BUN mg/dl: divide by 0.357
Serum creatinine µmol/l → mg/dl: divide by 88.4)

until Giordano's trials of dialdehyde starch (oxidized starch, oxystarch). Industrial uses of reactions between polyaldehydes and urea or ammonia had been utilized for some time in the preparation of plastics and resin adhesives. Giordano and coworkers (39, 40) reasoned that should polyaldehyde derivatives of starch prove to be nontoxic, and insoluble in intestinal fluids, then their affinity for urea might be valuable in renal insufficiency.

Clinical trials in uremic patients of both oxidized starch and oxidized cellulose, have been conducted. Starch derived from maize or potatoes is a natural polysaccharide composed of amylase, nonbranched chains of glucose residues containing maltose, a dissaccharide-4-l-glucopyranosil-D-pyranosil-D-pyranosium and amylopectin, a many branched glucose polymer. Cellulose, a natural linear-chain polysaccharide is the principal constituent of wood and is composed of repeating units of cellobiose, a dissaccharide 4-B-D-glucopyranosil-D-glucose. By reacting starch or cellulose in mole/mole concentrations with sodium periodate, their polyaldehyde derivatives are prepared. Both polyaldehydes are insoluble at acid pH, but become soluble at alkaline pH. At neutral pH, oxidized cellulose has negligible solubility, while a portion of oxidized starch will dissolve (41). Hence, only oxidized cellulose has been tested in regeneration of dialysate. Both ammonia and urea bind to oxystarch over a broad pH range at temperatures ranging from 25 °C to 70 °C. Giordano's original tedious process for synthesizing oxystarch from starch by reaction with an excess of sodium metaperiodate at 2 to 5 °C for 24 h, with subsequent centrifugation, washing, and a final acetone treatment, has been shortened by raising the reaction temperature to 32 °C for about 6 h. Oxystarch made from corn starch, potato starch or amylomaize (hybrid corn starch) shows identical behavior in binding ammonia and urea.

At body temperature and at pH of 7.4, each repeat unit of oxystarch binds 1.5 to 1.9 moles of ammonia *in vitro* from a 0.3 N ammonia solution; when present in excess, oxystarch will extract all of the ammonia from an identical solution. Oxystarch also binds urea and l-aspartic acid *in vitro*, but does not adsorb creatinine, uric acid, l-lysine or albumin. At room temperature each mole of oxystarch binds 0.87 moles of urea. Ingested ^{14}C-oxystarch is excreted in the feces with 81% of the radioactivity remaining, indicating that most oxystarch is not hydrolyzed or metabolized in man (41).

Oxystarch is relatively nontoxic. Weanling mice, fed 2% oxystarch in a casein diet, undergo normal development and growth. Rats, however, develop severe diar-

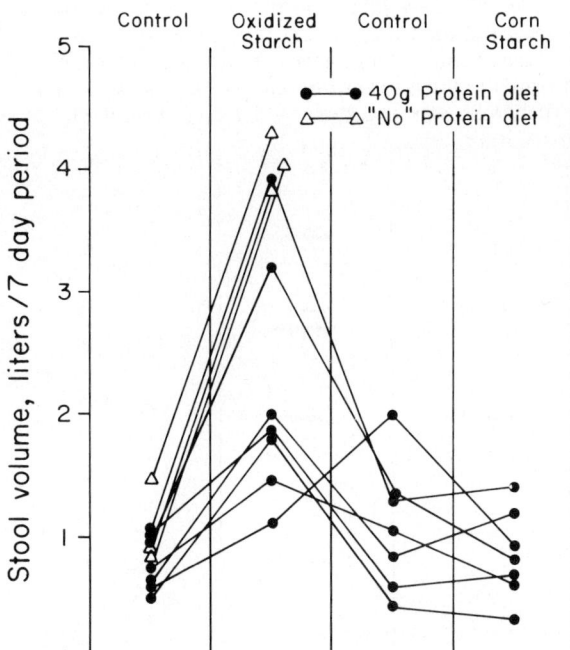

Figure 2. Uremic patients (creatinine clearance of 8 to 20 ml/min) given oxidized starch (35 g/day) increased stool bulk on either a 40 g protein or a no protein diet. An increased stool volume, however, does not in itself alter fecal nitrogen excretion.

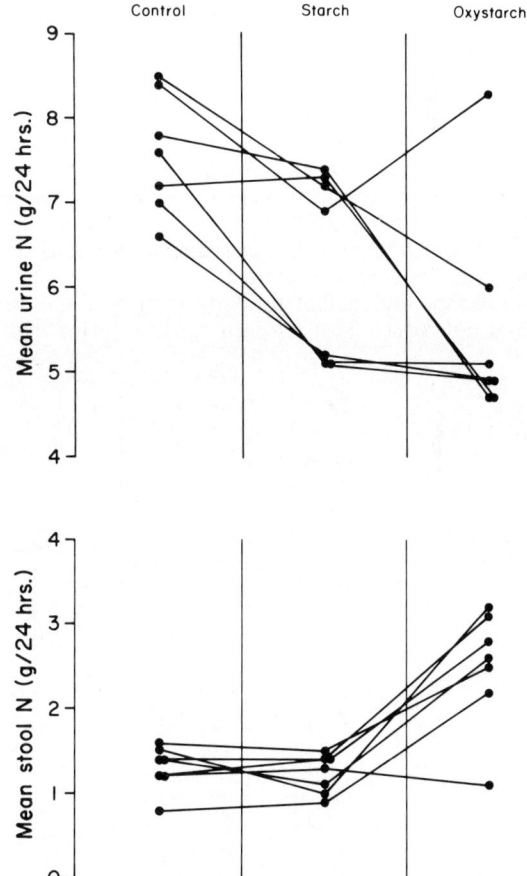

Figure 3. Uremic patients fed oxidized starch, 28 g/day, increased fecal nitrogen content by a mean of 1 g. Corn starch administered as a control did not alter fecal nitrogen content. Total nitrogen balance was unchanged due to a fall in urinary nitrogen content.

rhea on a 2% oxystarch diet while dogs tolerate as much as a 5% oxystarch diet. Explosive diarrhea and a cholera-like electrolyte and fluid depletion syndrome are noted in dogs fed more than 10% oxystarch in their diet (34). Uremic patients will accept 20 to 35 g oxystarch/day in divided doses. An increase in stool volume of 200 to 600 ml/day is usual as is an increased frequency of bowel movements without diarrhea (Figure 2).

In an effort to delay or omit hemodialysis treatments, Giordano and coworkers (39) fed 20 g oxystarch/day to uremic patients (creatinine clearances of 0.4 to 3.2 ml/min) inducing a significant fall in blood urea nitrogen level and a concomitant increase in fecal nitrogen content averaging 1.45 g (52 mmol N_2)/day (range of 0.7 to 8.0 g (25 to 286 mmol N_2) increase/day). Friedman and coworkers (42) performed a double blind starch-oxystarch full balance study in seven uremic patients (creatinine clearances of 6 to 30 ml/min) and confirmed Giordano's findings. In Friedman's study, oxystarch was fed in divided daily doses of 28 g added to a 40 to 50 g protein diet. Blood urea nitrogen levels fell 33% during oxystarch treatment from a mean of 93.1 mg/dl (33 mmol/l of urea) to a mean of 62.1 mg/dl (22 mmol/l of urea) without significant change in serum creatinine, plasma amino acid, uric acid or glucose concentrations. Fecal nitrogen increased significantly from a control mean of 1.4 g (50 mmol N_2)/24 h to 2.5 g (89.3 mmol N_2)/24 h (Figure 3). There was a simultaneous fall in urinary nitrogen excretion from a mean of 7.6 g/24 h to 5.5 g/24 h (271 mmol to 196 mmol N_2) preventing the development of negative nitrogen balance. Fecal potassium content increased by 5 to 22 mmol/day during oxystarch treatment, suggesting a possible role for the drug in acute renal failure.

Based on the finding that antibiotic sterilization of the gut does not reduce fecal nitrogen content during oxidized starch treatment, it has been inferred that either urea or ammonia can be bound equally. It may be hypothesized that the polyaldehydes in the unsterilized uremic gut adsorb urea in the stomach and ammonia in the colon. Patients fed a nitrogen-free diet increase fecal nitrogen content during oxystarch treatment to the same extent as those on a 40 g protein diet, indicating that the trapped nitrogen comes from luminal excretion, rather than undigested dietary components (Figure 3). Man and associated (43) also found an increase of 1.0 g (35.7 mmol N_2) in fecal nitrogen content in 12 uremic patients (mean creatinine clearance of 4.1 ml/min) fed 30 g of oxystarch daily. No such increase was noted when oxystarch was replaced by methylcellulose, an aperient which increased stool bulk to the same extent as did oxystarch. Although oxystarch treatment increases fecal nitrogen and potassium excretion, it should be noted that the clinical significance of this findings is still undefined.

Animal experimentation has not indicated a promising role of oxystarch in anephric rats. Though nephrectomized rats fed either oxystarch (1 g/day) or charcoal (1 g/day) live longer than controls (44), this increase is a consequence of delayed hyperkalemia (Figures 4 and 5). Rats who were potassium depleted prior to nephrectomy, lived longer than nondepleted nephrectomized controls, and did not have any extension of life attributable to oral sorbent therapy (45).

Esposito and Giordano (46) recently explored methods of increasing the efficiency of nitrogen sorbtion by dialdehyde compounds. They conducted the only trial, to date, of oxycellulose administration to uremic patients. In graded daily doses of 1 to 100 g of oxycellulose, they achieved a remarkable increase in fecal nitrogen content which rose from 0.8 g (29 mmol N_2) when 1 g oxycellulose was ingested, to 1.2 g (43 mmol N_2) at a

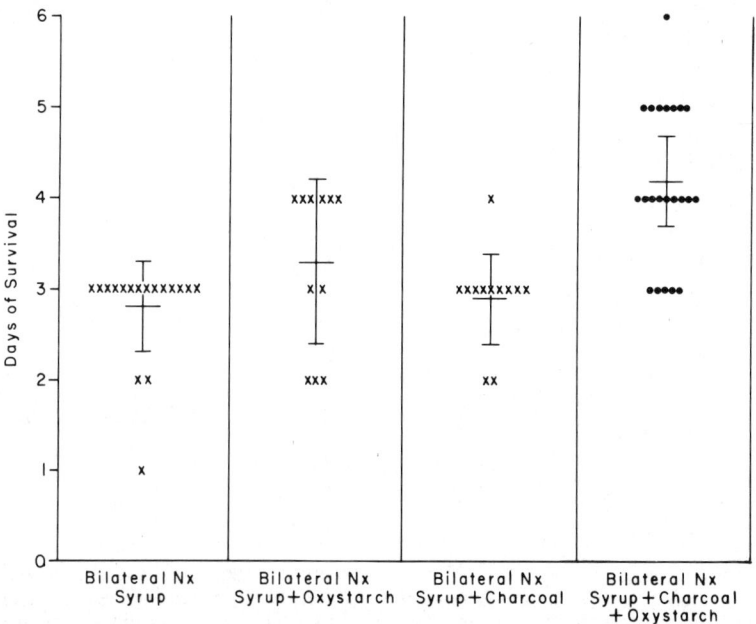

Figure 4. Bilaterally nephrectomized (NX) rats live longer when fed a mixture of corn syrup, oxidized starch, and charcoal than do control rats given only the sugar syrup.

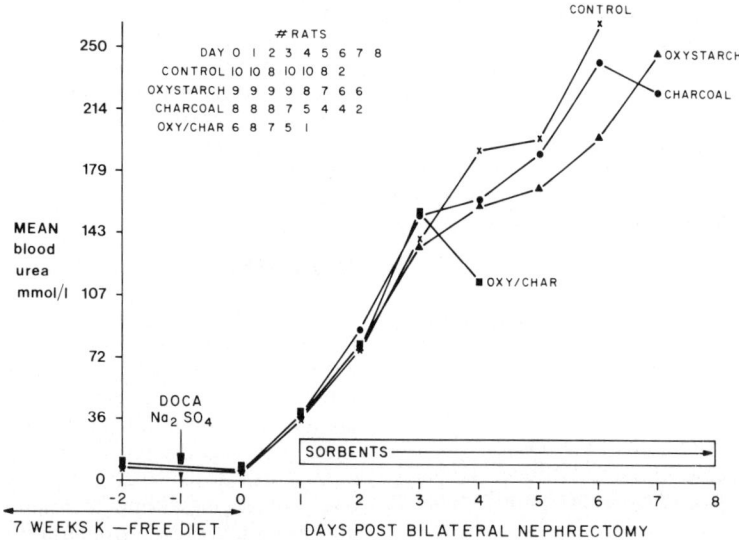

Figure 5. The mechanism of life prolongation in nephrectomized rats fed oxidized starch and charcoal is the prevention of lethal hyperkalemia. When rats were potassium depleted, by diet and DOCA treatment before nephrectomy, the benefit of sorbent therapy is no longer evident.
(Blood urea mmol/l → BUN mg/dl: divide by 0.357)

10 g dose of oxycellulose, and 5.2 g (186 mmol N_2) at the relatively high dose of 100 g of oxycellulose. There was no difference in patient preference of oxycellulose or oxystarch. Both were well accepted. Clearly, further clinical trials of higher doses of dialdehyde sorbents in uremic patients are appropriate to the quest for less expensive uremia therapy.

Locust bean gum

Yatzidis (47) investigated the sorbing capacities of several naturally occurring gums, including arabic, tragacanth, Karaya, psilium seed, and locust bean. Of these, only locust bean gum, a straight chain mannose polymer, molecular mass approximately 310,000 daltons, showed promise in uremia treatment, when reacted *in vitro* with recirculated hemodialysate, or the intestinal fluid obtained from a colostomy of a 'severely uremic patient'. Locust bean gum adsorbed more urea per gram than did oxystarch. In 100 ml of intestinal fluid 1.5 g of locust bean gum reacting at 37°C at pH 8.2 for 12 h, reduced the concentrations of urea from 31.0 to 20.5 mmol/l, creatinine from 0.3 to 0.18 mmol/l, uric acid from 0.30 to 0.17 mmol/l and ammonia from 20.0 to 10.0 mmol/l. Locust bean gum is not toxic. Bread made from the seeds of ceratonia siliqua, its source, was regularly ingested by the Greek population during the second World War without apparent ill effect. Locust bean gum is apparently not digested; blood galactose levels (a part of the gum molecule) do not rise within three hours of its ingestion.

Only a single report details the effect of locust bean gum treatment in uremic patients (48). Two patients, a 66 year old woman with polycystic kidneys, and a 45 year old man with renal tuberculosis in a solitary kidney, were given daily divided doses of 25 g of locust bean gum mixed with one tablespoon of cotton seed oil. Both patients tolerated the sorbent well, had a fall to normal of elevated blood pressures, and had 'slight but distinct' reductions of serum urea, creatinine and phosphate levels by the second week of treatment. Serum creatinine concentrations fell from 570 to 500 µmol/l in one and from 380 to 310 µmol/l in the other patient. Yatzidis concluded 'the observed clinical and biochemical results' justified further trials of 'locust bean gum as an agent for possible oral use in the treatment of uremia'.

Liquid membrane capsules

Conceptualized and developed by Asher and associates (49), the use of liquid membrane capsules hold promise as an alternative technique for intraintestinal sorption of nitrogenous solutes. Liquid membrane capsules consist of drops of a continuous oil emulsion suspended in an aqueous external phase which contains an active internal phase. For clinical application, Asher proposes a mixture of capsules which would release urease, converting urea to ammonia, and then bind ammonia to be passed out of the gut in feces.

In dogs made azotemic (blood urea nitrogen of 50 to 100 mg/dl [18 to 36 mmol/l of urea]) by 7/8 surgical ablation of their renal mass, liquid membrane capsules were administered into the jejunum through a previously inserted external catheter. Urease was introduced in one capsule formulation and citric acid, an ammonia reacting chemical in another. This experiment showed both that the enzyme urease retained activity within a liquid membrane capsule, converting to ammonia, which was then extracted by a second capsule. A calculated dose of 120 ml of capsules daily will remove 12 g (200 mmol) of urea. The significance of Asher's approach is that it provides another means of extracting nitrogenous solutes from the gut with virtually no toxic risk attributable to an inert sorbent shell. Liquid membrane capsules could be given in a mixture of sorbents and are currently being evaluated in this form.

OTHER APPLICATIONS OF ORAL SORBENTS

Antacids

Binding of dietary phosphate ions by antacids will prevent uremic hyperphosphatemia, reciprocal hypocalcemia and consequent secondary hyper-parathyroidism (discussed in Chapter 35).

Concerns in designing an aluminum-based gel for phosphate removal in the gut include the advantage of gelation at acid pH (50) which assures firm binding of phosphate due to its enhanced attraction to the gel by coordination with inner electrons. The choice of exchangeable counter ions for gel formulation include acetate, bicarbonate, chloride, sulfate, or nitrate. To avoid sulfate accumulation, this ion can be replaced after gelation by the acetate ion. Sparks and associates (50) found an aluminum sulfate gel to have the greatest sorbing capacity for phosphate, and are pursuing clinical trials of its long term use.

Dialysis dementia, a rare, usually fatal complication of maintenance hemodialysis, has been linked to aluminum containing antacids in a postulated syndrome of aluminum intoxication (51). The safety of aluminum containing phosphate binders is presently questioned (see also chapter 42). Alternatively this syndrome has been attributed to antacid induced phosphate depletion (52). Magnesium containing antacids should not be used in renal insufficiency as hypermagnesemia is usually present, though its clinical expression is masked by perturbations in calcium, potassium and sodium metabolism.

Hyperkalemia

Control of hyperkalemia in both acute and chronic renal failure may be effected by extraction of potassium from gut fluid. Sodium polystyrene sulfonate (Kayexalate) is a cation exchange resin which exchanges sodium for potassium on a mole for mole basis. Calcium and magnesium may also exchange for sodium. In a dose of 60 g daily (three doses of 20 g) the resin is about 33% effective, exchanging about 20 mmol of potassium for sodium. Simultaneous administration of 20 ml of 70% sorbitol syrup every 4 hours, will prevent constipation which may complicate treatment with Kayexalate. Oxystarch, which adsorbs both potassium and nitrogen, may also have a role in treating uremic hyperkalemia.

Mannitol induced diarrhea can also be utilized, not only to lessen hyperkalemia, but also, to extract fluid from volume overloaded dialysis patients, in the interdialytic interval. We have administered 50 g of mannitol in a 25% oral solution with a prompt diarrheal response (53).

Lipid reduction

During a clinical trial in which a mixture of oxidized starch, 35 g/day and activated charcoal, 35 g/day, were

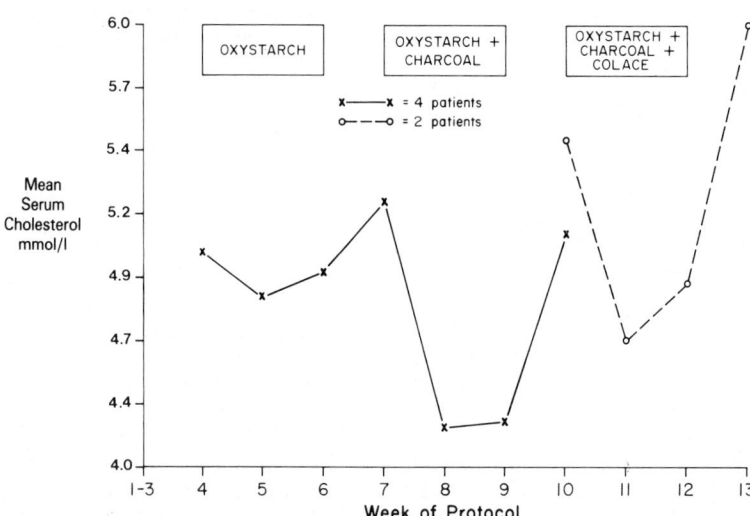

Figure 6. A fall in serum cholesterol concentration was observed in these and all other uremic patients fed charcoal in a dose of 20 to 35 g/day (+oxystarch). No effect was observed from oxystarch alone. Serum triglyceride level also declines promptly during charcoal treatment.
(Colace: proprietary name for dioctyl-Na-sulfasuccinate, a laxative).
(Serum cholesterol mmol/l → mg/dl: divide by 0.0259).

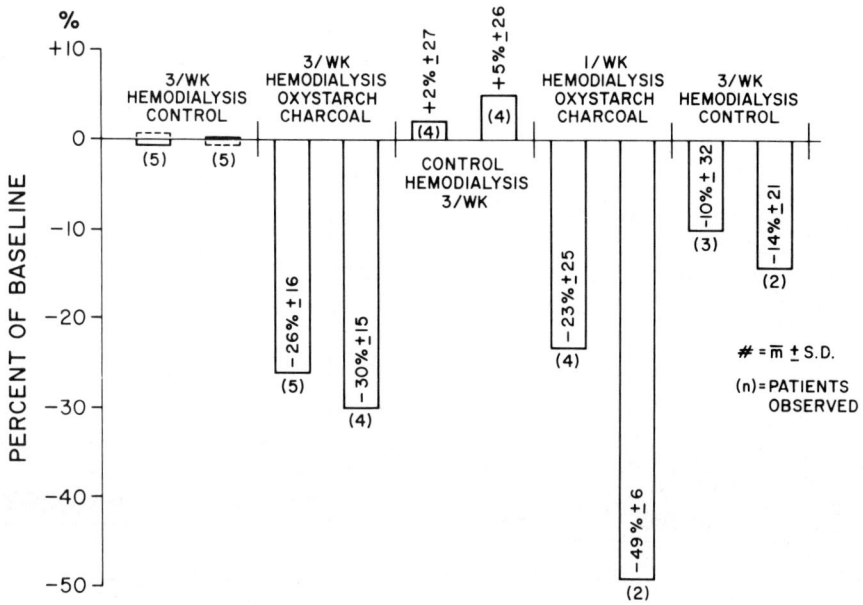

Figure 7. A marked decline in serum cholesterol concentration is induced in hemodialysis patients fed charcoal (+oxystarch), 35 g/day.

administered to uremic patients to quantitate fecal nitrogen excretion, a serendipitous sharp decline in serum cholesterol (Figure 6) and triglyceride was observed. A derivative study confirmed that it was the charcoal and not the oxidized starch which was binding lipids (54). Lemperi et al (55) confirmed this observation and extended the application of charcoal for lipid sorption to its incorporation in bread fed to patients in chronic renal failure. It is now apparent that charcoal is virtually inactive in the uremic gut as a nitrogen binder, but acts to reduce serum lipids with high efficiency.

Goldenhersch et al (56) provided an explanation of this puzzling observation in their investigations *in vitro* of the effect of plasma, duodenal fluid, gall bladder fluid and intestinal fluid on the adsorption of creatinine by charcoal. They found that small gut fluid inhibits 95% of creatinine adsorption at a 5 mg/dl (442 µmol/l) creatinine concentration, perhaps due to 'lipid-like substances in the intestine which compete with the toxin for some surface sites on the activated carbon'. That charcoal is, indeed, a powerful lipid binder, is shown by reduction in serum cholesterol in patients hemoperfused over charcoal. Subsequent studies have reproduced this sorbent induced reduction in plasma cholesterol in several groups of uremic patients. In one study, an unsuccessful attempt to decrease the frequency of hemodialy-

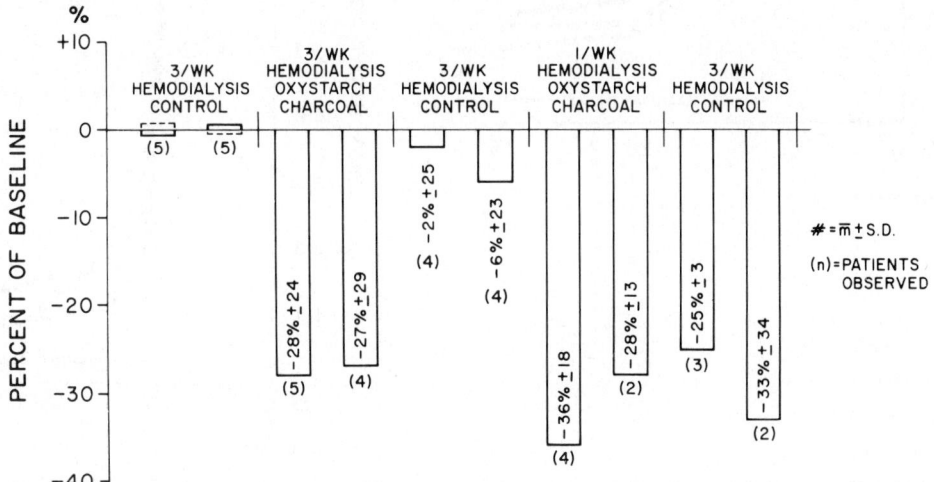

Figure 8. Patients on maintenance hemodialysis also have a sharp drop in serum triglycerides during oral charcoal (+oxystarch) treatment at a dose of 35 g/day.

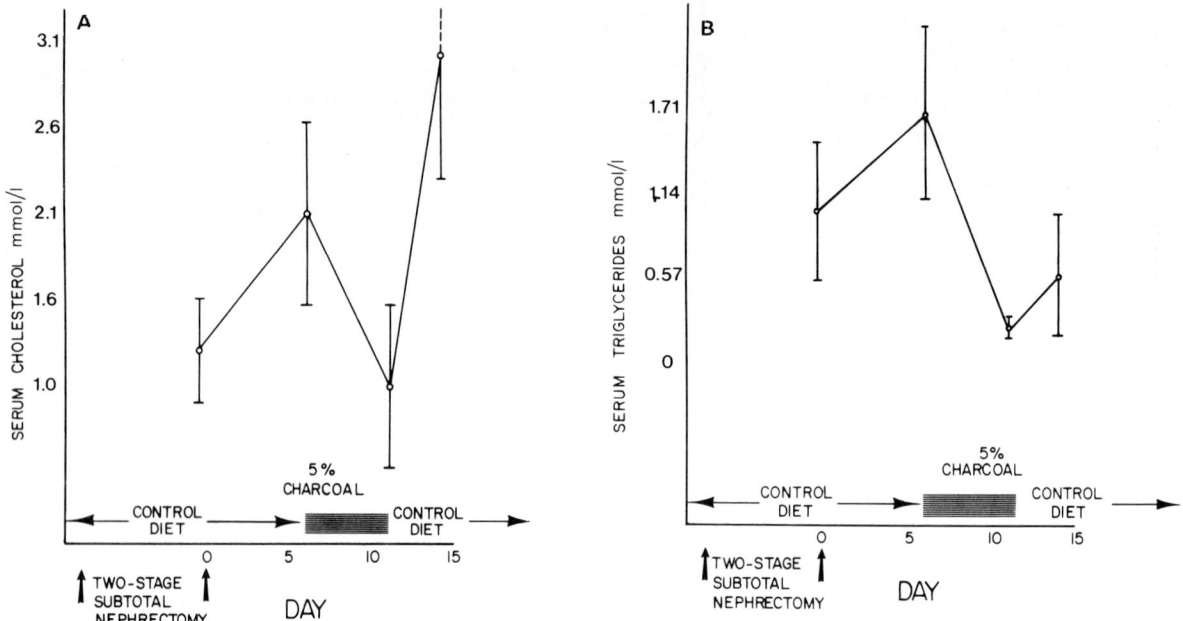

Figure 9. Charcoal effect in rats made azotemic by 5/6 nephrectomy: A. a decline in cholesterol during 5% charcoal ingestion; B. a fall in triglycerides of even greater degree during charcoal treatment.
(Serum cholesterol mmol/l → mg/dl: divide by 0.0259.
Triglycerides mmol/l → mg/dl: divide by 0.0114).

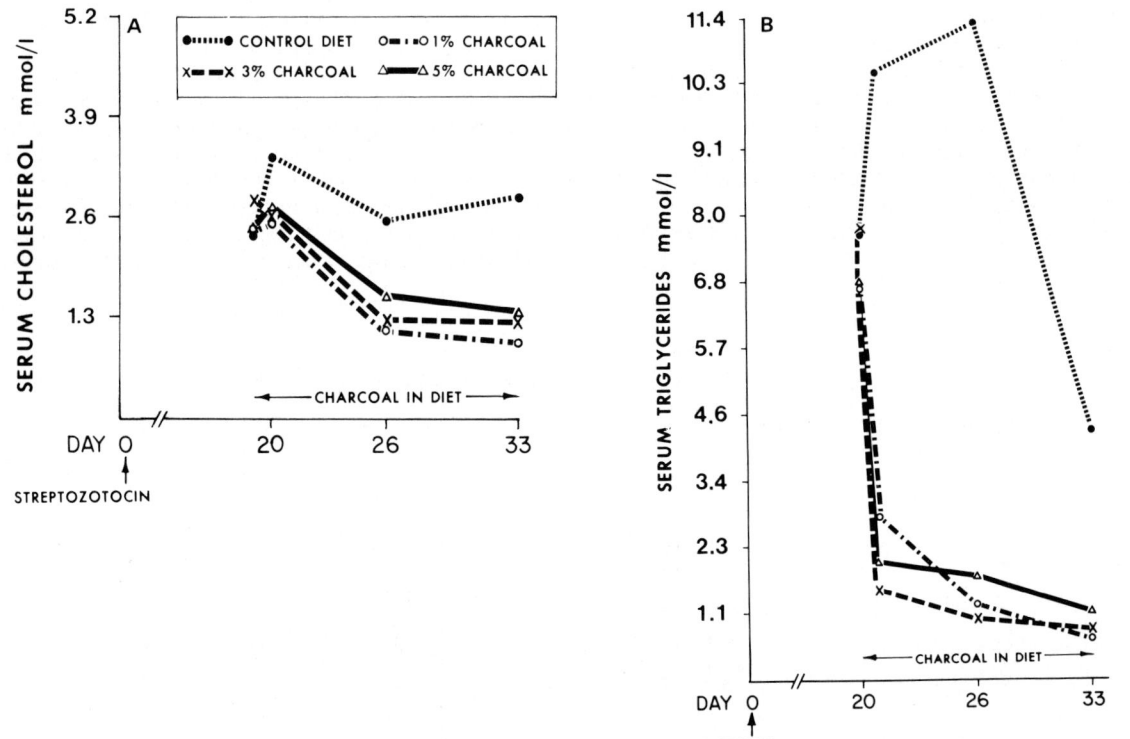

Figure 10. Sensitivity of streptozotocin induced diabetic rats to charcoal: A. as little as a 1% charcoal diet lowers cholesterol level; B. serum triglycerides also fall significantly and promptly during 1% charcoal feeding.
(Serum cholesterol mmol/l → mg/dl divide by 0.0259.
Serum triglycerides mmol/l → mg/dl divide by 0.0114).

sis from thrice to once weekly, cholesterol fell during oral charcoal plus oxystarch treatments of three weeks (Figure 7); a marked reduction in serum triglycerides values was also noted (Figure 8).

To explore the charcoal hypolipidemia effect in an animal model, Manis and colleagues (57, 58) fed a 25% charcoal diet to normal rats and produced a significant fall in fasting cholesterol and triglycerides. At a 10% dietary content, fasting triglyceride decreased but cholesterol level was unchanged. An enhanced hypolipidemic action was found in 5/6th nephrectomized azotemic rats which responded to a 5% charcoal diet (Figures 9a, b). The most sensitive rat model yet studied is the streptozotocin induced diabetic rat which responds to as little as 0.5% dietary charcoal. Thus, in six rats made diabetic, mean serum cholesterol concentration rose from a control of 68 ± 11.6 mg/dl (1.8 mmol/l) to 192 ± 63 mg/dl (5.0 mmol/l) and then fell on charcoal feeding to 43 ± 6.3 mg/dl (1.1 mmol/l) (Figure 10a). A marked reduction in serum triglycerides was also noted (Figure 10b). Radiocholesterol studies in induced diabetic rats show that there was no increase in fecal cholesterol when as much as 25% charcoal was incorporated in the diet (59). Thus, the mechanism of charcoal lipid lowering remains undefined and probably is not due to enhanced stool excretion.

To elucidate the genesis of serum lipid reduction, we are attempting to characterize metabolic lipoprotein alterations induced by charcoal. It is known that key enzymes in triglyceride and cholesterol metabolism (lipoprotein lipase and lecithincholesterol acyl transferase, respectively) are subject to major influence by various lipo-protein peptides whose activities may be altered. Decreased lipoprotein lipase activity, for example, is thought to underlie the hypertriglyceridemia of diabetic rats (59) and has been reported in human diabetics as well. More palatable forms of charcoal are being sought to facilitate further human investigations. Whether oral charcoal will some day be of clinical importance in the treatment of hyperlipidemic states is not clear. Certainly, the effect on serum lipids provides a useful and interesting investigational opportunity.

CONCLUSION

Persistence and tenacity of a handful of investigators, led by Yatzidis, Giordano, and Sparks, may one day make intragut sorption an important component of uremia therapy. Fewer than five oral sorbents have been carefully clinically evaluated to date. It should prove possible to formulate a mixture of absorbents, adsorbents, and ion exchange substances to extract any desired combination of solutes (Figure 11). For some nephrologists the image of the gut persists as a displaced, hypertrophied and available 'nephron' for substitutive therapy in uremia.

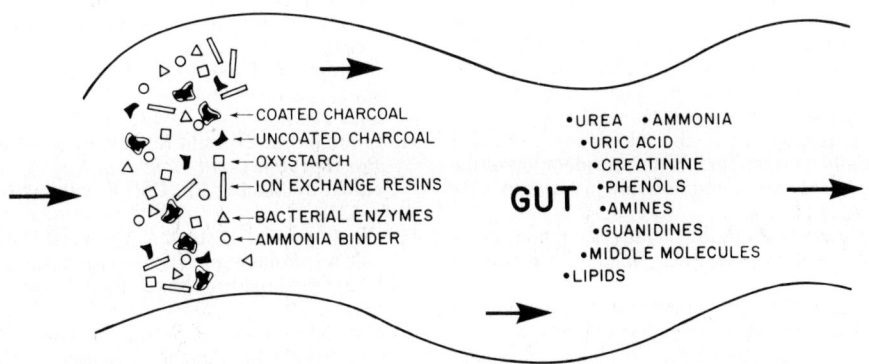

Figure 11. Multiple sorbents for use of bowel as a 'kidney'. A mixture of sorbents acting by differing mechanisms could extract sufficient nitrogenous solutes to replace missing renal function without dialytic therapy.

REFERENCES

1. Friedman EA, Delano BG: Can the world afford uremia therapy? *Proc 8th Int Congr Nephrol* (Athens), edited by Zurukzoglu W, Papadimitriou M, Pyrpasopoulos M, Sion M, Zamboulis C, Basel, S Karger 1981, p 577
2. Wing AJ, Selwood NH: Registry data, a collaborative exercise. *Proc 8th Int Congr Nephrol* (Athens), edited by Zurukzoglu W, Papadimitriou M, Pyrpasopoulos M, Sion M, Zamboulis C, Basel, S Karger 1981, p 571
3. Shapiro WB, Schilb TP, Porush JG, Waltrous CL, Oguagha C, Faubert PF and Chou S: Sobert regeneration in hemofiltration. *Proc 8th Int Congr Nephrol* (Athens), edited by Zurukzoglu W, Papadimitriou M, Pyrpasopoulos M, Sion M, Zamboulis C, Basel, S Karger 1981, p 414
4. Gelfand MC: Hemoperfusion in uremia at the crossroads: is there a true role? *Proc 8th Int Congr Nephrol* (Athens), edited by Zurukzoglu W, Papadimitriou M, Pyrpasopoulos M, Sion M, Zamboulis C, Basel, S Karger 1981, p 407
5. Salisbury PF, Briggs JN, Hamel NC, Cross CE, Rieben PA: Pulmonary lavage: The use of lung, in situ, as an 'artificial kidney'. *Trans Am Soc Artif Intern Organs* 5:32, 1959

6. Asher WJ: Introduction to sorbents. In: *Sorbents and Their Clinical Application.* Edited by Giordano C, New York, Academic Press, 1980, p 3
7. Sparks RE: Review of gastrointestinal perfusion in the treatment of uremia. *Clin Nephrol* 11:81, 1979
8. Bernard C: Sur les voies d'élimination de l'urée après extirpation des reins. (The pathways of elimination of urea after bilateral nephrectomy) *Archs Gen Méd,* Series 4, 13:449, 1847 (in French)
9. Auguste MC: Le drainage duodénal dans le traitement de l'urémie. (Drainage of the duodenum for the treatment of uremia). *Bull Mém Soc Méd Hôp Paris* 45:1313, 1929 (in French)
10. Pendleton WR, West FE: The passage of urea between the blood and the lumen of the small intestine. *Am J Physiol* 101:391, 1932
11. Hessel G, Pekelis E, Meltzer H: Untersuchungen über die Ausscheidung harnfähiger Stoffe in den Magendarmkanal bei nephrektomierten Hunden. (Investigations on the excretion of uremic substances in the gastro-intestinal tract of anephric dogs). I, II, III, IV, and V. *Z Ges Exp Med* 91:267, 1933 (in German)
12. Seligman AM, Frank HA, Fine J: Treatment of experimental uremia by means of peritoneal irrigation. *J Clin Invest* 25:211, 1946
13. Vermooten V, Hare DM: The use of continuous gastric lavage in the treatment of uraemia associated with prostatism. *J Urol* 59:907, 1948
14. Maluf N Sr: Intestinal and gastric perfusion in a patient with severe chronic uremia. *J Urol* 64:268, 1950
15. Kolff WJ: *New Ways of Treating Uraemia.* London, JA Churchill, 1947
16. Twiss EE, Kolff WJ: Treatment of uremia by perfusion of isolated intestinal loop. *JAMA* 146:1019, 1951
17. Schloerb PR: The management of uremia by perfusion of an isolated jejunal segment. *J Clin Invest* 37:1818, 1958
18. Quinton W, Dillard D, Scribner BH: Cannulation of blood vessels for prolonged hemodialysis. *Trans Am Soc Artif Intern Organs* 6:104, 1960
19. Schloerb PR: Enterodialysis in the management of renal failure: a metabolic balance study with consideration of the exchange rates of electrolytes and nonprotein nitrogen. *Clin Res Proc* 4:251, 1956
20. Sparks RE: Gastrosorbents in the therapy of uremia; inferences from intestinal loop dialysis. *Kidney Int* 7 (Suppl 3):S373, 1975
21. White BH, Harkins HN: The treatment of experimental uremia by intestinal lavage. *Surgery* 24:90, 1948
22. Thompson WS, Lewis JJ, Alving AS: Physiological changes during perfusion of the isolated intestinal loop in chronic uremia. *J Lab Clin Med* 39:69, 1952
23. Pyrah LN, Care AD: The use of an isolated loop of ileum as an auxiliary kidney. *Br J Urol* 29:45, 1957
24. Orlowski T, Ajewski Z, Rymkiewicz H, Sicinski A: A trial of treatment of chronic renal insufficiency by lavage of an isolated intestinal loop. *Pol Arch Med Wewn* 31:857, 1961
25. Rasanen T: The treatment of chronic renal failure with lavage of the separated intestinal loop. *Acta Chir Scand* 126:233, 1963
26. Clark JE, Templeton JY III, McCurdy DK: Perfusion of isolated loops in the management of chronic renal failure. *Trans Am Soc Artif Intern Organs* 8:246, 1962
27. Pateras VR, Dosseto JB, Gault MH, Helle SJ, Tagushi Y, MacKinnon KJ: The role of intestinal perfusion in the management of chronic uremia. *Trans Am Soc Artif Intern Organs* 10:292, 1964
28. Young TK, Lee SC, Tang CK: Diarrhea therapy of uremia. *Clin Nephrol* 11:86, 1979
29. Phillips RA, Huang CC, Lee SC, Young TK, Blackwell RQ: A new approach to the study of gastrointestinal functions in man by an oral lavage method. *Chin Med J* 23:85, 1976
30. Yatzidis H: Recherches sur l'épuration extrarénale à l'aide du charbon actif (Investigations on extrarenal purification with activated carbon). *Nephron* 1:310, 1964 (in French)
31. Winchester JF, Apiliga MT, Mackagy JM, Kennedy AC: Haemodialysis with charcoal haemoperfusion. *Proc Eur Dial Transpl Assoc* 12:526, 1975
32. Hagstam KE, Larsson LE, Thysell H: Experimental studies on charcoal haemoperfusion in phenobarbital intoxication and uraemia, including histopathologic findings. *Acta Med Scand* 180:593, 1966
33. Davis TA: Activated carbon fibers in hemoperfusion devices. *Kidney Int* 7 (Suppl 3):S406, 1975
34. Sparks RE, Mason NS, Meier PM, Litt MH, Lindan O: Removal of uremic waste metabolites from the intestinal tract by encapsulated carbon and oxidized starch. *Trans Am Soc Artif Intern Organs* 17:229, 1971
35. Yatzidis H and Oreopoulos D: Early clinical trials with sorbents. *Kidney Int* 10 (Suppl 7):S215-217, 1976
36. Denti E, Luboz MP, Tessore VA, Castino F, Gaglia PF: Adsorbents in hemoperfusion. *Kidney Int* 7 (Suppl 3):S401, 1975
37. Maxwell MH, Gordon A, Greenbaum M: Oral sorbents in medicine. In *Uremia,* edited by Kluthe R, Berlyne G, Burton B, Stuttgart, Georg Thieme Verlag, 1972, p 720
38. Gardner DL, Emmerling DC, Williamson KD, Baytos WC, Hassler CR: Encapsulated adsorbents for removal of nitrogenous metabolites via oral ingestion. *Kidney Int* 7 (Suppl 3):S393, 1975
39. Giordano C, Esposito R, Randazzo G, Oxystarch as a gastrointestinal sorbent in uremia. In *Uremia,* edited by Kluthe R, Berlyne G, Burton B, Stuttgart, Georg Thieme Verlag, 1972, p 231
40. Giordano C, Esposito R, Pluvio M: The effects of oxidised starch on blood and faecal nitrogen in uraemia. *Proc Eur Dial Transpl Assoc* 10:136, 1973
41. Giordano C, Esposito R: Studies on oxystarch and uremia. *Proc 8th Ann Contr Conf Artif Kidney Program NIAMDD,* edited by Mackey BB, DHEW publ no (NIH) 7-248, 1975, p 125
42. Friedman EA, Fastook J, Beyer MM, Rattazzi T, Josephson AS: Potassium and nitrogen binding in the human gut by ingested oxidized starch (OS). *Trans Am Soc Artif Intern Organs* 20:161, 1974
43. Man NK, Drueke T, Paris J, Elizalde Monteverde C, Rondon Nucete M, Zingraff J, Jungers P: Increased nitrogen removal from the intestinal tract of uraemic patients. *Proc Eur Dial Transpl Assoc* 10:143, 1973
44. Friedman EA, Laungani GB, Beyer MM: Life prolongation in nephrectomized rats fed oxidized starch and charcoal. *Kidney Int* 7 (Suppl 3):S377, 1975
45. Saltzman MJ, Beyer MM, Friedman EA: Mechanism of life prolongation in nephrectomized rats treated with oxidized starch and charcoal. *Kidney Int* 10 (Suppl 7):S343, 1977
46. Esposito R and Giordano C: Polyaldehydes. In: *Sorbents and their Clinical Applications,* edited by Giordano C, New York, Academic Press, 1980, p 131
47. Yatzidis H: Preliminary studies with locust bean gum: A new sorbent with great potential. *Kidney Int* 13 (Suppl 8):S150, 1978
48. Yatzidis H, Koutsicos D and Digenis P: Newer oral sorbents in uremia. *Clin Nephrol* 11:105, 1979
49. Asher WJ, Bovee KC, Vogler TC, Hamilton RW and Holtzapple PG: Liquid membrane capsules administered to the gastro-intestinal tract of dogs for removal of urea from the blood. *Clin Nephrol* 11:92, 1979

50. Sparks RE, Mason NS, Rutherford WE, Slatopolsky E: Maximizing phosphate capacity of aluminum-based gels. *Kidney Int* 13 (Suppl 8):S160, 1978
51. Jacobs C, Brunner FP, Chantler C, Donckerwolcke RA, Gurland HJ, Hathway RA, Selwood NH, Wing AJ: Combined report on regular dialysis and transplantation in Europe, VII, 1976. *Proc Eur Dial Transpl Assoc* 14:2, 1977
52. Pierides AM, Ward MK, Kerr DNS: Haemodialysis encephalopathy: possible role of phosphate depletion. *Lancet* 1:1234, 1976
53. Heneghan WF, Feldman J, Lundin AP and Friedman EA: Mannitol induced diarrhea for excessive weight gain in maintenance *hemodialysis* Abstracts *Am Soc Nephrol* 13:41A, 1980
54. Friedman EA, Saltzman MJ, Beyer MM, Josephson AS: Combined oxystrarch-charcoal trial in uremia: Sorbent-induced reduction in serum cholesterol. *Kidney Int* 10 (Suppl 7):S273, 1977
55. Lamperi S, Di Maio G, Benizzelli U, Icardi A: Activated charcoal and essential aminoacids as dietary supply in chronic uremia. In press
56. Goldenhersh KK, Huang W, Mason NS, Sparks RE: Effect of microencapsulation on competitive adsorption in intestinal fluids. *Kidney Int* 10 (Suppl 7):S251, 1977
57. Manis T, Zeig S, Lum GY, Friedman EA: Oral sorbents in uremia and diabetes: Charcoal-induced hypolipidemia. *Trans Am Soc Artif Intern Organs* 25:19, 1979
58. Manis T, Deutsch J, Feinstein EI, Lum GY, Friedman EA: Charcoal sorbent-induced hypolipidemia in uremia and diabetes. *Am J Clin Nutr* 33:1485, 1980
59. Manis T and Deutsch J: Hypolipidemic effect of activated charcoal. *Proc 8th Int Congr Nephrol* (Athens) edited by Zurukzoglu W, Papadimitriou M, Pyrpasopoulos M, Sion M, Zamboulis C, Basel, S Karger, 1981, p 422

19
URAEMIC TOXINS

JONAS BERGSTRÖM and PETER FÜRST

Introduction	354
Clinical signs of uraemic toxicity	354
The effect of various therapeutic modalities on toxic uraemic manifestations	355
In vitro effects of uraemic plasma	355
Toxicity of inorganic substances in uraemia	356
Water	356
Sodium	356
Potassium	356
Hydrogen ions	357
Magnesium	358
Phosphate	358
Sulphate	358
Trace elements	358
Toxicity of organic substances in uraemia	358
Urea	359
Creatinine	361
Guanidines	361
Methylguanidine	361
Guanidinosuccinic acid (GSA)	362
Other guanidines	362
Products of nucleic acid metabolism	363
Uric acid	363
Cyclic AMP	363
Pyridine derivatives	363
Amino acids and dipeptides	363
Amines	364
Aliphatic amines	364
Aromatic amines	365
Polyamines	365
Indoles	366
Phenols	366
Carbohydrate-derivatives	367
Myoinositol	367
Mannitol and sorbitol	367
Glucuronic acid and other compounds	367
Other metabolites	367
Middle molecules	368
The Middle Molecule Hypothesis	368
Isolation and characterisation of middle molecule substances	368
Accumulation and elimination of middle molecules	370
Toxicity of middle molecules	371
Lipochromes	372
The trade-off hypothesis	372
Parathyroid hormone (PTH)	372
Natriuretic hormone	373
Larger polypeptides, proteins, and other high-molecular weight compounds	373
Conclusions	374
Acknowledgements	374
References	374

INTRODUCTION

The chemical theory of the pathogenesis of the uraemic syndrome begins with Prévost and Dumas (1), who discovered in 1821 that removal of the kidneys leads to a rise in blood urea concentration. Since that time it has been assumed that the clinical features of uraemia are caused by retention of toxic substances in the body fluids which are normally excreted in the urine. With refinement of analytical techniques, an ever increasing number of substances have been found with elevated concentrations in uraemic plasma and many have been classified as an uraemic toxin or even *the* uraemic toxin. However, despite more than 150 years of research, it has not been possible to explain all uraemic toxic manifestations by accumulation of known compounds. Accordingly, the search for uraemic toxins continues.

It is now recognised that the functions of kidneys are not limited to the excretion of waste metabolites, electrolytes and water. We are increasingly aware of the importance of the kidneys for calcium homeostasis and as endocrine organs affecting blood pressure regulation and erythropoiesis. It is also established that the kidneys catabolise a number of peptide hormones (see Chapter 36). Accordingly, some of the symptoms and signs of uraemia may be due to endocrine disturbances, either of renoprival origin or secondary to impaired homeostasis. It may be impossible to separate such disturbances from direct effects of toxic compounds retained as a consequence of reduced renal function.

CLINICAL SIGNS OF URAEMIC TOXICITY

The clinical syndrome of uraemia is too well known to require more than a cursory description. Particularly striking are the neurological signs (see Chapter 37) and symptoms including mental changes, fatigue, muscle twitching, stupor, convulsions and coma. Symptomatic peripheral neuropathy is not uncommon, especially in patients treated with regular dialysis. The gastrointestinal symptoms such as anorexia, hiccup and vomiting (one of the earliest manifestations of uraemia), may be associated with stomatitis, glossitis, gastritis, pancreatitis and enterocolitis. Cardiovascular symptoms are also common, including those of heart failure, hypertension (disorders closely connected with salt and water retention), hyperkalaemia, pericarditis, myocarditis and atherosclerosis (see Chapters 28, 30, 31). Decreased production and increased destruction of red cells result in anaemia. Impaired haemostasis leads to bleeding from the mucous membranes and in the skin (caused by a defect in platelet aggregation). Fibrinolysis is inhibited as well (Chapters 9, 10 and 32). Pruritus and hyperpigmentation of the skin in chronic uraemia are also frequently encountered. Those who wish to pursue this subject further are referred to current textbooks and, in particular, to the monograph by Schreiner and Maher (2).

The immunological response is impaired in uraemic patients and the susceptibility to infections may be increased (see Chapter 33). Disturbances in calcium and phosphorus metabolism give rise to uraemic osteodystrophy (see Chapter 35) causing conditions such as osteomalacia, osteosclerosis, osteitis fibrosa with bone pain, fractures and, in children, retardation of growth (see Chapter 25).

A number of changes in intermediary metabolism are also encountered in uraemic patients, including abnormalities in lipid (see Chapter 29), carbohydrate (see Chapter 36) and protein metabolism (see Chapter 27).

It has been observed that certain cell membrane transport phenomena are abnormal in uraemia. The active sodium efflux is inhibited in uraemic red (3) and white blood cells (4). The transmembrane potential of skeletal muscle cells is decreased in patients with severe uraemia (5-7), signifying inhibition of the electrogenic sodium pump or increased membrane permeability for sodium. This abnormality is reversed by adequate dialysis (8). The 'sick cell syndrome' is not specific for uraemia for it is also observed in patients with other severe debilitating illnesses (6, 9).

In summary, uraemia seems to affect practically all organs and tissues of the body; mucous and serous membranes are affected, various transport phenomena in the cell membranes are inhibited and intermediary metabolic processes are impaired.

THE EFFECT OF VARIOUS THERAPEUTIC MODALITIES ON TOXIC URAEMIC MANIFESTATIONS

It has been known for some time that the clinical syndrome of uraemia, be it acute or chronic, is reversible. The evidence for this is based on observations that patients in renal failure can be kept alive and asymptomatic for years by means of intermittent haemodialysis. Daily prophylactic dialysis is also known to prevent the appearance of toxic symptoms in patients with acute renal failure (10). These results imply that dialysis leads to the removal of diffusible substances which, when present in raised concentrations in the tissue fluids of the body, produce the clinical syndrome of uraemia.

It is also well known that a protein-poor diet lessens uraemic signs and symptoms, especially gastrointestinal symptoms, as it reduces blood urea concentration. From this observation it can be concluded that at least some of the uraemic toxins are products of protein catabolism.

The bacterial flora of the gut appears to be involved in the pathogenesis of uraemic toxicity. It has been shown that germ-free rats with acute uraemia survive longer than those with normal intestinal flora (11, 12). A toxic role by the bacterial flora in the gut is further supported from observations that severely uraemic patients showed marked clinical improvement of asterixis, myoclonus and mental alertness following 'sterilisation' of the bowel with broad-spectrum antibiotics (13). Abnormal colonisation of the small intestine by both anaerobic and aerobic bacteria was recently reported (14). In fact, several metabolites retained in uraemic plasma arise from bacterial activity in the intestinal tract (*vide infra*).

IN VITRO EFFECTS OF URAEMIC PLASMA

Indirect evidence of uraemic toxicity has been obtained from many bioassay studies *in vitro*, which showed that plasma, serum, ultrafiltrate and dialysate from uraemic patients affect numerous biological processes. Toxic changes have been obtained in HeLa cells (15, 16). Calcification of rachitic cartilage is inhibited (17, 18). Uraemic sera also inhibit *in vitro* erythropoiesis (19-30), fibroblast growth (31, 32), lymphocyte transformation (33-37), mononuclear phagocytes (38) and platelet functions (39). Moreover autohaemolysis of normal red cells and proteolytic activity may be enhanced in the presence of uraemic serum (40, 41).

A variety of metabolic processes *in vitro* are impaired in the presence of uraemic serum; glucose utilisation and glycolysis are inhibited (42, 43) and gluconeogenesis is enhanced (liver) or inhibited (liver, brain tissue) (44-46). There is also inhibition of protein synthesis, mitochondrial metabolism, uncoupling of phosphorylation (47-50), inhibition of fibrinolysis (51) and lipolysis (52).

Several transmembrane transport systems in a variety of cells are also inhibited *in vitro* in the presence of uraemic serum or ultrafiltrate. These include transport of sodium in cell membranes (53-57), calcium in mitochondria (58), phosphate in red cells (59), uric acid in liver slices (60, 61), hippuric acid derivatives in kidney and liver tissue (62-66), amino acids in muscle (67) and folates in the Ehrlich ascites tumour cell (68).

In vitro inhibition of several enzymes by uraemic serum has also been reported. Among these are lactic dehydrogenase (69, 70), lipoprotein lipase (52, 71, 72), xanthine oxidase (61), phenylalanine hydroxylase (73), ATPase in brain and red cells (74, 75), thymidine kinase in lymphocytes (76), thiopurine methyltransferase (77), and transketolase in red cells (78-81) and nervous tissue (82) (but no inhibition was found in erythrocytes by other investigators [83]). Transketolase inhibiton has been suggested to play a role in peripheral neuropathy of uraemia. However, transketolase activity in liver, brain and erythrocytes of uraemic rats is not different from normals (84). The effects of uremic serum on transmembrane transport mechanisms and transport enzymes

(ATPase) are of special interest in view of Bricker's (85) hypothesis that a humoral factor, produced as a result of homeostatic adaptation to sodium retention and which decreases tubular sodium reabsorption, might be important in uraemia by inhibiting transmembrane transport in other cells as well.

In conclusion, there is evidence that a variety of clinical disturbances, such as anaemia, immunological deficiency, bleeding tendency, disorders of carbohydrate and lipid metabolism, may be related to toxins or inhibitors present in plasma or other body fluids in uraemic patients.

TOXICITY OF INORGANIC SUBSTANCES IN URAEMIA

Homeostatic control of water, inorganic ion and acid-base balance is mainly accomplished by the kidneys. When renal function deteriorates the kidneys are unable to exert full homeostatic control, resulting in disturbances in water and electrolyte metabolism. This is especially evident in patients with acute renal failure, who are anuric or oliguric, and also in the terminal stage of chronic uraemia. Some disturbances may also be present in patients with mild or moderate chronic renal failure. Water and electrolyte abnormalities contribute to the toxic symptomatology in the majority of uraemic patients and, if left unattended, may lead to a fatal outcome. With the advent of improved diagnostic methods, a better understanding of the principles of fluid and electrolyte balance and more effective therapeutic regimens (ion exchange resins, diuretics, dialysis), the problems of water and electrolyte disturbances in uraemia can be mastered to the extent that they only rarely cause death.

The abnormalities of water and electrolyte metabolism in uraemia will be briefly reviewed with emphasis on toxic effects. However, it is beyond the scope of this chapter to give a complete review of the subject. Those interested are referred to current textbooks of renal disease and of the physiology and pathology of fluid and electrolyte metabolism.

Water

Water overload may be either approximately isotonic, as in most oedematous conditions, or hypotonic, as in water intoxication. Since osmolality is not a reliable measure of tonicity in the uraemic patient, due to the high concentration of urea in the body fluids (urea being distributed approximately equally between the extra- and intra-cellular fluid), the best indication of water excess is a low plasma sodium concentration. A patient with acute renal failure is especially prone to develop water intoxication due to excessive water intake, either by inappropriate thirst or by iatrogenic infusion of an excess of electrolyte-poor solutions or both. Water excess in patients with renal failure may produce oedema and heart failure. More typically a variety of signs and symptoms such as mental confusion, restlessness, twitching, muscle cramps, convulsions and coma may occur. These are probably related to osmotic water transport into the central nervous system (86). In patients with chronic renal failure slight asymptomatic hyponatraemia is commonly encountered. Schreiner and Maher (2) list water intoxication among the conditions that mimic uraemia, considering that it can be avoided by better care of the patient.

Sodium

Patients with acute anuria or with terminal chronic uraemia cannot excrete a sodium load. Hence, inadequate excretion of administered sodium may give rise to hypertension, pulmonary oedema, heart failure and peripheral oedema.

Patients with chronic renal failure can usually maintain a satisfactory sodium homeostasis as fractional sodium reabsorption is decreased in surviving nephrons. This partially compensates for the decrease in glomerular filtration of sodium (85, 87, 88). The ability of the residual nephrons to adapt the sodium reabsorption to changes in sodium intake exceeds the ability of the normal nephron. This 'magnification phenomenon' in chronic renal disease implies that the excretory response per nephron to a change in sodium intake varies inversely with the number of surviving nephrons (89). However, the overall ability to adapt sodium excretion to a change in sodium load is limited, and sodium retention is frequently encountered in advanced chronic renal failure. Other patients may be 'salt losing' and may require sodium supplements to maintain the extracellular fluid volume.

Recently it has been shown that sodium vanadate is an inhibitor of Na^+, K^+-activated adenosine triphosphatase with a strong natriuretic effect (90). Serum vanadium levels are elevated in patients with chronic uraemia and it has been suggested that vanadium, which is a naturally occurring trace element, acts as a potential natriuretic material present in the plasma of patients with chronic renal failure (91). It has been suggested that the adaptation of fractional sodium reabsorption in chronic uraemia involves increased secretion of a natriuretic hormone, which may cause toxicity by inhibiting solute transport in the body cells (85), and that end organ responsiveness of the uraemic kidney to the natriuretic factor is enhanced (92).

Studies of total body exchangeable sodium (93, 94) did show an increase in oedematous uraemic patients, and in patients with terminal chronic uraemia. Muscle sodium has also been found to be increased in patients with acute and chronic renal failure (7, 95–99) and a high intra-cellular sodium concentration in muscle (6, 7), in red cells (3, 53) and in white cells (100) has been demonstrated.

Potassium

In renal insufficiency, failure to excrete potassium may result in hyperkalaemia, caused by oral intake or parenteral administration of potassium, or following release of

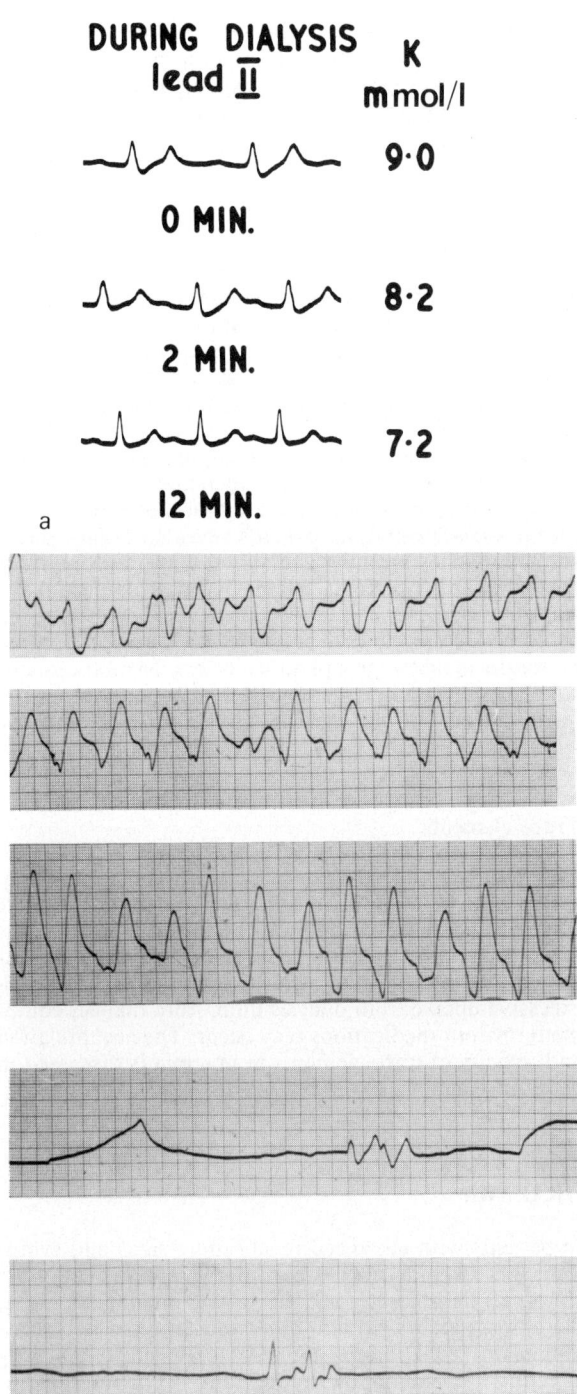

Figure 1. (a) Correction of hyperkalaemic ECG changes during haemodialysis (lead II).
(b) ECG during terminal hyperkalaemia, not corrected by haemodialysis ('dying heart' [plasma K 9.1 mmol/l]).

potassium from the tissues during endogenous catabolism. The risk of potassium intoxication is particularly high in patients with acute post-traumatic renal failure and with rapid tissue breakdown (101). Metabolic acidosis potentiates hyperkalaemia because potassium moves out of the cells as pH decreases (95, 102, 103). The inhibition of ion tansport and decrease in transmembrane potential found in uraemic and other severely ill patients (3, 5, 6) may also contribute to a rise in extracellular potassium concentration. The breakdown of liver and muscle glycogen also results in the release of potassium by the cells (104, 105).

Progressive hyperkalaemia is attended by neuromuscular and cardiovascular disturbances, ultimately leading to cardiac arrest or ventricular fibrillation. Typical ECG changes of hyperkalaemia are shown in Figures 1a and 1b.

There is ample evidence that the length of survival of a laboratory animal (e.g. the dog) following bilateral nephrectomy or ligation of both ureters is directly related to the extra-cellular potassium concentration (2). It is also interesting to note that experiments with the isolated frog heart and with mice *in vivo* indicated that the toxic action of potassium chloride was potentiated by urea (106, 107). Low potassium concentrations in muscle have been found in acute renal failure (108, 109).

Unlike the situation in acute renal failure, the patient with relatively stable chronic uraemia has a normal or only slightly raised plasma potassium concentration. To achieve normal elimination the potassium excretion per nephron in chronic uraemia must increase. This largely depends on increased tubular potassium secretion in the residual functioning nephrons (110). Increased faecal excretion of potassium also helps to maintain plasma potassium concentrations in these patients (111). However, potassium loading results in hyperkalaemia on account of the in toto reduced ability of the diseased kidney to excrete potassium (112). Muscle potassium in chronic renal failure has been found reduced (7, 113), normal (6, 97) or increased (95, 98, 99, 108, 109). According to our experience with more than 200 muscle biopsies in chronic renal failure, intracellular potassium depletion in muscle is exceptional and not a characteristic feature of chronic uraemia.

Hydrogen ions

Present views of hydrogen ion metabolism and excretion and of metabolic acidosis in uraemia have been published earlier (114, 115). Severe and prolonged metabolic acidosis results in major disturbances of a number of fundamental metabolic and physiological processes, causing central nervous system disorders, hyperventilation, hyperkalaemia, abnormalities in energy metabolism and bone mineral metabolism and other disorders.

It is now generally accepted that the hydrogen ions produced by body metabolism are buffered mainly by bicarbonate and that the kidney repletes the bicarbonate stores by tubular excretion of hydrogen ions. The widely held view is that hydrogen ions are released by oxidation of sulphur-containing amino acids, chiefly cystine and methionine, and incomplete oxidation of carbohydrates and lipids, as well as by hydrolysis of certain phospho-esters. The metabolic acidosis occurring in patients with renal failure results from the inability to excrete the amount of normally produced hydrogen ions (116). The turnover rate of hydrogen ion in a normal adult of average size is approximately 60 mmol/24 h (117). The reduced ability of the chronically diseased kidney to excrete acid is closely linked with a decreased excretion of ammonia (118, 119), in spite of increased ammonia production by each of the surviving nephrons (120, 121). Impaired renal bicarbonate reabsorption is also observed in many patients with chronic uraemia (122). It has been reported that parathyroid hormone (PTH) may play a pathogenic role in renal acidosis by impairing the ability of the kidney to eliminate fixed acids (123, 124).

There are uraemic patients whose plasma bicarbonate level remains unaltered in the presence of a positive hydrogen ion balance (125). This observation was explained by a buffering action of the skeleton in these patients. Indirect evidence favouring such a concept is also derived from the observations that in normal subjects given ammonium chloride and in patients with renal acidosis a negative calcium balance occurs (126-128). The role of acidosis in renal osteodystrophy is discussed in more detail in Chapter 35.

In patients with uraemic acidosis intracellular pH was found to be normal in skeletal muscle (128) and slightly increased in leucocytes (129).

Uraemic acidosis can be partly or fully corrected by dialysis which provides an excess of bicarbonate, acetate or lactate anions in the dialysis fluid, lactate and acetate being quantitatively metabolised to bicarbonate.

Magnesium

It is well established that the serum magnesium concentration is raised in most patients with severe renal insufficiency (130; see also 131-133). Toxic manifestations in uraemic patients, caused by magnesium administration, have been described (134).

Magnesium metabolism in chronic renal failure is discussed in Chapters 7, 35 and 49.

Phosphate

Phosphate is known to accumulate in patients with renal insufficiency. The plasma concentration rises when the glomerular filtration rate falls below 25% of normal (135).

The role of phosphate retention in causing increased parathyroid activity early in the course of renal failure and its contribution to various clinical and biochemical abnormalities observed in uraemic patients is reviewed in Chapter 35.

A high inorganic phosphate concentration in plasma carries the risk of calcium phosphate deposits in organs and tissues (136). Restriction of phosphate prevents deterioration of renal function in the remnant kidney model of chronic renal failure in the rat presumably by prevention of renal calcification (137) and has also a preservative effect in experimental glomerulonephritis (138). Phosphate restriction with decrease in plasma inorganic phosphate was suggested as an explanation why low protein diets may prevent the progression of deterioration of renal function in patients with chronic renal failure (139-141).

Sulphate

Inorganic sulphate excreted by the kidneys is derived mostly from oxidation of sulphur containing amino acids. The plasma concentration of sulphate is increased in uraemia proportional to acidosis, creatinine and inorganic phosphate concentrations and, inversely proportional, to the glomerular filtration rate (142-144). There is, however, little evidence that sulphate per se is toxic; when sulphate concentration increases it partly 'replaces' the chloride ion in the extracellular fluid (2). A recent study in dialysis patients revealed higher serum sulphate values in patients dialysed with the Redy-Sorb System than in patients treated with single-pass dialysis (145; see also Chapter 17). However, no toxic effects could be ascribed to high sulphate levels except for a rise in serum alkaline phosphatase. It has been speculated whether sulphate may be involved in the pathogenesis of renal osteodystrophy possibly by complex formation with calcium in the gut or in plasma (144).

Trace elements

Heavy metals and other trace elements are normal constituents of food and drinking water. Some of them are essential to man but some can be harmful. In uraemic patients accumulation of these elements has to be expected, because of reduced renal excretion. In addition, excessive uptake from dialysis fluid, from dialysis equipment or from medications may occur. The accumulation and toxicity of trace elements in uraemia is discussed in detail in Chapters 6, 41 and 42.

TOXICITY OF ORGANIC SUBSTANCES IN URAEMIA

In patients with advanced renal failure signs and symptoms of uraemia may occur in the absence of gross abnormalities of water and electrolyte metabolism. It is, therefore, widely held that other substances which accumulate in renal failure are also toxic, presumably by affecting transmembrane solute transport or intermediary metabolism. Numerous organic compounds accumulate in the body fluids of uraemic patients; the most important are listed in Table 1.

Correlations have been sought between the appearance of certain uraemic signs and the concentration of one or more particular substances in plasma. However, such correlations, if found, are no proof that one specific substance is responsible since a great number of substances excreted by the kidneys accumulate simultaneously as renal function deteriorates. Therefore, other criteria

Table 1. Organic compounds which accumulate in uraemia.

urea	acetoin
creatinine	2,3-butylene glycol
methylguanidine	middle molecules
guanidinosuccinic acid	lipochromes
other guanidines	insulin
uric acid	glucagon
cyclic AMP	parathyroid hormone
pyridine derivatives	natriuretic hormone (?)
amino acids	growth hormone
aliphatic amines	gastrin
aromatic amines	renin
polyamines	calcitonin
indoles	prolactin
phenols	β_2-microglobulin
myoinositol	lysozyme
mannitol	retinol-binding protein
glucuronic acid	β_2-glucoprotein
oxalic acid	ribonuclease

have been sought and toxicity tests have been performed. Substances known to be present in raised concentration in patients with uraemic signs and symptoms have been given either to experimental animals, or added to various tissues, cells or enzymes *in vitro* and toxic effects were observed. Many of these experiments are open to criticism since the concentrations used were often much higher than those encountered in the blood of uraemic patients.

Another criticism of the *in vitro* experiments is that they reflect only acute toxicity and, therefore, will be inadequate for assessing chronic toxicity, which occurs in uraemia. Even when investigations are performed correctly, with the compound present in concentrations comparable to those found in uraemic patients, it may be doubtful if these *in vitro* effects relate to *in vivo* toxicity.

Clinically there is a possibility that a number of compounds, each of which present in a concentration too low to be toxic, may act synergistically, to produce toxic effects. Mutual potentiation of inhibition of respiration of cerebral slices has been observed by combinations of metabolites (urea, magnesium, acetoin, 2,3-butylene-glycol, sulphate, creatinine, creatine, p-cresol and guanidine), each metabolite being present in a concentration not being inhibitory per se (146). However, no effect of ultrafiltrates of serum from patients with uraemic coma could be demonstrated. Combinations of metabolites (urea, creatinine, guanidino-succinic acid and methylguanidine) caused depressions in cardiac output and myocardial oxygen extraction in the isolated perfused heart, which could not be obtained with each of the compounds alone (147).

A solute could be considered as a uraemic toxin if it fulfils certain criteria:
1. The compound should be chemically identified. Specific and accurate quantitative analysis in biological fluids should be possible.
2. The plasma level and/or tissue concentrations of the compound should be higher in uraemic than in non-uraemic patients.
3. High concentrations should be related to specific uraemic symptoms which disappear when the concentration is reduced.
4. Toxic effects should be obtained in human subjects, experimental animals and/or in an appropriate *in vitro* system at concentrations comparable to those found in the body fluids of uraemic patients.

A survey follows of organic compounds known to accumulate in uraemic body fluids and toxic effects observed *in vitro* and *in vivo* will be described. The earlier literature on this subject has been extensively reviewed elsewhere (2, 108).

Urea

Urea is quantitatively the most important end product of nitrogen metabolism in mammals and accounts for about 85% of the urinary nitrogen excretion. The urea concentration increases in the body fluids when renal function deteriorates. The blood concentration of urea is, however, also dependent on the nitrogen intake and the balance between endogenous protein synthesis and breakdown. Thus, in conditions of hypercatabolism, e.g. after severe trauma and in sepsis, the urea production rate is grossly increased.

Urea is synthesised in the liver by the Krebs-Henseleit cycle. Several studies suggest that urea synthesis is increased in acute experimental uraemia (148–153) and that the activity of the urea cycle enzymes is increased in this condition (154). There is evidence that urea is decomposed to ammonia in the gastro-intestinal tract by bacteria containing urease (155–157). The ammonia thus formed is mainly converted to urea in the liver but some may also be utilised for synthesis of non-essential amino acids, provided that the nitrogen intake is low and the requirement of essential amino acids is fulfilled (158).

The intestinal breakdown of urea is, however, only slightly increased in uraemia, in spite of the high urea concentration in the body fluids (159), and the contribution of urea as a non-essential nitrogen source for protein synthesis is probably minimal even under optimal conditions.

Soon after the discovery that removal of the kidneys of dogs led to a rise in the blood urea concentration (1), it was recognised that in patients with Bright's disease 'urea exists in considerable quantity in the blood, when it is materially defective in the urine' (160, 161). It should be mentioned that in 1831 Richard Bright (162) had questioned the role of urea as a uraemic toxin. Evidence implicating urea as the toxic substance in uraemia was brought forward by a number of investigators who administered urea to experimental animals or to normal subjects (2). However, there are several objections to these experiments, the main one being that it may not be possible to distinguish toxic effects of urea per se from side effects such as dehydration, osmotic diuresis or water shifts between extra- and intracellular fluid. In fact, one of the earlier investigators (163) found that the toxic effect of a concentrated urea solution was similar to the effect of an equal volume of distilled water. Much of the early literature, however (2), is confusing and conflicting and does not contribute to any definite conclusion.

More relevant were the clinical experiments where urea was added to dialysis fluid. Nephrectomised dogs maintained by peritoneal dialysis developed toxic symptoms (vomiting, diarrhoea, intestinal haemorrhage and coma) when the blood urea concentration was 370 to 480 mg/dl (62 to 80 mmol/l) (164). However, dogs whose ureters had been transplanted into the ileum remained virtually free of toxic symptoms, even when the blood urea concentration rose to 800 mg/dl (133 mmol/l) (165). Dogs subjected to peritoneal dialysis against high concentrations of urea (1 g/dl [167 mmol/l]) or potassium isocyanate (15 mg/dl [1,9 mmol/l]) in the dialysis fluid showed shortened survival compared with dogs dialysed without these additions (166). The authors speculated whether isocyanate, which may be derived spontaneously from urea, may contribute to the uraemic syndrome by carbamoylation reactions with free amino acids and proteins. In fact there are recent observations that haemoglobin carbamoylation with increase in HbA_1 results from a condensation of urea-derived cyanate with the N-terminal amino group (167). There is also a possibility that decreased drug binding to albumin in uraemia may be due to carbamylation of albumin by cyanate (168). However, direct measurements of cyanide and thiocyanate in blood of normals and uraemic patients did not show any differences (169). Paradoxically the cognitive behaviour of dialysed uraemic rats improved when urea had been added to the dialysis fluid, suggesting that urea played no major role in impairment of mental function in uraemia (170).

Survival of bilaterally nephrectomised dogs could be prolonged threefold by reducing urea formation through inhibition of arginase by infusion of L-lysine (171). Both groups of animals died at the same blood urea concentrations. The therapeutic implications of these important observations await further elucidation.

Patients with acute renal failure dialysed against a solution containing sufficient urea to prevent a change in the plasma urea concentration, showed the same degree of clinical improvement in the uraemic syndrome during dialysis as patients in whom urea was removed (172). Chronic uraemic patients treated with haemodialysis improved despite maintaining the plasma urea concentration in the range 200 to 300 mg/dl [(33 to 50 mmol/l]) but the haemorrhagic diathesis persisted. At higher concentrations, however, toxic symptoms occurred such as headache, vomiting and fatigue (173). In similar experiments in patients with chronic renal failure high concentrations of urea in the blood were associated with malaise, lethargy, pruritus, headache, vomiting and bleeding tendencies (174). In these patients the lowest plasma concentrations of urea, at which symptoms began to appear, were 200 to 300 mg/dl (33 to 50 mmol/l). When urea loading was stopped, headache and vomiting subsided quickly. Furthermore, addition of urea to the dialysis fluid in uraemic subjects caused glucose intolerance (175).

Numerous *in vitro* studies have been performed using different test systems and media containing high concentrations of urea. A number of enzyme systems are inhibited by urea but only at concentrations that are much higher than those occurring in uraemic patients (176). Urea reduced the rate of oxygen consumption of brain tissue homogenate (177), and also inhibited the activity of kidney tissue mono-amino-oxidase (178) and serum lactate dehydrogenase (179). Urea also appears to be a selective inhibitor of argininosuccinate lyase at physiological levels and it was suggested that urea may exert regulatory control of its own production (180). However, as pointed out earlier, urea generation seems to be increased and not decreased in uraemia (148–154). According to several investigators the glucose uptake by the rat diaphragm and by red cells (*in vitro*) was inhibited (181–183); however, another group of investigators found no effect (184). Urea seems to have an effect on tissue respiration *in vitro* (brain and liver slices) at concentrations found in uraemic patients (146). However, no correlation was found between the accumulation of urea and the degree of mitochondrial respiratory inhibition in the liver of the uraemic rat (185). It has also been found that urea, at concentrations present in uraemic patients, inhibited protein synthesis in stimulated lymphocytes (186). An unexplained finding was that urea makes cell membranes more permeable to dyes and possibly to toxins (187). Interestingly, experiments with the isolated frog heart and with mice *in vivo* demonstrated that the toxic action of potassium chloride is potentiated by urea (106, 107). Inhibition of platelet aggregation by urea in concentrations of 100 to 300 mg/dl (17 to 50 mmol/l) has been observed (188) but, according to Somer et al. (189), urea alone cannot be held responsible for platelet abnormalities in uraemia.

In concentrations of 120, 60 and 15 mg/dl (20, 10 and 2,5 mmol/l) urea decreased the cardiac output response to increasing arterial pressure in the perfused isolated rat heart and this effect was potentiated by creatinine, guanidino-succinic acid and methylguanidine (147). In the isolated guinea pig heart, urea, in concentrations of 60 to 600 mg/dl (10 to 100 mmol/l), reduced contractility and increased oxygen consumption (190). However, no effect was seen on energy metabolism in the perfused isolated rat heart (191). It has also been reported that urea (but not creatinine, guanidines and phenolic acids) *in vitro* inhibits the aminopyrine demethylating system (192) and, therefore, may interfere with the metabolism of drugs. Bromosulfophthalein clearance by the isolated perfused rat liver was not changed by urea in the perfusate, indicating that urea has little or no effect on liver function on an acute basis (193).

In conclusion, there is overwhelming evidence that urea exerts toxic effects. Clinically high concentrations may induce headache, fatigue, nausea, vomiting, glucose intolerance and bleeding tendency. In addition, urea is one of the few substances which exerts *in vitro* toxic effects at concentrations found in the blood of uraemic patients. However, it should be emphasised that the most severe uraemic gastrointestinal, cardiovascular, mental and neurological changes were not observed in patients dialysed against high urea concentrations (172). Obviously it is not possible to explain the wide spectrum of uraemic symptoms and signs by urea intoxication only. Urea should be considered a 'mild' uraemic toxin.

Creatinine

Creatinine, which is formed from creatine phosphate mainly in skeletal musculature, is the major guanidine compound retained in patients with diminished glomerular filtration rate. Creatinine is routinely determined in plasma or serum as a measure of impairment of renal function and it might be expected that a variety of uraemic symptoms correlate with the plasma creatinine level; this does not, however, necessarily imply a causal but rather an effective relationship. In fact, creatinine seems to be relatively non-toxic. Large amounts of creatinine have been fed to healthy subjects without any adverse effects (194, 195) and animals also tolerate large doses (196). Enhanced in vitro haemolysis has been reported after ingestion of creatinine by normal man or when creatinine was added to normal blood in vitro (197). However, other investigators could not confirm these findings (198, 199). It was also found that ingestion of 30 to 40 g/day (266 to 354 mmol) of creatinine impairs glucose tolerance (183). In general, toxic effects in vitro on incubation in a medium containing creatinine have only been observed at concentrations much higher than those found in uraemic patients. It has been reported that creatinine inhibits glucose uptake by the rat diaphragm and human red cells (183) and inhibits oxygen uptake by cerebral slices (146). Creatinine was reported to inhibit red cell proliferation and maturation at concentrations found in uraemia (27); this was, however, not confirmed in another study (200).

There is a possibility that metabolites of creatinine formed by bacteria in the gut might be absorbed, accumulating in the body fluids of uraemic patients (201). In patients with decreased renal function extrarenal clearance is increased (202, 203). A larger quantity of creatinine is excreted into the gut and metabolised than in normal subjects (204) which may account for the fact that a portion of endogenously formed creatinine is not found in either the urine or as an increased body pool. The following metabolites have been identified: 1-methylhydantoin, creatine, sarcosine, mono-methylamine and glyoxylate-glycolate (205). There is also evidence that methylguanidine can be formed from creatinine (206, 207). There is no evidence that methylhydantoin, sarcosine and glyoxylate-glycolate have any toxic effects in uraemia. Both creatine and phosphocreatine have been reported to be elevated in the blood of patients with renal failure (208-211) but there is no evidence of toxicity of these substances. Mono-methylamine and methylguanidine both seem to be toxic in uraemia (vide infra).

Guanidines

Guanidines in high concentrations inhibit a wide variety of enzymes of biological interest (212). Guanidine derivatives are potent inhibitors of mitochondrial respiration in vitro (213) and, if albumin is added to the suspending medium, mitochondria from guinea pig skeletal muscle become many times more sensitive to inhibition by guanidine (214). Guanidines also interfere with mitochondrial calcium transport (215).

The early literature on guanidines in uraemia has been extensively reviewed by Schreiner and Maher (2). The first evidence of accumulation of guanidines (other than creatinine) in uraemia came in 1915, when Foster (216-218) extracted a toxic base from uraemic blood which, when injected into guinea pigs, caused dyspnoea, convulsions, coma and death. Subsequently, this material has been identified as guanidine (219). Later, numerous studies confirmed that guanidine or guanidine-like compounds are elevated in uraemia and hypertension (220-227). However, these early studies are difficult to evaluate due to the use of imprecise and unspecific methods of determination. Injection or infusion of guanidine in experimental animals produced severe toxic symptoms mimicking those of uraemic toxicity (228-230).

Methylguanidine

For 15 years investigators have been interested in the role of methylguanidine (MG) as a uraemic toxin. MG is provided by a diet rich in broth or in boiled beef, which contain large amounts of MG formed from the oxidation of creatinine during boiling (207). Endogenous production of MG occurs by conversion from creatinine (201, 206, 207, 231) and from arginine (231). From studies with germ-free rats, or rats treated with antibiotics, it became apparent that the gut bacterial flora plays no role in the conversion of creatinine to methylguanidine (206), and a non-enzymatic conversion has been suggested (207). Low protein diet and essential amino acid supply decrease the serum concentration and urinary excretion of methylguanidine in chronic renal failure (232) presumably due to decreased turnover of arginine. The increase in urinary excretion of MG in uraemia is related to the plasma creatinine concentration (233-235), which suggests increased production (236). For many years plasma concentrations of MG were found to be high in uraemic patients (237). However, the analytical methods, used were inaccurate, giving too high values (226, 238) as MG was formed from creatinine during the analytical procedure (239).

More recently specific methods for determination of MG and other guanidines became available using liquid ion-exchange chromatography (233, 235, 240-243). It was found that in most uraemic patients MG levels in plasma were below 0.2 mg/dl (2.7 µmol/l). By using a more sensitive specific technique (ion pair extraction and partition chromatography for determination of MG) we confirmed that the plasma concentration of MG in uraemic patients was usually below 0.2 mg/dl (244) and that there was also a good correlation between the MG and creatinine concentration in plasma. There is evidence from tissue determinations in experimental animals, from observations in postdialysis rebound and from injections of labelled MG, that MG, which is a strongly basic compound, accumulates preferentially in the intracellular fluid compartment (234, 236, 245-247).

A ten-fold increased concentration of MG in adrenal cortex and coeliac ganglion was found in cats injected with labelled MG (246). It has been suggested that toxic effects may be obtained in spite of relatively low plasma concentrations because the toxicity might be exerted within the cells where the concentrations are much higher (234). MG, which has not been detected in normal cerebrospinal fluid, was found to be present in the cerebrospinal fluid from patients with chronic uraemia. Rabbits with acute renal failure showed grossly elevated levels in cerebrospinal fluid (248).

Infusion of MG into dogs caused a syndrome resembling uraemia with anorexia, vomiting, diarrhoea, pruritus, anaemia, altered glucose tolerance, high plasma fibrinogen levels, reduced fibrinolytic activity, defective calcium absorption, stomach and duodenal ulceration, haemorrhage, convulsions and semi-coma (181, 182, 247). Intravenous injections of MG in rats caused a marked increase of urinary sodium excretion (249, 250). Salivary flow was markedly reduced in cats infused with MG (251) and external pancreatic secretion was reversibly inhibited in the isolated perfused pancreas (252). It should be pointed out that the these toxic effects in experimental animals have been obtained with plasma concentrations of MG considerably higher than found in uraemic patients.

Several *in vitro* effects of high MG concentrations have been described including autohaemolysis of red cells (197, which has not been confirmed by other investigators [198, 253]), enhancement of glucose utilisation in the rat diaphragm and human erythrocytes (183), inhibition of lymphocyte DNA synthesis (254), erythrocyte globin synthesis (255), inhibition of pancreatic Na^+-K^+-ATPase, Mg^{++}-ATPase and Ca^{++}-ATPase (252) and noradrenaline transport in sympathetic nerve synoptic vesicles (246). However, the concentrations of MG used were considerably higher than those found in uraemic sera. It has been suggested that MG might play a role in the sympathetic neuropathy of uraemia (246).

At concentrations found *in vivo* in uraemia, inhibition was observed of ^{59}Fe uptake by bone marrow cultures (27) and of diamine oxidase (histaminase) activity in serum (256). Energy production and utilisation by human platelets (257) and transepithelial sodium transport (258) were not impaired and erythrocyte cation content or transport were also not affected by high concentrations of MG (253).

Guanidinosuccinic acid (GSA)
GSA appears in much higher concentrations both in the plasma and urine of uraemic patients than in normal plasma and urine, suggesting increased production (259–263). Surprisingly the GSA concentration was found to be higher in patients dialysed three times a week than in patients dialysed twice a week (264). Low protein diet and essential amino acids diminished the serum concentration and urinary excretion of guanidinosuccinic acid in chronic renal failure (232). The metabolic pathway of the biosynthesis of this compound has been investigated with the perfused rat liver model (263). It appeared that GSA is formed in the liver by transamidation of arginine to aspartic acid. This is in agreement with the concept that a rise in plasma concentration of creatine and guanidinoacetic acid (GAA, both are elevated in renal failure) leads to suppression of glycine amidinotransferase, resulting in a decrease of GAA formation and the transfer of the amidino group of arginine to aspartic acid (261). These studies do not support the theory that GSA is formed from canavaninosuccinic acid (265, 266).

The excretion of GAA is decreased in uraemia despite an elevation in plasma concentration (259, 261, 267) and the urinary GAA/GSA ratio has been proposed as an indicator of kidney dysfunction (267).

No correlation was found between GSA levels and uraemic symptoms and signs including nerve conduction velocity (198, 199, 268). Chronic intoxication with GSA in rabbits failed to induce typical uraemic symptoms, such as neuropathy, anaemia, cardiac failure and haemorrhagic diathesis, but resulted in bradycardia, lowering of plasma uric acid and an increase in blood lactic acid (269). Infusion of GSA in dogs resulted in depression of cardiac function at concentrations comparable to those found in uraemic patients (270). However, isolated rat and guinea pig hearts perfused with GSA had the same metabolic and dynamic functions as control hearts (147, 190, 191).

It has been reported that GSA inhibits ADP activation of platelet factor 4 and platelet aggregation *in vitro* induced by ADP, adrenaline and collagen (271), but these observations were not confirmed by others (188). No inhibitory effects by GSA, methylguanidine and phenolic compounds were seen on anaerobic or aerobic ATP production or on utilisation of ATP (257). GSA has been found to inhibit transketolase activity in red cells and nervous tissue (78), an observation that also has not been confirmed by others (198, 199).

Increased autohaemolysis of red cells by high concentrations of GSA has been reported (197) but was not confirmed (198, 199). GSA had little inhibitory effect on DNA synthesis in lymphocytes (254). The addition of GSA in concentrations known to occur in uraemic plasma caused a marked inhibition of globin synthesis (255) but no effect on colony formation of erythroid bone marrow cells (200).

No effects of GSA were observed on glucose oxidation in white cells or glucose uptake by rat diaphragm (272, 273), erythrocyte cation transport (253), transepithelial sodium transport (258) and on bromosulfophthalein clearance by the isolated perfused rat liver (193).

Other guanidines
A number of other guanidine compounds have been found in increased concentrations in serum from uraemic patients: guanidinobutyric acid, guanidinopropionic acid and taurocyamine (262, 274).
Taurocyamine and guanidine were found elevated in cerebrospinal fluid from uraemic patients (248, 274). Ureter-ligated rabbits also had high concentrations of taurocyamine in serum and brain (274). There is no evidence that any of these compounds are toxic in uraemia

except for guanidinopropionic acid which inhibits glucose-6-phosphate dehydrogenase *in vitro* (262) and increases autohaemolysis of red cells (197).

In conclusion, the concentrations of various (toxic) guanidine compounds are higher in uraemic patients than in normal subjects. However, most *in vitro* and *in vivo* toxic effects have been observed at much higher concentrations than are found in uraemic patients and their exact roles as uraemic toxins are not established.

Products of nucleic acid metabolism

Uric acid
Uric acid, the end-product of purine metabolism in primates, is normally excreted in the urine, but to some extent it is also converted by bacteria in the gut (275). The daily production of urate is normal (276) or decreased (277) in patients with severe uraemia. Extrarenal elimination of uric acid increases in chronic renal disease and eventually becomes the major route of elimination. The principal uricolytic products are carbon dioxide and ammonia (urea).

Moderate hyperuricaemia frequently occurs early in the course of chronic renal disease but becomes marked only in the terminal stage of uraemia. Functional adaptation of the residual nephrons in chronic renal failure results in increased urate excretion per nephron due to both decreased tubular reabsorption and increased tubular secretion (278).

Hyperuricaemia occurs in advanced renal failure (2) but rarely results in manifest gout (279, 280) unless there is a predisposition to this clinical syndrome. Patients with uraemic pericarditis have been found to have uric acid concentrations in the blood exceeding those in uraemic patients without pericarditis (277) but it is not clear whether there is a causal relationship between raised uric acid concentrations and pericarditis. Intravenous infusion of 0.5 to 2 g (3 to 12 mmol) uric acid in normal man raised the serum level as high as 22.4 mg/dl (1.33 mmol/l) without any toxic effects (281). Urate ions are essentially freely filtrable and protein binding does not significantly impair dialysance (282). *In vitro* studies with uric acid have failed to show any toxic effects on glucose metabolism (183) or tissue respiration (146).

Cyclic AMP
Plasma cyclic AMP concentrations are elevated in renal failure and correlate with plasma creatinine concentration (283–287). It has also been suggested that this metabolically active substance was responsible for uraemic symptoms.

Cyclic AMP is the second messenger of a number of hormones and excretion of nephrogenic cyclic AMP has been taken as an index of hyperparathyroidism. The elevated plasma levels in uraemia may be the consequence of reduced excretion but also of increased production secondary to endocrine changes (see Chapter 36).

Cyclic AMP inhibits *in vitro* platelet aggregation (288–290) and a recent study shows that in uraemic patients the aggregation response correlates inversely with cyclic AMP concentration, suggesting that cyclic AMP may contribute to the platelet defect in uraemia (287). The concentration of cyclic AMP (329 daltons) is reduced by haemodialysis (284, 287). The decrease after dialysis is either sustained (283) or the level returns to predialysis concentration about 30 min after dialysis (287), the latter observation suggesting increased production rate.

Pyridine derivatives
Products of pyridine metabolism have also been isolated from haemodialysis fluid and estimated in uraemic plasma. N-methyl-2-pyridone-5-carboxamide (2-PY amide), N-methyl-2-pyridone-5-carboxylic acid (2-PY acid), and N-methyl-2-pyridone-5-formamidoacetic acid (2-PY hippurate) each products of pyridine metabolism have been isolated from haemodialysate (291, 292). Additionally, higher plasma levels of pseudouridine, 4-amino-5-imidazole carboxamide and 2-PY amide have been found in uraemic patients than in normals. Analysis before and after haemodialysis showed that the concentrations of the first two solutes were reduced approximately to the same degree as urea (293).

Protein synthesis in liver homogenates was found to be inhibited by 2-PY hippurate and 2-PY acid at much higher concentration than found in uraemic plasma, but 2-PY amide had no inhibiting effect (292).

Amino acids and dipeptides

Numerous abnormal amino acid concentrations in plasma have been found in uraemic patients (294–298). These include an increase in conjugated amino acid concentrations (299–303) and both increases and decreases of individual free amino acids. Among consistent findings are high concentrations of several non-essential amino acids, decreased concentrations of essential amino acids and a decreased ratio of phenylalanine/tyrosine and of valine/glycine. These changes are probably not the result of reduced urinary excretion of amino acids but more likely are caused by nutritional inadequacy or by toxic changes in protein metabolism (304–307).

Tryptophan, which is the only amino acid bound to plasma proteins, is abnormally low in uraemia in spite of a normal or raised free tryptophan concentration (308–311); a low free tryptophan concentration was, however, found in non-dialysed patients on low protein diet (312). This reduced binding (313) appears to be part of a more general abnormality in uraemia, since binding of a number of drugs, such as diphenylhydantoin, digitoxin, and sulphonamides is also reduced, probably because of competitive binding by other metabolites retained in uraemia (see Chapter 39). Competition for protein binding between tryptophan and indolic tryptophan metabolites was observed, when these metabolites were added *in vitro* to normal serum. This suggests that one cause of decreased protein binding of tryptophan in uraemia may be accumulation of its metabolites which compete for binding to albumin (311). The total tryptophan concentration increases following dialysis, due to increased protein binding, presumably because of removal of competing metabolites (295, 311, 314, 315).

It is well known that in renal failure the plasma concentration of tyrosine is low and the ratio phenylalanine/tyrosine is high, which has been attributed to inhibition of the formation of tyrosine from phenylalanine (73, 316–319). Specific abnormalities in uraemia are also reported of citrulline (320), valine (297, 321) and hydroxyproline (322). Hydroxyproline is found almost exclusively in collagen, which in man is largely confined to the skeleton. The plasma concentrations of free and bound hydroxyproline are increased in uraemia (322–324) correlating with creatinine concentrations (325). The hydroxyproline plasma concentrations also correlate significantly both with bone resorption and formation in bone biopsies (325) and might be an index of bone collagen turnover.

Hydroxylysine is also a typical component of collagen. Patients with chronic renal insufficiency have elevated plasma levels and increased urinary excretion of hydroxylysine glucosides and increased excretion of hydroxylysine bound in polypeptide and in small molecules of neutral or acidic character. The excretion of free hydroxylysine, however, was often within normal limits (326). The increased excretion of conjugated hydroxylysine may be another index of collagen turnover in uraemia.

Histidine, which is often low in uraemic plasma (327), appears to be an essential amino acid in uraemia (328–330) and possibly also in normal man (330). Concentrations of methylhistidines (1-methylhistidine and 3-methylhistidine) have been reported as increased in the plasma of severely uraemic patients (316, 331). 3-Methylhistidine, a constituent of actin and myosin of skeletal muscle (332, 333), is not reutilised for protein synthesis (334, 335) but excreted unchanged in the urine (336). In patients with reduced renal function a hyperbolic relationship was found between serum 3-methylhistidine concentration and inulin clearance (337). There is no evidence that any of these amino acids exerts toxic effects. Platelet aggregation was not affected by 1-methylhistidine and 3-methylhistidine even in concentrations higher than those found in uraemic plasma (338).

Certain sulphur-containing amino acids including cysteine-homocysteine, taurine and cystathionine have been shown to accumulate in patients with uraemia, treated with haemodialysis (339, 340). Interestingly, experimental chronic infusion of homocysteine in baboons produced atherosclerotic lesions after three months (341) and homocysteinuric children have also a high incidence of vascular disease. N-monoacetyl-cysteine was recently identified and found to be elevated in uraemic plasma (340).

As has been demonstrated β-aminoisobutyric acid is also elevated in uraemic plasma but there is no correlation with plasma levels of urea, creatinine and uric acid (342). Mice given pharmacological doses of β-aminoisobutyric acid showed twitching and cramps and some of them died, however, at plasma levels which were a hundred times higher than those encountered in uraemic patients.

It has been shown that the intracellular free amino acid pools in muscle tissue are changed in uraemic man. Low extra- and intracellular pools of threonine, valine, tyrosine and histidine were found to be typical features of chronic uraemia (317, 321, 343). Carnosine (β-alanyl histidine) is also low in uraemic muscle, which may be another sign of histidine depletion.

Intracellular isoleucine and leucine concentrations were normal in nondialysed uraemic patients and markedly increased in patients treated with peritoneal dialysis (317, 343); considering that this occurred in spite of intracellular concentrations of valine being low, it seems that there is an imbalance of the branched-chain amino acids (valine, isoleucine and leucine) in uraemia. Similar amino acid imbalances have been observed in experimental animals, exerting toxic effects by increasing amino acid requirements, impairing nitrogen utilisation and inhibiting growth (344).

Determination of amino acids and related compounds before and after hydrolysis of deproteinised plasma have revealed the presence of several conjugated amino acids. The concentration of bound amino acids is higher in uraemic than in normal plasma (301, 302, 314, 345). Some of them may represent dipeptides while others may be of a larger molecular size (see middle molecules). Much higher concentrations of β-aspartylglycine have also been detected in uraemic sera than in normal sera and toxicity has been assessed in mice with acute renal failure, receiving 1 g/kg body weight, resulting in alterations of behaviour, low activity and low response to stimuli, such as sound and shaking, an hour after the injection (346). Large quantities of β-aspartylglycine can be isolated from enzymatic digestion of collagen. Dietary gelatin significantly elevates the urinary excretion of this peptide in man (347). In view of the high doses required to obtain toxic symptoms *in vivo*, toxicity in uraemic man is not substantiated.

Amines

Aliphatic amines

Aliphatic amines are formed by bacterial action in the gut: 3-methylamine (TMA) from lecithine and choline, and 1-methylamine (MMA) from sarcosine and creatinine. Both TMA and MMA may act as precursors of 2-methylamine (DMA) (348).

Total aliphatic amines, DMA and TMA, are elevated in uraemic plasma and the concentrations are decreased by dialysis (348–350). Severely uraemic patients have raised duodenal concentrations of DMA (13). Sterilisation of the gut with broad-spectrum antibiotics decreases the blood concentrations of DMA and TMA with clinical improvement of asterixis, myoclonus and mental alertness. It was suggested that potentially toxic metabolites in the small intestine may have appreciable nutritional and toxic sequelae in uraemia. High duodenal amine levels are associated with abnormal colonisation of the small intestine by both anaerobic and aerobic bacteria (14, 351). A correlation has been found between serum concentrations of 3-methylamine and choice reaction time and EEG changes, and also between 2-

methylamine and choice reaction time (351). Both 2-methylamine and 3-methylamine have been identified in uraemic breath by gas chromatographic analysis and appeared to correlate with the classical fishy smell (352).

Faecal methylamine was found to be higher in uraemic subjects, being related to the degree of renal impairment (353). According to unpublished observations methylamine can be formed from creatinine when added to intestinal contents during anaerobic incubation *in vitro*. It has also been pointed out that commercial samples of methylguanidine, that has been described as a uraemic toxin, contain substantial quantities of methylamine as an impurity. This may have affected the results of toxicity studies (354). In chronic uraemic rats altered monoamine and diamine oxidase activities were observed in various tissues and body fluids, and it has been suggested that these alterations may affect the metabolism of many amines (350).

Very high concentrations of aliphatic amines (MMA, DMA and ethylamine) inhibit succinate oxidation and glutamic acid decarboxylase activity (355). High concentrations of aliphatic amines also reduce oxidative processes in brain slices (146, 356). Some haemolytic action has been found *in vitro* (357) and depression of oxidation in the brain and red cells was also demonstrated (358). Except in one investigation (146), far higher concentrations than are present in uraemic plasma were used in these *in vitro* studies.

The mean concentration of choline in plasma of azotaemic subjects receiving haemodialysis was found to be about twice that of normal subjects (359). The choline levels fell during the first two hours of dialysis but returned to predialysis values after six hours of treatment, suggesting the existence of a rapidly activated homeostatic control mechanism. The degree of peripheral neuropathy was inversely correlated with the levels of free choline in plasma, suggesting a causal relationship. Reduction of kidney mass may be responsible for the increase of free choline levels in uraemia, since the kidney has a role in the homeostatic regulation of plasma choline (360).

High serum concentrations of carnitine have been found in renal insufficiency (361) but it is unknown whether this is of any clinical significance. Of more clinical importance may be the observation that the plasma carnitine levels in dialysis patients are low and are further reduced after dialysis (362). Carnitine is required in fatty acid transport into mitochondria and depletion of carnitine may possibly be associated with lipid abnormalities in uraemia.

Aromatic amines
These substances are degradation products of the aromatic amino acids (phenylalanine and tyrosine) and are formed by decarboxylation. High concentrations of free and conjugated aromatic amines have been observed in uraemic plasma (363, 364).

A few aromatic amines were also identified in dialysate from uraemic patients (365). Tyramine, which is a product of bacterial action in the gut or is formed in the tissues from tyrosine, accumulates in the plasma following ligation of ureters in rabbits and in plasma and cerebrospinal fluid of uraemic patients (218, 366, 367).

It has been found that high concentrations of aromatic amines inhibit oxidative reactions in brain slices (366). High concentrations of phenylethylamine, tyramine and 3-hydroxytyramine inhibit succinate oxidation, glutamic acid carboxylase and dopa carboxylase to varying extents (364). Again it should be emphasised that these *in vitro* effects were only obtained with concentrations several times higher than are found in uraemic plasma.

Polyamines
Putrescine, spermidine and spermine are widely distributed in the human body. They are strongly basic, low molecular weight compounds, which appear to be a universal prerequisite for growth (368). Cadaverine, the next higher homologue of putrescine, was discovered as a product of putrefaction (369). Putrescine, spermidine and spermine are formed in animal tissues, cadaverine and putrescine are also formed by intestinal bacteria by decarboxylation of lysine and ornithine in the intestine.

Polyamines have been found to impair glucose transport in the rat jejunum *in vitro* (370–372).

The urinary excretion of polyamines is increased in cancer patients and in patients with infections (373).

It has been reported that free polyamines in plasma, expressed as spermine equivalents, are elevated in children with uraemia and that these elevated concentrations persist following institution of dialysis therapy (374).

The free spermidine concentration is much higher in cells than in plasma. Higher red cell levels of spermidine were found in uraemic patients compared to normal controls, whereas the spermine concentrations were not different (375). There was also a significant correlation between red cell spermidine values and both plasma urea and plasma creatinine concentrations. These findings, in combination with low urinary excretion of polyamines, suggest that impaired urinary excretion contributes to the accumulation of spermidine in red cells (375).

It appears that substantial quantities of polyamines can be obtained from serum and urine after acid hydrolysis at elevated temperatures, which has led to the postulate that polyamine conjugates play an important role in polyamine metabolism of man (376). It was recently reported that spermidine (measured by radioimmune assay) in uraemic serum was partly bound to a macromolecule not present in normal serum (377). In this context it is of interest that a strongly basic middle molecule peptide, containing spermidine has been isolated from uraemic body fluids (378).

The hypothesis was recently brought forward that the raised polyamine level in chronic dialysis patients could possibly contribute to accelerated cardiovascular disease observed in dialysis patients, by stimulating proliferation of arterial smooth-muscle cells, a central process in atherogenesis (379).

In a recent review of a potential role of polyamines as uraemic toxins similarities were brought forward between cancer and uraemia in causing anorexia, weight loss, wasting, carbohydrate intolerance, peripheral neuropathy, dysimmunity of the cellular type, elevated serum amine-oxidases, normocytic normochromic anaemia with moderate decrease in red cell survival time and similar bone marrow pictures (380). In an exciting new study, recently published, spermine was identified as an inhibitor of erythropoiesis in patients with chronic renal failure (380a). Evidence for this was that the inhibitor and radiolabelled spermine appeared in identical serum fractions, that *in vitro* inhibition took place at concentrations reported in uremic sera and that the inhibitory effect of uremic serum could be abolished by adding a specific antiserum to spermine.

Indoles

Largely as a result of bacterial action in the gut, tryptophan is deaminated and decarboxylated giving rise to a number of metabolites (tryptamine, indoleacetic acid, skatole, skatoxyl, indole, indoxyl, indican and others). By action of tryptophan hydroxylase and tryptophan pyrrolase, a number of biologically active compounds are produced, including 5-hydroxytryptamine (serotonin). An detailed discussion of the metabolic pathways of indolic compounds is presented by Ludwig and co-workers (381).

Various indoles have been found in increased concentrations in plasma or in dialysates of uraemic patients (365, 367, 381–387). These compounds are readily removed by dialysis (367, 381). High concentrations of indole acetic acid and N-acetyltryptophan suggest increased transamination of tryptophan and a possible defect in renal amino acid acylase in uraemia (387). The concentration of 5-hydroxyindoleacetic acid in brain tissue is high in uraemic rats (388–389).

Patients with chronic renal disease and uraemic encephalopathy had raised plasma free tryptophan and high cerebrospinal fluid concentrations of tryptophan, 5-hydroxyindoleacetic acid and homovanillic acid; these are precursor and metabolites of serotonine, which is a cerebral neurotransmitter (388).

High concentrations of indoles inhibit oxidation in brain slices (357) and decrease blood sugar by insulinase inhibition in rat liver and intact mice (390). It is also of interest that 3-carboxyanthralinic acid and kynurenate both inhibit gluconeogenetic pathways by action on phosphoenolpyruvatecarboxykinase (391–394). Indole-3-acetic acid causes 50% inhibition of leucocyte iodination potential at a concentration of 50 γ/l (0,3 µmol/l) (395).

There is, however, no evidence of toxic effects *in vitro* or *in vivo* of tryptophan metabolites in concentrations found in uraemic plasma.

Phenols

Phenols, phenolic acid and their conjugates have been found in increased concentrations in uraemic plasma, cerebrospinal fluid and dialysate, and it has been suggested that they play a primary role in the pathogenesis of the uraemic syndrome (396–411). Toxicity of phenolic compounds has been related particularly to cerebral depression (214, 400). An extensive review of the metabolic pathways of degradation of aromatic amino acids was given by Wootton (386). Phenols, phenolic acids and their conjugates are formed as a result of the deamination, decarboxylation and oxidation of the aromatic amino acids tyrosine and phenylalanine. Some of them are products of bacterial action in the gut. Phenolic compounds are conjugated in the liver with glucuronic or sulphuric acid. It has been found that haemodialysis reduced the concentration of phenols in plasma but the dialysance was about half that of creatinine (411–413). A post-dialysis rebound phenomenon has also been observed (407).

Earlier investigators (2) employed methods which assessed groups of aromatic compounds and were thus, unselective. Using paper chromatographic methods, a great number of aromatic compounds were observed in dialysate from patients with acute uraemia, of which many have been identified (365). It was found that both plasma and urinary concentrations of individual phenols (4-hydroxybenzoic acid and 4-hydroxyphenyllactic acid) were elevated in uraemic patients, suggesting increased production (or decreased degradation) in uraemia (408). Employing gas chromatography for measurement of individual phenols, it could be shown that p-cresol and phenol concentrations were higher in uraemic patients than in normals and that the p-cresol, but not the phenol concentration decreased when the dietary protein intake was reduced (414–416).

Using gas chromatography with mass spectrometry for identification of hydroxyphenolic acids in uraemic serum, Niwa and co-workers (414) described nine different compounds. Of these p-hydroxybenzoic acid and p-hydroxyphenylacetic acid were markedly increased in uraemic serum. Haemodialysis reduced their concentrations by 34–64% and it was concluded that haemodialysis was rather efficient in removing these acids. The concentration of aryl acids (hippuric acid, benzoic acid etc) as estimated by fluorometric assay was strikingly elevated when creatinine clearance fell below 10 ml/min.

Uraemic serum caused net flow secretion in isolated proximal tubules from rabbit kidneys, an effect also excerted by para-aminohippuric acid. The concentration of aryl acids in serum and urine as measured fluorometrically was related to the secretory activity in a direct linear fashion and hippuric acid determined by gas liquid chromatography accounted for approximately 1/4 of this activity. It was concluded that the secretory activity of uraemic serum is due to the accumulation of aryl acids, probably of the hippuric class, and, further, that relatively high levels of these biological active substances may contribute to general organ dysfunction in uraemia, owing to their potential to act as competitive inhibitors of organic anion transport (417).

A number of studies have shown that phenols may exert toxic effects in experimental animals and in *in vitro* systems. Dihydroxybenzoic acid induces neurotoxicity in rats (418). Infusion of phenol and p-cresol into dogs induced a variety of neurological symptoms (196).

Platelet aggregation *in vitro* is inhibited by another phenolic compound, p-hydroxyphenylalaninic acid (419) and by phenol itself (420). However, no effects of these compounds on anaerobic or aerobic ATP generation or on utilisation of ATP were observed (257). High concentrations of 4-aminobenzoic acid and 2-hydroxyphenylic acid inhibited Na^+-K^+-ATPase, Mg^{++}-ATPase and Ca^{++}-ATPase in the pancreas of the cat (252).

It has been reported that hydroxyphenylacetic acid and phenyllactic acid competitively inhibit red cell Na^+-K^+-activated ATPase but in concentrations considerably higher than are found in uraemic plasma (421).

More recently the action of phenols and phenolic acids, which may be high in the plasma of patients with either uraemic or hepatic coma, was studied on red cell membrane ATPase, platelet membrane ATPase and brain homogenate ATPase (422). At concentrations as low as 25 µg/ml (0,27 µmol/ml) phenol was a competitive inhibitor of red cell membrane Na^+-K^+-ATPase and also inhibited Mg^{++}-ATPase. Phenyl-glucuronide had no effect, whilst the action of hydroxyphenolic acids varied in the different systems. Even lower concentrations of phenols and phenolic acids affected whole cells systems such as ^{22}Na efflux from red cells and ^{32}P uptake. Among these compounds was also phenyl-glucuronide. These *in vitro* effects point to a toxic role of phenols in uraemia and suggest that conjugated phenols are toxic as well. Polymorphonuclear leucocyte function (iodination capacity) is also inhibited by phenol at a concentration of 0.5 mg/dl (5.3 µmol/l) but phenylglucuronide was without effect (395).

Aromatic compounds identified in dialysate from uraemic patients inhibit oxygen consumption in guinea pig brain slices, anaerobic glycolysis in rat brain and a variety of enzymes but only in concentrations several times higher than those found in uraemic plasma (386, 423). Aromatic acids, chiefly 2-hydroxy- and 3-hydroxyphenyl derivatives, inhibit malic dehydrogenase (424). P-cresol inhibits *in vitro* respiration in liver and brain slices but not in concentrations as found in uraemic plasma (146).

Several phenyl and phenolic acids inhibit mevalonate-5-phosphate kinase and mevalonate-5-pyrophosphate decarboxylase of the rat brain, thus possibly interfering with myelinisation (425).

In conclusion, there is evidence that phenolic compounds retained in uraemia may exert toxic effects, especially on membrane transport and metabolism, and that these effects may occur at concentrations present in uraemic plasma.

Carbohydrate-derivatives

Myoinositol

This member of the vitamin B complex is a natural constituent of food and is synthesized in muscle, liver, brain and kidneys (426–429). The major pathway for myoinositol catabolism requires initial oxidation to D-glycuronate in the renal cortex (430, 431). In patients with renal failure, the plasma and cerebrospinal fluid concentration and urinary excretion of myoinositol are elevated (432–436) suggesting that the production is increased or catabolism is decreased. Myoinositol concentrations were decreased after haemodialysis (433, 435, 436).

The cerebrospinal fluid concentration in uraemic patients was also higher than in normals (435). On the other hand, plasma 1,5-anhydroglucitol, an anhydride form of sorbitol, has been found lower in uraemia than in healthy subjects (434). The urinary excretion of myoinositol is also increased in diabetes mellitus, but the plasma levels are not different from normal (432, 437).

A striking decrease in sciatic nerve conduction velocity was found in normal rats given large amounts of myoinositol orally and intraperitoneally (433, 438). Dorsal root ganglion cells in tissue culture showed toxic changes in presence of myoinositol at concentrations known to occur in uraemic plasma (439). However, neither spinal fluid nor plasma myoinositol concentrations showed any correlation with nerve conduction velocities or EEG changes in uraemic patients (436).

Mannitol and sorbitol

The mannitol concentration in plasma, red cells and cerebrospinal fluid is also increased in uraemia. A relationship was demonstrated between the increase in sorbitol in cerebrospinal fluid and signs of peripheral neuropathy in non-dialysed uraemic patients (440).

Glucuronic acid and other compounds

High concentrations of glucuronic acid were found in serum and cerebrospinal fluid of patients with uraemic coma (367). The significance is unknown.

In a study which was mainly methodological, several aldoses, alditols, aldonolactones and Krebs cycle intermediates were identified in uraemic serum by chemical ionization mass spectrometry (441).

Other metabolites

Oxalic acid concentrations are elevated in uraemia, plasma concentrations varying proportionate to plasma urea concentrations (442). The whole blood oxalate concentration was higher in renal failure than the plasma concentration. Haemodialysis resulted in a reduction of the concentration to values within the normal range. Crystals of calcium oxalate have been identified in the kidneys and myocardium in patients who died from uraemia (443). Oxalic acid inhibits the activity of lactic acid dehydrogenase *in vitro* (444, 445) but it is not known if this has any relevance to uraemic toxicity *in vivo*.

It has been found that the concentrations of pyruvate, acetoin and 2,3,-butylene glycol are increased in uraemic patients with disturbed consciousness but no correlation was found between the degree of mental impairment and the blood concentrations (446). Serum levels of succinic acid, adipic acid, 3-methyladipic acid, pimelic acid, azelaic acid and of 2.4-dimethyladipic acid (a substance only recently identified) were considerably increased in uraemic plasma (447).

The organic acid fraction of haemofiltrates of uremic patients separated in the form of methyl esters by gas chromatography and mass spectrometry yielded a similar pattern of organic acid methylates as found in urine from normal individuals. More than 80 different organic compounds were identified (aromatic acids, aliphatic acids, dicarboxylic acids, phenols, amines, indoles, purines, pyridines, carbohydrates etc) and nine unknown compounds were also characterised according to their mass spectrometric data (448). N-phenylacetyl-α-aminoglutarimide was present in haemofiltrate at levels 50 to 100 times higher than in urine and the reduction in haemofiltrate concentration with time during treatment was far more rapid than for the other compounds.

An unidentified fluorescent substance in uraemic serum, haemofiltrate, dialysate, and in urine appeared to have a molecular weight of less than 1 000 (449).

Middle molecules

The Middle Molecule of Hypothesis
It has long been known that there is a poor correlation between some toxic manifestations of uraemia and the concentrations of creatinine, urea and uric acid in plasma. This discrepancy between the accumulation of small molecules and the occurrence of uraemic symptoms was most obvious in patients treated with long-term peritoneal dialysis who, in spite of the relatively poor dialysance of small molecules, were doing well and did not develop neuropathy (450, 451). In a discussion of a paper at a meeting in 1965, Scribner (452) made the following point:

'... there is a chance that because the peritoneal membrane is leaky, we are removing with peritoneal dialysis certain higher molecular weight substances more efficiently than with hemodialysis and this may account for the better results, and suggest that we need a leaky membrane for a hemodialyzer'.

The 'leakiness' of the peritoneal membrane to middle molecules (MM) was later confirmed by the Scribner group in carefully designed studies (453). Inadequate dialysis was supposed to result in retention of compounds with larger molecular weights which could be removed by prolonged dialysis with a thin membrane, but could not be removed by either short or prolonged dialysis with a thick membrane with a rather bad permeability for middle molecular weight compounds (454). The observation that prolongation of dialysis time can arrest or reverse peripheral neuropathy independently of the predialysis values of urea and creatinine (455), also suggested a toxic role of MM.

These clinical findings form the background of the *Square Meter-Hour Hypothesis* (456). This hypothesis relates the efficiency of dialysis in preventing the development of neuropathy to the numbers of hours of dialysis per week and the active membrane surface area. Results were obtained which supported the concept that MM were toxic (457, 460). It was, therefore, suggested that the term Square Meter-Hour Hypothesis should be changed to *Middle Molecule Hypothesis* (461).

Few new theories in nephrology have evoked so much interest and created so much confusion and generated so many conflicting opinions as the MM hypothesis. Numerous attempts were made to prove or disprove the hypothesis. Various dialysis strategies were specially designed to increase or decrease the presumed level of the MM in the body fluids, relating these changes to the symptomatology of the patient or to the *in vitro* toxicity of plasma or dialysate. Some of these results appeared to support the hypothesis (462–468) but others did not (469–474). No direct determinations of MM in plasma were performed in most of these studies.

Mathematical models were used to predict the accumulation and transfer of MM (475–481, see also Chapter 3). Common to all these calculations was the assumption that the generation rate of toxic MM was the same in normal and uraemic man.

The important role of residual renal function in the elimination of MM was emphasised (475, 482, 483). Based on B_{12} clearance studies of various dialysers and various dialysate flow rates, and assuming that the renal clearance of endogenous middle molecules equals glomerular filtration rate (endogenous creatinine clearance), a dialysis index was devised, which expressed the weekly clearance of MM (dialysis clearance + renal clearance), in relation to the minimum 'safe' weekly total clearance, which was assumed to be 30 l/wk for a standard man with a body surface area of $1.73 \, m^2$ (479).

The MM hypothesis has had a great impact on dialyzer and membrane technology and dialysis strategies even before any MM had been detected or identified. More permeable membranes were developed in conformity with the MM hypothesis and dialyzers with large membrane areas were designed and marketed with the purpose to enhance MM removal (see Chapters 4, 5 and 14). Favourable clinical results were reported with haemofiltration and charcoal haemoperfusion, both procedures suggesting very efficient removal of MM by these methods (see Chapter 12 and 16) and later with continous ambulatory peritoneal dialysis (CAPD) which is also a most efficient method for removal of MM (see Chapter 23).

Isolation and characterisation of middle molecule substances
Evidence of the existence of substances with MM characteristics was brought forward long before the MM hypothesis was developed. In 1938 Cristol and co-workers (484) reported that small polypeptides were present in increased concentrations in blood of uraemic patients, especially those with severe central nervous system disturbances and terminal uraemic coma. They also noticed that their concentrations were not related to nonprotein nitrogen and varied independently of creatinine, indoxyl and alkali-reserve. Ten years later studies by three other groups confirmed these observations (485–487). In 1958 Dési, Fehér and Szold (488, 489) were able to isolate a fraction from uraemic plasma by means of ion exchange resins. This fraction was extremely toxic in experimental animals and appeared to be a peptide of low molecular weight. Similar results were obtained by Yatzidis and co-workers (490) who found that the toxic peptides were efficiently absorbed on activated charcoal. No less than 38 ninhydrin positive peptides were isolated from dialysis fluid (491) and peptide bound amino

acids were found increased in uraemic plasma (301, 302, 314).

Next, quite independently of the discussion about MM, Dzúrik and co-workers reported in 1971 and 1972 that peptides, isolated by high-voltage electrophoresis and not detectable in healthy volunteers, were present in serum and urine of uraemic patients (492, 493).

Several groups have used gel filtration of plasma, plasma ultrafiltrate obtained *in vivo* (isolated ultrafiltration), dialysate and urine for separation of one or more fractions in the MM weight range which were in general detected by ultraviolet absorption at different wave lengths (494–592). Most of these studies showed that MM are present in higher concentrations in uraemic than in normal plasma.

The separation of MM by gel chromatography rests on the assumption that this technique discriminates different compounds according to their molecular size. However, this is only approximately true, since certain compounds may be retained on the column (especially certain cyclic compounds) and may be eluted even after the void volume of the column whereas other compounds are eluted earlier than expected according to their molecular weight (592). Thus, it appeared, that some acidic middle molecule fractions isolated in the expected molecular weight range of 1,000 to 2,000 have lower molecular weights (559, 570, 587, 590).

For preparation and concentration of larger amounts of material in the MM range, membrane technology has proved to be suitable. Reverse osmosis with subsequent lyophilisation, followed by desalting procedures have been used for isolation of peptidic compounds, which exhibit toxicity *in vitro* (532, 553, 562).

The MM-fraction isolated by gel filtration only represents a complex mixture of compounds, presumably with different molecular weights, with different generation rates, different optical densities and probably also with different biological activities (*vida infra*).

Some groups have attempted to separate and characterise the uraemic MM-fractions obtained by gel filtration further, by applying ion exchange chromatography, electrophoretic methods or high-pressure liquid chromatography (496, 503, 504, 506–508, 510, 512, 514, 516–518, 522, 524, 527, 530, 531, 535, 541–546, 548–550, 552, 556, 557, 559, 560, 563–565, 567, 569, 576, 577, 579–581, 586–590). These studies confirmed that the MM-fractions isolated by gel filtration consist of a mixture of different compounds. In one study using high-pressure liquid chromatography no less than approximately 100 MM peaks were separated (581).

The most commonly employed methodology for separation and quantitation of individual MM-fractions is now gel filtration followed by gradient ion exchange chromatography, by which uraemic serum, ultrafiltrate, dialysate and normal and uraemic urine can be separated in several UV absorbing subfractions (we called our subfractions 7a, 7b, 7c etc [517]). However, the chromatographically pure fractions obtained by ion exchange chromatography do not represent single compounds. This was shown by applying isotachophoresis to three of these fractions (7a, 7b, 7c) which could be further separated into subfractions (590).

So far only a few MM compounds have been isolated in pure form and of even fewer has the molecular structure been elucidated. Lutz and co-workers (378) isolated four basic peptides by partition chromatography and paper electrophoresis with a molecular weight of 1300 to 1800, and determined the molar ratios of the individual amino acids but not the amino acid sequences. One contained spermidine, another a guanidine group and an amino sugar derivative. They were strongly protein-bound and showed evidence of insulin stimulation of lipoprotein lipase (509).

Klein et al. (537) determined the chief peptide constituents of a fraction of middle-sized, ninhydrin-positive molecules in uraemic patients. The fraction was obtained from haemodialysate by chromatography on Dowex 50, and resolved upon thin-layer electrophoresis on Sephadex G-25 into nine ninhydrinpositive fractions and one staining only with tolidine reagent. All 10 electrophoretic fractions gave similar filtration profiles with Bio-Gel P-6 in the presence of sodium dodecyl sulphate and 2-mercaptoethanol. The chief peptide components common to each electrophoretic fraction have molecular weights of approximately 3000 and are especially abundant in lysine, glycine, glutamic acid and serine, while concentrations of aromatic amino acids are low.

Abiko and co-workers in Japan (532, 533, 543, 550) using ultrafiltration, gel filtration, and ion exchange chromatography, were able to isolate four peptides from plasma ultrafiltrate of severely uraemic patients: the peptides were subjected to amino acid sequence determination and were later synthesised, as were several analogues. A heptapeptide, corresponding to position 13 through 19 of β_2-microglobulin (533) and a tryptophan-containing pentapeptide (543), corresponding to position 123 through 127 of the β-chain of fibrinogen had an inhibiting effect on rosette formation between human lymphocytes and sheep erythrocytes *in vitro*, suggesting that they might cause or contribute to the impaired immune response in uraemia. A tripeptide (H-His-Gly-Lys-OH) was isolated from uraemic ultrafiltrate (532). Another tripeptide (H-Glu-Asp-Gly-OH), which was isolated from 'neurotoxic' dialysate inhibited LDH activity *in vitro* (550). These are the first publications, in which the complete structure of new biologically active MM peptides are reported, demonstrating that they consist of fragments of known proteins. However, these peptides were only obtained from single patients and it is not yet possible to evaluate their role as uraemic toxins *in vivo*.

The Necker group in Paris (516) is now in the process of isolating and identifying a middle molecule compound (b_{4-2}), which appears to be a carbohydrate with neurotoxic properties. In current studies it could be demonstrated that the b_{4-2} solute is a glucuronide with a molecular mass of 568 daltons corresponding to a glucuron conjugate of an aglycon (not yet identified) with molecular weight of 392 (561, 562).

Le Moel and coworkers (571) found that the gel chromatographic fraction containing b_{4-2} consists of three carbohydrate and three peptide subfractions, of which the three carbohydrate fractions contained glucuron conjugates.

Using high voltage electrophoresis, isotachophoresis, mass spectrometry and enzymatic hydrolysis one of the compounds of fraction 7c has now been identified in our laboratory. It appeared to be a β-glucuronidated conjugate of p-OH-benzoic acid and glycine (588, 589, 591). Other subfractions (7a, 7b) yielded several free amino acids after hydrolysis indicating that they contain peptidic material (588).

Some misleading artefacts have to be considered when evaluating plasma MM in uraemic patients. Haemolysates from normal and uraemic erythrocytes contain MM-fractions in high concentration (7c-7e). Therefore the serum has to be rapidly separated from the cells to avoid haemolytic contamination (559). Certain drugs such as theophylline, furosemide, methyldopa (559) and salicylic acid (unpublished observations) may interfer with endogenous middle molecule determination in peaks 7c-7f. This is of practical importance since many uraemic patients receive multiple drug therapy.

Accumulation and elimination of middle molecules
The newly acquired techniques in separation and quantitation of MM have been applied in a number of clinical studies.

It was shown that the plasma and urinary MM patterns are similar in individual uraemic patients. However, when comparing the excretion rates for each peak, very great differences were found between the patients, suggesting that the generation rate varied considerably from one patient to another (512, 557).

More of the plasma peaks of MM were low or absent when the creatinine clearance was 15 ml/min or more, but were elevated exponentially as renal function further deteriorated (512, 587). The clearance of different middle molecule fractions was strongly correlated to the creatinine clearance (512). Furthermore the ratio of the clearance of fractions 7a-7d to the clearance of inulin was about 1.0, thus indicating that no tubular reabsorption or secretion of middle molecules occurs in uraemic man (574). In the isolated rat kidney perfused with uraemic haemofiltrate fractions a slight reabsorption of 7b and 7d was found, where 7a and 7c were excreted in the amount of the filtered load. However, at low perfusate concentration 7c showed evidence of tubular secretion (582, 583).

Several investigators have found that dialysis treatment reduced the plasma concentration of MM, which were, in some studies, recovered from in dialysis fluid (497, 503, 504, 507, 522, 541, 542, 544-547, 557, 558, 575, 578, 587). This was also the case when a sorbent-based dialysate regeneration system was used (571).

In patients kept on stable dialysis schedules correlations were sought between predialysis plasma MM concentrations and the theoretical efficiency of dialysis with regard to MM, taking residual renal function into consideration. The MM dialysis index (D.I.) was calculated assuming a molecular mass of 1,000 daltons. The plasma concentrations of some of the middle molecules (7a, b, f and g) were negatively correlated with D.I. (most pronounced for peak 7b [$r = -0.73$]) and also with residual renal function (creatinine clearance) (544). Peaks 7c and d showed no significant correlation with D.I. and, therefore, appeared to vary more or less independently of residual renal function and efficiency of dialysis treatment. This probably reflects a larger variability in the net production rate of these fractions than of the other peaks, a factor not taken into consideration in most mathematical models. The concentration profile for 7a, 7b and 7c after dialysis was complex with an initial rebound and subsequent rapid decrease followed by an increase to predialysis levels.

From these data Gotch and Sargent (594) investigated possible kinetic relationships of MM in renal failure and dialysis therapy. They concluded that fractions 7b and 7g may be irreversible metabolic end products generated in and confined to a volume approximating extracellular fluid. In contrast, the concentration profiles reported for 7a, b and c suggested that they are metabolic intermediates and that a complex metabolic disturbance is brought on by dialysis, making modeling impossible without far more precise knowledge of the metabolic steps involved than currently is available.

Oulès and co-workers (578) were unable to demonstrate a correlation between plasma MM and small molecule accumulation on one hand and residual renal function on the other. They, however, reported correlations between the levels of peaks 7b, c, and d and serum PTH concentrations and suggested that the considerable variations in MM accumulation and their generation rate may be due to an 'extra-uraemic factor'. Comparison of serum MM levels in patients in a carefully controlled study of long (7.5 h) versus short (3.6 h) haemodialysis revealed higher plasma MM levels in the shorter dialysis schedule. The differences were, however, relatively small indicating that the MM have a higher dialysance and, therefore, lesser mass than the >1,000 daltons size of MM separated by gel filtration (558). Furthermore, based on *in vivo* clearance data obtained with capillary dialysers the mass of the MM-fractions 7a-7f appeared to range from 500 to 700 daltons (557). This is in keeping with clearance data presented earlier for 7c (542). These results would imply that the MM solutes filtered by hollow fiber dialysers have a higher dialysance and therefore, smaller size than the 1,000 to 2,000 daltons proposed for uraemic MM isolated by gel filtration on Sephadex G 15. This conclusion is in good agreement with recent results of chemical characterisation of MM (561, 572, 589, 592). The elimination of MM substances by a 1 m² cuprophane coil dialyser was found to be sufficiently effective as to prevent excessive increase of the plasma levels of MM in stabilised patients undergoing short-term regular dialysis treatment (587).

It was recently reported that patients who had been treated with chronic haemodialysis for more than 10 years had higher plasma MM concentrations than patients treated for about 5 years who in turn had higher plasma MM levels than conservatively treated patients (552).

Patients on continuous ambulatory peritoneal dialysis (CAPD) have been shown to have lower plasma MM levels than patients on intermittent peritoneal dialysis who, in turn, had lower MM plasma concentrations than patients treated with haemodialysis (558, 591). This confirmed that CAPD is presently the most effective dialytic method for MM removal.

Haemoperfusion over activated carbon reduces the plasma concentration of MM (490, 502, 522, 527, 542, 544, 545, 556). It has been claimed that MM removal by haemoperfusion is more efficient than by haemodialysis (490, 502, 556); this was, however, not confirmed by others (511, 522, 527, 529, 542). Following renal transplantation uraemic MM disappeared from plasma more rapidly than urea and creatinine (524).

Toxicity of middle molecules
The numerous clinical studies in dialysis patients designed to prove or disprove toxicity of MM (without actually measuring their concentration) have not given a definite answer (see 'Middle Molecule Hypothesis').

With direct measurements of MM in plasma, it was demonstrated that 'sick' uraemic patients (with pericarditis, peripheral neuropathy, malnutrition and severe fluid retention) tend to accumulate MM material either because of reduced excretion or increased production or both, whereas patients free of these complications (such as adequately dialysed haemodialysis and CAPD patients, or patients maintained on successful conservative treatment) had low MM peaks (514, 540, 551–553, 575, 578, 581). In most of these studies it was not possible to relate any specific uraemic symptom to accumulation of a specific uraemic MM-fraction. Only neuropathy was an exception, which seemed to correlate with MM accumulation (540, 553, 573).

There is evidence that MM are important for the pathogenesis of renal anaemia. In uraemic children there was an inverse relationship between the dialysis index on one hand and the transfusion requirement and concentration of MM in serum on the other hand, but no such relationship was demonstrated for serum creatinine (595). MM-fraction from uraemic children had an inhibiting effect on erythropoiesis of hypertransfused polycythaemic mice after injection of erythropoietin, which was not obtained with fractions from nonuraemic children (584). This fits the preliminary results of investigations showing that MM inhibits erythropoiesis in intact mice (513). Furthermore, the uraemic MM-fraction diminished the number of erythroid bone-marrow cells in intact mice by 47%, but did not effect other bone-marrow cells (585, 586).

Toxic effects of MM *in vitro* were observed in bone marrow measured as reduced incorporation of ^{3}H-thymidine (534, 555, 568), and ^{59}Fe incorporation into haeme (568). Two important steps in haemoglobin synthesis were inhibited in peripheral reticulocytes *in vitro*: globin synthesis (^{14}C-histidine incorporation (255) and porphobilinogen synthesis by δ-aminolaevulinic acid dehydrase (525). Osmotic fragility of erythrocytes *in vitro* is increased in presence of MM-fractions 7c and 7d (577), and increased oxidative haemolysis caused by a MM-fraction has also been demonstrated (538, 570). These results suggests that MM toxicity may play a role in uraemic anaemia, not only by inhibition of erythropoiesis and haemoglobin synthesis but also by enhancing red cell destruction.

There is also evidence that MM have a depressive effect on certain immunological functions. It was reported that infusion of MM-material in rodents delays the rejection of skin allografts (528). An inhibiting effect on graft versus–host reaction in irradiated mice was observed after injection of allogenic lymphocytes preincubated with MM (528, 576). Antibody production was, however, not affected by continuous infusion of MM in rats (576). Several *in vitro* studies showed inhibition of phytohaemagglutinine stimulated lymphoblast proliferation and mixed lymphocyte reaction (511, 514, 518, 521, 549, 576, 577). Reduced E-rosette formation by T-lymphocytes in the presence of sheep-erythrocytes after incubation with two defined MM-peptides was reported (533, 543). However, no inhibition of this reaction was found in presence of a crude MM-fraction (521). The latter result and the fact that significant lymphocyte killing was not obtained in the mixed lymphocyte reaction (523) excluded a rapid cytotoxic effect of MM on T-lymphocytes. More likely an inhibitor of cell-proliferation could be the common denominator of an *in vivo* as well as *in vitro* immunosuppressive effect, since MM-extract noticably inhibited the proliferation of various normal or tumorous cell lines (549). All these findings are consistent with a role for MM in inhibiting cell-mediated immunity in renal insufficiency, a well-known symptom of the uraemic state.

Phagocytic activity of whole blood as well as granulocyte phagocytic activity was found to be increased in presence of MM *in vitro* (501, 580). It was also reported that MM inhibit migration of unseparated leucocytes *in vitro* and cause morphological changes observed by scanning electron microscopy, but lymphocytes were not influenced (560). However, no effect of MM on proliferation and digestive capacity of human mononuclear phagocytes *in vitro* was observed, but a toxic effect was obtained with fractions of higher molecular weight (536).

Crude MM-fraction also inhibited aggregation of human platelets *in vitro* induced by various compounds (ADP, collagen, ristocetin, arachidonate, and adrenaline, all known to stimulate platelet aggregation (567, 573, an effect also obtained with desalted peak 7d and 7e material (567), suggesting that the platelet defect of uraemia is related to MM toxicity.

According to the original MM hypothesis peripheral neuropathy was thought to be a typical sign of uraemic toxicity caused by MM (461). However, these early studies of the influence of MM on nervous function were not verified by direct determinations of MM. The Necker group in Paris combined clinical observations of dialysis patients using a dialyser with a membrane highly permeable to MM (the polyacrylonitrile membrane, see chapter 14) (596) with biochemical studies of plasma and dialysate. They reported that effective dialysis of MM for more than 3 months improved the neurological status in six patients with severe neuropathy, who all had high plasma concentrations of a MM-fraction (b_{4-2}), which was isolated by chromatographic methods (500, 506, 566). This MM-fraction, which was isolated from dialysate, was found to exert toxic effects on the frog sural nerve *in vitro* (535, 575 [see also chapter 14]). A correlation between plasma concentration of b_{4-2} and motor nerve conduction velocity was observed in uraemic rats (554). The toxic substance in b_{4-2} is now partly identified (559 [see above]). Some further support for MM being involved in uraemic neurotoxicity comes from the observation of a definite degree of inverse correlation between crude MM accumulation and motor nerve conduction velocity in uraemic patients (553).

Kumegawa and co-workers (569) investigated the effect of MM-fractions on the spinal dorsal root ganglion in the embryo of the chick after 8 days of incubation in tissue culture. They could demonstrate by electron microscopy, that the MM-fraction had a direct effect on nerve fibres (which showed degeneration) but not on nerve cells. The activities of glucose-6-phosphate dehydrogenase and pyruvate kinase were inhibited in the ganglion. These findings suggest that MM have a direct action on nerve tissues.

Proliferation of undifferentiated cell lines is also affected by MM *in vitro*. ^{3}H-thymidine incorporation into DNA of HeLa and skin fibroblasts is inhibited (565) and in one study an inhibitory effect of uraemic ultrafiltrate and of a MM-fraction on fibroblast proliferation and ^{3}H-thymidine incorporation was only observed in the presence of whole plasma (normal or uraemic), suggesting an interaction of MM toxins with macromolecules (563).

Intermediary metabolism *in vitro* can also be affected by presence of MM. An inhibitory effect of MM on glucose utilisation in several tissues and cells has been observed (498, 499, 564, 570). This is of interest since one established symptom of uraemia is glucose intolerance.

It was recently reported that the desalted fraction 7c but no other MM subfraction inhibited mitochondrial respiration (548, 579). A MM-fraction isolated by gel chromatography and thin layer chromatography from uraemic ultrafiltrate produced hypotension and in higher doses cardiotoxic effects in rats when injected intravenously (530).

Some enzyme activities are also inhibited by MM-fractions *in vitro*, namely lactate dehydrogenase (505), adenylate cyclase (515), pyruvate kinase, Na^+-K^+-ATPase and glukokinase (523), insulin stimulation of lipoprotein lipase (520), α-aminolaevulinic acid dehydrase (525, 570) and catalase activity (570).

In most of these bioassay studies MM-fractions were present in the medium in approximately the same concentrations as found in uraemic plasma. The results suggest that MM contribute to many symptoms and signs in uraemia such as anaemia, susceptibility to infection, immunological incompetence, bleeding, neuropathy, glucose intolerance and lipid changes. However, in most of these studies the effect of the uraemic MM-fractions *in vitro* were not compared with the corresponding fractions, isolated from non-uraemic individuals, but only to buffer blanks. Many buffers such as tris-HCL, EDTA and ammonium acetate can have a strong effect on the bioassay systems, used for detecting uraemic toxicity, and this has to be taken into consideration. A high ionic strength may also have an inhibitory effect (573). There is also a possibility that normal plasma may contain substances which after isolation exert inhibitory effects on cells *in vitro*. A critical review shows that of all *in vitro* studies made with more or less purified MM-fractions only a few were conducted with appropriate control samples from non-uraemic subjects (563, 568, 573).

Lipochromes

It is known that uraemic man and animals accumulate lipochromes (597, 598). These are medium-sized molecules, so-called carotenoids, that darken on exposure to UV. It was suggested that these substances might be responsible for the hyperpigmentation often seen in cases of advanced chronic renal failure. The dialysis characteristics suggest that some unidentified lipochromes have a molecular mass in the range of 600 to 1,000 daltons (597) and should be considered as MM.

Histochemical examination of skin biopsies indicates that the increased pigmentation observed clinically is associated with an increased amount of melanin. With the methods employed lipochrome deposition could however not be ruled out (599).

The trade-off hypothesis

According to this hypothesis, which was originated by Bricker (85) in 1972, certain humoral factors which may exert toxic effects accumulate in uraemia, not as a consequence of reduced renal excretion but due to homeostatic adaptation to the reduced glomerular filtration rate.

Parathyroid hormone (PTH)

An example of a trade-off effect is the increased secretion of PTH seen in uraemia.

The increase of plasma PTH occurs in part as a consequence of phosphate retention which by decreasing ionised calcium, stimulates the parathyroid glands to increase PTH-secretion. This in turn tends to lower the phosphate threshold and to increase phosphate excretion, thereby creating a new steady state with normal plasma phosphate and calcium but elevated PTH-secretion. In end-stage renal failure the PTH-secretion is elevated to an extent that toxic effects are encountered. An important consequence of the increased PTH-levels in uraemia is the development of bone disease, characterised by osteitis fibrosa. For that reason PTH is by definition a uraemic toxin. For a more comprehensive discussion of this subject the reader is referred to chapter 35.

Massry and Goldstein (600, 601) have recently suggested that PTH may have several additional toxic effects in uraemia, some of which are mediated by exaggerated stimulation of cyclic AMP. They suggest that the following uraemic manifestations could be induced by excessive plasma levels of PTH: encephalopathy, neuropathy, dialysis dementia, bone disease, aseptic necrosis, soft tissue calcification, soft tissue necrosis, myopathy, pruritus, carbohydrate intolerance, hyperlipidemia, anaemia and sexual dysfunction. In support of their hypothesis they cite a number of their own and other investigations and anecdotal observations. However,

Slatopolsky et al. (602) reviewed the role of PTH as a uraemic toxin and came to the conclusion that the only confirmed toxic effects are bone disease and abnormal electroencephalographic patterns (603, 605), the latter being explained by a potential role of PTH in increasing the calcium content of brain (605). A direct relationship was found between N-terminal PTH-levels and EEG abnormalities in dialysis patients (606). Some studies showed a correlation between impairment in peripheral nerve function and increased plasma PTH concentrations in renal failure (603, 607, 608). However, a recent study (609) failed to show any correlation between plasma parathyroid hormone concentrations, nerve conduction velocity and serum lipids in haemodialysis patients.

Anaemia of chronic renal failure is also suggested to be a feature of hyperparathyroidism, either because of myelofibrosis or from a direct toxic effect of PTH (601). Improvement of anaemia has been observed in patients with renal failure after parathyroidectomy (610–612). No correlation between haematocrit levels and biochemical indices of secondary hyperparathyroidism was observed in 96 long-term haemodialysis patients, and because of a group patients did not show a significant change in haematocrit levels after parathyroidectomy (613), Slatopolsky concluded that:

'With regard to PTH as a pathogenetic factor for carbohydrate intolerance, hyperlipidemia and anaemia, outstanding clinical research is lacking and conclusive experimental data are practically nonexistent. Thus, it is still an open question whether PTH as a uraemic toxin has more generalised effects than its action on bone and perhaps on the central nervous system.'

Natriuretic hormone
Bricker (85) postulated that a natriuretic hormone, which is stimulated by volume expansion, accounts for decreased fractional reabsorption of sodium in chronic uraemia when the glomerular filtration falls. In the end-stage of renal failure natriuretic hormone activity is assumed to be excessively high, exerting an inappropriate (toxic) effect on the active transport of sodium and other substances in all body cells.

The plasma and urine of chronic uraemic patients with high fractional sodium excretion rates contain a fraction, isolated by gel filtration, which inhibits sodium transport in the frog skin and the toad bladder, and appears to be natriuretic in the rat (258, 495, 614, 615). Chemically, the natriuretic factor which has a low molecular weight (less than 1,000) seems to be a peptide containing at least 7 amino acids (616, 617), apparently being a typical MM. How this factor is related to the MM fractions isolated by other groups and to the toxic manifestation in uraemic patients remains to be elucidated.

Larger polypeptides, proteins and other high-molecular weight compounds

The normal kidney removes proteins of a molecular mass below 50,000 by both luminal and contraluminal uptake in the proximal tubular cells, where they are degraded (618, 619). It would, therefore, not be surprising if chronic uraemia with lack of renal tissue would lead to accumulation of biologically active and potentially toxic compounds with a higher molecular weight than middle molecules. Some small molecular weight proteins appearing in increased concentrations in renal failure are β_2-microglobulin, lysozyme, retinol-binding protein, β_2-glucoproteins and ribonuclease (RNase) (620–627). Ribonuclease is a glycoprotein with a molecular mass of 33,000 daltons. Plasma RNase levels are markedly increased in uraemic patients and show a close relationship to plasma creatinine levels. They are however unaffected by dialysis (627, 628). Purified RNase from human urine is capable of inhibiting ^{3}H-thymidine uptake by lymphocytes stimulated by various mitogens, and of inhibiting growth of red and white cells in bone marrow cultures and also adversely affect the growth of pancreatic fibroblastoid cells *in vitro* (627). RNase has also an inhibiting effect on virus multiplication (629, 630) and on tumour cell growth *in vitro* (631). It was therefore suggested that the ribonuclease glucoprotein represents a large number of nondialysable high molecular weight toxins (627).

High-molecular fractions with a molecular mass of more than 10,000 daltons isolated from normal and uraemic urine or from uraemic plasma ultrafiltrate or dialysate have been shown to exert several adverse effects *in vitro*. Such fractions inhibit ^{3}H-thymidine and ^{59}Fe-incorporation in bone marrow cells (534, 555, 632), gluconeogenesis of kidney and liver slices (633, 634) and inhibit phytohaemagglutinin-stimulated lymphocyte transformation (635). A fraction of uraemic plasma with a molecular mass higher than 10,000 daltons inhibited the proliferation and digesting capacity of human mononuclear phagocytes, whereas the corresponding fraction from normal serum was inactive (536). The toxic fraction could not be removed by conventional haemodialysis with Cuprophan or polyacrylonitrile membranes (636). A new combined haemofiltration and dialysis system was designed wich selectively removes small and large molecules but returns middle molecules to the patient, since it was though that MM are benificial and should not be removed (637). Clinical experiences with this system are still inconclusive (638).

The cited *in vitro* studies suggest a role for high-molecular weight compounds in causing uraemic toxicity. Considering that such compounds are not readily removed by conventional dialysis treatment and that uraemic patients can be kept alive and thriving on intermittent dialysis for decades probably means that they are not major uraemic toxins.

Among compounds degraded by the kidneys are also a number of peptide hormones such as growth hormone, corticotropin, PTH, insulin, glucagon and gastrin. Plasma concentrations of PTH, insulin, growth hormone, glucagon, prolactin, and gastrin are, therefore, high in uraemic patients. The metabolic and toxic effects of these hormonal disorders are reported in Chapters 36 and 35 High plasma renin levels in uraemia and their role in hypertension are discussed in Chapter 28. All these compounds, which are in the upper middle molecular weight range or larger, pass poorly through conventional dialysis membranes.

CONCLUSIONS

In the first edition we wrote 'It is today not possible to evaluate the exact role of the manifold compounds which accumulate in renal failure in causing or contributing to the various symptoms and biochemical abnormalities of uraemia'. Four years later this still holds true. The new information gathered in these years has shed further light on the complexity of the problem but not led yet to a break-through in our understanding of the nature of uraemic toxicity. A better understanding of the nature of uraemic toxicity can only be achieved by combined efforts of clinical nephrologists, endocrinologists and biochemists, and this will hopefully lead to improvement of the conservative treatment of uraemia and the development of more efficient and selective methods for purification of the body fluids.

ACKNOWLEDGEMENTS

This work was supported by grants from NIAMDD (contract no. N01-AM-2-2215), Bethesda, Maryland, USA and the Medical Research Board (contract no. B82-191-1002-17B), Sweden.

REFERENCES

1. Prevost JL, Dumas JA: Examen du sang et de son action dans les divers phénomènes de la vie. (Examination of the blood and its action in the different phenomena of life) *Ann Chim Phys* 23:90, 1821 (in French)
2. Schreiner GE, Maher JF: *Uremia: Biochemistry, Pathogenesis and Treatment.* Springfield, Illinois, USA, Charles C Thomas, 1961
3. Welt LG, Sachs JR, McManus TJ: An ion transport defect in erythrocytes from uremic patients. *Trans Assoc Am Physicians* 77:169, 1964
4. Edmondson RPS, Hilton PJ, Jones NF, Patrick J, Thomas RD: Leucocyte sodium transport in uraemia. *Clin Sci Mol Med* 49:213, 1975
5. Bolte HD, Riecker G, Röhl D: Measurements of membrane potential of individual muscle cells in normal men and patients with renal insufficiency. *Proc 2nd Int Congr Nephrol (Prague),* edited by Vostál J, Richet G, Basel, S Karger, 1963, p 114
6. Cunningham JN, Carter NW, Rector FC Jr, Selding DW: Resting transmembrane potential difference of skeletal muscle in normal subjects and severely ill patients. *J Clin Invest* 50:49, 1971
7. Bilbrey GL, Carter NW, White MG, Schilling JF, Knochel JP: Potassium deficiency in chronic renal failure. *Kidney Int* 4:423, 1973
8. Cotton JR, Woodard T, Carter NW, Knochel JP: Resting skeletal muscle membrane potential as an index of uremic toxicity. A proposed new method to assess adequacy of hemodialysis. *J Clin Invest* 63:501, 1979
9. Welt LG, Smith EKM, Dunn MJ, Szerwinski A, Proctor H, Cole C, Balfe JW, Gitelman HJ: Membrane transport defect; the sick cell. *Trans Assoc Am Physicians* 80:217, 1967
10. Teschan PE, O'Brien TF, Baxter CR: Prophylactic daily hemodialysis in the treatment of acute renal failure. *Clin Res* 7:280, 1959
11. Einheber A, Carter D: The role of the microbial flora in uremia. I. Survival times of germfree, limited-flora, and conventionalized rats after bilateral nephrectomy and fasting. *J Exp Med* 123:239, 1966
12. Carter D, Einheber A, Bauer H, Rosen H, Burns WF: The role of the microbial flora in uremia. II. Uremic colitis, cardiovascular lesions, and biochemical observations. *J Exp Med* 123:251, 1966
13. Simenhoff ML, Burke JF, Saukkonen JJ, Wesson LG, Schaedler RW: Amine metabolism and the small bowel in uraemia. *Lancet* 2:818, 1976
14. Simenhoff ML, Saukkonen JJ, Burke JF, Wesson LG, Schaedler RW, Gordon SJ: Bacterial populations of the small intestine in uremia. *Nephron* 22:63, 1978
15. Henkin RE, Byatt PH, Maxwell MH: Evidence for the presence of a dialyzable 'toxic' factor in the sera of uremic subjects. *Clin Res* 9:202, 1961
16. Henkin RE, Levine ND, Sussman HH, Maxwell MH: Evidence for the presence of substances toxic for HeLa cells in the serum and in the dialysis fluid of patients with glomerulonephritis. *J Lab Clin Med* 64:79, 1964
17. Yendt ER, Connor TB, Howard JE: In vitro calcification of rachitic rat cartilage in normal and pathological human sera with some observations on the pathogenesis of renal rickets. *Bull. Johns Hopkins Hosp* 96:1, 1955
18. Oreopoulos D, Pitel S, Husdan H, De Veber GA, Rapoport A: Contrasting effect of hemodialysis and peritoneal dialysis on the inhibition of in vitro calcification by uremic serum. *Can Med Assoc J* 110:43, 1974
19. Sacchetti C: Physiopathologie des érythroblastes dans l'anémie des azotémies chroniques (Physiopathology of the erythroblasts in the anaemia of chronic azotaemia). *Acta Haematol (Basel)* 9:97, 1953 (in French)
20. Markson JL, Rennie JB: The anaemia of chronic renal insufficiency: the effect of serum from azotaemic patients on maturation of normoblasts in suspension cultures. *Scott Med J* 1:320, 1956
21. Berman L, Powsner ER: Review of methods for studying maturation of human erythroblasts in vitro: evaluation of a new method of culture of cell suspensions in a clot-free medium. *Blood* 14:1194, 1959
22. Baldini M, Panacciulli I: The maturation rate of reticulocytes. *Blood* 15:614, 1960
23. Erslev AJ, Hughes JR: The influence of environment on iron incorporation and mitotic division in a suspension of normal bone marrow. *Br J Haematol* 6:414, 1960
24. Bozzini CE, Devoto FC, Tomio JM: Decreased responsiveness of hematopoietic tissue to erythropoietin in acutely uremic rats. *J Lab Clin Med* 68:411, 1966
25. Kuroyanagi T, Saito M: Presence of toxic substances which inhibit erythropoiesis in serum of uremic nephrectomized rabbits. *Tohoku J Exp Med* 88:117, 1966
26. Fisher JW, Hatch FE, Roh BL, Allen RC, Kelley BJ: Erythropoietin inhibitor in kidney and plasma from anemic uremic human subjects. *Blood* 31:440, 1968
27. Lamperi S, Bandiani G, Fiorio P, Muttini P, Scaringi G: Effects of some substances retained in uremia on erythropoiesis: the effect on bone marrow cell cultures. *Nephron* 13:278, 1974
28. Moriyama Y, Rege A, Fisher JW: Studies on an inhibitor of erythropoiesis. II. Inhibitory effects of serum from uremic rabbits on heme synthesis in rabbit bone marrow cultures. *Proc Soc Exp Biol Med* 148:94, 1975

29. Wallner SF, Vautrin RM, Kurnick JE, Ward HP: The effect of serum from patients with chronic renal failure on erythroid colony growth in vitro. *J Lab Clin Med* 92:370, 1978
30. Mitelman M, Levi J, Djaldetti M: Functional activity of uremic erythroblasts incubated in autologous and homologous plasma. *Blut* 38:467, 1979
31. Rachmilewitz M: Effect of uremic serum and urine on growth of fibroblasts in vitro. *Arch Intern Med* 67:1132, 1941
32. McDermott FT: The effect of 10% human uremic serum upon human fibroblastic cell cultures. *J Surg Res* 11:119, 1971
33. Silk MR: The effect of uremic plasma on lymphocyte transformation. *Invest Urol* 5:195, 1967
34. Kasakura S, Lowenstein L: The effect of uremic blood on mixed leucocyte reactions and on cultures of leucocytes with phytohemagglutinin. *Transplantation* 5:283, 1967
35. Newberry WM, Sanford JP: Defective cellular immunity in renal failure: depression of reactivity of lymphocytes to phytohemagglutinin by renal failure serum. *J Clin Invest* 50:1262, 1971
36. Slavin RG, Orlin JF, Fisher VW: The effect of uremic serum on normal human and guinea pig lymphocytes. *Proc Soc Exp Biol Med* 148:1229, 1975
37. Touraine JL, Touraine F, Revillard JP, Brocher J, Traeger J: T-lymphocytes and serum inhibitors of cell-mediated immunity in renal insufficiency. *Nephron* 14:195, 1975
38. Jørstad S, Viken KE: Inhibitory effects of plasma from Uraemic patients on human mononuclear inagocytes cultured in vitro. *Acta Path Microbiol Scand [Sect C]* 85:169, 1977
39. Horowitz HI, Cohen BD, Marinez P, Papayoanou MF: Defective ADP-induced platelet factor 3 activation in uremia. *Blood* 30:331, 1967
40. Giovannetti S, Balestri PL, Cioni L: Spontaneous in vitro autohaemolysis of blood from chronic uraemic patients. *Clin Sci* 29:407, 1965
41. Hörl WH, Heiland A: Enhanced proteolytic activity – cause of protein catabolism in acute renal failure. *Am J Clin Nutr* 33:1423, 1980
42. Morgan JM, Morgan RE: Study of the effect of uremic metabolites on erythrocyte glycolysis. *Metabolism* 13:629, 1964
43. Dzúrik R, Krajči-Lazáry B: The effect of uremic serum on carbohydrate metabolism in rat diaphragm. *Experientia* 23:798, 1967
44. Renner D, Heintz R: Oxygen consumption and utilization of carbohydrate and fat metabolites in kidney cortex slices and in brain homogenate using sera of chronic uraemic patients. *Proc Eur Dial Transpl Assoc* 2:128, 1965
45. Dzúrik R, Niederland TR, Černáček P: Abnormal carbohydrate metabolism in liver slices incubated in uremic serum. *Clin Sci* 37:409, 1969
46. Renner D, Heintz R: Der Einfluß urämischen Serums auf die Glucose-neubilding und auf die aktivierte Essigsäure in Gewebeschnitten. Untersuchungen zur urämischen Intoxikation (The influence of uraemic serum on gluconeogenesis and on activated acetic acid in tissue slides. Investigations on uraemic intoxication). *Klin Wochenschr* 51:82, 1973 (in German)
47. Delaporte C, Gros F, Anaguostopoulos T: Inhibitory effects of plasma dialysate on protein synthesis in vitro: influence of dialysis and transplantation. *Am J Clin Nutr* 33:1407, 1980
48. Heintz R, Renner D: Über Hemmwirkungen des Serums von Kranken mit hepatorenalem Syndrom und mit chronischer Urämie auf Sauerstoffverbrauch und Kohlenhydratstoffwechsel von Nieren- und Hirngewebe der Ratte (On inhibition by serum from patients with a hepato-renal syndrome and chronic uraemia of the oxygen consumption and carbohydrate metabolism of rat kidney and brain tissue). *Klin Wochenschr* 43:1167, 1965 (in German)
49. Glaze RP, Morgan JM, Morgan RE: Uncoupling of oxidative phosphorylation by ultrafiltrates of uremic serum. *Proc Soc Exp Biol Med* 125:172, 1967
50. Yamada T, Yoshida A, Koshikawa S: Alteration of oxidative phosphorylation in uremia. *Jpn Circ J* 33:59, 1969
51. Bennett NB, Ogston D: Inhibitors of the fibrinolytic enzyme system in renal disease. *Clin Sci* 39:549, 1970
52. Boyer JL, Scheig RL: Inhibition of postheparin lipolytic activity in uremia and its relationship to hypertriglyceridemia *Proc Soc Exp Biol Med* 134:603, 1970
53. Bittar EE: Maia muscle fibre as a model for the study of uraemic toxicity. *Nature* 214:310, 1967
54. Bittar EE: The effect of uremic plasma on the efflux of sodium from the toad oocyte. *Proc 4th International Congr Nephrol, Stockholm,* edited by Alwall N, Berglund F, Josephson B, Basel, S Karger, 1969, p 47
55. Buckalew VM Jr, Nelson DB: Natriuretic and sodium transport inhibitory activity in plasma of volume-expanded dogs. *Kidney Int* 5:12, 1974
56. Kramer HJ, Gospodinov D, Kruck F: Functional and metabolic studies on red blood cell sodium transport in chronic uremia. *Nephron* 16:344, 1976
57. Flanigan WJ, Anderson DS, Stout K, Koike TI: Site of action of an uremic serum fraction inhibiting sodium transport in frog skin. *Nephron* 22:117, 1978
58. Russell JE, Avioli LV: The effect of chronic uremia on intestinal mitochondrial activity. *J Lab Clin Med* 84:317, 1974
59. Kuroyanagi T, Kurisu A, Sugiyama H, Saito M: The ADP and ATP levels and the phosphorylating activity of erythrocytes in patients with uremia associated with chronic renal disease. *Tohoku J Exp Med* 84:105, 1964
60. Podevin R, Paillard F, Richet G: Action of uremic serum on uric acid 2-^{14}C transport by isolated renal tubules. *Proc 4th Int Congr Nephrol Stockholm,* edited by Alwall N, Berglund F, Josephson B, Basel, S Karger, 1969, p 49
61. White AG, Nachev P: Uremic inhibition of purine uptake by rat hepatic slices. *Am J Physiol* 228:436, 1975
62. White AG: Uremic serum inhibition of renal paraaminohippurate transport. *Proc Soc Exp Biol Med* 123:309, 1966
63. Bricker NS, Klahr S, Purkerson M, Schultze RG, Avioli LV, Birge SJ: In vitro assay for a humoral substance present during volume expansion and uraemia. *Nature* 219:1058, 1968
64. Ciccone JR, Keller AI, Braun SR, Murdaugh HV, Preuss HG: Azotemic inhibition of organic acid transport in the liver. *Biochim Biophys Acta* 163:108, 1968
65. Bourke E, Frindt G, Preuss H, Rose E, Weksler M, Schreiner GE: Studies with uraemic serum on the renal transport of hippurates and tetraethylammonium in the rabbit and rat: effects of oral neomycin. *Clin Sci* 38:41, 1970
66. Orringer EP, Weiss FR, Preuss HG: Azotaemic inhibition of organic anion transport in the kidney of the rat: mechanisms and characteristics. *Clin Sci* 40:159, 1971
67. Černáček P, Spustová V, Dzúrik R: Inhibitor(s) of Protein Synthesis in Uremic Serum and Urine: partial Purification and Relationship to Amino Acid Transport. *Biochem Med* 27:305, 1982
68. Jennette JC, Goldman ID: Inhibition of the membrane transport of folates by anions retained in uremia. *J Lab Clin Med* 86:834, 1975

69. Morgan JM, Morgan RE, Thomas GE: Inhibition of lactic dehydrogenase by ultrafiltrate of uremic blood. *Metabolism* 12:1051, 1963
70. Emerson PM, Withycombe WA, Wilkinson JH: Inhibition of lactate dehydrogenase by sera of uraemic patients. *Lancet* 2:571, 1965
71. Murase T, Cattran DC, Ubenstein B, Steiner G: Inhibition of lipoprotein lipase by uremic plasma, a possible cause of hypertriglyceridemia. *Metabolism* 24:1279, 1975
72. Bagdade JD, Shafrir E, Wilson DE: Mechanism(s) of hyperlipidemia in chronic uremia. *Trans Am Soc Artif Intern Organs* 22:42, 1976
73. Young GA, Parsons FM: Impairment of phenylalanine hydroxylation in chronic renal insufficiency. *Clin Sci Mol Med* 45:89, 1973
74. Cole CH, Balfe JW, Welt LG: Induction of a ouabain-sensitive ATPase defect by uremic plasma. *Trans Ass Am Physicians* 81:213, 1968
75. Minkoff L, Gaertner G, Darab M, Mercier C, Levin ML: Inhibition of brain sodium-potassium ATPase in uremic rats. *J Lab Clin Med* 80:71, 1972
76. Korz R, Loebnitz U, Brunner H, Heintz R: Lymphocyte enzymes of DNA-synthesis in chronic renal failure. *Proc Eur Dial Transpl Assoc* 13:528, 1977
77. Pazmino PA, Sladek SL, Weinshilboum RM: Thiol S-methylation in uremia: Erythrocyte enzyme activities and plasma inhibitors. *Clin Pharmacol Ther* 28:356, 1980
78. Lonergan ET, Semar M, Lange K: Transketolase activity in uremia. *Arch Intern Med* 126:851, 1970
79. Lonergan ET, Semar M, Sterzel RB, Treser G, Needle MA, Voyles L, Lange K: Erythrocyte transketolase activity in dialyzed patients. *New Engl J Med* 284:1399, 1971
80. McVicar M, Gauthier B, Goodman CT: Uremic neuropathy. Monitoring of transketolase activity inhibition in a child. *Am J Dis Child* 125:263, 1973
81. Kuriyama M, Mizuma A, Jokomine R, Igata A, Otuji J: Erythrocyte transketolase activity in uremia. *Clin Chim Acta* 108:169, 1980
82. Sterzel RB, Semar M, Lonergan ET, Treser G, Lange K: Relationship of nervous tissue transketolase to the neuropathy in chronic uremia. *J Clin Invest* 50:2295, 1971
83. Warnock LG, Cullum UX, Stouder DA, Stone WJ: Erythrocyte transketolase activity in dialysis patients with neuropathy. *Biochem Med* 10:351, 1974
84. Dirige OV, Jacob M, Wang M, Swendseid ME, Kopple JD: Transketolase activity in tissues of uremic rats. *J Nutr* 103:1723, 1973
85. Bricker NS: On the pathogenesis of the uremic state. An exposition of the 'trade-off hypothesis'. *New Engl J Med* 286:1093, 1972
86. Arieff AI, Guisado R: Effects on the central nervous system of hypernatremic and hyponatremic states. *Kidney Int* 10:104, 1976
87. Platt R: Sodium and potassium excretion in chronic renal failure. *Clin Sci* 9:367, 1950
88. Platt R: Structural and functional adaptation in renal failure. *Br Med J* 1:1313 and 1372, 1952
89. Bricker NS. Fine LG, Kaplan M, Epstein M, Bourgoignie JJ, Light A: 'Magnification Phenomenon' in chronic renal disease. *New Engl J Med* 299:1287, 1978
90. Balfour WE, Grantham JS, Glynn IM: Vanadate-stimulated natriuresis. *Nature* 275:768, 1978
91. Bello-Reuss EN, Grady T, Mazumdar EC: Serum vanadium levels in chronic renal disease. *Ann Internal Med* 91:743, 1979
92. Fine LG, Bourgoignie JJ, Weber H, Bricker NS: Enhanced end-organ responsiveness of the uremic kidney to the natriuretic factor. *Kidney Int* 10:364, 1976
93. Edelman IS, Leibman J, O'Meara MP, Birkenfeld LW: Interrelations between serum sodium concentration, serum osmolarity and total exchangeable sodium, total exchangeable potassium and total body water. *J Clin Invest* 37:1236, 1958
94. Comty CM: A longitudinal study of body composition in terminal uremics treated by regular hemodialysis: I. Body composition before treatment. *Can Med Assoc J* 98:482, 1968
95. Bergström J: Muscle electrolytes in man. Determined by neutron activation analysis in needle biopsy specimens. A study on normal subjects, kidney patients, and patients with chronic diarrhoea. *Scand J Clin Lab Invest* 14:(Suppl 68), 1962
96. Villamil MF, Yeyati N, Rubianes C, Taquini AC: Water and electrolyte of muscle in chronic renal failure. *Acta Physiol Lat Am* 13:184, 1963
97. Graham JA, Paton AM, Linton AL: Body water and electrolyte composition in acute renal failure. *Can Med Assoc J* 104:1000, 1971
98. Bergström J, Hultman E: Water, electrolyte and glycogen content of muscle tissue in patients undergoing regular dialysis therapy. *Clin Nephrol* 2:24, 1974
99. Broyer M, Delaporte C, Maziere B: Water, electrolytes and protein content of muscle obtained by needle biopsy in uremic children. *Biomedicine* 21:278, 1974
100. Patrick J, Jones NF: Cell sodium, potassium and water in uraemia and the effects of regular dialysis as studied in the leucocyte. *Clin Sci Mol Med* 46:583, 1974
101. Teschan PE, Post RS, Smith LH, Abernathy RS, Davis JH, Gray DM, Howard JM, Johnson KE, Klopp E, Mundy RL, O'Meara MP, Rush BJ: Post.traumatic renal insufficiency in military casualties. *Am J Med* 18:172, 1955
102. Keating RE, Weichselbaum TE. Alanis M, Margraf HW, Elman R: The movement of potassium during experimental acidosis and alkalosis in the nephrectomized dog. *Surg Gynec Obstet* 96:323, 1953
103. Scribner BH, Burnell JM: Interpretation of the serum potassium concentration *Metabolism* 5:468, 1956
104. Fenn WO: The deposition of potassium and phosphate with glycogen in rat livers. *J Biol Chem* 128:297, 1939
105. Bergström J, Beroniade V, Hultman E, Roch-Norlund AE: Relation between glycogen and electrolyte metabolism in human muscle. In: *Transport und Funktion Intracellulärer Elektrolyte,* edited by Kruck F, München-Berlin-Wien, Urban & Schwarzenberg, 1967, p 108
106. Pankow DZ: Einfluss des Harnstoffs auf die Kaliumchloridvergiftung bei Mäusen (The influence of urea on potassiumchloride intoxication in mice). *Klin Wochenschr* 46:1005, 1968 (in German)
107. Pankow D, Pohle K: Untersuchungen zur Frage einer Beeinflussung der bei Urämie drohenden K⁺-Vergiftung durch Harnstoff (Investigations on the effect of urea on imminent potassium intoxication in uraemia). *Z Klin Chem* 6:369, 1968 (in German)
108. Bergström J, Bittar EE: The basis of uremic toxicity, chapter 14. In: *The Biological Basis of Medicine,* edited by Bittar E, Bittar N, New York, Academic Press, 1969, vol 6, p 495
109. Bergström J, Hultman E: Muscle composition in chronic renal failure. *Minerva Nefrol* 16:1, 1969
110. Van Ypersele de Strihou C: Potassium homeostatis in renal failure. *Kidney Int* 11:491, 1977
111. Hayes CP, McLeod ME, Robinson RR, Stead EA: An extrarenal mechanism for the maintenance of potassium balance in severe chronic renal failure. *Trans Assoc Am Physicians* 80:207, 1967
112. Winkler AW, Hoff HE, Smith PK: The toxicity of orally

administered potassium salts in renal insufficiency. *J Clin Invest* 20:119, 1941
113. Campanacci L, Maschio G, Poli D, Mioni G, Rizzo A, Bazzato G, Riz G: Il muscolo nell'uremia cronica. Reperti morfologici e biochimici compiuti con l'ausilio dell'agobiopsia muscolare (The muscle in chronic uraemia. Morphological and biochemical investigations with the help of muscle needle biopsy). *G Clin Med* 48:1252, 1967 (in Italian)
114. Rector FC Jr: Renal acidification and ammonia production; chemistry of weak acids and bases; buffer mechanisms. In: *The Kidney*, edited by Brenner BR, Rector FC Jr, Philadelphia, London, Toronto, WB Saunders Company 1st edn, 1976, vol. 1, p 318
115. Sebastian A, McSherry E, Morris RC Jr: Metabolic acidosis with special reference to the renal acidoses. In: The Kidney, edited by Brenner BR, Rector FC Jr, Philadelphia, London, Toronto, WB Saunders Company 1st edn, 1976, vol. 1, p 615
116. Relman AS: The acidosis of renal disease. *Am J Med* 44:706, 1968
117. Elkinton JR, McCurdy DK, Buckalew BM Jr: Hydrogen ion and the kidney. In: *Renal Disease*, edited by Black DAK, Philadelphia, PA Davis Co, 2nd edn, 1967, p 110
118. Palmer WW, Henderson LJ: A study of the several factors of acid excretion in nephritis. *Arch Intern Med* 16:109, 1915
119. Van Slyke DD, Linder GC, Hiller A, Leiter L, McIntosh JF: The excretion of ammonia and titratable acid in nephritis. *J Clin Invest* 2:255, 1926
120. Buckalew VM Jr, Morrison AB: Chronic acidosis in subtotally nephrectomized rats. *Arch Pathol* 73:241, 1962
121. Simpson DP: Control of hydrogen ion hemeostasis and renal acidosis. *Medicine (Baltimore)* 50:503, 1971
122. Schwartz WB, Hall PW, Hays RM, Relman AS: On the mechanism of acidosis in chronic renal disease. *J Clin Invest* 38:39, 1959
123. Hellman DE, Au WY, Barter FC: Evidence for a direct effect of parathyroid hormone on urinary acidification. *Am J Physiol* 209:643, 1965
124. Muldowney FP, Donahoe JF, Carroll DV, Powell D, Freaney R: Parathyroid acidosis in uraemia. *Quart J Med* 163:321, 1972
125. Goodman AD, Lemann J Jr, Lennon EJ, Relman AS: Production, excretion of acid in health and disease. *J Clin Invest* 44:495, 1965
126. Lemann J Jr, Litzow JR, Lennon EJ: The effects of chronic acid loads in normal man. Further evidence of the participation of bone mineral in the defense against chronic metabolic acidosis. *J Clint Invest* 45:1608, 1966
127. Litzow JR, Lemann J Jr, Lennon EJ: The effect of treatment of acidosis on calcium balance in patients with chronic azotemic renal disease. *J Clin Invest* 46:280, 1967
128. Maschio G, Bazzato G, Beroglia E, Sardini D, Mioni G, D'Angelo A, Marzo A: Intracellular pH and electrolyte content of skeletal muscle in patients with chronic renal acidosis. *Nephron* 7:481, 1970
129. Levin GE, Baron DN: Leucocyte intracellular pH in patients with the metabolic acidosis of renal failure. *Clin Sci Mol Med* 52:325, 1977
130. Robinson RR, Murdaugh HV, Peschel E: Renal factors responsible for the hypermagnesemia of renal disease. *J Lab Clin Med* 53:572, 1959
131. Hamburger J: Electrolyte disturbances in acute uremia. *Clin Chem* 3:332, 1957
132. Wacker WEC, Vallee BL: Magnesium metabolism. *N Engl J Med* 259:431, 1958

133. Schwartz WB, Polak A: Electrolyte disorders in chronic renal disease. *J Chron Dis* 11:319, 1960
134. Randall RE Jr, Cohen MD, Spray CC Jr, Rossmeisl EC: Hypermagnesemia in renal failure. Etiology and toxic manifestations. *Ann Intern Med* 61:73, 1964
135. Goldman R, Bassett S: Phosphorus excretion in renal failure. *J Clin Invest* 33:1623, 1954
136. Editorial (Anonymous): Hyperphosphataemia and renal function. *Lancet* 1:753, 1978
137. Ibels LS, Alfrey AC, Haut L, Huffer WE: Preservation of function in experimental renal disease by dietary restriction of phosphate. *New Engl J Med* 298:122, 1978
138. Karlinsky ML, Haut L, Buddington B, Schrier NA, Alfrey AC: Preservation of renal function in experimental glomerulonephritis. *Kidney Int* 17:293, 1980
139. Walser M, Mitch WE, Collier VU: The effect of nutritional therapy on the course of chronic renal failure. *Clin Nephrol* 11:66, 1979
140. Barsotti G, Guiducci A, Ciardella F, Giovannetti S: Effects on renal function of a low-nitrogen diet supplemented with essential amino-acids and ketoanalogues and of hemodialysis and free protein supply in patients with chronic renal failure. *Nephron* 27:113, 1981
141. Maschio G: Long-term effects of dietary phosphate restriction in chronic renal failure (CRF). *Abstracts, 3rd Conference on Chronic Uremia*, Capri, Aug-Sep, 1980
142. Tallgren LG: Inorganic sulphates in relation to the serum thyroxine level and in renal failure. *Acta Med Scand* *[Suppl]*640, 1980
143. Hänze S: Serumsulfat und Sulfatclearance bei normaler und eingeschränkter Nierenfunktion (Serumsulphate and sulphate clearance in normal renal function and in renal failure). *Klin Wochenschr* 44:1247, 1966 (in German)
144. Michalk D, Klare B, Manz F, Schärer K: Plasma inorganic sulfate in children with chronic renal failure. *Clin Nephrol* 16:8, 1981
145. Freeman RM, Richards CJ: Studies on sulfate in end-stage renal disease. *Kidney Int* 15:167, 1979
146. Lascelles PT, Taylor WH: The effect upon tissue respiration in vitro of metabolites which accumulate in uraemic coma. *Clin Sci* 31:403, 1966
147. Scheuer J, Stezoski SW: The effect of uraemic compounds on cardiac function and metabolism. *J Mol Cell Cardiol* 5:287, 1973
148. Perez GO, Rietberg B, Owens B, Schiff ER: Effect of acute uraemia on arginine metabolism and urea and guanidino acid production by perfused rat liver. *Pflügers Arch* 372:275, 1977
149. Archibald RM: Determination of citrulline and allantoin and demonstration of citrulline in blood plasma. *J Biochem* 156:121, 1974
150. Bondy PK, Engel FL, Farrar B: Metabolism of amino acids and protein in adrenalectomized and nephrectomized rats. *Endocrinology* 44:476, 1949
151. Frohlich J, Scholmerich M, Hoppe-Seyler G, Maier KP, Falke H, Schollmeyer P, Gerok W: The effect of acute uraemia on gluconeogenesis in isolated perfused rat livers. *Eur J Clin Invest* 4:453, 1974
152. Lacy WW: Effect of acute uremia on amino acid uptake and urea production by perfused rat liver. *Am J Physiol* 216:1300, 1969
153. Sellers AL, Katz J, Marmorston J: Effect of bilateral nephrectomy on urea formation in rat liver slices. *Am J Physiol* 191:345, 1957
154. Hoppe-Seyler G, Maier KP, Schollmeyer P, Frohlich J, Falke H, Gerok W: Studies on urea cycle enzymes in rat liver during acute uraemia. *Eur J Clin Invest* 5:15, 1975
155. Chao FC, Tarver H: Breakdown of urea in the rat. *Proc*

Soc Exp Biol Med 84:406, 1953
156. Levenson SM, Crowley LV, Horowitz RE, Malm OJ: The metabolism of carbon-labeled urea in the germfree rat. J Biol Chem 234:2061, 1959
157. Walser M, Bodenlos LJ: Urea metabolism in man. J Clin Invest 38:1617, 1959
158. Richard P: Nutritional potential of nitrogen recycling in man. Am J Clin Nutr 25:615, 1972
159. Walser M: Urea metabolism in chronic renal failure. J Clin Invest 53:1385, 1974
160. Christison R: Observations on the variety of dropsy which depends on diseased kidneys. Edinburgh Med Surg 32:262, 1829
161. Christison R: On Granular Degeneration of the Kidneys and its Connection with Dropsy, Inflammation and other Diseases, Philadelphia, PA, A Waldie 1839, p 146
162. Bright R: Reports of Medical Cases, Selected with a View of Illustrating the Symptoms and Cure of Disease by a Reference to Morbid Anatomy, London, Longman, Rees, Orme, Brown and Green, vol 2, 1831
163. Bouchard quoted by Ascoli G: Vorlesungen über Urämie (Lectures on Uraemia), Jena, Fischer, 1903, p 296 (in German)
164. Grollman EF, Grollman A: Toxicity of urea and its role in the pathogenesis of uremia. J Clin Invest 38:749, 1959
165. Bollman JL, Mann FC: Nitrogenous constituents of blood following transplantation of ureters into different levels of intestine. Proc Soc Exp Biol Med 24:923, 1927
166. Gilboe DD, Javid MJ: Breakdown products of urea and uremic syndrome. Proc Soc Exp Biol Med 115:633, 1964
167. Flückiger R, Harmon W, Meier W, Loo S, Gabbay KH: Hemoglobin carbamylation in uremia. New Engl J Med 304:823, 1981
168. Bachmann K, Valentovic M, Shapiro R: A possible role for cyanate in the albumin binding defect of uraemia. Biochem Pharmacol 29:1598, 1980
169. Yatzidis H, Koutsicos D, Vlassopoulos D, Cristodoulos D, Yulis G: Studies on cyanide and thiocyanate in uraemia. Int J Artif Organs 4:60, 1981
170. Teschan PW: Studies in the pathogenesis of uremic encephalopathy, in Uremia, edited by Kluthe R, Berlyne GM, Burton B, Stuttgart, Georg Thieme Verlag, 1972, p 32
171. Sen DK: Uraemia and its treatment by arginase inhibitor. Nature 184:459, 1959
172. Merrill JP, Legrain M, Hoigne R: Observations on the role of urea in uremia. Am J Med 14:519, 1953
173. Johnson WJ, Hagge WW, Wagoner RD, Dinapoli RP, Rosevear JW: Effects of urea loading in patients with far-advanced renal failure. Mayo Clin Proc 47:21, 1972
174. Hegstrom RM, Murray JS, Pendras JP, Burnell JM, Scribner BH: two years experience with periodic hemodialysis in the treatment of chronic uremia. Trans Am Soc Artif Intern Organs 8:266, 1962
175. Hutchings RH, Hegstrom RM, Scribner BH: Glucose intolerance in patients on long-term intermittent dialysis. Ann Intern Med 65:275, 1966
176. Rajogopalan KV, Fridovich I, Handler P: Inhibition of enzyme activity by urea. Fed Proc 19:49, 1960
177. Giordano C, Crescenzi A: Riduzione del consumo di ossigeno di feetine ed omogenati di organo da parte dell'urea (Decrease of oxygen consumption of fetal bone tissue and of organ homogenates by urea). Boll Soc Ital Biol Sper 37:1199, 1961 (in Italian)
178. Giordano C, Bloom J, Merrill JP: Effects of urea on physiologic systems. I. Studies on monoamine oxidase activity. J Lab Clin Med 59:396, 1962

179. Emerson PM, Wilkinson JH: Urea and oxalate inhibition of the serum lactate dehydrogenase. J Clin Pathol 18:803, 1965
180. Menyhart J, Gróf J: Urea as a selective inhibitor of argininosuccinate lyase. Eur J Biochem 75:405, 1977
181. Balestri PL, Biagini M, Rindi P, Giovannetti S: Uremic toxins. Arch Intern Med 126:843, 1970
182. Giovannetti S, Balestri L, Biagini M, Menichini G, Rindi P: Implications of dietary therapy. Arch Intern Med 126:900, 1970
183. Balestri PL, Rindi P, Biagini M, Giovannetti S: Effects of uraemic serum, urea, creatinine and methylguanidine on glucose metabolism. Clin Sci 42:395, 1972
184. Perkoff GT, Thomas CL, Newton JD, Sellman JC, Tyler FH: Mechanism of impaired glucose tolerance in uremia and experimental hyperazotemia. Diabetes 7:375, 1958
185. Martinelli R, Rodrigues Lea, Machado AE, Rocha H: The effect of acute uremia on liver mitochondrial activity. Nephron 17:155, 1976
186. Schumacher K, Schneider W, Alzer G, Oerkermann H: The influence of urea on protein synthesis of stimulated lymphocytes. Klin Wochenschr 50:929, 1972
187. Baur M: Zur Pharmakologie des Harnstoffs (Beiträge zum Problem der Urämie) (On the pharmacology of urea [Contribution to the problem of uraemia]). Naynyn-Schmiedebergs Arch Exp Path Pharm 167:104, 1932 (in German)
188. Davis JW, Field MC Jr, Phillips PE, Graham BA: Effects of exogenous urea, creatinine and guanidino succinic acid on human platelet aggregation in vitro. Blood 39:388, 1972
189. Somer JB, Stewart JH, Castaldi PA: The effect of urea on the aggregation of normal human platelets. Thromb Diath Haemorrh 19:64, 1968
190. Kersting F, Brass H: The effects of uraemic compounds on oxygen consumption and mechanical activity of isolated guinea pig hearts. Proc Eur Dial Transpl Assoc 13:472, 1977
191. Penpargkul S, Kuziak J, Scheuer J: Effect of uraemia upon carbohydrate metabolism in isolated perfused rat heart. J Mol Cell Cardiol 7:499, 1975
192. Leber HW, Streitzig P, Kayser M, Schütterle G: Influence of uremia on drug-metabolizing enzymes in rat liver microsomes. In: Uremia, edited by Kluthe R, Berlyne GM, Burton B, Stuttgart, Georg Thieme Verlag, 1972, p 37
193. Liang MY, Toporek M, Schepartz B: Screening uremic 'toxins' using bromosulfophthalein clearance by the isolated perfused rat liver. Nephron 22:306, 1978
194. Rose WC, Dimmitt FW: Experimental studies on creatine and creatinine. VII. The fate of creatine and creatinine when administered to man. J Biol Chem 26:345, 1916
195. Shannon JA: The renal excretion of creatinine in man. J Clin Invest 14:403, 1935
196. Mason MF, Resnik H, Mino AS, Rainey J, Pilcher C, Harrison TR: Mechanism of experimental uremia. Arch Intern Med 60:312, 1937
197. Giovannetti S, Cioni L, Balestri PL, Biagini M: Evidence that guanidines and some related compounds cause haemolysis in chronic uraemia. Clin Sci 34:141, 1968
198. Dobbelstein H, Edel HH, Schmidt M, Schubert G, Weinzierl M: Guanidinbernsteinsäure und urämie: 1. Klinische Untersuchungen (Guanidino-succinic acid and uraemia. 1. Clinical investigations). Klin Wochenschr 49:348, 1971 (in German)
199. Dobbelstein H, Korner WF, Weinzierl M, Schmidt M, Schubert G, Grunst J, Edel HH: Pathophysiologic aspects of guanidinosuccinic acid (GSA) in uremia. In: Uremia, edited by Kluthe R, Berlyne GM, Burton B, Stuttgart, Georg Thieme Verlag, 1972, p 7

200. Ohno Y, Rege AB, Fischer JW, Barona J: Inhibitor of erythroid colonyforming cells (CFU-E and BFU-E) in sera of azotemic patients with anemia of renal disease. *J Lab Clin Med* 92:16, 1978
201. Jones JD, Burnett PC: Implication of creatinine and gut flora in the uremic syndrome: induction of 'creatininase' in colon contents of the rat by dietary creatinine. *Clin Chem* 18:280, 1972
202. Mitch WE, Collier VU, Walser M: Creatinine metabolism in chronic renal failure. *Clin Science* 58:327, 1980
203. Hankins DA, Babb AL, Uvelli DA, Scribner BH: Creatinine degradation II: mathematical model including the effect of extra-renal removal rates. *Int J Artif Organs* 4:68, 1981
204. Jones JD, Burnett PC: Creatinine metabolism in humans with decreased renal function: creatinine deficit. *Clin Chem* 20:1204, 1974
205. Jones JD, Burnett PC: Creatinine metabolism and toxicity. *Kidney Int* 7 (Suppl 3):S294, 1975
206. Perez G, Faluotico R: Creatinine: a precursor of methylguanidine. *Experientia* 29:1473, 1973
207. Gonella M, Barsotti G, Lupetti S, Giovannetti S: Factors affecting the metabolic production of methylguanidine. *Clin Sci Mol Med* 48:341, 1975
208. Abdon NO, Gisselsson L: On the appearance of phosphocreatine in blood at uraemia. *Acta Med Scand (Suppl)* 90:444, 1938
209. Bolliger A, Carrodus AL: Creatine retention in blood and cerebrospinal fluid. *Med J Aust* 1:69, 1938
210. Grimberg A: La phosphocréatinémie chez les urémiques (Phosphocreatinaemia in uraemic patients). *Rev Méd* 56:382, 1939 (in French)
211. Gross H, Sandberg M: The concentration of creatine in heart, diaphragm, and skeletal muscle in uremia. *Ann Intern Med* 16:737, 1942
212. Hollunger G: Guanidines and oxidative phosphorylations. *Acta Pharmacol Toxicol* (Copenh) 11:Suppl 1, 1955
213. Pressman BL: Ionophorous antibiotics as models in biological transport. *Fed Proc* 27:1283, 1968
214. Davidoff D: Effects of guanidine derivatives on mitochondrial function. Phenethyl-guanidine inhibition of respiration in mitochondria from guinea pig and rat. *J Clin Invest* 47:2331, 1968
215. Davidoff F: Effects of guanidine derivatives on mitochondrial function. Ca^{2+} uptake and release. *J Biol Chem* 249:6406, 1974
216. Foster NB: The isolation of a toxic substance from the blood of uremic patients. *Trans Ass Am Physicians* 30:305, 1915
217. Foster NB: Uremia. *Harvey Lect* 16:52, 1920
218. Foster NB: Uremia. *JAMA* 76:281, 1921
219. Harrison TR, Mason MF: The pathogenesis of the uremic syndrome. *Medicine* (Baltimore) 16:1, 1937
220. Bohn H, Schlapp W: Untersuchungen zum Mechanismus des blassen Hochdrucks; der guanidingehalt des Blutes beim blassen und roten Hochdruck (Investigations of the pathogenesis of the pale hypertension. The guanidine concentration in the blood in cases of pale and red hypertension). *Zbl Inn Med* 53:571, 1932 (in German)
221. De Wesselow OLV, Griffiths WJ: The blood guanidine in hypertension. *Br J Exp Path* 13:428, 1932
222. Bradley SE: Laboratory findings in blood and urine in health and disease. *Med Clin North Am* 29:1314, 1945
223. Olsen NS, Bassett JW: Blood levels of urea nitrogen, phenol, guanidine and creatinine in uremia. *Am J Med* 10:52, 1951
224. Boyd LJ, Papper EM, Handelsman MB, Levitt MB, Post J: Symposium and panel discussion. Coma and unconsciousness. *NY State J Med* 58:3616, 1958
225. Carr MH, Schloerb PR: Analysis for guanidine and methylguanidine in uremic plasma. *Ann Biochem* 1:221, 1960
226. Yatzidis H, Oreopoulos D, Tsaparas N, Voudiclari S, Stravroulaki A, Zestanakis S: Colorimetric determination of guanidines in blood. *Nature* 212:1498, 1966
227. Fürst P, Allgén LG, Bergström J, Ekborg S, Persson BA, Ryhage R, Zimmerman L: New bioanalytical methods for the study of uremic toxicity. In: *Uremia*, edited by Kluthe R, Berlyne G, Burton B, Stuttgart, Georg Thieme Verlag, 1972, p 42
228. Paton DN: The significance of guanidines in the animal body. *Glasgow Med J* 104:297, 1925
229. Minot AS, Dodd K: Guanidine intoxication: a complicating factor in certain clinical conditions in children. *Am J Dis Child* 46:522, 1933
230. Mason MF, Resnik H, Minot AS, Rainey Jn, Pilcher C, Harrison TR: Mechanism of experimental uremia. *Arch Intern Med* 60:312, 1937
231. Orita Y, Tsubakihara Y, Ando A, Nakata K, Takamitsu Y, Fukuhara Y, Abe H: Effect of arginine or creatinine administration on the urinary excretion of methylguanidine. *Nephron* 22:328, 1978
232. Ando A, Orita Y, Nakata K, Tsubakihara Y, Takamitsu Y, Ueda N, Yanase M, Abe H: Effect of low protein diet and surplus of essential amino acids on the serum concentration and the urinary excretion of methylguanidine and guanidinosuccinic acid in chronic renal failure. *Nephron* 24:161, 1979
233. Stein IM, Perez G, Johnson R, Cummings NB: Serum levels and urinary excretion of methylguanidine in chronic renal failure. *J Lab Clin Med* 77:1020, 1971
234. Giovannetti S, Balestri PL, Barsotti G: Methylguanidine in uremia. *Arch Intern Med* 131:709, 1973
235. Stein IM, Micklus MJ: Concentrations in serum and urinary excretion of guanidine, 1-methylguanidine, and 1,1-dimethylguanidine in chronic renal failure. *Clin Chem* 19:583, 1973
236. Orita Y, Ando A, Tsubakihara Y, Mikami H, Kikuchi T, Nakata K, Abe H: Tissue and blood cell concentration of methylguanidine in rats and patients with chronic renal failure. *Nephron* 27:35, 1981
237. Carr MH, Schloerb PR: Analysis for guanidine and methylguanidine in uremic plasma. *Ann Biochem* 1:221, 1960
238. Giovannetti S, Biagini M, Cioni L: Evidence that methylguanidine is retained in chronic renal failure. *Experientia* 24:341, 1968
239. Jones JD, Giovannetti S: Charcoal-catalyzed oxidation of creatinine to methylguanidine. *Biochem Med* 5:281, 1971
240. Baker LRI, Marshall RD: A reinvestigation of methylguanidine concentration in sera from normal and uraemic subjects. *Clin Sci* 41:563, 1971
241. Micklus MJ, Stein IM: The colorimetric determination of mono- and disubstituted guanidines. *Anal Chem* 54:545, 1973
242. Shainkin R, Berkenstadt Y, Giatt Y, Berlyne GM: An automated technique for the analysis of plasma guanidino acids, and some findings in chronic renal disease. *Clin Chim Acta* 60:45, 1975
243. Perez G, Rey A, Micklus M, Stein I: Cation-exchange chromatography of guanidine derivatives in plasma of patients with chronic renal failure. *Clin Chem* 22:240, 1976
244. Eksborg S, Persson BA, Allgén LG, Bergström J, Zimmer-

man L, Fürst P: A selective method for determination of methylguanidine in biological fluids. Its application in normal subjects and uremic patients. *Clin Chim Acta* 82:141, 1978
245. Giovannetti S, Barsotti G: Dialysis of methylguanidine. *Kidney Int* 6:177, 1974
246. Hennemann H: *Die Urämische Sympathicopathie* (Uraemic sympathicopathy). Stuttgart, Georg Thieme Verlag, 1976 (in German)
247. Balestri PL, Barsotti G, Camici M, Giovannetti S: High plasma fibrinogen levels and reduced fibrinolytic activity in dogs intoxicated with methylguanidine. *Clin Nephrol* 2:81, 1974
248. Yamamoto A, Saito A, Manji T, Nishi H, Ito K, Maeda K, Ohta K, Kobayashi K: A new automated analytical method for guanidino compounds and their cerebrospinal fluid levels in uremia. *Trans Am Soc Artif Intern Organs* 24:61, 1978
249. Hennemann H, Bloemertz B, Heidland A: Methylguanidine – the natriuretic factor of uremic toxemia? In: *Uremia*, edited by Kluthe R, Berlyne GM, Burton B, Stuttgart, Georg Thieme Verlag, 1972, p 12
250. Hennemann H, Bloemertz B, Heidland A: Studies on natriuretic properties of methylguanidine. *Res Exp Med* (Berl) 158:58, 1972
251. Heidbreder E, Ralla W, Heidland A: Methylguanidin und exokrine Pankreasfunktion – ein Modell der urämischen Pankreopathie? (Methylguanidine and exocrine pancreatic function – a model of uraemic pancreopathy) *Dtsch Med Wochenschr* 37:1829, 1974 (in German)
252. Wizeman V: Exocrine pancreatic function in chronic renal failure. *Proc Eur Dial Transpl Assoc* 13:585, 1977
253. Ingerowski RM, Ingerowski GH, Dunn MJ: The effects of guanidinosuccinic acid and methylguanidine on erythrocyte cation transport. *Proc Soc Exp Biol Med* 139:80, 1972
254. Ku G, Hird VM, Varghese Z, Ahmed KY, Fiter M, Ng CM, Moorhead JF: Inhibition of DNA synthesis by guanidine compounds in uraemia. *Proc Eur Dial Transpl Assoc* 11:427, 1974
255. Leber HW, Baumgarten C, Goubeaud G, Matthias R, Schütterle G: Globin synthesis in uraemia. *Proc Eur Dial Transpl Assoc* 12:355, 1975
256. Gäng V, Berneburg H, Hennemann H, Hevendehl G: Diamine oxidase (histaminase) in chronic renal disease and its inhibition in vitro by methylguanidine. *Clin Nephrol* 5:171, 1976
257. Carroll HJ: Energy production and utilization by human platelets in the presence of some guanidines and phenols (uremic toxins) that inhibit aggregation. *Thromb Diath Haemorrh* 34:63, 1975
258. Bourgoignie J, Klahr S, Bricker NS: Inhibition of transepithelial sodium transport in the frog skin by a low molecular weight fraction of uremic serum. *J Clin Invest* 50:303, 1971
259. Cohen BD, Stein IM, Bonas JE: Guanidinosuccinic aciduria in uremia: a possible alternate pathway for urea synthesis. *Am J Med* 45:63, 1968
260. Stein IM, Cohen BD, Kornhauser RS: Guanidinosuccinic acid in renal failure. Experimental azotemia and inborn errors of the urea cycle. *N Engl J Med* 280:926, 1969
261. Cohen BD: Guanidinosuccinic acid in uremia. *Arch Intern Med* 126:846, 1970
262. Shainkin R, Giatt Y, Berlyne GM: The presence and toxicity of guanidinopropionic acid in uremia. *Kidney Int* 7 (Suppl 3):S302, 1975
263. Perez G, Rey A, Schiff E: The biosynthesis of guanidinosuccinic acid by perfused rat liver. *J Clin Invest* 57:807, 1976
264. Kamoun PP, Pleau JM, Man NK: Semiautomated method for measurement of guanidinosuccinic acid in serum. *Clin Chem* 18:355, 1972
265. Takahara K, Nakanishi S, Natelson S: Cleavage of canavaninosuccinic acid by human liver to form guanidinosuccinic acid, a substance found in the urine of uremic patients. *Clin Chem* 15:397, 1969
266. Takahara K, Nakanishi S, Natelson S: Studies on the reductive cleavage of canavanine and canavaninosuccinic acid. *Arch Biochem Biophys* 145:85, 1971
267. Sasaki M, Takahara K, Natelson S: Urinary guanidinoacetate/guanidinosuccinate ratio: an indicator of kidney dysfunction. *Clin Chem* 19:315, 1973
268. Kopple JD, Gordon S, Wang M: Effect of chronic uremia, protein intake and hemodialysis (HD) on guanidinosuccinic acid (GSA) levels. *Abstracts Am Soc Nephrol*, 5:41, 1971
269. Dobbelstein H, Grunst J, Schubert G, Edel HH: Guanidinbernsteinsäure und Urämie. II. Tierexperimentelle Befunde (Guanidinosuccinic acid and uraemia. II. Results of animal experiments). *Klin Wochenschr* 49:1077, 1971 (in German)
270. Acquatella H, Perez-Rojas M, Burger B, Lozano JR: Modificaciones experimentales de la contractilidad miocardica producidas por toxico retenido en la uremia: el acido guanidinosuccinico (Experimental modification of myocardial contractility caused by toxins retained in uraemia: guanidinosuccinic acid). *Arch Inst Cardiol Mex* 44:624, 1974 (in Spanish)
271. Horowitz HI, Stein IM, Cohen BD, White JG: Further studies on the platelet-inhibitory effect of guanidinosuccinic acid and its role in uremic bleeding. *Am J Med* 49:336, 1970
272. Davidson MB: The effect of guanidinosuccinic acid on in-vitro carbohydrate metabolism. *Experientia* 26:1206, 1970
273. Davidson WD, Tanaka KR: Effect of uremia on phagocytosis-stimulated glucose oxidation (PSGO) in human granulocytes. *Clin Res* 19:416, 1971
274. Matsumoto M, Kishikawa H, Mori A: Guanidino compounds in the sera of uremic patients and in the sera and brain of experimental uremic rabbits. *Biochem Med* 16:1, 1976
275. Sorensen LB: Degradation of uric acid in man. *Metabolism* 8:687, 1959
276. Sorensen LB: Gout secondary to chronic renal disease: studies on urate metabolism. *Ann Rheumat Dis* 39:424, 1980
277. Clarkson BA: Uric acid related to uraemic symptoms. *Proc Eur Dial Transpl Assoc* 3:3, 1966
278. Steele TH, Rieselbach RE: The contribution of residual nephrons within the chronically diseased kidney to urate homeostasis in man. *Am J Med* 43:876, 1967
279. Sarre H, Mertz DP: Sekundäre Gicht bei Niereninsuffizienz. (Secondary gout in renal failure). *Klin Wochenschr* 43:113, 1965 (in German)
280. Richet G, Mignon C, Ardaillou R: Goutte secondaire des néphropathies chroniques (Secondary gout in chronic nephropathy). *Presse Méd* 73:633, 1965 (in French)
281. Folin O, Berglund H, Derick C: The uric acid problem. An experimental study of animals and man including gouty subjects. *J Biol Chem* 60:361, 1924
282. Farrell PC, Ward RA, Hone PW: Uric acid: binding levels of urate ions in normal and uraemic plasma and in human serum albumin. *Biochem Pharmacol* 24:1885, 1975
283. Kaminsky NI, Broadus AE, Hardman JG, Jones DJ Jr, Ball JH, Sutherland EW, Liddle GW: Effects of parathyroid hormone on plasma and urinary adenosine 3′,5′-monophosphate in man. *J Clin Invest* 49:2387, 1970

284. Bartelson NM, Basil T, Lavender AL: 3',5'-cyclic AMP levels in hemodialysis patients. *Abstracts Am Soc Nephrol,* 8:7, 1974
285. Schneider W, Jutzler GA: Implications of cyclic adenosine 3'-5'-monophosphate in chronic renal failure. *New Engl J Med* 291:155, 1974
286. Tomlinson S, Barling PM, Albano JDM, Brown BL, O'Riordan JLH: The effects of exogenous parathyroid hormone on plasma and urinary adenosine 3',5'-cyclic monophosphate in man. *Clin Sci Mol Med* 47:481, 1974
287. Wathen R, Smith M, Keshaviah P, Comty CM, Shapiro F: Depressed in vitro aggregation of platelets of chronic hemodialysis patients (CHDP): a role for cyclic AMP. *Trans Am Soc Artif Intern Organs* 21:320, 1975
288. Zucker MG: Unpublished observations. In: *Physiology of Blood Platelets,* edited by Marcus AJ, Zucker MG, New York, Grune and Stratton Inc, 1965, p 53
289. Salzman EW, Levine L: Cyclic 3',5'-adenosine monophosphate in human blood platelets. *J Clin Invest* 50:131, 1971
290. Mills DCB, Smith JB: The control of platelet responsiveness by agents that influence cyclic AMP metabolism. *Ann NY Acad Sci* 201:391, 1972
291. Kramer B, Seligson H, Seligson D, Baltrush H: Isolation of N-methyl-2-pyridone-5-carboxamide from hemodialysis fluid obtained from uremic patients. *Clin Chim Acta* 10:447, 1964
292. Clayton EM, Seligson D, Seligson H: Inhibition of protein synthesis by N-methyl-2-pyridone-5-formamidoacetic acid and other compounds isolated from uremic patients. *Yale J Biol Med* 38:273, 1965
293. Asatoor AM: Retention of pseudouridine and 4-amino-5-imidazolecarboxamide in uraemia. *Clin Chim Acta* 20:407, 1968
294. Giordano C, De Pascale C, De Santo NG, Esposito R, Cirilli C, Stangherlin P: Disorder in the metabolism of some amino acids in uremia. *Proc 4th Int Cong Nephrol Stockholm (1969),* edited by Alwall N, Berglund F, Josephson B, Basel, S Karger 1970, p 196
295. Gulyassy PF, Aviram A, Peters JH: Evaluation of amino acid and protein requirements in chronic uremia. *Arch Intern Med* 126:855, 1970
296. Young GA, Parsons FM: Plasma amino acid imbalance in patients with chronic renal failure on intermittent dialysis. *Clin Chim Acta* 27:491, 1970
297. Kopple JD, Swendseid ME: Protein and amino acid metabolism in uremic patients undergoing maintenance hemodialysis. *Kidney Int* 7 (Suppl 2):S64, 1975
298. Ganda OP, Aoki TT, Soeldner JS, Morrison RS, Cahill GF Jr: Hormone-fuel concentrations in anephric subjects. Effect of hemodialysis (with special reference to amino acids). *J Clin Invest* 57:1403, 1976
299. Thierfelder H, Sherwin CP: Phenylacetylglutamin und seine Bildung im menschlichen Körper nach Eingabe von Phenylessigsäure (Phenylacetylglutamine and its production in the human body after administration of phenylaceticacid). *Hoppe Seylers Z Physiol Chem* 94:1, 1915 (in German)
300. Salisbury PF, Dunn MS, Murphy EA: Apparent free amino acids in deproteinized plasma of normal and uremic persons. *J Clin Invest* 36:1227, 1957
301. Frimpter GW, Thompson DD, Luckey EH: Conjugated amino acids in plasma of patients with uremia. *J Clin Invest* 40:1208, 1961
302. Burzynski S: Bound amino acids in serum of patients with chronic renal insufficiency. *Clin Chim Acta* 25:231, 1969
303. Czerniak Z: N-substituted amino acids in serum of patients with chronic renal insufficiency. *Clin Chim Acta* 28:403, 1970
304. Arroyave G, Wilson D, De Funes C, Behar M: The free amino acids in blood plasma of children with kwashiorkor and marasmus. *Am J Clin Nutr* 11:517, 1962
305. Snyderman SE, Holt LE Jr, Norton PM, Roitman E, Phansalkar SV: The plasma aminogram. I. Influence of the level of protein intake and a comparison of whole protein and amino acid diets. *Pediatr Res* 2:131, 1968
306. Swendseid ME, Kopple JD: Nitrogen balance, plasma amino acid levels, and amino acid requirements. *Trans NY Acad Sci* 35:471, 1973
307. Smith SR, Pozefsky T, Chhetri MK: Nitrogen and amino acid metabolism in adults with protein-calorie malnutrition. *Metabolism* 23:603, 1974
308. Guylyassy PF, Peters JH, Lin SC, Ryan PM: Hemodialysis and plasma amino acid composition in chronic renal failure. *Am J Clin Nutr* 21:565, 1968
309. Gulyassy PF, Peters JH, Schoenfeld P: Transport and protein binding of tryptophan in uremia. In: *Uremia,* edited by Kluthe R, Berlyne GM, Burton B, Stuttgart, Georg Thieme Verlag, 1972, p 163
310. Sullivan PA, Murnaghan D, Callaghan N, Kantamaneni BD, Curzon G: Cerebral transmitter precursors and metabolites in advanced renal disease. *J Neurol Neurosurg Psychiatry* 41:581, 1978
311. Saito R, Niwa T, Maeda K, Kobayashi K, Yamamoto Y, Ota K: Tryptophan and indolic tryptophan metabolites in chronic renal failure. *Am J Clin Nutr* 33:1402, 1980
312. Cernacek P, Begvarova H, Gerova Z, Válek A, Spustová V: Plasma tryptophan level in chronic renal failure. *Clin Nephrol* 14:246, 1980
313. De Torrente A, Glazer GB, Gulyassy P: Reduced in vitro binding of tryptophan by plasma in uremia. *Kidney Int* 6:222, 1974
314. Peters JH, Gulyassy PF, Lin SC, Ryan PM, Berridge BJ Jr, Chao WR, Cummings JG: Amino acid patterns in uremia: comparative effect of hemodialysis and transplantation. *Trans Am Soc Artif Intern Organs* 14:405, 1968
315. Gulyassy PF, De Torrente A: Tryptophan metabolism in uremia. *Kidney Int* 7 (Suppl 3):S311, 1975
316. Giordano C, Deplascale C, De Cristofaro D, Capodicasa G, Balestrieri C, Baczyk K: Protein malnutrition in the treatment of chronic uremia, in *Nutrition in Renal Disease,* edited by Berlyne GM, Baltimore, Williams and Wilkins, 1968, p 23
317. Bergström J, Fürst P, Norée LO, Vinnars E: The effect of peritoneal dialysis on intracellular free amino acids in muscle from uraemic patients. *Proc Eur Dial Transpl Assoc* 9:393, 1972
318. Kopple JD, Wang M, Vyhmeister I, Baker N, Swendseid M: Tyrosine metabolism in uremia, in *Uremia,* edited by Kluthe R, Berlyne GM, Burton B, Stuttgart, Georg Thieme Verlag, 1972, p 150
319. Jones MR, Swendseid ME, Kopple JD: Phenylalanine and tyrosine metabolism in uremia. *Kidney Int* 8:459, 1975
320. Chan W, Wang M, Kopple JD, Swendseid ME: Citrulline levels and urea cycle enzymes in uremic rats. *J Nutr* 104:678, 1974
321. Bergström J, Fürst P, Norée LO, Vinnars E: Intracellular free amino acids in uremic patients as influenced by amino acid supply. *Kidney Int* 7:(Suppl 3) 345, 1975
322. Dubovsky J, Duboska E, Pacovsky V, Hrba J: Free and peptide hydroxyproline in chronic uremia. *Clin Chim Acta* 19:387, 1968
323. Blagg CR, Bradshaw RA, Beckley D, Fenton SSA: Serum

free hydroxyproline in chronic renal disease. *Clin Res* 18:192, 1970
324. Bishop MC, Smith R: Non-protein-bound hydroxyproline in plasma in renal bone disease. *Clin Chim Acta* 33:403, 1971
325. Hart W, Duursma SA, Visser WJ, Njio LKF: The hydroxyproline content of plasma of patients with impaired renal function. *Clin Nephrol* 4:104, 1975
326. Dubovsky J, Geary WT Jr, Chilcutt DA: Estimation of hydroxylysine in urine and serum of patients with chronic uremia. *Clin Chim Acta* 76:41, 1977
327. Giordano C, De Santo NG, Rinaldi S, Depascale G, Pluvio M: Histidine and glycine essential amino acids in uremia. In: *Uremia,* edited by Kluthe R, Berlyne GM, Burton B, Stuttgart, Georg Thieme Verlag, 1972, p 138
328. Bergström J, Fürst P, Josephson B, Norée LO: Improvement of nitrogen balance in a uremic patient by the addition of histidine to essential amino acid solutions given intravenously. *Life Sci* 9 part II: 787, 1970
329. Fürst P: ^{15}N-studies in severe renal failure. II. Evidence for the essentiality of histidine. *Scand J Clin Lab Invest* 30:307, 1972
330. Kopple JD, Swendseid ME: Evidence that histidine is an essential amino acid in normal and chronically uremic man. *J Clin Invest* 55:881, 1975
331. Condon JR, Asatoor AM: Amino acid metabolism in uraemic patients. *Clin Chim Acta* 32:333, 1971
332. Asatoor AM, Armstrong MD: 3-Methylhistidine, a component of actin. *Biochem Biophys Res Commun* 26:168, 1967
333. Trayer IP, Harris CI, Perry SV: 3-Methylhistidine and foetal forms of skeletal muscle myosin. *Nature* 217:452, 1968
334. Young VR, Haverberg LN, Bilmazes C, Munro HN: Potential use of 3-methyl-histidine excretion as an index of progressive reduction in protein catabolism during starvation. *Metabolism* 22:1429, 1973
335. Long CL, Hoverberg LN, Young VR, Kinney JM, Munro HN, Geiger JW: Metabolism of 3-methylhistidine in man. *Metabolism* 24:929, 1975
336. Young VR, Alexis SC, Baliga BS: Fate of administered 3-methylhistidine. Lack of muscle transfer, ribonucleic acid charging and quantitative excretion as 3-methylhistidine and its N-acetyl derivative. *J Biol Chem* 247:3592, 1972
337. Whitehouse S, Katz N, Schaeffer G, Kluthe R: Histidines and renal function. *Clin Nephrol* 3:24, 1975
338. Davis JW, Nininger RJ, Phillips PE: Failure of methylhistidine to inhibit platelet aggregation at concentrations found in uremic plasma. *Am J Clin Nutr* 28:930, 1975
339. Wilcken EEL, Gupta VJ, Reddy SG: Accumulation of sulphur-containing amino acids including cysteine-homocysteine in patients on maintenance haemodialysis. *Clin Sci* 58:731, 1976
340. Gejyo F, Ito G, Kinoshita Y: Identification of N-monoacetylcystine in uremic plasma. *Clin Sci* 60:331, 1981
341. Harker LA, Ross R, Slichter SJ, Scott CR: Homocystine-induced arteriosclerosis. The role of endothelial cell injury and platelet response in its genesis. *J Clin Invest* 58:731, 1976
342. Gejyo F, Kinoshita Y, Ikenaka T: Elevation of serum levels of β-amino-isobutyric acid in uremic patients and the toxicity of the amino acid. *Clin Nephrol* 8:520, 1977
343. Bergström J, Fürst P, Norée LO, Vinnars E: Intracellular free amino acids in muscle tissue of patients with chronic uremia. The effects of peritoneal dialysis and infusion of essential amino acids. *Clin Sci Mol Med* 54:51, 1978
344. Harper AE: Amino acid toxicities and imbalances. In: *Mammalian Protein Metabolism,* edited by Munro HN, Allison JB, New York, Academic Press, 1964, vol. 2, p 87
345. Kopple JD, Swendseid ME, Shinaberger JH, Umezawa CY: The free and bound amino acids removed by hemodialysis. *Trans Am Soc Artif Intern Organs* 19:309, 1973
346. Gejyo F, Kinoshita, Ito G, Ikenaka T: Identification of β-aspartylglycine in uremic serum and its toxicity. *Contrib Nephrol* 9:69, 1978
347. Pisano JJ, Prado E, Freedman J: β-Aspartylglycine in urine and enzymic hydrolyzates of proteins. *Arch Biochem Biophys* 117:394, 1966
348. Simenhoff ML: Metabolism and toxicity of aliphatic amines. *Kidney Int* 7 (Suppl 3):S324, 1975
349. Simmenhoff ML, Asatoor AM, Milne MD, Zilva JF: Retention of aliphatic amines in uraemia. *Clin Sci* 25:65, 1963
350. Wang M, Tam CF, Swendseid ME, Kopple JD: Monoamine and diamine oxidase activities in uremic rats. *Life Sci* 17:653, 1975
351. Simmenhoff ML, Glinn HE: Toxicity of aliphatic amines in uremia. *Trans Am Soc Artif Intern Organs* 23:560, 1977
352. Simenhoff ML, Burke JF, Saukkonen JJ, Ordinario AT, Doty R: Biochemical profile of uremic breath. *N Engl J Med* 297:132, 1977
353. Owens CWI, Padovan W: Faecal methylamine in normal and uraemic subjects. *Clin Sci* 56:509, 1979
354. Giovannetti S, Balestri PL, Barsotti G: Methyl-guanidine in uraemia. *Arch Intern Med* 131:709, 1973
355. Young DS, Wootton IDP: The retention of amines as a factor in uraemic toxaemia. *Clin Chim Acta* 9:503, 1964
356. Quastel JH, Wheatley AHM: The effects of amines on oxidations of the brain. *Biochem J* 27:1609, 1933
357. Führer H, Neubauer E: Hämolyse durch Substanzen homologer Reihen (Haemolysis by substances from homologous series). *Naunyn Schmiedeberg Archs Pharmacol* 56:333, 1907 (in German)
358. Graeffe E: Über die Wirkung von Ammoniak und Ammoniakderivaten auf die Oxydation Prozesse in Zellen (On the effect of ammonia and ammonia derivatives on the intracellular oxidation processes). *Hoppe Seyler Z Physiol Chem* 79:421, 1912 (in German)
359. Rennick B, Acara M, Hysert P, Mookerjee B: Choline loss during hemodialysis: homeostatic control of plasma choline concentrations. *Kidney Int* 10:329, 1976
360. Acara M, Rennick B: Regulation of plasma choline by the renal tubule: bidirectional transport of choline. *Am J Physiol* 225:1123, 1972
361. Chen SH, Lincoln SD: Increased serum carnitine concentration in renal insufficiency. *Clin Chem* 23:278, 1977
362. De Felice SL, Klein MI: Carnitine and hemodialysis – a minireview. *Current Ther Res* 28:195, 1980
363. Morgan RE, Morgan JM: Plasma levels of aromatic amines in renal failure. *Metabolism* 15:479, 1966
364. Young DS, Wootton IDP: Conjugation of aromatic amines in renal failure. *Clin Chim Acta* 22:403, 1968
365. Hicks JM, Young DS, Wootton IDP: Abnormal blood constituents in acute renal failure. *Clin Chim Acta* 7:623, 1962
366. Loeper M, Lemaire A, Cottet J: La tyraminémie dans l'imperméabilité rénale (Tyraminaemia in case of impermeability of the kidney). *Bull Soc Méd Hôp Paris* 54:1537, 1938 (in French)
367. Müting D: Studies on the pathogenesis of uremia. Comparative determinations of glucuronic acid, indican, free

and bound phenols in the serum, cerebrospinal fluid, and urine of renal diseases with and without uremia. *Clin Chim Acta* 12:551, 1965
368. Janne J, Poso H, Raina A: Polyamines in rapid growth and cancer. *Biochim Biophys Acta* 473:242, 1978
369. Herbst EJ, Bachrach U: Metabolism and biological function of polyamines. *Ann NY Acid Sci* 171:691, 1970
370. Mayhew E, Harlos JP, Juliano RL: The effect of polycations on cell membrane stability and transport processes. *J Membr Biol* 14:213, 1973
371. Peter HW, Wolf HU, Seiler N: Influence of polyamines on two bivalent cation activated ATPases. *Hoppe Seyler Z Physiol Chem* 354:1146, 1973
372. Arvanitakis S, Mangos J, McSherry NR, Rennert O: Effect of polyamines and cystic fibrosis serum on glucose transport. *Tex Rep Biol Med* 34:175, 1976
373. Dreyfuss F, Chayen R, Dreyfuss G, Dvir R, Ratan J: Polyamine excretion in the urine of cancer patients. *Israel J Med Sci* 11:785, 1975
374. Campbell RA, Talwalker YB, Harner MH, Bartos D, Bartos F, Musgrave JE, Puri H, Grettie DP, Dolney AM, Loggan B: Polyamines, uremia, and hemodialysis. In: *Advances in Polyamine Research,* vol 2, edited by Campbell RA, Morris DR, Bartos D, Daves GD Jr, Bartos F, New York, Raven Press, 1978, p 319
375. Swendseid ME, Panaqua M, Kopple JD: Polyamine concentrations in red cells and urine of patients with chronic renal failure. *Life Sci* 26:533, 1980
376. Russel DH, Durie BGM, Salmon SE: Polyamines as predictors of success and failure in cancer chemotherapy. *Lancet* 2:797, 1975
377. Campbell RA, Grettie DP, Bartos F, Bartos D, Marton LJ: Uremic polyamine dysmetabolism. *Proc Clin Dial Transpl Forum* 8:194, 1978
378. Lutz W: Chemical compositions and rate of passage across semipermeable membranes of basic peptides isolated from peritoneal dialysis fluid from patients with chronic renal failure. *Acta Med Pol* 17:137, 1976
379. Bagdade JD, Subbaiah PV, Bartos D, Bartos F, Campbell RA: Polyamines: An unrecognized cardiovascular risk factor in chronic dialysis? *Lancet* 1:412, 1979
380. Campbell R, Bartos F, Bartos D, Grettie D: The uremic hyperpolyaminemic perturbations: an hypothesis, in *Controversies in Nephrology, Proceedings of the First Conference,* edited by Schreiner GE, Washington, Nephrology Division, Georgetown University, 1979, p 435
380a. Radtke HW, Rege AB, LaMarche MB, Bartos D: Identification of Spermine as an Inhibitor of Erythorpoiesis in Patients with Chronic Renal Failure. *J Clin Invest* 67:1623, 1981
381. Ludwig GD, Senesky D, Bluemle LW Jr, Elkinton JR: Indoles in uremia: identification by countercurrent distribution and paper chromatography. *Am J Clin Nutr* 21:436, 1968
382. Obermayer F, Popper H: Über Urämie (On uraemia). *Z Klin Med* 2:332, 1911 (in German)
383. Haas G: Der Indikangehalt des menschlichen Blutes unter normalen und pathologischen Zuständen (The indican content of the human blood in normal and abnormal conditions). *Dtsch Arch Klin Med* 119:177, 1916 (in German)
384. Becher E: Über Indikanretention in den Geweben (On retention of indican in the tissues). *Dtsch Arch Klin Med* 129:8, 1919 (in German)
385. Townsend SR: Hyperindicanemia in renal insufficiency and the significance of the diazo reaction. *J Lab Clin Med* 23:809, 1938
386. Wootton IDP: Retention of aromatic compounds in acute renal failure, in *Sci Basis Med Ann Rev,* edited by the University of London, Athlone Press, 1963, p 235
387. Byrd DJ, Berthold HW, Trefz KF, Kochen W, Gilli G, Schärer K, Schuler HW, Asbach HW: Indolic tryptophan metabolism in uraemia. *Proc Eur Dial Transpl Assoc* 12:347, 1976
388. Siassi F, Wang M, Chan W, Swendseid ME: Brain serotonin metabolism in experimental uremia. *Fed Proc* 33:651, 1974
389. Bloxam DL, Warren WH: Error in the determination of tryptophan by the method of Denekla and Dewey. A revised procedure. *Anal Biochem* 60:621, 1974
390. Mirsky IA, Diengott D, Perisutti G: Insulinase-inhibitory action of metabolic derivatives of L-tryptophan. *Proc Soc Exp Biol Med* 95:154, 1957
391. Quagliariello E, Papa S, Saccone C, Alifano A: Effect of 3-hydroxyanthranilic acid on the mitochondrial respiratory system. *Biochem J* 91:137, 1964
392. Foster DO, Ray PD, Lardy HA: Activation of phosphoenolpyruvatecarboxykinase of rat liver by administration of L-tryptophan. *Fed Proc* 25:220, 1966
393. Ray PD, Foster DO, Lardy HA: Paths of carbon in gluconeogenesis and lipogenesis. IV. Inhibition by L-tryptophan of hepatic gluconeogenesis at the level of phosphoenolpyruvate formation. *J Biol Chem* 241:3904, 1966
394. Veneziale CM, Walter P, Kneer N, Lardy HA: Influence of L-tryptophan and its metabolites on gluconeogenesis in the isolated perfused liver. *Biochemistry* 6:2129, 1967
395. Wardle EN, Williams R: Polymorph leucocyte function in uraemia and jaundice. *Acta Haematol* (Basel) 64:157, 1980
396. Becher E: Studien über die Pathogenese der echten Urämie, insbesondere über die Bedeutung der retinierten Phenole und anderer Darmfäulnisprodukte (Investigations of the pathogenesis of uraemia in particular on the significance of retention of phenols and other intestinal decay products). *Z Gesamte Inn Med* 46:369, 1925 (in German)
397. Becher E, Litzner S: Über das Auftreten von freiem Phenol im Blut bei Niereninsuffizienz (On the appearance of free phenol in the blood in renal failure). *Klin Wochenschr* 5:147, 1926 (in German)
398. Becher E: Die Bedeutung des Liquor cerebrospinalis in die Pathogenese der Urämie (The significance of the cerebrospinal fluid in the pathogenesis of uraemia). *Münchener Med Wochenschr MMW* 72:146, 1926 (in German)
399. Mason MF, Resnik H, Minot AS, Rainey J, Pilcher C, Harrison TR: Mechanism of experimental uremia. *Arch Intern Med* 60:312, 1937
400. Dickes R: Relation between the symptoms of uremia and the blood levels of the phenols. *Arch Intern Med* 69:446, 1942
401. Roen PR: The chemical basis of uremia: blood phenol. *J Urol* 51:110, 1944
402. Nesbit RM, Burk LB, Olsen NS: Blood level of phenol in uremia. *Arch Surg* 53:483, 1946
403. Wallace SL, Little JM, Bobb JRR: The relation of phenol retention to uremia and the effect of phthalysulfathiazole and streptomycin on phenol production. *J Lab Clin Med* 33:845, 1948
404. Olsen NS, Bassett JW: Blood levels of urea nitrogen, phenol, guanidine and creatinine in uremia. *Am J Med* 10:52, 1951
405. Dunn I, Weinstein IM, Maxwell MH, Kleeman CR: Significance of circulating phenols in anemia of renal disease. *Proc Soc Exp Biol Med* 99:86, 1958
406. Kramer B, Seligson H, Baltrush H, Seligson D: The isolation of several aromatic acids from the hemodialysis

fluids of uremic patients. *Clin Chim Acta* 11:363, 1965
407. Jutzler GA, Kramer HJ, Keller HE, Kramer H, Doenecke F: Zum Verhalten der Phenole und des Kreatinins bei Niereninsuffizienz, insbesondere bei chronischen Dialyse-Patienten (On the relation between phenols and creatinine in renal failure, in particular in chronic dialysis patients). *Arch Klin Med* 214:214, 1968 (in German)
408. Kramer HJ, Kramer HK, Keller HE, Jutzler GA: Beitrag zur möglichen Bedeutung der Phenole in der Pathogenese des Urämiesyndroms (Contribution to the possible significance of the phenols for the pathogenesis of the uraemic syndrome). *Verh Dtsch Ges Inn Med* 74:1229, 1968 (in German)
409. Bajaj VR, Garg BB, Saini AS, Bhatt PS, Singh PC, Singh ID: Phenolic acid retention in chronic renal failure. *Indian J Med Sci* 27:235, 1973
410. Nagpaul RK, Mehta HC, Saini AS: Urinary phenolic acids of normal dogs and their retention in acute experimental uraemia. *Indian J Exp Biol* 13:193, 1975
411. Wardle EN, Wilkinson K: Free phenols in chronic renal failure. *Clin Nephrol* 6:361, 1976
412. Alwall N, Norviit L, Steins AM: Clinical extracorporeal dialysis of blood with artificial kidney. *Lancet* 1:60, 1948
413. Drivas G, Farb M, Kenward D: Small molecules in chronic renal failure. *Lancet* 2:367, 1980
414. Niwa T, Ohki T, Maeda K, Saito A, Ohta K, Kobayashi K: A gas chromatographic-mass spectrometric assay for nine hydroxyphenolic acids in uremic serum. *Clin Chim Acta* 96:247, 1979
415. Wengle B, Hellström K: A gas chromatographic technique for the analysis of volatile phenols in serum. *Scand J Clin Lab Invest* 28:477, 1971
416. Wengle B, Hellström K: Volatile phenols in serum of uraemic patients. *Clin Sci* 43:493, 1972
417. Porter RD, Cathcart-Rake WF, Wan SH, Whittier FC, Grantham JJ: Secretory activity and aryl acid content of serum, urine, and cerebrospinal fluid in normal and uremic man. *J Lab Clin Med* 85:723, 1975
418. Record BN, Princhard JW, Gallagher BB, Seligson D: Phenolic acids in experimental uremia. I. Potential role of phenolic acids in the neurological manifestations of uremia. *Arch Neurol* 21:387, 1969
419. Rabiner S, Molinas F: The role of phenol and phenolic acids on the thrombocytopathy and defective platelet aggregation of patients with renal failure. *Am J Med* 49:346, 1970
420. Zweifler AJ, Sanbar SS: Inhibition of platelet adhesiveness and aggregation by benzyl alcohol and phenol. *Thromb Diath Haemorrh* 21:362, 1969
421. Kramer HK, Gospodinov D, Kramer HJ, Krück F: Inhibition of transport-ATPase by uremic toxins. *Proc Eur Dial Transplant Assoc* 9:521, 1972
422. Wardle EN: Phenols, phenolic acids and sodium-potassium ATPases. *J Mol Med* 3:319, 1978
423. Hicks JM, Young DS, Wootton IDP: The effect of uraemic blood constituents on certain cerebral enzymes. *Clin Chim Acta* 9:228, 1964
424. Nordmann R, Arnaud M, Nordmann J: Retentissement de l'insuffisance rénale chronique sur les principaux acides du cycle tricarboxylique et metabolites voisins (Response effect of chronic renal failure on the principal acides of the tricarboxylic acid cycle and related metabolites). *Clin Chim Acta* 12:304, 1965 (in French)
425. Bhat CS, Ramasarma T: Effect of phenyl and phenolic acids on mevalonate-5-phosphate kinase and mevalonate-5-pyrophosphate decarboxylase of the rat brain. *J Neurochem* 32:1531, 1979

426. Daughaday WH, Larner J, Houghton E: The renal excretion of myoinositol in normal and diabetic human beings. *J Clin Invest* 33:326, 1954
427. Hauser G, Finelli VN: The biosynthesis of free and phosphatase myoinositol from glucose by mammalian tissue slices. *J Biol Chem* 238:3224, 1963
428. Dawson MC, Freincel N: The distribution of free myo-inositol in mammalian tissue slices. *J Biol Chem* 242:2599, 1967
429. Milhorat AT: Inositols: requirements of human beings. In: *The Vitamins*, edited by Sebrell WH Jr, Harris RS, New York, Academic Press 1971, vol 3, p 412
430. Howard CF Jr, Anderson L: Metabolism of myoinositol in animals. II. Complete catabolism of myoinositol-^{14}C by rat kidney slices. *Arch Biochem* 118:332, 1967
431. Wang YM, Van Eys J: The enzymatic defect in essential pentosuria. *N Engl J Med* 282:892, 1970
432. Pitkänen E: The serum polyol pattern and the urinary polyol excretion in diabetic and in uremic patients. *Clin Chim Acta* 38:221, 1972
433. Clements RS, De Jesus PV, Winegrad AT: Raised plasma myoinositol levels in uraemia and experimental neuropathy. *Lancet* 1:1137, 1973
434. Servo C, Pitkänen E: Variation in polyol levels in cerebrospinal fluid and serum in diabetic patients. *Diabetologia* 11:575, 1975
435. Servo C, Bardy A, Pasternack A, Pitkänen E: Plasma, red cell and cerebrospinal fluid concentrations of myoinositol in patients with severe chronic renal failure. *Ann Clin Res* 8:374, 1976
436. Blumberg A, Esslen E, Bürgi W: Myoinositol – a uremic neurotoxin? *Nephron* 21:186, 1978
437. Aloia JF: Monosaccharides and polyols in diabetes mellitus and uremia. *J Lab Clin Med* 82:809, 1973
438. De Jesus PV, Clements RS, Winegrad AI: Hypermyoinositolemic polyneuropathy in rats. A possible mechanism for uremic polyneuropathy. *J Neurol Sci* 21:237, 1974
439. Liveson JA, Gardner J, Bornstein MB: Tissue culture studies of possible uremic neurotoxins: myoinositol. *Kidney Int* 12:131, 1977
440. Pitkänen E, Bardy A, Pasternack A, Servo C: Plasma, red cell and cerebrospinal fluid concentrations of mannitol and sorbitol in patients with severe chronic renal failure. *Ann Clin Res* 8:368, 1976
441. Schoots AC, Leclercq PA: Chemical ionization mass spectrometry of trimethylsilylated carbohydrates and organic acids retained in uremic serum. *Biomed Mass Spectrom* 6:502, 1979
442. Zarembski PM, Hodgkinson A, Parsons FM: Elevation of the concentration of plasma oxalic acid in renal failure. *Nature* 212:511, 1966
443. Fanger H, Esparza A: Crystals of calcium oxalate in kidneys in uremia. *Am J Clin Path* 41:597, 1964
444. Emerson P, Wilkinson JH: Urea and oxalate inhibition of the serum lactate dehydrogenase. *J Clin Path* 18:803, 1965
445. Emerson P, Withycombe W, Wilkinson JH: Inhibition of lactate dehydrogenase by sera of uraemic patients. *Lancet* 2:571, 1976
446. Thölen H, Bigler F, Heusler A, Stauffacher W, Staub H: Zur Pathogenese des Urämiesyndroms, Brenztrauben-säure, Acetoin und 2,3-Butylenglykol in Blut von Patienten mit Nieren- und Leberkrankheiten (On the pathogenesis of the uraemic syndrome; pyruvate, acetocin and 2,3-butylenglycol in the blood of patients with kidney and liverdisease). *Experientia* 18:454, 1962 (in German)
447. Niwa T, Ohki T, Maeda K, Saito A, Kobayashi K: Pattern of aliphatic dicarboxylaic acids in uremic serum in-

cluding a new organic acid, 2,4-dimethyladipic acid. *Clin Chim Acta* 99:71, 1979
448. Pinkston D, Spiteller G, Von Henning H, Matthaei D: High-resolution gas chromatography – mass spectrometry of the methyl esters of organic acids from uremic hemofiltrates. *J Chromatogr* 223:1, 1981
449. Schwertner HA, Weintraub ST, Hawthorne SB: The unidentified fluorescent substance in serum of patients with chronic renal disease is also found in hemofiltrates, dialysis fluids, and urine. *Clin Chem* 26:1927, 1980
450. Tenckhoff H, Shilipetar G, Boen ST: One year's experience with home peritoneal dialysis. *Trans Am Soc Artif Intern Organs* 11:11, 1965
451. Tenckhoff H, Curtis FK: Experience with maintenance peritoneal dialysis in the home. *Trans Am Soc Artif Intern Organs* 16:90, 1970
452. Scribner BH: Discussion. *Trans Am Soc Artif Intern Organs* 11:29, 1965
453. Babb AL, Johansen PJ, Strand MJ, Tenckhoff H, Scribner BH: Bi-directional permeability of the human peritoneum to middle molecules. *Proc Eur Dial Transpl Assoc* 10:247, 1973
454. Shaldon S: Haemodialysis in chronic renal failure. *Postgrad Med J* (Suppl 42), 1966
455. Jebsen RH, Tenckhoff H, Hoult JC: Natural history of uremic polyneuropathy and the effects of dialysis. *New Engl J Med* 277:327, 1967
456. Babb AL, Popovich RP, Christopher TG, Scribner BH: The genesis of the square meter-hour hypothesis. *Trans Am Soc Artif Intern Organs* 17:81, 1971
457. Christopher TG, Cambi V, Harker LA, Hurst PE, Popovich RP, Babb AL, Scribner BH: A study of hemodialysis with lowered dialysate flow rate. *Trans Am Soc Artif Intern Organs* 17:92, 1971
458. Ginn HE, Bugel HJ, James L, Hopkins P: Clinical experience with small surface area dialyzers (SSAD). *Proc Clin Dial Transpl Forum* 1:53, 1971
459. Milutinovic J, Halar EM, Harker LA, Babb AL, Scribner BH: Further experience with hemodialysis at 100 ml/min dialysate flow rate. *Proc Clin Dial Transpl Forum* 1:48, 1971
460. Rosenzweg J, Babb AL, Vizzo JE, Scribner BH, Ginn HE: Clinical experience with small surface area dialyzers (SSAD). *Proc Clin Dial Transpl Forum* 1:56, 1971
461. Babb AL, Farrell PC, Uvelli DA, Scribner BH: Hemodialyzer evaluation by examination of solute molecular spectra. *Trans Am Soc Artif Intern Organs* 18:98, 1972
462. Millora AB, Woodruff MW, Kiley JE: Comparison of higher blood flow hemodialysis with lower blood flow in light of the square meter-hour hypothesis. *Trans Am Soc Artif Intern Organs* 18:85, 1972
463. Shinaberger JH, Miller JH, Rosenblatt MG, Gardner PW, Carpenter GW, Martin FE: Clinical studies of 'low flow' dialysis with membranes highly permeable to middle weight molecules. *Trans Am Soc Artif Intern Organs* 18:82, 1972
464. Manji T, Maeda K, Kawaguchi S, Kobayashi K, Ohta K, Saito A, Amano I, Shimoji T, Fujisaki Y: Short time dialysis with 2 m² hollow fibre kidney. *Proc Eur Dial Transpl Assoc* 11:153, 1974
465. Mirahmadi KS, Kay JH, Miller JH, Gorman JT, Rosens M: Clinical evaluation of patients dialysed with double Gambro 4 hours, three times per week. *Proc Eur Dial Transpl Assoc* 11:121, 1974
466. Rattazzi T, Wathen R, Comty C, Raij L, Leonard A, Shapiro F: The comparison of low flow (Q_D 200) to regular flow (Q_D 500) dialysis. *Trans Am Soc Artif Intern Organs* 20:402, 1974

467. Teschan PE, Ginn HE, Bourne JR, Walker PJ, Ward JW: Quantitative neurobehavioral responses to renal failure and maintenance dialysis. *Trans Am Soc Artif Intern Organs* 21:488, 1975
468. Milutinovic J, Babb AL, Eschbach JW, Follette WC, Graefe U, Strand MJ, Schribner BH: Uremic neuropathy; evidence of middle molecule toxicity. *Artif Organs* 2:45, 1978
469. Cambi V, Dall'Aglio P, Savazzi G, Arisi L, Rossi E, Migone L: Clinical assessment of haemodialysis patients with reduced small molecules removal. *Proc Eur Dial Transpl Assoc* 9:67, 1972
470. Kjellstrand CM, Petersen RJ, Evans RL, Shideman JR, Von Hartitzsch B, Buselmeier TJ: Considerations of the middle molecule hypothesis. II: Neuropathy in nephrectomized patients. *Trans Am Soc Artif Intern Organs* 19:325, 1973
471. Maiorca R, Castellani A, Migozzi G, Panzetta GO, Usberti M: Short time personalised dialysis: good results in spite of high levels of small and middle molecules. *Proc Eur Dial Transpl Assoc* 11:146, 1974
472. Hurst KS, Saldanha LF, Steinberg SM, Galen MA, Lowrie EG, Gagneux SA, Lazarus JM, Strom TB, Carpenter CB, Merrill JP: The effects of varying dialysis regimens on lymphocyte stimulation. *Trans Am Soc Artif Intern Organs* 21:329, 1975
473. Lowrie EG, Steinberg SM, Galen MA, Gagneux SA, Lazarus JM, Gottlieb MN, Merill JP: Factors in the dialysis regimen which contribute to alterations in the abnormalities of uremia. *Kidney Int* 10:409, 1976
474. Nakagawa S, Suenaga M, Sasaki S, Yoshiyama N, Takeuchi J, Kitaoka T, Koshikawa S, Yamada T: Comparison of dialysis programmes on different molecular prescriptions: a preliminary study. *Proc Eur Dial Transpl Assoc* 14:167, 1977
475. Kjellstrand CM, Evans RL, Petersen RJ, Rust LW, Shideman J, Buselmeier TJ, Rozelle LT: Considerations of the middle molecule hypothesis. *Proc Clin Dial Transpl Forum* 1:127, 1972
476. Popovich RP, Moncrief JW: The prediction of metabolite accumulation concomitant with renal insufficiency: the middle molecule anomaly. *Trans Am Soc Artif Intern Organs* 20:377, 1974
477. Sargent JA, Gotch FA: The study of uremia by manipulation of blood concentrations using combinations of hollow fiber devices. *Trans Am Soc Artif Intern Organs* 20:395, 1974
478. Popovich RP, Hlavinka DJ, Bomar JB, Moncrief JW, Decherd JF: The consequences of physiological resistances on metabolite removal from the patient-artificial kidney system. *Trans Am Soc Artif Intern Organs* 21:108, 1975
479. Babb AL, Strand MJ, Uvelli DA, Milutinovic J, Scribner BH: Quantitative description of dialysis treatment: a dialysis index. *Kidney Int* 7 (Suppl 2):S23, 1975
480. Frost TH, Kerr DNS: Kinetics of hemodialysis: A theoretical study of the removal of solutes in chronic renal failure compared to normal health. *Kidney Int* 12:41, 1977
481. Sargent JA, Gotch FA: Principles and biophysics of dialysis. In: *Replacement of renal function by dialysis* 1st ed, edited by Drukker W, Parsons FM, Maher JF, The Hague, Boston, London, Martinus Nijhoff Medical Division, 1978, p 322
482. Babb AL, Farrell PC, Strand MJ, Uvelli D, Milutinovic J, Scribner BH: Residual renal function and chronic hemodialysis therapy. *Proc Clin Dial Transpl Forum* 2:142, 1972
483. Milutinovic J, Strand M, Casaretto A, Follette W, Babb

AL, Scribner BH: Clinical impact of residual glomerular filtration rate (GFR) on dialysis time – a preliminary report. *Trans Am Soc Artif Intern Organs* 20:410, 1974
484. Cristol P, Jeanbrau E, Monnier P: La polypeptidémie en pathologie rénale (The polypeptidaemia in diseases of the kidney). *J Méd France* 27:24 1938 (in French)
485. Walker J: A study of the azotemia observed after severe burns. *Surgery* 19:825, 1946
486. Rosenthal O, McArthy MD: Postburn azotemia, its characteristics and relationship to the severity of terminal injury. *Am J Physiol* 148:365, 1947
487. Christensen HN, Decker DG, Lunch EL, Mackenzie TM, Powers JH: The conjugated, non-protein, amino acids of plasma. V. A study of the clinical significance of peptidemia. *J Clin Invest* 26:853, 1947
488. Dési I, Féher I, Weisz P, Szold E: Untersuchungen der Toxizität des mit Ionenaustauschharzen behandelten urämischen Blutes (Investigation on toxicity of uraemic blood treated with ion exchange resins). *Z Ges Inn Med* 12:1127, 1957 (in German)
489. Féher I, Dési I, Szold E: Isolation of a toxic fraction from uraemic blood. *Experientia* 14:292, 1958
490. Yatzidis H, Psimenos G, Mayopoulou-Symvoulidis D: Non dialysable toxic factor in uremic blood effectively removed by the activated charcoal. *Experientia* 25:1144, 1969
491. Lubash GD, Stenzel KH, Rubin AL: Nitrogenous compounds in hemodialysate. *Circulation* 30:848, 1964
492. Dzúrik R, Adam J, Valovičová E, Řezníček J, Zvara V: The effect of haemodialysis on blood peptide levels. *Proc Eur Dial Transpl Assoc* 8:167, 1971
493. Adam J, Dzúrik R, Valovičová E: Ninhydrin-positive substances in serum and urine of patients with chronic uraemia. *Clin Chim Acta* 36:241, 1972
494. Dzúrik R, Hupková V, Holomán J, Valovičová E: Abnormal carbohydrate metabolism in uraemia. *Int Urol Nephrol* 3:409, 1971
495. Bourgoignie JJ, Hwang KH, Espinel C, Klahr S, Bricker NS: A natriuretic factor in the serum of patients with chronic uremia. *J Clin Invest* 51:1514, 1972
496. Dall'Aglio P, Buzio C, Cambi V, Arisi L, Migone L: La rétention de moyennes molecules dans le sérum urémique (Retention of middle molecules in uraemic serum). *Proc Eur Dial Transpl Assoc* 9:409, 1972 (in French)
497. Dzúrik R, Božek P, Řezníček J, Oborníková A: Blood level of middle molecular substances during uraemia and haemodialysis. *Proc Eur Dial Transpl Assoc* 10:263, 1973
498. Dzúrik R, Hupkova V, Černáček P, Valovičová E, Niederland TR: The isolation of an inhibitor of glucose utilization from the serum of uraemic subjects. *Clin Chim Acta* 46:77, 1973
499. Gajdoš M, Dzúrik R: Erythrocyte glycolysis in uraemia; dynamic balance caused by the opposite action of various factors. *Int Urol Nephrol* 5:331, 1973
500. Man NK, Terlain B, Faris J, Werner G, Sausse A, Funck-Brentano JL: An approach to 'middle molecules' identification in artificial kidney dialysate, with reference to neuropathy prevention. *Trans Am Soc Artif Intern Organs* 19:320, 1973
501. Odeberg H, Olsson I, Thysell H: The effect of uremic serum on granulocyte iodination capacity. *Trans Am Soc Artif Intern Organs* 19:484, 1973
502. Chang TMS, Migchelsen M, Coffey JF, Stark A: Serum middle molecule levels in uremia during long term intermittent hemoperfusions with the ACAC (coated charcoal) microcapsule artificial kidney. *Trans Am Soc Artif Intern Organs* 20:364, 1974
503. Fürst P, Asaba H, Gordon A, Zimmerman L, Bergström J: Middle molecules in uraemia. *Proc Eur Dial Transpl Assoc* 11:417, 1974
504. Hanicki Z, Sarnecka-Keller M, Klein A, Slizowska K: Middlesized ninhydrin-positive molecules in uraemic patients treated by repeated haemodialysis. I. Preliminary characteristics. *Clin Chim Acta* 54:47, 1974
505. Lutz W, Markiewicz K, Klyszejko-Stefanowicz L: Investigations on the activity of lactic dehydrogenase and its inhibitors in the serum of uremic patients during hemodialysis. *Acta Med Pol* 15:97, 1974
506. Man NK, Cueille G, Zingraff J, Druecke T, Jungers P, Sausse A, Brillon JP, Funck-Brentano JL: Investigations on clinico-chemical correlations in uraemic polyneuritis. *Proc Eur Dial Transpl Assoc* 11:214, 1974
507. Peters JH, Gotch FA, Keen M, Berridge BJ Jr, Chao WR: Investigation of the clearance and generation rate of endogenous peptides in normal subjects and uremic patients. *Trans Am Soc Artif Intern Organs* 20:417, 1974
508. Gordon A, Bergström J, Fürst P, Zimmerman L: Separation and characterization of uremic metabolites in biologic fluids: a screening approach to the definition of uremic toxins. *Kidney Int* 7 (Suppl 2):S45, 1975
509. Lutz W: Studies on formation of complexes of insulin with basic peptides isolated from the plasma of uremic patients. *Acta Med Pol* 16:159, 1975
510. Migone L, Dall'Aglio P, Buzio G: Middle molecules in uremic serum, urine and dialysis fluid. *Clin Nephrol* 3:82, 1975
511. Touraine JL, Navarro J, Corré C, Traeger J: Inhibitory effect of mediumsized molecules from patients with renal failure on lymphocyte stimulation by phytohemagglutinin. *Biomedicine* 23:180, 1975
512. Asaba H, Bergström J, Fürst P, Oulès R, Zimmerman L: Accumulation and excretion of middle molecules. *Proc Eur Dial Transpl Ass* 13:481, 1976
513. Bergström J Fürst P, Zimmerman L: A study of uremic toxicology. *Annual Report of NIH Contract* N01-AM-2-2215, 57-59, 1976-75
514. Bergström J, Asaba H, Fürst P, Gordon A, Quadracci L, Zimmerman L: Middle molecules in uremia, in *Proc 6th International Congress of Nephrology (Florence)*, edited by Giovannetti S, Bonomini V, D'Amico G, Basel, S Karger, 1976, p 600
515. Cloix JF, Cueille G, Funck-Brentano JL: Inhibition of bovine renal adenylate cyclase by urinary products. *Biomedicine* 25:215, 1976
516. Funck-Brentano JL, Man NK, Sausse A, Zingraff J, Boudet J, Becker A, Cueille GF: Characterization of a 1100-1300 MW uremic neurotoxin. *Trans Am Soc Artif Intern Organs* 22:163, 1976
517. Fürst P, Zimmerman L, Bergström J: Determination of endogenous middle molecules in normal and uremic body fluids. *Clin Nephrol* 5:178, 1976
518. Gordon A, Lewin A, Rosenfeld J, Roberts M, Maxwell MH: Adsorption of uremic toxins, in *Proc 6th International Congress of Nephrology (Florence)*, edited by Giovannetti S, Bonomini V, D'Amico G, Basel, S Karger, 1976, p 612
519. Hanicki Z, Cichocki T, Sarnecka-Keller M, Klein A, Komorowska Z: Influence of middle-sized molecule aggregates from dialysate of uremic patients on lymphocyte transformation in vivo. *Nephron* 17:73, 1976
520. Lutz W: The influence of a strongly basic uremic peptide on liberation of lipoprotein lipase activity from human adipose cells. *Acta Med Pol* 17:55, 1976
521. Navarro J, Touraine JL, Corré C, Traeger J: Effect in vitro des moyennes molecules sur la prolifération lym-

phocytaire (In vitro effect of middle molecules on proliferation of lymphocytes). *Pathol Biol (Paris)* 24:189, 1976 (in French)
522. Winchester JF, Apiliga MT, Kennedy AC: Short-term evaluation of charcoal hemoperfusion combined with dialysis in uremic patients. *Kidney Int* 10 (Suppl 7):D315, 1976
523. Yamada T, Nakagawa S: Analysis of uremic ultrafiltrate: a possible coincidence of highly toxic small molecular fraction with guanidine derivatives. *Trans Am Soc Artif Intern Organs* 22:155, 1976
524. Asaba H, Bergström J, Fürst P, Gordon A, Groth CG, Oulès R, Zimmerman L: The effects of renal transplantation on middle molecules in plasma and urine. *Clin Nephrol* 8:329, 1977
525. Goubeaud G, Leber HW, Schott HH, Schutterle G: Middle molecules and haemoglobin synthesis. *Proc Eur Dial Transpl Assoc* 13:371, 1977
526. Grof J, Menyhart J: Non diffusible toxic polypeptides in uraemic sera: A new group of uremic toxins. *Acta Chir Acad Sci Hung* 18:283, 1977
527. Leber HW, Neuhäuser M, Goubeaud G: Chronic uremia: hemodialysis or hemoperfusion, in *Artificial Organs* edited by Kenedi RM, Courtney JM, Gaylor JDS, Gilchrist T. London, MacMillan Press Ltd, 1977, p 220
528. Navarro J, Touraine JL, Corré C, Traeger J: Prolongation of skin allograft survival and inhibition of graft versus host reaction in rodents treated with 'middle molecules'. *Cell Immunol* 31:349, 1977
529. Oulès R, Asaba H, Neuhäuser M, Yahiel V, Gunnarsson B, Bergström J, Fürst P: The removal of uremic small and middle molecules and free amino acids by carbon hemoperfusion. *Trans Am Soc Artif Inter Organs* 23:583, 1977
530. Pogglitsch H, Petek W, Waller J, Stübchen-Kirschner H: Hämodynamisch wirksame nieder- und mittelmoleculare Metabolite in Hämofiltrat niereninsuffizienter Patienten (Haemodynamically active low and middle molecular metabolites in haemofiltrate of patients with renal failure). *Wien Klin Wochenschr* 89:812, 1977 (in German)
531. Schneider H, Streicher E, Hachmann H, Chmiel H, v. Mylius U: Clinical experience with haemofiltration. *Proc Eur Dial Transpl Assoc* 14:136, 1977
532. Abiko T, Kumikawa M, Ishizaki M, Takahashi H, Sekono H: Identification and synthesis of a tripeptide in coecum fluid of an uremic patient. *Biochem Biophys Res Commun* 83:357, 1978
533. Abiko T, Kunikawa M, Higuchi H, Sekino H: Identification and synthesis of a heptapeptide in uremic fluid. *Biochem Biophys Res Commun* 84:184, 1978
534. Brunner H, Mann H, Essers U, Schulthesis R, Byrne T, Heintz R: Preparative isolation of middle molecular weight fractions from the hemofiltrate of patients with chronic uremia. *Artif Organs* 2:375, 1978
535. Funck-Brentano JL, Boudet J, Sausse A, Cueille G, Man NK: In vitro sural nerve test for the evaluation of middle molecule neurotoxicity in uraemia. In *Technical Aspects of Renal Dialysis*, edited by Frost TH, Tunbridge Walls, Kent, UK, Pitman Medical, 1978, p 256
536. Jörstad S, Kvernes S: Uraemic toxins of high molecular weight inhibiting human mononuclear phagocytes cultured in vitro. *Acta Path Microbiol Scand [C]* 86:221, 1978
537. Klein A, Sarnecka-Keller M, Hanicki Z: Middle-sized ninhydrin-positive molecules in uremic patients treated by repeated haemodialysis. II. Chief peptide constituents of the fraction. *Clin Chim Acta* 90:7, 1978
538. Leber HW, Spigelhalter R, Schütterle G: A new aspect concerning uremic hemolysis: increased susceptibility of erythrocytes to peroxidation. *Proc Eur Dial Transpl Assoc* 15:437, 1978
539. Lutz W, Madry K, Grande G: 'Middle molecules' in acute experimental uremia. *Acta Med Pol* 19:417, 1978
540. Man NK, Cueille G, Zingraff J, Drueke T, Jungers P, Sausse A, Boudet J, Funck-Brentano JL: Evaluation of plasma neurotoxin concentration in uraemic polyneuropathic patients. *Proc Eur Dial Transpl Assoc* 15:164, 1978
541. Ringoir S, Smet R: Serum chromatographic pattern in different dialysis strategies. *Int J Artif Organs* 1:218, 1978
542. Trznadel K, Walasek L, Kidava Z, Lutz W: Comperative studies on the effect of hemoperfusion and hemodialysis on the elimination of some uremic toxins. *Clin Nephrol* 10:229, 1978
543. Abiko T, Onodera I, Sekono H: Isolation, structures and biological activity of the Trp-containing pentapeptide from uremic fluid. *Biochem Biophys Res Commun* 89:813, 1979
544. Asaba H, Fürst P, Oulès R, Yahiel V, Bergström J: The effect of hemodialysis on endogenous middle molecules in uremic patients. *Clin Nephrol* 11:257, 1979
545. Gál CY, Gróf J: Die Elimination von Stoffen mit kleinen und mittlerem Molekulargewicht bei wiederholter Verwendung von C-DAK-Kapillärdialysatoren (Removal of low and middle molecular weight substances with reuse of CDAK capillary dialysers). *Z Urol Nephrol* 72:27, 1979 (in German)
546. Mamdani BH, Mashouf SM, Evenson MA, Dunea G: Chromatographic studies of uremic plasma. *Int J Artif Organs* 2:187, 1979
547. Mikkers F, Ringoir S, Smet R: Analytical isotachophoresis of uremic blood samples. *J Chromatogr* 162:341, 1979
548. Murisasco A, Saingra S, Crevat A, Rinaudo JB, Gallice P: Action des moyennes molécules en niveau de la respiration cellulaire chez les patients traités par hémodialyse (Effect of middle molecules on the cell respiration in haemodialysis patients). *Proc Soc de Néphrol* 1979, p 586 (in French)
549. Navarro J, Gerlier D, Touraine JL, Later R, Contreras P, Dore JF, Traeger J: A potent inhibitor of cell proliferation in 'middle molecules', isolated from the urine of uremic patients. *Biomedicine* 31:261, 1979
550. Abiko T, Onodera I, Sekino H: Characterization of an acidic tripeptide in neurotoxic dialysate. *Chem Pharm Bull (Tokyo)* 28:1629, 1980
551. Asaba H, Bergström J, Fürst P, Johnson C, Yahiel V: Plasma middle molecules in asymptomatic and 'sick' uremic patients. *Artif Organs* 4 (Suppl):137, 1980
552. Buzio C, Manari C, Calderini G, Montagna G, Migone L: Serum middle molecules in uremia. *Artif Organs* 4 (Suppl):143, 1980
553. Botella J, Gea T, Sanz-Guajardo D, Criado M, Thorres MT, Guardiola J: Blood levels of middle molecules and their effects on motor nerve conduction velocity. *Artif Organs* 4 (Suppl):151, 1980
554. Boudet J, Man NK, Cueille G, Legrain Y, Funck-Brentano JL: Relationship between plasma concentration of middle molecular weight fraction b, motor nerve conduction velocity, and plasma creatinine in experimental chronic renal failure rats. *Artif Organs* 4 (Suppl):115, 1980
555. Brunner H, Mann H, Essers U, Byrne T: Large-scale isolation of middle and higher molecular weight uremic toxins. *Artif Organs* 4 (Suppl):41, 1980
556. Chang TMS, Lister C: Middle molecules in hepatic coma

and uremia. *Artif Organs* 4 (Suppl):169, 1980
557. Chapman GV, Farrell PC: Size, composition and dialytic removal of uremic middle molecules (UMMs). *Abstracts Int Soc for Artif Organs Symposium on Present Status and Future Orientation of Research on the Importance of Middle Molecules in Uremia and other Diseases,* Avignon, Nov 28-29, 1980
558. Chapman GV, Farrell PC: Uremic middle molecules: separation and quantitation. *Artif Organs* 4 (Suppl):160, 1980
559. Chapman GV, Ward RA, Farrell PC: Separation and quantification of the 'middle molecules' in uremia. *Kidney Int* 17:82, 1980
560. Cichocki T, Hanicki Z, Klein A: Influence of middle-molecule-weight solutes from dialysate on the migration rate of leukocytes. *Kidney Int* 17:231, 1980
561. Cueille G, Man NK, Sausse A, Farges JP, Funck-Brentano JL: Characterisation of sub-peak b_{4-2}, middle molecule. *Artif Organs* 4 (Suppl):28, 1980
562. Cueille G, Man NK, Sausse A, Farges JP, Funck-Brentano JL: Technical aspects on middle molecules: separation, isolation, and identification. *Artif Organs* 4 (Suppl):8, 1980
563. Delaporte C, Gros F, Johnson C, Bergström J: In vitro cytotoxic properties of plasma from uremic patients. *Clin Nephrol* 17:247, 1982
564. Dzúrik R, Spustová V: Metabolic actions of middle molecules. *Artif Organs* 4 (Suppl):59, 1980
565. Ehrlich K, Holland F, Turnham T, Klein E: Osmotic concentration of polypeptides from hemofiltrate of uremic patients. *Clin Nephrol* 14:31, 1980
566. Funck-Brentano JL, Man NK: An overview of clinical implication of middle molecules and their kinetics in uremia. *Artif Organs* 4 (Suppl):125, 1980
567. Gallice P, Fournier N, Crevat A, Saingra S, Frayssinet R, Murisasco A, Sicardi F: In vitro inhibition of platelet aggregation by uremic middle molecules. *Biomedicine* 33:185, 1980
568. Gutman RA, Huang AT, Bouknight NS: Inhibitor of marrow thymidine incorporation from sera of patients with uremia. *Kidney Int* 18:715, 1980
569. Kumegawa M, Hiramatsu M, Yamada T, Yajima T: Effects of intermediatesized molecular components in uremic sera on nerve tissue in vitro. *Brain Res* 198:234, 1980
570. Leber HW, Debus E, Grulich U, Schütterle G: Potential role of middle molecular compounds in the development of uremic anemia. *Artif Organs* 4 (Suppl):63, 1980
571. Le Moel GE, Strecker G, Troupel S, Dolegeal M, Jacobs C, Galli A, Agneray J: Carbohydrate content of middle molecular weight substances (MMWS) in uraemic patients: preliminary results. *Artif Organs* 4 (Suppl):37, 1980
572. Le Moel GE, Strecker G, Cueille G, Boudet J, Man NK, Galli A, Agneray J: Uremic middle molecules: analytical study of middle molecular weight fractions subpeak b4.2. *Artif Organs* 4 (Suppl):17, 1980
573. Lindsay RM, Dennis BN, Bergström J, Johnson C, Fürst P: Platelet function as an assay for uremic toxins. *Artif Organs* 4 (Suppl):82, 1980
574. Lustenberger N, Schindhelm K, Nordmeyer C, Schurek HJ, Stolte H: Renal handling of middle molecules in uremic patients and in the isolated rat kidney. *Artif Organs* 4 (Suppl):110, 1980
575. Man NK, Cueille G, Zingraff J, Boudet J, Sausse A, Funck-Brentano JL: Uremic neurotoxin in the middle molecular weight range. *Artif Organs* 4:116, 1980
576. Navarro J, Contreras P, Touraine JL, Freyria AM, Later R, Traeger J: Effect of middle molecules on immunological functions. *Artif Organs* 4 (Suppl):76, 1980
577. Ota K, Sanaka T, Agishi T, Nakajama O: Influence of uremic middle molecules on blood cells. *Artif Organs* 4:113, 1980
578. Oulès R, Emond C, Claret G, Branger B, Mion H, Mion C: Middle molecule accumulation in uremia: an 'extra uremic factor'? *Artif Organs* 4 (Suppl):177, 1980
579. Rinaudo JB, Bernard P, Crest M, Moret JM, Murisasco A, Saingra S, Frayssinet R, Crevat A, Gallice P, Fournier N, Sicardi F: Some aspects of middle molecule toxicity. *Artif Organs* 4 (Suppl):90, 1980
580. Ringoir S, Landschoot N, Smet R: Inhibitor of phagocytosis by middle molecular fraction from ultrafiltrate. *Clin Nephrol* 13:109, 1980
581. Saito A, Kanazawa I, Chung TG, Maeda K: Analytical study for separation of middle molecules. *Artif Organs* 4 (Suppl):13, 1980
582. Schindhelm K, Schlatter E, Schurek HS, Stolte H: The isolated perfused rat kidney and uremic middle molecules. *Contrib Nephrol* 19:191, 1980
583. Schurek HS, Schindhelm K, Schlatter E, Stolte H: Renal handling of uremic middle molecules as studied in the isolated perfused rat kidney. *Renal Physiol* 2:163, 1980
584. Scigalla P, Gudim VI, Ivanova VS, Moskaleva GP, Noach CH, Devaux S, Gorbunova NA, Grossmann P: Die Mittelmoleküle als Erythropoesehemmfaktoren im Blut terminal niereninsuffizienter Kinder; einfluß der urämischen Mittelmoleküle auf die Fe^{59} einbaurate polyzythämischer Mäuse (Middle molecules as inhibitors of erythropoiesis in the blood of children with terminal renal failure; the influence of uraemic middle molecules on the rate of incorporation of Fe^{59} in polycythaemic mice). *Dtsch Gesundh Wesen* 35:1331, 1980 (in German)
585. Scigalla P, Gudim VI, Ivanova VS, Moskaleva GP, Noach CH, Devaux S, Gorbunova NA, Grossmann P: Die Mittelmoleküle als Erythropoesehemmfaktoren im Blut terminal niereninsuffizienter Kinder; über die Hemmwirkung von Mittelmolekülen aus dem Serum terminal niereninsuffizienter Kinder auf die Erytropoese intakter Mäuse (Middle molecules as inhibitors of erythropoiesis in the blood of children with terminal renal failure; on the inhibition of the erythropoiesis of normal mice by middle molecules from the blood serum of children in the terminal stage of renal failure). *Dtsch Gesundh Wesen* 35:1366, 1980 (in German)
586. Scigalla P, Gudim VI, Ivanova VS, Moskaleva GP, Noach CH, Devaux S, Gorbunova NA, Grossmann P: Die Mittelmoleküle als Erythropoesehemmfaktoren im Blut terminal niereninsuffizienter Kinder; Wirkung der Mittelmoleküle aus urämischem serum auf die pluripotenten Knochenmarkstammzellen in-vivo (The middle molecules as inhibitors of erythropoiesis in the blood of children with terminal renal failure; effect of middle molecules from uraemic serum on pluripotential bone marrow stem cells in-vivo). *Dtsch Gesundh Wesen* 35:1422, 1980 (in German)
587. Válek A, Dzúrik R, Spustová V, Válková D: Concentration of plasma middle molecular weight substances and clinical condition of patients undergoing short-time regular dialysis treatment. *Artif Organs* 4 (Suppl):173, 1980
588. Zimmerman L, Fürst P, Bergström J, Jörnvall H: A new glycine containing compound with a blocked amino group from uremic body fluids. *Clin Nephrol* 14:107, 1980
589. Zimmerman L, Jörnvall H, Bergström J, Fürst P, Sjövall J: Characterization of middle molecule compounds. *Artif Organs* 4 (Suppl):33, 1980
590. Zimmerman L, Baldesten A, Bergström J, Fürst P: Isota-

chophoretic separation of middle molecule peptides in uremic body fluids. *Clin Nephrol* 14:183, 1980
591. Bergström J, Asaba H, Fürst P, Lindholm B: Middle molecules in chronic uremic patients treated with peritoneal dialysis. In: *Advances in peritoneal Dialysis,* edited by Gahl GM, Kessel M, Nolph KD, Amsterdam, Oxford, Princeton, Excerpta Medica, 1981, p 47
592. Zimmerman L, Jörnvall H, Bergström J, Fürst P, Sjövall J: Characterization of a double conjugate in uremic body fluids: glucuronidated Ohydroxybenzolglycine. *FEBS Lett* 129:237, 1981
593. Shioya Y, Yoshida H, Nakajima T: A method for the M.W. estimation of peptides. In *Peptide Chemistry 1979,* edited by Yonehara H. Osaka (Japan), Protein Research Foundation, 1980, p 127
594. Gotch FA, Sargent JA: Modelling of middle molecules in clinical studies. *Artif Organs* 4 (Suppl):133, 1980
595. Scigalla P, Gudim VI, Noach CH, Devaux S, Grossmann P: Zur Bedeutung der Mittelmolekülenelimination aus dem Serum niereninsuffizienter Kinder für die Pathogenese der renalen Anämie (The significance of the elimination of middle molecules from the serum of children with renal failure for the pathogenesis of renal anaemia). *Dtsch Gesundh Wesen* 35:170, 1980 (in German)
596. Funck-Brentano JL, Sausse A, Man NK, Granger A, Rondon-Nucete M, Zingraff J, Jungers P: Une nouvelle méthode d'hémodialyse associant une membrane à haute perméabilité pour les moyennes molécules et un bain de dialyse en circuit fermé (A new haemodialysis technique employing a membrane highly permeable for middle molecules and a closed circuit dialysate supply system). *Proc Eur Dial Transpl Assoc* 9:55, 1972 (in French)
597. Tsaltas TT: Studies of lipochromes (urochromes) in uremic patients and normal controls. I. The elimination of plasma lipochromes by hemodialysis. *Trans Am Soc Artif Intern Organs* 15:321, 1969
598. Tsaltas TT: Studies of lipochromes in uremic patients and normal controls. II. Isolation and identification of carotenoids and lipochromes and their oxidation products in plasma. *Trans Am Soc Artif Intern Organs* 16:272, 1970
599. Comaish JS, Ashcroft T, Kerr DNS: The pigmentation of chronic renal failure. *Acta Derm Venereol (Stockh)* 55:215, 1975
600. Massry SG, Goldstein DA: Role of parathyroid hormone in uremic toxicity. *Kidney Int* 13 (Suppl 8):S39, 1978
601. Massry SG, Goldstein DA: The search for uremic toxin(s) 'X'. 'X' = PTH. *Clin Nephrol* 11:181, 1979
602. Slatopolsky E, Martin K, Hruska K: Parathyroid hormone metabolism and its potential as a uremic toxin. *Am J Physiol* 239 (1):F1, 1980
603. Cooper JD, Lazarowitz VC, Arieff AI: Neurodiagnostic abnormalities in patients with acute renal failure: evidence for neurotoxicity of parathyroid hormone. *J Clin Invest* 61:1448, 1978
604. Guisade R, Arieff AI, Massry SG: Changes in the electroencephalogram in acute uremia. *J Clin Invest* 55:738, 1975
605. Arieff AI, Massry SG: Calcium metabolism of brain in acute renal failure. *J Clin Invest* 53:387, 1974
606. Goldstein DA, Feinstein EI, Chui LA, Pattabhiraman R, Massry SG: The relationship between the abnormalities in electroencephalogram and blood levels of parathyroid hormone in dialysis patients. *J Clin Endocrinol Metab* 61:130, 1980
607. Avram MM, Feinfeld DA, Huatuco AH: Search for the uremic toxin: decreased motor-nerve conduction velocity and elevated parathyroid hormone in uremia. *N Engl J Med* 298:1000, 1978

608. Goldstein DA, Chui LA, Massry SG: Effect of parathyroid hormone and uremia on peripheral nerve calcium and motor nerve conduction velocity. *J Clin Invest* 62:88, 1978
609. Schaeffer K, Offermann G, Von Herrath D, Schröter R, Stölzel R, Arntz HR: Failure to show a correlation between serum parathyroid hormone, nerve conduction velocity and serum lipids in hemodialysis patients. *Clin Nephrol* 14:81, 1980
610. Avram MM, Alexis H, Rahman M, Son B, Iancu M: Decreased tranfusional requirement following parathyroidectomy in long term hemodialysis. *Abstracts Am Soc Nephrol* 5:5, 1971
611. Better OS, Shasha SM, Windver J, Chaimovitz C: Improvement in the anemia of hemodialysis patients following parathyroidectomy (PTX). *Abstracts Am Soc Nephrol* 9:1, 1976
612. Zingraff J, Tilman D, Marie P: Anemia and secondary hyperparathyroidism. *Arch Intern Med* 138:1650, 1978
613. Podjarny E, Rathaus M, Korzets Z, Blum M, Zevin D, Bernheim J: Is anemia of chronic renal failure related to secondary hyperparathyroidism? *Arch Intern Med* 141:453, 1981
614. Bourgoignie JJ, Hwang KH, Ipakchi E, Bricker NS: The presence of a natriuretic factor in urine of patients with chronic uremia. *J Clin Invest* 53:1559, 1974
615. Kaplan MA, Bourgoignie JJ, Rosecan J, Bricker NS: The effects of the natriuretic factor from uremic urine on sodium transport, water and electrolyte content, and pyruvate oxidation by the isolated toad bladder. *J Clin Invest* 53:1568, 1974
616. Bourgoignie JJ, Kaplan M, Eun C, Favre H, Hwang K, Blumenfeld O, Bricker NS: On the characterization of the natriuretic factor. *Clin Res* 23:429A, 1975
617. Bricker NS, Schmidt RW, Faure H, Fine L, Bourgoignie JJ: On the biology of sodium excretion: the search for a natriuretic hormone. *Yale J Biol Med* 48:293, 1975
618. Carone FA: Renal handling of proteins and peptides. *Ann Clin Lab Sci* 8:287, 1978
619. Hall CL, Hardwicke J: Low molecular weight proteinuria. *Annu Rev Med* 30:199, 1979
620. Berggård I, Bearn AG: Isolation and properties of a low molecular weight beta-2-globulin occurring in human biological fluids. *J Biol Chem* 243:4095, 1968
621. Bernier GM, Cohen RJ, Conrad ME: Microglobulinaemia in renal failure. *Nature* 218:598, 1968
622. Dall'Aglio P, Maiorca R, Scarpioni L, Migone L: Serum proteins and dialysis treatment. *Proc Eur Dial Transpl Assoc* 7:182, 1970
623. Hansen VE, Karle H, Andersen V: Lysozyme turnover in the rat. *J Clin Invest* 50:1473, 1971
624. Wibell L, Evrin PE, Berggård I: Serum beta-2-microglobulin in renal disease. *Nephron* 10:320, 1973
625. Kult J, Dragoun GP: Low molecular serum proteins in uremic patients. In: *Renal Insufficiency* Würzburg Symposium 1974), edited by Heidland A, Hennemann H, Kult J, Stuttgart, Georg Thieme 1976, p 115
626. Reddi KK: Serum ribonuclease of normal persons and patients with renal impairment. *Clin Biochem* 11:133, 1978
627. Rabin EZ, Algom D, Freedman MH, Geunthier L, Dardick I, Tattrie B: Ribonuclease activity in renal failure. *Nephron* 27:254, 1981
628. Rabin EZ, Tattrie B, Algom D, Freedman M, Saunders F, Roncari DAK: Ribonuclease activity in renal failure: evidence for toxicity. *Abstracts Am Soc Nephrol* 9:22, 1976
629. Leclerc J: Action of ribonuclease on the multiplication of influenza virus. *Nature* 177:578, 1956

630. Glukhov BN, Jerusalimsky AP, Canter VM, Salganik RJ: Ribonuclease treatment of tick-borne encephalitis. *Arch Neurol* 33:598, 1976
631. Bertholeyns J, Baudhuin J: Inhibition of tumor cell proliferation by dimerized ribonuclease. *Proc Natl Acad Sci USA* 72:573, 1976
632. Brunner H, Brunner A, Essers U, Heintz R: Inhibition of bone marrow cell proliferation by undialyzable fractions, in *Renal Insufficiency* (Würzburg Symposium 1974), edited by Heidland A, Hennemann H, Kult J, Stuttgart, Georg Thieme Publishers, 1976, p 90
633. Lamberts B, Brunner H, Ochs HG, Spellerberg P, Heintz R: Effect of urine metabolites from healthy and uremic subjects on gluconeogenesis in slices of rat kidney cortex and liver. *Clin Nephrol* 6:465, 1976
634. Dzúrik R, Spustová V, Černáček P: Inhibitor of renal gluconeogenesis (IGN): additional physiological modulator? *Int J Biochem* 12:103, 1980
635. Korz R, Hild D, Brunner H, Büssing A: Untersuchungen zur Pathogenese der urämischen Lymphozytentransformationshemmung. (Investigations on the pathogenesis of the inhibition of lymphocyte transformation in uraemia). *Klin Wochenschr* 58:1233, 1980 (in German)
636. Jörstad S, Smeby LC, Wideröe TE, Berg KJ: Transport of uremic toxins through conventional hemodialysis membranes. *Clin Nephrol* 12:168, 1979
637. Jörstad S, Smeby LC, Wideröe TE, Berg KJ: Removal of uremic toxins and regeneration of hemofiltrate by a selective dual hemofiltration artificial kidney (SEDUFARK) system. *Clin Nephrol* 13:85, 1980
638. Jörstad S, Smeby LC, Wideröe TE: Toxicity of middle molecules: Clinical evaluation using a selective filtration artificial kidney. *Artif Organs* (Suppl) 4:98, 1980

20
REGULAR DIALYSIS TREATMENT (RDT)

BARBARA G. DELANO

Introduction	391
Initiation of maintenance hemodialysis	391
Time to plan	392
No time to plan	392
Discontinuation of dialysis	393
The early phases of maintenance dialysis	393
Hemodialysis schedules	393
Adequacy of dialysis	393
'Adequacy' of a single dialysis	394
Short dialysis	394
Infrequent dialysis	395
The portable suitcase kidney	396
Routine monitoring of medical problems in dialysis patients	396
Evaluation of the long term dialysis patient	398
Regular hemodialysis treatment for high risk groups of patients	399
The elderly	399
Atherosclerotic heart disease	399
Coronary bypass surgery	399
Diabetes mellitus	400
Systemic lupus erythematosus	400
Diffuse scleroderma (progressive systemic sclerosis)	400
Multiple myeloma	400
Amyloidosis/Liver disease	401
Dialysis associated ascites	401
Heroin addicts	402
Sickle cell anemia	402
Pregnancy	402
References	402

INTRODUCTION

Today, throughout the world, close to 100,000 patients with end-stage renal disease are kept alive by maintenance hemodialysis therapy (1). As health care workers, it is incumbent upon us to be familiar with the many facets of this ubiquitous therapy. Important technical information such as selection of equipment for hemodialysis (dialyzers, monitors, etc.) is discussed elsewhere in this book. This chapter addresses the problems of when to initiate dialysis therapy, how to select a schedule, and special precautions and considerations for high risk patients. In addition to providing a scheme for routine monitoring of dialysis patients it also gives an assessment of 10 (or more) years veterans of dialysis.

INITIATION OF MAINTENANCE HEMODIALYSIS

There is no difficulty in deciding to begin dialysis in a severely symptomatic uremic patient. The asymptomatic patient, inexorably deteriorating in terms of measured renal function, does create a problem, however, as to when to abandon conservative therapy in favor of dialysis. Controversy exists over the optimal time to initiate regular dialysis therapy.

The most therapeutically aggressive view is held by Bonomini and co-workers (2), who believe that regular hemodialysis should begin when the patients' endogenous creatinine clearance falls to between 15 to 21 ml/min. In correlating survival rates of their patients with the creatinine clearance at which hemodialysis was begun (0 to 21 ml/min), Bonomini and co-workers found the best survival (85% over four years) in those patients who started dialysis with higher creatinine clearances. Bonomini (3) explained these results by suggesting that in patients whose endogenous creatinine clearances is no higher than 5 ml/min uremic complications are more pronounced and will irreversibly progress despite maintenance hemodialysis. Indeed, he suggests that by starting hemodialysis at a higher creatinine clearance the harmful effects of protein depletion can be eliminated, and renal and extrarenal hormone equilibrium may be better preserved (4).

Scribner (5) points out that Bonomini's patients may not be representative of general selection criteria. Survival of Bonomini's patients with a creatinine clearance of 0 to 5 ml/min, who were dialyzed 2 to 3 times per week for 5 to 10 hours, was inexplicably poor (only 40% were alive after 4 years). Depending on age and co-existing systemic diseases, annual mortality in regularly dialyzed patients ranges from 5 to 10% in most large centers around the world. Poor survival together with deterioration of motor nerve conduction velocities in Bonomini's patients were interpreted by Scribner as evidence of inadequate dialysis thereby invalidating the conclusions as to efficacy of the 'early' treatment schedule.

Substantial clinical experience indicates that maintenance hemodialysis is best initiated when the patients' creatinine clearance is approximately 5 ml/min. As residual renal function falls below this level, the patient becomes catabolic, loses weight, and develops complications such as motor neuropathy and pericarditis – all of which interfere with subsequent rehabilitation. Berlyne and Giovannetti (6) concur in advising beginning hemodialysis at a creatinine clearance of 5 ml/min. Admittedly with stringent dietary protein restriction, it is possible to postpone dialysis in some patients until glomerular filtration rate diminishes to as low as 2 ml/min. This is not to be advised unless both patient and physician are attuned to a regimen of frequent visits and close monitoring of the patients' overall condition. On the other hand, starting maintenance hemodialysis at a glomerular filtration rate in excess of 15 ml/min is not justified, except perhaps in malignant hypertension or intractable nephrotic syndrome. Not only would such early treatment overload presently available dialysis facilities, but patients would risk mortality and morbidity due to the dialysis procedure.

Maher (7) found that, depending on diagnosis, renal diseases progress at differing rates; occasionally, patients survive without dialysis for as long as 3 years after reaching a serum creatinine concentration of 10 mg/dl (884 µmol/l). By contrast accelerated deterioration in renal function over weeks to months is common in systemic sclerosis, malignant hypertension and rapidly progressive glomerulonephritis.

While at our institution we have generally subscribed to the 5 ml/min starting point for maintenance hemodialysis, the patient's clinical condition is more important than laboratory measurements of glomerular filtration rate. We have recently seen some patients with uremic symptoms (i.e. nausea, vomiting, lassitude) at a serum creatinine concentration of 5 mg/dl (442 µmol/l) (creatinine clearance of approximately 10 ml/min) who subjectively feel much improved after a dialysis. Usually, these patients have diabetes mellitus, or some other systemic illness. In such cases, a trial of dialysis may be warranted and if the patient feels better, it may be wise to begin maintenance dialysis at that time.

TIME TO PLAN

Ideally, with early recognition of renal disease and progressive renal failure, there is adequate opportunity to plan for smooth initiation of long term hemodialysis. As soon as it becomes clear that a patient has progressive renal failure, the patient, family and medical advisors should review the probable rate of deterioration and the types of treatment available. The suitability of hemodialysis, peritoneal dialysis or transplantation may vary according to the patient's age, diagnosis and preference. In our program every new patient meets with both the transplant surgeon and the nephrologist. Whenever possible and appropriate, the new patient should also meet someone who is leading an active life after many years of dialysis. Hurdling the barriers of psychological adjustment to regular dialysis is made easier by full and frank disclosure of all facts to the patient.

At the outset, management of renal failure should include provision of vascular access well in advance of need to allow an arteriovenous fistula to 'mature'. Elderly, obese, and diabetic patients may require two to four months before a fistula is ready for use. The Cimino-Brescia arteriovenous fistula (8) is the access of choice for most patients. Patients with small or thrombosed veins, diabetic patients or the very obese may have a bovine carotid heterograft performed as the procedure of choice ([9], see Chapter 8). We usually perform vascular access surgery when the creatinine clearance has fallen to approximately 10 ml/min. Patients who can be anticipated to have a 'slow access maturation', such as diabetic patients, should have surgery earlier (15 to 20 ml/min). In those individuals with slowly progressive diseases (e.g. polycystic kidney disease) we may delay vascular access until their clearance has fallen to 6 to 8 ml/min (which may take months to years).

NO TIME TO PLAN

Unfortunately, all too frequently patients present with far advanced uremia requiring immediate dialysis. These patients may be handled in the following ways:

1. Permanent access (a fistula or artery heterograft) is placed in the non-dominant arm (to permit self-puncture of the fistula if the patient is going to be on home or limited care dialysis). For immediate use a Scribner shunt is temporarily placed in the dominant arm or leg. In older or diabetic patients two arteriovenous anastomoses, however, may lead to high output cardiac failure (10, 11). A further drawback is that vessels in the shunt limb are permanently destroyed. Also, shunts have a recognized propensity for thrombosis and infection.

2. Permanent access may be placed in the non-dominant arm, and repetitive peritoneal dialysis performed until the access is mature. Occasionally, in patients with polycystic kidneys, pyelonephritis, obstructive uropathy, high urine volume, urinary tract infection, or extracellular dehydration, an occasional peritoneal dialysis may delay the need for maintenance hemodialysis for a long time. (A delay of 4 years has been observed after one peritoneal dialysis [12]). Intermittent peritoneal dialysis or continuous ambulatory peritoneal dialysis is an acceptable mode of long term therapy.

3. Permanent access is placed in the non-dominant arm and the patient sustained by repeated subclavian cannulation (13).

4. The plan we have found most useful, is to create permanent access in the non-dominant arm while sustaining the patient with hemodialysis via percutaneous femoral venous catheters until the fistula matures (14, 15). Our experience has been described previously (16). Repeated femoral catheter dialysis can be successfully performed over many months ([17]: one patient had 102 consecutive femoral catheterizations). We have found the procedure to be simple, safe, and easily performed by selected members of our nursing staff after suitable instruction (18). Femoral catheter dialysis is associated with infrequent but appreciable complications. These include bleeding at the catheter site, iliofemoral vein thrombosis with pulmonary embolism and perforation of the inferior vena cava (19).

Recently subclavian vein cannulation has been introduced to provide temporary vascular access for hemodialysis. The cannula which is specially designed for this purpose can remain in situ for a week and can be used repeatedly, causing minimal discomfort for the patient (20).

DISCONTINUATION OF DIALYSIS

Occasionally the physician is faced with the decision (when) to discontinue dialysis. We have observed the return of sufficient renal function to permit stopping dialysis in eight patients. Four of the eight had malignant hypertension, two had gouty nephropathy, one had chronic glomerulonephritis and one had cortical necrosis (21). Resumption of renal function in patients with malignant hypertension, once the blood pressure is controlled, is being reported with increasing frequency (22–26), particularly with minoxidil therapy (26). Reversal of renal failure has also been reported in scleroderma (27–29) and myeloma kidney (30). A pre-dialysis serum creatinine concentration equal to or lower than the previous post-dialysis creatinine concentration, and an increase in the patient's urine volume are important clues suggesting the return of renal function.

A much more difficult area to deal with is when to stop or withhold dialysis in a patient who for example is in coma due to dialysis dementia or is terminally ill with far advanced cancer. These are both economical and ethical issues (31). One view has been espoused by Beauchamp (32). He states that dialysis treatment is not obligatory when it offers no prospect of benefit. In addition, treatment may not be appropriate when its burdens outweigh its benefits for the patient. Beauchamp also discusses the irresponsible or 'no show' patient. He believes that a physician has at most a 'weak obligation' to dialyze a patient if he or she repeatedly misses treatments and shows up in an emergency room situation.

These issues are obviously not easy ones, they have not been extensively discussed (33) and at the moment, each physician must make his or her own decisions in these matters. There is a great need for some set of guidelines to follow.

THE EARLY PHASES OF MAINTENANCE DIALYSIS

There are few empirically determined guidelines as to how to begin regular dialysis therapy. When the first hemodialysis is a rapid and efficient one, patients may develop various problems: headache, nausea, vomiting, blurring of vision, muscle twitching, disorientation, tremors, seizures and rarely coma. This dialysis disequilibrium syndrome characteristically occurs towards the end of dialysis after rapid lowering of the blood urea nitrogen concentration (34). The most consistent finding in patients with dialysis disequilibrium is an elevated cerebrospinal fluid (CSF) pressure and cerebral edema. The exact cause of the cerebral edema is not known. One explanation is that urea is cleared more rapidly from the blood than from the CSF. Indeed, the urea concentration in the CSF during rapid dialysis is 14 to 19 mmol/kg of water (84 to 114 mg/dl) higher than in plasma, causing an appreciably higher osmolality. This presumably draws fluid in, and the CSF pressure rises (35, 36).

However, CSF pressure generally rises whether dialysis is slow or rapid, regardless of the presence of the disequilibrium syndrome (37).

Animal studies, however, have shown that the rate of clearance of urea from the CSF is the same as from the plasma (38). Other possible causes of dialysis disequilibrium are hypoglycemia (39), hyponatremia (40), and acidosis (41). Arieff and Massry (42) have experimentally demonstrated a fall in the CSF pH while arterial pH returned towards normal during rapid hemodialysis. A fall in the intracellular pH of the cerebral cortex and a rise in brain water content have also been demonstrated (43).

The solute that contributes to the observed rise of brain intracellular osmolality has not been identified. Changes in the measured solutes in the brain cannot account for the rise in osmolality (42). The fall in bicarbonate concentration of both cerebral spinal fluid and brain suggest the appearance of organic acids which could be the by-products of protein or polypeptide metabolism (44). These unidentified solutes have been termed idiogenic osmols (42).

Recognizing that each patient will require individualization of therapy, we attempt to prevent or minimize the disequilibrium syndrome by starting the patient with short, frequent, treatments (45). Using 'standard' coil, hollow fiber or plate dialyzers, we dialyze for 2 h on day one, 2 to 4 h on day two, no dialysis on day three, 4 h on day four, and then proceed with routine thrice weekly 4 to 5 h treatments.

Other methods of avoiding or reducing the disequilibrium syndrome have been suggested (46–49). These include adding osmotically active solutes (dextrose, glycerol, mannitol, etc.) to the dialysate or substituting bicarbonate for acetate in order to minimize rapid alterations in plasma osmolality or bicarbonate concentration during dialysis.

If the dialysis disequilibrium syndrome does occur, intravenous injection of 50 ml of 50% dextrose may improve the situation transiently, particularly if given within minutes of the onset of headache. Dextrose injections may be repeated two or three times over the next 2 hours. Dialysis should be discontinued, at least temporarily, if patient discomfort is severe.

HEMODIALYSIS SCHEDULES

Adequacy of dialysis

Because dialysis is time consuming and expensive, there is great interest in shortening the duration of the procedure. To accomplish this requires evaluation of differing dialysis protocols, but always in light of effective treatment or so-called adequacy of dialysis. Obviously, any worthwhile innovation in dialysis scheduling must assure that the patient will fare no worse and, hopefully, will actually be benefited.

After 15 to 20 years of studying treatment schedules, adequate dialysis is still a concept which is not easy to define (50). Statistical methods of assessing the adequacy of hemodialysis have been proposed (51), though not necessarily accepted. Babb and Scribner (52, 53) devised the dialysis index (DI) by which they feel the weekly amount of dialysis needed for a patient can be prescribed. In order to discern what is insufficient or 'underdialysis', measurements of motor nerve conduction velocity (MNCV), electroencephalogram, hematocrit (Hct), continuous performance test, diet log and activity index were used.

The retention of middle molecules, unknown substances with a molecular mass in the 500 to 2000 dalton range (see Chapter 19), is thought by many to be responsible for inadequate dialysis, particularly when manifested by the presence of peripheral neuropathy (54, 55). Several investigators have supported the middle molecule hypothesis (56, 57) while others doubt that these molecules are any more important than small molecules in determining adequacy of dialysis (58–61). Lowrie and co-workers, by varying dialysis regimens, found that abnormal alterations in parameters such as motor nerve conduction times and bleeding times correlated better with increased concentrations of small rather than 'middle' molecules. They also noted that some patients spontaneously and unconsciously attempted to reduce the level of metabolites like urea by reducing the dietary intake of proteins (62).

At the present time no one measure, chemical or clinical, has proven acceptable to measure adequacy of dialysis. Kopple and Swendseid (63), for example, stipulate that adequate dialysis must permit good nutrition, particularly the intake of protein and amino acids. Desforges (64) states that adequate dialysis improves but does not correct the anemia of uremia. Good dialysis reverses the bleeding tendency and may improve white cell function. Parker (65) believes adequate dialysis is that in which the resting muscle membrane potential returns to and remains normal. The status of the patients' bones (66) and cardiovascular system (67, 68) must also be considered in formulating an assessment of sufficient dialysis therapy.

In a study of 50 consecutive hemodialysis patients at our institution we found that a normal serum albumin and a hematocrit greater than 26% correlated best with patients clinically judged to be adequately dialyzed (69).

We believe the definition of adequate dialysis submitted by DePalma (70), though perhaps imprecise, is nevertheless useful until a specific quantifiable substitute is found. It is:

'Adequate dialysis is that which permits the patient to be rehabilitated, eat a reasonable diet, make blood, maintain a near normal blood pressure, and prevent the development or progression of neuropathy'.

'Adequacy' of a single dialysis

The biochemical changes that occur during a single dialysis depend on several factors. At any point during a stable dialysis the concentration of a substance (e.g. urea) depends on its rate of generation, its volume of distribution, the patients' residual renal function, the hemodialyzer clearance and the elapsed dialysis time (71).

Hemodialysis clearance depends on the type of membrane, the total dialyzer surface area and the flow rate of blood and dialysis fluid.

A 50 to 60% reduction in serum creatinine and urea concentrations is desirable during a single hemodialysis. If this is not obtained, the following questions must be asked:

1. Is the artificial kidney surface area adequate? A large muscular man may need a dialyzer with a 2.5 m² surface area, as compared to a 1.3 m² dialyzer for a small woman.
2. Is the blood flow adequate? In patients without heart disease and with good vascular access, blood flows of 250 to 300 ml/min may be maintained with impunity.
3. Are the hours of dialysis adequate? Most dialyses in our unit are 4 to 5 h in duration (see below).
4. Is blood recirculation occurring? At our institution, recirculation of blood has caused recurrent uremic symptoms with dialysis time that has previously been adequate (72). Recirculation can occur in the presence of normal venous pressure and good blood flow. The percentage of recirculation is calculated in the following way: the BUN is determined in the blood to the dialyzer (C_a), in the blood from the dialyzer (C_v) and in peripheral blood (C_p). Samples should be taken simultaneously and the following formula is used:

$$\frac{C_p - C_a}{C_p - C_v} \times 100 = \% \text{ recirculation.}$$

If more than 20% of the blood is found to be recirculating corrective access surgery should be strongly considered. Recirculation is a well recognized risk in single needle dialysis.

Short dialysis

Many attempts to shorten dialysis time have been published. Milutinovic and associates (73) suggest that in evaluating all reports of reduced dialysis time the patients' residual renal function must be taken into consideration. They studied 15 chronic dialysis patients in whom they reduced the hours of dialysis according to each patient's individual glomerular filtration rate (GFR). It was concluded that even a low residual GFR could permit time reductions of up to 60%. In one case as little as 2 hours of treatment, three times per week, was sufficient. They caution, however, that it may be years before we can properly evaluate any negative result of reduced dialysis times. Dialysis regimens which include no 'excess' treatment time, leave the patient no reserve to protect against stress, infection, trauma, or dietary protein indiscretion.

Indeed, Ahmad and co-workers (53) found that in a

group of five patients with glomerular filtration rates greater than 1.0 ml/min (mean 3.2 ml/min), dialysis time could be reduced from a mean of 16.4 to a mean of 6.7 h per week for up to 4 years. By contrast, in four additional patients with GFR's of less than 1.3 ml/min, reduced dialysis time was associated with the development of neuropathy. To reduce dialysis time safely in patients with a residual GFR of less than 1.0 ml/min, the following precautions are recommended (53):
(a) Use a potassium free dialysate;
(b) Increase oral phosphate binders;
(c) Consider the use of bicarbonate-containing dialysate;
(d) If intercurrent illness occurs, increase dialysis time temporarily.

Manji and co-workers (74) feel that to decrease dialysis time safely, blood flow through the dialyzer must be increased (something that may be difficult to do), the surface area of the dialyzer should be increased, or a more efficient membrane should be used. Alverez-Ude et al. (75) did reduce dialysis time from 6 to 8 h three times a week to 4 to 5 h thrice weekly by increasing blood flow. They found that when dialyzed for shorter hours, patients had a higher incidence of itching, tingling, numbness, impaired vibratory sense and difficulty in controlling blood pressure. However, shorter dialysis time also was associated with less postdialysis muscle weakness and dizziness.

In a more positive vein, Knoll et al. (76) found no change in median nerve conduction velocity, vibratory sense or hematocrit in a group of 48 patients followed for 23 months on a shortened dialysis schedule.

Manji and co-workers (74) also studied the effect of increased dialyzer surface area in permitting shorter treatment plans. They used a 2.0 m^2 or a 2.5 m^2 hollow fiber kidney, and were able to dialyze patients for 4 to 4.5 h thrice weekly. Clinically, the patients did not appear different from when they were dialyzed 6 to 7 hours thrice weekly with a 1.3 m^2 dialyzer. Similarly, Ari, Oren, and Berlyne (77) were able to halve the time of each treatment by using two Ultraflow coils in series. Others have suggested the importance of kinetic modeling in evaluating hemodialysis schedules (78).

In an important paper with practical implications, Martin et al. (79) compared a group of patients dialyzed 6 to 9 h thrice weekly on a 1.0 m^2 dialyzer with patients treated thrice weekly for 3 to 3 ½ h on a 1.5 m^2 dialyzer. Shortening treatment time in this fashion permitted an increase in the treatment capacity of their dialysis unit. There was also a decrease in the number of hours per month the unit was used, and fewer nurses and technicians were required. Although patients so treated had higher pre- and post-dialysis serum creatinine, blood urea nitrogen, and serum phosphate concentrations, the short dialysis regimen was not associated with symptoms in most patients. However, a cautionary note was added by two patients who developed uremic pericarditis of sufficient severity to require pericardiectomy.

In a large cooperative study in which we participated, the effect of the hours of dialysis and the blood urea nitrogen levels on morbidity and mortality were evaluated in four groups of patients:

Group I — time 4.5 h, mean BUN 51 mg/dl (18 mmol/l of urea)
Group II — time 4.5 h, mean BUN 88 mg/dl (31 mmol of urea)
Group III — time 3.3 h, mean BUN 54 mg/dl (19 mmol/l of urea)
Group IV — time 3.25 h, mean BUN 90 mg/dl (32 mmol/l of urea)

Because Group III experienced more hospitalization than Group I and Group IV experienced more than Group II, it was suggested that less time may contribute to morbidity. The effect of time was marginal, however, compared to the effect of higher blood urea nitrogen concentrations (80).

With regard to substances of molecular weight in the range 500 to 2000 ('middle molecules'), the use of a polyacrylonitrile (PA) membrane, which is more permeable than the standard Cuprophane or other cellulose-based membranes, has been advocated by some as a means of diminishing dialysis time (81). We have not been able to reduce the duration of dialyses when employing a dialyzer with a PA membrane. Clinical evidence of underdialysis was apparent in previously stable patients when dialysis time was halved from 6 to 3 h.

Sellars, Robson & Wilkinson (82) caution that patients dialyzed fewer hours have a higher exchangeable body sodium and may be at greater risk of hypertension.

By recirculating the dialysate, Cambi (83) found no deterioration in a group of patients treated for 2 h every other day with a standard Cuprophane dialyzer (1.0 to 1.5 m^2). He did, however, have to infuse molar sodium bicarbonate in order to maintain the pre-dialysis serum bicarbonate above 21 mmol/l.

Infrequent dialysis

In addition to experimentation with the number of hours per dialysis treatment, there have been trials of decreased numbers of treatments per week. Most centers dialyze patients three times per week. In a comparative study, we demonstrated that patients dialyzed three times per week, rather than the same number of hours twice a week, had higher hematocrits, lower pre-dialysis creatinine and urea concentrations, and a greater sense of well-being (84).

Dyck and co-workers (85) studied the effects of dialyzing a group of 11 patients once per week (8 h for men, 6 h for women) while maintaining them on a stringent diet. This was a crossover study and the same group of patients were dialyzed three times per week (8 h for men, 6 h for women) while on a more liberal diet. Only 5 of 11 patients completed the study. (There were three deaths, two transplants, and one withdrawal). All patients disliked the restricted protein diet and noticed an increase in weakness and fatigue, but between the two study periods there was no significant difference in cutaneous sensation, motor nerve conduction studies, or electromyograms. By contrast, Friedman and co-workers (86) were unsuccessful in an attempt to reduce dialysis frequency to once per week by giving patients intestinal sorbents (oxystarch and charcoal) although a severely restricted protein intake was not a part of the regimen.

Another interesting direction in seeking optimal dialysis was pursued first by Snyder and co-workers (87) and then by Manohar et al. (88). They increased the frequency of dialysis to five 2 h treatments per week. A single needle system was used for access. A group of 10 patients treated in this way for an average of 21 months had no significant difference from a control group of conventionally treated patients in terms of hematocrit, creatinine concentration, and parathyroid hormone levels. Motor nerve conduction velocities remained normal. They also had no hospitalizations, access failures or other complications during the study period. By increasing the frequency of dialysis, it has been postulated that there is a reduction in the magnitude of the metabolic and physiologic changes produced during each period of dialysis (89).

Caution must be used in evaluating these studies because different types and sizes of dialyzers were used. Strict cross-over studies were not followed nor was residual renal function clearly compared in various groups. At the moment, we feel that any attempt to reduce the frequency of dialysis to less than three times per week in the absence of significant residual renal function is fraught with danger. The number of hours per treatment will be based on the dialyzer selected, patient size, blood flow and residual renal function. For a patient with a creatinine clearance less than 1.0 ml/min each treatment should last 4 to 5 h.

THE PORTABLE SUITCASE KIDNEY

A development that will make dialysis time demands more tolerable for the patient is the portable suitcase kidney. This easily carried dialysis machine only requires a tap water source and a standard electric current supply. Patients have been able to vacation and use the machine in hotel rooms, friend's homes, or while camping. This may eliminate difficulty in scheduling guest dialyses in distant units (90) and enable Australia-antigen (HBsAg) positive patients to travel freely. The use of the suitcase kidney is, of course, limited to those patients trained in self dialysis.

ROUTINE MONITORING OF MEDICAL PROBLEMS IN DIALYSIS PATIENTS

Detailed discussion of the common medical problems of dialysis patients are covered in other sections of this book. We would like, however, to include a 'worksheet' type approach that serves as a general guide to dealing with these problems:

Table 1: Outlines management of hypertension, Table 2: Anemia; Table 3: Heart disease; Table 4: Peripheral neuropathy; and Table 5: Renal osteodystrophy.

Table 1. Hypertension (91–112) (see also Chapter 28).

Hypertension is a common complication of end-stage renal insufficiency and may persist despite the initiation of hemodialysis. In most patients (70%) the hypertension is sodium and volume dependent and can be controlled by ultrafiltration. In the remainder of patients, the hypertension appears to be angiotension-dependent and these patients usually have a high plasma renin activity (PRA) (91).

The use of a specific angiotension antagonist (Saralasin) can help differentiate between the two populations of patients; those who have a hypotensive response to Saralasin (and a high PRA) and those who do not (with a low PRA) (92).

I. *Mild* (70%)
   a) *Definition*
      1. Predialysis diastolic pressure 100 mm Hg or
      2. controllable by dialysis
      3. PRA usually normal
   b) *Treatment*
      1. Ultrafiltration
      2. Dietary salt and fluid control

II. *Moderate* (20%)
   a) *Definition*
      1. Predialysis diastolic pressure of 110 to 120 mm Hg
      2. Blood pressure possible to control with drugs
      3. PRA higher than Group I, but usually between normal limits.
   b) *Treatment*
      1. Dietary salt and fluid control
      2. Ultrafiltration during dialysis
      3. Medications (first try drugs on non-dialysis days and then every day if needed).
         a) Methyldopa 250 mg (up to 2 g/day) or
         b) Clonidine hydrochloride (up to 2.4 mg every other day) (93) or
         c) Propranolol hydrochloride 40 mg three times a day (94, 95) (to a total of 240 mg twice a day)
         d) Metoprolol (96)
      4. Hemofiltration (97, 98), particularly if dopamine β-hydroxylase (DBH) level is greater than 50 IU (98).

III. *Severe high blood pressure* (10%)
   a) *Definition*
      1. Diastolic pressure of 120 to 140 mm Hg or more, may be associated with visual problems, cachexia and wasting
      2. PRA usually high
      3. DBH may be high
      4. Failure of above drug regimens to control blood pressure
   b) *Treatment*
      1. Ultrafiltration
      2. Salt and fluid dietary control
      3. Minoxidil 2.5 mg by mouth, four times a day (to total of 40 mg every other day) (99–102)
         a) May have to add diuretic
         b) May have to add propranolol hydrochloride 40 mg twice daily
         c) Captopril 100 mg three times a day (103–105)
         d) Hemofiltration. (If blood pressure not controlled, or side effects become intolerable)
      4. Bilateral nephrectomy (106–108) (rarely if ever needed since introduction of minoxidil)

Table 2. Anemia (113–123) (see also Chapter 32).

Anemia is universal in hemodialysis patients and is due to several factors including decreased red cell survival, blood loss (from mucosal irritation, from iatrogenic blood testing and residual blood loss in the dialyzer) as well as decreased erythropoietin production. Effective hemodialysis will improve the hematocrit in several patients. An evaluation and treatment plan for those who remain severely anemic follows:

I. *Diagnosis*
   a) Hematocrit, hemoglobin, white blood cell count, sickle cell preparation, serum folate level, serum vitamin B_{12} level, serum histidine level (113).
   b) Serum iron, iron binding capacity, ferritin level. If low:
      1. Check stool for guaiac positive material
      2. Check frequency of blood tests
      3. Check amount of blood left in dialyzer
   c) Red blood cell indices:
      If evidence of hemolysis, eliminate the following possible causes: copper, nitrates or chloramine toxicity, improperly mixed dialysate or drugs.
   d) Bone marrow examination

II. *Treatment*
   a) If serum folate low, give folic acid 1 mg/day
   b) If vitamin B_{12} low, give vitamin B_{12}, 1000 µg (once, intramuscularly (114))
   c) If histidine low, give histidine 1 g/day
   d) If iron low:
      1. Ferrous sulfate 600 mg at bedtime (without phosphate binders) (115).
      2. If no response in 2 months: intravenous or intramuscular Inferon 2 ml once per week for 4 weeks, once every 2 weeks for 2 months and then once per month (pay attention to possible iron overload, see Chapter 32)
   e) If anemia persists prescribe androgens (116–119) nandrolone decanoate 3 mg/kg or testosterone enanthete 4 mg/kg once per week until a response is elicited, and then 200 mg per month thereafter.
   f) If hyperparathyroidism present, consider parathyroidectomy (120–121)
   g) Transfuse only:
      1. If patient is symptomatic from anemia
      2. In the elderly or patients with atherosclerotic heart disease and hematocrit of less than 25%
      3. If hematocrit is less than 15% for one month

Table 3. Heart disease (124–150) (see also Chapter 30).

As the dialysis population becomes less selected and older, the incidence of heart disease increases. We include an evaluation and treatment plan for some of the more common types encountered.

A. *Pericarditis* (124, 129)
   I. *Evluation*
      a) History and physical examination (chest pain, friction rub, fever, etc.) If signs of cardiac tamponade present do immediate pericardiocentesis.
      b) Electrocardiogram (ST-segment elevation, electrical alterans, low voltage)
      c) X-ray: rapid change in heart size and shape with normal lungs.
      d) Echocardiogram (130, 131)
      e) Bacterial, viral, fungal studies.

   II. *Treatment*
      a) Daily dialysis (132–134) with regional or 'tight' heparinization (135). If no response in 2 weeks:
      b) Indomethacin 50 mg, by mouth, four times a day (136). If no response in one week:
      c) Pericardiocentesis with or without installation of steroids, triamcinolone hexacetonide 50 mg four times a day (137, 138)
      d) Pericardiectomy (139)

B. *Congestive heart failure*
   I. *Evaluation*
      a) History and physical examination (blood pressure, shortness of breath, rales, gallop)
      b) EKG, chest x-ray
      c) Echocardiogram (140, 141)
      d) Check triglycerides, lipoproteins and cholesterol (142–143)
   II. *Treatment*
      a) If fluid overloaded;
         1. Improve ultrafiltration
         2. Restrict dietary salt
         3. Control hypertension
         4. Look for vascular or myocardial calcification from hyperparathyroidism (144)
      b) If cardiac output high:
         1. Improve anemia (145–146)
         2. Measure blood flow through arteriovenous fistula. If fistula flow is 20% or more of cardiac output, occlude temporarily. If there is improvement, surgically decrease size of fistula (147, 148)
      c) If cardiac output low:
         1. Intensive dialysis (149–152)
         2. Digoxin; normal digitalizing dose, 1/2 to 1/3 maintenance dose
         3. Check serum digoxin levels frequently
         4. Use dialysis solution with K = 3 mmol/l
         5. Consider continuous ambulatory peritoneal dialysis (CAPD) (see Chapter 23)
      d) Cardiac arythmias
         1. Holter monitoring during dialysis (153)
         2. Check potassium
         3. Quinidine 400 mg by mouth before dialysis (154).

C. *Bacterial endocarditis* (155–158)
   I. *Evaluation*
      a) History and physical examination, history of drug abuse
      b) Blood cultures (minimum of six)
      c) Examine access site for infection
   II. *Treatment*
      a) Appropriate antibiotics (4 to 6 weeks)
      b) Remove infected vascular access
      c) If necessary, valve replacement

Table 4. Peripheral neuropathy (159–172) (see also Chapter 37).

The cause of the peripheral neuropathy of uremia, a distal motor and polyneuropathy remains elusive. 'Middle molecules' and parathyroid hormone have been implicated by some. Other causes such as diabetes mellitus, alcoholism, systemic lupus erythematosus, amyloidosis and vitamin deficiency (particularly the water soluble B vitamins) should be excluded.

In recent years neuropathy appears less prevalent (perhaps because of the earlier use of dialysis) and we only do motor nerve conduction studies if there are clinical indications. The following tests are used to evaluate peripheral nerve function:

A. *Motor nerve conduction velocities* (MNCV), Normal values:
   1. Upper extremities
      a) Ulnar and median nerves: 45–75 m/sec.
   2. Lower extremities
      a) Peroneal and tibial nerve: 38–55 m/sec
B. *Vibratory threshold test*
I. *Mild neuropathy*
   1. Signs and symptoms: none
   2. MNCV
      a) Upper extremities: 40–45 m/sec
      b) Lower extremities: 33–38 m/sec
   3. Measure parathyroid hormone (168)
   4. Treatment
      a) Vitamin supplementation (Vitamin B)
      b) Increase dialysis time (minimum thrice weekly dialysis)
      c) Repeat MNCV in 3 months
II. *Moderate neuropathy*
   1. Signs and symptoms: Paresthesias, pins and needles, restless legs, decreased vibratory sense, decreased deep tendon reflexes.
   2. MNCV
      a) Upper extremities 30–40 m/sec
      b) Lower extremities 25–33 m/sec
   3. Treatment
      a) Increase dialysis schedule to four times/week (minimum) and increase total dialysis time/week
      b) Consider dialysis with membrane more permeable to middle molecules (169)
      c) Vitamin supplement
      d) Repeat MNCV in 2 months
      e) Consider parathyroidectomy (168)
III. *Severe neuropathy*
   1. Signs and symptoms: Parathesia, muscle weakness, absent deep tendon reflexes, foot drop
   2. MNCV
      a) Upper extremities < 30 m/sec
      b) Lower extremities < 25 m/sec
   3. Treatment
      a) Intensive dialysis: five to six times/week
      b) Dialyze with membrane highly permeable to middle molecules (?)
      c) Vitamin supplement
      d) Repeat MNCV in 1 month
      e) Consider hemoperfusion (?) (170)
      f) Consider transplant, if no improvement (171–173)
IV. *Carpal tunnel syndrome* may be related to access (174, 175)

EVALUATION OF THE LONG TERM DIALYSIS PATIENT

Since chronic hemodialysis became a possibility 20 years ago (197), there has accumulated a substantial number of patients who have been maintained by this therapy for 10 or more years. In Brooklyn, we have started a 'Decade Club' in which patients who have been on hemodialysis for at least 10 years are treated to dinner by their physicians. In June 1980 more than 50 patients were invited to the dinner.

Table 5. Renal osteodystrophy (176–196) (see also Chapter 35).

Renal osteodystrophy is one of the complications of uremia that became more apparent as hemodialysis prolonged life.

The methods of dialysis in the past may have aggravated bone disease by contributing to the negative calcium balance seen in these patients. Today, with attention to calcium and phosphorus levels, and with the active metabolites of vitamin D, it is possible to treat and control bone disease in many patients (176–179).

I. *Initial evaluation*
   1. *Biochemical*
      a) Calcium
         If high: Search for other causes, including multiple myeloma, solid tumor, vitamin D toxicity, sarcoid, immobilization.
         If low:
         1. Check serum albumin
         2. Adjust dialysate bath (at least 3 mEq/l [1,5 mmol/l])
         3. 1,25 dihydroxycholecalciferol 0.25–1.5 mg/d (180, 181)
         4. Ca supplements (182, 183)
      b) Phosphorus
         If high:
         1. Phosphate binders (i.e. amphojel) (184)
         2. Low phosphate diet
         If low:
         1. Diminish amount phosphate binders
      c) Check magnesium
      d) Alkaline phosphatase
         If high: Fractionate alkaline phosphatase to eliminate liver function abnormalities.
      e) Serum parathormone level
   2. *X-rays*
      Metabolic bone survey: hand films best (185, 186); skull, pelvis, hands, long bones, chest
   3. *Nuclear diagnostics*
      ^{99}Te polyphosphate bone scan (187, 188)
   4. *Pathology*
      Bone biopsy of iliac crest
II. *Management*
   1. Control phosphate (pre-dialysis 4–6) with aluminum hydroxide and diet
   2. Use dialysate with calcium of 6 to 7 mEq/l (3 to 3,5 mmol/l)
   3. Ca supplements, oral intake 1.5 to 2 g/day (189)
   4. 1,25 (OH)$_2$-vitamin D (190, 191), 0.25 to 1.5 mg/day or 1 alpha-OH-vitamin D (192, 193)
   5. 24, 25 (OH)$_2$-vitamin D particularly for osteomalacia [194, 195]
   6. Parathyroidectomy and re-implant of part of gland in forearm (196)

Despite Lindner's warning of accelerated atherosclerosis (198), evaluation of these 'long term' dialysis patients reveals that they stand a good chance of surviving a decade or more if their hypertension is controlled, if they refrain from smoking and their calcium and phosphorus product is kept normal (199).

We have evaluated the cardiovascular status of 10 long-term hemodialysis patients (treated more than 5 years [mean 8,4 years]) by treadmill stress testing according to the Bruce multistage protocol. Eight of the

10 patients had both VO₂Max and echocardiographic indices within the normal range established for their ages (200). The two patients with abnormal parameters had sustained hypertension.

We also evaluated the pituitary gland reserve in 11 long term patients (mean dialysis treatment 8.8 years) and found that while some had a diminished reserve of ACTH, TSH and prolactin secretion, the abnormalities of pituitary reserve were unaffected by the length of dialysis. Clinically significant endocrine defects have not been clearly identified in these patients (201).

Among the facts reported at a recent conference (202) devoted to survival of long term RDT patients (over 10 years on dialysis) were:
(a) Long term and short term patients have similar transfusion requirements;
(b) Eight of eleven patients in one study had severe restrictive lung function;
(c) Joint and bone pain increased with cumulative duration of dialysis;
(d) All patients had hypergammaglobulinemia;
(e) Psychologically, long term patients are independent, aloof to other patients, and described as a group that 'give ulcers rather than get them.'

REGULAR HEMODIALYSIS TREATMENT FOR HIGH RISK GROUPS OF PATIENTS

With increasing dialysis facilities and experience, regular dialysis treatment has been extended to groups of patients who in previous years were excluded.

Reported below are some guidelines to follow in dialyzing high-risk or unusual patients.

The elderly

Older patients, frequently excluded from early dialysis programs, now may enter with ease. Indeed the average age of the hemodialysis population in the U.S.A. has risen from age 40 in 1972 to 54 in 1979 (203).

While some studies suggest that older dialysis patients do as well as younger ones (204), there generally are some problems. Chester and co-workers (205) reviewed 45 patients over the age of 70 and compared them with a group of younger dialysis patients. The older patients had twice as many medical problems, had a higher incidence of gastrointestinal bleeding (22% vs. 7% in the control group), required more blood transfusions (6.9 units/year compared to 3.4 units/year) and many (69%) required digoxin. In addition, 30% of the elderly died within the first 9 months of dialysis. Other workers have also found a high mortality in the first year and a high incidence of infection (206, 207).

Several studies have commented on the fact that older patients have a lower serum phosphorus level and lower interdialytic weight gain (204, 205). This suggests better patient diet compliance.

When dialyzing the elderly, it is advisable to maintain the hematocrit above 25% to minimize myocardial anoxia. Patients on digoxin will require a higher potassium concentration in the bath, and vascular access must be carefully observed to make sure that it is not an excessive strain on the cardiac output.

Atherosclerotic heart disease

Patients with severe atherosclerotic heart disease (ASHD) may present difficult problems for the hemodialyzer, since the majority of deaths in chronic hemodialysis programs is caused by cardiovascular disease (208). Burke et al. (209) and Lundin et al. (199) have reported, however, that patients without significant risk factors or underlying heart disease have a low incidence of developing subsequent atherosclerotic complications. Rostand (210) reported that those patients with ischemic heart disease prior to the onset of hemodialysis had a poor prognosis. He also noted that only 39 of 320 patients without evidence of prior heart disease developed it during a 7 year follow-up and these patients were older, had higher blood pressure and higher triglyceride levels.

Hemodialysis may benefit uremic patients with congestive heart failure or cardiomyopathy by improving left ventricular function (149, 211).

Among the factors associated with uremia and dialysis that may aggravate ASHD are anemia (which may increase cardiac output (212), hypertension, fluid overload and vascular access (148). Delano et al. (145) and Neff and coworkers (146) have shown that correction of anemia can restore the cardiac output to normal in dialysis patients. Therefore, in dialyzing patients with atherosclerotic heart disease, we recommend maintaining the hematocrit above 25%.

Patients taking digoxin, studied by Holter monitoring have a high rate (39%) of serious arrythmias during dialysis (154). Such patients should be dialyzed against a bath containing 3.0-3.5 mmol/l of K and should receive quinidine sulfate (400 mg by mouth 45 minutes prior to dialysis).

We have seen several patients develop angina and hypotension during the latter hours of dialysis. In this group, shorter more frequent dialysis may be appropriate, or they may be suitable candidates for chronic ambulatory peritoneal dialysis.

Coronary bypass surgery

Coronary bypass surgery is possible in hemodialysis patients (213-215). This operation should be considered in patients who have a reasonable life expectancy with dialysis but whose survival or quality of life is threatened by a correctable surgical condition. Patients should be dialyzed one day prior to surgery and then frequently (5 of the first 7 days thereafter). Patients should have their hematocrit maintained around 30% pre and post operatively. Care should be taken to prevent excess fluid accumulation and hyperkalemia which may be corrected by dialysis (214). As there may be difficulty with vascular access (215) meticulous peri-operative fistula care should be maintained. Finally, extreme hemodilution during cardiopulmonary bypass should be avoided. The pump oxygenator should be primed with at least 50% whole blood.

Diabetes mellitus

Patients with renal failure due to diabetes mellitus were once virtually excluded from dialysis programs. Now they comprise a substantial portion of the hemodialysis population (216). Indeed 25% of patients started on hemodialysis in Brooklyn, NY during the year 1978 had diabetes mellitus as their primary diagnosis compared to less than 2% before 1973.

As the number of diabetic patients on dialysis grows, so do the problems. Survival in this particular group of patients is indeed improving (217, 218) but they are still a high risk group who live a shorter period of time than their nondiabetic counterparts. Avram et al. (219) report that only 14% of diabetic patients in their program were alive after 4 years of dialysis.

Complications during dialysis are many in the diabetic patients. Annually approximately 20% of such patients will have a myocardial infarction or an episode of congestive heart failure (220). Angina may be aggravated by the dialysis procedure. Vision, already marginal in many of these patients, may be compromised because of heparin use and rapid swings in blood pressure (221). There is a 35% yearly loss of vision due to progression of retinopathy or ocular hemorrhage (220).

Maintaining vascular access in diabetic patients is especially difficult (222). Goldstein and Massry (223) reported that 60% of diabetic patients followed for 44 months required access revision. Butt et al. (224) have been able to construct a workable access in all but 20% of diabetic patients during the first operation. No revision was needed for 35% of these patients during a 3 year follow-up. Sepsis, frequently originating in an access infection is prevalent (222, 223).

Hyperosmolar non-ketotic coma has been reported (225). Insulin requirements frequently increase in diabetic patients beginning dialysis (222, 223). The use of a dextrose free dialysate has been suggested (226), but, diabetic patients dialyzed against a non-dextrose bath may develop hypoglycemia (227). In our own institution we have demonstrated, by doing half hourly blood sugar determinations, that the blood sugar tends to approach the bath level during treatment (228).

Diabetic patients may have exaggerated weight gain between dialysis (229) probably due to increased thirst. It has been suggested that this is due to a raised intracellular sodium concentration (230), although others dispute this (231). Once the patients become fluid overloaded, it is difficult to remove fluid because of hypotension due to autonomic nervous dysfunction (232).

For the management of a diabetic patient on dialysis we suggest the following: Early intervention: start dialysis at a creatinine clearance of 8 to 10 ml/min and place access as soon as possible. We dialyze with a bath containing 200 mg/dl (10.1 mmol/l) of dextrose and provide a diet high in protein and vitamins (233). When indicated, we perform retinal photocoagulation early and use tight control of the heparin dose (see Chapter 10) in patients with retinopathy. A study as to the efficacy of rigid blood sugar control by self-monitoring and multiple insulin doses is currently being conducted. To avoid possible adverse effects of heparin on diabetic retinopathy, peritoneal dialysis (intermittent P.D. or C.A.P.D.) in cases of end-stage diabetic renal disease with retinopathy, is often preferred.

Systemic lupus erythematosus

Early reports of hemodialysis treatment in patients with systemic lupus erythematosus were discouraging (234). More recently, Coplon, Siegel and Fried (235) reported 10 patients with lupus who had been treated with hemodialysis for between 4 and 33 months. Four patients died, three of infections. Hypertension is a frequent problem, but it can be controlled by nephrectomy if necessary (235). As the systemic manifestations of systemic lupus tend to remit with dialysis (236, 237) steroids should be discontinued as soon as possible. Our experiences in treated patients with lupus, including three patients on home dialysis, reveal that few patients live longer than 3 years (238, 239). Among our patients is one in whom the diagnosis of systemic lupus erythematosus did not become apparent until several months after the initiation of dialysis. In this patient, profound anemia and difficulty in obtaining compatible blood for transfusions because of antibodies was a problem.

Diffuse scleroderma (Progressive systemic sclerosis)

Once renal insufficiency occurs in diffuse scleroderma, the survival time without renal replacement therapy can be measured in weeks (240). Early results of patients treated with dialysis were poor (241), however, our experience and expertise in treating these patients is increasing.

Although long-term management is frequently complicated by severe hypertension, cardiac and pulmonary problems (242), several authors suggest hemodialysis and bilateral nephrectomy may lead to reasonable survival in some patients (243, 244).

Simon et al. (245) collected 40 patients with scleroderma who were treated with dialysis. Thirteen patients, including four who did not have bilateral nephrectomy, survived for periods of up to 3 years. Resolution of the cutaneous manifestations of systemic sclerosis after the initiation of hemodialysis has occasionally been reported (246).

Difficulty in maintaining a patient's vascular access is frequently reported (243–245). Cheigh and Kim (247) suggest a Thomas shunt be used if a fistula cannot be maintained. The report of reversal of renal failure in some patients with scleroderma by control of hypertension even after extended periods of hemodialysis (248) should temper enthusiasm for early bilateral nephrectomy in favor of trials of conservative control of blood pressure.

We have treated seven patients with systemic sclerosis by dialysis in the past 3 years. Six died within 3 months. Our longest survival was 7 months; this patient had severe cardiac and pulmonary disease. Vascular access was a problem in all patients (242).

Multiple myeloma

Success with hemodialysis in patients with multiple

myeloma was limited. Dabir-Vaziri and co-workers (249) were able to improve survival in such patients by increasing dialysis from twice to three times weekly. Leech et al. (250) had two patients who were able to live productive lives for 25 months and 15 months, respectively, while on dialysis. Johnson, Kyle and Dahlberg (251) reported 11 patients placed on long term dialysis for periods of 2 to 64 months. Four patients returned to full time activity, although only two lived longer than 1 year. In these series, transfusion requirements were not excessive nor were infectious complications except during terminal stages. Avram (252) has treated six patients with multiple myeloma and four have lived longer than 3 years.

We have treated four patients with myeloma. No special problems in the delivery of dialysis treatment were noted, although three patients died after 14 months, 16 months and 32 months, respectively, of progression of the bone lesions. One patient is alive after 6 months of treatment, but requires frequent admissions to the hospital.

Randall and co-workers (253) dialyzing two patients with light chain disease found that these patients deposited the light chain in their heart, liver and other organs. They suggest that in such patients peritoneal dialysis may be the procedure of choice. They believe that the light chains were deposited in the organs because they were not removed by hemodialysis, whereas light chains may pass the peritoneal membrane.

Amyloidosis

Ari et al. (254) found very few differences in dialyzing ten patients with amyloidosis compared to ten control patients. Average shunt life, serum albumin and hematocrit were the same in both groups, and they encountered no difficulties in the hemodialysis procedure.

In addition, amelioration of the symptoms of familial Mediterranean fever in those patients with amyloidosis has been reported during dialysis (255). However, the 2 year cumulative survival for the 212 patients with amyloid on dialysis reported by the European Dialysis and Transplant Association was only 53% compared to 75.8% for all patients (256). Both Shapiro, Chou and Porush (257) and Avram, Lapinid and Lipner (258) reported difficulties in hemodialyzing patients with amyloidosis and the nephrotic syndrome. These difficulties included resistant edema because of hypoalbuminemia with hypovolemia leading to early clotting of arteriovenous fistulae, and frequent episodes of hypotension during dialysis. Both groups infused large amounts of albumin (150 g/wk to 600 g/2 wks) without benefit. Only bilateral surgical nephrectomy (257) or 'medical nephrectomy' (destruction of residual renal function by nephrotoxic metallic salts [258]) permitted the serum albumin to rise to a level where dialysis was no longer a problem.

Stone and co-workers (259) believe that patients with amyloidosis are not favorable candidates for hemodialysis for several reasons. Hearts with amyloid involvement may be unable to tolerate hemodynamic stresses and the hemodialysis membranes are impermeable to the amyloid fibril precursors, the immunoglobulin light chains. They suggest that peritoneal dialysis is preferable to hemodialysis in these patients because the paraprotein may be removed by this route.

In our program we have maintained one young man successfully on home hemodialysis for 2 years without any cardiovascular or access problems. Another young man with minimal hypertension recently had an intracranial hemorrhage which may have been due to amyloid deposition in the blood vessels of the brain.

Liver disease

Given the high incidence of liver disease that occurs in dialysis patients and transplant recipients (33% of 267 patients in one series [260]) it is surprising that there is not more in the literature about the techniques of dialyzing these patients. In one large study of 84 dialysis patients with liver disease, complications of hemodialysis were frequent, particularly in patients with cirrhosis. The problems included severe hypotension and gastrointestinal bleeding. In some patients hypotension was severe enough to halt the dialysis procedure (261).

Our experience in dialyzing patients with cirrhosis and ascites have been similar. In addition we have had difficulty removing fluid because of hypoalbuminemia. Our policy has been to infuse salt poor albumin (50 to 100 g) throughout the dialysis in an attempt to maintain the blood pressure. A novel approach has recently been applied at our institution. In this procedure ascitic fluid is extracorporeally dialyzed with a CDAK 2.5 m^2 kidney and then returned to the peritoneal cavity (262). During this procedure blood pressure and heart rate remain stable and there are no hemorrhagic complications as heparin is not required. Sixty minutes of extracorporeal ascites dialysis can eliminate 50% of urea and creatinine in 15 to 21 liters of ascites. This method also avoids large protein loss.

Dialysis associated ascites

Dialysis related ascites is an entity that develops in some patients once they are on hemodialysis. In some cases, the ascites is associated with cachexia and hypertension, and these patients may show improvement both in cachexia and clearing of ascites following bilateral nephrectomy (263, 264).

Etiologies are varied, and include previous peritoneal dialysis, cirrhosis, tuberculosis, overhydration, infections, peritonitis, hemosiderosis, hepatitis, Hodgkins disease, portal hypertension (due to polycystic liver) and nephrotic syndrome (265–269). Therapeutic approaches are also varied, and include salt and water restriction, osmotic ultrafiltration during dialysis, paracentesis, and the instillation of adrenal steroids intraperitoneally (270). Transplantation has been reported to control ascites in some cases (265–266). Arismendi et al. (267) believe, however, that an etiology for the ascites can be found in many patients, and that a 'healthy skepticism' should exist before declaring that the patient has idiopathic, refractory ascites.

Heroin addicts

There are few reports in the literature on dialysis of heroin addicts, although it is clear that many of addicts develop renal insufficiency, usually due to focal glomerulo-sclerosis (271).

Avram (258) reports on his experience with 15 patients, 1/3 of which died. There was a high incidence of sepsis (53%) and access problems (26%).

Our own experience in dialyzing 15 addicts or former addicts presented the following problems:

(a) It is difficult to establish vascular access because the patient's veins have frequently been destroyed by self-administration of drugs;
(b) Staphyloccocal septicemia occurs often and repeatedly in patients who injected heroin through their access;
(c) Bacterial endocarditis is a frequent occurrence (155);
(d) Due to sociopathic tendencies, such patients may prove to be disruptive in the dialysis unit. They also fail to comply with dialysis schedules or prescribed medication (272). We have also found them to habituate readily to almost any medication, especially tranquilizers and analgesics.

Sickle cell anemia

Renal failure is uncommon in patients with sickle cell anemia, although a few patients with this disorder have been maintained on chronic dialysis programs (273–275).

We have experience with 4 patients. Unlike other patients reported in the literature who have not required transfusions (276), our patients needed an average of 1.5 to 2.0 units of blood per month. Dialysis was performed in the standard way, and there were no adverse reactions to the dialysis procedure and no episodes of painful crises, hemorrhages, or thrombotic complications. All four patients required digitalis and had a limited cardiac reserve. In one patient, a brachioradial arterio-arterial bovine 'jump' graft was used to prevent strain on the heart (277). None of our patients lived longer than 19 months (278).

Pregnancy

It is now possible for a pregnant woman who develops acute renal failure to be maintained during the pregnancy with dialysis (279, 280). In addition, female patients with chronic renal failure may ovulate (281) and may even become pregnant. While these patients usually abort spontaneously or have their pregnancy therapeutically terminated, 14 chronic dialysis patients have had successful pregnancies (282).

If a dialysis patient becomes pregnant and wishes to continue the pregnancy, certain manipulations will increase the chances of having a healthy infant. The hours of hemodialysis should be increased in an attempt to keep the BUN less than 70 to 84 mg/dl (25 to 30 mmol/l of urea) and the creatinine to less than 7.9 mg/dl (0.7 mmol/l) (279). We would suggest a 5 day/wk schedule. The blood pressure should be rigorously controlled. The patients should be transfused to maintain the hematocrit at approximately 30%. A high protein (greater than 80 g) and calcium rich diet is recommended. 'Tight' or regional heparinization is desirable (Chapter 10).

Sheriff et al. (283) delivered their patients by caesarian section when the plasma estriol concentration reached a desirable level. Others have permitted spontaneous labor to occur.

REFERENCES

1. Maher JF: Dialysis. In: *Contemporary Nephrology*, edited by Klahr S, Massry SG, Plenum Publishing Corporation, vol 1, 1981, p 579
2. Bonomini V, Albertazzi A, Vangelista A, Botorotti GS, Stefoni A and Scolari MP: Residual renal function and effective rehabilitation in chronic dialysis. *Nephron* 16:89, 1976
3. Bonomini V: On optimal dialysis. *Kidney Int* 7 (Suppl 3):S365, 1975
4. Bonomini V: Long term early dialysis. *3rd International Conference Uremia Capri (Abstracts)* 7, 1980
5. Scribner BH: A critical comment. *Nephron* 16:100, 1976
6. Berlyne GM, Giovannetti S: When should entry into a regular hemodialysis program occur? *Nephron* 16:81, 1976
7. Maher JF: When should maintenance dialysis be initiated? *Nephron* 16:83, 1976
8. Brescia MJ, Cimino JE, Appel K, Hurwich BJ: Chronic hemodialysis using venipuncture and a surgically created arteriovenous fistula. *N Eng J Med* 275:1089, 1966
9. Butt KMH, Rao TKS, Maki T, Mashimo S, Manis T, Delano BG, Kountz SL, Friedman EA: Bovine heterograft as a preferential hemodialysis access. *Trans Am Soc Artif Intern Organs* 20:339, 1974
10. Ahearn DJ, Maher JF: Heart failure as a complication of hemodialysis arteriovenous fistula. *Ann Intern Med* 77:201, 1972
11. Bergrem H, Flatmark A, Simonsen S: Dialysis fistulas and cardiac failure. *Acta Med Scand* 204:191, 1978
12. Maher JF, Ahearn DJ, Bryan CW, Nolph KD: Prognosis of chronic renal failure – III Survival after one peritoneal dialysis. *Nephron* 15:8, 1975
13. Erben J, Kvanicka J, Bastecky J, Vortel V: Experience with routine use of subclavian vein cannulation in haemodialysis. *Proc Eur Dial Tranpl Assoc* 6:59, 1969
14. Arana VA: Percutaneous femoral vein catheterization in patients requiring hemodialysis. *J Urol* 106:492, 1971
15. Shaldon S, Silva H, Pomeroy J, Rao AI, Rosen SM: Percutaneous femoral venous catheterization and reusable dialyzer in the treatment of acute renal failure. *Trans Am Soc Artif Intern Organs* 10:133, 1964
16. Pascua LJ: Vascular access update. *Trans Am Soc Artif Intern Organs* 25:526, 1979
17. Matalon R, Nidus BD, Cantacuzino D, Eisinger RP: Intermittent hemodialysis with repeated femoral vein puncture. *JAMA* 214:1883, 1970
18. DoCampo DM, Rao TKS, Butt KMH, Friedman EA:

Nurse performed percutaneous femoral vein catheterizations for hemodialysis. *Abstracts Southeastern Dial Transpl Assoc* 11:35, 1976
19. Kjellstrand CM, Merino GE, Mauer SM, Casal R, Buselmeier TJ: Complications of percutaneous femoral vein catheterization for hemodialysis. *Clin Nephrol* 4:37, 1975
20. Uldall PR, Dyck RF, Woods F, Merchant N, Martin GS, Cardella CJ, Sutton D, DeVeber GA: A subclavian cannula for temporary vascular access for hemodialysis or plasmapheresis. *Dial Transpl* 8:963, 1979
21. Maxey RW, Rao TKS, Manis T, Delano BG, Friedman EA: Return of renal function after commencing maintenance hemodialysis. *Proc Clin Dial Transpl Forum* 5:12, 1975
22. Mamdani BH, Lim VS, Mahurkar SD, Katz AI, Dunea G: Recovery from prolonged renal failure in patients with accelerated hypertension. *N Engl J Med* 291:1343, 1974
23. Siegel EG: Recovery from anuria due to malignant hypertension. *JAMA* 215:1122, 1971
24. Luft FC, Bloch R, Szwed JJ, Grim CM, Grim CE: Minoxidil treatment of malignant hypertension. Recovery of renal function. *JAMA* 240:1985, 1978
25. Bacon BR, Ricanati ES: Severe and prolonged renal insufficiency. Reversal in a patient with malignant hypertension. *JAMA* 239:1159, 1978
26. Mitchell HC, Graham RM, Pettinger WA: Renal function during long term treatment of hypertension with minoxidil. *Ann Intern Med* 93:676, 1980
27. Lam M, Ricanati ES, Kusher I: Reversal of severe renal failure in systemic sclerosis. *Ann Intern Med* 89:642, 1978
28. Mitnick PD, Feig PU: Control of hypertension and reversal of renal failure in scleroderma. *N Engl J Med* 299:871, 1978
29. Graham MB, Kyser FA, Gashti EN: Resolution of renal failure with malignant hypertension in scleroderma. Case report and review of the literature. *Am J Med* 67:533, 1979
30. Brown WW, Hebert LA, Piering WF, Pisciotta AVJ, Jr., Garancis JC: Reversal of chronic end-stage renal failure due to myeloma kidney. *Ann Intern Med* 90:793, 1979
31. Anonymous: Ethics and the nephrologist. Editorial. *Lancet* 1:594, 1981
32. Beauchamp TL: Can we stop or withhold dialysis? In: *Controversies in Nephrology*, edited by Schreiner GE, Washington, Georgetown Univ., 1979, p 164
33. Diamond LH: Can we stop or withhold dialysis? In: *Controversies in Nephrology*, edited by Schreiner GE, Washington, Georgetown Univ, 1979, p 171
34. Kennedy AC, Linton AL, Eaton JC: Urea levels in cerebrospinal fluid after haemodialysis. *Lancet* 1:410, 1962
35. Rosen SM, O'Connor K, Shaldon S: Haemodialysis disequilibrium. *Br Med J* 2:672, 1964
36. Hampers CL, Doak PB, Callaghan MN, Tyler HR, Merrill JP: The electroencephalogram and spinal fluid during hemodialysis, I. *Arch Intern Med* 118:340, 1966
37. Arieff A: Neurological complications of uremia. In: *The Kidney*, edited by Brenner BM, Rector FC. Philadelphia, WB Saunders, Co, 1981, p 2325
38. Arieff AI, Massry SG, Barrientos A, Kleeman CR: Brain, water, and electrolyte metabolism in uremia: Effects of slow and rapid hemodialysis. *Kidney Int* 4:177, 1973
39. Riggs GA, Bereu BA: Hypoglycemia. A complication of hemodialysis. *N Engl J Med* 277:1139, 1967
40. Wakim KG: Predominance of hyponatremia over hypoosmolality in simulation of the dialysis disequilibrium syndrome. *Mayo Clin Proc* 44:433, 1969
41. Cowie J, Lambie AT, Robson JS: The influence of extracorporeal dialysis on the acid base composition of blood and cerebrospinal fluid. *Clin Sci* 23:397, 1962
42. Arieff AI, Massry SG: Dialysis disequilibrium syndrome. In *Clinical Aspects of Uremia and Dialysis*, edited by Massry SG, Sellers AL, Springfield Il, CC Thomas, 1976, p 36
43. Arieff AI, Guisado R, Massry SG, Lazarowitz VC: Central nervous system pH in uremia and the effects of hemodialysis. *J Clin Invest* 58:306, 1976
44. Bito LZ, Myers RE: On the physiological response of the cerebral cortex to acute stress. *J Physiol* (Lond) 221:349, 1972
45. Maher JF, Schreiner GE: Hazards and complications of dialysis. *N Engl J Med* 273:370, 1965
46. Porte FK, Johnson WJ, Klass OW: Prevention of dialysis disequilibrium syndrome by the use of high sodium concentration in the dialysate. *Kidney Int* 3:327, 1973
47. Rodrigo F, Shideman J, McHuch R, Buselmeier T, Kjellstrand C: Osmolality changes during hemodialysis. *Ann Intern Med* 86:554, 1977
48. Graefe U, Milutinovic J, Follette W, Vizzo J, Babb AL, Schribner BH: Less dialysis-induced morbidity and vascular instability with bicarbonate dialysis. *Ann Intern Med* 88:332, 1978
49. Rosen RA, Lazarowitz VC, Arieff AI: Dialysis disequilibrium syndrome prevention with glycerol. *Kidney Int* 14:683, 1978
50. Gotch F: (Adequacy of dialysis). Introduction: structure of the conference. *Kidney Int* 7 (Suppl 2):S2, 1975
51. Lowrie EG, Lazarus JM, Hampers CL, Merrill JP: Some statistical methods for use in assessing the adequacy of hemodialysis. *Kidney Int* 7 (Suppl 2):S 231, 1975
52. Babb Al, Scribner BH: Quantitative description of dialysis treatment. I: A dialysis Index. *Kidney Int* 7 (Suppl 2):S23, 1975
53. Ahmad S, Babb AL, Milutinovic J, Scribner BH: Effect of residual renal function on minimal dialysis requirements. *Proc Eur Dial Transpl Assoc* 16:107, 1979
54. Teschan PE: EEG and other neurophysiological abnormalities in the uremic syndrome. *Kidney Int* 7 (Suppl 2):S30, 1975
55. Funck-Brentano JL, Man NK, Sausse A: The effects of dialysis with PAN membrane on neuropathy and middle molecular weight toxins. *Kidney Int* 7 (Suppl 2):S 52, 1975
56. Hattler BG: The elusive middle molecule? *Proc Clin Dial Transpl Forum* 3:130, 1973
57. Man NK, Granger A, Rondon- Nurete M, Zingraff J, Jungers P, Sausse A, Funck-Brentano JL: One year follow-up of short dialysis with a membrane highly permeable to the middle molecule. *Proc Eur Dial Transpl Assoc* 10:236, 1973
58. Kjellstrand CM, Peterson RJ, Evans RL, Shideman JR, Von Hartitzsch B, Buselmeier TJ: Considerations of the middle molecule hypothesis II: neuropathy in nephrectomized patients. *Trans Am Soc Artif Intern Organs* 19:325, 1973
59. Bosl R, Shideman JR, Meyer RM, Buselmeier TJ, Von Hartitzsch B, Kjellstrand CM: Effects and complications of high efficiency dialysis. *Nephron* 15:151, 1975
60. Gotch FA, Sargent JA, Peters JH: Studies on the molecular etiology of uremia. *Kidney Int* 7 (Suppl 2):S176, 1975
61. Asaba H, Bergström J, Fürst P, Oulès R, Zimmerman L: Accumulation and excretion of middle molecules. *Proc Eur Dial Transpl Assoc* 13:481, 1976
62. Lowrie EG, Steinberg S, Galen MA, Gagneux SA, Lazarus JM, Gottlieb MN, Merrill JP: Factors in the dialysis regimen which contribute to alterations in the abnormalities

of uremia. *Kidney Int* 10:409, 1976
63. Kopple JD, Swendseid ME: Protein and amino acid metabolism in uremia patients undergoing maintenance hemodialysis. *Kidney Int* 7 *(Suppl* 2):S64, 1975
64. Desforges JR: A review of the effects of hemodialysis on the blood in uremia. *Kidney Int* 7 *(Suppl* 2):S123, 1975
65. Parker TF: Study of trans-membrane potential as an assessment of the adequacy of dialysis. *Proc 12th Annu Contractors Conf Artif Kidney Progam, NIAMDD*, edited by Mackey BB, NIH Publ No 81-1979, 1981, p 226
66. Slatopolsky E: Recommendations for treatment of renal osteodystrophy in dialysis patient. *Kidney Int* 7 *(Suppl* 2):S253, 1975
67. Lazarus JM, Lowrie EG, Hampers CL Merrill JP: Cardiovascular disease in uremic patients on hemodialysis. *Kidney Int* 7 *(Suppl* 2):S167, 1975
68. DelGreco F, Simon NM, Davies W: Hypertension in chronic renal failure. The role of sodium volume homeostasis and the renal pressor system. *Kidney Int* 7 *(Suppl* 2):S176, 1975
69. Feldman JN, Lundin AP, Delano BG, Friedman EA: Determination of adequate maintenance hemodialysis in clinical judgement. *Abstracts Am Soc Artif Intern Organs* 10:42, 1981
70. DePalma JR: Adequate hemodialysis schedule. *N Engl J Med* 285:353, 1972
71. Colton CK, Lowrie EG: Hemodialysis: Physical principles and technical considerations. In *The Kidney* edited by Brenner BM, Rector FC, Philadelphia PA, WB Saunders Co, 1981, p 2425
72. Seidman MS, Lundin AP, Brown CD, Friedman EA, Berlyne GM: Extent of blood recirculation during two needle hemodialysis. *Abstracts Am Soc Artif Intern Organs* 8:56, 1979
73. Milutinovic J, Strand M, Casaretto A, Follette W, Babb AL, Scribner BH: Clinical impact of residual glomerular filtration rate on dialysis time. A preliminary report. *Trans Am Soc Artif Intern Organs* 20:410, 1974
74. Manji T, Maeda K, Ohta K, Saito A, Amano A, Kawaguchi S, Kobayashi K: Short time dialysis. *Proc Eur Dial Transpl Assoc* 12:589, 1975
75. Alvarez-Ude F, Ward M, Elliot RW, Uldall PR, Wilkinson R, Appelton DR, Kerr DNS, Petrella E, Gentile M, Romagnoni M, Orlandini G, Luciani L, Ferrandes C, D'Amico G: A comparison of short and long haemodialysis. *Proc Eur Dial Transpl Assoc* 12:606, 1975
76. Knoll O, Loew H, Graefe U, Steinhausen D, Langer K, Alterhoff G: Neuropathy and short time haemodialysis. *Proc Eur Dial Transpl Assoc* 16:729, 1979
77. Ari BJ, Oren A, Berlyne GM: Short duration – high area regular dialysis using 2 UF coils in series. *Nephron* 16:74, 1976
78. Frost TH, Kerr DNS: Kinetics of hemodialysis: A theoretical study of the removal of solutes in chronic renal failure compared to normal health. *Kidney Int* 12:41, 1977
79. Martin AM, Oduro-Domirah A, Gibbins JK, Devapal D, Mitchell DC: Regular short haemodialysis in end stage renal failure. *Br Med J* 3:758, 1975
80. Lowrie EG, Laird NM, Parker TF, Sargent JA: The effect of the hemodialysis prescription on patient morbidity. Report from the National Cooperative Dialysis Study. *N Engl J Med* 305:1176, 1981
81. Funck-Brentano JL, Man NK, Sausse A: The effect of more porous dialysis membrane on neuropathic toxins. *Kidney Int* 7 *(Suppl* 3):S552, 1975
82. Sellars L, Robson V, Wilkinson R: Sodium retention and hypertension with short dialysis. *Br Med J* 1:520, 1979
83. Cambi V: Critical appraisal of hemofiltration and ultrafiltration. The development of ultra short dialysis. Preliminary results. *J Dial* 2:143, 1978
84. Delano BG, Goodwin NJ: Patient transfer from center to home hemodialysis. *Abstracts Am Soc Nephrol* 4:19, 1970
85. Dyck PJ, Johnson WJ, Lambert EH, Nelson RA, O'Brien RC: Uremic neuropathy-controlled study of restricted protein and fluid diet and infrequent hemodialysis versus conventional hemodialysis treatment. *Mayo Clinic Proc* 50:641, 1975
86. Friedman EA, Saltzman MJ, Delano BG, Frank WM, Hirsch SR, Beyer MM, Galonsky RS: Clinical efficacy of oxidized starch in uremia. *Proc 10th Annu Contractors' Conf Chronic Uremia Program of NIAMDD*, edited by Mackey BB, DHEW Publ no (NIH) 77-1442, 1977, p 112
87. Snyder D, Louis BM, Gorfien P, Mordujovich J: Clinical experience with long term brief 'daily' haemodialysis. *Proc Eur Dial Transpl Assoc* 11:128, 1974
88. Manohar ND, Louis BM, Gorfien P, Lipner HI: Success of frequent short hemodialysis. *Trans Am Soc Artif Intern Organs* 27:604, 1981
89. Kjellstrand CM, Evans RL, Peterson RJ, Shideman JR, Von Hartitzsch B, Buselmeier TJ: The 'unphysiology' of dialysis: A major cause of dialysis side effects? *Kidney Int* 7 *(Suppl* 2):S30, 1975
90. Briefel GR, Hutchisson JT, Galonsky RS, Hessert RL, Friedman EA: Compact travel hemodialysis system. *Proc Clin Dial Transpl Forum* 5:61, 1975
91. Lindner A, Douglas SW, Adamson JW: Propranolol effects in long term hemodialysis patients with renin-dependent hypertension. *Ann Intern Med* 88:457, 1978
92. Fadem SZ, Lifschitz MD: Use of saralasin in end stage renal disease. *Kidney Int* 15 *(Suppl* 9):S93, 1979
93. Peraino RA, Price CG: Efficacy of clonidine in patients treated with hemodialysis. *Proc Clin Dial Transpl Forum* 8:106, 1978
94. Maggiore Q, Biagini M, Zoccali C, Misefari M: Propranolol treatment of resistant arterial hypertension in patients on chronic haemodialysis. *Proc Eur Dial Transpl Assoc* 11:222, 1974
95. Smith EC, Dhar MD, Freedman P: Propranolol in management of hypertension in long term dialysis programs. *JAMA* 299:1777, 1974
96. DeFremont JF, Coevoet B, Andrejak M, Makdassi R, Quichaud J, Lambrey G, Gueris J, Caillens C, Harichaux P, Alexandre JM, Fournier A: Effects of antihypertensive drugs on dialysis-resistant hypertension, plasma renin, and dopamine betahydroxylase activities, metabolic risk factors and calcium phosphate homeostasis: Comparison of metoprolol, alphamethyldopa and clonidine in a crossover trial. *Clin Nephrol* 12:198, 1979
97. Henderson LW, Sanfelippo ML, Stone RA: Hemofiltration for long-term maintenance of patients with end stage renal disease: Impact of hypertension. *Adv Nephrol* 9:21, 1980
98. Henderson LW: Hemofiltration for the treatment of hypertension associated with end-stage renal failure. *Artif Organs* 4:103, 1980
99. Quellhorst E, Schuenemann B, Doht B: Treatment of severe hypertension in chronic renal failure by haemofiltration. *Proc Eur Dial Transpl Assoc* 14:129, 1977
100. Bennett WM, Golper TA, Muther RS, McCarron DA: Efficacy of minoxidil in treatment of severe hypertension in systemic disorders. *J Cardiovasc Pharmacol* 2 *(Suppl* 2):S142, 1980
101. Campese VM, Stein D, DeQuattro V: Treatment of severe hypertension with minoxidil: Advantages and limitations. *J Clin Pharmacol* 19:231, 1979

102. Mitchell HC, Pettinger WA: Long-term treatment of refractory hypertensive patients with minoxidil. *JAMA* 239:2131, 1978
103. Wauters JP, Waeber B, Brunner HR, Turini GA, Guignard JP, Gavras H: Captopril and salt subtraction to treat 'uncontrollable' hypertension in haemodialysis patients. *Proc Eur Dial Transpl Assoc* 16:610, 1979
104. Mimran A, Shaldon S, Barjon P, Mion C: The effect of an angiotensin antagonist (Saralasin) on arterial pressure and plasma aldosterone in hemodialysis-resistant hypertensive patients. *Clin Nephrol* 9:63, 1978
105. Ferguson RK, Vlasses PH, Koplin JR, Shirinian A, Burke JF, Alexander JC: Captopril in severe treatment resistant hypertension. *Am Heart J* 99:579, 1980
106. Lee C, Neff MS, Slifkin RF, Leiter E: Bilateral nephrectomy for hypertension in patients with chronic renal failure on a dialysis program. *J Urol* 119:20, 1978
107. Onesti G, Swartz C, Ramirez U: Bilateral nephrectomy for control of hypertension. *Trans Am Soc Artif Intern Organs* 14:361, 1968
108. Briggs WA: Nephrectomy in selected patients with severe refractory hypertension receiving dialysis. *Surg Gynecol Obstet* 141:251, 1975
109. Hull AR, Long DL, Prati RC, Pettinger WA, Parker TF: The control of hypertension in patients undergoing regular maintenance hemodialysis *Kidney Int* 7 (*Suppl* 2) S 184, 1975
110. Chester AC, Schreiner GE: Hypertension and hemodialysis. *Trans Am Soc Artif Intern Organs* 24:36, 1978
111. Zucchelli P, Auccala A, Santoro A, Sturani A, Esposti ED, Ligabue A, Chiarini C: Management of hypertension in dialysis. *Int J Artif Organs* 3:79, 1980
112. Kornerup HJ, Fredstad B, Pedersen RS: A longitudinal study of arterial blood pressure in chronic haemodialysis patients with different levels of plasma renin concentration. *Scand J Urol Nephrol* 12:161, 1978
113. Giordano C, De Santo NG, Rinaldi S, Acone D, Esposito R, Gallo B: Histidine for the treatment of uraemic anaemia. *Br Med J* 4:714, 1973
114. Bastron MD, Woods HF, Walls J: Persistant anemia associated with reduced serum B_{12} levels in patients undergoing regular hemodialysis therapy. *Clin Nephrol* 11:133, 1979
115. Parker PA, Izard MW, Maher JF: Therapy of iron deficiency anemia in patients on maintenance hemodialysis. *Nephron* 23:181, 1979
116. Williams JS, Stein JH, Ferris TF: Nandrolone decanoate therapy for patients receiving hemodialysis. A controlled study. *Arch Intern Med* 134:289, 1974
117. Hendler ED, Goffinet JA, Ross S, Longnecker RD, and Bakoric V: Controled study of androgen therapy in anemia of patients on maintenance hemodialysis. *N Engl J Med* 291:1046, 1974
118. Mirahmadi MK, Vaziri ND, Gorman JT: Controlled evaluation of hemodialysis patients on nandrolone decanoate vs testosterone enanthate. *Trans Am Soc Artif Intern Organs* 25:449, 1979
119. Neff MS, Goldberg J, Slifkin RF, Eiser AR, Calamia V, Kaplan M, Baez A, Gupta S, Mattoo N: A comparison of androgens for anemia in patients on hemodialysis. *N Engl J Med* 304:871, 1981
120. Zingraff J, Drueke T, Marie P, Man NK, Jungers P, Bordier P: Anemia and secondary hyperparathyroidism. *Arch Intern Med* 138:1650, 1978
121. Barbour GL: Effect of parathyroidectomy on anemia in chronic renal failure. *Arch Intern Med* 139:889, 1979
122. Castellani A, Cristinelli L, Mileti M, Brandi S, Mombelloni G, Mioni G, Gregorini R, Maiorca PU, Guerra G, Maira L: Beneficial and determined effects of hemodialysis in uremic anemia. *Kidney Int* 11:142, 1977
123. Erslev AJ: Anemia of chronic renal diseases. *Arch Intern Med* 128:774, 1970
124. Kumar S, Lesch M: Pericarditis in renal disease: *Prog Cardiovasc Dis* 22:387, 1980
125. Renfrew R, Buselmeier TJ, Kjellstrand CM: Pericarditis and renal failure. *Annu Rev Med* 31:345, 1980
126. Horton JD, Gelfand MC, Sherber HS: Natural history of asymptomatic pericardial effusions in patients on maintenance hemodialysis. *Proc Clin Dial Transpl Forum* 7:76, 1977
127. Kleiman JH, Motta J, London E, Pennell JP, Popp RL: Pericardial effusions in patients with end-stage renal disease. *Br Heart J* 40:190, 1978
128. Osanldo E, Shalhoub RJ, Cioffi RF, Parker RH: Viral pericarditis in patients receiving hemodialysis. *Arch Intern Med* 139:301, 1979
129. Goldstein DH, Nagar C, Srivastava N, Schacht RA, Ferris FZ, Flowers NC: Clinically silent pericardial effusions in patients on long-term hemodialysis. Pericardial effusions in hemodialysis. *Chest* 72:744, 1977
130. Feigenbaum H: *Echocardiography*. Philadelphia PA, Lea & Febiger 1976, p 419
131. Gilman JK, Luft FC, Weyman AE: Echocardiography in the diagnosis of pericarditis in patients with uremia. *Proc Clin Dial Transpl Forum* 8:121, 1978
132. Marin PV, Hull AR: Uremic pericarditis. A review of incidence and management. *Kidney Int* 7 (*Suppl* 2) S 163, 1975
133. Kwasnik EM, Koster K, Lazarus JM, Sloss LJ, Mee RB, Cohn L, Collins JJ: Conservative management of uremic pericardial effusions. *J Thorac Cardiovasc Surg* 76:629, 1978
134. El-Said W, Gabal IA: Treatment of uremic pericarditis and pericardial effusion by augmented hemodialysis. *Int Urol Nephrol* 10:53, 1978
135. Swartz RD, Port FK: Preventing hemorrhage in high-risk hemodialysis. Regional versus low-dose heparin. *Kidney Int* 16:513, 1979
136. Minuth ANW, Nottebohm GA, Eknoyan G, Suki NW: Indomethacin treatment of pericarditis in chronic hemodialysis patients. *Arch Intern Med* 135:807, 1975
137. Buselmeier TJ, Davin TD, Simmons RL, Hull AR, White MG, Duncan DA, Lynch RE, Mauer SM, Casali R, Sutherland DE, Howard RH, Najarian JS, Kjellstrand CM: Local steroid instillation versus pericardiectomy for intractable pericardial effusion: the problem revisited through a multi-institutional study. *Trans Am Soc Artif Intern Organs* 23:719, 1977
138. Buselmeier TJ, Davin TD, Simmons RL, Najarian JS, Kjellstrand CM: Treatment of intractable uremic pericardial effusion. Avoidance of pericardiectomy with local steroid instillation. *JAMA* 240:1358, 1978
139. Lornoy W, DeBroe M, Hilderson J, Boghaert A, Cuvelier J, Derom F, Ringoir S: Uremic pericarditis in chronic hemodialysis patients. Treatment by surgical pericardiostomy. *Acta Clin Belg* 32:230, 1977
140. Schott CR, LeSar JF, Kotler MN, Parry WR, Segal BL: The spectrum of echocardiographic findings in chronic renal failure. *Cardiovasc Med* 3:217, 1978
141. Acquatella H, Perez-Rojas M, Burger B: Left ventricular function in terminal uremia. A hemodynamic and echocardiographic study. *Nephron* 22:160, 1978
142. Sherrard DJ, Brunzell JD: Uremic hyperlipidemia: The nature of the problem. *Proc Clin Dial Transpl Forum* 7:176, 1977
143. Rapoport J, Aviram M, Chaimovitz C, Brook JG: Defective high-density lipoprotein composition in patients on chronic hemodialysis. A possible mechanism for acceler-

ated atherosclerosis. *N Engl J Med* 299:1326, 1978
144. Davidson RC, Pendras JR: Calcium related cardiorespiratory deaths in chronic hemodialysis. *Trans Am Soc Artif Intern Organs* 13:36, 1967
145. Delano BG, Nacht R, Friedman EA, Krasnow N: Myocardial anaerobiosis in anemia in uremic man. *Am J Cardiol* 29:39, 1972
146. Neff MS, Kim KE, Persoff M, Onesti G, Swartz C: Hemodynamics of uremic anemia. *Circulation* 43:876, 1971
147. Cerra FB, Shapiro R, Anthone R, Anthone S: Physiologic response patterns to occlusion of clinically significant arteriovenous fistulas. *J Dial* 1:665, 1977
148. Anderson CB: Cardiac failure and upper extremity arteriovenous dialysis fistula. *Arch Intern Med* 136:292, 1976
149. Hung J, Harris PJ, Uren RF, Tiller DJ, Kelly DT: Uremic cardiomyopathy-effect of hemodialysis on left ventricular function in end-stage renal failure. *N Engl J Med* 302:547, 1980
150. Friedman HS: Effect of hemodialysis on left ventricular function in uremic cardiomyopathy. *N Engl J Med* 303:524, 1980
151. Scharf S, Wexler J, Longnecker R, Blaufox MD: Effect of hemodialysis on left ventricular function in uremic cardiomyopathy. *N Engl J Med* 303:523, 1980
152. Verbeelen D, Bossuyt A: Effect of hemodialysis on left ventricular function in uremic cardiomyopathy. *N Engl J Med* 303:523, 1980
153. Edson J, Avram MM, Gan A, Edson JN: Cardiac arrhythmias in hemodialysis patients. *Proc Clin Dial Transpl Forum* 7:83, 1977
154. Morrison G, Michelson EL, Brown S, Morganroth J: Mechanism and prevention of cardiac arrhythmias in chronic hemodialysis patients. *Kidney Int* 17:811, 1980
155. Lavelle KJ, Dentino MM: Surgical treatment of infective endocarditis in hemodialysis patients. *Clin Nephrol* 9:6, 1978
156. Tobin M, Montes M, Mookerjee BK: Endocarditis in hemodialysis patients with systemic disease. *J Dial* 2:75, 1978
157. Gregoratos G, Karliner JS: Infective endocarditis. Diagnosis and management. *Med Clin North Am* 63:173, 1979
158. Leonard A, Raij L, Shapiro FL: Bacterial endocarditis in regularly dialyzed patients. *Kidney Int* 4:407, 1973
159. Bolton CF: Peripheral neuropathies associated with chronic renal failure. *Can J Neurol Sci* 7:89, 1980
160. Jebsen RH, Tenckhoff H, Honet JC: Natural history of uremic polyneuropathy and effects on dialysis. *N Engl J Med* 277:327, 1967
161. Nielsen VK: The peripheral nerve function in chronic renal failure VII. Longitudinal course during terminal renal failure and regular haemodialysis. *Acta Med Scand* 195:155, 1974
162. Kjellstrand CM, Petersen RJ, Evans RL, Shideman JR, von Hartitzsch B, Buselmeier TJ: Considerations of the middle molecule hypothesis II: neuropathy in the nephrectomized patients. *Trans Am Soc Artic Intern Organs* 19:325, 1973
163. Dyck PJ, Johnson WJ, Lambert ER, Bushek W, Pollock M: Detection and evaluation of uremic peripheral neuropathy in patients on hemodialysis. *Kidney Int* 7 (Suppl 2):S 201, 1975
164. Tenckhoff H, Jebsen RH, Honet JC: The effect of long term dialysis treatment on the course of uremic neuropathy. *Trans Am Soc Artif Int Organs* 13:58, 1967
165. Tyler HM: Neuropathy in uremic patients on dialysis. *New Engl J Med* 292:1075, 1975
166. Thomas PK: Peripheral neuropathy in dialysis patients. *Int J Artif Organs* 3:6, 1980
167. Daniel CR, Bower JD, Pearson JE, Holbert RD: Vibrometry and uremic peripheral neuropathy. *South Med J* 70:1311, 1977
168. Avram MM, Feinfeld DA, Huatuco AH: Search for the uremic toxin. Decreased motor-nerve conduction velocity and elevated parathyroid hormone in uremia. *N Engl J Med* 298:1000, 1978
169. Man NK, Cueille G, Zingraff J, Boudet J, Sausse A, Funck-Brentano JL: Uremic neurotoxin in the middle molecular weight range. *Artif Organs* 4:116, 1979
170. Otsubo O, Kuzuhara K, Simada Y, Yamauchi Y, Takahashi I, Yamada Y, Otsubo K, Inou T: Treatment of uraemic peripheral neuritis by direct haemoperfusion with activated charcoal. *Proc Eur Dial Transpl Assoc* 16:731, 1979
171. Bolton CF, Noltzon MA, Boltzon RB: Effects of renal transplantation on uremic neuropathy. *N Engl J Med* 284:1170, 1971
172. Oh ST, Clement RS, Lee YW, Diethelm AG: Rapid improvement in nerve conduction velocity following renal transplantation. *Ann Neurol* 4:369, 1978
173. Jain VK, Cestero RV, Baum J: Carpal tunnel syndrome in patients undergoing maintenance hemodialysis. *JAMA* 242:2868, 1979
174. Kenzora JE: Dialysis carpal tunnel syndrome: *Orthopedics* 1:195, 1978
175. Harding AE, LeFanu J: Carpal tunnel syndrome, related to antebrachial Cimino-Brescia fistula. *J Neurol Neurosurg Psychiatry* 40:511, 1977
176. Brautbar N, Kleeman CR: Disordered divalent ion metabolism in kidney failure. *Adv Nephrol* 8:179, 1979
177. Alvarez-Ude F, Feest TG, Ward MK, Pierides AM, Ellis HA, Peart M, Simpson W, Weightman D, Kerr DNS: Hemodialysis bone disease: Correlation between clinical, histologic, and other findings. *Kidney Int* 14:68, 1978
178. Goldsmith RS, Furszyfer J, Johnson WJ, Fournier AE, Arnaud CD: Control of secondary hyperparathyroidism during long term hemodialysis. *Am J Med* 50:692, 1971
179. Slatopolsky E, Rutherford WE, Hoffstein PS, Elkan IO, Butcher HR, Bricker NS: Non-suppressible secondary hyperparathyroidism in chronic progressive renal disease. *Kidney Int* 1:38, 1972
180. Baker LR, Muir JW, Cattell WR, Tucker KA, Sharman VL, Goodwin FJ, Marsh FP, Hately W, Morgan AG, DeSaintonge DM: Use of 1,25(OH)2-Vitamin D_3 in prevention of renal osteodystrophy: preliminary observations. *Contrib Nephrol* 18:147, 1980
181. Berl T, Berns AS, Hufer WE, Hammill K, Alfrey AC, Arnaud CD, Schrier RW: 1,25 Dihydroxycholecalciferol effects in chronic dialysis. A double-blind controlled study. *Ann Intern Med* 88:774, 1978
182. Coburn JW, Koppel MH, Brickman AS, Massry SG: Studies on intestinal absorption of calcium in patients with renal failure. *Kidney Int* 3:264, 1973
183. Oettinger CW, Merrill R, Blanton T, Briggs W: Reduced calcium absorption after nephrectomy in uremic patients. *New Engl J Med* 291:458, 1974
184. Llach F, Massry SG, Koffler A, Malluche HH, Singi FR, Brickman AS, Kurokawa K: Secondary hyperparathyroidism in early renal failure. Role of phosphate retention. *Kidney Int* 12:459, 1977
185. Sundaram M, Joyce PF, Shields JB, Riaz MA, Sagar S: Terminal phalangeal tufts: earliest site of renal osteodystrophy findings in hemodialysis patients. *Am J Roent* 133:25, 1979
186. Guerra LE, Amato JA, Maher JF: Inconsistency in radiographic evaluation of progressive renal osteodystrophy.

Clin Nephrol 11:307, 1979
187. Olgaard K, Madsen S, Heerfordt J, Hammer M, Jensen H: Scintigraphic skeletal changes in non-dialyzed patients with advanced renal failure. *Clin Nephrol* 12:273, 1979
188. Duursma SA, Visser WJ, Mees EJD, Njio L: Serum calcium, phosphate and alkaline phosphatase and morphometric bone examination in 30 patients with renal insufficiency. *Calcif Tissue Res* 16:129, 1974
189. Varghese Z, Farrington K, Moorhead JF: Renal osteodystrophy. Dietary influences and management. *Proc Nutr Soc* 38:337, 1979
190. Fischer JA, Binswanger U: 1,25-dihydroxycholecalciferol in dialysed patients with clinically asymptomatic renal osteodystrophy A controlled study. *Contrib Nephrol* 18:82, 1980
191. Brickman AS, Sherrard DJ, Jowsey J, Singer FR, Baylink DJ, Maloney N, Massry SG, Norman AW, Coburn JW: 1,25 dihydroxycholecalciferol: Effect on skeletal lesions and plasma parathyroid hormone levels in uremic osteodystrophy. *Arch Intern Med* 134:883, 1974
192. Fournier A, Bordier P, Gueris J, Sebert JL, Marie P, Ferriere C, Bedrossian J, DeLuca HF: Comparison of 1 alpha-hydroxycholecalciferol and 25-hydroxycholecalciferol in the treatment of bone mineralization. Greater effect of 25-hydroxycholecalciferol on bone mineralization. *Kidney Int* 15:196, 1979
193. Manji T, Kobayashi K: Effect of 1α OH D$_3$ on bone mineral content in the forearm of chronic hemodialyzed patients. *Contrib Nephrol* 22:39, 1980
194. Bordier P, Zingraff J, Guéris J, Jungers P, Marie P, Péchet M, Rasmussen H: The effect of 1α(OH)D$_3$ and 1α, 25(OH$_2$)D$_3$ on the bone in patients with renal osteodystrophy. *Am J Med* 64:101, 1978
195. DeLuca HF: Vitamin D endocrinology. *Ann Intern Med* 85:367, 1976
196. Swanson MR, Biggers JA, Remmers AR Jr, Sarles HE, Nelson RM, Fish JC: Results of parathyroidectomy for autonomous hyperparathyroidism. *Arch Intern Med* 139:989, 1979
197. Quinton W, Dillard D, Scribner BH: Cannulation of blood vessels for prolonged dialysis. *Trans Am Soc Artic Int Organs* 6:104, 1960
198. Lindner A, Charra B, Sherrard DJ, Scribner BH: Accelerated atherosclerosis in prolonged maintenance hemodialysis. *N Eng J Med* 290:697, 1974
199. Lundin AP, Adler AJ, Feinroth MV, Berlyne GM, Friedman EA: Maintenance hemodialysis survival beyond the first decade. *JAMA* 244:38, 1980
200. Lundin AP, Stein RA, Frank F, Berlyne GM, Krasnow N, Friedman EA: Cardiovascular status in long term hemodialysis patients. An exercise and echocardiographic study. *Nephron* 28:234, 1981
201. Roseman PM, Leu ML, Sacerdote A, Lundin AP, Delano BG, Friedman EA, Wallace EZ: Pituitary gland reserve in patients on long term hemodialysis. *Clin Res* 28:266A, 1980
202. Avram MM: Survival after 10 years of dialysis and prevention of renal disease. In: Proceedings edited by Avram MM, New York, London, Plenum Med Book Co, 1982
203. Becker EL: Finite resources and medical triage. *Am J Med* 6:549, 1979
204. Rathaus M, Bernheim JL: Are your elderly patients good candidates for dialysis? *Geriatrics* 33:56, 1978
205. Chester AC, Rakowski TA, Argy WP Jr, Giacalone A, Schreiner GE: Hemodialysis in the eight and ninth decades of life. *Arch Intern Med* 139:1001, 1979
206. Ghentons WN, Bailery GL, Zschaeck D, Hampers CL, Merrill JP: Long term hemodialysis in the elderly. *Trans Am Soc Artif Intern Organs* 17:125, 1971
207. Rao TKS, Nathanson G, Avram M, Manis T, Kountz SL, Friedman EA: Improved survival in older, sicker patients begun on maintenance hemodialysis. *Proc Clin Dial Transpl Forum* 6:62, 1976
208. Jacobs C, Brummer FP, Chantler C, Donckerwolcke RA, Gurland HJ, Hathway RA, Selwood NH, Wing AJ: Combined report of regular dialysis and transplantation in Europe VII. 1976 – *Proc Eur Dial Transpl Assoc* 14:3, 1977
209. Burke J, Francos G, Moore L: Accelerated atherosclerosis in chronic dialysis patients. Another Look. *Nephron* 21:181, 1978
210. Rostand SG: Ischemic heart disease in patients undergoing maintenance hemodialysis. *Kidney Int* 16:600, 1979
211. Vaziri ND, Prakash R: Echocardiographic evaluation of the effect of hemodialysis on cardiac size and function in end stage renal disease. *Am J Med Sci* 278:201, 1979
212. Scharf S, Wexler J, Longnecker RE, Blaufox MD: Cardiovascular disease in patients on chronic hemodialysis therapy. *Prog Cardiovasc Dis* 22:343, 1980
213. Chawla R, Gailiunas P Jr, Lazarus JM, Gottlieb MN, Lowrie EG, Collings JJ, Merrill JP: Cardiopulmonary bypass surgery in chronic hemodialysis and transplant patients. *Trans Am Soc Artif Intern Organs* 23:694, 1977
214. Byrd LH, Sullivan JF: Successful coronary artery bypass in a hemodialysis patient. *J Dial* 2:33, 1978
215. Crawford FA, Selby JH, Bewer JP, Lehan P: Coronary revascularization in patients maintained on hemodialysis. *Circulation* 56:684, 1977
216. Rao TKS, Hirsch S, Avram MM, Friedman EA: Prevalence of diabetic nephropathy in Brooklyn. In: *Diabetic Renal-Retinal Syndrome* edited by Friedman EA, L'Esperance FA. New York, Grune and Stratton, 1980, p 205
217. Comty CM, Kjellsen D, Shapiro FL: A reassessment of the prognosis of diabetic patients treated by chronic hemodialysis. *Trans Am Soc Artif Intern Organs* 22:404, 1976
218. Arieff AI: Kidney, water, and electrolyte metabolism in diabetes mellitus. In *The Kidney*, edited by Brenner BM, Rector FC, Philadelphia PA, WB Saunders Co, 1976, p 1268
219. Avram MM, Slater PA, Fein PA, Altman E: Comparative survival of 673 patients with chronic uremia treated with renal transplantation and maintenance hemodialysis. *Trans Am Soc Artif Intern Organs* 25:391, 1979
220. Friedman EA, Rubin JA: Dialysis and transplant of diabetics in the U.S. *Nephron* 18:309, 1977
221. Blagg CR: Visual and vascular problems in dialyzed diabetic patients. *Kidney Int* 6 (Suppl 1):S 27, 1974
222. Rassissieh SD, Yen MC, Lazarus JM, Lowrie EG, Goldstein HH, Takacs FJ, Hampers CL, Merrill JP: Hemodialysis-related problems in patients with diabetes mellitus. *Kidney Int* 6 (Suppl 1):S 100, 1974
223. Goldstein DA, Massry SG: Diabetic nephropathy: Clinical course and effect of hemodialysis. *Nephron* 20:286, 1978
224. Butt KMH, Ortega-Gayton M, Shirani K, Hong JH, Adamson RJ, Manis T, Friedman EA. Angioaccess in uremic diabetics. In *Diabetic-Renal Retinal Syndrome*, edited by Friedman EA, L'Esperance FA, New York, Grune & Stratton, 1980, p 209
225. Potter DJ: Death as a result of hyperglycemia without ketosis. A complication of hemodialysis. *Ann Intern Med* 64:399, 1966
226. Ma KW, Masler DS, Brown DC: Hemodialysis in diabetic patients with chronic renal failure. *Ann Intern Med* 83:215, 1975
227. Pitkanen E, Koivula T: Continuous blood glucose moni-

toring and characteristics of diabetes in patients on maintenance hemodialysis treatment. *Scand J Urol Nephrol* 12:309, 1979
228. Levitz CS, Hirsch S, Ross JM, Butt KMH, Friedman EA: Lack of blood glucose control in hemodialyzed and renal transplantation diabetics. *Trans Am Soc Artif Intern Organ* 26:362, 1980
229. Watkins PJ, Parsons V, Bewick M: The prognosis and management of diabetic nephropathy. *Clin Nephrol* 7:243, 1977
230. Jones R, Poston L, Hinestrosa H, Parsons V, Williams R: Weight gain between dialyses in diabetics: Possible significance of raised intracellular sodium content. *Br Med J* 280:153, 1980
231. Burn J, Gill GV, Flear CT: Weight gain between dialysis in diabetics. *Br Med J* 280:643, 1980
232. Lazarus JM, Kjellstrand CM: Dialysis: medical aspects. In: *The Kidney* edited by Brenner BM, Rector FC, WB Saunders Co, Philadelphia PA 1981, p 2521
233. Davis M, Comty C, Shapiro F: Dietary management of patients with diabetes treated by hemodialysis. *J Am Diet Assoc* 75:265, 1979
234. Gral T, Schroth P, Rosen V, Sellers A, Maxwell MH: Is chronic hemodialysis indicated in the treatment of terminal lupus nephritis? *Abstracts Am Soc Nephrol* 4:31, 1970
235. Coplon NS, Siegel RC, Fried JF: Hemodialysis in end stage lupus nephritis. *Abstracts Am Soc Artif Intern Organs* 2:14, 1973
236. Fries JF, Powers R, Kempson R: Late stage lupus nephropathy. *J Rheumatol* 1:166, 1974
237. Friedman EA: Lupus-nephritis. What to do until data arrives? *Nephron* 19:190, 1978
238. Maxey RW, Rao TKS, Ginzler E, Butt KMH, Kountz EA, Friedman FA: Course of treated uremia due to systemic lupus erythematosus. *Abstracts Am Soc Artif Intern Organs* 6:56, 1977
239. Delano BG, Feinroth MV, Feinroth M, Friedman EA: Home and medical center hemodialysis: Dollar comparison and payback period. *JAMA* 246:230, 1981
240. McKinney TD, McAllister CJ, Stone WJ, Johnson HK, Ginn HE: Hemodialysis and renal transplantation in progressive systemic sclerosis: report of two cases. *Clin Nephrol* 12:178, 1979
241. Cooper WL, Winer RL, Mira Hadi KS, Gorman JT: Hemodialysis for progressive systemic sclerosis with renal failure. *Abstracts Am Soc Nephrol* 9:29, 1976
242. Rao TKS: Hemodialysis and transplantation in systemic disease: the facts. In: *Strategy for Renal Failure*, edited by Friedman EA, New York, John Wiley & Co, 1978, p 321
243. Javier P, Dumler F, Levin NW: Renal scleroderma: Comparison of different modalities of treatment. *South Med J* 73:657, 1980
244. Leroy ED, Fleischmann RM: The management of renal scleroderma: Experience with dialysis, nephrectomy and transplantation *Am J Med* 64:974, 1978
245. Simon NM, Graham MB, Kyser FA, Gashti EN: Resolution of renal failure with malignant hypertension in scleroderma. Case report and review of the literature. *Am J Med* 67:533, 1979
246. Barker DJ, Farr MJ: Resolution of cutaneous manifestations of systemic sclerosis after haemodialysis. *Br Med J* 1:501, 1976
247. Cheigh JS, Kim SJ: Scleroderma kidney disease: A therapeutic approach with nephrectomy and hemodialysis. *J Dial* 1:349, 1977
248. Lam M, Ricanati ES, Khan MR, Kushner I: Reversal of severe renal failure in systemic sclerosis. *Ann Intern Med* 89:642, 1978
249. Dabir-Vaziri N, Goldman R, Schultze RG: Dialysis in myeloma kidney disease *Abstracts Am Soc Artif Int Organs* 3:15, 1974
250. Leech SH, Polesky HF, Shapiro FL: Chronic hemodialysis in myelomatosis. *Ann Intern Med* 77:239, 1972
251. Johnson WJ, Kyle RA, Dahlberg PJ: Dialysis in the treatment of multiple myeloma. *Mayo Clin Proc* 55:65, 1980
252. Avram MM: Survival in uremia due to systemic diseases. *Kidney Int (Suppl 8)* S 55, 1978
253. Randall RE, Williamson WC, Mullinax F, Tung MF, Still JS: Manifestations of systemic light chain deposition. *Am J Med* 60:293, 1976
254. Ari JB, Zlotnik M, Oren A, Berlyne GM: Dialysis in renal failure caused by amyloidosis of familial Mediterranean fever. *Arch Intern Med* 136:449, 1976
255. Rubinger D, Friedlaender MM, Popovtzer MM: Amelioration of familial Mediterranean fever during hemodialysis. *N Engl J Med* 301:142, 1979
256. Anonymous: Treatment of renal amyloidosis. Editorial. *Lancet* 1:1062, 1980
257. Shapiro W, Chou SY, Porush TC: Nephrectomy for intractable proteinuria secondary to severe nephrotic syndrome. *Abstracts Am Soc Nephrol* 8:24, 1975
258. Avram MM, Lipner H, Gan AC: Medical nephrectomy. The use of metallic salts for the control of massive proteinuria in the nephrotic syndrome. *Trans Am Soc Artif Intern Organs* 22:431, 1976
259. Stone WJ, Latos DL, Lankford PG, Baker AS: Chronic peritoneal dialysis in a patient with primary amyloidosis, renal failure and factor X deficiency. *South Med J* 71:764, 1978
260. Toussaint C, Dupont E, Vanherweghem JL, Cappel R, DeRoy G, Vereerstraeten P, Kinnaert P, Thiry L, Van Geertruyden J: Liver disease in patients undergoing hemodialysis and kidney transplantation. *Adv Nephrol* 8:269, 1979
261. Wilkinson SP, Weston MJ, Parsons V, Williams R: Dialysis in the treatment of renal failure in patients with liver disease. *Clin Nephrol* 8:287, 1977
262. Adler AJ, Feldman J, Friedman EA, Berlyne GM: Use of extracorporeal ascites dialysis in combined hepatic and renal failure. *Nephron* 30:31, 1982
263. Gotloib L, Servadis C: Ascites in patients undergoing maintenance hemodialysis. *Am J Med* 61:65, 1976
264. Feingold LN, Gutman RA, Walsh FX, Gunnels JC: Control of cachexia and ascites in hemodialysis patients by bilateral nephrectomy. *Arch Intern Med* 134:889, 1974
265. Wang F, Pillary VKG, Ing TS, Armbruster KFW, Rosenberg JC: Ascites in patients treated with maintenance hemodialysis. *Nephron* 12:105, 1974
266. Singh S, Mitra S, Berman L: Ascites in patients on maintenance hemodialysis. *Nephron* 12:114, 1974
267. Arismendi GS, Izard MW, Hampton WR, Maher JF: The clinical spectrum of ascites associated with maintenance dialysis. *Am J Med* 60:46, 1976
268. Craig R, Sparberg M, Ivanovich P, Rich L, Doidal E: Nephrogenic ascites. *Arch Intern Med* 134:276, 1974
269. Eknoyan G, Dichoso C, Hyde S, Yium J: 'Overflow ascites' – the safety valve of the volume-expanded patient on dialysis. *Proc Clin Dial Transpl Forum* 3:156, 1973
270. Buselmeier TJ, Simmons RL, Duncan DA: Local steroid treatment of intractable ascites in dialysis patients. *Proc Clin Dial Transpl Forum* 5:9, 1975
271. Rao TKS, Nicastri AD, Friedman EA: Natural history of heroin associated nephropathy. *N Engl J Med* 290:19, 1974
272. Friedman EA, Manis T, Delano BG: Response of psy-

chotic and sociopathic patients to maintenance hemodialysis. *Abstracts Am Soc Artif Intern Organs* 2:22, 1973
273. Friedman EA, Rao TKS, Sprung GL, Smith A, Manis T, Bellervue R, Butt KMH, Lenere RD, Holden DM: Uremia in sickle cell anemia treated by maintenance hemodialysis. *N Engl J Med* 291:431, 1974
274. Gold DD: Hemodialysis and transfusions for uremic patients with sickle cell disease. *N Engl J Med* 291:1361, 1974
275. Elberg AJ, Baker R, Koch K, Gorman H, Wenger AJ, Strauss J: Transfusion requirements in patients with sickle cell disease on hemodialysis. *N Engl J Med* 294:444, 1976
276. Pote HH Jr, Lyons H, Schwartz AB: Hemodialysis in sickle cell disease – 24 months experience. *Abstracts Am Soc Artif Intern Organs* 4:51, 1975
277. Butt KMH, Kountz SL: A new vascular access for hemodialysis, the arterial jump graft. *Surgery* 79:476, 1976
278. Manis T, Friedman EA: Sickle hemoglobinopathy and the kidney. *Contrib Nephrol* 7:211, 1977
279. Nemoto R, Sugiyama Y, Kuwahara M, Kato T, Tsuchida S: Successful delivery of a patient on hemodialysis for acute renal failure: a case report and review of the literature. *J Urol* 118:673, 1977
280. Naik RB, Clark AC, Warren DJ: Acute proliferative glomerulonephritis with crescents and renal failure in pregnancy successfully managed by intermittent haemodialysis. Case Report. *Br J Obstet Gynaecol* 86:819, 1979
281. Goodwin NJ, Valenti C, Hall JE, Friedman EA: Effect of uremia and chronic hemodialysis on the reproductive cycle. *Am J Obstet Gynecol* 100:528, 1968
282. Wing AJ, Brunner FP, Brynger H, Chantler C, Donckerwoloke RA, Gurland HJ, Hathway RA, Jacobs C, Selwood NH: Combined report on regular dialysis and transplantation in Europe. VIII 1977. *Proc Eur Dial Transpl Assoc* 15:2, 1978
283. Sheriff MH, Hardman M, Lamont CA, Shepherd R, Warren DJ: Successful pregnancy in a 44-year-old haemodialysis patient. *Br J Obstet Gynaecol* 85:386, 1978

21

PERITONEAL DIALYSIS: A HISTORICAL REVIEW

WILLIAM DRUKKER

Introduction: The invention of peritoneal lavage	410
Early studies of the peritoneum	412
The peritoneum as a semi-permeable membrane	412
Permeability of the peritoneum	413
Experimental peritoneal dialysis	414
The first attempt of intermittent peritoneal dialysis	414
Necheles' criticism	414
Continuous peritoneal dialysis	414
Other unsuccessful early attempts (1930–1940)	415
The turning of the tide: The investigations of fine and collaborators (1946–1948)	415
Successful treatment of acute renal failure with peritoneal dialysis	415
The composition of the peritoneal dialysis fluid	416
Sodium concentration	416
Dextrose concentration	416
Lactate and acetate vs. bicarbonate	417
Continuous vs. intermittent peritoneal dialysis	418
Peritoneal access	418
Different types of catheters	418
The stylet catheter	419
Standardising the technique	419
Development of 'hanging bottle' peritoneal dialysis	419
Commercial preparation of dialysis fluid and tubing	419
Closed administration systems	419
Semi-automatic peritoneal dialysis machines ('cyclers')	419
Further progress	421
Clearance studies	421
Significance of dialysate flow rates	421
The permeability of the peritoneum to larger solutes (so called middle molecules)	421
The first chronic case successfully treated with periodic peritoneal dialysis	422
Indwelling plastic conduits	422
Peritoneal access by repeated puncture	422
Periodical peritoneal dialysis in the home	423
Conservative treatment of acute renal failure vs. peritoneal dialysis	423
Haemodialysis vs. peritoneal dialysis in acute renal failure	423
Peritoneal dialysis becomes a 'good leaden bullet' in the treatment of acute uraemia, but remains a 'cinderella' treatment for chronic uraemia	423
Introduction of the Tenckhoff catheter	425
Cyclers	425
Introduction of closed loop, reverse osmosis, automatic peritoneal dialysis machines	425
Increasing utilisation of periodic peritoneal dialysis in the 1970's and 1980's	426
Enhancement of peritoneal dialysis efficiency	427
Hydrodynamical and physical methods	427
Pharmacological methods	428
Recirculation peritoneal dialysis	429
Reciprocating peritoneal dialysis	430
Fresh fluid semicontinuous peritoneal dialysis	430
Regeneration peritoneal dialysis	431
The evolution of a simple 'machine free' system via automatic cyclers into a complicated reverse osmosis closed loop system and back to a machine free methodology called CAPD (Continuous Ambulatory Peritoneal Dialysis)	432
CAPD and the peritonitis problem	433
Cost of CAPD	433
Undesirable effects of CAPD	433
Success of CAPD	433
Continuous cyclic peritoneal dialysis (CCPD) or automated long cycle peritoneal dialysis (ALCPD)	434
Summary and some unanswered questions	434
Acknowledgments	435
References	435

INTRODUCTION: THE INVENTION OF PERITONEAL LAVAGE

For several centuries the peritoneum has enchanted physiologists, pathologists, surgeons, gynaecologists and internists. More recently nephrologists joined the teams of clinical investigators.

The concept of peritoneal lavage goes back almost 150 years (1) when it served a purpose totally different from removal of toxins.

Actually the idea came from a clergyman, the Reverend Stephen Hales, a man with great interest in biology (Figure 1). It so happened that the reverend gentleman in the year 1744 during his pastorate at Teddington in the London District of Richmond, attended a Thursday meeting of the Royal Society of Medicine in London and learned about a new – rather drastic – method of treating recurrent ascites, presented by Christopher Warrick, a surgeon from Truro in Cornwall, England (2).

Mr. Warrick was called to the assistance of a lady named Jane Roman, near 50 years old, who was confined to bed by recurrent ascites. He performed paracentesis and drew 36 pints[1] of fluid from her abdominal cavity, being aware that this would not be an absolute cure for the ascites of the lady. Therefore he took some part of the extracted 'lymph' to his own home and started a number of experimental investigations with the withdrawn fluid, looking for a method whereby the 'ruptured lymphatics must close their mouths' so as to prev-

---

[1] 1 pint = 0,568 l.

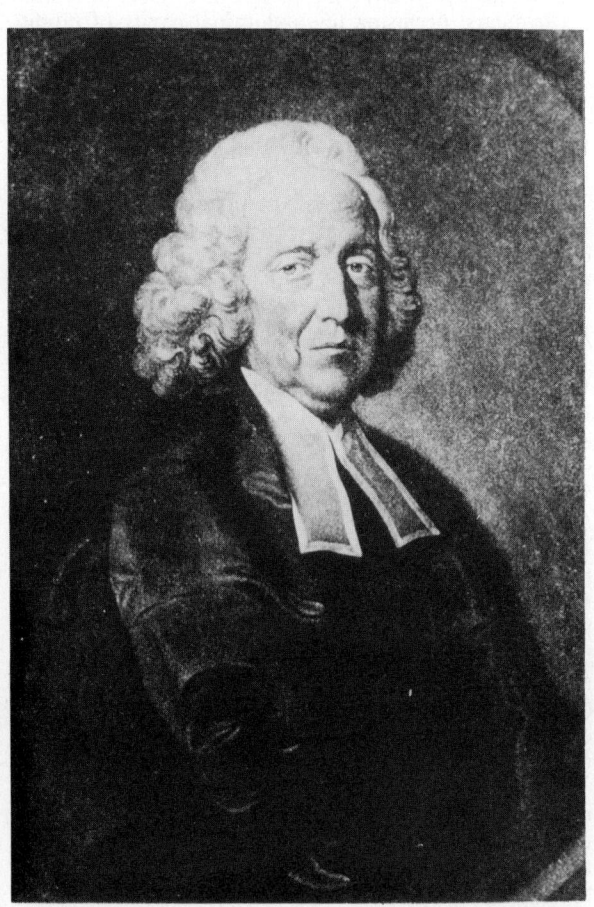

Figure 1. The REV. STEPHEN HALES: 'A Method of conveying Liquors into the Abdomen during the Operation of Tapping; ... communicated in a Letter to Cromwell Mortimer, M.D. Secr. R.S. (Febr. 12, 1744)'. (From the Library of the Royal Society of Medicine, London, England).

IV. *A Method of conveying* Liquors *into the* Abdomen *during the Operation of* Tapping; *proposed by the Reverend* Stephen Hales, *D. D. and F. R. S. on Occasion of the preceding Paper*; *communicated in a Letter to* Cromwell Mortimer, *M. D. Secr. R. S.*

SIR,   Feb. 22. 1743-4.

Read Feb. 23. 1743-4.
IT occurred to me, on your reading, *Thursday* last, before the Society, the Case of the Woman at *Truro* in *Cornwall*, who was cured of a Dropsy, by injecting into the *Abdomen Bristol* Water and *Cohore* Wine, after having drawn off a good Quantity of the dropsical *Lympha*; that, in case of further Trial, that, or any other Liquor, shall be found effectual to the Purpose, it might be more commodiously injected in the following Manner; *viz.*

By having Two *Trochars* fixed at the same time, one on each Side of the Belly; one of them having a Communication with a Vessel full of the medicinal Liquor by means of a small leathern Pipe: This Liquor might flow into the *Abdomen*, as fast as the dropsical *Lympha* passed off through the other *Trochar*; whereby the dropsical *Lympha* might be conveyed off, to what Degree it shall be thought proper; and that without any Danger of a *Syncope* from Inanition; because the *Abdomen* would, through the whole Operation, continue distended with Liquor, in such a Degree as shall be found proper, by raising or lowering the Vessel with the medicinal Liquor in it.

It is probable, that, if the Surface of the medicinal Liquor be about a Foot higher than the *Abdomen*, it may be sufficient for the Purpose.

It were easy to find the Force with which the *Abdomen* is distended by the dropsical *Lympha*, by seeing to what Height it arose in a Glass Tube fixed to the *Trochar*; which Tube being taken away, it might, I suppose, be sufficient to have the medicinal Liquor flow in from a lesser perpendicular Height, than that to which the dropsical *Lympha* arose in the Glass Tube. I am,

SIR,

Your humble Servant,

Stephen Hales.

Figure 2. The Rev. Stephen Hales' letter to the Secretary of the Royal Society (3).

ent recurrence of the ascites. As expected the relief of the lady was only of short duration: 10 days after the first paracentesis 'an inundation alarmed her again' and within 14 days the patient again desired Mr. Warrick's assistance for relief. By this time he had drawn some conclusions from his experimental work and resolved to try their efficiency. With another paracentesis he removed more than 20 pints of clear briny lymph as before, which quantity did not exceed 2/3 of the whole. Then he replaced the 'ascitic lymph' by a bloodwarm mixture of equal parts of fresh Bristol water and cohore claret (a Bordeaux wine). After injection of 10-12 pints of the claret-water mixture the patient collapsed and apparently went into an alarming condition. She recovered however and Mr Warrick, who had interrupted the injection, and expected that this partial instillation of the therapeutical fluid would not be effective enough, asked the lady if she thought herself capable of undergoing the procedure a second time. She was apparently a courageous patient and she answered him 'in the affirmative'. He then prepared a stronger mixture for the second injection, the claret being in a double proportion of the water and drew off the whole contents of the abdomen and repeated the injection as before. The patient complained of 'heavy pungent pain, darting through all the viscera' and Warrick became alarmed because her breathing became difficult, her pulse faltered, the syncope returned and the patient became speechless. He withdrew the cannula, ended the procedure and much to his relief the patient recovered.

During a 1 month follow-up the ascites did not recur. 'Apparently the mouths of the lymphatics had been closed'.

The Reverend Stephen Hales (3) obviously felt pity for the poor lady and wrote a letter to the secretary of the Royal Society, Dr. Cromwell Mortimer, which was published in the Philosophical Transactions, suggesting a more gentle modification of Mr. Warrick's method for 'an absolute cure for an ascites'. By

> 'having two trochars fixed at the same time, one on each side of the belly; one of them having a communication with a vessel full of the medicinal liquor by means of a small leathern pipe: this liquor might flow into the abdomen, as fast as the dropsical lympha passed off through the other trochar; by which the dropsical lympha might be conveyed off to what degree it shall be thought proper; and that without any danger of a syncope from inanition; because the abdomen would, through the whole operation, continue distended with liquor, in such a degree as should be found proper; by raising or lowering the vessel with the medicinal liquor in it'.

This first description of peritoneal lavage was essentially identical with continuous peritoneal lavage, later to be used for the treatment of uraemia.

In retrospect Mr. Warrick's method 'for an absolute cure' of recurrent ascites obviously served the purpose of obliterating the abdominal cavity, something that should definitely be avoided in peritoneal dialysis... At Mr. Warrick's last visit to the patient he 'left her in pursuit of that health which she soon acquired and continued to enjoy...'

EARLY STUDIES OF THE PERITONEUM

Nothing is known of the fate of subsequent patients with recurrent ascites; the next publication on experimental peritoneal lavage was published more than 130 years later and came from Wegner (4), a German investigator, who published in 1877 the results of a series of animal experiments, perfusing the abdominal cavity of rabbits with cold saline solution, observing a decrease of the animals' body temperature.

The peritoneum as a semi-permeable membrane

The results of other animal experiments of Wegner were more important: he observed an increase in volume of concentrated sugar solutions or glycerol during a dwell period in the abdominal cavity.

This phenomenon was studied again by a group of English physiologists, headed by Starling in 1894 and 1895. Starling and his co-workers (5, 6) confirmed Wegner's observations and also demonstrated a decrease in volume of a hypotonic solution, whereas the volume of isotonic solutions or serum remained unaltered for several hours.

Similar observations were reported by Orlow (7) from Germany: solutions with a low sodium chloride concentration (0.3% [51 mmol/l]) when injected in the peritoneal cavity, decreased in volume with an increase of the salt concentration. Hypertonic salt solutions (1.5% [256 mmol/l] or more) caused transfer of fluid from the blood and an increase of plasma chloride. Solutions with sodium chloride concentrations between 0.4 and 1.5% (68 and 256 mmol/l) decreased slowly in volume, the chloride concentrations equilibrating with the chloride concentration of the blood serum.

The experimental work of Clark (8) showed that after introduction of a sodium chloride solution first absorption occurs and later slower diffusible substances enter the peritoneal fluid from the blood with an increase of the osmotic pressure of the peritoneal fluid, slowing the absorption. When dextrose was introduced (8, 9), making the fluid hypertonic and preventing absorption of fluid, water and crystalloids entered the peritoneal fluid. Because of the slow diffusion of dextrose this effect was rather long lasting. Dextrose appeared therefore an excellent substance to remove fluid from the blood into the peritoneal cavity.

Finally Clark (8) showed that the rate of absorption through the peritoneum was increased by elevating the temperature of the solution and decreased by introducing a cold solution. A similar effect was noted by application of heat to the abdominal wall, which apparently increased the permeability of the peritoneum. Cooling the abdominal wall had the opposite effect (10).

Other investigators (11) noted an increase in absorption from the peritoneal cavity by increasing intestinal mobility (e.g. by means of physostigmin). When intesti-

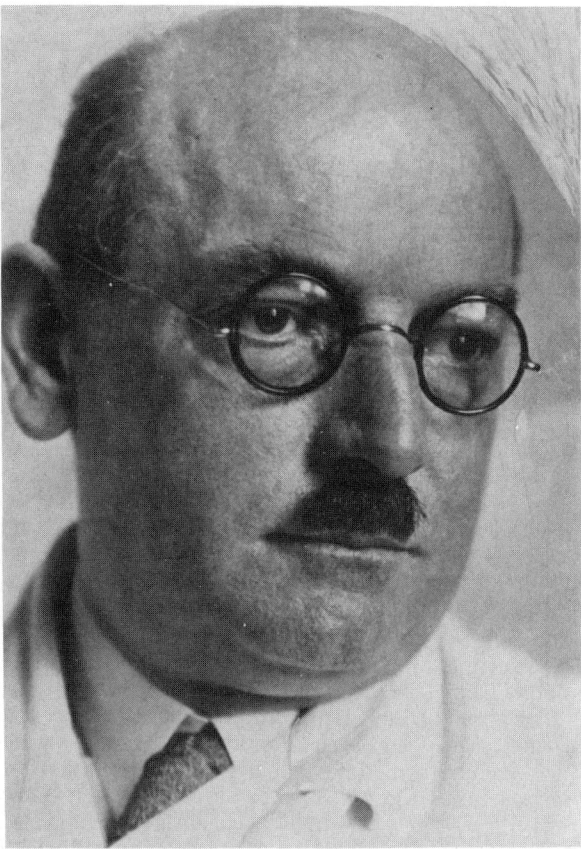

Figure 3. G. GANTER, M.D. (1885-1940), professor of medicine at Würzburg, Germany, who introduced the concept of intermittent peritoneal dialysis (1923 [24]).

nal peristalsis was inhibited with opiates absorption was delayed.

Putman (12) demonstrated that his experimental animals tolerated the intraperitoneal introduction of sodium chloride solutions of less than 1% (170 mmol/l) reasonably well, being initially uncomfortable but rapidly recovering. However solutions of more than 1% sodium chloride were tolerated poorly: the animals frequently died within a few hours.

Permeability of the peritoneum

Many of these early investigations and other experimental data from ancient literature (9, 10, 12–14) presented convincing evidence that the peritoneal membrane is permeable in two directions, acting *in vivo* in a similar way as a pig's bladder membrane *in vitro* or a membrane of nonbiological material like parchment (15). Starling and Tubby (5) and several other investigators (10, 16) also demonstrated a bidirectional permeability of the peritoneum for larger solutes in the range of the so called middle molecules (see chapters 2, 12, 19 and 22). Methylene blue (molecular weight 374), indigo carmine (M.W. 466) or eosin (M.W. 624), when introduced in the peritoneal fluid, pass rapidly into the blood and appear subsequently in the urine.

When these substances are injected intravenously, they pass rapidly through the peritoneum in the opposite direction to appear promptly in the peritoneal fluid. The permeability of the peritoneum for molecules in the middle molecular weight range was rediscovered in 1965 and plays presently an important role in the clinical application of the peritoneum as a dialysis membrane in uraemia.

As early as 1923 Putman (12) described the living peritoneum as a membrane with holes punched in it, permitting the passage of larger molecules than ordinary, non-living dialysis membranes do.

In addition, a living membrane like the peritoneum is subject to inflammation which changes the permeability drastically (17–19), permitting the passage of protein molecules.

Comprehensive surveys of the earlier literature and historical studies on the physiology and permeability of the peritoneum have been published previously. The reader who is interested in these early investigations is referred to these reviews (20–22).

Further progress and practical application of the acquired knowledge was relatively slow, mainly because most work was undertaken by scientists. The clinical investigators had not appreciated a medical application so far.

Furthermore World War I delayed and interrupted progress in medical work. In 1918 two American paediatricians, Blackfan and Maxcy (23), were the first to utilise the peritoneal cavity for the administration of fluids to dehydrated children. The first attempt to use the peritoneal membrane the other way, namely to remove uraemic substances from the body of a human patient, dates back to 1923.

EXPERIMENTAL PERITONEAL DIALYSIS

Ganter (24), a German clinical investigator, is traditionally credited with the first attempts of peritoneal dialysis in a human being. Originally (in 1918) he removed a pleural effusion from a uraemic man, replacing the fluid with 0,75 l of a sodium chloride solution. He observed some improvement of the patient's condition during the next two days.

Subsequently he performed a series of experimental peritoneal dialyses in rabbits and guinea pigs, made uraemic by ligation of the ureters. Injecting 40 to 60 ml of saline into the peritoneal cavity of a guinea pig, Ganter removed the remaining fluid after approximately 3 h and then instilled fresh salt solution. The procedure was repeated every 3 h, up to 4 times, thereby sometimes 'rinsing' the peritoneal cavity several times without a dwell time.

Actually Ganter performed in his animals what later became intermittent peritoneal dialysis.

He observed an almost complete equilibration of the nonprotein nitrogen content of the peritoneal fluid with the blood in 3 h and noted that some 2/5 to 4/5 of the injected quantity was absorbed: often only 10 ml could be recovered.

Ganter noted a definite improvement of the animal's condition after each session of peritoneal lavage.

THE FIRST ATTEMPT OF INTERMITTENT PERITONEAL DIALYSIS

Finally Ganter instilled 1,5 l of physiological saline in the peritoneal cavity of a patient who became rather acutely uraemic from a bilateral obstruction of the ureters caused by a uterine carcinoma. He observed a slight, transient improvement in the patient's condition (1923).

In another patient who was deeply comatous from diabetic keto-acidosis 3 l of saline was injected into the peritoneal cavity: a striking but transient improvement was noted, the patient waking up, temporarily communicating with this relatives

After these observations Ganter published his investigations in the Münchener Medizinische Wochenschrift in December 1923, but ended his work for unknown reasons.

In the years after World War I several German investigators were active in the field of replacement of renal function either with still experimental extracorporeal haemodialysis (so called 'external dialysis' [22, 25-27]) or with peritoneal dialysis (so called 'internal dialysis" [22]), probably because of the numerous cases of trench nephritis observed during the war with a rapid progressive course leading to fatal uraemia and, on the other hand, because of the numerous victims of acute renal failure complicating battle field injuries, also usually dying from uraemia.

Necheles' criticism

One of these investigators, Heinrich Necheles (25, 26) from Hamburg, Germany, who was in touch with John Jacob Abel in Baltimore, the inventor of the vividiffusion apparatus (see chapter 2), read Ganter's paper and repeated his animal experiments with negative results. Apparently, not very happy with Ganter's work he wrote to John Abel in June 1924 (without mentioning Ganter's name):

'zZ Berlin 16/6, 1924... Ich habe jetzt seine Methode nachgeprüft, die unter Kritik meiner Arbeiten vor einigen Monaten in der Münchener Medizin. Wochenschrift erschienen ist; hier wurde als physiologischerer Weg vorgeschlagen, das Peritoneum der Bauchhöhle als Dialysiermembran zu benutzen und zu durchspülen; in einigen klinischen Fällen will er vorübergehend Erfolg gesehen haben, in Tierexperimenten nicht. Ich habe diese Frage an einem grösseren Material nephrectomierter Katzen und Hunde nachgeprüft, ohne irgend einen Erfolg gesehen zu haben. In der Tat stellt sich das Peritoneum eine ausgedehnte Fläche vor, es findet auch Dialyse statt, der Reststickstoff der Durchspülungsflüssigkeit ist erhöht, der klinische Erfolg ist aber eher als negativ zu bezeichnen, wahrscheinlich weil der Eingriff ein zu schweren ist.' [2]

Necheles abandoned his peritoneal experiments and returned to his own experimental work with a dialyser with semi-permeable conical tubes prepared from visceral animal peritoneum (gold-beaters' skin), which apparently was a good dialysis membrane (25, 26, see also chapter 2).

CONTINUOUS PERITONEAL DIALYSIS

Three years later, in 1927, two other German investigators reported their attempts to save the lives of three

---

[2] Translation: 'Temporarily in Berlin, June 16, 1924... I have now tried a method which was published a few months ago in the Münchener Medizin. Wochenschrift simultaneously criticising my own work. The author suggests using the peritoneum as a dialysis membrane and to perfuse the peritoneal cavity because this would be more physiological. The author states that he, in a few clinical cases transient favourable results has observed, but not in his animal experiments. I repeated these experiments on a rather large number of bilaterally nephrectomised cats and dogs without any result. The peritoneum has indeed a large surface area and dialysis does occur for the nitrogen in the perfusion fluid is increased, but the clinical results are negative. Probably because the intervention is too drastic.'

uraemic patients with acute renal failure, caused by mercury bichloride, with peritoneal dialysis (Heusser and Werder [28], 1927). They modified Ganter's technique, inserting two catheters and perfusing the peritoneal cavity continuously, using one catheter (located between the diaphragm and the liver) for the inflow and the other one (placed in the pelvic area) for the outflow. They observed that not only nitrogenous substances were extracted but also mercury and noted some protein loss in the dialysis fluid. Their attempts were unsuccessful.

OTHER UNSUCCESSFUL EARLY ATTEMPTS (1930–1940)

In the late twenties and early thirties peritoneal dialysis remained a new and relatively unknown method of treatment: seven years passed before another report was published by Balazs and Rosenak (1934, [29]). They also dialysed three cases of acute renal failure with anuria, caused by mercury bichloride, using a similar technique. Their attempts were also futile: obviously those groups of clinical investigators used too little dialysis fluid and their rinsings were too short.

At that time experience with the new procedure was minimal. Nothing was known about the efficiency of peritoneal dialysis, about optimal flow rate of the dialysis solution or peritoneal clearances. In the 1930's peritoneal dialysis remained an ill investigated, experimental, more or less 'hit and miss' treatment of uraemia.

Somewhat more successful were Wear and co-workers (30) in 1938. They treated five patients, dialysed longer (2 to 5 h) and noted a fall in serum creatinine and non protein nitrogen. One patient improved enough to tolerate surgical removal of bladder stones. This patient recovered.

In the same year Rhoads (31) treated two uraemic patients with chronic renal failure with peritoneal dialysis, using for the first time the intermittent method, as used by Ganter in his animal experiments 14 years earlier. He instilled 1,5 l of dialysate through a single catheter, removing the fluid after a 'dwell' time of approximately 15 min through the same tube, repeating the procedure several times. The outflow fluid contained significant amounts of urea.

During World War II thousands of cases of acute renal shutdown caused by severe trauma both in the military and in the civilian population in Europe, the Far East and in other scenes of war, harshly alerted surgeons, internists and nephrologists (at that time a new budding specialism) to the problem.

In this context it is worth quoting the remark made by Dr. Edward D. Churchill from Boston MA at a meeting of the American Surgical Association held in April 1946, in Hot Springs VA after Dr. Fine (32) presented his classical paper on the treatment of acute renal failure by peritoneal dialysis:

... 'despite all the optimistic reports on the successful management of shock in this war, renal shutdown was the stonewall against which we butted our heads many times. ... The surgeons caring for these patients with anuria tried many forms of treatment: high spinal anesthesia; alkalies to the point of severe alkalosis; and many other measures. Still the patients died in uraemia. Dr. Fine's methods represent one more procedure, that may be applicable to men suffering from renal shutdown following severe trauma. I hope it will prove successful...'.

THE TURNING OF THE TIDE: THE INVESTIGATIONS OF FINE AND COLLABORATORS (1946–1948)

After an interval of 8 years (1938–1946) the method finally started catching up. The pioneering investigations of Fine, Frank and Seligman (32–35) from Boston MA were published in 1946 and 1948 and the experiences from the Mayo Clinic were made public by Odel and associates (22) in 1948.

The Boston investigators were convinced that the peritoneum was an efficient dialysis membrane, which, however so far had been utilised for the treatment of uraemia without success. They decided to determine systematically whether peritoneal dialysis could be made practical for clinical use. They made numerous studies on nephrectomised dogs before turning to peritoneal dialysis for the treatment of uraemic patients.

Emphasising the importance of a meticulous technique and observing a painstaking sterility, not only in human patients but also in experiments on the dog, they adopted the continuous flow-technique as Heusser and Werder in 1927 and Balazs and Rosenak in 1934 had done.

Their irrigation fluid, originally Ringer solution with dextrose was later changed to tyrode solution prepared in 5 gallon (appr. 19 l) Pyrex carboys. In the dog experiments they determined the optimal flow rates of the dialysate and achieved urea clearances ranging 5 to 11 ml/minute (depending on the position of the dog) with flow rates of 25 to 50 ml/minute. The survival of bilateral neprhectomised dogs was prolonged from 3 to 10 days and the animals did not die from uraemia, but from bacterial infection along the catheter tracts.

SUCCESSFUL TREATMENT OF ACUTE RENAL FAILURE WITH PERITONEAL DIALYSIS

In March 1946, Fine and his collaborators reported a successful application of peritoneal irrigation in a patient with severe uraemia from sulphathiazol induced anuria. The patient survived after 4 days of continuous peritoneal lavage. The investigations of the Boston team were the first in the field of peritoneal lavage, to be based on sound scientific evidence; they attracted considerable interest and should be considered as a landmark in the history of treatment of uraemia. From then on the tide turned.

In 1948, Odel and co-workers collected a total of 53 uraemic patients previously reported in the literature and treated by peritoneal dialysis. In this group they noted 27 cases with reversible, and 13 with irreversible lesions. Thirteen others had undetermined kidney disease. Seventeen survived, the majority being cases with acute renal failure, caused by incompatible blood transfusions, sulphonamide intoxications or toxaemia of pregnancy.

Muehrcke (36) found in the literature until 1948 a total of 101 uraemic patients treated by peritoneal dialysis: 63 were diagnosed as having acute renal failure, 32 had irreversible, chronic lesions and 6 were cases of poisoning. Of those with acute renal failure 32 survived. In the Netherlands, an early series of 21 patients was reported by Kop (37), who worked with Kolff in Kampen between July 1945 and November 1947. Five had acute renal failure; three of them survived.

Nevertheless in the early 1950's peritoneal dialysis was still an experimental procedure, considered by many to be used as a last resort in cases with terminal uraemia. Side effects and complications were observed during and after treatment. They were often dangerous, frequently leading to death from pulmonary oedema or peritonitis.

THE COMPOSITION OF THE PERITONEAL DIALYSIS FLUID

Other complications and undesirable side effects were often observed and in retrospect they can be readily explained by the unsuitable compositions of many different dialysis fluids used by various investigators until the mid 1960's.

Odel and associates (22) reviewed the literature until 1948, and calculated the electrolyte composition of dialysate solutions reported by a number of clinical investigators, as far as data were available. When studying Table 1 (which is partly derived from Odel and associates [22]), it is not surprising that hyperchloraemic metabolic acidosis was a frequently observed side effect of peritoneal dialysis with Locke-Ringer and modified Tyrode solutions and 'normal' or 'twice normal' saline. Obviously these fluids contained excessive chloride concentrations and were deficient in bicarbonate (or acetate and lactate, which also serve as a source for fixed base) or even did not contain bicarbonate at all.

Sodium concentration

Peripheral oedema, pulmonary oedema and hypertension frequently accompanied peritoneal dialysis in the earlier days of its use (until the early fifties): high dialysate sodium concentrations up to 156 mmol/l, were used rather commonly. Reid and co-workers (38) who performed the first peritoneal dialysis in England (in March 1946) used a rinsing fluid consisting of 'twice normal saline'. The patient, a lady of 36 suffering from acute renal failure caused by a mismatched blood transfusion, tolerated bilateral renal decapsulation and two days of peritoneal dialysis with a dialysate containing 306 mmol sodium and chloride per liter. She survived and made a full recovery.

In the late fifties and early sixties it became apparent that lower dialysate sodium and chloride values were indicated and that appropriate amounts of bicarbonate (or acetate or lactate) were indicated to avoid (or to correct) electrolyte abnormalities in the patients (39, 40) see also Table 1).

Dextrose concentration (See footnote to table 1)

For adequate dehydration of the patients the osmolality of the rinsing fluid was often increased by adding dextrose in different concentrations (up to about 6 g/100 ml). It appeared however that the sodium concentration of the excess fluid removed from the extracellular fluid compartment was much lower than the normal concentration in the extracellular fluid (80 to 115 mmol [mean 110 mol/l] versus 140 mmol/l, Moriarty and Parsons [41], 1966. See also Chapter 22).

The sodium concentration in the ultrafiltrate is dependent on the dwell time of the dialysate in the peritoneal cavity (Parsons FM & Moriarty MV personal communication). In rats (Figure 4) using hypertonic, dehydrating glucose dialysis solution the sodium concentration in the dialysis fluid falls reaching the lowest value in about 45 min. After a 2.5 h dwell time sodium has equilibrated across the peritoneum (Figure 4) but by this time some of the ultrafiltered water has started to be reabsorbed. In

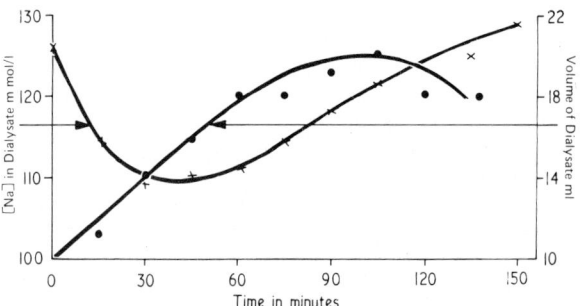

Figure 4. The change in volume (● ●) and sodium concentration (× ×) in hypertonic peritoneal dialysis fluid with time in the rat. Initially 10 ml of dialysis fluid was injected. (Parsons and Moriarty, unpublished observation).

order to remove not only water but also an adequate amount of sodium during 'hypertonic' pertitoneal dialysis with the conventional hourly exchange time the sodium content of the dialysate should be below the normal extracellular concentration of 140 mmol/l, e.g. 110–125 mmol/l, depending on the glucose content of the dialysate (41).

These observations have been confirmed more recently by Nolph and associates (42–44). Obviously the disadvantage of glucose to achieve water removal by osmotic ultrafiltration is the absorption of this solute from the peritoneal cavity.

Other solutes have been used for increasing dialysis fluid osmolality without the risk of causing hyperglycaemia: dextran, fructose, sorbitol, xylitol and gelatin (42, 45). All had disadvantages, either being toxic or

Table 1. Composition of solutions for peritoneal dialysis used by some previous investigators[1]. (Partly derived from Odel and associates [22] with permission).

	Na mmol/l	K mmol/l	Cl mmol/l	Ca mmol/l	bicarb mmol/l	acet/ lact. mmol/l	glucose[2] g/100 ml	osmolal m osm/l		Ref nr
Ganter 1923	136	0	136	0	0	0	0	272	—	24
Balasz, Rosenak 1934	136 0	0 0	136 0	0 0	0 0	0 0	0 4.2	272 233	—	29
Wear, Sisk, Trinkle 1938	130 156	4 3	110 165	2 4	28 2	0 0	0 0.09	274 326	Hartmann sol Locke/Ringer sol	30
Fine, Frank, Seligman 1946	151	3	145	1	12	0	1.5	321	Mod. Tyrode	32
Reid, Penfold, Jones 1946	306	0	306	0	0	0	0	612	Twice normal saline	38
Kop 1946-1947	135	5.4	109	2.5	23	0	1–3	330–440	—	37
Odel, Ferris, Power 1948	151 139 140	3 3 3	145 109 109	1 1 1	12 36 24	0 0 13	1.5 1–2 1–2	321 344–400	Mod. Tyrode 'P' solution Mod. 'P' sol	22
Maxwell, Rockney, Kleeman, Twiss 1959	140	0–4	101–105	2	0	45	1.5	372–380	—	40
Doolan and coworkers 1959	128	as indicated	100	parenterally	28	0	3.25	400	—	39
Moriarty, Parsons 1966	141	0	101	1.8	0	45	1. 36–6.36	372–667	—	41
Presently	130–135	0	99–101	1.75–2.0	0	35–45	1.5–4.25	334–350	—	42

[1] Magnesium values in these fluids fluctuate between 0 and 1½ mmol/l
Na, K, Cl, bicarbonate, acetate, lactate: mmol/l = mEq/l
Ca, Mg: mmol/l × 2 = mEq/l, Ca mmol/l × 4 = mg/dl, Mg mmol/l × 2.4 = mg/dl.

[2] Glucose = dextrose monohydrate; 1.5 g/dl of dextrose monohydrate = $\frac{180 \times 1.5}{198}$ = 1.36 g/dl anhydrous dextrose.

Presently for most commercially made peritoneal dialysis fluids the term dextrose (which is anhydrous) is used.

too expensive or both. Glucose (dextrose monohydrate), usually in concentrations of 1,5–4,25% is still preferred.

Even presently the optimal composition of peritoneal dialysis solution is a matter of debate. In 1959 Doolan and co-workers (39) used a dialysis solution with a low sodium concentration of 128 mmol/l, a chloride concentration equal to the blood (100 mmol/l) and a bicarbonate concentration of 28 mmol/l. By administering calcium parenterally and omitting calcium from the dialysis fluid they avoided the precipitation of calcium carbonate. The potassium content was adapted to the clinical setting and the plasma potassium values of the patient. Maxwell and co-workers, also in 1959 (40), utilised a fluid with 140 mmol/l sodium and 101–105 mmol/l chloride, depending on the amount of potassium chloride to be added and 2 mmol/l calcium.

Lactate and acetate vs. bicarbonate

Others (32) sterilised bicarbonate solution separately, which then was added aseptically to the rinsing fluid, after cooling. Acetate poses problems when sterilised together with glucose, because caramelisation takes place. Presently other dialysis solutions are prepared, however, either with lactate or acetate at a pH adjusted to below 5.5, which prevents caramelisation. In this context it should be mentioned that lactate, if the racemic mixture is used, will only partly be metabolised into bicarbonate: the laevo-isomer will be converted only (21). Strict sterility of course is obligatory and because large amounts of fluid (40 l/day) are required, problems may occur when peritoneal rinsing fluid is prepared in bottles of 1 or 2 l, which have to be replaced every 1 or 2 h. Obviously the disconnections endanger the sterility of the circuit. Fine and co-workers (32) prepared the dialysis fluid in 20 l Pyrex carboys. This made the creation of a closed administration system possible. Two elevated carboys were joined by a Y-tube and the fluid flowed by gravity through syphon tubes into the peritoneal cavity (Figure 5). This system – presumably because of the many technical problems – never gained popularity.

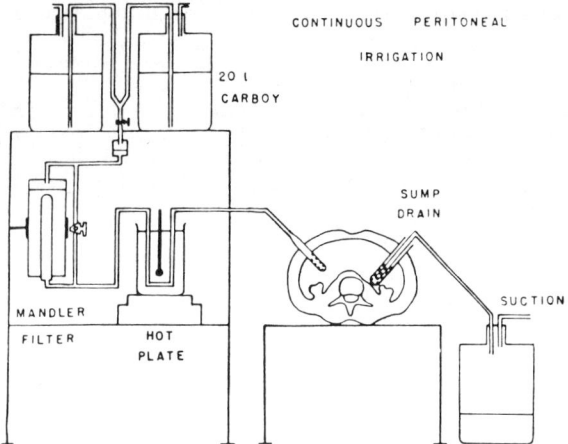

Figure 5. Flow diagram of Dr. Fine's closed circuit for continuous peritoneal irrigation. Dialysis fluid supply came from two 20 l Pyrex carboys (1946 [32]). (With permission of the publishers of *Ann Surg*.)

Maxwell and associates (40) circumvented these problems by introducing commercially prepared solutions in 1 l infusion bottles, which came together with sterile Y-type administration tubing (1959). Obviously the continuity of this system had to be broken hourly; for every

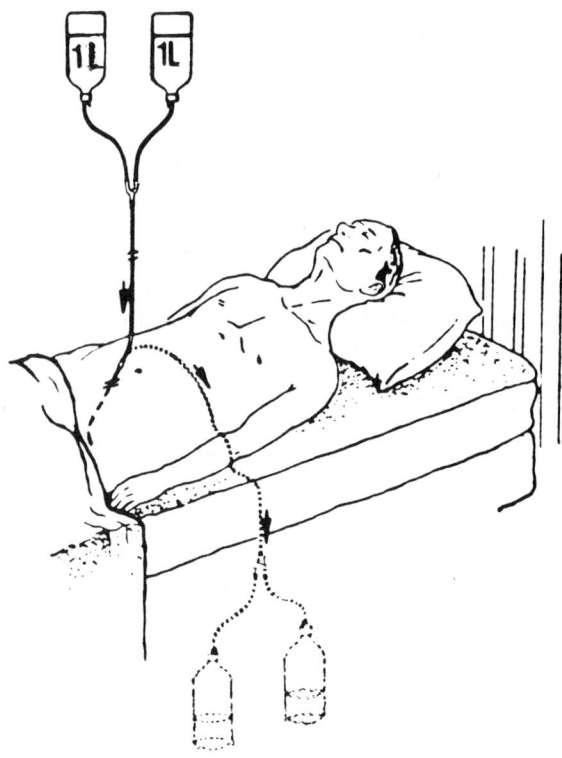

Figure 6. 'Hanging bottle' peritoneal dialysis (Maxwell et al, 1959 [40]). (With permission of the authors and the publishers of the *JAMA*).

exchange two fresh bottles had to be connected. This endangered sterility every hour.

CONTINUOUS vs. INTERMITTENT PERITONEAL DIALYSIS

Another controversy concerned the technique of peritoneal dialysis. Many early investigators (3, 4, 30, 32, 34, 45) were advocates of the continuous flow method. This method involved the (surgical) insertion of two catheters: one in the right upper quadrant (between liver and diaphragm) and the other in either lower quadrant of the abdomen, often being located in the cul de sac. Continuous lavage was then instituted: the dialysis fluid was instilled through one catheter, leaving the peritoneal cavity through the other (Figure 5). Channelling of the dialysis fluid between the inflow and outflow catheters was predictable and common. Leakage occurred frequently and obviously the risk of peritonitis was appreciably greater than with the 'one catheter, intermittent' technique. With this method, advocated by Rhoads (31), Reid, Penfold and Jones (38), Grollman and associates (46, 47) and others, only one catheter is inserted in the peritoneal cavity, the rinsing fluid being instilled and drained after a certain dwell time through the same catheter, usually by the syphon effect.

In the 1950's the continuous method was gradually abandoned and in 1959 the matter was settled in favour of the intermittent method by the introduction of a nylon non-irritating flexible catheter by Maxwell and co-workers (40), which was relatively easily introduced through the linea alba with a trocar.

PERITONEAL ACCESS

Different types of catheters

Actually the access to the peritoneal cavity has been a problem for years (48) and a multitude of access devices has been used: Foley catheters (38), mushroom tip catheters, whistle tip catheters (34), polyethylene tubes (45), stainless steel sump drains (similar to the metal-perforated suction tubes, used in operating theatres (32) and even glass drains. Also simple soft rubber tubes with or without side holes were utilised.

Leakage was a common problem, opening the way for infection and often mattress sutures were applied to eliminate this problem. Rosenak and Oppenheimer (49) introduced a rigid catheter with a collar which was sewn in the subcutis to prevent leakage.

Obstruction was common because of kinking of the catheter or from blood clots or plugging of the outflow tube with tiny bits of omental fat, sucked into the lumen through the side perforations (40). Another common cause of catheter failure was the wrapping of the omentum around the catheter blocking outflow, sometimes causing inflow obstruction.

Doolan (39) described in 1959 a new PVC catheter, constructed by his associate Murphy. This catheter, which had multiple small side holes, was transversely

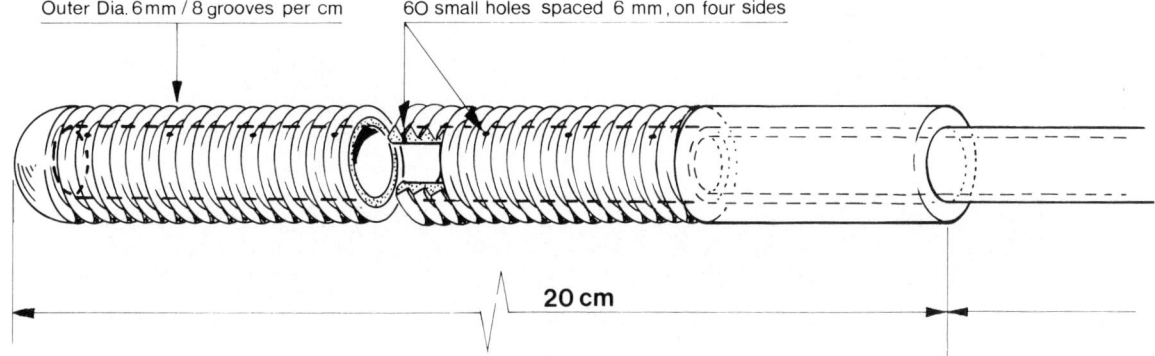

Figure 7. Murphy-Doolan implantable peritoneal lavage tube, made from transversely ridged polyvinylchloride, with 60 small hand-punched holes (1959 [39]). (With permission of the authors and the publishers of the *Am J Med*).

ridged with spiral grooves. The ridging helped to prevent blockage by the omentum and kinking. Introduction, however, was somewhat laborious and had to be performed either with a # 22 gall bladder trocar or by laparotomy. It did not become widely used (Figure 7).

The stylet catheter

A major advance was made by Weston and Roberts (50), who improved the Maxwell catheter (1965). Roberts, a research biochemist, happened to visit Dr. Weston at the Cedars-Sinai Medical Center in Los Angeles in 1964 and saw him struggling to pierce the abdominal wall of a sick patient with a 17F trocar to insert a Maxwell catheter. Roberts made a simple modification by inserting a pointed stylet within the Maxwell catheter (Figures 8a, b and c), thus eliminating the need for a trocar and sutures. The stylet catheter (Trocath) soon became commercially available. It simplified temporary peritoneal access considerably. The use of the stylet catheter is now standard practice for acute dialysis and for temporary access in case of cathether failure in chronic patients treated with periodic peritoneal dialysis.

STANDARDISING THE TECHNIQUE

In the late fifties and early sixties intermittent peritoneal dialysis became gradually a safe and standardised procedure, in particular by the work of Doolan and his coworkers (39) and Maxwell and associates (40). Both groups contributed much to the improvement and perfection of peritoneal dialysis technique.

DEVELOPMENT OF 'HANGING BOTTLE' PERITONEAL DIALYSIS

Commercial preparation of dialysis fluid and tubing

The Maxwell and Doolan groups both used commercially prepared rinsing fluids which considerably simplified the procedure and also contributed appreciably to the popularisation of peritoneal dialysis in the hospital setting. Both groups of investigators used the 'hanging bottle system' which had to be operated manually. Usually two bottles each containing 1 l of dialysis fluid were used with a Y type of administration tubing connected to the catheter (Figure 6). The rinsing solution flowed into the peritoneal cavity by gravity as rapidly as possible (usually taking 5 to 10 minutes). After a dwell time (30 min to 1 h), the inflow tubing was clamped and the fluid was drained from the abdomen by syphon effect, into the original bottles which were lowered to the floor besides the patient's bed. The system could easily be operated by nurses but obviously carried the risk of bacterial contamination and peritonitis because the inflow circuit had to be broken every hour.

Closed administration systems

Years before (in 1946) Fine and co-workers (32) created a closed dialysate administration system by introducing 5 gallons (appr. 19 l) Pyrex carboys for sterilising the rinsing solution. Two of these large bottles made a peritoneal dialysis possible lasting 20 hours. The Seattle group used these carboys later (1962) with an automatic peritoneal cycling machine (51). However the need for special requirements (a large autoclave, special caps, special Pyrex bottles) made this system expensive. Later 12 gallon (45 l) carboys were used permitting a single carboy for each dialysis (51). Cost, transport problems and explosion risks of the large carboys restricted the use of these large bottles to local use in Seattle.

SEMI-AUTOMATIC PERITONEAL DIALYSIS MACHINES ('CYCLERS')

Bosch et al. (52) constructed a semi-automatic supply system, consisting of 15 or more, commercially available 3 l bottles with sterile dialysis solution, interconnected by sterile polyethylene tubes and wide bore needles. A somewhat similar commercially produced apparatus made in West-Germany was modified by the author (1967). Instead of multiple 3 l bottles 6 interconnected

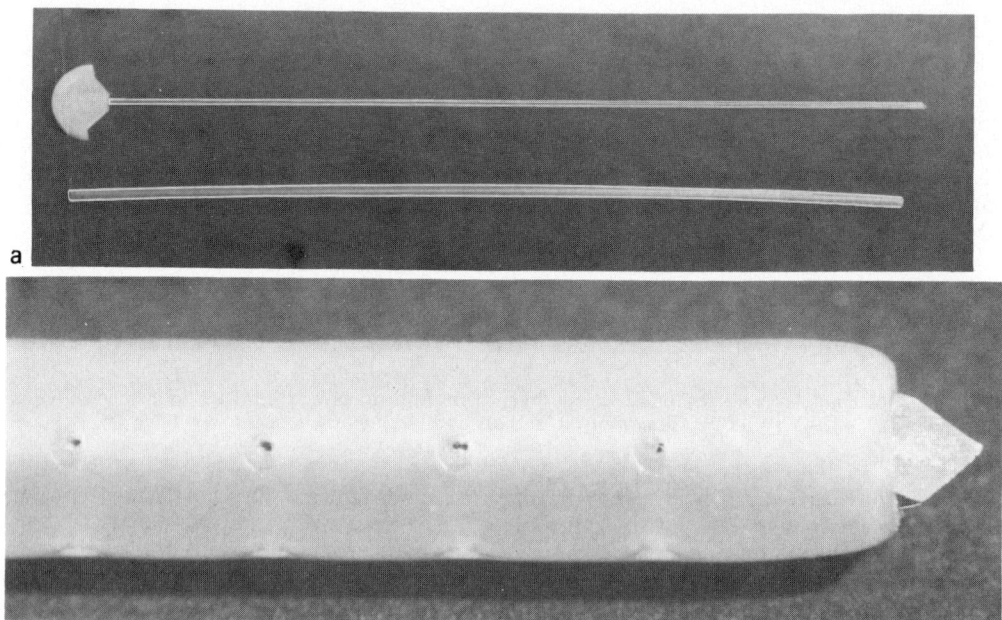

Figure 8 (a and b). Stylet catheter ('Trocath') (Weston and Roberts, 1965 [50]).

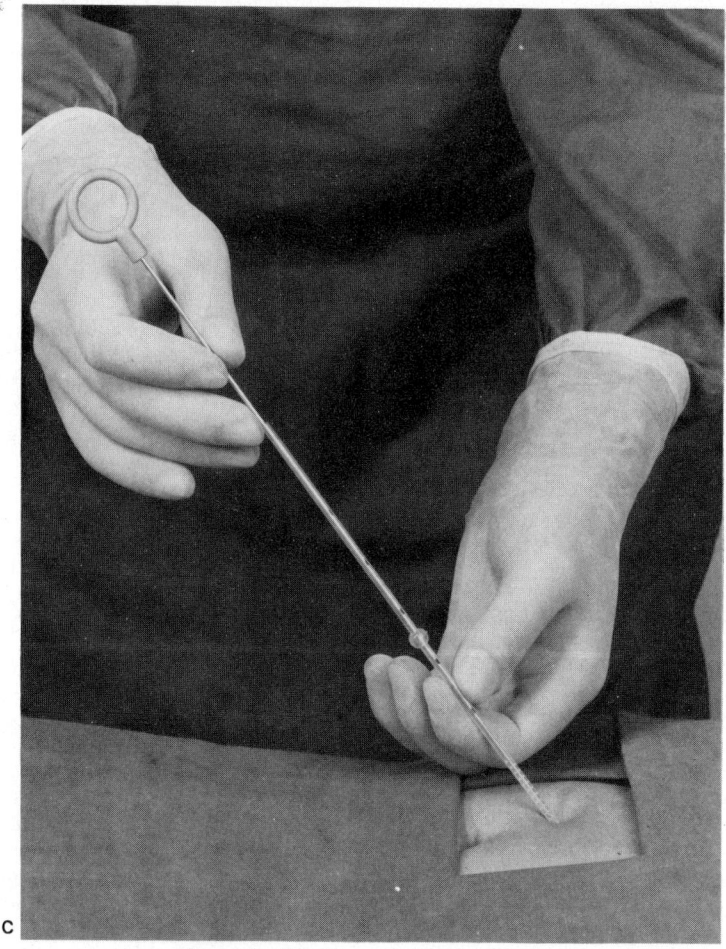

Figure 8c. Insertion of a stylet catheter.

21: Peritoneal dialysis: a historical review

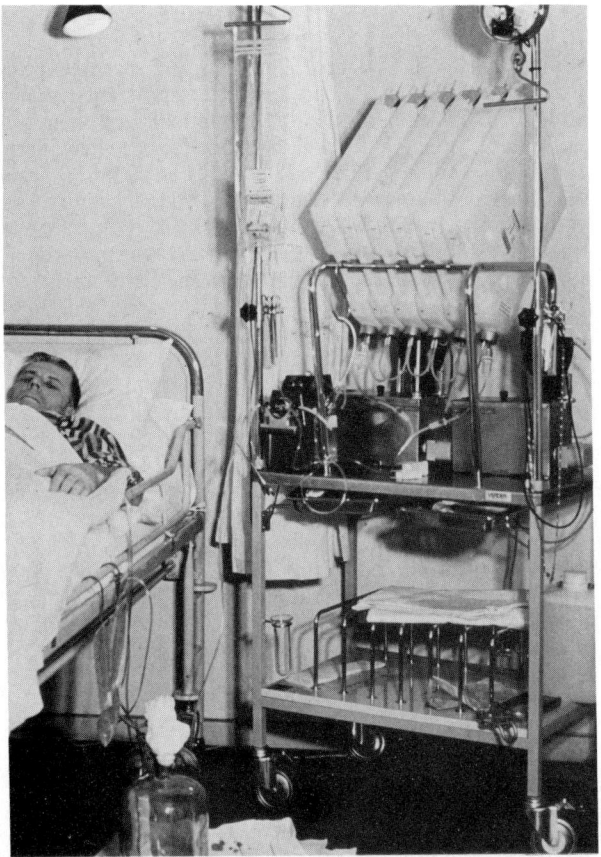

Figure 9. Cycler with 6 interconnected 10 l plastic containers.

10 l plastic containers, also commercially produced, were utilised (Figure 9).

These semi-automatic peritoneal dialysis systems, called cyclers, were bacteriologically much safer than the hanging bottle systems, which however are presently still popular in smaller hospitals.

The 'cycler' (53) was the precursor of the modern automatic peritoneal dialysis machines which were introduced in the mid sixties for home peritoneal dialysis (54). Obviously, peritoneal dialysis technique and practical application of the procedure made considerable progress in the 1950's and 1960's.

FURTHER PROGRESS

Clearance studies

The kinetics and biophysics have been studied by several groups of investigators; their work significantly improved the effectiveness of the procedure.

In 1945–46 Seligman, Frank and Fine (32–35) studied the effect of irrigation flow rate on peritoneal urea clearance in dogs.

Grollman and co-workers (46, 47) determined, also in dogs, the rapidity with which substances like urea passed into the peritoneal cavity. They noted that after intraperitoneal injection of 1 l of fluid, equilibrium was complete in about 2 h. An identical period of time appeared to be necessary in the human subject when 2 or 3 l were introduced in the peritoneal cavity. They also determined in dog experiments the disappearance rate of dextrose from the peritoneal fluid and the amount of fluid that was removed from the extracellular space with different concentrations of dextrose.

Significance of dialysate flow rates

Boen (20, 21) investigated the relationship between dialysate flow rates and peritoneal clearances of urea and several other substances. Optimal clearances were obtained with a flow rate of 3.5 l/h. For practical purposes he advised 2.5 l/h, the gain with higher flow rates being only minimal. Tenckhoff and associates (55) repeating Boen's original investigations obtained different results: the peritoneal clearance of urea could be increased 2 to 3 fold by increasing the dialysate flow rate from 2 to 12 l/h, which was well tolerated by the patient. Several other groups of investigators (42, 56–58) studied peritoneal clearances and mass transfer kinetics and factors influencing peritoneal dialysis efficiency.

So far these investigators limited their studies with a few exceptions to so called small molecules up to the size of uric acid (molecular weight 168).

THE PERMEABILITY OF THE PERITONEUM TO LARGER SOLUTES (SO CALLED MIDDLE MOLECULES)

Scribner (59) noticed in 1965, that patients on chronic periodic peritoneal dialysis, which controls plasma chemistries of small molecules less efficiently haemodialysis does often feel better than when treated by haemodialysis. Notwithstanding a certain amount of 'underdialysis' of small molecules, peripheral neuropathy either did not develop, or did not progress. He presented the hypothesis that the peritoneum, that is more permeable for proteins, is also more permeable for substances of higher molecular weight than the artificial membranes commonly used for haemodialysis. He suggested that peritoneal dialysis removed larger molecules (molecular weight 300–2000), the so called 'middle molecules', more efficiently than haemodialysis. Scribner's hypothesis was confirmed by the work of Babb et al. (60) who in 1973 reported on the mass transfer characteristics of the human peritoneum during peritoneal dialysis with special respect to solutes with different molecular weights. They demonstrated that clearances of small molecules were only 1/4 to 1/6 of those with haemodialysers. Higher molecular weight solutes (e.g. vitamin B_{12} [1355], inulin [5200]) were removed at relatively higher rates than urea and other small molecules compared with haemodialysis using conventional membranes. The longer peritoneal dialysis times served primarily to reduce small molecule concentrations to acceptable levels.

THE FIRST CHRONIC CASE SUCCESSFULLY TREATED WITH PERIODIC PERITONEAL DIALYSIS

The successful application of intermittent peritoneal dialysis in cases with acute renal failure (38–40) lead to a trial of repeated peritoneal dialysis in a patient with terminal, chronic, irreversible renal failure shortly before Scribner and collaborators in Seattle, WA (61) initiated intermittent haemodialysis treatment in their first two chronic patients (March 1960, see chapter 2). The patient, Willie Mae Stewart, a 33 year old black female, was first seen by Dr. R.F. Ruben at the Mount Zion Hospital in San Francisco, CA as an outpatient who came back for a post partum check-up. She was not doing too well and was found to be uraemic. Dr. Ruben, who was an assistant resident of Dr. Paul Doolan at the US Naval Hospital at Oakland CA, admitted the patient to the Clinical Investigation Center at the Naval Hospital. The decision was made to perform an initial peritoneal dialysis to improve her condition and a Murphy-Doolan peritoneal catheter was inserted. After the first dialysis further examination revealed bilateral shrunken end-stage kidneys and, obviously, the patient was a case of end-stage chronic renal failure. But after the first dialysis she thrived so well that it was decided to leave the tube in, to clamp it and await events. She deteriorated in a week or so and a second dialysis was done. And after the second dialysis Ruben and Doolan wondered why not a third, not a fourth and after the fourth why not a fifth...? They decided to start what became later 'periodic' peritoneal dialysis and dialysed her as an outpatient every time the blood creatinine level reached 20 mg/dl (appr. 1770 µmol/l). The dialyses were terminated when creatinine was around 13 mg/dl (1150 µmol/l). The patient went home after each dialysis and remained in a symptom free condition, somewhat restricting her physical activities to housework, shopping and helping with the care of her children and enjoying television.

After 3 months and 12 peritoneal dialyses the catheter failed and a new catheter was inserted through a small laporatomy. Periodic peritoneal dialysis was continued, but by the end of April 1960 pericarditis developed with fever and a psychotic syndrome. The patient refused further treatment and died on the 4th of June 1960, after 6 months of periodic peritoneal dialysis. The post mortem revealed pericarditis, peritonitis, bilateral bronchopneumonia and chronic glomerular nephritis with contracted kidneys.

This was actually the first chronic patient successfully treated with periodic (peritoneal) dialysis. The case report has never been published in the literature; it was presented for publication but a reviewer rejected it, probably because it was a single case and survival was relatively short.[3]

---

[3] The author is indebted to Dr. Paul Doolan, presently at St. Mary's Hospital, Waterbury, CT and Dr. Richard M. Ruben, presently in San Francisco, CA who provided a detailed case history and further particulars of this historical patient.

INDWELLING PLASTIC CONDUITS

Merrill and collaborators (62) attempted repeated peritoneal irrigation in four patients with end-stage irreversible renal failure and also in one patient with acute renal failure, utilising a plastic conduit for repeated insertion of the catheter. They had little success: a number of technical problems necessitated revision or removal of the conduits in periods from 2 weeks to 4 months. In one patient the use of the device however permitted peritoneal irrigation to be carried out temporarily at home.

The successful introduction of intermittent haemodialysis for terminal irreversible chronic renal failure in April 1960 by Scribner and co-workers (61) lead the Seattle team to attempt periodic peritoneal dialysis in a patient who clotted all his cannulae and eventually ran out of cannulation sites. By the end of January 1965, periodic peritoneal dialysis was started. Originally, an indwelling plastic conduit was implanted, to facilitate repeated insertion of a plastic or silastic catheter.

The condition of the patient, a 28 year old male with end-stage chronic glomerulonephritis, remained good during 4 months. Thereafter infections started around the plastic conduit and recurrent peritonitis and adhesions became more and more of a problem. The patient died 9 months after the first peritoneal dialysis.

In the early 1960's many centres attempted periodic peritoneal dialysis for end-stage chronic renal failure using various implanted devices for repeated access to the peritoneal cavity. The reports, however, were discouraging (63), the main problem being peritonitis from infection along the channel of the indwelling devices and from manually changing of bottles. Repeated episodes of peritonitis were often followed by the development of adhesions with partial or more extensive obliteration of the peritoneal cavity, decreasing the dialysis efficiency. Most patients died within a few months to a year.

The approach of the Seattle group was different: instead of the hanging bottle method they reintroduced 20 l Pyrex carboys (originally used by Fine and co-workers [32–35]), which soon were replaced by larger bottles with a volume of 45 l [21, 63]). In addition Boen and co-workers used the automatic cycling machine, constructed by Mr. James Sisley (21, 53) of the Medical Instrument Facility of the University of Washington, Seattle. Later an improved cycling machine was designed and constructed by Boen and Curtis et al. (53, 63), which was easily transportable. This improved system facilitated uninterrupted cycling without breaking the continuity of the closed sterile fluid administration circuit. In addition, the problem of nursing time was largely solved.

PERITONEAL ACCESS BY REPEATED PUNCTURE

Because of the bad results obtained with implanted 'buttons' or other conduits, the Seattle group changed to a so called repeated puncture technique, introducing a catheter in the peritoneal cavity for each dialysis and removing it at the end of each treatment (53, 63, 64). Satisfactory results were obtained with this technique in a 28 year old woman with end-stage chronic pyelonephritis and a residual creatinine clearance of 0.7 ml/min. She was rehabilitated with once weekly ambulatory peritoneal dialysis, originally lasting 14 h, later 22 h (53).

PERIODICAL PERITONEAL DIALYSIS IN THE HOME

Using similar equipment and repeated puncture access Tenckhoff, Shilipetar and Boen (64) trained a 32 year old housewife for periodic peritoneal dialysis in the home. She started home treatment in May 1964 with once weekly, later twice weekly dialysis. Forty 1 carboys were shipped in special crates from the hospital to the patient's home, and obviously, a doctor's visit, once or twice weekly was necessary to insert the peritoneal catheter. Initially, this was performed by using a trocar described by McDonald (65); later the stylet catheter ('Trocath' [50]) was utilised. The treatment was reasonably successful but frequent bleeding episodes from the abdominal wall occurred. The treatment caused apparently considerable stress: the husband reacted with two depressive episodes for the first time in his life.

Because of the many technical problems, the workload of preparing large amounts of sterile rinsing fluid, the transport problems of the heavy carboys filled with dialysis fluid and the peritoneal access problem in the home setting, requiring regualr doctor's visits, periodic peritoneal dialysis remained for the time being an experimental procedure, not only in the home but also in the hospital (64). On the other thand Boen, Mion and other members of Scribner's team (53, 54) had convincingly demonstrated that periodic peritoneal dialysis as replacement of renal function for end-stage chronic kidney disease was feasible and could basically be further developed into an acceptable alternative for regular haemodialysis treatment.

CONSERVATIVE TREATMENT OF ACUTE RENAL FAILURE vs. PERITONEAL DIALYSIS

After many years of quite irrational conservative treatment of uraemia (in particular of uraemia caused by acute renal failure) the Bull-Joekes-Lowe regimen developed in the UK and the Borst treatment based on the same principle developed in the Netherlands (66, 67) seemed to provide in the late 40's a rational and rather easy conservative means of treating acute renal failure.

In many centres these regimens became standard practice with occasional use of the artificial kidney, which was developed some years before by Kolff and Berk (see chapter 2) and of peritoneal dialysis.

Notwithstanding the successes reported by Fine and coworkers (32–35) and by Grollman et al. (46, 47) and the work reported from Scribner's group in Seattle (51, 53, 55, 63, 64), peritoneal dialysis was only slowly and hesitatingly accepted as treatment for acute renal failure in centres which had no artificial kidney available.

The use of peritoneal dialysis in cases of acute renal failure became, however, more wide spread as it became clear, with increasing experience, that the conservative regimen in cases with prolonged oliguria or (and) severe catabolism failed. In addition the application of peritoneal dialysis was facilitated by the introduction of commercially prepared dialysis solutions and the stylet catheter.

HAEMODIALYSIS vs. PERITONEAL DIALYSIS IN ACUTE RENAL FAILURE

On the other hand it became apparent that even peritoneal dialysis failed in highly catabolic cases of acute renal failure, requiring early and frequent (daily) haemodialysis (68). But in numerous cases of acute renal failure peritoneal dialysis became the treatment of choice, in others haemodialysis was preferred. The choice often depended on personal preference and experience, on available equipment and of course on contra-indications to either method.

PERITONEAL DIALYSIS BECOMES A 'GOOD LEADEN BULLET' IN THE TREATMENT FOR ACUTE URAEMIA, BUT REMAINS A 'CINDERELLA' TREATMENT FOR CHRONIC URAEMIA

With growing experience indications and contra-indications both for peritoneal and haemodialysis became gradually clear. Peritoneal dialysis appeared to be particularly useful in patients with recent wounds and where there was a haemorrhagic risk because systemic heparinisation was not required and also in cases where slower chemical change than that brought about by the artificial kidney was required (e.g. in advanced uraemia with very high levels of blood urea, in which haemodialysis may cause severe disequilibrium).

The Editor of the Lancet (69) stated in 1959:

'Peritoneal dialysis is obviously no "silver bullet" for renal failure, but in suitable cases it is a good leaden bullet, which should perhaps be more commonly fired'.

Peritoneal dialysis was also utilised as a 'holding procedure' for patients waiting for a place in a chronic haemodialysis programme or while waiting for vascular access to mature and as a holding procedure whilst waiting for a kidney transplant (70). But the rapid technical improvement of haemodialysis and the increasing success of renal transplantation made these treatments in the past twenty years the 'Glamour Stars' of the medical world (71) and periodic peritoneal dialysis remained the 'Cinderella' treatment for chronic renal failure. Long-term treatment was frequently associated with recurrent episodes of peritonitis, with protein loss, malnutrition, progressive wasting and poor rehabilitation.

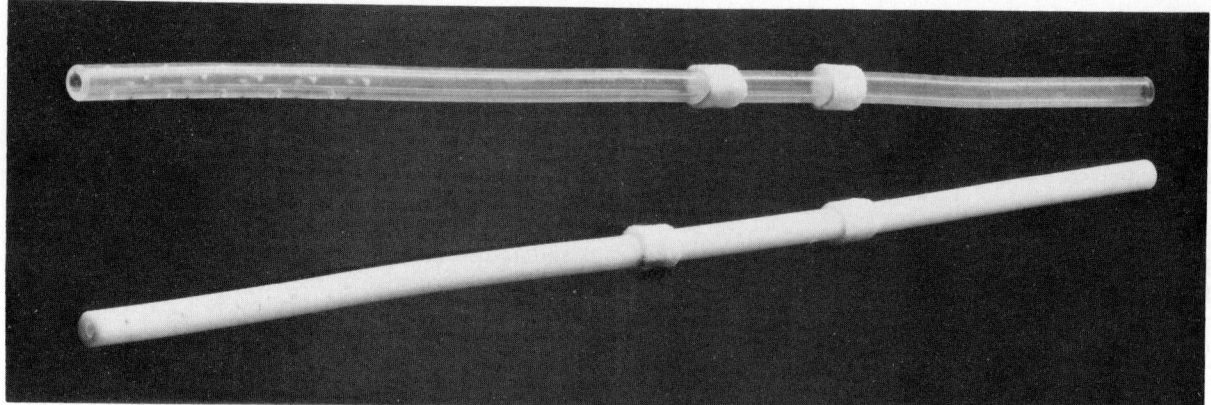

Figure 10a. Tenckhoff catheter, clear and radio-opaque model (1968 [79]).

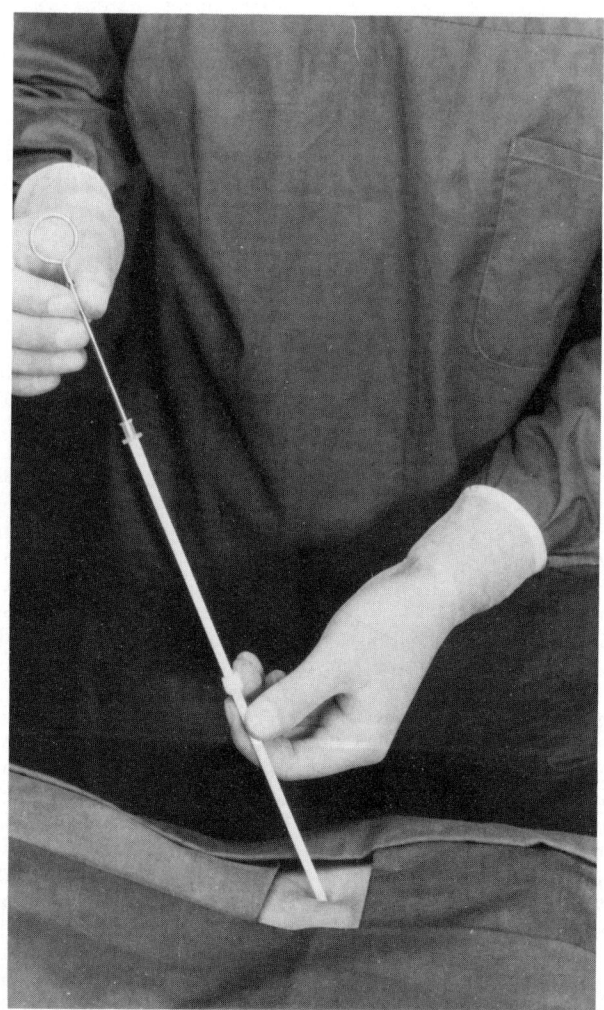

Figure 10b. Introduction of a modified, single cuff Tenckhoff catheter with a pointed stylet inserted (85).

In the late sixties and early seventies, however, two technical developments changed the 'Cinderella' aspect of periodic intermittent peritoneal dialysis, dramatically.

So far peritoneal access was one of the bottle necks of long-term peritoneal dialysis. The stylet catheter, mentioned before, was an important technical step forwards, but was impractical for longterm periodic peritoneal dialysis in chronic cases.

INTRODUCTION OF THE TENCKHOFF CATHETER

Numerous indwelling devices, both access conduits (51, 62, 72-74) and catheters (75-78), had been designed. None appeared to be completely satisfactory: either dislocations or obstruction (by kinking or by the omentum) caused problems and sooner or later infection occurred leading to loss of the device and usually to peritonitis.

The Tenckhoff catheter (79), introduced in 1968, did much better and is still faring well. This catheter or its subsequent modifications are now accepted as the only practical access devices. The original Tenckhoff catheter is made from silastic (Figure 10) and is basically a modification of the curled Palmer catheter (77). It has an open end and numerous side holes in its terminal part of 15 cm (6 inch). Two Dacron felt cuffs protect against infection along the subcutaneous tract: one just outside the peritoneum, the other in the subcutaneous tissue. The curled section of the Palmer catheter was replaced by a straight intra-abdominal part. The Tenckhoff catheter is inserted either surgically through a mini-laparotomy or with local anaesthesia and the aid of a special trocar at the bedside.

The Tenckhoff catheter appeared to be a major advance for periodic peritoneal dialysis. It allows longterm access to the abdominal cavity and the incidence of infection is low. Still, dislocation and obstruction may occur[4] and therefore several investigators modified the design (80-83). Goldberg and Hill (82) designed a catheter somewhat similar to the Tenckhoff catheter, but with a blunt formed tip, facilitating the introduction with an internal obturator and provided the catheter with an inflatable cuff, some distance from the distal end. After insertion the cuff was inflated with sterile saline to prevent occlusion of the drainage holes by the peritoneal contents (omentum) and to keep the catheter down in the pelvis. For the same reason the catheter developed by Oreopoulos (84) has two silastic discs near the distal end of the intra-abdominal part. The Goldberg catheter can be introduced with a trocar; the Oreopoulos device, however, has the disadvantage that it requires surgical implantation. Still another modification (85)

combines the stylet of the Weston-Roberts catheter (50) with a slightly altered version of the Tenckhoff catheter, making insertion by simple puncture at the bedside possible (Figure 10b).

The choice of the type of indwelling device usually depends on personal preference and experience. The original Tenckhoff catheter is still widely used.

CYCLERS

Another major advance which made periodic peritoneal dialysis much more dependable was the introduction of automatic cycling machines by Boen and co-workers in 1962 (51-53). These cyclers were later (1972) combined with automatic machines which produce sterile rinsing fluid from concentrate and pre-treated water.

Several models of automatic 'cyclers' have been described in previous years (1962-1968 [51-54, 86-89]). These peritoneal cyclers are relatively simple apparatus with timers which are set for inflow time, dwell period and outflow, freeing nurses from manual operation. Premixed sterile dialysis fluid is either supplied from 19 to 45 l Pyrex carboys (51, 53) or small (1-2 l) interconnected bottles (52, 87) or from interconnected plastic containers with 10 l sterile dialysis fluid each. These containers and the cycling machine are commercially available from Messrs. Braun A.G., Melsungen, Western Germany. The Lasker system (86, 87) is also commercially produced (American Medical Products, Fairfield, NJ, USA). Other cyclers are marketed by Gambro Inc., Lund, Sweden, an English firm named RA Scientific in London and other firms. In the McDonald machine (88), non-sterile rinsing fluid is pumped through a Millipore filter to obtain sterility. A similar system, also incorporating a Millipore filter was constructed by Vercellone in 1968 (89).

These cycling machines are simple to operate and relatively cheap. But because large quantities of sterile rinsing fluid have to be stored and transported, the operating cost is relatively high. The most serious objection however is that sterility of the system cannot be guaranteed, because containers or bottles have to be changed or (and) interconnected manually. In addition systems depending for sterility on bacterial filters do not seem very reliable and safe.

INTRODUCTION OF CLOSED LOOP, REVERSE OSMOSIS, AUTOMATIC PERITONEAL DIALYSIS MACHINES

A prototype of proportioning peritoneal dialysis system was constructed and described by Tenckhoff and co-workers in 1969 (90). Sterile dialysate was prepared from a concentrate and locally produced distilled water with an occlusive roller pump. Because of the necessity of a water still and a rather large stainless steel water sterilisation tank it was a bulky system, requiring a considerable amount of floor space.

An automatic peritoneal dialysis system using reverse osmosis (RO) for tapwater purification and sterilisation

---

[4] Evaluation of the cause of obstruction is facilitated by using a radio-opaque model (Quinton Instrument Co, Seattle, WA, USA). This obviates filling with contrast fluid, which may be harmful for the peritoneum, but obviously has the disadvantage that filling defects caused e.g. by fibrin clots (which can be removed by urokinase) cannot be demonstrated.

was designed years later also by Tenckhoff and co-workers (1972 [91]). The purified sterile water was mixed with sterile concentrate at a ratio of 20 to 1, also by an occlusive roller pump. A commercial model of this system (with different proportioning pumps) was manufactured by Physio-Control Corporation of Seattle, WA and was marketed in 1973. A similar machine of somewhat different design was marketed by Drake-Willock Corporation from Portland, OR (Figures 11 and 12). Both systems deionise, sterilise and polish the water by reverse osmosis. They have both a proportioning ratio of about 1 to 19, the Drake-Willock machine using roller pumps and the other machine piston pumps. Both use more or less identical cycling and monitor systems. The machines are bacteriologically and technically safe but both have the disadvantage of cold sterilisation with formaldehyde solution, which carries the risk of accidental infusion of the disinfectant in the peritoneal cavity.

The reverse osmosis machines are expensive but running cost is relatively low being limited to the cost of sterile concentrate and concentrated dextrose solutions, sterile administration tubing sets and electrical power for driving the reverse osmosis compressor and proportioning pumps and the heater.

These machines have the important advantage that the fluid factory and the peritoneal circuit form a closed system and that this continuity is not broken during the dialysis procedure, in contrast with the simpler (and

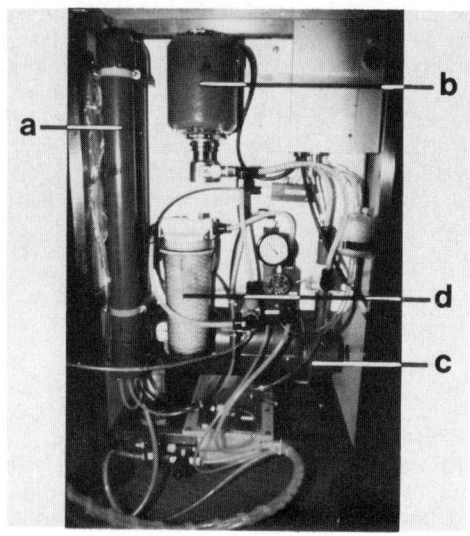

Figure 12. Reverse osmosis unit of automatic peritoneal dialysis machine. a. R.O. filter, b. high pressure pump, c. heat exchanger, d. water filter.

cheaper) cyclers. The risk of bacteriological contamination of the sterile circuit or the rinsing fluid is practically eliminated. The incidence of peritonitis with these machines is therefore minimal. On the other hand they are much more complicated, requiring training for adequate operation and maintenance. These machines became increasingly popular for periodic maintenance peritoneal dialysis until the late seventies, in particular in the United States, Canada and in European countries.

Presently our knowledge of the (patho-)physiology of the peritoneum and of the peritoneal transport, the introduction of the new indwelling catheters and the new automatic R.O. proportioning-cycling machines have doubtless made periodic peritoneal dialysis a safe and efficient method for long-term replacement of renal function. Rehabilitation and quality of life and presumably survival rates are comparable with those obtained with extracorporeal haemodialysis (92), in particular when peritoneal dialysis is performed overnight in the home.

INCREASING UTILISATION OF PERIODIC PERITONEAL DIALYSIS IN THE 1970's AND 1980's

The present state of the art and the advantages of periodic peritoneal dialysis (simplicity, safety, lack of anticoagulation, its excellent potential for self training) led understandably to increased interest in the use of peritoneal dialysis for the treatment of patients with terminal chronic renal failure.

In the Northwest Kidney Center in Seattle, WA the number of chronic peritoneal dialysis patients increased from 11 (7% of the total number of dialysis patients) in 1970 to 59 (13%) in 1978 (see table 2). The total number of peritoneal dialyses at this centre increased from 121

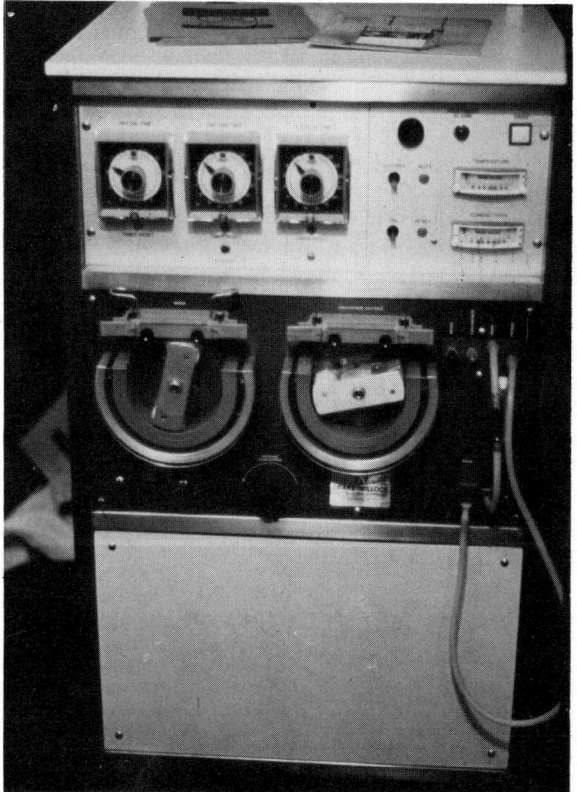

Figure 11. Reverse osmosis automatic peritoneal machine, 1973.

Table 2. Peritoneal dialysis population at the Northwest Kidney Center, Seattle, WA, USA, 1970-1978.

Year	Total nr of patients	Perit. dial. patients	Percentage
1970	156	11	7.1
1971	159	15	9.4
1972	186	24	12.9
1973	229	20	8.7
1974	263	20	7.6
1975	291	24	8.2
1976*	344	47	13.7
1977	418	66	15.8
1978	456	59	12.9

From: Blagg (92 [1979]) with permission from the author and the publisher of Dial Transpl.
* Introduction of automatic equipment.

Table 3. Chronic peritoneal dialysis population in Europe, 1971-1980.

	Total nr of chron. dialysis patients in Europe	Total nr of chron. perit. dial. patients in Europe	% of total
Mrt. 31, 1971	5 133	102	2.0
Dec. 31, 1971	7 499	159	2.1
Dec. 31, 1972	10 496	175	1.7
Dec. 31, 1973	14 171	196	1.4
Dec. 31, 1974	17 927	268	1.5
Dec. 31, 1975	22 757	336	1.6
Dec. 31, 1976	27 779	436	1.6
Dec. 31, 1977	31 842	545	1.7
Dec. 31, 1978	35 840	839	2.3
Dec. 31, 1979	42 228	1583	3.9
Dec. 31, 1980	51 157	2749	5.4

From: Annual EDTA Statistical Reports, I-XI, Proc Eur Dial Transpl Assoc 18, 1981 (94) and preceding years.

in 1972 to 2406 in 1978 (92). The number of chronic patients on periodic peritoneal dialysis increased dramatically around 1976, when automatic equipment became available.

In Europe the number of chronic peritoneal dialysis patients was 159 in 1971 and increased slowly until 1978. In that year a rather sharp rise occurred, doubtless because of the advent of the Tenckhoff catheter and its modifications and the closed loop automatic RO machines.

With these innovations periodic peritoneal dialysis came of age both in the USA and in Europe, and presumably also in other areas of the world.

In 1978 the number of chronic peritoneal dialysis patients increased to 839 (2.3% of the total number of chronic dialysis patients), in 1979 to 1583 (3.9%) and in 1980 to 2749 (5.4%) (93, 94, table 3).

Doubtless the considerable increase in recent years has to be explained, at least partly, by the introduction and the surprisingly fast acceptance of continuous ambulatory peritoneal dialysis. The main disadvantage of maintenance (periodic) peritoneal dialysis is still the discrepancy between the present duration of haemodialysis sessions (3× weekly 6 hours or less) and peritoneal dialysis (3× weekly 12-14 hours). This has become even more pronounced when so called short and ultra short haemodialysis protocols were introduced in recent years. This disadvantage however maybe nullified by performing peritoneal dialysis in the evening and during the night with automatic RO equipment.

ENHANCEMENT OF PERITONEAL DIALYSIS EFFICIENCY

With peritoneal dialysis, clearances of small molecules (urea, creatinine, uric acid) are appreciably lower than with the artificial membranes of haemodialysers, even when the clearances of so called middle molecules are more or less similar (95, 96 [see table 4]).

Understandably, much work has been done to enhance the efficiency of peritoneal dialysis, in particular to increase the removal of small solutes.

Hydrodynamical and physical methods

Different approaches have been summarised by Gutman (97, see table 5).

Ad 1. The influence of dialysis fluid flow and exchange volumes have been studied by several early investigators in the 1940's and 50's (20, 21, 34, 40, 55). Fine and coworkers (1946 [32]), while using the continuous flow method found maximum clearances of urea with dialysis

Table 4. Comparison of typical haemodialysis and peritoneal dialysis clearance values.

	Exchange area	C_{urea} ml/min	C_{creat} ml/min	C_{inulin} ml/min	Q_B ml/min	Q_D ml/min
Haemodialysis	1-2 m²	150	110	5	200-250	350-500
Peritoneal dialysis	1.5-2 m² (?)	20-26	15	5	?	30-70

From: Barbour (95) and Nolph et al (96).
Urea: 60 daltons.
Creatinine: 113 daltons.
Inulin: 5200 daltons.

Table 5. Enhancement of the effectiveness of peritoneal dialysis.

1. Increase of dialysate flow
2. Optimalisation of dialysate temperature
3. Increase of solute transfer by diffusion by optimalisation of 'dwell' time and 'dwell' volume
4. Increase of solute transfer by convection (increase of ultrafiltration)
5. Vasodilatation
   Increase of peritoneal blood flow?
   Opening of peritoneal capillaries?
6. Increase of membrane permeability

From: Gutman (97) 1979 with permission (slightly modified).

fluid flow rates of 40–60 ml/min (2.4–3.6 l/h); using the intermittent technique Boen (1959–1961 [20, 21, 98]) found optimal clearances with exchange volumes of 3–4 l/h (50–67 ml/min), admitting that these figures could be wrong. Later Tenckhoff and co-workers, including Boen (55), using automated equipment demonstrated that the urea clearance could be doubled (to 40 ml/min) with a dialysis fluid flow rate of 200 ml/min, i.e. an exchange volume of 12 l/h. Obviously these high flow rates led to better mixing diminishing stagnant dialysate layers.

Nevertheless, the small solute clearances obtained with these very high flow rates fall far short of the clearances obtained with extracorporeal haemodialysis (95, 96 [table 4]). In addition these high exchange volumes are expensive and often uncomfortable for the patients.

Robson and co-workers (99) recently confirmed a substantial increase in small solute clearances with exchange volumes up to 6 l/h (see table 6). Since patients could not tolerate a flow rate of 6 l/h or 100 ml/min, a volume of 4 l/h was considered a satisfactory compromise and this is presently accepted as the standard exchange volume with automatic RO equipment, yielding urea clearance values of 24–28 ml/min (see table 7).

Ad 2. The effect of temperature has been studied by Gross and McDonald (56) in 1967. Lowering dialysate temperature decreases peritoneal clearance values (and may be uncomfortable to the patient). Obviously, the

Table 6. Small solute clearances with different peritoneal dialysate flow rates.

Mean clearances, ml/min (2 l exchange volume)

Flow rate l/h	Creat.	Urea	Uric acid
2	13	22	10
3	14	22	10
4	19	26	14
6	23	30	17

From: Robson et al (99, with permission).

Table 7. Mean peritoneal clearances ± SEM in ml/min at a flow rate of 4 l/h and an exchange volume of 2 l.

Creatinine	18.6 ± 3.2
Urea	26.2 ± 2.4
Uric acid	13.2 ± 2.8
Phosphate	14.0 ± 2.7
Potassium	20.4 ± 2.2

From: Robson et al (99) with permission.

upper limit is close to 38 °C at the abdominal inflow point.

Ad 3. Optimalisation of dwell time. Several investigators have demonstrated that complete equilibration of small molecules between peritoneal fluid and the blood occurs in 2–3 h (20, 21, 99). Dwell times with 4 l hourly exchanges are necessarily much shorter (15–20 min), optimal extraction of waste metabolites therefore does not occur; maximum extractions being only accomplished with dwell times of 4 h and longer, as occur in chronic ambulatory peritoneal dialysis. Data of Robson (99) and Gutman (97) suggest that some enhancement is obtained by using two exchanges of 2 l/h, with a residual fluid volume of 1 l remaining in the peritoneal cavity between two exchanges, which is well tolerated by the patient.

Ad 4. Increase of solute transfer by convection was studied by Henderson and Nolph (101, 102). They demonstrated that hypertonicity of the peritoneal fluid not only increases ultrafiltration but also enhances clearances of small and middle molecules (e.g. inulin). This has to be explained by the solvent drag effect of (osmotically induced) ultrafiltration (see also chapter 12). This phenomenon has been used for augmentation of pritoneal dialysis efficiency in animal experiments by Zelman and associates (103). In practice increased ultrafiltration by more liberal use of hypertonic rinsing fluid for more efficient solute clearing could be compensated by increasing fluid intake and a more liberal salt intake by the patient.

Ad 5 and 6. Increase of solute clearances by increasing peritoneal blood flow and membrane permeability has been achieved with various drugs.

Pharmacological methods

Although some early investigations date back to some 10 years ago or more (104, 105), the classic investigations on this subject from Nolph, Maher and collaborators (106–112) and others (113–114) are from recent years. The aim of these investigations was to study the effect of small amounts of vaso-active drugs in the dialysis solution. This provides relatively high concentrations of the pharmacological agent adjacent to and within the peritoneal membrane with minimal systemic effects. Slow resorption and passage through the liver via the portal venous circulation also results in minimal concentrations in the systemic circulation (106). Several drugs were studied; two (diazoxide and nitroprusside) increased creatinine clearances by 20-25%, which could reduce dialysis time by 6-8 h; with nitroprusside a doubling of inulin clearance was observed. It is unlikely that the enhancing effects can be explained by simple vasodilatation and an increase of peritoneal blood flow rate. A direct effect on the permeability of the peritoneal membrane is more likely.

Other drugs (ethacrynic acid, frusemide and others) have been studied both in rabbits and patients. Some are effective in the dialysis solution. Others work only on the blood side (glucagon). These investigations are also helpful in clarifying some issues about mesenteric blood flow, mechanisms of transport and to identify which drugs are deleterious, e.g. norepinephrine, which causes vasoconstriction. For similar reasons peritoneal dialysis clearances are very low in shock, i.e. when there is generalised vasoconstriction.

Investigations are continuing, but so far drug enhancement of peritoneal dialysis efficiency has not (yet) found clinical application.

RECIRCULATION PERITONEAL DIALYSIS

Recently interest in recirculation dialysis originally described in 1965, another approach to enhance peritoneal dialysis efficiency, has been revived by Kolff's group (83). For reasons discussed previously continuous flow peritoneal dialysis was gradually replaced by intermittent dialysis in the 1950's. But in 1965 Shinaberger, Shear and Barry (115) reported urea- and creatinine clearances which were two to three times greater with recirculation peritoneal dialysis than with standard intermittent lavage. With this method (peritoneal-extracorporeal recirculation dialysis) 3 to 4 l of sterile peritoneal dialysis fluid were recirculated through a twin coil dialyser; this apparently appreciably increased the efficiency of peritoneal dialysis (Figure 13). A similar system was described by Lange, Freser and Mangalet from Western Germany in 1968 (116). Stephen and co-workers (83) using a newly developed ⊓-shaped two way implantable peritoneal catheter, modified the Shinaberger design. The sterile (primary) dialysate was recirculated through the blood path of a hollow fibre dialyser. The 'secondary' (non-sterile) dialysate was recirculated from a 20 l reservoir through a charcoal module for (incomplete) regeneration (Figures 14 and 15). This non-sterile bath fluid had to be changed at least once during dialysis. The peritoneal flow rates had to be limited to 200 ml/min or less, higher flow rates resulting in abdominal pain. Clearance values were somewhat higher than with conventional intermittent peritoneal dialysis, but the results were slightly disappointing. Apparently streaming or recirculation of the dialysis fluid sometimes occurred in the peritoneal cavity. In addition, problems of infection, often with peritonitis occurred with the two way subcutaneous catheter.

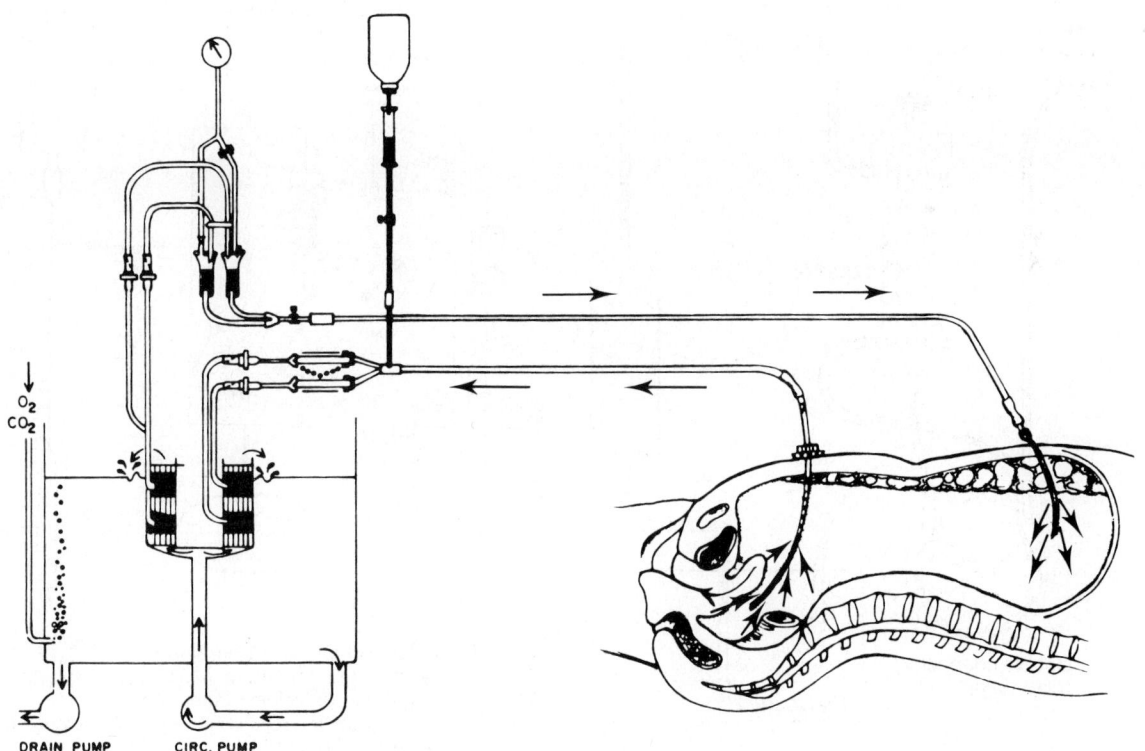

Figure 13. Peritoneal-extracorporeal recirculation dialysis (Shinaberger, 1965 [115]), using Twin Coil artificial kidney. (With permission of the authors and the publishers of the *Trans Am Soc Artif Intern Organs*).

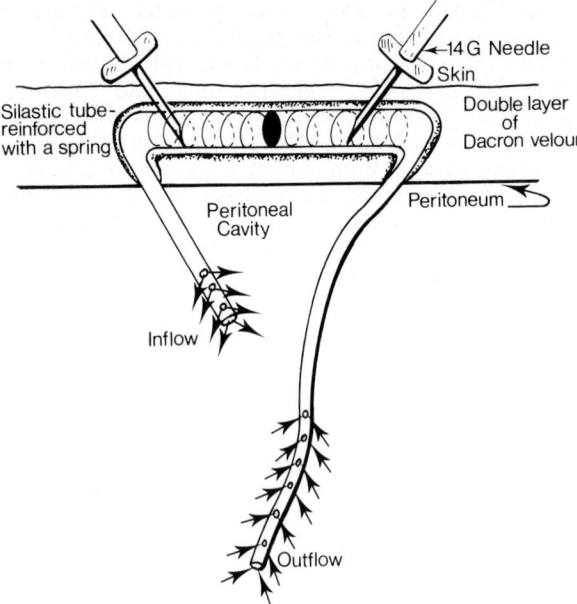

Figure 14. Two way subcutaneous catheter used for recirculation peritoneal dialysis (Stephen et al, 1976 [83, 117]).

These, per se, ingenious methods did not gain application in other centres.

RECIPROCATING PERITONEAL DIALYSIS

Another approach to augmentation of peritoneal clearances was called reciprocating peritoneal dialysis (117, 118): the peritoneal cavity is primed with appr. 1 l of fresh dialysis fluid. A preset volume (appr. 200 ml) reciprocates with a high flow rate between peritoneal catheter and a transpak bag, via the blood path of a dialyser. The secondary (non-sterile) dialysis fluid recirculates through the dialyser from the 20 l reservoir through the charcoal module in a similar way as described previously in the recirculating system, constructed by the same investigators. The urea clearance increased some 29 % over urea clearances obtained with conventional intermittent peritoneal dialysis. However, in this procedure catheter problems (plugging, infection) were frequent.

FRESH FLUID, SEMICONTINUOUS PERITONEAL DIALYSIS

A simpler system of 'semicontinuous' peritoneal dialysis (without regeneration of the dialysate through a dia-

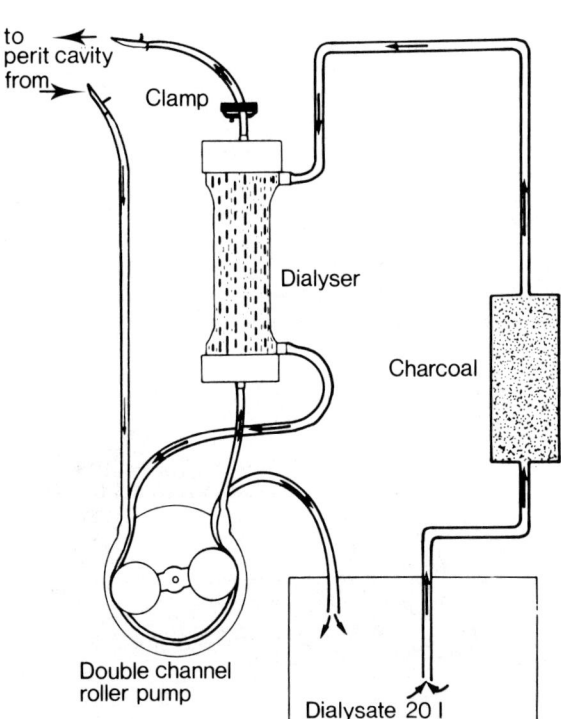

Figure 15. Peritoneal-extracorporeal recirculation dialysis with partial regeneration of dialysis fluid (Stephen et al, 1976 [83]).

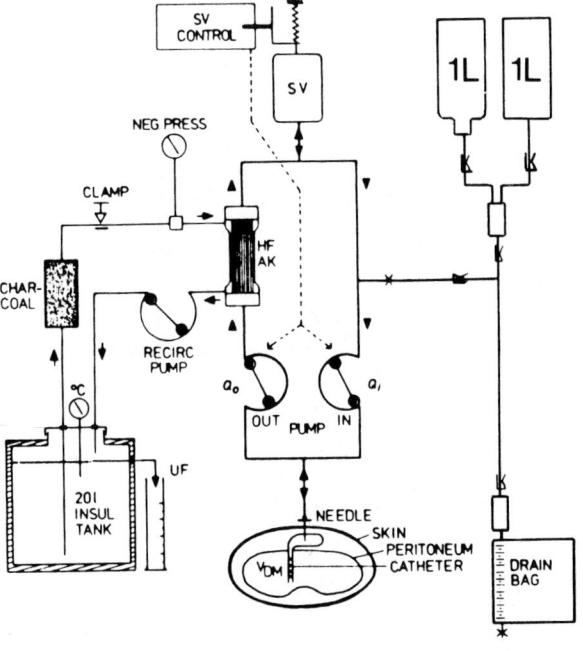

Figure 16. Reciprocating peritoneal dialysis (1978 [117,118]).
SV: Transpak bag containing preset stroke volume
VDM: intraperitoneal volume (appr. 2 l)
CLAMP: screw clamp for regulating negative pressure of secondary dialysis fluid.

(Figures 14, 15 and 16 are reproduced with permission of the authors and the publishers of the *Trans Am Soc Artif Intern Organs* and *Dial Transpl.*)

lyser), using a simple single needle device was constructed by Di Paolo (119) in 1978. After priming the peritoneal cavity with 1 to 1.5 l dialysis fluid 100 ml dialysate is drained every minute and an equal amount of fresh rinsing fluid is introduced. In 8 h approximately 50 l are exchanged and several litres of ultrafiltrate are simultaneously drained. Total dialysis time could be shortened by 50%: with three 8 h 'semi-continuous' peritoneal dialysis sessions per week, serum levels of urea, creatinine and uric acid were similar to the levels obtained with twice weekly 24 hours of 'conventional' intermittent peritoneal dialysis.

Commercial closed loop RO delivery machines can be converted to 'fresh fluid' semicontinuous systems, delivering a stroke volume of 200 ml fresh dialysis solution (118). Because the peritoneal cavity is initially 'primed' with 2 l rinsing fluid, a certain amount of dialysate remains in the abdomen during the dialysis procedure. Dialysate flow rates are obtained of 160 ml/min (approx. 10 l/hour) and urea clearance is boosted to appr. 40 ml/min.

Obviously it is presently possible to enhance peritoneal dialysis efficiency by 25–50% both by pharmacological or hydrodynamical methods, which makes shortening of total dialysis hours per week possible. But one of the problems resulting from increasing efficiency of peritoneal dialysis by drugs or high flow rates (and also from high dextrose concentrations to correct overhydration) is the inevitable increase of loss of plasma proteins which can cause a state of protein malnutrition (Dr. F.M. Parsons, personal communication).

The different procedures to enhance peritoneal clearances are still in an experimental stage and are not yet accepted for practical application. The pro's and con's should be carefully balanced: shortening of dialysis time versus the frequency of technical break-downs, catheter problems, the risk of infection, the increased loss of plasma proteins and the possibility of discomfort for the patient. In addition these new technologies are taking away the simplicity, which has always been one of the advantages and attractions of peritoneal dialysis compared with extracorporeal haemodialysis.

Further development and practical application have been overshadowed by the introduction of CAPD.

REGENERATION PERITONEAL DIALYSIS

Regeneration of peritoneal dialysate has been attempted by Gordon and Maxwell and co-workers (120, 121) and by Lai and collaborators (122). Both systems employ urease, charcoal and ion exchange resins and have been tested in series of animal experiments. The former system has been utilised in a number of clinical trials (121, 123); 4 l of fresh dialysis fluid are used and the outflowing perfusate is regenerated by recirculation through a gamma-ray sterilised sorbent cartridge as used in the Redy system (see chapter 17) and after passage through a bacterial filter re-introduced in the peritoneal cavity. Several problems were encountered, such as adequate sterilisation of the dialysate pathway including the

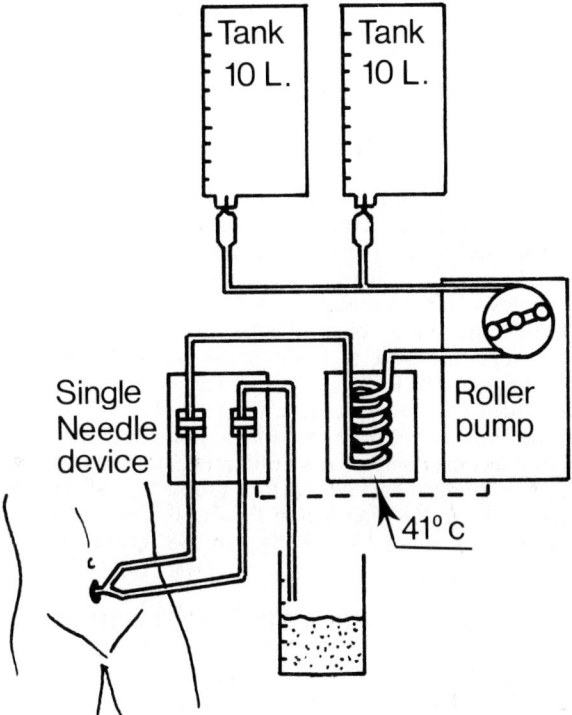

Figure 17. Fresh fluid, semicontinous peritoneal dialysis (1978 [119]).

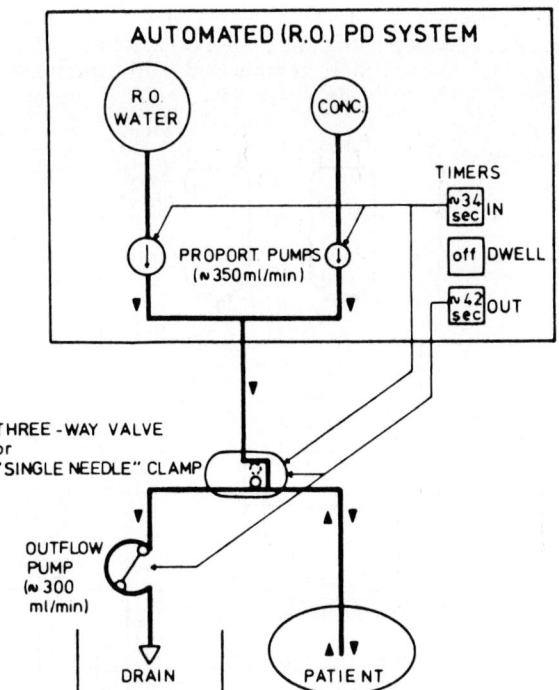

Figure 18. Fresh fluid, semicontinous peritoneal dialysis with a reverse osmosis dialysis fluid delivery machine (118).

cartridge, ensuring a sterile rinsing fluid, the preparation of pyrogen free urease and the production of regenerated rinsing fluid with an adequate, non-irritating pH. According to Lewin (123) these problems have been successfully solved.

Since fluid quantities with this system are not a problem, it seems possible to produce dialysate flow rates of 6 l/h or more, which should provide augmented small molecule clearances compared with conventional intermittent peritoneal dialysis. The system has the advantage of portability, like the original Redy system for haemodialysis. Transportability e.g. for travelling purposes, will be more of a problem. For each dialysis 4 l of sterile fresh dialysate and a fresh sterile sorbent cartridge (weighing several kg) are required. For one week of travelling (three dialyses) an extra weight of about 20 kg plus the machine have to be carried on. For additional protection against bacterial contamination it seems wise to insert a photochemical reactor, producing ultraviolet light in the inflow line before the indwelling peritoneal catheter as described by Eisinger in 1980 (124).

THE EVOLUTION OF A SIMPLE 'MACHINE FREE' SYSTEM VIA AUTOMATIC CYCLERS INTO A COMPLICATED REVERSE OSMOSIS CLOSED LOOP SYSTEM AND BACK TO A MACHINE FREE METHODOLOGY CALLED CAPD (CONTINUOUS AMBULATORY PERITONEAL DIALYSIS)

Manual hanging bottle peritoneal dialysis of the 1960's and 1970's has moved away from a simple 'machine free' system via automatic cyclers and more complicated closed loop automatic peritoneal systems with RO machines to even more complicated, still experimental regeneration systems derived from haemodialysis technology. It has been suggested that back to nature activists, conservationists, pollution fighters and similar groups also have influenced the nephrologic mind particularly in the field of replacement of renal function (Diaz Buxo [125]). The way back to a simple, machine free, power free, natural membrane mediated replacement of renal function originated in Austin, Texas and was pointed out by Popovich and colleagues (126). Their paper was originally not accepted for presentation at the San Francisco ASAIO meetings in 1976, but the method, by the originators called 'continuous ambulatory peritoneal dialysis (CAPD)' was briefly described in an abstract (126) and later in 1978 published in full (127). Their method aroused considerable interest in many centres in North America, Canada, Europe and Australia. Basically this treatment modality resembles intermittent 'hanging bottle' peritoneal dialysis. Dwell periods however are extended to 4 to 6 h by day and 8 h overnight (allowing the patient uninterrupted sleep). In place of glass bottles 3 l capacity plastic bags containing 2 l of peritoneal dialysis solution became available commercially. With completion of the inflow the empty bag and administration set are folded in a small container or a cloth waist pocket. When the dwell time has elapsed the used dialysate is drained into the empty plastic bag by gravity, which is then discarded and replaced by a bag with fresh dialysis fluid, the Tenckhoff catheter or one of its modifications being used for peritoneal access.

Treatment is carried out 7 days a week and most patients exchange four or five bags a day at intervals of 4 h, extending the interval to eight hours during the night.

CAPD does not require major capital investment for a machine or special plumbing and other (often expensive)

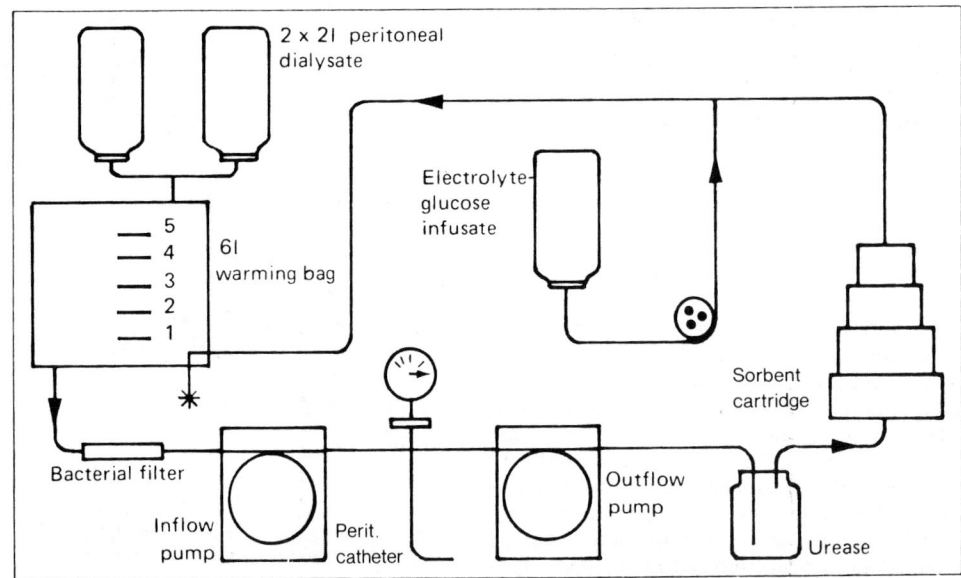

Figure 19. Flow diagram of the Sorbsystem (Redy) regenerating peritoneal dialysis system (1974 [120], 1978 [121, 123]).

provisions in the house as for haemodialysis. It is performed as self-treatment and training time is short (1-3 weeks).

Removal of small molecules (urea) with CAPD is approximately 1/3 less efficient than with haemodialysis (15 h/week), but more efficient than with intermittent peritoneal dialysis (40 h/week) (see table 8).

Removal of middle molecules with CAPD however (as illustrated by B_{12} and inulin) is much more efficient as compared with intermittent peritoneal dialysis and haemodialysis.

But all that glitters is not gold: the advantages of CAPD (128-137) have been overshadowed by a number of complications (134, 135) and three major disadvantages: a high incidence of peritonitis, a high rate of protein loss (10-20 g/day) and the cumbersome and the time consuming nature of the technique (131), each exchange taking about 45 minutes. Four exchanges therefore take away 3 h of working time each day.

So far protein loss seems to be a lesser problem, which can be overcome by an adequate protein intake (134).

CAPD and the peritonitis problem

Peritonitis is still a major drawback. Even in a centre particularly dedicated to CAPD peritonitis developed in 50% of the patients.

Recent surveys report an incidence ranging from one episode per approximately 5 patient months (135, 136) to one episode every 7.4 or 7.6 patient months (137, 138). With painstaking care and optimal training of patients, however, frequency will be much less and some centres report one episode per 11.3 and 12.6 patient months (134, 138, 139).

Doubtless the risk of peritonitis is commensurate with the number of times that the closed circuit has to be broken for changing bags. Actually this has to be done 35 times per week for five exchanges per day, against six times for thrice weekly closed loop automatic (intermittent) peritoneal dialysis. Also adherence to a strict sterile technique may be difficult for a patient who has to change bags three to five times a day, seven days a week, throughout the year. A certain amount of neglect has to be expected psychologically (140). Potential candidates for CAPD should undergo a careful selection and patients' characteristics should be thoroughly evaluated before a decision is made and training is started (141). Obviously patients who are unable to learn or to accept a fastidious sterile technique are unsuitable for this mode of treatment.

Another critical step in the change of the tubing, which is done every 2 weeks if the patient changes his own tubing.

Presently this is preferably done by a nurse every 4 weeks either at a return visit of the patient to the hospital or at the patient's home (142).

Cost of CAPD

According to several clinical investigators, cost of CAPD is considerably less than of regular haemodialysis, either at the hospital or at the home (133, 135, 143). According to Robson and Oreopoulos (133) the expenses of CAPD are (in Canada) only one third of the yearly cost of intermittent peritoneal dialysis with an automatic cycler.

It has therefore been suggested that CAPD could potentially be a mode of treatment to alleviate the staggering and still escalating cost of treatment for end-stage renal failure (128, 143, 144). In addition, it does not require major capital investment for a machine. The short training period and the treatment outside hospital are also cost saving elements. As has been mentioned before no special plumbing and other costly provisions at the patient's home are required. But cost calculations in other centres have been different: in the USA maintenance cost of CAPD was approximately equivalent to the cost of home haemodialysis (128). However, in Canada, in Australia and the UK CAPD seems to be the cheapest form of all types of dialysis treatment.

CAPD is applicable to a much wider range of patients than haemodialysis including the elderly and the diabetic uraemic patients. This element may outweight the cheaper maintenance cost of CAPD, because a much greater number of patients can (and will) be treated (144).

Undesirable effects of CAPD

With increasing experience undesirable side effects have been noted like hypertriglyceridaemia, hyperglycaemia in diabetics and excessive weight gain. These side effects have doubtless to be ascribed to the absorption of dextrose from the rinsing fluid: four exchanges per day of dialysis fluid containing 1.5% dextrose may generate some 350 calories (1470 kJ). Four 4.25% dextrose exchanges could produce 850 calories (3570 kJ) per day (145). Investigations are underway to generate osmolar pressure gradients across semi-permeable membranes, with other compounds than dextrose; an 1.4% mixture of amino acids has been tried and impermeant polymer ions have been experimentally utilised (146).

Success of CAPD

CAPD gained surprisingly fast popularity: by the end of 1980 51.157 patients were treated in Europe with dialysis and some 2700 were treated by peritoneal dialysis. Of all patients treated by dialysis on December 31, 1980 1229 (2.4%) were treated by CAPD (93). In 1981 the total number of dialysis patients on CAPD in Europe more than doubled to 2992 (147).

The sudden increase of the percentage of chronic patients treated with peritoneal dialysis in Europe between 1977 and 1981 (from 1.7 to 5.4%) is undoubtedly due to CAPD (94 [see Table 3]).

The success of CAPD on the one hand and the high incidence of peritonitis and the inconvenience of multiple daily exchanges on the other hand, stimulated further research.

CONTINUOUS CYCLIC PERITONEAL DIALYSIS (CCPD) OR AUTOMATED LONG CYCLE PERITONEAL DIALYSIS (ALCPD)

Two groups of investigators (148–150) introduced a modified CAPD technique, called continuous cyclic peritoneal dialysis (CCPD) or automated long cycle peritoneal dialysis (ALCPD).

Both methods (which are identical) reintroduce a machine: a cycler is programmed to deliver three or four exchanges of 2 l over 9 to 10 hours during the night. At disconnection in the morning 2 l dialysis fluid remain in the peritoneal cavity for 12 to 14 h.

The results (see table 8) are comparable to CAPD and better than with intermittent peritoneal dialysis. Only one connection at night and one disconnection in the morning are required, which according to the originators should 'significantly reduce the incidence of peritonitis" (148, 149).

Although at the time of writing the place of CAPD for short and medium term treatment of end stage renal disease seems rather secure (144), the long-term success rate is still unknown. There has been too little time and experience to form an opinion on newer techniques like CCPD (or ALCPD).

SUMMARY AND SOME UNANSWERED QUESTIONS

Peritoneal dialysis is the oldest modality of replacement of renal function. The first primitive attempt of a peritoneal dialysis in a human being was performed by a German doctor early in 1923 (24), one and a half year before the first human extracorporeal haemodialysis was carried out, also in Germany, in October 1924 (27).

Peritoneal dialysis evolved slowly and did not gain very much practical application until the work of Doolan (39) and Maxwell (40) in the USA in 1959. In particular the introduction of commercially prepared dialysis solution and tubing and the disposable stylet catheter by Weston and Roberts in 1965 (50) were major steps forward and in the 1960's peritoneal dialysis gained ground for treatment of acute renal failure.

It was however overshadowed by haemodialysis which made rapid technical and practical progress in the late 1950's and early 1960's, in particular when Scribner and co-workers (61) reported their successful haemodialysis treatment of chronic irreversible uraemia in the early 1960's.

Many considered chronic intermittent peritoneal dialysis as a less efficient, time consuming, cheap, second class treatment of chronic uraemia. It was more or less the 'Cinderella treatment' of chronic patients used temporarily for patients on the waiting list for haemodialysis treatment or transplantation (151). Only a few mastered the painstaking technique of chronic peritoneal dialysis and were able to provide patients with irreversible end-stage kidney disease a good quality of life. Many other patients who were treated by chronic peritoneal dialysis in the 1960's faced a treatment which only delayed death. In 1965 Scribner (59) stirred the dialysis world again: he had noted that patients on chronic peritoneal dialysis which controlled traditional blood chemistries less well than haemodialysis often felt better. In addition peripheral neuropathy did not occur or did not progress despite a certain amount of 'underdialysis'. Scribner then presented the hypothesis that the peritoneal membrane was more permeable than Cuprophan and that peritoneal dialysis removed substances of higher molecular weight more efficiently than haemodialysis. This hypothesis led to the middle molecule hypothesis (152) which greatly influenced dialysis strategy and technology and led to a growing interest in chronic intermittent peritoneal dialysis.

The break-through came also from Seattle when Tenckhoff and co-workers (79) in the late '60's introduced the indwelling Silastic catheter, which solved the problem of repeated peritoneal access and when the closed loop reverse osmosis dialysis fluid factories with automatic cyclers became available in 1972 (91). With these innovations chronic intermittent peritoneal dialysis came of age (153). Presently chronic intermittent peritoneal dialysis with a 'closed loop, reverse osmosis automatic system' is widely accepted as an adequate mode of replacement of renal function, offering satisfactory rehabilitation. Morbidity and mortality compare well with regular haemodialysis and the economics seem to be competitive.

The main indications are lack of vascular access, diabetes and advanced age, in particular when myocardial reserve is impaired with cardiovascular instability. Automatic peritoneal dialysis is also preferred in the home setting when no suitable partner is available.

In recent years a new, machine and power free meth-

Table 8. Clearances (l/week) for different solutes by various dialysis techniques.

	Haemodialysis 15 h/week	IPD 40 h/week	CAPD continuous	CCPD Nocturnal	Diurnal	Total	Normal kidney
Urea (60 daltons)	135	60	76–84	54	12.7	66.7	604
Creatinine (113 daltons)	90	28	58	46.2	12.5	58.7	1200
B_{12} (1350 daltons)	30	15–16	50	34.8	10.1	44.9	1200
Inulin (5200 daltons)	5	12	30	—	—	—	1200

From: Moncrief et al (130) and Diaz-Buxo et al (149). With permission (slightly modified).
IPD : Intermittent peritoneal dialysis.
CAPD : Continuous ambulant peritoneal dialysis.
CCPD : Continuous cyclic peritoneal dialysis (see text).

od of maintenance peritoneal dialysis, called CAPD, rapidly gained popularity (125–131).

Strong advocates have enthusiastically highlighted its advantages (132–138).

It is very likely that the relatively sudden increase of the percentage of chronic peritoneal patients in the European statistics (93, 94) has to be ascribed to the (increasing) popularity of CAPD. However, there are also other reasons. More and more patients in the older age groups are accepted for maintenance dialysis treatment (93, 144). Peritoneal dialysis for these patients is often the treatment of choice.

But, in the future, will that be CAPD?

Many questions remain presently unanswered. Has CAPD really come of age (137)? Will the greatest problem, the high frequency of peritonitis be overcome (134, 135, 139, 140, 154)? Will the dialysis capacity of the peritoneal cavity and the membrane be irreversably damaged by recurrent attacks of peritonitis or (and) frequent (daily) exchanges with hypertonic dialysis fluid (containing 4.25% glucose)?

What will be the long-term survival rate of the patients on the one hand and the long-term survival of the technique on the other hand? Some European figures became recently available. According to these figures 2 year survial rate of CAPD patients was only 60% and the two year 'technique survival' was only 28% (147).

Is CAPD really superior to all other forms of peritoneal dialysis (155) or is it a step backwards compared with automatic, closed loop, intermittent modality?

Will CAPD supersede the closed loop, automatic mode of peritoneal dialysis? Will it even displace regular haemodialysis? It has been claimed that CAPD will become the treatment of choice for up to 50% of patients with end stage renal disease (137, 138, 156). But is the present enthusiasm perhaps due to the common overreaction, which often follows a new therapy and will it be followed by a swinging back of the balance to the negative side until it finds its equilibrium with all the advantages on one scale and all the disadvantages on the other?

Critical opinions are already sounding: Friedman, Lundin and Butt (157) report a drop-out rate of CAPD patients of 50% in the first year.

Maher (158) asked when chairing a panel on peritoneal dialysis in New York in 1979:

'Can the role of continuous ambulatory peritoneal dialysis be defined at present or must it await further kinetic studies, long-term observation of a limited number of patients and evidence of a lower incidence of peritonitis even when employed by those less dedicated than the pioneers of this technique?'

Two more crucial and final questions: is CAPD becoming the 'silver bullet' for treatment of end-stage chronic renal disease?

Will CAPD be another milestone in the history of dialysis or will it be a fading 'glamorous star' on the firmament of medicine?

A critical statement was sounded at a recent symposium in Norwich, UK:

...'CAPD was greeted with much enthousiasm as a relatively cheap and effective form of dialysis, but there are serious doubts as to whether it will be a viable long-term treatment, comparable with haemodialysis – the "gold standard"... (159)'.

Obviously many questions remain:

'At the present time (Spring 1981) CAPD represents a veritable metabolic Pandora's Box, with many important questions but few answers as yet.' (Schmidt and Blumenkrantz (160).

We are still eagerly waiting for the missing answers.

ACKNOWLEDGEMENTS

The author gratefully acknowledges the courtesy of Mr D.W.C. Stewart, librarian, The Royal Society of Medicine, London UK, for the picture of the Rev. Stephen Hales *(Figure 1)* and the facsimile of the reverend's letter to the secretary of the Royal Society of Medicine *(Figure 2)*.

Mr. David Hamilton, PhD, FRCS, consultant surgeon Dept. of Surgery, Western Infirmary, Glasgow, Scotland, kindly provided the author with a photocopy of the original letter from Heinrich Necheles to John Jacob Abel, dated June 16, 1924, which the author gratefully acknowledges. The original letter is in the archives of the Johns Hopkins Hospital, Baltimore MD, USA.

Dr. Ganter's picture *(Figure 3)* and his biographical data were kindly supplied by the editors of the Münchener Medizinische Wochenschrift (Mr. H. Lichtenstern).

Figure 4 was kindly supplied by Dr. F.M. Parsons, Leeds UK.

The author gratefully acknowledges the courtesy of Dr. Paul D. Doolan, St. Mary's Hospital, Waterbury CT and Dr. Richard F. Ruben, San Francisco CA, USA who sent him a photocopy of the case history report and further particulars of the first chronic patient maintained with periodic peritoneal dialysis.

Figure 8c and 10b are reproduced from photographs made available by B. Braun Melsungen AG, W. Germany and kindly supplied by Messrs. Soho BV, Purmerend, The Netherlands.

Figure 10a is reproduced from a photograph made available by Messrs. Quinton Instrument Co., Seattle WA, USA, which is gratefully acknowledged.

REFERENCES

1. Earle DP: An eighteenth century suggestion for peritoneal dialysis? *Int J Artif Organs* 3:67, 1980
2. Warrick Ch: An improvement on the practice of tapping; by which that operation instead of a relief for symptoms, becomes an absolute cure for an ascites. *Philos Trans R Soc Lond* (Biol) 43:5, 1744-1745
3. Hales S: A method of conveying liquors into the abdomen during the operation of tapping. *Philos Trans R Soc Lond* (Biol) 43:8, 1744-1745
4. Wegner G: Chirurgische Bermerkungen über die Peritonealhöhle mit besonderer Berücksichtigung der Ovariotomie (Surgical considerations regarding the peritoneal cavity with special attention to ovariotomy). *Langenbecks Arch Chir* 20:51, 1877 (in German)
5. Starling EH, Tubby EH: On absorption from and secretion into the serous cavities. *J Physiol (Lond)* 16:140, 1894
6. Leathes JB, Starling EH: On the absorption of salt solutions from the pleural cavities. *J Physiol (Lond)* 18:106, 1895

7. Orlow WN: Einige Versuche über die Resorption in der Bauchhöhle (Some experiments on the resorption in the peritoneal cavity). *Pflügers Arch* 59:170, 1895 (in German)
8. Clark AJ: Absorption from the peritoneal cavity. *J Pharmacol Exp Ther* 16:415, 1921
9. Cunningham RS: Studies on absorption from serous cavities. *Am J Physiol* 53:488, 1920
10. Klapp R: Über Bauchfellresorption (On resorption by the peritoneum). *Mitt Grenzgeb Med Chir* 10:254, 1902 (in German)
11. Clairmont P, von Haberer H: Experimentelle Untersuchungen zur Physiologie und Pathologie des Peritoneums (Experimental investigations on the physiology and pathology of the peritoneum). *Langebecks Arch Chir* 76:1, 1905 (in German)
12. Putnam T: The living peritoneum as a dialyzing membrane. *Am J Physiol* 63:548, 1922-1923
13. Hertzler AE: *The Peritoneum Structure and Function in Relation to Principles of Abdominal Surgery.* St Louis, CV Mosby Company, 1919, vol I, p 379
14. Schechter AJ, Cary MK, Carpentieri AL, Darrow DC: Changes in composition of fluids injected into the peritoneal cavity. *Am J Dis Child* 46:1015, 1933
15. Graham T: Liquid diffusion applied to analysis. *Philos Trans R Soc Lond* (Biol) 151:183, 1861
16. Prima C: Über die Resorptionsfähigkeit des Bauchfells bei gesteigerten Darmperistaltik (On the resorption activity of the peritoneum during increased intestinal peristalsis). *Mitt Grenzgeb Med Chir* 36:678, 1923 (in German)
17. Fleisher MS, Loeb L: Studies in edema II. The influence of adrenalin on absorption from the peritoneal cavity, with remarks on the influence of calcium chloride on absorption. *J Exp Med* 12:288, 1910
18. Fleischer MS, Loeb L: Studies in edema VII. The influence of nephrectomy and other surgical operations and of the lesions produced by uranium-nitrate upon resorption from the peritoneal cavity. *J Exp Med* 12:487, 1910
19. Fleischer MS, Loeb L: Studies in edema VIII. The influence of caffeine on absorption from the peritoneal cavity and the influence of diuresis on edema. *J Exp Med* 12:510, 1910
20. Boen ST: *Peritoneal dialysis. A Clinical Study of Factors Governing its Effectiveness.* MD Thesis 1959 Univ of Amsterdam, Assen, van Gorcum and Comp NV – Dr. HJ Prakke and HMG Prakke
21. Boen ST: *Peritoneal Dialysis in Clinical Medicine.* American Lecture series, Springfield IL, Charles C Thomas, 1964
22. Odel HM, Ferris DO, Power MH: Clinical considerations of the problem of extrarenal excretion: peritoneal lavage. *Med Clin North Am* 32:989, 1948
23. Blackfan KD, Maxcy KF: The intraperitoneal injection of saline solution. *Am J Dis Child* 2:1257, 1918
24. Ganter G: Über die Beseitigung giftiger Stoffe aus dem Blute durch Dialyse (On the elimination of toxic substances from the blood by dialysis). *MMW* 70:1478, 1923 (in German)
25. Necheles H: Über dialysieren des strömenden Blutes am Lebenden (On dialysis of the circulating blood in vivo). *Klin Wochenschr* 2:1257, 1923 (in German)
26. Necheles H: Erwiderung zu vorstehender Bermerkung (Commentary on the above remark). *Klin Wochenschr* 2:1888, 1923 (in German)
27. Haas G: Dialysieren des strömenden Blutes am Lebenden (Dialysing the circulating blood). *Klin Wochenschr* 4:13, 1925 (in German)
28. Heusser H, Werder H: Untersuchungen über die Peritonealdialyse (Investigations on peritoneal dialysis). *Brun's Beitr Klin Chir* 141:38, 1927 (in German)
29. Balazs J, Rosenak S: Zur behandlung der Sublimatanurie durch peritoneale Dialyse (On the treatment of anuria caused by mercury bichloride with peritoneal dialysis). *Wien Klin Wochenschr* 47:851, 1934 (in German)
30. Wear JB, Sisk IR, Trinkle AJ: Peritoneal lavage in the treatment of uremia. *J Urol* 39:53, 1938
31. Rhoads JE: Peritoneal lavage in the treatment of renal insufficiency. *Am J Med Sci* 196:642, 1938
32. Fine J, Frank HA, Seligman AM: The treatment of acute renal failure by peritoneal irrigation. *Ann Surg* 124:857, 1946
33. Frank HA, Seligman AM, Fine J: Treatment of uremia after acute renal failure by peritoneal irrigation. *JAMA* 130:703, 1946
34. Seligman AM, Frank HA, Fine J: Treatment of experimental uremia by peritoneal irrigation. *J Clin Invest* 25:211, 1946
35. Fine J, Frank HA, Seligman AM: Further experiences with peritoneal irrigation for acute renal failure. *Ann Surg* 128:561, 1948
36. Muercke RC: *Acute Renal Failure,* Saint Louis, The CV Mosby Company, 1969, p 274
37. Kop PSM: *Peritoneaal Dialyse* (Peritoneal Dialysis). MD Thesis Groningen, Kampen (The Netherlands), JH Kok NV, 1948 (in Dutch, with summaries in English, French and German)
38. Reid R, Penfold JB, Jones RN: Anuria treated by renal decapsulation and peritoneal dialysis. *Lancet* 2:749, 1946
39. Doolan PD, Murphy WP, Wiggins RA, Carter NW, Cooper WC, Watten RH, Alpen EL: An evaluation of intermittent peritoneal lavage. *Am J Med* 26:831, 1959
40. Maxwell MH, Rockney RE, Kleeman CR, Twiss MR: Peritoneal dialysis. *JAMA* 170:917, 1959
41. Moriarty MV, Parsons FM: Intermittent peritoneal dialysis. *Proc Eur Dial Transpl Assoc* 3:359, 1966
42. Nolph KD, Hano JE, Teschan PE: Peritoneal sodium transport during hypertonic peritoneal dialysis: physiologic mechanism and clinical implications. *Ann Intern Med* 75:253, 1971
43. Ahearn DJ, Nolph KD: Controlled sodium removal with peritoneal dialysis. *Trans Am Soc Artif Intern Organs* 18:423, 1972
44. Nolph KD: Peritoneal dialysis in *Replacement of Renal Function by Dialysis,* edited by Drukker W, Parsons FM, Maher JF, The Hague, Boston London, Martinus Nijhoff, Medical Division, 1st edition, 1978, p 285
45. Rosenak S, Siwon P: Experimentelle Untersuchungen über die peritoneal Ausscheidung harnpflichtiger Substanzen aus dem Blut (Experimental investigations on peritoneal excretion of uraemic products from the blood). *Mitt Grenzgeb Med Chir* 39:391, 1925 (in German)
46. Grollman A, Turner LB, McLean JA: Intermittent peritoneal lavage in nephrectomized dogs and its application to the human being. *Arch Int Med* 87:379, 1951
47. Grollman A: *Acute renal Failure.* Springield IL, Charles C. Thomas, 1954
48. Blumenkrantz MJ, Roberts M: Progress in peritoneal dialysis: a historical prospective. *Contrib Nephrol* 17:101, 1979
49. Rosenak SS, Oppenheimer GD: An improved drain for peritoneal lavage. *Surgery* 23:832, 1948
50. Weston RE, Roberts M: Clinical use of stylet catheter for peritoneal dialysis. *Arch Int Med* 15:659, 1965

51. Boen ST, Mulinari AS, Dillard DH, Scribner BH: Periodic peritoneal dialysis in the management of chronic uremia. *Trans Am Soc Artif Intern Organs* 8:256, 1962
52. Bosch E, De Vries LA, Boen ST: A simplified automatic peritoneal dialysis system. *Proc Eur Dial Transpl Assoc* 3:362, 1966
53. Boen ST, Mion CM, Curtis FK, Shilipetar G: Periodic peritoneal dialysis using repeated puncture technique and an automatic cycling machine. *Trans Am Soc Artif Intern Organs* 10:409, 1964
54. Tenckhoff H, Boen ST: Long term peritoneal dialysis in the home, the first one and one half years. *Proc Eur Dial Transpl Assoc* 2:104, 1965
55. Tenckhoff H, Ward G, Boen ST: The influence of dialysate volume and flow rate on peritoneal clearance. *Proc Eur Dial Transpl Assoc* 2:113, 1965
56. Gross M, McDonald HP Jr: Effects of dialysate temperature and flow rate on peritoneal clearance. *JAMA* 202:215, 1967
57. Nolph KD, Stoltz ML, Maher JF: Altered peritoneal permeability in patients with systemic vasculitis. *Ann Intern Med* 75:753, 1971
58. Henderson LW: Peritoneal dialysis. In *Clinical Aspects of Uremia and Dialysis* (chapter 19), edited by Massry SG, Sellers AL, Springfield IL, Charles C Thomas, 1976, p 561-568
59. Scribner BH: Discussion. *Trans Am Soc Artif Intern Organs* 15:87, 1965
60. Babb AL, Johansen PJ, Strand MJ, Tenckhoff H, Scribner BH: Bi-directional permeability of the human peritoneum to middle molecules. *Proc Eur Dial Transpl Assoc* 10:247, 1973
61. Scribner BH, Buri R, Caner JEZ, Hegstrom R, Burnell JM: The treatment of chronic uremia by means of intermittent dialyses. *Trans Am Soc Artif Intern Organs* 6:114, 1960
62. Merrill JP, Sabbaga E, Welzant W, Crane C: The use of an indwelling plastic conduit for chronic peritoneal irrigation. *Trans Am Soc Artif Intern Organs* 8:252, 1962
63. Boen ST, Curtis FK, Tenckhoff H, Scribner BH: Chronic hemodialysis and peritoneal dialysis. *Proc Eur Dial Transpl Assoc* 1:221, 1964
64. Tenckhoff H, Shilipetar G, Boen ST: One year's experience with home peritoneal dialysis. *Trans Am Soc Artif Intern Organs* 11:11, 1965
65. McDonald HP Jr: A peritoneal dialysis trocar. *J Urol* 89:946, 1963
66. Bull GM, Joekes AM, Lowe KG: Conservative treatment of anuric uraemia. *Lancet* 2:229, 1949
67. Borst JCG: Protein katabolism in uraemia. *Lancet* 1:824, 1948
68. Teschan PE, Baxter MD, O'Brien TF, Freyhof JN, Hall WH: Prophylactic hemodialysis in tne treatment of acute renal failure. *Ann Intern Med* 53:992, 1960
69. Leading article (anonymous): Intermittent peritoneal lavage. *Lancet* 2:551, 1959
70. Mowbray JF: Peritoneal dialysis for pre- and postoperative management in a cadaveric transplantation program. *Trans Am Soc Artif Intern Organs* 13:46, 1967
71. Matthews DE: Beyond survival. *Dial Transpl* 9:657 1980
72. Barry KG, Shambaugh GE, Goler D: A new flexible cannula and seal to provide prolonged access for peritoneal drainage and other procedures. *J Urol* 90:125, 1963
73. Malette WG, MacPaul JJ, Bledsoe F, MacIntosh DA, Koegel E: A clinical successful subcutaneous peritoneal access button for repeated peritoneal dialysis. *Trans Am Soc Artif Intern Organs* 10:396, 1964
74. Jacob GB, Deane N: Repeated peritoneal dialysis by the catheter replacement method: description of technique and a replaceable prosthesis for chronic access to the peritoneal cavity. *Proc Eur Dial Transpl Assoc* 4:136, 1967
75. Gutch CF: Peritoneal dialysis. *Trans Am Soc Artif Intern Organs* 10:406, 1964
76. Gutch CF, Stevens SC: Silastic catheter for peritoneal dialysis. *Trans Am Soc Artif Intern Organs* 12:106, 1966
77. Palmer RA, Quinton WE, Gray JE: Prolonged peritoneal dialysis for chronic renal failure. *Lancet* 1:700, 1964
78. McDonald HP Jr, Gerber N, Mischra D, Wolm L, Peng B, Waterhouse K: Subcutaneous Dacron and Teflon cloth adjuncts for silastic arterio venous shunts and peritoneal dialysis catheters. *Trans Am Soc Artif Intern Organs* 15:176, 1968
79. Tenckhoff H, Schechter H: A bacteriologically safe peritoneal access device. *Trans Am Soc Artif Intern Organs* 14:181, 1968
80. Lewkonia RM: Simple indwelling cannula for repeated peritoneal dialysis. *Lancet* 2:134, 1970
81. Heal MR, England AG, Goldstein HJ: Four years experience with indwelling silastic cannulae for long-term peritoneal dialysis. *Br Med J* 4:596, 1973
82. Goldberg EM, Hill W: A new peritoneal access prosthesis. *Proc Clin Dial Transpl Forum* 3:122, 1973
83. Stephen RL, Atkin-Thor E, Kolff WJ: Recirculation peritoneal dialysis with subcutaneous catheter. *Trans Am Soc Artif Intern Organs* 22:575, 1976
84. Oreopoulos DG: Overall experience with peritoneal dialysis. *Dial Transpl* 7:783, 1978
85. Gahl GM, Kessel M: The indwelling stylet catheter for peritoneal dialysis. *Clin Nephrol* 6:414, 1976
86. Lasker N, McCauley EP, Passarotte CT: Chronic peritoneal dialysis. *Trans Am Soc Artif Int Organs* 12:94, 1966
87. Jarrel B, Lasker N, Roberts M: A simple system of automated peritoneal dialysis. *Dial Transpl* 3 (nr 2):36, 1974
88. McDonald H Jr: An automatic peritoneal dialysis machine: preliminary report. *Trans Am Soc Artif Intern Organs* 11:83, 1965
89. Vercellone A, Piccoli G, Cavalli PL, Ragni R, Alloatte S: A new automatic peritoneal dialysis system. *Proc Eur Dial Transpl Assoc* 5:344, 1968
90. Tenckhoff H, Shilipetar G, van Paasschen WH, Swanson E: A home peritoneal dialysate delivery system. *Trans Am Soc Intern Artif Organs* 15:103, 1969
91. Tenckhoff H, Meston B, Shilipetar G: A simplified automatic peritoneal dialysis system. *Trans Am Soc Artif Intern Organs* 18:436, 1972
92. Blagg CR: Peritoneal dialysis and the Medicare ESRD program. *Dial Transpl* 8:1081, 1979
93. Brynger H, Brunner FP, Chantler C, Donckerwolcke RA, Jacobs C, Kramer P, Selwood NH, Wing AJ: Combined report on regular dialysis and transplantation X, 1979. *Proc Eur Dial Transpl Assoc* 17:4, 1980
94. Jacobs C, Broyer M, Brunner FP, Brynger H, Donckerwolcke RA, Kramer P, Selwood NH, Wing AJ, Blake PH: Combined report on regular dialysis and transplantation in Europe, XI, 1980. *Proc Eur Dial Transpl Assoc* 18:38, 1981
95. Barbour GL: The kinetics of peritoneal dialysis. *Dial Transpl* 8:1055, 1979
96. Nolph KD, Popovich RP, Ghods AJ, Twardowski Z: Determinants of low clearances of small solutes during peritoneal dialysis. *Kidney Int* 13:117, 1978
97. Gutman RA: Toward enhancement of peritoneal clearance. *Dial Transpl* 8:1072, 1979

98. Boen ST: Kinetics of peritoneal dialysis. *Medicine* 40:243, 1961
99. Robson M, Oreopoulos DG, Izatt S, Ogilvie R, Rapoport A, DeVeber GA: Influence of exchange volume and dialysate flow rate on solute clearance in peritoneal dialysis. *Kidney Int* 14:486, 1978
100. Giordano C: Studies on peritoneal dialysis. *Dial Transpl* 7:828, 1978
101. Henderson L: Peritoneal ultrafiltration dialysis. Enhanced urea transfer using hypertonic peritoneal dialysis fluid. *J Clin Invest* 45:950, 1964
102. Henderson L, Nolph KD: Altered permeability of the peritoneal membrane after using hypertonic peritoneal dialysis fluid. *J Clin Invest* 48:992, 1969
103. Zelman A, Gisser D, Whitam PJ, Parsons RH, Schuyler R: Augmentation of peritoneal dialysis efficiency with programmed hyper/hypo-osmotic dialysates. *Trans Am Soc Artif Intern Organs* 23:203, 1977
104. Hazel HG, Valtin H, Gosselin RE: Effects of drugs on peritoneal dialysis in the dog. *J Pharmacol Exp Ther* 145:122, 1964
105. Henderson LW, Kintzel JE: Influence of antidiuretic hormone on peritoneal membrane area and permeability. *J Clin Invest* 50:2437, 1971
106. Nolph KD, Ghods AJ, van Stone JC, Brown P: Effect of intraperitoneal vasodilators on peritoneal clearances. *Proc 9th Ann Contractors Conf Artif Kidney-Chronic Uremia Program of NIAMDD* edited by Mackey BB, DHEW publ nr (NIH) 77, 1167:118, 1976
107. Nolph KD, Ghods AJ, van Stone J, Brown PA: The effects of intraperitoneal vasodilators on peritoneal clearances. *Trans Am Soc Artif Intern Organs* 22:586, 1976
108. Maher JF, Hirszel P, Abraham JE, Galen MA, Chamberlin M, Hohnadel DC: The effect of dipyrimadole on peritoneal transport. *Trans Am Soc Artif Intern Organs* 23:219, 1977
109. Maher JF, Hohnadel DC, Shea CD, Sanzo F, Cassetta M: Effect of intraperitoneal diuretics on solute transport during hypertonic dialysis. *Clin Nephrol* 7:96, 1977
110. Hirszel P, Maher JF, LeGrow W: Increased peritoneal mass transport with glucagon acting at the vascular surface. *Trans Am Soc Artif Intern Organs* 24:136, 1978
111. Maher JF, Hirszel P, Lasrich M: Modulation of peritoneal transport rates by prostaglandins. *Adv Prostaglandin Thromboxane Res* 7:695, 1980
112. Maher JF: Peritoneal transport rates: mechanisms, limitations, and methods for augmentation. *Kidney Int* 18, (Suppl 10):S117, 1980
113. Raja RM, Kramer SM, Rosenbaum JL: Enhanced clearance with intraperitoneal nitroprusside in high flow recirculation peritoneal dialysis. *Trans Am Soc Artif Intern Organs* 24:133, 1978
114. Hirszel P, Lasrich M, Maher JF: Augmentation of peritoneal mass transport by dopamine. Comparison with norephinephrine and evaluation of pharmacologic mechanism. *Lab Clin Med* 94:747, 1979
115. Shinaberger J, Shear L, Barry KG: Increasing efficiency of peritoneal dialysis: experience with peritoneal-extracorporeal recirculation dialysis. *Trans Am Soc Artif Intern Organs* 11:76, 1965
116. Lange K, Freser G, Maigalat J: Automatic continuous high flow rate peritoneal dialysis. *Arch Klin Med* 214:201, 1968
117. Stephen RL: Reciprocating peritoneal dialysis with a subcutaneous peritoneal catheter. *Dial Transpl* 7:834, 1978
118. Kablitz C, Stephen RL, Duffy DP, Jacobsen SC, Zelman A, Kolff WJ: Technological augmentation of peritoneal urea clearance. Past, present, future. *Dial Transpl* 9:741, 1980
119. Di Paolo N: Semicontinuous peritoneal dialysis. *Dial Transpl* 7:839, 1978
120. Gordon A, Greenbaum M, Maxwell MH: Sorbent regeneration of peritoneal dialysate. *Trans Am Soc Artif Intern Organs* 20A:130, 1974
121. Blumenkrantz MJ, Lewin AJ, Gordon A, Roberts M, Pecker EA, Coburn JW, Maxwell MH: Development of a sorbent peritoneal dialysate regeneration system – a progress report. *Proc Eur Dial Transpl Assoc* 15:213, 1978
122. Lai F, Scott R, Tankersley R, Wayt H, Green L, Rhodes R, Zelman A: Third generation artificial kidney. *Trans Am Soc Artif Intern Organs* 21:346, 1975
123. Lewin AJ: Sorbent based regenerative peritoneal dialysis system. *Dial Transpl* 7:831, 1978
124. Eisinger AJ: A simple method of lessening the incidence of peritonitis in peritoneal dialysis using a photochemical reactor. *Clin Nephrol* 14:42, 1980
125. Diaz Buxo JA: Introduction: Peritoneal dialysis 1979. *Dial Transpl* 8:1054, 1979
126. Popovich RP, Moncrief JW, Decherd JB, Bomar JB, Pyle WK: The definition of a novel portable/wearable equilibrium peritoneal dialysis technique. *Abstracts Trans Am Soc Artif Intern Organs* 5:64, 1976
127. Popovich RP, Moncrief JW, Nolph KD, Ghods AJ, Twardowski ZJ, Pyle WK: Continuous ambulatory peritoneal dialysis. *Ann Intern Med* 88:449, 1978
128. Leading article (anonymous): Chronic ambulatory peritoneal dialysis. *Br Med J* 2:229, 1979
129. Thomson NM, Walker RG, Whiteside C, Scott DF, Atkins RC: Continuous ambulatory dialysis (CAPD) in the treatment of end stage renal failure. *Proc Eur Dial Transpl Assoc* 16:171, 1979
130. Moncrief JW, Nolph KD, Rubin J, Popovich RP: Additional experience with continuous ambulatory peritoneal dialysis (CAPD). *Trans Am Soc Artif Intern Organs* 24:476, 1978
131. Oreopoulos DG, Robson M, Izatt S, Clayton S, DeVeber GA: A simple and safe technique for continuous ambulatory peritoneal dialysis (CAPD). *Trans Am Soc Artif Intern Organs* 24:482, 1978
132. Moncrief JW: Continuous ambulatory peritoneal dialysis. *Dial Transpl* 7:809, 1978
133. Robson MD, Oreopoulous DG: Continuous ambulatory peritoneal dialysis. A revolution in the treatment of chronic renal failure. *Dial Transpl* 7:999, 1978
134. Khanna R, Oreopoulos DG, Dombros N, Vas S, Williams P, Meema HE, Husdan H, Ogilvie R, Zellerman G, Roncari DAK, Clayton S, Izatt S: Continuous ambulatory peritoneal dialysis (CAPD) after three years: still a promising treatment. *Peritoneal Dialysis Bull* (Publ Toronto Western Hosp, Can) 1:24, 1981
135. Gokal R, McHugh M, Fryer R, Ward MK, Kerr DNS: Continuous ambulatory peritoneal dialysis: one year's experience in a UK dialysis unit. *Br Med J* 281:474, 1980
136. Chan MK, Chuah P, Raftery MJ, Baillod RA, Sweny P, Varghese Z, Moorhead JF: Three years' experience of continuous peritoneal dialysis. *Lancet* 1:1409, 1981
137. Oreopoulos DG: The coming of age of continuous ambulatory peritoneal dialysis (CAPD). *Dial Transpl* 8:460, 1979
138. Moncrief JW: Continuous ambulatory peritoneal dialysis. *Dial Transpl* 8:1077, 1979
139. Nolph KD, Prowant B, Sorking MI, Gloor H: The incidence and characteristics of peritonitis in the fourth years of a continuous ambulatory peritoneal dialysis program. *Peritoneal Dialysis Bull* (publ Toronto Western Hosp, Can) 1:50, 1981
140. Mion C, Slingemeyer A, Liendo-Liendo C, Perez C, Despaux E: Reduction in incidence of peritonitis (P) asso-

ciated with continuous ambulatory peritoneal dialysis (CAPD). *Proc Clin Dial Transpl Forum* 9:9, 1979
141. Perras S, Zappacosta AR: Identifying candidates for continuous ambulatory peritoneal dialysis. *Dial Transpl* 10:10, 1981
142. Clayton S, Quinton C, Oreopoulos DG: Update of the Toronto Western Hospital technique of continuous ambulatory peritoneal dialysis (CAPD). *Peritoneal Dial Bull* (Publ Toronto Western Hosp, Can) 1:38, 1981
143. Anonymous: Renal failure – who cares? *Lancet* 1:1011, 1982
144. Anonymous: CAPD for chronic renal failure. *Lancet* 2:1172, 1980
145. Nolph KD: Peritoneal dialysis: physiology, current applications and future directions. *Proc Eur Dial Transpl Assoc* 16:277, 1979
146. Nolph KD: Polymer induced ultrafiltration in dialysis: high osmotic pressure due to impermeant polymer sodium. *Trans Am Soc Artif Intern Organs* 24:162, 1978
147. Kramer P, Broyer M, Brunner FP, Brynger H, Donckerwolcke RA, Jacobs C, Selwood NH, Wing AJ: Combined report on regular dialysis and transplantation in Europe, XII, 1981. *Proc Eur Dial Transpl Assoc* 19:4, 1982 1982
148. Diaz-Buxo JA, Walker PJ, Farmer CD, Chandler JT, Holt KL: Continuous cyclic peritoneal dialysis (CCPD). *Kidney Int* (Abstract) 19:145, 1981
149. Diaz-Buxo JA, Farmer CD, Walker PJ, Chandler JT, Holt KL: Continuous cyclic peritoneal dialysis: a preliminary report. *Artif Organs* 5:157, 1981
150. Adams FF, Brunt JR, Pucker CT, Williams AV: Automated long cycle peritoneal dialysis (ALCPD). *Kidney Int* (Abstract) 19:144, 1981
151. Mowbray JF: Human cadaveric transplantation: report of twenty cases. *Br Med J* 2:1387, 1967
152. Babb AL, Farrell PC, Uvelli DA, Scribner BH: Hemodialysis evaluation by examination of solute molecule spectra. *Trans Am Soc Artif Intern Organs* 18:98, 1972
153. Diaz Buxo JA, Haas VF: The influence of automated peritoneal dialysis on an established dialysis system. *Dial Transpl* 8:531, 1979
154. Bazzato G, Landini S, Coli BL, Lucatello S, Fracasso A, Moracchiello M: A new technique of continuous ambulatory peritoneal dialysis (CAPD): double-bag system for freedom to the patient and significant reduction of peritonitis. *Clin Nephrol* 13:251, 1980
155. Robson MD, Oreopoulos DG, Izatt S, Rapoport A, DeVeber GA: Comparison of intermittent with continuous peritoneal dialysis. *Proc Eur Dial Transpl Assoc* 15:197, 1978
156. Villarroel F: Future of intracorporeal dialysis. *Contrib Nephrol* 17:111, 1979
157. Friedman EA, Lundin AP, Butt KMH: Rushed judgment in uremia therapy (Editorial). *Artif Org* 5:97, 1981
158. Maher JF, Deane N, Henderson LW, Lasker N, Nolph KD, Popovich R, Roxe D: Peritoneal dialysis: can we overcome its current limitations? *Trans Am Soc Artif Intern Organs* 25:523, 1979
159. Parsons FM, Ogg C (editors): *Renal Failure – Who cares? (Symposium proceedings).* Lancaster UK, MTP, Medical and Technical Publ Co Ltd, 1982
160. Schmidt RW, Blumenkrantz MJ: IPD, CAPD, CCPD, CRPD – peritoneal dialysis past, present and future. *Int J Artif Org* 4:124, 1981

22

PERITONEAL ANATOMY AND TRANSPORT PHYSIOLOGY

KARL D. NOLPH

The anatomy and histology of the peritoneal dialysis system	440
The peritoneum and the peritoneal cavity	440
The parietal peritoneum	440
The visceral peritoneum	441
Membrane resistances to solute movement	441
Anatomy and permeability characteristics of the peritoneum	441
Assessment of dialysis efficiency	442
Net solute removal rate (mass transfer)	442
Clearances	442
Dialysance, instantaneous clearance, and mass transfer coefficient	442
Factors affecting dialysis efficiency	442
Flow-rate and other physical characteristics of the dialysis solution	442
Dialysate flow rate	442
Dialysis solution distribution	443
Temperature	443
pH	443
The addition of protein to dialysis solution	443
Osmolality	443
Microcirculatory factors	443
Evidence that peritoneal capillary blood is the major source of solutes and fluid removed	443
Peritoneal capillary blood flow	445
Capillary permeability	446
Interstitial factors and fluid films	446
Mesothelial factors	448
Mesothelial permeability	448
Total pore area across mesothelium	448
Ultrafiltration factors	448
Hypothesis to explain solute sieving during ultrafiltration	448
Other factors	449
Body solute distribution volumes, protein binding of solutes, and intracellular trapping	449
Body solute distribution volumes	449
Protein binding of solutes	449
Intracellular trapping	449
Lipid solubility	450
Comparisons with hollow-fiber dialyzers	450
Capillary dimensions, configurations, and permeability	450
Dialysate flow characteristics	451
Comparisons of different resistances for large and small solutes during hollow-fiber dialysis and peritoneal dialysis	452
Blood flow comparisons	452
Manipulating peritoneal transport	452
Cycling time	452
Vasoactive substances	453
Manipulating the interstitium	453
Other drug effects	454
Surface-acting agents	454
References	454

THE ANATOMY AND HISTOLOGY OF THE PERITONEAL DIALYSIS SYSTEM

The peritoneum and the peritoneal cavity

The peritoneum is a living membrane that covers visceral organs, forms the visceral mesentery that connects loops of bowel, and reflects over the inner surface of the abdominal wall (1, 2) (Figure 1). The peritoneum is continuous and forms a closed sack, which, because the space within contains only small amounts of fluid (probably less than 100 ml), usually is nearly collapsed. In an adult of normal size, the space can be enlarged by instillation of fluid; two or more liters of fluid can be accommodated without causing discomfort. The surface of the membrane is a shiny layer of mesothelial cells, beneath which lies supporting interstitium containing extracellular fluid, connective tissue fibers, blood vessels, and lymphatics. The visceral peritoneum is that part of the membrane that courses over the surface of visceral organs. As visceral peritoneum reflects from loops of bowel to form the visceral mesentery (connecting adjacent loops of bowel), the interstitium becomes interspersed between adjacent mesothelial layers. The parietal peritoneum is that portion of the membrane that covers the inner surface of the abdominal wall. The total surface area of the peritoneal mesothelium (parietal and visceral) is believed to approximate the surface area of skin (which, in most adults, is 1 to 2 m^2) (3).

The parietal peritoneum

The parietal peritoneum represents only a small portion of the total mesothelial surface area and receives its blood supply from the vasculature of the abdominal wall. The exact ratio of parietal to visceral peritoneal surface area is unknown, but the many folds of visceral mesentery obviously represent a larger fraction of the total peritoneal surface area; therefore, parietal peritoneum participation in solute transport during peritoneal dialysis usually is considered to be less than the participation of visceral peritoneum. Portions of the parietal peritoneum, however, may be more vascular than some of the nearly avascular sections of mesentery, and the true fractional contributions of parietal and visceral per-

440

22: *Peritoneal anatomy and transport physiology*   441

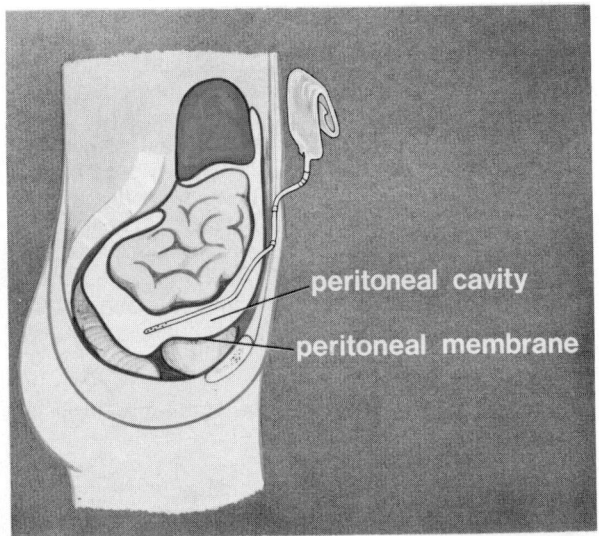

Figure 1. A diagrammatic sketch of the peritoneal cavity and the membrane lining the cavity. A peritoneal catheter is in place.

itoneum to solute transport during peritoneal dialysis have not yet been determined.

During peritoneal dialysis, solutes moving from capillaries in the parietal peritoneum must traverse capillary endothelial walls, parietal peritoneal interstitium, and the parietal peritoneal mesothelial layer (4, 5). Relative contributions of parietal lymphatics versus capillaries to net transport during peritoneal dialysis are unknown, but it is assumed that blood vessels are a more important source because of the relatively slow flow through lymphatics (4, 5).

The visceral peritoneum

The visceral mesentery contains many relatively large blood vessels on their way to visceral organs. Arteriolar and capillary beds capable of participating in exchange of solutes during peritoneal dialysis are located primarily where mesentery and large blood vessels reflect over loops of bowel and then divide into smaller (less than 10 microns in diameter) arterioles and capillaries on the bowel surface (6). Lymphatics also are plentiful in the visceral mesentery, but their participation in peritoneal dialysis is unknown.

As in the parietal peritoneum, solutes moving from the visceral peritoneal microcirculation into dialysis solution must cross capillary endothelium, interstitium, and mesothelium.

Membrane resistances to solute movement

Pathways for solute movement from peritoneal capillaries into the peritoneal cavity can be subdivided into at least six resistance sites (5): R_1: stagnant fluid films within peritoneal capillaries, R_2: capillary endothelium, R_3: capillary basement membranes, R_4: interstitium, R_5: mesothelium, R_6: stagnant fluid films within the peritoneal cavity. These sites and their hypothesized dimensions are diagramatically shown in Figure 2.

Anatomy and permeability characteristics of the peritoneum

The exact route taken by solutes traversing the peritoneal cellular layers has not been established. Some reports suggest that solutes up to a molecular mass of 30,000 daltons diffuse across biological membranes, primarily through intercellular channels, as indicated in Figure 2 (7, 8). The results of a study of isolated rat mesentery, however, indicate that transcellular movement of some solutes may occur, at least across mesothelium (9). Capillary endothelial cells in the human peritoneum are not known to be fenestrated as are glomerular capillaries (10).

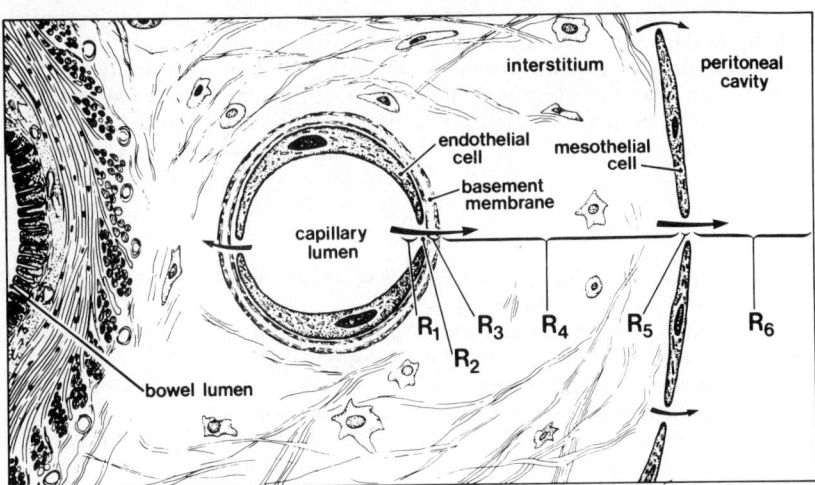

Figure 2. Resistances ($R_1 - R_6$) to solute movement during peritoneal dialysis (see text). (From Nolph et al. [5] with permission of the publisher).

The basement membrane seems to offer little resistance to solute diffusion when molecular mass is less than 30,000 daltons (7, 8). Mesothelium appears to be more permeable than endothelium, possibly because of the larger intercellular gaps between mesothelial cells (11). The permeability of the peritoneal mesothelium apparently is not uniform; it has been suggested that the visceral portion is more permeable than the parietal portion (12).

ASSESSMENT OF DIALYSIS EFFICIENCY

Net solute removal rate (mass transfer)

For solutes not present in instilled dialysis solution, the amount removed can be determined by multiplying drainage volume by solute concentration in dialysate. Net removal of solutes in the instilled fluid can be calculated by subtracting the amount instilled (instillation volume × concentration in the instilled fluid) from the total amount removed. Net solute removal rates can be expressed as the amount removed between the time dialysis solution is instilled and the time drainage is completed. Such a cycle usually is referred to as one exchange, and the removal rate per exchange or per minute can be expressed in milligrams, milliequivalents, or millimoles. The net removal rate often is referred to as the *mass transfer rate*.

The rate of net solute diffusion into dialysis solution, however, is a function of the concentration gradient from blood to dialysis fluid. The instilled dialysis solution approximates normal diffusible plasma concentrations of electrolytes, and thus net electrolyte removal (in the absence of ultrafiltration) is small when plasma values are normal. The initial dialysate concentration of other solutes such as urea and creatinine is zero, and the initial concentration gradient for diffusion depends on the plasma concentration, assuming that peripheral blood reflects concentrations in peritoneal capillary inflow. (The latter may not be so for solutes such as lipids or glucose in the process of being absorbed from gastrointestinal tract or dialysate [13, 14]). Because net solute removal rates of nonelectrolytes depend primarily on blood concentrations, the quantities removed per unit time are not good indices of peritoneal dialysis efficiency.

Clearances

The efficiency index most commonly used (at least by clinicians) is the *clearance rate* of a solute from the plasma. This is calculated by dividing the amount of solute removed per unit time, the mass transfer rate, by the concentration of solute in plasma. This calculation expresses the volume of plasma cleared of that solute per unit time (usually expressed in milliliters per minute). The clearance term is independent of the blood solute concentration and expresses the efficiency of removal.

Clearance, so calculated, represents the mean clearance rate per exchange. The *instantaneous clearance* is highest at the beginning of an exchange when the dialysis solution solute concentration is near zero and the diffusion gradient is maximum. The instantaneous clearance approaches zero exponentially as the dialysis solution concentration approaches equilibrium with blood.

The mean clearance rate, though independent of blood solute concentration, is influenced by effective peritoneal membrane area, blood flow rate to the peritoneum, flow rate of dialysis fluid, the physical characteristics of the dialysis solution, the size and number of distribution spaces of the solute, fluid films adjacent to endothelium and mesothelium, and the permeability characteristics of the peritoneal membrane.

Dialysance, instantaneous clearance, and mass transfer coefficient

Estimates of the theoretical instantaneous clearance at the beginning of an exchange have been developed. Such a derivation (often called a *dialysance, or a mass transfer coefficient*) is thought to be primarily or solely a function of peritoneal diffusive permeability (cm/min) and the effective surface area (cm^2) (15-17). Henderson and Nolph (16) have proposed that ratios of dialysance or mass transfer coefficients for different solutes are the same as ratios of respective permeability coefficients when effective membrane pore area is the same for both solutes. For example:

$$\frac{\text{dialysance inulin}}{\text{dialysance urea}} =$$

$$= \frac{\text{Membrane area} \times \text{inulin permeability coefficient}}{\text{Membrane area} \times \text{urea permeability coefficient}}$$

The use of such terms often incorporates assumptions as to the movement of solutes within body spaces, contributions of convective transport, absence of blood flow limitations on solute movement, and simplifications relative to inflow time and drainage time. These primarily research terms are used to determine more precisely the effective area and permeability characteristics of the peritoneal membrane. Clinically, the mean clearance rate is a direct calculation of what is actually accomplished, is more readily understood, and is more commonly used. The discussion of factors affecting peritoneal dialysis efficiency will deal primarily with their relation to peritoneal clearances.

FACTORS AFFECTING DIALYSIS EFFICIENCY

Flow-rate and other physical characteristics of dialysis solution

Dialysate flow rate
During peritoneal dialysis in adults when dialysis solution is instilled and drained by gravity rather than by automated equipment, it is customary to use 2.0 l exchanges with an inflow duration of 10 min, a dwell time of 30 min, and a drainage period of 20 to 30 min. Thus,

dialysate flow rate is a potential limitation on peritoneal dialysis clearance of small highly diffusible solutes. With 1.5% dextrose* dialysis solution (which is usually slightly hypertonic to azotemic plasma), a typical drainage volume is 2100 to 2200 ml per exchange. With a 70 min exchange, this represents an average dialysate turnover rate near 30 ml/min. If a solute equilibrated totally between plasma and dialysate during such an exchange (and even urea does not), the maximum clearance possible would be 30 ml/min. Urea clearance usually is 18 to 20 ml/min with this type of exchange.

Clearances of small solutes can be increased by more rapid exchanges. As dwell time is shortened, however, the portion of exchange time occupied by inflow and drainage increases. During inflow and drainage, there is less volume in the peritoneal cavity, which reduces clearances during those times and so reduces the final average clearance per exchange. Thus, although clearances can be increased by increasing dialysate flow, with the usual manual method a point of diminishing gains is eventually reached. Boen (18, 19), using a 10 min inflow, 5 min dwell time, and 15 min drain cycle, has shown that urea clearance decreases at flow rates above 3.5 l/h. Studies by Penzotti and Mattocks (20) support this finding. Tenckhoff, Ward, and Boen (21), using automated cycling equipment, later showed that urea clearance may increase to over 40 ml/min with dialysate flow rates of 12 l/h. By using automatic peritoneal dialysis equipment to cut down on inflow and drainage time, short exchanges may be more efficient. The nursing time required for more rapid exchanges (when performed manually) also is a major limiting factor.

It is possible to achieve higher dialysis solution flow rates without increasing inflow and drainage times by continuous flow through two catheters or a double-lumen catheter (22–27). Clearances of urea may approach 40 ml/min using an 18 l/h dialysate flow (24). Dialysis solution may be utilized single pass (23) or be recycled after passage through an extracorporeal dialysis system (24, 26). A danger limiting this approach is channeling, whereby dialysis solution streams from lumen to lumen. Abdominal pain is common at flow rates above 12 l/h, presumably due to mechanical irritation (24).

Another way to increase the dialysate flow rate is to increase the volume per exchange. Dialysis solutions are marketed primarily in 2 l containers, making this an easy choice for manual methods. Many adults, however, find intraperitoneal volumes greater than 2 l uncomfortable, and some patients cannot even tolerate 2 l exchanges.

Reciprocating peritoneal dialysis (see also Chapter 21) involves rapid in-and-out cycling of dialysate (100 to 200 ml, in one min and out the next), with an intraperitoneal residual dialysate reservoir of usually 2 l (28, 29). This can accommodate net flow rates of 6 l/h or more with better patient tolerance and without the manipulations of patient position often required for complete drainage. Urea clearances of 30 to 40 ml/min may be achieved. Dialysate regeneration (with sorbents or by dialysis of used dialysate) is often attempted at high dialysate flow rates (30).

Dialysis solution distribution
Manipulations of dialysate flow rate minimally affect the clearances of larger solutes that are limited by membrane area and permeability; however, the mechanics of moving dialysis solution in and out of the peritoneal cavity may improve the clearances of larger solutes when optimal distribution of dialysis solution is assured (so as to minimize large pools and distribute the solution in thin layers with maximum membrane contact). Total membrane resistance also includes blood and dialysate films adjacent to the membrane. Currently there are no techniques that assure optimal intraperitoneal distribution of dialysate, and good catheter placement and patient positioning often are achieved only after trial and error.

Temperature
Dialysis solution temperature influences solute movement into the peritoneal cavity, and higher temperatures presumably enhance solute diffusion (31). It is customary to heat peritoneal dialysis solution to body temperature before instillation.

pH
A high dialysate pH may increase net clearances of anions of weak acids such as urate and barbiturate. As these acids diffuse into more alkaline dialysate, fractions are converted to the charged, less diffusible anionic salts. This helps keep the diffusible acid concentration low on the dialysate side and tends to 'trap' the solute in less diffusible form (32–34).

The addition of protein to dialysis solution
For solutes bound to protein, the addition of protein to dialysis solution may enhance clearances (34). The diffusible free solute binds to protein in the dialysate maintaining a very low dialysate water concentration of the free diffusible form and a high efflux gradient.

Osmolality
Peritoneal dialysis solutions made hypertonic with dextrose increase clearances (16). This is partly accounted for by the solvent drag effects of osmotically induced ultrafiltration during such exchanges. But clearances often remain elevated when less hypertonic exchanges are resumed, which may be due to vasodilatory effects of the hyperosmolar solutions.

Microcirculatory factors

Evidence that peritoneal capillary blood is the major source of solutes and fluid removed
Peritoneal capillary blood may be the major source of solutes, cells, and water removed during peritoneal dial-

---

* 1.5% dextrose dialysis solution equals 15 g/l of dextrose monohydrate or 13.6 g/l of anhydrous dextrose (d-glucose) which equals 76 mmol/l.

ysis. Most evidence for this is indirect and can be summarized as follows (also, see Table 1).

1. Hypertonic peritoneal dialysis solution (4.25% dextrose monohydrate) can generate net ultrafiltration in excess of 500 ml/h (35). Many liters per day of ultrafiltration can be tolerated with the rapid resolution of edema. If hypertonic exchanges are used intermittently, so avoiding severe hyperglycemia or hypotension, net ultrafiltration per hypertonic exchange remains consistent (36). It seems unlikely that mesothelial cells, interstitium, or lymphatics could yield so much ultrafiltrate over short periods of time; it is more reasonable to assume that ultrafiltrate comes from the capillaries.

2. Dramatic reductions in blood pressure can sometimes be observed after one or two hypertonic exchanges, which suggests that ultrafiltration without adequate mobilization of extravascular fluid can jeopardize blood volume.

3. Hypotension can decrease peritoneal clearances (37). Although such clearance reductions often are modest, even in severe shock (for reasons discussed below), the findings suggest that solute clearances are affected by peritoneal capillary blood flow (4).

4. Intraperitoneal or systemic use of vasoconstrictors reduces peritoneal clearances (38–41) and decreases both the number of peritoneal capillaries perfused and peritoneal capillary blood flow (6, 42, 43), which supports the conjecture that the status of the microcirculation influences peritoneal clearances.

5. Peritoneal clearances increase with intraperitoneal administration of vasodilators (38, 44–52). These agents increase peritoneal capillary blood flow, as well as the number of capillaries perfused (42, 45). Vasodilation and/or direct effects of these agents may increase capillary permeability (53). The point, however, is that vasoactive agents affect peritoneal clearances in the expected direction if clearances relate directly to blood flow, number of capillaries, and vascular permeability.

6. Histamine topically applied to the rat peritoneum widens the intercellular gaps in small venules (54), as assessed by serial section studies of the peritoneum with electron microscopy, computerized reconstruction of venular intercellular gaps, and direct observations of fluorescein-tagged albumin movement across the walls of small vessels in the rat mesentery, using a laser beam microscope. Miller and co-workers (55) have observed a similar extravasation of albumin with nitroprusside. In clinical studies, nitroprusside added to peritoneal dialysis solution also markedly increased protein losses (42–46).

7. Patients with severe systemic vasculitis, presumably involving the peritoneal microcirculation, can have significantly reduced peritoneal clearances (56, 57). To date, there are reports of reduced clearances in patients with systemic lupus erythematosus, diffuse scleroderma (progressive systemic sclerosis), and malignant hypertension.

8. Some patients with widespread diabetic vascular disease have significantly reduced clearances (56). This is not a universal finding in all diabetics, but may be related to capillary basement membrane thickening and to vascular disease as it exists in the peritoneum.

9. The concentration of potassium in the intracellular fluid of mesothelial cells is near 140 mEq/l (58–60); dialysis solution in the peritoneal cavity, however, approaches Gibbs-Donnan equilibrium with the potassium concentration in serum water (61, 62). Because the composition of dialysis solution is similar to that of extracellular fluid, it is not surprising that the mesothelial cells can maintain their normal internal milieu even though bathed with dialysis solution. The fact that intracellular electrolytes do not participate in peritoneal dialysis exchange to any great extent, however, does not exclude the possibility that some creatinine and urea are removed from the intracellular fluid.

10. Solutes can be removed by convection in the absence of a diffusion gradient when hypertonic solutions induce ultrafiltration (63–65). The net removal of potassium by convection per liter of ultrafiltrate does not exceed potassium concentration in extracellular fluid (61, 66), and therefore even hypertonic exchanges do not appear to mobilize much, if any, intracellular potassium.

11. Diffusible solutes probably are removed from peritoneal interstitium and perhaps to some extent from mesothelial intracellular fluid (4, 5, 65, 67). Ultrafiltrate would of course involve water movement through the interstitium and perhaps to some extent through or from mesothelial cells (64). Mesothelial cells can tolerate only a modest degree of dehydration, however, and interstitial pools of water and solute would be exhausted quickly without rapid replacement from peritoneal capillaries. Hence, most of the water and solutes removed during peritoneal dialysis must represent water and solute movement from peritoneal capillaries into the peritoneal cavity via pathways *through* the interstitium and mesothelial layer.

Table 1. Indirect evidence that peritoneal capillary blood is a major source of solutes, cells, and water removal during peritoneal dialysis.

1. Sustained ultrafiltration with repeated hypertonic exchanges
2. Hypotension with repeated hypertonic exchanges
3. Decreased clearances with hypotension
4. Decreased clearances with vasoconstrictors
5. Increased clearances with vasodilators
6. Drugs known to increase protein leaking from venules increase protein losses during peritoneal dialysis
7. Decreased clearances with vasculitis
8. Decreased clearances with diabetic vascular disease
9. Dialysate potassium concentrations approach Gibbs-Donnan equilibrium with plasma, not with intracellular fluid
10. Convective removal of potassium per liter of ultrafiltrate does not exceed extracellular concentrations
11. Limited pools of fluid and solutes in peritoneal mesothelium and interstitium are quickly exhausted unless rapidly replaced
12. Lymphatic flow presumably quite low; drainage not chylous
13. Dialysate leukocyte counts and fibrin increase rapidly with inflammation

12. Solutes and water could move into the peritoneal interstitium from peritoneal lymphatics (68). The portions of removal of solutes or water that come from peritoneal lymphatics are unknown, but have been assumed to be minimal because lymphatic flow rates are presumably low and drainage usually is not chylous. We have followed one patient on continuous ambulatory peritoneal dialysis whose drainage contained lymph for nearly 3 years after an episode of streptococcal peritonitis. Drainage was milky, particularly after meals, and contained high triglyceride concentrations. There was no evidence of inflammation (dialysate white counts were low and there were no symptoms). This finding, however, is extremely unusual.

13. The finding that dialysate leukocyte counts in the presence of infection can increase over several hours from less than 100 to many thousands of white cells per cubic millimeter is additional evidence that peritoneal capillary blood can rapidly and significantly contribute to what is removed in peritoneal dialysis solution (69, 70). In the presence of inflammation, an outpouring of fibrinogen with formation of fibrin in dialysate apparently often occurs quickly.

Thus, indirect evidence supports the hypothesis that peritoneal dialysis represents fluid and solute exchange between peritoneal capillary blood and dialysis solution in the peritoneal cavity. The capillary, the endothelium, the peritoneal interstitium, and the mesothelium represent the resistance sites that fluid and solutes must cross if exchange is to take place.

Peritoneal capillary blood flow

The absolute peritoneal capillary blood flow that participates in peritoneal dialysis exchange is not known. Total splanchnic blood flow in adult humans may exceed 1,200 ml/min (71). Most of this blood, however, is on its way to visceral organs, not to small vessels of the peritoneum. In fact, our observations of the rat peritoneum suggest that the mesentery itself is not particularly vascular and that most of the small vessels capable of participating in exchange may be located at sites where peritoneum reflects over loops of bowel (72, 73).

Maximum urea clearances in adult humans usually do not exceed 30 ml/min, even with the most rapid cycling (21, 24, 74). A possible explanation may be that maximum urea clearances are approaching effective peritoneal capillary blood flow and that this blood flow does not exceed 30 to 40 ml/min. Abundant indirect evidence, however, suggests that such is not the case. Rather, indirect evidence suggests that maximum peritoneal urea clearances are not primarily blood flow–limited. This evidence (summarized in Table 2) is as follows:

1. Animal studies have shown that urea clearances remain above 70% of control values even with severe shock and 38% reductions in splanchnic blood flow (37). This observation suggests that although the magnitude of change in peritoneal capillary flow from control to shock conditions is not known, effective peritoneal capillary flow is well above urea clearance in the control state and falls into a modest flow-limiting range only in the presence of severe hypotension.

Table 2. Indirect evidence that maximum* peritoneal urea clearances are not primarily blood-flow-limited.

1. Urea clearances remain 70% of control even in shock
2. Urea clearances increase <20% with vasodilators
3. Vasodilators increase clearances of larger solutes more than urea clearances
4. Clearances of CO_2 and H_2 gases are nearly three times maximum urea clearances
5. Urea clearances, if only 1/3 of effective capillary blood flow (as gas clearances suggest), would be minimally flow-limited according to kinetic modeling analyses and *in vitro* simulations

* Very high dialysate flow, >4 l/h, yields urea clearances in man <40 ml/min.

2. Urea clearances increase only modestly (usually less than 20%) with intraperitoneal vasodilators (42–47). Vasodilators influence the number of capillaries perfused, induce venodilation, and alter vascular permeability, directly (6, 72, 73). Because these latter effects could account for the modest increases in small solute clearances observed with vasodilator use any increases in effective capillary flow so induced have little or no effect on urea clearances and this indicates that there is no major blood flow limitation on urea clearances.

3. In fact, vasodilators primarily increase clearances of larger solutes (43, 44), and such increases may exceed 100% for solutes above 5,200 daltons. Although these observations would support the contention that vasodilator effects may be related more to venodilation and alterations in permeability than to effects on blood flow *per se* (54, 73, 75), they do not negate the very likely possibility that vasodilators increase effective peritoneal capillary flow. However, if this was the major effect of the drugs, and if urea clearances were flow-limited, then proportionally greater increases should occur in urea clearances than in clearances of larger solutes.

4. Peritoneal clearances of CO_2 gas in humans and hydrogen gas in rabbits are two-to-three times the maximum urea clearances (4, 76). Gas clearances also should be limited by effective peritoneal capillary flow and should not exceed urea clearances to any great extent if capillary flow was the main determinant of urea clearance; on the other hand, gases should diffuse across all membrane resistances more rapidly. Gases also might use transcellular routes, whereas the path taken by nongaseous solutes is primarily through intercellular gaps and extracellular pathways (25, 26, 77). The fact that gas clearances can be two-to-three times urea clearances suggests that urea clearances are limited by total membrane resistances, including fluid films, rather than by peritoneal capillary flow.

5. If it is true that urea clearances are only one-third to one-half of the effective capillary blood flow, then kinetic modeling analyses and *in vitro* simulations of peritoneal dialysis suggest that under such conditions effective capillary flow would exert only modest limitations on peritoneal urea clearances and that the relationship between urea clearance and effective capillary flow would be in the 'plateau' portion of the clearance-to-

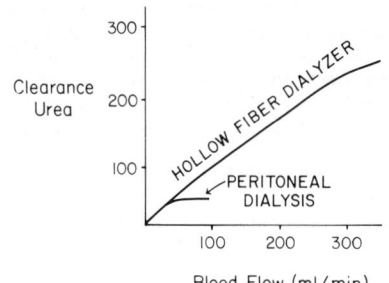

Figure 3. Urea clearances are related to blood flow in a hollow-fiber dialyzer and during peritoneal dialysis (at high dialysis solution flow rates). Peritoneal blood flow values are theoretical, based on gas diffusion studies.

blood flow relationship (4). Figure 3 shows a hypothetical relationship of urea clearance to blood flow at high dialysis solution flow rates for peritoneal dialysis, compared with typical findings with a hollow-fiber artificial kidney. With the hollow-fiber kidney, dialysate flow would be near 500 ml/min; with peritoneal dialysis, flow rates would exceed 4 l/h. If effective peritoneal capillary flow rate is near 70 ml/min (as CO_2 gas diffusion studies suggest), then urea clearances would show a nearly 'plateau' relationship with effective blood flow. This plateau presumably represents effects of membrane and fluid film resistances. On the other hand, the hollow-fiber dialyzer fluid film and membrane resistances to urea transport are so low that the system is primarily blood-flow-limited. Urea clearance remains at a very high fraction of blood flow up to very high blood flows.

Capillary permeability

In contrast to the situation for small solutes, where interstitial and fluid films appear to be major determinants of maximum clearances, the permeability of the microcirculation appears to be a major influence on clearances of larger solutes (43, 47, 75). The evidence for this is summarized below and in Table 3.

Table 3. Evidence that vascular permeability is a major resistance for large solutes.

1. Increased protein losses with agents known to increase venular permeability
2. Proportionately larger increases in inulin clearances (compared with urea clearances) with vasoactive drugs
3. Increased protein losses with peritoneal inflammation
4. Laser studies with fluorescein-tagged albumin in the rat microcirculation

1. As previously mentioned, protein losses increase when agents known to increase venular permeability are topically applied to the mesentery (54). Intraperitoneal nitroprusside, for example, markedly increases protein losses.
2. Vasoactive drugs cause proportionally larger increases in inulin clearances than in urea clearances (43–47). Evidence suggests that vasoactive drugs alter vascular permeability (54, 55), which would explain the proportionally greater effects on larger solutes, where vascular permeability has a major effect on clearances.
3. Protein losses increase with peritoneal inflammation (78–81). Peritoneal inflammation from any cause stimulates an outpouring of white blood cells into the peritoneal dialysis solution (70). Inflammation in other tissues of the body usually is associated with vasodilation; therefore, it would be reasonable to assume that this also would occur in the peritoneum. Thus, the protein losses with inflammation may merely reflect endogenous mechanisms that induce vasodilation. Vasodilation *per se* may result in perfusion of more permeable capillaries (53). Local release of histamine may increase vascular permeability.
4. After injection of fluorescein-tagged albumin into the rat, the albumin remains within the microcirculation over many minutes of observation without obvious leaking into the interstitium (54). There is an almost explosive outpouring of albumin from the microcirculation into the interstitium within seconds after agents that alter vascular permeability are topically applied peritoneally.

Interstitial factors and fluid films

Indirect evidence suggests that fluid films and interstitial resistance are important in limiting urea clearances during peritoneal dialysis (Table 4).

Table 4. Indirect evidence that fluid films and/or interstitial resistance limit urea clearances during peritoneal dialysis.

1. Maximum urea clearances near 30 ml/min even with rapid cycling or with vasodilators
2. Dialysate relatively stagnant
3. Probably very wide dialysate channels
4. Interstital solute path; potentially long distance
5. *In vitro* simulations of peritoneal dialysis demonstrate high fluid film resistances
6. Little evidence to support blood flow limitation
7. Vascular resistance appears low for small solutes.

1. As previously mentioned, maximum urea clearances usually do not exceed 30 ml/min, even with rapid cycling or use of intraperitoneal vasodilators (21, 24, 74). The rapid cycling should minimize limitations due to dialysis solution flow rate. Vasodilators, which presumably increase the number of capillaries perfused and alter capillary permeability, should minimize endothelial resistance. Studies in isolated mesentery suggest that mesothelial intercellular gaps are greater than 500 Å wide and offer very little resistance (9–12, 82, 83). Thus, under the conditions of rapid cycling and use of intraperitoneal vasodilators (and assuming that effective peritoneal capillary flow is not limiting), major resistance sites that explain the limits on urea clearances should be the interstitium and the stagnant fluid films in the peritoneal cavity.
2. Dialysate in the peritoneal cavity within the many folds of the mesentery always remains relatively stagnant, even with rapid cycling (21, 24, 74).

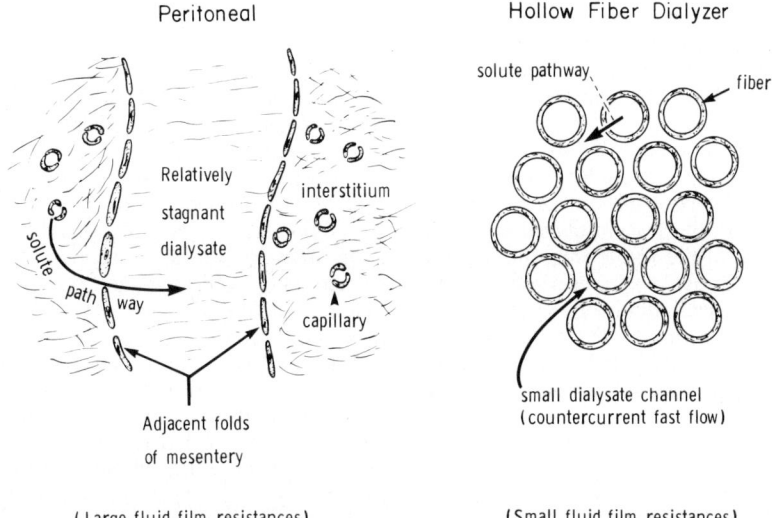

Figure 4. Dialysate channel configurations in peritoneal and hollow-fiber dialysis.

3. Dialysate channels probably are relatively wide (74). Figure 4 is a comparison between dialysate channel dimensions during peritoneal dialysis and those in a man-made hollow-fiber dialyzer. Note that in the hollow-fiber dialyzers much of the cross-section represents blood path. In small dialysate channels there is rapid counter-current flow and minimal fluid film resistance (84, 85). In contrast, in the peritoneal system the interstitium and stagnant pools of fluid between folds of mesentery represent substantial fluid film resistances.

4. The interstitial solute path probably represents a relatively long distance (5), and, as shown in Figure 2, may be 100 microns or more. Figure 5 shows that the situation may be even more complex. Wayland (54) suggests that the interstitium may represent a network of aqueous channels through mucopolysaccharide and collagenous gels. Hypertonic peritoneal dialysis solutions may dehydrate the interstitium and, although the total distance may be shortened, the aqueous network of channels could become more tortuous and the resistance to solute movement could actually increase (73, 86).

5. *In vitro* simulations of peritoneal dialysis (using hollow-fiber dialyzers with the outer shell removed placed in stagnant pools of fluid) demonstrate rapid deterioration in urea clearances attributable to high fluid film resistances (4, 87). Even with the most rapid cycling in and out of the simulated peritoneal cavity, clearances cannot be restored. Vigorous shaking of the cavity and improved mixing diminish the effects of fluid film resistances to some extent, but never approach the perfor-

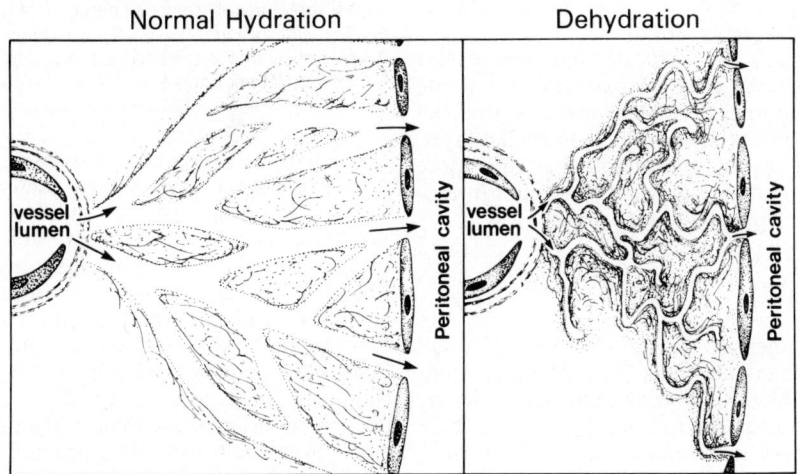

Figure 5. Hypothetical changes in interstitial aqueous channel dimensions during peritoneal dialysis and interstitial dehydration.

mance that can be achieved with rapid counter-current flow of dialysis fluid in the usual manner (87).

6. As mentioned previously, because there is little evidence in support of a blood flow limitation, the importance of fluid film is implied.

7. Wayland (54) suggests that endothelium offers very little resistance to small solute movement from peritoneal capillary blood into peritoneal dialysis solution. When rats are injected with fluorescein-tagged small solutes, extensive migration of the solute into the interstitium is observed. This contrasts with observations after injection of fluorescein-tagged albumin, where movement of albumin across vascular walls is not obvious over many minutes unless agents that increase vascular permeability are administered in solutions bathing the peritoneum (54).

Mesothelial factors

Mesothelial permeability

Results of functional and morphological studies in isolated mesentery suggest that gaps between adjacent mesothelial cells may form very loose junctions, particularly over the diaphragmatic surface (11). Intercellular gaps 500 Å wide have been observed. Transport studies in isolated mesentery also suggest the presence of pores of similar dimensions (82, 83). Some mesothelial intercellular junctions may be tighter, however, and may influence peritoneal transport. Diuretics (88) and inhibitors of cellular metabolic pathways (9) may influence diffusion rates through isolated mesentery and during peritoneal dialysis. Alterations in mesothelial metabolic functions may alter dimensions of intercellular gaps or cell surface charges; both factors could influence the permeability characteristics of the mesothelium to passive solute movement. Cell surface charges in particular might influence the movement of charged solutes. Whether the active transport of electrolytes across mesothelial cell walls influences net electrolyte removal or uptake during peritoneal dialysis remains unknown.

Total pore area across mesothelium

Studies by Karnovsky (7, 77) indicate that intercellular gaps between mesothelial cells are pathways for solute movement; if so, the total pore area would be well below the total gross surface area of the mesothelial layer, and the magnitude of the transmesothelial total pore area could be influenced by the extent of solution/mesothelial contact within the abdominal cavity.

Ultrafiltration factors

Ultrafiltration can increase solute clearances (16, 63). Solutes may accompany the bulk flow of water from peritoneal capillary blood into the peritoneal cavity by convection. Most solutes do not accompany the bulk flow of water in proportions comparable to the concentrations of solute in extracellular water (16, 45, 61, 65). Thus, the concentration gradient for net diffusion of a solute from blood to dialysis solution may be enhanced by ultrafiltration. With longer dwell times, the sieving effects of disproportionate water removal would be obliterated by greater net diffusion into the peritoneal dialysis solution. Even at equilibrium, greater amounts of solute would be removed because of the increased drainage volumes (89).

Convective net removal of sodium and potassium per liter of ultrafiltrate usually is well below respective extracellular fluid concentrations (61, 65). The convective component of sodium and potassium removal can be calculated by subtracting net removal accountable to diffusion from the net total removal. Another way to estimate convective transport is to instill solutions with sodium and potassium concentration in Gibbs-Donnan equilibrium with serum water. Although a sieving effect creates a concentration gradient for some diffusion, net electrolyte removal per liter of ultrafiltrate remains far below that in extracellular fluids with 1 to 2 h cycles (89). Severe hypernatremia can result from overly zealous peritoneal ultrafiltration and removal of water without amounts of sodium equal to extracellular concentrations (90, 91; see also Chapter 21).

Hypothesis to explain solute sieving during ultrafiltration

How is it possible that a membrane as permeable as the peritoneum (which, in terms of protein losses, is more permeable than the membrane of hollow-fiber dialyzers [92, 93]) can hinder convective movement of electrolytes with ultrafiltration? The answer to this question is not known. Possible mechanisms for the net electrolyte sieving effect with peritoneal ultrafiltration are summarized in Table 5 and Figure 6.

Table 5. Possible mechanisms for the net electrolyte sieving effect with peritoneal ultrafiltration.

1. Ultrafiltration through narrow intercellular gaps in proximal capillaries
2. Endothelial cell surface charges in intercellular gaps
3. Transendothelial cell water movement
4. Interstitial gel surface charges along aqueous channels
5. Mesothelial cell surface charges in intercellular gaps
6. Transmesothelial cell water movement
7. Dextrose interaction with cations in intercellular gaps or interstitial channels

1. There is substantial evidence that the width of intercellular gaps progressively increases from proximal to distal portions of the capillaries, with the most permeable portions being in the small venules (54). The capillaries of the peritoneum may differ from man-made fibers in having a progressive increase in pore width along the capillary, whereas man-made fibers are more homogenous. At the proximal end of the capillaries, hydrostatic pressure should be higher (53). Glucose should be more osmotically effective across this tighter portion of the capillary than in the distal portion, where glucose may be readily absorbed and exert little osmotic pressure. Thus, combined hydrostatic and osmotic pressure could induce maximum ultrafiltration rates across portions of the capillary that are least permeable.

2. If most of the water flows through the intracellular gap where junctions are rather narrow, then endothelial cell surfaces in close proximity and their respective charges could impede electrolyte movement through the gap.

3. Perhaps when transmembrane hydrostatic and osmotic pressures are high enough, some transendothelial cell water movement does occur (64). Such net movement of water across the cell may occur without proportional movement of electrolytes through the very complex internal cell milieu.

4. Surface charges on the capillary basement membrane or on the surfaces of interstitial gels may impede the movement of charged solutes, which would be akin to the charge interference by polar molecules in the glomerulus (94). That passage of albumin is restrained more by charge than by pore dimensions has been suggested (94).

5. Mesothelial cell surface charges in intercellular gaps could influence electrolyte movements; however, if it is true that mesothelial permeability is much greater than endothelial permeability, then this could be less important than the same phenomenon in the endothelium.

6. The movement of ultrafiltrate from the interstitium into the peritoneal cavity could occur by hydrostatic pressure, with the build-up of fluid in the interstitium and with some osmotic pressure induced by glucose gradients across the mesothelium. If the mesothelium is indeed more permeable than the endothelium, then the major glucose gradient could be across the vessel wall, with only a modest glucose gradient maintained across the mesothelium. Nevertheless, if water does move through mesothelial cells, this could interfere with the convective transport of electrolytes.

7. We have reported studies showing that even neutral molecules may not accompany ultrafiltration induced by glucose osmotic pressure in the same proportions as when ultrafiltration is induced by hydraulic pressure across the same membrane (95). This is not an effect of osmotic pressure *per se,* but perhaps is due to the use of a solute (e.g. glucose) that can enter the membrane and move upstream against the flow of ultrafiltrate (96). We have hypothesized that molecular interaction within the membrane may alter net sieving effects (96).

Figure 6 summarizes these ultrafiltration characteristics during peritoneal dialysis. We have previously presented a hypothesis to explain the net sieving effects reported (97). The primary assumption is that most ultrafiltration is across the proximal capillary where the effective pore width is small compared to that in the distal capillary.

OTHER FACTORS

Body solute distribution volumes, protein binding of solutes, and intracellular trapping

Body solute distribution volumes
Larger body fluid spaces (e.g., when body size is large) are associated with less rapid decreases in blood solute concentrations during dialysis (for solutes that can diffuse readily from extravascular pools into blood [98]). When concentrations decrease rapidly, clearances calculated by using a pre-exchange blood sample rather than a midpoint sample will be spuriously low. Blood concentration changes following an hourly exchange usually are small and within the limits of the laboratory methods. On the other hand, large patients also have greater peritoneal surface area. They may have more fluid-membrane contact per exchange volume and may have higher clearances.

Protein binding of solutes
Total clearances of solutes bound to plasma proteins such as calcium are lower than their molecular size

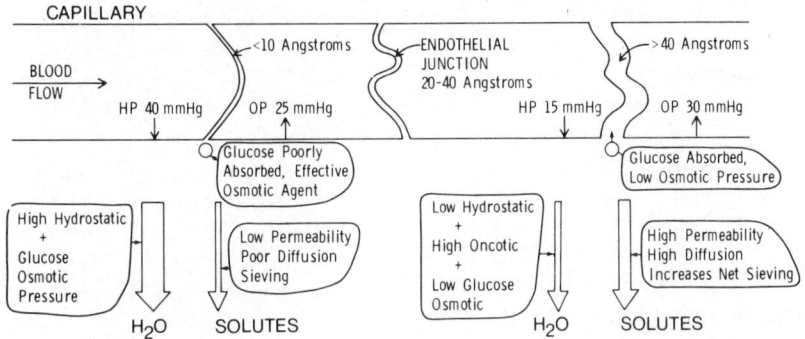

Figure 6. Hypothetical diagrammatic summary of factors influencing ultrafiltration during peritoneal dialysis (see text). (From Nolph et al. [97], with permission of the publisher).
HP = Hydrostatic pressure
OP = Osmotic pressure

would suggest (18). Total clearance may change if fractions of bound and free solute are altered.

Intracellular trapping

Some solutes are not readily mobilized from the intracellular space. This may represent slow diffusion across cell membranes or binding to intracellular constituents. Plasma clearances usually are not affected, but plasma concentrations may rapidly increase immediately post-dialysis for such solutes. With diffusion disequilibrium, plasma clearances overestimate the true clearance from the total space of distribution. Also, if blood samples are allowed to set for any time prior to serum or plasma separation, concentrations in serum or plasma may increase as *in vitro* re-equilibration occurs. Calculated plasma or serum clearances will be lower than actual plasma clearances *in vivo* if separation is delayed.

Lipid solubility

Lipid-soluble substances may be removed in peritoneal dialysis drainage at concentrations higher than in serum (99). Possible explanations include facilitated transport through lipid layers of the cell wall or direct removal of lipid substances from cell surfaces of the peritoneum and cells of the mesentery.

COMPARISONS WITH HOLLOW-FIBER DIALYZERS

Capillary dimensions, configurations, and permeability

Figure 7 shows cross-sections of a peritoneal capillary and a synthetic fiber in a hollow-fiber dialyzer. The

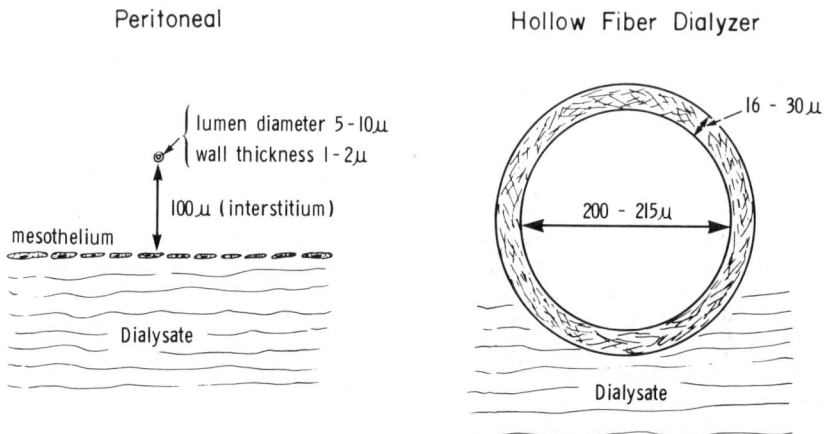

Figure 7. Scaled comparison of peritoneal and hollow-fiber capillaries.

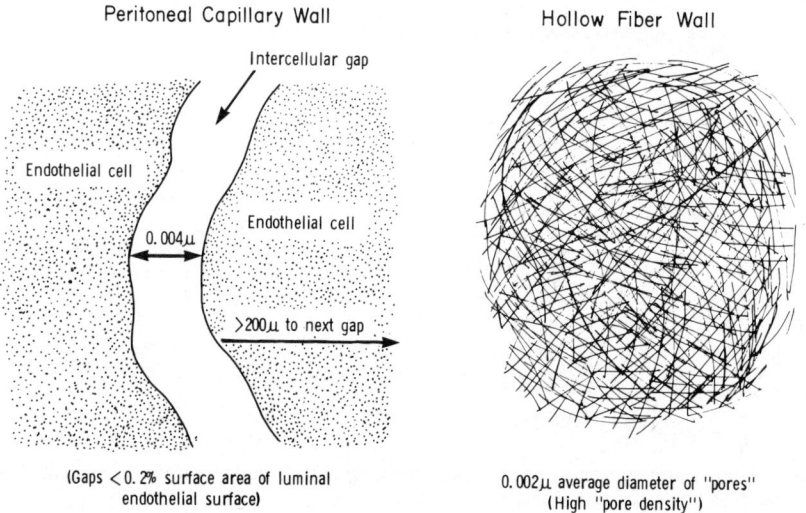

Figure 8. Luminal view of transcapillary pathways for solute movement.

22: *Peritoneal anatomy and transport physiology* 451

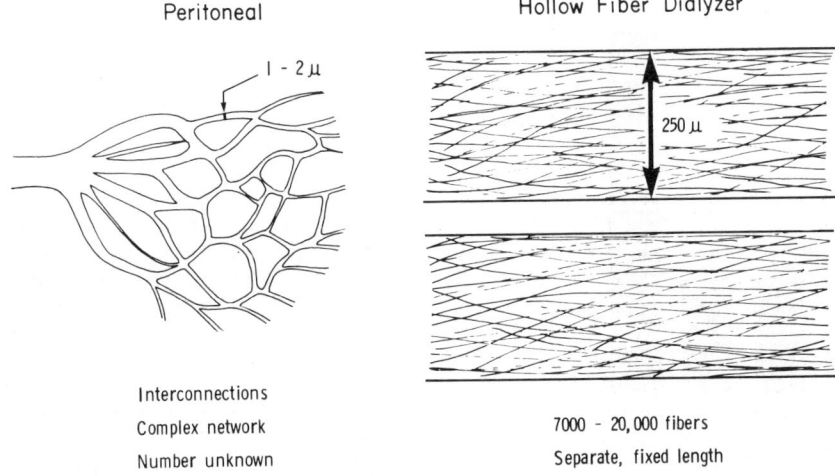

Figure 9. Lateral view of capillaries in peritoneal and hollow-fiber dialysis.

dimensions are drawn to scale, as indicated. Even though the synthetic fiber wall is much thicker, a high fraction of the wall luminal surface may represent 'pore' area. The fiber wall is a mesh synthetic material with many spaces between interstices. In contrast, the peritoneal capillary may have not only a very small relative total luminal surface, but only a small fraction (less than 0.2%, according to Pappenheimer [100]) of that luminal surface may represent 'pore' area. This is true, of course, only if intercellular gaps are indeed the major pathways for solute and water movement from the capillary.

Figure 8 shows lateral views of the fiber walls. This demonstrates even more clearly the great distance that may exist between intercellular slits in capillary endothelium and in contrast, the high fraction of synthetic fiber walls representing space available for solute exchange between the molecules, composing the wall.

Figure 9 shows lateral views of the course of capillaries in the peritoneal membrane and synthetic fibers in a hollow-fiber dialyzer. Notice that the capillary network in the peritoneal system is complex, with many interconnections. The total number of capillaries participating in exchange is unknown. In contrast, each fiber in the hollow-fiber dialyzers is a separate entity. There are no interconnections and the numbers are well known, depending on the type of hollow-fiber dialyzer. In the peritoneal system, only a portion of capillaries may be perfused at any one time, as others may essentially be closed down by precapillary sphincter tone (5). In contrast, most fibers in the hollow-fiber dialyzer are perfused simultaneously in the absence of fiber plugging (101).

Dialysate flow characteristics

Figure 10 compares typical dialysate flow rates in milliliters per minute and in liters per week for dialysis with a hollow-fiber dialyzer (12 h per week), intermittent per-

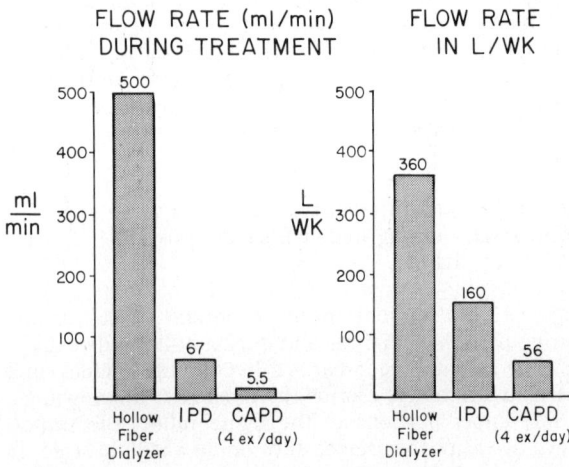

Figure 10. Dialysate flow rates for hollow-fiber dialyzers, intermittent peritoneal dialysis (IPD) and continuous ambulatory peritoneal dialysis (CAPD) are compared in ml/min and l/wk.

itoneal dialysis (40 h per week), and continuous ambulatory peritoneal dialysis (four 2-liter exchanges per day). This figure does not include ultrafiltration rates that have little impact on the values for hollow-fiber dialysis and intermittent peritoneal dialysis but add substantially to total flow for continuous ambulatory peritoneal dialysis.

With hollow-fiber dialysis, urea clearances are primarily blood-flow-limited; with intermittent peritoneal dialysis, urea clearances during treatment probably are limited primarily by fluid film resistances, for the reasons discussed above; with continuous ambulatory peritoneal dialysis, the urea clearances are limited by dialysis solution flow rate and are nearly identical to dialysis solution flow rate.

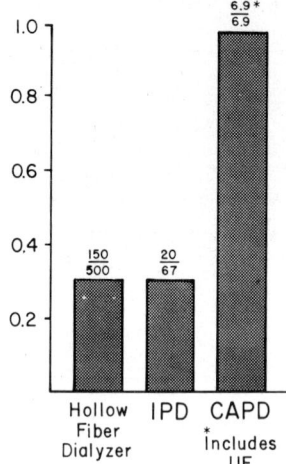

Figure 11. The ratios of urea clearance/dialysate flow for different techniques are compared, as in Figure 10.

Figure 11 shows that typical urea clearances during treatment sessions are nearly one-third of the dialysis solution rate for both hollow-fiber dialysis and intermittent peritoneal dialysis. During continuous ambulatory peritoneal dialysis, the ratio of urea clearance to flow rate of dialysis solution approaches 1.0 (101–107).

Comparisons of different resistances for large and small solutes during hollow-fiber dialysis and peritoneal dialysis

Figure 12 is a summary of the important resistance sites during peritoneal dialysis and during hollow-fiber dialysis. The height of each bar is a hypothetical value, since the actual numbers are for the most part unknown.

The upper portions of the figure reflect the importance of various resistance sites on an absolute scale. In peritoneal dialysis, the vascular wall probably offers substantial resistance only to the solutes larger than

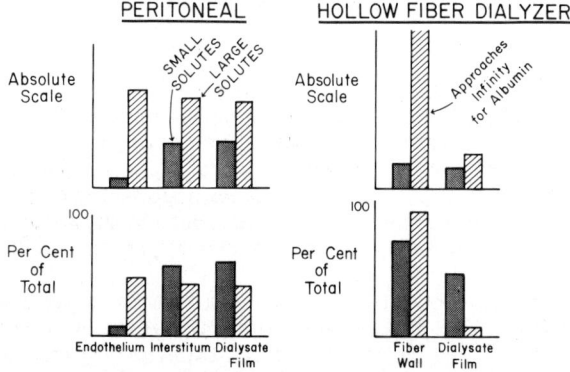

Figure 12. Hypothetical absolute and relative magnitudes of various resistances in peritoneal dialysis and hollow-fiber dialysis for small (<100 daltons) and large (>5000 daltons) solutes (see text). Blood film resistances are not compared but are especially important in extracorporeal dialyzers.

1000 daltons (54). For smaller solutes, this is a short distance to traverse with a relatively large mean pore size (perhaps greater than 40 Å in width at the venular end of the capillary) (7, 8, 77). The interstitial resistance is substantial for both small and large solutes. Again, this would be an even greater resistance for large solutes, since they must diffuse across this distance, and greater hindrance by the dimensions of the aqueous channels (if such truly exists) would be expected. The fluid films in the peritoneal cavity offer substantial resistance to both small and large solutes. The resistance to the latter would be greater because of the distances involved and their poorer diffusibility. Mesothelial resistance is not shown, since intercellular gaps may be 500 Å or more in diameter and there is little evidence to suggest that mesothelium is a major resistance site (9, 82, 83). Intracapillary stagnant fluid films and capillary basement membranes are not shown, since they also are not known to be major resistance sites.

Below these hypothetical absolute resistance values for peritoneal dialysis are figures showing relative resistances. In the case of urea clearance, the interstitium and the fluid films are proportionately greater resistances. Because the vascular wall is a major resistance site for large solutes, interstitial and dialysis solution fluid films are proportionally shown as less important.

In the hollow-fiber dialyzer, there are only two major resistance sites: the fiber wall and fluid films. The mean pore size of the fiber wall may be 20 Å or less (108). Synthetic fiber resistance to very large solutes such as albumin approach infinity, since fibers are impermeable to solutes of such a size. The thickness of the fiber wall makes the fiber an important resistance site for urea, primarily, perhaps, because of the distance involved. Dialysis solution fluid film resistances are much smaller than in peritoneal dialysis for reasons discussed. Thus, on a relative scale, the fiber wall would offer a high proportion of the total resistance to movement of both small and large solutes.

Blood flow comparisons

Figure 3 relates the clearance of urea to blood flow during hollow-fiber dialysis and to hypothetical effective peritoneal capillary blood flow during peritoneal dialysis. Hollow-fiber dialyzers are so efficient that urea clearance is limited markedly by blood flow. Gas diffusion studies previously mentioned suggest that effective peritoneal capillary blood flow during peritoneal dialysis in adults of a normal size is near 60 to 70 ml/min and do not explain maximum urea clearances during rapid cycling peritoneal dialysis of only near 30 ml/min (4, 76).

MANIPULATING PERITONEAL TRANSPORT

Cycling time

Figure 13 shows the effects of dialysate flow rates on peritoneal clearances of urea. At rates above 4 l/h, peri-

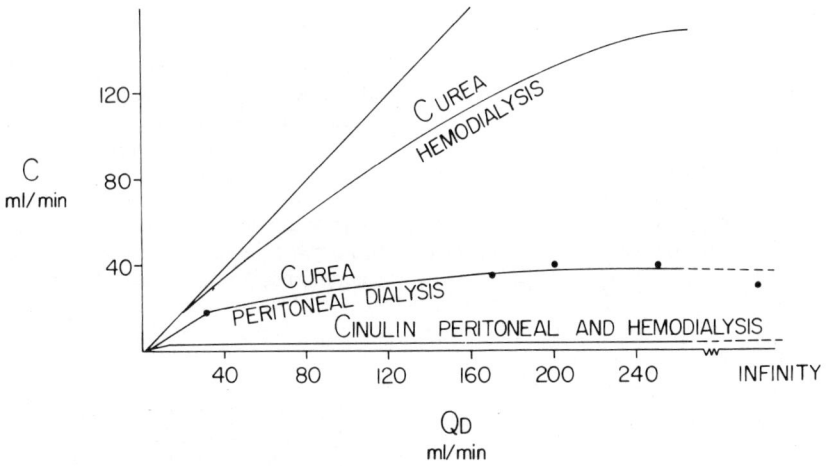

Figure 13. Typical clearances of urea and inulin during peritoneal and hemodialysis related to dialysate flow rate (Q_D). (From Nolph et al. [4] with permission of the publisher).

toneal clearances are only moderately dialysate flow rate-limited and approach maximum clearances. Many techniques for increasing dialysis solution flow rate have been described (78). Although studies suggest that clearances relate to flow rate in a fairly fixed manner regardless of the cycle or residual volumes used, further investigation is needed.

Vasoactive substances

Table 6 summarizes all substances that reportedly alter the status of the peritoneal microcirculation by intraperitoneal or systemic administration (49, 50). Vasodilatory drugs presumably increase clearances by increasing the number of capillaries perfused, opening more permeable capillaries, and minimizing blood flow limitations, if present. Vasoconstrictors tend to decrease the number of capillaries perfused and close down more permeable capillaries, and may introduce some blood flow limitations on small solute clearances.

All commercial peritoneal dialysis solutions appear to cause a transient constriction of the microvasculature of the parietal peritoneum (lasting 1 to 3 min), but subsequently cause a marked (150 to 200%), sustained vasodilation of parietal, as well as visceral, peritoneal vessels (43). The vasoconstrictive component of the solutions has not been identified, but does not appear to be the pH (43). Studies in rats strongly suggest that the vasodilatory components of solutions are the hyperosmolality and nonbicarbonate anions (72). Very high molecular weight vasodilators may not be effective if administered intraperitoneally. Glucagon, for example, increases clearances only when given intravenously unless dosage is very high by the intraperitoneal route (109). It has been suggested that glucagon is too large to effectively cross the mesothelium and interstitium and achieve high concentrations at vascular receptor sites (109). (Very large doses overcome the slow absorption from the peritoneum and are effective.) Whether other agents exert their vasodilatory effects by reaching receptor sites from the luminal side of the vessel or from the extraluminal side when administered intraperitoneally is unclear.

Table 6. Substances reportedly affecting peritoneal clearances.

Nitroprusside (IP)
Dopamine (IP, IV)
Norepinephrine (IV)
Bradykinin (IP)
Diazoxide (IP)
Dipyridamole (PO, IP, IV)
Ethacrynic acid (IP)
Furosemide (IP)
Glucagon (IP, IV)
Histamine (IP)
Tolazoline (IP)
Isoproterenol (IP)
Secretin (IV)
Prostaglandins (IP)
Dioctyl sodium succinate (IP)

( ) = route of administration
IP = intraperitoneal
IV = intravenous
PO = by mouth

Manipulating the interstitium

Preliminary studies suggest that hypo-osmolar solution may reduce interstitial resistance and increase protein losses (86). Figure 5 demonstrates the hypothesis to explain such an observation. The number and dimensions of aqueous channels through the interstitium may be increased by better hydration, since hyperosmolar solutions could cause interstitial dehydration leading to an increased resistance to passive solute movement through the interstitium.

Other drug effects

Diuretics seem to have a slight influence on the net removal of electrolytes during peritoneal dialysis (88). The mechanisms to explain this are not known, but possibly relate to alterations in mesothelial cell surface charges.

Surface-acting agents

Surface-acting agents such as dioctyl sodium sulfosuccinate reportedly increase clearances when administered intraperitoneally (110). Whether these agents alter the status of the microcirculation or influence the other components of resistance in the peritoneal membrane is not known. And whether the dimensions of aqueous channels through the interstitium or fluid films adjacent to the mesothelium could be changed by altering surface tensions also is not known.

REFERENCES

1. Cunningham RS: The physiology of the serous membranes. *Physiol Rev* 6:242, 1926
2. Putnam TJ: The living peritoneum as a dialyzing membrane. *Am J Physiol* 63:547, 1922-1923
3. Henderson LW: Peritoneal dialysis. In: *Clinical Aspects of Uremia and Dialysis,* edited by Massry SG, Sellers AL, Springfield IL, Charles C Thomas, 1976
4. Nolph KD, Popovich RP, Ghods AJ, Twardowski Z: Determinants of low clearances of small solutes during peritoneal dialysis. *Kidney Int* 13:117, 1978
5. Nolph KD, Miller F, Rubin J, Popovich RP: New directions in peritoneal dialysis concepts and applications. *Kidney Int* 18, (Suppl 10):S111, 1980
6. Nolph KD, Ghods AJ, Brown P, Van Stone J, Miller FN, Wiegman DL, Harris PD: Factors affecting peritoneal dialysis efficiency. *Dial Transpl* 6:52, 1977
7. Karnovsky MJ: The ultrastructural basis of capillary permeability studied with peroxides as a tracer. *J Cell Biol* 3:213, 1967
8. Cotran RS: The fine structure of the microvasculature in relation to normal and altered permeability. In: *Physical Bases of Circulatory Transport: Regulation and Exchange,* edited by Reeve EB, Guyton AC, Philadelphia, PA, WB Saunders Co, 1967
9. Rasio EA: Metabolic control of permeability in isolated mesentery. *Am J Physiol* 276:962, 1974
10. Miller F: The peritoneal microcirculation. In: *Peritoneal Dialysis,* edited by Nolph KD, The Hague, Boston, London, Martinus Nijhoff, 1981
11. Tsilibary EC, Wissig SL: Absorption from the peritoneal cavity: SEM study of the mesothelium covering the peritoneal surface of the muscular portion of the diaphragm. *Am J Anat* 149:127, 1977
12. Cascarano J, Rubin AD, Chick WL, Sweifach BW: Metabolically induced permeability changes across mesothelium and endothelium. *Am J Physiol* 206:373, 1964
13. Nolph KD, Rosenfeld PS, Powell JT, Danforth E Jr: Peritoneal glucose transport in hyperglycemia during peritoneal dialysis. *Am J Med Sci* 259:272, 1970
14. Maher JF: Principles of dialysis and dialysis of drugs. *Am J Med* 62:475, 1977
15. Bomar JB, Decker JS, Dechard JF, Hlavinka DJ, Moncrief JW, Popovich RP: The elucidation of maximum efficiency minimum cost peritoneal dialysis protocols. *Trans Am Soc Artif Intern Organs* 20:120, 1974
16. Henderson LW, Nolph KD: Altered permeability of the peritoneal membrane after using hypertonic peritoneal dialysis fluid. *J Clin Invest* 48:992, 1969
17. Babb AL, Johansen PJ, Strand MJ, Tenckhoff H, Scribner BH: Bi-directional permeability of the human peritoneum to middle molecules. *Proc Eur Dial Transpl Assoc* 10:247, 1973
18. Boen ST: *Peritoneal Dialysis in Clinical Medicine,* Springfield IL, Charles C Thomas, 1964
19. Boen ST: Kinetics of peritoneal dialysis, comparison with artificial kidney. *Medicine* 40:243, 1961
20. Penzotti SC, Mattocks AM: Effects of dwell time, volume of dialysis fluid, and added accelerators on peritoneal dialysis of urea. *J Pharm Sci* 60:1520, 1971
21. Tenckhoff H, Ward G, Boen ST: The influence of dialysate volume and flow rate on peritoneal clearance. *Proc Eur Dial Transpl Assoc* 2:113, 1965
22. Lange K, Treser G: Automatic continuous high flow peritoneal dialysis. *Trans Am Soc Artif Intern Organs* 13:164, 1967
23. Lange K, Treser H, Managalap J: Automatic continuous high flow rate peritoneal dialysis. *Arch Klin Med* 214:201, 1968
24. Stephen RL, Atkin-Thor E, Kolff WJ: Recirculating peritoneal dialysis with subcutaneous catheter. *Trans Am Soc Artif Intern Organs* 22:575, 1976
25. Lewin AK, Greenbaum MA, Gordon A, Maxwell MH: Sorbent based regenerating delivery system for use in peritoneal dialysis. *Trans Am Soc Artif Intern Organs* 20:130, 1974
26. Shinaberger JH, Shear L, Barry KG: Increasing efficiency of peritoneal dialysis-experience with peritoneal extracorporeal recirculation dialysis. *Trans Am Soc Artif Intern Organs* 11:76, 1965
27. Kablitz C, Stephen RL, Duffy DP: Technological augmentation of peritoneal urea clearance: past, present and future. *Dial Transpl* 9:741, 1980
28. Finkelstein FO, Kliger AS: Enhanced efficiency of peritoneal dialysis using rapid, small-volume exchanges. *asaio J* 2:103, 1979
29. Warden GD, Maxwell JG, Stephen RL: The use of reciprocating peritoneal dialysis with a subcutaneous peritoneal catheter in end-stage renal failure in diabetes mellitus. *J Surg Res* 24:495, 1978
30. Blumenkrantz MJ, Gordon A, Roberts M: Applications of the Redy sorbent system to hemodialysis and peritoneal dialysis. *Artif Organs* 3:230, 1979
31. Gross M, McDonald HP Jr: Effects of dialysate temperature and flow rate on peritoneal clearance. *JAMA* 202:215, 1967
32. Knochel JP, Mason AD: Effect of alkalinization on peritoneal diffusion of uric acid. *Am J Physiol* 210:1160, 1966
33. Deger GE, Wagoner RD: Peritoneal dialysis in acute uric acid nephropathy. *Mayo Clin Proc* 47:189, 1972

34. Campion DS, North JP: Effect of protein binding of barbiturates on their rate of removal during peritoneal dialysis. *J Lab Clin Med* 66:549, 1965
35. Rubin J, Nolph KD, Popovich RP, Moncrief J, Prowant B: Drainage volumes during CAPD. *asaio J* 2:2, 1979
36. Popovich RP, Moncrief JW, Nolph KD, Ghods AJ, Twardowski ZJ, Pyle WK: Continuous ambulatory peritoneal dialysis. *Ann Intern Med* 88:449, 1978
37. Erbe RW, Greene JA Jr, Weller JM: Peritoneal dialysis during hemorrhagic shock. *J Appl Physiol* 22:131, 1967
38. Hare HG, Valtin H, Gosselin RE: Effects of drugs on peritoneal dialysis in the dog. *J Pharmacol Exp Ther* 145:122, 1964
39. Henderson LW, Kintzel JE: Influence of antidiuretic hormone on peritoneal membrane area and permeability. *J Clin Invest* 50:2437, 1971
40. Chan MK, Varghese Z, Baillod RA, Moorhead JF: Peritoneal dialysis: effect of intraperitoneal dopamine. *Dial Transpl* 9:382, 1980
41. Gutman RA, Nixon WP, McRae RL, Spencer HW: Effect of intraperitoneal and intravenous vasoactive amines on peritoneal dialysis: study in anephric dogs. *Trans Am Soc Artif Intern Organs* 22:570, 1976
42. Miller FN, Nolph KD, Harris PD, Rubin J, Wiegman DL, Joshua IG: Effects of peritoneal dialysis solutions on human clearances and rat arterioles. *Trans Am Soc Artif Intern Organs* 24:131, 1978
43. Miller FN, Nolph KD, Harris PD, Rubin J, Wiegman DL, Joshua IG, Twardowski ZJ, Ghods AJ: Microvascular and clinical effects of altered peritoneal dialysis solutions. *Kidney Int* 15:630, 1979
44. Nolph KD, Ghods AJ, Van Stone J, Brown PA: The effects of intraperitoneal vasodilators on peritoneal clearances. *Trans Am Soc Artif Intern Organs* 22:586, 1976
45. Nolph KD, Ghods AJ, Brown PA, Miller FN, Harris P, Pyle K, Popovich R: Effects of nitroprusside on peritoneal mass transfer coefficients and microvascular physiology. *Trans Am Soc Artif Intern Organs* 23:210, 1977
46. Nolph KD, Ghods AJ, Brown PA, Twardowski ZJ: Effects of intraperitoneal nitroprusside on peritoneal clearances with variations in dose, frequency of administration, and dwell times. *Nephron* 24:114, 1979
47. Nolph KD: Effects of intraperitoneal vasodilators on peritoneal clearances. *Dial Transpl* 7:812, 1978
48. Hirszel P, Lasrich M, Maher JF: Augmentation of peritoneal mass transport by dopamine. *J Lab Clin Med* 94:747, 1979
49. Gutman RA: Toward enhancement of peritoneal clearances. *Dial Transpl* 8:1072, 1979
50. Maher JF: Acceleration of peritoneal mass transport by drugs and hormones. *Artif Organs* 3:224, 1979
51. Felt J, Richard E, McCaffrey C: Peritoneal clearance of creatinine and inulin during dialysis in dogs: Effect of splanchnic vasodilators. *Kidney Int* 16:459, 1979
52. Maher JF, Hirszel P, Lasrich M: Modulation of peritoneal transport rates by prostaglandins. *Adv Prostaglandin Thromboxane Res* 7:695, 1980
53. Renkin EM: Exchange of substances through capillary walls: Circulatory and respiratory mass transport. In: *Ciba Foundation Symposium,* edited by Wolstenholme GEW, Boston, Little Brown, 1969, p 50
54. Wayland H: Transmural and interstitial molecular transport. Action of histamine. In: *Continuous Ambulatory Peritoneal Dialysis,* edited by Legrain M, Amsterdam, Excerpta Medica, 1980, p 20
55. Miller FN, Joshua IG, Harris PD, Wiegman DL, Jauchem JR: Peritoneal dialysis solutions and the microcirculation. *Contrib Nephrol* 17:51, 1979
56. Nolph KD, Stoltz M, Maher JF: Altered peritoneal permeability in patients with systemic vasculitis. *Ann Intern Med* 78:891, 1973
57. Brown ST, Ahearn DJ, Nolph KD: Reduced peritoneal clearances in scleroderma increased by intraperitoneal isoproterenol. *Ann Intern Med* 78:891, 1973
58. Manery JF: Water and electrolyte metabolism. *Physiol Rev* 34:334, 1954
59. Tarail R, Hacker ES, Taylor R: The ultrafilterability of potassium and sodium in human serum. *J Clin Invest* 31:23, 1952
60. Folk BP, Zierler KL, Lilienthal JL: Distribution of potassium and sodium between serum and certain extracellular fluids in man. *Am J Physiol* 153:381, 1948
61. Brown ST, Ahearn DJ, Nolph KD: Potassium removal with peritoneal dialysis. *Kidney Int* 4:67, 1973
62. Kelton JG, Vlan R, Stiller C, Holmes E: Comparison of chemical composition of peritoneal fluid and serum. *Ann Intern Med* 89:67, 1978
63. Henderson LW: Peritoneal ultrafiltration dialysis: Enhanced urea transfer using hypertonic peritoneal dialysis fluid. *J Clin Invest* 45:950, 1966
64. Ahearn DJ, Nolph KD: Controlled sodium removal with peritoneal dialysis. *Trans Am Soc Artif Intern Organs* 18:423, 1972
65. Nolph KD, Hano JE, Teschan PE: Peritoneal sodium transport during hypertonic peritoneal dialysis: Physiologic mechanisms and clinical implications. *Ann Intern Med* 70:931, 1969
66. Nolph KD, Sorkin MI, Moore H: Autoregulation of sodium and potassium removal during continuous ambulatory peritoneal dialysis. *Trans Am Soc Artif Intern Organs* 26:334, 1980
67. Nolph KD: CAPD – A logical approach to peritoneal dialysis limitations (A comparison of the peritoneal dialysis system and hollow fiber kidneys). *Int J Nephrol Urol Androl* 1:5, 1980
68. Wayland H, Silberberg A: Blood to lymph transport. *Microvasc Res* 15:367, 1978
69. Nolph KD, Prowant B: Complications during continuous ambulatory peritoneal dialysis. In: *Continuous Ambulatory Peritoneal Dialysis,* edited by Legrain M, Amsterdam, Excerpta Medica, 1980, p 258
70. Rubin J, Rogers WA, Taylor HM, Everett ED, Prowant BP, Fruto LV, Nolph KD: Peritonitis during continuous ambulatory peritoneal dialysis. *Ann Intern Med* 92:7, 1980
71. Wade OL, Combes B, Childs AW, Wheeler HO, Dournand D, Bradley SE: The effect of exercise on the splanchnic blood flow and splanchnic blood volume in normal man. *Clin Sci* 15:457, 1956
72. Miller FN, Nolph KD, Joshua IG: The osmolality component of peritoneal dialysis solutions. In: *Continuous Ambulatory Peritoneal Dialysis,* edited by Legrain M, Amsterdam, Excerpta Medica, 1980, p 12
73. Nolph KD: Introductory remarks: Anatomy, physiology and kinetics of peritoneal transport during peritoneal dialysis. In: *Continuous Ambulatory Peritoneal Dialysis,* edited by Legrain M, Amsterdam, Excerpta Medica, 1980, p 7
74. Goldschmidt ZH, Pote HH, Katz MA, Shear L: Effect of dialysate volume on peritoneal dialysis kinetics. *Kidney Int* 5:240, 1975
75. Miller FN, Wiegman DL, Joshua IG, Nolph KD, Rubin J: Effects of vasodilators and peritoneal dialysis solution on the microcirculation of the rat cecum. *Proc Soc Exp Biol Med* 161:605, 1979
76. Aune S: Transperitoneal exchange. II. Peritoneal blood

flow estimated by hydrogen gas clearance. *Scand J Gastroenterol* 5:99, 1970
77. Karnovsky MJ: The ultrastructural basis of transcapillary exchanges. In: *Biological Interfaces: Flows and Exchanges,* Boston, Little Brown, 1968, p 64
78. Nolph KD: Peritoneal dialysis. In: *Replacement of Renal Function by Dialysis,* edited by Drukker W, Parsons FM, Maher JF, The Hague, Boston, London, Martinus Nijhoff, First edition, 1978, p 277
79. Blumenkrantz MJ, Roberts CE, Card B: Nutritional management of the adult patient undergoing peritoneal dialysis. *J Am Diet Assoc,* 73:351, 1978
80. Giordano C, De Santo NG: Dietary management of patients on peritoneal dialysis. *Contrib Nephrol* 17:77, 1979
81. Kobayashi K, Manji T, Hiramatsu S: Nitrogen metabolism in patients on peritoneal dialysis. *Contrib Nephrol* 17:93, 1979
82. Nagel W, Kuschinsky W: Study of the permeability of isolated dog mesentery. *Eur J Clin Invest* 1:149, 1970
83. Gosselin RE, Berndt WO: Diffusional transport of solutes through mesentery and peritoneum. *J Theor Biol* 3:487, 1962
84. Maher JF, Nolph KD: Factors affecting optimal performance of coil dialyzers. *Proc 6th Int Congr Nephrol,* edited by Giovannetti S, Bonomini V, D'Amico G, Basel, S Karger 6:657 1976
85. Maher JF, Nolph KD: Resistance to diffusion in dialyzers. *Clin Nephrol* 1:333, 1974
86. Rubin J, Nolph KD, Arfania D, Miller FM, Wiegman DL, Joshua IG, Harris PD: Studies on non-vasoactive peritoneal dialysis solutions. *J Lab Clin Med* 93:910, 1979
87. McGary TJ, Nolph KD, Rubin J: In vitro simulations of peritoneal dialysis: A technique for demonstrating limitations on solute clearances due to stagnant fluid films and poor mixing. *J Lab Clin Med* 96:148, 1980
88. Maher JF, Hohndel DC, Shea C, Di Sanzo F, Cassetta M: Effects of intraperitoneal diuretics on solute transport during hypertonic dialysis. *Clin Nephrol* 7:96, 1977
89. Nolph KD, Twardowski ZJ, Popovich RP, Rubin J: Equilibration of peritoneal dialysis solutions during long dwell exchanges. *J Lab Clin Med* 246:256, 1979
90. Boyer J, Gill GN, Epstein FH: Hyperglycemia and hyperosmolality complicating peritoneal dialysis. *Ann Intern Med* 67:568, 1967
91. Smith RJ, Block MR, Arieff AI, Blumenkrantz MJ, Coburn JW: Hypernatremic, hyperosmolar coma complicating chronic peritoneal dialysis. *Proc Clin Dial Transpl Forum* 4:96, 1974
92. Nolph KD, New DL: Effects of ultrafiltration on solute clearances in hollow fiber artificial kidneys. *J Lab Clin Med* 88:593, 1976
93. Nolph KD, Stoltz ML, Maher JF: Electrolyte transport during ultrafiltration of protein solutions. *Nephron* 8:473, 1971
94. Glassock RJ: The nephrotic syndrom. *Hosp Pract* 14:105, 1979
95. Nolph KD, Hopkins CA, New D, Antwiler GD, Popovich RP: Differences in solute sieving with osmotic vs. hydrostatic ultrafiltration. *Trans Am Soc Artif Intern Organs* 22:618, 1976
96. Twardowski ZJ, Nolph KD, Popovich RP, Hopkins CA: Comparison of polymer, glucose, and hydrostatic pressure induced ultrafiltration in a hollow fiber dialyzer: Effects on convective solute transport. *J Lab Clin Med* 92:619, 1978
97. Nolph KD, Miller FN, Pyle K, Popovich RP, Sorking MI: A hypothesis to explain the characteristics of peritoneal ultrafiltration. *Kidney Int* 20:543, 1981
98. Nolph KD, Whitcomb ME, Schrier RW: Mechanisms for inefficient peritoneal dialysis in acute renal failure associated with heat stress and exercise. *Ann Intern Med* 71:317, 1969
99. Maher JF, Hirszel P, Hohnadel DC, Abraham J, Lasrich M: Fatty acid removal during peritoneal dialysis: mechanisms, rates and significance. *asaio J* 1:8, 1978
100. Pappenheimer JR: Passage of molecules through capillary walls. *Physiol Rev* 33:387, 1953
101. Nolph KD, Ahearn DJ, Esterly JA, Maher JF: Irreversible morphological and functional changes in hollow fiber kidneys with a single dialysis. *Trans Am Soc Artif Intern Organs* 20:604, 1974
102. Nolph KD: Peritoneal clearances. *J Lab Clin Med* 94:519, 1979
103. Nolph KD, Popovich RP, Moncrief JW: Theoretical and practical implications of continuous ambulatory peritoneal dialysis. *Nephron* 21:117, 1978
104. Popovich RP, Moncrief JW: Kinetic modeling of peritoneal transport. *Contrib Nephrol* 17:59, 1979
105. Popovich RP, Pyle WK, Moncrief JW: Peritoneal dialysis. *Am Inst Chem Eng Symp Series* 75:31, 1979
106. Popovich RP, Pyle WK, Hiatt MP, McCollough WS, Moncrief JW: Metabolite transport kinetics in peritoneal dialysis. In: *Continuous Ambulatory Peritoneal Dialysis,* edited by Legrain M, Amsterdam, *Excerpta Medica,* 1980, p 28
107. Popovich RP, Moncrief JW, Nolph KD, Ghods AJ, Twardowski ZJ, Pyle WK: Continuous ambulatory peritoneal dialysis. *Ann Intern Med* 88:449, 1978
108. Green DM, Antwiler GD, Moncrief JW, Decherd JF, Popovich RP: Measurement of the transmittance coefficient spectrum of cuprophan. *Trans Am Soc Artif Intern Organs* 22:627, 1976
109. Hirszel P, Maher JF, LeGrow W: Increased peritoneal mass transport with glucagon acting at the vascular surface. *Trans Am Soc Artif Intern Organs* 24:136, 1979
110. Mattocks AM, Penzotti SC: Acceleration of peritoneal dialysis with minimum amounts of dioctyl sodium sulfosuccinate. *J Pharm Sci* 61:475, 1972

23
PRACTICAL USE OF PERITONEAL DIALYSIS

CHARLES M. MION

Introduction	457
Technical aspects of peritoneal dialysis	458
Access to the peritoneal cavity	458
A mandatory prerequisite: sterility and aseptic techniques	458
Disposable versus permanent catheters	458
Recommendations for placement of peritoneal catheters and preparation of the patient	458
Deane's prosthesis	459
Complications related to insertion of stylet catheters	459
The permanent Silastic Tenckhoff catheter	460
Implantation of the Tenckhoff catheter	460
Catheter care	461
Other indwelling catheters	461
Complications related to placement of indwelling silastic catheters	462
Catheter revision: removal and replacement	463
Catheter survival	464
Dialysis solutions	464
Composition of dialysis solutions	464
Delivery and storage of dialysis solutions	465
Concentrated solutions	465
Peritoneal dialysis equipment and automatic machines	465
Automatic cyclers	466
Reverse osmosis machines	466
Manual technique	467
Sorbent peritoneal dialysate regeneration system	468
The peritoneal dialysis procedure	468
Maintenance of sterility	468
Exchange cycles	468
Periodic peritoneal dialysis	468
Continuous ambulatory peritoneal dialysis (CAPD)	468
Side effects and complications of peritoneal dialysis	469
Side effects	469
Metabolic disturbances	469
Haemodynamic and cardiorespiratory side effects	470
Gastro-intestinal side effects	470
Thirst	470
Complications of peritoneal dialysis	470
Pain	470
Peritonitis	470
Metabolic complications	475
Miscellaneous complications	475
Indications for peritoneal dialysis	476
Peritoneal dialysis in acute renal failure	476
Peritoneal dialysis in chronic renal failure	476
Peritoneal dialysis in treatment of poisoning	477
Peritoneal dialysis in miscellaneous conditions (in the adult)	477
Special indications in children	477
Contra-indications to peritoneal dialysis	477
Maintenance peritoneal dialysis	478
Periodic peritoneal dialysis	478
Dialysis schedules	478
Effect of residual renal function on dialysis requirements	478
Clinical results	478
Home versus hospital peritoneal dialysis	479
Long term results and actuarial survival rates	479
Continuous ambulatory peritoneal dialysis	479
Dialysis schedules	479
Clinical and biochemical results with CAPD	479
Survival of CAPD patients	479
Periodic versus continuous ambulatory peritoneal dialysis	480
Special indications for peritoneal dialysis	480
End stage diabetic nephropathy	480
Maintenance peritoneal dialysis and transplantation	480
Maintenance peritoneal dialysis in children	480
The future of peritoneal dialysis	480
Decay of the peritoneal membrane	481
Maintenance peritoneal dialysis versus haemodialysis	481
Future role of peritoneal dialysis in the treatment of terminal chronic renal failure	481
References	481

INTRODUCTION

The modern era of clinical peritoneal dialysis started in 1959 with the introduction of the single catheter method and of commercially prepared dialysis solution (1). Peritoneal dialysis then became an established method for the treatment of acute renal failure, but many clinicians were reluctant to use it despite its technical simplicity, because of a high incidence of associated peritonitis, a lower efficacy in comparison with haemodialysis and the rather high cost of commercially prepared dialysis solutions. From 1961 to 1972, these shortcomings were partly overcome due to many conceptual and technological advances including: a better understanding of solute peritoneal transfer kinetics which gave a rational basis for improving peritoneal clearances (2, 3); the development of automated closed circuit dialysate delivery systems which strikingly reduced the incidence of peritoneal infection (4); the introduction of a bacteriologically safe peritoneal access device which eliminated the difficulties and hazards of the repeated puncture technique (5); and finally simplified logistics and reduced costs which were obtained when the reverse osmosis machines became available for the continuous production of sterile, apyrogenic dialysis fluid at the bedside (6). Despite these improvements and early clinical studies demonstrating its feasibility and efficiency in patients with chronic uraemia (7-10), peritoneal dialysis was long regarded as having little place in the treatment of end stage renal disease, except in a few dedicated dialysis centres. In 1976, the concept of a 'portable wearable equilibrium' peritoneal dialysis technique was introduced (11). This new approach resulting in steady low blood levels of uraemic metabolites was later developed as continuous ambulatory peritoneal dialysis (CAPD), the technique being simplified with the introduction of dialysis solutions in plastic bags (12, 13). Continuous ambulatory peritoneal dialysis stimulated a wave of enthusiasm among nephrologists and the number of end stage uraemic patients treated with this method has increased rapidly in Europe as well as in the U.S.A. (14). Today, there is no doubt that peritoneal dialysis will remain an accepted treatment of end-stage renal disease (15). The return to the original simplicity of the open dialysis system, however, has brought back on the front page the problem of peritoneal infection and its prevention (16).

In this chapter, the practical aspects of peritoneal dialysis will be discussed. The aim is to provide detailed information on the available techniques and also to present a balanced view on the advantages and shortcomings of peritoneal dialysis.

TECHNICAL ASPECTS OF PERITONEAL DIALYSIS

Access to the peritoneal cavity

A mandatory prerequisite:
sterility and aseptic technique
When starting peritoneal dialysis, the physician should keep in mind that bacterial contamination of the peritoneum is a permanent risk. Peritonitis should be seen as a life threatening complication (17) and every effort should be made to prevent it. Asepsis is the safest and most cost effective approach for prophylaxis of infection (18). Aseptic procedures are too often neglected by physicians who wrongly prefer to rely upon antibiotics in case of peritoneal infection; the importance of aseptic procedures in reducing peritoneal infection rate to an acceptable level has been demonstrated (19). It is the physician's responsibility to monitor very frequently aseptic techniques lest patients and nurses become negligent. The use of iodine compounds for chemical 'sterilisation' is recommended to prepare the patient and the equipment and in all connect-disconnect procedures of peritoneal dialysis. It should be kept in mind that a five minute delay is necessary for effective contact disinfection with povidone-iodine solutions (Betadine) which are commonly used because of a good skin tolerance.

Peritoneal dialysis is done almost universally with the single catheter method (1), which permits the tidal irrigation of the peritoneum without channelling, and being the technique of choice for its simplicity and safety. Two main types of peritoneal catheters are currently available: the disposable stylet catheter (Trocath) (20) and the permanent Silastic catheter (5).

Disposable versus permanent catheters
Permanent (indwelling) Silastic catheters, besides being bacteriologically safer when used with a closed dialysate delivery circuit (6, 7) have many advantages over disposable catheters. The advantages include avoidance of repeated puncture, ease of instituting dialysis, excellent irrigation characteristics independent of the patient's position, no pain during or between dialyses, few restrictions in physical or recreational activities leading to excellent patient acceptance and suitability for self dialysis (21). Therefore, Silastic indwelling peritoneal catheters are preferred in most circumstances. However, there are still some specific indications for the use of disposable catheters, e.g. in acute poisoning when only one dialysis session is contemplated, in the setting of severe extracellular volume overload and severe hyperkalaemia when acute dialysis has to be considered, because of one-way obstruction of a Silastic catheter with abdominal distension (drainage of the peritoneal cavity can be accomplished through a stylet catheter), or during antibiotic treatment of a skin infection of the abdominal wall before implanting a permanent Silastic catheter.

Recommendations for placement of peritoneal catheters and preparation of the patient
Before inserting a peritoneal catheter, the bladder should be emptied. If the patient cannot void, urethral catheterisation should be done. Surgical preparation of the abdominal wall includes shaving from xyphoid to symphysis pubis and a large area of skin disinfected. The physician should examine carefully the patient's abdomen for complications which may cause difficulties (e.g. skin infection, previous surgery, or organomegaly).

The operator wears mask, cap, sterile gown and gloves; the sterile field is shielded to isolate the patient; all assistants and bystanders should wear masks and caps. If the patient is conscious the physician should give a description of the procedure to the patient to relieve anxiety and to obtain his cooperation. As the procedures progresses, each step of the operation has to be explained. This will allow catheter implantation under mild sedation (diazepam 10 mg IM, atropine 0.25 mg IM) and local anaesthesia (1% procaine) in most patients. General anaesthesia is necessary in children and may be preferable in obese patients and in patients with previous extensive abdominal surgery and a suspicion of intraabdominal adhesions.

When a 'blind' procedure (stylet or Trocath) is used for implanting the catheter, the abdomen must be filled with prewarmed dialysis solution. Enough fluid is infused to distend the abdomen moderately without causing discomfort or respiratory embarrassment to the patient. The volume of infused dialysate varies with the patient's size and abdominal distensibility. Priming may be done prior to implantation through a large bore (14 to 15 gauge), short bevel spinal needle (8 to 10 cm long) or during the procedure itself after introducing the perforated segment of the catheter within the peritoneal cavity. Priming the abdomen with fluid increases the safety of introducing the Trocath (18, 22); it creates a fluid cushion which maintains the parietal peritoneum against the abdominal wall, it reduces the risk of bowel perforation and facilitates catheter positioning as the intestinal loops are floating freely in a fluid medium.

The (disposable) stylet catheter consists of two parts: a plastic catheter of approximately 3 mm overall diameter and 25 to 30 cm long with multiple small holes on its distal 8 cm and a metal stylet protruding from the end of the catheter and providing a sharp cutting tip to penetrate the abdominal wall (see Figure 8a, b and c, chapter 21).

The usual insertion site is on the midline 3 to 6 cm below the umbilicus. The catheter may also be located in either iliac fossa. After local anaesthesia, a 2 mm skin incision is made with a n° 11 blade: the catheter should fit snugly in the wound to prevent leakage and to reduce the risk of infection. Nicking the fascia of the linea alba with the blade reduces the force needed to carry the catheter through. The stylet catheter is inserted perpendicular to the abdominal wall, while the patient tightens his abdominal musculature: a sudden decrease in resistance occurs when the stylet catheter passes the parietal peritoneum and enters the peritoneal cavity. The stylet is then withdrawn about 2 cm to sheathe its cutting tip. If the abdomen has not been primed with fluid prior to the procedure, the catheter should be advanced until all perforations are within the peritoneal cavity; the stylet should then be withdrawn and 2,000 ml of dialysis fluid instilled into the abdominal cavity. At this point, the catheter, with the reinserted stylet but with shielded cutting tip is advanced at 45° into the true pelvis; the stylet is then removed. The dialysis fluid should well up into the catheter lumen confirming that the catheter is in the peritoneal space; the administration set is attached to the catheter and the dialysate is allowed to drain out. Careful positioning of the catheter is essential to achieve a technically satisfactory dialysis. Final placement is made by assessing drainage and by positioning the tip of the catheter according to the patient's comfort. The catheter is fixed to the abdominal wall with non allergenic surgical tape and the entry site is protected with several sterile 10 cm gauze squares cut to fit around the catheter and are then taped to the skin.

When dialysis is completed, the peritoneal cavity is drained and the catheter is removed under strict aseptic conditions. Occasionally, catheter withdrawal may be uncomfortable and painful to the patient due to the incarceration of omental fringes into the holes in the distal segment of the catheter. When this occurs, the catheter should be gently mobilised and freed by a slow axial rotation after infusing 2 ml of 1% procaine into the lumen of the catheter. After withdrawing the catheter, the stab wound is closed with surgical tape strips and dressed for 48 h.

Deane's prosthesis
Instead of repeated use of the Trocath catheter the Deane's prosthesis may be used to maintain a sinus tract from the exterior to the peritoneal cavity (23–25). This prosthesis consists of a flexible solid plastic bar connected to a round mesa-shaped rigid plastic head; the bar, inserted into the abdominal wall after termination of dialysis, keeps the sinus tract open until a new catheter is introduced into the peritoneal cavity for the next dialysis.

Other prostheses have also been described for repeated insertion of disposable plastic catheters (26, 27). These prostheses have also been used in periodic peritoneal dialysis for end-stage renal disease: two funnel shaped subcutaneous prostheses were inserted in the abdominal wall and used alternatively for the introduction of the stylet catheter for twice weekly dialyses (28).

Complications related to insertion of stylet catheters
Numerous complications have been described with the use of the stylet catheter (22, 29–31). Most of them are due to inexperience, and can be avoided by following accurately the correct implantation procedure.

Bleeding is frequently observed after catheter implanting and clears spontaneously after a few dialysate exchanges. The addition of heparin (500 U/l) to the dialysis solution is recommended to prevent early catheter clotting. Major bleeding is diagnosed when effluent dialysate is grossly bloody (haematocrit > 5%). In most circumstances, the site of bleeding is in the abdominal wall, the blood seeping into the peritoneal cavity at the peritoneal entry site. Attempts to stop bleeding include the following: pressure dressing, placement of a deep purse string around the catheter, injection of epinephrine solution in the tissues surrounding the catheter, and discontinuation of heparin in the dialysis fluid (with the associated risk of catheter plugging by blood clots). It is often difficult to assess the efficiency of such measures since bleeding has a tendency to stop spontaneously. A transfusion is rarely needed and the necessity for laparotomy is exceptional.

Bowel perforation is a rare complication; its incidence is estimated between 0.1 (31) and 1.3% of all dialyses (32). This accident is best prevented by priming the abdomen with fluid prior to catheter insertion; during placement, the catheter should never be forced into the peritoneal cavity whenever intra-abdominal resistance occurs. Previous abdominal surgery (with peritoneal adhesions), distension of the bowel with gas, or a scaphoid abdomen are the usual predisposing factors. The risk of perforation is also high when the patient is unconscious or cachectic. In these circumstances, surgical placement should be preferred to blind implantation. A perforation of the gut has to be suspected in case of failure of dialysate to drain, cloudy, malodorous or frankly faeculent returning fluid or watery diarrhoea (32), the stool has then a strongly positive Clinistix test for glucose. Early signs of peritoneal irritation are common. Two therapeutic approaches have been equally successful: firstly conservative management with local and systemic antibiotics and continued peritoneal dialysis through another abdominal entry site (31–33), secondly laparotomy and surgical repair of the perforation, followed by continuous antibiotic lavage to prevent formation of peritoneal adhesions and loss of peritoneal surface area (21).

Perforation of the bladder has also been reported (32, 34, 35); after continuous drainage of the bladder with a Foley catheter and inserting a new peritoneal catheter, the dialyses were continued uneventfully.

Leakage of dialysis fluid around the catheter is a consequence of too large an incision of the skin and/or the peritoneum. This apparently benign complication should be prevented as leaking interferes with accurate fluid balance, causes abdominal wall and scrotal edema and carries the risk of infection. Catheter re-insertion through a new small incision and avoidance of abdominal overdistension with dialysis fluid are effective measures.

Inadequate drainage of peritoneal fluid is often encountered when a hurried operator does not take the necessary time to position the catheter properly and to check the adequacy of the drainage at the time of implantation. Other possible causes of inadequate drainage are: disruption of the syphon effect due to air gaining access into the peritoneal cavity, blockage of side-holes by omentum, intraperitoneal pooling of fluid by adhesions, and fibrin or blood clots plugging the catheter lumen (22, 30). Manipulating (or) flushing the catheter may restore a proper drainage; in case of failure, catheter replacement is mandatory. When plugging of the catheter by blood clots is suspected, catheter disobstruction may be achieved by instilling a fibrinolytic agent (streptokinase 250,000 U) in the catheter lumen and waiting one hour before resuming dialysis (36, 37).

Pain in a localised area (e.g. rectum, vagina), may result from mechanical trauma by the catheter tip. Relief will be obtained by withdrawing slowly the semirigid catheter a few centimeters.

Skin infection at the site of the stylet catheter (22) implantation is seldom reported, but is rather common. It should be prevented by careful cleansing of the skin stab wound after catheter removal; if successive catheter placements are necessary, repeated puncture at the same site should be avoided.

Other complications related to catheter placement include loss of catheter into the peritoneal cavity (22, 30), preperitoneal catheter placement with creation of a preperitoneal space due to not perforating the linea alba and peritoneum with the stylet (30), and accidental pulling out of the catheter during dialysis by an agitated patient (22).

The permanent Silastic Tenckhoff catheter

This catheter (see also Figures 10a, b, Chapter 21) is fitted with one or two Dacron felt cuffs which fix the catheter inside the abdominal wall and provide a barrier against the bacterial invasion of the peritoneum along the outside of the catheter (5).

Two types of standard adult catheters are available: the 'acute' type has one Dacron felt cuff, the 'chronic' type has two cuffs. The catheter has three segments: the intraabdominal portion which is provided with side holes, the subcutaneous segment and the external part. The Dacron felt cuffs of the 'chronic' catheter are 7 cm apart and separate the three segments. The inner (distal) cuff is placed between the linea alba and the peritoneum and the outer (proximal) cuff should be located 1 or 2 cm inside the skin exit; the segment of the catheter between the two cuffs lies in a tunnel of subcutaneous tissue (figure 1). Many centres use only the single cuff catheter because it is simpler to implant and to remove (29, 38, 39). We prefer the double cuff catheter: the inner felt cuff stimulates the formation of a fibrous block near the peritoneal entry point of the catheter and prevents the progression of subcutaneous tunnel infection to the peritoneum (40). It also prevents widening of the catheter sinus tract and subsequent herniation of the bowel or omentum at this site (21).

Implantation of the Tenckhoff catheter

Silastic catheters may be implanted at the bedside (18). The abdomen must be filled with warm dialysis solution as described previously (see section on placement of the Trocath catheter). Under local anaesthesia, a 4 to 6 cm midline skin incision is made below the umbilicus. The linea alba is exposed by blunt dissection with a haemostat. A special trocar with a bivalved tip is used. Trocar insertion is made easier by a stab incision of the fascia and is performed perpendicular to the abdominal wall, asking the patient to tighten his musculature. The permanent catheter, stiffened by an obturator, is then introduced in the peritoneal space using the trocar which is directed in a caudal direction; for this manoeuvre, the obturator should not protrude at the tip of the catheter to prevent injury to intra abdominal structures. The catheter should be gently advanced toward the pelvis without strain; if progression of the catheter is impeded by elastic resistance, omental entanglement of the catheter tip must be suspected. The catheter should then be withdrawn and reinserted at a different angle. When the catheter tip reaches the deeper pelvis, the patient notes a sense of pressure at the rectum. At this point, the obturator is withdrawn and the catheter is checked for ease of irrigation. In case of persisting pain, indicating that the intraabdominal catheter portion is too long or too far in, the catheter is pulled back on a few centimeters or removed and reinserted after trimming away up to 5 cm of its distal end. Careful attention should be given to obtain a satisfactory catheter position allowing painless, easy irrigation lest continuing pain necessitates early catheter replacement or leads to the patient's refusal of peritoneal dialysis. The trocar is then removed. The deeper cuff is tightly anchored to the peritoneum and to the linea alba in a 45° position maintaining the intraabdominal catheter segment in a caudal direction. A lateral subcutaneous tunnel with an arcuate course should be created; a 5 mm stab incision is made at its external end to give way to the external catheter segment. The exit site should be properly dimensioned to fit nicely around the Silastic tube. If the exit site is to large infection may develop or if it is to small sloughing may occur. The subcutaneous Dacron felt cuff should be placed at about 1 to 2 cm inside the skin exit to prevent skin erosion. The catheter is then placed into the subcutaneous tunnel and its external segment pulled through the skin exit with the aid of a metal guide. The catheter should be irrigated with heparinised saline and closed with a rubber cap. The midline incision is closed and dressed. Dialysis should be started as soon as possible adding hepa-

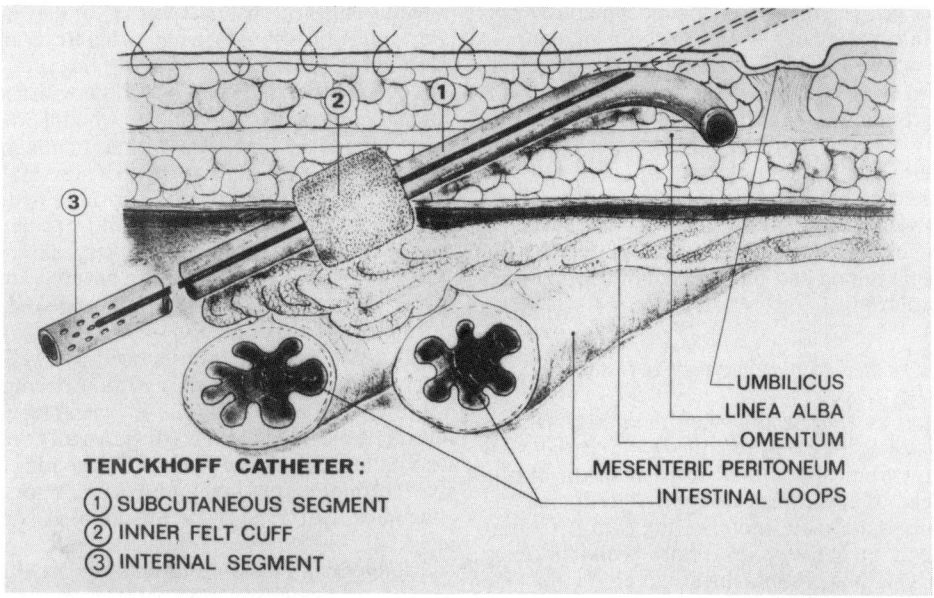

Figure 1. Surgical implantation of a 'chronic' Tenckhoff catheter (see text). When closing the peritoneal cavity, the peritoneum is attached to the inner Dacron cuff: the catheter is positioned at a 45° angle, to maintain the intraperitoneal segment in a caudal direction (Courtesy Dr. A. Slingeneyer).

rin (500 U/l) to the dialysis fluid.

The procedure for surgical implantation of the permanent Silastic catheter is similar to the bedside technique. We prefer the surgical technique for the following reasons: priming the abdomen with fluid is usually not necessary, catheter positioning under direct vision is easier, and entanglement of the catheter tip with the omentum is easily prevented by pulling up the omentum towards the upper abdomen with a finger or a smooth haemostat during catheter insertion. After incision of the skin and linea alba, the peritoneum is identified, incised and marked with haemostats. The catheter is previously moistened with heparinised saline and gently inserted in the depth of the true pelvis. Proper positioning and easy irrigation are checked. The peritoneum is tightly closed around the catheter and the distal Dacron felt cuff to prevent leakage. The last steps are similar to those described for the bedside technique. Following catheter placement, dialysis should be started without delay using small volumes of heparinised dialysis solution. Recently, placement of the Tenckhoff peritoneal dialysis catheter under peritoneoscopic visualisation has been proposed as an alternative to blind introduction with a trocart or surgical placement (41). A single cuff Tenckhoff catheter may be inserted by means of a pointed stylet in a similar way as the 'Frocath' catheter (see Figure 10b, Chapter 21).

Catheter care
The exit site of the catheter should be kept clean and dry at all times. It should be protected by a 8 × 8 cm sterile gauze dressing which also prevents direct contact of the catheter with the skin. Before and after each dialysis, the exit site is cleaned with sterile applicators dipped into povidone-iodine (Betadine) or hydrogen peroxide. When the wound and exit site are healed, a daily shower is recommended after removing the dressing; after the shower, the exit site is carefully dried and cleaned with Betadine and redressed. Careful attention to this procedure will help keep the exit site free of infection; yet, some patients remain uninfected for long periods despite omitting protective dressings at the exit site (42).

Other indwelling catheters
Other types of permanent Silastic catheters have been developed in an attempt to avoid some of the shortcomings of the Tenckhoff catheter. To minimise the problem of omental obstruction and catheter dislodgement, a catheter with large draining holes and a balloon near its intraabdominal end has been designed (43); the balloon, inflated with saline, serves two purposes: to act as a 'stand off' for the bowel and omentum and to keep the catheter in the lower part of the abdomen. The Toronto Western Hospital catheter (44) is similar to the 'acute' Tenckhoff catheter except for two or three silicone rubber discs (1 mm thick, 30 mm diameter) bounded perpendicularly to the intraabdominal catheter segment. The silicone rubber discs minimise catheter dislodgement and outflow obstruction by fixing the catheter between the lower bowel loops. More recently, another disc catheter (45) and the disc column peritoneal catheter (46) have been described. Clinical experience with these alternatives to the Tenckhoff catheter is still too limited to draw any conclusion as to their possible advantages.

A subcutaneous peritoneal catheter was designed with the aim to circumvent the inconvenience of the external catheter segment and to minimise the risk of infection (47). This device consists of a subcutaneous reservoir and an intraperitoneal extension, both made from silicone rubber (see Figure 14, Chapter 21). The reservoir is covered with a layer of Dacron velour to facilitate tissue ingrowth and fixation of the prosthesis. A 14 gauge needle is inserted into the subcutaneous reservoir at each dialysis. The results obtained with the subcutaneous peritoneal catheter during a two and a half year experience in 48 patients did not show a clear superiority over standard Silastic catheters, except for the absence of external tubing and more freedom during interdialytic intervals (48).

Complications related to placement of indwelling silastic catheters
Leakage of dialysis fluid occurs when the peritoneum is not tightly closed at the point of entry of the catheter. It may also result from abdominal overdistension during dialysis because of incomplete drainage. Reducing the volume of infused dialysate and ensuring complete drainage at the end of each cycle usually seals the leak. Should it persist, postponing further dialysis for one week will usually be sufficient for the leak to seal off spontaneously (29).

Bleeding is observed occasionally during the first few exchanges following catheter implantation. Abundant haemorrhage is exceptional; its persistence despite omission of heparin in the dialysis solution may require a laparotomy to ligate an injured mesenteric vessel.

Bowel perforation is exceptional and is prevented by avoiding forceful insertion against intraabdominal resistance and by making sure the obturator is sheathed within the Silastic tube before introducing the catheter into the peritoneal cavity.

Subcutaneous bleeding with hematoma formation can occur from a small vessel injured during blunt dissection of the subcutaneous tissue.

Reflex ileus following catheter implantation is common but rarely persists beyond 24 to 36 h. In an occasional patient, a persistent paralytic ileus with major abdominal distension will occur, even when implantation has been uneventful. Oral mannitol in a 10% solution and hypertonic enemas help to restore intestinal motility.

Complications occurring during long-term use of indwelling peritoneal catheters
Skin exit infection is most commonly due to *Staph aureus* or *epidermidis* and is observed in 15 to 30% of the patients (39, 40). Its early detection is, if it occurs, essential to prevent infection of the subcutaneous Dacron cuff which requires catheter replacement. Tenderness, sloughing and redness of the skin around the catheter, associated with discharge may be observed. The patient should be trained to inspect carefully the exit site, in order to recognise asymptomatic skin exit inflammation. When infection is suspected, cultures should be taken and antistaphylococal antibiotic therapy (Vancomycin 1 g IV, Oxacillin) should be started without delay and maintained for at least 10 to 15 days (and adapted according to microbiologic data). Infection of the subcutaneous cuff necessitates removal of the catheter. Preferably infection should be cured before implanting a new permanent catheter (18).

To cure the skin exit infection without interrupting the patient's peritoneal dialysis schedule, we combine an aggressive local treatment with systemic antibiotics: after excision of the skin at the exit site, the subcutaneous cuff is thoroughly freed from surrounding tissues and the Dacron felt is carefully peeled off from the silastic tube; the open wound is irrigated every day with Betadine until cultures of the wound are negative on three consecutive days; the catheter is then removed and replaced during the same operation (49).

Tunnel infection manifests itself by swelling, pain and fever. Tunnel infection may extend deeply into the abdominal wall and may cause persisting peritonitis by intraperitoneal bacterial seeding, usually seen with single Dacron cuff Silastic catheters (21). In addition to aggressive antibiotic treatment and surgical drainage of the cubcutaneous tunnel, catheter removal is always necessary.

Catheter cuff erosion and prolapse are due to pressure necrosis of the skin at the catheter exit site. This early complication is best prevented by making the subcutaneous catheter tunnel of an appropriate length at the time of placement; the subcutaneous Dacron cuff should lie into the subcutaneous tissue at about 1 cm from the exit site. Cuff erosion and prolapse require elective catheter replacement (18).

Catheter malfunction presents itself most often by failure to drain at the start of dialysis. Inflow obstruction from subcutaneous catheter kinking is a rare complication. The common causes of outflow obstruction are the following (18): 1) catheter encasement by adhesions due to torpid peritoneal infection and (or) recurrent peritonitis; 2) catheter malposition due to poor implantation technique, 3) catheter entanglement in the omentum and (or) migration of the intraperitoneal catheter segment out of the pelvis due to intestinal peristalsis (44); 4) catheter obstruction by incarceration of tissue into the catheter side holes. Fluoroscopy or X-ray after dye injection is a helpful diagnostic procedure; these causes of catheter malfunction are best remedied by catheter revision.

Intraluminal catheter obstruction is often caused by fibrin clots that can be dislodged by forceful irrigation with a large syringe (21), dissolved by instillation of fibrinolytic agents, or removed by the 'Italian clot screw' (50).

Failure to drain may be of functional, reversible origin. It is the most frequent complication of chronic peritoneal dialysis. It responds readily to bowel stimulation by oral administration of mannitol or by enema. This treatment should always be tried before looking for a mechanical cause of catheter failure (21).

Other complications include migration of the distal cuff out of the rectus sheath allowing the perforated part of the catheter to move partially into the subcutaneous tissue causing fluid accumulation in the abdominal wall (51); hernia formation at the point of entry of the catheter into the peritoneal cavity (51); and rupture of the subcutaneous Silastic tube segment from an acciden-

23: *Practical use of peritoneal dialysis* 463

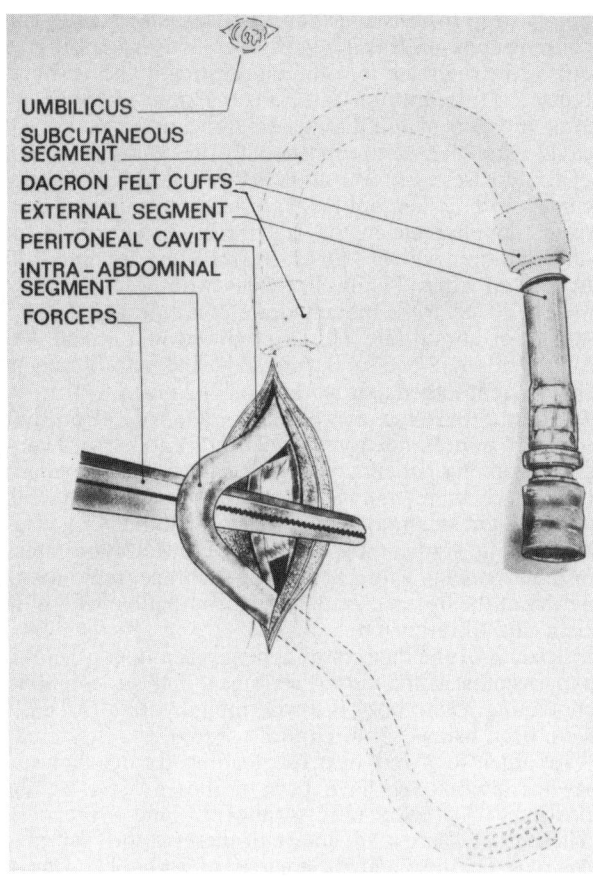

Figure 2. Revision of the 'chronic' Silastic catheter. The intraperitoneal segment is removed from the peritoneal cavity with a smooth haemostat (or a finger); it is subsequently reintroduced and repositioned. The subcutaneous segment remains *in situ*. (Courtesy Dr A. Slingeneyer).

tal brisk pull to the dialysate line during dialysis (personal observation).

Catheter revision: removal and replacement
Catheter revision is often necessary when malfunction occurs. Under local anaesthesia, the original midline incision is reopened; the abdominal wall is dissected down through the fascia to the point of entry into the peritoneal cavity; below this point, the peritoneum is incised over about 3 to 4 cm; the intraperitoneal segment is pulled out from the peritoneal space with a finger or a forceps and freed from surrounding adhesions or incarcerated tissues (Figure 2). The intraperitoneal segment is then properly positioned into the true pelvis (21).

Catheter removal is indicated in case of exit infection not responding to antibiotic therapy, formation of a tunnel abcess, irreversible catheter failure, transfer of the patient to another treatment modality (e.g. haemodialysis, transplantation) or when renal function has improved and dialysis is no longer required. Single cuff catheters are easily removed by a single skin incision around the catheter exit site. Two skin incisions are required for removal of double cuff catheters (one incision for each cuff); to reduce the risk of peritoneal infection, it is preferable to dissect down first to the deep cuff, remove the catheter from the peritoneal cavity, and then close this first incision before approaching the potentially contaminated subcutaneous cuff (21).

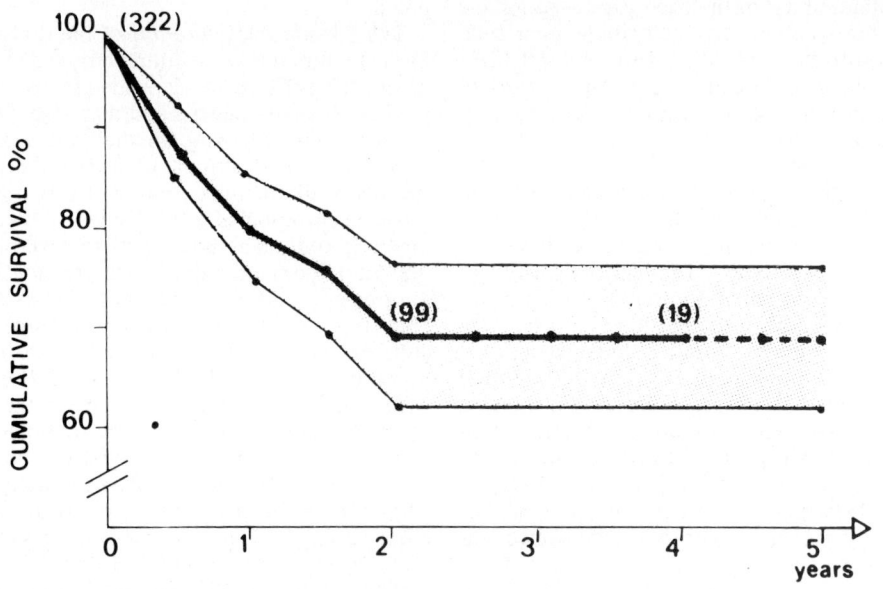

Figure 3. Cumulative survival of the 'chronic' Tenckhoff catheter in 270 patients receiving maintenance peritoneal dialysis for end stage renal failure. (Courtesy Dr A. Slingeneyer).

Catheter replacement is a procedure similar to first implantation. However, careful attention should be paid to the possible persistence of infectious foci on or in the abdominal wall. In case of doubt, the new catheter should be implanted at least 5 cm away from the suspected area (18). Implantation in the epigastrium has given satisfactory results in some patients who needed frequent catheter replacements (49).

Catheter survival
Despite various complications that may restrict its life expectancy, the permanent Silastic catheter has an average life of 10 to 12 months, with reports of a single catheter remaining functional for as long as 5.5 (52) and 7 years (53). In a recent review of the patients in our unit (322 'chronic' Tenckhoff catheters implanted in 270 patients) an actuarial analysis of the cumulative catheter survival showed a one year survival of 80% and a five year survival of 70% (Figure 3) (49).

Dialysis solutions

Composition of dialysis solutions
Despite recommendations for limiting to a minimum the formulations of peritoneal dialysis solutions (54, 55) there is still a great variety of formulae among commercially available solutions. These dialysis solutions contain approximately the following (in mmol/l)*: dextrose monohydrate 76 (1.5 g/dl), 126 (2.5 g/dl) or 215 (4.25 g/dl); sodium 130 to 140; chloride 98 to 108; acetate or lactate 35 to 45; calcium 1.5 to 2 (6 to 8 mg/dl); magnesium 0.75 (1.8 mg/dl). Potassium is usually not included, but may be added if necessary at the time of utilisation. Sodium bisulphite is added in small quantities to limit caramelisation of dextrose during autoclaving: its final concentration is below toxic levels (56, 57). Aluminium contamination of the chemicals used for the preparation of the solution may contribute to a final aluminium concentration exceeding 10 to 12 µg/l (0.37 to 0.44 µmol/l) which represents a potential hazard of chronic aluminium intoxication with long term use (59; see also Chapter 44). The final pH of sterile apyrogenic solutions is in the range of 5.2 to 6.2.

The aluminium concentration in the solution used in CAPD should not exceed 10 µg/l (0,37 mmol/l).

Dialysate dextrose concentration determines water removal by osmotic ultrafiltration. The higher the concentration of dextrose, the greater the amount of ultrafiltrate. Water is removed from the plasma at a faster rate than sodium, so that the ultrafiltrate is hyponatric, lowering the sodium concentration in dialysate in the initial phase of diffusion (60, 61); eventually, during prolonged dwell time of dialysis solutions, sodium concentration equilibrates between plasma and dialysate due to the transfer of sodium from the blood (62, 63). Ultrafiltration in peritoneal dialysis is a self limited process, because dextrose diffuses readily across the peritoneal capillary wall; there is an exponential decrease in dialysate concentration of dextrose with time as dextrose diffuses out of the dialysate into the blood stream and is metabolised. Ultrafiltration rates are maximal immediately after infusion of the dialysis solution in the peritoneal cavity, then decrease proportionally due to the reduction of the dextrose concentration (64, 65). During a 2 l exchange with a 76 mmol/l (1,5 g/dl) concentration of dextrose monohydrate in the dialysis fluid the volume of ultrafiltration will be 50 to 100 ml after 1 h and 150 to 200 ml after 2 h dwell times; with a 215 mmol/l (4.25 g/dl) dextrose monohydrate concentration 300 to 400 ml of ultrafiltrate will be produced in 1 h, and 400 to 600 ml in 2 h (66). Beyond 3 h, the ultrafiltrate is slowly reabsorbed at a rate of 4.2 ml/min with a 76 mmol/l dextrose concentration and of 3.7 ml/min with 215 mmol/l dextrose (67). Ultrafiltration rates vary greatly among patients, because of marked interpatient differences in membrane permeability. Some patients with a 'tight' membrane maintain a high dialysate plasma osmotic gradient and have high ultrafiltration rates; in other patients with an 'open' membrane, rapid dissipation of the osmotic gradient is incompatible with efficient ultrafiltration (68).

Because of the dangers of hyperglycaemic non ketotic hyperosmolar coma during peritoneal dialysis, solutions containing 354 mmol/l dextrose monohydrate (7.0 g/dl) have been banned from clinical use (69).

In order to avoid dextrose loading during dialysis, several alternatives have been proposed: gelatin (70), dextran (71), fructose (72), sorbitol (73) and xylitol (74). The lack of clearcut advantage of these various substances over dextrose and the toxicity of sorbitol (75) have precluded their routine use. More recently, amino acids have been proposed as osmotic agents in dialysis solutions (76). A preliminary report confirms their efficiency (77) but their long term tolerance has yet to be evaluated.

The *sodium concentration* of the dialysis solution affects the amount of sodium removed. Sodium transfer across the peritoneum depends greatly on the diffusion gradient between plasma and dialysate. Sodium removal is enhanced by lowering the dialysate sodium concentration (78, 79). For periodic peritoneal dialysis, the recommended sodium concentration is 130 mmol/l (54). Sodium concentration of 118 mmol/l has been proposed to facilitate sodium removal and to avoid the usual postdialytic hypernatraemia, which frequently causes thirst after osmotic ultrafiltration (80). The availability of two dialysis solutions with different sodium concentrations (130 and 140 mmol/l) gives greater flexibility in regulating sodium removal (66). During a 60 min, 2 l exchange with a dialysis solution containing 130 mmol/l sodium, the net sodium removal is approximately 30, 50 and 80 mmol, respectively, with dextrose concentrations of 76, 126 and 215 mmol/l; when the dialysate sodium is 140 mmol/l, the net sodium removal per exchange is reduced to 10, 30 and 50 mmol/l, respectively, with the same dextrose concentrations (66).

Potassium is usually omitted from most dialysate solutions because of the low peritoneal clearance (81). Addition of potassium chloride may be necessary in pa-

---

* A dialysis solution with 1.5% dextrose monohydrate ($C_6H_{12}O_6 \cdot H_2O$) equals 1.36 g/dl of anhydrous dextrose (180 daltons) or 75.6 mmol/l.

tients treated with digitalis glucosides, in cases of hypokalaemia due to intestinal losses and inadequate intake, in anorectic subjects with peritonitis and during prolonged peritoneal lavage. Potassium concentration in dialysis fluid should not exceed a normal plasma potassium concentration of 4.5 mmol/l.

Acetate or lactate are the usual 'alkaline' anions of dialysis solutions because insoluble calcium and magnesium salts will form in the presence of bicarbonate. Optimal concentration of these buffers is in the range of 38 to 40 mmol/l (54); the frequently used concentration of 35 mmol/l of acetate and of lactate does not compensate for the obligatory bicarbonate loss during peritoneal dialysis and does not allow for complete correction of metabolic acidosis. Higher concentrations of buffers (e.g. 45 mmol/l) may lead to metabolic alcalosis (82). There are many theoretical advantages for using acetate instead of lactate: due to the higher pK (4.7), acetate solutions have a final pH in the range of 5.8 to 6.2, whereas the pH of lactate solutions is usually below 5.4. Acetate is a more effective source of bicarbonate (83) and is metabolised even in case of lactic acidosis (84), and finally, dialysis solutions containing acetate have been shown to be bacteriostatic under certain experimental conditions (85, 86). However, lactate is often chosen by manufacturers because dextrose caramelisation during autoclaving is less marked with this anion due to its pK of 3.9.

Bicarbonate has been used in calcium- and magnesium-free solutions (62, 87); intravenous calcium infusion is then necessary to compensate for calcium losses during dialysis.

Divalent cations, (calcium and magnesium) in dialysate solutions exist for the major part in ionised form. Calcium and magnesium in dialysis solutions should be nearer to the plasma diffusable concentrations rather than to the total plasma concentrations. With a calcium concentration of 1.75 mmol/l (7.0 mg/dl) a positive calcium balance is obtained during dialysis; calcium transfer from dialysate to blood is impeded by ultrafiltration when using 215 mmol/l dextrose solutions (88). With a calcium concentration of 1.5 mmol/l, calcium balance will be negative when plasma calcium levels exceed 2.05 mmol/l (8.2 mg/dl) (89) and aggravation of renal osteodystrophy has been observed in patients using this low calcium concentration in dialysis solutions (90).

Most peritoneal dialysis solutions contain 0.75 mmol/l (1.8 mg/dl) magnesium. Recent observations suggest that the magnesium concentration should be lowered to 0.52 mmol/l (1.25 mg/dl) to allow for a better control of serum magnesium concentration in patients with end stage renal failure (88, 91).

Heparin is added to dialysis solutions after catheter implantation (18) or during peritoneal lavage for peritonitis (21). The usual dose is 200 to 500 IU/l. Heparin may also be added to dialysis solutions using the acetate formulation before autoclaving at 115 °C for 1/2 h in a rapid cooling steriliser (92).

Antibiotics are added to dialysis solutions during the treatment of peritoneal infections (18). Kanamycin added to fresh dialysate loses 30% of its activity in 24 h (93); antibiotic decay in dextrose/electrolyte concentrate used for automatic peritoneal dialysis was demonstrated for gentamicin, nafcilin, cephalothin and penicillin (39). When heparin and aminoglycosides are simultaneously added, both anticoagulant and antibiotic activities are retained provided that the two drugs are added separately in a dilute solution and no precipitate forms in the dialysate (94, 95).

Sodium hydroxide has been added to increase the pH of dialysis solution, to prevent abdominal pain (52). Various pharmacologically active substances have also been added to dialysate in order to modify mass transfer rates across the peritoneal membrane (96–105), but there are no reports concerning their routine use in clinical practice. Finally, amino acid enriched dialysate has been used to prevent aminoacid losses (106).

Insulin addition to dialysate prevents hyperglycaemia in diabetic patients during dialysis (107, 108) and may be used as the sole route of insulin administration in diabetic patients on continuous ambulatory peritoneal dialysis (109).

Delivery and storage of dialysis solutions
Commercial ready to use dialysis solutions are available in 1 or 2-litre glass bottles, 0.5, 1 and 2-litre plastic bags and 10-litre plastic containers. Glass bottles should be considered as the only containers guaranteeing absolute sterility and apyrogenicity. Plastic bags, made of transparent polyvinyl-chloride, which allow checking the clearness of the solution before use, should be used with caution as contamination of their content can occur during storage (110). Rigid 10-litre plastic containers are not transparent and the clarity of their content is difficult to check even with transillumination; although rare, fungal contamination of dialysis solutions may occur through pin holes and/or small cracks formed during transportation and storage (111).

Concentrated solutions
Two types of concentrate are necessary for use with automatic reverse osmosis machines: 1) a dextrose-electrolyte solution close to saturation with a concentration ratio of 20 to 1 consisting of a 50% dextrose solution which also contains a 20 fold electrolyte concentration giving a final dextrose concentration of 126 mmol/l (2.5 g/dl); 2) 126 to 313 mmol/l (2.5 to 6.2 g/dl) dextrose concentrates used to complement the previous solution in order to adjust the final dextrose concentration according to the patient's needs. Both concentrates are available in 2-litre glass bottles or in 2.5-litre plastic bags. Because of heavy caramelisation during autoclaving of the dextrose electrolyte concentrate, the preparation of a dextrose free concentrate has been suggested (91).

Peritoneal dialysis equipment and automatic machines

With the introduction, in 1962, of the first automatic equipment for the delivery of sterile premixed dialysis solutions via a closed circuit (4), it soon became apparent that with this innovation the peritoneal infection rate decreased drastically; with this technical improve-

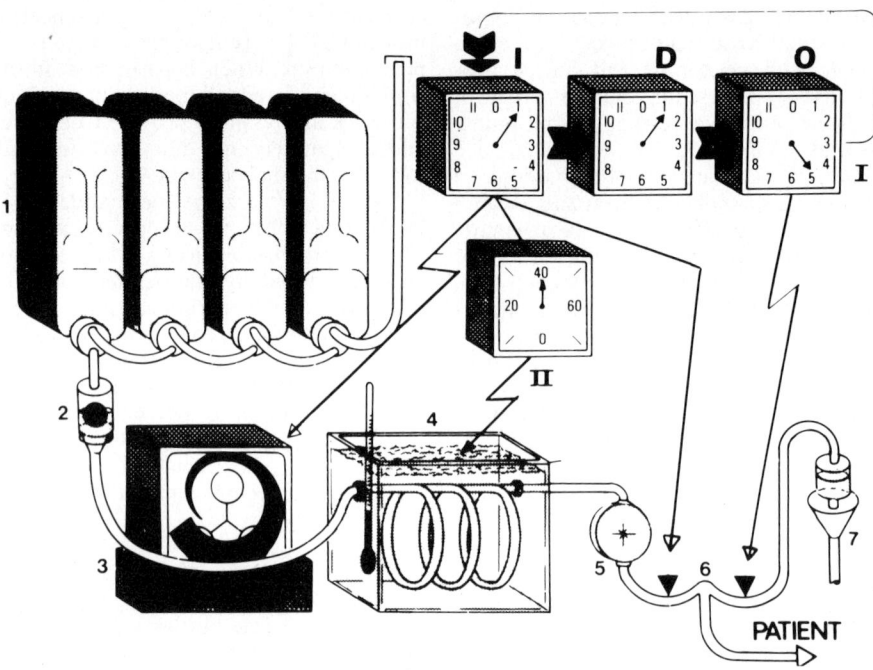

Figure 4. Schematic representation of an automatic cycler for closed circuit intermittent peritoneal dialysis. 1) dialysate in 10-litre plastic containers assembled in series; 2) bubble trap; 3) roller pump; 4) rewarming bath with thermostat (II); 5) bacteriological filter; 6) electric clamps; 7) drainage tubing isolated from drain by an air break with a fluid level. I Electric timers. I: inflow timer; D: diffusion 'dwell' timer; O: outflow timer. (Courtesy Dr A. Slingeneyer).

ment peritoneal dialysis gained in safety what it lost in simplicity (52).

Automatic cyclers

Cyclers are automatic devices which regulate instillation and drainage of the dialysis solution. They consist of two or three electric timers activating two electric clamps and controlling the succession of an unlimited number of peritoneal dialysis cycles comprising three periods, one for instillation, one for diffusion (dwell period) and one for drainage of the dialysis fluid (Figure 4). Infusion is by gravity or by a peristaltic pump through an infusion line including a dialysate rewarming device; drainage is by gravity or with a negative pressure pump. Each period of the cycle is controlled by one of the electric timers which may be set independently to determine the duration of a given period. Cyclers utilised previously hospital prepared dialysate in 40-litre glass containers (112). Usually commercial solutions are used and a stock of sterile dialysate is created by inter connecting a number of 2-litre bags or bottles or 10-litre containers (113–123). The dialysate supply for each dialysis varies from 10 to 60 l depending on the dialysate flow and the planned duration of the dialysis session. The delivery circuit, including interconnecting tubings for bags or containers and the disposable sets for instillation and drainage of dialysis fluid are commercially available.

Reverse osmosis machines

In 1972, the development of automatic, so called reverse osmosis RO peritoneal dialysis systems capable of producing unlimited quantities of sterile pyrogen-free dialysate from tap water and sterile concentrate (6) opened a new era in peritoneal dialysis. With this equipment, sterile, apyrogenic water is obtained by reverse osmosis; dialysis solution is prepared by mixing one volume of dextrose/electrolyte concentrate and 19 volumes of reverse osmosis treated, sterile water; to this mixture, a variable amount of dextrose concentrate is added to adapt the dextrose concentration of the final dialysis fluid to the patient needs. A schematic diagram of a reverse osmosis peritoneal dialysis system is shown in Figure 5. Several automatic peritoneal dialysis systems are currently commercially available. They are produced in France by ABG Semca, Paris, and in the United States by Becton and Dickinson – Drake Willock, Portland, Oregon, and Physiocontrol Corp., Redmond, Washington. The ABG Semca and Physiocontrol machines are provided with automatic disinfection and rinsing procedures saving patient and/or nursing time and ensuring strict sterility of the dialysate circuit. In fact, the safety of these systems depends on the perfect quality of the reverse osmosis modules, including intactness of the (acetate cellulose or nylon) hollow fiber membranes and the tightness of the assembled permeators (124). It has been shown that occasionally bacteria from supply water may cross most currently available reverse osmosis modules and may colonise the downstream portion of the system (125). Accordingly, the safe use of reverse osmosis modules for the production of sterile pyrogen free

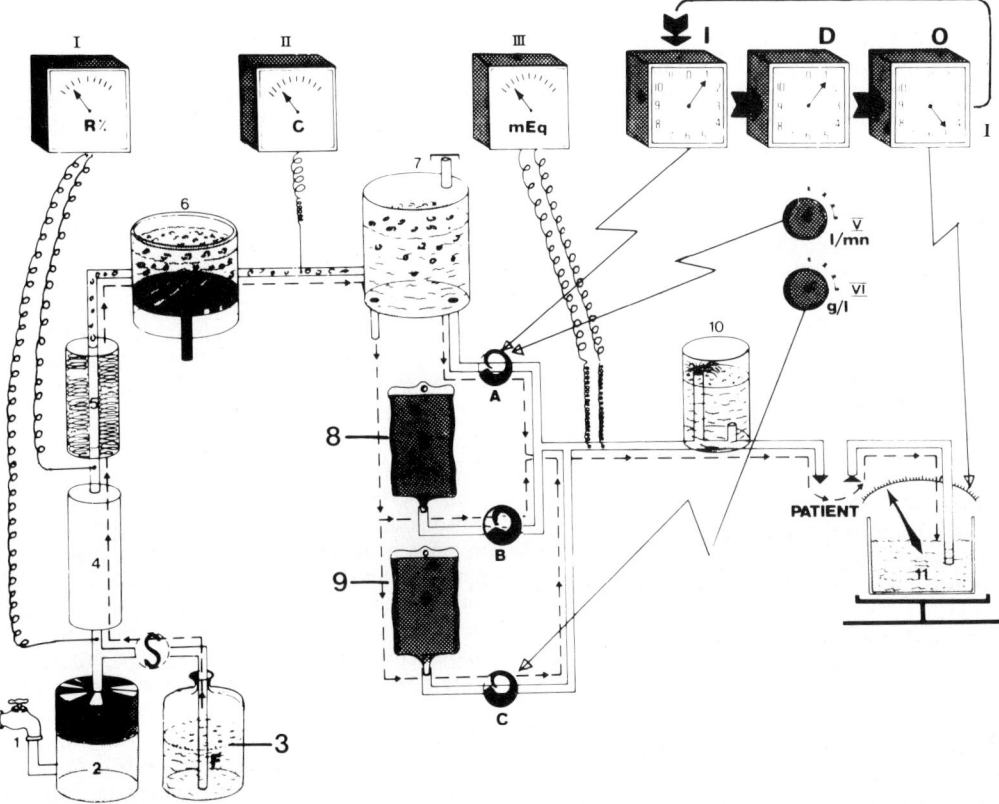

Figure 5. Schematic representation of a reverse osmosis peritoneal dialysis system. 1) water feed; 2) water reservoir; 3) formaldehyde (F) reservoir for automatic sterilisation; 4) reverse osmosis module with resistance (R%) meter (I). 5) rewarmer; 6) de-aeration device with temperature (C) control (II) 7) sterile water reservoir; 8) and 9) dialysis fluid concentrate and dextrose concentrate in plastic bags; 10) bubble trap; 11) drainage reservoir with scale for measuring the volume drained. ABC: proportioning pumps for water (A) dextrose-electrolyte (B) and dextrose concentrate (C) with conductivity meter (mEq) (III). I: Electric timers, for inflow (I), diffusion (D) and outflow (O). (Courtesy Dr A. Slingeneyer).

water includes the following requirements: 1) the pretreatment of tap water should be exactly in accordance with the recommendations of the manufacturers of the reverse osmosis module; pre-treatment devices such as carbon filters, softeners, pre-filters and storage tanks may promote bacterial growth (125); 2) use of back-up devices (bacterial filters, ultraviolet lamp, heaters) to insure downstream sterility during dialysis fluid production (6); 3) routine disinfection of the reverse osmosis modules and dialysate circuit with 3% formalin after each dialysis (126); and 4) changing without delay of the reverse osmosis modules when their ion rejection capability decreases (126). The effectiveness of these measures and the safety of the RO machines have been proven in most published series (39, 127, 128), except in one report where a persistently high incidence of peritonitis was observed with the use of a certain type of RO machine (129). Apparently a combination of a faulty construction of the RO modules in this type of machine together with inappropriate water pretreatment and a bacteriological unsafe water supply were responsible for the bacteriological contamination of the dialysate.

Manual technique (versus cyclers and reverse osmosis machines)

Periodic peritoneal dialysis was quickly adopted in most intensive care units because of the simplicity of the original manual technique (1). However, the frequent openings of the dialysate delivery circuit with each bottle exchange resulted in a high incidence contamination of the dialysis fluid and of peritonitis (22, 30). Automatic peritoneal dialysis with a closed dialysate delivery circuit reduced dramatically the incidence of peritonitis (19). It also reduces the work load of the nursing staff and facilitates the irrigation of the peritoneal cavity at fixed intervals, thereby improving peritoneal dialysis efficiency. Therefore, automatic peritoneal dialysis should have the absolute preference for periodic peritoneal dialysis instead of manual technique when the equipment is available. Cyclers offer the advantages of simplicity, moderate capital cost and easy and inexpensive maintenance. Their main drawback is the need for commercial solutions, which are expensive, bulky and may become contaminated during storage. Automatic machines produce at the bedside unlimited amounts of low cost dialysis solutions; on the other hand, they are complex, maintenance is less easy and more expensive and they are still too noisy and bulky; their capital cost is still high (130). However, most of these shortcomings may be overcome by technical improvements.

Sorbent peritoneal dialysate regeneration system
The concept of regeneration of peritoneal dialysate by a sorbent cartridge (Redy-Sorbsystem, Organon Teknika, Turnhout, Belgium, see chapter 17) has been introduced (131–135). In this system 2 l of spend dialysate recirculate through a urease column and a sorbent cartridge containing activated carbon, zirconium oxide and zirconium phosphate (136). A sterile infusion system reinfuses dextrose (which diffuses into the patient) in the dialysis fluid and calcium and magnesium, because both are removed by the sorbent cartridge (see chapter 17). The regenerated dialysate is instilled in the peritoneal cavity by a pump.

This seems a promising concept, which is still in an experimental stage.

Early clinical application has given encouraging results (133–135).

The present sorbent cartridge, however, contains considerable amounts of aluminium oxide and such aluminium is released by the cartridge when the dialysate is either acid or alkaline (137, 138). Therefore, the presently available cartridge should be considered as potentially hazardous for use in peritoneal dialysis. A new, low aluminium sorbent cartridge has been prepared and will be available before long (see chapter 17).

The peritoneal dialysis procedure

Maintenance of sterility during preparation for dialysis and connect-disconnect procedures
Careful attention to sterile techniques should aim at maintaining absolute sterility of the lumen of the peritoneal catheter and of the dialysis solutions; without special care, contamination is likely to occur during the following manoeuvres: 1) connection and disconnection of the dialysate circuit to the Tenckhoff catheter; 2) preparation of automatic equipment, when assembling the dialysate circuit; 3) exchange of bottles or plastic bags containing dialysis solutions, particularly when temperature of the solutions is maintained in a rewarming bath (33, 139–142). These procedures should be done in a clean environment, after meticulous preparation of the necessary supplies; Betadine should be used generously for disinfecting all surfaces before inserting needles or spikes in stoppers of containers with dialysis solutions and luer connectors into the peritoneal catheter lumen. The operator should wash his hands carefully with Betadine soap solution (a surgical scrub takes time but is recommended), wear a cap and mask (as should all other attendants) and sterile gloves and sterile drapes should be used when handling the peritoneal catheter. The practical aspects of all these procedures have been thoroughly described by Tenckhoff (18, 21).

Peritoneal irrigation and dialysate exchange cycles
During dialyses with the single catheter technique (intermittent peritoneal dialysis), irrigation of the peritoneal cavity by dialysis solution is carried out by exchange cycles comprising three phases: inflow, diffusion (dwell) and outflow.

Most adults will tolerate an inflow volume of 2 l. The exchange volume can be adjusted, however, from 1 to 3 l, according to patient's size, abdominal volume and cardiopulmonary tolerance, without any major reduction in effectiveness (143, 144). On the other hand, peritoneal clearances increase linearly with increments in dialysate exchange rates (145). Intermittent peritoneal dialysis can be accomplished according to two main protocols: *periodic peritoneal dialysis* and *continuous ambulatory peritoneal dialysis*.

Periodic peritoneal dialysis
This mode of peritoneal dialysis alternates dialyses of various duration (10 to 48 h or longer) with inter-dialytic phases lasting for one or more days according to patient's needs (i.e., protein catabolism, residual renal function, body size, etc). A standard protocol uses exchange cycles with 5–10 min infusion time (200–400 ml/min), 0 to 15 min dwell time, 10 to 20 min drainage time. With dialysate exchange rates of 3 to 4 l/h urea and creatinine clearances are maintained around 20 to 25 ml/min and 12 to 20 ml/min respectively (146). Faster dialysate exchange rates result in higher peritoneal clearances but are often associated with abdominal pain (145, 146). It is difficult to maintain a dialysate exchange rate higher than 2 l/h when manual techniques are used for peritoneal irrigation. The introduction of automated techniques (cyclers or reverse osmosis machines) has not only increased the safety (by reducing the infectious risk), but also the effectiveness of peritoneal dialysis by insuring the regularity of exchange cycles. In a cost-effectiveness analysis of various peritoneal dialysis protocols, increasing dwell-times appeared to result in a considerable saving of dialysate with little reduction of net urea transfer (147), a fact of major economic consequence when pre-mixed commercial solutions are used (148).

Technical modifications of intermittent peritoneal dialysis have been proposed to obtain higher urea clearances and to shorten the dialysis duration. They include *peritoneal extracorporeal re-circulation dialysis* (149), *automatic high flow rate peritoneal dialysis* (150), *semi-continuous peritoneal dialysis* (151) and *reciprocating dialysis* (152) (see chapter 21).

Continuous ambulatory peritoneal dialysis (CAPD)
The basic principle of CAPD is a permanent bathing of the peritoneal cavity by dialysis solutions which are exchanged every 4 to 10 h. Originally five exchanges per day of 2 h were recommended (12); this required 10 disconnect/connect procedures per day for infusion and drainage, and was associated with an unacceptably high peritoneal infection rate (16). The introduction of dialysate in plastic bags simplified the procedure (13). The bags are connected to the permanent peritoneal catheter

by short connecting tubing with special connectors at each end. After inflow, the bag, still attached to the connecting tube, is carried rolled up in a waist purse under the clothing. At the end of the diffusion period, the dialysate is drained into the same bag which is then discarded and a fresh bag is attached to the same connecting line. Therefore, the number of dialysate circuit openings is reduced to one per bag exchange with less risk for microbial contamination of the circuit. The same connecting line, initially used for one week and changed by the patient under sterile conditions (12), is now usually changed once a month by a nurse in order to decrease the risk of peritoneal infection (153). Several models of peritoneal catheter connectors (154–158) and a connecting tube with an in-line bacterial filter (159) have been proposed to increase the safety of continuous ambulatory peritoneal dialysis.

The long dwell times used in CAPD allow for complete equilibration of solutes between plasma and dialysate; therefore, urea clearance values approximate dialysate exchange rates (12).

In CAPD, each exchange takes about 30 to 45 min. The time lost every day by the patient due to bag exchanges is about 3.5 to 5 h per day (160). To overcome this waste of time, *continuous cyclic peritoneal dialysis* (CCPD) has been introduced (161, 162); this modification also incorporates prolonged dwell-times. Three nocturnal exchanges of 2 l (each lasting 3 h) are administered by an automatic cycler while the patient sleeps and a fourth exchange also of 2 l is left in the abdomen during the day. The patient disconnects himself after instillation of the fourth exchange (in the early morning).

This minimises the number of disconnections and the risk of peritoneal infection. In addition more freedom is provided to the patient.

The clearances are similar to those with CAPD.

SIDE EFFECTS AND COMPLICATIONS OF PERITONEAL DIALYSIS

Peritoneal dialysis is basically a simple procedure. However, using the peritoneal cavity as an artificial kidney does not go without hazard. Undesirable effects and complications of peritoneal dialysis have been described in many papers and reviews (22, 30, 163–171). The side effects, that are inherent in the dialysis procedures as practiced today, and the complications, that should be definitely prevented, as they cannot only render dialysis intolerable to the patient, but also threaten his life, will be discussed separately.

Side effects

There are four main categories of undesired side effects: metabolic disturbances, cardiorespiratory consequences, digestive symptoms, and thirst.

Metabolic disturbances
Protein losses are inherent in peritoneal dialysis due to the high permeability of the peritoneal membrane (2, 172, 173). The protein loss per dialysis depends on the nature and type of peritoneal catheter (174, 175), the length of the dwell time, the osmolality and the temperature of dialysis solutions (176), and the duration of dialysis; during periods of peritoneal infection, protein losses may increase 3 to 10 fold (176–178). Protein concentration is usually highest in the first drainage (173, 176, 177); this wash-out phenomenon may be explained by the remaining 'ascites' in the peritoneal cavity during interdialytic intervals (173). The protein loss may also be explained by the presence of an extravascular albumin pool adjacent to the peritoneum, because there is a tendency of the residual peritoneal fluid or ascites to equilibrate with plasma protein as has been demonstrated in studies on transfer kinetics of labelled albumin across the peritoneum (179, 180). An increase in protein concentration in the dialysate has also been noted at the end of dialysis (181); this late rise has been attributed to mechanical or chemical irritation of the peritoneum. Figures on total protein losses during peritoneal dialyses as presented in the literature are widely divergent. This is explained by wide variations between individual patients, although protein losses tend to be rather constant in the same patient (177). It also depends on different techniques of peritoneal dialysis. In early studies of periodic peritoneal dialysis when disposable plastic catheters and the repeated puncture technique were common, the average total protein losses reported in literature ranged from 38.5 to 72.9 g per dialysis in the absence of peritonitis (175–177). In more recent studies when peritoneal dialysis was performed with a permanent silastic catheter and 40 l of dialysate per session, the average total protein losses were reportedly ranging from 4 to 22.3 g per dialysis (181–183). In CAPD protein losses varied from 5.4 to 6.9 g and from 6.2 to 11.5 g per day in patients with or without previous peritonitis (184). All protein fractions present in blood plasma are found in the peritoneal fluid, albumin being the most abundant, representing 65 to 71% of the total protein content of the peritoneal fluid (182–185) or 8.5 to 12 g per dialysis (184). Losses of immunoglobulins have been reported varying from 17.9 g, 3.8 g and 0.78 g (186) to 1.9 g, 0.35 g and 0.12 g (182), respectively, for IgG, IgA and IgM; complement fractions (C_3, C_4) and transferrin have also been found in appreciable amounts (182, 183).

Amino acid losses during peritoneal dialysis average 4.96 g per 27¼ l (187); the concentrations of most amino acids in dialysate were proportional to their plasma concentrations (188). In CAPD, daily mean amino acid losses are between 2 g and 3.5 g/day, 30% of the total amino acid removed consisting of essential amino acids (189).

Protein losses of varying magnitude can result in protein malnutrition. However, metabolic studies have shown that a positive nitrogen balance is maintained in patients treated by maintenance peritoneal dialysis provided the dietary protein intake exceeds 1.2 g/kg body weight per day (172). Protein supplementation of the diet with egg yolks (187) or amino acids (188), intravenous infusion of amino acids during dialysis (187) or addition of amino acids to the dialysis fluid (106) and high protein diets have been recommended to prevent protein depletion. With peritoneal extracorporeal recirculation dialysis, the protein losses were drastically reduced by reinfusing the fluid contained in the extracorporeal circuit into the peritoneal cavity at the end of dialysis (149).

The absorption of *dextrose* from dialysis fluid is a function of dextrose concentration and of dialysate flow rate (190). The total amount of dextrose absorbed per dialysis varies with the duration of dialysis and the type of dialysis solution used (76, 126 or 215 mmol/l dextrose), and varies from 300 to 720 g per day in periodic peritoneal dialysis (190, 191) and from 91 to 214 g per day in continuous ambulatory peritoneal dialysis (192). This dextrose load can induce hyperglycaemia (190, 191, 193, 194) and probably contributes to the high triglyceride levels observed in patients on maintenance peritoneal dialysis (195) and to the obesity observed in some patients on CAPD.

Other metabolic consequences of peritoneal dialysis include hyperlactacidaemia (196, 197) and fatty acid removal (198).

Haemodynamic and cardiorespiratory side effects
Instillation of 2 or 3 l of dialysis solution into the peritoneal cavity induces a 140% increase in intraabdominal pressure and 98% increase of the inferior vena cava pressure (199). There are conflicting data, however, as to the haemodynamic consequences of these changes and how the pulmonary artery pressure and cardiac output are affected. The first of these parameters increased and the second decreased in two studies (200, 201). However, both remained stable according to two other reports (199, 202). The different results of these studies may be explained by differences in the amount of dialysate relative to the patient's body weight. In another study with exchanges volumes of 15 to 26 ml/kg body weight, the intraabdominal pressure was in the range of 5 cm of water and peritoneal dialysis remained free of serious haemodynamic side effects (203).

Vagal induced bradycardia leading to severe hypotension or cardiac standstill can occur during dialysate infusion and should immediately be treated with atropine (30, 164, 204).

Distension of the peritoneal cavity with dialysis fluid results in an upward displacement of the diaphragm and a decrease in vital capacity (205). However, in another more recent report, the only parameter of pulmonary function affected by the infusion of 2 l of dialysis fluid was a reduction of the functional residual capacity; the vital capacity remaining normal (206). A decrease in arterial PO_2 occurs when fluid is run into the peritoneal cavity but changes in PCO_2, usually in the opposite direction from those of PO_2, are less consistent (207). Oxygen transport during an entire peritoneal dialysis has also been studied (208). A slight increase in arterial PO_2 accompanied the negative fluid balance obtained; 2,3-disphosphoglycerate erythrocyte content decreased slightly from high initial values, but there was no change in haemoglobin oxygen affinity.

Gastro-intestinal side effects
Impaired appetite is normally noticed during peritoneal dialysis (181); the performance of overnight dialysis minimises this effect. Nausea and vomiting during the first dialysate exchange was noted in 35% of 54 patients treated by home intermittent peritoneal dialysis (209). Anorexia and vomiting are also observed among the patients treated with CAPD (77, 210, 211), resulting in dietary protein intakes lower than recommended to the patients (212).

Thirst
Thirst is a common complaint in patients dialysed with 10 to 15 min dwell-times and dextrose dialysate concentrations of 126 mmol/l or over. The removal of ultrafiltrate with a low sodium concentration results in post dialytic hypernatraemia and hyperosmolality, and causes thirst. Lowering dialysate sodium concentration to 118 mmol/l during periodic peritoneal dialysis is effective in thirst prevention (80). The long dwell-times of CAPD permit isonatric removal of extracellular fluid and thirst is not observed with this form of peritoneal dialysis (12).

Complications of peritoneal dialysis

Pain
Although much less common with the permanent Silastic catheter than with the disposable catheter (213), pain occurring during dialysis is always distressing to the patient. Localisation and timing of pain should be carefully studied.

Pain occurring during inflow can be caused by low temperature of the dialysis solution and also by a low pH of dialysis solutions requiring adequate sodium hydroxyde buffering (21); pain can be caused by pulsatile dialysate inflow due to infusion by a peristaltic pump. This pain may be alleviated by infusion by gravity or by using special flow dampeners (214); pain can also be caused by a high inflow rate, particularly in case of peritoneal catheter encasement. Pain may be also a symptom of low grade peritonitis and peritoneal adhesion formation (18). Painful abdominal distension at the end of infusion should be relieved by immediate drainage and reduction of exchange volumes.

Outflow pain is much less common. It may be due to entrapment of omentum in the catheter lumen during drainage; incomplete emptying of the abdominal cavity, longer dwell-times and analgesics will help the patient.
Permanent pain occurring after several hours of dialysis is suggestive of mechanical or chemical peritoneal irritation and improves quickly with oral indomethacin (50–100 mg). Constant pain persisting after dialysis completion is almost always indicative of peritonitis (except during the period following catheter implantation). Catheter related pain has been discussed previously (see page 260).

Peritonitis
Peritonitis continues to be the major complication of peritoneal dialysis.

Peritoneal infection entails many harmful and sometimes lethal consequences (17, 169, 171). In the acute phase, protein losses increase (176-178, 180-183); ultrafiltration decreases due to a lower osmotic gradient caused by augmented dextrose absorption (178, 215); ileus and bowel distension can aggravate the pulmonary consequences of peritoneal dialysis (205), resulting in hypoxaemia because of upward diaphragmatic displacement and reflex rigidity of the abdomen (216); nitrogen balance becomes negative because of decreased protein intake, increased protein breakdown and protein losses into the dialysate (217); adhesion formation often occurs (218) resulting in peritoneal multi-location with catheter obstruction (21) and abcess formation; and finally, although seldom reported in peritoneal dialysis patients, death can ensue from uncontrolled sepsis (17). On the long term, peritoneal adhesions may decrease the active surface area of the peritoneal membrane, leading to inadequate dialysis necessitating transfer of the patient to haemodialysis. Sclerotic thickening of the peritoneum (219) and fibroplastic encapsulating peritonitis with intestinal occlusion (220) or persistent fever (221) have also been observed.

The main *routes of peritoneal contamination* are: 1) through the lumen of the peritoneal catheter; 2) across the abdominal wall, through the sinus tract around the catheter; 3) across the wall of an intraperitoneal hollow viscus; 4) from the blood stream; 5) via the peritoneal lymphatics; 6) and finally via the female genital tract.

Exogenous contamination of the peritoneal cavity occurs mainly through the catheter because of breaks in sterility during connection and disconnection of the dialysate delivery circuit to the peritoneal catheter or to the dialysate reservoir, or from dialysis solutions contaminated during storage, particularly when kept in plastic bags (110) or in 10 l plastic containers (111). Dialysate in a plastic bag may be contaminated during immersion in a rewarming bath (33, 139-147). Unsterile dialysate may be produced by an inadequately maintained reverse osmosis machine (120) and infection can occur from defective tubing or accidental disconnection of the dialysate circuit during dialysis. Infection can also occur via the sinus tract around the catheter in case of dialysate leak after catheter placement (21), with the use of the Deane prosthesis (24, 25) or because of infection of the distal segment of the catheter sinus tract, seeding the peritoneal cavity (18).

Endogenous infection of the peritoneum can complicate acute visceral inflammation such as appendicitis, diverticulitis, cholecystitis or perforation of the bowel (17, 222). Transmural migration of bacteria has been inferred from animal experiments (223), but there is no clearcut evidence that bacteria can cross an intact intestinal wall. Transient intestinal ischemia has been shown to cause bacterial peritonitis (224). Endogenous contamination can also occur in cases of septicaemia (17) and from organisms residing in the female genital tract (171).

The *diagnosis of peritonitis* is often more difficult in patients treated with peritoneal dialysis because the usual symptoms and signs of acute peritoneal inflammation are modified by peritoneal irrigation. In most circumstances, however, close attention to the patient's complaints and the aspect of dialysate effluent permit an early diagnosis. Diagnostic criteria have been defined including at least two of the following: 1) symptoms and signs of peritonitis; 2) cloudy dialysis effluent; 3) positive culture of peritoneal fluid (171). In two recent reports (125, 171) signs and symptoms of dialysis associated peritonitis were analysed. Abdominal pain, occurred in 80%, nausea and vomiting in 30%; diarrhoea in 7%. Fever was reported between 29 and 53%, abdominal tenderness in 70% with rebound tenderness in 53%. Cloudy dialysate effluent was observed at least once in each peritonitis episode.

Asymptomatic episodes of peritoneal infection are also possible, requiring special alertness. They can cause one way obstruction of the catheter, loss of appetite, decreasing volumes of dialysate returns, weight gain and oedema and ill defined abdominal discomfort (18, 225).

Careful microbiological examination of the peritoneal fluid is essential for the diagnosis and proper management of peritonitis: peritoneal fluid cultures, Gram staining and white cell counts of the effluent have all been advocated. Effluent fluid cultures are the keystone of the diagnosis, provided an adequate methodology is used.

The following procedures are recommended (171): 1) immediate transfer to the microbiology laboratory of the peritoneal fluid specimens aseptically collected using a vacutainer or an intact dialysate bag: 2) use of appropriate media for aerobic (blood agar and McConkey plates, brain-heart infusion broth), anaerobic (prereduced chopped meat-carbohydrate broth) and fungal (Sabouraud) medium cultures; 3) concentration of specimens by filtration with standard bacteriological filters (16) or more conveniently using the Addi-Check System (Millipore Corp., Bedford, MA, U.S.A.) (171, 226); and 4) minimum observation periods of 7 days for aerobic and 2 weeks for anaerobic cultures because of slow growth of fastidious organisms. Routine cultures in the absence of signs of peritonitis have been proposed for early recognition of infection. In fact, the significance of organisms in the dialysate is not clear (227) as clinical peritonitis seldom follows the appearance of organisms in the dialysate effluent (2, 16, 228, 229); the possibility of specimen contamination when taking cultures on a routine basis (230) can cause confusion and should therefore be discouraged. Gram staining of peritoneal fluid smears is a useful diagnostic adjunct at the time of patient's admission: organisms are seen on direct examination in 30 to 40% of cases and this is helpful in making the choice of an antibiotic before knowing the results of cultures.

Cell counts of the peritoneal fluid are of little value for the diagnosis of peritonitis because the number of cells – normally in the range of 0 to 50 per ml – can fluctuate markedly in a matter of hours (16, 231) and also because cloudiness of the fluid occurs when there are 50 to 100 cells or more per ml of fluid (21, 231). The same limitations exist for the test strip (Cytur-test, Boehringer Mannheim GmbH, Fed Rep Germany), recently proposed for the early detection of high leucocytes counts (232, 233). Differential cell count shows more than 50% polymorphonuclear neutrophils in the acute phase of peritonitis, and its return to normal has been proposed to monitor the effectivity of the antibiotic treatment (16, 231). It also permits the identification of unusual cell patterns in cloudy dialysate, such as peritoneal eosinophilia (234, 235) or a lymphocytosis pointing to tuberculous peritonitis (236).

Aetiologically two types of peritonitis can be identified: 1) infectious peritonitis and 2) cryptogenic (or sterile, aseptic or no growth) peritonitis.

Infectious peritonitis should always be suspected until otherwise proven, as the percentage of infection in large series of patients with peritonitis is over 80% in periodic peritoneal dialysis (237) and usually over 60% in continuous ambulatory peritoneal dialysis (238).

Infection is commonly caused by Gram positive cocci (*Staph. epidermidis, Staph. aureus, Streptococcus viridans, Enterococcus*) or Gram negative bacteria (*Enterobacteriacae, Pseudomonas sp., Acetobacter sp.*) which account respectively for 50 to 60% and 20 to 40% of all infections (16, 171, 237). Uncommon causes of peritonitis include anaerobes, fungi, higher bacteria and *Vibrio*. Anaerobic peritonitis is a rare entity and the presence of *Bacterioides fragilis* or *Clostridium sordelli* should be considered as a sign of leakage from the bowel (171). Fungal peritonitis is less exceptional: *Candida* species account for 1 to 4% of infections. *C. albicans, C. tropicalis, C. parapsilosis* and *C. krusei* have all been identified in some cases (239–244). Infections caused by a lipophylic yeast (245), by environmental fungi such as *Aspergillus sp.* (246) *Dreschlera specifera* (111, 247) and *Fusarium sp.* (171), by higher bacteria (*Actinomyces sp.* (248), *Nocardia bacterioides* (244) and *Vibrio Alginolyticus* (249)) have also been described.

Tuberculous peritonitis often presents as a sterile peritonitis which, does not respond to treatment (250, 251). A deteriorating general condition and signs of systemic toxicity should raise suspicion; in a case observed by the author a differential cell count with 90% lymphocytes was an important diagnostic clue. Stains for acid-fast bacilli are usually negative, peritoneal biopsy is required for early diagnosis.

Sterile peritonitis may be diagnosed only after carefully excluding a microbiological aetiology. Less frequent in periodic than in continuous ambulatory peritoneal dialysis, its incidence varies from 4 to 50% of all peritonitis episodes (238). The aetiology of this condition remains obscure. Physicochemical irritation of the peritoneum by dialysate has been suggested as a possible cause. The low pH (52) and high osmolality (252) of dialysis solutions have been incriminated.

Other possible causes are 5-methoxyfurfural and bisulfite (92), particulate matter (253) in the dialysis fluid or accidental contamination with endotoxins (126, 254, 255), or with formalin (39) or povidone-iodine (256). Negative cultures can also result from a poor microbiological methodology, including delayed transfer of the

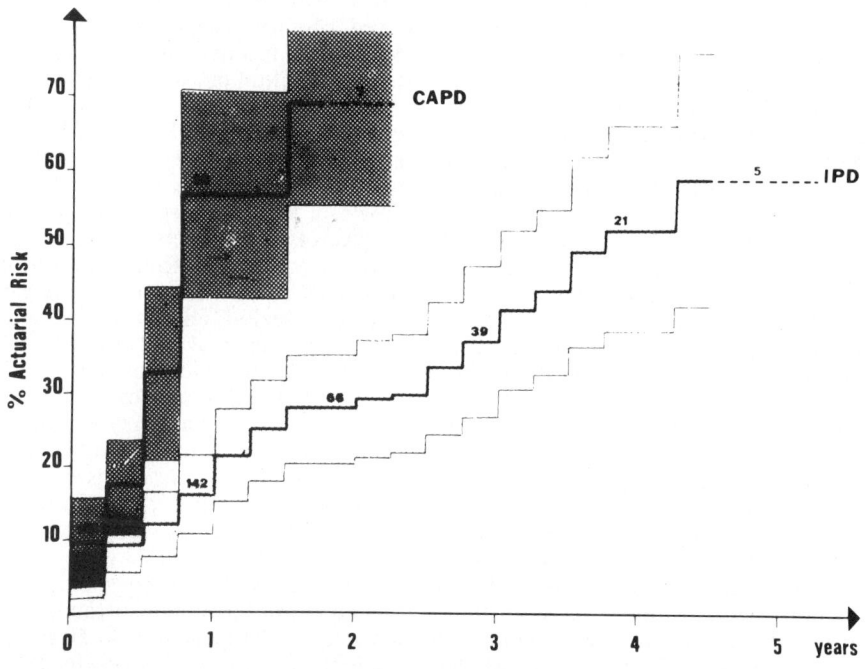

Figure 6. Actuarial analysis of the risk of having a first episode of peritonitis in patients treated with maintenance peritoneal dialysis. CAPD (continuous ambulatory peritoneal dialysis): 57% of the exposed patients had a peritonitis episode at the end of the first year of treatment. IPD (periodic peritoneal dialysis): 50% of the patients had a first episode of peritonitis after 3.6 years of exposure. (Confidence limits represented by dotted area; difference statistically significant, $p<0.001$). (Courtesy Dr A. Slingeneyer).

specimens to the laboratory, inoculation of culture media with an insufficient amount (0.1 ml) of non concentrated peritoneal fluid, and the presence of antibiotics in the peritoneal effluent (16, 171). Pseudo-membranous colitis associated with aseptic peritonitis has recently been described (257).

Peritoneal eosinophilia (234, 235) has been described in patients with a cloudy peritoneal effluent, usually without pain. The white cell count was over 100 cells per mm^3 and the differential count consisted of less than 50% polymorphonuclear leucocytes with more than 10% eosinophils. The natural course of this condition appeared benign not necessitating any therapy. Peritoneal eosinophilia can occur during the treatment of bacterial peritonitis (16, 234).

The *incidence of peritonitis* has been reported as a percentage of all dialyses, ranging from 0.2 to 1.9% (19); it has also been presented for groups of patients as the number of episodes per year of treatment, ranging from 0.23 to 6.3 peritonitis episodes per year (171) or as the mean time interval between two peritonitis episodes which, according to data presented in the literature, range from 10 weeks (12) to 4.7 years (111). These methods of presenting the incidence of peritonitis have been critisised however and are unsuitable for statistical evaluation (158). The use of the actuarial life table method (259) is preferable (260). The actuarial analysis of peritoneal infection in patients treated by the author's group with periodic or continuous ambulatory peritoneal dialysis is presented in Figure 6.

The most sensible approach to the problem of peritoneal dialysis associated peritonitis is *an efficient prevention programme,* which requires a team approach actively involving both the patient and the nursing staff. Protocols should be designed for the care of the catheter including preventing dialysate leakage from early abdominal distension, the use of povidone-iodine and adherence to meticulous sterility with connect/diconnect procedures (18). A closed dialysate delivery circuit should be preferred whenever possible and plastic bags should be used rather than bottles for manual techniques. Rewarming baths should be abandoned. The use of bacteriologic filters in the dialysate infusion line has significantly reduced the risk of infection from a contaminated dialysate (261, 262). Careful maintenance of reverse osmosis machines should include routine sterilisation of the reverse osmosis membranes after each dialysis and frequent checks of membrane integrity (39). Shortening of a single dialysis to less than 72 h (263) and the use of a special quick connect/disconnect device (Betacap, Quinton Instruments Corp. Seattle WA U.S.A.) (264) have also contributed to a decreased infection rate. Peritoneal disinfection with a saline iodine flush technique has been proposed (265) but its efficiency and safety have recently been questioned because the iodine concentration in the irrigating solution has to be in the toxic range to be bactericidal (266). The use of a photochemical reactor in the dialysate infusion line has also been suggested (267).

Antibiotic prophylaxis has been attempted either with oral neomycin (263, 268) or with intraperitoneal antibiotics (228, 269), but the results of these studies have been inconclusive. A recent double blind randomised trial with oral cephalexin in patients on CAPD showed no benefit from prophylactic antibiotics (270).

The management of peritonitis should aim at controlling the peritoneal infection, preserving the integrity of the peritoneal membrane and sustaining the patient's general condition during the acute phase of the disease. Early recognition of the peritoneal infection and prompt initiation of therapy are both necessary to increase the chances of complete cure. A widely accepted therapeutic regimen includes peritoneal lavage and antibiotic treatment (18, 40, 59, 167, 237, 271). Continuous peritoneal lavage removes fibrin and cellular debris and should be promptly instituted after completion of the diagnostic procedures. Heparin should be added to the dialysate (500 IU/l) to reduce fibrin clot formation and to prevent subsequent adhesions (272). Peritoneal lavage should be continued until negative cultures have been obtained on three consecutive days; thereafter, the usual dialysis schedule can be resumed. The efficacy and innocuity of peritoneal lavage have been recently questioned (273): this procedure may interfere with normal defence mechanisms of the peritoneum (274). In patients on continuous ambulatory peritoneal dialysis, good results have

Table 1. Antibiotic dosage for peritonitis complicating dialysis (from Maher JF (169) with permission).

Drug	Systemic dosage mg/kg/day	Safe plasma concentration µg/ml	Plasma water concentration µg/ml	Intraperitoneal dosage mg/l
Cephalothin	40–80	50–100	15–30	10–50
Ampicillin	50–100	50–100	40–80	20–50
Methicillin	50–100	100–200	65–130	100
Oxacillin	50–100	50–100	5–10	10
Carbenicillin	50–100	200	100	200
Penicillin G	80,000 (U)	50,000 (U)	25,000 (U)	10,000 (U)
Gentamicin	1–2/3	10–12	8–10	8
Kanamycin	7.5/3	10–15	10–15	10
Lincomycin	10–15	2–5	0.5	2–5
Clindamycin	5–15	2	0.2	1–2
Chloramphenicol	5–10	40–60	20–30	20–30
Amphotericin	0.5–1.0	0.5–3.5	0.1–0.5	3

been obtained with 6 h exchanges following three initial rapid dialysate exchanges (16, 275).

Antibiotics can be prescribed intraperitoneally, systemically and by both routes simultaneously. Most authors recommend the addition of antibiotics to the dialysate; data concerning appropriate concentrations and the stability of antibiotics in dialysis solutions are presented in Table 1 (169). Aminoglycosides can be added to heparin containing dialysate without losing their efficiency (95). Most antibiotics administered intraperitoneally diffuse readily into the blood and can attain bactericidal serum levels provided that the concentration in the dialysis solution is adequate. However, an initial loading dose should often be given parenterally to obtain effective plasma concentrations quickly (93). Numerous studies are available concerning the pharmacokinetics and dosages of antibiotics in patients treated with peritoneal dialysis (276-291); these data have been obtained in uninfected patients however and the transfer rates occurring in infected subjects may actually be higher.

A practical antibiotic regimen includes the addition of 200 mg cephalothin per litre of dialysis fluid as the initial treatment; if Gram stains and/or cultures detect Gram negative bacteria in the peritoneal effluent, tobramycin (16 mg/l dialysate) should also be added (although cephalothin and tobramycin should not be mixed in the same syringe, they can be added safely to the same dialysate bag [18, 171]). This antibiotic combination has a broad antibacterial spectrum and will be effective against most bacteria; however, the choice of antibiotic(s) may have to be modified later, according to the *in vitro* sensitivity of the isolated organisms. Trimethoprim-sulfamethoxazole has also been advocated as the first choice antibacterial agent (271); vancomycin can play a major role in case of penicillinase forming *Staphylococcus* species (292, 293).

The clinical course of peritonitis should be monitored by daily cultures and serial white cell counts of the peritoneal effluent (16, 231). In periodic peritoneal dialysis, oral or parenteral antibiotics are empirically continued for 10 to 15 days after stopping peritoneal lavage. In CAPD, intraperitoneal antibiotics are continued until clinical, microbiological and cytologic criteria of cure are satisfactory. When aminoglycosides are used, the duration of treatment should not exceed two weeks to reduce the risk of nephrotoxicity and ototoxicity (171).

Fungal peritonitis has been successfully managed with 5-fluorocytosine and kinetics studies of this antifungal drug have been carried out in infected patients (239). Cure has also been obtained with intraperitoneal and/or intravenous amphotericin B (242-244), although intraperitoneal administration in one series caused severe abdominal pain (244). The experience with miconazole (243) and ketoconazole is still limited.

Catheter removal during the course of peritonitis may be indicated when peritoneal fluid cultures remain positive after one week of adequate antibiotic treatment. Resistance to treatment can result from an infected indwelling catheter, from the formation of an intraperitoneal abscess or from a perforated intraabdominal viscus. Catheter removal has also been recommended in cases of fungal peritonitis (243, 244).

When secondary perforation peritonitis is suspected, a laparatomy should be carried out without delay. The bowel and other viscera should be carefully inspected because minute lesions may be responsible for persisting multibacterial infections. The decision to abandon peritoneal dialysis because of spreading of the infection over the entire peritoneal cavity at this stage can be difficult, but transfer of the patient to haemodialysis often has been preferred.

Supportive treatment is essential for an ultimate successful cure of peritonitis. Total parenteral nutrition is required in the anorectic patient for the maintenance of a good nutritional status. Ambulation and breathing exercises (294) help to prevent pulmonary complications. Extracorporeal ultrafiltration can be used as an adjunct to peritoneal dialysis when control of extracellular volume becomes difficult as a consequence of reduced peritoneal ability to ultrafilter and (or) when intravenous infusion of liberal amounts of fluid is indicated to increase the caloric intake. In severe cases, early transfer to haemodialysis is often the only alternative to satisfactory control of uraemia and electrolyte and water balance.

Cryptogenic peritonitis is usually milder and of shorter duration than infectious peritonitis; it may heal spontaneously or with simple peritoneal lavage with heparinised dialysate (238).

Tuberculous peritonitis should be treated with at least two bactericidal antituberculous drugs, preferably isoniazid and rifampicin, for at least nine months (295).

Outcome and prognosis of peritonitis associated with peritoneal dialysis have improved since the introduction of the Tenckhoff catheter. Since then peritonitis became a benign disease with no death attributable to this complication (40, 126). In fact, a favourable outcome occurs in a large majority of patients. They can continue on peritoneal dialysis without apparent reduction in peritoneal clearances (52, 296). However, there is growing evidence in the literature that peritoneal dialysis associated infectious peritonitis can also be a life threatening disease with an unpredictable course. Deaths related to peritonitis, either from uncontrolled infection or from secondary cardiovascular, neurologic or pulmonary complications are reported with an increasing frequency (17, 220, 256, 297). As in other types of peritonitis, the source of contamination, the patient's age and the existence of associated diseases are important prognostic factors (216).

Catheter outflow failure necessitating catheter replacement occurs frequently in peritonitis. Inadequate peritoneal dialysis following peritonitis is not rare, because of peritoneal adhesion formation, reducing the effective surface area of the peritoneum (18, 298, 299). Recent studies with longer follow-ups have detected a significant progressive reduction in peritoneal mass transfer coefficients in patients who had peritonitis previously (300). Extracellular volume excess has also been attributed to reduced peritoneal ultrafiltration following infection (170, 301). Finally, relapsing episodes of partial intestinal occlusion necessitating abdominal surgery caused by the development of chronic fibrous peritoneal thickening and induration has been reported (220, 252) with a course similar to practolol peritonitis (302). This new entity has been observed both after sterile and microbial peritonitis. The surgical removal of the neoformed peritoneal membrane is indicated, but this surgery has been complicated by lethal septic peritonitis (252).

Metabolic complications
Peritoneal dialysis interferes with the metabolism of water and electrolytes and of carbohydrates. Electrolyte imbalance due to renal failure is usually satisfactorily corrected by peritoneal dialysis, however, difficulties with dialysate outflow, excessive administration of dialysis solutions with high osmolality or unusual permeability characteristics of the peritoneal membrane observed in certain patients (68) may all induce metabolic complications.

Hypovolaemia resulting in acute hypotension and even shock because of excessive ultrafiltration has been observed. To prevent this, it is wise to test the ultrafiltration capacity of each patient by measuring the ultrafiltration obtained in a certain period of time with different dialysate formulations avoiding more than two or three consecutive highly hypertonic exchanges.

Hypervolaemia can be caused by the accumulation of dialysate in the peritoneal cavity due to poor drainage or to a peritoneal fluid leak into the subcutaneous tissue caused by a rupture of the peritoneal membrane in particular after recent abdominal surgery. The subsequent extracellular fluid overload can lead to hypervolaemia with pulmonary oedema or (and) hypertension (22, 30). In this situation, extracorporeal ultrafiltration is mandatory.

Hypernatraemia with plasma sodium concentrations over 150 mmol/l has been reported in 3 to 10% of dialyses (22, 303). It results from osmotic ultrafiltration with the production of a low sodium ultrafiltrate (60, 61). It can be prevented by giving to the patient adequate amounts of free water orally or 5% dextrose solution intravenously depending on his clinical status (see also chapter 21 and 22). Hypernatraemia can also result from the accidental instillation of hypernatric dialysate due to a malfunctioning reverse osmosis machine (170).

Hypokalaemia has been observed in 10 to 19% of peritoneal dialyses (22, 303): it is usually moderate and without clinical significance, but may cause severe arrhythmias in a digitalised patient. Severe hypokalaemia can occur with prolonged peritoneal lavage in the anorectic patient (e.g. with peritonitis) and may be aggravated by dextrose loading and correction of acidosis. To prevent this risk 2 to 4 mmol/l KCl should be added to dialysis solutions.

Hyperkalaemia results from the inappropriate use of potassium containing dialysate (30) or from ineffective dialysis in a highly catabolic patient. A sudden rise of serum potassium concentration has been noted shortly after termination of peritoneal dialysis and has been attributed to the breakdown of glycogen (22, 62); it never reached levels requiring the resumption of dialysis.

Metabolic alkalosis with serum bicarbonate level over 30 mmol/l has been attributed to the use of dialysate containing 42 to 45 mmol/l lactate and possibly to 'contraction alkalosis' due to the rapid removal of water and slow diffusion of bicarbonate from the plasma (82, 163). Peritoneal dialysis with lactate containing dialysis solutions has been associated with persistent metabolic acidosis in patients with liver failure (163). This can be corrected by intravenous bicarbonate or continuation of dialysis with dialysis solution containing acetate (30).

Blood sugar levels over 11 mmol/l (200 mg/dl) have been observed in 10 to 15% of dialyses (22, 303). *Severe hyperglycaemia* may occur even in the non diabetic patient with the prolonged use of 215 mmol/l (4.25%) or 354 mmol/l (7%) concentrations of dextrose monohydrate in dialysis solutions because of rapid loading with dextrose, absence of glycosuria and uraemic carbohydrate intolerance (191, 193). This rare complication (occurring in 1 to 3% of dialyses) can result in hyperosmolar (non ketotic) coma with convulsions and death. Close monitoring of blood sugar levels is mandatory when serial exchanges with high dextrose concentrations are needed and insulin should be given intraperitoneally (107–109) or subcutaneously to maintain blood sugar levels below 16.5 mmol/l (300 mg/dl). A major risk of post-dialytic *hypoglycaemia* exists in patients receiving insulin during dialysis, and convulsions with irreversible brain damage can complicate such hypoglycaemic episodes (30). Prevention is best accomplished by omitting intraperitoneal insulin for the last four exchanges or by leaving a final volume of 500 ml of 215 mmol/l (4.25 g/dl) dextrose monohydrate dialysate in the peritoneal cavity at the end of dialysis (59); with subcutaneous insulin, the last injection should be administered at least six hours before the termination of dialysis.

Miscellaneous complications
Cardiovascular complications, including arrhythmias, with occasional fatalities due to acute digitalis toxicity, myocardial infarction or cardiac arrest have been noted in 15 to 66% of peritoneal dialyses (22, 303).

Pulmonary complications include pneumonitis following basal atelectasis (205) and pneumonia due to aspiration of gastric contents (22); both carry a significant mortality. Rare cases of acute massive hydrothorax have been reported. In seven cases (304, 305) it occurred on the right side and caused severe dyspnea, appearing during the first 24 h of dialysis, which was relieved by thoracocentesis and cessation of peritoneal dialysis. In a case of post-traumatic acute renal failure, acute hydrothorax was due to the seeping of fluid through a rent in the diaphragm (165). Bilateral pleural effusions seem more common and are often asymptomatic (205, 306).

Neurologic complications including confusion, headache, neuromuscular irritability, transient cerebral abnormalities or seizures have been noted in 6 to 18% of dialyses (22, 303). They have been attributed to the dialysis disequilibrium syndrome, but metabolic disturbances (hyperosmolality, hypoglycaemia, alkalosis) may cause similar manifestations and should be excluded. Post-dialytic convulsions have also been observed 6 to 12 h after termination of dialysis (22, 303); in one series, this was associated with an impaired lactate metabolism (196).

Asymptomatic pneumoperitoneum results from the introduction of small amounts of air during dialysis procedures; it usually goes unnoticed, except if visualised on a chest X-ray showing air under the diaphragm. Acute pneumoperitoneum may be observed after accidental air infusion at the end of dialysis when an automatic cycler with a roller pump is used for dialysate infusion or when a reverse osmosis machine is fed with poorly deaerated water. Acute pneumoperitoneum may cause persistent epigastric and shoulder pain in the upright position; air removal should be attempted by infusion 1 or 2 l of dialysis fluid followed by the Trendelenburg or chest-knee position (18).

Wound dehiscence with evisceration is a real hazard when peritoneal dialysis is performed following recent abdominal surgery (30, 169). This should be prevented by sealing tightly the abdominal incision at the termination of the surgical procedure and by using small volume exchanges (170, 307); it is often safer to treat the patient with haemodialysis until the abdominal wound heals (308).

Increase in size of a pre-existing hernia can occur, but this seldom interferes with the dialysis procedures (21) except in some patients with wide open scrotal hernias where discomfort may result from accumulation of a large volume of dialysis fluid.

Infusion of *inadequately rewarmed dialysate* has been a cause of severe complications. Infusion of cold dialysate can induce acrocyanosis or cardiac arrhythmias (169). This resulted in a cardiac arrest in two children (21). Overheated dialysate is a cause of severe intraabdominal pain that may be quickly relieved by immediate drainage of the dialysate, however, it has been followed in one occasion by a persistent paralytic ileus and metabolic acidosis (170). Fail safe temperature monitoring is mandatory for automatic and semi-automatic peritoneal dialysis equipment.

In patients undergoing maintenance peritoneal dialysis, *malnutrition* may become a problem which is often unrecognised (309). It has been described as the 'depletion syndrome' (310) and is characterised by a progressive loss of lean body mass, often masked by overhydration giving a false impression of stable body weight. The diagnosis of this 'failure to thrive' syndrome, which is often associated with peripheral neuropathy (21) is difficult because it resembles closely signs and symptoms of chronic uraemia.

The *recurrent ascites syndrome* is another complication of periodic peritoneal dialysis, occurring in patients transferred to haemodialysis (18, 311). Low serum albumin is a constant finding and is associated with hypovolaemia and frequent hypotensive episodes during dialysis causing difficult ultrafiltration. Fibrosis and chronic inflammatory changes have been seen in peritoneal biopsies.

INDICATIONS FOR PERITONEAL DIALYSIS

The numerous indications for peritoneal dialysis can be classified under five different headings: 1) acute renal failure; 2) chronic renal failure; 3) poisoning; 4) miscellaneous conditions in the adult; and 5) special indications in children.

Peritoneal dialysis in acute renal failure

This has always been a major indication for peritoneal dialysis. Today, most nephrologists agree that the first dialysis should be peritoneal when dialysis is required for acute renal failure (312). The various factors influencing the choice between peritoneal or haemodialysis have been amply reviewed (313–315).

In many dialysis units, peritoneal dialysis is preferred because it can be started easily and without delay. Its technical simplicity favours easy acceptance by the nursing staff. Because heparin is unnecessary peritoneal dialysis is particularly suitable in bleeding and traumatised patients. Despite reduced peritoneal clearances in hypotensive patients (316), peritoneal dialysis remains efficient. Furthermore, when the patient is treated with peritoneal dialysis invasive diagnostic procedures (e.g. a kidney biopsy) can be performed with less risk than in a haemodialysed patient. However available staff and equipment are also important determinants in making the choice (315). Recently, satisfactory results were reported with continuous equilibration peritoneal dialysis (CAPD) in 20 patients with oliguric acute renal failure (317).

Peritoneal dialysis may, however, not be adequate in hypercatabolic patients because of its low efficiency; this can be compensated by instituting dialysis early ('prophylactic' dialysis) and by maintaining peritoneal urea clearances in the range of 25 to 30 ml/min with an appropriate dialysate flow (318). Peritoneal dialysis has been used with success after recent abdominal surgery (319) although an increased incidence of peritoneal infection has been reported in this setting (164). In cases of secondary peritonitis, peritoneal dialysis has been used preferably to treat both uraemia and peritoneal infection.

In acute renal failure following X-ray contrast procedures, iodinated contrast material was efficiently removed by peritoneal dialysis (320). Similarly, substantial amounts of monoclonal immunoglobulins have been removed by peritoneal dialysis in cases of multiple myeloma with renal failure (321). Whether removal of these solutes affects the clinical course is unknown.

Peritoneal dialysis in chronic renal failure

Peritoneal dialysis has been used both as a temporary treatment and as a long term maintenance therapy of irreversible end stage renal disease.

As a *temporary treatment*, peritoneal dialysis is indicated: 1) in cases of acute renal failure superimposed on chronic renal insufficiency, in particular in patients with chronic pyelonephritis or polycystic kidneys, where long term remissions may be obtained after a few dialyses (322, 323); 2) during the clinical observation of a patient without previous history of chronic renal disease; 3) in preparation for blood access surgery in the bleeding uraemic patient and during maturation of a recently created arteriovenous fistula; 4) as a holding procedure until a place becomes available in a haemodialysis unit; and 5) in conjunction with an active transplantation programme, both to maintain the patient before transplantation and to manage post-transplant acute renal failure (324, 325).

Long term peritoneal dialysis is indicated on medical grounds in patients unsuitable for haemodialysis (52, 59, 301) such as: 1) older patients, age usually over 65 years, 2) patients with preexisting cardiovascular diseases (socalled high cardio-vascular risk patients) e.g. patients with angina pectoris, with previous myocardial infarction, cardiomyopathies, arrhythmias, or a previous cerebrovascular accident, 3) insulin and non-insulin dependent diabetic patients, 4) those with frequent blood access failures, 5) children, 6) patients with severe bleeding risks, 7) and Jehovah's witnesses. Maintenance peritoneal dialysis has also been proposed for home dialysis (326, 327); because of the absence of extracorporeal blood circulation, peritoneal dialysis can be safely used in the home even for patients living alone and is often more acceptable than haemodialysis for parents dialysing an uraemic child in the home setting (328). With the introduction of continuous ambulatory peritoneal dialysis, the indications for peritoneal dialysis in chronic renal failure have been enlarged, and some groups consider it the first choice of treatment (153, 297, 329).

Peritoneal dialysis in the treatment of poisoning
Peritoneal dialysis is one of the accepted modalities for treatment of acute exogenous intoxications with drugs or poisons. Recent reviews have amply analysed the numerous intoxications treated by peritoneal dialysis (330–333). The effectiveness of peritoneal dialysis in removing toxic substances is only 5 to 30% of haemodialysis or haemoperfusion (332). Attempts to enhance peritoneal clearances of drugs have been made by manipulation of dialysate pH to facilitate anionic diffusion of weak acids or bases (334, 335), and the addition of albumin to the dialysate to prevent back diffusion of toxic substances such as phenobarbital or salicylates (336, 337) by binding to albumin. The use of pharmacologic additives has also been suggested to increase the effectiveness of peritoneal dialysis in poisoning, but clinical experience is still lacking (332).

Peritoneal dialysis may be advantageous in patients with marked hypotension or hypothermia or both, in young children where haemodialysis can be technically difficult, and in patients too ill to be transported to a centre where haemodialysis is available (333). The role of peritoneal dialysis in the management of acute intoxications is presently very limited: haemoperfusion is usually the treatment of choice. Obviously the drug or toxic substance should be dialysable (see Chapter 16 and 39).

Peritoneal dialysis in miscellaneous conditions (in the adult)

Peritoneal dialysis has been applied to patients with various morbid states even in the absence of renal failure. Its usefulness appears well established in the following predominantly non-renal conditions: 1) intractable heart failure with diuretic resistant oedema, wherein diuretic responsiveness can be restored by osmotic ultrafiltration (338–340), 2) severe hyperuricaemia and acute gouty nephropathy (341–343); 3) profound hypothermia where peritoneal dialysis permits safe progressive core rewarming (344, 345); 4) severe hypercalcaemia which has been successfully treated by peritoneal dialysis with a calcium free dialysis fluid (346, 347), and 5) prolonged hypoglycaemia due to an overdose of an oral hypoglycaemic agent (348, 349).

Beneficial results of peritoneal dialysis have also been reported in acute pancreatitis (350, 351), hepatic coma (352), and severe psoriasis (353). The reported series are, however, uncontrolled and too small to draw definite conclusions.

Special indications in children

Peritoneal dialysis has been safely used in infants and children with acute renal failure and poisoning (354, 355) and more recently in the treatment of end-stage chronic renal disease (328, 356–360). Peritoneal dialysis has also been helpful in the treatment of a wide range of different disorders, including cystic fibrosis with congestive heart failure (361), the respiratory distress syndrome (362, 363), severe hydrops foetalis (364) and Reye's syndrome (365, 366). Encouraging results have also been obtained in the treatment of maple syrup urine disease (367), of propionic acidaemia (368) and with the removal of unconjugated bilirubin (with albumin containing dialysis solutions) (369).

CONTRAINDICATIONS FOR PERITONEAL DIALYSIS

There is no absolute contraindication to peritoneal dialysis (18). However, extracorporeal dialysis seems to be preferable in acute and chronic respiratory insufficiency, when infusion of dialysis fluid may aggravate hypoxaemia and respiratory acidosis leading ultimately to cardiac arrest. Haemodialysis also is preferred in patients with drains in the peritoneal cavity, an enterostomy or ureterostomy, with spreading infection or cellulitis of the abdominal wall (which increase the risk of peritoneal infection), with a past history of repeated abdominal surgery, and with diffuse peritoneal malignancy which increases the risk of perforation of a viscus. Peritoneal dialysis is also contraindicated in patients with intestinal obstruction with gross abdominal distention and in patients with a large hernia with a wide open hernial sack. Adequate dialysate inflow, drainage and maintenance of the fluid balance may all be difficult. Serious obesity may make catheter implantation difficult and even hazardous. These conditions may be regarded as relative contraindications. The limitations of peritoneal dialysis in the hypercatabolic patient have previously been discussed (318).

MAINTENANCE PERITONEAL DIALYSIS

Despite growing interest (370) the application of periodic peritoneal dialysis in the last decade remained limited. By the end of 1977 only 545 patients with end stage renal failure were treated by this dialysis modality in Europe (371).

On the other hand by the end of 1979 the total number of patients in Europe on treatment with peritoneal dialysis had increased by more than 70% compared to 1978, mainly because the fast growth of the number of patients treated by continuous ambulatory peritoneal dialysis (CAPD). In many of them CAPD was the treatment of first choice (372).

By the end of 1980, 1,728 patients, representing 2.4% of the total dialysis population in Europe, were treated by CAPD (373).

In the USA this treatment modality was applied to 2,170 patients in 1980 (374).

Periodic peritoneal dialysis

In recent years this treatment modality became less popular as the method of first choice for patients with end-stage chronic renal disease, partly because of a better understanding of its limitations (375, 376) and partly because of the introduction of CAPD.

Dialysis schedules
In the early years of periodic peritoneal dialysis, using the repeated puncture technique, 36 to 40 h dialyses were performed once a week (7–10) or even once every 21 to 28 days in combination with restricted protein intake (377). The introduction of the permanent indwelling catheter made more frequent dialysis possible. Since then a great variety of dialysis schedules has been proposed: 10 to 12 h 2 to 3 times a week (40), 10 h 4 times a week (127, 378), 9 h 3 times a week (379), 5 to 7 overnight dialyses (380) and short daily dialyses (381). The weekly amount of dialysate used with these schedules ranged from 70 to 240 l at a dialysate flow rate of 2 to 4 l/h.

Table 2. Effect of residual renal function (KCr) on overall creatinine clearance (C) and dialysis requirements (td) of a patient started on periodic peritoneal dialysis with *an initial schedule of 36 h per week*. The measured peritoneal creatinine clearance (KdCr) is 18 ml/min.

KCr (ml/min)	C (ml/min)	Required td adjustment * (hr/week)
3	6.8	—
2	5.8	+ 9.3
1	4.8	+18.6
0	3.8	+27.9

* Increases in td required to maintain C to its initial value.

Effect of residual renal function on dialysis requirements
Most reports on results obtained with periodic peritoneal dialysis do not include detailed information on important parameters such as body size and surface area, protein and total caloric intake and residual renal function. Consequently, often no meaningful conclusions can be drawn from these studies as to the optimal dialysis schedule for a given patient.

Recently, the concept of an *overall creatinine clearance* has been proposed as an index for chronic peritoneal dialysis to aim at a clearance of 4 to 5 ml/min (382), which is compatible with adequacy of peritoneal dialysis. This index can be calculated according to the equation:

$$C = \frac{KdCr \times td}{10{,}080} + KCr$$

where, C   = overall creatinine clearance
KdCr = measured peritoneal creatinine clearance in ml/min
td   = dialysis time in minutes per week
KCr = endogenous creatinine clearance in ml/min
10,080 = total minutes in one week.

This equation underlines the major contribution of the residual renal function, KCr, on the total amount of creatinine cleared per week in a given patient. As shown in Table 2, in a patient dialysed 36 h per week C will decline from 6.8 ml/min to 3.8 ml/min when KCr decreases from 3 ml/min to zero. To maintain C at its initial value, an increase of 28 h of dialysis per week would be required since 1 ml/min of KCr is equivalent to 9.3 h per week of periodic peritoneal dialysis (383). However, such an adjustment would not be accepted by most patients, who are reluctant to accept the burden of 40 or more hours of periodic peritoneal dialysis per week.

Measurement of residual GFR in dialysis patients (384). The clearance period should be 2½ to 3 days e.g. over a weekend if the patient undergoes dialyses on Monday, Wednesday and Friday (if the patient has a urine volume of 500 ml or more/24 h the clearance period could be limited to 24 to 36 h). The urine collection begins with voiding after dialysis as soon as possible (but not later than 1.0 h). That first specimen should be discarded. All urine is collected thereafter and final voiding should be as close to the next dialysis as possible.

Arterial blood samples for measuring creatinine concentration are obtained at the end of the dialysis preceeding the clearance measurement and an 'on dialysis' sample at the dialysis which terminates the collection period.

The clearance is calculated in the usual way, using the mean of the 'on' and 'off' blood samples.

Clinical results
Excellent control of uraemia has been observed with periodic peritoneal dialysis in most patients observed for short periods (40, 127, 379–381, 385–388). A low incidence of peritonitis has been obtained in most series (19). Better cardiovascular stability, higher haematocrit, a lesser frequency of pericarditis (385), and improved platelet functions (390, 391) have been claimed as advantages of periodic peritoneal dialysis. Negative aspects have also been reported. Thirst, resulting in excessive drinking and weight gain, is a frequent cause of

poor blood pressure control (392). Serum albumin levels are usually low (183) and the control of hyper phosphataemia requires high doses of phosphate binding agents. Renal osteodystrophy and neuropathy have been observed (59). Inadequate dialysis often only becomes apparent after 12 to 18 months of periodic peritoneal dialysis, requiring transfer to haemodialysis. Underdialysis, often goes long unrecognised because of a subtle clinical picture characterised by anorexia, muscle wasting and general malnutrition. The usual signs of the uraemic syndrome like mucositis, pericarditis and neuropathy are often absent (383, 393). In addition the syndrome developes insidiously.

Home versus hospital peritoneal dialysis
Periodic peritoneal dialysis has been used in the hospital as well as in the home. However, home peritoneal dialysis is usually preferred because of simplicity and safety which allow unattended overnight dialysis even if the patient is living alone; the risk of peritoneal infection is lower; hepatitis B outbreaks in the nursing staff and in other dialysis patients caused by contaminated peritoneal fluid from chronic HBsAg carriers is prevented (394, 395). In addition, occupying a hospital dialysis station for more than 40 h per week is costly both in staff time, bed occupancy and total expense (393).

Hospital periodic peritoneal dialysis facilities should be reserved for training patients for home dialysis and for temporary treatment of patients with medical and social problems (396).

Long term results and actuarial survival rates
Data on long term patient survival with periodic peritoneal dialysis are scarce. Most published series cover follow-up periods too short to allow for objective statistical analysis of patient survival (40, 379–381, 385–388). In the available literature, only four papers discuss cumulative patient survival data (127, 299, 393, 397). Three years survivals of 40 to 55% were observed when all patients were included, the 3 year survival was 65% for patients less than 60 years old (299, 393): these data are comparable to cumulative survival observed in patients of similar age groups treated with haemodialysis (398). However, a large number of patients had to be converted to haemodialysis. 'Technique survival', comparable to graft survival following transplantation, was therefore proposed as a better measure of success of peritoneal dialysis (393). In two groups (299, 393) such an analysis showed a disappointing 25 to 30% technique survival at three years. Causes for conversion to haemodialysis were inadequate dialysis, frequent infections, loss of familial support and abdominal pain. These data confirm that periodic peritoneal dialysis has important limitations for long term treatment of end stage renal failure.

Continuous ambulatory peritoneal dialysis

This low dialysate flow technique achieves lower clearances than periodic peritoneal dialysis of urea and other small molecule substances but this is partially compensated by increasing total dialysis time from 40 to about 168 h per week (64, 374). Defined as a portable wearable equilibrium peritoneal dialysis technique (11), it has stimulated a tremendous interest because of its continuous action and its simplicity.

Dialysis schedules
Peritoneal urea clearance is equal to the drained volume. The frequency of daily dialysate exchanges should be prescribed to obtain a desirable blood urea level taking into account protein intake, urea generation, and residual renal function (309). Five exchanges per day were initially recommended (12), but presently most patients practise 4 daily exchanges (77, 153). In a few patients, satisfactory results were obtained with 3 daily exchanges, but the residual renal creatinine clearance was over 1 ml/min (399).

A method of estimating the relationship between protein intake and urea generation has been described that can be used to determine the number of exchanges per day or per week to achieve a total urea clearance (peritoneal urea clearance + renal urea clearance) required to maintain a certain level of blood urea (generally 20 to 30 mmol/l, [120 to 180 mg/dl]) (309).

Clinical and biochemical results with CAPD
Short term clinical experiences (12, 77, 155, 400) have reported excellent control of blood pressure despite more liberal sodium and water intakes, higher haemoglobin levels (without a proven increase in total red cell mass [401]), and excellent control of serum chemistries, with phosphate maintained near normal values despite a lower dose of phosphate binding agents. Longer follow-ups have confirmed these data (153, 402, 403). Nevertheless continuous ambulatory peritoneal dialysis certainly causes problems (403, 404). Initially high peritoneal infection rates have been reduced with various techniques (13, 16, 262). Numerous medical complications have been noted such as initial orthostatic hypotension, the development of different types of herniae including hiatus hernia; gastrointestinal symptoms with anorexia and low protein intake, backache, foot gangrene in patients with arteriitis, obesity and hypertriglyceridaemia. Some complaints such as inability to perform job or household activities and shortness of breath were noted with a discouraging frequency as the duration of continuous ambulatory peritoneal dialysis increased (403). Finally, loss of the ultrafiltration capacity has been recently described in an increasing number of patients (405–407).

Survival of CAPD patients
Survival data of patients treated with continuous ambulatory peritoneal dialysis are even more scarce than for periodic peritoneal dialysis obviously because the method has been introduced only recently. Cumulative patient and technique survival were discussed in two papers, showing a 77% patient survival and 58% technique survival at three years in one group (403) and a 55% patient survival with a 30% technique survival at 2½ year in another group (405). Recurrent peritonitis,

patient's preference or loss of ultrafiltration capacity were the main causes for transfer to haemodialysis.

Periodic versus continuous ambulatory peritoneal dialysis

The limitations of periodic peritoneal dialysis are well recognised (298, 376, 383). CAPD appears to solve most of these problems (408) at the price of a higher infectious risk and a never ending manual labour (409). However, it is still too early to appreciate in full what will ultimately be the place of either technique in the treatment of end stage renal failure. It is highly probable that the indication for periodic peritoneal dialysis primarily will be limited to patients of small body size and small surface area (less than 55 kg and 1.40 m^2) who are able to dialyse at home and who dislike the rituals of CAPD (383). A secondary indication will arise from complications, particularly the loss of capacity to ultrafiltrate, occurring during CAPD in patients judged medically unsuitable for haemodialysis. In the author's view, the two methods of peritoneal dialysis are complementary to each other (405) and any doctor interested in maintenance peritoneal dialysis should master both periodic and continuous ambulatory peritoneal dialysis as the former still remains the standard of reference for the prevention of peritoneal infection (299).

Special indications for maintenance peritoneal dialysis

End stage diabetic nephropathy
Early experiences with regular haemodialysis in diabetic patients were marred by a rapid deterioration of vision, accelerated neuropathy, gangrene of the inferior limbs (410, 411); it was suggested that peritoneal dialysis with slow exchange rates, absence of heparinisation and cardiovascular stability during treatment would prevent many of these complications and obtain better clinical results.

Experience with peritoneal dialysis in diabetic patients is still limited to a rather small number of patients followed only for short periods of time (412–422). Claims for more frequent stabilisation of retinopathy, less dialysis related morbidity, slower progression of neuropathy, less frequent pericarditis and foot gangrene than in haemodialysed patients should be accepted with caution. Interestingly there was no difference in the incidence of peritonitis and in peritoneal clearances of urea and creatinine between diabetic and non diabetic patients (415). Adequate blood sugar control can be obtained by insulin supplementation during dialysis given via the intraperitoneal route, by adding 4 to 6 units of crystalline insulin per litre of 76 mmol/l dextrose monohydrate dialysis fluid (1.5 g/dl) and 8 to 10 units per litre of 215 mmol/l (4.25 g/dl) dextrose monohydrate dialysis solution (421). Insulin can also be given subcutaneously at a dose of 4 to 5 units of regular insulin for 101 mmol/l (2 g/dl) dextrose, 8 to 10 units for 152 mmol/l (3 g/dl) dextrose and 12 to 15 units for 215 mmol/l (4.25 g/dl) dextrose concentrations in the dialysis fluid (383, 419).

In three reports (418, 420, 422) peritoneal and haemodialysis were compared in non randomised studies in small groups of patients: progression of retinopathy and neuropathy were slower with peritoneal dialysis, but survival was similar with both techniques; one report recommended peritoneal dialysis as the first choice dialytic therapy in insulin dependent diabetics awaiting transplantation (420).

CAPD offers two advantages to the diabetic patient: permanent infusion of insulin via the peritoneum functioning as an artificial pancreas (109) and the possibility of self treatment even in the blind patient (423).

However, a striking improvement in the results obtained with haemodialysis in diabetics since 1976 by a Minneapolis group (424), makes it hazardous to speculate on the possible advantages of periodic and continuous ambulatory peritoneal dialysis versus haemodialysis.

Maintenance peritoneal dialysis and transplantation
Renal transplantation can be done without restriction in uraemic adults maintained on any mode of peritoneal dialysis (59, 324, 325, 425–427). Early experiences reported an increased infection rate after transplantation (428), but with the use of permanent indwelling catheters, peritoneal dialysis was also reported as a safe procedure to treat episodes of acute renal failure following transplantation (301).

Maintenance peritoneal dialysis in children
Periodic peritoneal dialysis was used in children with favourable results (347, 356–360). No blood access problems and no venapunctures, easy overnight home dialysis permitting normal family life and better school attendance were noted as advantages over haemodialysis. Slow growth is observed in about 50% of the young patients, and usually no catch-up growth is noted. Puberty occurs at a later age than normal (347, 357, 360).

Peritoneal dialysis may be an obstacle in children of small size where intraperitoneal kidney implantation is considered (359). In children of larger size, extraperitoneal transplantation is no problem and an end-stage renal disease programme integrating transplantation and peritoneal dialysis is considered by many as first choice approach to the problem of treatment of end stage renal failure in children (359, 360).

The future of peritoneal dialysis

Recent reviews have thoroughly discussed the future of maintenance peritoneal dialysis (15, 405, 408, 429). Obviously many medical and non-medical considerations (e.g. socioeconomic factors, availability of alternative treatment methods) are important determinants of the utilisation of maintenance peritoneal dialysis (or any other alternative) for the treatment of end-stage chronic renal failure (430). Therefore, the discussion of this subject will be limited in this chapter to the medical factors influencing the use of maintenance peritoneal dialysis.

Decay of the peritoneal membrane
Limited data are available on the long term effects of the dialysis procedure on the peritoneal membrane. Two studies of sequential peritoneal clearance measurements in patients treated with periodic peritoneal dialysis (431) or CAPD (296) showed conflicting results. In another study, repeated mass transfer coefficients were measured in 12 patients treated by CAPD for 12 months or more. Three patients showed a significant decrease in mass transfer coefficients after several months of treatment (300).

On the other hand, there is a growing literature on the development of organic peritoneal lesions such as adhesions, sclerotic thickening of the peritoneum and chronic plastic peritonitis (219-221, 252, 298, 405-407); these lesions lead gradually to inadequate dialysis, decreased ability to ultrafilter or episodes of partial intestinal obstruction which necessitate conversion of the patient to haemodialysis and sometimes repeated surgery. How long the peritoneal membrane will last and in how many and which patients, remain the central questions. The answers will determine the future of peritoneal dialysis in chronic renal failure.

Maintenance peritoneal dialysis versus haemodialysis
Controlled evaluation of maintenance peritoneal dialysis permitting an objective comparison with haemodialysis is not yet available; a long term randomised study is presently going on in the United States, but the results are not yet released (432). In a 3 year prospective study recently completed, there was no major difference in the morbidity and the survival in two comparable groups of patients treated either with haemodialysis or peritoneal dialysis. However, in the latter group, lower serum urea nitrogen and albumin values and higher haematocrit and serum triglyceride levels were noted (422).

On the basis of presently available data, the conclusion that peritoneal dialysis is a proved equivalent alternative to maintenance haemodialysis should be considered as misleading (433). The results obtained in a few thousands patients with terminal renal failure treated with peritoneal dialysis for an average duration of less than of 18 months can in no way be compared with the enormous amount of information obtained in large cohorts of patients treated for more than ten years with haemodialysis (434, 435).

The main medical advantage of peritoneal dialysis is the *cardiovascular stability* obtained during treatment; orthostatic hypotension, frequently observed in CAPD (77) is probably preventable by increasing the dialysate sodium concentration and sodium dietary intake (66). These characteristics and advantages of peritoneal dialysis should be weighed against the limitations of the method when peritoneal dialysis is considered for long term replacement of renal function. In that respect, it seems to be useful to evaluate the relative advantages and disadvantages of both peritoneal dialysis and haemofiltration (436), as the latter is also associated with excellent cardiovascular stability.

THE FUTURE ROLE OF PERITONEAL DIALYSIS IN THE TREATMENT OF TERMINAL CHRONIC RENAL FAILURE

Maintenance peritoneal dialysis can be seen as an adjunct for any end stage renal disease programme (405). Two major indications will remain for its use in chronic renal failure: in children, integrated with an active transplantation programme and in patients aged 65 or older in whom survival may be comparable to that obtained with haemodialysis (437). Between the ages of 15 and 65, peritoneal dialysis may be the first choice in diabetic patients and in those with severe cardiovascular disease. However, in patients without complicating risk factors, peritoneal dialysis should be considered as a temporary treatment (438). It may be convenient to start maintenance therapy with peritoneal dialysis in particular when home dialysis has priority. However, physicians and patients should be aware that transfer to haemodialysis may sooner or later become necessary. Therefore, haemodialysis equipment should be available at anytime permitting transfer to haemodialysis without any delay that could threaten the patient's health.

REFERENCES

1. Maxwell MH, Rockney RE, Kleeman CR, Twiss MR: Peritoneal dialysis. 1. Technique and application. *JAMA* 170:917, 1959
2. Boen ST: Kinetics of peritoneal dialysis. A comparison with the artificial kidney. *Medicine* 40:243, 1961
3. Henderson LW: Peritoneal ultrafiltration dialysis: enhanced urea transfer using hypertonic dialysis fluid. *J Clin Invest.* 49:950, 1966
4. Boen ST, Mulinari AS, Dillard DH, Scribner BH: Periodic peritoneal dialysis with the management of chronic uremia. *Trans Am Soc Artif Intern Organs* 8:256, 1962
5. Tenckhoff H, Schechter H: A bacteriologically safe peritoneal access device for repeated peritoneal dialysis. *Trans Am Soc Artif Intern Organs* 14:181, 1968
6. Tenckhoff H, Meston B, Shilipetar RG: A simplified automatic peritoneal dialysis system. *Trans Am Soc Artif Intern Organs* 18:436, 1972
7. Boen ST, Mion CM, Curtis FK, Shilipetar G: Periodic peritoneal dialysis using the repeated puncture technique and an automatic cycling machine. *Trans Am Soc Artif Intern Organs* 10:409, 1964
8. Gutch CF, Stevens SC, Watkins FL: Periodic peritoneal dialysis in chronic renal insufficiency. *Ann Intern Med* 60:289, 1964
9. Palmer RA, Quinton WE, Gray JE: prolonged peritoneal dialysis for chronic renal failure. *Lancet* 1:700, 1964
10. Schumacher RR, Ridolfo AS, Martz BL: Periodic peritoneal dialysis for chronic renal failure. A case study of sixteen months experience. *Ann Intern Med* 60:296, 1964
11. Popovich RP, Moncrief JW, Decherd JB, Bomar JB, Pyle WK: The definition of a novel portable/wearable equilibrium peritoneal dialysis technique. *Abstracts Am Soc Artif*

Intern Organs 5:64, 1976
12. Popovich RP, Moncrief JW, Nolph KD, Ghods AJ, Twardowski ZJ, Pyle WK: Continuous ambulatory peritoneal dialysis. *Ann Intern Med* 88:449, 1978
13. Oreopoulos DG, Robson M, Izatt S, Clayton S, DeVeber GA: A simple and safe technique for continuous ambulatory peritoneal dialysis (CAPD). *Trans Am Soc Artif Intern Organs* 24:484, 1978
14. Anonymous: CAPD for chronic renal failure. *Lancet* 1:1172, 1980
15. Oreopoulos DG: Peritoneal dialysis is here to stay. *Nephron* 24:7, 1979
16. Rubin J, Rogers WA, Taylor HM, Everett ED, Prowant BF, Fruto LV, Nolph KD: Peritonitis during continuous ambulatory peritoneal dialysis. *Ann Intern Med* 92:7, 1980
17. Slingeneyer A, Mion C, Béraud JJ, Oulès R, Branger B, Balmes M: Peritonitis, a frequently lethal complication of intermittent and continuous ambulatory peritoneal dialysis. *Proc Eur Dial Transpl Assoc* 18:212, 1981
18. Tenckhoff H: Home peritoneal dialysis. In: *Clinical Aspects of Uremia and Dialysis,* edited by Massry SG, Sellers AL, Springfield IL, Charles C Thomas, 1976, p 583
19. Boen ST: Overview and history of peritoneal dialysis. *Dial Transpl* 6 (no 2):12, 1977
20. Weston RE, Roberts M: Clinical use of stylet catheter for peritoneal dialysis. *Arch Intern Med* 115:659, 1965
21. Tenckhoff H: *Chronic peritoneal dialysis manual.* Univ of Washington School of Medicine, Seattle WA, 1974
22. Vaamonde CA, Michael UF, Metzger RA, Carroll KE: Complications of acute peritoneal dialysis. *J Chronic Dis* 28:637, 1975
23. Jacob GB, Deane N: Repeated peritoneal dialysis by the catheter replacement method: description of technique and a replaceable prosthesis for chronic access to the peritoneal cavity. *Proc Eur Dial Transpl Assoc* 4:136, 1967
24. Vidt DG, Somerville J, Schultz RW: A safe peritoneal access device for repeated peritoneal dialysis. *JAMA* 214:2293, 1970
25. Bigelow P, Oreopoulos DG, deVeber GA: Use of the Deane prosthesis in patients on long term peritoneal dialysis. *Can Med Assoc J* 109:999, 1973
26. Malette WG, McPhaul JJ, Bledsoe F, McIntosh DA, Koegel E: A clinically successful subcutaneous peritoneal access button for repeated peritoneal dialysis. *Trans Am Soc Artif Intern Organs* 10:396, 1964
27. Gotloib L, Galili N, Nisencorn I, Servadio C, Garmizo AL, Sudarsky M: Subcutaneous intraperitoneal prosthesis for maintenance peritoneal dialysis. *Lancet* 1:1318, 1975
28. Gotloib L, Mines M, Garmizo AL, Rodoy J: Peritoneal dialysis using the subcutaneous intraperitoneal prosthesis. *Dial Transpl* 8:217, 1979
29. Oreopoulos DG: Maintenance peritoneal dialysis. In: *Strategy in Renal Failure,* edited by Friedman EA, New York, John Wiley and Sons, 1978, p 393
30. Ribot S, Jacobs MG, Frankel HJ, Bernstein A: Complications of peritoneal dialysis. *Am J Med Sci* 35:505, 1966
31. Henderson LW: Peritoneal dialysis. In: *Clinical Aspects of Uremia and Dialysis,* edited by Massry SG, Sellers AL, Springield IL, Charles C Thomas, 1976, p 555
32. Simkin EP, Wright FK: Perforating injuries of the bowel complicating peritoneal catheter insertion. *Lancet* 1:64, 1968
33. Rubin J, Oreopoulos DG, Lio TT, Mathews R, deVeber GA: Management of peritonitis and bowel perforation during chronic peritoneal dialysis. *Nephron* 16:220, 1976
34. Lopez de Novales E, Hernando L: Risks of peritoneal catheter insertion. *Lancet* 1:473, 1968
35. Mackenzie JC, Rutherford CW, Cattell WR: Risks of peritoneal catheterisation. *Lancet* 1:1373, 1968
36. Thompson N, Uldall R: A problem in peritoneal dialysis. *Lancet* 2:602, 1969
37. Ladefoged J, Steiness I: Intra-abdominal bleeding complicating peritoneal dialysis. *Lancet* 1:190, 1970
38. Brewer TE, Caldwell FT, Patterson RM, Flanigan WJ: Indwelling peritoneal (Tenckhoff) dialysis catheter. Experience with 24 patients. *JAMA* 219:1011, 1972
39. Gutman RA: Automated peritoneal dialysis for home use. *Q J Med* 47:261, 1978
40. Tenckhoff H, Curtis FK: Experience with maintenance peritoneal dialysis in the home. *Trans Am Soc Artif Intern Organs* 16:90, 1970
41. Ash SR, Wolf GC, Bloch R: Placement of the Tenckhoff peritoneal dialysis catheter under peritoneoscopic visualization. *Dial Transpl* 10:383, 1981
42. Rae A, Pendray M: Advantages of peritoneal dialysis in chronic renal failure. *JAMA* 225:937, 1973
43. Goldberg EM, Hill W: A new peritoneal access prosthesis. *Proc Clin Dial Transpl Forum* 3:122, 1973
44. Oreopoulos DG, Izatt S, Zellerman G, Karanicolas S, Mathews RE: A prospective study of the effectiveness of three permanent catheters. *Proc Clin Dial Transpl Forum* 6:96, 1976
45. Moulopoulos S, Ziroyanis P, Vita L, Papadoyanakis N: A new catheter for chronic peritoneal dialysis. *Proc Eur Soc Artif Organs* 5:185, 1979
46. Ash SR, Johnson H, Hartman J, Granger J, Koszuta J, Sell L, Dhein C, Blevins W, Thornstill JA: The column disc peritoneal catheter: a peritoneal access device with improved drainage. *asaio J* 3:109, 1980
47. Stephen RL, Atkin-Thor E, Kolff WJ: Recirculating peritoneal dialysis with subcutaneous catheter. *Trans Am Soc Artif Intern Organs* 22:575, 1976
48. Kablitz C, Kessler T, Dew PA, Stephen RL, Kolff WJ: Subcutaneous peritoneal catheter: 2½ years experience. *Artif Organs* 3:210, 1979
49. Slingeneyer A, Charpiat A, Balmes M, Mion C: Is an alternative to the Tenckhoff catheter necessary? In: *Advances in Peritoneal Dialysis,* edited by Gahl GM, Kessel M, Nolph KD, Amsterdam, Oxford, Princeton, Excerpta Medica, International Congress series 567, 1981, p 179
50. Giovanetti S, Cioni L, Maggiore QL, Balestri PL, Biagini M: A 'clot score' for the winged in-line shunt. *Proc Eur Dial Transpl Assoc* 4:363, 1967
51. Scott DF, Marshall VC: Insertion and complications of Tenckhoff catheters – surgical aspects. In: *Peritoneal Dialysis,* edited by Atkins RC, Thomson NM, Farrell PC, Edinburgh, Churchill Livingstone, 1981, p 61
52. Tenckhoff H: Peritoneal dialysis today: a new look. *Nephron* 12:420, 1974
53. Oreopoulos DG: Peritoneal dialysis is reinstated. *J Dial* 2:295, 1978
54. Tenckhoff H: Choice of peritoneal dialysis solutions. *Ann Intern Med* 75:313, 1971
55. Vidt DG: Recommendations on choice of peritoneal dialysis solutions. *Ann Intern Med* 78:144, 1973
56. Halaby SF, Mattocks AM: Absorption of sodium bisulfite from peritoneal dialysis solutions. *J Pharm Sci* 54:52, 1965
57. Wilkins JW, Greene JA, Weller JM: Toxicity of intraperitoneal bisulfite. *Clin Pharmacol Ther* 9:328, 1968
58. Gilli P, De Bastiani P, Fagioli F, Buoncristiani U, Carobi C, Stabellini N, Squerzanti R, Rosati G, Farinelli A: Positive aluminium balance in patients on regular peritoneal

treatment: an effect of low dialysate pH? *Proc Eur Dial Transpl Assoc* 17:219, 1980
59. Oreopoulos DG: Chronic peritoneal dialysis. *Clin Nephrol* 9:165, 1978
60. Nolph KD, Hano E, Teschan PE: Peritoneal sodium transport during hypertonic peritoneal dialysis. *Ann Intern Med* 70:931, 1969
61. Raja RM, Cantor RE, Beoryko C, Busherhi H, Kramer MS, Rosenbaum JL: Sodium transport during ultrafiltration peritoneal dialysis. *Trans Am Soc Artif Intern Organs* 18:429, 1972
62. Boen ST: *Peritoneal dialysis in clinical medicine* Springfield IL, Charles C Thomas, 1964
63. Canaud B, Liendo-Liendo C, Claret G, Mion H, Mion C: Etude 'in situ' de la cinétique de l'ultrafiltration en cours de dialyse péritonéale avec périodes de diffusion prolongée ('In situ' studies of ultrafiltration kinetics during peritoneal dialysis with periods of prolonged diffusion). *Néphrologie* 1:126, 1980 (in French)
64. Popovich RP, Moncrief JW: Kinetic modeling of peritoneal transport. *Contrib Nephrol* 17:59, 1979
65. Nolph KD, Twardowski ZJ, Popovich RP, Rubin J: Equilibration of peritoneal dialysis solutions during long-dwell exchanges. *J Lab Clin Med* 93:246, 1979
66. Canaud B, Mimran A, Liendo-Liendo C, Slingeneyer A, Mion C: Blood pressure control in patients treated by continuous ambulatory peritoneal dialysis. In: *Continuous Ambulatory Peritoneal Dialysis,* edited by Legrain M, Amsterdam, Excerpta Medica, 1980, p 212
67. Rubin J, Nolph KD, Popovich RP, Moncrief JW, Prowant B: Drainage volumes during continuous ambulatory peritoneal dialysis. *Am Soc Artif Intern Organs J* 2:54, 1979
68. Randerson DH, Farrell PC: Mass transfer properties of the human peritoneum. *asaio J* 3:140, 1980
69. Vidt DG: Hazards of hyperosmolar solutions. *Ann Intern Med* 79:599, 1973
70. Frank HA, Seligman AM, Fine J: Further experiences with peritoneal irrigation for acute renal failure. *Ann Surg* 128:561, 1948
71. Gjessing J: The use of dextran as a dialyzing fluid in peritoneal dialysis. *Acta Med Scand* 185:237, 1969
72. Robson M, Rosenfeld JB: Fructose for dialysis. *Ann Intern Med* 75:975, 1971
73. Yutuc W, Ward G, Shillipetar G, Tenckhoff H: Substitution of sorbitol for dextrose in peritoneal irrigation fluid. A preliminary report. *Trans Am Soc Artif Intern Organs* 13:168, 1967
74. Yen T: Experimental study on peritoneal dialysis using xylitol containing solutions. *J Formosan Medical Association* (Taipei) 69:292, 1970
75. Bischel MD, Barbour BH: Peritoneal dialysis with sorbitol versus dextrose dialysate. *Nephron* 12:449, 1974
76. Oreopoulos DG, Crassweller P, Katirtzoglou A, Ogilvie R, Zellerman G, Rodella H, Vas SI: Amino acids as an osmotic agent (instead of glucose) in continuous ambulatory peritoneal dialysis. In: *Continuous Ambulatory Peritoneal Dialysis,* edited by Legrain M, Amsterdam, Excerpta Medica, 1980, p 335
77. Oreopoulos DG, Clayton S, Dombros N, Zellerman G, Katirtzoglou A: Nineteen months experience with continuous ambulatory peritoneal dialysis. *Proc Eur Dial Transpl Assoc* 16:178, 1979
78. Papadoyanakis N, Papadakis E, Malamos B: Sodium changes in peritoneal dialysis. *Proc Eur Dial Transpl Assoc* 6:289, 1969
79. Ahearn DJ, Nolph KD: Controlled sodium removal with peritoneal dialysis. *Trans Am Soc Artif Intern Organs* 18:423, 1972
80. Shen FH, Sherrard DJ, Scollard D, Merritt A, Curtis FK: Thirst, relative hypernatremia, and excessive weight gain in maintenance peritoneal dialysis. *Trans Am Soc Artif Intern Organs* 24:142, 1978
81. Brown ST, Ahearn DJ, Nolph KD: Potassium removal with peritoneal dialysis. *Kidney Int* 4:67, 1973
82. Gault MH, Fergusson EL, Sidhu JS, Corbin RP: Fluid and electrolyte complications of peritoneal dialysis. *Ann Intern Med* 75:253, 1971
83. La Greca G, Biasioli S, Chiaramonte S, Davi M, Fabris A, Feriani M, Pisani E, Ronco C, Zen F: Acid-base balance in peritoneal dialysis. *Clin Nephrol* 16:1, 1981
84. Hayat JC: The treatment of lactic acidosis in the diabetic patient by peritoneal dialysis using sodium acetate. A report of cases. *Diabetologia* 10:485, 1974
85. Richardson JA, Borchardt KA: Adverse effect on bacteria of peritoneal dialysis solutions that contain acetate. *Br Med J* 3:749, 1969
86. Leahy TH, Sullivan MJ, Slingeneyer A, Mion C: The efficiency of microbial retention by peritoneal dialysis filters. *Trans Am Soc Artif Intern Organs* 26:225, 1980
87. Vaziri ND, Ness R, Wellikson L, Barton C, Greep N: Bicarbonate-buffered peritoneal dialysis. An effective adjunct in the treatment of lactic acidosis. *Am J Med* 67:392, 1979
88. Parker A, Nolph KD: Magnesium and calcium mass transfer during continuous ambulatory peritoneal dialysis. *Trans Am Soc Artif Intern Organs* 26:194, 1980
89. Garrett JJ, Cuddihe RE: Calcium absorption during peritoneal dialysis. *Trans Am Soc Artif Intern Organs* 14:372, 1968
90. Oreopoulos DG, deVeber GA: Peritoneal dialysis and blood chemical changes. *Ann Intern Med* 72:781, 1973
91. Tenckhoff H: Solutions and equipment. *Dial Transpl* 6 (no 2):24, 1977
92. Wing WT, Uldall R: Simplified peritoneal dialysis. *Lancet* 1:297, 1970
93. Atkins RC, Mion C, Despaux E, Van-Hai N, Jullien C, Mion H: Peritoneal transfer of kanamycin and its use in peritoneal dialysis. *Kidney Int* 3:391, 1973
94. Koup JR, Gerbracht L: Combined use of heparin and gentamicin in peritoneal dialysis. *Drug Intell Clin Pharm* 9:389, 1975
95. Koup JR, Gerbracht L: Reduction in heparin activity by gentamicin. *Drug Intell Clin Pharm* 9:568, 1975
96. Nolph KD, Ghods AJ, Van Stone J, Brown PA: The effects of intraperitoneal vasodilators on peritoneal clearances. *Trans Am Soc Artif Intern Organs* 22:586, 1976
97. Gutman RA, Nixon WP, McRae RL, Spencer HW: Effect of intraperitoneal and intravenous vasoactive amines on peritoneal dialysis: study in anephric dogs. *Trans Am Soc Artif Intern Organs* 22:570, 1976
98. Maher JF, Hohnadel DC, Shea C, DiSanzo F, Cassetta M: Effect of intraperitoneal diuretics on solute transport during hypertonic dialysis *Clin Nephrol* 7:96, 1977
99. Nolph KD, Ghods A, Brown P, Miller F, Harris P, Pyle K, Popovich R: Effects of nitroprusside on peritoneal mass transfer coefficients and microvascular physiology. *Trans Am Soc Artif Intern Organs* 23:210, 1977
100. Hirszel P, Maher JF, LeGrow W: Increased peritoneal mass transport with glucagon acting at the vascular surface. *Trans Am Soc Artif Intern Organs* 24:136, 1978
101. Hirszel P, Lasrich M, Maher JF: Augmentation of peritoneal mass transport by dopamine. Comparison with norepinephrine and evaluation of pharmacologic mechanisms. *J Lab Clin Med* 94:747, 1979
102. Nolph KD, Ghods AJ, Brown PA, Twardowski ZJ: Effects of intraperitoneal nitroprusside on peritoneal clearances in man with variations of dose, frequency of ad-

ministration and dwell times. *Nephron* 24:114, 1979
103. Maher JF, Hirszel P, Lasrich M: Effects of gastrointestinal hormones on transport by peritoneal dialysis. *Kidney Int* 16:130, 1979
104. Hirszel M, Lasrich M, Maher JF: Divergent effects of catecholamines on peritoneal mass transport. *Trans Am Soc Artif Intern Organs* 25:110, 1979
105. Maher JF, Hirszel P, Lasrich M: Modulation of peritoneal transport rates by prostaglandins. In: *Advances in Prostaglandin and Thromboxane research* vol 7, edited by Samuelsson B, Ramwell PW, Paoletti R, New York NY, Raven Press, 1980 p 695
106. Gjessing J: Addition of aminoacids to peritoneal dialysis fluid. *Lancet* 2:812, 1968
107. Crossley K, Kjellstrand CM: Intraperitoneal insulin for control of blood sugar in diabetic patients during peritoneal dialysis. *Br Med J* 1:269, 1971
108. Shapiro DJ, Blumenkrantz MJ, Levin SR, Coburn JW: Absorption and action of insulin added to peritoneal dialysate in dogs. *Nephron* 23:174, 1979
109. Flynn CT, Hibbard J, Dohrmann B: Advantages of continuous ambulatory peritoneal dialysis to the diabetic with renal failure. *Proc Eur Dial Transpl Assoc* 16:184, 1979
110. Stewart WK, Anderson DC, Wilson MI: Hazard of peritoneal dialysis: contaminated fluid. *Br Med J* 1:606, 1967
111. Slingeneyer A, Mion C, Despaux E, Perez C, Duport J, Dansette AM: Use of a bacteriologic filter in the prevention of peritonitis associated with peritoneal dialysis: long term clinical results in intermittent and continuous ambulatory peritoneal dialysis. In: *Peritoneal Dialysis* edited by Atkins RC, Thomson NM, Farrell PC, Edinburgh, Churchill Livingstone, 1981, p 301
112. Tenckhoff H, Boen ST, Shilipetar G: Preparation of peritoneal dialysis fluid. *Hosp Pharmacy* 2:7, 1967
113. Curtis FK, Boen ST: Automatic peritoneal dialysis with a simple cycling machine. *Lancet* 2:620, 1965
114. McDonald HP Jr: An automatic peritoneal dialysis machine: preliminary report. *Trans Am Soc Artif Intern Organs* 11:83, 1965
115. Bosch E, deVries LA, Boen ST: A simplified automatic peritoneal dialysis system. *Proc Eur Dial Transpl Assoc* 3:362, 1966
116. Mallick NP, Coles GA, Rees JKH, Agosti J: An automatic peritoneal dialysis system. *Lancet* 1:1303, 1967
117. Vercellone A, Piccoli G, Cavalli PL, Alloatti S, Segoloni GP: A new semi-automatic peritoneal dialysis system. *Proc Eur Dial Transpl Assoc* 6:341, 1969
118. Tenckhoff H, Shilipetar G, Van Paasschen WH, Swanson E: A home peritoneal dialysate delivery system. *Trans Am Soc Artif Intern Organs* 15:103, 1969
119. McDonald HP Jr: An automatic peritoneal dialysis machine for hospital or home peritoneal dialysis: preliminary report. *Trans Am Soc Artif Intern Organs* 15:108, 1969
120. Haapanen E, Tirkkonen T: A new simplified peritoneal dialyser. *Proc Eur Dial Transpl Assoc,* 8:468, 1971
121. Parker AS, Witcher JW, Barrett RH, Mackenzie JC, Iles RN, Shaw AF: A new automatic peritoneal dialyser. *Proc Eur Dial Transpl Assoc* 9:107, 1972
122. Jarrell B, Lasker N, Roberts M: A simple system of automated peritoneal dialysis. *Dial Transpl* 3 (no 2):36, 1974
123. Bergström J, Marklund M, Olofsson S, Tysk J: An automated apparatus for peritoneal dialysis with volumetric fluid balance measurement. *Dial Transpl* 5 (no 4):58, 1976
124. Kabei N, Kolff WJ, Foux A: Evaluation of hollow-fiber reverse osmosis permeators for use in peritoneal dialysis. *Dial Transpl* 6 (no 1):59, 1977
125. Petersen NJ, Carson LA, Favero MS: Microbiological quality of water in an automatic peritoneal dialysis system. *Dial Transpl* 6 (no 2):38, 1977
126. Gutman RA, Shelburne JD: An outbreak of cryptogenic peritonitis: implications for reverse osmosis production of biologically safe water. *Dial Transpl* 6 (no 2):35, 1977
127. Karanicolas S, Oreopoulos DG, Pylypchuk G, Fenton SSA, Cattran DC, Rapoport A, deVeber GA: Home peritoneal dialysis: three years' experience in Toronto. *Can Med Assoc J* 116:226, 1977
128. Diaz-Buxo JA, Chandler JT, Farmer CD, Smith DL: Chronic peritoneal dialysis at home – a comparison with hemodialysis. *Trans Am Soc Artif Intern Organs* 23:191, 1977
129. Furman KI, Koornhof HJ, Frizelle K, Block C, VanWyck H, Allcock R: Unsafe automatic peritoneal dialysis in Johannesburg. *Kidney Int* (Abstract) 16:86, 1979
130. Blagg CR: Seattle experience with peritoneal dialysis. *Dial Transpl* 7:790, 1978
131. Lewin AJ, Gordon A, Greenbaum MA, Maxwell MH: Sorbent based regenerating delivery system for use in peritoneal dialysis. *Proc Clin Dial Transpl Forum* 5:126, 1973
132. Raja RM, Kramer MS, Rosenbaum JL: Recirculation peritoneal dialysis with sorbent Redy cartridge. *Nephron* 16:134, 1976
133. Blumenkrantz MJ, Lewin AJ, Gordon A, Roberts M, Pecker EA, Coburn JW, Maxwell MH: Development of a sorbent peritoneal dialysate regeneration system – a progress report. *Proc Eur Dial Transpl Assoc* 15:213, 1978
134. Giordano C, Esposito R, Bello P, Wuarto E: A resin-sorbent system for regeneration of peritoneal fluid for daily dialysis. *Dial Transpl* 8:351, 1979
135. Blumenkrantz MJ, Gordon A, Roberts M, Lewin AJ, Pecker EA, Moran JK, Coburn JW, Maxwell MH: Applications of the Redy sorbent system to hemodialysis and peritoneal dialysis. *Artif Organs* 3:230, 1979
136. Gordon A, Better OS, Greenbaum MA. Marantz LB, Gral T, Maxwell MH: Clinical maintenance hemodialysis with a sorbent-based low-volume dialysate regeneration system. *Trans Am Soc Artif Intern Organs* 17:253, 1971
137. Branger B, Ramperez P, Marigliano N, Mion H, Shaldon S, Mion C: Aluminium transfer in bicarbonate dialysis using a sorbent regenerative system: an in vitro study. *Proc Eur Dial Transpl Assoc* 17:213, 1980
138. Mion C, Branger B, Issautier R, Ellis HA, Shaldon S: Dialysis fracturing osteomalacia without hyperparathyroidism in patients treated with HCO_3 rinsed Redy cartridge. *Trans Am Soc Artif Intern Organs* 27:634, 1981
139. Abrutyn E, Goodhart GL, Roos K, Anderson R, Buxton A: Acinetobacter calcoaceticus outbreak associated with peritoneal dialysis. *Am J Epidemiol* 107:328, 1978
140. Mader JT, Reinarz JA: Peritonitis during peritoneal dialysis. The role of the preheating water bath. *J Chronic Dis* 31:635, 1978
141. Kilmos HJ, Anderson KEH: Peritonitis with pseudomonas aeruginosa in hospitalized patients treated with peritoneal dialysis. *Scand J Infect Dis* 11:207, 1979
142. Gauntner WC, Feldman HA, Puschett JB: Peritonitis in chronic peritoneal dialysis patients. *Clin Nephrol* 13:255, 1980
143. Pirpasopoulos M, Lindsay RM, Rahman M, Kennedy AC: A cost-effectiveness study of dwell times in peritoneal dialysis. *Lancet* 2:1135, 1972
144. Goldschmidt ZH, Pote HH, Katz MA, Shear L: Effect of dialysate volume on peritoneal dialysis kinetics. *Kidney*

Int 5:240, 1974
145. Tenckhoff H, Ward G, Boen ST: The influence of dialysate volume and flow rate on peritoneal clearance. *Proc Eur Dial Transpl Assoc* 2:113, 1965
146. Robson M, Oreopoulos DG, Izatt S, Ogilvie R, Rapoport A, deVeber GA: Influence of exchange volume and dialysate flow rate on solute clearance in peritoneal dialysis. *Kidney Int* 14:486, 1978
147. Bomar JB, Decherd JF, Hlavinka DJ, Moncrief JW, Popovich RP: The elucidation of maximum efficiency-minimum cost peritoneal dialysis protocols. *Trans Am Soc Artif Intern Organs* 20:120, 1974
148. Mani MK, Raibagi MH, Dingankar AD: The economics of peritoneal dialysis. A cost-efficiency study. *Nephron* 17:130, 1976
149. Shinaberger JH, Shear L, Barry KG: Increasing efficiency of peritoneal dialysis: experience with peritoneal-extracorporeal recirculation dialysis. *Trans Am Soc Artif Intern Organs* 11:76, 1965
150. Lange K, Treser G: Automatic continuous high flow rate peritoneal dialysis. *Trans Am Soc Artif Intern Organs* 13:164, 1967
151. Di Paolo N, Acconcia A, Manganelli A: Acceleration of peritoneal dialysis with simple device. *Nephron* 19:271, 1977
152. Kablitz C, Stephen RL, Jacobsen SC, Kirkham R, Kolff WJ: Reciprocating peritoneal dialysis. *Dial Transpl* 3:211, 1978
153. Nolph KD, Sorkin M, Rubin J, Arfania D, Prowant B, Fruto L, Kennedy D: Continuous ambulatory peritoneal dialysis: three years experience at one center. *Ann Intern Med* 92:609, 1980
154. Oreopoulos DG, Zellerman G, Izatt S: The Toronto Western Hospital permanent peritoneal catheter and continuous ambulatory peritoneal dialysis connector. In: *Continuous Ambulatory Peritoneal Dialysis* edited by Legrain M, Amsterdam, Excerpta Medica, 1980, p 79
155. Moncrief JW, Rutherford CE, Sorrels PAJ, Bailey A, Popovich RP: Technical aspects of continuous ambulatory peritoneal dialysis new connection devices developed by Baxter Travenol Laboratories. In: *Continuous Ambulatory Peritoneal Dialysis,* edited by Legrain M, Amsterdam, Excerpta Medica, 1980, p 79
156. Fuchs C, Koppensteiner G: Evaluation of a continuous ambulatory peritoneal dialysis connecting system on the basis of hygiene. In: *Continuous Ambulatory Peritoneal Dialysis,* edited by Legrain M, Amsterdam, Excerpta Medica, 1980, p 82
157. Bazzato G, Landini S, Coli U, Lucatello S, Fracasso A, Moracchiello M: A new technique of continuous ambulatory peritoneal dialysis (CAPD): Double-bag system for freedom to the patient and significant reduction of peritonitis. *Clin Nephrol* 13:251, 1980
158. Buoncristiani U, Bianchi P, Cozzari M, Carobi C, Quintaliani G, Barbarossa D: A new safe simple connection system for CAPD. *Int J Nephrol Urol Androl* 1:50, 1980
159. Slingeneyer A, Liendo-Liendo C, Mion C: Continuous ambulatory peritoneal dialysis with a bacteriological filter on the dialysate infusion line. In: *Continuous Ambulatory Peritoneal Dialysis,* edited by Legrain M, Amsterdam, Excerpta Medica, 1980, p 59
160. Randerson DH, Farrell PC: Clinical assessment of CAPD. *Dial Transpl* 10:389, 1981
161. Price CG, Suki WN: Newer modifications of peritoneal dialysis: Options in the treatment of patients with renal failure. *Am J Nephrol* 1:97, 1981
162. Diaz-Buxo JA, Farmer CD, Walker PJ, Chandler JT, Holt KL: Continuous cyclic peritoneal dialysis: a preliminary report. *Artif Organs* 5:157, 1981
163. Burns RO, Henderson LW, Hager EB, Merrill JP: Peritoneal dialysis *N Engl J Med* 267:1060, 1962
164. Hager EB, Merrill JP: Peritoneal dialysis and acute renal failure. *Surg Clin North Am* 43:883, 1963
165. Maher JF, Schreiner GE: Hazards and complications of dialysis. *N Engl J Med* 273:370, 1965
166. Barry KG, Schwartz FD, Hano JE, Schrier RW, Canfield C: Peritoneal dialysis: current applications and recent developments. *Proc 3rd Int Cong Nephrol* (Washington), edited by Heptinstall RH, Basel, Karger, 1966, vol 3, p 288
167. Miller RB, Tassitro CR: Peritoneal dialysis. *N Engl J Med* 281:945, 1969
168. Boen ST: Undesirable effects of peritoneal dialysis. *Contrib Nephrol* 17:72, 1979
169. Maher JF: Peritonitis complicating peritoneal dialysis. *Proc Northeastern Meeting Renal Physicians Assoc* 3:47, 1980
170. Oreopoulos DG, Khanna R: Complications of peritoneal dialysis other than peritonitis. In: *Developments in Nephrology 2: Peritoneal Dialysis,* edited by Nolph KD, The Hague, Boston MA, London, Martinus Nijhoff, 1981, p 309
171. Vas SI, Low DE, Oreopoulos DG: Peritonitis. In: *Developments in Nephrology 2: Peritoneal Dialysis,* edited by Nolph KD, The Hague, Boston MA, London, Martinus Nijhoff, 1981, p 344
172. Henderson LW: The problem of peritoneal membrane area and permeability. *Kidney Int* 3:409, 1973
173. Berlyne GM, Jones JH, Manc MB, Wales MB, Hewitt V, Nilwarangkur S: Protein loss in peritoneal dialysis. *Lancet* 1:738, 1964
174. Gutch CF: Peritoneal dialysis. *Trans Am Soc Artif Intern Organs* 10:406 1964
175. Gutch CF, Stevens SC: Silastic catheter for peritoneal dialysis. *Trans Am Soc Artif Intern Organs* 12:106, 1966
176. Strauch M, Walzer P, v Henning GE, Roettger G, Christ H: Factors influencing protein loss during peritoneal dialysis. *Trans Am Soc Artif Intern Organs* 13:172, 1967
177. Gordon S, Rubini ME: Protein losses during peritoneal dialysis. *Am J Med Sci* 253:283, 1967
178. Rubin J, McFarland S, Hellems EW, Bower JD: Peritoneal dialysis during peritonitis. *Kidney Int* 19:460, 1981
179. Bianchi R, Mariani G, Masini S, Matera F, Zucchelli GD: Radioimmunoassay of human serum albumin in peritoneal dialysate. *Nuklearmedizin* 18:112, 1974
180. Bianchi R, Mariani G, Pilo A, Carmassi F: Mechanisms of albumin loss during peritoneal dialysis in man. *Eur J Clin Invest* 5:409, 1975
181. Lindner A, Tenckhoff H: Nitrogen balance in patients on maintenance peritoneal dialysis. *Trans Am Soc Artif Intern Organs* 16:255, 1970
182. Scarpioni L, Poisetti P, Ballocchi S, Bergonzi G, Mistraletti C: Protein loss and compensation in uremic patients during peritoneal dialysis. *Int J Artif Organs* 1:76, 1979
183. Blumenkrantz MJ, Gahl GM, Kopple JD, Kamdar AV, Jones MR, Kessel M, Coburn JW: Protein losses during peritoneal dialysis. *Kidney Int* 19:53, 1981
184. Katirzoglou A, Oreopoulos DG, Husdan H, Leung M, Ogilvie R, Dombros N: Reappraisal of protein losses in patients undergoing continuous ambulatory peritoneal dialysis. *Nephron* 26:230, 1980
185. Berlyne GM, Hewitt V, Jones JH, Nilwarangkur S, Ralston AJ: Patterns of protein loss in peritoneal dialysis. *Proc Eur Dial Transpl Assoc* 1:177, 1964
186. McKelvey EM, Yeoh HH, Schuster GA, Sharma B, Levin

NW: Immunoglobulin and dextran losses during peritoneal dialysis. *Arch Intern Med* 134:266, 1974
187. Berlyne GM, Lee HA, Giordano C, dePascale C, Esposito R: Amino acid loss in peritoneal dialysis. *Lancet* 1:1339, 1967
188. Young GA, Parsons FM: The effect of peritoneal dialysis upon the amino acids and other nitrogenous compounds in the blood and dialysates from patients with renal failure. *Clin Sci* 37:1, 1969
189. Giordano C, DeSanto NG, Capodicasa G, Di Leo VA, Di Serafino A, Cirillo D, Esposito R, Fiore R, Damiano M, Buonadonna L, Cocco F, Dilorio B: Amino acid losses during CAPD. *Clin Nephrol* 14:230, 1980
190. Nolph KD, Rosenfeld PS, Powell JT, Danforth E, Jr: Peritoneal glucose transport and hyperglycemia during peritoneal dialysis. *Am J Med Sci* 259:272, 1970
191. Boyer J, Gordon NG, Epstein FH: Hyperglycemia and hyperosmolality complicating peritoneal dialysis. *Ann Intern Med* 67:568, 1967
192. Lindholm B, Ahlberg M, Alvestrand A, Fürst P, Karlander SG, Bergström J: Nutritional aspects of continuous ambulatory peritoneal dialysis. In: *Continuous Ambulatory Peritoneal Dialysis* edited by Legrain M, Amsterdam, Excerpta Medica, 1980, p 199
193. Mion C, Jullien C, Mirouze J: Les hyperglycémies majeures au cours des dialyses péritonéales (Severe hyperglycaemia during peritoneal dialyses). *Gaz Méd France* 75:3165, 1968 (in French)
194. Robson MD, Levy J, Rosenfeld JB: Hyperglycaemia and hyperosmolarity in peritoneal dialysis. Its prevention by the use of fructose. *Proc Eur Dial Transpl Assoc* 6:300, 1969
195. Cattran DC, Fenton SSA, Wilson DR, Steiner G: Defective triglyceride removal in lipemia associated with peritoneal dialysis and hemodialysis. *Ann Intern Med* 85:29, 1976
196. Lee HA, Hill LF, Hewitt V, Ralston AJ, Berlyne GM: Lacticacidaemia in peritoneal dialysis. *Proc Eur Dial Transpl Assoc* 4:150, 1967
197. Dixon SR, Irvin ROH: Blood lactate levels after peritoneal dialysis with fluid containing lactate ions. *Proc Eur Dial Transpl Assoc* 6:293, 1969
198. Maher JF, Hirzel P, Hohnadel DC, Abraham J, Lasrich M: Fatty acid removal during peritoneal dialysis: mechanisms, rates and significance. *asaio J* 1:8, 1978
199. Schurig R, Gahl G, Schartl M, Becker H, Kessel M: Central and peripheral haemodynamics in longterm peritoneal dialysis patients. *Proc Eur Dial Transpl Assoc* 16:165, 1979
200. Pacifico AD, Lasker N, Frank MF, Levinson GE: Cardiovascular function in peritoneal dialysis. *Trans Am Soc Artif Intern Organs* 11:86, 1965
201. Swartz C, Onesti G, Mailloux L, Neff M, Ramirez O, Germon P, Kazem I, Brady LW: The acute hemodynamic and pulmonary perfusion effects of peritoneal dialysis. *Trans Am Soc Artif Intern Organs* 15:367, 1969
202. Acquatella H, Perez-Roja M, Bruger B, Guinand-Baldo A: Left ventricular function in terminal uremia. A hemodynamic and echocardiographic study. *Nephron* 22:160, 1978
203. Gotloib L, Mines M, Garmizo L, Varka I: Hemodynamic effects of increasing intraabdominal pressure in peritoneal dialysis. *Perit Dial Bull* (Toronto, Can) 1:41, 1981
204. Rutsky EA: Bradycardic rhythms during peritoneal dialysis. *Arch Intern Med* 128:445, 1971
205. Berlyne G, Lee HA, Ralston AJ, Woolcock JA: Pulmonary complications of peritoneal dialysis. *Lancet* 2:75, 1966
206. Ahluwalia MPS, Sekar T, Moorthi DS, Gelman ML, Shah T, Doherty GB, MacDonnell KF: Pulmonary function testing during peritoneal dialysis. *Kidney Int* (Abstract) 19:140, 1981
207. Goggin MJ, Joekes AM: Gas exchange in renal failure. I. Dangers of hyperkalaemia during anaesthesia. II. Pulmonary gas exchange during peritoneal dialysis. *Br Med J* 2:244, 1971
208. Hirszel P, Maher JF, Tempel GE, Mengel CE: Influence of peritoneal dialysis on factors affecting oxygen transport. *Nephron* 15:438, 1975
209. Mion C, Slingeneyer A, Huchard G, Deschodt G, Polito C, Issautier R, Florence P: Traitement de suppléance chez l'insuffisance rénal chronique à haut risque: hémodialyse ou dialyse péritonéale? (Replacement treatment in high risk cases of chronic renal failure: haemodialysis or peritoneal dialysis?) In: *Actualités Néprhologiques de l'Hôpital Necker* edited by Grünfeld JP, Paris, Flammarion Médecine Sciences, 1979, p 71 (in French)
210. Oreopoulos DG, Vas S, Zellerman G, Meema HD, Blair GR, Khanna R, McCready W: Is continuous ambulatory peritoneal dialysis still a promising dialysis treatment? *Proc Clin Dial Transpl Forum* 9:5, 1979
211. Mion C, Slingeneyer A, Canaub B: Continuous ambulatory peritoneal dialysis in France: results of a national survey and two years' experience at one centre. In: *Peritoneal Dialysis* edited by Atkins RC, Thomson NM, Farrell PC, Edinburgh, Churchill Livingstone, 1981, p 126
212. Farrell PC, Randerson DH: Long-term nutritional and clearance status in CAPD patients. *Contemporary Dial* (Reseda, CA) 1:45, 1980
213. Pauli HG, Büttikofer E, Vorburger Ch: Clinical experience with peritoneal dialysis. *Helv Med Acta* 1:51, 1966
214. Ivanovich P, Jones KM, Borsanyi A: Relief of pain associated with automated peritoneal dialysis. *Proc Eur Dial Transpl Assoc* 12:156, 1976
215. Raja RM, Kramer MS, Rosenbaum JL, Bolisay C, Krug M: Contrasting changes in solute transport and ultrafiltration with peritonitis in CAPD patients. *Am Soc Artif Intern Organs* 27:68, 1981
216. Hau T, Ahrenholz DH, Simmons RC: Secondary bacterial peritonitis: the biologic basis of treatment. *Curr Probl Surg* 16:3, 1979
217. Grodstein GP, Blumenkrantz MJ, Kopple JD: Effect of intercurrent illnesses on nitrogen metabolism in uremic patients. *Trans Am Soc Artif Intern Organs* 25:438, 1979
218. Mion C, Boen ST, Scribner P: An analysis for the factors responsible for the formation of adhesions during chronic peritoneal dialysis. *Am J Med Sci* 250:675, 1965
219. Gandhi VC, Humayun HM, Ing TS, Daugirdas JT, Jablokow VR, Iwatsuki S, Geis WP, Hano JE: Sclerotic thickening of the peritoneal membrane in maintenance peritoneal dialysis patients. *Arch Intern Med* 140:201, 1980
220. Heale WF, Letch KA, Dawborn JK, Evans SM: Long term complications of peritonitis. In: *Peritoneal Dialysis* edited by Atkins RC, Thomson NM, Farrell PC, Edinburgh, Churchill Livingstone, 1981, p 284
221. Denis J, Paineau J, Potel G, Fontenaille C, Guenel J: Continuous ambulatory peritoneal dialysis. *Ann Intern Med* 93:508, 1980
222. Mion C, Slingeneyer A, Beraud JJ, Oulès R, Balmes M: Peritonitis in home maintenance peritoneal dialysis: Incidence, diagnostic problems and prognosis. *J Dial* 2:426, 1978
223. Schweinburg FB, Seligman AM, Fine J: Transmural migration of intestinal bacteria. A study based on the use of

radioactive Escherichia Coli. *N Engl J Med* 242:747, 1950
224. Stephen CG, Meadows JG, Kerkering RM, Markowitz SA, Nisman RM: Spontaneous peritonitis due to hemophilus influenzae in an adult. *Gastroenterology* 77:1088, 1979
225. Prowant BF, Nolph KD: Clinical criteria for diagnosis of peritonitis. In: *Peritoneal Dialysis* edited by Atkins RC, Thomson NM, Farrell PC, Edinburgh, Churchill Livingstone, 1981, p 355
226. Stec F, Slingeneyer A, Perez C, Despaux E, Mion C: Large volume filtration of peritoneal fluid in intermittent and continuous ambulatory peritoneal dialysis. In: *Advances in Peritoneal Dialysis* International Congress Series 567, edited by Gahl GM, Kessel M, Nolph KD, Amsterdam, Oxford, Princeton, Excerpta Medica, 1981, p 158
227. Montgomerie JG, Kalmanson GM, Guze LB: Renal failure and infection. *Medicine* 47:1, 1968
228. Axelrod J, Meyers BR, Hirschman SZ, Stein R: Prophylaxis with cephalothin in peritoneal dialysis. *Arch Inter Med* 132:368, 1973
229. Black HR, Finkelstein FO, Lee RV: The treatment of peritonitis in patients with chronic indwelling catheters. *Trans Am Soc Artif Intern Organs* 20:115, 1974
230. Zaruba K, Oliveri M: Early diagnosis of peritoneal infection during continuous ambulatory peritoneal dialysis by the dialysate-digest medium-tube method. *Lancet* 2:1226, 1980
231. Williams P, Pantalony D, Vas ST, Khanna R, Oreopoulos DG: The value of dialysate cell count in the diagnosis of peritonitis in patients on continuous ambulatory peritoneal dialysis. *Perit Dial Bull* (Toronto, Can) 1:59, 1981
232. Chan LK, Oliver DO: Simple method for early detection of peritonitis in patients on continuous ambulatory peritoneal dialysis. *Lancet* 2:1336, 1979
233. Vas SI, Low DE, Layne S, Khanna R, Dombros N: Microbiological diagnostic approach to peritonitis in continuous ambulatory peritoneal dialysis patients. In: *Peritoneal Dialysis* edited by Atkins RC, Thomson NM, Farrell PC, Edinburgh, Churchill Livingstone, 1981, p 264
234. Hymayun HM, Ing TS, Gandhi VC, Chen WT, Hano JE. Daugirdas JT: Peritoneal fluid eosinophilia during the first months of maintenance peritoneal dialysis. *Kidney Int* (Abstract) 19:149, 1981
235. Splinowitz B, Golden R, Rascoff J, Charytan C: Eosinophilic peritonitis in continuous ambulatory peritoneal dialysis patients. *Abstracts Am Soc Artif Intern Organs* 10:59, 1981
236. Glickman RM, Isselbacher KJ: Abdominal swelling and ascites. In: *Harrison's Principles of Internal Medicine* edited by Isselbacher KJ, Adams RD, Braunwald E, Petersdorf RG, Wilson JD, 9th edition, New York (etc), McGraw Hill Book Company, 1980, Chapter 40, p 211 and 212 (Int Student edition)
237. Golper TA. Bennett WM, Hones SR: Peritonitis associated with chronic peritoneal dialysis. A diagnostic and therapeutic approach. *Dial Transpl* 7:1173, 1978
238. Atkins RC, Humphery T, Thomson NM, Williamson J, Hooke D, Davidson A: Bacterial and sterile peritonitis. In: *Peritoneal Dialysis,* edited by Atkins RC, Thomson NM, Farrell PC, Edinburgh, Churchill Livingstone, 1981, p 272
239. Holdsworth SR, Atkins RC, Scott DG, Jackson R: Management of Candida peritonitis by prolonged peritoneal lavage containing 5-fluorocytosine. *Clin Nephrol* 4:157, 1975
240. Barnes R, Brown D, Silva J, Easterling R: Candida peritonitis complicating peritoneal dialysis. *Kidney Int* (Abstract) 8:413, 1975
241. Bayer AS, Blumenkrantz MJ, Montgomerie JZ, Galpin JE, Coburn JW, Guze LB: Candida peritonitis. Report of 22 cases and review of the English literature. *Am J Med* 61:832, 1976
242. Mandell IN, Ahern MH, Kliger AS, Andriole VT: Candida peritonitis complicating peritoneal dialysis: successful treatment with low dose amphotericin B therapy. *Clin Nephrol* 6:492, 1976
243. Khanna R, Oreopoulos DG, Vas S, McCready W, Dombros N: Fungal peritonitis in patients undergoing chronic intermittent or continuous ambulatory peritoneal dialysis. *Proc Eur Dial Transpl Assoc* 17:291, 1980
244. Arfania D, Everett ED, Nolph KD, Rubin J: Uncommon causes of peritonitis in patients undergoing peritoneal dialysis. *Arch Intern Med* 141:61, 1981
245. Wallace M, Bagnall H, Glen D, Averill S: Isolation of lipophilic yeasts in 'sterile' peritonitis. *Lancet* 2:956, 1979
246. Ross DA, Anderson DC, Macnaughton MC, Stewart WK: Fulminating disseminated aspergillosis complicating peritoneal dialysis in eclampsia. *Arch Intern Med* 121:183, 1968
247. O'Sullivan FX, Wiegmann TB, Patak RV, Lynch JM, Hodges GH, Brandsberg JW, Barnes WG: An unusual case of peritonitis in CAPD due to a plant parasite. *Abstracts Am Soc Artif Intern Organs* 9:57, 1980
248. De Santo NG, Altucci P, Giordano C: Actinomyces peritonitis associated with dialysis. *Nephron* 16:236, 1976
249. Taylor R, McDonald M, Russ G, Carson M, Lukaczynski E: Vibrio alginolyticus peritonitis associated with ambulatory peritoneal dialysis *Br Med J* 283:275, 1981
250. Tucker T, Adams FF, Moffatt T, Dodds H, Dodds K: Tuberculous peritonitis in home peritoneal dialysis patients. *Kidney Int* (Abstract) 16:900, 1979
251. Khanna R, Fenton SS, Cattran D, Thompson D, Deitel M, Oreopoulos DG: Tuberculous peritonitis in patients undergoing continuous ambulatory peritoneal dialysis. *Perit Dial Bull* (Toronto, Can) 1:10, 1980
252. Thomson NM, Atkins RC, Hooke D, Maydom B, Scott DF: Long term clinical experience with CAPD in Australia. In: *Peritoneal Dialysis,* edited by Atkins RC, Thomson NM, Farrell PC, Edinburgh, Churchill Livingstone, 1981, p 93
253. Lasker N, Burke JF Jr, Patchefsky A, Haughey E: Peritoneal reactions to particulate matter in peritoneal dialysis solutions. *Trans Am Soc Artif Intern Organs* 21:342, 1975
254. Karanicolas S, Oreopoulos DG, Izatt S, Shimizu A, Manning RF, Sepp H, de Veber GA: Epidemic of aseptic peritonitis caused by endotoxin during chronic peritoneal dialysis. *N Engl J Med* 296:1336, 1977
255. Gandhi VC, Kamadana MR, Ing TS, Daugirdas JT, Viol GW, Robinson JA, Geis WP, Hano JE: Aseptic peritonitis in patients on maintenance peritoneal dialysis. *Nephron* 24:257, 1979
256. Yee E, Foss K, Schmidt RW: Use of povidone iodine in continuous ambulatory peritoneal dialysis – a technique to reduce the incidence of infectious peritonitis. *Trans Am Soc Artif Intern Organs* 26:223, 1980
257. Handa SP, Greer S, Tewari HD: Pseudomembranous colitis and cloudy peritoneal drainage in patients on peritoneal dialysis. *Kidney Int* (Abstract) 19:148, 1981
258. D'Apice AJF, Atkins RC: Analysis of peritoneal dialysis data. In: *Peritoneal Dialysis,* edited by Atkins RC, Thomson NM, Farrell PC, Edinburgh, Churchill Livingstone, 1981, p 440
259. Kaplan EL, Meier P: Non parametric extractions from incomplete observations. *J Am Stat Assoc* 53:457, 1958
260. Randerson DH, Farrell PC: Analysis of peritonitis data in

CAPD. In: *Advances in Peritoneal Dialysis* International Congress Series 567, edited by Gahl GM, Kessel M, Nolph KD, Amsterdam, Oxford, Princeton, Excerpta Medica, 1981, p 265
261. Sarles HE, Lindley JD, Fisch JC, Biggers JA, Cottom DL, Cotton JR, Mader JT, Dunaway JE, Remmers AR Jr: Peritoneal dialysis utilizing a Millipore filter. *Kidney Int* 9:54, 1976
262. Mion C, Slingeneyer A, Liendo-Liendo C, Perez C, Despaux E: Reduction in incidence of peritonitis associated with continuous ambulatory peritoneal dialysis. *Proc Clin Dial Transpl Forum* 9:9, 1979
263. Schwartz FD, Kallmeyer J, Dunea G, Kark RM: Prevention of infection during peritoneal dialysis. *JAMA* 199:115, 1967
264. Sherman RA, Longnecker RE, Davis V: Initial experience with a quick connect/disconnect device for chronic peritoneal dialysis. *Dial Transpl* 9:665, 1980
265. Stephen RL, Kablitz C, Kitahara M, Nelson JA, Duffy DP, Kolff WJ: Peritoneal dialysis peritonitis: saline-iodine flush. *Dial Transpl* 8:584, 1979
266. Furman KI, Kündig H, Ninen DT, Block JD: Reason for failure of saline-iodine flushes. In *Advances in Peritoneal Dialysis,* International Congress Series 567, edited by Grahl GM, Kessel M, Nolph KD, Amsterdam, Oxford, Princeton, Excerpta Medica 1981, p 281
267. Eisinger AJ: A simple method of lessening the incidence of peritonitis in peritoneal dialysis using a photochemical reactor. *Clin Nephrol* 14:42, 1980
268. Sharma BK, Smith EC, Rodriguez H, Pillay UKG, Gandhi VC, Dunea G: Trial of oral neomycin during peritoneal dialysis. *Am J Med Sci* 262:175, 1971
269. Eremin J, Marshall VC: The place of prophylactic antibiotics in peritoneal dialysis. *Australasian Ann Med* 18:264, 1969
270. Low DE, Vas SI, Oreopoulos DG, Manuel MA, Saiphoo MM, Finer C, Dombros N: Prophylactic cephalexin ineffective in chronic ambulatory peritoneal dialysis. *Lancet* 2:753, 1980
271. Rottembourg J, Jacq D, Singlas E, Nguyen M: Medical management of peritonitis. In: *Continuous Ambulatory Peritoneal Dialysis,* edited by Legrain M, Amsterdam, Excerpta Medica, 1980, p 248
272. O'Leary JP, Malik FS. Donahoe RR, Johnston AD: The effects of a minidose of heparin on peritonitis in rats. *Surg Gynecol Obstet* 148:571, 1979
273. Williams P, Khanna R, Vas SI, Oreopoulos DG, Layne S, Pantalony D: Treatment of peritonitis: to lavage or not? *Perit Dial Bull* (Toronto, Can) 1:14, 1980
274. Vas SI, Duwe A, Weatherhead J: Natural defence mechanisms of the peritoneum: the effect of peritoneal dialysis fluid on polymorphonuclear cells. In: *Peritoneal Dialysis,* edited by Atkins RC, Thomson NM, Farrell PC, Edinburgh, Churchill Livingstone, 1981, p 41
275. Williams P, Khanna R, Oreopoulos DG: Treatment of peritonitis in patients on CAPD: no longer a controversy. *Dial Transpl* 10:272, 1981
276. Bulger RJ, Bennett JV, Boen ST: Intraperitoneal administration of broad spectrum antibiotics in patients with renal failure. *JAMA* 194:1198, 1965
277. Greenberg PA, Sanford JP: Removal and absorption of antibiotics in patients with renal failure undergoing peritoneal dialysis. *Ann Intern Med* 66:465, 1967
278. Ruedy J: The effects of peritoneal dialysis on the physiological disposition of oxacillin, ampicillin, tetracycline in patients with renal disease. *J Can Med Assoc* 94:257, 1966
279. Perkins RL, Smith EJ, Saslaw S: Cephalothin and cephaloridine: comparative pharmacodynamics in chronic uremia. *Am J Med Sci* 257:116, 1969
280. Ahern MJ, Finkelstein FO, Andriole VT: Pharmacokinetics of cefamandole in patients undergoing hemodialysis and peritoneal dialysis. *Antimicrob Agents Chemother* 10:457, 1976
281. Kaye D, Wenger N, Agarwall B: Pharmacology of intraperitoneal cefazolin in patients undergoing peritoneal dialysis. *Antimicrob Agents Chemother* 14:318, 1978
282. Local FK, Munro AJ, Kerr DNS, Sussman M: Pharmacokinetics of intravenous and intraperitoneal cefuroxine in patients undergoing peritoneal dialysis. *Clin Nephrol* 16:40, 1981
283. Wise R, Reeves DS, Parker AS: Administration of Ticarcillin, a new antipseudomonal antibiotic, in patients undergoing dialysis. *Antimicrob Agents Chemother* 5:119, 1974
284. Reinarz JA, McIntosch DA: Lincomycin excretion in patients with normal renal function, severe azotemia, and with hemodialysis and peritoneal dialysis. *Antimicrob Agents Chemother* 10:232, 1976
285. Smithivas T, Hyams PJ, Matalon R, Simberkoff MS, Rahal JJ: The use of gentamicin in peritoneal dialysis. I. Pharmacologic results. *J Infect Dis* 124:S77, 1971
286. Hyams PJ, Smithivas T, Matalon R, Katz L, Simberkoff MS, Rahal JJ: The use of gentamicin in peritoneal dialysis. II. Microbiologic and clinical results. *J Infect Dis* 124:S84, 1971
287. Malacoff RF, Finkelstein FO, Andriole VT: Effect of peritoneal dialysis on serum levels of tobramycin and clindamycin. *Antimicrob Agents Chemother* 8:574, 1975
288. Regeur L, Colding H, Jensen H, Kampmann JP: Pharmacokinetics of amikacin during hemodialysis and peritoneal dialysis. *Antimicrob Agents Chemother* 11:214, 1977
289. Ayus JC, Eneas JF, Tong TG, Benowitz NL, Schoenfeld PY, Hadley KL, Becker CE, Humphreys MH: Peritoneal clearance and total body elimination of vancomycin during chronic intermittent peritoneal dialysis. *Clin Nephrol* 11:129, 1979
290. Adam WR, Brown DJ, Hales P, Dawborn JK: The use of sulphadimidine (sulphamezathine) in patients with renal failure. *Med J Aust* 12:936, 1973
291. Bennett WM, Muther RS, Parker RA, Feig P, Morrison G, Golper TA, Singer I: Drug therapy in renal failure: dosing guidelines for adults. Part I: Antimicrobial agents analysis. *Ann Intern Med* 93:62, 1980
292. Atkins RC, Humphery T, Thomson N, Hooke D, Williamson J, Davidson A: Efficacy of treatment in CAPD peritonitis. The problem of staphylococcal antibiotic resistance. In: *Peritoneal Dialysis,* edited by Atkins RC, Thomson NM, Farrell PC, Edinburgh, Churchill Livingstone, 1981, p 333
293. Nielsen HE, Sorensen I, Hansen HE: Peritoneal transport of vancomycin during peritoneal dialysis. *Nephron* 24:274, 1979
294. Berqvist Poppen M, von Sydow U: Pulmonary complications of peritoneal dialysis. *Lancet* 2:752, 1966
295. Stead NW, Bates JA: Tuberculosis. In: *Harrison's Principles of Internal Medicine,* edited by Isselbacher FJ, Adams RD, Braunwald E, Petersdorf RG, Wilson JD, 9th edition New York etc, McGraw Hill Book Company, 1980, p 583 and 707 (Int Student edition)
296. Rubin J, Nolph K, Arfania D, Brown P, Prowant B: Follow-up of peritoneal clearances in patients undergoing continuous ambulatory peritoneal dialysis. *Kidney Int* 16:619, 1979
297. Oreopoulos DG, Khanna R, Williams P, Dombros N, Carmichael D: Efficacy of clinical experience with contin-

uous ambulatory peritoneal dialysis in Canada. In: *Peritoneal Dialysis,* edited by Atkins RC, Thomson NM, Farrell PC, Edinburgh, Churchill Livingstone, 1981, p 114
298. Ghantous WN, Salkin MS, Adelson BH, Ghantous S, McGinnis K, Valenziano A, Cronin M: Limitations of peritoneal dialysis in the treatment of ESRD patients. *Trans Am Soc Artif Intern Organs* 25:100, 1979
299. Mion C: Introductory remarks: Maintenance haemodialysis versus intermittent peritoneal dialysis versus continuous ambulatory peritoneal dialysis. In: *Continuous Ambulatory Peritoneal Dialysis,* edited by Legrain M, Amsterdam, Excerpta Medica, 1980, p 317
300. Randerson DH, Farrell PC: Long-term peritoneal clearance in CAPD. In: *Peritoneal Dialysis,* edited by Atkins RC, Thomson NM, Farrell PC, Edinburgh Churchill Livingstone, 1981, p 22
301. Tenckhoff H: Advantages and shortcomings of peritoneal dialysis in the treatment of chronic renal failure. In: *Séminaires d'Uro-Néphrologie Pitié-Salpêtrière,* edited by Küss R, Legrain M, Paris, Masson, 1977, p 197
302. Marshall AJ, Baddeley H, Barritt DW, Davies JD, Lee REJ, Low-Beer TS, Read AE: Practolol peritonitis. A study of 16 cases and a survey of small bowel function in patients taking beta-adrenergic blockers. *Q J Med* 46:135, 1977
303. Valk TW, Swartz RD, Hsu CH: Peritoneal dialysis in acute renal failure: analysis of outcome and complications. *Dial Transpl* 9:48, 1980
304. Rudnick MR, Coyle JF, Beck LH, McCurdy DK: Acute massive hydrothorax complicating peritoneal dialysis, report of 2 cases and a review of the literature. *Clin Nephrol* 12:38, 1979
305. Kuehnel E: Massive pleural effusion secondary to CAPD. Abstract. *Kidney Int* 19:152, 1981
306. Alquier P, Achard J, Bonhomme R: Hydrothorax aigu au cours de dialyses péritonéales (Acute hydrothorax in the course of peritoneal dialyses). *Nouv Presse Méd* 4:192, 1975 (in French)
307. Berne TW, Barbour BH: Acute renal failure in general surgical patients. *Arch Surg* 30:814, 1971
308. Thomson WB, Buchanan A, Doak PD, Peart WS: Peritoneal dialysis *Br Med J* 1:932, 1964
309. Blumenkrantz MJ, Schmidt RW: Managing the nutritional concerns of the patient undergoing peritoneal dialysis. In: *Developments in Nephrology 2: Peritoneal Dialysis,* edited by Nolph KD, The Hague, London, Boston MA, Martinus Nijhoff, 1981, p 275
310. Palmer RA, Newell JE, Gray ES, Quinton WE: Treatment of chronic renal failure by prolonged peritoneal dialysis. *N Engl J Med* 274:248, 1966
311. Rodriguez HJ, Walls J, Slatopolsky E, Klahr S: Recurrent ascites following peritoneal dialysis. A new syndrome? *Arch Intern Med* 134:283, 1974
312. Levinsky NG, Alexander EA, Vankatachalam MA: Acute renal failure. In *The Kidney,* edited by Brenner BM, Rector FC, 2nd edition, Philadelphia, WB Saunders Co, 1981, p 1181
313. Derot M, Legrain M, Jacobs C: Indications respectives du rein artificiel et de la dialyse péritonéale dans le traitement de l'insuffisance rénale aiguë (à propos de 537 observations). (Indications for haemodialysis vers. peritoneal dialysis in the treatment of acute renal failure). *Proc Eur Dial Transpl Assoc* 2:44, 1965 (in French)
314. Firmat J, Zucchini A: Peritoneal dialysis in acute renal failure. *Contrib Nephrol* 17:33, 1979
315. Mathew TH: Comparison of peritoneal and haemodialysis in acute renal failure. In *Peritoneal Dialysis,* edited by Atkins RC, Thomson NM, Farrell PC, Edinburgh, Churchill Livingstone, 1981, p 80
316. Erbe RW, Greene JA Jr, Weller JM: Peritoneal dialysis during haemorrhagic shock. *J Appl Physiol* 22:131, 1967
317. Posen GA, Luisello J: Continuous equilibration peritoneal dialysis in the treatment of acute renal failure. *Perit Dial Bull* (Toronto, Can) 1:6, 1980
318. Cameron JS, Ogg C, Trounce JR: Peritoneal dialysis in hypercatabolic acute renal failure. *Lancet* 1:1188, 1967
319. Tzamaloukas AH, Garella S, Chazan JA: Peritoneal dialysis for acute renal failure after major abdominal surgery. *Arch Surg* 106:639, 1973
320. Brooks MH, Barry KG: Removal of iodinated contrast material by peritoneal dialysis. *Nephron* 12:10, 1973
321. Yium J, Martinez-Maldonado M, Eknoyan G, Suki WN: Peritoneal dialysis in the treatment of renal failure in multiple myeloma. *South Med J* 64:1403, 1971
322. Mirouze J, Mion C, Jullien C: Place de la dialyse péritonéale dans le traitement de l'insuffisance rénale chronique évoluée (The place of peritoneal dialysis in the treatment of end stage renal failure). *Proc Eur Dial Transpl Assoc* 4:156, 1967 (in French)
323. Maher JF, Ahearn DJ, Bryan CW, Nolph KD: Prognosis of chronic renal failure. III. Survival after one peritoneal dialysis. *Nephron* 15:8, 1975
324. Mowbray JF: Peritoneal dialysis for pre- and postoperative management in a cadaveric transplantation program. *Trans Am Soc Artif Intern Organs* 13:46, 1967
325. Brulles A, Caralps A, Andreu J, Masramon J, Lloveras J, Gil-Vernet JM: Long-term peritoneal dialysis. *Lancet* 1:624, 1974
326. Fenton SSA. Cattran DC, Barnes NM, Waugh KJ: Home peritoneal dialysis a major advance in promoting home dialysis. *Trans Am Soc Artif Intern Organs* 23:194, 1977
327. Diaz-Buxo JA, Walker PH, Chandler JT, Farmer CK, Holt KL: Impact of peritoneal dialysis on renal replacement therapy. *Dial Transpl* 8:1061, 1979
328. Counts S, Hickman R, Garbaccio A, Tenckhoff H: Chronic home peritoneal dialysis in children. *Trans Am Soc Artif Intern Organs* 19:157, 1973
329. Moncrief JW, Popovich RP, Nolph KD, Rubin J, Robson M, Dombros N, deVeber GA, Oreopoulos DG: Clinical experience with continuous ambulatory peritoneal dialysis. *asaio J* 2:114, 1979
330. Nolph KD: Peritoneal dialysis. In: *Replacement of Renal Function by Dialysis* edited by Drukker W, Parsons FM, Maher JF, The Hague, Boston MA, London, Martinus Nijhoff, 1st edition, 1978, p 277
331. Winchester JF, Gelfand MC, Knepshield JH, Schreiner GE: Dialysis and hemoperfusion of poisons and drugs. Update. *Trans Am Soc Artif Intern Organs* 23:762, 1977
332. Maher JF: Principles of dialysis and dialysis of drugs. *Am J Med* 62:475, 1977
333. Rubin J: Comments on dialysis solutions composition, antibiotic transport, poisoning and novel uses of peritoneal dialysis. In: *Developments in Nephrology 2: Peritoneal Dialysis,* edited by Nolph KD, The Hague, Boston MA, London, Martinus Nijhoff, 1981, p 240
334. Knochel JP, Clayton LE, Smith WL, Barry KG: Intraperitoneal THAM: an effective method to enhance phenobarbital removal during peritoneal dialysis. *J Lab Clin Med* 64:257, 1964
335. Knochel JP, Mason AD: Effect of alkalinization on peritoneal diffusion of uric acid. *Am J Physiol* 210:1160, 1966
336. Campion DS, North JDK: Effect of protein binding of barbiturates on their rate of removal during peritoneal dialysis. *J Lab Clin Med* 66:549, 1965
337. Etteldorf JN, Dobbins WT, Summitt RL, Rainwater WT,

Fischer RI: Intermittent peritoneal dialysis using 5% albumin in the treatment of salicylate intoxication in children. *J Pediatr* 58:226, 1961
338. Mailloux LU, Swartz CD, Onesti GO: Peritoneal dialysis for refractory congestive failure. *JAMA* 199:873, 1967
339. Cairns KB, Proter GA, Kloster FE, Bristow JD, Griswold HE: Clinical and hemodynamic results of peritoneal dialysis for severe cardiac failure. *Am Heart J* 76:227, 1968
340. Raja RM, Krasnoff SO, Moros JG, Kramer MS, Rosenbaum JL: Repeated peritoneal dialysis in treatment of heart failure. *JAMA* 213:2268, 1970
341. Barry KG, Hunter RH, Davis TE, Crosby WH: Acute uric acid nephropathy. *Arch Intern Med* 111:452, 1963
342. Weintraub LR, Penner JA, Meyers MC: Acute uric acid nephropathy in leukemia. *Arch Intern Med* 113:111, 1964
343. Maher JF, Rath CE, Schreiner GE: Hyperuricemia complicating leukemia. Treatment with allopurinol and dialysis. *Arch Intern Med* 123:198, 1969
344. Reuler JB, Parker RA: Peritoneal dialysis in the management of hypothermia. *JAMA* 240:2289, 1978
345. Zawada ET Jr: Treatment of profound hypothermia with peritoneal dialysis. *Dial Transpl* 9:255, 1980
346. Stoltz ML, Nolph KD, Maher JF: Factors affecting calcium removal with calcium free peritoneal dialysis. *J Lab Clin Med* 78:389, 1971
347. Counts SJ, Baylink DJ, Shen FH, Sherrard DJ, Hickman RO: Vitamin D intoxication in an anephric child. *Ann Intern Med* 82:196, 1975
348. Skoutakis VA, Black WD, Acchiardo SR, Wood GC: Peritoneal dialysis in the treatment of acetohexamide induced hypoglycemia. *Am J Hosp Pharm* 34:68, 1977
349. Lampe WT: Hypoglycemia due to acetohexamide. *Arch Intern Med* 120:239, 1967
350. Wall AJ: Peritoneal dialysis in the treatment of severe acute pancreatitis. *Med J Aust* 2:281, 1965
351. Gjessing J: Peritoneal dialysis in severe acute hemorrhagic peritonitis. *Acta Chir Scand* 133:645, 1967
352. Siedek M, Sieberth HG, Schmitz G, Redlich A: Extrarenal indications for peritoneal dialysis (report of 2 cases). *Proc Eur Dial Transpl Assoc* 3:355, 1966
353. Twardowski ZJ, Nolph KD, Rubin J, Anderson PC: Peritoneal dialysis for psoriasis. An uncontrolled study. *Ann Intern Med* 88:349, 1978
354. Segar WE, Gibson RK, Rhamy R: Peritoneal dialysis in infants and small children. *Pediatrics* 27:603, 1961
355. Chan JCM, Campbell RA: Peritoneal dialysis in children, a survey of its indications and applications. *Clin Pediatr* 12:131, 1973
356. Gagnadoux MF, Hernandez MA, Broyer M, Vacant J, Royer P: La dialyse péritonéale chronique; alternative à l'hémodialyse itérative chez l'enfant (Chronic peritoneal dialysis; an alternative to regular haemodialysis in the child). *Arch Fr Pediatr* 34:860, 1977 (in French)
357. Hickman RO: Nine years experience with chronic peritoneal dialysis in childhood. *Dial Transpl* 7:803, 1978
358. Brouhard BH, Berger M, Cunningham RJ, Petrusick T, Allen W, Lynch RE, Travis LB: Home peritoneal dialysis in children. *Trans Am Soc Artif Organs*, 25:90, 1979
359. Potter DE, McDaid TK, Ramırez JA: Peritoneal dialysis in children. In: *Peritoneal Dialysis* edited by Atkins RC, Thomson NM, Farrell PC, Edinburgh, Churchill Livingstone, 1981, p 356
360. Williamson Balfe J, Vigneux A, Willumsen J, Hardy BE: The use of CAPD in the treatment of children with endstage renal disease. *Perit Dial Bull* (Toronto Can) 1:35, 1981

361. Stamm SJ, Doctor J, Rose R, Isbister I, Hickman RO: Peritoneal dialysis in the treatment of cystic fibrosis with congestive heart failure. *Clin Pediatr* 5:575, 1966
362. Collipp PJ: Peritoneal dialysis for the respiratory distress syndrome. *JAMA* 203:169, 1968
363. Boda D, Muranyi L, Veress I, Pataki L, Streitmann K, Hencz P: Peritoneal dialysis in the treatment of hyaline membrane disease of newborn premature infants. *Acta Paediatr Scand* 60:90, 1971
364. Nathan E: Severe hydrops foetalis treated with peritoneal dialysis and positive-pressure ventilation. *Lancet* 1:1393, 1968
365. Pross DC, Bradford WD, Krueger RP: Reye's syndrome treated by peritoneal dialysis. *Pediatrics* 45:845, 1970
366. Samaha FJ, Blau E, Berardinelli JL: Reye's syndrome. Clinical diagnosis and treatment with peritoneal dialysis. *Pediatrics* 53:336, 1974
367. Samma SE, Cottom D: Peritoneal dialysis in maple syrup urine disease. *Lancet* 2:1423, 1969
368. Russell G, Thom H, Tarlow MJ, Gomperz D: Reduction of plasma proprionate by peritoneal dialysis. *Pediatrics* 53:281, 1974
369. Hobolth N, Devantier M: Removal of induced reacting bilirubin by albumin binding during intermittent peritoneal dialysis in the newborn. *Acta Paediatr Scand* 58:171, 1969
370. Oreopoulos DG: Renewed interest in chronic peritoneal dialysis. *Kidney Int* 13 (suppl 8):S117, 1978
371. Wing AJ, Brunner FP, Brynger H, Chantler C, Donckerwolcke RA, Gurland HJ, Hataway RA, Jacobs C, Sellwood NH: Combined report on regular dialysis and transplantation in Europe, VIII, 1977. *Proc Eur Dial Transpl Assoc* 15:2, 1978
372. Brynger H, Brunner FP, Chantler C, Donckerwolcke RA, Jacobs C, Kramer P, Selwood NH, Wing AJ: Combined report on regular dialysis and transplantation in Europe, X, 1979. *Proc Eur Dial Transpl Assoc* 17:69, 1980
373. Jacobs C, Broyer M, Brunner FP, Brynger H, Donckerwolcke RA, Kramer P, Selwood NH, Wing AJ: Combined report on regular dialysis and transplantation in Europe. XI, 1980 *Proc Eur Dial Transpl Assoc* 18:38, 1981
374. Moncrief JW, Popovich RP: Continuous ambulatory peritoneal dialysis. Worldwide experience. In: *Developments in Nephrology 2. Peritoneal Dialysis* edited by Nolph KD, The Hague, Boston MA, London, Martinus Nijhoff, 1981, p 178
375. Maher JF: Peritoneal dialysis update. *Trans Am Soc Artif Intern Organs* 24:774, 1978
376. Maher JF, Deane N, Henderson LW, Lasker N, Nolph KD, Popovich R, Roxe DM: Peritoneal dialysis: can we overcome its current limitations? *Trans Am Soc Artif Intern Organs* 25:523, 1979
377. Levin S, Winkelstein JA: Diet and infrequent peritoneal dialysis in chronic anuric uremia. *N Engl J Med* 277:619, 1967
378. Blumenkrantz MJ, Shapiro DJ, Miller JH, Barshay M, Kopple JD, Shinaberger JO, Friedler RM, Coburn JW: Chronic peritoneal dialysis for the management of chronic renal failure. *Proc Clin Dial Transpl Forum* 3:117, 1973
379. von Hartitzsch B, Hill AVL, Medlock TR: Nine-hour peritoneal dialysis three times weekly – an alternative to conventional haemodialysis. *Proc Eur Dial Transpl Assoc* 13:306, 1976
380. Sherrard DJ, Curtis FK, Lindner A, Scollard D, Merritt A: Peritoneal dialysis, a feasible alternative. *Proc Clin Dial Transpl Forum* 3:114, 1973
381. Giordano C, De Santo NG, Cirillo D: Short daily peritoneal dialysis: 3 years' experience. *Nephron* 21:131, 1978

382. Boen ST, Haagsma-Schouten WAG, Birnie RJ: Long-term peritoneal dialysis and a peritoneal dialysis index. *Dial Transpl* 7:377, 1978
383. Ahmad S, Shen FH, Blagg CR: Intermittent peritoneal dialysis as renal replacement therapy. In: *Developments in Nephrology 2: Peritoneal dialysis,* edited by Nolph KD, The Hague, Boston MA, London, Martinus Nijhoff, 1981, p 144
384. Milutinovic J, Cutler RE, Hoover P, Meijsen B, Scribner BH: Measurement of residual glomerular filtration rate in the patient receiving repetitive hemodialysis. *Kidney Int* 8:185, 1975
385. Tenckhoff H, Blagg CR, Curtis FK, Hickman RO: Chronic peritoneal dialysis. *Proc Eur Dial Transpl Assoc* 10, 363, 1973
386. Scribner BH, Giordano C, Oreopoulos DG, Mion C, Buoncristiani U, Dawids SG, Gahl GM, Jones KM: Long term peritoneal dialysis. *Proc Eur Dial Transpl Assoc* 12:131, 1975
387. Schuenemann B, Quellhorst E, Fuchs CH: Introduction into the problems of chronic peritoneal dialysis. *Int J Artif Organs* 1:5, 1979
388. Walker RG, Thomson NM, Scott DF, Atkins RC: Intermittent peritoneal dialysis in the treatment of end stage renal failure. *Med J Aust* 15:3, 1979
389. Silverberg S, Oreopoulos DG, Wise DJ, Uden DE, Meindok H, Jones M, Rapoport A, deVeber GA: Pericarditis in patients undergoing long-term hemodialysis and peritoneal dialysis. Incidence, complications and management. *Am J Med* 63:874, 1977
390. Lindsay RM, Friesen M, Koens F, Linton AL, Oreopoulos DG, deVeber GA: Platelet function in patients on long term peritoneal dialysis. *Clin Nephrol* 6:335, 1976
391. Nenci GG, Berrettini M, Agnelli G, Parise P, Buoncristiani U, Ballatori E: Effect of peritoneal dialysis, haemodialysis and kidney transplantation on blood platelet function. I. Platelet aggregation by ADP and epinephrine. *Nephron* 23:287, 1979
392. Sherrard DJ, Curtis FK, Hanson P, Terao S, Harris H, Laris L, Klahn M, Thompson B: Infection and other complications of peritoneal dialysis. *Dial Transpl* 6:(no 2) 28, 1977
393. Ahmad S, Gallagher N, Shen F: Intermittent peritoneal dialysis status reassessed. *Trans Am Soc Artif Intern Organs* 25:86, 1979
394. Oreopoulos DG: Hepatitis and treatment of chronic renal failure by peritoneal dialysis. *Lancet* 2:1256, 1972
395. Spector D: Hepatitis B miniepidemic in a peritoneal dialysis unit. *Arch Intern Med* 137:1030, 1977
396. Oreopoulos DG, Khanna R, McCready W, Vas S, Izatt S, Zellerman G: Intermittent peritoneal dialysis in the hospital. *Dial Transpl* 9:231, 1980
397. Price JD, Ashby KM, Reeve CE: Results of 12 years' treatment of chronic renal failure by dialysis and transplantation. *Can Med Assoc J* 118:263, 1978
398. Brynger H, Brunner FP, Chantler C, Donckerwolcke RA, Jacobs C, Kramer P, Selwood NH, Wing AJ: Combined report on regular dialysis and transplantation in Europe X 1979. *Proc Eur Dial Transpl Assoc* 17:36, 1980
399. Forbes AMW, Reed VL, Goldsmith HJ: The adequacy of six litre daily continuous ambulatory peritoneal dialysis. *Proc Eur Dial Transpl Assoc* 17:276, 1980
400. Henderson LW: Ultrafiltration with peritoneal dialysis. In: *Developments in Nephrology 2 Peritoneal Dialysis,* edited by Nolph KD, The Hague, Boston MA, London, Martinus Nijhoff, 1981, p 124
401. Goldsmith HG, Forbes A, Gyde DHB, Summerfield G: Hematological aspects of continuous ambulatory peritoneal dialysis. In: *Continuous Ambulatory Peritoneal Dialysis,* edited by Legrain M, Amsterdam, Excerpta Medica, 1980, p 302
402. Chan MK, Chuah P, Raftery M, Baillod RA, Sweny P, Varghese Z, Moorhead JF: Three years' experience of continuous ambulatory peritoneal dialysis. *Lancet* 1:1409, 1981
403. Khanna R, Oreopoulos DG, Dombros N, Vas S, Williams P, Meema HE, Husdan H, Ogilvie R, Zellerman G, Roncari DAK, Clayton S, Izatt S: Continuous ambulatory peritoneal dialysis after three years: still a promising treatment. *Perit Dial Bull* (Toronto, Can) 1:24, 1981
404. Nolph KD, Prowant B: Complications during continuous ambulatory peritoneal dialysis. In: *Continuous Ambulatory Peritoneal Dialysis,* edited by Legrain M, Amsterdam, Excerpta Medica, 1980, p 258
405. Mion C: A review of seven years' home peritoneal dialysis. *Proc Eur Dial Transpl Assoc* 18:91, 1981
406. Faller B, Marichal JF: Loss of ultrafiltration in CAPD: clinical data. In: *Advances in Peritoneal Dialysis* International Congress series 567, edited by Gahl GM, Kessel M, Nolph KD, Amsterdam, Oxford, Princeton, Excerpta Medica, 1981, p 227
407. Verger C, Brunschvicg O, Le Charpentier Y, Lavergne A, Vantelon J: Structural and ultrastructural peritoneal membrane changes and permeability alterations during continuous ambulatory peritoneal dialysis. *Proc Eur Dial Transpl Assoc,* 18:199, 1981
408. Nolph KD: Continuous ambulatory peritoneal dialysis. *Am J Nephrol* 1:1, 1981
409. Shaldon S: A cynical critique of continuous ambulatory peritoneal dialysis. In: *Continuous Ambulatory Peritoneal Dialysis,* edited by Legrain M, Amsterdam, Excerpta Medica, 1980, p 137
410. Ghavanian M, Gutch CF, Kopp KF, Kolff WJ: The sad truth about diabetic nephropathy. *JAMA* 222:1386, 1972
411. Shapiro FL, Leonard A, Comty CM: Mortality, morbidity and rehabilitation results in regularly dialysed patients with diabetes mellitus. *Kidney Int* 6 (Suppl 1):S8, 1974
412. White N, Snowden SA, Parsons V, Sheldon J, Bewick M: The management of terminal renal failure in diabetic patients by regular dialysis therapy. *Nephron* 11:261, 1973
413. Blumenkrantz MJ, Shapiro DJ, Mimura N, Oreopoulos DG, Friedler RM, Levin S, Tenckhoff H, Coburn JW: Maintenance peritoneal dialysis as an alternative in the patient with diabetes mellitus and end-stage uremia. *Kidney Int* 6:(Suppl 1) S108, 1974
414. Finkelstein FO, Kliger AS, Bastl C, Yap P, Goffinet J: Chronic peritoneal dialysis in diabetic patients with end-stage renal failure. *Proc Clin Dial Transpl Forum,* 5:142, 1975
415. Blumenkrantz MJ, Kamdar A, Coburn JW: Peritoneal dialysis for diabetic patients with end-stage nephropathy. *Dial Transpl* 6:(no 2) 47, 1977
416. Mitchell JE: End stage renal failure in juvenile diabetes mellitus: a five year follow-up of treatment. *Mayo Clinic Proc* 52:281, 1977
417. Rubin JE, Friedman EA: Dialysis and transplantation in diabetics in the United States. *Nephron* 18:309, 1977
418. Quellhorst E, Schuenemann B, Mietzsch G, Jacob I: Haemo- and peritoneal dialysis treatment of patients with diabetic nephropathy – a comparative study. *Proc Eur Dial Transpl Assoc* 15:205, 1978
419. Mion C, Slingeneyer A, Oulès R, Selam JL, Delors J, Mirouze J: Home peritoneal dialysis in diabetics with end-stage renal failure. *Contrib Nephrol* 17:120, 1979
420. Hood SA, Frohnert PP, Mitchell JC, Kurtz SB: Home

peritoneal dialysis: dialysis therapy of choice in chronic renal failure of juvenile onset diabetes mellitus. *Dial Transpl* 9:843, 1980
421. Katirtzoglou A, Izatt S, Oreopoulos DG, Dombros N, Blair GR, Chisholm L, Meema HE, Ogilvie R, Vas S, Leibel B, McCreedy W: Chronic peritoneal dialysis in diabetics with end-stage renal failure. In: *Diabetic Renal Retinal Syndrome*, edited by Friedman EA, L'Esperance FA, New York, Grune and Stratton, 1980, p 317
422. Roxe DM, Del Greco F, Hughes J, Krumlovsky F, Ghantous W, Ivanovich P, Quintanilla A, Salkin M, Stone NJ, Reins M: Hemodialysis vs. peritoneal dialysis: results of a 3-year prospective controlled study. *Kidney Int* 19:341, 1981
423. Strosahl VS, Waldorf PV: Visual impairment-not a contraindication for continuous ambulatory peritoneal dialysis. *Dial Transpl* 10:371, 1981
424. Shapiro FL, Comty CM: Hemodialysis in diabetics – 1979 update. In: *Diabetic Renal Retinal Syndrome*, edited by Friedman EA, L'Esperance FA, New York, Grune and Stratton, 1980, p 333
425. Cardella CJ: Renal transplantation in patients on peritoneal dialysis. *Perit Dial Bull* (Toronto Can) 1:12, 1980
426. Evans DH, Sorkin MI, Nolph KD: CAPD and transplantation. *Abstracts Am Soc Artif Intern Organs* 10:72, 1981
427. Gokal R, Ramos JM, Veitch P, Proud G, Taylor RMR, Ward MK, Wilkinson R, Kerr DNS: Renal transplantation in patients on continuous ambulatory peritoneal dialysis. *Proc Eur Dial Transpl Assoc* 18:222, 1981
428. Leigh DA: Peritoneal infections in patients on long-term peritoneal dialysis before and after human cadaveric renal transplantation. *J Clin Path* 22:539, 1969
429. Legrain M, Jacobs C: Place of chronic ambulatory peritoneal dialysis in the treatment of end-stage renal failure. In: *Continuous Ambulatory Peritoneal Dialysis*, edited by Legrain M, Amsterdam, Excerpta Medica, 1980, p 347
430. Shapiro FL: Hemodialysis and alternative treatments. A look into the near future. *Nephron* 24:2, 1979
431. Finkelstein FO, Kliger AS, Bastl C, Yap P: Sequential clearance and dialysance measurements in chronic peritoneal dialysis patients. *Nephron* 18:342, 1977
432. Blumenkrantz MJ (Cooperative dialysis study) Controlled evaluation of maintenance peritoneal dialysis. *Dial Transpl* 7:797, 1978
433. Mion C: Discussion. *Proc Eur Dial Transpl Assoc* 13:313, 1976
434. Friedman EA, Lundin AP, Butt KMH: Rushed judgment in uremia therapy. *Artif Organs* 5:97, 1981
435. Lundin AP: Alternatives to diffusion dialysis: is there a need for a better 'mousetrap'? *Nephron* 27:7, 1981
436. Shaldon S, Deschodt G, Beau MC, Claret G, Mion H, Mion C: Vascular stability during high flux haemofiltration. *Proc Eur Dial Transpl Assoc* 16:695, 1979
437. Chester AC, Rakowski TA, Argy WP Jr, Giacalone A, Schreiner GE: Haemodialysis in the eighth and ninth decades of life. *Arch Intern Med* 139:1001, 1979
438. Vantelon J, Verger C, Glennie N, Hatt D, Becker A: Pour ou contre la dialyse péritonéale continue ambulatoire (Pro's and con's of continuous ambulatory peritoneal dialysis). In: *Actualités Néphrologiques Hôpital Necker*, edited by Grünfeld JP, Paris, Flammarion Med Sciences, 1981, p 353 (in French)

24

HOME DIALYSIS

ROSEMARIE A. BAILLOD

Introduction	493
Patient selection	494
Availability of home dialysis	494
Medical considerations	494
Age	494
Married and single status	495
Anxiety	495
Learning ability	495
Financial status	497
Accommodation	497
Special advantages of home dialysis	497
Technical and medical features of home haemodialysis	497
Blood access	497
Dialysers	498
Dialysis fluid preparation	498
Water preparation	498
Monitoring	498
Cleansing and disinfection of equipment	498
Ultrafiltration	498
Control of hypertension	499
Disequilibrium	499
Anticoagulation	499
Blood loss, prevention of anaemia	499
Psychology	499
Who does dialysis in the home?	499
Training	450
Setting the scene	450
CAPD training	501
The teacher	501
Assessment of haemodialysis training	504
Choice and arrangement of haemodialysis equipment in the home	505
Maintenance support in the home	508
Medical follow-up	508
Management of medical problems and role of the local doctor	509
Advisory service for the management of dialysis problems	509
Technical maintenance and emergency repairs of haemodialysis equipment	509
Updating of dialysis technique and detection of recurrent errors	510
Supply of disposables	510
Role and value of social workers and community support	510
Analysis of results	510
Advantages to patient	510
Advantages to the nephrology service	511
Failure of patient and the hospital	511
Home dialysis in children	512
Conclusions	512
Acknowledgement	512
References	512

INTRODUCTION

Viewed in retrospect, the idea of haemodialysis taking place in the home in the early sixties seemed audacious. The practice not only set a medical precedent but it occurred at a very early stage in the development of haemodialysis for treatment of chronic renal failure. Even today, although over 20,000 patients and their families have mastered the techniques of home dialysis, the medical profession still regards it with apprehension and wonder.

The early literature described the success of regular dialysis treatment and revealed the considerable variation in survival rates. By 1965 (1) 80% of all European centres lacked space, staff and adequate finance. A similar situation existed in the United States (2). These problems were obviously greater in the centres which achieved the best treatment results. The demand for treatment combined with the conviction that there was a satisfactory alternative to death from renal failure, provided motivation to initiate and pursue home dialysis. The home offered space, the family staff and both features cut costs to all concerned.

The first home dialysis is reported to have taken place in Japan in 1961 (3). Early in 1964 three pioneers of regular haemodialysis, Scribner (Seattle), Merrill (Boston) and Shaldon (London) (4–6) devised and successfully implemented home dialysis. The work was greeted with surprise and adverse criticism but due to the needs described above, other centres tentatively introduced home dialysis. Each new centre modified the techniques to suit its own ideas and needs.

Many of the initial rapid advances in the development of equipment and changes in dialysis techniques must be attributed to their adaptation for home dialysis use. Unattended overnight dialysis of 10 h or longer demanded fail-safe monitoring devices in order to promote confidence in the patient and family (6, 7).

The pressing financial and patient need for self-care in the home environment has been made manifest by the rapidly developed interest in continuous ambulatory peritoneal dialysis (CAPD) both in Europe and North America (8, 9). Its relationship to home haemodialysis will be incorporated into this Chapter, which is intended to give practical guidance on techniques and highlight some of the problems involved rather than review the literature of home dialysis.

PATIENT SELECTION

Great emphasis has always been placed on the selection of suitable patients for a home dialysis programme (6, 7). As dialysis techniques and patient health improved much of the 'original selection debate' (10-15) has become out-moded. Facilities for home treatment still remain limited in many countries. Additionally today's patients are more diverse in age and medical complications all of which makes selection at the present time as appropriate as ever. However, regardless of the apparent complications, desire and motivation for treatment at home remain the most important factors for successful treatment.

Availability of home dialysis

The use of home dialysis varies from country to country and from centre to centre depending on national policies and local medical opinion. This is illustrated by review of its availability and use in relation to other treatments which are discussed in detail in Chapter 44 of this book.

Home dialysis is in fact used for only 10% of all patients receiving haemodialysis treatment thoughout the world, the largest proportion of whom live in English speaking countries. European statistics (16) show the percentage of haemodialysis patients on home treatment in the United Kingdom and Ireland to be 64% and 33% respectively compared to the European average of 17.5%.

Legislation in the USA (Public Law 92 - 603) in 1972 caused a rapid decline in the percentage of patients doing home haemodialysis, but because of the enormous increase in the total number of patients treated, the actual number of patients treated at home continued to rise. Presently 13% of patients are on home haemodialysis. Newer legislation (Public Law 95 - 292) is designed to motivate more home care thereby hoping to reduce the huge financial cost of the USA Renal Failure Programme (17).

The number of European countries with home dialysis facilities has steadily increased and all countries with well established renal failure programmes have home dialysis. The increase in the home programmes reflect the general increase and activity of the renal failure programme in individual countries. Fifty per cent of countries registered with the European Dialysis and Transport Association (EDTA) Registry do not have home dialysis facilities; these are either just setting up a renal failure service or are from the Eastern parts of Europe. Another exception is Japan which has a very extensive and experienced renal failure programme in which only 1% of patients receive their treatment at home.

CAPD has exploded into the 'home – self-care' location in the last 3 years. Its long-term reliability has not yet been proven. Presently it is making a great contribution and is becoming rapidly and widely available (8, 9, 18).

Some centres use home dialysis as the treatment of choice for highly selected patients, others find it an economic necessity. For example, in the United Kingdom where central government's tight budgetary control rarely allows new hospital or dialysis facilities to be built, a relatively small number of hospital centres with limited facilities are used as a nucleus for an active transplantation and home dialysis programme. In the extreme situation, when transplantation fails if hospital dialysis is not available and death is the only alternative, motivation for home dialysis is high. In 1975 the EDTA Registry analysed the use and failure of home haemodialysis (14). When a patient failed to take the opportunity of home dialysis, inspite of adequate facilities, training and organisation, this was shown to be largely due to lack of interest and little motivation. Medical contra-indications to home dialysis and lack of accommodation accounted for only 11% and 12% respectively, whereas refusal from lack of motivation for training or failure to learn was as high as 21% and 18% respectively; 28% of patients turned down for home dialysis were considered unsuitable because there was no suitable partner. In our experience this does not apply if self-dialysis is taught (12).

However, if adequate facilities for either home or hospital treatment are available, and if there is freedom of choice for both medical staff and patient, then past experience can provide clear guidelines for the selection of patients who would best benefit from home dialysis.

Medical considerations

Clearly patients with secondary medical problems such as severe cardio-vascular disease, which may be exacerbated by the actual haemodialysis procedure, should be excluded from a home haemodialysis programme, although they may be acceptable for a supervised hospital haemodialysis. However, we have shown that young adults with severe physical handicap such as blindness, deafness and immobility can be accommodated on home dialysis (19, 20). This type of patient has already adapted to his first handicap before being faced with the problems of renal failure. It is very unlikely that patients faced with two handicaps simultaneously such as severe diabetic retinopathy and nephropathy could cope with the responsibility of self-care dialysis in the home.

CAPD, once established in a patient, has few medical contraindications to home care since it has almost no immediate physical changes which could be life threatening (8).

The greatest medical contraindication to home treatment both for haemodialysis and peritoneal dialysis is evidence of persistent lack of discipline and inability to comply for, even with CAPD, unsupervised inadequately motivated patients get into serious medical trouble.

Age

Three age groups need special attention when considering home dialysis, very small children, adolescents and the elderly. Haemodialysis of children weighing less than 20 kg requires skill and home dialysis may not be satisfactory if the child is uncooperative or parents have less than average expertise. Past experience has clearly shown that parents invariably do excellent home care and if the necessity arises most children and families are able to perform the treatment reliably (21). Children positively benefit from home haemodialysis, being able to enjoy the continuity of home life. However, it is noticable that children thrive at the expense of anxiety in the parents (22). CAPD is able to display all its great advantages when applied to children. It frees the child from anxiety and the uncomfortable feelings experienced during the haemodialysis procedure. The diet, although not totally liberal, is less restricted, especially for potassium, which is always a cause of concern in children. The improvement in haemoglobin is most beneficial. Since loving parents are careful and aware of their responsibility the bag changes rarely lead to infection (23).

Adolescents do well on home haemodialysis (24) but as they reach the age for leaving home for work or further education, it is necessary to break the very strong bond created by parental supervision of dialysis. Transfer to a limited care centre should be considered. The possibility of CAPD should be presented to all adolescents for if they are able to make the psychological adjustment to the physical presence of the peritoneal catheter, CAPD would prove a great bonus making the break from home easier and giving freedom and the extra time needed at this stage of their lives.

The elderly present the greatest problem when considering home or self-care. Chronological age is not absolute, there being young 70 year olds and elderly 55 year olds. Dialysis itself is more risky as time progresses and patients age at an even faster rate than those with normal renal function. A patient trained for selfcare in their late 50's may be doing extremely well at home 10 years later but other medical conditions may develop in both the patient and spouse. The supposedly fit companion may become seriously ill and in need of care or even die. The loneliness of old age demands the absolute necessity of hospital contact and regular support both for the patient and spouse. Even fit and loving relatives of the same generation often find they cannot cope with the concepts of dialysis and diet, and also the obstinacy and perversity often displayed by the elderly patient. The relatives may even become ill from the anxiety and responsibility.

The development of immobility in the home or difficulty in making outside contact with friends or even getting to the hospital frequently becomes an insurmountable handicap requiring the patient to be permanently in a nursing home. Younger relatives rarely find they can support the elderly indefinitely whether the treatment is haemodialysis or CAPD as both can lead to serious disruption in the younger generation's family life.

When planning home or self-care for the elderly the unit must be prepared to give greater support at all levels and to constantly review the family situation, being prepared to revert to central unit care.

Married and single status

A relevant issue is 'does the patient have a close, caring partner; if so, is this within a family group or formal marriage?' For the single patient it is important to know the relationship to others within the home or whether it is a solitary existence.

In happy, stable relationships, the introduction of home haemodialysis rarely leads to a breakdown. However, home dialysis will highlight areas of contention. Previous problems are intensified, stressing the relationship and even disrupting it. It is never easy to assess relationships, but if there is any clear evidence of previous disharmony, 'self dialysis' at home, or limited care centre dialysis should be recommended.

Single patients are able to undertake home haemodialysis, even if they live and dialyse entirely alone (12). The single patient living with family or friends can also dialyse at home without dependency on a trained partner. In fact, the single patient may in the long term resent being dependent. However, there is no doubt that a single person living alone, or even with the family, is at risk should loneliness becomes a problem and cause depression. Such patients become careless and this can lead to errors in dialysis technique. The problems are usually retrievable but morbidity is increased and rehabilitation decreased (25). Sympathetic understanding of their problems is essential, and an occasional hospital dialysis may be helpful. Obviously CAPD has an important role for the independent patient or those leading a solitary existence.

Anxiety

The inherent anxiety of a patient with end-stage renal failure must be greatly increased by the introduction of the initial complex procedures of haemodialysis. This can make it difficult to ascertain mental stability and might therefore hinder appropriate selection.

The simplicity of CAPD makes it much more acceptable as a first choice treatment even if it is intended to convert to haemodialysis at a later date. The treatment when well supervised, is so simple that it can rapidly allay fears and replace confidence to such an extent that the patient can master new ideas and regain control of his life. The self-care education and acquired techniques of CAPD are invaluable in facilitating smoother and quicker home haemodialysis training.

Anxiety can often be greatly allayed by successful dialysis at home. But even with good training and personal ability, anxiety can become a crippling factor leading to so much distress and irritability in the household that it may be necessary to reconsider the continuation of home treatment especially home haemodialysis.

Learning ability

The level of literacy has poor correlation with learning and adaptation to new routines and disciplines. The original assessment of potential achievement can be entirely wrong. Having started to teach patients occasionally one is encountered who is apparently intelligent but has a poor grasp of the basic educational achievements of reading, writing and calculation. However, although aca-

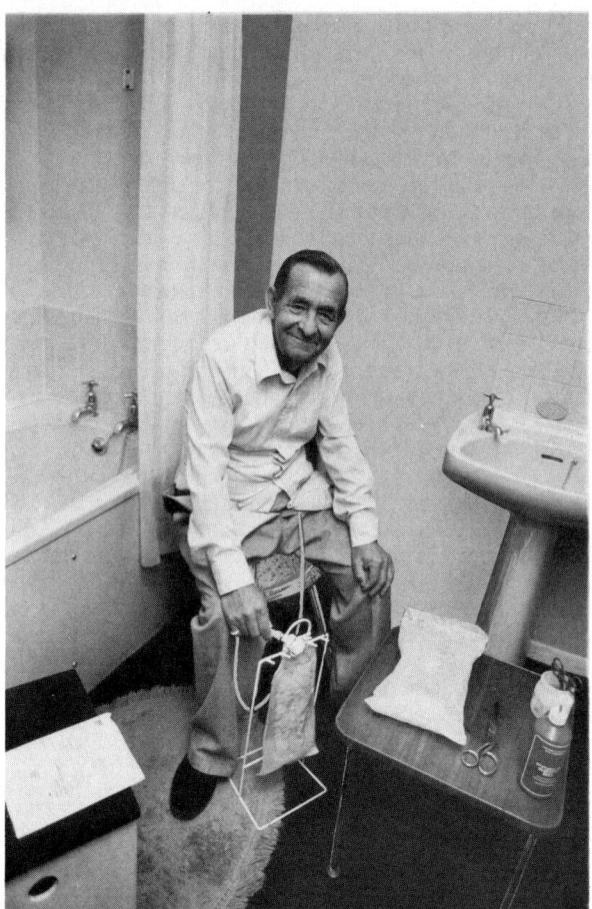
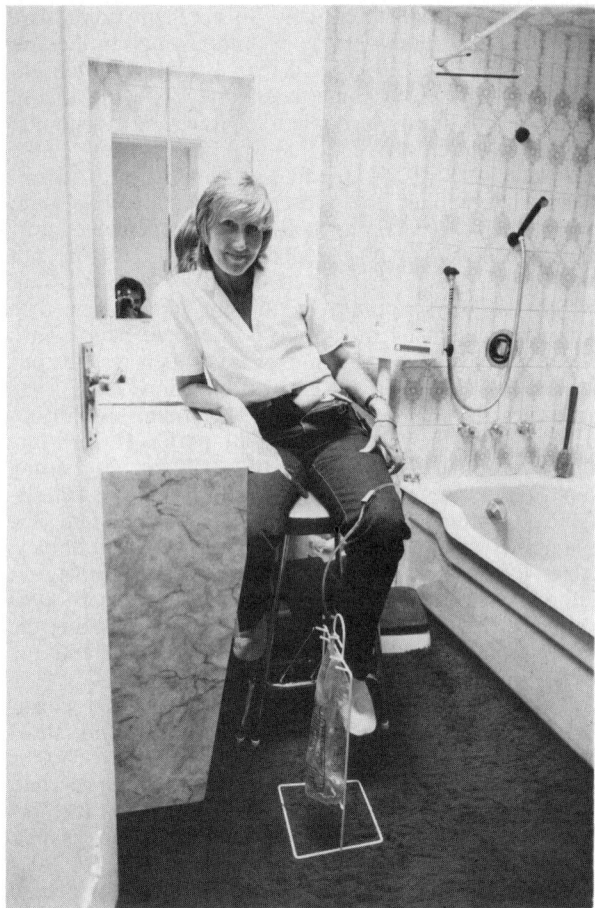
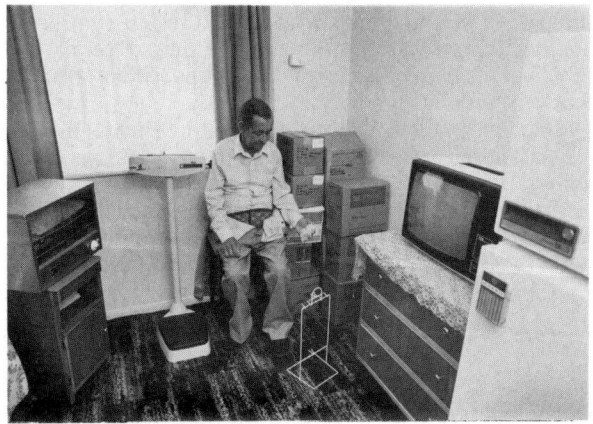
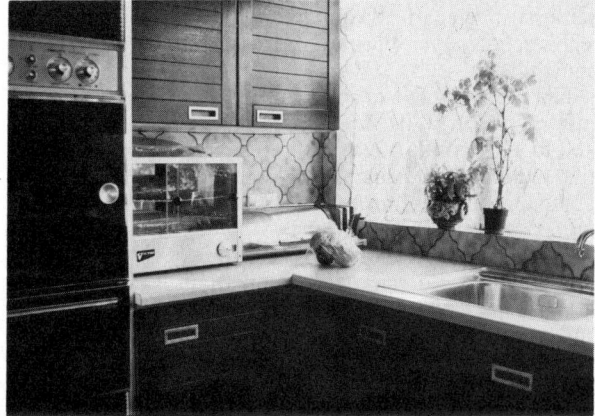

Figure 1-4. 1. (top, left) Elderly CAPD patient performing his bag exchange in the bathroom. 2. (bottom, left) Same CAPD patient sitting in his spare bedroom where he keeps his stores. 3. (top, right) CAPD patient in her bathroom demonstrating her arrangement for peritoneal bag exchange. Also in the bathroom are weighing scales and a clothes hanger for hanging up the bag on any hook in the house. 4. (bottom, right) The kitchen of patient in Figure 3 showing a small heating cabinet used for heating the bags of peritoneal dialysis fluid.

demic achievements might be useful, the uneducated but motivated patient can be equally, if not more, successful in acquiring the routine procedures of home dialysis. Intelligent but mechanically inept patients are often difficult to teach. It is also important to note that the problems of acquiring the necessary new skills and adaptation to new ideas multiply with age.

Financial status

Although most western countries provide social benefits as part of their medical care these are not always adequate. Personal money, a secure and flexible job, a car and a good home certainly makes home dialysis more comfortable and easier (26) but are not essential prerequisites.

Accommodation

Household cleanliness or lack of it does not necessarily influence the quality of home haemodialysis or the health of the patient, but dirty, ill kept equipment deteriorates very fast. However, household cleanliness or general tidiness does play a role in the success of CAPD. Home haemodialysis is usually confined to a specially prepared treatment room whereas it is normal practice, and indeed one of CAPD's greatest advantages, that it does not require a separate room and can normally be accommodated in any type or size household.

Two examples of the accommodation of CAPD into the home are shown in a number of photographs. Figure 1 shows an elderly CAPD patient performing his bag change in his bathroom. Figure 2 shows the same gentleman after finishing the exchange, sitting in his spare bedroom among his stores, deep freeze and household spares. CAPD equipment is small and portable and various spaces around the home can usually be found with ease. Figures 3, 4 and 5 show a household in which the patient, a young mother, changes her bag on a stool in the bathroom, keeps her heating cabinet in the kitchen and her boxes of peritoneal dialysis fluid in the garage.

When considering home haemodialysis even though new, smaller equipment, not requiring special adaptations or much space, is available (27) it is important to realise that most people find it irritating to incorporate the treatment aspects into their bedroom or living room on anything but a temporary basis. Children in particular dislike the equipment visibly intruding into their non-dialysis time. House moves are unpleasant to the family because it entails changing jobs, school, neighbours and losing security. Various methods of tackling the problem of accommodation will be described later in this chapter.

Special advantages of home dialysis

Home dialysis was devised by doctors to provide space and cut costs. This has proved to be correct when done successfully. Whether home haemodialysis or CAPD is used two patients can be treated for the same cost as one centre treated patient. Apart from this home dialysis also provides some very definite advantages, not least the control of large outbreaks of hepatitis, especially before accurate identification of carriers could be made. Uninfected patients treated at home have been spared from possible infection whilst carrier patients doing self treatment at home reduce the possibility of outbreaks of hepatitis amongst staff and patients (28, 29).

Home dialysis is specifically advantageous for patients living long distances from a treatment centre. For independent persons it provides freedom from organisation and forced communication with people not necessarily compatible with the patient. Home comforts, presence of family and friends and flexibility of dialysis regimen extends to the patient the best potential for rehabilitation. Skilled patients personalise their treatment and appreciate the control they have over the quality of their health and life style.

TECHNICAL AND MEDICAL FEATURES OF HOME HAEMODIALYSIS

The technical and medical aspects of chronic haemodialysis are covered extensively in other chapters of this book. However, there are some special features to be considered in relation to home dialysis. No selection of equipment mentioned in this chapter is attempted since several countries have successfully developed and produced their own models. In general it is wisest to choose those pieces of equipment which have proved reliable in personal experience, providing they can be used safely in the home.

Blood access

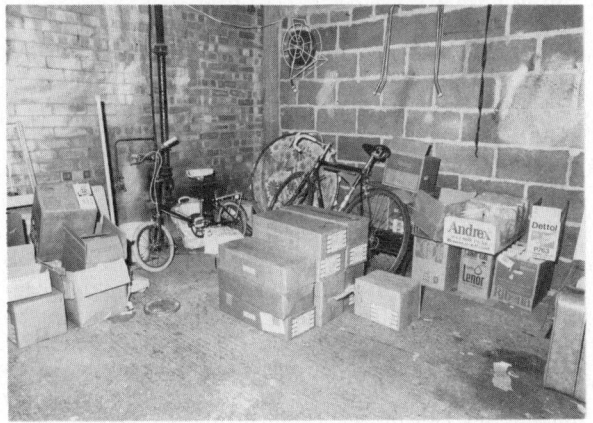

Figure 5. The garage of the patient in Figure 3, with her stock of 4 weeks peritoneal fluid.

Easy blood access for repetitive haemodialysis holds the key to success or failure in the home. The use of the external Quinton-Scribner shunt was quick and easy to teach. However, the internal arteriovenous fistula has proved its advantages of longevity of function and lack of complications (30, 31). These aspects outweigh the initial problems of teaching patients to acquire the skill of self insertion of needles into their own veins (32). A fistula can be said to be inadequate if it is not suitable for easy self venepuncture. Because of the dangers of venepuncture through infected or unhealed previous puncture sites it is important that the patient has multiple choice of sites to insert the needles. If necessary revision of the existing fistula or forming fistulae in both arms may be required.

The external shunt still remains useful for certain selected patients. Pre-puberty children and the occasional adult are emotionally unable to accept repeated venepuncture, although in a hospital unit skilled personnel can overcome this problem. For the parent at home the problem of acquiring the skill of venepuncture is compounded by lack of confidence of both parent and child and the changed role from the child's protector to the inflictor of pain. Children can be taught self venepuncture but this is frequently associated with delaying tactics, often with regressive behaviour, at the start of each dialysis. A similar response may occur when a parent undertakes venepuncture. Fistulae are usually acceptable later, often at the patient's request. Should the problem of blood access dominate then the value of the use of CAPD is obvious.

Dialysers

There is now an endless choice of dialysers. Safety, small volume, easily controlled and flexible ultrafiltration and reliable connections should be guiding features. Extremely efficient dialysers are potentially dangerous for home use. Disposable dialysers are best but their advantages have to be balanced against cost. The cheaper Kiil dialyser proved particularly successful in the home but is rarely used today as space and help are required for reassembly.

Dialysis fluid preparation

Equipment for the preparation of dialysis fluid should be chosen for its reliability, compactness, easy cleaning and maintenance with minimal patient care.

Water preparation

Chapter 6 is devoted to water preparation for dialysis.

Small ion exchange or reverse osmosis units are available. Although reverse osmosis units are expensive they appear to give the safest water supply, particularly if town mains water is not of constant composition.

Problems in the home can arise if there is not sufficient water pressure for reliable function of water preparation units.

Again, reliability, compactness with minimal care should be the objective when selecting equipment.

Monitoring (See also Chapter 11)

Monitoring is the essence of home haemodialysis. Automated equipment with fixed programmes requiring minimal manual attention result in fewer mistakes. There is, however, a growing tendency to make the equipment more sophisticated increasing both the sensitivity and the number of parameters recorded (33). The value of this has to be carefully weighed against the increased number of components which can go wrong and unnecessary complexity leading to confusion. When the systems become so sensitive that they are activated by entirely safe variations, unnecessary alarms will irritate the patient who will then find ways to 'beat the system'. This usually results in eliminating the whole alarm system thus producing a much more dangerous situation. In principle safety depends on simplicity.

Cleansing and disinfection of equipment

Many centres find it is uneconomical to use new disposable dialysis equipment for each dialysis. They reuse after cleaning and sterilise with formalin or other agents as necessary (see Chapter 15). Reuse is safer in the home than in the hospital centre as the possibility of mixing up other patients' dialysers and blood lines is eliminated. Pyrogen reactions occur less frequently at home because of direct connection to mains water instead of tank storage often found in hospital units. Particular attention should be paid to the cleaning, disinfection and maintenance of water preparation equipment, such as softeners, deionisers and reverse osmosis units because stagnation of water occurs between dialysis. This also applies to the dialysis fluid supply system. When equipment is temporarily out of regular use it should be left primed with formalin or an equivalent sterilising fluid.

Ultrafiltration

The techniques for fluid removal from patients whether by positive pressure in the blood compartment or negative pressure on the dialysate side or changes in membrane permeability needs careful planning and control in the home. Today better equipment is available which allows direct visual measurement of the ultrafiltrate, however there is often the temptation to ultrafilter excessively.

Most problems during dialysis relate to excessive or too rapid removal of fluid leading to profound hypotension or cramps. When this happens the patient may be physically incapacitated and unable to control his dialysis and is therefore in danger of making further errors. For example, a patient who has severe cramp in the leg towards the end of dialysis might be tempted to stand on the leg to relieve the cramp. Standing up at this late stage in a dialysis can cause severe hypotension, the patient faints and while falling hits his head on the equipment or the floor. The patient at this point is also fully heparinised. Thus a simple cramp from excessive ultrafiltration can become compounded into a series of accidents which could end with concussion and a subdural haemorrhage. Dependable ultrafiltration characteristics of both dialyser and monitor are required to minimise such problems, as is the cooperation of the patient to reduce inter-dialytic weight gain.

Control of hypertension

The use and the choice of hypotensive drugs in home dialysis patients must be very cautiously considered, as the procedure of haemodialysis can be made exceedingly hazardous in patients receiving such treatment. Profound falls in blood pressure, unresponsive to saline infusion or other routine measures, can occur when antihypertensive drugs are prescribed which is dangerous in a home dialysis setting. The control of severe hypertension by rapid ultrafiltration is also dangerous in the home. In principle, both hypotensive drugs and rapid ultrafiltration should be avoided in home dialysis treatment. The patient's weight should be gradually lowered until the desired postdialysis weight and blood pressure is achieved. This may take several dialyses. The patient should be advised to reduce fluid intake to a minimum to reduce inter-dialytic weight gain and to undertake frequent short dialyses for achieving control of blood pressure in home dialysis.

Disequilibrium

In order to prevent disequilibrium regular biochemical checks and good maintenance of the equipment should be carried out to ensure the reliability of the dialysis solution. It is essential to avoid long infrequent dialyses since the greater the change in the patient's biochemistry and ultrafiltration the more likely the danger of headache, vomiting and possible convulsions. This point must be clearly explained to patients and, according to the equipment used, they must be instructed not to exceed the appropriate number of hours for a dialysis at home and also the maximum safe period between dialyses, should the normal routine be interrupted.

Anticoagulation

Technical problems rapidly develop if heparin dosage is too low and conversely medical problems increase if dosage is too high. Thus the equipment chosen should be accurate and reliable for infusion of heparin. It is not satisfactory in the home to rely on patients giving bolus doses as one or more may be forgotten. Errors of over or under dosage are usually made by the patient selecting the wrong strength of heparin, and the supply of only one, or at the most two, strengths of heparin helps to prevent this problem.

Blood loss, prevention of anaemia

Today's dialysers are better designed and the siting of the blood pump and blood compartment monitors allows shorter blood lines. These features improve the blood return at the end of dialysis. Careful monitoring of individual patients to assess blood retained in the dialyser is necessary if dialysers are reused because some patients have more blood loss when the number of reuses increase.

Of paramount importance in preventing blood loss is good effective training and attention to details both when selecting equipment and in its use. Patients can be taught to administer intravenous haematinics when necessary whilst on haemodialysis at home.

Psychology

The psychological aspects of chronic haemodialysis are best coped with by a flexible approach to problems both during training and when at home. In this context good training is also vital if unnecessary anxiety is to be prevented. Recognition of each patient's natural behaviour when faced with a problem will demonstrate the best approach. Those patients who can relax and sleep on dialysis may do their treatment overnight and have more personal free time, whilst patients who remain anxious on treatment are best treated during the day or evening.

WHO DOES THE DIALYSIS IN THE HOME?

Before progressing further, the question 'who is actually going to do the haemodialysis in the home?' must be clarified. In CAPD the answer is usually patently obvious – the patient. For haemodialysis, however, this is not the commonly accepted answer. The concept of home haemodialysis was based on the institute of marriage: i.e. a home to give space for the equipment and a permanent partner to do the treatment. As already indicated, partners may not be permanent nor necessary.

In the early sixties, when home haemodialysis was instigated, it was considered necessary to have a trained nurse continuously in attendance with a doctor immediately available even for routine hospital dialysis. Therefore, it is not surprising that it was felt necessary to have a fit, able person to dialyse the patient in the home. However, the situation has changed radically. Today, patients are much fitter, equipment has been improved, dialysis times are shorter, treatment is less traumatic, and experience has shown that home dialysis can be done safely and effectively by the patient alone.

In spite of this, physicians still place maximum emphasis on the need for a partner and often exclude those patients who have none. Over the years there has been considerable concern regarding the stress placed on the helper, but almost everyone continues to presume that the spouse is the automatic choice of helper. A realistic appraisal of the need, choice and role of the helper has to be made, since much of the success of home haemodialysis and happiness of the persons involved will depends on this. In order to do this the author has, over the years, found it necessary to consider the following points.

Dominance, distribution of work, decision making and dependency vary infinitely amongst marriage partnerships. The introduction of home dialysis with a leader appointed by the hospital may automatically disrupt the previous well established order (34).

Rehabilitation is not just the return of physical health, but the return to former status within the family and society. It is inconceivable that a wife be held responsible for accurate safe dialysis of a dominant, self-willed man, who may have been apathetic during his illness but after successful treatment recovers his mental as well as physical well being. Alternatively, the dominant spouse invariably takes away the patient's initiative, which has already been eroded by unreliable health, thereby preventing full rehabilitation. Designation of a helper by the centre invariably means two people instead of one having their lives controlled indefinitely by the treatment regimen. The patient may not necessarily have confidence in the spouse or appointed helper and agitation caused by anxiety leads to aggression, with shouting of orders and obvious irritation. This behaviour might well be alien to their normal relationships. The spouse or helper are fit and therefore learn more quickly and easily over-shadow the patient, who may then be protected from scrutiny, resulting in large areas being unlearnt or not understood.

Within the author's experience, the responsibility for home haemodialysis has evolved as follows. From 1964 to 1965 the spouse dialysed the patient; in 1966 the patient was responsible, but had substantial help from the spouse. In 1967 the patient was taught self dialysis and had lesser help from the spouse who was formally trained separately from the patient. Since 1968, patients have been taught self dialysis alone and have been left responsible to train a volunteer relative or friend if help is desired.

The result of teaching the patient independent self dialysis, but allowing them to make the choice of involving others in their treatment has produced the following results (12): Some patients prefer to do everything for themselves and especially like to be left alone when starting and finishing dialysis. However, the majority of patients do have help from the family, usually in the form of preparing the room and switching on the equipment. Thereafter, the patient takes over the preparation and control of the dialysis. Most help is given at the end of dialysis when everyone wants to clear up the equipment and remove the fistula needles as quickly as possible so that the family can retire to bed. Some patients have a very close relationship with their partner and the whole procedure is equally divided into areas of responsibility. It is not always the spouse who becomes interested in the dialysis procedure; often children, other relatives or neighbours like and get satisfaction from helping, and several persons can act as substitutes.

Regardless of the arrangements made between the patient, his family and friends, the patient must take final responsibility.

These can only be guidelines, not rules. In the situation of dialysing children in the home, the parents are responsible for the treatment. Parents can and do suffer great humiliation from their children, who invariably learn quicker. It takes experience to present the parent in a favourable light to the child, who on the one hand will expose the parents' weakness whilst on the other hand wants and needs to feel secure and dependent. Needless to say, the adolescent illustrates this problem pre-eminently.

The elderly patient, whether doing haemodialysis or CAPD, frequently needs help and the rule of independent self dialysis training should be relaxed to incorporate the spouse in the training sessions. Without this formal training the spouse often becomes exceedingly anxious.

TRAINING

Formal teaching programmes for home haemodialysis or CAPD incorporating details of all methods and equipment currently available would be rapidly outdated so only general topics will be discussed.

Setting the scene

No definite training period or programme can be stipulated especially for haemodialysis as the subject matter is unusual and the pupils are so varied. Several features frustrate the first few weeks of any training programme. Physical handicaps can be an embarrassment to the patient initially. General physical weakness and impairment of fine movements may result from neuropathy or a prolonged period of inactivity. Defective eyesight, particularly as an aftermath of malignant hypertension, can prove particularly troublesome. Even the reading of a thermometer and dials on the monitor unit or the inability to connect two sterile plastic lines without contamination may prove an insurmountable task. These and other disabilities may throw doubt and uncertainty on whether patient selection has been correct and inevitably increase the anxiety of the patient.

The teaching of home dialysis is the most effective form of rehabilitation. At the end of their haemodialysis training the patients have achieved entirely new skills and confidence which allows them considerable control over their health and life. Casual day clothes should always be worn during the training period as the dressed mobile patient is more able to identify himself as a pupil rather than a patient and the medical and nursing staff become more identified as teachers. This change from patient to pupil allows a more positive approach to life.

Whenever possible a separate dialysis training area should be made available. The teaching rehabilitation programme should be like a school (35). As patients must attend the centre regularly during the day, they should be discouraged from attempting any other work during the intensive first half of their training period. Their total physical and mental attention is required on the premise that complete mastery of the subject saves time and gives freedom in the long term.

Experienced teachers are aware of a well recognised pattern of achievements in these patients. In the first month of haemodialysis training patients tend to acquire knowledge steadily for periods of a few days, followed by longer periods of regression when previous accomplishments are totally forgotten. These periods are filled with depression and despair. In the second month knowledge is retained and consolidated as more and more facts fall into place. An average of 2 months training is usually needed, 6 weeks being the minimum with the occasional patient taking as long as 6 months.

CAPD training

There is a great fallacy regarding training for CAPD. The impression given by most centres is that shortness of training programmes is admirable. Whilst one of the aims of CAPD is to reduce costs, particularly by reducing hospital or centre care, the patients' renal failure is the same life threatening problem, whether treated by haemodialysis or peritoneal dialysis.

Physicians with long experience of the management of renal failure know that euphoria and physical well-being follow the initial dialysis treatment, but that this is followed by a period of bereavement. For the CAPD patients who are summarily discharged from hospital after 2 to 3 weeks total care and training, the full impact of the seriousness and permanency of their condition does not impinge on them until they are at home and no longer have the immediate support of the centre.

Obviously the repetitive teaching of joining two connectors together in a sterile manner seems simple compared to the procedure of haemodialysis. However, training for independent self haemodialysis was never just the instruction of the practical aspects but a continuous conversation and education on the understanding of the patients' disease and how best to fit it into their original lifestyle.

For the CAPD patient there must be more regular telephone contact, more frequent hospital attendence and home visits by the nurse to compensate for the shorter centre contact. The teaching of fluid balance within the context of dry body weight, fluid weight gain, flesh weight gain and blood pressure control has always been the most difficult aspect to grasp, even after years of successful home and self-care haemodialysis. For CAPD patients it is no less difficult to learn.

It has, unfortunately, been assumed that the basic simplicity of the procedure of CAPD can be directly transferred to the management of end stage renal failure without recognition of the complexity of the disease and its impact on the patient and family.

The teacher

There is no doubt that certain people have a special aptitude of being able to transfer their knowledge regardless of the diverse abilities of the pupil. They may be from any discipline, doctors, nurses or technicians within the sphere of dialysis and their value is immeasurable. Their most important attribute is their sensitivity to the pupils' needs which allows them to adjust their teaching methods appropriately. For example, it may be necessary to teach using direct orders and lists of instructions with no explanations being given; other patients can only retain information if clear explanations are given. In the situation of home haemodialysis training, other individual features must be considered; for example some patients need reassurance that nothing can go wrong, on the other hand others need to learn that carelessness can be exceedingly dangerous. A good teacher will see that one pupil does not have his confidence destroyed by accidents or problems, but will allow another pupil to make the error in order that the unpleasant experience will prevent rash behaviour in the future. A good teacher knows his subject so well that teaching becomes an effortless procedure with time available to choose the most descriptive words for each individual patient. Gradually the commonly used words can be changed into the correct terminology. Once the correct terminology is acquired, then the patient can discuss problems with anyone familiar with the subject. A good teacher knows that the use of appropriate praise is invaluable to these patients as is the judicial use of discipline. It is important to be realistic and exclude from the teaching staff the intelligent experienced person who does not have a teaching gift for they become impatient and irritated, and the patients become unhappy and are hence unable to learn.

Many teaching and revision aids are available (slide, tape, film and instruction manuals) all aimed to teach dialysis to staff and patients (36-39). They have a role to play but no mechanical apparatus, picture or written word can replace the infinite flexibility of the human voice to describe and emphasise the subject being taught. These adjuncts to teaching should, when possible, be available but care should be taken to adjust the programmes to fit the pupils comprehension. Instruction books are often blindly followed and given the status of 'the law'. Sections taken out of context and applied to inappropriate situations can lead to danger. Instruction books often use words, not just technical ones, which some patients may find unfamiliar. This makes the whole book meaningless. If, on the other hand, the patient makes his own notes and builds up his own manual, then his words clearly indicate what he has learnt and how he reasoned the problems.

Slide and tape visual aids allow the partly trained patient to replay visual scenes until he fully understands the problems. It saves embarrassment to the patient who often feels he should be able to understand immediately and spares annoyance on the part of the teacher who may become irritated on repeating the same thing many times. Another valuable teaching aid is a videotape recording of the patient during either preparation for or during dialysis which can then be played back to the patient to show how and where mistakes were made. Patients when making mistakes often claim they have not been taught certain tasks or that they were taught in

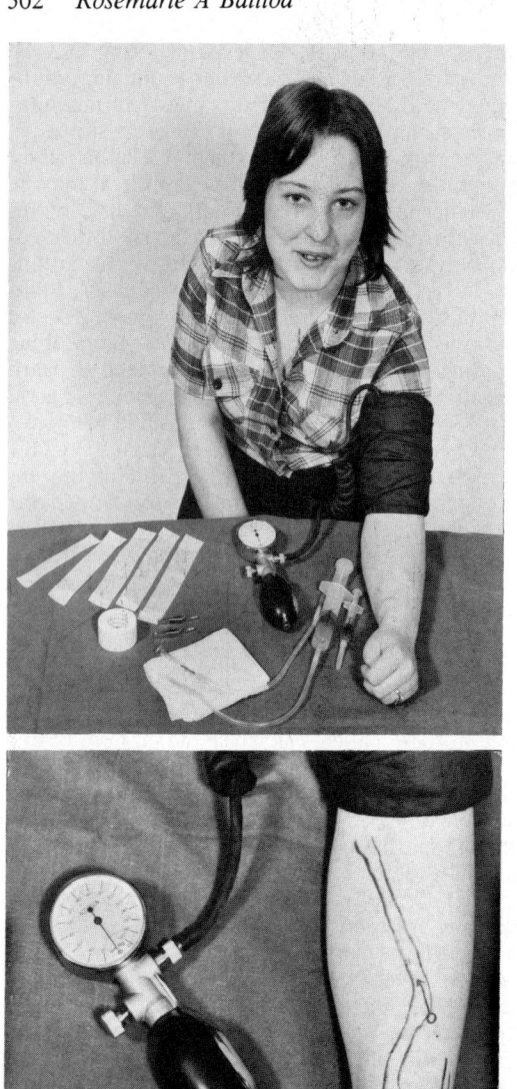
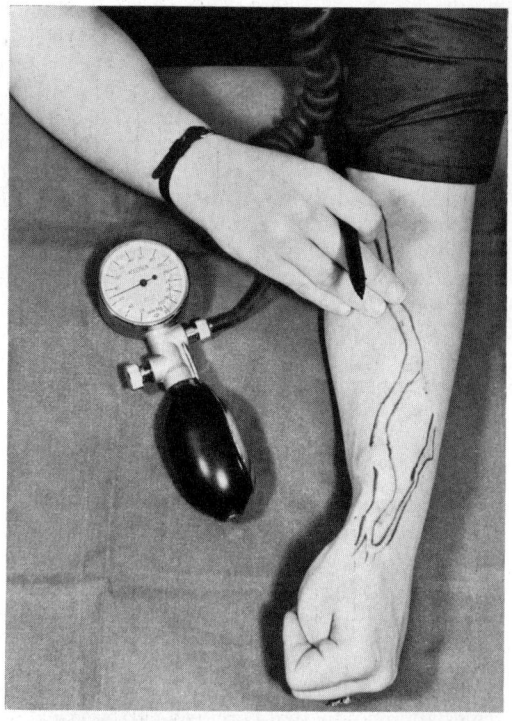
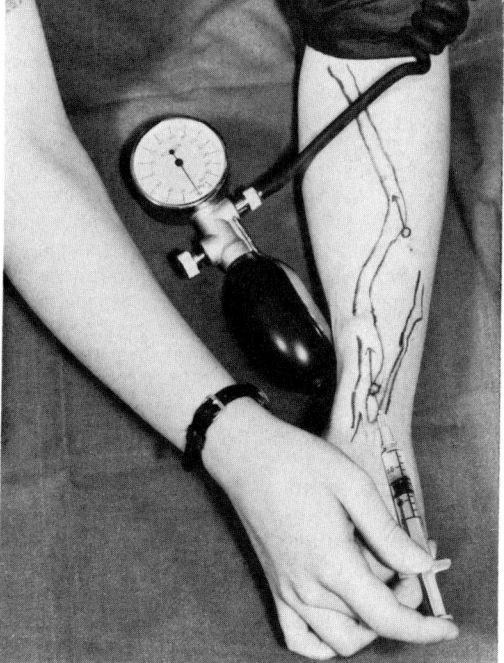

Figures 6-9. 6. (top, left) Patient assembles all necessary items – local anaesthetic, loading dose of heparin, needles, small clamps, strips of paper tape, and sits at a suitable work top. A blood pressure cuff with manometer is used for venous occlusion. It provides accurate measurement of pressure which is also visible and easily controlled. Local anaesthetic is used during training. It may be discarded later if patient chooses. 7. (top, right) Venous occlusion of 60-80 mmHg is applied. The patient is taught to feel the distended veins and draw as many as possible. This must be done at every dialysis in order to teach transfer of touch into 'visible' vessels which have three dimentional shape and depth under the skin. 8. (bottom, left) Having drawn the vessels a suitable insertion site is chosen. The area for the local anaesthetic is ringed and the direction of needle insertion drawn and arrowed. The choice of site is obvious in this picture for after outling the veins, clear angles allowing straight insertion of needles are seen. 9. (bottom, right) The local anaesthetic is introduced. No bleeding will occur from needle prick if no venous occlusion is applied.

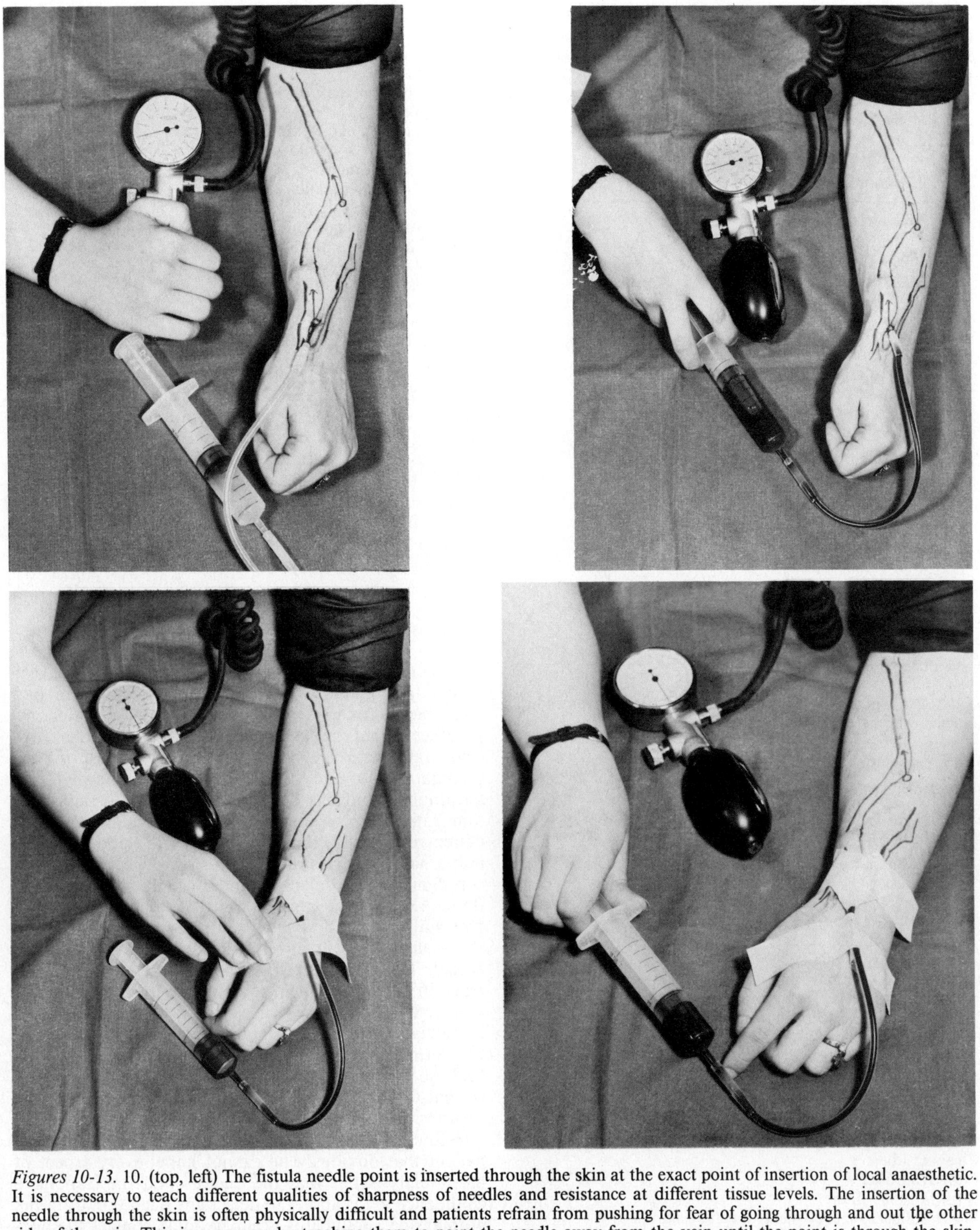

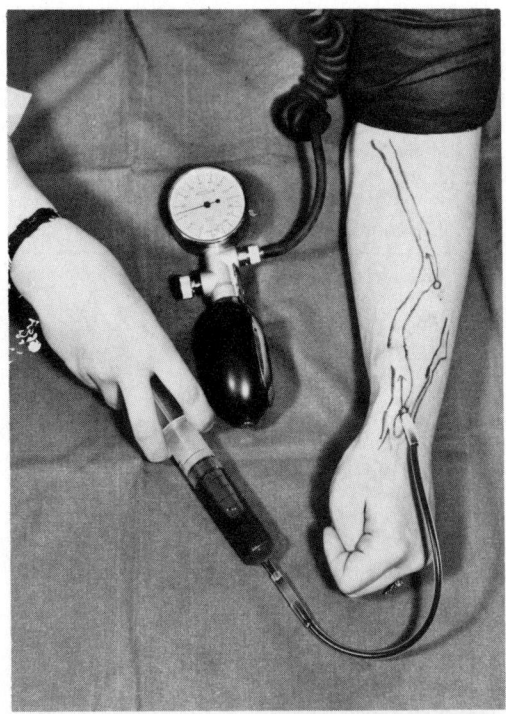
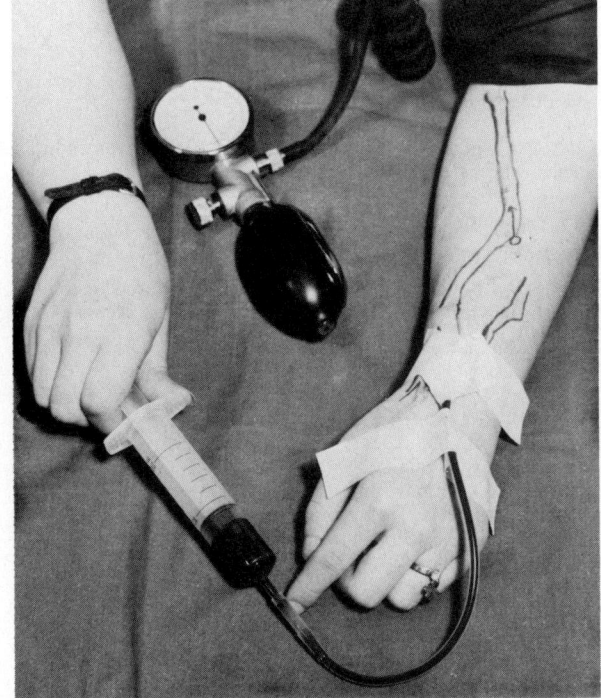

Figures 10-13. 10. (top, left) The fistula needle point is inserted through the skin at the exact point of insertion of local anaesthetic. It is necessary to teach different qualities of sharpness of needles and resistance at different tissue levels. The insertion of the needle through the skin is often physically difficult and patients refrain from pushing for fear of going through and out the other side of the vein. This is overcome by teaching them to point the needle away from the vein until the point is through the skin. After insertion of the needle point the venous cuff is inflated again. 11. (top, right) The needle is pushed along the drawn line at the appropriate depth. The flow of blood from needle to syringe is checked and some blood and heparin returned. The venous pressure is released. 12. (bottom, left) With the prepared strips of tape the needle is carefully strapped single handed. 13. (bottom, right) The flow of blood is checked after strapping to ensure good needle position in vein.

a different way. This is best overcome by assigning the patient to the same teacher whenever possible and keeping a check list of teaching points. The check list states the date when a patient is shown a task and a date when considered competent. Tables 1 and 2 show typical check lists for haemodialysis, and Table 3 is a list for CAPD.

Table 1. Routine haemodialysis training check list.

Temperature
Pulse
Blood pressure
Weight
Filling of data forms
Water testing
Concentrate tank filling
Commencing sterilising cycle
Connections and clamps
Priming the dialyser
Heparin preparation
Starting
Machine gauges
Blood and heparin pumps
Clotting times
Finishing
Rinsing and re-formalinising
Collecting blood samples
Dialysate samples
Drugs:
   Intravenous vitamins and iron, oral vitamins, Aludrox and antibiotics
Filling in home charts

Table 2. Typical list of important *non* routine procedures taught to home dialysis patients.

During dialysis

Hypotension and administration of saline

Joining blood lines of dialyser together to recirculate blood through dialyser whilst patient is temporarily disconnected.

Recognition and what to do in case of:
  Blood leak
  Mains electricity failure
  Mains water failure
  Pyrogen reaction
  Formaldehyde reaction
  Protamine reaction
  Hard water danger and symptoms
  Returning blood to patient under gravity
  Changing bubble catcher
  Burst blood pump rubber
  Ruptured lines
  Blood clotting times

Maintenance

Cleaning filters
  (a) Wall filter
  (b) Machine filter
Water softener or equivalent; reverse osmosis unit
  (a) Regenerating
  (b) Cleaning
  (c) Disinfection with formaldehyde
Rinsing system and reuse of the dialyser.

Table 3. CAPD training points.

Temperature
Pulse
Blood pressure
Weight
Use of home charts
Selection of peritoneal fluid
Use of clamps
Use of preparation kit
Care of peritoneal catheter
Bag changing technique
Observation of fill and drain times
Symptoms of peritonitis
Use of antibiotics
Diet
Drugs

The most difficult skill to acquire is the insertion of needles for dialysis. Particular attention must be paid to teaching this, since home dialysis will certainly fail or become extremely traumatic both physically and mentally if the patient does not attain the required skill or lacks confidence. Figures 6 to 13 show the steps involved in self venepuncture. Patients should follow this routine, especially drawing on the skin the situation of the vein at every dialysis until confidence is achieved.

Assessment of haemodialysis training

It is impossible to prepare the patient for every eventuality and in fact it would be unkind and frightening to create accidents to demonstrate a point. Of major importance is that the patient knows 'the norm', has sufficient training to detect any faults (especially during the preparation for dialysis), has a working knowledge of terminology and has been taught accurate verbal communication. These are points to be checked before the patient is allowed home. To do this the patient is put into a haemodialysis room on his own. The teacher can communicate via telephone or by standing outside the door. At this stage simple problems can be set to interfere with preparation, for example water turned off at the main supply or an electrical plug taken out of its socket. These very simple abnormalities can reveal the reaction of the patient to something new. Some patients will note the problem, check the probable causes and immediately correct the fault. Others panic pushing all the buttons and bells in sight. A third group of patients find the fault and describe the problem sufficiently well so that the teacher can make the diagnosis and give the appropriate instructions.

Before going home it is important to explain to the patient that obviously he cannot know every aspect of haemodialysis but that the doctors and the staff have confidence in his ability to detect any deviation from the normal and should this occur he must contact the hospital centre at all times for advice. Seeking such advice is expected and not thought of as failure, for learning in the home is a continuation of hospital tuition. Efforts to struggle along alone at home must be discouraged.

Transfer to the home is made easy by the use of a home dialysis nurse (40). Her duty is to be present for the first dialysis. On the average one week of her time is allocated to each new patient, but longer periods of support and teaching in the home environment may be necessary for some patients. The presence of the home dialysis nurse is of considerable help both practically and psychologically. During the transitional period she is able to check every procedure, demonstrate the equipment to the family, giving tuition if requested. She can advise on the best arrangement for equipment, particularly small items, stores and those items that require refrigeration. During the home visits there is time to discuss many problems, large and small, technical and emotional, which the patient may have longed to discuss but had been unable to find the appropriate time or atmosphere earlier. The home dialysis nurse should provide the patient with a list of suitable telephone numbers and extensions for medical, technical or other emergency situations. In addition she teaches record keeping, ordering of stores, sending blood and dialysate samples and dialysis records to the hospital. During the first few months the patient appreciates occasional visits from the nurse to check progress and assess confidence.

CHOICE AND ARRANGEMENT OF HAEMODIALYSIS EQUIPMENT IN THE HOME

It is of paramount importance to remember that a home essentially comprises two features, the family and the place in which they live. The introduction of the equipment, and with it the procedure of dialysis, into the home is nothing less than the intrusion of an unwanted guest. Although it can never aspire to become welcome, somehow the guest must be made as acceptable as possible. To achieve this it may be necessary to compromise on ideal standards and allow for flexibility of choice and arrangement of equipment.

Investigation into the feasibility of home dialysis requires a visit to the home, not just to check space and plumbing etc. but to assess atmosphere and relationships within the family. At this initial visit it is wise to arrange for every member of the family to be present not forgetting the patient, if he is still a hospital in-patient. It is necessary to check every room for size and possible use and, surprisingly, one may find that a grandparent or a lodger also lives in the house but no one thought it necessary to mention them. The home visit should not be used solely to collect knowledge of house and family but also to give advice and information to the family to help allay fears and clarify their attitude to home dialysis and the equipment. In addition to the assessment of the family and the available space other essential aspects to be examined are the water supply, drainage and power supply. An adequate sustained water pressure is necessary for the water treatment equipment and not, as frequently thought, for the dialysis fluid proportioning device. In old houses the water pipes may have to be replaced. The main problems in relation to the water supply and drainage system are accessibility and the cost of installation to the site chosen for the equipment. In most newly constructed homes the water pressure is usually adequate but the plumbing may be quite inaccessible, being situated in conduits or concrete floors, so that provision of drains and water for dialysis equipment is very expensive.

Since the visit to the home combines social assessment with the technical aspects of the treatment it must be done by a person totally familiar with the treatment requirements and procedures as well as being sympathetic to the needs and personal wishes of the patient and family. The person who does the initial home assessment obviously should co-ordinate with the medical and technical teams and when necessary pay further visits with the appropriate members of the team. Notwithstanding the need to ensure safe dialysis treatment, 'home dialysis' does not mean turning the home into a 'mini' hospital. The idea of walking into a home with a team of experts, selecting a room regardless of the family needs, knocking down walls and disrupting the home just to move in set pieces of equipment arranged in a standard manner must be severely criticised. It may give standard dialysis treatment but it will not rehabilitate the patient and his family psychologically and will lead to unhappiness and failure of home dialysis.

In established home dialysis centres there is usually a person whose main function is to assess the home and supervise the home adaptations. The title of this person is the *Home Dialysis Administrator.* Qualifications for the post are variable but are usually administration, dialysis knowledge and sympathetic understanding of people.

When selecting the room for installation of the home dialysis equipment the following points must be considered:
1. It is extremely rare for a home to have a spare room as most families use all available space. In particular, modern homes are usually smaller, with fewer rooms of lesser size, than older dwellings. Whatever choice is made some person in the home will be deprived of some privilege.
2. Never take the best room in the home even if offered; it is usually done with genuine feeling at the time but often resented later. The immediate fear of death of the patient makes people offer more than they can emotionally afford to give in the long term.
3. If possible never make the bedroom the dialysis room, as medical equipment constantly seen can become a psychological burden. This may not apply if the room is large enough to build a cupboard in which the equipment can be stored out of sight when not in use.
4. The advice to move to larger accomodation has to be considered with great care for this costs more initially and in up-keep. Furthermore, appropriate accommodation may be difficult to find. Above all it is extremely disruptive to the family especially if they have to move to another district. If, however, a family have decided to move for any reason, then a move to a larger house may be an excellent solution.

The eventual choice of the space in which to assemble

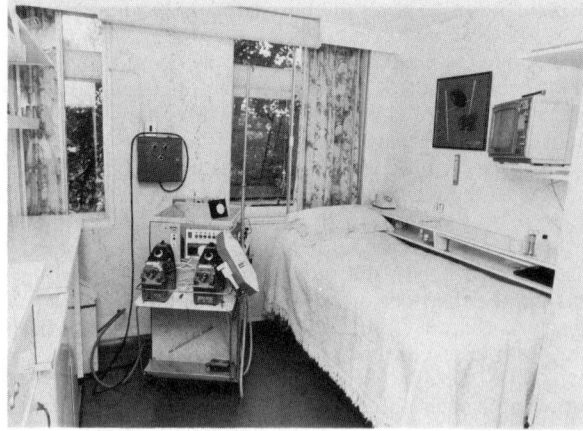

Figure 14. Ideal room converted for haemodialysis.

the haemodialysis equipment should cause minimal inconvenience to the family provided the space is big enough to assemble and to use the equipment safely. It should be convenient for plumbing purposes. The minimum size of the treatment room is 9 m² which would provide space for water preparation equipment, the dialysis machine, the dialyser, a bed, standing scales (though bed scales are necessary for young children), storage facilities and a sink unit. Floors, walls and shelves should be constructed for ease of cleaning but the patient should be allowed to choose colours for walls and curtains and floor covering. Good lighting is essential. The ideal room is shown in Figure 14. This room, 4 m × 3 m, was converted for haemodialysis in 1970 and although in continuous use since then it still appears new. Its meticulous cleanliness reflects the patient, a man now aged 67, who is very fastidious and gadget minded. Any part of the equipment which could be improved for practical purposes or aesthetic effect he had redesigned and had made. For example, to enable him to see dials and fuses on the side of the machine without having to move equipment he has fitted mirrors on the wall. In addition, he has installed an automatic switch to an emergency generator installed in his garage. Figures 15 and 16 show two views of a very small dialysis room, 3 m × 3 m, once used as a pantry in a hundred year old house. The patient can be seen standing at the sliding door of the glass partition separating it from the kitchen.

The room shows everything essential to home dialysis, especially the television. On the wall are shelves for a small stock of items, the main storage area being elsewhere in the house. There is a small heating unit on the

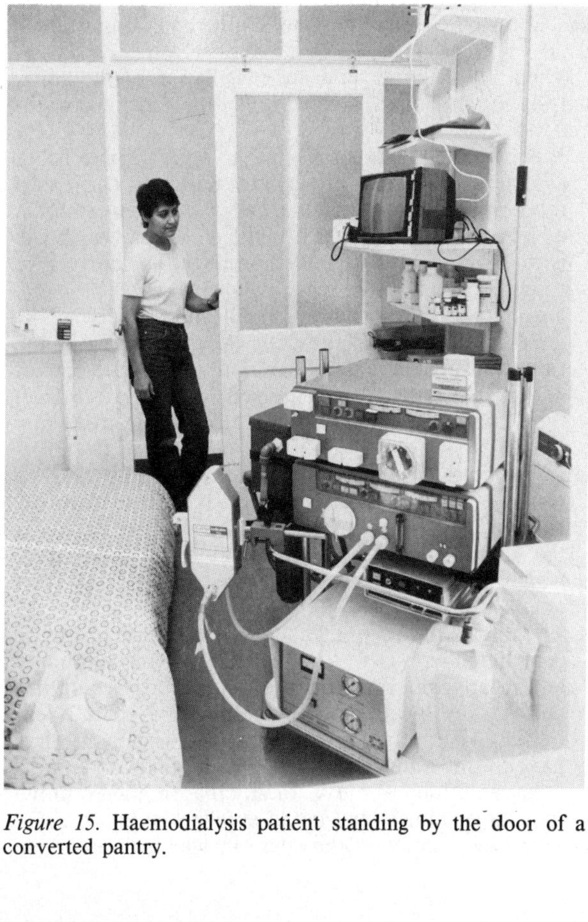

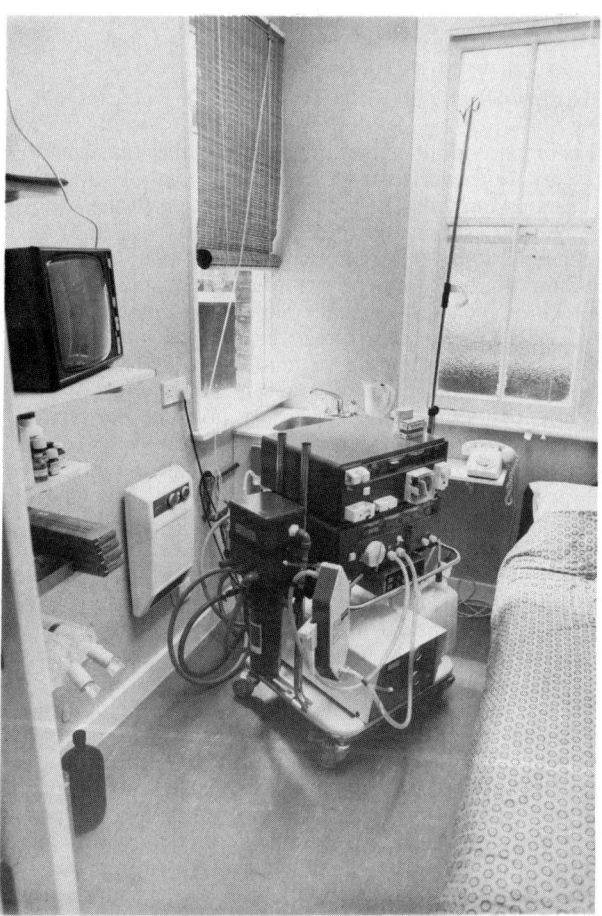

Figure 15. Haemodialysis patient standing by the door of a converted pantry.

Figure 16. As Figure 15, the mobile trolley holds the monitor, reverse osmosis unit, dialyser and dialyser re-use equipment.

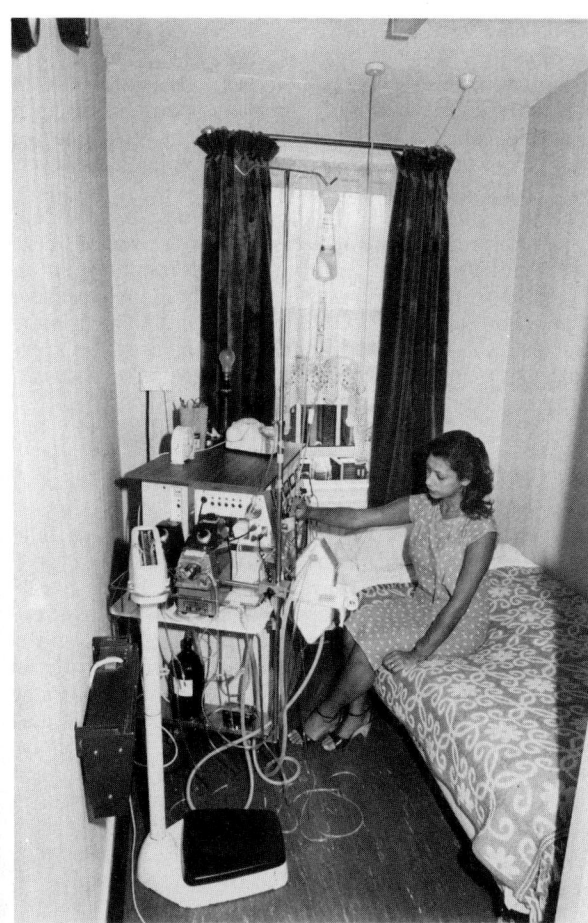
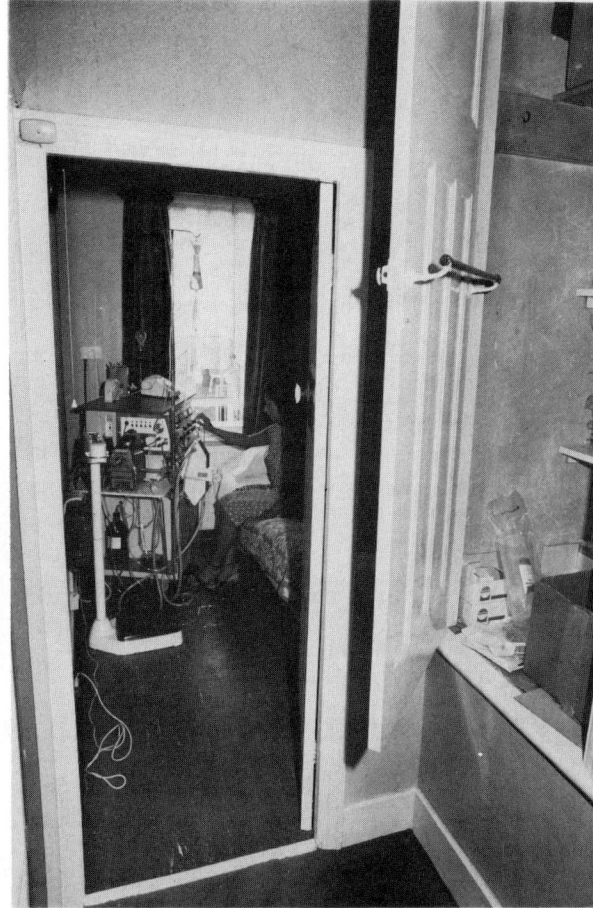

Figure 17. Very small home haemodialysis room with equipment suitable for re-use of dialyser and lines.

Figure 18. As Figure 17, showing storage of disposable equipment.

wall, taking up minimal space. All the necessary equipment is assembled on one mobile trolley – this includes the dialysis monitor, water filter with reverse osmosis unit and dialyser re-use facility. Nothing needs detaching. The telephone is by the bed and the vital telephone numbers – always to hand – are stuck on the side of the sink unit near the head of the bed.

In most homes, besides the standard rooms, there is usually one very small bedroom or box storage room, frequently this is the only available space. Figures 17 and 18 show such a room 2 m × 3 m, which has very little space once the bed is installed. The patient can be seen sitting on her bed adjusting the monitor, which also has an automatic system for re-using the dialyser and blood lines. Once prepared the dialyser and lines are re-used for 2 weeks (i.e. five times). It does give the impression of a jungle of lines, but the machine is simple to use and cuts out recurrent preparation procedures which is greatly appreciated. Out of sight behind the door is the remaining essential equipment, a very small water softener and hand-washing sink. Just outside the room a cupboard provides adequate storage space for all disposable items.

Figures 19 and 20 illustrate what can be done when space is not available for conventional dialysis purposes. The patient, his wife and two sons aged 18 and 20, occupy their own private apartment which has two reasonable sized bedrooms, a large kitchen and medium sized living room. The family was reluctant to move to larger premises. Two large cupboards were built in the bedroom to match existing furniture (Figure 19). They were designed to hold a Redy system or Sorb System (see Chapter 17) in one and the stores for 6 weeks in the other. The patient prepares the Redy System in the kitchen and in Figure 20 the patient is shown sitting in his usual dialysis position with the Redy apparatus standing on a removable plastic floor covering in the sitting room. The patient dialyses three times weekly in the evening immediately after work and is joined by his family, including the dogs.

The series of photographs illustrate not only the variety of choice of equipment for home haemodialysis, but the diversity of households accommodating the equipment. In addition, one can see the different attitudes of the patient to their dialysis rooms. All are clean, but the level of tidiness or adaption to improve convenience of

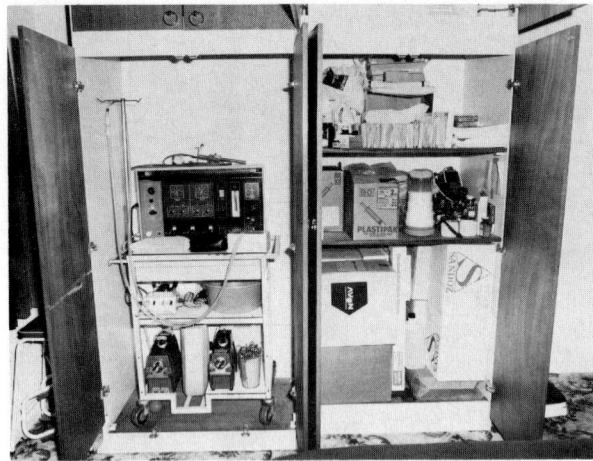

Figure 19. Storage of Redy machine (Sorb System) and equipment in the bedroom at home.

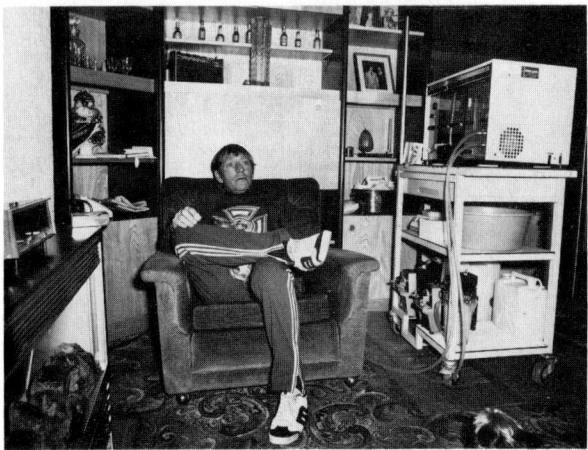

Figure 20. Redy machine (Sorb System) moved to living room for home dialysis.

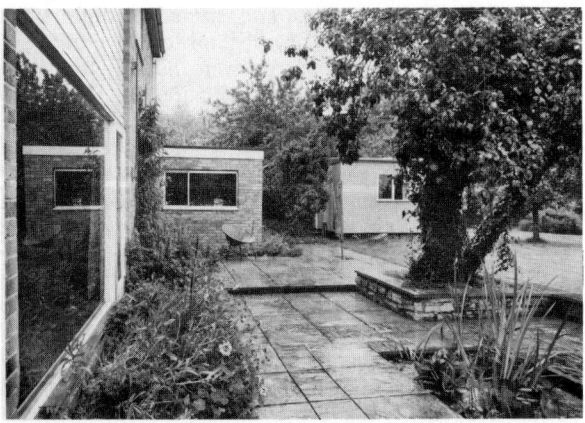

Figure 21. A portable cabin, equipped for home dialysis, situated in a garden. Note also the single storey extension to the house also of suitable size for dialysis equipment.

their dialysis rooms are as different as their personalities.

Another alternative to overcome the problem of limited space is to install the dialysis equipment in a portable cabin when there is sufficient space in the grounds of the house (Figure 21). The patients, however, often feel isolated during dialysis as it is not always possible to connect the cabin to the house. In very cold weather adequate heating is essential to prevent a 'freeze up'. Another method is to build an additional room on to the patient's house but this is usually more expensive than a portable cabin. If either a cabin or an extension is erected then some additional delay is usually experienced as planning permission has usually to be obtained from the municipal authority.

MAINTENANCE SUPPORT IN THE HOME

Patients established on home dialysis who have full-time jobs and a satisfactory family life find they have very little spare time. They appreciate an efficiently run organisation which provides medical and technical services for both routine and emergency problems and a reliable, regular delivery of supplies. Since most patients live more than an hour travelling time from the hospital (many may live several hours journey away) hospital visits should be kept to the minimum and the telephone used whenever possible. Loss of time and work – either of the patient or a member of his family – may occur if delivery of stores or arrival of a technician for repairs requires someone to remain in the home. To overcome this problem, patients often give keys to the hospital or neighbours.

These dialysis associated activities lead to frustration especially when emergencies change schedules with further loss of time. An appreciation of these points should influence the planning of the maintenance support in the home.

These comments, which were originally intended for a haemodialysis programme, are also entirely relevant to a CAPD programme.

Medical follow-up

On starting home dialysis patients should be seen at monthly intervals to discuss their dialysis data, particularly the correct dry body weight according to blood pressure measurements. Any non-urgent problems encountered during dialysis can be discussed at the same time. Thereafter, haemodialysis patients can be assessed by review of dialysis records, blood and machine samples for biochemistry sent regularly by post each month to the centre or local hospital. Full review with extensive biochemistry and X-rays related to known on-going medical aspects discussed in other parts of this book are undertaken at regular intervals. Apart from the attention to immediate emergencies, well established stable patients only need physical review every six months.

CAPD patients need to attend the centre for regular line changes and they are at the moment subject to more follow-up care since this is a new procedure and has general interest in addition to research activities.

Obviously some patients need more supervision than others. Since dialysis records of weight and blood pressure can be faked by less sensible patients, a policy of spot checks is recommended whereby every patient visiting the centre has weight and blood pressure recorded, regardless of the purpose of the visit. Our records show that 90% of patients require little or no supervision and care but the remaining 10% provide 90% of the centre's work. As patients settle into the routine of home dialysis, the dialysis procedure becomes increasingly efficient and the patient's health improves. These patients are contented, rarely miss going to work and develop minor illnesses no more often than the normal healthy community.

Management of medical problems and role of the local doctor

The role of the local doctor is limited on several accounts. In the first instance the development of any serious medical complications is usually associated with increased catabolism and disturbance of biochemical parameters. The patient is then best treated by the hospital centre where back up dialysis is available with a medical staff trained to recognise interrelated problems. There is no indication for the hospital doctor to go to the home; instead the patient should come to the hospital. Secondly, most local doctors have insufficient knowledge of the medical aspects and technicalities of dialysis and despite interest usually do not have sufficient time to learn. Apart from this most non-nephrologically trained doctors do not seem to realise the patient is equivalent to an anephric patient and the action of drugs may be modified whilst the dose may have to be altered accordingly (see Chapter 39). An unusual situation can arise whereby the patient proves to be more knowledgable than his local doctor and unless both patient and doctor take a realistic appraisal of each other, ridiculous situations may arise. The local doctor can, however, make useful contributions to the medical care of these patients if he is prepared to make home visits to assess situations and then discuss them in detail with the hospital medical team.

Medical problems related to haemodialysis which the local doctor might encounter at home are: overt or occult haemorrhage in relation to the use of anticoagulants, excessive ultrafiltration with hypotension and cramps, pyrogen reactions or bacteraemia with hypotension and fever, air embolus, hyponatraemia and hypercalcaemia.

Dialysis errors rarely lead to death at home. In general these complications are managed adequately by simple telephone directions from the centre and immediate transfer to hospital if necessary.

CAPD appears a simple treatment in the absence of complications. However, should peritonitis occur it is best supervised by the patient's centre, for two reasons. Firstly, growth and identification of the infecting organisms is often very difficult and secondly, it would be exceedingly dangerous to assume that peritonitis has arisen as a result of a technical error and fail to recognise an intra-abdominal emergency such as a perforated diverticulum or appendix.

Advisory service for the management of dialysis problems

Apart from medical complications of dialysis already mentioned, most dialysis problems result from minor technical faults either in patients technique or from component failure of the equipment. A telephone advisory service provided by the centre can solve most problems. The service should be available at all times when patients are allowed to haemodialyse at home. Home haemodialysis patients should be firmly instructed not to dialyse outside of the hours provided. Most centres can easily provide a 24 h service. The advice is given by trained nurses who coordinate with technicians and doctors as indicated. It is important to teach the nurses how to extract accurate information and to give precise directions. Included in this is accurate identification of the patient, and their self-care experience. The nurse must ensure that they and the patient understand each other precisely. All the calls should be logged in a book for reference. This is especially helpful if there is a recurring problem. The easiest advice to give is to ask the patient to come to the centre, but the patient might live a long distance away and transport could be difficult and costly. Careful discussion can often solve the problem to everyone's satisfaction.

Technical maintenance and emergency repairs of haemodialysis equipment

The regular use of the equipment in the home makes it particularly easy to plan maintenance servicing. The timing of the regular servicing depends on the particular equipment used. On average it takes two years of clinical use for any newly designed piece of equipment to be thoroughly tested, after which the times to replace components and adjust sensitivities can be defined and incorporated into the servicing manual. Occasionally a well designed but poorly constructed model, giving endless faults, is delivered. If this equipment is put into the home, dialysis is doomed to immediate failure. To avoid such problems, it is wise to give all home machines a period of continuous use and observation in the hospital centre before installation in a home.

Most centres provide emergency repairs using their own technicians. Home visits for repairs should normally be made within 24 h. It is rarely necessary to work outside routine hours as most patients can postpone a dialysis for 24 h. Today most equipment is modularised. This allows quick on the site repair of the machine by exchanging the defective module and less urgent repair of the faulty module in the workshop. Some machines are also small enough to be exchanged at home by a technician working single handed. Occasionally, technical visits outside routine hours are needed for young children on home dialysis and for the solving of 'spurious' problems occurring after several hours of normal dialysis.

Obviously, if a centre uses only one type of equipment, the services can become more streamlined, both in detection of faults and maintenance of spares; but limitation to one type of equipment for all patients would not allow flexibility.

Updating of dialysis technique and detection of recurrent errors

Over the years, the dialysis techniques in most units have changed many times. However, not all patients welcome new ideas, even if more economic and time saving. If they have an old fashioned but reliable technique, there must be very good reasons for asking the patient to change. Many of the patients will be able to change methods if given clearly written instructions; others may need additional telephone advice. Some patients will need individual retraining, if necessary in the hospital. If a centre has a home dialysis nurse, then the retraining can take place at home. Sometimes a patient apparently makes recurrent errors which are not reproducible in the hospital. The home dialysis nurse can make a valuable contribution by being present to watch, detect the fault and follow up with re-education.

Supply of disposables

Many centres buy, store and distribute all disposable items and drugs. As the home dialysis programme increases, the storage area and distribution transport has to increase correspondingly. For large centres this task can easily be transferred to a commercial firm. It is important to have close agreement with this firm in order to control the type of items, numbers needed and frequency of delivery. According to storage facilities in the home, deliveries should be 6 weekly, 2 monthly, sometimes extending to 6 monthly. To save patient time one organisation should deliver all items together.

Role and value of social workers and community support

People on haemodialysis are thought of as 'poor brave things' who must be given every possible aid and succour. There may be patients who do need support, but there are many others who lead independent lives and regard social workers and others as interfering and time wasting. Unless the social worker, and other community helpers are familiar with dialysis they may have difficulties in understanding the frustrations of the patient and are unable to give constructive help and in fact may give dangerous advice. Certainly some patients feel the need to express themselves to people independent from their direct medical care but is important that social and community workers co-ordinate with the dialysis centre.

The apparently effortless process of CAPD hides the reality that these patients also have terminal renal failure and are entitled to sympathy and understanding. However some CAPD patients feel deprived for they have no dramatic equipment to demonstrate the seriousness of their medical state.

Friendships made amongst patients in hospital while training are valuable and often provide mutual support over the years. The mothers of children on dialysis take great strength and courage from each other, they appear to have a 'hot line' to each other. They rightly know that no one else understands their problems quite so well as another mother in a similar position.

ANALYSIS OF RESULTS

Advantages to patient

Since the yearly statistical reports on dialysis and transplantation in Europe included survival figures on home dialysis, it has been noted that home dialysis gives the highest survival rates, both in the short and long term (14, 16, 41, 42) (See also Chapter 47). This is especially so for children. Although the results are distorted by more stringent selection criteria and the omission of the initial difficult hospital treatment, one should consider the excellent home dialysis figures obtained in the United Kingdom over the past 15 years since 1966. Limited facilities there have pressurised the doctors to put 60-75% of all patients treated, on home haemodialysis at some stage of management of their renal failure. The fact that home patients not only have the highest survival rates but also the highest rehabilitation rates (42) demonstrates that treatment at home is as good, if not of a consistently higher standard than the average hospital centre can achieve.

Home dialysis allows patients freedom to integrate dialysis into their lives and to personalise the treatment to give consistency of performance (43). It cannot be over emphasised how important it is for the physically rehabilitated patient to be able to earn a living for himself and his family. To be self reliant in maintaining their health gives patients great confidence.

Having dialysis treatment at home cuts out travelling time to a hospital centre, which is often far in excess of the time spent by an experienced patient preparing for dialysis. Preparation time in the home is usually reduced to short visits to the treatment room whilst the equipment is going through its automatic cycle. Certainly for patients living considerable distances from the hospital centre, home dialysis is the only answer unless the patient and family move home. Provided that good communication by telephone or telex and regular air service are all available, patients can dialyse at any distance from a dialysis centre. Several centres in the United Kingdom have many years experience of training and supervising patients abroad. A London centre has had up to 25 patients living in countries such as Pakistan, Persia, Saudi Arabia, Zambia, Nigeria and Trinidad (RE

Crockett National Kidney Centre, London personal communication, 1981). Extensive training and planning for emergencies is needed for these patients.

Advantages to the nephrology service

Where energy and motivation are put into a home dialysis training programme, which includes patient self reliance, the advantages are immense. This is especially so if transplant facilities are poor or if patients are unsuitable for transplantation. Dialysis facilities remain available for new patients and the trained patient at home requires minimal medical or nursing supervision. Most home haemodialysis training centres can train four patients per dialysis station per year. Some beds must be retained for hospitalisation of home patients, but the need for this facility has remained constant over the past 12 years being 10 to 12 dialyses per patient per year for a centre caring for 100 home patients (12, 44). Technical faults requiring extra time to repair, admissions to hospital for treatment of non-renal diseases, or illness of the patient or relatives are the usual reasons for temporary hospital dialysis. Confidence in their own dialysis ability is often shown by the patient's reluctance to use hospital facilities if the problem, once diagnosed, can be managed at home. Children, in particular, refuse to stay in hospital a moment longer than necessary. Even so, the number of beds for hospitalisation will increase as the dialysis population ages. Although CAPD needs a shorter training programme, episodes of peritonitis need longer periods of hospitalisation than technical haemodialysis problems. The number of days in hospital per patient per year appears to be three to five times greater than home haemodialysis. However, experience is limited and with improved techniques this may fall.

Even with active, more successful transplant programmes, the numbers of patients on dialysis will continue to increase (14, 42). Few countries can allow unlimited increase of hospital dialysis facilities. After the initial high investment of training and equipment, the running costs of home haemodialysis falls rapidly. When a patient no longer needs dialysis, the equipment can be transferred to a new patient. Well cared for equipment has an average 7 year life span and this makes the initial purchase economic. The figures quoted for the cost of hospital and home dialysis differ widely from country to country (6, 28, 45) but in the United Kingdom, where medical care both in hospital and home is known to be one of the cheapest, home dialysis costs less than a third of centre treatment. Any patient treated longer than 6 months in the home becomes an economic asset.

However, it is not just the monetary savings which have to be considered. Even today, many centres continue to have problems in acquiring trained staff. It is, therefore, extremely important to utilise available medical and nursing expertise in the most advantageous way (10, 19).

Figure 22 is a schematic representation of the patients and their management at the author's own centre where only 16 dialysis stations are available. Between 40 to 45 new patients start treatment each year. There are always

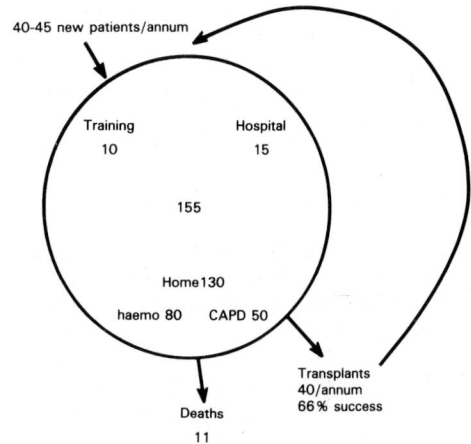

Figure 22. Schematic representation of the annual movement of patients through the author's 16 bedded centre (see text).

ten patients in training for either home haemodialysis or CAPD. Fifteen patients are categorised as hospital patients, five need nursing care, but ten are on limited care treatment overnight. One hundred and thirty patients, a still increasing number, are on home care, 80 do haemodialysis and 50 CAPD. Transplantation remains constant at about 40 per annum.

Failure of patient and the hospital

The incidence of home dialysis failure is considerably less than might be expected in view of the complexity of the procedure (12–14): the European figure for 1976 was 6.2%. More up to date statistics are not available. Recent review of the author's own data (46) shows that of 110 patients who started their treatment between 1963 and 1970, 97 were treated by home haemodialysis of which only 8 patients failed to continue home treatment (46). Anxiety with lack of confidence is the major problem and if, as in the early days of home treatment, a centre too easily allows the patient to return for temporary hospital dialysis when problems arise, the patient will never develop self reliance. Lonely people, whilst they may be extremely competent in their own dialysis, appreciate the community spirit of centre dialysis. Sympathetic understanding is always needed, but constructive guidance is the correct management. Not all patients whose marriages break down wish to return to hospital dialysis (12). The development of serious secondary medical problems or just growing old may require a return to permanent hospital dialysis, as might the illness or death of a spouse of an older patient. Some patients appreciate short periods of centre dialysis, between relatively long periods of home dialysis.

Patients or families who have decided they really do not want home dialysis have been known to sabotage their equipment. However, more frequently, the reason for the return to permanent hospital dialysis is due to failure of the hospital service rather than the patient's dialysis skills. A bad piece of equipment or a poor blood access, neither being the fault of the patient, leads to extreme frustration with the system and personnel involved. Patients will tolerate the occasional disturbance of their routine, but not the disruption of the whole family which occurs if the dialysis is frequently delayed. The smaller the problem, the more irritated the patient becomes, examples being minor changes in disposable items or failure to deliver sufficient stores to last until the next delivery.

Failure of an expert technician to repair a fault on the first or recurrent visits, leads to doubt about his skill and loss of confidence in the equipment. To restore confidence, it may prove necessary to change the offending equipment, even if all faults have been corrected, for experience has proved this to be very valuable in relieving patient's anxieties. Above all, failure to provide easy access for communication with doctors and nursing or technical staff leads to strained relations with the hospital dialysis centre and loss of confidence.

Home dialysis in children

Home haemodialysis has proved very successful for children, although the skills needed for dialysis of very small children, i.e. less than 20 kg, are very high. The parents make a 'fine art' of personalising the treatment, making most experienced staff look like beginners as far as their child is concerned. It is not surprising, therefore, that children with competent parents overwhelmingly prefer treatment at home. Short dialysis for 3 h, four or five times each week, either immediately after school or just before bedtime, allows a full day's activity and a full night's sleep for the whole family, and a more liberal diet. The short dialysis is relatively atraumatic, the child being able to get up and play immediately. If the treatment room is next to the living area, the child can easily be observed while the parents follow their routine home activities (22, 24). CAPD must be developed especially for the very young and small paediatric patient. For infants it could change their whole prognosis. Experienced centres need to be encouraged to obtain information on growth and development in patients treated by CAPD as soon as possible. CAPD in the paediatric group reduces anxiety not only of the patient but of the whole family. It allows a more liberal diet, full schooling and a better family and social life style, and haemoglobin values are higher.

CONCLUSIONS

Home haemodialysis has made a contribution far beyond its original concept of keeping patients with end-stage renal failure alive at a reduced and realistic cost. It has stimulated the development of safe and reliable equipment and obliged dialysis personnel to make their dialysis techniques fail safe. The result is an improved survival rate and a higher quality of dialysis which has allowed rehabilitation of patients to a level whereby they are productive within the society in which they live. Home haemodialysis has found a permanent place within the renal service, especially for patients proven unsuitable for transplantation and for centres with limited space and staff. CAPD will also find a place within the service but may not fulfil the initially high hopes of unlimited application as all home treatments need disciplined, co-operative patients. When home dialysis is undertaken in a well organised, motivated manner, the patients appreciate the independence and control they have over their own health and life style.

ACKNOWLEDGEMENT

Figure 21 is reproduced by permission of Omar Mobile Homes, Shortmead Street, Biggleswade, U.K.

REFERENCES

1. Alberts C, Drukker W: Report on regular dialysis treatment in Europe. *Proc Eur Dial Transpl Assoc* 2:82, 1965
2. Eschbach JW, Wilson WE, Peoples RW, Wakefield AW, Babb AL, Scribner BH: Unattended overnight home haemodialysis. *Trans Am Soc Artif Intern Organs* 12:346, 1966
3. Nose Y: Discussion. *Trans Am Soc Artif Intern Organs* 11:15, 1965
4. Curtis FK, Cole JJ, Fellows BJ, Tyler LL, Scribner BH: Hemodialysis in the home. *Trans Am Soc Artif Intern Organs* 11:7, 1965
5. Merrill JP, Schupak E, Cameron E, Hampers CL: Hemodialysis in the home. *JAMA* 190:468, 1964
6. Baillod RA, Comty C, Ilahi M, Konotey-Ahulu FID, Sevitt L, Shaldon S: Overnight haemodialysis in the home. *Proc Eur Dial Transpl Assoc* 2:99, 1965
7. Baillod RA, Comty CM, Crocket RE, Shaldon S: Experience with regular haemodialysis in the home. *Proc Eur Dial Transpl Assoc* 3:126, 1966
8. Nolph KD: Continuous ambulatory peritoneal dialysis. *Am J Nephrol* 1:1 1981
9. Jacobs C, Broyer M, Brunner FP, Brynger H, Donckerwolcke RA, Kramer P, Selwood NH, Wing AJ: Combined report on regular dialysis and transplantation in Europe X1. *Proc Eur Dial Transpl Assoc* 18:3, 1981
10. Shaldon S, Oakley JJ: An independent specialist home haemodialysis training and support unit. *Proc Eur Dial Transpl Assoc* 4:24, 1967
11. Baillod RA, Crockett RE, Ross A: Social and psychological aspects of regular haemodialysis treatment. *Proc Eur Dial Transpl Assoc* 5:97, 1968
12. Baillod RA, Moorhead JF: Review of 10 years home dialysis. *Proc Eur Dial Transpl Assoc* 11:68, 1974
13. Baillod RA, Moorhead JF: Therapeutic and social interactions of treatment of renal failure. In: *Proc 6th Int Congr Nephrol* Florence 1975, edited by Giovannetti S, Bonomini V, D'Amico G, Basel, München, New York, S Karger 1976, p 663
14. Gurland HJ, Brunner FP, Chantler C, Jacobs C, Schärer K, Selwood NH, Spies G, Wing AJ: Combined report on regular dialysis and transplantation in Europe, V1, 1975. *Proc Eur Dial Transpl Assoc* 13: 3, 1976

15. Sand P, Livingston G, Wright RG: Psychological assessment of candidates for a hemodialysis program. *Ann Intern Med* 64:602, 1966
16. Brynger H, Brunner FP, Chantler C, Donckerwolcke RA, Jacobs C, Kramer P, Selwood NH, Wing AJ: Combined report on regular dialysis and transplantation in Europe X. *Proc Eur Dial Transpl Assoc* 17:4, 1979
17. Fox RC: Exclusion from dialysis: A sociologic and legal perspective. *Kidney Int* 19:739, 1981
18. Johnson RS: Home dialysis: the competition between CAPD and hemodialysis. *JAMA* 245:1511, 1981
19. Roberts CM, Davis B, Pavitt L, Selsby M, Baillod RA, Moorhead JF: Home dialysis training in a blind patient and a deaf patient. *Proc Eur Dial Transpl Nurses Assoc* 1:41, 1973
20. Roberts CM: Home dialysis in a haemophiliac paraplegic patient. *Proc Eur Dial Transpl Nurses Assoc* 7:62, 1979
21. Barratt TM, Baillod RA: Chronic renal failure and regular dialysis. In: *Paediatric Urology*, 2nd edn, edited by Innes Williams D, Johnston JH, London, Boston MA, Sydney, Wellington Toronto, Durban, Butterworth Cy Ltd, 1982, p 37
22. Wass VJ, Barratt TM, Howarth RV, Marshall WA, Chantler C, Ogg CS, Cameron JS, Baillod RA, Moorhead JF: Home haemodialysis in children. *Lancet* 1:242, 1977
23. Williamson Balfe J, Irwin MA: Continuous ambulatory peritoneal dialysis in pediatrics. In: *Continuous Ambulatory Peritoneal Dialysis*, edited by Legrain M, Amsterdam, Oxford, Princeton, Excerpta Medica 1980, p 131
24. Baillod RA, Ku G, Moorhead JF: Home dialysis in children and adolescents. *Proc Eur Dial Transpl Assoc* 9:335, 1972
25. Pavitt L, Roberts C: The selection or non-selection of patients for a chronic renal failure programme. *Proc Eur Dial Transpl Nurses Assoc* 5:52, 1977
26. Gordon PM, Cattell WR: Blind spots in home dialysis. *Proc Eur Dial Transpl Assoc* 9:33, 1972
27. Mansell MA, Wing AJ: Long term experience of home dialysis with sorbent regeneration of dialysate. *Proc Eur Dial Transpl Assoc* 13:275, 1976
28. Scribner BH, Blagg CR: Maintenance dialysis. In: *Renal Diseases*, edited by Black D, Oxford, Blackwell Scientific Publications, 1972, p 495
29. Knight AH, Fox RA, Baillod RA, Niazi SP, Sherlock S, Moorhead JF: Hepatitis-associated antigen and antibody in haemodialysis patients and staff. *Br Med J* 3:603, 1970
30. Baillod RA, Knight AH, Crockett RE, Naish PF: Comparative assessment of arterio-venous shunts and Cimino Brescia fistulae. *Proc Eur Dial Transpl Assoc* 6:65, 1969
31. Shaldon S: In: Round table discussion: The Cimino-Brescia fistula. *Proc Eur Dial Transpl Assoc* 5:396, 1968
32. Shaldon S: The use of the arterio-venous fistula in home haemodialysis. *Proc Eur Dial Transpl Assoc* 6:94, 1969
33. Carmody M, Cattell WR, Baillod RA, Gambi V, Koch KM: Round table discussion: Dialysis – petrified or progressive? *Proc Eur Dial Transpl Assoc* 11:537, 1974
34. Shambaugh PW, Hampers CL, Bailey GL, Snyder D, Merrill JP: Hemodialysis in the home. Emotional impact on spouse. *Trans Am Soc Artif Intern Organs* 13:41, 1967
35. Baillod RA, Crockett RE, Lee BN, Moorhead JF, Stevenson CM: Establishment of home dialysis training centre with continuation of improved nocturnal hospital dialysis. *Proc Eur Dial Transpl Assoc* 4:30, 1967
36. Pavitt L, Chapple M, Herbert B, Oag D, Sanderson M, Smith A, Winder E: A team approach to patient education. *Proc Eur Dial Transpl Nurses Assoc* 4:58, 1976
37. Florkemeier V, von Bayer H, Finke K, Schadlich HJ, Sieberth HG: An audio-visual teaching programme for training home dialysis patients. *Proc Eur Dial Transpl Assoc* 10:538, 1973
38. Maiorca R, Castellani A, Cristinelli L, Migoyzi G, Mileti M, Mombelloni S, Usberti M: A video box colour film for home dialysis training. *Proc Eur Dial Transpl Assoc* 10:545, 1973
39. Blagg CR, Daly SM, Rosenquist BJ, Jensen WM, Eschbach JW: Home hemodialysis: the importance of patient training. *Ann Intern Med* 73:841, 1970
40. Roberts CM, Pavitt L: The value of a home dialysis nurse to a renal unit. *Proc Eur Dial Transpl Nurses Assoc* 5:27, 1977
41. Drukker W, Haagsma-Schouten WAG, Alberts C, Spoek MH: Report on regular dialysis treatment in Europe V. 1969. *Proc Eur Dial Transpl Assoc* 6:99, 1969
42. Parsons FM, Brunner FP, Burck HC, Gräser W, Gurland HJ, Härlen H, Schärer K, Spies GW: Statistical report. *Proc Eur Dial Transpl Assoc* 11:3, 1974
43. Roberts CM: Adapting dialysis to conform with individual needs and an active life. *Proc Eur Dial Transpl Nurses Assoc* 3:94, 1975
44. Moorhead JF, Baillod RA, Hopewell JP: Home dialysis. *Proc 4th Int Congr. Nephrol*, Stockholm 1969, edited by Alwall N, Berglund F, Josephson B, Basel, München, New York, S Karger 3:131, 1970
45. Burton BT: Socio-economic aspects of hemodialysis. *Proc 4th Int Congr Nephrol*, Stockholm 1969, edited by Alwall N, Berglund E, Josephson B, Basel, München, New York, S Karger 3:141, 1970
46. Baillod RA, Varghese Z, Fernando ON, Moorhead JF: Review of 71 patients receiving renal replacement for greater than 10 years. *Proc Third Capri Uremia Conf: Uremia-Pathobiology of Patients Treated for 10 Years or More*, edited by Giordano C, Friedman EA, Milan, New York NY, Wichtig Editore, 1981, p 35

25
PAEDIATRIC DIALYSIS

RAYMOND A. DONCKERWOLCKE, CYRIL CHANTLER and MICHEL J.C. BROYER

Acute renal failure in infancy and childhood	514
Introduction	514
Aetiology	515
Assessment and initial therapy	515
Conservative management	516
Complications	516
Treatment of acute renal failure by dialysis	517
Peritoneal dialysis in acute renal failure	517
Equipment	517
Procedure	517
Complications	517
Peritonitis	517
Catheter malfunction	518
Perforation of a viscus (bowel or bladder)	518
Bleeding	518
Neurological complications	518
Hyperglycaemia and hypernatraemia	518
Failure of peritoneal dialysis to correct hyperkalaemia	518
Haemodialysis in acute renal failure	518
Vascular access	518
Technique of haemodialysis	518
Conclusions	519
Chronic renal failure in infancy and childhood	519
Incidence and age of onset	519
Primary renal disease in children	519
Organisation of services and facilities required for the treatment of children	520
Regular haemodialysis	521
Vascular access for regular dialysis treatment	521
Choice of the dialyser and bloodlines	521
Management of regular dialysis	522
Complications	522
Home dialysis	522
Regular peritoneal dialysis	523
Intermittent peritoneal dialysis (IPD)	523
Technique	523
Results	524
Complications	524
Indications	524
Continuous ambulatory peritoneal dialysis (CAPD)	524
Technique	524
Results	524
Complications	524
Indications	524
Survival rates and causes of death	525
Medical problems	525
Growth failure and endocrine disorders	525
Osteodystrophy	526
Anaemia	527
Cardiovascular complications	528
Diet	528
Psychosocial problems	529
The child and his disease	529
The families	530
The dialysis team	530
Rehabilitation	530
Practical directives for haemodialysis in children	531
Preparation for dialysis	531
Dialysis techniques	531
Treatment of complications during dialysis	532
References	533

ACUTE RENAL FAILURE IN INFANCY AND CHILDHOOD

Introduction

Successful management of renal failure in children, particularly infants, requires knowledge of the functional characteristics of the kidney during development and an understanding of the metabolic balance of the growing child. The newborn kidney is immature containing only 17% of its adult cellular complement; at six months postnatally cell division is complete and further growth is due to an increase in cell size. Nephron formation is complete before birth but the superficial cortical nephrons are not functionally mature so that at birth the more mature juxtamedullary nephrons contribute a greater proportion of total glomerular filtration than in the adult. This is associated with a proportional increase in juxtamedullary blood flow but total renal blood flow is small because of the high renal vascular resistance (1). Glomerular filtration rate (GFR) at birth averages about 20 ml/min/1.73 m^2 but the rapid postnatal increase in renal blood flow is associated with a rapid rise in GFR to 48 ml/min/1.73 m^2 at 1 month and to 80 ml/min/1.73 m^2 by 6 months of age (2). The functional limitations of the newborn kidney are manifest by a higher blood urea and phosphate and a lower plasma bicarbonate concentration. It is likely that the low GFR is determined by the immaturity of tubular function to prevent overperfusion of nephrons and wasting of salt and water (3); fractional reabsorption of filtered sodium in the proximal tubule is reduced with greater reabsorption in the distal tubule. Excessive urinary sodium loss is present in very immature infants between 28 and 32 weeks gestation and sodium wasting is also common in infants with obstructive uropathy and distal tubular damage.

The functional demands on the newborn full term

kidney are greater than on the adult kidney because the metabolic rate of the infant related to body weight is considerably greater. Insensible water loss even at rest in a neutral thermal environment is five times greater, energy demands in relation to body weight about three times and normal fluid intake four times larger. At least as important is the absence of normal thirst control in an individual who is unable spontaneously to take more water when fluid depleted or sodium overloaded. Therefore, it is not surprising that renal vascular causes of acute renal failure are especially prominent in the newborn, that dehydration leading to acute tubular necrosis is prevalent in infants, and that uraemia, acidosis, and hyperkalaemia can develop with astonishing rapidity in the small child.

GFR related to surface area is comparable in children and adults from the age of two years and food intake is roughly comparable when related to surface area but not to body weight (2). This is important when considering the amount of dialysis, size of dialyser, fluid and food intake of the uraemic child and will be referred to later. Blood pressure rises steadily throughout childhood with an upper normal limit of 110/65 mm Hg at birth to 130/80 mm Hg at 13 years. Care must be taken to use a blood pressure cuff of sufficient size to avoid erroneously high readings: the inflatable bladder should be centred over the brachial artery encircling at least three quarters of the circumference of the arm and the width of the cuff should be at least two thirds of the length of the upper arm.

Aetiology

The incidence and causes of acute renal failure vary in different countries depending on the general quality of health care and environmental conditions. Table 1 itemises the diagnosis in 99 children referred to Guy's Hospital, London, over a seven year period (4); 20% were less than 6 weeks old. Poor renal perfusion accounted for nearly a third of all referrals; the cause was usually obvious and included gastroenteritis, pyloric stenosis, cardiac failure, post surgery especially after cardiovascular operations, burns and renal vascular catastrophes in the newborn. Sudden relapse of nephrotic syndrome was commonly associated with hypovolaemia due to the rapid loss of salt and water into the extracellular space as the plasma albumin concentration fell. This may cause tubular necrosis and uraemia and may also be associated with circulatory arrest. Most important is the determination of haemoglobin which may reveal haemoconcentration, for pulse and blood pressure may be surprisingly well maintained by peripheral vasoconstriction, which is reflected by a wide gap between the rectal and peripheral temperature. As previously noted, the newborn kidney is especially susceptible to vascular damage. Medullary or papillary necrosis may accompany severe cases of acute tubular necrosis. Hyperosmolar solutions used as contrast media for renal radiology may cause medullary damage. Cortical necrosis occurs after severe fluid loss, birth asphyxia, haemorrhage, or burns; focal necrotising lesions in other organs are common. Renal venous thrombosis is especially common in infants and 70% of cases present in the first month of life (5), antecedent events include shock, perinatal asphyxia, cyanotic heart disease and hyperosmolar dehydration and disseminated intravascular coagulation.

Urinary tract infection in newborns is often associated with septicaemia perhaps because of the low concentration of circulating immunoglobulin at this age; accordingly it may present with generalised symptoms and signs such as vomiting, lethargy and jaundice. Congenital obstructive uropathy is frequently complicated by inability to concentrate the urine and by sodium wasting due to distal nephron damage and it is not, therefore, surprising that these infants may present severely fluid depleted.

Assessment and initial therapy

Children, especially infants, with acute renal failure, are usually dangerously ill and for the reasons outlined the metabolic derangements are rapid in onset and severe. Therefore, treatment and investigation must proceed simultaneously. Whilst the indications for dialysis are

Table 1. Causes of acute renal failure in children treated at Guy's Hospital 1971-1975 (modified from Counahan et al. [4]).

Diagnosis	n	Treatment				Result			
		Con	PD	PD-HD	HD	Recovered	CFR	RDT+T	Dead
Renal hypoperfusion	41	21	13	2	5	29	3	0	9
Haemolytic uraemic syndrome	18	4	10	3	1	9	5	2	2
Glomerulonephritis	9	5	2	1	1	6	1	1	1
Septicaemia and/or urinary tract infection	13	4	6	3	3	5	0	0	8
Congenital obstructive or dysplastic uropathy	8	7	0	1	1	1	4	1	2
Acute on chronic renal disease	8	0	0	2	2	0	2	6	0
Poisoning	2	0	2	0	0	2	0	0	0
Total	99	41	33	12	13	62	15	10	22

Con = conservative
PD = peritoneal dialysis
HD = haemodialysis
CRF = chronic renal failure
RDT = regular dialysis treatment
T = transplantation

similar to those in adults, the increased metabolism and energy demands necessitate more frequent dialysis for it is difficult to manage an anuric catabolic infant on a conservative regimen. The initial assessment includes a clinical evaluation of the degree of fluid loss, blood pressure measurement if necessary using Doppler ultrasonography (6), central and peripheral temperature measurement to gauge tissue perfusion (7), haemoglobin and plasma and urinary electrolyte concentrations. Urinary sodium and urea concentrations are especially useful to determine the adequacy of renal perfusion (4). From these determinations the necessary amount of IV fluid required to restore extracellular volume can be calculated, but careful continuous monitoring is essential to prevent overload. The blood volume of a child can be calculated as 80 ml per kg body weight. Thus an initial transfusion of whole blood or plasma of 20 ml/kg in a shocked child is usually safe. An obviously saline depleted infant will have lost about 10% of body weight as water, so again the rapid infusion of 20 ml/kg of physiological saline can be undertaken whilst more precise calculations are being undertaken.

If peripheral circulation is not restored by adequate fluid replacement even though blood pressure and venous pressure are normal then the careful use of a peripheral vasodilator (hydralazine [dosage see below], or chlorpromazine 0.1 mg/kg IV) may be associated with a resumption of urine flow.

Hypernatraemia should be corrected only slowly, over 48 h, to avoid neurological damage; the calculated water deficit being supplied by solutions with a sodium content of 25 to 40 mmols/l providing not more than 100 ml/kg of *free* water per 24 h. Hypertension usually responds to IV or IM hydralazine, 0.5 to 1.0 mg/kg or IV diazoxide, 5 mg/kg body weight.

Hyperkalaemia, if life threatening, should be treated with IV 2.5% calcium gluconate 2 ml/kg, correction of acidosis and an ion exchange resin in the calcium phase, 1 g/kg orally or rectally.

Hypocalcaemia in the neonate presents with jittery movements or convulsions and should be treated with IV calcium gluconate.

Hypoglycaemia requires intravenous administration of dextrose 1 g/kg. Metabolic acidosis can be corrected with 8.4% sodium bicarbonate (1 mmol/ml) diluted before use; 2 mmol/kg will raise plasma bicarbonate by about 6 mmol/l in the infant. It is not advisable to correct the acidosis completely because of the risk of hypokalaemia and the high sodium load involved in the treatment. Intensive treatment of possible septicaemia should be undertaken after blood cultures have been obtained. Care must be exercised when drugs whose excretion is dependent on renal function are used and the dosage should be reduced, accordingly, and the plasma concentration measured at intervals.

Further investigation involving renal radiology, ultrasonography, dynamic renal scintillography (gamma scan) and renal biopsy should only be undertaken when the condition of the child has been stabilised, if necessary by dialysis. Nonetheless, urgency is imperative, for an obstructed infected urinary tract may require immediate surgery to establish adequate drainage. The gamma scan using ^{99m}Tc DTPA (diethylene triamino pentacetic acid) is particularly useful because it often gives information comparable to intravenous urography but is much less hazardous as it involves no osmotic load. Furthermore, it can provide a useful measure of renal perfusion and function.

Conservative management

Whilst dialysis is usually undertaken at an early stage, careful control of fluid, electrolyte and nutritional intake is required. After the fluid deficit has been corrected, intake should be reduced to the level of the insensible loss (minus water of oxidation), 22 ml per kg/24 h between birth and 1 year then falling to 9 ml/kg/24 h at 12 years, plus an allowance for pyrexia, abnormal losses, urine output and loss by ultrafiltration during dialysis. Electrolyte requirements are difficult to estimate and should be kept as low as possible with sodium and potassium intake not exceeding 2 mmol/kg/24 h unless the child receives dialysis. An adequate calcium intake of 500 mg/24 h (25 mmol) should be ensured if necessary by feeding supplements. The high energy intake of infants has been mentioned and at least 100–150 Cal (420 to 630 kJ) per kg per day is required at birth. About 2 g per kg of first class protein should be provided at birth falling to 1 g per kg at 1 year and thereafter. Suitable oral feed which take account of all these requirements can be made up using low solute of humanised cows milk preparations (S.M.A., S$_{26}$, Ostermilk new, Cow and Gate baby milk plus) but unmodified cows milk or evaporated milk are not suitable. Extra energy can be provided with double cream (4 Cal [16,8 kJ] per ml) and with a glucose polymer such as caloreen or calonutrin. Alkali can be added as sodium bicarbonate (1 to 2 mmol/kg/24 h). The osmolality of the food should be measured and slowly increased to prevent diarrhoea and vomiting.

With older children the help of an experienced dietician is essential so that account can be taken of the child's taste preferences. The most important point is to ensure that the diet prescribed is actually eaten and this can only be done with the child's co-operation.

Maintaining adequate nutrition in infants with renal failure who cannot be maintained on an oral intake is extremely difficult. Even with the most concentrated IV feeding regimens utilising fat emulsions, frequent dialysis is essential to remove the excess water involved. Detailed description is beyond the scope of this discussion but reviews are available (2, 8, 9).

Complications

The complications and cause of death in acute renal failure are primarily related to the condition which caused the renal failure and to the complications of dialysis, most of which can be avoided.

Convulsions commonly complicate renal failure especially in infants and are usually attributed to a combination of factors such as uraemia, hyponatraemia, hypocalcaemia and hypertension though the primary disorder causing the renal failure e.g. the haemolytic syndrome may be implicated (10). Again, good management can minimise the risk.

Treatment of acute renal failure by dialysis

Peritoneal dialysis is the most common mode of treatment of acute renal failure in childhood because of its simplicity, availability, its relative safety and its effectiveness. In acute renal failure in newborns and infants it is the treatment of choice.

Children weighing more then 20 kg with a prolonged period of oliguria are often treated with haemodialysis after one or two peritoneal dialyses. Available facilities and expertise will often determine the choice between peritoneal and haemodialysis in older children.

There is no evidence that outcome is better with either technique. In haemodynamically unstable cardiovascular patients or in those with a generalised coagulopathy, peritoneal dialysis may be preferable.

Peritoneal and haemodialysis are also used in the treatment of poisoning and of some metabolic derangements and in those disturbances of fluid and electrolyte metabolism that are not controllable by conservative treatment. Recently developed treatment methods such as haemoperfusion over resin or charcoal and haemofiltration have decreased the need of dialysis in the treatment of these disorders.

Peritoneal dialysis in acute renal failure
(see also Chapter 23)

The general outline of peritoneal dialysis in children is similar to that in adults. Some differences will be discussed.

Equipment
Dialysis solutions containing 7% dextrose monohydrate (or 6.36% anhydrous dextrose) should be avoided in paediatric dialysis because of the risk of hyperglycaemia and excessive ultrafiltration. A 4.25% solution of dextrose monohydrate is used to achieve ultrafiltration and this can be made by mixing commercially available solutions.[1] In newborns and infants the replacement of acetate or lactate by bicarbonate in the dialysis solution has been advocated, especially if metabolic derangements are to be treated. Unfortunately, the calcium in the dialysis solution precipitates out under these circumstances and has to be provided separately by intravenous administration. Special plastic peritoneal catheters for children are commercially available (McGaw, Pharmaceal, Vygon, Baxter laboratory, Wallace) and for intermittent long term peritoneal dialysis paediatric Silastic catheters are available (Abbott, Evergreen, Cobe). To avoid bacterial contamination a closed system for administration of the dialysis fluid is required.

Regular weight control during dialysis is imperative even if cumulative fluid balances are recorded. In the acutely ill patient fluid loss by vomiting and diarrhoea may be very important and should be replaced accurately. Volumetric fluid balance measurements are a prerequisite for the use of automatic cycling machines in children. If a manual system is used, accurate fluid balances must be recorded and the volume of the spent dialysate should be measured.[2]

Procedure
Premedication with diazepam, 0,25 mg/kg intravenously; chlorpromazine, 0.5 mg/kg intramuscularly or with chloral hydrate 30 mg/kg by rectal administration is recommended in an anxious child. After local anaesthesia with procaine, the abdomen should be primed with 20 ml dialysis solution/kg body weight, through a small bore needle or cannula prior to the insertion of the peritoneal catheter. This is necessary to avoid the catheter plunging into an intra-abdominal organ such as the inferior vena cava for the small infant is unable to tense the abdominal muscles when the catheter is inserted.

The stylet catheter is then inserted through a small skin incision, a few centimeters below the umbilicus in the midline; when the peritoneum is entered, the stylet is removed and the catheter advanced to the left side of the pelvis. (See Figures 8a, b and 8c in Chapter 21).

When midline insertion is not possible, the catheter can be inserted in the flank area, outside the line of the inferior epigastric artery.

Dialysis solution is delivered to the abdomen in amounts of 40 to 60 ml/kg in infants and small children and 30 to 40 ml/kg in older children (not exceeding 2000 ml) with each cycle. The fluid is infused by gravity flow and allowed to remain for 30 min and then also withdrawn by gravity. The cycle requires 1 h. Total dialysis time is limited to 36 h, but if renal failure continues the procedure has to be repeated 48 h later. At the start of dialysis more rapid cycling is recommended until any contamination of the dialysis fluid by blood has disappeared.

Five hundred units of heparin/litre of dialysate are added to the first three cycles. Since hyperkalaemia is often present, dialysis is started with no potassium added to the dialysate; after three to six cycles KCl, 3 mmol/l, is added to the dialysis solution.

In the unconscious patient a gastric tube is introduced and the stomach emptied. This will avoid aspiration of stomach contents when vomiting occurs due to diaphragmatic irritation.

Complications
Peritonitis. This is a most dangerous complication and scrupulous attention to asepsis is mandatory. If intermittent dialysis in patients with acute renal failure is carried out, a reduction of dialysis treatment to 36 h considerably reduces the risk of infection of the peritoneum.

It is better to dialyse for a few days and then to

---

[1] Equal quantities of 6.36% and 1.36% of anhydrous dextrose give a final concentration of 3.8%, which equals a solution of 4.25% dextrose monohydrate.

[2] One should be aware that commercially prepared bags (or bottles) often not contain precisely the specified amount of dialysis solution. Often they contain a slight overfill.

remove the cannula, allowing a period of conservative treatment, than to leave the cannula in place for long periods of time. When peritoneal dialysis is resumed a new catheter is inserted. If, however, peritonitis occurs, it should be treated with antibiotics and continuation of peritoneal dialysis.

One should be aware that even when infection of the peritoneum has subsided the efficiency of dialysis may be reduced, making haemodialysis necessary.

Catheter malfunction. Obstruction of the catheter may be caused by omental fat, fibrin or blood clots.

Extravasation of fluid into the abdominal wall is a frequent complication of peritoneal dialysis in children. The use of a suitable catheter, which should be correctly inserted with all perforations inside the peritoneal cavity will avoid this problem. In any event, the cannula must be removed if any leakage occurs in the abdominal wall.

If a long period of peritoneal dialysis is envisaged we insert a cuffed Silastic cannula with a long tunnel in the abdominal wall under general anaesthesia, after an initial period of conventional peritoneal dialyses with a stylet catheter.

Perforation of a viscus (bowel or bladder). This is a rare complication. The catheter should be removed and reinserted; usually the perforation closes spontaneously.

Bleeding. Bleeding after insertion of the catheter, continuing during the first few cycles is not uncommon.

Exceptionally the haemorrhage is considerable, leading to hypotension and shock.

Neurological complications. These sometimes occur and are caused by sudden changes in the body fluid composition (disequilibrium). They are related to an inappropriate dialysis procedure and can be avoided.

Hyperglycaemia and hypernatraemia. Both can be caused by dialysis solutions containing high dextrose concentrations. But even a dialysis fluid with 1.5% hydrous dextrose (= 1.36% anhydrous dextrose) may cause these complications in newborns and small infants.

Hyperglycaemia is also related to the glucose intolerance associated with the overall catabolic state of uraemia and infection. Hyperglycaemia should be treated with small doses insuline (0.1 U/kg IV).

Hypernatraemia may occur from more rapid removal of water than sodium and will usually respond to prolonging of dialysis cycles or the substitution of the dialysis fluid by a solution with a sodium concentration of 130 mmol/l (see also chapters 21, 22, 23).

Failure of peritoneal dialysis to correct hyperkalaemia. This has been reported in infants with acute renal failure following cardiac surgery (11), perhaps because of poor peripheral circulation from inadequate cardiac output.

Haemodialysis in acute renal failure

Vascular access

For emergency haemodialysis there is a need for a simple, immediately usable vascular access. Methods for cannulation of the superior and inferior vena cava have been developed (12). Superior vena cava catheterisation is effected through cannulation of the subclavian or jugular vein, and subclavian cannulation with a 9 French caliber [3] catheter with 5 peripheral side ports has been reported in patients older than 5 years (13).

The catheter is inserted under local anaesthesia with fluoroscopic guidance using the Seldinger technique via the subclavian approach and then advanced into the right atrium and customised to the size of the child. Dialysis is performed using a single needle system.

Acute haemodialysis using one or two percutaneous femoral vein catheters is possible even in small children and the use of a single needle device allows dialysis through a single femoral vein catheter. When two catheters are to be inserted in small children, it is easier to catheterise both femoral veins instead of insertion of both catheters on the same side (14). The catheter should be of at least 8 French caliber to provide an adequate bloodflow.

Percutaneous catherisation is useful when only a few dialyses are necessary, but for prolonged treatment an arteriovenous shunt is required; to avoid haemorrhage at the shunt site, dialysis should be delayed for at least 12 h after operative insertion.

Technique of haemodialysis

The technique of haemodialysis in acute renal failure is not different from that in chronic renal failure. However, patients with acute renal failure often have an unstable cardiovascular system, making dialysis more hazardous (15). Therefore special guidelines for haemodialysis in acute renal failure are required. Patients with acute renal failure often are critically ill so careful monitoring of vital functions is essential. Continuous cardiac monitoring with frequent blood pressure control and monitoring of central venous pressure is necessary.

Measurements of central/peripheral temperature gradients to detect peripheral vasoconstriction is useful in assessing the adequacy of cardiac output and circulating blood volume (7). Heating blankets are useful to prevent hypothermia in small children. Continuous weight recording is necessary to avoid sudden changes in blood volume and body fluids. The dialyser should be primed with saline or blood to prevent circulatory collapse at the start of dialysis.

In acute dialysis vigorous ultrafiltration is often required but the efficiency of dialysis has to be reduced to avoid the dialysis disequilibrum syndrome. Therefore a less efficient dialyser (BUN clearance less than 1.5 ml/kg body weight/min) and a shorter dialysis time (3 h or less) are required. To avoid circulatory collapse a dialyser allowing careful regulation of ultrafiltration and with reduced compliance during application of negative pressure for ultrafiltration is preferred. Sequential haemodia-

---

[3] 1 French = 0.3 mm.

lysis and ultrafiltration is recommended in volume overloaded patients.

The Rhône Poulenc dialyser RP6 with its variable surface area combined with an ultrafiltration regulation device, is particularly useful in acute dialysis in children. Mannitol (1 g/kg body weight) may be infused during dialysis to avoid an excessive decrease in serum osmolality.

The dose of mannitol infused is twice as much during the first hour of dialysis as during each of the remaining hours. Substitution of bicarbonate for acetate in the dialysate may be important in patients with severe metabolic disturbances. Low dose heparin infusion or regional heparinisation may be necessary in patients with acute renal failure to avoid haemorrhage following surgery.

Conclusions

The prognosis of acute renal failure due to primary kidney disease is relatively good (Table 1) and a majority of the children when properly managed make a full recovery. In contrast, there is a poor survival of patients when acute renal failure complicates severe infections or major operations, because death in these instances is due to the primary disease (11, 15, 16). The services required for adequate treatment are formidable, however, requiring skilled paediatric nursing, 24 h chemical pathology and haematology, paediatric radiology and nuclear medicine, paediatric dieticians and social workers, nephrologists familiar with paediatric problems and experienced paediatric urologists as well as the general nephrology and dialysis expertise. Accordingly, such services tend to be concentrated in a few units serving a large population.

CHRONIC RENAL FAILURE IN INFANCY AND CHILDHOOD

Incidence and age of onset

Marked differences in the incidence of end stage renal disease (ESRD) in childhood have been reported. Figures ranging from 4 to 15 new cases per year per million child population (agegroup 0–15 years), have been published. The 1980 Report of the Registry of the European Dialysis and Transplant Association (EDTA) shows that in countries with well developed facilities for the treatment of children four to five paediatric patients per million child population started initial treatment in 1978, 1979 and 1980 (17–23). In France there are striking regional differences in the number of paediatric patients starting renal replacement treatment. In some areas ten new paediatric patients per million children started treatment per year, while only 4.9 patients per million children started treatment in France as a whole. Less than three children per million started treatment in 1980 in Europe. This probably indicates that many children still die from chronic renal failure either due to a lack of treatment facilities, or to selection policies. Early diagnosis and advances in treatment will reduce the incidence of ESRD in childhood. This only relates to ESRD due to malformations of the urinary tract and possibly glomerulonephritis. Unfortunately, in more than 50% of the patients, ESRD is due to a genetically transmitted disease or to malformation of the kidneys for which no therapeutic approach seems possible.

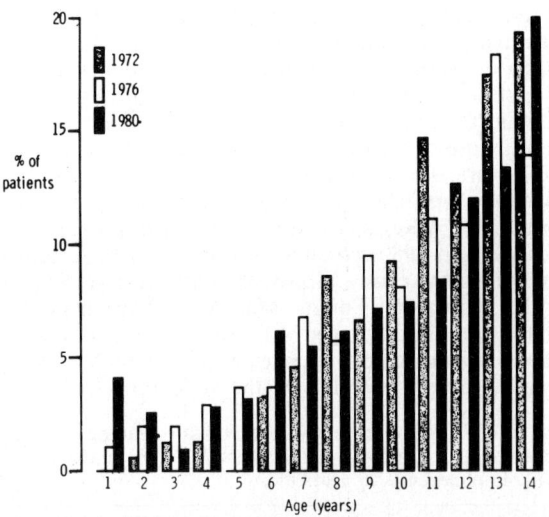

Figure 1. Distribution of patients according to age in the year of initial treatment (1972-1976-1980) (EDTA Registry 1980 [23], with permission of the publishers).

The age distribution of children accepted for treatment in Europe is shown in Figure 1 for the years 1972, 1976 and 1980 (23). At the start of treatment the majority of the patients were 10 to 14 years old (67%) and only 8.3% were less than 5 years old. The incidence of ESRD is certainly underestimated for the age group 0 to 5 years. In countries with no age discrimination for the treatment of ESRD, 17% of all patients starting treatment are less than 5 years old. An increase in the number of patients less than 5 years old at the start of treatment has also been noticed in Europe during the last few years.

Primary renal disease in children

Glomerulopathies, hereditary or genetically determined diseases, pyelonephritis, generally associated with urinary tract abnormalities and hypoplasia and (or) dysplasia

Table 2. Frequency of different causes of chronic paediatric renal disease (PRD) (EDTA Registry 1980 [23]).

	All patients on Registry *	New cases 1980 *
Glomerulonephritis	32.3	25.2
Pyelonephritis	21.9	23.3
Hereditary-familial	16.1	20.4
Hypoplasia	12.1	15.4
Other diagnosis	12.5	11.8
Uncertain	5.1	3.9

* Expressed as % of total number of patients.

of the kidney account for more than 80% of the cases of terminal renal failure in childhood. Hypoplasia and dysplasia of the kidney and such hereditary renal diseases, as cystinosis, are more important causes of renal failure in children than in adults. The relative frequency of the main causes of ESRD in children as recorded by the EDTA are shown in Table 2. The changing pattern of causes of renal diseases found in all paediatric patients on the EDTA Registry and in the new cases accepted for treatment in 1980 remains unexplained (23). A detailed analysis of the causes of primary renal disease observed at the Hôpital des Enfants Malades in Paris from 1969 to 1981 in children aged 0 to 16 years old is given in Table 3. The relative frequency of different causes of renal disease is similar to the data reported by the EDTA Registry in 1980. Age differences were apparent: haemolytic uraemic syndrome and cortical necrosis are more frequent in patients in the age group 0 to 5. In this age group glomerular disease was related to diffuse mesangial sclerosis, congenital nephrotic syndrome and anti glomerular and tubular basal membrane nephropathies. In boys below the age of 5 years hypoplasia of the kidney is an important cause of renal failure (24).

The knowledge of the primary renal disease in children with chronic renal failure is of crucial importance for several reasons. The speed of progression towards the end-stage of renal disease varies according to the aetiology. This progression is slow in patients with hypoplastic kidneys and sometimes very fast in patients with glomerular diseases. This has to be taken into account in timing the decision of fistula creation in preparation for dialysis. Moreover the risk of recurrence of the disease in the transplanted kidney makes the diagnosis of primary renal disease important. Therefore, a minimal delay of 1 year between the start of dialysis and transplantation is proposed for diseases like rapidly progressive glomerulonephritis and Schoenlein-Henoch glomerular disease. Finally, the discovery of a genetically transmitted disease necessitates genetic counselling and requires early investigations in siblings.

Table 3. Causes of primary renal disease leading to ESRD, observed at the Hôpital des Enfants Malades in Paris, 1969-1981, in children 0-16 years old.

Malformations of the kidney and of the urinary tract (33.1%)		
Malformative uropathies + pyelonephritis	61	(15.6%)
'Segmental hypoplasia'	16	(4.0%)
Hypoplastic and dysplastic kidneys	52	(13.3%)
Glomerular diseases (26.4%)		
Idiopathic nephrotic syndrome with hyalinosis	46	(11.7%)
Diffuse mesangial sclerosis	6	(1.5%)
Congenital nephrotic syndrome (Finnish type)	4	(1.0%)
Membrano-proliferative glomerulonephritis (of which dense deposits disease 7)	22	(5.6%)
Glomerulonephritis with mesangial IgA deposits	5	(1.3%)
Other type or unclassified GN	15	(3.8%)
Genetically transmitted disease (25.8%)		
Nephronophthisis	56	(14.3%)
Cystinosis	21	(5.3%)
Alport's syndrome	12	(3.0%)
Oxalosis	6	(1.5%)
Infantile polycystic disease	2	(0.5%)
Nail patella syndrome	1	
Acroosteolysis with nephropathy	1	
Familial mediterranean fever	1	
Bartter's syndrome	1	
General diseases (5.6%)		
Schoenlein-Henoch glomerulonephritis	20	(5.1%)
Systemic lupus erythematosus	1	
Peri-arteritis nodosa	1	
Vascular diseases (4.8%)		
Haemolytic uraemic syndrome	15	(3.8%)
Cortical necrosis	2	(0.5%)
Renal vein thrombosis	1	
Unclassified	1	
Miscellaneous		
Bilateral Wilm's tumour	5	(1.3%)
Surgical loss of a solitary kidney (post traumatic)	3	(0.75%)
Spina bifida and neurological bladder	3	(0.75%)
Unclassified (1.5%)	6	(1.5%)

Organisation of services and facilities required for treatment of children

The relatively small number of children starting dialysis each year results in logistics which are different from those in adult patients. It has, therefore, been suggested that a limited number of specialised children's centres should be established to cope with the problem rather than to treat the occasional child who presents with chronic renal failure in a local adult centre. Treatment of children in adult centres often results in complications due to inappropriate dialysis technique; moreover treatment of children on the same ward as adults may create additional psychological problems in both categories.

One paediatric centre per million child population per country is sufficient to provide treatment for all children with end stage renal disease. These centres will have to care for four to six new paediatric patients per year. By the end of 1980, 76 paediatric centres had been established in Europe but these centres treated only 42% of paediatric patients undergoing renal replacement therapy in Europe (23). The cost of paediatric dialysis is higher than for adult patients. Paediatric units which should be separated from the adults treatment area are usually small with a relatively high staff-to-patient ratio and they must provide a number of services not required for adult patients. The basic requirements for such centres are a paediatric nephrologist, nurses experienced in dialysis of children, a dietician, a hospital school and a social worker. Paediatric surgery and urology are required. They also need psychiatry services and the support of a general paediatric unit. In some countries, with sparse populations, such centralisation of facilities may require children and families to travel long distances for dialysis. Nevertheless, such centres are recommended at least for the initiation of treatment, when feasible.

Regular haemodialysis

The basic principles and procedures of haemodialysis in children are the same as in adults. However, haemodialysis of (small) children is associated with complications such as shunt and fistula failures, hypertension, cardiac failure, pulmonary oedema and encephalopathy caused by disequilibrium, when equipment and methods designed for adults are used.
Several modifications in technique and equipment are required for paediatric purposes.

Vascular access for regular dialysis treatment
Blood access is a major problem in paediatric patients. Some guidelines concerning placement of arteriovenous (AV) shunts and fistula can be offered. Application of adult type shunt material at proximal shunt sites (upper arm or groin) is often required for long-term access, but the use of adult size shunt material and shunt placement in proximal vessels leads to a high blood flow (500 ml/min or more) and increases the haemodynamic stress. A special paediatric shunt, using a smaller caliber vessel tip and Silastic tubing was developed by Kjellstrand (25). This shunt can be used in distal shunt sites. However, shunt survival in children is often reduced if paediatric shunt material is used, seldom exceeding 4 months. In very small children, weighing less than 10 kg, a proximal AV shunt or vein to vein cannulation are both useful alternatives (26). Newborns can be dialysed via the umbilical vessels.

In children weighing more than 20 kg, an AV fistula is the preferred vascular access for long-term haemodialysis; Brescia-Cimino fistulae, saphenous vein autografts (27), bovine carotid heterografts and polytetrafluoroethylene (PTFE) grafts have been used successfully (28). Brescia-Cimino fistulae in children require several months of maturation following surgery before they can be used for dialysis. Other fistulae are usable within a few days. If a Scribner shunt has to be placed in these children, adult shunt material can be used in distal shunt sites (peripheral radial artery, posterior tibial artery).

For smaller children, weighing less than 20 kg, construction of arteriovenous fistulae using microsurgical techniques is possible. Although excellent results with distal as well as proximal fistulae in small children have been reported, most centres are still reluctant to use arteriovenous fistulae in small children (29). Saphenous vein grafts placed between brachial artery and cephalic vein often lead to enormous vessel dilatation and aneurysm formation after long term use and the high blood flow through the fistula can induce congestive heart failure.

Choice of the dialyser and bloodlines
The dialyser should be carefully adapted to the size of the patient. Selection relates to the blood volume of the dialyser and blood lines and to the efficiency of the dialyser. The volume of the extracorporeal blood circuit should never exceed 10% of the patient's blood volume (BV = 80 ml/kg body weight). Larger shifts of blood between dialyser and patient will lead to hypotension during dialyses and fluid overload due to return of the extracorporeal blood after dialysis. Dialysers allowing careful regulation of ultrafiltration and with low compliance during application of negative pressure for ultrafiltration are preferred (30).

Special paediatric bloodlines with volumes varying between 35 and 75 ml are commercially available (Cobe, Gambro). Paediatric blood lines with 3 mm diameter tubing will restrict bloodflow to less than 75 ml/min. If higher blood flows are required special short blood lines with larger inner diameter will reduce extracorporeal blood volume (available from Bellco, Italy).

Although blood flow rates must be individually determined for each patient, general guidelines are proposed based on patient's weight. In very small children, weighing less than 10 kg, blood flow rates should not exceed 75 ml/min. In children weighing 10 to 20 kg blood flow rates should be less than 150 ml/min and in children weighing more than 20 kg blood flow rates up to 250 ml/min can be used. The patient's body weight or surface area and clinical condition should determine the clearance characteristics of the dialyser to be used.

To avoid the dialysis disequilibrium syndrome the urea clearance of the dialyser should not exceed 4 ml/min/kg.

To obtain efficient clearances of small molecules like urea and creatinine a ratio dialyser surface area/patient surface area of 0.75 has been proposed (31). In Table 4 characteristics of paediatric dialysers are summarised (the reader is also referred to Table 6 in chapter 5).

Table 4. Characteristics of disposable paediatric dialysers.

Dialysers	Priming volume (ml)	Compliance (ml/100 mg Hg)	Membrane surface area (m^2)	Urea clearance at Q_B of: 50 / 75 / 100 / 150 / 200 (ml/min) *
Gambro mini-minor PL	20	6	0,23	30 / 37 / 51 / — / —
Gambro minor PL	30	10	0,41	43 / 59 / 67 / 77 / 100
Secon 132	20	9	0,75	— / 61 / 82 / 110 / 125
Gambro Lundia 0,82 PL	70	—	0,68	— / 70 / 90 / 115 / 127
RP 5 (all layers)	170	17	1,03	— / 50 / 75 / 100 / 115
CDAK 0.6	53	0	0,60	— / 50 / 83 / 105 / 118
Asahi AM 09	55	0	0,60	38 / 41 / 58 / 71 / —
RP 6 (all layers)	150	—	1,00	— / — / 88 / 109 / —

* Data collected with *in vivo* studies at Q_D = 500 ml/min.

Management of regular dialysis in children
In patients weighing 10 to 15 kg and without marked fluid retention (less than 2.5% of body weight) between dialysis, the priming fluid is often transfused into the patient at the beginning of the procedure. In very small children weighing less than 10 kg, transfusion of the priming fluid into the patient is always required. Regular monitoring of body weight is needed and in very small children continuous weight recording during dialysis is imperative. Weighing equipment readings should be unaffected by normal movements of patients or dialysis equipment. Ultrafiltration should be planned carefully and any excessive fluid loss should be replaced all through the dialysis. For this purpose 0.9% saline, 20% mannitol or albumin solution should be used.

Therefore careful observation of the patient during dialysis is necessary, because in small children critical changes may appear, indicated by changes in vital signs. Regular control of vital signs is extremely important.

General heparinisation can be effected by administration of a bolus of 50 U heparin/kg body weight at the beginning of dialysis, followed by continuous infusion of 50 U heparin/kg/h. At the end of dialysis the blood is transfused back to the patient. Only small amounts of saline (less than 50 ml) are used for the washback procedure to reduce volume shifts between dialyser and patient.

The relatively high need for calories, protein and fluids related to the body weight will require more dialysis in children than in adults. Therefore, patients without significant residual kidney function are dialysed three times weekly or more. The duration of dialysis required to obtain a sufficient removal of small and middle molecules has empirically been determined and is based on arbitrary indices. Also the time required for adequate fluid removal using dialysers with small ultrafiltration coefficients influences dialysis prescription.

More recently urea kinetic modelling and the use of a dialysis index were proposed for the determination of dialysis schedules in children (32, 33). Urea kinetic modelling relates to the patient's urea generation and dialysis time is adapted in order to obtain predetermined levels of predialysis urea concentration. Using this method a significant reduction in dialysis time was obtained while adequacy of dialysis was maintained (32).

A dialysis index to assess dialysis time has also been proposed (33). The weekly hours of dialysis required are determined by the formula:

$$\text{Hours per week} = \frac{\text{D.S.A.}}{\text{B.S.A.}} \times \text{Index}.$$

The index lies between 13 and 18.
D.S.A.: Dialyser Surface Area in m^2
B.S.A.: patient's Body Surface Area in m^2
Individual adjustment of the dialysis time is influenced by regular determination of predialysis plasma urate levels.

Complications
If inappropriate dialysers are used, side effects related to 'unphysiology' of dialysis develop. Too efficient dialysis leads to a rapid fall in extracellular osmolality with shifting of water into the cells, especially the brain cells. This causes nausea, vomiting, headache and convulsions (disequilibrium syndrome). Convulsions are a relatively frequent complication of paediatric dialysis but can be avoided by restricting the efficiency of the dialyser and reducing the rate in fall of serum osmolality. Dialysers with poor compliance characteristics will cause large shifts of blood between dialyser and patient. During dialysis this may result in hypotension and shock preventing ultrafiltration and after dialysis acute volume overload with hypertension and pulmonary oedema may occur. Ultrafiltration during conventional dialysis has to be reduced to less than 5% of the total body weight to avoid side effects such as vomiting, abdominal pain, muscle cramps and hypotension, but sequential ultrafiltration and dialysis will allow greater ultrafiltration without side effects (34). Persistence or increase of hypertension during dialysis, despite adequate ultrafiltration is occasionally seen. The response of hypertension to ultrafiltration improves in most cases after bilateral nephrectomy.

Hyperkalaemia occurs more frequently in small children then in adults during catabolic states or from high potassium intake. The importance of high energy intake to suppress hyperkalaemia in these patients needs to be emphasised. Potassium cardiotoxicity is an important cause of death in paediatric dialysis patients. Recurrent pericarditis, despite adequate dialysis, is occasionally seen in children. These children are mostly hypertensive and are usually overhydrated. Cardiac tamponade seldom occurs.

Home dialysis

The estimated cost of home dialysis is about half the cost of hospital haemodialysis (35); in spite of this few children in Europe are placed on this mode of treatment and the numbers have been relatively constant over the last few years; 34, 42 and 34 children started home haemodialysis in 1977, 1978, and 1979 respectively. At the end of 1979, 148 of 1469 children in Europe receiving treatment for end stage renal failure were haemodialysed at home, 45% of the 148 were in the UK, 20% in France and 16% in the Fed. Republic of Germany (36). In one large centre in the UK, 28 of 75 children treated over a 10 year period had received home haemodialysis but the number starting treatment each year fell from 6 in the middle of the 10 year period to 1 each year at the end (37). The fall was thought to represent the increasing awareness that successful transplantation provided a better quality of life than long term haemodialysis which was reserved mainly for children in whom transplantation had failed. In many instances short term haemodialysis whilst awaiting transplant is easier and cheaper in hospital because expensive home alterations do not need to be undertaken. It is likely that continuous ambulatory peritoneal dialysis (CAPD) will further reduce the popularity of home haemodialysis even in those countries where home haemodialysis is currently practised.

The advantages of home dialysis are that it is much less expensive, especially if non disposable dialysers are used; the high initial dialyser cost is offset by many years of use, the dialyser being rebuilt every 1 to 2 weeks after three to six re-uses. Re-uses of disposable dialysers (38) clearly reduces this cost difference between disposable and nondisposable dialysers. Alterations in the home (see Chapter 24) also contribute to the initial cost and if the period on dialysis is likely to be short, a portable dialysis system (Redy System, see Chapter 17) which does not require expensive plumbing, may be preferable. The other main advantage for the patient is that it enables the child to receive his treatment at home with his family and to participate fully in family life which is clearly of fundamental importance for his social and emotional development. The psychological stress on the child is therefore reduced. Survival figures of children on home haemodialysis (84.6% at 5 years) are better than of children on hospital haemodialysis (66.3%) (EDTA registry 1979 [36]). This difference, however, can be attributed to selection though the quality of dialysis provided by well trained motivated parents to their individual child may be a factor along with better nutrition and physical rehabilitation in an child who is less anxious and leading a more normal life.

The rehabilitation of a child on home haemodialysis measured by frequency of school attendance at a normal school is superior on home haemodialysis (39, 40) because hospital dialysis must necessarily interfere with ordinary schooling unless arrangements are made for evening dialysis. Whilst growth on haemodialysis is generally less good than after transplantation, some children, at least on home dialysis, can grow normally and indeed catch up growth (37). The initial cost of conversion of the home is high and the other major disadvantage is the stress on the family (40). Twelve of 24 families with a child on home dialysis after one year exhibited signs of stress compared with 5, all with pre-existing other problems in addition to the child's illness, at the start of dialysis (40). In contrast, only 5 of the home patients were emotionally disturbed at the end of the first year compared with 14 of the 24 at the start. Nevertheless the families do not appear to be more disturbed than those with a child with another chronic disabling disease such as leukaemia (40). Clearly, the initial selection for home haemodialysis must include a careful evaluation of the family's ability to cope with the treatment and to support the youthful patient. It is also important that the relatives know that if the stress becomes too great an alternative to home dialysis will be available. Many children and their families including siblings, adapt very well to home dialysis and in one large series no instances of marital breakdown were recorded (40).

The dialysis room in the home should be near the centre of activity such as the living area. It should not be a remote bedroom, and the dialysis should preferably be undertaken in the late afternoon and evening. Overnight dialysis is best avoided because the child feels better and is more likely to go to school if he is able to sleep for some hours after dialysis (40). An important point is that the composition of domestic water (in particular the aluminium content) should be checked regularly. The composition of the water at the home is not necessarily the same as the water supplied to the hospital dialysis unit. Regular attendance, usually once a month, at the centre are required for medical assessment, advice and support. A telephone advisory service should be available at all times either by a senior nurse or a doctor. Technical support should be available during normal working hours.

In case of problems or complications admission to the dialysis centre is advisable. Arrangements for holidays with or without the family can make a considerable contribution to psychological well being. The full supporting facilities of a children's unit such as a paediatrician, a social worker, a dietician and a paediatric psychiatrist are important both in selecting and supporting children on home haemodialysis. Generally, single parent families are unsuitable because of the strain involved; a good marital relationship is vital. Usually, one parent and the child are trained in hospital, but in time both parents contribute to the treatment. The insertion of fistula needles cause problems though many children will undertake this themselves. Home haemodialysis can be undertaken easily by most paediatric units and provides an efficient, safe and rewarding treatment for many children, their families and the staff of the unit.

Regular peritoneal dialysis

Regular peritoneal dialysis has been extensively used in the treatment of ESRD in children and has been shown as effective as regular haemodialysis for control of uraemia and its complications (41–43). Only a small number of children were treated by this method up to 1979. This number increased with the use of CAPD: in 1980 5% of all children on regular dialysis in Europe were undergoing CAPD (44).

Intermittent peritoneal dialysis (IPD)
Technique. IPD is performed through an indwelling Silastic catheter, tailored to the size of the child. This catheter has one or two Dacron cuffs. The catheter is inserted surgically through a small laparotomy. Omentectomy is performed at the time of cannula insertion in small children because they are more susceptible to obstruction of the catheter by omental fringes. After insertion of the catheter, dialysis is started immediately and continued without interruption for 4 to 6 days in order to avoid early catheter obstruction by fibrin plugs. Dialysis is subsequently performed two or more times per week with a duration of 40 to 60 h per week according to blood chemical concentrations and fluid balance.

The volume for one exchange is calculated on a body weight basis: 20 to 30 ml/kg at the start, progressively increasing to 40 to 50 ml/kg. Automatic or semi-automatic cycling machines performing at least one cycle per hour are used. Dialysis solution contains sodium 135 to 140 mmol/l, chloride 100 to 110 mmol/l, calcium 1 to 1.75 mmol/l (4–7 mg/dl), acetate 30 to 45 mmol/l, and dextrose (anhydrous) 83 mmol/l (1.5%). Potassium is added (2 mmol/l) to the solution if the predialysis serum potassium level is less than 4 mmol/l. A hypertonic solution containing 235 mmol/l of anhydrous dextrose (4.25%) is used for one or more exchanges if required for adequate extracellular fluid volume control. Dietary recommendations include a normal intake of protein (1 to 2.5 g/kg BW according to age) and a limitation of sodium, potassium and water intake.

Results. Relatively few reports on children treated by IPD are available (41–43). These data show that IPD is an effective form of therapy for chronic uraemia in children but it requires a much longer dialysis time than haemodialysis. However, the low dialysance avoids any disequilibrium syndrome. BUN and serum creatinine values remain higher with peritoneal dialysis than with haemodialysis. Plasma proteins usually remain normal, but in small children substantial protein loss leading to moderate hypoalbuminaemia has been noticed. Haematocrits tend to be higher in children on IPD than in those on haemodialysis. Linear growth seems to be similar on IPD and on haemodialysis (42, 43).

Complications. During treatment with IPD complications may occur and include obstruction of the catheter which may be reversible and can sometimes be remedied by changing the patients position, by using small enemas and by flushing the catheter with heparin solutions. But often the obstruction is permanent and the catheter has to be replaced. Mean catheter survival has been reported as short as 10 weeks (42) and as long as 16 months (43). Other technical complications include dialysate leakage around the catheter and extrusion of the catheter. Massive recurrent hydrothorax, a rare complication, constitutes a contra-indication to continue IPD.

Infection of the peritoneum is the major complication. Infection is more frequent and severe in patients treated at the hospital than in the home (42). This point suggests that long term IPD ought to be performed only at home. Progressive fibrosis of the peritoneum had been reported in adult patients after infections, with loss of permeability of the peritoneal membrane (45). One of us (M.B.) has observed personally a child with fibrosis of the peritoneal membrane, without previous peritonitis but possibly related to the frequent use of hypertonic dialysate solution.

Indications. IPD is an acceptable alternative to haemodialysis when vascular access is not available for a prolonged period of time.

Continuous ambulatory peritoneal dialysis (CAPD)

Only recently has CAPD been applied to children. In 1980, 56 children treated by CAPD in Europe were reported to the Registry of the EDTA (23).

Technique. CAPD is performed through an indwelling catheter surgically inserted as described above for IPD. Immediately following the insertion, the patient is dialysed with an automatic cycling machine for 4 to 6 days and subsequently CAPD is started on the basis of four exchanges per day. Exchange volume is progressively increased from 30 to 50 ml/kg within a few weeks. The parents are trained to perform CAPD at home (see also Chapter 24). Regular attendances, at least once a month, at the dialysis centre are required.

The patients are instructed in the need of a high protein intake (120% of recommended dietary allowances) and of restriction of fluid and sodium intake (at least at the start of treatment).

Results. Clearances of small and middle molecules with CAPD are higher than with IPD (see Chapter 21), but BUN and plasma creatinine values are higher than in patients on regular haemodialysis. Patients on CAPD need less phosphate binders and exchange resins than those on haemodialysis. Haematocrits are also higher than in regular haemodialysis patients. The peritoneal protein loss is particularly marked in small children and often leads to hypoproteinaemia and hypoalbuminaemia. Fluid removal with hypertonic solutions is also less efficient in very young children; this is probably due to enhanced dextrose absorption (46). Shortening of dwell times when hypertonic solutions are used and an increase of the number of exchanges per day may improve fluid removal.

Decreased plasma parathormone levels and improvement of osteodystrophy was found in CAPD patients receiving 25(OH)D$_3$ medication (47, 48). Normal growth was found in some patients but catch-up was lacking (49). Rehabilitation of children on CAPD is excellent and full time school attendance is frequently achieved. Physical activity could be almost normal, but some limitations, in order to protect the cutaneous exit site of the catheter, are recommended. The burden of bag exchange is important but is easier to tolerate when both parents are involved in the procedure, and for this reason there are in children very few examples of abandonment.

Complications. Leakage around the catheter, extrusion and obstruction of the catheter are relatively rare complications of CAPD. The primary complication of CAPD is recurrent peritonitis. An incidence of one episode per 8 to 12 months has been reported. Early recognition and treatment generally leads to prompt recovery. Some patients are more susceptible to infection than others. Technical progress and a better selection of patients could certainly decrease the incidence of infection.

Indications. CAPD should be considered as the treatment of choice in selected patients (and selected families). In these patients it should be effected only during a limited period of time (1 to 2 years), e.g. while waiting for a kidney transplant. A strong motivation and full cooperation of well informed parents is required for successful CAPD treatment. CAPD is also an alternative if regular haemodialysis is no longer possible. It should be considered in patients with no vascular access site left, in patients with poor dialysis tolerance and in children with severe psychological problems related to the haemodialysis procedure or to dietary restrictions.

CAPD should be considered as the treatment of choice for patients with haemorrhagic diseases and for patients at risk for increased intracranial pressure.

Peritoneal dialysis is sometimes the only possible treatment method for end stage renal failure in very small children (less than 18 months). However CAPD does not allow adequate regulation of body fluids in these children and for this purpose IPD is probably more efficient.

Although CAPD allows sufficient control of biochemical abnormalities and full rehabilitation it is still too early to predict the longterm results of this treatment in children.

SURVIVAL AND CAUSES OF DEATH

Dialysis in combination with transplantation has evolved from an experimental treatment to an accepted form of treatment of end stage renal disease in children. A recent report of the Paediatric Registry of the EDTA recorded a 3 year survival of 75.5% for hospital- and 90.8% for home-haemodialysis (36).

Age differences are apparent: At 3 years, survival on hospital dialysis was 63%, 70% and 78% for the age groups 0 to 5, 5 to 10 and 10 to 15 years respectively.

For long term survivors who were treated with renal replacement therapy for 8 years or more, survival was 51%. Patient survival on hospital dialysis was significantly better in centres specialised in the treatment of children (Figure 2 [49]).

Most causes of death (70%) in haemodialysed children are cardiovascular in origin. Improvement of treatment will further reduce mortality due to cerebrovascular accidents and hypertensive cardiac failure.

The more favourable results in specialised centres are due to a decrease of causes of death such as hyperkalaemia, cardiac arrest, cerebrovascular accidents and cachexia. Careful integration of dialysis and transplantation will further improve survival in children with end stage renal disease.

MEDICAL PROBLEMS

Growth failure and endocrine disorders

Growth retardation is a common though not inevitable consequence of chronic renal failure. Normal growth is observed in some pre- and more post-pubertal children both before and whilst being maintained on chronic dialysis (37), though this is rare. Figure 3 shows the height percentiles of children starting dialysis and it is clear that many children are already small by the time dialysis is initiated (50). Figure 4 shows the change in height

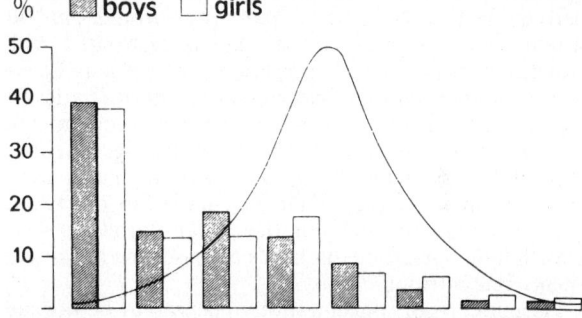

Figure 3. Height percentiles (PERC) at start of haemodialysis or at first transplant. The curve indicates the distribution of normal percentiles (EDTA Registry 1974 [50], with permission).

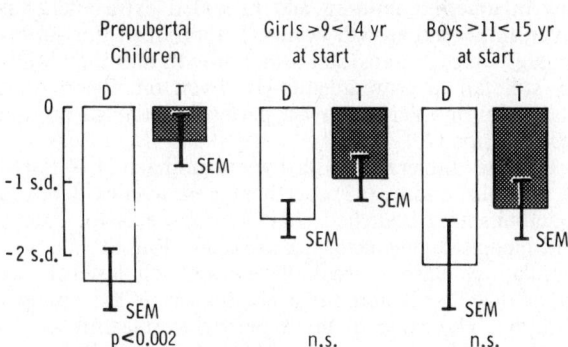

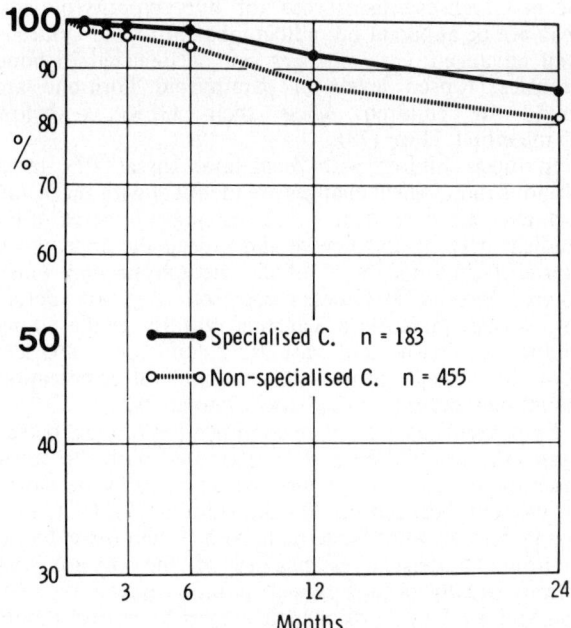

Figure 2. Patient survival on hospital haemodialysis (1976-1978) in specialised paediatric centres compared with non-paediatric centres (EDTA Registry 1978 [49], with permission).

Figure 4. Change in standard deviation of height from mean of normal children of the same chronological age, during treatment by haemodialysis (D) or transplantation (T) in children treated for more than 5 years (EDTA Registry 1978 [49], with permission).
Plain bars indicate before treatment, stippled bars after treatment.
s.d. = standard deviation from normal
SEM = standard error of the mean of the group

with dialysis or transplantation in children treated for more than 5 years: the poor growth on dialysis is obvious (49). Many of these children will reach adult life dwarfed (36) and this causes considerable psychological stress both to the children and their parents. Skeletal maturation is often retarded by at least 2 to 6 years and should be assessed regularly (51, 52). Pubertal development is delayed (23, 53) and should also be charted regularly (54); pubertal delay correlates with the retardation in bone age (39, 55). This delay in bone age is of some practical importance because these children continue to grow, albeit slowly, at an age when normal children have ceased to grow and final height may be better than anticipated (39). Height must be measured accurately using a precise apparatus (56).

The possible causes of growth retardation have been reviewed (57-59) and there are striking anthropometric and biochemical similarities between protein energy malnutrition and chronic azotaemia. There is little evidence that uraemia itself inhibits growth, though nitrogen retention and the accumulation of uraemic toxins derived from protein intake may affect protein anabolism (60-62). Renal osteodystrophy is associated with growth retardation and hyperparathyroidism may be especially important (see below). Growth hormone levels are generally high in renal failure (63) but somatomedin concentrations are reduced (64) though the figures partly depend on the methodology and normal figures have also been reported (65). Following initiation of regular dialysis somatomedin levels rise which correlates with growth (66). Somatomedin levels are also low in protein energy malnutrition.

Plasma cortisol concentration appeared to be normal in children with renal failure (67). FSH and LH levels appear adequate in uraemic children. Thyroid function is within the low normal range with depressed TSH levels (68), except in children with cystinosis who frequently develop hypothyroidism with increased TSH levels (69).

There is evidence that spontaneous energy intake is low in uraemic children and provided extra energy is given improved growth occurs (58) although this unfortunately does not ensure normal growth and the majority still fail to grow adequately. Even on liberal diets plasma amino acids show a pattern similar to protein malnutrition (70).

Glucose intolerance with hyperinsulinaemia is found in uraemic children (63) and there is indirect evidence of metabolism of branched chain amino acids for energy and increased gluconeogenesis (62, 66). Raised values of circulating plasma triglycerides and cholesterol are found (63, 71, 72) and these are higher in the younger children. The cause of the hypertriglyceridaemia is obscure but there is evidence of both deficient clearing of plasma triglycerides and increased production. There is no evidence that the use of liberal diets is associated with increased hyperlipidaemia but rather that an adequate nutritional status lowers the circulating lipids. It has been suggested that the hypertriglyceridaemia results in part from the inability to metabolise carbohydrates (63) as in diabetes mellitus and this suggests the need to ensure energy requirements adequately from fat, particularly polyunsaturated fat, rather than giving carbohydrate supplements (73).

Protein turnover is reduced in uraemic children with both reduced synthesis and breakdown, though the latter may be increased with the stress of fasting or infection (60, 62); net protein anabolism is reduced. This may be partially linked to altered energy metabolism, though there is evidence for a direct effect of uraemic toxins on protein synthesis. Adequate dialysis is associated with improvement in protein turnover (74) and nitrogen balance improves also in uraemic undialysed children placed on very low protein diets supplemented with essential amino acids or keto acids (62).

Anabolic steroids have been used in a pilot study of boys on regular haemodialysis and improved growth occurred without causing a rapid advance in bone maturation and without evidence of other toxic effects apart from hepatic dysfunction in one child which was readily reversible when the treatment was withdrawn. Further studies of the use of low dose anabolic steroids to improve protein synthesis in uraemic children on dialysis would appear reasonable.

Osteodystrophy

Renal osteodystrophy is common in children with chronic renal failure (75, 76). The occurrence is probably enhanced by the rapid turnover rate of bone associated with remodelling and growth. In addition to the changes which occur in adults (see Chapter 35) the metaphyseal growth zone is affected and abnormalities similar to genuine (nutritional) rickets are seen on radiographs. Osteodystrophy is especially common in children with congenital renal disease leading to renal insufficiency early in life (77). Whilst evidence of osteomalacia (or rickets) and osteitis fibrosa (or hyperparathyroidism) may not be apparent on radiographs until renal failure is well advanced, early changes can be detected in bone biopsies. Raised levels of parathyroid hormone are found in children when their GFR is below 45 ml/min/1.73 m^2 (78).

In most children with renal bone disease the most obvious radiological changes are identical with the X ray changes caused by rickets, but secondary hyperparathyroidism may be also severe and indeed the appearance of rickets in radiographs of the metaphysis may mask osteitis fibrosa (79). Unless recognised early, bone deformities can appear with alarming rapidity in the young infant. Soft tissue and vascular calcifications are less common though corneal and conjunctival calcification sometimes occur (76) (See also Chapter 38).

Epiphyseolysis is a severe complication of renal osteodystrophy in children and is associated with the accumulation of woven bone and fibrous tissue in the radiolucent zone between ossification centres (79). It is associated with advanced osteitis fibrosa. When treated with vitamin D derivatives healing of the metaphyseal lesions usually occurs, though parathyroidectomy may be required. Later, orthopaedic surgery to correct deformities of the metaphyseo-diaphyseal region may be required. Attempts to stabilise slipped epiphysis by screws etc. should be discouraged even though the epiphysis, especially in the femoral region, may consolidate outside the normal position (79).

Avascular necrosis of bone, especially of the head of the femur is a well recognised complication occurring after renal transplantation but can also occur in children on dialysis. It is clearly undesirable to perform femoral head replacement operations in small children but a femoral osteotomy is often succesful in alleviating pain and abolishing the limping in children with symptoms. Early mobilisation after surgery is desirable and the operation is tolerated well as long as it is undertaken after the osteodystrophy has been suppressed with vitamin D derivatives. Long terms results of the operation are not yet established. Whilst renal osteodystrophy can be controlled in children on long term dialysis and the radiological abnormalities of rickets disappear with vitamin D derivatives, residual metaphyseal irregularities and periosteal erosions are common (53).

Treatment of renal osteodystrophy in children on regular dialysis requires supplementation with vitamin D derivatives to heal rickets and suppress hyperparathyroidism and implicates the control of plasma phosphate by dialysis, diet and oral phosphate binders. Daily doses of 0.15 to 1 µg of $1,25(OH)_2D_3$ or 1 to 3 µg of $1\alpha(OH)D_3$ in children with chronic renal failure will promote normalisation of plasma calcium and parathyroid hormone concentrations and heal the bone lesions (80, 81). Hypercalcaemia is a major risk but usually responds rapidly when the treatment is stopped. Whilst $1,25(OH)_2D_3$ may be more effective than $25(OH)D_3$ in suppressing hyperparathyroidism, there is some evidence that it is less effective in promoting bone mineralisation and in the treatment of rickets (82); in fact osteomalacia may progress in an occasional child on dialysis being treated with $1,25(OH)_2D_3$. Healing then may occur when $25(OH)D_3$ is added. Doses of 50 to 200 µg/day of $25(OH)D_3$ promote healing of osteodystrophy but when hypercalcaemia occurs it is more prolonged and therefore more dangerous than with $1,25(OH)_2D_3$ or $1\alpha(OH)D_3$. In addition to vitamin D therapy an adequate intake of calcium (0,5 to 1 g per day) should be ensured by diet manipulations or by oral supplements of calcium gluconate. Commercially available supplements include Calcium Sandoz syrup which is preferable to the effervescent tablets which contain sodium. Phosphate intake should be restricted and with adequate dialysis, predialysis plasma phosphate concentrations can be maintained within the normal range. Phosphate binders such as aluminium hydroxide or calcium carbonate are often not required. However, it may be that phosphate restriction should be more rigorous when attempting to ameliorate secondary hyperparathyroidism and to lower plasma parathyroid hormone concentrations to normal, though evidence for this is not yet clear.

The dialysate calcium concentration chosen is usually 1.75 mmol/l (7 mg/dl) but this depends on a number of factors such as dietary calcium intake, plasma calcium concentration and vitamin D intake. Parathyroidectomy is sometimes required to control osteitis fibrosa if suppression with vitamin D fails and may be considered even in infants. Auto transplantation of a small portion of parathyroid tissue into the brachioradialis muscle has been recommended so that some parathyroid function is maintained and long term vitamin D supplements can be avoided (83). It is not yet clear whether vitamin D supplements should be given in the absence of radiological evidence of renal osteodystrophy.

While bone biopsy changes are always evident and raised parathyroid hormone levels are frequent, the risk of inducing hypercalcaemia has to be considered. It does, however, seem rational to attempt suppression of parathyroid hormone levels especially if they are very high and therefore low dose treatment with $1\alpha(OH)D_3$ or $1,25(OH)_2D_3$ seems rational even in the absence of radiological changes; bone biopsies are not routinely recommended because of the unavoidable trauma of the intervention. Clearly when maintenance treatment with vitamin D is undertaken plasma calcium concentrations should be monitored at regular intervals. There is no doubt that renal osteodystrophy is a potent cause of growth retardation in children on regular haemodialysis. Adequate treatment with vitamin D supplements is often associated with increased growth (84) though this is not invariably the case (85). Continued poor growth in the presence of unsuppressible hyperparathyroidism may respond favourably to parathyroidectomy.

Anaemia (see also Chapter 32)

Children on regular haemodialysis are often profoundly anaemic and require regular transfusions to maintain haemoglobin levels above 5 g/dl; the mean haematocrit in children on haemodialysis was $19.3\% \pm 2.9$ (40). The transfusion requirements may in the past have been responsible for the better graft survival in children compared with adults (39). Prepubertal children are more anaemic than pubertal children (Table 5) and require

Table 5. Anaemia in paediatric patients treated with regular haemodialysis (EDTA Registry 1979 [36]).

	Prepubertal			Pubertal		
	Number	Hb/g/dl*	mmol/l	Number	Hb/g/dl*	mmol/l
Total	67	6.4±1.01	3.95	92	7.20±1.91	4.44
Not transfused	12 (17%)	6.8±0.89	4.20	32 (35%)	8.20±2.12	5.06 $p<0.05$
Nephrectomy	16	6.3±1.18	3.89	14	6.80±2.13	4.19
No nephrectomy	43	6.5±0.97	4.01	72	7.25±1.91	4.47 $p<0.02$

* Mean (±1 SD).

more transfusions. At these low levels of haemoglobin no effect of nephrectomy was noted in the EDTA Registry survey but this does not exclude the possibility that nephrectomy will further aggravate anaemia in the individual child.

Many factors probably contribute to the severe anaemia in children but the most important is probably the loss of blood in the dialyser; as noted previously the volume of the dialyser and the blood lines in relation to blood volume of the patient is greater in a child and therefore the blood losses are relatively larger.

Intestinal losses are also an important contributing factor and 70% of calculated blood loss in a child on dialysis occurs via this route (86); in the same study a close inverse correlation was found between daily blood loss and the packed red cell volume. It is, therefore, important to restrict losses from repeated blood sampling, and the blood left in the dialyser and blood lines should be carefully returned to the patient. One of the main advantages of CAPD in children may well be the less severe anaemia.

Occasionally a haemolytic anaemia has occurred due to copper, nitrite or chloramines in the water supply (87). Hypersplenism can occur (88) and a persistent low white cell and platelet count and a palpable spleen (though this sign is not invariably present) suggest the need for red cell survival and splenic uptake studies; splenectomy can lead to an increase in haemoglobin (2). While bilateral nephrectomy should be avoided when possible, severe hypertension necessitating vigorous fluid removal with dialysis can lead to anorexia and malnutrition. In these circumstances bilateral nephrectomy can lead to correction of hypertension, a better nutritional status and a rise in haemoglobin. Iron supplements should not be given routinely in children receiving frequent transfusions because of the danger of iron overload. They should only be considered if the iron stores or serum ferritin levels are low (89, 90). No response to anabolic steroids was noted in a study of growth promotion by anabolic steroids (91).

Cardiovascular complications

Hypertension in children on regular haemodialysis usually responds to increased salt and water removal by ultrafiltration during dialysis. Inadequate dialysis with dialysers that are too small or too large (leading to hypotension during dialysis and hypertension after wash back) is the commonest cause of persistent hypertension in children treated by regular dialysis.

Sequential ultrafiltration and dialysis (see Chapters 19 and 28) usually allows sufficient fluid removal during dialysis without hypotension in a child who persistently develops hypotension during conventional dialysis, necessitating saline or plasma infusion to stabilise blood pressure and leading to hypertension after the dialysis.

Nonetheless the occasional child does tend to develop hypotension during dialysis with nausea and abdominal pain. The mechanism of this hypotension is incompletely understood but too rapid reduction in plasma and extracellular fluid osmolality leading to shifting of fluid into the cells and hypovolaemia seem to be causal factors. Failure of normal peripheral vasoconstriction to maintain blood pressure during dialysis may be due to defective catecholamine or renin release. Rapid removal of renin or pressoramines or loss of response to these hormones may also contribute. Acetate toxicity has also been incriminated.

A vicious circle of hypertension between dialyses, high predialysis blood urea concentrations, excessive salt and water intake but poor food intake leading to malnutrition, hypercatabolism and hypotension during dialysis associated with the need for increased salt and water removal, can easily develop. This can be managed by extra attention to nutrition using energy supplements and even nasoenteric feeding combined with frequent short dialysis sessions with sequential ultrafiltration and dialysis until the patient's condition stabilises.

In occasional children severe hypertension is due to renal ischaemia and hyperreninaemia. This is especially common in children with renal failure due to the haemolytic uraemic syndrome. Even excessive salt and water removal does not control blood pressure but results in nausea, anorexia and lethargy. Bilateral nephrectomy may be required to improve the child's health, appetite and activity.

Alternatively, if possible recovery of renal function is envisaged, blood pressure may be controlled with vasodilators such as minoxidil and beta blocking agents or with captopril, though smooth dialysis is more difficult in children on hypotensive medication. Nonetheless such measures may be useful, for recovery of renal function after 14 months on haemodialysis has been reported in a child with the haemolytic uraemic syndrome (37).

Chronic hypertension, uraemia and malnutrition all contribute to impaired cardiac performance in children on haemodialysis but anaemia and, in some children, hypercirculation caused by arteriovenous fistulae, are of especial importance (92). Systolic time intervals and echocardiography have been used in infants to assess myocardial function. They disclosed appreciably reduced myocardial performance in children on dialysis (93).

Cardiac arrest, pulmonary oedema and other cardiac catastrophies are among the causes of death in children on dialysis and, therefore, frequent cardiac assessment is an important part of the management in paediatric dialysis.

Good dialysis, correction of hypertension, management of anaemia, attention to nutrition with reduction of hyperlipidaemia, and monitoring of the cardiac effects of shunts and fistulae are all of importance for prevention of cardiovascular complications.

DIET

The high energy requirements relative to body weight of children have been discussed earlier and it is tempting to speculate that the impact of uraemia on the nutritional status of the child is more drastic because the energy

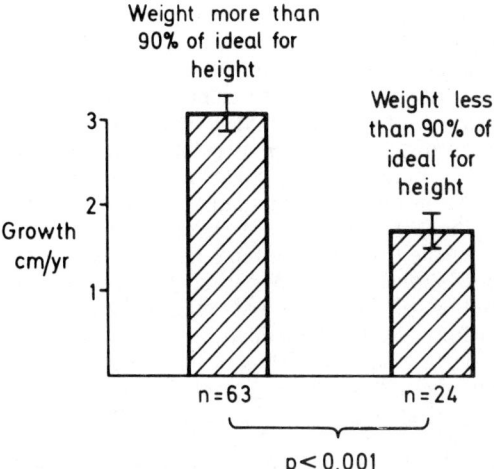

Figure 5. Growth in dialysed prepubertal children in relation to weight (mean ±1 SEM) (EDTA Registry 1977 [39], with permission).

deficit caused by the anorexia of renal failure is greater (94). It is important to ensure whenever possible an adequate food intake in children on dialysis. Figure 5 shows the difference in growth between prepubertal children on dialysis in whom weight was normal for height compared with children who were undernourished (39).

Protein intake should be at least 1 g per kg body weight per day of first class protein, if possible more (95). Total nitrogen intake can be reduced by feeding essential amino acid supplements (61, 96) but this is expensive and involves prescription of special diets. There is little or no evidence as yet that amino acid supplements added to an adequate protein intake in children contribute either to biochemical improvement or increased growth (97). Unfortunately, children do not respond well to special diets and if their eating habits are to stringently limited, the response is often a refusal to eat.

If the child is dialysed adequately (37), at least three times per week, a more or less normal diet can be permitted. Nutritional intake of each individual child should be evaluated at intervals and compared with recommended intakes (96) for children of the same age together with assessment of the clinical condition and the biochemical data.

An experienced dietician taking care of the patient can individually encourage the child to make necessary adjustments in protein, sodium, and potassium, intake within the limits of a normal family diet and in accordance with the child's own preferences. Extra energy supplements consisting of fat (double cream, polyunsaturated oil emulsions) and carbohydrate (caloreen, calonutrin) flavoured to taste and consumed between the meals are useful both to increase total energy intake and to diminish appetite: this prevents the urge to eat other foods with an undesirable high content of salt and water. Plasma lipids should be monitored and if undesirably raised the diet should be adjusted. Adequate energy and protein intake should be maintained whilst reducing the proportion of carbohydrate in the diet. Only fluid intake is strictly limited, though excessive weight gain between dialyses is usually primarily due to excessive sodium intake. This should be suspected if the child is normonatraemic. If excessive thirst and hypertension are encountered, in the presence of a reasonable sodium intake the possibility of hyperreninaemia should be suspected.

An adequate calcium intake should be ensured and, with adequate dialysis and proper dietary policy, hyperphosphataemia will rarely be encountered so that oral phosphate binders are usually not necessary to maintain normal plasma phosphate concentrations. Whether a very strict control of phosphate intake would lower plasma parathyroid hormone concentrations and be associated with better growth is not yet known.

Little information concerning trace metals is available but copper levels appeared to be adequate; plasma zinc concentrations are low in some patients (98), though they appeared to be normal in the paediatric haemodialysis population in the unit of one of the authors.

No study linking plasma zinc and growth in uraemic children has been published as yet.

In conclusion, low somatomedin levels, hyperparathyroidism with renal osteodystrophy and protein energy malnutrition have been implicated of causing uraemic growth retardation, but without definite evidence: the cause is still uncertain and may be multifactorial.

The latter two can be influenced by careful management of the child on dialysis. Special attention has to be given to adequate nutrition and to adequate protein intake in particular. When this is achieved, worthwhile growth is obtainable in at least some patients (98, 99).

PSYCHOSOCIAL PROBLEMS

Optimal functioning of a dialysis programme for children not only necessitates appropriate medical and technical knowledge but simultaneous attention must be paid to the emotional and social impact of the treatment on the juvenile patients and their families. A team including physicians, nurses, social workers, teachers and a psychologist should be available to cope with the problems relating to the child and his disease (100–105).

The child and his disease

Even before the beginning of regular dialysis treatment the behaviour of young patients is influenced by their longstanding disease. At this stage the children are invariably depressed. Mutilation in conception and representation of their body image frequently prevail. The children are preoccupied with their illness and show evidence of a clear consciousness of death. They resent having their lives full of unpleasant restrictions.

The relationships of these children are characterised by withdrawal from social contacts and increasing dependence on their parents. Dialysis adds another important stress to the patient and adaptation at the beginning of treatment is often difficult. Anxiety, that may be either obvious or repressed will influence adaptation to the treatment. When the child's health improves drastic changes in attitudes and behaviour are frequently seen. The child becomes more active and less frightened. However, during the following months frequently recurring patterns of maladjustment emerge characterised by passivity, refuge in sleep, inaccessibility to others, anorexia and vomiting.

Some children react with excessive dependence, others become over-demanding or react with aggressive behaviour. Complications and necessary surgical procedures will influence the incidence of these setbacks.

The families

The parents, depressed by the problems of a child with chronic life threatening disease, often put too high expectations on the effect of dialysis. Therefore, if problems increase or even persist important reactions may occur, such as aggressive behaviour to the staff, lack of cooperation and unreasonable demands on the medical team. Faced with the problems of repetitive dialysis, the entire family is confronted with a series of stresses and demands that will influence the relationships both within and beyond the family. Daily life will be disturbed by the demanding programme: dialysis, diet, medication, restrictions of activity and hospitalisations of the child. The stresses and burdens that this situation places upon the family will accentuate personal problems of members of the family such as psychosomatic diseases, danger of family breakdown and relational problems of the parents at their work. The other children in the family may experience various degrees of emotional deprivation.

The dialysis team

The dialysis team participates with parents and children in all emotional problems generated during treatment. The demands of meeting the emotional needs of the patients and their families, however, often extend beyond the capacity of the team members. This sometimes leads to reactions of withdrawal into regressive patterns in members of the team and disruption of communications within the group. Assistance by a paediatric psychiatrist will be necessary in crisis situations. Team discussions may be helpful to place problems in perspective and will allow team members to support each other at times of stress.

REHABILITATION

The aim of regular dialysis treatment of paediatric patients is not only to prolong life but also to provide a basis for normal, physical, social and intellectual development. Rehabilitation should already be initiated during conservative treatment of the youthful chronic renal failure patient. In order to calm down the patient and his relatives, to prevent anxiety and to provide the basis for a normal life as much as possible, the child and his parents should receive adequate guidance. Successful rehabilitation during dialysis largely depends on this support. Competent guidance is already essential before the onset of the final stage of renal failure arises. Full information should be given during this period and there should be sufficient time and facilities for constant communication. Adequate guidance can only be given by a harmonious team consisting of paediatric nephrologists, nurses, dieticians, a childrens psychiatrist or a psychologist, social workers, teachers and other educational personnel.

Proper school facilities and arrangements for leisure times and holidays should be provided. A normal school programme should be attained whenever possible. However, the time lost on recurrent dialysis may be a hindrance. In this respect home dialysis should be encouraged.

A teacher should be attached to the hospital team to provide tutoring during dialysis treatment. At the same time he should establish a direct liaison between the hospital and the school in order to achieve the best possible educational program for each child. Instruction during dialysis also emphasises the importance of a proper educational programme.

Physical activities need not be restricted during leisure time although anaemia may be a limiting factor. Normal leisure times should be encouraged within the child's own possibilities to overcome the natural resistance of overprotective relatives.

School attendance has to be assessed regularly. The EDTA Registry reported in 1980 on school attendance of 317 children treated by dialysis in specialised centres (24). Details of this analysis are shown in Table 6. Hospital dialysis obviously interferes with full time school attendance. It is true that full time school attendancy increased from 17% after one year to 55% after 3 years of dialysis in the hospital. But in this respect home dialysis should be preferred: full time school attendance in this group was as high as 89%. Rehabilitation of long-term dialysis patients is more difficult to assess because all surveys include a combination of dialysed and transplanted patients. Nevertheless interesting results have

Table 6. School attendance of children treated in specialised paediatric centres in Europe (EDTA Registry 1980 [23]).

	Hospital dialysis	Home dialysis
Full time schooling	31%	89%
Regular part-time schooling	41%	8%
Irregular part-time schooling	16%	1.5%
Tuition at home	4%	1.5%
No schooling	7%	—
Unable to receive schooling	1%	—

been reported from a recent study carried out by the EDTA on rehabilitation of patients less than 15 years of age at the start of treatment who were restudied ten years later (104). It appeared that 70% of the survivors had a satisfactory employment and that a large number had left their parental homes to live their own lives, even raising their own families. An analogous study led to similar conclusions (105). Nevertheless even better rehabilitation was obtained after succesfull transplantation. Social failures were especially related to poor school attendance in the primary school period (103). This last point emphasises that adequate attention to teaching and education should have high priority. Teaching programmes should be undertaken at an early stage.

PRACTICAL DIRECTIVES FOR HAEMODIALYSIS IN CHILDREN

Preparation for dialysis

Before the initiation of dialysis the procedure has to be explained to the child by drawings and by attending a dialysis session of other children.

Blood access in the form of an AV fistula is created several months prior to the start of dialysis. Serum creatinine values are frequently used to determine the time of fistula creation and subsequently the start of dialysis (Table 7).

The rate of deterioration of renal function must also be considered when deciding on the time of fistula creation. In children selected for maintenance peritoneal dialysis an AV fistula is also constructed in order to create an immediately usable vascular access for haemodialysis if peritoneal dialysis fails.

Preparations for home dialysis are initiated at the time of fistula creation if the patient and his family are willing to perform the treatment at home.

Dietary prescriptions and controls for adequate nutrition are essential. The aim of nutritional therapy is to supply adequate calories and restrict intake of protein, sodium, potassium and phosphorus. Recommended intakes for children on dialysis treatment (106) are presented in Table 8.

Regular assessment of the nutritional status of the child is required. Cumulative interdialytic weight gain from excessive fluid intake should be distinguished from 'real' weight gain from an increase of the child's body mass.

The child should learn his own responsibility for his interdialytic weight increase. Calorie and protein intakes are assessed using diet surveys recorded during similar interdialytic periods at monthly intervals. Calculation of the urea generation rate can be used to check adherence to the prescribed protein intake (107, 108).

Dialysis techniques

Fistula needles. Gauge 18 to 14 are required to obtain an adequate bloodflow. Single needle technique allows adequate dialysis even in small children with only a short vessel area available for needle insertion (2–3 cm).

Primary nursing improves the quality of care for paediatric patients. Individual nurse-patient allocation not only provides more efficient technical work, but also improves patient's adaptation to treatment (109, 110).

The play-leader and teacher have to plan a playing and educational programme for each patient during the time spent on dialysis.

A basic rule: adjust each dialysis according to the individual requirement of each child.

Estimation of 'dry or ideal' body weight is essential. Percentile cards should be used to determine the ideal weight according to the body height and build of the child. If the patient thrives and grows and the muscle mass increases, the ideal body weight also increases.

Table 7. Fistula creation and start of dialysis.

Age (yrs)	Fistula creation Serum creatinine	Start of dialysis Serum creatinine
1–5	354 µmol/l–530 µmol/l (40–60 mg/l)	620 µmol/l–708 µmol/l (70–80 mg/l)
5–10	442 µmol/l–620 µmol/l (50–70 mg/l)	708 µmol/l–797 µmol/l (80–90 l)
10–15	530 µmol/l–708 µmol/l (60–80 mg/l)	797 µmol/l–885 µmol/l (90–100 ml/l)

Creatinine µmol l → mg/dl: multiply by 0.0113.

Table 8. Recommended food and electrolyte intake for paediatric dialysis patients (106).

Body weight kg	Protein g/kg body weight	Sodium g/day	Sodium mmol/day	Potassium g/day	Potassium mmol/day	Calories per kg body weight
<15	2	0.5–1	8.5–17	0.5–1	7–13	100
15–40	1.5–1	1–2	17–34	1–2	13–26	90–65
>40	1	2–3	34–51	2	26	65–40

Assessment of dry weight is sometimes difficult in children with hypertension. Measurements of extracellular water and plasma renin activity are used to determine if ultrafiltration is required.

The choice of the correct size of the dialyser is based on a simple formula:

$$\frac{DSA}{PSA} = 0.75$$

(DSA = Dialyser Surface Area, m²)
(PSA = Patient's body Surface Area, m²)

If dialysers with highly permeable membranes are considered this ratio should be reduced.

The bloodvolume of the extracorporeal circuit (volume of bloodlines and dialyser, including the additional volume due to compliance of dialyser) should not exceed 10% of child's circulating bloodvolume (bloodvolume = 80 ml/kg body weight).

The dialyser should have a BUN clearance of 3–4 ml/min/kg BW. Those characteristics also depend on bloodflow rates. Examples of paediatric dialysers for children weighing 10 to 30 kg are given in Table 9 (see also chapter 5). Individual differences in dialysis tolerance are often observed. Regular recurrence of headache, dizziness, nausea, abdominal pain and vomiting during the dialysis procedure indicate that the choice of the dialyser has to be reconsidered.

The amount of ultrafiltration during dialysis depends on the interdialytic weight gain. Excessive weight gain between dialyses is usually due to high sodium intake with secondary excessive water intake; limitation of dietary sodium intake should then be encouraged.

Fluid loss by ultrafiltration in excess of 5% body weight will induce symptoms of hypotension. Precise and continuous monitoring of ultrafiltration is required. Special devices for monitoring and regulation of ultrafiltration presently marketed are very useful in paediatric patients. Continuous weight recording is less reliable: weight changes may be caused by food and fluid intake, fluid loss by vomiting and by shifting of blood into (or out of) the dialyser, due to volume changes caused by compliance of the membrane. Sequential ultrafiltration and dialysis improve tolerance of ultrafiltration, even in small children (34). Substitution of acetate by bicarbonate as the alkalinising buffer in the dialysate decreases cardiovascular instability during ultrafiltration in 10% of the patients. Small amounts of saline are usually sufficient for the correction of hypotension during dialysis.

In paediatric patients dialysis two times a week may allow satisfactory rehabilitation but three dialyses a week are recommended allowing a more liberal dietary and fluid intake and reducing the side-effects during dialysis and vigorous ultrafiltration. In young children (<5 years) the higher metabolic rate and poor compliance to the diet often requires three dialyses per week.

Individual determination of total dialysis time per week will prevent overdialysis and may save time for the unit and the patient. Adapting dialysis time to obtain predialysis blood urea values less than 20 mmol/l (120 mg/dl) and urate levels below 0.40 mmol/l (6.7 mg/dl) will provide adequate dialysis.

Close supervision of the patient is required during dialysis. Careful observation will reveal agitation, color changes and abdominal pain. These clinical signs often preceed hypotension (109).

Regular determination of body weight and blood pressure pre- and postdialysis is required.

Treatment of complications during dialysis

Institution of dialysis often results in a marked improvement of hypertension, but many children will remain hypertensive despite dialysis with ultrafiltration.

Hypertensive emergencies are treated by diazoxide, 5 mg/kg IV or by hydralazine 0.25–0.50 mg/kg IV (106). For prolonged treatment of hypertension beta-adrenergic blockings agents are preferred to methyldopa because of less frequent occurrence of adverse reactions. In cases of severe and refractory hypertension the administration of captopril has to be considered. In dialysed children the initial daily dose (administered in one single dose) is shown in Table 10.

Unilateral nephrectomy may be performed in dialysed patients with persistent hypertension and removal of the second kidney may be effected during the transplantation procedure. Persistence of severe hypertension in dialysed patients will require bilateral nephrectomy.

Table 9. Examples of disposable paediatric dialysers for children weighing 10 to 30 kg.

Body weight kg	Disposable dialysers	Blood volume (ml)	BUN clearance at Q_B (ml/min)	(ml/min)	$\frac{DSA *}{PSA}$
10	Gambro mini-minor PL	20	30	50	0.51
15	Gambro mini-minor PL	20	51	100	0.35
	Gambro minor PL	30	43	50	0.63
20	Gambro minor PL	30	59	75	0.51
	RP 5 (8 layers)	85	57	150	0.62
25	Gambro minor PL	30	77	150	0.43
	RP 5 (10 layers)	110	70	150	0.66
30	Gambro lundia 0,82 PL	70	90	100	0.62
	Secon 132	20	82	100	0.68
	RP 5 (14 layers)	154	100	150	0.77
	CDAK 0.6	53	105	150	0.54

* DSA: Dialyser Surface Area, m².
PSA: Patient's body Surface Area, m².

Table 10. Initial daily dose of Captopril in paediatric dialysis patients.

Body weight kg	Captopril initial dose mg
0–10	1
10–18	5
18–30	12.5
30	25

Ultrafiltration with an inappropriate dialyser is the most common cause of hypotension during dialysis. Saline, mannitol and albumen solutions are commonly use to treat hypotension.

Convulsions during dialysis should be treated by administration of diazepam (5 to 10 mg according to body weight). During the first dialysis diazepam (2 to 5 mg IV) is given prophylactically. Alternatively mannitol may be administered to reduce osmolality changes (1 g/kg body weight). Recurrent convulsions are either due to cerebral abnormalities or inappropriate dialysis technique.

REFERENCES

1. Edelmann CM: Physiological adaptations required of a newborn kidney. *Contrib Nephrol* 15:1, 1975
2. Chantler C.: Renal Failure in Childhood. In: *Renal Disease,* edited by Black D. and Jones NF., 4th edition Oxford, London, Edinburgh, Melbourne, Blackwell Scientific publications, 4th ed., 1979, p 825
3. Thurau K, Boylan JW: Acute renal success. The unexpected logic of oliguria in acute renal failure. *Am J Med* 61:308, 1976
4. Counahan R, Cameron JS, Ogg C, Spurgeon P, Williams DG, Winder E, Chantler C: The presentation, management, complications and outcome of acute renal failure in childhood, Guy's Hospital 1971-1975. *Br Med J* 1:599, 1977
5. Arneil GC, MacDonald AM, Murphy AV, Sweet EM: Renal venous thrombosis, *Clin Nephrol* 1:119, 1973
6. Elseed AM, Shinebourne EA, Joseph MC: Assessment of techniques for measurement of blood pressure in infants and children. *Arch Dis Child* 48:932, 1973
7. Aynsley-Green A, Pickering D: Use of central and peripheral temperature measurements in the care of the critically ill child. *Arch Dis Child* 49:477, 1974
8. Harries JT: Intravenous feeding in infants. *Arch Dis Child* 46:855, 1971
9. Shaw JCL: Parental nutrition in the management of sick low birth weight infants. *Pediatr Clin North Am* 20:333, 1973
10. Donckerwolcke RA, Kuijten RH, Tiddens RA, van Gool TD: Haemolytic uraemic syndrome. *Paediatrician* 8:378, 1979
11. Hodson EM, Kjellstrand CM, Mauer SM: Acute renal failure in infants and children: outcome of 53 patients requiring hemodialysis treatment. *J Pediatr* 83:756, 1978
12. Raja RM, Kramer MS, Rosenbaum JL: Hemodialysis with single femoral vein catheter. *Dial Transpl* 6(5):53, 1977
13. Harmon WE, Meyer A, Grupe WE: Substitution of a percutaneous vascular access for repeated hemodialysis in children. *Nieren- und Hochdruckkrankheiten* 10:91, 1981
14. Ahola T, Bjorkman H, Mäkelä, Popila M, Vilska J, Hallman N: The low-weight groups and hemodialysis. *Acta Paediatr Scand* 61:1, 1972
15. Kjellstrand CM, Lynch RE, Mauer SM, Buselmeier TJ: Acute renal failure in children: conservative and dialysis management. In: *Pediatric Nephrology* vol 4, edited by Strauss J, New York NY, London, Garland STP in press, 1978, p 89
16. Chesney RW, Kaplan BS, Freedman RM, Haller JA, Drummond KN: Acute renal failure: an important complication of cardiac surgery in infants *J Pediatr* 87:381, 1975
17. Meadow SR, Cameron JS, Ogg CS: Regional service for acute and chronic dialysis in children. *Lancet* 2:707, 1970
18. Schärer K: Die behandlung der chronischen Niereninsuffizienz in der Bundesrepublik Deutschland (Treatment of chronic renal failure in the Fed Republic of Germany). *Monatsschr Kinderheilkd* 123:745, 1975 (in German)
19. Mc Crory WW, Shibuya M, Yano K: Recent trends in the mortality rate from renal disease in children and young adults in New York City, *J Pediatr* 47:928, 1975
20. Potter D: Management of the child on chronic dialysis. In: *Clinical Pediatric Nephrology,* edited by Lieberman E, Philadelphia, PA Lippingcott, 1976, p 439
21. Leumann EP: Die chronische Niereninsuffizienz im Kindesalter. (Chronic renal failure in children.) *Schweiz Med Wochenschr* 106:244, 1976 (in German)
22. Helin I and Winberg J: Chronic renal failure in Swedish children *Acta Paediatr Scand* 69:607, 1980
23. Broyer M, Donckerwolcke RA, Brunner FP, Brynger H, Jacobs C, Kramer P, Selwood NH, Wing AJ, Blake PH: Combined report on regular dialysis and transplantation of children in Europe 1980. *Proc Eur Dial Transpl Assoc* 18:59, 1981
24. Broyer M: The European experience with treatment of ESRD in young children, *NIH Conference on Renal Disease,* Washington DC 1981
25. Kjellstrand CM, Santiago EA, Buselmeier TJ: Development of a special paediatric shunt. *Proc Eur Dial Transpl Assoc* 8:505, 1971
26. Buselmeier TJ, Kjellstrand CM: AV shunts and fistulae in neonates, infants and children. *Proc Eur Dial Transpl Assoc* 10:511, 1973
27. D'Apuzzo VC, Gruskin CM, Brennan CP, Stiles GR, Fine RN: Saphenous vein autograft arteriovenous fistula for extended hemodialysis in children. *Acta Paediatr Scand* 62:28, 1973
28. Applebaum H, Shashikumar L, Somers LA, Buluarte HJ, Gruskin AB, Grossman M, Mc Garvey MJ, Weintraub WH: Improved hemodialysis access in children. *Pediatr Surg* 15:764, 1980
29. Gagnadoux MF, Pascal B, Bronstein M, Bourquelot P, Degoulet P, Broyer M: Arteriovenous fistulae in small children. *Dial Transpl* 9:318, 1980
30. Mauer SM, Lynch RE: Hemodialysis techniques for infants and children *Pediatr Clin North Am* 23:843, 1976
31. Donckerwolcke RA: Regular dialysis treatment in children. *The Capsule* 10:29, 1979 (Excerpta Medica, Amsterdam)
32. Harmon WE, Spinozzi N, Meyer A, Grupe WE: The use of protein catabolic rate to monitor pediatric hemodialysis. *Dial Transpl* 10:324, 1981
33. Gardiner AOP, Sawyer AN, Donckerwolcke RA, Haycock GB, Murphy A, Ogg CS, Winder EA, Chantler C: Assessment of dialysis requirement for children on regular haemodialysis. *Dial Transpl* 11:754, 1982
34. Gusmano R, Perfumo F, Basile G, Formicucci L: Dialysis strategy in children. *Dial Transpl* 7:361, 1978
35. Office of Health Economics: *Renal failure, a priority in health?* Office of Health Economics, 162 Regent Street, London WIR 6 DD Report No 62, 1978
36. Donckerwolcke RA, Chantler C, Broyer M, Brunner FP, Brynger H, Jacobs C, Kramer P, Selwood NH, Wing AJ: Combined report on regular dialysis and transplantation of children in Europe 1979. *Proc Eur Dial Transpl Assoc* 17:87, 1980
37. Chantler C, Carter JE, Bewick M, Counahan R, Cameron JS, Ogg CS, Williams DG, Winder E: Ten years experience with regular haemodialysis and renal transplantation.

Arch Dis Child 55:435, 1980

38. Wing AJ, Brunner FB, Brynger H, Chantler C, Donckerwolcke RA, Gurland H, Jacobs C, Selwood NH: Mortality and morbidity of re-using dialysers. *Br Med J* 111:853, 1978
39. Donckerwolcke RA, Chantler C, Brunner FP, Brynger H, Gurland HJ, Hathway RA, Jacobs C, Selwood NH, Wing AJ: Combined report on regular dialysis and transplantation of children in Europe 1977. *Proc Eur Dial Transpl Assoc* 15:77, 1978
40. Wass VJ, Barratt TM, Howarth RV, Marshall WA, Chantler C, Ogg CS, Cameron JS, Baillod RA, Moorhead JF: Home haemodialysis in children. *Lancet* 1:242, 1977
41. Counts S, Hickman R, Garbaccio A, Tenckhoff H: Chronic home peritoneal dialysis in children. *Trans Am Soc Artif Intern Organs* 19:157, 1973
42. Gagnadoux MF, Hernandez MA, Broyer M, Vacant J, Royer P: La dialyse péritonéale chronique: alternative de l'hémodialyse itérative chez l'enfant. Chronic peritoneal dialysis: an alternative to regular haemodialysis in children. *Arch Fr Pediatr* 34:860, 1977 (in French)
43. Hickman R: Peritoneal dialysis in children. *Dial Transpl* 6:42, 1977
44. Guillot M, Clermont MJ, Gagnadoux MF, Broyer M: Nineteen months experience with continuous ambulatory peritoneal dialysis in children: main clinical and biological results. In: *Advances in Peritoneal Dialysis*. International Congress Series 567, edited by Gahl GM, Kessel M, Nolph KD, Amsterdam, Oxford, Princeton, Excerpta Medica, 1981, p 203
45. Gandhi VC, Humayun HM, Ing TS, Daugirdas JT, Jablokow VR, Iwatsuki S, Geis P, Hano JE: Sclerotic thickening of the peritoneal membrane in maintenance peritoneal dialysis patients. *Arch Intern Med* 140:1201, 1980
46. Kohout EC, Alexander S: Ultrafiltration in the young patient on CAPD. In: *CAPD Update: Continuous Ambulatory Peritoneal Dialysis*, edited by Moncrief JW, Popovich RP, New York, Paris, Barcelona, Milan, Mexico City, Rio de Janeiro, Masson Publ USA Inc 1981, p 221
47. Guillot M, Lavocat C, Garabedian M, Sachs C, Balsan S, Gagnadoux MF, Broyer M: Evaluation of 25 (OH) D$_3$ loss in dialysate of children on continuous ambulatory peritoneal dialysis. *Proc Eur Dial Transpl Assoc* 18:290, 1981
48. Guillot M, Clermont MJ, Gagnadoux MF, Broyer M: Continuous ambulatory peritoneal dialysis in pediatrics: preliminary results of a 18 months experiences. In: *Renal Insufficiency in Children,* edited by Bulla M, New York NY Springer Verlag, 1982, p 197
49. Chantler C, Donckerwolcke RA, Brunner FP, Brynger H, Hathway RA, Jacobs C, Selwood NH, Wing AJ: Combined report on regular dialysis and transplantation of children in Europe, 1978. *Proc Eur Dial Transpl Assoc* 16:74, 1979
50. Schärer K, Chantler C, Brunner FP, Gurland HJ, Jacobs C, Parsons FM, Seyffart G, Wing AJ: Combined report on regular dialysis and transplantation of children in Europe, 1974. *Proc Eur Dial Transpl Assoc* 12:65, 1975
51. Tanner JM, Whitehouse RH, Marshall WA, Healy MJR, Goldstein H: *Assessment of Skeletal Maturity and Prediction of Adult Height (T.W.2 Method)*. London, New York, San Francisco, Academic Press, 1975
52. Greulich WW, Pyle SI: *Radiographic Atlas of Skeletal Development of Hand and Wrist*, 2nd Edn, Stanford Univ Press, Palo Alto, CA, 1975
53. Schärer K, Chantler C, Brunner FP, Gurland HJ, Jacobs C, Selwood NH, Wing AJ: Combined report in regular dialysis and transplantation of children in Europe 1975. *Proc Eur Dial Transpl Assoc* 13:59, 1976
54. Marshall WA, Tanner JM: Variations in pattern of pubertal changes in boys. *Arch Dis Child* 44:13, 1970
55. Broyer M, Kleinknecht C, Loirat C, Marti Henneberg C, Roy MP: Maturation osseuse et développement pubertaire chez l'enfant et l'adolescent en dialyse chronique. Skeleton maturation and pubertal development of the child and adolescent on chronic dialysis. *Proc Eur Dial Transpl Assoc* 9:181, 1972 (in French)
56. Tanner JM, Whitehouse RH, Hughes PCR, Vince FP: Effect of human growth hormone treatment for 1 to 7 years on growth of 100 children with growth hormone deficiency, low birth weight, inherited smallness, Turner's syndrome and other complaints, *Arch Dis Child* 46:745, 1971
57. West CD, Smith WC: An attempt to elucidate the cause of retardation in growth in renal disease. *Am J Dis Child* 91:460, 1956
58. Chantler C, Holliday MA: Growth in children with renal disease with particular reference to the effects of calorie malnutrition: a review. *Clin Nephrol* 1:230, 1973
59. Jones RWA, El Bishti M, Chantler C: The promotion of anabolism in children with chronic renal failure. In: *Topics in Paediatrics*, edited by Wharton B, Pitman Medical, Tunbridge Wells, UK, 1980, p 90
60. Chantler C, El Bishti M, Counahan R: Nutritional therapy in children with chronic renal failure. *Am J Clin Nutr* 33:1682, 1980
61. Jones RWA, Dalton N, Start K, El Bishti M, Chantler C: Oral essential amino acid supplements in children with advanced chronic renal failure. *Am J Clin Nutr* 33:1696, 1980
62. Chantler C, Jones RWA, Dalton N: Amino acid and protein metabolism in chronic renal failure. In: *Pediatric Nephrology, Proc. 3rd International Congress of Pediatric Nephrology, Philadelphia*, edited by Gruskin A, Norman ME, The Hague, Boston and London, Martinus Nijhoff 1981, p 310
63. El Bishti M, Counahan R, Bloom SR, Chantler C: Hormonal and metabolic response to intravenous glucose in children on regular haemodialysis. *Am J Clin Nutr* 31:1865, 1978
64. Saenger R, Wiedeman E, Schwartz E, Kortn-Schutz S, Lewy JE, Riggio RR, Rubin AL, Stensel KH, New M: Somatomedin and growth after renal transplantation. *Pediatr Res* 8:163, 1974
65. Lewy JE, Van Wyk JJ: Somatomedin and growth retardation in children with chronic renal insufficiency. *Kidney Int* 14:361, 1978
66. Pennissi AJ, Phillips LS, Uittenbogaart C, Ettenger RB, Malekzadeh MH, Fine RN: Nutritional intake, somatomedin activity and linear growth in children undergoing hemodialysis. *Kidney Int* 10:523, 1976
67. Betts PR, Howse PM, Morris R, Rayner PHW: Serum cortisol concentrations in children with chronic renal insufficiency. *Arch Dis Child* 50:245, 1975
68. Czernichow P, Dauzet MC, Broyer M, Rappaport R: Abnormal T.S.H., P.R.L. and G.H. response to T.S.H. releasing factor in chronic renal failure. *J Clin Endocrinol Metab* 43:630, 1976
69. Burke J, El Bishti M, Maisey MN, Chantler C: Hypothyroidism in children with cystinosis. *Arch Dis Child* 53:947, 1978
70. Counahan R, El Bishti M, Cox BD, Ogg CS, Chantler C: Plasma amino acids in children and adolescents on haemodialysis. *Kidney Int* 10:471, 1976

71. El Bishti MM, Counahan R, Stimmler L, Jarrett RJ, Wass VJ, Chantler C: Abnormalities in plasma lipids in children on regular haemodialysis. *Arch Dis Child* 52:932, 1977
72. Broyer M, Tete MJ, Laudat MH, Dartois AM: Plasma lipid abnormalities in children on chronic haemodialysis: relationship to dietary intake. *Proc Eur Dial Transpl Assoc* 13:385, 1977
73. Sanfelippo ML, Swenson RS, Reaven GM: Plasma triglyceride and insulin responses to diet in dialysed subjects with end stage renal failure. *Kidney Int* 10:525, 1976
74. Conley SB, Rose GM, Robson AM, Bier DM: The effects of dietary intake and hemodialysis on protein turnover in uremic children. *Kidney Int.* 17:837, 1980
75. Fine RN, Isaacson AS, Payne V: Renal osteodystrophy in children. The effect of hemodialysis and renal homotransplantation. *J Pediatr* 80:239, 1972
76. Mehls O, Krempian B, Ritz E, Schärer K, Schuler HW: Renal osteodystrophy in children on maintenance haemodialysis. *Proc Eur Dial Transpl Assoc* 10:197, 1973
77. Broyer M: Chronic renal failure. In: *Paediatric Nephrology* edited by Royer P, Habib R, Mathieu H, Broyer M, Philadelphia PA, WB Saunders, 1974, p 358
78. Norman ME, Mazin AT, Borden S, Gruskin A, Anast C, Baron R, Rasmussen H: Early diagnosis of renal osteodystrophy. *J Pediatr* 97:226, 1980
79. Mehls O, Ritz E, Krempien B, Gilli G, Link K, Wulich E, Schärer K: Slipped epiphyses in renal osteodystrophy. *Arch Dis Child* 50:545, 1975
80. Balsan S: Vitamin D metabolites in paediatrics. In: *Paediatric Diseases Related to Calcium*, edited by De Luca HF, Anast CS, Oxford, London, Edinburgh, Melbourne, Blackwell Scientific Publications, 1980, p 248
81. Postlethwaite RJ, Houston IB: Bone disease in children with chronic renal failure; therapy with $1\alpha(OH)$ Vit D_3 *Clin Endocrin* 7:suppl 117s, 1977
82. Fournier A, Bordier P, Gueris J, Sebert JL, Marie P, Ferriers C, Bedrossian J, De Luca H: Comparison of 1α OH cholecalciferol and 25(OH)cholecalciferol in the treatment of renal osteodystrophy greater effect of 25 OH cholecalciferol on bone mineralisation. *Kidney Int* 15:196, 1979
83. Talwalkar YB, Puri HC, Hawker CC, Tseng C, Campbell JR, Campbell RA: Parathyroid autotransplantation in renal osteodystrophy. *Am J Dis Child* 133:901, 1979
84. Chesney RW, Moorthy V, Eisman JA, Jax DK, Mazess R, De Luca HF: increased growth after longterm oral $1\alpha(OH_2)$ 25 Vit D_3 in childhood renal osteodystrophy. *New Engl J Med* 298:238, 1978
85. Bulla M, Delling G, Benz-Bohm G, Stock GJ, Sanchezue Reutter A, Ziegler R, Iuhmann H, Severin M, Kalbitzer E, Manegold C: Renale Osteodystrophie bei Kindern: Therapieversuch mit 1,25 dihydroxy-cholecalciferol. (Renal osteodystrophy in children: Therapeutic trial with 1,25 (OH)$_2$ cholecalciferol.) *Klin Wochenschr* 58:511, 1980 (in German)
86. Muller-Wiefel D, Sinn H, Gilli G, Schärer K: Hemolysis and blood loss in children with chronic renal failure. *Clin Nephrol* 8:481, 1977
87. Kjellstrand CM, Eaton JW, Yawata Y, Swofford H, Kolpin C, Buselmeier TJ, Von Hartitzsch B, Jacob HS: Haemolysis in dialysed patients caused by chloramines. *Nephron* 13:427, 1974
88. Ersler AJ: Management of anemia of chronic renal failure. *Clin Nephrol* 2:174, 1974
89. Bell JD, Kincaid WR, Morgan RG, Bunce H, Alperin JB, Sarles HE, Remmers AR: Serum ferritin assay and bone marrow iron stores in patients on maintenance hemodialysis. *Kidney Int* 17:237, 1980
90. Lynn KL, Mitchell TR, Sheppard J: Serum ferritin concentration in patients receiving maintenance hemodialysis. *Clin Nephrol* 14:124, 1980
91. Jones RWA, El Bishti M, Bloom SR, Burke J, Carter J, Counahan RC, Dalton N, Morris MC, Chantler C: The effects of anabolic steroids on growth, body composition and metabolism in boys on regular hemodialysis. *J Pediatr* 97:559, 1980
92. Ullmer HE, Greiner H, Schuler HW, Schärer K: Cardiovascular impairment and physical working capacity in children with chronic renal failure. *Acta Paediatr Scand* 67:43, 1978
93. Ullmer HE, Gilli G, Schärer K: Assessment of uremic cardiomyopathy in childhood by systolic time intervals. *Pediatr Res* 10:897, 1976
94. Holliday MA: Calorie deficiency in children with uremia: Effect upon growth. *Pediatrics* 50:590, 1972
95. Abitol CI, Holliday MA: Total parenteral nutrition in anuric children. *Clin Nephrol* 5:151, 1976
96. Aronson AS, Fürst P, Kylenstierna BO, Nyberg G: Essential amino acids in the treatment of advanced uremia: 22 months experience in a 5 year old girl. *Pediatrics* 56:538, 1975
97. Counahan R, El Bishti M, Chantler C: Oral essential amino acids in children in regular hemodialysis. *Clin Nephrol* 9:11, 1978
98. Tsukamoto Y, Iwanami S, Marumo F: Disturbances of trace element concentrations in plasma of patients in chronic renal failure. *Nephron* 6:174, 1980
99. Department of Health and Social Security. *Report No. 120: Recommended Intakes of Nutrients for the United Kingdom.* London, Her Majesty's Stationery Office, 1969
100. Wass VJ, Barratt TM, Howarth RV, Marshall WA, Chantler C, Ogg CS, Cameron JS, Baillod RA, Moorhead JF: Home haemodialysis in children. *Lancet* 1:242, 1977
101. Korsch BM, Fine RN, Gruskin CM, Negrete VF: Experience with children and their families during extended hemodialysis and kidney transplantation. *Pediatr Clin N Am* 18:625, 1971
102. Wolters WMG, Bonekamp ALM, Donckerwolcke RA: Experiences in the development of a haemodialysis centre for children. *J Psychosom Res* 17:271, 1973
103. Steinhauer RD, Mushin DN, Roe-Grent G: Psychosocial aspects of chronic illness. *Pediatr Clin North Am* 21:825, 1974
104. Chantler C, Broyer M, Donckerwolcke RA, Brynger H, Brunner FP, Jacobs C, Kramer P, Selwood NH, Wing AJ: Growth and rehabilitation of long term survivors of treatment for end stage renal failure in childhood. *Proc Eur Dial Transpl Assoc* 18:329, 1981
105. André JL, Picon G: Aspects psychosociaux du traitement de l'insuffisance rénale terminale. In: *26e Congrès des Pédiatres de Langue Française.* (Psycho-social aspects of the treatment of end stage renal failure.) Toulouse, Fournié, 1981, p 611 (in French)
106. Potter DE: Pharmacologic management of the pediatric patient with ESRD. *Dial Transpl* 8:65, 1979
107. Bennett N: Urea kinetics: a dietician's clinical tool in the nutritional management of patients with end stage renal disease. *Dial Transpl* 10:332, 1981
108. Comty CM, Davis M: Nutritional assessment in end-stage renal disease. *Dial Transpl* 10:130, 1981
109. Irwin MA: Working toward quality patient care in paediatric dialysis unit using primary nursing. *Dial Transpl* 8:1192, 1979
110. Hunter MB, Cole BR, Robson AM: Tactics for caring for children during hemodialysis. *Dial Transpl* 10:147, 1981

Table 2. Suggested treatment for some forms of primary acute renal disease.

Diagnostic category	Suggested treatment
"Nonspecific" subacute gomerulonephritis	Cyclophosphamide Azathioprine Prednisone Anticoagulation Combination ("Triple-therapy") Plasmapheresis
Lupus nephritis	Prednisone Azathioprine Cyclophosphamide Anticoagulation Plasmapheresis
Goodpasture's syndrome	Plasmapheresis Pulse-prednisone Immunosuppression (Nephrectomy for pulmonary bleeding)
Wegener's granulomatosis, Polyarteritis, systemic vasculitis	Cyclosphophamide/-prednisone Azathioprine, ALG (anti-lymphocytic globulin)
Acute interstitial nephritis a) drug induced b) "viral?"	Prednisone (Prednisone?)
Malignant hypertension Scleroderma	Intense anti-hypertensive therapy
Hemolytic- uremic syndrome	Anticoagulation Plasmapheresis
Thrombotic thrombocytopenic purpura	Anticoagulation, antiplatelet drugs Plasma infusion Plasmapheresis

in patients with chronic renal failure treated by dialysis. Table 2 summarizes some of the treatments for these disorders. Astounding successes have been achieved in individual cases but mortality has also resulted from the treatment in every single diagnostic category.

The rest of this chapter will be devoted to acute tubular necrosis. However, the sections regarding symptomatic and supportive treatment apply to all patients with acute renal failure.

DIFFERENTIAL DIAGNOSIS

In most instances, tubular necrosis is easily distinguished from prerenal failure and obstruction. The differential diagnosis is made by history, review of the patient's charts, clinical investigation and frequently confirmed by a series of radiological and laboratory tests.

The history and the patient's records often reveal clues to identify the correct diagnosis. For example, patients with prerenal failure may have had water and electrolyte losses from diarrhea and have received insufficient fluid in relation to losses. If body weight has been recorded, it will show a decrease. A previous history of stones or cancer in or near the genitourinary tract should raise the suspicion of urinary obstruction. Joint pain, rashes, or other organ involvement should suggest such diagnoses as lupus erythematosus, vasculitis, anaphylactoid purpura or acute interstitial nephritis. Catastrophic surgical events, sepsis, shock and oliguria, in spite of marked weight gain due to inappropriate fluid management, often precede tubular necrosis.

It used to be believed that urinary volume was a good indicator of kidney function and that acute tubular necrosis was usually signalled by oliguria. It has been increasingly recognized, however, that polyuria is common in acute tubular necrosis, particularly when caused by antibiotics. Even more confusing is the finding that patients with severe (ischemic) prerenal failure may continue to make large amounts of urine (42). Patients with partial urinary tract obstruction also may have a normal or increased urinary output. However, absolute anuria, particularly when interspersed with episodes of polyuria, suggests obstruction.

On physical examination, the patient with marked prerenal failure shows sunken eyes, central venous and pulmonary wedge pressures are low, skin turgor is decreased and orthostatic hypotension is present. These classical findings of extracellular fluid volume depletion may be absent, however, in some patients who have prerenal azotemia due to a decreased cardiac output (with markedly increased total body water because of edema). This is most commonly encountered in patients with heart failure secondary to myocardial infarction or after heart surgery for valve replacement or coronary artery bypass. A septic patient also may suffer from a sudden decrease in effective blood volume secondary to decreased tone of capacitance vessels without a decrease in total body fluid volume.

There is no typical physical finding in patients with acute tubular necrosis. Many such patients, however, have signs of fluid overload (peripheral edema, fluid lung, or frank pulmonary edema) secondary to inappropriate fluid management. Patients with urinary obstruction may have a large urinary bladder and (or) a pelvic mass.

Radiological procedures are often helpful, particularly in the diagnosis of obstruction. Thus, ultrasonography, intravenous pyelography, computerized axial tomography or radioisotope renography with or without furosemide administration demonstrate a dilated renal pelvis, particularly when delayed imaging is also used.

Ultrasonography of the obstructed kidney gives particularly accurate diagnostic information. It has a low incidence of false positive and false negative findings. Some cases, however, will require cystoscopy and retrograde or antegrade pyelography for a definite diagnosis (17–20).

Radiologic tests are less useful in differentiating between prerenal failure and acute tubular necrosis. The kidneys tend to be small in prerenal failure and enlarged in acute tubular necrosis, but this is an unreliable sign. Radiologic examination of the chest is very important, however, for the diagnosis of fluid overload in the lungs.

Table 3. Differential diagnosis between pre-renal failure and acute tubular necrosis.

Test	Pre-renal failure	Acute tubular necrosis
Urinary specific gravity	> 1.030	< 1.020
Urinary osmolality	> 500 mOsm/kg/H_2O	< 350 mOsm/kg/H_2O
Urine/plasma osmolal ratio	> 1.1	< 1.1
Urine/plasma creatinine ratio	> 20	< 20
Urine/plasma urea ratio	> 7	< 7
Serum urea N/creatinine ratio	> 10	⩽ 10
Urinary sodium concentration	< 30 mmol/l	> 30 mmol/l
Excreted/filtered sodium (FE_{Na})	< 1%	> 2%
Renal failure index	< 1	> 1
Free water clearance	< − 20 ml/hr	Rising to > − 15 ml/hr
2 h creatinine clearance	Stable	Falling
Urinary sediment	Hyaline or finely granular casts	Tubular cell casts
		Coarse granular casts
Proteinuria	0+ to 1+	1+ to 2+

These tests for distinguishing between pre-renal failure and acute tubular necrosis are nonspecific and should be used only as a part of the global clinical evaluation of the patient.

Some patients have a low cardiac output but a marked increase in total body water so that, paradoxically, they suffer both a fluid excess and prerenal failure.

The numerous diagnostic tests used to differentiate prerenal failure from acute tubular necrosis are listed in Table 3. The physiologic hypothesis is that with prerenal failure, glomerular filtrate is modified considerably by the intact tubules under maximum ADH and aldosterone stimulation. To the contrary, with acute tubular necrosis or urinary tract obstruction (21), the renal tubule modifies the glomerular filtrate, very little.

The literature regarding the accuracy of these tests is confusing. When first described, many of these tests were considered highly accurate, but later were found to be of very limited or no use, a frequent fate of medical tests (22). There is also no unanimity regarding the values that differentiate acute tubular necrosis from prerenal failure. For example, the urine sodium concentration or the urine to plasma creatinine concentration ratio reported to be suggestive of acute tubular necrosis varies almost ten-fold (23–42).

Recently, it has been stressed that the fractional excretion of sodium (FE_{Na}) differentiates between acute tubular necrosis and prerenal failure (28, 31–33). Practical experience, however, suggests that this test is of limited value in differentiating the patient who will need dialysis from the one who will recover renal function, when given fluids (34–37). Serial free water and creatinine clearances may be the best tests differentiating prerenal failure from acute tubular necrosis (38–41). Prerenal failure is a very common precursor of acute tubular necrosis. Often therefore, a specific diagnosis of either tubular necrosis or prerenal failure can not be made definitively; many patients have findings that lie in between the two entities.

The urinary sediment should be a good test to differentiate between acute tubular necrosis and prerenal failure but has not been rigorously evaluated in recent years. Early urine from patients with obstruction tends to have a chemical composition similar to urine from patients with prerenal failure. After 2 or 3 days it resembles urine from patients wiht acute tubular necrosis.

The studies summarized in Table 3 are all easy to perform and should be available in any hospital dealing with patients with acute renal failure. They should be done on these patients, with the understanding that the results should be interpreted as only one part of the total clinical picture. No test is infallible; most are only clues to the correct diagnosis.

PATHOGENESIS OF ACUTE TUBULAR NECROSIS AND TREATMENT

Review of experimental work

The etiology, pathogenesis and pathophysiology of acute tubular necrosis are of intense interest in experimental research. Ideally, an animal model should meet several criteria. The initiating factors should be identical to those operating in acute tubular necrosis in humans, a situation where multiple factors are usually involved. Secondly, it should be possible to determine the transition point from subclinical renal illness to clinical acute renal failure, the point of 'no return'. Five models presently used frequently are: renal artery constriction, intrarenal artery norepinephrine, intramuscular glycerol, mercuric chloride and uranyl nitrate. None of these models mimics accurately most situations causing acute tubular necrosis in humans and the interpretation of the results is still a matter of debate.

The pathogenesis of acute renal failure could involve perpetuated renal ischemia, decreased filtration through a changed glomerular membrane or tubular dysfunction with backleak of normally filtered tubular fluid, alone or in various combinations. Acute renal failure can occur with morphologically preserved but functionally damaged tubules, or involve frank necrosis of the tubular epithelium. When tubular cell necrosis occurs, the tubular cell may be shed off its basement membrane and potentially cause obstruction with increased intraluminal hydrostatic pressure.

Almost any of these events can be found at one point or another in the various models described above. It has become clear that none of them very faithfully mimic the human situation, that seems to evolve through many stages (43–51).

Common clinical etiologic factors

Figure 1 summarizes the factors precipitating acute renal failure. There seem to be two principal initiating events: ischemia and nephrotoxicity. Clinically, there is almost always a mixture of these factors. Thus, nephrotoxic proteins such as myoglobin and hemoglobin may cause not only direct tubular damage but also ischemia or obstruction. Conversely, factors that cause ischemia may lead to release of nephrotoxic substances such as myoglobin or nephrotoxic drugs may be given to the patient.

A number of factors cause renal ischemia without necessarily decreasing systemic blood pressure. These include dehydration secondary to burns, edema into nontraumatized tissue, diarrhea, vomiting and sequestration of extracellular fluid due to ileus or retroperitoneally in such conditions as acute pancreatitis or after surgery. Similarly, any reduction in cardiac output following myocardial dysfunction or reduction of the circulating blood volume or of the ratio of blood volume to capacitance of the vascular system such as may occur in bacterial gram negative sepsis, endotoxemia or anaphylactic reactions can also cause acute tubular necrosis. Surgery under general anesthesia uniformly decreases renal blood flow.

Almost no critically ill patient escapes being treated with drugs that are potentially nephrotoxic. Aminoglycosides and cephalosporin antibiotics are used especially frequently in this circumstance. Increasingly, diagnostic procedures also cause problems such as nephropathy following contrast radiography (52). Self inflicted intoxication with such substances as ethylene glycol and carbon tetrachloride is less frequent. Certain endogenously produced substances such as uric acid, calcium, myoglobin and hemoglobin, are also potentially nephrotoxic.

Patients developing tubular necrosis are usually exposed to several pathogenic factors. For example, after cardiovascular surgery, where both the operation and the anesthesia contribute to decreased renal blood flow, cardiac output may be decreased and nephrotoxic drugs may be administered. After cross clamping the aorta for repair of an abdominal aneurysm, nephrotoxic antibiotics are frequently used, sequestration of fluid may decrease cardiac output, internal hemorrhage may occur and myoglobin may be released from ischemic muscle.

Treatment of acute tubular necrosis based on pathogenesis

Figure 1 summarizes a possible scheme for the etiology, pathogenesis and pathophysiology of acute tubular necrosis. In the clinical situation, as noted above, there are almost always several factors operative. The key element in the ischemic pathway leading to acute tubular necrosis is decreased renal blood flow and a final common pathway for acute renal failure independent of nephrotoxicity or ischemia is a decrease in tubular fluid flow. Changes in the rate of delivery of salt and water to the distal tubule, sensed at the macula densa, also can stimulate renin release, inducing renal ischemia. A decrease in renal medullary vasodilator prostaglandin activity can also contribute to the decrease in renal blood flow. These factors may also perpetuate renal ischemia (43–51). Drugs that increase renal blood flow could thus theoretically influence the development of acute tubular necrosis.

Loop diuretics increase both renal blood flow and tubular fluid flow rates. Mannitol, ethacrynic acid and furosemide have each been used clinically a) prophylactically b) as a treatment for aborting incipient acute tubular necrosis or shortening its clinical course and c) to change oliguria to non-oliguria. Several clinical trials of these drugs have been undertaken; few of these have been controlled or randomized. Controlled trials have shown that furosemide, which has been investigated recently is either ineffective (53), can change oliguric acute tubular necrosis to non-oliguric, this easing management (54–56), or will appreciably shorten both the anuric period and the time it takes for the plasma creatinine concentration to fall to normal values (57). These drugs are effective only when used early during the development of acute renal failure (55, 58). In many patients they induce diuresis. Levinsky, Bernard and Johnston (59), reviewing the reports of treatment of acute

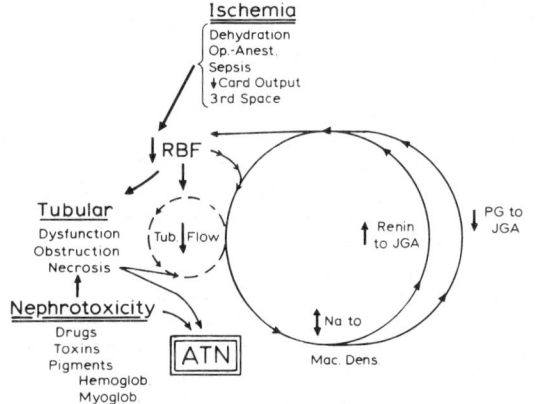

Figure 1. Scheme of events leading to acute tubular necrosis in patients. Ischemia or nephrotoxicity cause tubular dysfunction leading to a decrease in tubular fluid flow and a decrease in renal blood flow, possibly through activation of the renin angiotensin system or a decrease of prostaglandin activity. Frequently, many events co-exist or succeed each other in the same patient.

RBF	= Renal blood flow
ATN	= Acute tubular necrosis
JGA	= Juxtaglomerular apparatus
PG	= Prostaglandin
Op-Anest	= Operation + anesthesia
Mac. Dens.	= Macula densa

tubular necrosis with diuretics and mannitol, also found suggestive evidence that in the patients who responded by changing from oliguria to a diuresis, mortality rate was decreased. There is much uncertainty about these conclusions, however, as most of the studies have been uncontrolled.

Preliminary clinical and experimental data suggest that low-dose intravenous dopamine infused at a rate of 1 µg/kg/min may also change oliguria to diuresis (60, 61). Experimental studies suggest that a combination of dopamine and furosemide may be more effective (62).

Abel and coworkers (63) found that intravenous amino acids and high dose dextrose shortened the period of hypercreatininemia and lowered mortality in patients with acute tubular necrosis when treatment was started within 4 days after the onset of renal insufficiency. Leonard, Luke and Siegel (64), Asbach et al (65) and Baek and coworkers (66), however, could find no improvement in renal functional recovery during hyperalimentation with amino acids, although Baek et al (66), unlike the others (64, 65) found an improvement in survival. Experimental work on the influence of parenteral amino acids on the course of acute tubular necrosis is also contradictory (67, 68).

Experimentally, infusions of nucleotides and magnesium chloride can shorten the duration of acute tubular necrosis. It is clear that this cannot be used in patients because of the risk of magnesium intoxication (69, 70). Intravenous inosine has been effective in preventing renal injury during surgery (71).

Despite these controversies, a common clinical approach has been to use rapidly increasing doses of furosemide up to 10 mg/kg (30 µmol/kg) slowly infused over 30 to 60 min as well as 12 to 25 g (67 to 134 mmol) of mannitol intravenously in patients with suspected acute tubular necrosis provided that serum creatinine concentration is below 5 mg/dl (442 µmol/l). Dopamine (1 µg/kg/min, intravenously) can also be used. If diuresis is achieved, it may be maintained by small supplemental intravenous doses of furosemide. When there is no response, all such treatment should be discontinued. The risks of high dose furosemide include deafness, gastrointestinal bleeding and pancreatitis (72, 73). These occur rarely, however, and the possible benefits of shortening the oliguric period probably outweigh these potential complications. Mannitol, in particular, may cause severe intoxication secondary to hyperosmolality and extracellular fluid volume expansion when continued despite severe renal failure (74). Once the patient's electrolyte and fluid status is stabilized, intravenous hyperalimentation is begun with amino acids, dextrose and fat emulsions, as will be described later.

GENERAL PLAN OF WORK-UP, MORTALITY, AND THERAPEUTIC APPROACH

General approach

Figure 2 outlines the basic approach when a patient develops acute renal failure. Immediate dangers in such

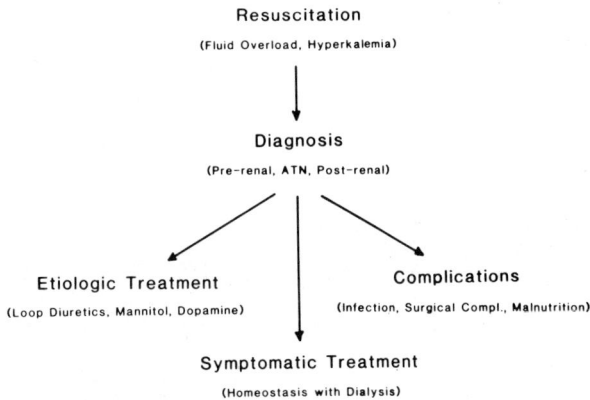

Figure 2. Schedule of approach to management of patients with acute renal failure.

patients include fluid overload with pulmonary edema and hyperkalemia with cardiac arrest. After guarding against these occurrences, diagnosis takes place, differentiating pre- and post-renal failure from acute tubular necrosis. Treatment with fluids or cardiotonics or both in the patients with pre-renal failure, removal of obstruction in those with post-renal failure, and a possible trial of renal vasodilator-diuretics in the patient with acute tubular necrosis is then undertaken. Should these efforts fail, homeostasis is maintained with dialysis, and a constant watch for specific complications is instituted.

Primary diseases and mortality

Table 4 summarizes the disorders leading to acute tubular necrosis during the 35 years between 1945 and 1980 while hemodialysis treatment has been clinically available. Surgery and trauma have always been the most common causative incidents preceding acute tubular necrosis. Medical causes account for between one-fourth to one-third of the cases. Although not expressed in the Table, there has been a marked decline in acute tubular necrosis complicating obstetrical and gynecological disease during the 35 years that dialysis has been available for these patients.

These figures apply only to highly technologically developed countries. In other parts of the world, acute renal failure is mostly secondary to acute infections, snake bites and abortions (75, 76). Thus, Chugh (75) reviewing 577 cases of acute renal failure in India, found that 63% were secondary to medical diseases, mostly due to gastrointestinal infections, 23% complicated obstetrical/gynecological disorders and only 14% followed surgery. When he reviewed figures from Asia and Africa, the findings were similar and markedly different from those published from North America and Europe, where in over 50% of the cases surgical complications were causative.

There has been no tendency for improvement in the mortality rate with time, nor has there been an increase in the patient's mean age in the later series (4–10). Analyses of the influence of age on mortality among patients

Table 4. Outcome and mean age of patients with acute tubular necrosis in the early, middle and late years of acute dialysis.

Initiating disorder	Univ. of Minnesota 1968-1979 n	Mortality %	Mean age	Glasgow Royal Infirmary 1959-1970 n	Mortality %	Mean age	Univ of Lund, Sweden 1945-1961 n	Mortality %	Mean age
Medical diseases, intoxications	140	63	41	56	36	48	225	35	50
Gastrointestinal surgery	95	78	55	97	58	51	87	56	54
Cardiovascular surgery	135	73	52	6	—	—	12	83	44
Obstetrical, gynecologic, other surgery, trauma	62	68	45	92	—	—	236	46	49
Total	432	69	48	251	44	—	560	44	50

Results of dialysis treatment of acute renal failure from the early years (1945-61), the middle years (1959-70), and recent years of acute dialysis (1968-79). Surgical disease has always been the most common cause of acute tubular necrosis. The mortality rate has not improved, nor has the mean age of the patients increased.

with acute renal failure done in the early years of dialysis usually found an inverse correlation of age with survival (4-9). More recent studies do not show such a correlation (10, 77, 78) however, the mortality rate is particularly high in children and in the elderly.

Thus, of 432 patients dialyzed between 1968 and 1979 at the University of Minnesota for acute renal failure, approximately 70% of those below the age of 20 or above the age of 50 died. On the contrary, patients between 20 and 50 years of age had a 50% survival rate (10, 77). Many more young and old patients are now being treated by dialysis for acute renal failure (10, 77), which may unfavorably influence overall survival statistics.

It is difficult to compare patients who are treated by dialysis now to those dialyzed almost 40 years ago. One of us, however, has participated in the analysis of the very first patients dialyzed for acute tubular necrosis (University of Lund 1945-1961) and a recent series (University of Minnesota 1968-1979). It seems clear that patients with acute tubular necrosis now have much more serious underlying disorders in each etiological category. Milder disorders such as gastroenteritis no longer give rise to acute tubular necrosis because of improved resuscitation and electrolyte and fluid management. Presently, cancer, catastrophic septicemia and major surgery are increasingly more common antecedents of acute tubular necrosis.

The comparative survival rate of groups of patients that are well defined as to age and basic disease, such as young men with acute renal failure sustained during war, is not encouraging. Teschan et al (6) reported a 32% overall survival in soldiers dialyzed for acute tubular necrosis during the Korean war (1950 to 1953). The survival rate for such soldiers in Viet Nam in the 1960's was 23 to 37% (79-91). Barsoum and coworkers (82) reported a 37% survival rate in young soldiers dialyzed for acute renal failure during the six-day war in the Middle East in 1973. These figures do not show any substantial improvement in survival. It is believed, however, that improved resuscitation and transportation enabled much more severely traumatized soldiers to reach dialysis units during the Viet Nam and Middle East Wars, than during the Korean conflict. Thus, subtle shifts in patient population towards more severely traumatized cases may conceal actual improvements in the management of acute tubular necrosis.

Table 4 shows that surgical complications remain the most common cause of acute tubular necrosis. A dramatic increase in the frequency of cardiovascular surgery as an antecedent of acute tubular necrosis is also apparent. Mean age and mortality have not changed, but, as noted above, in all probability, small children and very old patients are dialyzed for acute tubular necrosis more often now than before.

Some patients who sustain non-oliguric acute tubular necrosis and have preserved urine volume are believed to have lower mortality rates (24), as do patients in whom oliguria can be converted to diuresis (59). It is unclear whether this improved survival results from the diuresis itself or whether such patients have less severe disease. On the contrary, hypercatabolism carries an extremely poor prognosis. Thus, in one series of almost 600 patients (M. Bullock, Hennepin Co. Med. Center, Minneapolis, MN, unpublished), almost no patients survived who were over 40 years old and who had increments in blood urea nitrogen level exceeding 30 mg/dl/day (10.7 mmol/l of urea/day). It seems as if, at this rate of urea generation, patients deteriorate rapidly. Endogenous protein breakdown may be so fast that it prevents any reparative processes such as wound healing, cell production or sufficient leukocytosis for defense against infections. It is unknown whether increasing removal of urea by hyperefficient dialysis or decreasing protein breakdown through the use of hyperalimentation and anabolic steroids have any effect on such abnormalities.

Causes of death

The most common cause of death in patients with acute tubular necrosis treated by dialysis is infection. The survival rate of a patient relates directly to the number of infections, ranging from 85% survival in patients showing no infections to 20% in those with four or more infections (78, 33).

Other general ill effects of surgery and maximal stress, to which these patients are subjected, include myocardial infarction, pancreatitis, pulmonary emboli, stress ulcers and bleeding. Patients with acute tubular necrosis following gastrointestinal surgery have always shown the highest death rate (4–10, 82–85). Overlying all these effects of the primary disease are those of uremia, including the bleeding tendency and decreased immune defenses and such complications of the dialysis procedure as intermittent cerebral edema, cardiovascular stress with hypotension and arrhythmias and complications of anticoagulation.

Finally, there are difficulties in supplying calories and protein to these patients, without causing fluid overload. Thus, malnutrition is common and associated with a decrease in wound healing and immunological deficiencies. All these factors interact in subtle, poorly understood ways to cause the formidable mortality of these patients.

All in all, infections are directly responsible for death in between one-third and two-thirds of the patients. Myocardial infarctions and congestive heart failure cause between 5 and 30% of the deaths. Pulmonary emboli are much more common in the older patients and account for 1 to 5% of the fatalities. Gastrointestinal hemorrhage causes between 5 and 30% of the deaths but shows a marked decrease with more intense dialysis (4–10, 82–90).

Intracerebral bleeding and sequela of brain trauma are rarely causes of death; other rare causes of death include digitalis intoxication, hyperkalemia and technical problems of the dialysis procedure such as erroneous dialysate, air embolization or dialyzer rupture and shock. Several of the causes of death probably represent incurable underlying disease. These include cardiac failure following coronary artery bypass and other heart operations, irreversible brain damage secondary to brain trauma and devitalized bowel and peritonitis (4–10, 82–91). A number of these problems will now be discussed in more detail.

GENERAL MANAGEMENT

Resuscitation phase

Immediately after the onset of acute renal failure, two main threats to the patient's life arise. One is fluid overload, almost always iatrogenic, as excessive fluids are given in the mistaken belief that oliguria and uremia result from dehydration. The second problem is hyperkalemia, due both to the release of potassium from traumatized, damaged tissue and hematomata, as well as from shifts from the intracellular to the extracellular space, because of the acidosis that is almost uniformly present in such patients.

Fluid overload
Assessment of a patient's fluid state requires daily measurements of body weight, an accurate review of intake and output and continuous monitoring of fluid balance. Even when all these data are available, it is difficult to deal with such patients because of the impossibility of quantifying third spaced (sequestered) fluid volume accurately.

The most dangerous complication of fluid overload is fluid lung (pulmonary edema, uremic 'pneumonitis').

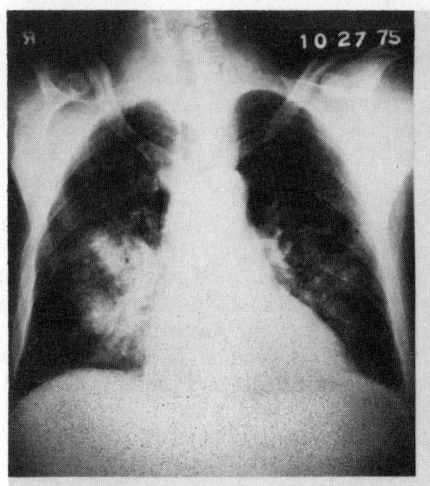
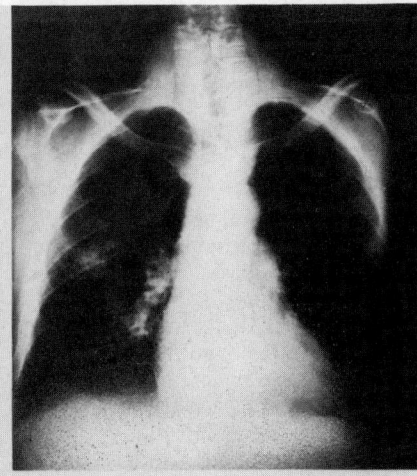
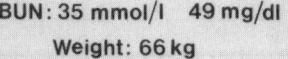

Figure 3. Classical appearance of fluid overload in a uremic patient. Note the occurrence of the central (butterfly or bat wing pattern) pulmonary edema. The infiltration rapidly clears with fluid removal by ultrafiltration in this patient. The first chest x-ray taken in the morning before dialysis, the second one on the evening of the same day after dialysis with a 3 kg fluid removal (from Kjellstrand et al [94] with permission of the publishers).

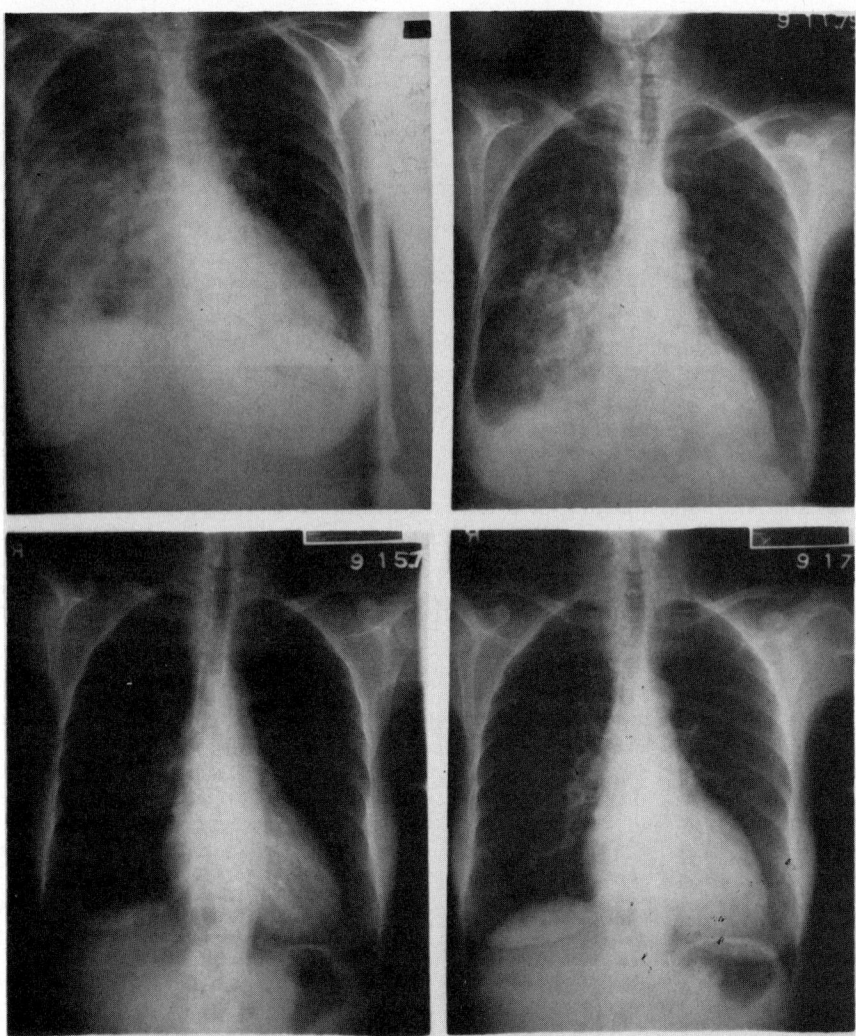

Figure 4. Lobar pulmonary edema in a patient with renal failure. Top left picture was taken immediately before dialysis, the second top right picture 5 hours later after a 5 kg fluid removal with dialysis. The lower left picture was taken the next morning with a further 1 kg weight loss induced by diarrhea. The bottom right picture was taken 3 days after dialysis with no further fluid removal.

Patients with acute renal failure frequently have a decreased plasma oncotic pressure, an increased hydrostatic pressure in pulmonary capillaries because of fluid overload and subtle capillary injury in their lungs, particularly in the perihilar region. All these factors make such patients susceptible to pulmonary edema (4, 92, 93). Figure 3 shows the typical perihilar x-ray localization of fluid. The edema may be atypical, is often impossible to differentiate from infections or pulmonary emboli (4, 94) and may cause hemoptysis (95). The x-rays of one such patient with lobar pulmonary edema, indistinguishable from pneumonia, are shown in Figure 4.

During the acute resuscitation phase, the patient's blood pressure and central venous pressure (CVP) should be monitored frequently. It is often helpful to measure cardiac output and pulmonary arterial and wedge pressures (96, 97).

A mild degree of fluid overload can sometimes be treated simply by not replacing ongoing output. In more urgent situations, oral sorbitol (70% solution, 2 ml/kg) or rectal sorbitol (20% solution, 10 ml/kg) can be used provided that the gastrointestinal tract is functionally intact (4, 98). Furosemide may contribute to clearing of the pulmonary edema even in oliguric patients (84). Severe fluid overload is one of the classical indications for emergency dialysis with ultrafiltration.

Hyperkalemia

The second lethal threat to a patient with acute renal failure is hyperkalemia. It is frequently associated with acidosis. Hyperkalemia causes cardiac conduction defects leading to asystole unless ectopic rhythms ending in ventricular fibrillation supervene. Figure 5 illustrates the electrocardiographic changes encountered in hyperkalemia and the approximate plasma potassium levels at

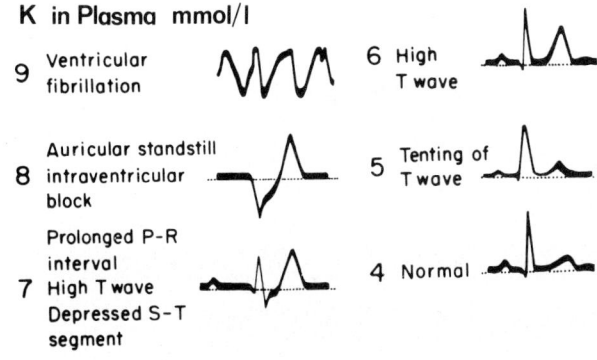

Figure 5. Electrocardiographic changes seen at various plasma-potassium levels. Note that the plasma levels are only approximate and electrocardiographic changes only roughly correlate to the plasma potassium levels (From Kjellstrand et al [94] with permission of the publishers).

which they occur. (See also Figures 1a and 1b in Chapter 19). Rarely, hyperkalemic electrocardiographic changes are indistinguishable from those of myocardial infarction.

The treatment of hyperkalemia consists of antagonizing the effects on the myocardium, shifting potassium to the intracellular space and removing it (92).

Both calcium and sodium ions directly antagonize the cardiotoxic effect of potassium. Calcium should be infused under electrocardiographic monitoring. In less urgent situations, infusion of a mixture of glucose, insulin, calcium, and sodium lactate (bicarbonate cannot be mixed with calcium) is started. This will favor movement of the potassium ion from the extracellular to the intracellular space. Lactate is converted (in patients not suffering from lactic acidosis) to bicarbonate in the body. Removal of potassium is achieved through the oral or rectal administration of exchange resins or by dialysis. Table 5 summarizes the treatment for hyperkalemia and Figure 6 exemplifies the usage of all treatment modalities.

Late routine general treatment

Once the restoration phase in a patient with acute tubular necrosis is over, treatment directed against commonly occurring complications is instituted. Included are prophylaxis against infection, gastrointestinal bleeding and malnutrition.

Infection prophylaxis
The urinary tract is infected in almost 80% and the lungs are infected in over 60% of patients with acute tubular necrosis. Clinical septicemia is present in approximately 30% and blood cultures may be positive in as many as 15% of the patients (4).

Most patients with acute tubular necrosis are oliguric, or develop oliguria when started on dialysis. An indwelling urinary catheter is not necessary in oliguric patients. As soon as it is clear that the patient is oliguric, the catheter should be removed and the bladder palpated and percussed daily. Straight catheterization can be performed if retention of urine is suspected. If a catheter is deemed necessary, a condom catheter should be tried. A closed system should always be utilized. Almost all bladders with indwelling catheters are infected after 4 days. Pyelonephritis and sepsis may result (99-103).

As soon as the restoration phase is over, all intravascular catheters not absolutely necessary for hemodynamic monitoring should be removed. There is almost never a reason to measure intra-arterial blood pressure

Table 5. Treatment of hyperkalemia.

Urgency	Treatment	Dose	Mechanism	Time for effect
Hyperacute	Calcium intravenously	10 ml 10% calcium gluconate/1-5 min. until EKG improves May need 100 ml	Antagonism	Immediate
Acute	A. Insulin-glucose-lactate-calcium intravenously B. Bicarbonate intravenously	500 ml 30% dextrose 30 units insulin +100 mmol Na-lactate +30 ml 10% calcium gluconate; 100 ml in 1st h then 20 to 30 ml/h	Shifts K$^+$ to intracellular space	30 min
Less urgent	A. Exchange resin	50 g Kayexalate orally in 100 ml 20% sorbitol solution or 60 g Kayexalate as an enema in 500 ml 10% sorbitol solution	Removes K$^+$ from body	1 to 2 h
	B. Dialysis	–	Removes K$^+$ from body	Immediate

From: Kjellstrand et al. (94) with permission of the publishers.

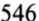

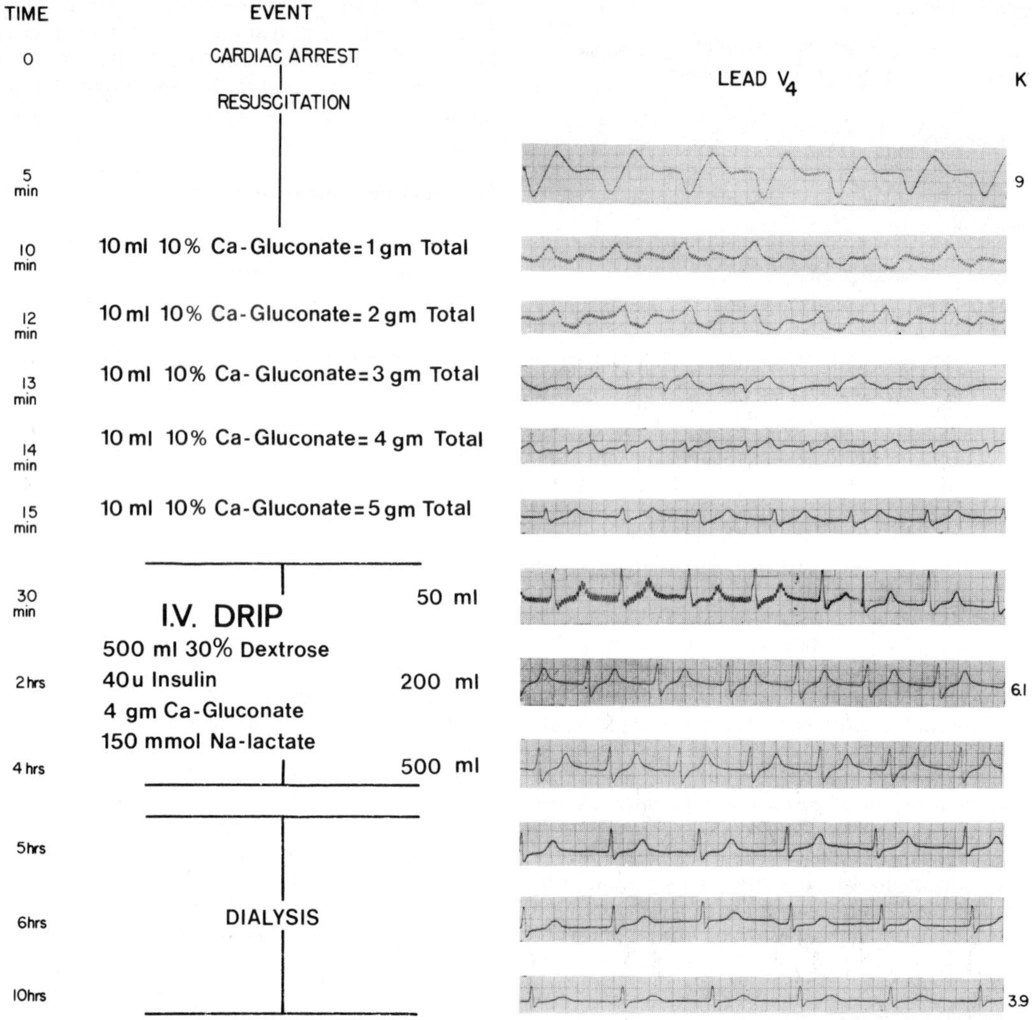

Figure 6. Electrocardiographic changes in a patient with hyperkalemia treated with rapid infusion of calcium gluconate, antagonizing potassium toxicity, followed by shifting of potassium to intracellular space through insulin, glucose, calcium and lactate infusion, and finally by dialysis (from reference [94] with permission).

in any patient. Nor should there be any need for continued measurements of central venous or wedge pressures. Clinical examination and chest x-ray suffice. Intravascular catheters become infected with increased frequency beyond the 4th day (104). A central catheter may be necessary for hyperalimentation but it may be safer to administer hyperalimentation fluids through the arteriovenous shunt. We have successfully hyperalimented many patients through their shunts and believe that infections are infrequent and easier to diagnose with this approach (105).

As the lungs so often become the site of infection, patients should be extubated as soon as possible, and mobilized. Physical therapy, breathing and coughing exercises are instituted, although the value of these is controversial (106, 107).

Indwelling catheters and treatment with broad spectrum antibiotics are often complicated by fungal complications, particularly candida, but others are also common. Prophylaxis is indicated with nystatin or clotrimazole (swish and swallow) every 4 hours or administered through a nasogastric tube (108–111). Specimens for culture should be obtained frequently. Isolation of the patient probably is of little help (112, 113).

Prophylaxis against gastrointestinal bleeding
Gastrointestinal stress ulcers are a risk in patients with acute tubular necrosis (88–90). These patients are frequently maximally stressed and have elevated gastrin levels (114–116). Aluminum hydroxide suspension (15 to 60 ml several times a day) should be used and gastric acidity titrated to a pH above 3.5 (117, 118). Aluminum hydroxide decreases gastric acidity, the absorption of phosphorus and hydrogen ions and the risk of peptic ulcer. If the patient has a nasogastric tube, it is instilled through the tube, diluted with normal saline and sorbi-

26: *Acute renal failure*   547

tol and left in place for half an hour. Adverse effects include formation of a medication bezoar with small and large bowel ischemia, perforation and death (119, 121). Small amounts of sorbitol, given with the aluminum hydroxide should prevent impaction and its consequences. Metabolic complications of aluminum hydroxide use include hypophosphatemia, so serum phosphorus must be monitored. Magnesium containing antacids must not be used lest magnesium intoxication ensue.

Cimetidine should also prevent stress ulceration, although it appears to be less effective than antacids (122–127). The dose of cimetidine must be reduced to half of the normal dose when used in patients on hemodialysis (128). Adverse effects of this drug include potential nephrotoxicity, decreased hepatic blood flow, and mental confusion (129–135). One suggestion has been to combine small doses of antacids and cimetidine and titrate gastric acidity. There are no clinical trials yet of such a combination treatment (136–139).

Prophylaxis against malnutrition
Many patients with acute tubular necrosis are critically ill and under maximal stress. They may utilize 5,000 calories and 200 g of protein per day (140).

Malnourished patients suffer from increased postoperative complications including deficient wound healing, immunological defects and increased rates of infections. It is therefore important to supply adequate calories and protein to such patients (141–144).

For feeding, the gastrointestinal route is much safer than intravenous hyperalimentation and should be used whenever possible. New techniques include small diameter soft nasogastric tubes, operative and percutaneous gastrostomy and ileostomy. An elemental oral diet is no more effective than regular homogenized high calorie, high quality protein, normal food. To the contrary, use of the elemental diet, because of the higher osmotic load, is complicated by diarrhea more often (145–147).

Intravenous hyperalimentation causes a number of clinical problems. Plasma electrolyte concentrations

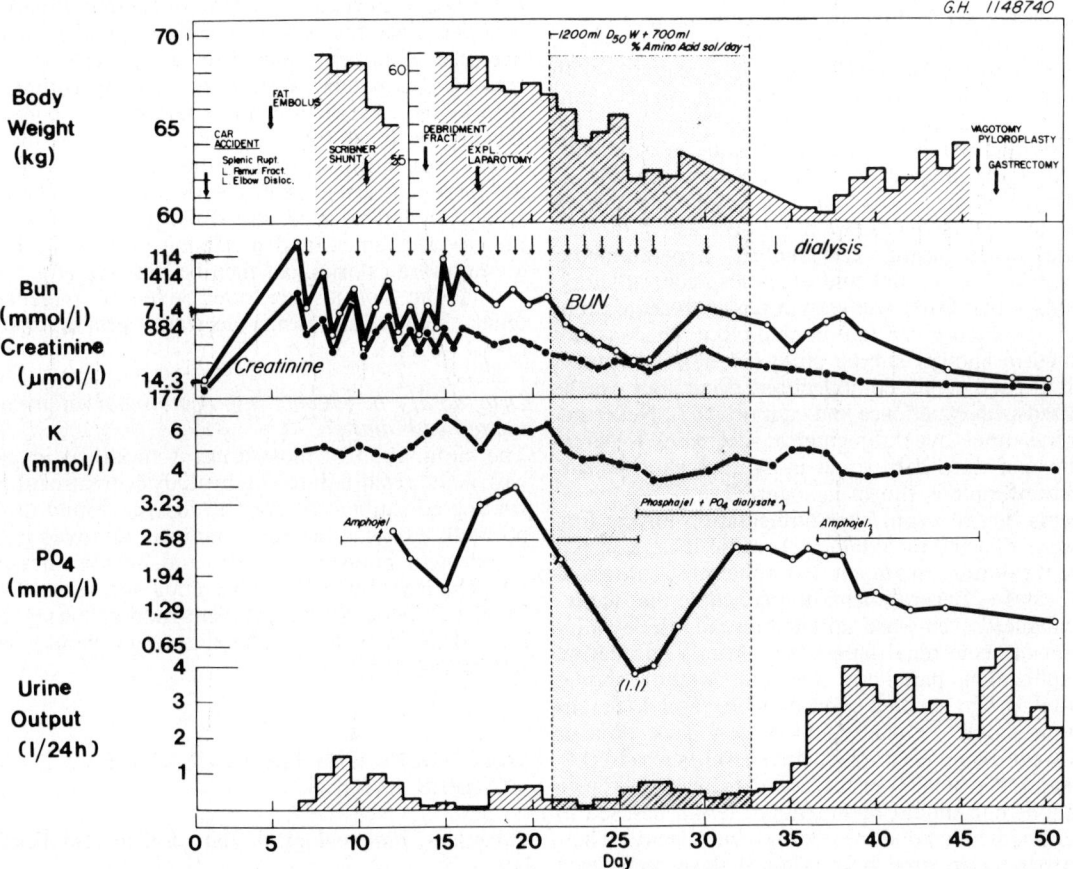

Figure 7. The influence of hyperalimentation and of catabolism in a patient requiring dialysis for acute renal failure following trauma. Before hyperalimentation, BUN ranged from 36 to 54 mmol/l despite daily dialysis. Plasma potassium varied between 5 and 7 mmol/l and phosphorus remained between 3.3 and 5.5 mmol/l. During hyperalimentation these values decreased and supplements of both potassium and phosphorus were required. (From [94], with permission).
(BUN mmol/l → mg/dl: multiply by 2.8
creatinine μmol/l → mg/dl: multiply by 0.0113
PO$_4$ mmol/l → mg/dl: multiply by 3.1).

may change rapidly and need to be measured frequently. Hypoglycemia and hyperglycemia can occur, contributing to water shifts and intracellular edema or dehydration. Finally, even with new concentrated solutions, hyperalimentation invariably causes periodic fluid overload and full hyperalimentation in the oliguric patient almost always necessitates daily hemodialysis to remove the 'carrier water'. Present regimens of hyperalimentation include 0.5 to 1.5 g/kg body weight/day of an amino acid solution. The patients also receive between 40 and 100 calories/kg/day (148): ten percent of the calories are supplied by the amino acid solution, 50% by dextrose and the remaining 40% by intravenous fat. The 20% fat solution contains more calories/volume and less osmoles/calorie than any other intravenous solution.

It should be understood that the exact needs, dangers and benefits of intravenous hyperalimentation for the patient with acute tubular necrosis are not yet fully evaluated. Feinstein, Blumenkrantz and Healy (140) for example, could not find any definite advantage of dextrose plus essential amino acids over dextrose plus essential and non-essential amino acids or over dextrose alone, a finding also noted by Leonard, Luke and Siegel (64).

Abel et al (63), however, found more rapid recovery of renal function and increased survival in patients with acute renal failure when given essential amino acid containing hyperalimentation solutions. Baek et al (66) found no difference in renal recovery rate but better survival in hyperalimental patients than in those not receiving hyperalimentation. Others have found neither an increase in renal recovery rate nor a decrease in mortality rate when using intravenous hyperalimentation (64, 65, 148). Animal studies are also contradictory. One study found faster recovery in rats with acute tubular necrosis when given amino acids, but this was not confirmed in another similar study (67, 68). Traumatic, thrombotic and septic complications occur, but can be minimized with experience and caution (147). Nevertheless, intravenous hyperalimentation decreases hypercatabolism and does help some individual patients survive. An example is shown in Figure 7.

It seems best to avoid hyperalimentation for the first 3 or 4 days of acute renal failure, because it can complicate the restoration treatment. Even the most enthusiastic advocates of hyperalimentation conclude that recovery is enhanced even when initiated on the 4th day after the onset of acute renal failure (63). After resuscitation and stabilization, parenteral hyperalimentation should be started if oral feeding is impossible. Full hyperalimentation should be reached in 3 to 4 days. Smaller amounts can be given through peripheral veins (145).

Sargent and Gotch (149) suggest that urea appearance (generation) rate should be measured. It can be used to titrate individual hyperalimentation requirements. Their data in patients treated by chronic dialysis show that protein catabolic rate = 6.4 × BUN generation + 11, and are similar to those of patients with acute renal failure (6.75 × BUN generation + 5.1) reported by Feinstein, Blumenkrantz and Healy (140). The factors (11 or 5.1) are obligatory extrarenal nitrogen losses in the feces and elsewhere in g/day and are equal to that generated by breakdown of 11 or 5.1 g of protein. The

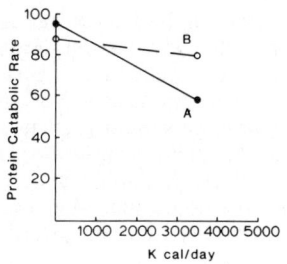

Figure 8. Protein catabolic rate (as grams of protein catabolized daily) plotted versus calorie infusion into patients with acute renal failure. In patient A, there is a clear decrease in protein catabolic rate in response to calorie infusion. Much less decrease is seen in patient B. (Modified from Sargent and Gotch [149]).

urea generation rate can easily be calculated by multiplying total body water of a patient, derived from clinical examination and tables, by the change in blood urea nitrogen concentration, measured at two different times, e.g., after a 24 h interval. When plotting protein catabolic rate against caloric intake in acutely ill patients, it becomes clear that some patients respond with a large decrease in protein catabolism as the calories are increased (e.g., patient A in Figure 8), whereas others (e.g., B in Figure 8) show much less response. In clinical use, this approach can be simplified to calculating the rise in blood urea nitrogen concentration each 24 h, while giving increasing amounts of calories. Whether the protein sparing achieved in an individual patient is worth the increased technical and metabolic problems caused by giving more calories can then be determined.

Anabolic steroids are often given to patients with renal failure and can decrease protein catabolic rate (150, 151).

Drug dosage in patients with acute renal failure and treated with dialysis

The elimination of most drugs is modified in patients with acute renal failure and by dialysis treatment, necessitating adjustment of normal dosages. Many drugs are normally excreted in urine, many are removed by dialysis. Protein binding of drugs, and hepatic metabolism may change in patients with uremia and sepsis. Chapter 39 of this book or two excellent monographs (152, 153) as well as frequently updated reviews should be consulted (154, 155).

DIAGNOSIS AND TREATMENT OF COMPLICATIONS

Infectious, immunological, and surgical complications

Renal failure leads to a global decrease in immune defense (156–158), as does major surgery (159, 160). In addition, infection is a major risk in patients with acute renal failure. Many patients suffer from malnutrition that also impairs the immune defense (141–144). Hyperalimentation with intense daily or alternate day dialysis may decrease this risk factor. A hematocrit value of

32% also seems to be most favorable in the postoperative period, and this value should be maintained in these patients (161). Infection prophylaxis, as described above, frequent cultures, and treatment with narrow-spectrum antibiotics are indicated. Daily to weekly cultures of urine, feces, sputum, blood and drainage fluids should be performed.

Infections can be difficult to diagnose in uremic patients who will not show a normal febrile response because urea is a potent antipyretic (162). Even moderate elevations of temperature are thus alarming signs in these patients. The severely traumatized patient also often fails to show the usual clinical signs of infection such as pain and tenderness, or rigidity in peritonitis. The most reliable sign is probably the white blood cell count, but even leukocytosis does not occur regularly. The white blood cell count should not be checked during dialysis, however, because of the dialysis associated leukopenia (163, 164).

Almost all patients who develop tubular necrosis after abdominal operations have neglected complications of surgery. Thus, Marshall (165) describing post-operative acute renal failure, reexplored 18 of 118 such patients; 17 had a gross surgical complication. All nine patients who developed acute tubular necrosis after large bowel surgery had developed a fecal leak. Post-operative shock was common in these patients. Kornhall (166) reviewing 298 surgical patients with acute tubular necrosis found that 98 patients (33%) had neglected surgical complications; 81 of these 98 (83%) died. An aggressive surgical approach to these patients is necessary. Marshall (165) comments: '... these patients are invariably too ill not to be operated on, rather than the reverse...' Investigations with x-rays, ultrasonography, gallium and indium scans, as well as computerized axial tomography are often indicated (165–172).

Metabolic and endocrine problems

The onset of acute uremia causes several endocrine-metabolic problems (see Chapter 36). Peripheral insulin sensitivity is decreased in uremia and many such patients have hyperinsulinemia. Furthermore, glucose metabolism tends to be decreased. If septicemia occurs, hyperglycemia often occurs. Glucose levels, therefore, must be carefully monitored to prevent marked fluid shifts (148).

Shortly after the onset of acute renal failure, plasma calcium levels start to decrease. This is not due to increased excretion but reflects a shift of calcium out of the extracellular space. Calcitonin increases to extremely high levels (173), and secondary to the decline in plasma calcium concentration, parathyroid hormone levels rise (174, 175). Calcium and magnesium levels in the brain increase which may contribute to the stupor and confusion often observed in such patients (176). Plasma phosphorus levels usually rise and may also contribute to the secondary hyperparathyroidism, the decline in plasma calcium concentration and the increase in calcitonin levels. The hypocalcemia and hyperphosphatemia can be particularly marked in patients with rhabdomyolysis and acute renal failure. When uremia subsides, some patients with acute renal failure develop marked hypercalcemia; this is also particularly pronounced in patients who suffered from rhabdomyolysis (177–182). Many other hormonal abnormalities occur, but are insufficiently studied. Plasma gastrin levels increase and may contribute to the stress ulcers that these patients develop (114–116).

Anemia develops quickly, possibly secondary to a decreased erythropoietin level or decreased peripheral sensitivity to erythropoietin. As mentioned above, these patients should be transfused to a hematocrit of approximately 32% (161). Plasma uric acid levels rise; particularly high levels are seen in patients with neoplasms or rhabdomyolysis (177–185). Excess uric acid may precipitate the acute renal failure by precipitating in renal tubules (184). In such patients, the ratio of uric acid to creatinine in urine exceeds 1.0 (186). Many of these metabolic problems, e.g., plasma calcium, phosphorus and uric acid levels improve with dialysis.

Other organ system abnormalities

Every organ system sustains dysfunction during acute uremia; most of these problems improve with dialysis. Many however, are made worse by inappropriate conservative management leading e.g., to electrolyte abnormalities.

Stupor, confusion, myoclonus and, in severe cases, seizures are consequences of acute severe uremia. They should never be allowed to develop and can be prevented by dialysis before the urea nitrogen level exceeds 100 to 120 mg/dl (35.7 to 42.8 mmol/l). Hyponatremia secondary to water intoxication may aggravate the clinical syndrome.

In patients with acute uremia, increased capillary permeability can cause pulmonary edema with only moderate fluid overload (see above). Other complications such as shock lung, acute respiratory distress syndrome and pulmonary emboli are consequences of the basic disease more than of uremia. Hemodialysis is also associated with moderate acute transient pulmonary dysfunction (see Chapter 32).

Cardiovascular problems rarely are due to uremia per se, but most often are caused by unskilled management. Thus, pericarditis, a complication of advanced uremia, almost never occurs when patients are dialyzed early. Arrythmias may occur secondary to underlying myocardial disease and may be provoked or aggravated by dialysis.

Uremic patients develop anorexia and, in severe cases, nausea and vomiting may occur. These can be treated symptomatically but are best prevented by early and frequent dialysis. Phenothiazines should be avoided because of the high incidence of extrapyramidal side effects in uremic patients. These drugs also aggravate hypotension during dialysis. Stress ulcers, as discussed above, should be prevented by antacids and cimetidine. In the rare patient who develops diffuse gastritis with severe bleeding gastrectomy may be necessary as illustrated in Figure 7. However, if major bleeding vessels can be identified through angiography, pitressin infusion or induced embolization by injection into the vessel may avoid this rather drastic operation (187, 188).

Coagulation abnormalities may also occur in acute uremia. The most well-known defect is platelet dysfunction, secondary to guanidino succinic acid accumulation. This abnormality is rapidly reversed by dialysis (189). Other abnormalities consist of a decrease of several clotting proteins and an increased level of prostacyclin in the capillaries (190). These factors do not improve with dialysis and contribute to the hemorragic diathesis of uremic patients. Fresh frozen plasma may improve some of these defects. Paradoxically some patients may also develop intravascular coagulation because of certain abnormalities, such as a decrease in antiplasmin level (191).

DIALYSIS: WHEN AND BY WHICH METHOD?

Indications for initiating dialysis

Dialysis effectively removes small molecular weight substances and efficiently corrects electrolyte abnormalities and excess of body water. But dialysis cannot synthesize or catabolize protein as the normal kidneys do.

In addition, all dialysis procedures are time consuming and take the (acute) patient away from other therapeutic and diagnostic procedures.

Hemodialysis may cause cardiovascular instability and transient pulmonary dysfunction and requires anticoagulation. Peritoneal dialysis interferes with diaphragmatic movements and carries the risk of peritonitis.

The indications for dialysis include: uremia, severe fluid overload, acidosis and hyperkalemia.

Electrolyte and fluid disturbances, often due to inappropriate conservative treatment, should not progress until they are so severe as to precipitate the need for emergency dialysis. In the well-managed patient with acute tubular necrosis the decision to start dialysis will be based on the degree of azotemia that the physician considers appropriate to treat.

The general trend has been towards early and more frequent dialysis. This strategy should protect the patient with acute renal failure, who is often struggling with extremely severe underlying basic problems, from taking on the additional burden of severe uremia and electrolyte and fluid disturbances.

Urgent indications for dialysis in acute renal failure are plasma potassium concentrations above 7 mmol/l, plasma bicarbonate levels of 15 mmol/l or less, blood urea nitrogen concentrations over 150 mg/dl (54 mmol/l of blood urea) and plasma creatinine values above 10 mg/dl (or 885 µmol/l). *Dialysis should be started long before such concentrations occur.*

In catabolic patients it may be helpful to calculate the mean BUN concentration around which pre- and post-dialysis values will vary, utilizing the formula:

1. Production of urea nitrogen = removal at a steady state

2. Removal = mean blood concentration of urea nitrogen × clearance of the dialyzer × fraction of time dialysis is applied.

For example, a 70 kg man, breaking down 70 g protein/day (i.e. producing about 11.5 g of urea nitrogen/day) and utilizing a dialyzer with a urea clearance of 150 ml/min for a 4 hour dialysis every other day would have a total urea clearance 36 l/48 h, i.e. 18 l/day. The calculated mean concentration of blood urea nitrogen would be 64 mg/dl (23 mmol/l of blood urea) using the formula:

3. Urea nitrogen production = total body water × (predialysis − postdialysis blood urea nitrogen concentration)

the decrease in BUN concentration during dialysis and the increment in the interdialytic interval can be calculated.

In the example given above, the decrease in BUN concentration approximates 54 mg/dl (19 mmol/l of blood urea) and the patient's BUN concentration would vary from a high 91 $(64 + \frac{54}{2})$ mg/dl (33 mmol of blood urea) to a low of 37 $(64 - \frac{54}{2})$ mg/dl (13 mmol/l of blood urea). This example suggests that it is not worthwhile starting dialysis before the BUN concentration has reached 90 to 100 mg/dl (32 to 36 mmol/l of blood urea) (unless electrolyte or fluid problems require earlier intervention).

Such quantitative approaches, however, as also described by Sargent and Gotch (149), do provide a rational way of managing such problems.

Hemodialysis versus peritoneal dialysis

Several authors have compared hemodialysis and peritoneal dialysis for treatment of acute renal failure. The survival data are similar regardless of which method is applied (86, 89, 193). Hemodialysis has the advantage of efficiency and shorter duration, so the patient can be free for other therapeutic and diagnostic procedures. It is technically more complicated, requires anticoagulation, and the rapid biochemical changes may induce side effects such as hypotension and disequilibrium. Peritoneal dialysis is simple, but carries the risk of peritonitis, and takes a long time. Peritoneal dialysis is probably best for patients with marked cardiovascular instability as hemodialysis may cause further problems or even death. Peritoneal dialysis is also preferable in patients with head trauma (91), and in patients with grossly contaminated abdominal cavities. The mechanical cleaning and removal of necrotic tissue and clots from the peritoneal cavity and the local action of antibiotics that can be added may be advantageous and improve survival (194–200). Peritoneal dialysis is contra-indicated in patients without peritonitis who have open wounds or a stoma in their abdomen. It should not be used in patients with recent intestinal anastomosis or when the peritoneal membranes are not intact. Finally, it is not always efficient enough for hypercatabolic patients. Some patients benefit from combined hemodialysis and peritoneal dialysis. For example, in many catabolic patients, continuous peritoneal dialysis may be supplemented by intermittent hemodialysis. In other patients, hemodialysis may be preferred initially when the patient is highly catabolic and peritoneal dialysis may be better at a later stage when the metabolic response has abated.

HEMODIALYSIS TECHNIQUES AND COMPLICATIONS

Vascular access (See also Chapter 8)

Percutaneous catheterization of the femoral or subclavian vein or the Scribner shunt are the vascular access procedures ordinarily used for acute hemodialysis. An arteriovenous fistula has no place in acute dialysis but can be performed later in those patients who do not regain renal function.

Two punctures can be performed in the femoral or the subclavian vein or a Y-connecter may be used with a single needle device. In the patient with accessible veins, a fistula needle can also be placed in a peripheral vein for the return line. The femoral vein has the advantage of being technically easier and anatomically safer than the subclavian vein. It has the disadvantage of being a 'dirtier' area, close to the perineum. Catheters can, therefore, not be left in place because of risk of infection. Complications of femoral vein catheterization consist of femoral vein thrombosis with pulmonary emboli when the catheter is left in situ more than 24 h, infections and inadvertent arterial punctures with hematoma and rarely arteriovenous fistula formation. Accidental perforation of the femoral vein by the Seldinger wire and then by the catheter, a rare occurrence, can cause a massive retroperitoneal hematoma and shock on initiation of hemodialysis. Yet, skilled operators have used repeated puncture of the femoral vein for several years. It is contraindicated to leave the catheter in situ more than 24 to 36 h (201).

The subclavian vein catheter is now being used with increasing frequency and is enthusiastically advocated by some. It can be left in place for several weeks with a moderate risk of infection. Technical complications include brachial plexus lesions, hemothorax and pneumothorax. Insertion is also more difficult than femoral vein puncture. It is almost exclusively used with a single catheter and a Y-connecter for the single needle technique (202–206).

The Scribner arteriovenous shunt remains the main stay for acute dialysis. Short term, it is relatively free of complications and can also be used for blood gas determinations, and hyperalimentation (105). It has the disadvantage of potentially sacrificing two vessels. The Scribner shunt rarely becomes infected or clotted during the brief period it is needed for acute dialysis. If the patient does not recover renal function, it can later be changed into an arteriovenous fistula (207).

A satisfactory arteriovenous shunt can usually be achieved in small children, weighing more than 3 to 4 kg, utilizing special pediatric shunt material to connect the radial artery and cephalic vein in the forearm. Children smaller than 3 kg can either undergo dialysis with an arteriovenous shunt in the groin or in the upper arm, or preferably can be dialyzed with vein-to-vein access. Hickman or Broviack catheters can be used for the return of blood to the patient but are sometimes difficult to use for outflow lines to the dialyzer.[1] A semi-rigid polyethylene catheter with a 9 French[2] diameter placed with the tip centrally, functions better as a blood outflow line. In children smaller than 3 kg, a blood flow rate of 15 ml/min can achieve effective dialysis (see below).

Almost any mode of vascular access can be used with the single needle technique with only very little loss of efficiency. It is difficult to use the single needle technique with hollow fiber dialyzers, however, because they have almost no compliance. Therefore, exchange volumes are small and pressures are extremely high.

Choice of dialysis equipment and procedures

Dialyzers
There is no great difference in efficiency or priming volumes between plate and hollow fiber dialyzers. Hollow fiber dialyzers tend to cause less thrombocytopenia; dialysis with plate dialyzers requires less heparin (208). Coil dialyzers tend to contain somewhat more blood and also have a higher compliance. It is difficult to use hollow fiber dialyzers with single needle technique because of the very low compliance. All in all, the choice between the different dialyzers is somewhat arbitrary except in very small children where special, small volume dialyzers must be used. A dialyzer and its blood lines should not contain more than 10% of the patient's blood volume. For a newborn child weighing 3½ or 4 kg, the whole system should not contain much more than 30 to 40 ml (209–212). (See also Chapters 5 and 25.)

Dialysis solution
The composition of the dialysis fluid should be adjusted to the patient's individual needs. Routine standard dialysis fluid, such as that used for patients with chronic renal failure, is not suitable for the acutely ill patient.

Sodium. Sodium concentration of the dialysis solution should be 140 mmol/l. A lower sodium concentration, as is used in treating hypertension in chronic uremic patients, is unsuitable for patients with acute renal failure. Every study comparing a lower to a higher concentration in the dialysis solution shows that the lower sodium concentration is associated with a much higher incidence of hypotension, disequilibrium and other complications (213–217). A method of slowly decreasing the

---
[1] Hickman and Broviack catheters are made by: *Ever-med Company, P.O. Box 296 Medina, Washington 98039, USA.*
[2] 1 French = 0.3 mm.

sodium concentration in the dialysis fluid during a dialysis session has recently been described. It results in more stable dialysis but is difficult to achieve with currently available equipment (218). If a patient has had hypernatremia for more than one day before dialysis, it is probably best to use a higher than normal dialysate sodium concentration. A concentration of sodium in the dialysis fluid approximately half way between that of the patient's plasma sodium concentration and the normal value is appropriate for the first one or two dialyses. When plasma sodium concentration is reduced too quickly, the patient develops cerebral edema because the brain accumulates idiogenic osmoles to compensate for hypernatremia and these are removed slowly (219).

Potassium. It is often necessary to use a dialysis fluid with a low potassium concentration, particularly for traumatized and hypercatabolic patients who can rapidly develop hyperkalemia. A low concentration of potassium in dialysis fluid must not be used in the digitalized patient, because severe digitalis intoxication can result if the potassium level is decreased too quickly. Furthermore, the rapid correction of the acidosis by dialysis may cause very sudden and marked shifts of potassium from the extra- to the intracellular space that may result in severe or even fatal hypokalemia (220).

Calcium. The most appropriate concentration in dialysate is probably identical to or slightly higher than that of normal plasma ionized calcium, i.e., 2.5 to 3.5 mEq/l (1.25 to 1.75 mmol/l or 5 to 7 mg/dl). Some patients with hypercalcemia must be dialyzed against a dialysis fluid containing no calcium (221). Patients with hypoproteinemia usually should not have a low calcium concentration in the dialysis solution because their ultrafilerable calcium concentration in plasma is normal. Patients with marked hyperphosphatemia should also have a lower than normal calcium concentration in the dialysis fluid until the plasma phosphorus concentration has been reduced to nearly normal levels. This situation may be particularly common in patients who have developed acute tubular necrosis complicating rhabdomyolysis, lymphoma or leukemia (184). A higher calcium concentration has been recommended in selected instances to maintain a higher blood pressure during dialysis (185).

Magnesium. It is customary to use a dialysis fluid with a magnesium concentration close to the normal plasma value, i.e., 1.5 to 1.7 mEq/l (0.75 to 0.85 mmol/l, 1.83 to 2.07 mg/dl) although a small fraction of plasma magnesium is protein bound. Patients with alcoholism and successfully hyperalimented patients may be hypomagnesemic and need higher concentrations. Magnesium intoxicated patients, usually resulting from errors in management, may need to be dialyzed against a dialysis solution containing no magnesium.

Bicarbonate or acetate. Acetate is widely used instead of bicarbonate in the dialysate. It is technically much easier to use as it does not precipitate with calcium and magnesium, unlike bicarbonate. Acetate containing dialysis fluid is also less expensive to prepare. Its buffering action occurs as it consumes a hydrogen ion, when metabolized to acetyl-coenzyme A. A number of problems may be associated with the usage of acetate. Some patients with chronic renal failure do not metabolize acetate at a normal rate. The acetate infusion rate from dialysis fluid even during standard flux dialysis may temporarily aggravate the metabolic acidosis in such patients. This abnormality may also occur in some patients with acute renal failure. The removal of large amounts of bicarbonate by dialysis could be catastrophic should the patient metabolize acetate slowly.

Some studies suggest that the use of acetate causes more dialysis hypoxemia than occurs with bicarbonate. Acetate decreases peripheral resistance more than bicarbonate does. In some patients, this may be beneficial because of decreasing afterload and preload. In septic patients with dilated vasculature and borderline blood pressure, however, such an occurrence could lead to further catastrophic falls in blood pressure (222).

At least three clinical studies have compared acetate to bicarbonate dialysis in patients with acute renal failure. Two of those, investigating eight and nine seriously ill patients respectively, came to the conclusion that more mannitol and albumin infusions were necessary to maintain blood pressure during acetate than during bicarbonate dialysis (223, 224). In a larger study with a double-blind, cross-over format in 120 dialyses of 30 acute patients, no difference was found between acetate and bicarbonate dialysis solution in blood pressure maintenance or other clinical dialysis problems (225). In this study, a dialysis solution sodium concentration of 140 mmol/l, as well as slow dialysis and mannitol infusion were used. Wehle et al (226) found that blood pressure fell more during acetate than during bicarbonate dialysis only when a low sodium concentration (133 mmol/l) was used. It did not occur when a normal sodium concentration (145 mmol/l) was used in the dialysis solution.

An empirical approach seems reasonable until more data have accumulated. Bicarbonate dialysis should be used for the most critically ill patients and in those who appear to have trouble with acetate dialysis.

Dextrose. Some dextrose should be used in the dialysis fluid. When dextrose-free dialysis is used, negative nitrogen balance occurs during the dialysis, suggesting gluconeogenesis (227). Furthermore, there are more subjective complaints and more episodes of hypotension when patients undergo dialysis without dextrose in the bath fluid (228). The minimum dextrose level in the dialysis solution should be 100 mg/dl (5.6 mmol/l). A much higher dextrose level (approximately 700 mg/dl [39 mmol/l]) during the initial dialysis may prevent disequilibrium. Slightly increased dextrose concentrations, such as 250 mg/dl (14 mmol/l), will supply some calories and still not raise the blood glucose levels more than 20 to 30 mg/dl, i.e., 1.1 to 1.7 mmol/l (209, 229).

Phosphorus. Most patients with acute renal failure have hyperphosphatemia. But, certain disorders such as heat stroke and some burns are associated with hypophosphatemia (230, 231). Hypophosphatemia may also be the result of successful hyperalimentation as illustrated in Figure 7. In these cases, phosphorus, in physiologic concentration, approximately 4 mg/dl (1.3 mmol/l) should be added to the dialysis solution. It cannot be added to the concentrate but must be diluted before mixing with the dialysis solution, which contains calcium, to prevent precipitation.

Chloride. Chloride concentration simply makes up the difference between cation and anions in dialysis fluid. In some patients with profound metabolic alkalosis, usually secondary to nasogastric drainage, a lower than normal acetate or bicarbonate and a higher than normal chloride concentration may be beneficial (232).

Method of dialysis
The first few dialyses in a patient are ordinarily associated with more side effects than later ones (192). The early part of each dialysis is also associated with more dialysis complications. For this reason, dialysis should be started slowly, and blood flow should be limited for the first 30 to 60 min. Most adult patients tolerate blood flow through a dialyzer that results in a urea clearance of 150 to 200 ml/min. In a normal sized adult, this means a dialyzer urea clearance of 2.5 to 3 ml/kg/min (209, 233–237). Such clearance should be uniformly used on all patients. Thus, in a newborn 3 kg baby, one wishes to achieve a urea clearance of only approximately 10 ml/min, but in a 100 kg adult, a urea clearance of approximately 250 to 300 ml/min should be achieved in order to lower blood urea nitrogen levels effectively. Because urea nitrogen distributes in total body water, a correction should be made for excessive fat.

Acutely uremic patients should be dialyzed slowly, but daily, with a urea clearance of only 1 to 2 ml/kg/min for the first one to four dialyses, by restricting dialyzer size or flow rates or both. A urea clearance of 3 ml/kg/min should not be used until the fifth dialysis. The subsequent frequency and efficiency of the dialyses can then be gauged empirically, based on clinical response, blood nitrogen levels and the need for other therapeutic and diagnostic interventions. In hypercatabolic patients, this rule cannot be strictly followed, because such a regimen may not be efficient enough to control uremia in such patients.

In addition to slowing the dialysis rate during each dialysis, symptoms can be further decreased by infusing mannitol (1.0 g/kg during the first two dialyses and 0.5 g/kg during the subsequent two dialyses). Other therapeutic measures, such as a higher dextrose or sodium concentration in the dialysis solution to avoid disequilibrium syndrome and hypotension, have been discussed above (209, 229, 238, 239).

Anticoagulation
Dialysis patients are routinely anticoagulated with heparin. Prostaglandins, presently in experimental use for anticoagulation, may induce less thrombocytopenia and bleeding, but more hypotension (240–243).

The usual bolus dosage of heparin is not suitable for patients with acute renal failure, many of whom are at risk of bleeding. Heparin should be given by constant infusion. For a 60 to 70 kg patient, approximately 4,000 units of heparin will suffice with modern hollow fiber or parallel plate dialyzers during a 5 hour dialysis (244, 245).

In actively bleeding patients or those where bleeding would be particularly hazardous, an even more cautious approach must be utilized. The heparin can be neutralized at the outlet of the dialyzer by the simultaneous infusion of protamine. This method, however, is complicated, requiring two synchronized pumps. Furthermore, once dialysis is over, protamine is metabolized faster than the heparin and a rebound increase in clotting time with bleeding may occur (246–248). It is, therefore, preferable to use low-dose heparin infused into the arterial line and let the patient neutralize it (249, 250). During such treatment, much smaller doses of heparin are infused into the arterial line. The clotting time should be kept below twice normal. It is not necessary to exceed 1,500 to 2,500 units of heparin in most patients. Some patients with clotting abnormalities may require much less heparin. No rebound phenomenon occurs with this method and even actively bleeding patients can safely be treated if managed by personnel skilled in the usage of this method (249, 250). Drip chambers tend to clot much more easily than the dialyzer. Once the dialysis is over, protamine, calculated to neutralize half of the infused heparin may be given intravenously to the patients. More sophisticated supervision with activated clotting times and determination of individual heparin requirements may further decrease the already low risk of bleeding with the use of low dose heparin (251, 252). Chapter 10 provides more detailed information.

Complications of hemodialysis and their treatment

Blood pressure problems
The most common and also dangerous problem occurring during hemodialysis is acute hypotension (192, 253, 254). Table 6 and Figure 9 outline factors contributing to or causing hypotension. Hypotension (a blood pressure fall exceeding 25%) occurs in approximately 20 to 50% of all acute dialyses (225, 254).

Ultrafiltration alone rarely causes hypotension because the body's defense mechanisms to compensate for sudden volume reduction, function efficiently unless dialysis is also performed simultaneously (255–257). In markedly fluid overloaded patients with labile blood pressure, isolated ultrafiltration can, therefore, be used. During ultrafiltration, potassium and hydrogen ion removal is inhibited, however, because of the Donnan equilibrium, attenuating correction of acidosis and hyperkalemia. The use of sequential ultrafiltration-dialysis seems to be of limited use in patients with acute renal failure. During this treatment, the first half of an artificial kidney treatment is spent ultrafiltering the patient's blood without any dialysis fluid perfusing the dialyzer. Thereafter, the hydrostatic and osmotic pressures are equalized across the dialysis membrane and no fluid is removed while dialysis fluid flows promoting diffusion.

Table 6. Factors potentially causing or contributing to hypotension during acute dialysis.

Pathogenesis	Mediator	Underlying pathology
Ultrafiltration	Hypovolemia	Autonomic dysfunction
Osmolality fall	Cell dysfunction? ↓ ADH??	Myocardial dysfunction
Dialysis removal of vasoactive amines	↓ Epinephrine, norepinephrine	(Destabilizing middle molecules?)
Membrane/blood incompatibility	Cell/protein damage ↑ prostacyclin	Drugs, infection, pain
Acetate infusion	↓ PaO$_2$	Slow acetate metabolism
"Toxin" infusion	?	—

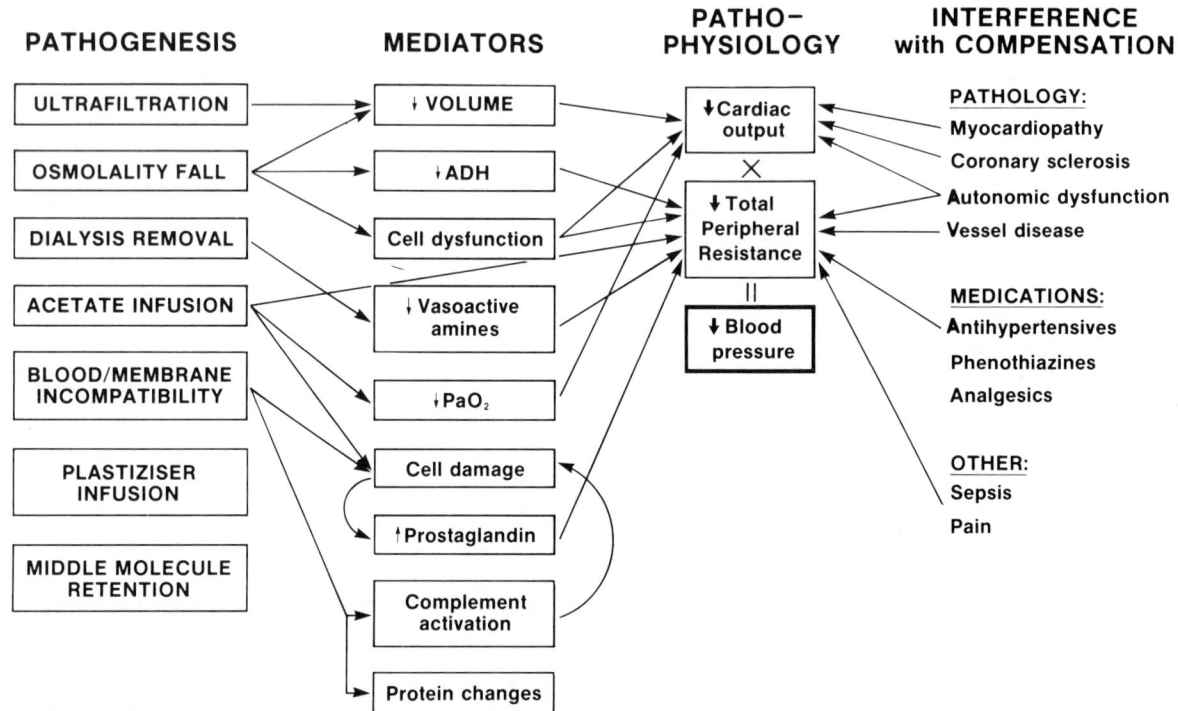

Figure 9. Known and postulated causes of hypotension during dialysis. It is important to differentiate these factors into 'pathogenesis' (how does dialysis trigger hypotension), 'mediators' (through what pathways do the dialysis triggered factors operate), and 'pathophysiology' (are cardiac output or total peripheral resistance or both involved?). Underlying these events are many factors that interfere with the compensation of cardiac output for falls in total peripheral resistance and vice versa. Thus, cardiomyopathy or coronary sclerosis may prevent increases in cardiac output when total peripheral resistance falls. Autonomic dysfunction and vascular disease may prevent increases in total peripheral resistance when cardiac output falls. A number of medications and other factors also act directly on cardiac output and total peripheral resistance. Several pathogenetic factors may affect many mediators, and some mediators affect both cardiac output and total peripheral resistance. Most factors seem to affect total peripheral resistance.

Keshaviah et al (258) have shown that there is no difference in the decrement in plasma volume at the end of simultaneous compared to sequential dialysis-ultrafiltration in dogs. Large clinical trials have shown that hypotension during the dialysis period of sequential ultrafiltration-dialysis is equal to that of simultaneous dialysis-ultrafiltration (258–261). In patients with acute renal failure it may be preferable to perform ultrafiltration one day and dialysis the next, rather than using sequencing. The induced hypovolemia can also be combated by infusion of colloid solutions, or if much fluid removal is needed, by concentrated colloid, such as 25% albumin solution. Theoretically, such a solution mobilizes fluid from the extracapillary, extracellular space into the intravascular space but the exact role of hyperoncotic albumin remains controversial (262).

The acute decrease in plasma osmolality that occurs during dialysis obviously contributes importantly to the pathogenesis of hypotension (239, 263). All studies to date, comparing dialysis solutions of varied sodium concentrations, have shown a decreased incidence and severity of hypotension with higher sodium concentrations (213–217, 264). The infusion of mannitol also attenuates the decrease in plasma osmolality and hypotension as, to a lesser extent, does the addition of dextrose to the dialysis solution (228, 238, 239, 263). Glycerol infusion has also been used for this purpose. The mechanism whereby the decrease in plasma osmolality causes hypotension is unknown; the cellular edema associated with decreased plasma osmolality may interfere with the body's response to hypotension. Other possible explanations, including prostaglandin release, decrease of plasma antidiuretic hormone activity and loss of vasoactive amines through the dialysis membrane, have been studied (265–280).

Interactions of blood components with the dialyzer membrane, e.g., complement activation resulting in leukocyte adherence and sequestration of leukocytes in the lungs, may lead to decreased PaO_2, potentially contributing to hypotension (281–284). Hypoxia occurring in patients dialyzed for acute renal failure should be treated with an increased oxygen content in the inspired air. New non-cellulosic membranes which are more biocompatible are presently being tested; one such membrane is used in hemofiltration devices. This may explain reported decreases in hypotension with this procedure (285).

Underlying pathology in severely ill acute renal failure patients may prevent them from compensating for dialysis induced hypotension. Autonomic dysfunction is sometimes present in uremic patients and vasoactive amines are infused empirically to prevent or treat dialysis induced hypotension (286–289).

In some patients, notably the elderly and those with prior cardiac surgery or heart disease, myocardial dysfunction may impair their ability to increase cardiac output in response to the fall of peripheral resistance that occurs during dialysis.

It should be kept in mind that patients may use antihypertensive agents or other drugs that cause hypotension. Such drugs (e.g., β blockers, methyldopa, phenothiazines) should be discontinued.

Patients with sepsis are also more susceptible to blood pressure problems, as are those under vasovagal stimulation by severe pain. Antimicrobials or analgesics may stabilize hemodynamics in such patients.

Cardiac arrythmias

In the acutely ill patient, underlying cardiac problems may contribute to the genesis of arrhythmias, as may the marked electrolyte shifts that often occur during dialysis. As noted above, patients who are receiving digitalis should not undergo dialysis against lower than normal potassium concentration in the dialysis fluid unless exceptional circumstances exist. Constant cardiac monitoring must be employed. When arrythmias occur, they should be treated appropriately remembering that certain drugs may have more prolonged effects in patients with renal failure.

Electrolyte abnormalities

In acute renal failure electrolyte disturbances are common. During dialysis numerous changes occur depending on composition of the dialysis fluid and associated non dialytic management. These aspects are discussed in the section on composition of dialysis fluid (see p. 551).

Disequilibrium

Dialysis almost invariably causes some degree of cerebral edema because of intracellular water migration into brain cells. This is most pronounced during the early phase of dialysis, accompanying a pronounced fall in plasma osmolality. It can be combated and avoided as mentioned above by higher sodium and dextrose concentrations in the dialysis fluid or by mannitol or glycerol infusion. Small children, those with previous brain damage and older patients are most susceptible to cerebral edema during dialysis. Children and patients with brain damage tend to convulse; older patients frequently develop psychosis. Families should be alerted to the possibility of transient psychosis during dialysis. Because disequilibrium occurs most frequently when starting dialysis in patients with advanced uremia, initiation of dialysis should not be delayed until the patient is severely uremic. The patient's BUN ordinarily should not be allowed to exceed 100 mg/dl (35.7 mmol/l of urea). However, patients are frequently severely uremic with very high BUN levels when first admitted. As previously discussed treatment should start with short dialyses, with low clearance technique, which should be repeated daily until uremia has been partly corrected.

Cell destruction

Hemodialysis influences the formed blood elements. Ten to fifteen minutes after start of dialysis, the leukocyte count falls to very low values (281–285). The leukopenia is attributed to increased leukocyte margination and sequestration in the pulmonary capillaries mediated by complement activation. This theory, however, has been challenged because some membranes markedly activate complement but do not cause leukopenia whereas the reverse is true for other membranes (285). There is presently no satisfactory explanation for the leukopenia. An adverse effect of the leukopenia is the associated hypoxemia, which should be treated with supplemental oxygen.

Platelets also decrease during dialysis. A mean decrement of 15% can be expected, but catastrophic falls can occur for unexplained reasons. Plate dialyzers may cause more thombocytopenia than hollow fiber dialyzers, although this observation remains unconfirmed. The cause of the thrombocytopenia is unknown (208).

Patients should not show any evidence of hemolysis during dialysis (285). Marked hemolysis should alert the physician to errors in the dialysis procedure. Such errors include grossly aberrant composition or dialysis fluid contamination with zinc, copper, chloramine or formaldehyde or overheating of the dialysis solution (see also Chapter 32).

Hypoxemia

During hemodialysis, PaO_2 will fall 10 to 20 mm Hg. In a patient with a normal oxygen tension before dialysis, this is of no consequence as it changes the blood oxygen saturation very little. However, in a seriously ill patient with a low initial PaO$_2$, this may be catastrophic. These patients should be given supplemental oxygen.

The exact mechanism for the decrease in PaO$_2$ is not known. Craddock et al (281, 283) attribute the hypoxemia to complement activation and complement-mediated leukostasis in the pulmonary capillaries, but other factors may also contribute (283–292).

Aurigemma et al (291) do not accept this explanation because complement activation, leukopenia and decreases in PaO$_2$ can be disassociated (285, 291). They believe that the decrease in PaO$_2$ is due to removal of CO$_2$ during dialysis. The resultant decrease of the respiratory drive, lowers PaO$_2$. They base this postulate on the evidence that bubbling of CO$_2$ through the dialysis solution can greatly ameliorate the fall in PaO$_2$. Finally, the metabolism of acetate into acetyl-coenzyme A requires CO$_2$ and oxygen, so oxygen consumption may be increased during acetate dialysis (292, 293). This phenomenon has not been carefully quantitated. The decreased arterial oxygen tension during dialysis is probably multifactorial. Whatever the ultimate cause, it is clear that critically ill patients with acute renal failure should receive oxygen supplementation during hemodialysis.

New methods

Ultrafiltration without dialysis and sequential ultrafiltration-dialysis are discussed under 'blood pressure problems' in this chapter (see p. 553).

Hemofiltration (see Chapters 12 and 13) may find wide applicability in the acutely ill patients (294). Hypotension is less common during hemofiltration than during hemodialysis. The exact reason is not known. It may be due to the slower removal of urea nitrogen by hemofiltration, but preliminary studies by Shaldon and associates (295) suggests this is not the sole explanation. It is also possible that more sodium is infused during hemofiltration than during hemodialysis. Thus, intracellular water migration may be less, as suggested by Gotch (296). Finally, better blood compatibility of the hemofiltration membrane may minimize any disturbances of blood pressure that relate to blood cell or protein trauma (285).

Continuous hemofiltration is another new development. Small amounts of hemofiltrate are removed continuously and replaced by a balanced salt solution. In some centers in Germany almost all patients with acute renal failure are treated by this method (297, 298). The experience in West Germany now exceeds 200 patients. The filters are connected either to special femoral artery to femoral vein catheters (297) or to ordinary Scribner shunts (298). No blood pumps are used. Filtration is that achieved by the patient's blood pressure, sometimes augmented by placing the filtration collection bag low below the patient. The negative hydrostatic pressure will augment the filtration rate. Filtration/infusion rates of approximately 9 (5 to 35) ml/min or 13 (7 to 50) l/24 h have been used. Approximately 10 units/h/kg body weight of heparin (17,000 units per day to 70 kg patients) are used. This results in approximately a doubling of heparin concentration and partial thrombin and thrombin times (298). Good control of uremia and avoidance of the acute side effects of intermittent hemodialysis, and good control of water and electrolytes are claimed. The procedure is said to markedly decrease the problem with hyperalimentation in that carrier volumes for hyperalimentation can easily be removed. The filters are changed approximately every other day.

PERITONEAL DIALYSIS IN ACUTE RENAL FAILURE

Peritoneal dialysis is discussed in detail in chapters 21, 22 and 23.

There is no difference in the mortality rate of acute renal failure whether the patient is treated with peritoneal or hemodialysis (86, 89, 193). Certain patients, such as those with head trauma, marked cardiovascular instability and contaminated abdominal cavities should preferentially be treated by peritoneal dialysis (84, 90, 91, 299). Patients with a stoma or contamination in or near the abdominal wall, hypercatabolic patients and those who need to be treated briefly to allow time for other therapeutic or diagnostic procedures should undergo hemodialysis. Peritoneal dialysis also cannot be used in patients with a large disruption of the peritoneal space such as occurs after surgery for an aortic aneurysm. It should also be avoided in patients who have had recent intestinal surgery, as a catheter close to the bowel suture lines impairs healing (300).

The new technique of continuous slow peritoneal dialysis (CAPD) may be particularly beneficial for critically ill patients with acute renal failure: correction of body chemistries proceeds smoothly allowing the body's compensatory mechanisms to adjust. It is presently the only practical method of continuous dialysis that avoids cycling of plasma chemistry and osmolality.

Peritoneal access (see also Chapters 21 and 23)

Peritoneal access can be obtained either with a stiff Teflon or soft Silastic catheter. Either can be placed by a percutaneous puncture technique or through a mini-laparotomy. The soft Silastic catheter, because of its longer subcutaneous tunnel, decreases the incidence of peritonitis caused by bacterial migration along the catheter. This catheter is tolerated better and seems to allow more efficient drainage of dialysate than the stiff catheter. A mini-laparotomy avoids bowel perforation, a possible complication of the percutaneous technique in these patients, who frequently have paralytic ileus or a mechanically distended bowel.

Choice of fluids and additives

Presently available commercial peritoneal dialysis solutions contain electrolytes in their usual extracellular concentrations. Exceptions are potassium, which is usually not added and lactate, which is used instead of bicarbonate. The dextrose monohydrate concentration is varied between 1.5 and 4.25 g/dl (76 to 215 mmol/l).

Because of the slow nature of peritoneal dialysis, there is less need for individual adjustment of the electrolyte composition of the dialysis solution. Potassium is added as indicated, depending on the patient's plasma potassium level. A dextrose concentration of 1.5 g/dl usually induces little net fluid removal from a patient. The more concentrated solution (4.25 g/dl) removes 250 to 500 ml of fluid per hour depending on cycling techniques (see Chapters 22 and 23). Heparin is no longer added routinely to the dialysis solution. Some will use heparin for the first few exchanges in a concentration of 500 to 1,000 units per liter of dialysis fluid. Heparin is added to the dialysis fluid, however, in patients with peritonitis, to prevent obstruction of the catheter by fibrinous exudate. At least in the patient with an intact peritoneum, there is negligible absorption of heparin from the dialysate (301, 302).

Antibiotics are of no value prophylactically (303–305). They should be added to the dialysate, and also used systemically, however, in patients with pre-existing peritonitis or those who develop peritonitis. Peritoneal lavage with antibiotics improves survival in patients with peritonitis (306–312). Antibiotics are added to the dialysis fluid to achieve a level equal to the desired plasma water concentration. Once the patient has received a loading dose there is often no need to give more systemic antibiotics. Plasma levels obviously should be measured.

A number of vasodilating pharmacological agents can be added to peritoneal dialysis fluid to increase the efficiency of the procedure. They include dopamine, glucagon, isoproterenol, tolazoline, nitroprusside, dipyridamole, prostaglandins and prostaglandin precursors (313–316, see also Chapter 23). Moderate increases in dialysis efficiency can be achieved, but none have been widely used clinically. The most frequently used agent for this purpose is probably nitroprusside, in a concentration of 4 to 5 µg (15 to 19 nmol)/l dialysis fluid. It has little or no systemic effect when used in this fashion (314).

Peritoneal dialysis technique

Intermittent peritoneal dialysis can be performed using 1 to 2 l exchanges per hour. As has already occurred in chronic dialysis, this technique may be replaced by slow continuous ambulatory dialysis (CAPD). Intermittent peritoneal dialysis has the disadvantages of prolonged treatment time and the risk of peritonitis and like hemodialysis, it is an intermittent procedure that requires specially trained personnel and expensive equipment. In slow continuous peritoneal dialysis, up to 2 l, or about 40 ml/kg, are instilled into the peritoneum every 3 to 6 h depending on the patient's blood chemistries, body size and rate of catabolism. If the patient needs other therapeutic or diagnostic procedures, a small amount of peritoneal dialysis fluid with heparin added is infused into the peritoneal cavity, the catheter is clamped and peritoneal dialysis is resumed when the patient returns to the ward. The training of personnel is simple, but meticulous aseptic technique is necessary to avoid peritonitis. Because of the smoothness of this technique, it can be utilized even in the most seriously ill and unstable patients. We have successfully employed the technique in several older patients with marked cardiovascular instability. Others have similar favorable anecdotal experiences (317). It appears to be a promising technique for patients with acute renal failure but there is no rigorous analysis as yet of the results.

Complications of peritoneal dialysis

The complications of peritoneal dialysis are outlined in Table 7. They have been described by several authors (318, 319) and are discussed in detail in Chapter 23. They will be only briefly discussed here.

Technical problems

The first technical problems of peritoneal dialysis include perforation of the intestine or bladder when the catheter is inserted by percutaneous puncture. Most authors suggest that when the intestine is perforated, the catheter should be replaced. Peritoneal dialysis with antibiotics added to the dialysis solution should then be instituted as it augments cleaning of the abdominal cavity and decreases the risk of peritonitis. Most such puncture wounds of the intestine heal spontaneously (320, 321).

Drainage problems during peritoneal dialysis are ordinarily due to dislodging or plugging of the catheter. Sometimes, the problem can be solved by the use of a Fogarty embolectomy catheter to remove a fibrin plug

Table 7. Complications of peritoneal dialysis.

I. Mechanical:	Pain
	Hemorrhage
	Puncture of intraabdominal organ
	Leakage
	Inadequate drainage
	Dissection of fluid
	Wound/bowel suture problems
	Intraperitoneal catheter loss
II. Metabolic:	Hypo/hyperglycemia
	Hypo/hypernatremia
	Hypo/hyperkalemia
	Acidosis/alkalosis
	Protein/amino acid loss
III. Cardiovascular/ pulmonary:	Fluid overload/pulmonary edema
	Hypotension
	Hypertension
	Arrythmia/cardiac arrest
	Atelectasis
	Pneumonia
	Aspiration
	Hydrothorax
IV. Infectious complications:	Abscess at puncture site
	Bacterial/fungal peritonitis
	(Sterile peritonitis)

See text (and Chapter 23) for details.

from the peritoneal catheter. Changing the patient's position sometimes improves drainage. Often, the catheter needs to be replaced (322, 323).

Metabolic complications
Hyperglycemia can occur with any form of peritoneal dialysis as large amounts (100 to 200 g/day) of dextrose are absorbed from the dialysis solution (322). This is a greater problem if the patient also receives hyperalimentation. Frequent glucose determinations are then necessary. The addition of small amounts of insulin to the peritoneal dialysis solution (such as 20 units to the 1.5% solution and 2 to 3 times that amount of the 4.25% solution) may stabilize the glucose levels even in diabetic patients (323).

Hypernatremia may occur during osmotic ultrafiltration because water traverses the peritoneum more easily than sodium (see chapters 21 and 23). The addition of furosemide to the dialysate has been suggested to increase sodium transport (324). Hyponatremia is a rare complication of dialysis usually due to inappropriate composition of dialysis solution.

Hypokalemia may occur because of potassium removal or a shift intracellularly, resulting from correction of acidosis and dextrose infusion.

Some patients with lactic acidosis cannot be dialyzed using solutions containing lactate as they do not metabolize it rapidly enough to correct their acidosis. Special solutions containing bicarbonate must be used in such patients (325).

Large amounts of protein and amino acids may be lost in the dialysate, particularly when peritonitis exists. Plasma concentrations of these substances should be monitored and repletion intravenously is often necessary (326, 327).

Cardiovascular and pulmonary complications
Arrhythmias and hypotension can occur during the instillation of the dialysis solution. This should be avoided by slowing the inflow rate or decreasing the infusion volume (328). Atelectasis and hypostatic pneumonia may complicate peritoneal dialysis, but can be partially counteracted by physical therapy. Hydrothorax occurs in 5 to 10% of patients with acute renal failure treated by peritoneal dialysis. It can obviously be a disastrous complication in an acutely ill patient (329-331).

Infectious complications
The most common complication of any form of peritoneal dialysis is peritonitis. The incidence should decrease when a long subcutaneous tunnel with a soft peritoneal dialysis catheter and a closed system of dialysis fluid delivery are used. Peritonitis can be diagnosed promptly by inspecting the dialysate for turbidity and by daily microscopic examination. More than 500 leukocytes/ml signifies peritonitis (332). A test-strip for leukocytes has also been used (333). When peritonitis is suspected, antibiotics should be added to the dialysate after fluid has been sent for culture. Sometimes parenteral administration of antibiotics is also necessary. Routine daily cultures of peritoneal fluid in such patients may detect an infection early.

Pleural dialysis
Pleural dialysis has been used in rare instances where other dialysis techniques were contraindicated (334, 335).

IMPROVING SURVIVAL

It is clear that the mortality of acute renal failure depends mainly on the underlying disease. Thus, in patients dialyzed acutely for primary kidney disease, the mortality is only 24%, whereas in acute tubular necrosis, a complication of various medical and surgical insults, it approaches 70% (Table 1). In the patient with acute tubular necrosis, the mortality rate correlates with the primary disease. In obstetric-gynecologic cases, the mortality is usually only between 10 and 20%, whereas when tubular necrosis follows major cardiovascular or gastrointestinal surgery, it can rise to almost 80% (Table 2). Improved survival rates, therefore, must depend mostly on improved management of the underlying disease. Aggressive surgery and a high index of suspicion for surgical complications are necessary (165, 166). Because infectious complications are so commonly the proximate cause of death for these patients, improved antibiotic treatment based on frequent cultures and sensitivity tests to guide the choice of antibiotic and dosage adjustment and use of some of the newer antibiotics also may help decrease mortality. Antibiotic barrage, such as suggested for immunosuppressed patients with cancer has not been studied in patients with acute renal failure and should be investigated. Increasing usage and an increased understanding of hyperalimentation could also contribute to a decrease in mortality rate by improving recovery from surgery and immune defense.

Many attempts have been made to improve the dialysis treatment itself. Earlier start, more frequent and more efficient dialysis have all been suggested as means of improving survival for patients with acute renal failure (4, 6-9, 89, 336-341). Results have been contradictory except when comparing very early to very late dialysis (89, 336-338). Most centers now utilize dialysis before the BUN reaches 100 to 110 mg/dl (36 to 39 mmol/l of urea) and use almost daily dialysis. Any further improvement would thus depend on the development of a continuous form of dialysis. Presently, continuous hemodialysis is not possible. Preliminary investigations of these methods are extremely interesting but the problems of anticoagulation and permanent angioaccess are not yet solved (297, 298). The only currently available technique allowing continuous dialysis is slow continuous peritoneal dailysis (CAPD) and slow continuous hemofiltration for acute renal failure. These methods deserve continuation of clinical trials in patients with acute renal failure.

RECOVERY OF RENAL FUNCTION; NEED FOR CONTINUED DIALYSIS

The clinical course of acute tubular necrosis is rapid. This is illustrated in Figure 10. In patients dialyzed for acute renal failure at the University of Minnesota the

26: *Acute renal failure* 559

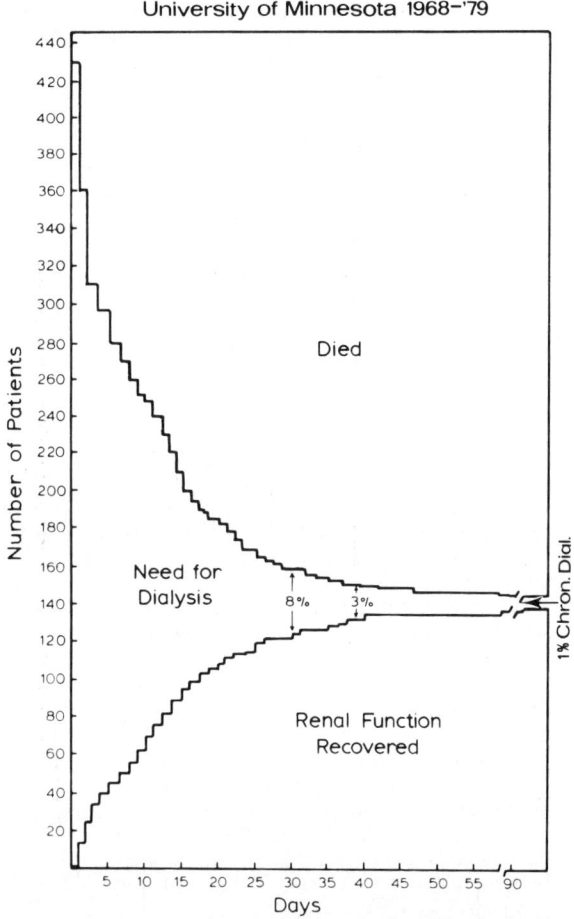

Figure 10. Clinical course of 432 patients with acute tubular necrosis dialyzed at the University of Minnesota in 1968-1979.
By 30 days, 92% of the patients have recovered renal function or died, and at 40 days only 3% of the patients remain on dialysis. (From Kjellstrand, Ebben and Davin [77], with permission of the Am Soc Artif Intern Organs).

median interval between initiation of dialysis and recovery of renal function of the survivors was 12 days. The median time between start of dialysis and death was 5 days. By 1 month 92% and by 1½ months 97% of the patients had either regained renal function or had died. After 45 days of acute renal failure 1/3 of the remaining patients died, 1/3 recovered renal function and 1/3 needed regular dialysis. The longest time a patient was dialyzed and recovered renal function was 88 days (77).

These data are similar to those collected from comparable groups of patients during the past few decades. Thus, Alwall (4) reported that in the early years of dialysis patients with acute tubular necrosis needed dialysis for an average of 15 days. One patient in his series did not recover renal function until 65 days after initiation of dialysis. In the Glasgow experience between 1959 and 1970, the mean duration of dialysis for acute renal failure was 11 days and the longest time to recovery of kidney function was 42 days (8). Obviously, these figures have not changed over the years. Thus, these patients have a swift clinical course and although they require an enormous investment in care and equipment, few patients require dialysis and intensive care for more than 4 weeks.

Renal function usually continues to improve for approximately one month after the last dialysis. Approximately one-third of the patients are left with moderate renal dysfunction (plasma creatinine level 1.5 to 3 mg/dl [133 to 265 μmol/l]) and 10% have residual chronic renal failure with plasma creatinine concentration exceeding 3 mg/dl ((265 μmol/l) (10, 77, 342-350). The duration of dialysis for acute tubular necrosis does not correlate with the ultimate plasma creatinine concentration. Thus, patients who were dialyzed only once eventually had the same plasma creatinine concentration (more than 1 month after the last dialysis) as those who needed dialysis for more than 1 month (10, 77). One patient needed dialysis for almost 3 months but ultimately reached a serum creatinine level of 1.2 mg/dl (106 μmol/l). Age, however, is directly related to the final serum creatinine concentration (Table 8). Older patients progress to chronic renal failure more often than younger patients. Isolated cases of severe irreversible renal failure have been reported (350-352).

Table 8. Ultimate serum creatinine vs age of patient.

Age (yrs)	Serum creatinine μmol/l	n
<10	53± 26.5	6
10-20	80± 17.7	5
20-30	106± 44.2	11
30-40	106± 8.8	5
40-50	115± 26.5	7
50-60	133± 70.7	13
60-70	177± 97.3	22
≪70	195+1123.8	13

The serum creatinine concentration obtained after recovery from acute renal failure is listed according to age group. It is clear that the older patients regained less renal function than the younger. (Modified from Kjellstrand et al [77] with permission of the Am Soc Artif Intern Organs)

Conversion of serum creatinine μmol/l to conventional units (mg/dl): multiply by 0.0113.

Six among approximately 500 patients have remained on chronic hemodialysis after they developed what was thought to be acute tubular necrosis. Three of them sustained acute renal failure after operations for aortic aneurysms. Cholesterol embolization, a known cause of chronic renal failure, may have contributed to their need for chronic hemodialysis. One patient had undergone methoxyflurane anesthesia, also a known cause of irreversible renal failure. In two patients, however, no known cause of chronic renal failure complicating the acute tubular necrosis could be identified (10, 77, 350). Bilateral renal cortical necrosis also begins acutely and results in irreversible renal failure requiring chronic dialysis.

Thus, of the patients who come to dialysis for acute tubular necrosis, approximately two-thirds will die, usually quite fast. Of the one-third who survive, almost 60% have complete return of renal function. Approximately 25% will be left with moderate renal insufficiency (creatinine < 3 mg/dl), 10% will have severe chronic renal failure (creatinine > 3 mg/dl [265 μmol/l]), and 5% will need chronic dialysis (10, 77).

CONCLUSIONS

Most patients with acute renal failure suffer from acute tubular necrosis. The mortality rate in this group of patients remains between 20 and 80% and has not improved with time. This is probably due to improvement in conservative management that leaves more severely ill patients in need of acute dialysis than before. Acute hemodialysis remains the main stay of treatment for these patients. Exciting new developments include continuous peritoneal dialysis and continuous hemofiltration. The ultimate problems and advantages of these procedures remain conjectural at this time. Improved treatment of the basic disease, particularly aggressive surgery, improved hyperalimentation and improved antibiotic treatment seem to offer the best chances for improving survival.

The patients with acute tubular necrosis have a very rapid clinical course. Moderate, clinically significant renal dysfunction is not an uncommon sequel. Severe chronic renal failure is unusual and the persistent need for maintenance hemodialysis is rare.

REFERENCES

1. Kolff WJ: First clinical experience with the artificial kidney. *Ann Intern Med* 62:608, 1965
2. Alwall N: On the artificial kidney. I. Apparatus for dialysis of the blood in vivo. *Acta Med Scand* 128:317, 1947
3. Murray G: Development of an artificial kidney; experimental and clinical experiences. *Arch Surg* 55:505, 1947
4. Alwall N: *Therapeutic and Diagnostic Problems in Severe Renal Failure*. Copenhagen, Munksgaard, 1963
5. Merrill JP, Smith S, Callahan EJ, Thorn GW: Use of artificial kidney: clinical experience. *J Clin Invest* 29:425, 1950
6. Teschan PE, Post RS, Smith LH, Abernathy RS, Davis JH, Gray DM, Howard JM, Johnson KE, Dlopp E, Mundy RL, O'Meara MP, Rush BF: Post-traumatic renal insufficiency in military casualties. I. Clinical characteristics. *Am J Med* 18:172, 1955
7. Balslov JT, Jorgensen HE: A survey of 499 patients with acute anuric renal insufficiency, causes, treatment, complications and mortality. *Am J Med* 34:753, 1963
8. Kennedy AC, Burton JA, Luke RG, Briggs JD, Lindsay RM, Allison MEM, Edward N, Dargie HJ: Factors affecting the prognosis in acute renal failure, A survey of 251 cases. *Q J Med* 42:73, 1973
9. Kirkland K, Edwards KDG, Whyte HM: Oliguric renal Failure: A report of 400 cases including classification, survival and response to dialysis. *Austral Ann Med* 14:275, 1965
10. Kjellstrand CM, Gornick C, Davin T: Recovery from acute renal failure. *Clin Exp Dial Apheresis* 5:143, 1981
11. Brunner FP, Brynger H, Chantler C, Donckerwolcke RA, Hathway RA, Jacobs C, Selwood NH, Wing AJ: Combined report on regular dialysis and transplantation in Europe, IX, 1978. *Prod Eur Dial Transpl Assoc* 16:2, 1979
12. Lundberg M: Dialysbehandling vid akut njurinsufficiens. *Lakartidningen* (Dialysis treatment in acute renal failure) 67:487, 1970 (in Swedish)
13. Eliahou HA, Boichis H, Bott-Kanner G, Barell V, Bar-Noach N, Modan B: An epidemiologic study of renal failure, II. Acute renal failure. *Am J Epidemiol* 101:281, 1975
14. Karatson A, Juhasz I, Koves S, Balogh F: Estimated frequency of acute and chronic renal insufficiencies in a transdanubian region of Hungary. *Int Urol Nephrol* 7:321, 1975
15. Lachhein L, Kielstein R, Sauer K, Reinschke P, Muller V, Krumhaar I, Falkenhagen D, Schmidt R, Klinkmann H: Evaluation of 433 cases of acute renal failure. *Proc Eur Dial Transpl Assoc* 14:628, 1977
16. Vaughan G: Acute renal failure. *Br Med J* 1:1333, 1980
17. Older RA, Van Moore A, Foster WL, Ladwig SH: Urinary tract obstruction, current methods of evaluation. *JAMA* 245:1854, 1981
18. Ellenbogen P, Scheible F, Talner L: Sensitivity of gray scale ultrasound in detecting urinary tract obstruction. *Am J Roentgenol* 130:731, 1978
19. Pfister R, Newhouse J: Interventional percutaneous pyeloureteral techniques: Antegrade pyelography and ureteral perfusion. *Radiol Clin North Am* 17:314, 1979
20. McClennan B: Current approaches to the azotemic patient. *Radiol Clin North Am* 17:197, 1979
21. Wilson DR: Renal function during and following obstruction. *Annu Rev Med* 28:329, 1977
22. Ransohoff DF, Feinstein AR: Problems of spectrum and bias in evaluating the efficacy of diagnostic tests. *N Engl J Med* 299:926, 1978
23. Chisholm GD, Charlton CAC, Orr WM: Urine-urea/blood-urea ratios in renal failure. *Lancet* 1:20, 1966
24. Anderson RJ, Linas SL, Berns AS, Henrich WL, Miller TR, Gabow PA, Schrier RW: Nonoliguric acute renal failure. *N Engl J Med* 296:1134, 1977
25. Sporn NI, Lancestremere RG, Papper S: Differential diagnosis of oliguria in aged patients. *N Engl J Med* 267:130, 1962
26. Mathew OP, Jones AS, James E, Bland H, Groshong T: Neonatal renal failure: usefulness of diagnostic indices. *Pediatrics* 65:57, 1980
27. Harrington JT, Cohen JJ: Measurement of urinary electrolytes; indications and limitations. *N Engl J Med* 293:1241, 1975
28. Miller TR, Anderson RJ, Linas SL, Henrich WL, Berns AS, Gabow PA, Schrier RW: Urinary diagnostic indices in acute renal failure. *Ann Intern Med* 88:47, 1978
29. Eliahou HE, Bata A: The diagnosis of acute renal failure. *Nephron* 2:287, 1965
30. Handa SP, Morrin PAF: Diagnostic indices in acute renal failure. *Can Med Assoc J* 96:78, 1967
31. Espinel CH: The FE_{Na} test; use in the differential diagnosis of acute renal failure. *JAMA* 236:579, 1976
32. Espinel CH, Gregory AW: Differential diagnosis of acute renal failure. *Clin Nephrol* 13:73, 1980
33. Espinel CH, Gregory AW: Acute renal failure in shock: the critical point. *Clin Res* 28:44A, 1980
34. Pru C, Kjellstrand CM: On the clinical usefulness of the

'FE$_{Na}$' test in acute renal failure: a critical analysis. *Proc Clin Dial Transpl Forum* 10:240, 1980
35. Jones LW, Weil MH: Water, creatinine and sodium excretion following circulatory shock with renal failure. *Am J Med* 51:314, 1971
36. Zager RA, Rubin NT, Ebert T, Maslow N: Rapid radioimmunoassay for diagnosing acute tubular necrosis. *Nephron* 26:7, 1980
37. Fang LS, Sirota RA, Ebert TH, Lichtenstein NS: Low fractional excretion of sodium with contrast media-induced acute renal failure. *Arch Intern Med* 140:531, 1980
38. Baek SM, Makabali GG, Shoemaker WC: Free-water clearance patterns as predictors and therapeutic guides in acute renal failure. *Surgery* 77:632, 1975
39. Landes RG, Lillehei RC, Lindsay WG, Nicoloff DM: Free-water clearance and the early recognition of acute renal insufficiency after cardiopulmonary bypass. *Ann Thorac Surg* 22:41, 1976
40. Shin B, Isenhower NN, McAslan TC, Mackenzie CF, Helrich M: Early recognition of renal insufficiency in postanesthetic trauma victims. *Anesthesiology* 50:262, 1979
41. Brown R, Babcock R, Talbert J, Gruenberg J, Czurak C, Campbell M: Renal function in critically ill postoperative patients: sequential assessment of creatinine, osmolar and free water clearance. *Crit Care Med* 8:68, 1980
42. Miller PD, Krebs RA, Neal BJ, McIntyre DO: Polyuric prerenal failure. *Arch Intern Med* 140:907, 1980
43. Reubi FC: The pathogenesis of anuria following shock. *Kidney Int* 5:106, 1974
44. Lucas CE: The renal response to acute injury and sepsis. *Surg Clin North Am* 56:953, 1976
45. Hermreck AS, Ruiz-Ocana FM, Proberts KS, Meisel RL, Crawford DG: Mechanisms for oliguria in acute renal failure. *Surgery* 82:141, 1977
46. Levinsky NG: Pathophysiology of acute renal failure. *N Engl J Med* 296:1453, 1977
47. Solez K, Morel-Maroger L, Sraer JD: The morphology of 'acute tubular necrosis' in man: Analysis of 57 renal biopsies and a comparison with the glycerol model. *Medicine* 58:362, 1979
48. Myers BD, Carrie BJ, Yee RR, Hilberman M, Michaels AS: Pathophysiology of hemodynamically mediated acute renal failure in man. *Kidney Int* 18:495, 1980
49. Olbricht CHJ: Experimental models of acute renal failure. *Contrib Nephrol* 19:110, 1980
50. Conger JD, Schrier RW: Renal hemodynamics in acute renal failure. *Annu Rev Physiol* 42:603, 1980
51. Smolens P, Stein JH: Pathophysiology of acute renal failure. *Am J Med* 70:479, 1981
52. Harkonen S, Kjellstrand C: Contrast nephropathy. *Am J Nephrol* 1:69, 1981
53. Kleinknecht D, Ganeval D, Gonzalez-Duque LA, Fermanian J: Furosemide in acute oliguric renal failure; a controlled trial. *Nephron* 17:51, 1976
54. Epstein M, Schneider NS, Befeler B: Effect of intrarenal furosemide on renal function and intrarenal hemodynamics in acute renal failure. *Am J Med* 58:510, 1975
55. Schrier RW: Acute renal failure: pathogenesis, diagnosis, and management. *Hosp Pract* March 1981, p 93
56. Brown CB, Ogg CS, Cameron JS: High dose furosemide in acute renal failure: a controlled trial. *Clin Nephrol* 15:90, 1981
57. Cantarovich F, Galli C, Benedetti L, Chena C, Castro L, Correa C, Loredo JP, Fernandez JC, Locatelli A, Tizado J: High dose furosemide in established acute renal failure. *Br Med J* 4:449, 1973
58. Kjellstrand CM: Ethacrynic acid in acute tubular necrosis. *Nephron* 9:337, 1972
59. Levinsky NG, Bernard DB, Johnson PA: Enhancement of recovery of acute renal failure: effect of mannitol and diuretics. In: *Acute Renal Failure* edited by Brenner BM, Stein JH, Edinburgh, London, New York, Churchill Livingstone Inc 1980, p 163
60. Henderson IS, Beattie TJ, Kennedy AC: Dopamine hydrochloride in oliguric states. *Lancet* 2:827, 1980
61. Neiberger RE, Passmore JC: Effects of dopamine on canine intrarenal blood flow distribution during hemorrhage. *Kidney Int* 15:219, 1979
62. Lindner A, Cutler RE, Goodman WG: Synergism of dopamine plus furosemide in preventing acute renal failure in the dog. *Kidney Int* 16:158, 1979
63. Abel RM, Beck CH, Abbott WM, Ryan JA, Barnett GO, Fisher JE: Improved survival from acute renal failure after treatment with intravenous essential L-amino acids and glucose. *N Engl J Med* 288:695, 1973
64. Leonard CD, Luke RG, Siegel RR: Parenteral essential amino acids in acute renal failure. *Urology* 6:154, 1975
65. Asbach HW, Stoeckel H, Schuler HW, Conradi R, Wiedemann K, Mohring K, Rohl L: The treatment of hypercatabolic acute renal failure by adequate nutrition and haemodialysis. *Acta Anaesth Scand* 18:255, 1974
66. Baek SM, Makabali GG, Bryan-Brown CW, Kusek J, Shoemaker WC: The influence of parenteral nutrition on the course of acute renal failure. *Surg Gynecol Obstet* 141:405, 1975
67. Oken DE, Sprinkel FM, Kirschbaum BB, Landwehr DM: Amino acid therapy in the treatment of experimental acute renal failure in the rat. *Kidney Int* 17:14, 1980
68. Toback FG: Amino acid enhancement of renal regeneration after acute tubular necrosis. *Kidney Int* 12:193, 1977.
69. Osias MB, Siegel NJ, Chaudry IH, Lytton B, Baue AE: Postischemic renal failure, accelerated recovery with adenosine triphosphate-magnesium chloride infusion. *Arch Surg* 112:729, 1977
70. Siegel NJ, Glazier WB, Chaudry IH, Gaudio KM, Lytton B, Baue AE, Kashgarian M: Enhanced recovery from acute renal failure by the postischemic infusion of adenine nucleotides and magnesium chloride in rats. *Kidney Int* 17:338, 1980
71. Wickham JEA, Fernando AR, Hendry WF, Watkinson LE, Whitefield HN, Armstrong DMG, Griffiths JR: Inosine in preserving renal function during ischaemic renal surgery. *Br Med J* 2:173, 1978
72. Kristensen BO, Skov J, Peterslund NA: Furosemide-induced increases in serum isoamylases. *Br Med J* 2:978, 1980
73. Quick CA, Hoppe W: Permanent deafness associated with furosemide administration. *Ann Otol Rhinol Laryngol* 84:94, 1975
74. Borges H, Hocks J, Kjellstrand C: Mannitol intoxication in patients with renal failure. *Arch Intern Med* 142:63, 1982
75. Chugh KS: Clinicopathological spectrum of acute renal failure in India. *Proc First Asian Pacific Congress Nephrology*, Nihon University, Sec Dept of Medicine, Tokyo 173, Japan, 1979, p 133
76. Sitprija V: The kidney in acute tropical disease. *Abstracts 8th Int Congress Nephrol* 1981, p 279
77. Kjellstrand CM, Ebben J, Davin T: Time of death, recovery of renal function, development of chronic renal failure and need for chronic hemodialysis in patients with acute tubular necrosis. *Trans Am Soc Artif Intern Organs* 27:45, 1981
78. McMurray SD, Luft FC, Maxwell DR, Hamburger RJ,

Szwed JJ, Lavelle KJ, Kleit SA: Acute tubular necrosis; a multifactorial analysis of variables. *Proc Clin Dial Transpl Forum* 6:110, 1976
79. Lordon RE, Burton JR: Post-traumatic renal failure in military personnel in Southeast Asia: experience at Clark USAF Hospital, Republic of the Philippines. *Am J Med* 53:137, 1972
80. Fischer RP: High mortality of post-traumatic renal insufficiency in Vietnam: a review of 96 cases. *Am Surg* 40:172, 1974
81. Stone WJ, Knepshield JH: Post-traumatic acute renal insufficiency in Vietnam. *Clin Nephrol* 2:186, 1974
82. Barsoum RS, Rihan ZEB, Baligh OK, Hozayen A, El-Ghonaimy EHG, Ramzy MF, Ibrahuim AS: Acute renal failure in the 1973 Middle East War; experience of a specialized base hospital: effect of the site of injury. *J Trauma* 20:303, 1980
83. McMurray SD, Luft FC, Maxwell DR, Hamburger RJ, Futty D, Szwed JJ, Lavelle KJ, Kleit SA: Prevailing patterns and predictor variables in patients with acute tubular necrosis. *Arch Intern Med* 138:950, 1978
84. Matas AJ, Payne WD, Simmons RL, Buselmeier TJ, Kjellstrand CM: Acute renal failure following blunt civilian trauma. *Ann Surg* 185:301, 1977
85. Elmgren DT, Cheung LY, Bloomer A, Maxwell JG: Acute renal failure after abdominal surgery — the importance of sepsis. *Am J Surg* 128:743, 1974
86. Stott RB, Ogg CS, Cameron JS, Bewick M: Why the persistently high mortality in acute renal failure? *Lancet* 2:75, 1972
87. Kumar R, Hill CM, McGeown MG: Acute renal failure in the elderly. *Lancet* 1:90, 1973
88. Baek S-M, Makabali GG, Shoemaker WC: Clinical determinants of survival from postoperative renal failure. *Surg Gynecol Obstet* 140:685, 1975
89. Kleinknecht D, Jungers P, Chanard J, Barbanel C, Ganeval D: Uremic and non-uremic complications in acute renal failure: evaluation of early and frequent dialysis on prognosis. *Kidney Int* 1:190, 1972
90. Casali R, Simmons RL, Najarian JS, von Hartitzsch B, Buselmeier TJ, Kjellstrand CM: Acute renal insufficiency complicating major cardiovascular surgery. *Ann Surg* 181:370, 1975
91. Sipkins JH, Kjellstrand CM: Severe head trauma and acute renal failure. *Nephron* 28:36, 1981
92. Zimmerman JE: Respiratory failure complicating post-traumatic acute renal failure: etiology, clinical features and management. *Ann Surg* 174:12, 1971
93. Lucas CE, Ledgerwood AM, Shier MR, Bradley VE: The renal factor in the post-traumatic 'fluid overload' syndrome. *J Trauma* 17:667, 1977
94. Kjellstrand CM, Davin TJ, Matas AJ, Buselmeier TJ: Postoperative acute renal failure: diagnosis, etiologic and symptomatic treatment and prognosis. In: *Critical Surgical Care*, edited by Najarian JS, Delaney JP, New York, Stratton, Intercontinental Med Book Corp, 1977, p 309
95. Schwartz EE, Teplick JG, Onesti G, Schwartz AB: Pulmonary hemorrhage in renal disease: Goodpasture's syndrome and other causes. *Radiology* 122:39, 1977
96. Holliday RL, Doris PJ: Monitoring the critically ill surgical patient. *Can Med Assoc J* 121:931, 1979
97. Bland R, Shoemaker WC, Shabot MM: Physiologic monitoring goals for the critically ill patient. *Surg Gynecol Obstet* 147:833, 1978
98. Anderson CC, Shahvari MBG, Zimmerman JE: The treatment of pulmonary edema in the absence of renal function-a role for sorbitol and furosemide. *JAMA* 241:1008, 1979
99. Turck M, Stamm W: Nosocomial infection of the urinary tract. *Am J Med* 70:651, 1981
100. Burke JP, Garibaldi RA, Britt MR, Jacobson JA, Conti M, Alling DW: Prevention of catheter-associated urinary tract infections. *Am J Med* 70:655, 1981
101. Hirsh DD, Fainstein V, Musher DM: Do condom catheter collecting systems cause urinary tract infection? *JAMA* 242:340, 1979
102. Editorial (anonymous): Catheter-associated urinary tract infections. *Lancet* 2:1033, 1978
103. Warren JW, Platt R, Thomas RJ, Rosner B, Kass EH: Antibiotic irrigation and catheter-associated urinary-tract infections. *N Engl J Med* 299:570, 1978
104. Michael L, March HM, McMichan JC, Southorn PA, Brewer NS: Infection of pulmonary artery catheters in critically ill patients. *JAMA* 245:1032, 1981
105. Buselmeier TJ, Najarian JS, Simmons RL, Rattazzi LC, Toledo LH, Fortuny IA, Leonard AS, Kjellstrand CM: An A-V shunt for long term hyperalimentation in azotaemic patients. *Proc Eur Dial Transpl Assoc* 10:516, 1973
106. Editorial (anonymous): Chest physiotherapy under scrutiny. *Lancet* 2:1241, 1978
107. Graham WGB, Bradley DA: Efficacy of chest physiotherapy and intermittent positive-pressure breathing in the resolution of pneumonia. *N Engl J Med* 299:624, 1978
108. Carpentieri U, Haggard ME, Lockhart LH: Clinical experience in prevention of Candidiasis by nystatin in children with acute lymphocytic leukemia. *J Pediat* 92:593, 1978
109. Pizzuto J, Conte G, Ambriz R: Nystatin prophylaxis in leukemia and lymphoma. *N Engl J Med* 298:279, 1978
110. Kirkpatrick CH, Alling DW: Treatment of chronic oral Candidiasis with clotrimazole troches; a controlled clinical trial. *N Engl J Med* 299:1201, 1978
111. Agger WA, Maki DG: Mucormycosis; a complication of critical care. *Arch Intern Med* 138:925, 1978
112. Caplan ES, Hoyt N: Infection surveillance and control in the severely traumatized patient. *Am J Med* 70:638, 1981
113. Nauseef WM, Maki DG: A study of the value of simple protective isolation in patients with granulocytopenia. *N Engl J Med* 304:448, 1981
114. Skillman JJ, Silen W: Stress ulceration in the acutely ill. *Annu Rev Med* 27:9, 1976
115. Le Gall JR, Mignon FC, Rapin M, Redjemi M, Harari A, Bader JP, Soussy CJ: Acute gastroduodenal lesions related to severe sepsis. *Surg Gynecol Obstet* 142:377, 1976
116. Terry RB, Turner MD: Effect of acute hemorrhage on gastrin secretion rate and blood levels of gastrin and insulin in normal dogs and in dogs after vagotomy. *Surg Gynecol Obstet* 142:353, 1976
117. Hastings PR, Skillman JJ, Bushnell LS, Silen W: Antacid titration in the prevention of acute gastrointestinal bleeding; a controlled, randomized trial in 100 critically ill patients. *N Engl J Med* 298:1041, 1978
118. White FA, Clark RB, Thompson DS: Preoperative oral antacid therapy for patients requiring emergency surgery. *South Med J* 71:177, 1978
119. Korenman MD, Stubbs MB, Fish JC: Intestinal obstruction from medication bezoars. *JAMA* 240:54, 1978
120. Welch JP, Schweizer RT, Bartus SA: Management of antacid impactions in hemodialysis and renal transplant patients. *Am J Surg* 139:561, 1980
121. Salmon R, Aubert PH, David R, Guedon J: Aluminum gel causing large-bowel perforation. *Lancet* 1:875, 1978
122. La Brooy SJ, Taylor RH, Hunt RH, Golding PL, Laidlaw JM, Chapman RG, Pounder RE, Vincent SH, Colin-Jones DG, Milton-Thompson GJ, Misiewicz JJ: Controlled

comparison of cimetidine and carbenoxolone sodium in gastric ulcer. *Br Med J* 1:1308, 1979
123. Strauss RJ, Stein TA, Mandell C, Wise L: Cimetidine, carbenoxolone sodium, and antacids for the prevention of experimental stress ulcers. *Arch Surg* 113:858, 1978
124. Belliveau P, Vas S, Himal HS: Septic induced acute gastric erosions: the role of cimetidine. *J Surg Res* 24:264, 1978
125. Levine BA, Sirinek KR, McLeod CG, Teegarden DK, Pruitt BA: The role of cimetidine in the prevention of stress induced gastric mucosal injury. *Surg Gynecol Obstet* 148:399, 1979
126. Burland WL, Parr SN: Experiences with cimetidine in the treatment of seriously ill patients. *Excerpta Medica* 32:345, 1977
127. Martin LF, Staloch DK, Simonowitz DA, Dellinger EP, Max MH: Failure of cimetidine prophylaxis in the critically ill. *Arch Surg* 114:492, 1979
128. Jones RH, Lewin MR, Parsons V: Therapeutic effect of cimetidine in patients undergoing haemodialysis. *Br Med J* 1:650, 1979
129. Schentag JJ, Calleri G, Rose JQ, Cerra FB, DeGlopper E, Bernhard H: Pharmacokinetic and clinical studies in patients with cimetidine-associated mental confusion. *Lancet* 1:177 and 626, 1979
130. Weddington WW, Muelling AE, Moosa HH, Kimball CP, Rowlett RR: Cimetidine toxic reactions masquerading as delirium tremens. *JAMA* 245:1058, 1981
131. Schlippert W: Cimetidine-H₂ receptor blockade in gastrointestinal disease. *Arch Intern Med* 138:1257, 1978
132. Finkelstein W, Isselbacher KJ: Cimetidine. *N Engl J Med* 299:992, 1978
133. Feely J, Wilkinson GR, Wood AJJ: Reduction of liver blood flow and propranolol metabolism by cimetidine. *N Engl J Med* 304:692, 1981
134. Mogelnicki SR, Waller JL, Finlayson DC: Physostigmine reversal of cimetidine-induced mental confusion. *JAMA* 241:826, 1979
135. Nichols TW: Phytobezoar formation. A new complication of cimetidine therapy. *Ann Intern Med* 95:70, 1981
136. Priebe HJ, Skillman JJ, Bushnell LS, Long PC, Silen W: Antacid versus cimetidine in preventing acute gastrointestinal bleeding; a randomized trial in 75 critically ill patients. *N Engl J Med* 302:426, 1980
137. Editorial (anonymous): Prevention or cure for stress-induced gastrointestinal bleeding? *Br Med J* 281:631, 1980
138. Halter F: Cimetidin versus Antazida. *Schweiz Med Wochenschr* 109:497, 1979
139. Bivins BA, Rogers EL, Rapp RP, Sachatello CR, Hyde GL, Griffen WO: Clinical failure with cimetidine. *Surgery* 88:417, 1980
140. Feinstein EI, Blumenkrantz MJ, Healy M: Clinical and metabolic response to parenteral nutrition in acute renal failure. A controlled double blind study. *Medicine* 60:124, 1981
141. Daly JM, Dudrick SJ, Copeland EM: Intravenous hyperalimentation; effect on delayed cutaneous hypersensitivity in cancer patients. *Ann Surg* 192:587, 1980
142. Dionigi R, Zonta A, Dominioni L, Gnes F, Ballabio A: The effects of total parenteral nutrition on immunodepression due to malnutrition. *Ann Surg* 185:467, 1977
143. Champault G, Fabre F, Patel JC: Hyperalimentation des opérés digestifs: Influence sur l'état immunitaire et sur le pronostic. (Hyperalimentation after gastro-intestinal surgery. Influence on the immune status and prognosis). *Nouv Presse Méd* 9:1559, 1980 (in French)
144. Mullen JL, Buzby GP, Matthews DC, Smale BF, Rosato EF: Reduction of operative morbidity and mortality by combined preoperative and postoperative nutritional support. *Ann Surg* 192:604, 1980
145. Michel L, Serrano A, Malt RA: Nutritional support of hospitalized patients. *N Engl J Med* 304:1147, 1981
146. Editorial: Current status of peripheral alimentation. *Ann Intern Med* 95:114, 1981
147. Padberg FT, Ruggiero J, Blackburn GL, Bistrian BR: Central venous catheterization for parenteral nutrition. *Ann Surg* 193:264, 1981
148. Abel RM: Acute renal failure, role of parenteral nutrition. *Contemp Surg* 13:21, 1978
149. Sargent JA, Gotch FA: Nutrition and treatment of the acutely ill patient using urea kinetics. *Dial Transpl* 10:314, 1981
150. Blagg CR, Parsons FM: Earlier dialysis and anabolic steroids in acute renal failure. *Am Heart J* 61:287, 1961
151. Gjorup S, Thaysen JH: Anabolic steroids in the treatment of uraemia. *Lancet* 2:886, 1958
152. Anderson RJ, Gambertoglio JG, Schrier RW: *Clinical Use of Drugs in Renal Failure.* Springfield IL, Charles C. Thomas, 1976
153. Bennett WM, Porter GA, Bagby SP, McDonald WJ: *Drugs and Renal Disease.* Edinburgh, London, New York, Churchill Livingstone, 1978
154. Winchester JF, Gelfand MC, Knepshield JH, Schreiner GE: Dialysis and hemoperfusion of poisons and drugs–update. *Trans Am Soc Artif Intern Organs* 23:762, 1977
155. Bennett WM, Muther RS, Parker RA, Feig P, Morrison G, Golper TA, Singer I: Drug therapy in renal failure: dosing guidelines for adults. *Ann Intern Med* 93:62, 1980
156. Wilson WEC, Kirkpatrick CH, Talmage DW: Suppression of immunologic responsiveness in uremia. *Ann Intern Med* 62:1, 1965
157. Byron PR, Mallick NP, Taylor G: Immune potential in human uraemia. *J Clin Path* 29:770, 1976
158. Dobbelstein H: Immune system in uremia. *Nephron* 17:409, 1976
159. Slade MS, Simmons RL, Yunis E, Greenberg LJ: Immunodepression after major surgery in normal patients. *Surgery* 78:363, 1975
160. Christou NV, Meakins JL: Delayed hypersensitivity in surgical patients: a mechanism for anergy. *Surgery* 86:78, 1979
161. Czer LSC, Shoemaker WC: Optimal hematocrit value in critically ill postoperative patients. *Surg Gynecol Obstet* 147:363, 1978
162. Wolk PJ, Apicella MA: The effect of renal function on the febrile response to bacteremia. *Arch Intern Med* 138:1084, 1978
163. Kaplow LS, Goffinet JA: Profound neutropenia during the early phase of hemodialysis. *JAMA* 203:133, 1968
164. Goldblum SE, Reed WP: Host defenses and immunologic alterations associated with chronic hemodialysis. *Ann Intern Med* 93:597, 1980
165. Marshall V: Secondary surgical intervention in acute renal failure. *Aust NZ J Surg* 44:96, 1974
166. Kornhall S: Acute renal failure in surgical disease with special regard to neglected complications *Acta Chir Scand* (Suppl) 419:3, 1971
167. Jensen F, Pedersen JF: The value of ultrasonic scanning in the diagnosis of intra-abdominal abscesses and hematomas. *Surg Gynecol Obstet* 139:326, 1974
168. Patel R, Tanaka T, Mishkin F, Savage A, Das M: Gallium-67 scan: aid to diagnosis and treatment of renal and perirenal infections. *Urology* 16:225, 1980
169. Koehler PR, Moss AA: Diagnosis of intra-abdominal and

pelvic abscesses by computerized tomography. *JAMA* 244:49, 1980
170. Polk HC, Shields CL: Remote organ failure : a valid sign of occult intra-abdominal infection. *Surgery* 81:310, 1977
171. Fry DE, Pearlstein L, Fulton RL, Polk HC: Multiple system organ failure; the role of uncontrolled infection. *Arch Surg* 115:136, 1980
172. Eiseman B, Beart R, Norton L: Multiple organ failure. *Surg Gynecol Obstet* 144:323, 1977
173. Ardaillou R, Beaufils M, Nivez M-P, Isaac R, Mayaud C, Sraer J-D: Increased plasma calcitonin in early acute renal failure. *Clin Sci Mol Med* 49:301, 1975
174. Weinstein RS, Hudson JB: Parathyroid hormone and 25-hydroxycholecalciferol levels in hypercalcemia of acute renal failure. *Arch Intern Med* 140:410, 1980
175. Hartenbower DL, Stella FJ, Norman AW, Friedler RM, Coburn JW: Impaired vitamin D metabolism in acute uremia. *J Lab Clin Med* 90:760, 1977
176. Arieff AI, Massry SG: Calcium metabolism of brain in acute renal failure; effects of uremia, hemodialysis and parathyroid hormone. *J Clin Invest* 53:387, 1974
177. Grossman RA, Hamilton RW, Morse BM, Penn AS, Goldberg M: Nontraumatic rhabdomyolysis and acute renal failure. *N Engl J Med* 291:807, 1974
178. de Torrente A, Berl T, Cohn PD, Kawamoto E, Hertz P, Schrier RW: Hypercalcemia of acute renal failure; clinical significance and pathogenesis. *Am J Med* 61:119, 1976
179. Akmal M, Goldstein DA, Telfer N, Wilkinson E, Massry SG: Resolution of muscle calcification in rhabdomyolysis and acute renal failure. *Ann Intern Med* 89:928, 1978
180. Feinstein EI, Akmal M, Goldstein DA, Telfer N, Massry SG: Hypercalcemia and acute widespread calcifications during the oliguric phase of acute renal failure due to rhabdomyolysis. *Mineral Electrolyte Metab* 2:193, 1979
181. Feinstein EI, Akmal M, Telfer N, Massry SG: Delayed hypercalcemia with acute renal failure associated with nontraumatic rhabdomyolysis. *Arch Intern Med* 141:753, 1981
182. Chugh KS, Nath IVS, Ubroi HS, Singhal PC, Pareek SK, Sarkar AK: Acute renal failure due to non-traumatic rhabdomyolysis. *Postgrad Med J* 55:386, 1979
183. Schiller WR, Long CL, Blakemore WS: Creatinine and nitrogen excretion in seriously ill and injured patients. *Surg Gynecol Obstet* 149:561, 1979
184. Kjellstrand CM, Campbell DC, von Hartitzsch B, Buselmeier TJ: Hyperuricemic acute renal failure. *Arch Intern Med* 133:349, 1974
185. Zawada ET, Bennett EP, Stinson JB, Ramirez G: Serum calcium in blood pressure regulation during hemodialysis. *Arch Intern Med* 141:657, 1981
186. Kelton J, Kelley WN, Holmes EW: A rapid method for the diagnosis of acute uric acid nephropathy. *Arch Intern Med* 138:612, 1978
187. Katzen BT, McSweeney J: Therapeutic transluminal arterial embolization for bleeding in the upper part of the gastrointestinal tract. *Surg Gynecol Obstet* 141:523, 1975
188. Athanasoulis CA, Baum S, Waltman AC, Ring EJ, Imbembo A, Vander Salm TJ: Control of acute gastric mucosal hemorrhage, intra-arterial infusion of posterior pituitary extract. *N Engl J Med* 290:597, 1974
189. Horowitz HI, Stein IM, Cohen BD: Further studies on the platelet inhibitory effect of guanidinosuccinic acid and its role in uremic bleeding. *Am J Med* 49:336, 1970
190. Remuzzi G, Marchesi D, Cavenaghi AE, Livio M, Donati MB, De Gaetano G, Mecca G: Bleeding in renal failure: A possible role of vascular prostacyclin. *Clin Nephrol* 12:127, 1979

191. Kanfer A, Vandewalle A, Beaufils M, Delarue F, Sraer JD: Enhanced antiplasmin activity in acute renal failure. *Br Med J* 339:195, 1975
192. Rosa AA, Dryd DS, Kjellstrand CM: Dialysis symptoms and stabilization in long-term dialysis, practical application of the CUSUM plot. *Arch Intern Med* 140:804, 1980
193. Marshall VC: Acute renal failure in surgical patients. *Br J Surg* 58:17, 1971
194. Bolooki H, Gliedman ML: Peritoneal dialysis in treatment of acute pancreatitis. *Surgery* 64:466, 1968
195. Aune S, Normann E: Diffuse peritonitis treated with continuous peritoneal lavage. *Acta Chir Scand* 136:401, 1970
196. Peloso OA, Gloyd VT, Wilkinson LH: Treatment of peritonitis with continuous postoperative peritoneal lavage using cephalothin. *Am J Surg* 126:742, 1973
197. Tzamaloukas AH, Garella S, Chazan JA: Peritoneal dialysis for acute renal failure after major abdominal surgery. *Arch Surg* 106:639, 1973
198. Sharbaugh RJ, Rambo WM: Cephalothin and peritoneal lavage in the treatment of experimental peritonitis. *Surg Gynecol Obstet* 139:211, 1974
199. Tolhurst-Cleaver CL, Hopkins AD, Kee Kwong KCN: The effect of post-operative peritoneal lavage on survival, peritoneal wound healing and adhesion formation following fecal peritonitis: an experimental study in the rat. *Br J Surg* 61:601, 1974
200. Perkash I, Satpati P, Agarwal KC: Prolonged peritoneal lavage in fecal peritonitis. *Surgery* 68:842, 1970
201. Kjellstrand CM, Merino GE, Mauer SM, Casali R, Buselmeier TJ: Complications of percutaneous femoral vein catheterizations for hemodialysis. *Clin Nephrol* 4:37, 1975
202. Schwarzbeck A, Brittinger WD, Strauch M: Percutaneous cannulation of subclavian vein for acute haemodialysis. *Proc Eur Dial Transpl Assoc* 15:575, 1978
203. Erben J, Kvasnicka J, Bastecky J, Groh J, Zahradnik J, Rozsival V, Bastecka D, Fixa P, Kozak J, Herout V: Long-term experience with the technique of subclavian and femoral vein cannulation in hemodialysis. *Artif Organs* 3:241, 1979
204. Schwarzbeck A, Brittinger WD, v Henning GE, Strauch M: Cannulation of subclavian vein for hemodialysis using Seldinger's technique. *Trans Am Soc Artif Intern Organs* 24:27, 1978
205. Gerhardt VW, Raliege R, Stein G, Richter G: Erfahrungen mit dem Subklaviakatheterismus bei der Hämodialyse. (Experience with cannulation of subclavian vein for hemodialysis). *Zschr Urol* 67:777, 1974 (in German)
206. Vaz AJ: Subclavian vein Single-needle dialysis in acute renal failure following vascular surgery. *Nephron* 25:102, 1980
207. Buselmeier TJ, Rynasiewicz JJ, Howard RH, Sutherland DE, Davin TD, Lynch RE, Hodson EH, Simmons RL, Najarian JS, Kjellstrand CM: Fistulisation of shunt vasculature: a unique approach to fistula development. *Br Med J* 2:933, 1977
208. Lynch RE, Bosl RH, Streifel AJ, Ebben JP, Ehlers SM, Kjellstrand CM: Dialysis thrombocytopenia: parallel plate vs hollow fiber dialyzers. *Trans Am Soc Artif Intern Organs* 24:704, 1978
209. Kjellstrand CM, Shideman JR, Santiago EA, Mauer M, Simmons RL, Buselmeier TJ: Technical advances in hemodialysis of very small pediatric patients. *Proc Clin Dial Transpl Forum* 1:124, 1971
210. Kjellstrand CM, Mauer SM, Buselmeier TJ, Shideman JR, Meyer RM, von Hartitzsch B, Simmons RL, Michael A, Vernier RL, Najarian JS: Haemodialysis of premature

and newborn babies. *Proc Eur Dial Transplant Assoc* 10:349, 1973
211. Kjellstrand CM: Hemodialysis for children. In: *Strategy in Renal Failure*, edited by Friedman EA, New York, J Wiley & Sons Inc 1977, p 149
212. Hodson EM, Kjellstrand CM, Mauer SM: Acute renal failure in infants and children: Outcome of 53 patients requiring hemodialysis treatment. *J Pediat* 93:756, 1978
213. Levine J, Falk B, Henriquez M, Raja RM, Dramer MS, Rosenbaum JL: Effects of varying dialysate sodium using large surface area dialyzers. *Trans Am Soc Artif Intern Organs* 24:139, 1978
214. Boquin E, Parnell S, Grondin G, Wollard C, Leonard D, Michaels R, Levin NW: Crossover study of the effects of different dialysate sodium concentrations in large surface area, short-term dialysis. *Proc Clin Dial Transpl Forum* 7:48, 1977
215. Gurich W, Mann H, Stiller S, Hacke W: Sodium elimination and alterations of the EEG during dialysis. (*Abstracts*) *Artif Organs* 3 :15, 1979
216. Van Stone JC, Cook J: Decreased postdialysis fatigue with increased dialysate sodium concentrations. *Proc Clin Dial Transpl Forum* 8:152, 1978
217. Ogden DA: A double blind crossover comparison of high and low sodium dialysis. *Proc Clin Dial Transpl Forum* 8:157, 1978
218. Chen WT, Ing TS, Daugirdas JT, Humayun HM, Brescia DJ, Gandhi VC, Hano JE, Kheirbek AO: Hydrostatic ultrafiltration during hemodialysis using decreasing sodium dialysate. *Artif Organs* 4:187, 1980
219. Feig PU, McCurdy DK: The hypertonic state. *N Engl J Med* 294:1444, 1977
220. Wiegand CF, Davin TD, Raij L, Kjellstrand CM: Severe hypokalemia induced by hemodialysis. *Arch Intern Med* 141:167, 1981
221. Eisenberg E, Gotch FA: Normocalcemic hyperparathyroidism culminating in hypercalcemic crisis, treatment with hemodialysis. *Arch Intern Med* 122:258, 1968
222. Kjellstrand CM, Pru C, Borges H: Acetate versus bicarbonate dialysis: a review of biochemical and clinical side effects. *Controv Nephrol* 3:92, 1981
223. Barcenas CG, Olivero J, Ayus J: Bicarbonate dialysis is hemodynamically superior to acetate dialysis. *Abstracts Am Soc Nephrol* 14:111A, 1979
224. Raja RM, Henriquez M, Kramer MS, Rosenbaum RL: Improved dialysis tolerance using Redy sorbent system with bicarbonate dialysate in critically ill patients. *Dial Transpl* 8:241, 1979
225. Borges HF, Fryd DS, Rosa AA, Kjellstrand CM: Hypotension during acetate and bicarbonate dialysis in patients with acute renal failure. *Am J Nephrol* 1:24, 1981
226. Wehle B, Asaba H, Castenfors J, Fürst P, Grahn A, Gunnarsson B, Shaldon S, Bergström J: The Influence of dialysis fluid composition on the blood pressure response during dialysis. *Clin Nephrol* 12:62, 1978
227. Wathen R, Keshaviah P, Hommeyer P, Cadwell K, Comty C: Role of dialysate glucose in preventing gluconeogenesis during hemodialysis. *Trans Am Soc Artif Intern Organs* 23:393, 1977
228. Leski M, Niethammer T, Wyss T: Glucose-enriched dialysate and tolerance to maintenance hemodialysis. *Nephron* 24:271, 1979
229. Rodrigo F, Shideman J, McHugh R, Buselmeier T, Kjellstrand C: Osmolality changes during hemodialysis. Natural history, clinical correlations, and influence of dialysate glucose and intravenous mannitol. *Ann Intern Med* 86:554, 1977
230. Nordstrom H, Lennquist S, Lindell B, Sjöberg HE: Hypophosphataemia in severe burns. *Acta Chir Scand* 143:395, 1977
231. Knochel JP, Caskey JH: The mechanism of hypophosphatemia in acute heat stroke. *JAMA* 238:425, 1977
232. Ayus JC, Olivero JJ, Adrogue HJ: Alkalemia associated with renal failure. *Arch Intern Med* 140:513, 1980
233. Bosl R, Shideman JR, Meyer RM, Buselmeier TJ, von Hartitzsch B, Kjellstrand CM: Effects and complications of high efficiency dialysis. *Nephron* 15:151, 1975
234. Kjellstrand CM: Reflections on dialysis side effects. *Rein Foie* 16B:327, 1974
235. Kjellstrand CM, Shideman JR, Bosl R., Buselmeier TJ: Theoretical aspects and complications of frequent or ultra-efficient short dialysis. *Rein Foie* 16B:375, 1974
236. Kjellstrand CM, Evans RL: Considerations of new dialysis schedules: theoretical evaluation and review of literature. *Opuscula Medico-Techn Lundensia* 16:26, 1975
237. Kjellstrand CM, Evans RL, Petersen RJ, Shideman JR, von Hartitzsch B, Buselmeier TJ: The 'unphysiology' of dialysis: a major cause of dialysis side effects? *Kidney Int* 7 (Suppl 2):S30, 1975
238. Rosa AA, Shideman J, McHugh R, Duncan D, Kjellstrand CM: The importance of osmolality fall and ultrafiltration rate on hemodialysis side effects. *Nephron* 27:134, 1981
239. Kjellstrand CM, Rosa AA, Shideman JR: Hypotension during hemodialysis: osmolality fall is an important pathogenetic factor. *asaio J* 3:11, 1980
240. Woods HF, Ash G, Weston MJ, Bunting S, Moncada S, Vane JR: Prostacyclin can replace heparin in haemodialysis in dogs. *Lancet* 2:1075, 1978
241. Turney JH, Williams LC, Fewell MR, Parsons V, Weston MJ: Use of prostacyclin in regular dialysis therapy. *Proc Eur Dial Transpl Assoc* 17:318, 1980
242. Turney JH, Williams LC, Fewell MR, Parsons V, Weston MJ: Platelet protection and heparin sparing with prostacyclin during regular dialysis therapy. *Lancet* 2:219, 1980
243. Zusman RM, Rubin RH, Cato AE, Cocchetto DM, Crow JM, Tolkoff-Rubin N: Hemodialysis using prostacyclin instead of heparin as the sole antithrombotic agent. *N Engl J Med* 304:934, 1981
244. Streifel A, Ebben J, Sahr C, Meyer R, Shideman J, Lynch R, Kjellstrand CM: Evaluation of three dry-sterilized hollow fiber artificial kidneys. *J Dial* 2:347, 1978
245. Ebben J, Wilson R, Hanna D, Burau M, Kjellstrand CM: Four new dialyzers. *J Dial* 4:147, 1980
246. Hampers CL, Blaufox MD, Merrill JP: Anticoagulation rebound after hemodialysis. *N Engl J Med* 275:776, 1966
247. Lindholm DD, Murray JS: A simplified method of regional heparinization during hemodialysis according to a predetermined dosage formula. *Trans Am Soc Artif Intern Organs* 10:92, 1964
248. Maher JF, Lapierre L, Schreiner GE, Geiger M, Westervelt FB Jr: Regional heparinization for hemodialysis: Technic and clinical experiences. *N Engl J Med* 268:451, 1963
249. Lindqvist B, Fritz H, Hagstam KE, Lecerof H, Liljenberg B: Short clotting-time during haemodialysis by heparinization with an infusion apparatus. *Acta Med Scand* 175:241, 1964
250. Kjellstrand CM, Buselmeier TJ: A simple method for anticoagulation during pre- and postoperative hemodialysis, avoiding rebound phenomenon. *Surgery* 72:630, 1972
251. Shapiro WB, Faubert PF, Porush JG, Chou S: Low-dose heparin in routine hemodialysis monitored by activated

partial thromboplastin time. *Artif Organs* 3:73, 1979
252. Farrell PC, Ward RA, Schindhelm K, Gotch FA: Precise anticoagulation for routine hemodialysis. *J Lab Clin Med* 92:164, 1978
253. Degoulet P, Roulx J-P, Aime F, Berger C, Bloch P, Goupy F, Legrain M: Programme dialyse-informatique III. Données épidémiologiques stratégies de dialyse et résultats biologiques. (Dialysis program information. Epidemiological data of different dialysis strategies and biological results). *J Urol Nephrol* (Paris) 82:1001, 1976 (in French)
254. Kjellstrand CM: Can hypotension during dialysis be avoided? *Controv Nephrol* 2:12, 1980
255. Ing TS, Ashbach DL, Kanter A, Oyama JH, Armbruster KFW, Merkel FK: Fluid removal with negative-pressure hydrostatic ultrafiltration using a partial vacuum. *Nephron* 14:451, 1975
256. Bergström J, Asaba H, Fürst P, Ouleès R: Dialysis, ultrafiltration, and blood pressure. *Proc Eur Dial Transpl Assoc* 13:293, 1976
257. Gerhardt RE, Abdulla AM, Mach SJ, Hudson JB: Isolated ultrafiltration in the treatment of fluid overload in cardiogenic shock. *Arch Intern Med* 139:358, 1979
258. Keshaviah P, Ilstrup K, Constantini E, Berkseth R, Shapiro F: The influence of ultrafiltration and diffusion on cardiovascular parameters. *Trans Am Soc Artif Intern Organs* 26:328, 1980
259. Pierides AM, Kurtz SB, Johnson WJ: Ultrafiltration followed by hemodialysis. A longterm trial and acute studies. *J Dial* 2:325, 1978
260. Jones EO, Ward MK, Hoenich NA, Kerr DNS: Separation of dialysis and ultrafiltration-does it really help? *Proc Eur Dial Transpl Assoc* 14:160, 1977
261. Glabman S, Geronemus R, von Albertini B, Kahn T, Moutoussis G, Bosch JP: Clinical trial of maintenance sequential ultrafiltration and dialysis. *Trans Am Soc Artif Intern Organs* 25:394, 1979
262. Marty AT: Hyperoncotic albumin therapy. *Surg Gynecol Obstet* 139:105, 1974
263. Henrich WL, Woodard TD, Blachley JD, Gomez-Sanchez C, Pettinger W, Cronin RE: Role of osmolality in blood pressure stability after dialysis and ultrafiltration. *Kidney Int* 18:480, 1980
264. Dumler F, Grondin G, Levin NW: Sequential high/low sodium hemodialysis: an alternative to ultrafiltration. *Trans Am Soc Artif Intern Organs* 25:351, 1979
265. Leithner C, Sinzinger H, Stummvoll HK, Klein K, Silberbauer K, Peskar BA: Enhanced 6-OXO-PGF$_{1\alpha}$ levels in plasma during hemodialysis. *Prostaglandins Med* 5:425, 1980
266. Borges H, Shideman J, Kjellstrand C: Hypotension during chronic hemodialysis: on the effects of prostaglandin inhibition. *Abstracts Am Soc Artif Intern Organs* 10:39, 1981
267. Vaziri ND, Skowsky R, Warner A: Effect of isoosmolar volume reduction during hemofiltration on plasma antidiuretic hormone in patients with chronic renal failure. *Int J Artif Organs* 3:322, 1980
268. Caillens H, Pruszczynski W, Meyrier A, Ang K-S, Rousselet F, Ardaillou R: Relationship between change in volemia at constant osmolality and plasma antidiuretic hormone. *Mineral Electrolyte Metab* 4:161, 1980
269. Nord E, Danovitch GM: Vasopressin response in hemodialysis patients. *Kidney Int* 16:234, 1979
270. Schrier RW, Berl T, Anderson RJ: Osmotic and nonosmotic control of vasopressin release. *Am J Physiol* 236:F321, 1979
271. Padfield PL, Brown JJ, Lever AF, Morton JJ, Robertson JIS: Blood pressure in acute and chronic vasopressin excess; studies of malignant hypertension and the syndrome of inappropriate antidiuretic hormone secretion. *N Engl J Med* 304:1067, 1981
272. Vaziri ND, Skowsky R, Saiki J: Antidiuretic hormone in endstage renal disease. *J Dial* 4:73, 1980
273. Van Stone JC, Carey J, Meyer R, Murrin C: Hemodialysis with glycerol containing dialysate. *asaio J* 2:119, 1979
274. Arieff AI, Lazarowitz VC, Guisado R: Experimental dialysis disequilibrium syndrome: prevention with glycerol. *Kidney Int* 14:270, 1978
275. Korchik WP, Brown DC, DeMaster EG: Hemodialysis induced hypotension. *Int J Artif Organs* 1:151, 1978
276. Korchik WP, DeMaster EG, Brown DC: Plasma norepinephrine and hemodialysis. *Kidney Int* 12:484, 1977
277. Ksiqzek A: Dopamine-beta-hydroxylase activity and catecholamine levels in the plasma of patients with renal failure. *Nephron* 24:170, 1979
278. Zuccelli P, Catizone L, Esposti ED, Fusaroli M, Ligabue A, Zuccala A: Influence of ultrafiltration on plasma renin activity and adrenergic system. *Nephron* 21:317, 1978
279. Cannella G, Picotti GB, Mioni G, Cristinelli L, Maiorca R: Blood pressure behaviour during dialysis and ultrafiltration. A pathogenic hypothesis on hemodialysis-induced hypotension. *Int J Artif Organs* 1:69, 1978
280. Brecht HM, Ernest W, Koch KM: Plasma noradrenaline levels in regular hemodialysis patients. *Proc Eur Dial Transpl Assoc* 12:281, 1976
281. Craddock PR, Fehr J, Daimasso AP, Brigham KL, Jacob HS: Hemodialysis leukopenia: pulmonary vascular leukostasis resulting from complement activation by dialyzer cellophane membranes. *J Clin Invest* 59:879, 1977
282. MacGrigor RR: Granulocyte adherence changes induced by hemodialysis, endotoxin, epinephrine, and glucocorticoids. *Ann Intern Med* 86:35, 1977
283. Craddock PR, Fehr J, Brigham KL, Kronenberg RS, Jacob HS: Complement and leukocyte-mediated pulmonary dysfunction in hemodialysis. *N Engl J Med* 296:769, 1977
284. Agar JW, Hull JD, Kaplan M, Pletka PG: Acute cardiopulmonary decompensation and complement activation during hemodialysis. *Ann Intern Med* 94:792, 1981
285. Aljama P, Bird PAE, Ward MK, Feest TG, Walker W, Tanboga H, Sussman M, Kerr DNS: Haemodialysis-induced leucopenia and activation of complement: effects of different membranes. *Proc Eur Dial Transpl Assoc* 15:144, 1978
286. McGrath BP, Tiller DJ, Bune A, Chalmers JP, Horner PI, Uther JB: Autonomic blockade and the valsalva maneuver in patients on maintenance hemodialysis: a hemodynamic study. *Kidney Int* 12:294, 1977
287. Ewing DJ, Winney R: Autonomic function in patients with chronic renal failure on intermittent haemodialysis. *Nephron* 15:424, 1975
288. Nies AS, Robertson D, Stone WJ: Hemodialysis hypotension in not the result of uremic peripheral autonomic neuropathy. *J Lab Clin Med* 94:395, 1979
289. Kersh ES, Kronfield SJ, Unger A, Popper RW, Cantor S, Cohn K: Autonomic insufficiency in uremia as a cause of hemodialysis-induced hypotension. *N Engl J Med* 290:650, 1974
290. von Hartitzsch B, Carr D, Kjellstrand CM, Kerr DNS: Normal red cell survival in well dialyzed patients. *Trans Am Soc Artif Intern Organs* 19:471, 1973
291. Aurigemma NM, Feldman NT, Gottlieb M, Ingram RH, Lazarus JM, Lowrie EG: Arterial oxygenation during hemodialysis. *N Engl J Med* 297:871, 1977
292. Oh MS, Uribarri JV, DelMonte ML, Friedman EA, Car-

roll HJ: Consumption of CO_2 in metabolism of acetate as an explanation for hypoventilation and hypoxemia during hemodialysis. *Abstracts Am Soc Nephrol* 13:125, 1980
293. Eiser AR, Jayamanne D, Koksong C, Che H, Slifkin RF, Neff MS: Contrasting alterations in oxygen consumption and respiratory quotient during acetate and bicarbonate hemodialysis. *Abstracts Am Soc Nephrol* 13:38, 1980
294. Pierides AM, Schniepp B, Johnson WJ: Hemofiltration in the treatment of acute and chronic renal failure. *Proc Clin Dial Transpl Forum* 9:50, 1979
295. Shaldon S, Beau MC, Deschodt G, Ramperez P, Mion C: Vascular stability during hemofiltration. *Trans Am Soc Artif Intern Organs* 26:391, 1980
296. Gotch FA: Net sodium flux in post-dilution hemofiltration. *Abstracts Am Soc Nephrol* 13:39A, 1980
297. Neff M, Slifkin R, Eiser A, Sadjadi S: A wearable artificial glomerulus. *Proc Clin Dial Transpl Forum* 9:23, 1979
298. Kramer P, Böhler J, Kehr A, Gröne HJ, Schrader J, Matthaei D, Scheler F: Intensive care potential of continuous arterio-venous hemofiltration. *Trans Am Soc Artif Intern Organs* 28:28, 1982
299. Olbricht C, Mueller C, Schurek HJ, Stolte H: Treatment of acute renal failure in patients with multiple organ failure by continuous spontaneous hemofiltration. *Trans Am Soc Artif Intern Organs* 28:33, 1982
300. Tolhurst Cleaver CL, Hopkins AD, Kee Kwong KC NG, Raftery AT: The effect of postoperative peritoneal lavage on survival, peritoneal wound healing and adhesion formation following fecal peritonitis: an experimental study in the rat. *Br J Surg* 61:601, 1974
301. Furman KI, Gomperts ED, Hockley J: Activity of intraperitoneal heparin during peritoneal dialysis. *Clin Nephrol* 9:15, 1978
302. Thayssen P, Pindborg T: Peritoneal dialysis and heparin. *Scand J Urol Nephrol* 12:73, 1978
303. Shear L, Shinaberger JH, Barry KG: Peritoneal transport of antibiotics in man. *N Engl J Med* 272:666, 1964
304. Axelrod J, Meyers BR, Hirschman SZ, Stein R: Prophylaxis with cephalothin in peritoneal dialysis. *Arch Intern Med* 132:368, 1973
305. Schwartz FD, Kallmeyer M, Dunea G, Kark RM: Prevention of infection during peritoneal dialysis. *JAMA* 199:79, 1967
306. Editorial (anonymous): Antibiotic lavage for peritonitis. *Br Med J* 2:691, 1979
307. Stewart DJ, Matheson NA: Peritoneal lavage in appendicular peritonitis. *Br J Surg* 65:54, 1978
308. Perkash I, Satpati P, Agarwal KC, Chakravarti RN, Chhuttani PN: Prolonged peritoneal lavage in fecal peritonitis. *Surgery* 68:842, 1970
309. Peloso OA, Floyd VT, Wilkinson LH: Treatment of peritonitis with continuous postoperative peritoneal lavage using cephalothin. *Am J Surg* 126:742, 1973
310. Atkins RC, Scott DF, Holdsworth SR, Davidson AJ: Prolonged antibiotic peritoneal lavage in the management of gross generalized peritonitis. *Med J Aust* 1:954, 1976
311. Aune S, Normann E: Diffuse peritonitis treated with continuous peritoneal lavage. *Acta Chir Scand* 136:401, 1970
312. Mandell IN, Ahern MJ, Kliger AS, Andriole VT: Candida peritonitis complicating peritoneal dialysis: successful treatment with low dose amphotericin B therapy. *Clin Nephrol* 6:492, 1976
313. Gutman RA, Nixon WP, McRae RL, Spencer HW: Effect of intraperitoneal and intravenous vasoactive amines on peritoneal dialysis: study in anephric dogs. *Trans Am Soc Artif Intern Organs* 22:570, 1976
314. Nolph KD, Ghods AJ, Van Stone J, Brown PA: The effects of intraperitoneal vasodilators on peritoneal clearances. *Trans Am Soc Artif Intern Organs* 22:586, 1976
315. Hirszel P, Lasrich M, Maher JF: Arachidonic acid increases peritoneal clearances. *Trans Am Soc Artif Intern Organs* 27:61, 1981
316. Maher JF: Characteristics of peritoneal transport; physiological and clinical implications. *Mineral Electrolyte Metab* 5:201, 1981
317. Posen GA, Luiselto J: Continuous equilibration peritoneal dialysis in the treatment of acute renal failure. *Peritoneal Dial Bull* (Toronto, Can.) 1:6, 1980
318. Vaamonde CA, Michael UF, Metzger RA, Carroll KE: Complications of acute peritoneal dialysis. *J Chron Dis* 28:637, 1975
319. Roxe DM, Argy WP, Frost B, Kerwin J, Schreiner GE: Complications of peritoneal dialysis. *South Med J* 69:584, 1976
320. Rubin J, Oreopoulos DG, Lio TT, Mathews R, de Veber GA: Management of peritonitis and bowel perforation during chronic peritoneal dialysis. *Nephron* 16:220, 1976
321. Simkin EP, Wright FK: Perforating injuries of the bowel complicating peritoneal catheter insertion. *Lancet* 1:64, 1968
322. Grodstein GP, Blumenkrantz MJ, Kopple JD, Moran JK, Coburn JW: Glucose absorption during continuous ambulatory peritoneal dialysis. *Kidney Int* 19:564, 1981
323. Crossley K, Kjellstrand CM: Intraperitoneal insulin for control of blood sugar in diabetic patients during peritoneal dialysis. *Br Med J* 1:269, 1971
324. Maher JF, Hohnadel DC, Shea C, DiSanzo F, Cassetta M: Effect of intraperitoneal diuretics on solute transport during hypertonic dialysis. *Clin Nephrol* 7:96, 1977
325. Vaziri ND, Ness R, Wellikson L, Barton C, Greep N: Bicarbonate-buffered peritoneal dialysis an effective adjunct in the treatment of lactic acidosis. *Am J Med* 67:392, 1979
326. Blumenkrantz MJ, Gahl GM, Kopple JD, Kamdar AV, Jones MR, Kessel M, Coburn JW: Protein losses during peritoneal dialysis. *Kidney Int* 19:593, 1981
327. Rubin J, McFarland S, Hellems EW, Bower JD: Peritoneal dialysis during peritonitis. *Kidney Int* 19:460, 1981
328. Gotloib L, Mines M, Garmizo L, Varka I: Hemodynamic effects of increasing intraabdominal pressure in peritoneal dialysis. *Peritoneal Dial Bull* (Toronto, Can) 1:41, 1981
329. Finn R, Jowett EW: Acute hydrothorax complicating peritoneal dialysis. *Br Med J* 2:94, 1970
330. Edwards SR, Unger AM: Acute hydrothorax; a new complication of peritoneal dialysis. *JAMA* 199:853, 1967
331. Lorentz WB: Acute hydrothorax during peritoneal dialysis. *J Pediat* 94:417, 1979
332. Hurley RM, Muogbo D, Wilson GW, Ali MAM: Peritoneal effluent cellularity: predictor of bacterial peritonitis. *Kidney Int* 8:427, 1975
333. Chan LK, Oliver DO: Simple method for early detection of peritonitis in patients on continuous ambulatory peritoneal dialysis. *Lancet* 2:1336, 1979
334. Lindholm T: Pleural dialysis in a case of acute renal failure. *Acta Med Scand* 165:239, 1959
335. Sheth KJ, Glicklich M: Pleural dialysis in acute renal failure. *Clin Nephrol* 6:370, 1976
336. O'Brien TF, Baxter CR, Teschan PE: Prophylactic daily hemodialysis. *Trans Am Soc Artif Intern Organs* 5:77, 1959
337. Teschan PE, Baxter CR, O'Brien TF, Freyhof JN, Hall WH: Prophylactic hemodialysis in the treatment of acute renal failure. *Ann Intern Med* 53:992, 1960
338. Conger JD: A controlled evaluation of prophylactic dialy-

sis in posttraumatic acute renal failure. *J Trauma* 15:1056, 1975
339. Fischer RP, Griffen WO, Reiser M, Clark DS: Early dialysis in the treatment of acute renal failure. *Surg Gynecol, Obstet* 123:1019, 1966
340. Conger JD: The use of prophylactic dialysis in acute renal failure. *Contemp Dial* Oct, 1980, p 41
341. Teschan PE, Ahmad S, Hull AR, Nolph KD, Shapiro FI: Daily dialysis; applications and problems. *Trans Am Soc Artif Intern Organs* 26:600, 1980
342. Bull GM, Joekes AM, Lowe KG: Renal function studies in acute tubular necrosis. *Clin Sci* 8:379, 1950
343. Finkenstaedt JT, Merrill JP: Renal function after recovery from acute renal failure. *N Engl J Med* 254:1023, 1956
344. Edwards KDG: Recovery of renal function after acute renal failure. *Aust Ann Med* 8:195, 1959
345. Price JDE, Palmer RA: A functional and morphological follow-up study of acute renal failure. *Arch Intern Med* 105:90, 1960
346. Briggs JD, Kennedy AC, Young LN, Luke RG, Gray M: Renal function after acute tubular necrosis. *Br Med J* 3:513, 1967
347. Hall JW, Johnson WJ, Maher FT, Hunt JC: Immediate and long-term prognosis in acute renal failure. *Ann Intern Med* 73:515, 1970
348. Lewers DT, Mathew TH, Maher JF, Schreiner GE: Long-term follow-up of renal function and histology after acute tubular necrosis. *Ann Intern Med* 73:523, 1970
349. Fuchs HJ, Thelen M, Wilbrandt R: Die Nierenfunktion nach akutem Nierenversagen-Eine Langzeitstudie an 70 Patienten (Renal function after acute renal failure — a long term study). *Dtsch Med Wochenschr* 99:1641, 1974 (in German)
350. Merino GE, Buselmeier TJ, Kjellstrand CM: Postoperative chronic renal failure: a new syndrome? *Ann Surg* 182:37, 1975
351. Levin ML, Simon NM, Herdson PB, del Greco F: Acute renal failure followed by protracted, slowly resolving chronic uremia. *J Chron Dis* 25:645, 1972
352. Siegler RL, Bloomer HA: Acute renal failure with prolonged oliguria; an account of five cases. *JAMA* 225:133, 1973

27

NUTRITION IN DIALYSIS PATIENTS

REINHOLD K.A. KLUTHE

Introduction	569
Evaluation of nutritional status	569
Acute renal failure	569
Chronic renal failure	570
Nutrition in the early stage of regular dialysis	571
Nutrition in the stable dialysis stage	572
Protein	572
Vitamins	572
Iron	573
Water and electrolytes	573
Histidine supplementation	573
Nutrition during episodes of metabolic instability	573
Nutrition in patients treated with continuous ambulatory peritoneal dialysis (CAPD)	573
Nutrition in diabetic dialysis patients	573
References	573

INTRODUCTION

Nutritional management of patients with renal failure has three major objectives:
1. To minimise the production of toxic metabolites of protein metabolism (urea, guanidines, middle molecules etc.), by limiting the protein intake and changing dietary protein composition to emphasise essential amino acids.
2. To normalise the 'milieu intérieur' by adjusting water and mineral intake.
3. to restore and maintain a good nutritional status, thereby decreasing the likelihood of such problems as serious infections.

Nutritional management of dialysed patients is important both in acute renal failure and in chronic renal failure. Regrettably, nutrition is often ignored once dialysis is undertaken and becomes the major treatment modality. Failure to provide adequate nutrition can lead to increased morbidity, however. Indeed, malnutrition and wasting are frequently observed in patients treated by dialysis.

EVALUATION OF NUTRITIONAL STATUS

Adequacy of nutrition should be assessed by dietary history, such physical findings as muscle circumference, skinfold thickness and such laboratory tests as urea, nitrogen appearance rate and serum protein concentrations. One of the most important methods for defining nutritional status as a basis for nutritional therapy is the physical examination. It should include inspection of the skin, hair and nails as well as determination of muscle mass (measurement of the circumference of the upper arm) and skin fold thickness (using a Lange-caliper and usually assessing the triceps area) (1–3). For children, measurement of height and estimation of bone age are obviously important (4). Impaired nutrition renal osteodystrophy or uraemia can impede growth. The weight/height ratio is also an important anthropometric parameter. Absolute and relative body weight must be interpreted considering fluid balance. Since we do not yet know the ideal weights for uraemic patients, we currently use as a guideline the individual's weight prior to the onset of renal failure or the patient's relative body weight (RBW) according to Broca (height in cm − 100 = kg body weight). Plasma protein (total protein, albumin, transferrin or C3-complement) and plasma lipid concentrations should also be determined because these are indices of nutritional adequacy. Recently, attention has also been directed toward the urea generation rate as a marker of protein intake. The daily production rate of urea is directly proportional to the amount of protein catabolised. When the patient is in nitrogen balance, this reflects the protein intake. (See also chapters 3 and 26).

ACUTE RENAL FAILURE

The nutritional requirements of patients with acute renal failure depend in part on how often dialysis is performed and what sort of dialysis is applied. Table 1 presents a schematic overview of nutrition in different stages of acute renal failure. This outline is applicable for uncomplicated ('non-hypercatabolic') patients treated with twice weekly haemodialysis. In patients who are unable to eat enough the application of special formula diets or the administration of amino acids is required, if necessary, by tube feeding to prevent negative caloric balance. It is important to recall that once diuresis is sufficient to obviate the need for dialysis, water, electrolyte and caloric needs increase considerably.

Complications, such as increased catabolism or infection, and increased nutrient removal by more frequent dialysis require the use of more intensive hyperalimentation (5). In addition, when peritoneal dialysis is utilised, compensation for protein losses (between 0.2 and 1.0 g/l dialysis fluid) is indicated. If adequate nourish-

Table 1. Nutrition in different stages of acute renal failure.

	Predialysis stage	Dialysis stage	Postdialysis stage
Water	depends on water loss	depends on water loss	unlimited
Calories	>147 kJ/kg >35 Cal/kg	unchanged	unchanged
Protein	0.35 to 0.4 g/kg (selected)	0.5 to 0.6 g/kg (on basis of 2 dialyses/week)	0.5 to 0.6 g/kg
Potassium	<30 mmol/day	30 to 60 mmol/day	rich
Sodium	10–20 mmol/day	10–20 mmol/day	unlimited

ment cannot be achieved through the gastrointestinal tract, partial or total parenteral nutrition should be instituted. In these cases amino acids mixtures with a high content of essential amino acids, including histidine, seem to be advantageous. Parenteral, high calorie feeding is easily possible using 70% dextrose monohydrate or an appropriate substitute and 10 to 20% fat suspensions infused into a large vein. The beneficial results of hyperalimentation in patients with acute renal failure were demonstrated by Abel et al. (6) in 1973. They noted a substantial decrease in death rate and a faster recovery from the kidney lesion with an earlier return of diuresis in patients treated with hyperalimentation.

CHRONIC RENAL FAILURE

In contrast with the acute renal failure patient, a long term nutritional strategy is indicated for the patient with chronic renal failure. Nutritional instructions should start before dialysis treatment is initiated. The nutritional status of the patient at the start of dialysis, the length, the technique and efficiency of the dialyses, and pertinent complicating diseases, should be considered in nutritional planning. Because of the close relationship between protein metabolism and uraemic intoxication, the protein intake is of special importance in the dietary prescription. The complexity of factors influencing protein requirements in maintenance dialysis patients is presented in Figure 1. The figure demonstrates that nutritional therapy must be individualised based on numerous considerations. For practical reasons nutritional therapy of regular dialysis patients should be divided into three stages (7):

1. The *early stage of adaption* to dialysis lasts about half a year. A major difference between haemodialysis and peritoneal dialysis is the necessity to compensate for protein loss induced by peritoneal dialysis. There is, however, a scarcity of available data on nutrition in this adaptive stage although this phase seems to be especially important in patients who have not been regularly controlled or adequately treated in the predialysis period.
2. Most data available on nutrition in chronic dialysis patients have been collected during the *stage of stabilisation*. The patient is well balanced metabolically and should be under good nutritional control during this stage.
3. The state of metabolic stability may be interrupted, however, with varying frequency, by *episodes of met-*

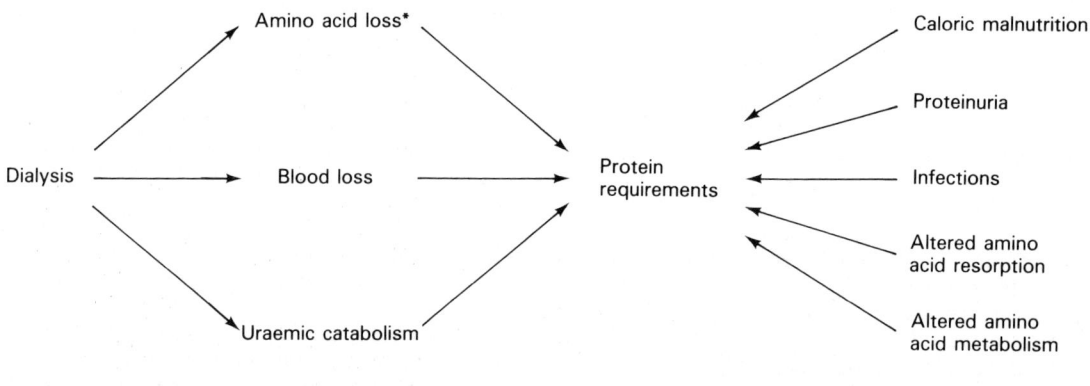

*plasma protein loss in peritoneal dialysis

Figure 1. Factors influencing protein requirements in regular dialysis patients.

abolic instability, provoked by dialysis complications, infections or surgical interventions which may or may not be associated with uraemia. Surgical interventions often require total parenteral nutrition.

Nutrition in the early stage of regular dialysis

The characteristics of the early stage of adaptation to regular dialysis treatment are presented in Table 2. The low protein diet commonly prescribed before initiating regular dialysis usually has reduced the protein stores to a greater or lesser extent. In the case of patients with advanced renal failure that have not previously been treated by protein restriction, uraemic hypercatabolism and insufficient nutrition, caused by lack of appetite resulting from the uraemic intoxication, may have led to the same condition. Protein malnutrition, of course, can also be the consequence of inadequate calorie intake. To diagnose this condition, determination of serum levels of transferrin and of the third component of the complement system are helpful. Since protein depletion increases the potential risks of complications, careful repletion is indicated. The nutritional recommendations for the stable phase, as presented in Table 3, are also applicable in this early stage of adaptation, but they should be considered as a *minimum* intake.

Sometimes repletion can be hindered because it is difficult to obtain full cooperation of the patient who has accommodated to a low protein diet. It often requires special attention and persuasiveness to get the cooperation of such patients. Often patients seem to be unable to consume enough protein and calories in the form of common food. In such cases prescription of special formula diets, which are commercially available, can be helpful. Suitable indicators for satisfactory repletion of protein stores are serum levels of transferrin and the C3 component of the complement system.

Many patients also have problems adhering to a prescribed fluid intake. The problems encountered will vary depending on when regular dialysis treatment was initiated. Problems mainly occur when dialysis treatment is started early, while the patient still produces appreciable amounts of urine and consequently has to drink substantial amounts of fluid to replace urinary and ultrafiltrate losses. In contrast, the anuric patient must limit the fluid intake.

Oral nutrition may clearly be a problem because of early side effects of dialysis procedures. In this early phase of regular dialysis treatment, the management of the patient before initiating dialysis is of importance.

Table 2. Nutritional problems in the early phase of regular dialysis treatment (before adaptation occurs).

1. Depleted 'protein stores'
2. Changing from low to high protein nutrition
3. Increasing caloric intake
4. Reduced intake of water
5. Poor tolerance of dialysis procedures causing inappetence, sickness, vomiting

This was recently confirmed by an evaluation of treatment preceding dialysis and survival rate of all patients entering a chronic dialysis programme (8). Patients were divided into two groups, one regularly controlled and carefully treated in an outpatient clinic (SCP group = Schematically Controlled Patients) and another heterogeneous group comprising patients who were admitted directly from practitioners or other hospitals, usually severely uraemic (NSCP group = Non Schematically Controlled Patients). Figure 2 presents the cumulative patient survival in both groups, calculated from the start of dialysis. The two groups were comparable with regard to primary renal disease, age and residual renal function at the time of the first dialysis. During the observation period 43 out of the NSCP group (numbering 141 patients) died (31%) compared to only 24 of the SCP group, consisting of 127 patients (19%). To evaluate the effectiveness of careful predialysis treatment, the analysis of the time of death is also of importance: Out of the 43 fatalities in the NSCP group, 22 died in the first half year after initiation of dialysis, half of them with the diagnosis of uraemic catabolism or septicaemia or both. From the SCP group, no patient died in the first half year. The difference could not be ascribed to hypertension because blood pressure control was similar in both groups of patients. There was a high frequency of hypercatabolism in the NSCP group, however, in contrast to the SCP group of patients in whom uraemia was con-

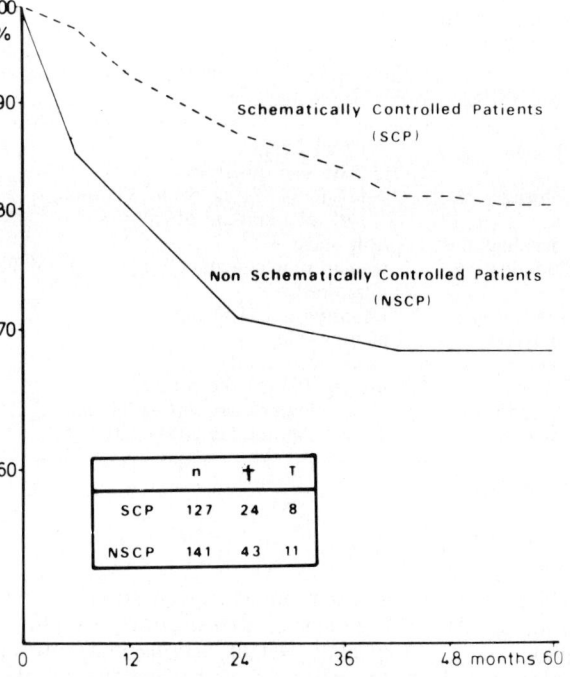

Figure 2. Cumulative survival of patients regularly controlled and treated in an outpatient clinic (before regular dialysis treatment was started: SCP group) and of patients admitted in severe uraemic condition from practitioners or other hospitals (inadequately pretreated: NSC group). See text. (From: Kluthe et al [8]).

trolled by a selective low protein, high caloric diet in the predialysis period. The lack of controlled dietary treatment in the late predialysis stage seems to be responsible for the bad prognosis in the NSCP group.

When subdividing the SCP group of patients, who had a better survival rate and who were adequately treated in the predialysis phase, into a group with optimal dietary adherence (consuming about 25 g protein in the form of a potato-egg-diet, which is the German modification of the Giordano-Giovannetti-diet) and into another group consuming about 45 g of protein per day, the patients with low protein intake appeared to have better survival chances than those with a higher protein intake. A negative influence of long-term protein restriction on the prognosis in the early dialysis stage, which has been suggested by some authors (9), can be ruled out from these results. Patients treated with a selective low protein diet, who entered the dialysis programme with a creatinine clearance below 4 ml/1.73 m^2, had even a better survival rate than patients with a higher protein intake. The four year cumulative survival in the non optimal (NOD) group was appreciably less than in the optimal dietary (OD) group who optimally adhered to the diet (Figure 3).

Nutrition in the stable dialysis stage

Recommendations for nutritional management during the stable stage of regular dialysis therapy are based on several recent studies (Table 3).

Table 3. Recommended nutrients for stabilised regular dialysis patients (twice weekly haemodialysis).

Protein	>1 to 1.2 g/kg (2/3 of high quality)
Calories	>126 to 147 kJ/kg (30 to 35 Cal/kg)
Fat	1/3 of total amount of calories
Carbohydrates	little sugar
Vitamins	regular supplementation of water soluble vitamins *
Iron	1.8 mmol/day (100 mg)
Potassium	60 mmol/day
Sodium	50 to 60 mmol/day
Water	usually 750 to 1000 ml/day
Phosphorus	19 to 39 mmol/day (600–1200 mg)
Calcium	25 to 50 mmol/day (1000-2000 mg)

* See Table 4.

Proteins
The protein recommendation, as appears from observations by different groups of investigators, should be more than 1.0 g/kg body weight. Kluthe and coworkers (11) and other groups have demonstrated that 1.0 g/kg is not enough, even when 2/3 of the protein is given in the form of high biologic value protein. In addition, total caloric intake must be considered and should be adjusted to the physical activities of the patient. Since total caloric intake, the quantity and the type of fat and the amount of monomere carbohydrates ingested in-

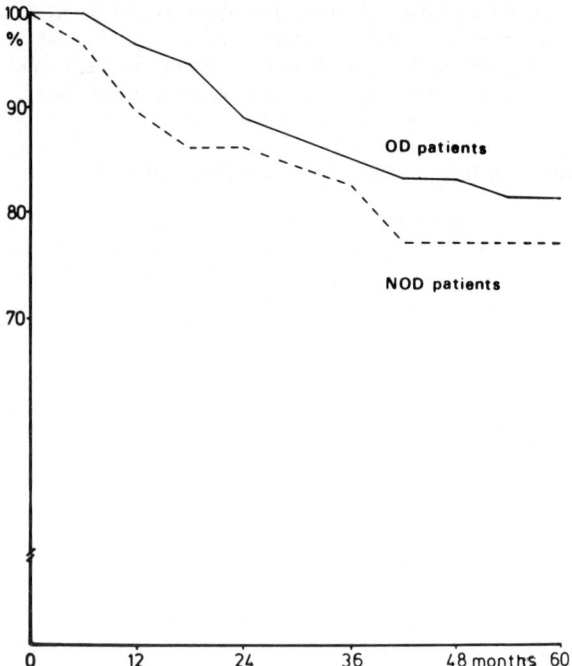

Figure 3. Cumulative survival rates of predialytically schematically controlled patients (SCP), divided in optimal dietary patients (OD) and non optimal dietary patients (NOD).

fluence plasma cholesterol and triglyceride levels, more attention is currently paid to more specific dietary recommendations (12).

Vitamins
Supplementation of water soluble vitamins should be performed (see Table 4) because the intake of water soluble vitamins is reduced due to the dietary restriction of fruits and vegetables. In addition, water soluble vitamins are removed during dialysis (13–15), although protein binding limits the removal of most B vitamins. It is, however, undesirable to substitute vitamin A because it has been demonstrated that vitamin A may be toxic in cases of chronic uraemia (16, 17). High levels of

Table 4. Water soluble vitamin substitution in regular dialysis patients.

	Recommended dose per day	
Vitamin	(Ref. 14)	(Ref. 10)
C (Ascorbic acid)	100 mg	200 mg
Folic acid	1	4
Niacin	20	100
B$_2$ (Riboflavin)	1,8	16
B$_1$ (Thiamin)	1,5	16
B$_6$ (Pyridoxine)	10	20
Pantothenic acid	5	20

vitamin A were found in the serum of patients who were supplemented with tablets containing vitamin A and there was a close positive relationship between serum lipid levels and serum vitamin A concentrations. Vitamin A has been incriminated as being responsible for premature atherosclerosis in dialysis patients. Vitamin D or its active dihydroxymetabolite also may be required as discussed in Chapter 35.

Iron
Iron substitution is necessary since even with an optimal dialysis technique blood loss can be minimised but not prevented. Blood losses induced by regular dialysis treatment may vary between 900 and 2600 ml per year, depending on fistula puncture technique, blood sampling and residual blood volume in the dialyser. In addition, gastrointestinal blood loss may contribute to iron deficiency in some patients. Cumulative annual blood loss in chronic dialysis patients may be as high as 6 to 8 l (19).

Water and electrolytes
Potassium, sodium and water intake have to be adjusted to the patient's individual needs. The values in Table 3 are guidelines for patients on twice weekly regular dialysis treatment.

Histidine supplementation
Giordano (20) obtained appreciable improvement of anaemia by administering 1.0 g histidine daily. Others, however, have observed no such effect (21). In a recent controlled study a definite positive effect of supplemental histidine on the anemia was observed in all patients having a histidine deficiency, as demonstrated by amino acid analysis of the blood (22). In these patients histidine supplementation (1.5 g histidine-HCl) resulted in a substantial decrease in the frequency of blood transfusions.

Nutrition during episodes of metabolic instability

During episodes with reduced appetite, malnutrition may occur in chronic dialysis patients particularly if their course is complicated by such problems as infections or surgical interventions. In these circumstances hyperalimentation should be considered. The intake of food should be regularly checked and the amount of calories ingested should be calculated (23). The increased needs of nutrients must be met and if enteral nutrition is no longer possible or only a limited amount can be achieved, parenteral nutrition is indicated. Eventually, total parenteral feeding may be necessary. The same amount of calories as would be given enterally is required and 1/3 of the calories should be in the form of fat.

Nutrition in patients treated with continuous ambulatory peritoneal dialysis (CAPD)

Basically similar nutritional recommendations apply to patients treated by continuous ambulatory peritoneal dialysis as for those undergoing regular haemodialysis treatment. The protein intake should reach at least 1.0 g/kg body weight (24, 25) since several grams of protein are lost daily into peritoneal dialysate. Peritonitis increases these losses as well as metabolic demands and decreases appetite. The daily loss of amino acids with peritoneal dialysis is comparable to that resulting from hemodialysis. Regarding sodium intake, there seems to be some difference in the two dialysis techniques. A higher intake of sodium (about 100 mmol Na/day than in regular haemodialysis patients seems to be permissable in most patients treated by continuous peritoneal dialysis (25). Higher salt and water intakes increase the need for hypertonic dextrose dialysis solution which may induce hyperlipaemia and obesity, requiring reduction in the carbohydrate intake.

Nutrition in diabetic dialysis patients

Nutritional requirements for diabetic patients treated by chronic dialysis are usually similar to those for nondiabetic patients. Some diabetic patients, who previously had a nephrotic syndrome, have gastric neuropathy or have extensive vascular disease, and hence, will enter the dialysis programme in a state of protein undernutrition. In these cases careful protein repletion is indicated. Of course, insulin requirements may decrease as renal failure progresses, but often increase as dialysis restores nutritional adequacy and provides additional dextrose.

REFERENCES

1. Blumenkrantz MJ, Kopple JD, Gutman RA, Chan YK, Barbour GL, Roberts CH, Shen FH, Gandhi VC, Tucker C, TH, Curtis FK, Coburn JW: Methods for assessing nutritional status of patients with renal failure. *Am J Clin Nutr* 33:1567, 1980
2. Kopple JD, Swenseid ME: Protein and amino acid metabolism in uremic patients undergoing maintenance hemodialysis. *Kidney Int* 7 (Suppl 2):S64, 1975
3. Zimmerman W, Schaeffer G, Schäfer B, Katz N, Südhoff A, Kluthe R: Anthropometrische Untersuchungen bei chronisch-hämodialysierten Patienten als Maß für den Ernahrungszustand (Anthropometric investigations in chronic haemodialysis patients as a measure of their nutritional status). *Nieren- u Hochdruckkrankheiten* 5:72, 1976 (in German)
4. Holliday MA: Calorie intake and growth in uremia. *Kidney Int* 7 (Suppl 2):S73, 1975
5. Spreiter SC, Myers BD, Swenson RS: Protein energy requirements in subjects with acute renal failure receiving intermittent hemodialysis. *Am J Clin Nutr* 33:1433, 1980
6. Abel RM, Beck CH Jr, Abbott WM, Ryan JA Jr, Barnett GO, Fischer JE: Improved survival from acute renal failure after treatment with intravenous essential amino acids and glucose. *New Engl J med* 288:695, 1973

7. Kluthe R: Nutritional management of patients treated with dialysis with special reference to RDT-patients. *Acta Chir Scand* (Suppl) 498:102, 1980
8. Kluthe R, Lüttgen FM, Heinze V, Findeisen M: Predialysis strategy and long term prognosis of RDT-patients. *Proc 2nd Prague Symposium on Renal Failure* Lund, Sweden, Gambro Publ, 1979, p 47
9. Ritz E, Mehls O, Gilli G, Heuck CC: Protein restriction in the conservative management of uremia. *Am J Clin Nutr* 31:1703, 1978
10. Quirin H, Schaeffer G: Vitaminzufuhr in der Nahrung und Substitution von Vitaminen bei Hämodialysepatienten. (Vitamin supply in food and substitution of vitamins in haemodialysis patients. In: *Aktuelle Fragen der Ernahrungstherapie in Nephrologie und Gastroenterologie*, edited by Canzler H, Georg Thieme Verlag Stuttgart FRG, 1978, p 58, (in German)
11. Kluthe R, Lüttgen FM, Capetianu T, Heinze V, Katz N, Südhoff A: Protein requirements in maintenance hemodialysis. *Am J Clin Nutr* 31:1812, 1978
12. Gokal R, Mann JT, Oliver DO, Ledingham JGG: Dietary treatment of hyperlipidemia in chronic hemodialysis patients. *Am J Clin Nutr* 31:1915, 1978
13. Berlyne GM: Dietary treatment of chronic renal failure. In: *Strategy in renal failure,* edited by Friedman EA, New York, Wiley J and Sons, 1978, p 175
14. Kopple JD, Swenseid ME: Vitamin nutrition in patients undergoing maintenance hemodialysis. *Kidney Int* 7 (Suppl 2):S79, 1975
15. Weinsier RL, Butterworth CE Jr: *Handbook of Clinical Nutrition. Clinical Manual for the Diagnosis and Management of Nutritional Problems.* St. Louis, Toronto, London, The CV Mosby Company, 1981
16. Yatzidis H, Digenis P, Fondas P: Hypervitaminosis A accompanying advanced chronic renal failure. *Br Med J* 3:352, 1975
17. Werb R, Clark WF, Lindsay RM, Jones EOP, Linton AL: Serum vitamin A levels and associate abnormalities in patients on regular dialysis treatment. *Clin Nephrol* 12:63, 1979
18. Hecking E, Köhler H, Zobel R, Lemmel EM, Mader H, Opferkuch W, Prellwitz W, Keim JM, Müller D: Treatment with essential amino acids in patients on chronic hemodialysis: a double blind cross-over study. *Am J Clin Nutr* 31:1821, 1978
19. Longnecker RE, Goffinet JA, Hendler ED: Blood loss during maintenance hemodialysis. *Trans Am Soc Artif Intern Organs* 20:135, 1974
20. Giordano C, de Santo NG, Rinaldi S, Acone D, Esposito R, Gallo B: Histidine supplements in the treatment of uraemia. *Proc Eur Dial Transpl Assoc* 10:161, 1973
21. Blumenkrantz MJ, Shapiro D, Swenseid ME, Kopple JD: Histidine supplementation for treatment of anaemia of uraemia. *Br Med J* 2:53, 1975
22. Lindenau K, Schmicker R, Cernaček P, Precht K, Spustova V, Dzúrik R: Indications for histidine substitution in RDT-patients. In: *Histidine II,* edited by Partsch G, Batsford S, Stuttgart, Georg Thieme, (Fed Rep Germany), 1980
23. Harvey KB, Blumenkrantz MJ, Levine SE, Blackburn GL: Nutritional assessment and treatment of chronic renal failure. *Am J Clin Nutr* 33:1586, 1980.
24. Armstrong VW, Striebel JP, Thalacker F: Einfluß der Dauer-Peritoneal-dialyse (CAPD) auf die Plasma-Aminosäuren-Konzentrationen von Patienten mit chronischer Niereninsuffizienz (Influence of CAPD on plasma amino acids in patients with chronic renal failure). *Nieren- u Hochdruckkrankheiten* 8:198, 1978 (in German)
25. Schuenemann G, Falda Z, Mergerian H, Quellhorst E: Klinische Erfahrungen mit der Dauerperitonealdialyse (Clinical experience with CAPD). *Nieren- u Hochdruckkrankheiten* 8:193, 1979 (in German)

BLOOD PRESSURE CONTROL IN CHRONIC DIALYSIS PATIENTS

ROBERT P. WHITE and ALBERT L. RUBIN

Introduction	575
Hypertension	575
Pathogenesis	575
Fluid volume	576
Renin	576
Pathophysiology of renin secretion	576
Neurogenic	576
Search for a marker of sympathetic activity	577
Other causes	577
Treatment of hypertension	577
Diuretics	577
Renin-angiotensin inhibition	578
Neurogenic agents	579
Vasodilators	580
Treatment of accelerated hypertension	580
Pharmacological agents	580
Bilateral nephrectomy	581
Hypotension	581
Pathogenesis	581
Treatment	582
Conclusions	582
References	583

INTRODUCTION

Proper blood pressure control is an essential prerequisite to longevity for patients on maintenance dialysis. Over the last decade, the refinement of extracorporeal hemodialysis and peritoneal dialysis techniques, the development of continuous ambulatory peritoneal dialysis and the release of a number of new pharmacological agents have allowed for greater ease of modification of blood pressure abnormalities.

Hypertension is an important predisposing factor to accelerated atherosclerosis and to the high incidence of cardiovascular and cerebral vascular disease in dialysis patients (1-3). In a recent study of 50 non-diabetic maintenance hemodialysis patients undergoing renal transplantation, 90% of patients with moderate or severe atherosclerosis had previous and concomitant hypertension (4). All patients between the ages of 25 and 40 years who had atherosclerosis had previous hypertension. (This study was done by both interoperative observation of and histologic evaluation of iliac vasculature and was significant in comparison to non-hypertensives with a p value <0.02.) Recurrent or persistent hypotension prevents adequate dialysis and patient rehabilitation and when severe, may lead to alterations of life style and even wasting and death (5, 6). Although not all the causative factors of either hypertension or symptomatic hypotension are well understood, both can usually be corrected or appreciably modified when appropriate treatment is initiated early (7).

Table 1. Factors in blood pressure regulation.

I	Salt + H_2O
II	Renin — Angiotensin
III	Neurogenic factors

For brevity not every aspect of blood pressure control is discussed in this chapter in detail. For enlargement of specific points, the reader is referred to the cited references.

Hypertension

Approximately 80% of patients with progressive renal failure approaching dialysis have hypertension, as arbitrarily defined by a diastolic pressure greater than 90 mm Hg or a systolic pressure over 150 mm Hg (8, 9). The percentage of dialysis patients considered to have dialysis-resistant hypertension requiring anti-hypertension medications varies considerably depending on the approach of the specific dialysis unit or the individual physician. Figures range from 5% to more than 30%. Demographic differences, different kinds of primary disease, variable policies of dialysis, differences in defining hypertension in dialyzed patients and ease of acceptance of medication by the patient population all may contribute to reported differences. In our experience, the various modalities of dialysis specifically applied alone control blood pressure in about 75% of the total dialysis population and 25% require at least one antihypertensive medication in addition to regular dialysis. Only as the exception is bilateral nephrectomy currently employed to control blood pressure.

Pathogenesis

Of the many factors that contribute to the hypertension seen in uremia, three are of paramount significance (see Table 1). Firstly the major pathogenetic factor for hypertension in all dialysis surveys is *increased body water* (8-14). Secondly if volume is corrected and hypertension persists, an absolute or relative *hyper-reninemia*, originating from the diseased kidney may be responsible (13, 15-21). Thirdly a significant factor that causes or accentuates hypertension in uremia is the *nervous system*, both central and autonomic (22-28). With the proper use of dialysis and medication these three principal determinants for blood pressure control in uremia can be modified. A rational and individual regimen can be developed for each hypertensive patient that will be associated with minimal side effects and expense and will be successful in normalizing blood pressure in almost all of the cases.

Fluid volume
Excessive fluid volume usually connotes increased salt and water volumes, although the two components can vary independently (14, 29). In certain patients, especially debilitated ones, the use of dialysis solution containing bicarbonate as the predominant buffer anion reportedly allows blood pressure stabilization during ultrafiltration and concomitant dialysis (30, 31). While salt (i.e. sodium) can be independently removed during dialysis by lowering the sodium content of the dialysis fluid below 130 m mol/l, cramps usually ensue and commercially available dialysis is fluid with a sodium content of 130 m mol/l or more is used at most centers (see chapter 7).

A special form of volume dependent hypertension is seen in the anephric patient. Although both sympathetic tone and a remnant or surrogate of the renin-angiotension system may influence blood pressure in anephric patients the predominant factor remains fluid volume (6, 9, 32-35).

Renin
While hypertension is controlled in most dialysis patients by salt and water manipulation, a significant number remain hypertensive despite adequate dialysis and ultrafiltration (8-15). These patients may have abnormal renin levels and thus pathologically active angiotensin levels. Whether this elevation of renin is absolute or relative in regard to salt and water content is difficult to document.

Pathophysiology of renin secretion. Release of renin from the juxtaglomerular apparatus is governed by at least three mechanisms. These are *neurogenic*, including circulatory catecholamines and direct sympathetic innervation (36-38), *intra-renal baroreceptor impulses* (39, 41) and, finally *sodium responsive intra-renal chemoreceptors* (41, 42). In patients with endstage kidney disease treated with hemodialysis, a relative dilutional hyponatremia, resulting from excess water intake or dialysis related excess sodium removal, delivers hyponatremic blood to the kidneys and stimulates renin release. Even though the overall arterial pressure may be normal or even elevated, renal blood flow through diseased blood vessels of end stage kidneys may be low and may be a further stimulus to renin release. An abnormal sympathetic tone, thought by many investigators to be present in uremia, also may cause renin release. Thus, abnormal renin secretion in progressive renal failure may be due to any of the three known mechanisms of renin release. Evidence for delayed destruction of renin and angiotensin in uremia is lacking.

With the prior development of the experimentally used competitive inhibitor of angiotension II (Saralasin) and the experimentally used converting enzyme inhibitor teprotide (Squibb 20881), the physiologically active component of renin could be identified regardless of whether this renin level increase was relative or absolute (43-45, [see under 'Treatment']).

Patients approaching the need for chronic dialysis and referred to nephrologists, are frequently already on a combination of anti-hypertensive agents. Determinations of plasma renin activity *in vitro* can be done in these patients, but this may not reveal the *in vivo* role of angiotensin II. In this setting, use of saralasin, teprotide or the recently released oral converting enzyme inhibitor, captropril, may be more informative.

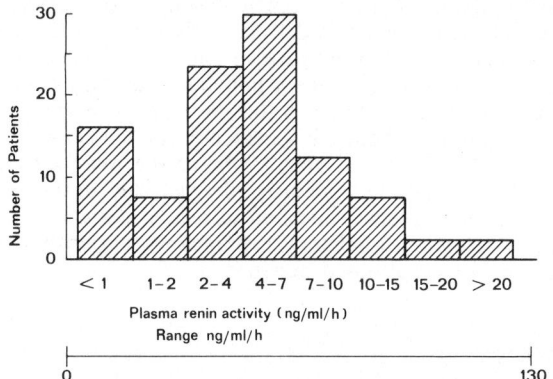

Figure 1. Distribution of predialysis plasma renin levels in 100 uremic patients, some of whom are receiving antihypertensive medication. Normal value for salt repleted non uremic patients is 5 ng/ml/h. Due to the large number of patients with near normal renin levels, the clinical roll of angiotensin II may not be discerned from renin determination alone. (See text).

Neurogenic
While most examples of hypertension seen among patients treated by dialysis are caused by the effects of excessive volume and sodium or renin activity or both, another important etiology is the nervous system, both central and autonomic. Hypertension that is enhanced by, or derived from, neurogenic sources is usually responsive to appropriate medication. With the exception of the hypertension associated with pheochromocytoma, understanding of neurogenically derived hypertension is still in its infancy. There is a great deal of investigative effort being made to determine the role of the central nervous system in causing and modifying hypertension, yet little of clinical significance is now agreed upon (46-48). There is more acceptance of the role of the autonomic nervous system, especially the sympathetic system. Not only are the catecholamines direct pressors themselves, but they also stimulate the renin system and in turn their production and release is stimulated by angiotensin (36-38, 49-52).

Search for a marker of sympathetic activity. While there is increasing evidence for the important role of the sympathetic nervous system in effecting and causing hypertension, to date there is no simple laboratory determination to quantitate this system. While urinary and/or plasma catecholamines are useful in evaluating potential pheochromocytoma, they do not correlate well with other forms of hypertension (53-60). With the discovery of the enzyme dopamine-β-hydroxylase (DBH) in the 1960's, its association with catecholamine release in the 1970's coupled with its ease of assay and greater stability than catecholamines, a new tool was believed available to quantitate sympathetic activity (61-65). Although the normal range of DBH levels in humans is wide, some observers found that subjects with labile and essential hypertension had appreciably higher levels than normals (66, 67). Some studies have revealed DBH levels to be positively correlated with hypertension in dialysis patients (6, 68) and one observer has noted a change (decrease) in DBH when blood pressure was lowered with hemofiltration (69). Other observers have found no such associations (25, 26).

While the discovery of a universally accepted simple and reliable test of sympathetic tone is still in the future, most investigators agree that selective modification of sympathetic tone will directly affect blood pressure.

The anemia of progressive renal failure may alter sympathetic tone and increase cardiac output (70, 71). This finding is not unique to hypertensive patients and correction of the anemia may lower cardiac output but may not necessarily lower blood pressure (72). Uremic sympathetic neuropathy is another possible cause of abnormal blood pressure response (73), although one observer has demonstrated that altered tone alone cannot be responsible (74).

Other causes
Another cause of hypertension in dialysis patients may be abnormal prostaglandin production from the diseased kidney. Prostaglandins, so named because they were originally found in seminal fluid, are a family of unsaturated cyclic fatty acids with a common 20 carbon skeleton (prostanoic acid) (75). These physiologically active substances are found in most body tissues and fluids and have widespread and varied effects including alterations of blood pressure (76).

Certain prostaglandins (PGA, PGE, PGF) are known to be synthesized by renal tissue (77). Specific prostaglandins have been implicated in modifying blood pressure by various mechanisms including a direct effect on blood vessel tone, modification of renal response to ischemia and activation of the renin-angiotensin system.

Recent work has shown that indomethacin and other anti-inflammatory agents inhibit prostaglandin production by interfering with prostaglandin synthetase (78). While the role of prostaglandins on blood pressure control in uremic patients is not yet known, prostaglandin modification may have a significant clinical application in the future (79).

Increased peripheral resistance from a number of etiologies is seen in uremic patients (14, 72). Increased salt and fluid volume, angiotensin II activity and sympathetic activity all directly increase peripheral resistance (80). Increased serum calcium concentration, especially when acute (81, 82), and altered prostaglandin production may also increase peripheral resistance (83, 84). The importance of this resistance in the resultant blood pressure elevation varies, depending on its severity and etiology.

Other causes of hypertension in patients treated with intermittent dialysis are conceivable. Great vessel and intra-renal baroreceptor alteration, anatomical distortion of vascular wall elasticity, uptake of dialyzer substance acting as pressure agents or dialyzer absorption of indigenous depressor substances and even pathophysiological changes of the brain, endorphin secretion, and cerebrospinal fluid are possible.

Treatment of hypertension

The major initial effort in treating hypertension in progressive renal failure is to restrict excessive salt and water intake of the predialysis patient (Table 2). Strict adherence to a low salt, low fluid diet often results in normalizing arterial pressures. Patient acceptance of this Spartan regimen is low, however, and additional measures must be employed.

Table 2. Anti-hypertensive agents.

$Na + H_2O$	Renin	Neurogenic	Direct vasodilator
Ultrafiltration	Captopril	(Propranolol) Prazosin Aldomet Clonidine Reserpine Guanethidine α-Blockers β-Blockers new	Hydralazine Minoxidil Diazoxide

Diuretics
The use of potent diuretics alone or in combination with other drugs in renal insufficiency often controls blood pressure when dietary measures fail. Furosemide (Lasix) in doses exceeding 200 mg are frequently required with falling urine output and renal function (84-86). Direct intravenous administration may sometimes be the only effective route (87). In patients with normal renal function, 70 to 100% of furosemide is rapidly removed by glomerular filtration and tubular excretion (half-life approximately 30 min) (88). Furosemide is rapidly cleared from anephric patients as well by extra-renal mechanisms. However, when creatinine clearance falls below 10 ml/min, even massive doses of furosemide are ineffective and may lead to deafness and other toxicities such as gastrointestinal irritation, hyperglycemia and hyperuricemia (89).

The other potent loop diuretic, ethacrynic acid, may occasionally be effective when furosemide is not. The pharmacokinetics of this drug are less well understood. Its potential for irreversible ototoxicity, however, is well recognized and the drug should be used only in selected situations (90).

Other common diuretics are usually ineffective as saluretics in progressive renal failure although a direct anti-hypertensive effect of the thiazides may still be beneficial (91, 92).

Eventually as renal failure progresses, unresponsiveness to all diuretics occurs and dialysis with fluid removal is required. Although some clinicians still use large dose potent loop diuretics to supplement water removal in recalcitrant patients, this should be minimized in order to preserve the residual renal function from potential nephrotoxic injury.

Renin-angiotensin inhibition

When diet and diuretics are unsuccessful, or only partially successful in controlling pressure, evaluation and modification of the renin-angiotensin system is warranted. Renin, an enzyme produced by the renal juxtaglomerular cells, acts on an alpha-2 globulin synthesized in the liver (renin substrate, angiotensinogen) to form angiotensin I, a decapeptide with little or no pressor activity. The levels of renin substrate in uremic patients do not appear to be a rate limiting step (93-95). Angiotensin I is converted to an octapeptide, angiotensin II, by 'converting enzyme' (see Figure 2). This potent pressor agent acts directly on arteriolar smooth muscle to increase arterial pressure. Other forms of angiotension (III, IV, etc.) are being documented, but for clinical significance, angiotensin II suffices.

Two types of experimental agents have been used to interfere with the renin-angiotensin system *in vivo* and thereby evaluate the clinical role of renin in supporting blood pressure (43, 44). The first type of agent, a competitive inhibitor of angiotensin II is typified by *Sar-ala-angiotensin II (P113, Saralasin)*. This agent, an octapeptide, has a greater affinity for angiotensin receptor sites than angiotensin II itself. In a high renin, high angiotensin II state, it lowers blood pressure by displacing angiotensin II (Figure 2). It is a weak pressor (agonist) owing to its structural similarities to angiotensin II (96). This competitive inhibitor has been used successfully to lower blood pressure and also to evaluate the role of renin in various forms of clinical hypertension, including hypertension associated with dialysis (43, 97-100).

The second type of agent is an inhibitor of converting enzyme. This stops the production of angiotensin II. *"Squibb 20881" or Teprotide* is such an agent (Figure 2). Recent work has revealed that this converting enzyme inhibitor has no agonistic effects and is superior to the competitive inhibitor in evaluating the clinical role of renin in low or normal renin situations (101). We have used this converting enzyme inhibitor in uremic patients prior to dialysis and have observed a renin effect in patients only mildly hypertensive (138/88 mm Hg) and with plasma renin values less than 3 ng/ml/h (normal values less than 5 ng/ml/h for salt repleted normal patients) (102). Squibb 20881 also inhibits the degradation of bradykinin and this may also explain a portion of its action (103, 104).

Saralasin is metabolized within minutes and is given by continuous intravenous infusion (105). Squibb 20881 has a longer pharmacological half-life and is given by slow intravenous injection. The dosage of either drug does not have to be modified for use in dialysis patients. While the intravenous converting enzyme inhibitor is not commercially available, Saralasin infusion is now easily performed when indicated.

The orally active converting enzyme inhibitor *captopril* was developed in 1977 (106). This rapidly active oral agent (60-90 min) can be used in the same manner as Saralasin or Teprotide in evaluating the contribution of the renin system to the hypertension. Numerous evaluations have revealed that captopril's blood pressure lowering effects correlate well with assayed renin activity (107-110). While the precise pharmacokinetics are not yet known its major action is clearly as a blockade of the renin-angiotensin system (see Figure 2). Preliminary reports have shown captopril to be extremely useful in lowering blood pressure both between and during dialyses (110). Some observers feel it will soon occupy the major role in dialysis resistant hypertension.

When renin inhibition tests reveal the hypertension to be due to relative or absolute increased renin activity, treatment should be begun with either Captopril, if available, or a β blocking agent -, *propranolo* being the

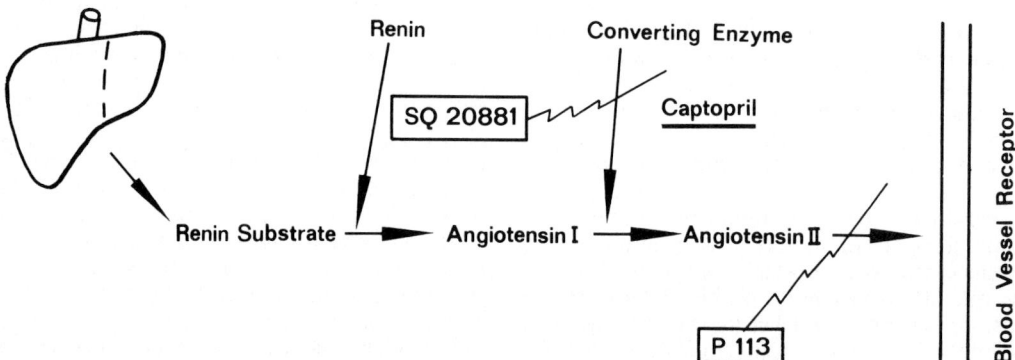

Figure 2. A scheme of the renin-angiotensin system and sites where inhibition can be achieved. The single agent currently available commercially is Captopril. (See text).

bench-mark agent by which others are judged (111-118).

Captopril has been already associated with certain undesirable effects, including renal failure (119), but physiologically it is the best and most direct agent for the treatment of hypertension mediated by abnormal renin activity.

Propranolol is metabolized by the liver and its major metabolite 4-hydroxypropranolol, is equally potent but has a shorter half-life (120, 121). The metabolism of the drug is only mildly altered in renal failure and dosage adjustment is unnecessary (122-124) (see Chapter 39). Propranolol may be administered twice daily on a chronic basis (120, 125, 126) or, with other medications, three or four times daily. An appreciable number of patients with essential hypertension exhibited an unexpected rise in blood pressure with propranolol treatment (127). For this reason, renin levels should be followed and correlated with blood pressure response, especially if there is no therapeutic effect. Propranolol has also been associated with hypoglycemia and Raynaud's phenomenon in dialysis patients (128).

Neurogenic agents
In the absence of fluid overload and when inappropriate renin activity has been ruled out by the previously mentioned inhibition tests or corrected by appropriate agents (or where severe bradycardia is present) other agents may be used either primarily or in addition to propranolol and Captopril (Table 3). Currently, our first choice of other agents would be the α blocker, prazosin hydrochloride (Table 2). *Prazosin (Minipress)* is a post synaptic α-adrenoreceptor blocker that has now been extensively used to treat hypertension, including the dialysis resistant hypertension of chronic renal failure (129-132). It is a weak basic drug which is highly bound to plasma proteins (~95 percent) and metabolized by the liver. In both renal and cardiac failure, the plasma free fraction and half-life are extended. Furthermore, in a certain number of patients (approximately 15% by our observations) an overt hypotensive episode occurs with the first dose of prazosin (133). In spite of this and perhaps due to the wide therapeutic dosage schedule, prazosin has been well accepted by dialysis patients with dosages easily adjusted as necessary (131, 132).

Alternate neurogenic agents include *methyldopa* and *clonidine* (Tables 2 and 3). Methyldopa (Aldomet) is a decarboxylase inhibitor that interferes with the conversion of dopa to dopamine with its metabolites stimulating central α-receptors. Although the plasma half-life of methyldopa is inversely proportional to creatinine clearance, (see Chapter 39), the usual therapeutic dosages are well tolerated after an initial period of adaptation characterized by lethargy (134). Dialysis patients may require up to 2 to 3 g daily. Aldomet also lowers plasma renin when used alone. Two precautions must be recognized: the dose prior to dialysis should be omitted to prevent hypotension during dialysis and, since the agent is dialyzable to a degree, blood pressure may rise following dialysis because of drug removal (135). Other undesirable effects include impotence and postural hypotension.

Clonidine (Catapress) is a direct α-adrenergic stimulator and consequently inhibits β sympathetic outflow. Dosage need not be altered for uremic patients, but the common side effects of drowsiness, dry mouth and withdrawal rebound hypertension may limit its use in dialysis patients (136, 137). The agent is effective, when appropriately administered, in lowering blood pressure in dialysis patients (138).

Agents to be avoided in dialysis patients include *guanethidine* and *reserpine*. Guanethidine, a potent adrenergic blocker (Table 2), may be prescribed without alteration of dosage in uremic patients even though the metabolized products are largely eliminated by the kidneys (139). It frequently causes severe postural hypotension and impotence. Cardiac output and renal blood flow are significantly decreased and compensatory reflexes during fluid removal with dialysis are inhibited. It should, therefore, be avoided whenever possible (140). Chronic reserpine therapy in dialysis patients is contraindicated because of frequent side effects and the availability of better tolerated, more effective agents. Newer β-sympathetic blocking agents have yet to reveal advantages over propranolol in dialysis patients. The

Table 3. Proposed stepwise pharmacological treatment of hypertension in dialysis. See text for discussion.

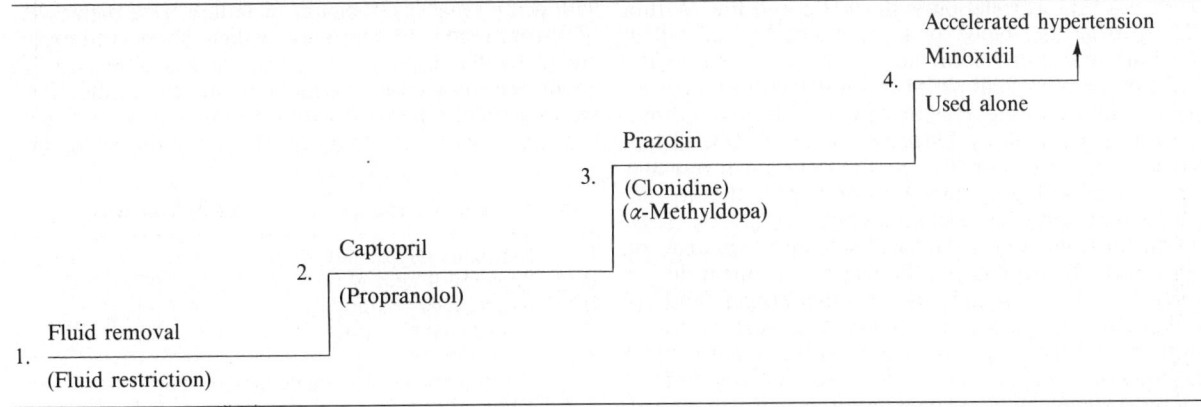

use of the α blockers *phenoxybenzamine (Dibenzyline)* or *phentolamine (Regitine)* in uremic patients is limited to special rare situations (141, 142).

Vasodilators

Once a drug choice has been made to modify the primary factor causing hypertension, addition of a drug causing direct vasodilation may minimize side effects and enhance drug effect. The oral direct vasodilators include *hydralazine* and *minoxidil* (Tables 2 and 3).

Hydralazine has been widely used and is well tolerated by dialysis patients especially when the hyperdynamic effects of the drug are minimized by concomitant therapy with propranolol. The need for frequent (4 times daily) doses and the growing acceptance of prazosin has caused the routine use of hydralazine to fall; however, its short action make it a good short term additional agent in renal failure, where needed. The incidence of a lupus-like syndrome is not increased in uremic patients and the dosage schedule does not have to be modified (see chapter 39), even though plasma hydralazine levels are reportedly higher in uremia (143). The drug is metabolized by hydroxylation, conjugation and acetylation, but there is some accumulation of the drug with renal failure. Since only a very small fraction is normally excreted in the urine, it has been suggested that there is slower metabolic breakdown of the drug in uremia. A peripheral neuropathy, responsive to pyridoxine, occasionally occurs when this medication is used.

Minoxidil (Loniten) is a very potent oral direct vasodilator that has ever-increasing success in controlling severe and moderate dialysis resistant hypertension (144-150). Initially, right atrial lesions developing in canines caused this promising agent to be used with caution in humans and for severe refractory hypertension only. Further study revealed that the incidence of pericardial disorders appearing in 477 minoxidil treated patients with severe hypertension was so low as to exonerate the drug (151). Resistance to minoxidil's effectiveness is so rare as to be reportable (152). Although there are hazards of hypotension and myocardial ischemia, the agent is well tolerated and its effects are dramatic (153-155). Minoxidil is predominantly metabolized by the liver (90%) and there is no evidence of accumulation in patients with renal failure (156). The agent is widely distributed throughout the body and its antihypertensive effect has little correlation with its 3 h half-life. Within 72 h of drug use, blood pressure is usually controlled. Maximal reductions occur after 3 months. Due to the direct decrease in total peripheral resistance with consequent reflux induced rise in cardiac rate and output, concomitant use of a β-blocker is required. Use of minoxidil leads to rise in renin and aldosterone levels that is controlled with propranolol or captopril, although surgical nephrectomy has also been employed (22, 34, 151). Hirsutism is an almost universal side effect that can be controlled with depilatories. Patient management during treatment with minoxidil also requires proper fluid removal during dialysis to counter the fluid retentive properties of the drug. Not only does this agent control the blood pressure of the maintenance dialysis patient, but by normalizing blood pressure in the severely hypertensive patient with renal insufficiency, it also stabilizes renal function and can delay or obviate the need for dialysis. There are increasing reports of cessation of dialysis and return of renal function with the use of this agent (157).

Treatment of accelerated hypertension

Pharmacological agents

For accelerated severe forms of hypertension, prompt utilization of *diazoxide* may be life-saving (Tables 2 and 4). Diazoxide is a potent direct vasodilator with an onset of action within minutes following rapid bolus injection. It is excreted in an active form by the kidney. Protein binding is decreased in uremia and its biological half-life increased (158). While others recommend the usual dosage in renal failure, we would suggest reducing the initial dose to 150 mg intravenously over 10 to 20 sec (1/2 ampule) (159). A second administration may be made with a higher dose if the blood pressure is not promptly decreased. For dialysis patients who become acutely hypertensive prior to or during dialysis, diazoxide may be used to return the blood-pressure to safer levels preferably before heparin is administered. Cardiac output may increase 75% by sympathetic reflex following diazoxide administration and β blocking may be required.

If available, both converting enzyme inhibitors and renin blockers may be used to treat severe hypertension, simultaneously assessing renin activity (43, 160). Both orally active captopril and minoxidil (119, 157) have been successfully used for accelerated hypertension.

Because of the simplicity of the use of diazoxide, this drug has largely replaced both the ganglionic blocker, *trimethephan (Arfonad)* and *nitroprusside (Nipride)* for hypertension control. These latter two agents are still used by titration when more precise control of blood pressure is required for special circumstances, i.e. surgery, stroke, aortic aneurysm with hemorrhage, intractable cardiac failure or when diazoxide fails. In the dialysis setting, however, due to the rapidity of response, diazoxide remains the predominant choice.

Recently, nitroprusside has been used to decrease the after load in cardiogenic shock with severe congestive failure following myocardial infarction or open heart surgery (161-163). Usually these cases are associated with acute renal insufficiency or failure. One metabolite of nitroprusside is thiocyanate, which is removed exclusively by the kidneys. *Thiocyanate* has a half-life of about one week under normal circumstances; therefore, the drug should be used with caution and for brief periods only, when renal failure exists. Prolonged therapy

Table 4. Agents for malignant (accelerated) hypertension.

I	Diazoxide (Hyperstat) [1,2]
II	Captopril (Capoten) [1]
III	Nitroprusside (Nipride) [1]
IV	Trimethaphan (Arfonad) [1]

[1] Concomitant use of furosemide may be indicated.
[2] β-Blockade advisable.

(over three days) under these conditions or large dose therapy requires daily assessment of thiocyanate levels. Deaths have been reported (164).

Bilateral nephrectomy
The growing successful use of minoxidil in dialysis resistant hypertension has greatly decreased the need for surgical bilateral nephrectomy. There are rare cases of intolerance and drug failure including patient's noncompliance (165). In these instances, nephrectomy may still be employed in spite of undesirable side effects.

Removal of all renal tissue may lead to lower 1,25 (OH)$_2$ vitamin D$_3$ levels with worsening of renal osteodystrophy. to a lower hematocrit because of reduced erythropoietin levels and to intra- and interdialysis hypotension due to lower plasma renin levels (5, 6, 166-169). In spite of this, bilateral nephrectomy may lead to dramatic rehabilitation of the hypertensive patient who is wasting on dialysis.

Medical or embolic ablation of renal tissue for blood pressure control has rarely been used in the past (170-172) but the proven efficacy of current oral agents have made this therapy even less desirable.

In summary, evaluation of the underlying etiology of blood pressure elevation in dialysis patients is essential in the formulation of a medical management plan. Once salt and volume overload are corrected, drug therapy is indicated in patients remaining even mildly hypertensive. The initial drug therapy should be a trial of converting enzyme inhibitor to evaluate the clinical significance of the renin angiotensin system followed, it indicated, by captopril or propranolol. If an additional agent is required, (e.g. because of a low pulse rate or the absence of a renin contribution to blood pressure elevation) then the α-blocker, prazosin should be employed (or clonidine or hydralazine). Resistant hypertension should be promptly treated with minoxidil. Alternate modalities of dialysis or hemofiltration may be employed, where available, to control pressure and no arbitrary or rigid guideline of how much the pressure should be lowered in the dialysis setting can yet be made.

Hypotension
Hypotension, although less frequent than hypertension, can impair rehabilitation of patients with renal failure. When hypotension occurs between dialyses, the patient's life style is further compromised. Hypotension during dialysis may impede fluid removal and may lead to congestion and inadequate correction of uremia. This initiates a vicious cycle of progressive clinical deterioration (56) if the hypotension goes uncorrected in subsequent dialyses.

Pathogenesis
Significant hypotension may occur in certain dialysis patients both with and without kidneys. Identification of the cause of the low blood pressure usually allows at least partial correction of the problem.

Dialysis patients may use analgesics and psychopharmacotherapeutic agents (opiates, phenothiazines and benzodiazepines) that may alter blood pressure levels substantially. These sources are usually readily identifiable and correctable.

Blood volume deficits are an important cause of hypotension both during and following dialysis. This cause is especially pronounced in small (pediatric) patients, poorly nourished patients and in the elderly. When the patient's blood flow is low, compensatory mechanisms may be insufficient to maintain adequate blood pressure as dialysis is instituted and blood is pooled in the extracorporeal circuit. Coexisting factors such as anemia and intrinsic heart disease aggravate the hypotension. Uremic pericardial effusions may precipitate hypotension early in dialysis (173). Some dialysis patients acquire hepatitis and may develop chronic liver disease with cirrhosis, intractable ascites and consequent hypotension (174-176).

Numerous reports have implicated acetate as an etiologic agent in hemodialysis induced hypotension (7, 31, 178, 179). One study of 27 patients with 102 hemodialyses against an acetate bath revealed that the episodes of hypotension were associated with a much higher average serum acetate level (4.5 ± 1.2 µmoles/l versus 1.4 ± 0.5 µmoles/l [$P < 0.05$], [179]). The precise mechanisms of this hypotension are not yet clear (see chapter 7).

After bilateral nephrectomy, plasma renin activity is low but any extrarenal renin-like activity that remains may influence blood pressure (6, 179-183). When nephrectomy is done for a reason other than severe hypertension, the postoperative blood pressure may be quite low.

The renin-angiotensin system is normally the major regulator of aldosterone secretion (184). In anephric patients, there is a minimal response of aldosterone secretion to high serum potassium levels and ACTH (185-187). Even infusion of angiotensin II and saralasin lead to a depressed response of plasma aldosterone levels in anephric patients compared to non-nephrectomized dialysis patients (188-191). The adrenal cortex appears to require a maintenance level of renin-angiotensin for normal aldosterone secretion in response to other stimuli (192). Without aldosterone mediated potassium loss via the colon, anephric patients may have more severe episodes of hyperkalemia.

Altered neurogenic (especially sympathetic) tone in uremia may decrease compensatory responses to hypotension during dialysis (73, 193). In one report, six of eight dialysis patients who had hypotensive episodes during dialysis had peripheral neuropathy and evidence of autonomic dysfunction when their response to a Valsalva maneuver and amyl-nitrite was studied (193). Another report correlated efferent sympathetic activity, baroreceptor arc and dialysis induced hypotension (73). In comparing 10 uremic patients with dialysis induced hypotension to 10 with no dialysis hypotension, there was an abnormality of the baroreceptor arc in those with dialysis induced hypotension. This group also had increased efferent sympathetic activity as measured by dopamine-β-hydroxylase levels and a higher mean arterial pressure between dialyses than the 10 without dialysis induced hypotension. This blood pressure abnormality would be similar to experimental hypertension in animals following baroreceptor denervation. Hemofiltration has been reported to control dialysis resistant hypertension, perhaps by decreasing 'middle molecule' levels and improving the degree of autonomic neuropathy (194). Low dopamine-β-hydroxylase levels have been associated with frequent problems with hypotension in anephric dialysis patients (6). Sympathetic neuropathy complicating metabolic diseases such as diabetes or vitamin deficiencies can also contribute to hypotension. Abnormal vitamin D metabolism in uremia with its resultant hypocalcemia may also be a factor (195).

There remain some compelling reasons, other than severe hypertension, for bilateral nephrectomy. These include malignancy, recurrent infections and significant ureteral reflux prior to renal transplantation. With continuing graft rejections requiring transplant nephrectomy, the future number of anephric dialysis patients will remain substantial.

Treatment

Treatment of hypotension occurring in dialysis patients should compensate for or eliminate the specific causes of the low blood pressure. The most pragmatic method is to treat the most easily correctable cause first.

Hypotension inducing drugs should be discontinued and electrolyte and vitamin deficiencies repleted. Heart failure may be minimized by fluid restriction, correction of any arrhythmias and the occasional use of digoxin in reduced doses. When hypotension is due to a restricted cardiac output from pericardial effusion, removal of the effusion becomes essential (see chapter 30).

Patient size and blood volume must be carefully correlated with the extracorporeal volume in the dialyzer and tubing. Coil dialyzers require a greater filling volume than e.g. hollow fiber dialyzers. The filling volume of the blood lines may be up to 180 ml. In small adults, the elderly, and children, smaller bore tubing should be used.

Appropriate use of blood products at the beginning of and during dialysis can help maintain adequate blood pressure. Packed red blood cells can be administered when anemia contributes to hypovolemia. Priming the dialyzer with saline plus plasma will minimize acute hypovolemic hypotension. Albumin and hypertonic saline administration during dialysis can increase blood volume by their osmotic effects.

Where an acetate bath is implicated in hemodialysis induced hypotension, a therapeutic trial of bicarbonate dialysis is indicated (31, 178). Additionally, where hypotension results from clinically mandated intradialysis aggressive fluid removal, 'sequential ultrafiltration' has been shown to be beneficial (196, 197).

Finally, although many patients with intradialysis hypotension on hemodialysis are stabilized within the initial month of therapy (198), a change in the modality of dialysis may be considered in those that have persistent difficulties. Intermittent peritoneal dialysis and continuous ambulatory peritoneal dialysis (CAPD) are by design less drastic and less challenging procedures to the cardiovascular system. As these two modalities gain in patient acceptance and application, the options of modifying clinically significant hypotension are increased.

Severe hypotension that prevents routine dialysis may be overcome by femoral vein cannulation for inflow to the dialyzer as the central venous core blood volume may be adequate for dialysis (199). In addition, intravenous pressor agents may sometimes permit dialysis in difficult situations. Use of these agents requires continuous monitoring of vital signs and clinical status during dialysis and they are usually used only for critically ill patients. If blood pressure is supported by an active vasoconstrictive agent, appropriate solute and fluid removal may be hampered due to decreased exchange between the intravascular and interstitial compartments during dialysis.

For resistant hypotension due to intractable ascites, the placement of peritoneo-venous shunt may be considered (200). When effective, this can replete the intravascular volume with the pooled intraperitoneal protein and fluid and thus allow adequate hemodialysis. This technique has not yet been systematically evaluated for dialysis patients, however.

CONCLUSIONS

Over the past decade, the application of maintenance dialysis has undergone major quantitative and qualitative changes. There has been a resurgence in the use of peritoneal dialysis including a rapid and unpredicted growth of continuous ambulatory peritoneal dialysis (CAPD). In the United States alone, the number of dialysis patients as of this writing is approaching 70,000 with an age range from infancy to the 9th decade.

With this bipolar expansion, problems peculiar to certain age groups have become commonplace to the practicing nephrologist. Chronic congestive failure, accelerated atherosclerosis, dialysis related hypotension, to name but a few, have narrowed the range of acceptable blood pressure levels for dialysis patients. Methods still must be developed to prevent complications of abnormal arterial pressure. Early treatment of hypertension, especially in the predialysis stage of renal disease associated with hypertension (glomerulonephritis, nephrosclerosis, diabetes), is warranted. Intensive treatment of even mild blood pressure elevation (over 90 mm diastolic) during maintenance dialysis is justified by the devastating effects of hypertensive and atherosclerotic complications.

REFERENCES

1. Lindner A, Charra B, Sherrard DJ, Scribner BH: Accelerated atherosclerosis in prolonged maintenance hemodialysis. *N Engl J Med* 290:697, 1974
2. Lowrie EG, Lazarus JM, Hampers CL, Merrill JP: Cardiovascular disease in dialysis patients. *N Engl J Med* 290:737, 1974
3. Merrill JP: Cardiovascular problems in patients on long-term hemodialysis (editorial). *JAMA* 228:1149, 1974
4. Vincenti F, Amend WJ, Abele J, Feduska NJ, Salvatierra O: The role of hypertension in hemodialysis-associated atherosclerosis. *Am J Med* 68:363, 1980
5. Rao TKS, Manis T, Delano BG, Friedman EA: Continuing high morbidity during maintenance hemodialysis consequent to bilateral nephrectomy. *Trans Am Soc Artif Intern Organs* 19:340, 1973
6. White RP, Sealey J, Reidenberg M, Stenzel KH, Sullivan JF, David DS, Laragh JH, Rubin AL: Mechanisms of blood pressure control in anephrics: Plasma renin and dopamine-β-hydroxylase activity. *Trans Am Soc Artif Intern Organs* 22:420, 1976
7. Henderson LW: Symptomatic hypotension during hemodialysis (editorial). *Kidney Int* 17:571, 1980
8. Lazarus JM, Hampers CL, Merrill JP: Hypertension in chronic renal failure. *Arch Intern Med* 133:1059, 1974
9. Wilkinson R, Scott DF, Uldall PR, Kerr DNS, Swinney J, Robson V: Plasma renin and exchangeable sodium in hypertension of chronic renal failure. The effect of bilateral nephrectomy. *Q J Med* 39:377, 1970
10. Stoker GS, Mani MK, Stewart JH: Relevance of salt, water and renin to hypertension in chronic renal failure. *Br Med J* 3:126, 1970
11. Comty CM, Baillod RA, Crockett R, Shaldon S: Forty months experience with a nurse-patient operated chronic dialysis unit. *Proc Eur Dial Transpl Assoc* 3:98, 1966
12. Weidman P, Maxwell MH: Hypertension. In: *Clinical Aspects of Uremia and Dialysis*, edited by Massry SG, Sellers AL, Springfield IL, Charles C Thomas, 1976, p 100
13. Dathram JRE, Goodwin FJ: The relationship between body fluid compartment volume, renin and blood pressure on chronic renal failure. *Clin Sci* 42:29, 1972
14. Kim KE, Onesti G, DelGuercio ET, Greco J, Fernandes M, Eidelson B, Swartz C: Sequential hemodynamic changes in end-stage renal disease and the anephric state during volume expansion. *Hypertension* 2:102, 1980
15. Weidman P, Maxwell MH, Lupu AN, Lewin AJ, Massry SG: Plasma renin activity and blood pressure in terminal renal failure. *N Engl J Med* 285:757, 1971
16. Vertes V, Cangiano JL, Berman LB, Gould A: Hypertension in end-stage renal disease. *N Engl J Med* 280:978, 1971
17. Brown JJ, Curtis JR, Lever AF, Robertson JIS, de Wardener HE, Wing AJ: Plasma renin concentration and control of blood pressure in patients on hemodialysis. *Nephron* 6:329, 1969.
18. Levinsky NG: The renal kallikrein-kinin system. *Circ Res* 44:441, 1979
19. Carretero OA, Scicli AG: The renal kallikrein-kinen system (editorial). *Am J Physiol* 238:F247, 1980
20. Kaneda H, Tashiro M, Murata T, Matsumoto J, Takeuchi M, Haruyama T: Factors influencing the release of renin in patients under chronic dialysis treatment. *Tohoku J Exp Med* 129:177, 1979
21. Huysmans F TH M, Thien TH, Koene RAP: Renin-angiotensin system and blood volume in patients with dialysis-resistant hypertension. *Neth J Med* 23:74, 1980
22. De Quattro V, Chan S: Raised plasma catecholamines in some patients with hypertension. *Lancet* 1:806, 1972
23. Atuk N, Roman J, Westervelt F: Catecholamines, renin and hypertension in terminal renal failure. *Abstracts Fifth Int Congr Nephrol*, p 115, 1972
24. Röckell A, Hennemann H, Sternagel-Haase A, Heidland A: Uraemic sympathetic neuropathy after haemodialysis and transplantation. *Eur J Clin Invest* 9:23, 1979
25. Ban M, Matsuno T, Ogawa K, Satake T: Plasma norepinephrine and dopamine-beta-hydroxylase activity in chronic renal failure. *Jpn Circ J* 43:627, 1979
26. Kobayashi K, Miura Y, Tomioka H, Sakuma H, Adachi M, Furuyama T, Yoshinaga K, Ishizaki M, Sekino H: Plasma catecholamines and dopamine-beta-hydroxylase activity in chronic renal failure. *Clin Chim Acta* 95:317, 1979
27. Bach C, Iaina A, Eliahou HE: Autonomic nervous system disturbance in patients on chronic hemodialysis. *Israel J Med Sci* 15:761, 1979
28. Tajiri M, Aizawa Y, Yuasa Y, Ohmori T, Nara Y, Hirasawa Y: Autonomic nervous dysfunction in patients on long-term hemodialysis. *Nephron* 23:10, 1979
29. Blumberg A, Nelp WB, Hegstrom RM, Scribner BH: Extracellular volume in patients with chronic renal disease treated for hypertension by sodium restriction. *Lancet* 2:69, 1967
30. Olinger GN, Werner PH, Bonchek LI, Boerboom LE: Vasodilator effects of the sodium acetate in pooled protein fraction. *Ann Surg* 190:305, 1979
31. Graefe U, Milutinovich J, Follette WC, Vizzo JE, Babb AL, Scribner BH: Less dialysis-induced morbidity and vascular instability with bicarbonate in dialysate. *Ann Intern Med* 88:332, 1978
32. Merrill JP, Schupak E: Mechanisms of hypertension in renoprival man. *Can Med Assoc J* 90:328, 1964
33. Dustan HP, Page IH: Some factors in renal and renoprival hypertension. *J Lab Clin Med* 64:948, 1964
34. Onesti O, Swartz C, Ramirez O, Brest AN: Bilateral nephrectomy for control of hypertension in uremia. *Trans Am Soc Artif Intern Organs* 14:361, 1968
35. Badder EM, Dagher F, Seaton JF, Harrison TS: Catecholamine responses to orthostatic stimulation in anephric man. *J Surg Res* 26:348, 1979
36. Vander AJ: Effect of catecholamines and the renal nerves on renin secretion on anesthetized dogs. *Am J Physiol* 209:659, 1965
37. Johnson JA, Davis JO, Witty RJ: Effects of catecholamines and renal nerve stimulation on renin release in the nonfiltering kidney. *Circ Res* 29:646, 1971
38. Reid IA, Schrier RW, Earley LE: An effect of extra renal beta adrenergic stimulation on the release of renin. *J Clin Invest* 51:1861, 1972
39. Tobian L, Tomboulian A, Janecek J: Effect of high perfusion pressures on granulation of juxtaglomerular cells in isolated kidney. *J Clin Invest* 38:605, 1959
40. Skinner SL, McCubbin JW, Page IH: Control of renin secretion. *Circ Res* 15:64, 1964
41. Thurau K, Schnermann J, Nagel W, Harstu M, Wahl M: Composition of tubular fluid in the macula densa segment as a factor regulating the function of the juxtaglomerular apparatus. *Circ Res* 20-21 (suppl 2):79, 1967
42. Freeman RM, Davis JO, Gotshall RW, Johnson JA, Spielman WS: The signal perceived by the macula densa during changes in renin release. *Circ Res* 35:307, 1974
43. Brunner HR, Gavras M, Laragh JH, Kennan R: Angiotensin II blockade in man by sar-ala-angiotensin II for understanding and treatment of high blood pressure. *Lancet* 2:1045, 1973

44. Gavras M, Brunner HR, Laragh JH, Sealey JS, Gavras I, Vukovich RA: An angiotensin-converting enzyme inhibitor to identify and treat vasoconstrictor and volume factors in hypertensive patients. N Engl J Med 291:817, 1974
45. Patel R, Ansari A: Serum angiotensin converting enzyme activity in patients with chronic renal failure on long term hemodialysis. Clin Chim Acta 92:491, 1979
46. Reis DJ, Duba N: The central nervous system and neurogenic hypertension. Prog Cardiovasc Dis 17:51, 1974
47. Folkow B: Central neurohormonal mechanisms in spontaneously hypertensive cats compared with human essential hypertension. Clin Sci 48:2055, 1975
48. Kerr DNS, Clinical and pathophysiologic changes in patients on chronic dialysis: The central nervous system. Adv Nephrol 9:109, 1980
49. Ferrario CM, Gildenburg PL, McCubbin JW: Cardiovascular effects of angiotensin mediated by central nervous system. Circ Res 30:257, 1972
50. Feldberg W, Lewis GP: The action of peptides on the adrenal medulla: Release of adrenaline by bradykinin and angiotensin. J Physiol (London) 171:98, 1964
51. Peach MJ, Cline WH Jr, Watts DT: Release of adrenal catecholamines by angiotensin II. Circ Res 19:571, 1969
52. Peach MJ: Adrenal medullary stimulation induced by angiotensin I, angiotensin II and analogues. Circ Res 28, 29 (suppl II):107, 1971
53. Brunjes S: Catecholamine metabolism in essential hypertension. N Engl J Med 271:120, 1964
54. Nestel PJ, Esler MD: Patterns of catecholamine excretion in urine in hypertension. Circ Res 26, 27 (suppl II):75, 1970
55. De Quattro V: Evaluation of increased norepinephrine excretion in hypertension using L-dopa-^{3}H. Circ Res 28:84, 1971
56. Engelman K, Portnoy B: A sensitive double isotope derivative assay for norepinephrine and epinephrine: Normal resting human plasma levels. Circ Res 26:53, 1970
57. Louis WJ, Doyle AE, Anavekar S: Plasma norepinephrine levels in essential hypertension. N Engl J Med 288:599, 1974
58. Atuk NO, Westervelt FB Jr, Roman J: The role of endogenous catecholamines on the plasma renin activity and hypertension in renal failure. Clin Res 21:94, 1973
59. Atuk NO, Bailey CJ, Turner S, Peach MJ, Westervelt FB Jr: Red blood cell catechol-o-methyl transferase, plasma catecholamines and renin in renal failure. Trans Am Soc Artif Intern Organs 22:195, 1976
60. Sparano F, Giaquinto G, Odoardi A, Mercuri MA, Tosti-Croce C, Sulon J, Sciarra F: 18-hydroxyl-11-deoxycorticosterone in hypertensive uremic patients during hemodialysis. Horm Res 10:282, 1979
61. Levin EY, Levenberg B, Kaufman S: The enzymatic conversion of 3,4 dihydroxyphenylethylamine to norepinephrine. J Biol Chem 235:2080, 1960
62. Creveling CR, Daly JW, Witkop B, Udenfriend S: Substrates and inhibitors of dopamine-β-hydroxylase. Biochim Biophys Acta 64:125, 1972
63. Craine JE, Daniels GH, Kaufman S: Dopamine-β-hydroxylase. The subunit structure and anion activation of the bovine adrenal enzyme. J Biol Chem 248:7838, 1973
64. Weinshilboum RM, Thoa NB, Johnson DB, Kopin IJ, Axelrod J: Proportional release of norepinephrine and dopamine-β-hydroxylase from sympathetic nerves. Science 174:1349, 1971
65. Geffen L: Serum dopamine-β-hydroxylase as an index of sympathetic function. Life Sci 14:1593, 1974
66. Schanberg SM, Stone RA, Kirshner N, Gunnells JC, Robinson RR: Plasma dopamine-β-hydroxylase: A possible aid in the study and evaluation of hypertension. Science 183:523, 1974
67. Stone RA, Gunnells JC, Robinson RR, Schanberg SM, Kirshner N: Dopamine-β-hydroxylase in primary and secondary hypertension. Circ Res (suppl) 1:34, 1974
68. De Fremont JF, Coevoet B, Andrejak M, Makdassi R, Quichaud J, Lambrey G, Gueris J, Caillens C, Harichaux P, Alexandre JM, Fournier A: Effects of antihypertensive drugs on dialysis-resistant hypertension, plasma renin and dopamine betahydroxylase activities, metabolic risk factors and calcium phosphate homeostasis: Comparison of metoprolol, alphamethyldopa and clonidine in a crossover trial. Clin Nephrol 12:198, 1979
69. Henderson LW: Hemofiltration for the treatment of hypertension associated with end-stage renal failure. Artif Organs 4:103, 1980
70. Duke M, Abelman WH: The hemodynamic response to chronic anemia. Circulation 39:503, 1969
71. Neff MS, Kim KE, Persoff M, Onesti G, Swartz C: Hemodynamics of uremic anemia. Circulation 43:876, 1971
72. Kim KE, Onesti G, Schwartz AB, Chinitz JL, Swartz C: Hemodynamics of hypertension in chronic end-stage renal disease. Circulation 46:456, 1972
73. Lilley JJ, Golden J, Stone RA: Adrenergic regulation of blood pressure in chronic renal failure. J Clin Invest 57:1190, 1976
74. Nies AS, Robertson D, Stone WJ: Hemodialysis hypotension is not the result of uremic peripheral autonomic neuropathy. J Lab Clin Med 94:395, 1979
75. McGilvery RW: Biochemistry a Functional Approach. Philadelphia PA, Saunders Co, 1970, p 571
76. Anderson RJ, Berl T, McDonald KM, Schrier RW: Prostaglandins: Effects on blood pressure, renal blood flow, sodium and water excretion (editorial review), Kidney Int 10:205, 1976
77. Lee JB, Covino BG, Takman BH, Smith ER: Renomedullary vasodepressor substance, medullin. Isolation, chemical characterization and physiological properties. Circ Res 17:57, 1965
78. Flower R, Gryglewski R, Herbaczynska-Cedro K, Vane JR: Effects of anti-inflammatory drugs on prostaglandin biosynthesis. Nature (New Biol) 238:104, 1972
79. Lee JB, Mookerjee BK: The renal prostaglandins as etiologic factors in human essential hypertension: fact or fantasy? Cardiovasc Med 1:302, 1976
80. Safar M, Fendler JP, Weil B, Beuve-Mery P, Brisset JM, Idatti JM, Meyer P, Milliez P: Hypertension in patients on maintenance haemodialysis. Rev Eur Etud Clin Biol 15:740, 1970
81. Coburn JW, Massry SG, DePalma JR, Shinaberger JH: Rapid appearance of hypercalcemia with initiation of hemodialysis. JAMA 210:2276, 1969
82. Weidman P, Massry SG, Coburn JW, Maxwell MH, Atleson J, Kleeman CR: Blood pressure effects of acute hypercalcemia. Studies in patients with chronic renal failure. Ann Intern Med 76:741, 1972
83. Fichman MP, Littenberg G, Brooker G, Horton R: The effect of prostaglandin A (PGA) on renal and adrenal function in man. Circ Res (suppl) 31:19, 1972
84. Gregory LF, Durrett R, Robinson RR, Clapp JR: The short term effect of furosemide on electrolyte and water excretion in patients with severe renal disease. Ann Intern Med 126:69, 1970
85. Rastogi SP, Volans G, Elliot RW, Eccleston DW, Ashcroft R, Webster D, Kerr DNS: High dose furosemide in the

treatment of hypertension in renal insufficiency and of terminal renal failure. *Postgrad Med J* 47:45, 1971
86. Allison MEM, Kennedy AL: Diuretics in chronic renal disease: A study of high dosage furosemide. *Clin Sci* 41:171, 1971
87. Rado JP, Juhos E, Szends L, Marosi J, Tako J, Salmon F: Acute renal effects of high doses of furosemide administered intravenously in patients with advanced renal insufficiency. *J Med* 4:219, 1973
88. Kelly MR, Cutler RE, Christopher TG, Forrey AW: Pharmacokinetics of furosemide in normal subjects and anephric patients. *Clin Res* 21:470, 1973
89. Mitchell JR, McMurty RJ, Statham CN, Nelson SD: Molecular basis for several drug-induced nephropathies. *Am J Med* 62:518, 1977
90. Pillay VKG, Schwarz FD, Aimi K, Kark RM: Transient and permanent deafness following treatment with ethacrynic acid in renal failure. *Lancet* 1:77, 1969
91. Jones B, Nanra RS: Double-blind trial of antihypertensive effect of chlorothiazide in severe renal failure. *Lancet* 2:1258, 1979
92. Langford HG: Thiazides for hypertension with renal failure. *Lancet* 1:203, 1980
93. Kotchen TA, Knight EL, Kashgarian M, Mulrow PJ: A study of the renin-angiotensin system in patients with chronic renal insufficiency. *Nephron* 7:317, 1970
94. Kotchen TA, Rice TW, Walters DR: Renin activity in normal, hypertensive and uremic plasma. *J Clin Endocrinol Metab* 34:928, 1972
95. Sealy JE, White RP, Laragh JH, Rubin AL: Prorenin and renin substrate in plasma from nephrectomized man. *Clin Sci Mol Med* (abstract) 24:411a, 1976
96. Case DB, Wallace JM, Keim HJ, Sealey JE, Laragh JH: Usefulness and limitations of Saralasin, a partial competitive agonist of angiotensin II, for evaluating the renin and sodium factors in hypertensive patients. *Am J Med* 60:825, 1976
97. Donker AJM, Leenan FHM: Infusion of angiotensin II analogue in two patients with unilateral renovascular hypertension. *Lancet* 2:1535, 1974
98. Brunner HR, Gavras H, Laragh JH: Specific inhibition of the renin-angiotensin system: A key to understanding blood pressure regulation. *Prog Cardiovasc Dis* 17:87, 1974
99. Mimran A, Shaldon S, Mathieu MN, Polito C, Barjon P, Mion C: The hypertension of long term hemodialysis patients: Studies with angiotensin II antagonist (P113). *Trans Am Soc Artif Intern Organs* 22:9, 1976
100. Fadem SZ, Lifschitz MD: Use of saralasin in end-stage renal disease. *Kidney Int* 15 (Suppl 9):S93, 1979
101. Case DB, Wallace JM, Keim HJ, Weber MA, Drayer JIM, White RP, Sealey JE, Laragh JH: Estimating renin participation in hypertension: Superiority of converting enzyme inhibitor over Saralasin. *Am J Med* 61:790, 1976
102. White RP, Byrd LH, Case DB, Sullivan JF, Laragh JH, Rubin AL: Testing for angiotensin dependency with converting enzyme inhibition compared to renin levels in hypertensive hemodialysis patients. *Abstracts Am Soc Nephrol* 10:56a, 1977
103. Ferreira SH, Bartelt DC, Green LJ: Isolation of bradykinin-potentiating peptides from Bothrops jararaca venom. *Biochemistry* 9:2583, 1970
104. Needleman P, Douglas JR Jr, Jakshik BA, Blumberg AL, Isakson PC, Marshall GR: Angiotensin antagonists as pharmacological tools. *Fed Proc* 35:2488, 1976
105. Needleman P, Johnson EM Jr, Vine W, Flanigan E, Marshall GR: The pharmacology of antagonists of angiotensin I and II. *Circ Res* 31:862, 1972
106. Ondetti MA, Rubin B, Cushman DW: Design of specific inhibitors of angiotensin converting enzyme: New class of orally active antihypertensive agents. *Science* 196:411, 1977
107. Brunner HR, Gavras H, Waeber B, Turini GA, Wauters JP: Captopril: An oral angiotensin converting enzyme inhibitor active in man. *Arch Int Pharmacodyn Ther* (Suppl) 1980, p 188
108. Case DB, Atlas SA, Laragh JM: Clinical experience with blockade of the renin-angiotensin-aldosterone system by an oral converting enzyme inhibitor (SQ14226 captopril) in hypertensive patients. *Prog Cardiovasc Dis* 21:196, 1978
109. Case DB: Antirenin drugs in diagnosis and treatment: An alternative to plasma renin activity measurements. *Cardiovasc Rev Reports* 9:679, 1980
110. Vaughan ED Jr, Carey RM, Ayers CR, Peach MJ: Hemodialysis-resistant hypertension: Control with an orally active inhibitor of angiotensin-converting enzyme. *J Clin Endocrinol Metab* 5:869, 1979
111. Buhler FR, Laragh JH, Vaughan ED Jr, Brunner HR, Gavras H, Baer L: Antihypertensive action of propranolol. *Am J Cardiol* 32:511, 1973
112. Buhler FR, Laragh JH, Baer L, Vaughan ED Jr, Brunner HR: Propranolol inhibition in renin secretion. *N Engl J Med* 287, 1209, 1972
113. Winer N, Choski DS, Yoon MS, Freedman AD: Adrenergic receptor medication of renin secretion. *J Clin Endocrinol Metab* 29:1168, 1969
114. Michelakis AM, McAllister RG: The effect of chronic adrenergic receptor blockade on plasma renin activity in man. *J Clin Endocrinol Metab* 34:386, 1972
115. Hollinfield JW, Sherman K, Vander Swagg R, Shand DG: Proposed mechanisms of propranolol's antihypertensive effect in essential hypertension. *N Engl J Med* 295:68, 1978
116. Lewis P: The essential action of propranolol in hypertension. *Am J Med* 60:837, 1976
117. Stumpe KO, Kolloch R, Vetter H, Gramann W, Kruck F, Rersel CH, Higuchi M: Acute and long-term studies of the mechanisms of action of beta-blocking drugs in lowering blood pressure. *Am J Med* 60:853, 1976
118. Davies R, Slater JDM: Is the adrenergic control of renin release dominant in man? *Lancet* 2:594, 1976
119. Grossman A, Eckland D, Price P, Edwards CRW: Captopril: reversible renal failure with severe hyperkalaemia. *Lancet* 1:712, 1980
120. Evans GH, Shand DG: Disposition of propranolol. Drug accumulation and steady state concentrations during oral administration in man. *Clin Pharmacol Ther* 14:487, 1973
121. Nies AS, Shand DG: Clinical pharmacology of propranolol. *Circulation* 52:6, 1975
122. Thompson FD, Joekes AM, Foulkes: Pharmacodynamics of propranolol in renal failure. *Br Med J* 2:434, 1976
123. Thompson FD, Joekes AM: Beta blockade in the presence of renal disease and hypertension. *Br Med J* 2:555, 1974
124. Holland OB, Kaplan NM: Propranolol in the treatment of hypertension. *N Engl J Med* 294:930, 1976
125. Berglund G, Andersson O, Hansson L, Olander R: Propranolol given twice daily in hypertension. *Acta Med Scand* 194:513, 1973
126. Wilkinson PR, Dixon N, Hunter KR: Twice daily propranolol treatment for hypertension. *J Int Med Res* 2:220, 1974
127. Drayer JIM, Keim HJ, Weber MA, Case DB, Laragh JM: Unexpected pressor responses to propranolol in essential hypertension. *Am J Med* 60:897, 1976
128. Poulter N, Gabriel R: Raynaud's phenomenon in hyper-

tensive dialysis patients taking a sustained-release propranolol formulation. *Curr Med Res Opin* 6:207, 1979
129. Jaillon P: Clinical pharmacokinetics of prazosin. *Clin Pharmacokinet* 5:365, 1980
130. Harter HR, Delmez JA: Effects of prazosin in the control of blood pressure in hypertensive dialysis patients. *J Cardiovasc Pharmacol* 1 (suppl):S43, 1979
131. Stokes GS, Monaghan JC, Frost GW, MacCarthy EP: Responsiveness to prazosin in renal failure. *Clin Sci* 57:383, 1979
132. Lowenthal DT, Hobbs D, Affrime MB, Twomey TM, Martinez EW, Onesti G: Prazosin kinetics and effectiveness in renal failure. *Clin Pharmacol Ther* 27:779, 1980
133. Moulds RFW, Jauernig RA: Mechanisms of prazosin collapse. *Lancet* 1:200, 1977
134. Myhre E, Brodwell EK, Stenback O, Hansen T: Plasma turnover of methyldopa in advanced renal failure. *Acta Med Scand* 191:343, 1972
135. Yeh BK, Dayton PG, Waters WC III: Removal of α-methyldopa (Aldomet) in man by dialysis. *Proc Soc Exp Biol Med* 135:840, 1970
136. Onesti G, Schwartz AB, Kim KE: Antihypertensive effect of clonidine. *Circ Res* 28 (suppl 2):53, 1971
137. Hansson L, Hunyor SN, Julius S, Hoobler SW: Blood pressure crisis following withdrawal of clonidine (Catapres, Catapresan), with special reference to arterial and urinary catecholamine levels and suggestions for acute management. *Am Heart J* 85:605, 1973
138. Garrett BN, Kaplan NM: Clonidine in the treatment of hypertension. *J Cardiovasc Pharmacol* 2 (suppl):S61, 1980
139. McMartin C, Simpson P: The absorption and metabolism of guanethedine in hypertensive patients requiring different doses of the drug. *Clin Pharmacol Ther* 12:73, 1971
140. Boura ALA, Green AF: Adrenergic neurone blocking agents. *Annu Rev Pharmacol* 5:183, 1965
141. Sandler G, Leishman AWD, Humberston PM: Guanethidine-resistant hypertension. *Circulation* 38:542, 1968
142. Ross EJ, Prichard BNC, Kaufman L, Robertson AIG, Harries BJ: Preoperative and operative management of patients with phaeochromocytoma. *Br Med J* 1:191, 1967
143. Reidenberg MM, Drayer D, De Marco AL, Dello CT: Hydralazine elimination in man. *Clin Pharmacol Ther* 14:970, 1973
144. Pettinger W: Introduction: The Brook Lodge Conference on Minoxidil. *J Cardiovasc Pharmacol* 2 (suppl):S91, 1980
145. Campiere C, Stefoni S, Martinelli S, Feliciangeli G, Bonomini V: Severe hypertension in chronic renal failure treated with minoxidil *Clin Exp Hypertension* 6:801, 1979
146. Bauer JH, Alpert MA: Rapid reduction of severe hypertension with minoxidil. *J Cardiovasc Pharmacol* (suppl) 2:S189, 1980
147. Tenschert W, Studer A, Zaruba K, Reuteler H, Siebenschein R, Siegenthaler W, Vetter W: Minoxidil in hypertension. *Arch Int Pharmacodyn Ther* 104 (suppl), 1980
148. Mitchell HC, Pettinger WA: Renal function in long-term minoxidil-treated patients. *J Cardiovasc Pharmacol* 2 (suppl):S163, 1980
149. Camel GH, Carmody SE, Perry HM Jr: Use of minoxidil in the azotemic patient. *J Cardiovasc Pharmacol* (suppl) 2:S173, 1980
150. Felts JH, Charles J: Minoxidil in refractory hypertension. *J Cardiovasc Pharmacol* 2 (suppl):S114, 1980
151. Martin WB, Spodick DH, Zins GR: Pericardial disorders occurring during open-label study of 1,869 severely hypertensive patients treated with minoxidil. *J Cardiovasc Pharmacol* 2 (suppl):S217, 1980
152. Wells JO: Unusual cases of resistance to minoxidil therapy. *J Cardiovsc Pharmacol* 2 (suppl):S228, 1980
153. Javier R, Dumler F, Park JH, Bok DV, Riley RW, Levin NW: Longterm treatment with minoxidil in patients with severe renal failure. *J Cardiovasc Pharmacol* 2 (suppl):S149, 1980
154. Campese VM, Stein D, DeQuattro V: Treatment of severe hypertension with minoxidil: Advantages and limitations. *J Clin Pharmacol* 19:231, 1979
155. Kern T, DeQuattro V, Bornheimer JF, DeQuattro E, Kolloch RE: Long-term effects of minoxidil therapy on renal function of patients with refractory hypertension: The significance of albuminuria. *J Cardiovasc Pharmacol* 2 (suppl):S156, 1980
156. Lowenthal DT, Affrime MB: Pharmacology and pharmacokinetics of minoxidil. *J Cardiovasc Pharmacol* 2 (suppl):S93, 1980
157. Wood BC, Sharma JN, Crouch TT: Oral minoxidil in the treatment of hypertensive crisis. *JAMA* 241:163, 1979
158. O'Malley K, Velasco M, Pruitt A, McNay JC: Depressed plasma binding of diazoxide in uremia. *Clin Pharmacol Ther* 18:53, 1975
159. Koch-Weser J: Drug Therapy: Diazoxide. *N Engl J Med* 294:1271, 1976
160. Muirhead EE, Brooks B, Aurora KK: Prevention of malignant hypertension by the synthetic peptide SQ 20881. *Lab Invest* 30:129, 1974
161. Franciosa FA Jr, Guiha NH, Limas CJ, Rodriguera E, Cohn JN: Improved left ventricular function during nitroprusside infusion in acute myocardial infarction. *Lancet* 1:650, 1972
162. Ross G, Cole PV: Cardiovascular actions of sodium nitroprusside in dogs. *Anaesthesia* 28:400, 1973
163. Palmer RF, Lasseter KC: Sodium nitroprusside. *N Engl J Med* 292:294, 1975
164. Montoliu J, Botey A, Pons JM, Revert L: Fatal hypotension in normal-dose nitroprusside therapy. (letter to the editor) *Am Heart J* 97:541, 1979
165. Martin WB, Zins GR, Greyburger WA: The use of minoxidil in 510 patients with refractory hypertension. *Clin Sci Mol Med* 48:1895, 1975
166. Cheigh JS, Rubin Al, Stenzel KM, Whitsell JC: Hypocalcemia following bilateral nephrectomy. *Urology* 2:121, 1973
167. Stenzel KH, Cheigh JC, Sullivan JS, Tapia L, Riggio RR, Rubin AL: Clinical effects of bilateral nephrectomy. *Am J Med* 58:69, 1975
168. van Ypersele de Strihou C, Stragier A: Effect of bilateral nephrectomy on transfusion requirement of patients undergoing chronic dialysis. *Lancet* 2:705, 1969
169. Kominami N, Lowrie EG, Ianberg LE, Skaren A, Hampers CL, Merill JP, Lange RD: The effect of total nephrectomy on hematopoiesis in patients undergoing chronic hemodialysis. *J Lab Clin Med* 78:524, 1971
170. McCarron DA, Rubin RJ, Barnes BA, Harrington JT, Millan VG: Therapeutic bilateral renal infarction in end stage renal disease. *N Engl J Med* 294:502, 1976
171. Avram MM, Lipner HI, Gan AL: Medical nephrectomy. The use of metallic salts for the control of massive proteinuria in the nephrotic syndrome. *Trans Am Soc Artif Intern Organs* 22:431, 1976
172. Morland JJ, Rottembourg J, Jardin A, Thibault P, Rouby JJ, Jacobs C, Legrain M: Selective bilateral renal artery embolization (RAE) as treatment of malignant hypertension in two repetitive dialysis patients. *Kidney Int* (Abstract) 10:338, 1976

173. Alfrey AC, Goss JE, Ogden DA, Vogel JHK, Holmes JH: Uremic hemopericardium *Am J Med* 45:391, 1968
174. Szmuness W, Prince AM, Grady GF, Mann MK, Levine RW, Friedman EA, Jacobs MS, Josephson A, Ribat S, Shapiro FL, Stenzel KH, Suki WN, Vyas G: Hepatitis B infection a joint prevalence study in 15 US hemodialysis centers. *JAMA* 227:901, 1974
175. Hindman SH, Gravelle CR, Murphy BL, Bradley DW, Budge WR, Maynard JE: 'e' antigen, Dane particles, and serum DNA polymerase activity in HB_s Ag carriers. *Ann Intern Med* 85:458, 1976
176. Grady GF: Collaborative study: Relationship of e antigen to infectivity of HB_sAg positive inoculations among medical personnel. *Lancet* 2:492, 1976
177. Kirkendol RL, Devia CJ, Bower JD, Holbert RD: A comparison of the cardiovascular effects of sodium acetate and sodium bicarbonate and other potential sources of fixed base in hemodialysis solutions. *Trans Am Soc Artif Intern Organs* 23:399, 1977
178. Kishimat T, Tanaka H, Yamakama M, Mizutani Y, Yamanoto T, Hirata S, Horiuchi N, Maekawa M: Morbidity, instability and serum acetate level during Hemodialysis. (abstracts) *Artif Organs* 3A:22, 1979
179. Deheneffe J, Cuesta V, Briggs JD, Brown JJ, Leckie BJ, Lever AF, Morton JJ, Robertson JIS, Semple PF, Tree M: The renin-angiotensin system in anephric man. *Proc Eur Dial Transpl Assoc* 13:495, 1976
180. Weinberger MH, Aoi W, Wade MB, Usa T, Grim CE, Dentino ME, Luft F: Renin-like activity in anephric man. Abstracts *Am Soc Nephrol* 9:51, 1976
181. Ganten D, Schelling P, Vecsei P, Ganten U: Iso-renin of extra-renal origin. The tissue angiotensinogenase system. *Am J Med* 60:760, 1976
182. Sealey JE, Moon C, Laragh JH, Alderman M: Plasma prorenin: Cryoactivation and relationship to renin substrate in normal subjects. *Am J Med* 61:731, 1976
183. Sealey JE, White RP, Laragh JH, Rubin AL: Plasma prorenin and renin in anephric patients. *Circ Res* 41 (suppl II):17, 1977
184. Davis JO, Carpenter CCJ, Ayers CR, Halman JE, Bahn RC: Evidence for secretion of an aldosterone-stimulating hormone by the kidney. *J Clin Invest* 40:684, 1961
185. McCaa RE, McCaa CS, Read VH, Bower JD, Guyton AL: Increased plasma aldosterone concentration in response to hemodialysis in nephrectomized man. *Circ Res* 31:473, 1972
186. McCaa RE, McCaa CS, Read VH, Bower JD: Influence of hemodialysis on plasma aldosterone concentration in nephrectomized patients. *Trans Am Soc Artif Intern Organs* 18:239 and 248, 1972
187. Vetter W, Zaruba K, Armbuster H, Beckerhoff R, Reck G, Siegenthaler W: Control of plasma aldosterone in supine anephric man. *Clin Endocrinol* (Oxf) 3:411, 1974
188. Woods TJC, McCaa RE, Bower JD, McCaa CS: Aldosterone response to angiotensin II in patients with terminal renal failure and after bilateral nephrectomy. *Trans Am Soc Artif Intern Organs* 20:154, 1974
189. Goodwin TJ, James VHT, Peart WS: The control of aldosterone secretion in nephrectomized man. *Clin Sci Mol Med* 47:235, 1974
190. Dekeneffe J, Cuesta V, Roberson J: The control of aldosterone in anephric man. *Clin Sci Mol Med* 48:465, 1975
191. Sealey JE, White RP, Laragh JH: Virtual absence of plasma aldosterone in anephric patients. *J Clin Endocrinol Metab* 47:52, 1978
192. Weidman P, Maxwell MH, Rowe P, Winer R, Massry SG: Role of the renin-angiotensin-aldosterone system in the regulation of plasma potassium in chronic renal disease. *Nephron* 15:35, 1975
193. Kersh ES, Kronfield SJ, Unger A, Popper RW, Cantor S, Cohn K: Autonomic insufficiency in uremia as a cause of hemodialysis-induced hypotension. *N Engl J Med* 290:650, 1974
194. Henderson LW, Lilley JJ, Ford CA, Stone RA: Hemodiafiltration. *J Dial* 1:211, 1977
195. Chaimovitz C, Abinader B, Benderly A, Better OS: Hypocalcemic hypotension. *JAMA* 222:86, 1972
196. Bergström J: Ultrafiltration without dialysis for removal of fluids and solutes in uremia. *Clin Nephrol* 9:156, 1978
197. Rouby JJ, Rottembourg J, Durande JP, Basset JY, Degoulet P, Glaser P, Legrain M: Hemodynamic changes induced by regular hemodialysis and sequential ultrafiltration hemodialysis: A comparative study. *Kidney Int* 17:801, 1980
198. Rosa AA, Fryd DS, Kjellstrand CM: Dialysis symptoms and stabilization in long-term dialysis. Practical application of the CUSUM plot. *Arch Intern Med* 140:804, 1980
199. Nidus B, Matalon R, Katz L, Cabaluna C, Pan C, Esinger R: Hemodialysis using femoral vein cannulation. *Nephron* 13:416, 1974
200. Le Veen HH, Wapnick S, Grosberg S, Kinney MJ: Further experience with peritoneo-venous shunt for ascites. *Ann Surg* 184:574, 1976

29

HYPERLIPIDEMIA AND ATHEROSCLEROSIS IN CHRONIC DIALYSIS PATIENTS

JOHN D. BAGDADE

Hyperlipidemia	588
Frequency of hyperlipidemia in renal failure patients	588
Pathogenesis of hyperlipidemia in renal failure	589
Abnormalities of lipoprotein lipase (LPL) mediated removal	589
Other factors	589
The possible role of carnitine deficiency	589
Drugs	589
Acetate	589
Dextrose	590
Acidosis	590
Treatment	590
Whether to treat	590
Assessing liproprotein changes	590
Diet	590
Drugs	590
Clofibrate	590
Physical training	591
Atherosclerosis	591
Accelerated atherosclerosis?	591
The evidence	591
Risk factors	591
Smoking, hypertension	591
Pathogenesis	591
References	593

HYPERLIPIDEMIA

Hyperlipidemia has been recognized in patients with renal disease for over a century. Only with the advent of dialysis treatment, however, has it been possible to determine why, in some chronically uremic patients, large lightscattering triglyceride-rich fat particles may accumulate in sufficient numbers to cause plasma lactescence.

Frequency of hyperlipidemia in renal failure patients

It now appears that about one-third of both maintenance peritoneal (1) and hemodialysis (2) patients have increases in the very-low-density plasma lipoprotein class (VLDL) which result in an isolated elevation in basal plasma triglyceride (TG) concentrations. As consequences of the impairment causing this increase in TG, there is an associated reduction of the plasma cholesterol to low-normal concentrations (3, 4), a reduction of high-density lipoprotein cholesterol levels (HDL), and a disproportionate increase in the ratio of cholesterol in the plasma low-density lipoprotein (LDL) class compared to that contained in the HDL fraction (5). The fact that undialyzed patients also demonstrate similar disturbances in TG transport indicates that these changes result from renal failure and not from dialysis treatment. In addition, the three major lipoprotein classes (VLDL, LDL, and HDL) contain an increased proportion of triglyceride in all patients with renal failure, both those with normal and those with increased fasting lipid concentrations. (2, [Figure 1]). This enrichment of all lipoprotein classes and accumulation of partially catabolized 'remnants' of VLDL in dialysis patients (6) provides strong evidence that impaired removal of VLDL is the principal mechanism contributing to TG elevation in dialysis patients. These abnormalities appear to be clinically significant because they have been shown to be sensitive indicators of coronary risk in non-renal populations (7). The decrease in HDL may be particularly important, since it appears to modulate the normal cellular uptake and egress of cholesterol by interacting with cell surface receptors for LDL. The reduction in HDL appears to result from an absolute deficiency of protein and not due to an alteration in cholesterol content, as its major apoprotein constituent, apo-AI, has been found to

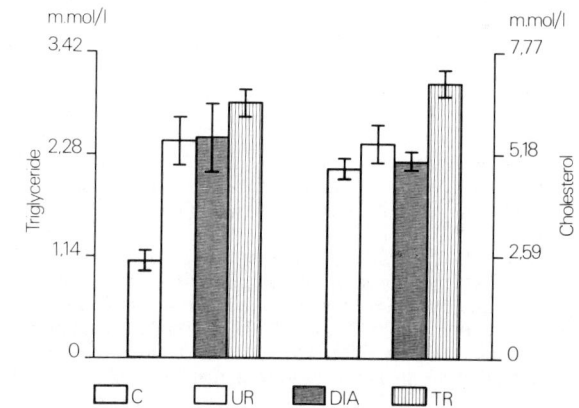

Figure 1. Basal concentrations of whole plasma triglyceride and cholesterol in 38 normolipidemic control subjects (C), 13 undialyzed (UR), and 14 dialyzed chronically uremic patients (DIA), and 23 patients who have undergone successful renal transplantation (TR).

SI units → conventional units
triglycerides: multiply by 88 (= mg/dl)
total cholesterol: multiply by 38.6 (= mg/dl)

be reduced (1). The vital role HDL plays in LDL transport is emphasized by the inverse relationship shown between plasma HDL cholesterol levels and tissue cholesterol pools (8).

Pathogenesis of hyperlipidemia in renal failure

While the precise mechanism(s) causing these changes have not yet been fully elucidated, most investigations indicate that impaired catabolism rather than increased production is primarily responsible for TG elevation in renal failure. Because early workers found that circulating insulin levels correlated with rates of endogenous TG production and basal insulin levels were increased in uremic patients (9) it was suspected that at least hepatic VLDL synthesis might be increased. Kinetic studies in both uremic patients (10) and animal models (11), however, indicated that in most renal failure patients VLDL production is not increased. In addition, the demonstration that elevated insulin levels in some uremic patients result from a disproportionate increase of proinsulin (12) makes this insulin-TG synthesis hypothesis less tenable.

Abnormalities of lipoprotein lipase (LPL)-mediated removal
Despite the technical difficulties inherent in assessing TG-removal mechanisms, it now is well established that both qualitative and quantitative abnormalities in lipoprotein lipase (LPL), the tissue enzyme system which mediates TG removal, are present in renal failure patients. Very low plasma lipolytic activity levels in dialysis patients after the injection of heparin (PHLA), an indirect and imprecise method used earlier to measure tissue LPL, were the first evidence to suggest that TG-removal was disturbed in uremia (9). The confusing combination of findings of markedly reduced PHLA and only slightly increased TG has been shown to result from a selective depression of hepatic lipase which quantitatively constitutes the majority of the PHLA response (13, 14), but is less important in TG removal than adipose tissue LPL. This reduction in hepatic LPL still may be extremely important in chronic uremia, since it contributes to the accumulation of so-called 'remnant' particles in dialysis patients (6).

With newer laboratory methods to quantitate LPL in tissues directly, Goldberg, Sherrard, and Brunzell (15) have shown that basal adipose tissue LPL activity is reduced in hypertriglyceridemic uremic patients and fails to increase normally post-prandially, but is normal in dialysis patients with normal TG. Other factors also appear to compromise LPL functionally in uremia. These include an LPL inhibitor which has been found in serum of hemodialysis patients (10) and both acute and chronically uremic rats (11). In humans this substance(s) is a poorly dialyzable solute of 'middle-molecule' size (see Chapter 19), the class of substances which have been shown to inhibit other important physiological processes such as glucose utilization, fibroblast proliferation, phagocytic activity of leukocytes, and lymphocyte transformation.

Disturbances in the apolipoprotein co-factors carried in HDL that normally modulate LPL function also may impair TG removal in uremia. It has been shown that the important C-II LPL activator peptide is decreased, and the inhibitory C-III apoprotein is increased in the HDL of chronic hemodialysis patients (16). The fact that clofibrate treatment can lower TG and correct these changes in LPL in hyperlipidemic dialysis patients supports the view that abnormalities in the TG-removal system is the major mechanism contributing to their TG elevation.

Other factors
The possible role of carnitine deficiency. A great deal of attention has recently been directed toward the possibility that an impairment in the cellular oxidation of fatty acids resulting from carnitine deficiency also might contribute to hyperlipidemia in uremic patients treated by dialysis. The fact that during dialysis treatment carnitine appears in the dialysate and levels fall in plasma (17) suggests that tissue carnitine levels may become depleted and that a deficiency state may develop in some patients and as a result their capacity to transport and oxidize fatty acids may be reduced. Low plasma levels of the dialyzable aminoacid and carnitine precursor lysine support the likelihood that triglyceride metabolism may be perturbed at this oxidative step in some chronically uremic patients. Despite some success in short-term treatment (18) it is premature at this time to recommend carnitine therapy as a modality of treatment for hyperlipidemic dialysis patients.

Drugs. A number of modalities in dialysis treatment also may alter plasma lipids. Androgens, sometimes administered to treat anemia in uremic patients, may increase TG when given in large doses (19). At lower doses, these anabolic agents have been shown in both non-uremic man (20) and experimental animals (21) to lower lipids, an effect which appears to result from improved LPL-related TG removal. Both propranolol, and the thiazide diuretics (1), anti-hypertensive medications regularly employed in a number of dialysis patients, also increase TG levels.

Acetate. Because the carbonates of calcium and magnesium were found to be poorly soluble in concentrated bicarbonate solutions during the early development of hemodialysis systems, acetate has been substituted successfully as a dialysate buffer anion. The theoretical possibility that acetate loads during dialysis might contribute to hyperlipidemia and atherosclerosis through conversion to long chain fatty acids and cholesterol in the liver and vascular tissues, has been a source of concern. There are few data, however, indicating that acetate has any deleterious effect on either plasma lipids or vascular tissues in dialysis patients. In one clinical study, no difference was observed when the effects of acetate and bicarbonate in dialysis fluid on TG and cholesterol levels were compared in hemodialysis patients (22). In addition, a kinetic study in uremic dogs has failed to show any evidence of enhanced lipogenesis during dialysis with acetate (23).

Dextrose. The possibility that high dextrose concentrations in dialysis fluid also might stimulate hepatic VLDL production, a normal effect of increased dietary carbohydrate, never has been conclusively shown. In addition the use of more physiologic dextrose concentrations in the dialysis bath has reduced this theoretical risk. It must be remembered that any increment in TG that might result from increased hepatic VLDL production during dialysis, would occur concomitant with the administration of large amounts of heparin which stimulates LPL and normally lowers TG. Since it has been shown that parenterally administered dextrose evokes lower TG responses than the same amount of dextrose given orally, concern about dextrose in dialysis solution on TG does not seem warranted. Furthermore, TG levels have been shown to fall during heparin-dialysis in the presence of both high and low concentrations of dextrose in the dialysis solution.

Acidosis. On the basis of the experimental observation that rats made uremic and acidotic developed similar changes in TG and LPL, attention has been given to the possibility that acidosis itself might adversely influence TG transport in dialysis patients. Preliminary data indicate that substitution of bicarbonate for acetate in the dialysis bath is associated with a beneficial effect on plasma lipids including HDL (Graefe U, University of Muenster, W. Germany, unpublished data). There is as yet insufficient evidence to recommend such a change, and further studies in this area are required.

Treatment

Whether to treat
Treating the forms of hyperlipidemia associated with premature cardiovascular disease is based on the assumption that lowering the elevated lipid class and elevating HDL reduces cardiovascular risk. While reports have appeared to indicate that established arterial lesions may regress with lipid-lowering treatment in the non-uremic population (24), no data of this type exist in chronic dialysis patients. Surprisingly, analysis of survival data in the Seattle dialysis population show that the risk associated with hyperlipidemia is less than that posed by the conventional risk factors of age, hypertension, and particularly cigarette smoking (25) which make a striking contribution to premature death.

Nevertheless, because of the risk associated with the disturbances in lipoprotein metabolism, it seems judicious that after secondary causes of hyperlipidemia such as hypothyroidism and diabetes have been excluded, to treat this problem in dialysis patients particularly those with more than one risk factor. It must be emphasized that the potential benefits of lowering TG and raising HDL are likely to be less than those derived from assiduous management of hypertension and the discontinuation of cigarette smoking.

Assessing lipoprotein changes
Some therapies which successfully lower total lipid levels at the same time may adversely affect other lipoprotein and apoprotein concentrations. Lowering the TG level may for example decrease HDL and/or increase plasma LDL. Therefore, in order to assess the efficacy of treatment it is necessary to monitor changes in both of the total plasma lipoprotein lipids. (The normal ratio of $Chol_{LDL}/Chol_{HDL}$ is 2.4 ± 1.2). A formula may be employed to estimate lipoprotein cholesterol levels when the routinely performed measurements of whole plasma TG (less than 500 mg/dl; [5.7 mmol]), cholesterol and HDL cholesterol are available (5).

Total plasma cholesterol

$$= \frac{TG}{5} = Chol_{LDL} + Chol_{HDL}$$

Diet
Compliance rates for even the most liberal renal diets rarely exceed 50% (26). Consequently strict adherence is unreasonable to expect, and this factor makes interpretation of the few past studies on dietary effects on hyperlipidemia in dialysis patients difficult. Since impaired removal appears to be the principal mechanism contributing to TG elevation in hemodialysis patients, the prolonged ingestion of a high-fat diet, which would overload an already stressed removal system, appears to be atherogenic because it promotes the accumulation of VLDL remnants and causes more marked degrees of post-prandial TG elevation (27). For this reason a diet which limits the intake of saturated fat and cholesterol and liberalizes carbohydrate is recommended (Table 1). Theoretically alcohol ingestion might increase hepatic TG synthesis, but since it appears to raise HDL levels in the non-uremic population (28), wine, for example, can provide a pleasing and potentially beneficial food and caloric source for dialysis patients.

Table 1. A dietary regimen for the treatment of hyperlipidemia in hemodialysis patients *.

Protein (% of total Cal/day)	15
Carbohydrate (% of total Cal/day)	50
Fat (% of total Cal/day)	35
Polyunsaturated to saturated fat ratio	0.87
Cholesterol (mg/day)	300 (0.78 mmol)
Cal/kg/day	35 (= 147 kJ)

* Goldberg et al (32).

Drugs
Clofibrate. Because of its 'anti-atherogenic' effects on lipoprotein transport, clofibrate treatment should be considered in hypertriglyceridemic dialysis patients. Even when administered at a markedly reduced dosage (1.0 to 2.0 g/week) because of its impaired renal excretion and markedly prolonged half-life in dialysis patients (29), clofibrate lowers TG, raises HDL cholesterol, lowers the plasma ratio of LDL to HDL cholesterol, and increases adipose tissue LPL and PHLA. This combination of salutary effects appears to result from improved TG removal (30). Concerns have been raised about possible gastrointestinal neoplasms resulting from treatment

with clofibrate based on a W.H.O. European multicentre study (31). Since patients treated by dialysis already have an increased incidence of malignancy, the risk attendant to clofibrate treatment must be weighed against that of accelerated cardiovascular morbidity.

Physical training
By promoting more efficient utilization of available substrate and oxygen by working tissues through peripheral enzyme and vascular adaptations, physical training has provided a useful new adjunct to the treatment of a number of chronic diseases. Goldberg and co-workers (32) have demonstrated that a program of graded exercise on a treadmill favorably affected a number of abnormalities in dialysis patients. Exercise-induced improvements included a 40% reduction in TG (exceeding that observed with clofibrate alone), a 20% increase in HDL-cholesterol, improved glucose tolerance and reduced insulin resistance. In addition, reduced blood pressure, and increased hematocrits and hemoglobin concentrations were observed in the majority of the patients. These observations indicate that the single therapeutic modality of exercise training in suitable dialysis patients provides a useful means of modifying several risk factors for coronary heart disease.

ATHEROSCLEROSIS

Accelerated atherosclerosis?

It has been widely accepted that atherosclerosis is accelerated and mortality from coronary heart disease increased in patients with end stage renal disease. While survival data from the United States (33) and Europe (34) have established that cardiovascular disease is the most common cause of death in chronic hemodialysis patients, many of these studies have failed to specify the disease type or to consider the presence of heart disease which antedated maintenance dialysis treatment.

The evidence
In the first study which called attention to the frequency of cardiovascular morbidity in dialysis patients, investigators in Seattle (33) found that survival in their small series of dialysis patients was sharply limited by coronary heart disease. Subsequently, somewhat different data from other centers (35, 36) emphasized the importance of pre-dialysis risk factors in predicting symptomatic cardiovascular disease, particularly during the first 5 years of treatment. In a study of the 6 year survival of a large group of dialysis patients who were matched with nondialysis subjects with the same risk factors (35), no increase in the incidence of ischemic heart disease (IHD) was observed. Female dialysis patients, however, were found to have a two-to-three fold increase in IHD above the incidence found in the Framingham study, indicating that the male predominance of IHD seen in the general population is not maintained in renal failure. Similar to the findings in a non-uremic population, blacks were found to have ischemic heart disease only half as frequently as whites (12.5% vs 25%), despite the presence of higher diastolic blood pressures and ECG evidence of ventricular hypertrophy, showing that racial factors also influence the development of IHD during hemodialysis treatment.

The answer to the important question of whether atherogenesis is accelerated in patients who are free of significant atherosclerotic disease prior to entering dialysis programs awaits the completion of long-term survival studies. Since the majority of patients have one or more acknowledged risk factors, there is not yet sufficient information about the long-term outcome of the smaller number of risk-free dialysis patients. Such data should soon become available, though patient ranks in recent years have increased significantly with older, higher risk patients. While the paucity of data limits establishing firmly a cause-effect relationship between chronic uremia and dialysis treatment and accelerated atherogenesis, recent reports of the European Dialysis and Transplant Registry and longterm survival data from the Seattle group (Lindner A, University of Washington, Seattle WA: personal communication) continue to support this association.

Risk factors
Smoking, hypertension. If dialysis patients do have risk factors and atheroma formation prior to dialysis treatment, it is clear that their survival is shortened even though important risk factors such as hypertension may be better controlled. Thus the clinical outcome and geometric increase in cardiovascular events in most dialysis patients is analogous to that of non-uremic patients who have a combination of risk factors, such as diabetics or women who take oral contraceptive preparations and who also are hypertensive, smoke cigarettes, or have hyperlipidemia (37).

Because of this apparent acceleration of cardiovascular disease during dialysis treatment, attention has been given to the treatment of risk factors. In one such study, hypertension and cigarette smoking appear to be more important risks than hyperlipidemia (25). Half the dialysis patients who smoked died within 5 years of starting treatment; whereas 78% of non-smokers survived 10 years. Dialysis patients with hypertension alone have a similarly ominous prognosis: a 57% two-year survival; normotensive patients had a 92% survival during the same time interval. In the absence of overt diabetes, glucose intolerance does not appear to be an important risk factor in chronic uremia.

Pathogenesis
Virchow's 'response to injury' hypothesis, based on the observation that atherosclerotic lesions resemble the response of arteries to injury to the vascular wall provides a useful model to examine how various risk factors in chronic uremia may influence lesion formation (Table 2). According to this hypothesis (38), all lesions are initiated by an injury to the artery's innermost endothelial cell layer, such as mechanically-induced changes (ballon catheter), a hemodynamic stress force such as hypertension or injury from prolonged exposure to toxins such as the amino acid homocystine, or other substances which accumulate in renal failure.

Table 2. Cardiovascular risk factors in chronic dialysis patients.

Certain
Hypertension
Cigarette smoking
Diabetes mellitus

Less certain
Hyperlipidemia
Glucose intolerance
Hyperuricemia

Intriguing possibilities
Polyamines (middle molecules)
Hyperparathyroidism
Immunologic injury
Accelerated platelet destruction

Antigen — antibody complexes also may contribute to endothelial injury by binding to membrane structures and involving other molecules such as complement, histamine, and kinins, and cells such as macrophages and polymorphonuclear leukocytes. This mechanism of endothelial cell injury may be important in patients who have an underlying immunologically related cause for their renal insufficiency. A mechanism of this type has been elucidated by Craddock et al. (39) in their studies of the pathogenesis of hemodialysis-induced angina pectoris. In these they showed that activation of the complement system (C5a) by cellophane coils of the hemodialyzer results in clumping of leukocytes in alveolar capillaries where they interfere with normal gas exchange (see also chapter 32) and produce free-oxygen radicals which could damage endothelial cells. Platelets also play an important role in the response of the arterial wall to endothelial injury. When endothelial cells are actually lost or when their vital functions are compromised, platelets rapidly adhere, aggregate, and release the contents of their granules at the injury site (Figure 2). Plasma lipoproteins and other mitogenic substances such as hormones can then infiltrate the arterial wall at these sites where they stimulate the replication and migration of arterial smooth muscle cells from the media into the intima. That endothelial injury is sustained in uremia and platelets are active in the repair process is supported by the fact that platelets are activated, their survival shortened (40), and endothelial cell turnover is increased in a mildly uremic animal model.

With tissue culture techniques it is now possible to assess factors in uremia which influence the central step of smooth muscle cell proliferation in atherogenesis. Since serum from dialysis patients enhances smooth muscle cell proliferation (41), humoral factors appear to play some role though their identity is unclear. Elevated levels of platelet factor 4 and beta-thromboglobulin (42), two peptides contained in the platelet α-granule, suggest that platelet-derived growth factor (PDGF) or other humoral factors such as polyamines (43), that promote cell growth, may be important. Since normal low density

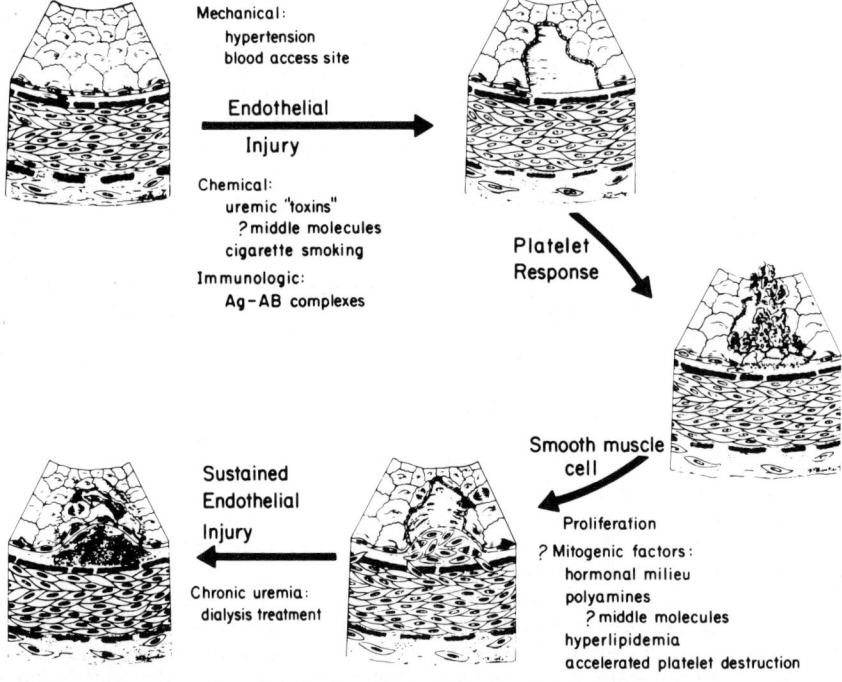

Figure 2. Cycle of events in the Response-to-Injury Hypothesis in chronic uremia. Endothelial injury resulting in actual desquamation or to alterations of the normal structure-function relationship of the arterial intimal cells may activate platelets which promote smooth muscle cell proliferation. Repeated or chronic endothelial injury in uremia may lead to lipid deposition, continued smooth muscle cell proliferation, and the development of a complicated lesion containing newly formed connective tissue and lipids which readily calcify in the setting of hyperparathyroidism.

lipoprotein (LDL) has been shown to stimulate smooth muscle proliferation in tissue culture, it is possible that LDL in these renal failure patients may act similarly through its apoprotein structure or (an)other mitogenic substance(s) bound to it.

Little information is available about factors in uremia that influence lipid and connective tissue accumulation within the arterial wall during atherogenesis. Cholesterol deposition in renal failure patients is favored by the low levels of high density lipoprotein which slow the normal egress of cholesterol from tissues, and possibly also by an impairment in the normal lysosomal degradation of internalized cholesterol.

As intriguing as these preliminary findings are, a number of compelling questions remain unanswered. What are the factors (likely several) that contribute to endothelial injury in chronic uremia? Which 'uremic toxins' could possibly damage endothelial cells? Could the hypoxemia created by the combination of anemia and cigarette smoking be 'toxic' and also stimulate smooth muscle cell growth? Are the same or other immune mechanisms which are operative in some forms of nephritis contributing to endothelial cell injury during dialysis treatment? It is likely that the answers to these questions will provide not only a better understanding of the altered pathophysiology of chronic uremia, but will offer insights into the pathogenesis of atherosclerosis in the non-uremic population as well.

REFERENCES

1. Brunzell JD, Albers JJ, Haas LB, Goldberg AP, Agadoa L, Sherrard DJ: Prevalence of serum lipid abnormalities in chronic hemodialysis. *Metabolism* 26:903, 1977
2. Bagdade JD, Casaretto A, Albers JJ: Effects of chronic uremia, hemodialysis and renal transplantation on plasma lipids and lipoproteins in man. *J Lab Clin Med* 87:37, 1976
3. Daubresse JC, Lerson G, Plomteux G, Rorive G, Luycks AS, Lefebvre PJ: Lipids and lipoproteins in chronic uraemia: a study of the influences of regular haemodialysis. *Eur J Clin Invest* 6:159, 1976
4. Ibels LS, Simons LA, King JO, Williams PF, Neale FC, Stewart JH: Studies on the nature and causes of hyperlipidaemia in uraemia, maintenance dialysis and renal transplantation. *Q J Med* 44:601, 1975
5. Bagdade JD, Albers JJ: Plasma high density lipoprotein concentrations in chronic hemodialysis and renal transplant patients. *N Engl J Med* 296:1436, 1977
6. Minamisono T, Wada M, Akamutsu A, Okabe M, Handa Y, Morita T, Asagami C, Naito HK, Nakamoto S, Lewis LA, Mise J: Dyslipoproteinemia (a remnant lipoprotein disease) in uremic patients on hemodialysis. *Clin Chim Acta* 84:163, 1978
7. Castelli WP, Doyle JT, Gordon T, Hames CG, Hjortland MC, Hulley SB, Kagan A, Zukel WJ: HDL cholesterol and other lipids in coronary heart disease. The cooperative lipoprotein phenotyping study. *Circulation* 55:767, 1977
8. Miller GJ, Miller NE: Plasma high density lipoprotein concentration and development of ischaemic heart disease. *Lancet* 1:16, 1975
9. Bagdade JD, Porte D Jr, Bierman EL: Hypertriglyceridemia: a metabolic consequence of chronic renal failure. *N Engl J Med* 269:181, 1968
10. Cattran DC, Fenton SA, Wilson DR, Steiner G: Defective triglyceride removal in lipemia associated with peritoneal dialysis and hemodialysis. *Ann Intern Med* 85:29, 1976
11. Bagdade JD, Yee E, Shafrir E, Wilson DE: Hyperlipidemia in renal failure: studies of plasma lipoproteins, hepatic triglyceride production and tissue lipoprotein lipase in a chronically uremic rat model. *Metabolism* 25:533, 1977
12. Mako M, Block M, Starr J, Nielsen E, Friedman EA, Rubenstein A: Proinsulin in chronic renal and hepatic failure: a reflection of the relative contribution of the liver and the kidney to its metabolism. *Clin Res* 21:631A, 1973
13. Mordasini R, Frey F, Flury W, Klose G, Greten H: Selective deficiency of hepatic triglyceride lipase in uremic patients. *N Engl J Med* 297:1362, 1977
14. Appelbaum-Bowden D, Goldberg AP, Hazzard WR, Sherrard DJ, Brunzell JD, Huttunen JK, Nikkila EA, Ehnholm C: Postheparin plasma triglyceride lipase in chronic hemodialysis: evidence for a role of hepatic lipase in lipoprotein metabolism. *Metabolism* 28:917, 1979
15. Goldberg AP, Sherrard DJ, Brunzell JD: Adipose tissue lipoprotein lipase in chronic hemodialysis: Role in plasma triglyceride metabolism. *J Clin Endocrinol Metab* 47:1173, 1978
16. Rapoport J, Aviram M, Chaimovitz C, Brook JG: Defective high-density lipoprotein composition in patients on chronic hemodialysis. *New Engl J Med* 299:1326, 1978
17. Bohmer T, Bergrem H, Eiklid K: Carnitine deficiency induced during intermittent haemodialysis for renal failure. *Lancet* 1:126, 1978
18. Lacour B, DiGiulio S, Chanard J, Ciancioni C, Haguet M, Lebkiri B, Basile C, Drueke T, Assan R, Funck-Brentano J-L: Carnitine improves lipid abnormalities in haemodialysis patients. *Lancet* 2:763, 1980
19. Choi ESK, Chung T, Morrison R, Meyers C, Greenberg M: Hypertriglyceridemia in hemodialysis patients during oral dromostanolone therapy for anemia. *Am J Clin Nutr* 27:901, 1974
20. Glueck CJ, Scheel D, Fishback J, Steiner R: Progestastegens, anabolic-androgenic compounds, estrogens: effects on triglycerides and post heparin lipolytic enzymes. *Lipids* 7:110, 1972
21. Bagdade JD, Livingston R, Yee E: Effects of the synthetic androgen fluoxymesterone on triglyceride secretion rates in the rat. *Proc Soc Exp Biol Med* 149:452, 1975
22. Davidson WD, Morin RJ, Rorke SJ, Guo LSS: The role of acetate in dialysate for hemodialysis. *Proc 10th Annu Contr Conf Artif Kidney Progr NIAMDD DHEW* edited by Mackey BB, publ no (NIH) 77-1442, 1977, p 15
23. Wathen RL, Keshaviah P, Comty C: Acid-base regulation in hemodialysis. *Proc 10th Annu Contr Conf Artif Kidney Progr NIAMDD DHEW* edited by Mackey BB, publ no (NIH) 77-1442, 1077, p 17
24. Basta LL, Williams C, Kioschos JM, Spector AA: Regression of atherosclerotic stenosing lesions of the renal arteries and spontaneous cure of systemic hypertension through control of hyperlipidemia. *Am J Med* 61:420, 1976
25. Haire H, Sherrard D, Scardapane D, Curtis FK, Brunzell JD: Smoking, hypertension and mortality in a maintenance dialysis population. *Cardiovasc Med* 3:1163, 1978
26. Wahlqvist ML, Hurley BP: Hyperlipoproteinemia and dietary fat modification in hemodialysis and renal transplant patients. *Med J Aust* 2:207, 1977
27. Zilversmit DB: Atherogenesis: A postprandial phenomenon. *Circulation* 60:473, 1979

28. Castelli WP, Doyle JT, Gordon T, Hames CG, Hjortland MC, Hulley SB, Kagan A, Zukel WJ: Alcohol and blood lipids: The cooperative lipoprotein phenotyping study. *Lancet* 2:153, 1977
29. Goldberg AP, Sherrard D, Haas L, Brunzell JD: Control of clofibrate toxicity in the treatment of uremic hypertriglyceridemia. *Clin Pharmacol Ther* 21:314, 1977
30. Goldberg AP, Appelbaum-Bowden DM, Bierman EL, Hazzard WR, Haas LB, Sherrard DJ, Brunzell JD, Huttunen JK, Ehnholm C, Nikkila EA: Increase in lipoprotein lipase during clofibrate treatment of hypertriglyceridemia in patients on hemodialysis. *N Eng J Med* 301:1073, 1979
31. A cooperative trial in the primary prevention of ischaemic heart disease using clofibrate. Report from the Committee of Principal Investigators. *Brit Heart J* 40:1069, 1978
32. Goldberg AP, Hagberg J, Delmez JA, Haynes ME, Harter HR: Metabolic effects of exercise training in hemodialysis patients. *Kidney Int* 18:754, 1980
33. Lindner A, Charra B, Sherrard DJ, Scribner BH: Accelerated atherosclerosis in prolonged maintenance dialysis. *New Engl J Med* 290:697, 1974
34. Cameron JS, Ellis FG, Ogg CS, Bewich M, Boulton-Jones JM, Robinson RD, Harrison J: A comparison of mortality and rehabilitation in regular dialysis and transplantation. *Proc Eur Dial Transpl Assoc* 7:25, 1970
35. Rostrand SG, Gretes JC, Kirk KA, Rutsky EA, Andreoli JE: Ischemic heart disease in patients with uremia undergoing maintenance hemodialysis. *Kidney Int* 16:600, 1979
36. Nicholls AJ, Catto GR, Edward N, Engeset J, Macleod M: Accelerated atherosclerosis in long-term dialysis and renal transplant patients: fact or fiction. *Lancet* 1:276, 1980
37. Editorial (anonymous): Cardiovascular risks and oral contraceptives. *Lancet* 1:1063, 1979
38. Ross R, Glomset JA: The pathogenesis of atherosclerosis. *N Engl J Med* 295:369 and 420, 1976
39. Craddock PR, Fehr J, Dalmasso AP, Brigham KL, Jacob HS: Hemodialysis leukopenia: pulmonary vascular leukostasis resulting from complement activation by dialyzer cellophane membranes. *J Clin Invest* 59:879, 1977
40. George CR, Slichter SJ, Quadracci LJ, Striker GE, Harker LA: A kinetic evaluation of hemostasis in renal disease. *N Eng J Med* 291:1111, 1974
41. Bagdade JD: Chronic renal failure and atherogenesis: serum factors stimulate the proliferation of human arterial smooth muscle cells. *Atherosclerosis* 34:243, 1979
42. Guzzo J, Niewiarowski S, Musial J, Bastl C, Grossman RA, Rao AK, Berman I, Paul D: Secreted platelet proteins with antiheparin and mitogenic activities in chronic renal failure. *J Lab Clin Med* 96:102, 1980
43. Bagdade JD, Subbaiah PV, Bartos D, Bartos F, Campbell RA: Polyamines: an unrecognized cardiovascular risk factor in chronic dialysis? *Lancet* 1:412, 1979

30

CARDIAC COMPLICATIONS OF REGULAR DIALYSIS THERAPY

CHRISTINA M. COMTY and FRED L. SHAPIRO

Introduction	595
Pericarditis	596
Pathology	596
Incidence and mortality	596
Pathogenesis	597
Clinical features	598
Differential diagnosis	599
Complications	599
Management	600
Digitalis	600
Anti-inflammatory drugs	601
Surgical management	601
Cardiac failure	602
Pathogenesis	602
Management of heart failure	604
Management of myocardial infarction	605
Bacterial endocarditis	605
Cardiac arrhythmias	606
References	607

INTRODUCTION

Since the introduction of regular hemodialysis treatment in 1960 (1), prolongation of useful life has been achieved for many thousands of patients. Long term hemodialysis, however, does not prevent cardiovascular disease. Indeed, cardiac complications on the basis of atherosclerosis are considered to be the commonest cause of death of long term dialysis patients. A recent report from Seattle indicates that 60% of deaths at the end of 13 years could be attributed to arteriosclerotic complications (myocardial infarction, stroke, congestive heart failure), occurring in patients who initially were selected because of the absence of vascular disease (2).

An analysis of survey data (Table 1) indicates an impressive mortality from cardiovascular disease, particularly cardiac disorders (3–11). It is difficult to attribute all these cardiac deaths to coronary artery disease because the causes of heart failure are not defined in these reports and patients with simple fluid overload and those with valvular disease may be included. It is also difficult to attribute all causes of sudden death to intrinsic, cardiac diseases, since cardiac arrest may result from many metabolic aberrations including fluid overload, shifts in serum potassium levels and changes in acid base balance.

In our own program, a total of 687 patients have been accepted for chronic hemodialysis since 1965 and there have been 293 deaths (Table 2). Heart disease due to coronary artery diseases (ASHD) was diagnosed only on

Table 1. Mortality from cardiovascular disease in Europe and USA.

Authors Europe	Year	Age group	% of deaths due to Hemorrhagic pericarditis	Myocardial infarction	Heart failure	Sudden death
Drukker et al (3)	1966	<55	—	3.7	30.0	—
Drukker et al (4)	1967	<55	—	3.0	26.0	—
Drukker et al (5)	1968	?	—	4.0	32.0	12.0
Drukker et al (6)	1969	<75	6.0	3.1	—	3.4
Drukker et al (7)	1970	<67	5.5	9.5	20.2	7.3
Brunner et al (8)	1972	?	5.6	5.6	25.3	4.7
Gurland et al (9)	1973	<70	6.0	6.0	25.0	
Brunner et al (10)	1978	all ages	3.8	11.2	13.4	14.5
USA						
Burton et al (11)	1971	?	—	(heart disease: 25.0)		
Present authors	1976	<81	3.1	20.5*	—	1.4

* Myocardial infarction and atherosclerotic heart disease.

Table 2. Incidence of cardiovascular deaths in Regional Kidney Disease Program, Minneapolis, Minnesota.

Year	No of deaths	Age at death	% deaths due to: Hemorrhagic pericarditis	Myocardial infarction	ASHD [1]	Sudden death	SBE [2]	CVA [3]
1965–76	293	12–81	3.1	13.7	6.8	1.4	1.7	7.2
Nondiabetics	236	12–81	3.4	5.5	5.5	1.7	2.7	7.2
Diabetics	57	24–68	1.8	21.1	10.5	0	0	7.0

[1] ASHD = Atherosclerotic heart disease.
[2] SBE = Subacute bacterial endocarditis.
[3] CVA = Cerebrovascular accident.

the basis of a history of myocardial infarction or angina pectoris, and/or definite ischemic changes on the electrocardiogram. Myocardial infarction was accepted as a cause of death when it was preceded by the classical clinical picture of acute myocardial infarction or where sudden death occurred with autopsy evidence of acute myocardial necrosis. Sudden deaths include those that result from hyperkalemia and from acute arrhythmias not clearly due to acute myocardial infarction. If diabetic patients are excluded, only 11% of the deaths were due to coronary artery disease. However, potentially preventable cardiac causes of death (hemorrhagic pericarditis, bacterial endocarditis) account for another 6.1% of all fatalities. Cumulative survival studies (Figure 1) show that in patients with a history of ASHD, the first year mortality was in excess of 25%, compared to less than 10% in those without such a history. Approximately 60% of patients with a history of ASHD died of cardiac problems.

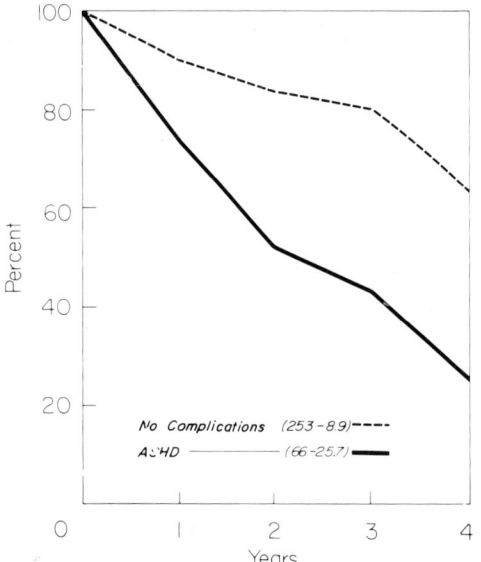

Figure 1. Cumulative survival of chronic dialysis patients with a history of coronary artery heart disease (ASHD) and without such a history.

PERICARDITIS

Pathology

The initial lesion in the typical case of uremic pericarditis is an aseptic inflammatory process with fibrin formation. The inflammatory process can be more severe with extensive thickening of parietal and visceral layers of the pericardium and areas of hemorrhage and fibrinous adhesions between both layers of the pericardium. Pericardial effusion is usually present and may be serous, serosanguinous or frankly hemorrhagic and frequently is loculated. The histological appearance is that of an acute inflammatory process with thickening of the pericardium by fibrin deposition and formation of highly vascular granulation tissue.

Subacute constrictive pericarditis closely resembles the relapsing seroconstrictive pericarditis seen in nonuremic individuals, representing a midpoint in the spectrum of pericardial disease extending from pericardial effusion with tamponade at one end to constrictive pericarditis at the other (12). On gross examination there may be active pericarditis with fibrin formation, hemorrhage, vascularization of the pericardium and pericardial fibrosis may be marked. Chronic constrictive pericarditis is a rare complication of uremic pericarditis where both layers of the pericardium are thickened by fibrosis and adherent to each other and to the underlying epicardium. So far calcification has not been reported in constrictive uremic pericarditis. As with pericarditis from other causes, associated myocarditis may occur (13).

Incidence and mortality

The incidence of pericarditis in acute renal failure has fallen progressively coincident with the widespread availability of hemodialysis for prophylactic therapy and the increased use of peritoneal dialysis. In 1954 Wacker and Merrill reported an incidence of 18% (14). Currently the incidence of pericarditis in acute renal failure is probably less than 5% and it occurs predominantly in patients who are highly catabolic as a result of trauma or sepsis.

In chronic renal failure there has again been a steady decline in the incidence of pericarditis in terminally

Table 3. Incidence of pericarditis in patients with chronic renal failure prior to the initiation of dialysis.

Year of study	Authors	Incidence
1954	Wacker and Merrill (14)	50.0%
1960–67	Bailey et al (17)	41.0%
1964–71	Drueke et al (16)	15.4%
1966–70	Comty et al (19)	13.1%
1960–74	Ribot et al (18)	1.7%
1971–75	Comty et al (20)	8.9%
1971–75	Wray and Stone (15)	16.0%
1972–76	Drueke et al (16)	12.1%

uremic patients (Table 3), probably reflecting improved conservative management by diet therapy and earlier elective initiation of chronic hemodialysis (15). In the dialyzed patient the incidence of clinical pericarditis has remained fairly stable in the United States, compared to European studies where a substantial reduction has been observed (Table 4).

Table 4. Incidence of clinical pericarditis in dialyzed patients.

Years	Authors	Incidence	
1960–67	Bailey et al 1968 (17)	14.0%	
1966–74	Ribot et al 1974 (18)	17.0%	
1966–70	Comty et al 1971 (19)	14.8%	difference not significant $p > 0.1$
1971–75	Comty et al 1975 (20)	18.4%	
1974–75	Wray & Stone 1976 (15)	15.3%	
1964–71	Drueke et al (16)	10.5%	difference significant $P < 0.1$
1972–76	Drueke et al (16)	5.8%	

Prospective echocardiographic studies suggest that the high incidence of dialysis-associated pericarditis is unrelated to pericardial disease antedating the initiation of chronic dialysis (15). Yet, echocardiography has revealed the presence of pericardial effusions in 53% of patients before the initiation of dialysis, and 51% of patients on long term dialysis.

Death as a direct result of pericarditis was initially as frequent as 20% (17–20). The incidence is now between 2.5 and 5% and pericarditis has accounted for 4.1% of deaths in European centers in 1977 and 3.1% of deaths in our experience (Table 1). Immediate causes of death have been tamponade, cardiac arrhythmias and heart failure. Factors adversely affecting survival include age (73% greater than 50 years), previous episodes of pericarditis (36%), delay in admission to hospital, and underlying ischemic heart disease (64% [20]).

Pathogenesis

Richard Bright in 1836 described an aseptic pericarditis in eight patients dying of uremia and attributed it to a generalized involvement of the serous membranes as a result of uncontrolled uremia (21). Most observers now believe that the initiating factor in uremic pericarditis is a serositis which is exacerbated and perpetuated by the hemorrhagic problems of the uremic patient and by continued trauma to the inflamed pericardial surfaces by myocardial contraction. Restoration of normal renal function in patients with acute renal failure and biochemical control by regular hemodialysis or successful transplantation in patients with chronic renal failure results in a resolution of pericarditis in the majority of cases without complication (16–20).

The development of pericarditis on a biochemical basis, however, does not explain the failure of the lesion to resolve in some patients following the control of uremia, nor why pericarditis should develop in stable patients treated by chronic hemodialysis for months or even years (19, 20). Furthermore, clinical observations indicate that pericarditis in the patient on chronic hemodialysis differs in several respects from that seen in patients with uncontrolled uremia. In the dialyzed patient pericarditis is associated with more severe constitutional symptons, is frequently unresponsive to conservative management, tends to involve the underlying myocardium by the inflammatory process more commonly, and has a higher incidence of acute and chronic complications (18, 19).

Several factors have been suggested as being of etiological importance in the pathogenesis of pericarditis in dialyzed patients (Table 5). The lack of significant difference in the plasma concentrations of urea, creatinine, or uric acid in patients who develop pericarditis compared to those who do not, does not exclude the possibility that other uremic toxins may be responsible (16, 19). Studies by Bergström and Fürst (22) suggest that middle molecular weight compounds may be involved. They observed that dialyzed patients with malnutrition or pericarditis had marked increases of the plasma concentrations of middle molecular weight compounds similar to patients with uremic polyneuropathy. Since clearance of compounds of such molecular weight is closely related to duration and adequacy of dialysis, it raises the question of the role of inadequate dialysis in the patho-

Table 5. Etiology of uremic pericarditis.

Etiological factor	Reference
Inadequate dialysis	17, 19, 31
Hypercatabolic states	
Sepsis	19
Surgery	17
Young females	16, 19, 20
Poor nutrition	19, 20
Hypercalcemia	16, 19, 23
Hyperparathyroidism	16, 18
Heparin	24–26
Cholesterol	26
Uric acid	27
Diabetes	
? related to infection	29
Infection	
CMV	30
Bacterial	31–33
Viral	19, 35
Fluid overload	16
Immunological?	—

genesis of pericarditis. That inadequate dialysis is of importance has been suggested by the decline in the incidence of pericarditis following the institution of thrice weekly dialysis routinely in the majority of centers, the response of pericarditis to augmentation of dialysis in 70% of the cases, and the development of pericarditis in hypercatabolic states. Our own observations and those of others (16, 19) suggest an association between severe secondary hyperparathyroidism and dialysis associated pericarditis. The plasma concentrations of calcium, phosphorus and PTH were significantly higher in dialyzed patients with pericarditis than in those without pericarditis (16). The mechanism is, however, unclear and other factors such as malnutrition, and possibly inadequate dialysis, may be implicated. Heparin is probably not an initiating factor in the development of pericarditis in dialyzed patients, although it may perpetuate the inflammatory process by causing repeated bleeding from the inflamed pericardial surfaces. The high incidence of acute and often fatal tamponade occurring both during and immediately after hemodialysis is probably not due to heparinization, but is rather a mechanical effect of ultrafiltration reducing blood volume and venous return thereby abolishing compensation of cardiac compression (28).

The role of infection in the development of uremic pericarditis is uncertain. In our own program the incidence of pericarditis is significantly higher in diabetic patients treated by chronic dialysis, (Table 5 [29]). The incidence of bacterial infection has also been shown to be significantly higher in the diabetic patient (see Chapter 33) and the development of pericarditis appears to be related to infection in 43% of diabetics (29). Cytomegalovirus was a direct causative agent in one study (30), and isolated cases of purulent pericarditis have been reported after transplant rejection, in severely debilitated patients with generalized sepsis (31, 32) and more recently in a patient who underwent coronary artery bypass surgery (33).

In other studies it has not been possible to exclude microbial contamination of the pericardium or secondary invasion after pericardiocentesis (32). Since bacterial infection had either preceeded or was associated with the development of aseptic pericarditis in between 31 and 80% of dialyzed patients (20), an immunological mechanism may be involved as with the aseptic pericarditis seen during the convalescent stages of meningococcal infection (34).

In some instances serological studies have confirmed the viral etiology of pericarditis, and Coxsackievirus A or B, influenza viruses A or B and echoviruses have been implicated (35). Fluid overload has been suggested but not clearly established as a precipitating factor in the development of pericarditis (16, 36). Echocardiographic studies have demonstrated an association between left ventricular failure as a result of fluid overload and pericarditis both before and after the initiation of dialytic therapy. Nevertheless, hypotension precedes the onset of chest pain or a friction rub in most patients with pericarditis. Hence fluid overload could be a result of the inability to maintain systemic blood pressure during dialysis, rather than a causative factor of pericarditis.

Finally, the incidence of pericarditis in patients being treated by chronic dialysis, and its absence after successful transplantation raise the possibility of a serositis possibly immunologically mediated, with a sensitive end organ, namely the pericardium.

Clinical features

Chest pain, which is a presenting complaint in 60 to 70% of patients with pericarditis, is frequently severe, requiring narcotics for relief (16, 18, 19). In over 90% of patients a friction rub is present.

Diagnostic problems occur in those patients who never develop chest pain or acquire it late in their course (Table 6). In the patient with advanced chronic renal failure (creatinine clearance less than 10 ml/min), other problems such as hypertension requiring drug therapy, fluid overload, and primary myocardial disease are frequently present. Nevertheless, pericarditis should be considered in patients with increasing cardiomegaly, right heart failure, or those with hypotension despite weight gain. Mental confusion and deterioration of renal function have also been reported as manifestations of pericardial effusion (26, 32).

Table 6. Clinical manifestations of uremic pericarditis.

Undialyzed patient (creatinine clearance < 10 ml/min)	Dialyzed patient
Chest pain, friction rub	Chest pain, friction rub
Cardiomegaly	Fever
Unexplained deterioration of renal function	Hypotension
	Rapid weight gain
Alteration in blood pressure control	Intolerance of ultrafiltration during hemodialysis
Mental confusion	Cardiac arrhythmias
	Cardiomegaly
	Mental confusion
	Clotting of vascular access

In the dialyzed patient, fever is present at the time of diagnosis in 76 to 96% of attacks (16, 18, 19). It may precede the clinical onset in 50% of patients.

Hypotension may be manifest in several ways (18). A low blood pressure may be present before dialysis despite weight gain due to salt and fluid retention. Attempts to remove the excess fluid by ultrafiltration are not tolerated. Weight gain may also occur as a result of frequent hypotensive episodes during dialysis that require saline infusion. Although Spodick (37) has emphasized the rarity of cardiac arrhythmias in nonuremic patients with acute pericarditis, arrhythmias, usually atrial fibrillation or flutter, have been presenting manifestations in between 19 and 28% of cases of uremic pericarditis (18, 19).

Mental confusion, lethargy and episodic disorientation have been reported in several patients with a large pericardial effusion. When present, these symptoms require differentiation from other causes of mental confusion such as cerebrovascular diseases, subdural hematoma, disequilibrium syndrome and other metabolic problems.

Pleural effusions, when accompanying pericarditis, may be unilateral or bilateral. They are common in uremic patients and complicate other conditions such as fluid overload, primary myocardial failure and pulmonary disease and do not assist in the differential diagnosis. Attempts to document the presence of pericardial effusion should be made in all patients with clinical pericarditis or cardiomegaly. The most sensitive currently available test is the echocardiogram which can detect as little as 30 ml of fluid in the pericardial sac.

Differential diagnosis

The differentiation of an aseptic pericarditis from a purulent pericarditis due to bacterial or fungal invasion may cause diagnostic problems. Purulent pericarditis is a serious disease with a high mortality and should be suspected in patients with severe debilitating diseases, in generalized sepsis, and in immunosuppressed patients. The diagnosis is frequently missed because of the absence of pain, the characteristic friction rub or EKG changes (38). Severe hypotension occurring during dialysis as a result of pericarditis must be differentiated from pyrogen reaction, bacteremia, hypovolemia and increasing congestive heart failure.

The differentiation of pericarditis from myocardial infarction and unstable angina may also cause diagnostic problems. The presence of a loud friction rub at the onset of pain strongly suggests primary pericardial disease. Cardiomegaly without pulmonary vascular congestion is also highly suggestive. The EKG and enzyme changes, although nonspecific in primary pericardial disease, can be diagnostic in myocardial infarction. Frequently, however, they are of little help in unstable angina. Other conditions that cause chest pain must be differentiated from pericarditis including pleurisy and spontaneous pneumothorax.

Complications (Table 7)

With the use of echocardiography, a pericardial effusion can be demonstrated in the majority of patients with uremic pericarditis. The hemodynamic significance of a pericardial effusion requires critical evaluation since a very large pericardial effusion accumulating slowly may cause less compression than the rapid accumulation of 150 ml of fluid in the pericardial sac. An effusion accumulating in a previously healthy distensible pericardial sac also has less hemodynamic effect than that of an effusion occurring in a previously diseased noncompliant sac. A loud friction rub with easily audible heart sounds is often present and does not exclude significant tamponade. A paradoxical pulse occurs frequently, but its presence is not diagnostic of a hemodynamically significant effusion. A paradoxical pulse may be absent in the presence of tamponade if the patient is severely hypotensive (28).

Congestive heart failure may cause considerable diagnostic difficulties since pericarditis and congestive heart failure frequently coexist and congestive heart failure may complicate the course of acute pericarditis either during conservative management or after surgery. Measurement of central venous pressure does not differentiate progressive heart failure or fluid overload from pericardial effusion since it is elevated in all three conditions and frequently exceeds 140 mm H_2O. A rapid increase in heart size, detected radiographically, particularly with clear lung fields, is suggestive of a pericardial effusion. The EKG is not diagnostic unless the P, QRS and T complexes all show alternans. The use of the Swan-Ganz catheter to obtain serial measurements of pulmonary artery, pulmonary capillary wedge and right ventricular pressures can be of the greatest value in differentiating hypotension due to cardiac tamponade from that caused by hypovolemia or increasing heart failure (39).

Hemorrhagic effusion frequently occurs as a complication of uremic pericarditis in both undialyzed and dialyzed patients (16, 18, 19, 32, 39, 40). Hemopericardium may also complicate pericardiocentesis as a result of laceration of the heart, or a coronary vessel, or trauma to the inflamed pericardial surfaces.

Cardiac arrhythmias frequently complicate uremic pericarditis and may occur early in the disease process (18, 19). Multiple causative factors for arrhythmias may be present in uremic patients including myocarditis, primary myocardial disease and changes in serum potassium levels. Cardiac arrhythmias and cardiac arrest may also develop with the onset of cardiac tamponade and they have frequently been noted during or after pericardiocentesis (18).

Myocarditis is a serious complication that is occasionally seen in association with uremic pericarditis and manifested by hypotension, intractable heart failure and serious arrhythmias. Drainage of the pericardial sac, pericardiectomy and corticosteroid therapy have been unsuccessful in alleviating this condition (19). A reversible cardiomyopathy characterized by pericarditis, massive cardiomegaly, gallop rhythm, hypotension, arrhythmias and sensitivity to digitalis has been described in uremic patients treated by severe protein restriction for prolonged periods of time (41, 42).

Heart failure may complicate the course of uremic pericarditis as a manifestation of myocarditis or preexisting heart disease. Acute left ventricular failure may occasionally occur during the treatment of uremic peri-

Table 7. Complications of uremic pericarditis.

Acute	Chronic
Pericardial effusion and tamponade	Subacute constrictive pericarditis
Hemopericardium	Constrictive pericarditis
Arrhythmias	
Myocarditis	
Heart failure	

carditis as the pericardial effusion disappears as a result of medical or surgical measures. This phenomenon in the dialyzed patient closely resembles the 'pericardial shock syndrome' reported by Spodick (37) in nonuremic patients, and is attributed to a sudden increase in venous return with relief of restriction in the presence of severe fluid overload.

Subacute constrictive pericarditis may follow after apparent resolution of an acute attack (18, 40). Patients complain of weight gain, fatigue, dyspnea and increased abdominal girth. Physical signs include hypotension, ascites, increasing peripheral edema, hepatomegaly and venous distention. A friction rub is frequently absent although it may be heard intermittently. Chest pain is infrequent. Radiologically, the heart size may be slightly enlarged or normal and pulmonary vascular congestion is absent. Echocardiography may show the presence of a small pericardial effusion and pericardial thickening.

Chronic constrictive pericarditis is a late complication that has been described with increasing frequency as more patients survive for longer periods of time on chronic hemodialysis after an episode of uremic pericarditis (19, 43–45). It must be differentiated from subacute and chronic constrictive pericarditis due to other causes (especially tuberculosis), and from congestive heart failure. Calcification has not been reported in uremic pericarditis to date. The diagnosis of constrictive pericarditis and differentiation from other lesions are made by angiocardiography and cardiac catheterization.

Management (Table 8)

Many centers treat pericarditis by augmentation of dialysis therapy although there are no laboratory studies to evaluate efficacy of such treatment. From the practical point of view, the role of hemodialysis therapy should be related to the patients' previous status. In the undialyzed uremic patient who is already on severe protein restriction, the development of pericarditis should indicate initiation of regular dialysis, which will cause resolution of pericarditis in 70% of cases. In the catabolic patient or patients without evidence of inadequate dialysis, it is customary to increase weekly dialysis time, preferably by increasing the frequency. Many centers perform daily dialysis for periods of 4 to 5 h on any of the currently available disposable dialyzers and continue such a regimen until the pericardial effusion decreases in size. Nevertheless, intensive dialysis should be abandoned in the face of increasing cardiac embarrassment and should not preclude the use of anti-inflammatory drugs if improvement does not occur during the first 2 to 3 days of therapy.

Peritoneal dialysis avoids the use of parenteral heparin and has been claimed to reduce the incidence of tamponade (24). Peritoneal dialysis has many advantages over hemodialysis apart from the avoidance of heparin. These include more gradual dehydration and avoidance of acute changes in intravascular volume. The decision to use peritoneal dialysis depends to a considerable extent on the facilities available to the physician. In untreated patients peritoneal dialysis avoids the dangers of heparinization in the presence of a hemorrhagic problem from uncontrolled uremia.

Problems with intensive dialysis, such as hypotension and dehydration, are particularly liable to occur during the dialysis procedure, when rapid changes in intravascular volume may precipitate clinical signs of cardiac tamponade (see preceeding paragraph on pathogenesis). It is preferable to restrict sodium and fluid intake between dialyses to avoid excessive weight gain and reduce the need for ultrafiltration. In stable patients who are normo- or hypotensive, with absent or small effusions, control of hydration presents few problems provided excessive or too rapid ultrafiltration is not attempted. Patients with unstable blood pressures or frank hypotension associated with large effusions, cardiac arrhythmias or evidence of severe fluid overload or myocardial failure require continuous monitoring using either a central venous pressure catheter or a Swan-Ganz catheter. Heart failure from fluid overload may necessitate gradual ultrafiltration by daily hemodialysis or by peritoneal dialysis. Surgical intervention should not be delayed when there are repeated problems with hypotension: an elective surgical procedure is preferable to emergency intervention.

Table 8. Management of pericarditis.

1. General
   Bed rest, monitor body weight, blood pressure, paradoxical pulse.
2. Maintain nutrition
   Adequate calories and protein, essential amino acid supplements.
3. Improve biochemical control of uremia
   Initiate dietary protein restriction.
   Initiate dialysis. Augment dialysis.
4. Control hydration and heart failure
   Salt and water restriction.
   Gentle ultrafiltration, small volume dialyzer.
   Digitalis.
   Central venous pressure monitor or Swan-Ganz catheter.
5. Prevent bleeding
   Discontinue oral anticoagulants.
   Regional heparinization.
   Peritoneal dialysis.
6. Anti-inflammatory drugs
   Indomethacin 25 mg three to four times daily.
   Prednisone 40 mg orally daily.
   Reduce dosage after 1 week, discontinue after 4 weeks.

Digitalis

The use of digitalis and related drugs in the management of pericarditis is disputed because of the theoretical possibility of a further reduction of venous return leading to decreased venous pressure (46). Nevertheless there is no reason to withhold digitalis when arrhythmias require its use, or when there is evidence of progressive heart failure. Drug dosage must be modified in the presence of renal failure and careful attention paid to potassium levels (see Chapter 39).

Anti-inflammatory drugs

Indomethacin is an anti-inflammatory drug which has been widely used in doses of 25 mg four times a day to treat nonuremic recurrent pericarditis without effusion (47). Dosage modification is not required in renal failure. Experience with indomethacin in uremic pericarditis is limited, although some observers have noted a good response in 50% of patients (20,48). Although there has been no mortality with its use, side effects such as nausea, vomiting, abdominal pain, headaches, occasional duodenal ulceration and gastrointestinal bleeding have required withdrawal of the drug in 20% of patients (20). The incidence of surgical intervention is similar to that of patients treated with prednisone. There are certain advantages to its usage in diabetic patients since it does not affect glucose homeostasis.

Experience with the use of prednisone in uremic pericarditis is limited (19, 20, 49), but it has been used successfully for many years for the treatment of idiopathic pericarditis (46). In one study the oral administration of 40 mg of prednisone daily to patients with high fever, severe pain and moderate or large pericardial effusion in the absence of sepsis, was followed by dramatic subsidence of pain and fever, diminution of friction rub and reduction in heart size within a week in 72% of patients (20). Thirty eight percent of patients failed to respond to prednisone or relapsed while prednisone was being withdrawn and were submitted to elective pericardiectomy. No complications have occurred with short term steroid therapy.

The administration of very large doses of nonabsorbable steroids (200 to 900 mg triamcinolone) into the pericardial sac after preliminary pericardiocentesis has achieved success in a limited number of patients (50). It is unclear, however, whether pericardiocentesis, per se, may have played a part in the relief of pain and subsidence of the effusion. Although the healthy pericardium may be impervious to nonabsorbable steroids, it is possible that, as with other serous membranes, significant absorption occurs across the inflamed pericardial surface. Hence, much of the beneficial effect may be a systemic steroid effect.

Surgical management (Table 9)

The role of pericardiocentesis in the management of uremic pericarditis is highly controversial, some investigators reporting a low mortality with either repeated pericardiocentesis or pericardiocentesis with catheter drainage (16, 17) while others have reported a mortality as high as 75% which they have attributed to the procedure (47, 48). Diagnostic pericardiocentesis may be necessary where there is a possibility that the effusion might be purulent or tuberculous. Pericardiocentesis can be life saving in the patient who develops acute tamponade. However the procedure should be undertaken with full precautions, with a surgeon available to perform emergency thoracotomy if complications occur. When the effusion is serous a simple aspiration may offer definitive cure. An open surgical procedure is preferable if the effusion is frankly hemorrhagic, or where clinical improvement fails to occur immediately, or when fluid reaccumulates.

A subxiphoid window has been used with some success by some investigators. These windows frequently close, however, allowing recurrent tamponade and there is a risk of incarceration or strangulation of the heart. Subacute and chronic constrictive pericarditis continue to be long term complications. Nevertheless, a subxiphoid window should be considered in patients who are unfit for a more extensive procedure, since it can be performed quickly under local anesthesia.

Pericardiectomy may vary from that of an anterior window with direct visualization of the pericardial sac, a partial pericardiectomy where more extensive resection is performed, to a total pericardiectomy where the heart is completely denuded of its pericardial covering. Many investigators consider that a large anterior window or even a partial pericardiectomy are treatments of choice for acute tamponade and large pericardial effusions which fail to respond to intensive hemodialysis and anti-inflammatory drugs (20, 51–53). Some cases of subacute constrictive pericarditis may benefit from a partial pericardiectomy if the patient is incapacitated by hypotension and fluid retention. An anterior pericardiectomy is mandatory for patients with a purulent pericarditis, in addition to full antibiotic therapy.

Table 9. Surgical management of pericarditis.

Procedure	Indication	Complications
Pericardiocentesis		
Simple aspiration	Diagnostic	Laceration of heart or coronary vessel
Intermittent aspiration	Emergency relief of tamponade	Failure to relieve tamponade
Catheter drainage		Recurrence of tamponade
		Arrhythmias
		Cardiac arrest
Subxiphoid window	Poor risk patients	Window closure, incarceration and strangulation of heart
Pericardiectomy		
Anterior window	Acute tamponade	Pulmonary infection
	Persistent or recurrent effusions after intensive dialysis and anti-inflammatory drugs	Acute heart failure
	Purulent pericarditis	
Partial pericardiectomy	Subacute constrictive pericarditis	
Total pericardiectomy	Constrictive pericarditis	

CARDIAC FAILURE

Pathogenesis

Cardiac function has been shown to be abnormal in patients with renal failure and many factors appear to be involved (Table 10). Although pulmonary edema (uremic lung) has long been recognized as a complication of acute and chronic renal failure, its pathogenesis is still in doubt. Left ventricular failure, increased pulmonary capillary permeability and fluid overload have all been invoked either singly or in combination. Although fluid overload appears to be of importance in the pathogenesis of pulmonary edema (54, 55), the absence of clearly elevated right aterial and pulmonary vascular pressures suggest that pulmonary capillary permeability is increased in acute and chronic renal failure (52, 53, 56, 57) and that fluid overload merely facilitates the appearance of uremic lungs (55).

Table 10. Factors affecting cardiac function in renal failure patients.

Etiological factor	Effect on cardiac function	Reference
Uremia	Increased pulmonary capillary permeability ('uremic lung')	56, 57
	Altered myocardial muscle metabolism	58–60
	Altered ATPase activity	61
	Uremic cardiomyopathy?	16, 41, 42
	Abnormal baroreceptor response	90, 95
Anemia	High output, low peripheral resistance	69–71
	Increased peripheral O_2 extraction	72
A-V fistula	High output, low peripheral resistance	77–79
Fluid overload	High cardiac output Normal or raised peripheral resistance	72
Hypertension	High cardiac output Raised peripheral resistance Low or high renin secretion	87, 90–92
Calcific cardiomyopathy	Heart failure, arrhythmias	101–105
ASHD*	Reduced stroke volume, cardiac output and ejection fraction	100
Scleroderma	Pericarditis (14%) Arrhythmias Heart block Cardiomegaly Systemic and pulmonary hypertension	
Beri-beri	High output congestive heart failure Peripheral neuritis	

* ASHD = atherosclerotic heart disease.

Experimental work suggests that the myocardium may be specifically damaged by uremia (58–61), but the existence of a specific uremic myocardiopathy is controversial at the present time. A reversible cardiomyopathy, characterized by pericarditis, massive cardiomegaly, hypotension, arrhythmias and increased sensitivity to digitalis, has been described in patients maintained for prolonged periods of time on low protein diets (41, 42). The condition is completely reversed by the initiation of regular hemodialysis alone without any change in dietary protein intake (41). These syndromes may be a direct result of uremia. Other observers have reported irreversible cardiomyopathy in dialyzed patients characterized by ventricular dilatation and myocardial hypokinesis (16). However malnutrition, vitamin deficiency, anemia, hypertension, heart failure, pericarditis, and preexisting atherosclerotic heart disease may all be contributing factors. Vitamin B_1 deficiency (beri-beri) can cause a similar clinical picture and may only be differentiated on the basis of red cell transketolase activity and therapeutic response to the administration of thiamine (62). Severe congestive cardiomyopathy may also result from decreased serum phosphate levels (63) and possibly from iron deficiency (64).

Renal failure is frequently associated with an increased cardiac output which has been attributed to anemia (65–68). Studies on anemic patients with normal renal function show that the increase in cardiac output is proportional to the degree of anemia (69, 70). The increased cardiac output has been attributed to a diminished peripheral resistance, resulting from decreased blood viscosity (71) and local peripheral vasodilation attributed to inadequate oxygen delivery to the tissues (69, 70). The increased cardiac output and peripheral blood flow coupled with increased oxygen extraction may be insufficient to supply adequate oxygen to tissues such as the heart muscle, hence pain may ensue. When the degree of anemia is extremely severe, anginal pain may be precipitated by exercise, tachycardia, or when blood volume and hence cardiac output are acutely reduced such as occurs during dialysis particularly when ultrafiltration is performed. In patients with ischemic heart disease, coronary blood supply is already compromised and anginal episodes may be precipitated at much less severe degrees of anemia. Even in the absence of uremia and of antecedent heart disease, the development of high output congestive heart failure in severely anemic patients (hemoglobin concentration below 5 g/dl) is well documented (70). Such heart failure can be aggravated when the usual hypovolemic state is changed to hypervolemia. The contribution of anemia to the development of heart failure in uremic patients is probably considerable, especially in the presence of hypervolemia. Nevertheless, when patients treated by chronic dialysis are transfused up to a normal hematocrit, while maintaining a constant blood volume, cardiac output decreases, reaching a normal value when the hematocrit is 30%. Despite a constant blood volume, blood pressure and peripheral resistance rise as in nonuremic patients (72). These observations suggest that the anemia of chronic renal failure may fortuitously protect patients from the effects of severe hypertension by reducing peripheral resistance. In acute renal failure cardiac function is also abnormal and the hyperkinetic circulation is considered to be unrelated to anemia or extracellular volume expansion. Diminished peripheral resistance has been attributed to impaired vasoconstrictive activity, but the precise mechanism is uncertain (69).

The development of the Brescia-Cimino arteriovenous (AV) fistula (73) has been a major advance in the field of long term hemodialysis and has diminished the problems of infection and clotting that were associated with the use of the AV shunt. Whereas blood flow rates through a Scribner AV shunt vary from 200 to 300 ml/min and tend to be stable during the life span of the cannula system, blood flow rates through the simple AV fistula are more variable, and hemodynamic studies show that the fistula may contribute up to 28% of the resting cardiac output (74–76). The hemodynamic effects of an AV fistula have been studied extensively in nonuremic patients, and closely resemble those seen in anemia (77–80), namely a decrease in the peripheral resistance, and a compensatory increase in cardiac output to maintain arterial blood pressure. The increase is achieved by a tachycardia. Later, compensatory hypervolemia increases stroke volume and maintains the raised cardiac output as the heart rate falls. Cardiomegaly and high output congestive heart failure are well recognized complications of AV fistulae in nonuremic patients and may occur even in the healthy heart. Although isolated cases of heart failure resulting from the presence of a Brescia-Cimino fistula (74–76) have been reported, many observers are reluctant to attribute heart failure to the presence of a fistula alone in the majority of cases (80, 81). Provided fistula flows are small, changes in cardiac output are insignificant at rest and only become substantially elevated at a level of exercise not usually attained by the chronic hemodialysis patient (82). Deterioration of cardiac function most often relates to hypertension, fluid overload, anemia and underlying ischemic heart disease. However, the increased work load introduced by even a small peripheral fistula may precipitate heart failure in patients with severely compromised cardiac function.

Whether or not the AV fistula is causing deterioration in cardiac function can be assessed using two clinical tests. A temporary occlusion of an AV fistula frequently results in a bradycardia referred to as a Nicoladini-Branham sign (82, 83), which is a reflex action blocked by atropine. A positive sign is highly indicative of compromised cardiac function. Measurements of blood flow velocity through the intact skin are also now feasible utilizing the Doppler technique. The volume of flow can be determined if the diameter of the fistula is known.

Some degree of extracellular volume expansion is present in the majority of patients with renal failure despite the absence of overt edema and may contribute to the appearance of well-being of many patients despite clinical and biochemical evidence of malnutrition (84). The well documented post transplant diuresis is attributed to extracellular volume expansion that is not apparent clinically. Fluid overload, by increasing venous return to the right heart, may participate in the increased cardiac output observed in patients with renal failure (85–87).

Clinical and experimental studies suggest that extracellular volume expansion is intimately linked to the high incidence of hypertension in renal failure. In the majority of dialyzed patients hypertension can be controlled by correcting extracellular volume (88, 89). Hemodynamic studies have yielded variable results on the mechanism involved. In the absence of heart failure the main effect of hemodialysis is to reduce cardiac output, right atrial and mean pulmonary artery pressures (68, 69, 86, 89, 90). However, no change in cardiac output or plasma volume occurs if fluid is not removed during dialysis (89). During dialysis peripheral resistance tends to rise, and the variable change in blood pressure during dialysis appears to be causally related to this phenomenon. In the dialysis patient with heart failure hemodynamic changes are somwhat different in that cardiac output tends to increase by a combination of mechanisms including reduction of extracellular fluid overload, and reduction in total peripheral resistance in parallel with a decrease in blood volume (86). Increased peripheral resistance rather than increased cardiac output appears to be responsible for the development of hypertension since normalization of cardiac output by raising the hematocrit to 40% is paralleled by an increase in peripheral resistance and blood pressure (72).

In some patients hypertension may not respond to extracellular volume depletion and may actually worsen (90). These patients frequently exhibit marked generalized weakness and refractory heart failure and attempts to reduce extracellular volume expansion by ultrafiltration during dialysis are offset by frequent episodes of severe hypotension. Plasma renin levels are high and hemodynamic studies show a raised cardiac output and increased peripheral resistance (67, 72, 89). Bilateral nephrectomy has been repeatedly demonstrated to be effective in reducing hypertension and decreasing peripheral vascular resistance (90–94). Thereafter, hypertension may still occur but has become responsive to extracellular volume depletion (see also Chapter 28). Although it has been suggested that hypertension in the patient with chronic renal failure is due to a resetting of baroreceptor control (95), more recent studies suggest that most uremic patients regardless of whether hypertensive or not have a blunted baroreceptor response, in that changes in blood pressure are not accompanied by the normal changes in heart rate. An increase in blood pressure is not associated with a bradycardia, and more importantly uremic patients may not show the expected tachycardia when the blood pressure is acutely lowered (89, 96–100). Neuropathy of the autonomic nervous system has been implicated, and the presence of preexisting hypertension, myocardial disease and anemia may be contributing factors.

In ischemic heart disease, cardiac function may be affected to varying degrees. Reductions in stroke volume, cardiac output and mean systolic ejection fraction while present at rest, are more marked during exercise. Increased venous return may cause a decrease in stroke volume and increase in heart rate rather than the usual response of increased stroke volume with little change in heart rate (99, 100). In renal failure, many factors affect-

Table 11. Cardiac manifestations of systemic disease causing renal failure.

Systemic disease	Cardiac manifestations
Diabetes mellitus	Generalized atherosclerosis Coronary artery insufficiency Myocardial infarction Hypertension, postural hypotension
Amyloidosis	Mild cardiomegaly Valvular stenosis and insufficiency Restrictive cardiomyopathy Low cardiac output, low blood pressure Postural hypotension Myocardial infarction
Systemic lupus erythematosus	Endocarditis Pericarditis → tamponade Aortic and mitral murmurs Arrhythmias, atrial fibrillation, A-V block
Periarteritis nodosa hypersensitivity angiitis	Hypertension Refractory heart failure Myocardial infarction Arrhythmias

ing cardiac function are associated with an increase in venous return (anemia, AV fistula, fluid overload) and adversely affect patients with chronic ischemic heart disease. Severe anemia, and acute intravascular volume changes, in the absence of a compensatory increase in cardiac output, may cause ischemic cardiac pain and may precipitate acute myocardial infarction.

Severe myocardial involvement by calcium deposition manifest by heart block, arrhythmias, intractible heart failure and acute cardiac arrest, has been well documented in the dialyzed patient (101–105). The condition is attributed to a persistently elevated calcium × phosphate product in plasma as a result of either hyperparathyroidism, vitamin D administration, failure to normalize serum phosphorus, or the use of a high calcium dialysate. Calcium phosphate deposition may be facilitated by a postdialysis alkalemia (106). Radiological signs of renal osteodystrophy and soft tissue metastatic calcification have been notably absent. Autopsy findings include marked calcium deposition in the atrioventricular node, intraventricular septum and the ventricular myocardium. Contiguglia and coworkers (107) have shown a correlation between skeletal and myocardial calcium content, which may prove of value in diagnosing the condition during life.

Many centers are accepting patients with systemic disease affecting the kidneys and which may involve the heart and other organs (Table 11). In diabetes mellitus, generalized atherosclerosis is common and is responsible for the high mortality of diabetic patients treated by chronic hemodialysis (28). The heart is frequently affected by coronary artery disease and by hypertension, and the clinical picture is frequently complicated by an autonomic neuropathy with attendent problems of postural hypotension. Systemic lupus erythematosus may involve the heart with endocarditis, pericarditis, aortic and mitral murmurs, and arrhythmias. Amyloidosis frequently involves the heart with infiltration of the myocardium and conducting tissue and involvement of the heart valves simulating valvular heart disease. Loss of myocardial distensibility results in a constrictive cardiomyopathy which must be distinguished from constrictive pericarditis. Other conditions including polyarteritis nodosa and scleroderma may affect both kidneys and heart.

Management of heart failure

Management of heart failure in the dialysis patient consists of alleviating conditions known to increase cardiac work load, and removal of possible precipitating factors. Careful evaluation including the use of echocardiography and radionuclide left ventriculography (108, 109) may identify patients with anatomically significant valvular lesions and evaluate the effect of vasodilator drug therapy. Right or left heart catheterization and coronary artery arteriography can be performed safely with low morbidity and mortality in dialyzed patients (109). Surgical intervention has been shown to be of benefit in patients with aortic or mitral valve disease as in nonuremic patients (110). Coronary artery bypass surgery may alleviate angina and possibly prolong survival in selected patients (110). In the prevention of heart failure (Table 12), emphasis is placed on reducing the degree of fluid overload by dialyzing thrice weekly, restricting sodium and fluid intake between dialysis and by adjusting the post dialysis weight to be commensurate with the patient's nutritional state. Acute pulmonary edema may occur unexpectedly after many weeks of poor dietary

Table 12. Management of heart failure.

Prevention
  Adequate hemodialysis thrice weekly.
  Sodium and fluid restriction between dialysis.
  Adjust post dialysis weight to nutritional status.
  Control hypertension by volume depletion, nephrectomy, antihypertensive drugs.
  Minimize anemia—diet, iron, anabolic steroids, reduce blood loss.

Acute heart failure
  Rest, nasal oxygen, aminophylline, venesection.
  Immediate hemodialysis or hemofiltration.
  Gradual ultrafiltration to appropriate weight.
  Treat precipitating causes—tachycardia, tachyarrhythmias, infection, pulmonary emboli, bacterial endocarditis.
  Digitalize if uncontrolled by fluid removal.

Chronic heart failure
  Sodium and water restriction, ultrafiltration.
  Maintain systolic pressure—3% saline, plasma, I.V. metaraminol (Aramine).
  Consider chronic peritoneal dialysis.
  Digitalis glycosides.
  Assess fistula flow.
  Vasodilation drug therapy.

intake. Older patients with underlying heart disease, particularly coronary artery disease, are intolerant of further extracellular volume expansion and tend to go into overt heart failure with small increments of excess volume. Hypertension adds a pressure load to the volume load of the heart and therefore, prevention of fluid overload is essential. In about 10 to 20% of patients, progressive ultrafiltration cannot achieve adequate control of hypertension and plasma renin levels are extremely high before dialysis. These patients benefit from bilateral nephrectomy. Anemia increases the myocardial work load if the hematocrit is less than 30%. The degree of anemia should be minimized by an adequate diet, with judicial iron and anabolic steroid therapy, and the avoidance of biliateral nephrectomy unless absolutely indicated for uncontrollable hypertension or infection. Blood transfusion may be necessary when the hematocrit falls to a level at which congestive heart failure is intractable or angina develops.

Acute heart failure (acute pulmonary edema) requires emergency treatment. It usually results from fluid overload as a result of dietary salt and fluid indiscretions or intravenous therapy but may occur in patients eating poorly. Acute myocardial infarction, pulmonary embolization, resolving pericarditis, tachyarrhythmias, severe infection, and bacterial endocarditis may also cause this complication. The basic therapeutic principles consist of nasal oxygen, aminophylline and emergency venesection. Hemodialysis is a very effective method of performing an immediate venesection followed by a more gradual reduction of blood volume by ultrafiltration during the remainder of the dialysis. Similar results can be obtained by hemofiltration. Peritoneal dialysis is less effective for the emergency treatment of acute heart failure since ultrafiltration is slower and patients may be intolerant of diaphragmatic splinting.

Chronic heart failure may be a recurrent problem in older patients with severe underlying coronary artery disease or hypertensive heart disease, or where the heart is involved by systemic disease. These patients are characteristically intolerant of minor degrees of fluid overload and develop hypotension, arrhythmias and angina pectoris when ultrafiltration is attempted. Prevention of fluid overload by careful restriction of sodium and water between dialysis, and by slow ultrafiltration are appropriate. Hypotension occurring at the initiation of hemodialysis can be avoided in many patients by using a low blood flow rate during the early stages of dialysis and by using small volume dialyzers. Occasionally, it may be necessary to prime the dialyzer with saline or plasma which is infused into the patient to avoid rapid changes in blood volume at the commencement of dialysis. Although hypotension may improve as ultrafiltration during dialysis alleviates heart failure, often the degree of hypotension may be so severe as to reduce cerebral and coronary blood flow. Infusions of hypertonic saline (150 ml of 3%) and plasma (if the plasma albumin concentration is low) may be utilized to maintain blood pressure while ultrafiltering. In patients with impaired peripheral vasoconstriction small doses of pressor agents may be helpful in achieving adequate ultrafiltration. In some patients with chronic congestive heart failure, peritoneal dialysis should be considered as an alternative to hemodialysis since ultrafiltration is more gradual and produces less acute changes in intravascular volume. As in nonuremic patients, use of digitalis glycosides is of benefit. Attention should be paid to the degree of anemia in these patients and blood flow rates should be evaluated if a simple fistula is being used. Intractable heart failure must be differentiated from constrictive pericarditis and requires right heart catheterization.

Management of myocardial infarction

The immediate management of dialysis patients after myocardial infarction is similar to that of nonuremic patients, emphasis being placed on prevention of serious arrhythmias, relief of pain, anxiety and heart failure. Fluid restriction becomes of paramount importance in this situation to prevent extracellular volume expansion contributing to the development of heart failure. Whenever possible hemodialysis should be delayed for 24 h after myocardial infarction, especially in patients with severe hypotension and arrhythmias. Nevertheless, the development of acute pulmonary edema, particularly in the patient who is obviously fluid overloaded, may require more urgent hemodialysis or peritoneal dialysis. If digitalis is prescribed the dosage must be adapted in accord with the severity of renal failure, the use of dialysis and with potassium abnormalities (see also Chapter 39).

The long term management of dialysis patients after myocardial infarction is aimed at alleviating or preventing conditions that increase cardiac work load namely extracellular volume expansion, hypertension and anemia. Coronary arteriography is of value in determining the extent of disease and whether surgical revascularization would be of value, as in nonuremic patients (110). Anticoagulants are of benefit in the acute phase of myocardial infarction. For chronic coronary insufficiency vasodilators may be helpful. Nitroglycerin, isosorbide dinitrate (Isordil) and propranolol are widely used to relieve angina and also to improve coronary blood flow, although propranolol should be avoided in patients with heart failure. In large doeses Isordil may produce hypotension. Propranolol, a beta-adrenergic blocker, reduces coronary vasoconstriction, improves blood pressure control in the dialyzed patient and effectively relieves angina especially when combined with moderate doses of Isordil. Otherwise, the management of the patient after myocardial infarction is similar to the management of those with chronic heart failure, namely reduction of the cardiac work load where possible by controlling factors such as anemia, hypertension and fluid overload.

BACTERIAL ENDOCARDITIS

Bacterial endocarditis has been reported as a complication of cannula and fistula infections, of peritoneal dialysis, and after renal transplantation (111-117). In our own program bacterial endocarditis accounted for 1.7%

of deaths and osteomyelitis was present in association with bacterial endocarditis in several cases (118).

The diagnosis of bacterial endocarditis frequently may be missed until late in the course of the disease, since many of the classical clinical findings are either absent or attributed to other causes. Fever is always present in bacterial endocarditis, but in dialysis patients it may be attributed to problems such as cannula infections and pyrogenic reactions. However, bacterial endocarditis should always be excluded in patients with prolonged fever. Splenomegaly may occur with endocarditis, but in the dialysis patient it may be due to red cell sequestration, or the spleen may have been removed in patients awaiting transplantation. Neurological manifestations have been reported, sometimes being prominent early symptoms and may include seizures and disturbances in the level of consciousness. Nevertheless neurological changes are frequently due to other causes including subdural hematoma, disequilibrium syndrome, cerebrovascular accident and aluminum intoxication (119).

Heart murmurs are frequent in dialysis patients. In many cases these are systolic flow murmurs usually attributed to anemia and a high cardiac output. In bacterial endocarditis the aortic valve is usually involved, either singly or in combination with other valves and the appearance of an aortic diastolic murmur de novo should always arouse suspicion of bacterial endocarditis. Functional diastolic murmurs have been described in uremic patients, and have been attributed to the presence of severe congestive heart failure and hypertension. The murmurs disappear with control of these factors (120, 121). A pericardial effusion was demonstrated by echocardiography in 5 out of 6 patients investigated by Barratt and his colleagues (121) who felt that in some instances, the so-called diastolic murmur was a sound of pericardial origin. The functional diastolic murmur associated with renal failure differs in location and quality from that of aortic incompetence. It is usually localized in the apical area rather than the left sternal edge, and is of maximum intensity with the patient supine rather than sitting. Failure of the diastolic murmur to disappear with control of uremia and fluid overload and in the absence of pericarditis should be followed by hemodynamic and bacteriological studies to exclude bacterial endocarditis. The usual cause of death from bacterial endocarditis is valvular perforation and heart failure. Underlying heart disease is frequent in these patients and may facilitate the appearance of congestive heart failure. Treatment consists of a six week course of parenteral antibiotic therapy, the type of antibiotic used being dependent on the organism isolated. It must be emphasized that antibiotic therapy alone may be unsuccessful and early valve replacement appears to be the treatment of choice for prolonged survival (112, 122–124).

CARDIAC ARRHYTHMIAS

All the arrhythmias including the so-called benign rhythm disturbances carry some risk of converting to lethal arrhythmias. In the dialyzed patient cardiac arrhythmias may be precipitated by many factors (Table 13). Arrhythmias occurring during dialysis must be differentiated from pseudoarrhythmias related to the use of a blood pump (125). Cardiac arrhythmias due to inappropriate ventilation are well documented in the literature (126) and are equally liable to occur in dialyzed patients. Dialysis induced increases in plasma bicarbonate and pH (106, 127–132) probably induce arrhythmias by alterations in intracellular potassium levels, since a linear inverse relationship between potassium and extracellular pH exists during both respiratory and metabolic alterations of hydrogen ion concentration (132). In patients with atherosclerotic heart disease, arrhythmias frequently develop in association with hypotension and acute volume changes during dialysis or when anemia is severe (hematocrit less than 20%).

Calcium and potassium have a profound effect on cardiac activity, not only in terms of serum and tissue levels, but also in relationship to each other, whether digitalis is being given or not. The patient with renal failure who has hyperkalemia and hypocalcemia together is more likely to develop an acute arrhythmia, and a cardiac arrest, than the patient with either problem alone. Hypomagnesemia may facilitate the development of digitalis induced toxicity. Hypercalcemia may occur in dialysed patients as a result of severe hyperparathyroidism or excessive administration of calcium and vitamin D derivatives. Hypercalcemia causes increased myocardial contractility and shortening of the QT interval when levels are 13 mg/dl (3.2 mmol/l) or higher. Hypercalcemia in the digitalized patient may lead to early digitalis toxicity and arrhythmias. Serum potassium changes during dialysis are affected both by acid base balance and by removal of potassium across the dialyzer. A dialysate potassium concentration of 1.5 mmol/l used on stable patients has not been associated with potassium depletion (131) despite the presence of mild hypokalemia after each dialysis. Nevertheless in our own experience this level of dialysate potassium has been associated with a significant number of arrhythmias in debilitated and malnourished patients especially in the older age groups. The use of a dialysate potassium concentration of 2 to 3 mmol/l has eliminated arrhythmias in sus-

Table 13. Factors precipitating arrhythmias.

1. Pericarditis
2. ASHD*: Severe anemia, acute myocardial infarction acute volume changes, congestive heart failure
3. Hyper- and hypokalemia
4. Hyper- and hypovolemia
5. Hypoxemia
6. Hypocapnia
7. Acidosis, alkalosis
8. Hyper- and hypocalcemia
9. Hyper- and hypomagnesemia
10. Calcific cardiomyopathy
11. Systemic diseases (Table 11)

* ASHD = Atherosclerotic heart disease.

ceptible patients. The rate of change of plasma potassium concentration rather than the absolute level appears to be important. Particular attention must be given to maintaining a stable plasma potassium concentration when patients are receiving digitalis.

Severe hyperkalemia produces characteristic electrocardiographic changes and ventricular fibrillation or asystole may result from high levels (7.0 mmol/l or more [see Chapters 19 and 26]). Acute hyperkalemia may be responsible for many cases of sudden death occurring in dialyzed patients. Hyperkalemia is preventable by adjustment of potassium intake and dialysate potassium.

REFERENCES

1. Scribner BH: The treatment of chronic uremia by means of intermittent hemodialysis. *Trans Am Soc Artif Intern Organs* 6:114, 1960
2. Lindner A, Charra B, Sherrard DJ, Scribner BH: Accelerated atherosclerosis in prolonged maintenance hemodialysis. *N Engl J Med* 290:697, 1974
3. Drukker W, Alberts C, Odé A, Roosendaal KJ, Wilmink JM: Report on regular dialysis treatment in Europe. *Proc Eur Dial Transpl Assoc* 3:90, 1966
4. Drukker W, Schouten WAG, Alberts C: Report on regular dialysis treatment in Europe. *Proc Eur Dial Transpl Assoc* 4:3, 1967
5. Drukker W, Schouten WAG, Alberts C: Report on regular dialysis treatment in Europe. *Proc Eur Dial Transpl Assoc* 5:3, 1968
6. Drukker W, Haagsma-Schouten WAG, Alberts C, Spoek MG: Report on regular dialysis treatment in Europe. *Proc Eur Dial Transpl Assoc* 6:99, 1969
7. Drukker W, Haagsma-Schouten WAG, Alberts C, Baarda B: Report on regular dialysis treatment in Europe. *Proc Eur Dial Transpl Assoc* 7:3, 1970
8. Brunner FP, Gurland HJ, Härlen H, Schärer K, Parsons FM: Combined report on regular dialysis and transplantation in Europe. *Proc Eur Dial Transpl Assoc* 8:3, 1972
9. Gurland HJ, Brunner FP, v Dehn H, Härlen H, Parsons FM, Schärer K: Combined report on regular dialysis and transplantation in Europe 1972. *Proc Eur Dial Transpl Assoc* 10:17, 1973
10. Brunner FP, Giesecke B, Gurland HJ, Jacobs C, Parsons FM, Schärer K, Seyffart G, Spies G, Wing AJ: Combined report on regular dialysis and transplantation in Europe 1974. *Proc Eur Dial Transpl Assoc* 12:3, 1975
11. Burton BT, Krueger KK, Bryan JA: National registry of long term dialysis patients. *JAMA* 218:718, 1971
12. Radel EI, Bloomfield DA, Haller JD, Defer W: A case of relapsing seroconstrictive pericarditis: Definition of a syndrome. *Am J Cardiol* 28:221, 1971
13. Langendorf R, Pirani CL: The heart in uremia — An electrocardiographic and pathologic study. *Am Heart J* 33:282, 1974
14. Wacker W, Merrill JP: Uremic paricarditis in acute and chronic renal failure. *JAMA* 156:764, 1954
15. Wray TM, Stone WJ: Uremic pericarditis: A prospective echocardiographic and clinical study. *Clin Nephrol* 6:295, 1976
16. Drueke T, Le Pailleur C, Zingraff J, Jungers P: Uremic cardiomyopathy and pericarditis. *Adv Nephrol* 9:33, 1980
17. Bailey GL, Hampers CL, Hager EB, Merrill JP: Uremic pericarditis, clinical features and management. *Circulation* 38:582, 1968
18. Ribot S, Frankel HJ, Gielchinsky I, Gilbert L: Treatment of uremic pericarditis. *Clin Nephrol* 2:127, 1974
19. Comty CM, Wathen R, Shapiro FL: Pericarditis in chronic uremia and its sequels. *Ann Intern Med* 75:173, 1971
20. Comty CM, Wathen R, Shapiro F: Incidence, mortality and effects of treatment on uremic pericarditis. *Abstracts Am Soc Nephrol* 8:28, 1975
21. Bright R: Tabular view of the morbid appearances of 100 cases connected with albuminous urine: with observations. *Guy Hosp Rep* 1:338, 1836
22. Bergström J, Fürst P: Uremic middle molecules. *Clin Nephrol* 5:143, 1976
23. Freeman RM, Lawton RL, Chamberlain MA: Hard water syndrome. *N Engl J Med* 276:1113, 1967
24. Cohen GF, Burgess JH, Kaye M: Peritoneal dialysis for the treatment of pericarditis in patients on chronic hemodialysis. *Can Med Assoc J* 102:1365, 1970
25. Skov SE, Hansen HE, Spencer ES: Uremic pericarditis. *Acta Med Scand* 186:421, 1969
26. Alfrey AC, Goss JE, Ogden DA, Vogel JHK, Holmes JH: Uremic hemopericardium. *Am J Med* 45:391, 1968
27. Clarkson BA: Uric acid related to uraemic symptoms. *Proc Eur Dial Transpl Assoc* 3:3, 1976
28. Spodick DH: Acute cardiac tamponade: Pathologic physiology, diagnosis and management. *Prog Cardiovasc Dis* 10:64, 1967
29. Comty CM, Kjellsen D, Shapiro FL: A reassessment of the prognosis of diabetic patients treated by chronic hemodialysis (CHD). *Trans Am Soc Artif Intern Organs* 22:404, 1976
30. Pabico RC, Hanshaw JB, Talley TE: Cytomegalovirus infection in chronic hemodialysis patients. *Abstracts Western Dial Transpl Soc* 1971
31. Harris CL, Benchimol A, Desser KB: Bacteroides pericardial effusion and cardiac tamponade in a patient with chronic renal failure. *Am Heart J* 89:629, 1975
32. Hager EB: Clinical observations of five patients with uremic pericardial tamponade. *N Engl J Med* 273:304, 1965
33. Bulkley BH, Humphries JO, Hutchins GM: Purulent pericarditis with asymmetric cardiac tamponade: A cause of death months after coronary artery bypass surgery. *Am Heart J* 93:776, 1977
34. Morse JR, Oretsky MI, Hudson JA: Pericarditis as a complication of meningococcal meningitis. *Ann Intern Med* 74:212, 1971
35. Osanloo E, Shalhoub RJ, Cioffi RF, Parker RH: Viral pericarditis in patients receiving hemodialysis. *Arch Intern Med* 139:301, 1979
36. Silverberg S, Oreopoulos DG, Wise DJ, Uden DE, Meindok H, Jones M, Rapoport A, Deveber GA: Pericarditis in patients undergoing long-term hemodialysis and peritoneal dialysis. Incidence, complications and management. *Am J Med* 63:874, 1977
37. Spodick DH: Arrhythmias during acute pericarditis. *JAMA* 235:39, 1976
38. Rubin RH, Moellering RC Jr: Clinical, microbiologic and therapeutic aspects of purulent pericarditis. *Am J Med* 59:68, 1975
39. Burton JR, Wands JR, Voigt GC, Sterioff S Jr, Caralis DG, Zachary JB, Smith GW: An approach to pericardial effusion in hemodialysis patients. *Johns Hopkins Med J* 133:312, 1973

40. Beaudry C, Nakamoto S, Kolff WJ: Uremic pericarditis and cardiac tamponade in chronic renal failure. *Ann Intern Med* 64:990, 1966
41. Bailey GL, Hampers CL, Merrill JP: Reversible cardiomyopathy in uremia. *Trans Am Soc Artif Intern Organs* 13:263, 1967
42. Lanhez LE, Lowen J, Sabbaga E: Uremic myocardiopathy. *Nephron* 15:17, 1975
43. Wolfe SA, Bailey GF, Collins JJ Jr: Constrictive pericarditis following uremic effusion. *J Thorac Cardiovasc Surg* 63:540, 1972
44. Lindsay J Jr, Crawley IS, Callaway GM: Chronic constrictive pericarditis following uremic hemopericardium. *Am Heart J* 79:390, 1970
45. Esmond WG, Lee YC, Hernandez F: Successful pericardiectomy in chronic constrictive uremic pericarditis. *South Med J* 64:533, 1971
46. McMichael J, Sharpey-Schafer EP: Action of intravenous digoxin in man. *Q J Med* 37:123, 1945
47. Hatcher CR, Logue RB, Logan WD, Symbas PN, Mansour KA, Abbott OA: Pericardiectomy for recurrent pericarditis. *J Thorac Cardiovasc Surg* 62:371, 1971
48. Minuth ANW, Nottebohm GA, Eknoyan G, Suki WN: Indomethacin treatment of pericarditis in chronic hemodialysis patients. *Arch Intern Med* 135:807, 1975
49. Eliasson G, Murphy FF: Steroid therapy in uremic patients: A report of three cases. *JAMA* 229:1634, 1974
50. Buselmeier TJ, Simmons RL, von Hartitzsch B, Najarian JS, Kjellstrand CM: Persistent uremic pericardial effusion: Pericardial drainage and localized steroid instillation as definitive therapy. *Abstracts Am Soc Nephrol* 6:17, 1973
51. Ghavamian M, Gutch CF, Hughes RK, Kopp KF, Kolff WJ: Pericardial tamponade in chronic hemodialysis patients: Treatment by pericardiectomy. *Arch Intern Med* 131:249, 1973
52. Singh S, Newmark K, Ishikawa I, Mitra S, Berman LB: Pericardiectomy in uremia: The treatment of choice for cardiac tamponade in chronic renal failure. *JAMA* 228:1132, 1974
53. Wray TM, Humphreys J, Perry JM, Stone WJ, Bender WH Jr: Pericardiectomy for treatment of uremic pericarditis. *Circulation* (Suppl II), 49 and 50:268, 1974
54. Alwall N, Lunderquist A, Olsson O: Studies on electrolyte – fluid retention; uremic lung – fluid lung? On pathogenesis and therapy (prelim. report). *Acta Med Scand* 146:157, 1953
55. Merrill JP: *The Treatment of Renal Failure. Therapeutic Principles in the Management of Acute and Chronic Uremia.* 2nd edn. New York, Grune and Stratton, 1965, p 113
56. Gibson DG: Haemodynamic factors in the development of acute pulmonary oedema in renal failure. *Lancet* 2:1217, 1966
57. Mostert JW, Evers JL, Hobika GH, Moore RH, Murphy GP: Cardiac evaluation in renal and pulmonary insufficiency. *NY State J Med* 70:1196, 1970
58. Raab W: Cardiotoxic substances in the blood and heart muscle in uremia (their nature and action). *J Lab Clin Med* 29:715, 1944
59. Knowlan DM, Platnek DA, Olson RE: Myocardial metabolism and cardiac output in uremia. *Clin Res* 9:941, 1960
60. Scheuer J, Stezoski S: The effects of uremic compounds on cardiac function and metabolism. *J Mol Cell Cardiol* 5:287, 1973
61. Pakkarimen A, Ilsalo E: Excretion of vanilmandelic acid (VMA) in patients with renal insufficiency. *Ann Intern Med* 54:175, 1965
62. Gotloib L, Servadio C: A possible case of beri-beri heart failure in a chronic hemodialyzed patient. *Nephron* 14:293, 1975
63. Darsee JR, Nutter DO: Reversible severe congestive cardiomyopathy in three cases of hypophosphatemia. *Ann Intern Med* 89:867, 1978
64. Jacobs A: The non-haematological effects of iron deficiency. *Clin Sci Mol Med* 53:105, 1977
65. DeFazio V, Christensen RC, Regan TJ, Baer LJ, Morita Y, Hellems HK: Circulatory changes in acute glomerulonephritis. *Circulation* 20:190, 1959
66. Agrest A, Finkielman S: Hemodynamics in acute renal failure: Pathogenesis of hyperkinetic circulation. *Am J Cardiol* 19:213, 1967
67. Goss JE, Alfrey AC, Vogel JHK, Holmes JH: Hemodynamic changes during hemodialysis. *Trans Am Soc Artif Intern Organs* 13:68, 1967
68. Bower JD, Coleman TG: Circulatory function during chronic hemodialysis. *Trans Am Soc Artif Intern Organs* 15:373, 1969
69. Richardson TQ, Guyton AC: Effects of polycythemia and anemia on cardiac output and other circulatory factors. *Am J Physiol* 197:1167, 1959
70. Graettinger JS, Parsons RL, Campbell JA: Correlation of clinical and hemodynamic studies in patients with mild and severe anemia with and without congestive failure. *Ann Intern Med* 58:617, 1963
71. Sharpey-Schafer EP: Cardiac output in severe anemia. *Clin Sci* 5:125, 1944
72. Neff MS, Kim KE, Persoff M, Onesti G, Swartz C: Hemodynamics of uremic anemia. *Circulation* 43:876, 1971
73. Brescia MJ, Cimino JE, Appel K, Hurwich BJ: Chronic hemodialysis using venipuncture and a surgically created arteriovenous fistula. *N Engl J Med* 275:1089, 1966
74. Ahearn DJ, Maher JF: Heart failure as a complication of hemodialysis arteriovenous fistula. *Ann Intern 'Med* 77:201, 1972
75. Anderson CB, Codd JR, Craff GM, Harter HR, Newton WT: Cardiac failure and upper extremity arteriovenous dialysis fistulas. *Arch Intern Med* 136:292, 1976
76. McMillan R, Evans DB: Experience with three Brescia-Cimino shunts. *Br Med J* 3:781, 1968
77. Holman E: Abnormal arteriovenous connections – Great variability of effects with particular reference to delayed development of cardiac failure. *Circulation* 32:1001, 1965
78. Pate JW, Sherman RT, Jackson T, Wilson H: Cardiac failure following traumatic arteriovenous fistula: A report of fourteen cases. *J Trauma* 5:398, 1965
79. Binak K, Regan TJ, Christensen RC, Hellems HK: Arteriovenous fistula: Hemodynamic effects of occlusion and exercise. *Am Heart J* 60:495, 1960
80. Dotremont G, Piessens J, Verberckmoes R: Hemodynamic studies in patients on chronic hemodialysis by venipuncture of a peripheral arteriovenous fistula. *Acta Cardiol* (Brux) 25:230, 1970
81. Payne RM, Soderblom RE, Lobstein PH, Hull AR, Mullins CB: Exercise-induced hemodynamic effects of arteriovenous fistulas used for hemodialysis. *Kidney Int* 2:344, 1972
82. Nicoladini C: Phlebarteriectasie der rechten oberen Extremtät. (Phlebarteriectasia of the right upper extremity) *Arch Klin Chir* 18:252, 1875 (in German)
83. Branham HH: Aneurysmal varix of the femoral artery and vein following a gunshot wound. *Internat J Surg* 3:250, 1890

84. Comty CM: Factors influencing body composition in terminal uraemics treated by regular haemodialysis. *Proc Eur Dial Transpl Assoc* 4:216, 1967
85. Gutkin M, Levinson GE, King AS, Lasker N: Plasma renin activity in end-stage kidney disease. *Circulation* 40:563, 1969
86. del Greco F, Simon NM, Roguska J, Walker C: Hemodynamic studies in chronic uremia. *Circulation* 40:87, 1969
87. Hampers CL, Zollinger RM, Skillmen JJ, Gumpert RW, Bailey GL, Merrill JP: Hemodynamic and body composition changes following bilateral nephrectomy in chronic renal failure. *Circulation* 40:367, 1969
88. Comty CM, Rottka H, Shaldon S: Blood pressure control in patients with end-stage renal failure treated by intermittent haemodialysis. *Proc Eur Dial Transpl Assoc* 1:209, 1964
89. Hampers CL, Skillman JJ, Lyons JH, Olson JE, Merrill JP: A hemodynamic evaluation of bilateral nephrectomy and hemodialysis in hypertensive man. *Circulation* 35:272, 1967
90. Lazarus JM, Hampers CL, Bennet AH, Vandam LD, Merrill JP: Urgent bilateral nephrectomy for severe hypertension. *Ann Intern Med* 76:733, 1972
91. Kolff WJ, Nakamoto S, Poutasse EF, Straffon RA, Figueroa JE: Effect of bilateral nephrectomy and kidney transplantation on hypertension in man. *Circulation* II (Suppl 2):23, 1964
92. Onesti G, Swartz C, Ramirez O, Brest AN: Bilateral nephrectomy for control of hypertension in uremia. *Trans Am Soc Artif Intern Organs* 14:361, 1968
93. Wilkinson R, Scott DF, Uldall PR, Kerr DNS, Swinney J: Plasma renin and exchangeable sodium in the hypertension of chronic renal failure. *Q J Med* 34:377, 1970
94. Weidman P, Maxwell MA, Lupu AN, Lewin AJ, Massry SG: Plasma renin activity and blood pressure in terminal renal failure. *N Engl J Med* 285:757, 1971
95. McCubbin JW, Green JH, Page IH: Baroreceptor function in chronic renal hypertension. *Circ Res* 4:204, 1956
96. Mostert JW, Evers JL, Hobika GH, Moore RH, Kenny GM, Murphy GP: The haemodynamic response to chronic renal failure as studied in the azotaemic state. *Br J Anaest* 42:397, 1970
97. Dustan HP, Page JA: Some factors in renal and renoprival hypertension. *J Lab Clin Med* 64:948, 1964
98. Goldenberger S, Thompson A, Guha A: Autonomic nervous dysfunction in chronic renal failure. *Circ Res* 19:531, 1971
99. Lowenthal DT, Reidenberg MM: The heart rate response to atropine in uremic patients, obese subjects before and during fasting, and patients with other chronic illnesses. *Proc Soc Exp Biol Med* 139:390, 1972
100. Hurst JW, Logue RB: *The Heart* 2nd ed, New York, McGraw-Hill Book Co, 1970
101. Arora KK, Lacy JP, Schacht RA, Martin DG, Gurch CF: Calcific cardiomyopathy in advanced renal failure. *Arch Intern Med* 135:603, 1975
102. Terman DS, Alfrey AC, Hammond WS, Donndelinger T, Ogden DA, Holmes JH: Cardiac calcification in uremia. A clinical, biochemical and pathologic study. *Am J Med* 50:744, 1971
103. Lewin K, Trautman ᵀ: Ischaemic myocardial damage in chronic renal failure. *Br Med J* 4:151, 1971
104. Davidson RC, Pendras JP: Calcium-related cardio-respiratory death in chronic hemodialysis. *Trans Am Soc Artif Intern Organs* 13:36, 1967
105. Sokol A, Gral T, Edelbarum DN, Rosen V, Rubini ME: Correlation of autopsy findings and clinical experience in chronically dialyzed patients. *Trans Am Soc Artif Intern Organs* 13:51, 1967
106. Ernst DE, Sadler JH, Ingram RH, Macom J: Acid-base balance in chronic hemodialysis. *Trans Am Soc Artif Intern Organs* 14:434, 1968
107. Contiguglia SR, Alfrey AC, Miller NL, Runnels DE, LeGeros RZ: Nature of soft tissue calcification in uremia. *Kidney Int* 4:229, 1973
108. Hung J, Harris PJ, Uren RF, Tiller DJ, Kelly DT: Uremic cardiomyopathy – Effect of hemodialysis on left ventricular function in end-stage renal failure; *N Engl J Med* 302:447, 1980
109. Schott CR, LeSar JF, Kotler MN, Parry WR, Segal BL: The spectrum of echocardiographic findings in chronic renal failure. *Cardiovasc Med* 217, 1978
110. Francis GS, Sharma BIM, Collins AJ, Helseth HK, Comty CM: Coronary-artery surgery in patients with end-stage renal disease. *Ann Intern Med* 92:499, 1980
111. Wang K, Sako Y, Hall WH, Gobel FF: Staphylococcal endocarditis in a renal arteriovenous fistula following nephrectomy. *Arch Intern Med* 130:418, 1972
112. Ribot S, Gilbert L, Rothfeld EL, Parsonnet V, Jacobs MG: Bacterial endocarditis with pulmonary edema necessitating mitral valve replacement in a hemodialysis--dependent patient. *J Thorac Cardiovasc Surg* 62:59, 1971
113. Lansing AM, Leb DE, Berman LB: Cardiovascular surgery in end-stage renal failure. *JAMA* 204:682, 1968
114. Rifkind D, Marchioro TL, Schneck SA, Hill RB Jr: Systemic fungal infections complicating renal transplantation and immunosuppressive therapy. Clinical, microbiologic, neurologic and pathologic features. *Am J Med* 43:28, 1967
115. Myerwitz RL, Medieros AA, O'Brien TF: Bacterial infection in renal homotransplant recipients. A study of fifty-three bacteremic episodes. *Am J Med* 53:308, 1972
116. Leonard A, Raij L, Shapiro FL: Bacterial endocarditis in regularly dialyzed patients. *Kidney Int* 4:407, 1973
117. Goodman JS, Crews DH, Gin HE, Koenig MG: Bacterial endocarditis as a possible complication of chronic hemodialysis. *N Engl J Med* 280:876, 1969
118. Leonard A, Comty CM, Shapiro FL, Raij L: Osteomyelitis in hemodialysis patients. *Ann Intern Med* 78:651, 1973
119. Alfrey AC, LeGendre GR, Kaehny WD: The dialysis encephalopathy syndrome: possible aluminum intoxication. *N Engl J Med* 294:184, 1976
120. Adam WR, Dawborn JK, Rosenbaum J: Transient early diastolic murmurs in patients with renal failure. *Med J Aust* 2:1085, 1970.
121. Barratt LJ, Robinson MA, Whitford JA, Lawrence JR: The diastolic murmur of renal failure. *N Engl J Med* 295:121, 1976
122. Wilcox BR, Proctor HJ, Rackley CE, Peters RM: Early surgical treatment of valvular endocarditis. *JAMA* 200:820, 1967
123. Wise JR Jr, Cleland WP, Hallidie-Smith KA, Bentall HH, Goodwin JF, Oakley CM: Urgent aortic-valve replacement for acute aortic regurgitation due to infective endocarditis. *Lancet* 2:115, 1971
124. English TAH, Ross JK: Surgical aspects of bacterial endocarditis. *Br Med J* 4:598, 1972
125. Matalon R, Nidus BD, Eisinger RP: Pseudoarrhythmias during hemodialysis. *N Engl J Med* 278:1439, 1968
126. Ayres SM, Grace WJ: Inappropriate ventilation and hypoxemia as causes of cardiac arrhytmias. The control of arrhythmias without antiarrhythmic drugs. *Am J Med*

46:496, 1969
127. Cowie J, Lambie AT, Robson JS: The influence of extracorporeal dialysis on the acid-base composition of blood and cerebrospinal fluid. *Clin Sci* 23:397, 1962
128. Blumberg A, Marti HR: Mechanism of post dialysis hyperventilation in patients with chronic renal insufficiency. *Clin Nephrol* 5:119, 1976
129. Graziani G, Ponticelli C, di Filippo G, Redaelli B: Acid-base changes in haemodialysis. *Br Med J* 3:163, 1970
130. Rosenbaum BJ, Coburn JW, Shinaberger JH, Massry SG: Acid-base status during the interdialytic period in patients maintained with chronic hemodialysis. *Ann Intern Med* 71:1105, 1969
131. Morgan AG, Burkinshaw L, Robinson PJA, Rosen SM: Potassium balance and acid base changes in patients undergoing regular haemodialysis therapy. *Br Med J* 1:779, 1970
132. Adler S, Roy A, Relman AS: Intracellular acid-base regulation. The response of muscle cells to changes in CO_2 tension or extracellular bicarbonate concentration. *J Clin Invest* 44:8, 1965

31
ACUTE COMPLICATIONS ASSOCIATED WITH HEMODIALYSIS

CHRISTOPHER R. BLAGG

Introduction	611
Disequilibrium, hypotension and related symptoms	612
Disequilibrium syndrome	612
Clinical manifestations	612
Pathogenesis	612
Prevention and treatment of disequilibrium	613
Hypotension	613
Hypotension association with sodium and fluid depletion	613
The role of sequential ultrafiltration and bicarbonate dialysis in the prevention of dialysis hypotension and nonspecific symptoms related to dialysis	614
The effects of ultrafiltration	614
The effect of acetate	614
Hypotension associated with hemorrhage	615
Complications associated with biochemical changes	615
Hyponatremia	615
Hypernatremia	616
Hyperkalemia	616
Hypokalemia	616
Hypercalcemia and hypermagnesemia	617
Miscellaneous dialysate-related problems	617
Fever and endotoxemia	617
Infections and pyrogen reactions	617
Overheated dialysate	618
Air embolism	618
Causes	618
Signs and symptoms of air embolism	618
Treatment	619
Prevention of air embolism	619
Hemorrhage	620
Gastrointestinal bleeding	620
Subdural hematoma	620
Uremic hemopericardium	620
Retroperitoneal hematoma	621
Hemorrhagic pleural effusion	621
Subcapsular liver hematoma	621
Hemorrhages into the skin	621
Miscellaneous problems associated with dialysis	621
Restlessness and insomnia	621
Hypoglycemia due to beta-blocking agents	621
Dermatologic abnormalities associated with hemodialysis	622
Pruritus	622
Muscle cramps	623
Priapism	623
Pulmonary function during dialysis	623
Joint and tendon abnormalities associated with hemodialysis	624
Spontaneous tendon rupture	624
Carpal tunnel syndrome	624
Uremic bursitis	624
Septic arthritis	624
Hearing loss	624
Hepatic friction rub	624
Recurrent abdominal pain associated with digoxin	625
First use syndrome	625
Leachables	625
Membrane sensitivity	625
Anti-N-like antibodies	625
Comment	625
References	626

INTRODUCTION

In 1960 maintenance hemodialysis was a new and experimental procedure, performed on a few highly selected patients by a team of physicians and other staff who were uncertain of the complications which might ensue, both during hemodialysis and as a result of prolonging life by this new treatment. Today, 21 years later, there are some 150,000 patients treated by maintenance dialysis throughout the world, the great majority of whom have their dialysis supervised by nurses or technicians; and there is also a significant number of patients, perhaps as many as 15% of the total, who provide their own dialysis treatment at home. These numbers suggest that hemodialysis is essentially a relatively safe procedure. Complications occurring during dialysis have been documented carefully and it is unlikely that many significant new major complications occuring during hemodialysis will be described in the future.

This chapter is a brief review of the major complications occurring during hemodialysis and, in particular, those not dealt with at length in other chapters of this book. It excludes complications occurring in the dialysis patient which are not related directly to the dialysis procedure. The subjects discussed are not an exhaustive list of all those complications that have been described as occurring or that relate to dialysis but rather those that the author considers to be most important or interesting. Similarly, when therapy is described, the emphasis is generally on treatment which is felt most appropriate in the light of his experience.

Dialysis patients present with all the same emergency and semiemergency situations that may occur in any other type of patient, and the treatment may be that used in the nondialysis patient or may be modified because of concurrent dialysis treatment. In addition, there are certain complications which are specific to the patient undergoing dialysis. For an exhaustive discussion of the risks and hazards associated with dialysis equipment, the reader is referred to the report by Keshaviah and coworkers (1) and to Chapter 11.

DISEQUILIBRIUM, HYPOTENSION AND RELATED SYMPTOMS

Numerically, the most frequently encountered problems are related to hypotension occurring during dialysis, nonspecific symptoms during and after dialysis apparently unrelated to hypotension or disequilibrium, and the dialysis disequilibrium syndrome, which remains a potential problem in patients with acute renal failure and in patients starting treatment by maintenance dialysis. Disequilibrium is discussed first because this enters into the differential diagnosis of many of the other problems encountered during dialysis, and a great deal is known about its pathophysiology.

Disequilibrium syndrome

Clinical manifestations
While no longer a frequent complication of maintenance dialysis, the disequilibrium syndrome is still a potential hazard for patients with acute renal failure and for patients commencing treatment with maintenance hemodialysis, particularly with use of large surface area high flux dialyzers and shorter dialysis times.

Mild disequilibrium may result only in restlessness and headache during dialysis, sometimes with nausea, vomiting, blurring of vision and muscle twitching. Blood pressure may be elevated, and there may be disorientation and tremor. Seizures occur in more severe cases (2) and may be accompanied by cardiac arrhythmias (3, 4). Both grand mal and petit mal seizures may occur, but focal signs are more often associated with preexisting neurologic disease (3). Most patients recover with appropriate care, but occasionally seizures lead to coma and death (5, 6).

Pathogenesis
Cerebral edema is regarded as the major cause of disequilibrium symptoms because of the consistent finding of elevated cerebrospinal fluid pressure and the occurrence of cerebral edema in patients dying with this syndrome. Kennedy and associates (7) first noted that during dialysis, the urea concentration and osmolality in cerebrospinal fluid fell more slowly than in the blood and that there was a concomitant rise in cerebrospinal fluid pressure – the so-called reverse urea shift. These findings were soon confirmed in both man and animals (8-10). However, after rapid hemodialysis in the uremic dog, urea concentration is only marginally higher in the brain than in plasma (11). Consequently, the rate of urea clearance from the brain more or less parallels that from plasma and there is a delay in clearance of urea from cerebrospinal fluid during dialysis. This is associated with a paradoxical acidosis in the cerebrospinal fluid and a fall in cerebrospinal fluid pH during dialysis, despite correction of systemic metabolic acidosis and rise in arterial pH (11). The alteration in cerebrospinal fluid pH may produce impaired mentation, and the intracellular acidosis in the brain can increase intracellular osmolality by altering osmotic activity of intracellular cations, resulting in brain edema (12).

The mechanism of the paradoxical cerebrospinal fluid acidosis during correction of metabolic acidosis depends on more rapid diffusion of carbon dioxide than bicarbonate across the blood-brain barrier, so that during dialysis cerebrospinal fluid PCO_2 is rapidly corrected while bicarbonate concentration remains low (12). However, in maintenance dialysis, arterial PCO_2 does not increase at the end of dialysis or shortly thereafter (13); and in rapidly hemodialyzed patients, no difference is found in PCO_2 or bicarbonate concentration in plasma or lumbar cerebrospinal fluid, whether disequilibrium occurs or not (14).

Other suggested causes for disequilibrium have included hypoglycemia (15) and hyponatremia (16). There is little evidence that hypoglycemia plays any significant role clinically in the development of disequilibrium, but mild hyponatremia associated with use of dialysate of low sodium concentration may play a minor role.

Brain edema causing disequilibrium symptoms may result from generation of idiogenic osmoles in the brain during dialysis (17, 18). This theory is based on experiments in uremic dogs showing occurence of a significant osmotic gradient between brain and blood during dialysis not due to changes in the concentrations of sodium, potassium, chloride, calcium, magnesium, or urea in the brain. The nature of these idiogenic osmoles remains unclear, but their genesis may relate to changes in intracellular binding of sodium and potassium caused by their displacement by ammonium ions resulting from the equilibrium between glutamine and glutamic acid. Thus, an increase in glutamic acid concentration in the brain could cause a fall in intracellular pH, loss of hydrogen ion into the cerebrospinal fluid, and so a fall of cerebrospinal fluid pH and rise in brain osmolality due to accumulation of acid osmoles.

The characteristic EEG findings of disequilibrium are an increase of slow wave activity, increased spike wave activity, and bursts of delta wave activity with loss of normal alpha rhythm (17). The cerebrospinal fluid pressure is normal in the uncomplicated nondialyzed uremic patient, but generally rises during dialysis whether disequilibrium occurs or not. This does not necessarily indicate brain edema, but could be due to an increase in cerebrospinal fluid volume or an increase in cerebral blood flow. However, autopsy of patients who have died during dialysis has shown brain swelling, often with tentorial herniation (19); and computerized tomographic (CT) scanning associated with densitometric analysis of brain tissue in patients undergoing dialysis has shown a significant decrease in density especially in the region of the basal ganglia and in keeping with a buildup of fluid in the brain parenchyma (20).

The differential diagnosis of disequilibrium includes a number of conditions discussed in Chapter 37. These include hypotension, nonspecific malaise associated with rapid dialysis, subdural hematoma, cerebrovascular accident, the uremic syndrome, hypertensive encephalopathy, dialysis dementia, cardiac arrhythmias, hyponatremia, hypernatremia, and hypoglycemia.

Prevention and treatment of disequilibrium
Prevention of disequilibrium in patients with acute renal failure was based originally on addition of an osmotically active solute to the dialysate because of demonstration of the 'reverse urea' effect (7), the aim being to prevent the fall in plasma osmolality resulting from urea removal by passage of osmotically active solute from dialysate to plasma so reducing the brain-plasma osmolality gradient. Solutes used for this purpose have included urea (21), dextrose (22), fructose (7), mannitol (23), sodium chloride (24), and glycerol (18, 25), but results generally have not been as good as anticipated. Because disequilibrium occurs most commonly during rapid hemodialysis, the simplest preventative measure is to slow the rate of biochemical change by shorter and more frequent dialyses, with or without reduction in blood flow rate (14, 26). This approach is useful in patients with acute renal failure and in the initial phase of maintenance dialysis, particularly in patients with severe overhydration, metabolic acidosis, or very high BUN levels. Alternatively, peritoneal dialysis with resulting slower biochemical changes may be effective, although disequilibrium has also been described with peritoneal dialysis.

While use of shorter more frequent hemodialyses is preferable, anticonvulsant drugs also have an important role in prevention and treatment of disequilibrium, although they have no effect on cerebral edema. Phenytoin is of particular value in prevention used as a loading dose of 1,000 mg (4 mmol) at least one day before commencing dialysis, followed by a maintenance dose of 300 to 400 mg daily. Phenytoin is of little value during seizure activity as, although it enters the brain rapidly, the brain level also declines very rapidly unless continued administration occurs. Intravenous diazepam (Valium) produces high brain levels within minutes and is the most effective agent for suppression of acute seizure activity. The effect of intravenous injection lasts 30 to 60 min and respiratory depression is less than with barbiturates (27). Short-acting barbiturates, such as thiopental or pentobarbital, also are effective within minutes but are more dangerous because of greater respiratory depression.

Hypotension

Episodes of hypotension are among the most common complications during hemodialysis, occuring in 20 to 30% of all dialyses (28-30). The development of large surface area compliant dialyzers and reduction in treatment time, together with increasing patient loads and decreased attention to individual patients during dialysis, all tend to increase the frequency of symptoms during dialysis. When not due to a specific cause such as cardiac arrhythmia, myocardial infarction, other cardiac problems or septicemia, hypotension generally is secondary to acute reduction in blood volume due either to excessive ultrafiltration during dialysis or to acute hemorrhage. Symptoms are similar, whatever the cause, and include unexplained anxiety, nausea and pallor, possibly associated with vomiting which may result in temporary relief. On sitting up, the patient becomes dizzy, develops tachycardia, and may become unconscious.

Hypotension associated with sodium and fluid depletion
Hypotension as a result of sodium and fluid depletion may occur at any time during or shortly after dialysis, and the time of onset may give a clue to the cause. Hypotension developing on connection to the dialyzer usually occurs in patients with a low blood volume prior to dialysis as a result of previous vomiting, diarrhea, fever, or reduced dietary sodium intake. In such a patient, the predialysis weight is low. Many patients have mild symptoms of hypotension on connection to the dialyzer during their early dialyses, but generally this is not a persistent problem.

Hypotension occurring during the course of dialysis usually is due to excessive ultrafiltration. This may result from too short a dialysis with consequent rapid ultrafiltration, an incorrect estimate of the ultrafiltration rate required to remove accumulated fluid, or in a patient with an arteriovenous shunt, may be due to a failing venous cannula with consequent increased pressure within the dialyzer and excessive ultrafiltration. Hypotension during dialysis may also be an early indication of the presence of a pericardial effusion.

Occasionally, hypotension may occur shortly after dialysis. Again, the most likely cause is excessive ultrafiltration, symptoms occurring when the patient becomes active following termination of dialysis.

Prevention of hypotension during dialysis includes accurate assessment of the patient's dry weight, monotoring of dietary sodium intake, knowledge of whether the patient is taking antihypertensive medications and consideration of the type of dialyzer, blood flow, ultrafiltration rate and duration of dialysis. The use of sequential ultrafiltration and bicarbonate dialysis is discussed below.

The treatment of hypotension occurring during dialysis includes lying the patient flat and reducing negative pressure to zero to prevent further ultrafiltration. Other causes of hypotension, particularly cardiac complications, pericardial effusion, or septicemia, must be excluded. With mild symptoms, intake of a salty food such as soup or potato chips may be all that is required. If hypotension persists or becomes more severe, an appropriate volume of saline must be administered via the venous drip chamber or the venous blood line. The infusion must be monitored, particularly in patients dialyzing with a blood pump, to insure the saline container does not empty and permit entrance of air into the blood circuit. Preferably, all infusions should be administered from collapsible plastic bags, rather than from glass bottles. The volume and rate of saline infusion must be based on the response of symptoms and blood pressure.

The role of sequential ultrafiltration and bicarbonate dialysis in the prevention of dialysis hypotension and nonspecific symptoms related to dialysis

During the 1960's in the United States, some centers preferred the Kiil dialyzer for maintenance dialysis while many others used a coil dialyzer which had a larger surface area and obligatory ultrafiltration. In addition to hypotension during dialysis, nonspecific symptoms, including headache and malaise during dialysis and a postdialysis syndrome characterized by a 'washed-out' feeling, appeared to be more common with the 4 to 6 h of dialysis twice weekly favored by users of coil dialyzers than with the 8 to 12 h of dialysis three times weekly preferred by those using the Kiil dialyzer. This lesser morbidity with a slower dialysis was one reason for the preference for the Kiil dialyzer for maintenance dialysis. Much of this difference in symptoms was attributable perhaps to disequilibrium and hypotension resulting from faster dialysis and increased ultrafiltration with the coil dialyzer, although this did not appear to be the full explanation for all symptomatic problems occurring during dialysis.

With development of larger surface area disposable dialyzers, and with the increased use of shorter dialysis time that followed the proposal of the square meter/hour (31) and middle molecule hypotheses (32), these symptoms appear to have become more common, even though disequilibrium itself is less likely with increased use of three-times-weekly dialysis. It would now appear that hypotension and many of these symptoms relate to ultrafiltration rate and changes in osmolality and possibly to the use of acetate rather than bicarbonate in dialysate.

The effect of ultrafiltration
(See also Chapters 12 and 13)

Patients vary widely in their tolerance of ultrafiltration and the rate at which fluid can be removed during dialysis. Too rapid ultrafiltration for the individual patient may result in hypotension with symptoms occurring during and after dialysis. Sensitivity to ultrafiltration is also affected by other factors such as presence of cardiovascular and peripheral vascular disease and autonomic neuropathy (33). Ultrafiltration without dialysis, when dialysate is bypassed from the dialyzer during the 1st hour or so of dialysis, makes possible removal of large volumes of fluid while maintaining blood pressure, despite profound weight loss, and even in patients who have the tendency to develop hypotension during routine dialyses (34-36). Because of the absence of dialysate flow, only ultrafiltration occurs from the plasma. The plasma osmolality remains constant during the weight loss because dialysis is not occurring. The rate of fluid removal with ultrafiltration alone can be as high as 3 l/h. Following sufficient fluid removal, dialysate flow is started through the dialyzer and normal dialysis (without ultrafiltration) is completed.

The mechanism of rapid ultrafiltration without symptoms has been investigated in order to evaluate why the blood pressure remains stable during fluid removal by ultrafiltration only. Studies using a high sodium dialysate have shown that relatively constant plasma osmolality may play a role in the stability of blood pressure during ultrafiltration (37), but the importance of other factors such as the serum potassium and plasma norepinephrine levels has also been suggested. This has been investigated in stable, normotensive, nonnephrectomized dialysis patients with normal autonomic nervous systems, without a history of episodes of hypotension on dialysis, and who were not receiving antihypertensive medications (38). Ultrafiltration alone, as compared with regular dialysis under standardized conditions, showed comparable supine blood pressures after comparable weight loss, but on standing following ultrafiltration alone, blood pressure did not fall and none of the patients became symptomatic, while 50% of the patients became symptomatic after regular dialysis. Addition of potassium to the dialysate to maintain a constant serum potassium level during the procedures did not prevent development of orthostatic symptoms following regular dialysis, and the increase in plasma norepinephrine concentration was not significantly different following the two procedures. In further experiments, constant osmolality was maintained by infusion of hypertonic mannitol; and in marked contrast to the results with isokalemic dialysis, no orthostatic decrease in blood pressure was noted in patients after a 2.6% decrease in body weight, and no patient became symptomatic upon standing whether treated by ultrafiltration alone or by regular dialysis. In the case of regular dialysis, blood pressure remained stable despite a fall in serum potassium and no significant increase in catecholamines. Infusion of hypertonic mannitol, in addition to producing constant osmolality, also results in expansion of circulating plasma volume, and so studies were performed in which the volume given in the hypertonic mannitol studies was matched with a volume of isotonic mannitol infusion, therefore maintaining volume while permitting osmolality to decline. As a result, blood pressure fell following a decrease in body weight and the isotonic volume infusion, and the increase in hematocrit and plasma proteins was comparable with the two mannitol solutions, suggesting comparable decrements in plasma volume. These studies suggest that an important mechanism for blood pressure protection during ultrafiltration is through an effect of osmolality on vascular reactivity, although the possibility of an additional effect on extracellular fluid volume distribution remains uncertain as there could also be volume flux occurring during the experiments.

This technique of removal of fluid by ultrafiltration alone has proved to be of considerable clinical use in the management of dialysis patients, particularly those who have episodes of vascular instability during rapid ultrafiltration during normal dialysis.

The effect of acetate

Acetate as a substitute for bicarbonate in dialysate was developed in response to the problem of the low solubility of calcium and magnesium carbonates in the concentrated dialysate required for use with proportioning dialysate systems (39). Acetate is metabolized rapidly to bicarbonate in the body with consequent repletion of the plasma bicarbonate level during and after dialysis. The maximum utilization rate of acetate for man has been calculated as 3.5 mmol/h/kg body weight (40), and this rate was not exceeded until development of larger surface area hemodialyzers and use of higher blood flow rates. In some uremic patients, acetate is not metabolized rapidly to bicarbonate (41), and the acetate load presented to a hemodialysis patient may approach 300 mmol/h (42) with a resulting appreciable rise in blood acetate levels in some patients. Recent studies have further clarified the relative roles of dialyzer efficiency and rate of acetate metabolism, and have shown that the maximum utilization rate is greater than previously recognized, but confirmed that some patients are acetate intolerant (43).

Graefe and colleagues (44) demonstrated by a double blind study that substitution of bicarbonate for acetate in dialysate reduced the morbidity associated with short dialysis using a large surface area dialyzer. They also showed that substitution of bicarbonate for acetate reduced vascular instability during dialysis (45), an effect similar to that observed by Bergström et al (35) using ultrafiltration without dialysis. This suggests that the acetate ion may be responsible for some of the morbidity occurring during rapid dialysis, presumably because of the peripheral vasodilating effect and greater cardiodepressant effect of acetate (46, 47).

Hypotension and symptoms during dialysis thus may be relieved by both ultrafiltration alone and by bicarbonate dialysis (48), and so a more serious consideration may be a long-term effect of acetate rather than bicarbonate. Hemodialysis with acetate does not optimally correct the metabolic acidosis of uremia, as manifested by the presence of lower predialysis bicarbonate concentrations using acetate dialysate (49). It is well known that chronic metabolic acidosis has a number of adverse effects (50, 51), including mobilization of bone calcium (52) and inhibition of bone growth in children (53), and these risks may be more important than development of symptoms during dialysis. Furthermore, in uremic dogs, ^{14}C-acetate may be incorporated into lipids in plasma, liver, and aorta (54), and the serum acetoacetate concentration is increased during acetate dialysis (55) raising the question of the role of acetate dialysis in lipid deposition.

Dialysis using bicarbonate dialysate, although it results in more optimal correction of acidosis and is not associated with rapid rebound of the bicarbonate level postdialysis, nevertheless is technically more cumbersome and increases the cost of dialysis. The possibility that bicarbonate dialysis may have long-term patient benefits requires continued evaluation, but newer dialysate supply systems have features permitting both dialysate bypass to permit ultrafiltration alone and use of bicarbonate rather than acetate dialysate. The ultimate role of both sequential ultrafiltration and the use of bicarbonate dialysis in minimizing the occurence of hypotension and other symptoms during dialysis remains to be determined, but both these techniques have proved invaluable in the management of patients who do develop such symptoms. It should be remembered, however, that use of a smaller dialyzer and attention to dialysis details, such as blood flow rate and duration of dialysis in relation to body size and residual renal function, also may help to reduce the incidence of such symptoms. Finally, when using short dialysis with large surface area dialyzers, it is important that attention be given to tailoring the dialysis process to the needs of the individual patient (see chapters 3 and 5). It should also be remembered that attention to the patient by staff during dialysis can help in minimizing these problems.

The possibility of hypotension due to causes other than salt and fluid depletion must always be considered and, in particular, the possibility of hemorrhage.

Hypotension associated with hemorrhage

Hypotension can result from bleeding, either internally in the patient or externally; for example, from a leak in the blood circuit. More common causes of the former are discussed elsewhere in this chapter. Hypotension due to blood loss is much less common than is hypotension due to excessive ultrafiltration.

Overt blood loss usually is due to either line separation or to a major membrane leak. The risk of line separation can be minimized by careful attention to connection of tubing and by use of tape bridges to reinforce connections. Membrane leaks may result from a faulty dialyzer, or may occur during dialysis, especially when a high transmembrane pressure is used.

Line separation is treated by reconnection and a serious membrane rupture by cessation of dialysis. Minor membrane leaks may be treated by clamping the arterial line and returning blood in the dialyzer to the patient, because pressure in the blood compartment of the dialyzer is greater than pressure in the dialysate compartment so minimizing the risk of contamination during the brief time required to return blood to the patient. However, a major membrane leak should be treated by immediate clamping of both arterial and venous lines, prompt cessation of dialysis, and sacrifice of blood remaining in the dialyzer. Transfusion should be given if indicated by the general status of the patient. The technique of blood leak detection in dialysate is discussed in Chapter 11.

COMPLICATIONS ASSOCIATED WITH BIOCHEMICAL CHANGES

Incorrect proportioning in the preparation of dialysate may occur as a result of both technical and human errors, the most important consequences being development of acute hyponatremia or hypernatremia depending upon the error. Both of these conditions may result in confusion, lethargy, muscle weakness, myoclonus, seizures, coma, and death (56).

Hyponatremia

When plasma is allowed to equilibrate with hypotonic dialysis fluid, hyponatremia occurs. With a batch-mix dialysis unit, hyponatremia and hypoosmolality can occur at the start of dialysis or following a bath change as a result of failure to add concentrate, failure to test dialysate prior to use, or use of the wrong quantity of concentrate or water. In proportioning systems, failure to connect to the concentrate container and to note or (and) set the conductivity limits (and failure to follow the check list for initiation of dialysis) will produce hyponatremia at the start of dialysis. Hyponatremia can also occur during the course of dialysis with a proportioning system, if the concentrate container runs dry and the conductivity limits are not set appropriately (see also remarks on monitoring of conductivity in Chapter 11).

Acute hypoosmolality causes the abrupt onset of hemolysis (57) with transient marked hyperkalemia which, assuming the patient survives the acute episode, rapidly subsides as potassium distributes throughout the body compartments. In addition, any residual renal function may be jeopardized by complicating acute renal failure. At the same time as the acute hemolysis occurs, the massive infusion of water from the hypotonic dialysate results in hypervolemia, hemodilution of all plasma constituents, acute water intoxication, and cerebral edema (58).

Symptoms include pain in the vein receiving the hypotonic, hemolyzed blood from the dialyzer, anxiety, restlessness, and headache. Pulse rate decreases initially then increases, and the patient develops precordial pain, cold, clammy skin, and distended neck veins, the latter associated with myocardial dysfunction. Severe lumbar pain and abdominal cramps have also been observed, perhaps due to ischemia.

Treatment consists of clamping the blood lines; the hemolyzed blood must not be returned from the dialyzer to the patient. When clinically indicated, 100% oxygen should be administered and the patient placed on a cardiac monitor with a defibrillator available. In the event of seizures, intravenous diazepam should be given. Blood should be obtained for baseline hematocrit, plasma hemoglobin, electrolytes, crossmatching, and enzyme levels. At the same time, a further batch of dialysate should be prepared, or in the case of a proportioning system, this should remain in bypass with appropriate concentrate until the dialysis fluid composition is up to normal levels. Then dialysis should be restarted without delay, using a new dialyzer. Once dialysis is recommenced, high transmembrane pressure is necessary to remove water excess, and it may be necessary to infuse saline, colloid, or blood to maintain blood pressure. Following dialysis the hematocrit, serum hemoglobin and electrolyte concentrations should be repeated and the patient hospitalized for 24 to 48 h for serial enzyme studies and observation for possible myocardial damage.

Prevention of acute hyponatremia and hypoosmolality depends upon meticulous attention to detail in preparing for dialysis. The final step before connecting dialyzer and patient should be checking the dialysate in a batch system or checking the conductivity meter and its setting in a proportioning system.

Hypernatremia

Hypernatremia and hyperosmolality due to use of inappropriate dialysate (59) may occur inadvertently with a batch-mix system if the wrong concentrate or wrong volume of concentrate or water is used and no check of the dialysate is made prior to dialysis. It may also occur when water and concentrate are incompletely mixed. With a proportioning system, this problem can occur only if the conductivity meter malfunctions or the alarm points are not set appropriately and the proportioning system is maladjusted; the water treatment equipment malfunctions; or in a hydraulically driven proportioning system, such as the Drake-Willock, if the concentrate bottle is elevated so providing a head of pressure to the system.

The effects of hypernatremia include transfer of water from the intracellular to the extracellular space, resulting in intracellular water depletion and hyperosmolality. Depending upon the rapidity of the shifts of sodium and water, the extracellular volume may be increased or decreased; but in any event, the extracellular fluid is hyperosmolar and cell volume is contracted. Symptoms include headache, nausea and vomiting, profound thirst, convulsions, coma, and death (56, 58, 60).

Treatment is cessation of dialysis and, if the patient can tolerate a rapid increase of extracellular volume, infusion of 5% dextrose in water to reduce plasma osmolality. Dialysis should be restarted with appropriate dialysate as soon as possible. Other treatment is symptomatic.

Hyperkalemia

Serious hyperkalemia is an uncommon problem in patients on maintenance dialysis except in those who are markedly underdialyzed or following significant dietary indiscretion. In patients using single needle dialysis, hyperkalemia may develop if recirculation occurs. This may be recognized by a disparity between urea concentration of blood from the dialysis inflow line and that from a peripheral vessel. The concentration of potassium in dialysate, usually between 1.0 and 3.0 mmol/l, results in net removal of potassium during dialysis. Potassium-free dialysate has been used but usually causes subnormal postdialysis plasma potassium levels which may contribute to postdialysis fatigue. Consequently, most patients now are dialyzed with dialysate potassium concentrations of at least 1.0 mmol/l.

In patients receiving digitalis, and particularly those with left ventricular hypertrophy, rapid lowering of the serum potassium level during dialysis may cause cardiac arrhythmias (61). Consequently, it is safer to dialyze such patients with dialysate potassium concentrations of between 2.0 and 3.5 mmol/l depending upon the patient's serum potassium level. Ventricular extrasystoles, sinus tachycardia, atrial fibrillation, and other arrhythmias may occur and can cause sudden death. Electrocardiographic monitoring should be used if serious problems are anticipated during dialysis of a digitalized patient.

Hypokalemia

Hypokalemia is not generally considered to be a problem in patients with chronic renal failure but may occur as a result of prolonged potassium loss secondary to nausea, vomiting, diarrhea, nasogastric suction, or use of diuretics. Although it is generally assumed that hypokalemia during dialysis is unlikely to be a significant problem, there is a recent report that lifethreatening levels of hypokalemia may develop in such patients despite use of dialysate containing potassium at a greater level than in the predialysis plasma (62). This problem can occur in association with marked predialysis acidosis such that, with institution of dialysis and rapid correction of the acidosis, a major transcompartmental shift of potassium occurs at a rate exceeding the capacity of potassium transfer across the dialysis membrane to compensate. As a result, severe hypokalemia may develop. Patients who may suffer from this problem have a history suggestive of potassium loss and a low or low-normal predialysis serum potassium level together with a low serum bicarbonate level and acidosis. Consideration should be given to use of a high potassium dialysate in such patients and to monitoring plasma potassium concentrations during dialysis.

Hypercalcemia and hypermagnesemia

In the early days of hemodialysis, dialysate was prepared using untreated tap water. However, it became obvious that in locations with high concentrations of calcium or magnesium in the tap water, and particularly when these levels fluctuated appreciably, water for dialysis fluid preparation required treatment prior to use. Currently it is recommended that all water for dialysate preparation be treated by deionization, reverse osmosis, or a combination of these processes (1, 63) in order to control levels of divalent cations and also to remove aluminum, fluoride and other trace minerals that may be present. In some areas the mineral content of the water is so high that considerable water treatment is necessary (see Chapter 6).

The 'hard water syndrome' is an acute syndrome occurring during dialysis, precipitated by hypercalcemia and hypermagnesemia and associated with failure of the water treatment process (64). Nausea and vomiting occur after the first hour of dialysis and may persist throughout the dialysis. Hypertension accompanies the vomiting even if there is significant weight loss due to ultrafiltration during dialysis, and the systolic blood pressure rise is greater than that of the diastolic pressure. This increase in blood pressure is attributed to the acute hypercalcemia. Acute pancreatitis may occur (65). Lethargy, muscular weakness, and headaches also have been reported with this syndrome, as has a burning sensation in the skin which may be due to hypermagnesemia.

With the occurrence of the hard water syndrome, dialysis should be terminated and should be restarted as soon as possible using appropriately treated water for the preparation of dialysate. Prevention depends upon regular maintenance and servicing of water treatment equipment.

Hypermagnesemia has been described in dialysis patients but is unlikely to be sufficient to cause symptoms unless the patient is taking magnesium-containing phosphate binders (66). However, although not an acute problem there is evidence that use of dialysate concentrate with 0.5 mmol/l of magnesium (1.0 mEq/l or 1.2 mg/dl) is associated with slight hypermagnesemia and an elevated bone magnesium content. Studies with dialysate containing 0.25 mmol/l (0.5 mEq/l or 0.6 mg/dl) of with magnesium-free dialysate have shown that this may be beneficial to bone disease, possibly by stimulating parathormone production and thereby increasing 1,25-dihydroxycholecalciferol production, calcium absorption from the gut and bone mineralization (67).

Miscellaneous dialysate-related problems

Acute copper intoxication and hemolysis secondary to leaching of copper from tubing in a dialysate supply system in association with a fall in pH of the dialysate following deionizer exhaustion has been reported (68). Chronic copper poisoning can also occur from dialysate made from untreated water supplied through copper pipes (69, 70).

Intoxications with other metals such as zinc (71, 72), lead (73), and nickel (74) may occur, and other trace elements such as fluoride may accumulate in dialysis patients. These problems are discussed in detail in Chapters 6, 7 and 41.

Hemolysis associated with nitrates (75) and with chloramines (76) in the water used for dialysate has also been reported. This, too, is discussed in Chapters 6 and 32.

FEVER AND ENDOTOXEMIA

Infections and pyrogen reactions

Febrile reactions during dialysis usually are associated with endotoxemia causing a 'pyrogen' reaction. Less commonly they are due to infection, and rarely they result from failure of temperature control of the equipment.

Fever due to infection is most likely to occur at the start of dialysis or shortly after the end of dialysis, while fever and chills developing during the course of dialysis are much more apt to be due to a pyrogen reaction in association with endotoxemia (77, 78).

Fever at the start of dialysis usually is due to contaminated equipment, and may be more likely to occur with a dialyzer which has been stored and reused if procedures are not followed carefully (see also Chapter 15). In the event of fever developing at the start of dialysis, the dialysis should be stopped, appropriate measures taken for investigation and treatment of infection, and dialysis restarted using fresh equipment.

When fever develops within an hour or so of termination of dialysis, this suggests infection occurring during the coming-off procedure. The most likely cause is the use of a contaminated hand pump for air-rinsing the dialyzer. The patient should be investigated and treated for possible infection.

Fever developing during the course of dialysis generally is thought to be due to a pyrogen reaction secondary to endotoxemia. Usually the fever is associated with chills, nausea, and sometimes hypotension. The severity of the episode varies from very mild to very severe but, in general, will respond promptly to treatment with antipyretics. Studies have shown the presence of circulating endotoxins or endotoxin-like activity in blood taken from patients during febrile episodes, and endotoxin has also been demonstrated in dialysate (77). High titres of antibodies against dialysate bacterial endotoxins have been found in dialysis patients (79), and although theoretically the pore size of the dialysis membrane is too small to allow passage of a molecule the size of endotoxin, small isolated defects could permit passage of sufficient endotoxin to result in a pyrogen reaction.

Treatment of a pyrogen reaction during dialysis is with antipyretic agents. The possibility of infection should always be considered (80), but the majority of febrile reactions occurring during the course of dialysis are associated with pyrogens.

Prevention of pyrogen reactions requires adequate cleaning and disinfection of dialysis equipment, as microbial contamination of water used for dialysis is frequent (81). This is particularly important for patients performing home dialysis as it has been found that an appreciable number of such patients use inadequately cleaned equipment (82).

Overheated dialysate

Failure of the thermostat in the dialysate temperature monitoring system may result in overheating of the dialysate. This can cause immediate severe hemolysis and lethal hyperkalemia, or if less severe, milder hemolysis may develop gradually. Thermostat failure causes a gradual rise in dialysate temperature, noted by the conscious patient as an increasing sensation of warmth. If undetected, heat-induced red cell damage may occur (83), but in most circumstances, if the patient is not obtunded, overheating will be detected before the temperature rise is extreme.

If the dialysate temperature rises above 51 °C, immediate and massive hemolysis can occur and may result in death from acute hyperkalemia (84). If the dialysate overheats to temperatures between 47 °C and 51 °C, the onset of hemolysis may be delayed for up to 48 h (85).

Prevention of this complication requires a high temperature monitor on the dialysis equipment set to alarm so as to prevent temperatures in excess of 42 °C.

In the event of a temperature rise to 51 °C dialysis must be stopped immediately, and the blood in the system should not be returned to the patient. The patient should be monitored closely for development of hyperkalemia, transfused if necessary, and have further dialysis using new equipment as soon as possible.

AIR EMBOLISM

Air embolism is an ever-present risk during dialysis because of the combination of a blood pump and the extended extracorporeal blood circuit (86). The frequency of significant air embolism during hemodialysis is uncertain and cases may go unreported. Nevertheless, with present-day equipment, the frequency is likely to be small.

Causes

Many causes of air embolism have been recognized (1). Air leakage may occur into that portion of the extracorporeal blood circuit which is under subatmospheric pressure, i.e., the prepump segment during fistula dialysis. Leakage can occur around the fistula needle at the needle hub as a result of arterial disconnection, through the heparin syringe at the connection to the tubing, or between barrel and plunger or through a crack in the barrel wall, at the arterial monitor line connection, in the arterial monitor, at a defective arterial drip chamber, through a split pump segment, or through a vented intravenous bottle. Air can pass in large quantities from dialysate to blood in the dialyzer. Refrigerated dialysate, as formerly used, could contain a large amount of dissolved air likely to come out of solution when dialysate was warmed by blood in the dialyzer. This is still seen when water used to make dialysate is very cold so allowing more air to be dissolved than the deaerating capacity of the equipment. A similar problem may be seen if the deaerator in the dialysis equipment is defective. With both fistula and cannula dialysis, air embolism may occur with an error in the procedure for returning blood to the patient after dialysis.

Signs and symptoms of air embolism

Death is said to have occurred with as little as 5 ml of air, although this must be extremely uncommon and would require very selective placement of the air.
The amount of air necessary to produce symptoms depends on several factors. For example, more air can be tolerated as microbubbles infused at a slow rate, thus allowing time for the air to go into solution in the blood. Arterial introduction of air can cause death by occlusion of a major cerebral or coronary artery. During hemodialysis, air usually enters the body through the venous end of the extracorporeal blood circuit, although air can be infused into an artery during a cannulation procedure.

The signs and symptoms of air embolism are in large part dependent upon position. If the patient is sitting or the head is elevated, air entering an arm vein will travel through the axillary and subclavian vein, then in retrograde fashion up the jugular vein to the cerebral venous system where it obstructs the venules in the brain resulting in brain cell damage. Death may ensue if a critical area of the brain is affected. Classically, the patient is said to cry out in alarm because of the sound of air rushing through the venous system to the brain then, depending upon the volume of air infused, convulse, lose consciousness, and possibly die.

The patient who is lying flat when air embolism occurs reacts differently. Air passes to the right atrium and right ventricle where it forms a foam, so interfering with the ability of the heart to pump. Especially if the patient is lying on his right side, air may pass through the pulmonary arteries to block the pulmonary capillary bed causing acute pulmonary hypertension, and some air may pass through the lungs to the left ventricle and systemic circulation. This results in arterial embolization with possible cardiac arrhythmias and neurological defects. In these circumstances, the patient develops acute dyspnea, cough and tightness in the chest, gasps for breath, becomes agitated and cyanosed, and can lapse into unconsciousness. Depending upon the volume of air, respiratory arrest may occur. Upon examination, pulse and blood pressure may be unobtainable and auscultation may reveal a churning sound caused by foaming of the blood within the heart.

It the event that the patient is in the Trendelenburg position because of hypotension at the time that air embolism occurs, air will pass to the lower extremities and cause patchy cyanosis associated with partial blockage of circulation. If infusion of air is stopped in time and the patient is kept in position so that the air remains trapped in the leg veins, there probably will be no serious sequelae.

Treatment

When air embolism is detected, the venous blood line should be clamped *immediately* before any other action is taken. The patient should be positioned with chest and head down and turned on the left side. It may be necessary to pull the patient off the bed, leaving hips and legs on the bed in order to maintain this position. The bed can then be put in the Trendelenburg position and the patient slid back on the bed, remaining on his left side throughout. If air embolism occurs during home dialysis, the patient can be pulled off the bed so that the left shoulder is on the floor and the hips are still on the bed and should remain in this position in the ambulance en route to the hospital. This position traps air at the apex of the right ventricle and away from the pulmonary valve so that the right ventricle acts as a bubble trap. Blood can then flow through the more dependent portion of the right ventricle to the pulmonary arteries and lungs.

If the patient is conscious, 100% oxygen by mask should be given. If unconscious, an airway or endotracheal tube should be placed and assisted respiration using 100% oxygen should be started.

If the patient is in cardiopulmonary distress and examination reveals foam in the right heart, percutaneous aspiration of foam may be necessary using an intracardiac needle and large syringe. Cardiac massage should not be commenced until foam has been removed from the right ventricle, so as to avoid passage of air into the pulmonary bed and left heart, so compounding the problem with arterial air embolization. The use of 100% oxygen is helpful in supplying oxygen to those parts of the lungs still being adequately perfused, and also because this increases the gas pressure gradient for nitrogen from bubble to blood and so increases diffusion. Other measures include intravenous administration of adrenal corticosteroids to reduce cerebral edema and infusion of heparin and low molecular weight dextran to increase microcirculation (86). However, if available, consideration should be given to putting the patient in a compression chamber so as to drive embolized air into solution. The patient can then go through decompression at a rate allowing the air to be expired through the lungs without coming out of solution (87).

Prevention of air embolism

Because air embolism is a life-threatening dialysis complication and treatment is difficult, often with poor results, prevention is of paramount importance. All intravenous fluid administered into the extracorporeal blood circuit should come from collapsible plastic bags only, as these can withstand pressures of at least 150 mm Hg without withdrawing air. This is particularly important if fluid is administered into the subatmospheric pressure area of the prepump segment of the blood circuit. Preferably, intravenous fluids should be administered through the venous drip chamber as rapidly as possible, with the blood pump turned off. Use of the prepump segment for fluid administration should be avoided. This also avoids puncturing the arterial drip chamber or blood line sleeve. Because of the risk, an attendant should be present whenever intravenous fluid is being administered during dialysis using a blood pump.

Heparin should be infused into the extracorporeal blood circuit at a point beyond the blood pump; i.e., infused against the positive pressure gradient. All needle-blood line connections must be tight, as must all arterial or prepump monitor line connections. An infusion sleeve on the prepump segment should not be used unless absolutely necessary. An air detector with a blood line clamp should be used on the venous blood line. Photocell air detectors are commonly used, but very fine microbubbles may not be detectable unless the detector sensitivity is set so as to give frequent false alarms. Additionally, clot on the side of the drip chamber may mask the photocell so permitting the bubble trap to empty undetected. Conductance type air detectors are better and depend on change in capacitance across the drip chamber when it empties to actuate a blood line clamp (see also Chapter 11).

Perhaps the most vulnerable time for air embolism to occur is when rinsing the dialyzer with air at the termination of dialysis. While air or air and saline rinsing is the most effective means of emptying the extracorporeal circuit of blood at the end of dialysis (88), the potential risk of air embolism is such that many physicians prefer to use saline alone. In the event that air is used, the proper procedure must be followed scrupulously. Both patient and assistant should have hemostats placed across the venous blood line so that either can clamp the tubing at the end of the rinse. Television or other distractions should not be permitted, and there should be no conversation so that the complete attention of patient and assistant is focused on the procedure. If the dialyzer is being emptied using air pumped through the blood pump, the assistant must keep one hand on the blood pump switch at all times. If blood is returned using a hand-squeezed pump, enough pressure must be used to keep the blood flowing freely into the venous drip chamber. If possible, the air detector and line clamp should stay on the venous line in the 'active' mode during the wash back procedure.

HEMORRHAGE

An increased incidence of spontaneous bleeding episodes has been reported in maintenance dialysis patients. These include gastrointestinal bleeding, subdural hematoma, uremic hemopericardium, retroperitoneal hematoma, hemorrhagic pleural effusion, spontaneous bleeding into the anterior chamber of the eye, subcapsular hematoma of the liver, and bleeding into the skin and other sites. The underlying cause is related to a number of factors including heparinization during dialysis, anticoagulant therapy, the functional platelet abnormalities of uremia (89) manifested by prolongation of bleeding time, and possibly increased prostacyclin (PGI_2) activity (90) (see also Chapters 9 and 10). The abnormalities in platelet function and PGI_2 activity are not always corrected by dialysis (91, 92). For these reasons, the maintenance dialysis patient is always at some risk of sudden bleeding. Petechial hemorrhages, blood blisters in the skin, and bruising around fistula punctures are not uncommon and usually have no significance except as a warning of the potential risk of bleeding. The possibility of internal bleeding must be considered in any case of unexplained hypotension during dialysis.

Gastrointestinal bleeding

Gastrointestinal bleeding in maintenance hemodialysis patients is related to the usual causes seen in nonuremic patients including peptic ulceration, aspirin ingestion, and hiatal hernia (93). Its occurrence is an indication for regional heparinization during dialysis or for dialysis using low-dose heparin (94) (see Chapter 10). The treatment of gastrointestinal bleeding is straightforward apart from the need to coordinate any surgery with the dialysis schedule.

Subdural hematoma (See also Chapter 37)

Subdural hematoma in maintenance hemodialysis patients, first described in 1969 (95), occurs in up to 3% of dialysis patients (96). It should be suspected in any patient presenting with headache or neurological symptoms resembling disequilibrium but which are not readily explained by this or other causes. Contributory factors include head trauma, excessive anticoagulation, excessive ultrafiltration, hypertension, and the increased cerebrospinal fluid pressure and brain swelling which may occur during dialysis. Frequent episodes of access-site infection or cannula clotting are said to be common in such patients.

The symptoms and signs of subdural hematoma may be nonspecific and often are confused with disequilibrium. However, the latter is unusual with maintenance dialysis except in new patients. The symptoms of disequilibrium usually do not fluctuate as much as those of subdural hematoma and, although headaches are common with disequilibrium, they usually disappear shortly after dialysis. If a previously stable maintenance dialysis patient presents with unexplained symptoms suggestive of disequilibrium, the diagnosis of subdural hematoma should always be considered. Headaches usually are severe, persisting through subsequent dialyses, and there may be focal or multifocal neurologic signs which may fluctuate. Usually neurologic signs are of no value in localizing the intracranial bleeding.

Lumbar puncture and electroencephalography are of little help in diagnosis as abnormalities of both occur with disequilibrium. Radioisotope scanning produces an appreciable percentage of false negative results. The most useful investigations include cerebral arteriography (97), echoencephalography, and computerized tomography of the brain.

When subdural hematoma is seriously considered, it is preferable to use peritoneal dialysis until the diagnosis is confirmed or rejected (98). Treatment is by surgical exploration and removal of clot. The results of surgery are disappointing with a reported patient survival of less than 50% (97, 99, 100). This is comparable to the results of treatment in nonuremic patients with acute subdural hematoma, where mortality is approximately 75% (101).

Uremic hemopericardium

Pericarditis is not uncommon in dialysis patients and may occur early in the course of treatment or at any time after the patient becomes stabilized on maintenance dialysis (102). While the former is commonly uremic in origin, pericarditis in a stable dialysis patient is more likely to be associated with cytomegalic or other virus infection or has no demonstrable cause (103) (see also Chapter 30). Pericarditis without effusion is an indication for more frequent dialysis, preferably with regional heparinization or low dose heparin (see Chapter 10), or for peritoneal dialysis avoiding the use of anticoagulants.

In a small number of patients, an obvious pericardial effusion may develop and this may be associated with bleeding into the pericardial sac. While relatively uncommon, pericardial effusion is important because of the potential risk of tamponade, which may escape early recognition. Such patients usually give a history of preceeding upper-respiratory infection and have symptoms of chest pain, respiratory distress, hypotension, and evidence of fluid overload, usually associated with fever and symptoms suggestive of a mild upper respiratory or gastrointestinal viral infection. In patients developing signs and symptoms suggestive of pericardial effusion, this diagnosis should be confirmed by X-ray, sonography, isotope scanning, or other means.

Treatment initially is by repeated pericardiocentesis (104) and the associated installation of a nonabsorbable steroid into the pericardial sac may be beneficial (105). If these measures fail, pericardectomy or pericardial fenestration usually is required (106).

Retroperitoneal hematoma

Spontaneous retroperitoneal hemorrhage with a resultant hematoma is an uncommon complication of dialysis, occurring in less than 1% of patients (107, 108). Diagnosis may be difficult in the absence of a history of trauma. There may be massive bleeding into the retroperitoneal space requiring transfusion of large volumes of blood, or the onset may be more insidious. Predisposing factors include minor trauma and anticoagulation; spontaneous retroperitoneal bleeding is a rare complication in nonuremic patients receiving anticoagulants. An iatrogenic retroperitoneal hematoma can occur from perforation of an iliac vein during insertion of a catheter into the femoral vein by the Seldinger technique (see Chapter 8).

Retroperitoneal bleeding presents with abdominal and flank or back pain, frequently associated with a distended abdomen and hypoactive or absent bowel sounds. An abdominal mass may be palpable and X-ray of the abdomen may show a soft tissue density and absence of psoas shadow, and a barium contrast meal may show a nonspecific ileitis. After significant bleeding, fever can occur without evidence of simultaneous infection. Bleeding around the pancreas may occur causing pancreatic injury and an increase of pancreatic enzymes. Neuropathy due to retroperitoneal bleeding and dissection around the femoral nerve has been described. Selective renal angiography may be helpful in diagnosing perirenal hemorrhage (109) and sonography is also useful diagnostically.

Treatment is usually conservative with replacement of blood loss and hemodialysis using minimal heparin or peritoneal dialysis. Anticoagulant therapy should be discontinued and the patient kept at rest. Surgical exploration usually is unnecessary.

Spontaneous retroperitoneal bleeding should be considered in any maintenance dialysis patient with unexplained acute abdominal distress and falling hematocrit and without obvious external blood loss.

Hemorrhagic pleural effusion

Pleuritis is a complication of uremia (110), and very occasionally hemorrhagic pleural effusion may occur in dialysis patients (111) probably related to anticoagulation in a patient with a fibrinous pleuritis. Treatment includes hemodialysis, avoiding heparin excess, or peritoneal dialysis, pleurocentesis, and possible use of nonabsorbable steroids as in the treatment of pericarditis. The possibility of development of pulmonary contraction in the patient who has had recurrent hemorrhagic pleuritis must be considered. Hemorrhagic pleural effusion should also suggest the possibility of cancer or of tuberculosis.

Subcapsular liver hematoma

Spontaneous subcapsular liver hematoma may occur in patients treated by dialysis and should be considered if a dialysis patient presents with right upper quadrant pain, rising alkaline phosphatase level, and decreasing hematocrit without evidence of external blood loss (112). Radioisotope scanning can provide supportive evidence. Management is dependent upon the extent and location of the liver injury and may require evacuation or partial hepatectomy.

Hemorrhages into the skin

Petechial hemorrhages and an increased frequency of blood blisters from bruising around fistula punctures are not uncommon in dialysis patients. There has also been a report of typical subungual splinter hemorrhages, identical with those of bacterial endocarditis, occurring in patients treated by maintenance hemodialysis (113).

MISCELLANEOUS PROBLEMS ASSOCIATED WITH DIALYSIS

Restlessness and insomnia

Restlessness and insomnia are frequent symptoms in patients with severe uremia, particularly in the months immediately prior to starting maintenance dialysis. Usually they are relieved within a few weeks of starting treatment.

When these symptoms develop in a stable patient on maintenance hemodialysis, causes such as anxiety are most likely, but the possibility of inadequate dialysis should always be considered. Consequently, any patient developing insomnia and restlessness should have a review of predialysis blood chemistry. Treatment is symptomatic. In the home dialysis patient suffering from insomnia, medication should be avoided, specifically in the period shortly before dialysis.

Hypoglycemia due to beta-blocking agents

Beta adrenergic-blocking agents are used in the treatment of the hypertension of chronic renal failure and, in particular, for treatment of persistent hypertension in maintenance dialysis patients. These drugs have hypoglycemic effects, and episodes of severe acute hypoglycemia in association with beta-blocking agents were first described in association with use of glucose-free dialysate in a single-pass system after patients had fasted for more than 18 h (114). Recently, episodes of profound hypoglycemia have been reported in nondiabetic dialysis patients receiving propranolol for hypertension who were not fasting (115). The effect of beta-blocking drugs on glucose metabolism is complex and may result in either hypoglycemia or hyperglycemia (116). Other contributory factors may include poor nutritional intake which may have caused decreased glycogen stores and other possible causes of liver dysfunction.

Symptoms and signs include a sharp rise of blood pressure, presumably due to release of catecholamines, vomiting, and unconsciousness occurring early in dialysis. This possibility should be considered when such symptoms develop in any dialysis patient receiving beta-blocking agents.

Because of the widespread use of beta-blockers for control of blood pressure, angina, or arrhythmias, it is possible that many dialysis patients, especially those with diabetes, liver dysfunction or poor nutrition, may develop transient episodes of hypoglycemia but do not manifest autonomic symptoms because these are prevented by the beta-blockers. Since use of a glucose-free dialysate may contribute to development of hypoglycemia, glucose-containing dialysate should be used for patients receiving beta-blockers. Alternatively, frequent blood sugar determinations may be made on maintenance hemodialysis patients taking beta-blockers.

Dermatologic abnormalities associated with hemodialysis

Xerosis and pruritus are extremely common in chronic renal failure and also occur in maintenance dialysis patients (117). Among the other dermatological problems reported in such patients are lesions resembling erythema multiforme, bullous dermatosis, and porphyria cutanea tarda. Lesions of bullous dermatosis are characterized by moderately painful bullae occurring on the dorsa of the hands and feet, unassociated with trauma (118). The cause is unknown and not related to medication, although there is a suggestion that sunlight may be a causative factor. Porphyria cutanea tarda has also been reported in dialysis patients (119), is associated with the preexisting inherited enzyme defect, and may be precipitated by iron overload (120).

Pruritus
Pruritus frequently complicates end-stage renal disease. This is usually much less of a problem in adequately treated maintenance dialysis patients but it still occurs sufficiently often to distress an appreciable number of patients (117). When pruritus is associated with hypercalcemia and secondary hyperparathyroidism, this shows a dramatic response to subtotal parathyroidectomy (121). For other patients, therapy is generally symptomatic with antihistamines and sedatives; a number of different treatments have been tried with varying degrees of success.

In a double-blind study, intravenous lidocaine, 100 mg (427 µmol), relieved pruritus completely in some patients and had a marked effect in others (122). Unfortunately, relief lasted only for a day following infusion, pruritus always recurring by the next day. Blood levels of lidocaine achieved were no greater than those used in treating cardiac arrhythmias, and if the drug was given at a rate no greater than 7 mg (30 µmol)/min, no adverse effects were noted other than occasional episodes of hypotension. Lidocaine has a normal plasma half-life in patients with chronic renal failure, suggesting that persistance of relief into the day after administration is due either to a metabolite normally excreted by the kidney being active as an antipruritic agent or because lidocaine is acting in a kinetic compartment from which the drug has a very slow rate of egress.

Administration of the nonabsorbable anion-exchange resin, cholestyramine, has also met with some success in treating uremic pruritus, 5 g twice daily in juice producing partial relief in most patients in a randomized 4-week double-blind study (123). Cholestyramine has the ability to bind organic acids, which may be a clue to the chemical cause of pruritus. It also relieves the itching of obstructive jaundice, possibly by binding of bile acids. Moreover, it reduces the itching of polycythemia vera. A second study, however, failed to show relief of uremic pruritus by cholestyramine (124), which may induce or aggravate metabolic acidosis (125) and is very difficult to present in a palatable form.

In 1977 Gilchrest and coworkers (126) reported good results with phototherapy for uremic pruritus. The beneficial effect of sunburn-spectrum ultraviolet (UVB) phototherapy using slightly below-minimum erythemal doses of ultraviolet B radiation has been reported (127). Gilchrest and colleagues (128) have treated patients by applying UVB phototherapy to one half of the body and placebo phototherapy to the other half and found that all patients noted generalized improvement without localization of benefit to the treated side, suggesting a systemic effect of UVB phototherapy. Remissions of up to several months were obtained, and a more rapid response occurred with more intensive schedules of treatment and with a second course of phototherapy. Possibly UVB phototherapy inactivates (a) circulating substance(s) present in uremia and responsible for pruritus; alternatively, a photoproduct with a long half-life may be capable of relieving pruritus without directly affecting the cause. Use of ultraviolet A (UVA) light in dialysis patients has also been reported to produce relief; and although this is not as dramatic as with UVB, this may prove to be preferable because UVA has a higher safety margin, is commercially available, and requires less stringent monitoring of the patient (129).

Relief of uremic pruritus has also been reported in a double-blind cross-over study using oral charcoal, 6 g daily for eight weeks (130). Charcoal is presumed to act as a sorbent of numerous organic and inorganic compounds. Heparin infusion has also been described as relieving pruritus (131); and in one case, reduction of dialysate magnesium concentration to 0.2 mmol/l (0.48 mg/dl), resulting in reduction of the predialysis serum magnesium concentration, produced relief (132).

As is usual in medicine, the wide range of measures available for treatment of uremic pruritus suggests that none is universally effective, and a better understanding of the cause of itching and its molecular basis is required. Meanwhile general measures should not be neglected, including antihistamines and tranquilizers (133), wearing of light clothing, and few bedclothes. Tepid baths or showers may help the patient who has difficulty in sleeping due to itching and may give sufficient, though temporary, relief to allow sleep. Cooling of the skin can be achieved by application of a lotion such as calamine, but local anesthetic or antihistamine creams and ointments should be avoided because of the risk of allergic contact sensitization.

Muscle cramps

Painful muscle cramps are common in nondialyzed and dialyzed uremic patients, both during and between dialyses, particularly in elderly patients. While not life-threatening, cramps may interfere seriously with patient well-being and rehabilitation.

Muscle cramps in dialyzed patients appear to be related to acutely induced plasma and extracellular volume contraction due to rapid extracellular volume removal or hypoosmolality. Cramps tend to occur late during dialysis, more frequently in the legs, and typically last about 10 min taking about 3 min to develop and 7 min to fully dissipate. In patients who develop muscle cramps, tonic EMG activity increases during the latter part of dialysis and appears to be useful as a predictor of the onset of cramp during dialysis (134).

We have used quinine sulfate empirically for relief of cramps for many years, and the effectiveness of this has been confirmed by a double-blind study (135) which showed that 320 mg (1.0 mmol) quinine sulfate prior to each dialysis was effective in reducing both the frequency and severity of cramps without hematologic, auditory, or visual side effects.

Relief or reduction in the frequency of cramps has been described with use of a higher dialysate sodium concentration (140 mmol/l), administration of sodium chloride by mouth (136), or with use of a bolus intravenous injection of 20 ml of hypertonic (17.5%) (3 mol/l) saline (137), a solution that must be appropriately labeled to avoid inadvertent use. However, use of hypertonic sodium chloride to relieve cramps is unsatisfactory because this partially cancels the effect of ultrafiltration in normalizing the patient's extracellular volume. As a result, hypertonic dextrose has also been used and double-blind studies have shown significant relief of cramps without complications using hypertonic (50%) dextrose injected intravenously (138, 139). Hypertonic dextrose results in an acute rise of the serum glucose level, but this returns to normal within one hour. Cramps during dialysis can also be prevented by sequential ultrafiltration (35).

Priapism

Priapism may occur at some time in as many as 2.5% of male patients between the ages of 14 and 42 on regular hemodialysis (140, 141). In the majority of cases, priapism develops during dialysis, is not related to sexual activity, and patients may be sleeping when awakened by a painful erection. Erections are known to occur during rapid-eye-movement sleep, irrespective of dream content, and this may be a precipitating factor. Most of the instances of priapism occur during heparinization while on dialysis and are not associated with general clotting problems, long-term anticoagulation, or androgen therapy. A high hematocrit and hypovolemia have been suggested as precipitating factors through increasing blood viscocity, and it has been recommended that if a male patient has a hematocrit greater than 25, androgen therapy should be stopped so as to avoid increased frequency of erections (142).

The prognosis for return of sexual function after priapism in dialysis patients is very poor despite venous bypass surgery. Following such surgery, only a small number of patients retain the capacity to sustain erection. Other treatments used have included spinal anesthetics and a variety of drugs such as phenothiazine, atropine, and ancrod. Recent developments in penile prostheses have made these the most effective treatment for patients with impotence following priapism.

Pulmonary function during dialysis

Transient and marked leukopenia during the first 15 to 30 min of hemodialysis, recognized for many years (143, 144), is associated with transient sequestration of neutrophils in the dialyzer and in the pulmonary capillary bed. The initiating mechanism of these phenomena is activation of complement through contact with the dialysis membrane and this is responsible for increased margination and sequestration of neutrophils in the pulmonary capillaries (145). Trapping of microaggregates of leukocytes has been said to lead to hypoxia. White cell studies and pulmonary function tests in patients before, during, and after hemodialysis have shown significant leukopenia and a fall in CO diffusing capacity within 15 min of the start of hemodialysis and development of hypoxia within 30 min. The white cell count returns to baseline level within 1 h but PO_2 and CO diffusing capacity remain low throughout dialysis and the fall in these is directly related to the initial fall in white cell count (146). Persistence of hypoxia, together with the fact that hypoxia can also occur using dialyzers that do not cause leukopenia (147) suggests that other mechanisms may cause the hypoxia. Jacob and Gavellas (148) studied dialyzers with cuprophane, regenerated cellulose, cellulose acetate, and polyacrylonitrile membranes in the same patients. Cuprophane and regenerated cellulose dialyzers produced profound leukopenia followed by rebound leucocytosis; this was less marked with cellulose acetate membranes, and the change was minimal with the polyacrylonitrile membrane. In spite of these differences, persistent hypoxia occurred during dialysis, independent of the membrane used, and progressed in severity even as the leukocyte count returned to or exceeded normal.

Thus leukopenia and hypoxia may be concurrent but unrelated phenomena. A possible explanation could be that the hypoxia is secondary to depression of ventilation due to loss of carbon dioxide across the membrane to dialysate during dialysis (149). Alternatively, the progressive improvement in acidosis during hemodialysis would decrease respiratory stimulation and therefore minute ventilation and arterial oxygen tension. Carbon dioxide would then either traverse the dialysis membrane or be used in acetate metabolism.

From the clinical point of view, these effects, including hypoxia, usually are insufficient to produce symptoms, although they could be significant in a patient with preexisting marginal cardiopulmonary function. In such patients, sequential ultrafiltration with subsequent use of bicarbonate dialysis could be beneficial (150, 151).

Joint and tendon abnormalities associated with hemodialysis

Hemodialysis patients have long been known to be prone to acute episodes of arthritis or periarthritis, and the appearance of soft tissue calcification in periarticular tissues is also well recognized. These problems are discussed in Chapter 35.

Spontaneous tendon rupture
There have been a number of reports of spontaneous tendon rupture in dialysis patients affecting the quadriceps and the hand. The cause is unclear. Chronic acidosis may lead to degeneration of tendons with changes in their tensile characteristics (152), but pathologic changes at the tendo-osseus junction due to secondary hyperparathyroidism may be more important (153). The latter view is supported by the description of quadriceps tendon rupture associated with X-ray evidence of hyperparathyroidism in five patients (154). Tendon ruptures occur after longer periods on dialysis and in young patients. Finger tendon ruptures usually are ignored by the patient because they are not significantly disabling. Patients with quadriceps tendon ruptures are treated by immobilization with plaster, physiotherapy, and frequently by parathyroidectomy.

Carpal tunnel syndrome
Carpal tunnel syndrome is being reported with increased frequency in dialysis patients and may be related to vascular access surgery and resulting ischemia or venous hypertension (155, 156) Jain and colleagues (157), in a survey of 62 patients treated by maintenance dialysis for at least 6 months, found 5 with carpal tunnel syndrome and another 5 with prolonged distal motor latencies. Synovial biopsy specimens from flexor tendons showed edema without inflammation, and it was felt that extracellular fluid volume excess in the presence of flexion and immobility during dialysis was important in development of the carpal tunnel syndrome. Treatment is surgical.

Uremic bursitis
Bursitis in uremic patients, with or without effusion, is a manifestation of uremic polyserositis. Most commonly, this presents as an olecranon bursal effusion resulting from trauma or from increased pressure in bursal vessels related to arteriovenous anastomosis together with the anticoagulant effects of heparin. As many at 6% of patients developed bursitis in one report (158) and all had arteriovenous fistulas and used cushions under their elbows for support. Bursitis usually occurred over the olecranon on the side with the vascular access, although effusions involving the trochanteric and achilles bursae also occurred. Treatment consists of aspiration and injection of nonabsorbable steroids. Although aspiration usually is sterile, septic bursitis may also occur.

Septic arthritis
Septic arthritis is a much more common complication in dialysis patients than in the general population (159). Because joint pain is not uncommon in dialysis patients, the possibility of septic arthritis always should be borne in mind. The most common causative organism is a staphylococcus, and the same microorganisms are often cultured simultaneously from joint, blood, and/or arteriovenous fistula, suggesting hematogenous spread. Unlike nonuremic septic arthritis, in addition to the usual joints such as knee, elbow, hip, and shoulder, other joints involved in the dialysis patient include the sternoclavicular, sacroiliac, and acromioclavicular joints, and the arthritis is more frequently multiarticular. Early diagnosis is mandatory in order to minimize the risk of disabling joint disease, but unfortunately, the diagnosis is not always easy because the occurrence of other types of acute arthritis is so frequent in dialysis patients. However, acute attacks of pseudogout usually are not associated with other systemic complaints. Septic arthritis should always be considered when a dialysis patient develops arthritis, especially if associated with fever or infection elsewhere, and an infectious cause must always be excluded by joint aspiration. Once an infection is identified, prompt and early treatment is required to prevent crippling joint damage.

Hearing loss

Hearing loss associated with dialysis has been described and is reviewed in a recent article by Rizvi and Holmes (160). Impairment may involve both vestibular and cochlear mechanisms and may be due to bleeding in the inner ear space as a consequence of heparinization or to cellular injury in the hair cells of the cochlea as a result of edema. However, the frequent use of ototoxic drugs in dialysis patients makes hearing loss difficult to evaluate, and a recent report found no evidence of an effect of dialysis on hearing after 1 to 5 years of dialysis (161).

Hepatic friction rub

A hepatic friction rub is an auscultatory finding most commonly associated with malignant neoplasm of the liver but recently described in two patients undergoing maintenance hemodialysis (162). Such a rub presumably is the equivalent of a uremic pericardial or pleural friction rub and theoretically should disappear with increased dialysis, although this did not occur.

Recurrent abdominal pain associated with digoxin

Recently an elderly male dialysis patient was described who had severe recurrent central abdominal pain, brought on by exertion, occurring shortly after dialysis, and especially after marked ultrafiltration (163). This was thought to be due to intestinal angina resulting from intestinal ischemia from reduced cardiac output or local vasoconstriction following intravascular volume depletion during dialysis. The patient's symptoms were relieved by discontinuing digoxin, probably because it is a mesenteric vasoconstrictor. This syndrome may occur in dialysis patients with calcified aortas who undergo rapid ultrafiltration and are taking digoxin and should be considered a possible cause of obscure abdominal pain in dialysis patients.

First-use syndrome

Reactions characterized by respiratory distress, with or without wheezing, malaise, and back or chest pain, and sometimes with chills and subsequent fever, occasionally occur within a few minutes of the start of dialysis using a new dialyzer. Usually such reactions are mild and self-limiting, although on occasion they may require the use of analgesics, antihistamines, or epinephrine (164). These reactions may be difficult to distinguish from pyrogenic reactions and other minor problems occurring during dialysis, although they are characterized by their immediate onset at the start of dialysis and the fact that they occur sporadically amongst patients in a center. A byproduct of sterilization with ethylene oxide gas, 2-chloroethanol, was identified in the blood compartment of a dialyzer of a patient who had a severe reaction on initiation of dialysis (165). Adequate rinsing of new dialyzers with 1 to 2 l of saline should eliminate this problem.

Leachables

Because dialyzers and tubing sets are made from plastic, there is always the likelihood of leaching polyvinyl chloride or plasticizers such as bis (2-ethylhexyl) phthalate into the blood. The latter probably is not very toxic, although it may affect various enzyme systems (166). Polyvinyl chloride has been associated with recurrent episodes of cutaneous necrotizing dermatitis in a dialysis patient (167), probably resulting from an immunologic process. The association between these and other chemicals leached from plastics and the occurrence of such effects as eosinophilia and itching during dialysis has not been clearly established. The occasional occurrence in dialysis patients of immediate reactions resembling IgE-mediated anaphylaxis has also been recorded and related to development of antibodies to phthalic anhydride and to diphenylmethane diisocyanate (168).

Membrane sensitivity

Episodes of asthma associated with leucopenia occurring during dialysis have been described in one patient, apparently associated only with use of cuprophane membrane dialyzers. The mechanism is thought to be either complement activation or pulmonary leucostasis with release of bronchoconstrictor substances from the impacted leucocytes. The latter explanation seems more likely as the patient did not have asthmatic reactions during dialysis with a polyacrylonitrile membrane which activates complement but does not cause pulmonary leucostasis (169).

Anti-N-like antibodies

Anti-N-like antibodies occurring in dialysis patients were first described in 1972 (170) and appear to be related to use of formaldehyde in sterilization of reused dialyzers. It has been shown that in these circumstances there can be alteration in red cell ATP content, indicating that red blood cell damage has occurred (171). Disposable dialyzers are no longer sterilized with formaldehyde by the manufacturer (as opposed to the Kiil dialyzer), but formaldehyde sterilization is still a usual part of the dialyzer reuse process. Recently it has been shown that anti-N-like antibodies are more common in home dialysis patients than in dialysis patients dialyzing at a facility, presumably because home dialysis patients tend not to rinse their dialyzers as well, with possible retention of small amounts of formaldehyde (172). Certainly when formaldehyde is used as a sterilizing agent, it is essential that it be removed by adequate rinsing (see also Chapter 15). Anti-N-like antibodies may increase hemolysis and so contribute to anemia in patients with renal failure but do not appear to have other significant actions.

COMMENT

Acute problems during hemodialysis range from the trivial and merely transient to the catastrophic and fatal. Nevertheless, the great majority of dialyses are uneventful, and each year, more than two million dialyses are performed in patients' homes around the world. Because most dialyses are uneventful, it is important that nursing and technical staff as well as patients learn of the acute complications of hemodialysis, their recognition, and the appropriate responses. Patient well-being, whether dialyzing at home or in a center, demands confidence in the treatment and its safety. This can only come from the example of staff who are themselves familiar with the acute complications of hemodialysis and are experienced in their management.

REFERENCES

1. Keshaviah PR, Luehmann D, Shapiro FL, Comty CM: *Investigation of the Risks and Hazards Associated with Hemodialysis Devices.* Technical report, Food and Drug Administration, Department of Health, Education and Welfare, 1980
2. Mawdsley C: Neurological complications of haemodialysis, *Proc R Soc Med* 65:871, 1972
3. Tyler HR: Neurologic disorders in renal failure. *Am J Med* 44:734, 1968
4. Wakim KG: The pathophysiology of the dialysis disequilibrium syndrome. *Mayo Clin Proc* 44:406, 1969
5. deC Peterson H, Swanson AG: Acute encephalopathy occurring during hemodialysis. *Arch Intern Med* 113:877, 1974
6. Kennedy AC: Dialysis disequilibrium syndrome. *Electroencephalogr Clin Neurophysiol* 29:206, 1970
7. Kennedy AC, Linton AL, Eaton JC: Urea levels in cerebrospinal fluid after haemodialysis. *Lancet* 1:410, 1962
8. Funder J, Wieth JO: Changes in cerebrospinal fluid composition following haemodialysis. *Scand J Clin Lab Invest* 19:301, 1967
9. Sitprija V, Holmes JH: Preliminary observations on the change in intracranial pressure and intraocular pressure during hemodialysis. *Trans Am Soc Artif Intern Organs* 8:300, 1962
10. Gilliland KG, Hegstrom RM: The effect of hemodialysis on cerebrospinal fluid pressure in uremic dogs. *Trans Am Soc Artif Intern Organs* 9:44, 1973
11. Arieff AI, Massry SG, Barrientos A, Kleeman CR: Brain water and electrolyte metabolism in uremia: effects of slow and rapid hemodialysis. *Kidney Int* 4:177, 1973
12. Posner JB, Plum F: Spinal fluid pH and neurologic symptoms in systemic acidosis. *N Engl J Med* 277:605, 1977
13. Rosenbaum BJ, Coburn JW, Shinaberger JH, Massry SG: Acid-base status during the interdialytic period in patients maintained with chronic hemodialysis. *Ann Intern Med* 71:1105, 1969
14. Hampers CL, Doak PB, Callaghan MN, Tyler HR, Merrill JP: The electroencephalogram and spinal fluid during hemodialysis. *Arch Intern Med* 118:340, 1966
15. Rigg GA, Bercu BA: Hypoglycemia: a complication of hemodialysis. *N Engl J Med* 277:1139, 1967
16. Wakim KG: Predominance of hyponatremia over hypoosmolality in simulation of the dialysis disequilibrium syndrome. *Mayo Clin Proc* 44:433, 1969
17. Arieff AI, Massry SG: Dialysis disequilibrium syndrome, in: *Clinical Aspects of Uremia and Dialysis*, edited by Massry SG, Sellers AL, Springfield IL, Charles C Thomas, 1976, p 34
18. Arieff AI, Lazarowitz UC, Guisado R: Experimental dialysis disequilibrium syndrome: prevention with glycerol. *Kidney Int* 14:270, 1978
19. Chazan BI, Rees SB, Balodimos MC, Younger D, Ferguson DB: Dialysis in diabetics. *JAMA* 209:2026, 1969
20. LaGreca G, Dettori P, Biasioli S, Fabris A, Feriani M, Pinna V, Pisani E, Ronco C: Brain density studies during dialysis. *Lancet* 2:582, 1980
21. Johnson WF, Hagge WW, Wagoner RD, Dinapoli RP, Rosevear JW: Effects of urea loading in patients with far-advanced renal failure. *Mayo Clin Proc* 47:21, 1972
22. Gutman RA, Hickman RO, Chatrian GE, Scribner BH: Failure of high dialysis-fluid glucose to prevent the disequilibrium syndrome. *Lancet* 1:295, 1967
23. Kjellstrand CM, Shideman JR, Santiago EA, Mauer M, Simmons RL, Buselmeier TJ: Technical advances in hemodialysis of very small pediatric patients. *Proc Clin Dial Transpl Forum* 1:124, 1971
24. Stewart WK, Flemming LW, Manuel MA: Benefit obtained by the use of high sodium dialysate during maintenance haemodialysis. *Proc Eur Dial Transpl Assoc* 9:111, 1972
25. Guisado R, Arieff AI, Massry SG: Dialysis disequilibrium syndrome: prevention by use of glycerol in the dialysate. *Clin Res* 22:207A, 1974
26. Maher JF, Schreiner GE: Hazards and complications of dialysis. *N Engl J Med* 273:370, 1965
27. Mattson RH: The benzodiazepines, in: *Antiepileptic Drugs*, edited by Woodbury DM, Penry KG, Schmidt, RP, New York, Raven, 1972, p 497
28. Degoulet P, Proulx J, Aime F, Berger C, Bloch P, Goupy F, Legrain M: Programme Dialyse – Informatique III – Données épidémiologiques. Stratégies de dialyse et résultats biologiques. (Dialysis programme. Epidemiological data. Dialysis strategies and biological results) *J Urol Néphrol* 82:1001, 1976 (in French)
29. Rubin LJ, Gutman RA: Hypotension during hemodialysis. *The Kidney* 11:21, 1978
30. Degoulet P, Rojas P, Boukari M, Aime F, Reach I: L'accident hypotensif au cours de la séance de dialyse. 1. Etude épidémiologique, la recherche des facteurs de risque, (Hypotensive episodes during dialysis sessions. 1 Epidemiological studies, investigations on risk factors). *Sem Uro-Néphrol*, Pitie-Salpétrière. Paris, Masson et Cie, 1978, p 164 (in French)
31. Babb AL, Popovich RP, Christopher TG, Scribner BH: The genesis of the square-meter hour hypothesis. *Trans Am Soc Artif Intern Organs* 17:81, 1971
32. Milutinovic J, Strand M, Casaretto A, Babb AL, Scribner B: Clinical impact of residual glomerular filtration rate on dialysis time. *Trans Am Soc Artif Intern Organs* 20:410, 1974
33. Kersh ES, Kronfield SJ, Unger A, Popper RW, Cantor S, Cohn K: Autonomic insufficiency in uremia as a cause of hemodialysis-induced hypotension. *N Engl J Med* 290:650, 1974
34. Kobayashi K, Shibata M, Kato K, Kato S, Nakamura S, Kurachi K, Yasuda B, Ota K, Maeda K, Imai T, Kawaguchi S, Tsutsui S, Shimizu K, Yamazaki C, Manji T, Nomura T: Studies on the development of a new method of controlling the amount and contents of body fluids (extracorporeal ultrafiltration method: ECUM) and the application of this method for patients receiving long-term hemodialysis. *Jap J Nephrol* 14:539, 1972
35. Bergström J, Asaba H, Fürst P, Oulès R: Dialysis, ultrafiltration and blood pressure. *Proc Eur Dial Transpl Assoc* 13:293, 1976
36. Man NK, Granger A, Rondon-Nucete M, Zingraff J, Jungers P, Sausse A, Funck-Brentano JL: One year follow-up of short dialysis with a membrane highly permeable to middle molecules. *Proc Eur Dial Transpl Assoc* 10:236, 1973
37. Wehle B, Asaba H, Castenfors J, Fürst P, Grahn A, Gunnarson B, Shaldon S, Bergström J: The influence of dialysis fluid composition on the blood pressure response during dialysis. *Clin Nephrol* 10:62, 1978
38. Henrich WL, Woodard TD, Blachley JD, Gomez-Sanchez C, Pettinger W, Cronin RE: Role of osmolality in blood pressure stability after dialysis and ultrafiltration. *Kidney Int* 18:480, 1980
39. Mion CM, Hegstrom RM, Boen ST, Scribner BH: Substitution of sodium acetate for sodium bicarbonate in the bath fluid for hemodialysis. *Trans Am Soc Artif Intern Organs* 10:110, 1964
40. Kveim M, Nesbakken R: Utilization of exogenous acetate

during hemodialysis. *Trans Am Soc Artif Intern Organs* 21:138, 1975
41. Novello A, Kelsch RC, Easterling RE: Acetate intolerance during hemodialysis. *Clin Nephrol* 5:29, 1976
42. Gonzalez FM, Pearson JE, Garbus SB, Holbert RD: On the effects of acetate during hemodialysis. *Trans Am Soc Artif Intern Organs* 20:169, 1974
43. Vreman HJ, Assomull VM, Kaiser BM, Blaschke TF, Weiner WM: Acetate metabolism and acid-base homeostasis during hemodialysis: influence of dialyzer efficiency and rate of acetate metabolism. *Kidney Int 18 (Suppl 10)*:S62, 1980
44. Graefe U, Milutinovic J, Follette W, Vizzo J, Scribner BH: Effect of high efficiency dialysis on acid-base balance and patient 'well-being'. *Abstracts Am Soc Nephrol* 9:31a, 1976
45. Graefe U, Milutinovic J, Follette WC, Vizzo JE, Babb AL, Scribner BH: Less dialysis morbidity and vascular irritability with bicarbonate in dialysate. *Ann Intern Med* 88:332, 1978
46. Kirkendol PL, Devia CJ, Bower JD, Holbert RD: A comparison of the cardiovascular effects of sodium acetate, sodium bicarbonate and other potential sources of fixed base in hemodialysate solutions. *Trans Am Soc Artif Intern Organs* 23:399, 1977
47. Aizawa Y, Ohmori T, Imai K, Matsuoka M, Hirasawa Y: Depressant action of acetate upon the human cardiovascular system. *Clin Nephrol* 8:477, 1977
48. Iseki K, Onoyama K, Maeda T, Shimamatsu K, Harada A, Fujimi S, Omae T: Comparison of hemodynamics induced by conventional acetate hemodialysis, bicarbonate hemodialysis and ultrafiltration. *Clin Nephrol* 14:294, 1980.
49. Lewis EJ, Tolchin N, Roberts JL: Estimation of the metabolic conversion of acetate to bicarbonate during hemodialysis. *Kidney Int 18 (Suppl 10)*:S51, 1980
50. Relman AS: Metabolic consequences of acid-base disorders. *Kidney Int* 1:347, 1972
51. Mitchell JH, Wildenthal K, Johnson RL Jr: The effects of acid-base disturbances on cardiovascular and pulmonary function. *Kidney Int* 1:375, 1972
52. Lemann JR Jr, Litzow JR, Lennon EJ: The effects of chronic acid loads in normal man: further evidence for the participation of bone mineral in the defense against chronic metabolic acidosis. *J Clin Invest* 45:1608, 1966
53. McSherry E, Morris RC Jr: Attainment of normal stature with alkali therapy in infants and children with classic renal tubular acidosis (RTA): evidence that acidosis is critical to the pathogenesis of impaired growth. *J Clin Invest* 61:509, 1978
54. Rorke SJ, Davidson WD, Guo SS, Morin RJ: Metabolic fate of 14C-acetate during dialysis. *Proc Eur Dial Transpl Assoc* 13:394, 1976
55. Tolchin N, Roberts JL, Hayashi J, Lewis EJ: Metabolic consequences of higher mass-transfer hemodialysis. *Kidney Int* 11:366, 1977
56. Weiner MW, Epstein FH: Signs and symptoms of electrolyte disorders, in: *Clinical Disorders of Fluid and Electrolyte Metabolism*, edited by Maxwell MH, Kleeman CR, New York, McGraw-Hill Book Company, 1972, p 629
57. Said R, Quintanilla A, Levin N, Ivanovich P: Acute hemolysis due to profound hypo-osmolality: a complication of hemodialysis. *J Dial* 1:447, 1977
58. Arieff AI, Guisado R: Effect on the central nervous system of hypernatremic and hyponatremic states. *Kidney Int* 10:104, 1976
59. Lindner A, Moskovtchenko JF, Traeger J: Accidental mass hypernatremia during hemodialysis. *Nephron* 9:99, 1972
60. Nickey WA, Chinitz VL, Kim KE, Onesti G, Swartz C: Hypernatremia from water softener malfunction during home dialysis. *JAMA* 214:915, 1970
61. Morrison G, Michelson EL, Brown S, Morganroth J: Mechanism and prevention of cardiac arrhythmias in chronic hemodialysis patients. *Kidney Int* 17:811, 1980
62. Wiegand CF, Davin TD, Raij L, Kjellstrand CM: Severe hypokalemia induced by hemodialysis. *Arch Intern Med* 141:167, 1981
63. Association for the Advancement of Medical Instrumentaiton: *Hemodialysis Systems Standards (proposed)*. Arlington, Virginia, 1978
64. Freeman RM, Lawton RL, Chamberlain MA: Hard-water syndrome. *N Engl J Med* 276:1113, 1967
65. Evans DB, Slapak M: Pancreatitis in the hard water syndrome. *Br Med J* 3:748, 1975
66. Govan JR, Porter CA, Cook JGH, Dixon B, Trafford JAP: Acute magnesium poisoning as a complication of chronic haemodialysis. *Br Med J* 2:278, 1968
67. Burnell JM: Acid-base chemistry in human bone. *Proc 10th Annu Contr Conf Artificial Kidney – Chronic Uremia Program, NIAMDD, edited by Mackey BB, DHEW publ (NIH) no 77-1442, 1977, p 35*
68. Klein WJ Jr, Metz EN, Price AR: Acute copper intoxication: a hazard of hemodialysis. *Arch Intern Med* 129:578, 1972
69. Blomfield J, Dixon SR, McCredie DA: Potential hepatotoxicity of copper in recurrent hemodialysis. *Arch Intern Med* 128:555, 1971
70. Lyle WH, Payton JE, Hui M: Haemodialysis and copper fever. *Lancet* 1:1324, 1976
71. Mansouri K, Halsted JA, Gombos EA: Zinc, copper, magnesium and calcium in dialyzed and nondialyzed uremic patients. *Arch Intern Med* 125:88, 1970
72. Gallery EDM, Blomfield J, Dixon SR: Acute zinc toxicity in haemodialysis. *Br Med J* 4:331, 1973
73. Beattie AD, Moore MR, Devenay WT, Miller AR, Goldberg A: Environmental lead pollution in an urban softwater area. *Br Med J* 2:491, 1972
74. Webster JD, Parker TF, Alfrey AC, Smythe WR, Kubo H, Neal G, Hull AR: Acute nickel intoxication by dialysis. *Ann Intern Med* 92:631, 1980
75. Carlson DJ, Shapiro GL: Methemoglobinemia from well water nitrates: a complication of home dialysis. *Ann Intern Med* 73:757, 1970
76. Eaton JW, Kolpin CF, Swofford HS, Kjellstrand CM, Jacob HS: Chlorinated water: a cause of dialysis-induced hemolytic anemia. *Science* 181:463, 1973
77. Raij L, Shapiro FL, Michael AF: Endotoxemia in febrile reactions during hemodialysis. *Kidney Int* 4:57, 1973
78. Peterson NJ, Boyer KM, Carson LA, Favero MS: Pyrogenic reactions from inadequate disinfection of a dialysis fluid distribution system. *Dial Transpl* 7:52, 1978
79. Gazenfield-Gazit E, Eliahou HE: Endotoxin antibodies in patients on maintenance hemodialysis. *Israel J Med Sci* 5:1032, 1969
80. Kolmos HJ, Moller S: The epidemiology of febrile reactions in haemodialysis. *Acta Med Scand* 203:345, 1978
81. Blagg CR, Tenckhoff H: Microbial contamination of water used for hemodialysis. *Nephron* 15:81, 1975
82. Favero MS, Carson LA, Bond WW, Peterson NJ: Factors that influence microbial contamination of fluids associated with hemodialysis machines. *Appl Microbiol* 28:822, 1974
83. Ham TH, Shen SC, Fleming FM, Castle WB: Studies on the destruction of red blood cells, IV, *Blood* 3:373, 1948

84. Fortner RW, Nowakowski A, Carter CB, King LH, Knepshield JH: Death due to overheated dialysate during dialysis. *Ann Intern Med* 73:443, 1970
85. Berkes SL, Kahn SI, Chazan JA, Garella S: Prolonged hemolysis from overheated dialysate. *Ann Intern Med* 83:363, 1975
86. Ward MK, Shadforth M, Hill AVL, Kerr DNS: Air embolism during haemodialysis. *Br Med J* 3:74, 1971
87. Baskin SE, Wozniak RF: Hyperbaric oxygenation in the treatment of hemodialysis associated air embolism. *N Engl J Med* 293:184, 1975
88. Ziegler EJ, Ogden DA, Cazee CR: Blood recovery from the Kiil artificial kidney: a comparison of three methods, in *Nephrology Symposium* presented by the AANNT, Philadelphia PA, *Am Assoc Nephrol Nurses and Technicians* 1972, p 92
89. Lindsay RM, Moorthy AV, Koens F, Linton AL: Platelet function in dialyzed and non-dialyzed patients with chronic renal failure. *Clin Nephrol* 4:52, 1975
90. Remuzzi G, Marchesi D, Cavenaghi AE, Livio M, Donati MB, DeGaetano G, Mecca G: Bleeding in renal failure: a possible role of vascular prostacyclin (PGI$_2$). *Clin Nephrol* 12:127, 1979
91. Harker LA, Slichter SJ: Bleeding time as a screening test for evaluation of platelet function. *N Engl J Med* 287:155, 1972
92. Remuzzi G, Marchiaro G, Mecca G, DeGaetano G: Bleeding in renal failure: altered platelet function in chronic uremia only partially corrected by hemodialysis. *Nephron* 22:347, 1978
93. Stewart JH, Tuckwell LA, Sinnett PF: Peritoneal and haemodialysis: a comparison of their morbidity and of the mortality suffered by dialyzed patients. *Q J Med* 35:407, 1965
94. Shapiro WB, Faubert PF, Chou S-Y, Porush JG: Low-dose heparin in the high-risk bleeding hemodialysis patient monitored by activated partial thromboplastin time. *Dial Transpl* 9:322, 1980
95. Leonard CD, Weil E, Scribner BH: Subdural hematoma in patients undergoing haemodialysis. *Lancet* 2:239, 1969
96. Leonard A, Shapiro FL: Subdural hematoma in regularly hemodialyzed patients. *Ann Intern Med* 82:650, 1975
97. Rosenbluth PR, Arias B, Quartetti EV: Current management of subdural hematoma. *JAMA* 197:759, 1962
98. Bidwell G, Sherrard D, Mathews M: Peritoneal dialysis: a temporizing means for hemodialysis patients with subdural hematomas. *Nephron* 18:352, 1977
99. Tallala A, Halbrook H, Barbour BH, Kurze T: Subdural hematoma associated with long-term hemodialysis for chronic renal disease. *JAMA* 212:1847, 1970
100. Bechar M, Lakke JPWF, van der Hem GK, Beks JWF, Penning L: Subdural hematoma during long-term hemodialysis. *Arch Neurol* 26:513, 1972
101. Richards T, Hoff J: Factors affecting survival from acute subdural hematoma. *Surgery* 75:253, 1974
102. Marini PV, Hull AR: Uremic pericarditis: a review of incidence and management. *Kidney Int 7 (Suppl 2)*:163, 1975
103. Beaudry C, Nakamoto S, Kolff WJ: Uremic pericarditis and cardiac tamponade in chronic renal failure. *Ann Intern Med* 64:990, 1966
104. Bailey GL, Hampers CL, Hager EB: Uremic pericarditis: clinical features and management. *Circulation* 38:582, 1968
105. Buselmeier TJ, Simmons RL, Najarian JS, von Hartitzsch B, Dietzman RH, Kjellstrand CM: Intractable uraemic pericardial effusion. *Proc Eur Dial Transpl Assoc* 10:289, 1973
106. Ghavamian M, Gutch CF, Hughes RK, Kopp KF, Kolff WJ: Pericardial tamponade in chronic-hemodialysis patients: treatment by pericardectomy. *Arch Intern Med* 131:249, 1973
107. Milutinovic J, Follette WC, Scribner BH: Spontaneous retroperitoneal bleeding in patients on chronic hemodialysis. *Ann Intern Med* 86:189, 1977
108. Bhasin HK, Dana CL: Spontaneous retroperitoneal hemorrhage in chronically hemodialyzed patients. *Nephron* 22:322, 1978
109. Tsai S, Shimizu AG: Spontaneous perirenal hemorrhage in patients on hemodialysis. *Urology* 5:523, 1975
110. Nidus BD, Matalon R, Cantacuzino D: Uremic pleuritis – a clinicopathologic entity. *N Engl J Med* 281:255, 1969
111. Galen MA, Steinberg SM, Lowrie EG, Lazarus JM, Hampers CL, Merrill JP: Hemorrhagic pleural effusion in patients undergoing chronic hemodialysis. *Ann Intern Med* 82:359, 1975
112. Bora S, Kleinfeld M: Subcapsular liver hematomas in a patient on chronic hemodialysis. *Ann Intern Med* 93:574, 1980
113. Blum M, Aviram A: Splinter hemorrhages in patients receiving regular hemodialysis. *JAMA* 239:47, 1978
114. Samii K, Ciancioni C, Rottembourg J, Bisseliches F, Jacobs C: Severe hypoglycemia due to beta-blocking drugs in haemodialysis patients. *Lancet* 1:545, 1976
115. Grajower MM, Walter L, Albin J: Hypoglycemia in chronic hemodialysis patients: association with propranolol use. *Nephron* 26:126, 1980
116. Holland OB, Kaplan NM: Propranolol in the treatment of hypertension. *N Engl J Med* 294:930, 1976
117. Young AW Jr, Sweeney EW, David DS: Dermatologic evaluation of pruritus in patients on hemodialysis. *NY State J Med* 73:2670, 1973
118. Gilchrest B, Rowe JW, Mikos MC: Bullous dermatosis of hemodialysis. *Ann Intern Med* 83:480, 1975
119. Brivet F, Drueke T, Guillemette J, Zingraff J, Crosnier J: Porphyria cutanea tarda-like syndrome in haemodialyzed patients. *Nephron* 20:258, 1978
120. Parilla JG, Ortega R, Pena ML, Rodicio JL, De Salamanca RE, Olmos A, Elder GH: Porphyria cutanea tarda during maintenance haemodialysis. *Br Med J* 2:1358, 1980
121. Hampers CL, Katz AI, Wilson RE, Merrill JP: Disappearance of 'uremic' itching after subtotal parathyroidectomy. *N Engl J Med* 279:695, 1968
122. Tapia L, Cheigh JS, David DS, Sullivan JF, Saal S, Reidenberg MM, Stenzel KH, Rubin AL: Pruritus in dialysis patients treated with parenteral lidocaine. *N Engl J Med* 296:261, 1977
123. Silverberg DS, Iaina A, Reisin E, Rotzak R, Eliahou HE: Cholestyramine in uraemic pruritus. *Br Med J* 1:752, 1977
124. Van Leusen R, Lojenga JCK, Ruben A Th: Is cholestyramine helpful in uraemic pruritus? *Br Med J* 1:918, 1978
125. Wrong OM: Cholestyramine in uraemic pruritus. *Br Med J* 1:1662, 1977
126. Gilchrest BA, Rowe JW, Brown RS, Steinman TI, Arndt KA: Relief of uremic pruritus with ultraviolet phototherapy. *N Engl J Med* 297:136, 1977
127. Schultz BC, Roenigk HH Jr: Uremic pruritus treated with ultraviolet light. *JAMA* 243:1836, 1980
128. Gilchrest BA, Rowe JW, Brown RS, Steinman TI, Arndt KA: Ultraviolet phototherapy of uremic pruritus: long-term results and possible mechanism of action. *Ann Intern Med* 91:17, 1979
129. Hindson C, Taylor A, Martin A, Downey A: UVA light

for relief of uraemic pruritus. *Lancet* 1:215, 1981
130. Pederson JA, Matter BJ, Czerwinski AW, Llach F: Relief of idiopathic generalized pruritus in dialysis patients treated with activated oral charcoal. *Ann Intern Med* 93:446, 1980
131. Yatzidis H, Digenis P, Tountas C: Heparin treatment of uremic itching. *JAMA* 222:1183, 1972
132. Graf H, Kovarik J, Stummvoll HK, Wolf A: Disappearance of uraemic pruritus after lowering dialysate magnesium concentration. *Br Med J* 2:1478, 1979
133. Tapia L: Pruritus on hemodialysis. *Int J Dermatol* 18:217, 1979
134. Howe RC, Wombolt DG, Michie DD: Analysis of tonic muscle activity and muscle cramps during hemodialysis. *J Dial* 2:85, 1978
135. Kaji DM, Ackad A, Nottage WG, Stein RM: Prevention of muscle cramps in haemodialysis patients by quinine sulphate. *Lancet* 2:66, 1976
136. Catto GRD, Smith FW, McLeod M: Treatment of muscle cramps during maintenance haemodialysis. *Br Med J* 3:389, 1973
137. Jenkins P, Dreher WH: Dialysis-induced muscle cramps: treatment with hypertonic saline and theory as to etiology. *Trans Am Soc Artif Intern Organs* 21:479, 1975
138. Milutinovic J, Graefe U, Follette WC, Scribner BH: Effect of hypertonic glucose on the muscular cramps of hemodialysis. *Ann Intern Med* 90:926, 1979
139. Neal CR, Resnikoff E, Unger AM: Treatment of dialysis-related muscle cramps with hypertonic dextrose. *Arch Intern Med* 141:171, 1981
140. Sale D, Cameron JS: Priapism during regular dialysis. *Lancet* 2:1567, 1974
141. Port FK, Fiegel P, Hecking E, Kohler H, Distler A: Priapism during regular haemodialysis. *Lancet* 2:1287, 1974
142. Fassbinder W, Frei U, Issantier R, Koch KM, Mion C, Shaldon S, Slingeneyer A: Factors predisposing to priapism in haemodialysis patients. *Proc Eur Dial Transpl Assoc* 12:380, 1975
143. Kaplow LS, Goffinet JA: Profound neutropenia during the early phase of hemodialysis. *JAMA* 203:1135, 1968
144. Brubaker LH, Nolph KD: Mechanisms of recovery from neutropenia induced by hemodialysis. *Blood* 38:623, 1971
145. Craddock PR, Fehr J, Brigham KL, Kronenberg RS, Jacob HS: Complement and leucocyte-mediated pulmonary dysfunction in hemodialysis. *N Engl J Med* 296:769, 1977
146. Mahajan S, Gardiner H, DeTar B, Desai S, Muller B, Johnson N, Briggs W, McDonald F: Relationship between pulmonary functions and hemodialysis-induced leukopenia? *Trans Am Soc Artif Intern Organs* 23:411, 1977
147. Bogue BA, Butruille Y, Ebert C, Gagneux SA, Strom J: Absence of cardiopulmonary dysfunction using AN-69 as compared with cellulosic membranes. *Proc Clin Dial Transpl Forum* 7:170, 1977
148. Jacob AI, Gavellas G, Zarco R, Perez G, Bourgoignie JJ: Leukopenia, hypoxia and complement function with different hemodialysis membranes. *Kidney Int* 18:505, 1980
149. Sherlock J, Ledwith J, Letteri J: Hypoventilation and hypoxemia during hemodialysis: reflex response to removal of CO_2 across the dialyzer. *Trans Am Soc Artif Intern Organs* 23:406, 1977
150. Brautbar N, Shinaberger JH, Miller JH, Nachman M: Hemodialysis hypoxemia: evaluation of mechanism utilizing sequential ultrafiltration-dialysis. *Nephron* 26:96, 1980
151. Kraut J, Gafter U, Brautbar N, Miller J, Shinaberger J: Prevention of hypoxemia during dialysis by the use of sequential isolated ultrafiltration-diffusion dialysis with bicarbonate dialysate. *Clin Nephrol* 15:181, 1981
152. Lotem M, Robson MD, Rosenfeld JB: Spontaneous rupture of the quadriceps tendon in patients on chronic haemodialysis. *Ann Rheum Dis* 33:428, 1974
153. Cirincione RJ, Baker BE: Tendon ruptures with secondary hyperparathyroidism. *J Bone Joint Surg* 57-A:852, 1975
154. Morein G, Goldschmidt Z, Pauker M, Seelenfreud M, Rosenfeld JB, Fried A: Spontaneous tendon ruptures in patients treated by chronic hemodialysis. *Clin Orthop* 124:209, 1977
155. Warren DJ, Otieno LS: Carpal tunnel syndrome in patients on intermittent hemodialysis. *Postgrad Med J* 51:450, 1975
156. Holtmann B, Anderson CB: Carpal tunnel syndrome following vascular shunts for hemodialysis. *Arch Surg* 112:65, 1977
157. Jain VK, Cestero RVM, Baum J: Carpal tunnel syndrome in patients undergoing hemodialysis. *JAMA* 242:2868, 1979
158. Handa SP, Uremic bursitis. *Ann Intern Med* 89:723, 1978
159. Mathews M, Shen F.-H, Lindner A, Sherrard DJ: Septic arthritis in hemodialyzed patients. *Nephron* 25:87, 1980
160. Rizvi SS, Holmes RA: Hearing loss from hemodialysis. *Arch Otolaryngol* 106:751, 1980
161. Mirahmadi MK, Vaziri ND: Hearing loss in end-stage renal disease-effect of dialysis. *J Dial* 4:159, 1980
162. Kothari T, Swamy A, Mangla JC, Cestero RVM: Hepatic friction rub in uremia. *Arch Intern Med* 140:419, 1980
163. Feinroth M, Feinroth MV, Lundin AP, Friedman EA, Berlyne GM: Recurrent abdominal pain associated with digoxin in a patient undergoing maintenance haemodialysis. *Br Med J* 281:838, 1980
164. Ogden DA: New-dialyzer syndrome. *N Engl J Med* 302:1262, 1980
165. Gutch CF, Eskelson CD, Ziegler E, Ogden DA: 2-Chloroethanol as a toxic residue in dialysis supplies sterilized with ethylene oxide. *Dial Transpl* 5:21, 1976
166. Lewis LM, Flechtner TW, Kerkay J, Pearson KH, Nakamoto S: Bis(2-ethylhexyl)phthalate concentrations in the serum of hemodialysis patients. *Clin Chem* 24:741, 1978
167. Bommer J, Ritz E, Andrassy K: Necrotizing dermatitis resulting from hemodialysis with polyvinyl chloride tubing. *Ann Intern Med* 91:869, 1979
168. Patterson R, Zeiss CR, Roxe D, Pruzansky JJ, Roberts M, Harris KE: Antibodies in hemodialysis patients against hapten-protein and hapten-erythrocytes. *J Lab Clin Med* 96:347, 1980
169. Aljama P, Brown P, Turner P, Ward MK, Kerr DNS: Haemodialysis-triggered asthma. *Br Med J* 3:251, 1978
170. Howell E, Perkins H: Anti-N-like antibodies in the sera of patients undergoing chronic hemodialysis. *Vox Sang* 23:291, 1972
171. Orringer EP, Mattern WD: Formaldehyde-induced hemolysis during chronic hemodialysis. *N Engl J Med* 294:1416, 1976
172. Lewis KJ, Dewar PJ, Ward MK, Kerr DNS: Formation of anti-N-like antibodies in dialysis patients: effect of different methods of dialyzer rinsing to remove formaldehyde. *Clin Nephrol* 15:39, 1981

32

HEMATOLOGIC PROBLEMS OF DIALYSIS PATIENTS

JOSEPH W. ESCHBACH

Anemia	630
Pathophysiology in progressive renal failure	630
Improvement from regular dialysis treatment	631
Complications of the dialysis procedure	631
Erythropoietic deficiency states	631
Acute hemolysis	632
Copper-induced acute hemolysis	632
Chloramine	632
Nitrates	632
Formaldehyde	632
Overheated dialysate	633
Hypotonic dialysate	633
Altered tissue-oxygen delivery	633
Complications unrelated to the dialysis procedure	634
Decreased erythropoiesis	634
Bilateral nephrectomy	634
Iron deficiency	634
Hyperparathyroidism	634
Transfusions	634
Infections	635
Histidine deficiency	635
Increased hemolysis	635
Hypersplenism	635
Hypophosphatemia	635
Drugs	635
Other causes of acute hemolysis	635
Iron overload	635
Increased erythropoiesis	636
Management	636
Initiation of dialysis	636
Iron balance	636
Folic acid and histidine	637
Approach to the "refractory" anemia	637
Androgens	637
Other possible stimulating agents	638
Hypersplenism and/or osteitis fibrosa	638
Changing to peritoneal dialysis	638
Transfusions	638
Bleeding abnormalities	638
Pathophysiology	638
Beneficial effects of regular dialysis therapy	639
Complications of the dialysis procedure	639
Leukocyte problems	639
Changes in chronic renal failure	639
Effects of the dialysis procedure	640
References	640

ANEMIA

The kidney has a unique relationship to red cell production because of its production of the hormone erythropoietin (ESF). The development of anemia in almost all patients with chronic renal failure, therefore, is not surprising and is a major factor in preventing total rehabilitation with maintenance dialysis therapy. Several detailed reviews of erythropoietin have been published recently (1–4).

Pathophysiology in progressive renal failure

Studies of the anemia of progressive renal failure have emphasized three mechanisms: 1) decreased ESF production by the diseased kidney, resulting in erythroid marrow hypoproliferation (5); 2) shortening of the red cell survival (6); and 3) toxic depression of erythroid proliferation and heme synthesis by inhibitors retained in the uremic state (7, 8).

Decreased ESF production is the most significant of these mechanisms. Earlier studies documented serum ESF levels that were either unmeasurable or low (9). More recently, up to 40% of non-anephric, uremic patients had normal or slightly elevated hormone levels as measured by a modified bioassay (10), but still lower levels than anticipated for a similar degree of anemia in non-uremic individuals. Extrarenal (particularly hepatic) sources of ESF have been described (11, 12) but contribute only a small amount under ordinary circumstances. Despite reduced ESF levels, erythropoiesis continues at a basal level as shown by ferrokinetics (13) and responds to hypoxic and hyperoxic stresses qualitatively, though not necessarily quantitatively, as occurs with the intact feedback mechanism in non-uremic patients (14–16). However, this feedback mechanism does not seem to be operative in the erythrocytosis occasionally observed in renal transplant recipients (17). Red blood cell survival (normally 120 days) is variable but generally shortened by one-half (6, 18) by the time advanced renal failure develops. Yet the degree of red cell destruction rarely exceeds the compensatory ability of the normal erythroid marrow. Major degrees of hemolysis (greater than 3 times normal) can be observed in the hemolytic-uremic syndrome (19), after ingestion of certain drugs, or as complications of dialysis (see below).

The relative importance of uremic inhibitors of ESF or erythropoiesis is difficult to assess. Such toxins have been suggested for many years (7, 8, 20) as shown in most, but not all (21) *in vitro* studies, but whether they are of physiological significance in the pathogenesis of the anemia of chronic renal failure is far from proven. The observation of increased ESF levels in some anemic dialysis patients (10) suggests the presence of inhibitors. However, it is difficult to postulate inhibitors in the severely uremic patients with the hemolytic-uremic syndrome who have markedly increased red cell production (19), or in those dialysis patients who normalize their hematocrit (22). In addition, ESF has been shown to be effective when infused into uremic animals (23-25). Recently, human erythropoietin has been purified (26) so that the development of a more specific and sensitive radioimmunoassay should help to clarify the role of inhibitors (27). Previous methods to measure ESF in serum have either utilized the standard bioassay which is unable to detect normal levels, the non-specific hemagglutination-inhibition assay (28), or a radioimmunoassay that also measures biologically inactive ESF (29). An additional mechanism occasionally contributing to the anemia is blood loss, which can occur in advanced renal failure secondary to a decrease in platelet factor 3 and diminished platelet adhesiveness and aggregation (30).

Improvement from regular dialysis treatment

Most forms of bleeding, such as ecchymoses, epistaxis, and pericardial and gastrointestinal bleeding, when associated with severe uremia, can be reduced or eliminated by the initiation of regular dialysis therapy. Hemo- and peritoneal dialysis improve platelet function (31). Although one study of well hemodialyzed patients disclosed normal red blood cell survival (32), other studies have indicated incomplete correction in the red cell life span with thrice-weekly hemodialysis (33-36). Serial studies of red cell survival indicate improvement but not normalization in red cell life span with maintenance hemodialysis (37, 38). One of these studies disclosed further worsening in red cell survival after the initial 8 weeks of hemodialysis with subsequent improvement (38). Erythropoiesis, on the other hand, often improves during the first 6 to 12 months of hemodialysis as measured by ferrokinetics (14). This spontaneous improvement occurs especially if transfusions are avoided. Hematocrit levels have risen with peritoneal dialysis as well, either with the intermittent (IPD) (39) or the continuous ambulatory (CAPD) method (40). There are recent reports suggesting that CAPD results in higher hematocrit levels than IPD (40, 41). Red cell survival improved in one patient, but quantitation of red cell production and destruction has not been done to explain the mechanism(s) for this improvement. The removal of larger molecular weight erythropoietic inhibitors by the more porous peritoneal membrane is an attractive hypothesis not yet supported with data. Most patients with chronic renal failure have hematocrit levels between 15 and 30% prior to the initiation of dialysis. These levels subsequently rise to between 20 and 35% in most iron-repleted dialysis patients and occasionally normalize (22). On the other hand, many anephric patients maintain hematocrit levels between 15 and 25%. It seems unlikely that, despite comparable dialyzer efficiency and hours of dialysis per week, these differences could be explained solely on the basis of retained toxic inhibitors. It is known that some severely diseased kidneys are able to secrete elevated amounts of ESF (17). Therefore, variations in hormonal output may be responsible for the wide variations in hematocrit levels, modified by inhibitors, if present.

Complications of the dialysis procedure

Although regular dialysis therapy may benefit the anemic end-stage renal failure patient, the dialysis procedure per se, particularly hemodialysis, has the potential to negate these benefits. Erythropoiesis can be further decreased through iron and folate deficiencies; hemolysis can develop abruptly; and the oxygen affinity of hemoglobin can be altered, resulting in an acute reduction in tissue oxygen delivery.

Erythropoietic deficiency states
Optimal erythropoiesis depends on an adequate reserve of at least two co-factors: iron and folic acid. Deficiencies in these factors can occur because the former is depleted by means of the unavoidable blood loss into the hemodialyzer, and the latter is dialyzable.

Iron deficiency is a very common complication for the hemodialysis patient and can develop within one-half to 2 years even in the absence of overt bleeding. Loss of blood into the dialyzer at the end of each treatment is unavoidable and only varies in amount, depending on the dialyzer and the blood-return rinsing technique. Isotope studies have quantified this blood loss to vary between 4 and 50 ml of whole blood per dialysis (42). Assuming an average loss of 20 ml per dialysis, an average hematocrit of 25%, thrice-weekly dialysis, and knowing that 1.0 ml of red cells contains 1.0 mg of iron, approximately 780 mg of iron is lost per year by dialyzer blood loss alone. In addition, blood loss from periodic laboratory tests, the occasional clotting of blood in the dialyzer, membrane ruptures and accidental blood losses from cannulas or fistulas at the initiation or termination of hemodialysis may double this amount. Since mobilizable body iron stores are between 1200 and 1500 mg (43), iron deficiency easily can develop unless periodic iron repletion occurs. Body iron stores can be estimated by bone marrow evaluation of reticuloendothelial iron granules (44), but quantitation is now possible by means of serum ferritin levels. A radioimmunoassay (45) of serum for ferritin is reliable, much less expensive, and simpler to do repeatedly than marrow sampling, thus making the serum ferritin assay the best way to diagnose iron deficiency and to quantify iron stores (46-52). Serum iron levels are unreliable indicators of iron deficiency in dialysis patients (47, 49, 50). The primary effect of iron deficiency is to decrease erythropoiesis, because most iron is utilized by red cells. However, there is recent interest in the effects of iron deficiency exclusive of anemia. Striated muscle dysfunction, decreased immune function predisposing to infection, and possibly altered behavior have been observed in iron depleted, red cell repleted animals (53). Iron deficiency is a rare complication in the peritoneal dialysis patient unless induced by non-dialysis mechanisms.

Folic acid is easily dialyzed so that serum levels decrease during the relatively more efficient hemodialysis (54), but have not decreased after peritoneal dialysis (55). Megaloblastic marrow changes characteristic of folate deficiency have been described in hemodialysis patients (56). Most studies suggest, however, that folic acid deficiency rarely develops in patients consuming 60 to 80 g of dietary protein daily (55, 57), which contains enough folic acid to replace easily that which is lost via dialysis. Serum folate should be measured by the Lactobacillus casei assay, a heat-extracted radioassay, since the elevated unsaturated serum folate-binding protein commonly observed in uremia falsely lowers the routine folate radioassay (58). Low red cell (i.e. tissue) levels of folic acid, in contrast to serum levels, are more indicative of folate deficiency since it takes more than 4 months of a dietary intake of less than the minimum daily requirement of 50 µg to lead to megaloblastic marrow changes and subsequently to macrocytic peripheral red cells. Therefore, patients whose dietary protein intake is chronically low, or who consume folate antagonists such as diphenylhydantoin, are prone to develop a macrocytic anemia superimposed on their existing anemia of chronic renal failure.

Acute hemolysis (See also Chapter 31)

The standard dialysis blood pumps have low shearing stresses and do not cause any significant hemolysis, nor is there any other evidence that current dialyzers interfere with red cell survival. Nevertheless, acute hemolysis occasionally occurs superimposed upon the stable, mild hemolysis that exists in most patients. Although most dialysis patients have a red cell survival between one-third of normal to near normal values, occasionally there is marked aggravation of this hemolysis with subsequent abrupt decrements in hematocrit levels.

At least five mechanisms of red cell injury can complicate the hemodialysis procedure. *Oxidant red cell destruction* can occur after exposure to dialysate containing copper, chloramine or nitrate. *Inhibition of red cell glycolysis* can occur from dialysate containing formaldehyde. *Thermal red cell injury* can occur from overheated dialysate, and *mechanical trauma* theoretically can be imposed on the red cell by a malfunctioning or improper blood pump or partial obstruction within the extracorporeal circuit. Finally, *osmolar trauma* can result from hypo- or hypertonic dialysate. Treatment of these conditions requires discontinuing dialysis immediately once the complication is recognized.

Copper-induced acute hemolysis occurred in the United States in 1968, leading to death of at least four dialysis patients (59-61). The pathogenesis is thought to be due to the release of ionized copper from copper tubing present in the inflow dialysis fluid circuit that resulted when the pH in this circuit either fell below 6.3 or became quite alkaline. This situation can occur when the deionizer anion resin bed becomes exhausted, resulting in inadequate neutralization of the usual hydrogen ion released from the unexhausted cation exchange column. Dialysate copper levels subsequently increase quickly and transfer into patients' plasma saturating circulating plasma ceruloplasmin, allowing free copper to diffuse into the red cells where, as an oxidant, it inhibits glycolytic enzymes, such as hexokinase, phosphofructokinase and pyruvatekinase (62), resulting in acute hemolysis. Although this syndrome has not occurred since copper tubing has been eliminated from dialysate circuits and the deionizers are more carefully maintained, it is an ever potential threat and should be suspected if skin flushing and chilling occur followed by vomiting, abdominal cramps and diarrhea while on dialysis. The plasma or serum will usually have a greenish hue due to the increased copper and ceruloplasmin levels.

Chloramine, formed by ammonia and chlorine that are bactericidal agents in urban water supplies, is an oxidant that, if present in dialysate, can result in methemoglobinemia and hemolysis. Initially, it was proposed that the plasma of many hemodialysis patients possessed an inhibitor that triggered the chloramined induced hemolysis (63). However, further studies failed to characterize this plasma substance as an inhibitor in that it had no abnormal effects on red cell metabolism (64). Chloramine can induce hemolysis, but its effect is probably no greater in uremia than in the non-uremic state.

The hemolytic effect of chloramine can be reduced by a deionizer in the water supply (65). Column deionization seems to remove some of the chloramine, however, complete removal requires passage through a carbon column, which is the method of choice when chloramines are present in appreciable concentrations.

Its effects can also be neutralized by addition of ascorbic acid to the dialysis fluid (66, 67 [see also chapter 6]).

Nitrates, if present in the water used to prepare dialysate, convert to nitrites, then diffuse into the blood circuit, resulting in oxidant red cell damage and methemoglobinemia. This has occurred once when nitrate contaminated well water was used in the dialysis fluid (68). Nausea, vomiting, lethargy and hypotension with cyanosis occur, and the blood in the venous blood line changes to a black color. Oxygen therapy results in no improvement in the color of the extracorporeal circuit.

Formaldehyde is a potent reducing agent, and at concentrations greater than 0.1 nM/l causes inhibition of red cell glycolysis leading to hemolysis. Installation into a dialysis unit of a new water filter containing a formaldehyde and melamine resin resulted in acute hemolysis (69). Formaldehyde's mechanism of action involves conversion of NAD (nicotinamide-adenine dinucleotide) to NADH. This results in the inhibition of glycolysis at the level of glyceraldehyde 3-phosphate dehydrogenase, which decreases the cellular energy stores of ATP. Although this brand of water filter has been removed from the commercial market, the threat of formaldehyde-induced hemolysis is always present, since this bactericidal and sporicidal agent is commonly used as a sterilizing agent for dialysis equipment. It is removed prior to each dialysis procedure by flushing procedures, but the Clinitest tablet, commonly used to detect residual formaldehyde before dialysis is begun, is relatively insensitive. This raises the question whether low grade, chronic formaldehyde exposure occurs in dialysis patients, and if so, whether it contributes to the underlying hemolysis that is observed. It has now been repeatedly shown that formaldehyde sterilization of the dialyzer and other dialysis equipment leads to the development of anti-N-like cold agglutinins in 3 to 45% of hemodialysis patients (70–73), usually, but not always (74, 75), after dialyzer reuse (see also Chapter 15). When chromium red cell survival is measured, it discloses slightly shorter life spans than anti-N-like negative hemodialysis patients (73). However, acute hemolytic episodes may occur and remit quite spontaneously in patients with these agglutinins (75). Anti-N-like cold agglutinins do not develop in all hemodialysis patients exposed to formaldehyde, and when hemolysis does occur it is either transient or mild. Therefore, the clinical significance of these cold agglutinins is still unresolved.

Overheated dialysate produces thermal red cell injury, resulting in spherocyte formation and increased osmotic fragility leading to hemolysis if the dialysate temperature is above 47 °C (76). If the temperature rises above 51 °C, marked hemolysis occurs with hyperkalemia and cardiac arrest (77). This complication should never happen as long as dialysis machines have visual and audible alarms activated when the dialysate temperature exceeds 38.6 °C.

Hypotonic dialysate can occur from malfunction of the proportioning pump or from improper composition of the concentrate or bath mixture. This should never happen with proper conductivity monitoring, yet human error in one case resulted in overriding the conductivity meter when the dialysis solution concentrate tank became empty, leading to acute hemolysis with a drop in hematocrit to 8% (78). More threatening to the patient than the acute hemolysis, however, is acute water intoxication resulting in acute swelling of the brain and causing encephalopathy and seizures. The hemolysis may be suspected by noting a bright red appearance to the blood returning from the dialyzer to the patient.

Altered tissue-oxygen delivery
Oxygen transport depends on the functioning of four components: pulmonary gas exchange, cardiac output, hemoglobin concentration and the hemoglobin molecule's affinity for oxygen (79). Since the hemoglobin concentration in advanced renal failure, and particularly in dialysis patients, is about one-half of normal, other compensatory adjustments are necessary in order for this complex regulatory system to maintain an adequate end-capillary oxygen tension. Increased cardiac output (80, 15) and increased oxygen release from the hemoglobin molecule at the tissue level account for the major compensatory adjustments to any anemia, including that in chronic renal failure. When the position of the hemoglobin oxygen dissociation curve is shifted to the right, as indicated by an increase in P_{50} (that partial pressure of oxygen at which 50% of the hemoglobin is saturated), there is extra oxygen release from hemoglobin to tissues. There are at least five different factors known to affect the shape of this curve: the configuration or structure of the four polypeptide hemoglobin chains, the temperature, the intracellular pH and carbon dioxide level (the Bohr effect), and the concentration of an intraerythrocytic organic phosphate, 2,3-diphosphoglycerate (DPG). The last two factors are of greatest importance in the anemia of dialysis patients. An increase in either intraerythrocytic hydrogen ion or carbon dioxide concentration shifts the oxygen dissociation curve rightward and tends to displace oxygen from the hemoglobin molecule. DPG lies in the central cavity of the hemoglobin molecule between the 2-α and 2-β polypeptide globin chains but combines with only two amino acid residues, histidine at position H-21 of the β chains in the desoxy- and not the oxy-form of hemoglobin (81). When DPG stabilizes hemoglobin in the desoxy form, more oxygen is released at the tissue level. Of these factors that affect DPG, inorganic serum phosphate levels appear to be the most important. Levels less than 0.32 mmol/l (1 mg/dl), as occasionally seen in parenteral hyperalimentation or rarely from excessive antacid therapy, can deplete many organic phosphates, including intraerythrocytic 2,3-DPG, leading to a leftward shift in the oxygen dissociation curve and therefore less hemoglobin oxygen release. Conversely it has been claimed that the hyperphosphatemia of growing children leads to increased DPG levels and decreased oxygen affinity, which in turn accounts for a 'physiologic' anemia (82).

In view of the known pH and inorganic phosphate shifts that occur during hemodialysis, and to a lesser extent, during peritoneal dialysis, changes in the hemoglobin oxygen dissociation curve might be anticipated. However, most studies have either failed to show any change in 2,3-DPG levels or have shown impaired tissue oxygenation based on studies of only part of the complete and complex system. The expected detrimental effect of dialysis on oxygen delivery is less than expected and when all factors are considered, there is a slight increase in oxygen consumption by the end of dialysis (83) despite a decrease in PAO_2 that may occur during either acetate (83–85) or bicarbonate (86) hemodialysis. The decrease in PAO_2 occurs early in hemodialysis and so has been missed by some investigators, but its cause is poorly understood. Leukocyte aggregation and sequestration in the pulmonary vascular bed secondary to complement activation has been suggested as causing the hypoxemia through ventilation perfusion mismatch (87). However, there may be little correlation between the early leukopenia and hypoxemia since hypoxemia occurs during dialyzer re-use (when leukopenia is absent or minimal) or during hemodialysis utilizing the polyacrylonitrile membrane which does not elicit the complement-induced leukopenia (88, 89). Changes in pH associated with acetate-hemodialysis have been associated with hypoxemia (90), but bicarbonate hemodialysis does not necessarily prevent the hypoxemia (86). Another mechanism leading to hypoxemia may be the loss of carbon dioxide into the dialysate which reduces PCO_2, thereby depressing respiratory center drive (91). However, when the respiratory effect of CO_2 depletion has been prevented by controlled mechanical ventilation during dialysis, PAO_2 values still fall during the first 30 min of dialysis (92), suggesting that some other factor(s) must be responsible for the hemodialysis-induced hypoxemia. There appears to be little adverse effect on oxygen delivery from peritoneal dialysis (93).

Complications unrelated to the dialysis procedure

There are some non-dialysis related complications that have an impact on the anemia of chronic renal failure. These processes can either reduce or, rarely, stimulate erythropoiesis, reduce RBC survival, or stimulate iron overload.

Decreased erythropoiesis
Red cell production is reduced in chronic renal failure, but can be further reduced under the following settings: bilateral nephrectomy, iron deficiency, osteitis fibrosa, transfusions, systemic infections and possibly histidine deficiency.

Bilateral nephrectomy results in a decrease in mean hematocrit levels from an initial mean value of 25% to 15% (94). Since red cell survival remains unaffected by bilateral nephrectomy (95, 96), this drop in red cell mass is entirely due to decreased ESF production. Ferrokinetic studies confirm a three-fold decrease in erythropoiesis after bilateral nephrectomy, and transfusion requirements may increase three-fold (96). This has also been quantitated by changes in plasma ESF levels as measured by a refined bioassay (10). Mean ESF levels in nephric, anemic patients treated with hemodialysis were 17.8 ± 1.5 mU/ml (normal, nonanemic values: 7.8 ± 3.6 mU/ml). Anephric hemodialysis patients had levels ranging from below 2.8 to 5.5 mU/ml. Therefore ESF levels were decreased approximately five-fold in anephric patients. This implies that even though there may be little or no excretory function in remnant kidneys, the endocrine function continues to contribute significantly to erythropoiesis. Even though an estimated 10% of ESF is produced by tissues other than the kidney, presumably the liver, under ordinary circumstances this is not enough to compensate for the removal of both kidneys. The persistence of severe anemia with its associated tissue hypoxia can result in incomplete rehabilitation and probable need for repetitive transfusions which can increase the risk of hepatitis, iron overload and the development of cytotoxic antibodies against a future transplant. Therefore, bilateral nephrectomy should be reserved only for those dialysis patients whose severe hypertension cannot be controlled with drugs or whose bilaterally infected kidneys do not respond to appropriate antibiotics. Bilateral nephrectomy as a means of preparing a patient for a cadaveric transplant is strongly discouraged, since there is little evidence that transplant survival improves by this procedure unless there are circulating antiglomerular basement membrane antibodies present.

Iron deficiency usually occurs as a result of chronic low grade blood loss, and eventually leads to decreased erythropoiesis. This is in contrast to acute blood loss, which can stimulate erythropoiesis in the dialysis patient similar to normal subjects, although the ability to respond is less because of a reduced ESF reserve. Studies in phlebotomized uremic sheep (15), as well as in isolated dialysis patients whose hematocrits have fallen below 15% by acute blood loss (97, 98), have shown evidence of increased endogenous ESF secretion and subsequent increase in red cell production if iron stores are adequate. Although the major reason for the chronic blood loss is associated with the dialysis procedure as detailed earlier, dialysis patients in general have a higher incidence of gastrointestinal, uterine, pericardial and tissue bleeding than normal subjects. The use of systemic anticoagulation by means of warfarin and aspirin-containing drugs can contribute to prolonged bleeding in hemodialysis patients. Correction of the blood loss with iron replacement and control of the bleeding will return erythropoiesis to its previous level.

Hyperparathyroidism has been associated with anemia in subjects with normal kidney function, and can aggravate the existing anemia in dialysis patients. Over 38 dialysis patients have had improvement in their anemia following parathyroidectomy (99–102). Some investigators consider parathyroid hormone (PTH) to be an uremic toxin that inhibits erythropoiesis (10, 103), but others have noted no difference in PTH levels between those who increase and those who do not increase their hematocrit after parathyroidectomy (102). The extent of marrow fibrosis, present on bone biopsy, seems to be the best correlate, and when reduced by parathyroidectomy results in a mean rise in hematocrit from 22 to 30%. Non-surgical control of secondary hyperparathyroidism with vitamin D analogues and phosphate control has also resulted in an improved hematocrit (100, 101). Although ferrokinetic studies have yet to be reported, it appears that the major effect of osteitis fibrosa is to decrease erythropoiesis by decreasing effective erythroid marrow mass. If marrow fibrosis becomes severe, myelofibrosis develops so that hematological compensation occurs by extramedullary hematopoiesis resulting in splenomegaly. This leads to shortening of red cell survival as well as pancytopenia (104).

Transfusions, by increasing tissue oxygenation, can theoretically suppress ESF release and lead to decreased erythropoiesis. There is a feedback mechanism between the kidney and erythroid marrow governed by hypoxia or hyperoxia. The normal kidney responds to transient hypoxia by increasing ESF production, which subsequently leads to increased erythropoiesis. As a result of an increase in red cell mass and therefore increased oxygen delivery, ESF production eventually decreases, which in turn reduces erythropoiesis to its previous level. When polycythemia is induced with transfusion, ESF production and erythropoiesis are suppressed. However, it is not necessary to produce polycythemia to demonstrate transfusion-induced marrow suppression, since a change in hemoglobin from 4 to 7 g/dl in a subject with normal renal funcion is enough to decrease urinary and plasma ESF levels (105). There is evidence that this feedback mechanism persists in chronic renal failure. Controlled manipulations of red cell mass in uremic, anemic sheep showed an inverse relationship between hematocrit levels and plasma iron turnover (15). Observations in repeatedly transfused dialysis patients have disclosed a spontaneous increase in the hematocrit after transfusions were stopped. Ferrokinetic studies also have documented suppression of erythropoiesis when hematocrits were artifically raised from 20 to 30% (14). Reduction in the erythroid iron turnover, red cell utilization and reticulocyte count all gave evidence of suppression. The per cent of marrow normoblasts also was found to decrease in seven anephric patients who were transfused from a hematocrit of 24 to 33% (97). When 1 unit of red cells is infused for symptoms of tissue hypoxia, it is unlikely that erythropoiesis is suppressed, but when 2 or more units are infused, resulting in a greater rise in hematocrit, erythroid suppression is more likely.

Infections. Clinical experience has shown that serious systemic infections in dialysis patients are often associated with a decrease in hematocrit. Mild, local infections, such as those involving cannula exit sites or infected fistula punctures, do not seem to affect the hematocrit adversely. The mechanism for the decrease in hematocrit associated with severe infections is due to reticuloendothelial blockade preventing iron from being released to circulating transferrin, thereby reducing the iron available for heme synthesis.

Histidine deficiency, if present, can accentuate the anemia of dialysis patients. Histidine is an essential amino acid in normal subjects and in patients with chronic renal failure (106), since histidine deficiency results in a significant drop in hemoglobin concentration in both groups.

Because histidine is one of the amino acids that link iron to the globin molecule, it is thought that histidine is essential for erythropoiesis; however, there have been no erythrokinetic studies documenting whether histidine deficiency affects erythropoiesis or red cell survival. Low levels of plasma histidine have been found in dialysis patients by several investigators; these levels subsequently rose with histidine supplementation (107). It appears that patients ingesting protein diets greater than 1 g/kg/day receive adequate histidine. However, those individuals who are on restricted protein diets probably are not ingesting enough histidine. Unfortunately, the presence of a low histidine blood level does not necessarily imply that there is deficient erythropoiesis secondary to histidine deficiency, since a number of hemodialysis patients treated with histidine have not shown improvement in their hematocrit (108, 109). Although there is some histidine lost during dialysis, this appears to be easily replaced by an adequate dietary intake of protein. Histidine supplementation is necessary only for those individuals who are on low protein diets and have low histidine levels, but their hematological response may be unpredictable (see also Chapter 27).

Increased hemolysis
Hypersplenism. In a small number of dialysis patients hematocrit levels may fall or transfusion requirements may rise in the absence of an obvious cause. Hypersplenism should be suspected in patients with a palpable spleen and markedly shortened red cell survival. The pathogenesis of this complication is probably multifactorial and includes such etiologies as chronic hepatitis (110), transfusion-induced hemosiderosis with splenomegaly (111), severe marrow fibrosis (104), and splenomegaly secondary to other causes of acute hemolysis such as chloramine induced hemolysis (112) or any oxidant-induced hemolysis (113). Splenectomy should not be performed, however, unless definite splenic sequestration can be documented by isotopic studies. Characteristically, ^{51}Cr red cell survival studies will show a T½ of 11 days or less with a 2:1 or greater uptake over the spleen in comparison to the heart or liver (114). Splenomegaly can usually be documented by palpation or by an isotopic scan. Some patients are able to maintain stable hematocrits despite this increased hemolysis because of marrow compensation (115).

Hypophosphatemia. Elevated plasma inorganic phosphate levels are common in dialysis patients unless there is dietary protein restriction or the ingestion of aluminum containing phosphate-binding gels. Occasionally, these measures result in marked reduction in plasma inorganic phosphate levels. If the level falls below 0.32 mmol/l (1 mg/dl), a failure-to-thrive syndrome may occur due to poor tissue oxygenation as a result of a depletion of red cell ADP and probably of 2,3-DPG levels (116). Marked hemolysis also can occur when the red cell is deprived of these inorganic phosphates (117). Although this degree of hypophosphatemia is rare in the dialysis patient, it is a possibility and a correctable cause of acute hemolysis.

Drugs. Dialysis patients in general are often treated with various antibiotics and antihypertensive agents, which have been shown to cause hemolysis in a small number of subjects without renal disease. Cephalosporins, penicillin, and alpha methyldopa may cause hemolysis characterized by the development of a positive Coombs' reaction, although the mechanism of developing antibodies is different in all three situations, and hemolysis is not necessarily present even when the Coombs' test is positive. In addition, sulfonamides and anti-malarials may act as oxidants and cause acute hemolysis in those individuals who have abnormal red cell hexosemonophosphate shunt metabolism. If a sudden fall in hematocrit occurs in any patient consuming these drugs, they should be discontinued until the cause of the drop in the hematocrit has been established.

Other causes of acute hemolysis. If the hematocrit falls in the absence of any of the above mentioned causes, hemolysis should be suspected if bone marrow examination shows normal or active erythropoiesis. Autoimmune factors can be implicated in the patient with lupus erythematosus and hemolytic crises can recur in the dialysis patient afflicted with sickle cell anemia.

Iron overload
Iron overload is a serious potential complication for the long term dialysis patient who either receives parenteral iron indiscriminately or whose erythroid function is so poor that frequent transfusions are required to prevent tissue hypoxia. Because iron deficiency develops easily in the hemodialysis patient from dialyzer blood losses, many patients have been subjected to routine programs of iron replacement, usually as intravenous iron-dextran

during each dialysis, weekly, monthly or quarterly. Iron stores vary between 1200 to 1500 mg and can easily be exceeded by routine iron-dextran administration (118, 119). Since one unit of red cells contains approximately 200 mg of iron, it does not require too many transfusions to exceed iron stores. The important question, however, is whether iron overload leads to hemochromatosis with its associated hepatic, cardiac, and endocrine dysfunctions. A recent study showed that in non-uremic anemic patients receiving 2 to 3 units of blood per month, within 4 years there was evidence of cardiac dysfunction, abnormal glucose tolerance tests with decreased insulin output, abnormal liver function tests and portal fibrosis on liver biopsy (120). Iron was present in both reticuloendothelial and parenchymal cells. Serum ferritin levels ranged to a high of 5000 µg/l with a mean of 2500 µg/l (normal values 10 to 300 µg/l). These changes are typical of early hemochromatosis. This amount of iron overload and elevated ferritin levels are occasionally encountered in dialysis patients and hemosiderosis of the liver and heart have been observed (49, 118, 119).

Proximal muscle myopathy has also been observed in iron overloaded dialysis patients whose serum ferritin levels exceed 1000 µg/l (121). Most of these patients had HLA-antigens as observed in patients with primary hemochromatosis, raising the possibility that possession of 'hemochromatosis alleles' may predispose the iron treated or transfused hemodialysis patient to iron overload. It seems inevitable that patients receiving large amounts of iron-dextran or blood will eventually develop functional impairment of the liver, heart, pancreas, pituitary or proximal muscles, although it has been implied that it cannot happen (119). One of the reasons why it may rarely happen is that repetitive dialyzer blood losses in the hemodialysis patient help prevent excessive iron overload. This is perhaps fortunate, since removal of iron by chelation during dialysis, although occasionally successful (118), usually is not ideal (49, 122). The best treatment is prevention, and now that iron stores can be followed by serial serum ferritin levels (48), iron overload secondary to iron-dextran therapy should never occur. The automatically scheduled routine use of iron-dextran should be discouraged. Serum ferritin should be measured periodically and iron therapy should be used when indicated by the findings of iron deficiency (see below). Treatment of transfusion induced iron overload is more difficult and includes measures to stimulate erythropoiesis (see Management, below), a reduction of transfusions to one at a time, and giving a transfusion only when symptoms of tissue hypoxia develop rather than at a set level of hematocrit.

Increased erythropoiesis
Active liver disease, either viral (viral hepatitis [123–125]) or toxic (drug induced [125, 126]), has been associated with a transient improvement in the anemia of dialysis patients. Hematocrit and reticulocyte levels increased at a time when hepatic regeneration occurred. This response has even occurred in anephric patients; in one patient, plasma erythropoietin levels increased significantly and subsequently fell when liver injury resolved. Individuals with chronic, active hepatitis sustain hematocrit increases for a longer time. This suggests that the liver maybe a significant potential source of extrarenal erythropoietin.

Management

The ideal management of the anemia of chronic renal failure is to replace the erythropoietic stimulating hormone that the damaged kidney fails to produce. Although human ESF has been purified (26), it is unlikely that sufficient quantities will be available for clinical use for many years. Preliminary studies in anemic, uremic sheep suggest that ESF is effective (25), but the role of possible inhibitors in human renal failure has yet to be resolved. Until hormone replacement is feasible and practical, it is important to optimize erythropoiesis, minimize blood loss and hemolysis and search for other means to stimulate the erythroid marrow.

Initiation of dialysis
Dialysis should be instituted prior to the development of serious complications, i.e., when the creatinine clearance falls to 5 to 7 ml/min. Severe protein restriction is not recommended since it can induce nutritional deficiencies and patients usually restrict protein spontaneously. Dialysis therapy should be scheduled on at least a three times a week basis allowing the patient to eat a minimum of 1 to 1.5 g/kg of protein per day. Three times a week hemodialysis has also resulted in higher hematocrit levels than dialysis twice a week (36). Characteristically, hematocrits often continue to fall after dialysis is initiated, but eventually stabilize, and if transfusions are avoided, there will be a spontaneous improvement in erythropoiesis during the first 6 to 12 months of maintenance hemodialysis (14). Transfusions, because of their potentially erythropoietic suppressing effects, as well as their known risk of transmitting hepatitis, should be limited only to situations where there is definite tissue hypoxia present, such as angina pectoris or cerebral vascular insufficiency. There are occasions when the quality of life, however, is so poor because of severe anemia that transfusion therapy may be indicated, but should be strictly limited until other measures, discussed below, have been tried. An exercise program should be encouraged for all new dialysis patients as soon as their uremic symptoms are reversed or controlled. A routine program of daily exercise by brisk walking, jogging, or excercising on a bicycle ergometer has resulted in a significant rise in the hematocrit (127).

Iron balance
In order to maintain optimal erythropoiesis, iron stores must be maintained. In the peritoneally dialyzed patient, iron (blood) losses are negligible, but for the hemodialyzed patient, blood loss occurs with each dialysis; the only variable is the amount. Most patients beginning dialysis therapy already have expanded iron stores, because as chronic renal failure progresses red cell utilization of iron slowly decreases so that red cell iron shifts to the reticuloendothelial system. If transfusions were

given, it is likely that iron stores are increased further. On the other hand, there are approximately 25% of uremic non-dialysis patients who have iron deficiency (128) because of blood loss associated with the qualitative platelet defect. Therefore, iron stores should be evaluated in all patients once they have become stabilized on maintenance dialysis. For the hemodialysis patient, because iron losses are unavoidable, iron balance must be quantitated serially. Serum ferritin levels correlate well with tissue iron stores and there is a linear decrease in serum ferritin levels in hemodialysis patients that can allow prediction of the onset of iron deficiency (50). It is recommended that serum ferritin levels be determined at least every 6 months. Normal iron balance as defined by serum ferritin levels varies considerably according to investigator and laboratory method, although the methods are basically the same (45). When serum ferritin has been related to bone marrow iron (a qualitative and not a quantitative assessment), values of less than 40, 108, 150, and 500 µg/l (46-49) have been associated with absent marrow iron. However, when serum ferritin levels are related to intestinal iron absorption (which is a physiologic indicator of iron stores), iron deficiency was present at ferritin levels of less than 30 and 50 µg/l (49, 50). Measurements of serum iron, total iron binding capacity, and percent transferrin saturation are not helpful in defining the status of iron stores (47-50). If iron stores are normal in the patient beginning routine dialysis, it may take 6 to 24 months before iron deficiency develops unless there are blood losses above and beyond that associated with uncomplicated routine hemodialysis. Iron deficiency takes longer to develop in the chronic peritoneal dialysis patient since blood losses are minimal with that technique, although there have been no longitudinal studies of iron balance in peritoneal dialysis patients. Once iron deficiency is diagnosed, it should be treated with oral ingestion of iron sulfate or iron gluconate, 300 mg one hour before or 2 h after a meal, three times a day, and without concomitant ingestion of phosphate binding gels, which can also bind iron (129). Studies of iron absorption in hemodialysis patients disclose that absorption is physiologic and is related to the magnitude of iron stores present, similar to that in nonuremic subjects; that is, there is an inverse relationship between iron absorption and iron stores. There is almost an identical absorption of dietary iron in hemodialysis patients compared to non-uremic subjects at a given level of serum ferritin (50). Low serum ferritin and hematocrit levels rise with proper administration of oral iron. Oral iron therapy has been shown to be as efficacious as parenteral iron in correcting and maintaining iron stores and hematocrit (130, 131). Parenteral iron-dextran should be reserved for the iron deficient patient who either cannot tolerate oral iron, cannot comply to its ingestion, or does not respond with an anticipated rise in hematocrit. If it has to be given, it is better to give it intravenously (during dialysis), than intramuscularly, because should an anaphylactic reaction occur, it can be immediately treated with appropriate intravenous medication. Since serious, (non-fatal) systemic reactions developed in 11% of 481 non-dialysis patients treated with intravenous iron-dextran (132), caution is advised in administering this drug. Another reason why iron-dextran should not be considered a primary method of iron replacement is that temporary iron overload can easily be created, which then suppresses the normal physiologic absorption of dietary iron. Some hemodialysis patients who eat well, have good dialyzer-blood rinse techniques, minimal blood samplings, and meticulous cannula or fistula care, can maintain normal iron stores in the absence of supplemental iron or transfusions for up to 2 years despite blood losses that exceed their known iron stores. This implies that more patients than realized have significant absorption of dietary iron provided their iron absorption mechanism is not suppressed by artificially maintaining high serum ferritin levels with intermittent iron-dextran therapy.

Folic acid and histidine
If dietary intake of protein continues below 1 g/kg despite adequate dialysis and relief of uremic symptoms, dietary supplementation with folic acid 1 mg/day and histidine 10 mg/day (133), should prevent deficiencies of these nutrients that could eventually affect erythropoiesis (see also Chapter 27).

Approach to the 'refractory' anemia
Most hemo- and peritoneal dialysis patients gradually will increase their hematocrit levels to above 25 through the management outlined above. Tissue oxygenation usually is adequate at this level because of compensatory increases in cardiac output and a shift to the right in the oxygen-hemoglobin dissociation curve. However, if the hematocrit fails to rise to a level preventing tissue hypoxia or if the anemia worsens despite adequate iron stores, the following approaches should be considered.

Androgens. Studies of various androgens in hemodialysis patients indicate that most (134-140), but not all patients (141, 142) respond by increasing their hematocrit by at least 5 vol. %. Recently, a controlled comparison study of four androgens disclosed that intramuscular nandrolone decanoate (3 mg/kg/wk) and intramuscular testosterone enanthate (4 mg/kg/wk) for 6 months resulted in significant hematocrit increases, whereas oral fluoxymesterone (0.4 mg/kg/d) and oral oxymetholone (1 mg/kg/d) were less effective (143). Anephric patients failed to respond in this study, whereas in some studies occasional responses were observed as evidenced by a rise in serum erythropoietin levels and/or hematocrits (134, 136, 139, 144, 145). Nandrolone decanoate should be the primary drug of choice and should be given for at least 6 months. If no response occurs, a 6 month trial with fluoxymesterone should be considered. The mechanism of action of these anabolic agents primarily involves the stimulation of remnant renal erythropoietin production and secondarily direct erythroid marrow stimulation (146). Increased hepatic synthesis of ESF probably occurs as well, particularly from fluoxymesterone, which can affect hepatic cellular function. Fluoxymesterone has had some hepatic side effects in non-uremic subjects: cholestasis, peliosis, hepatitis, and hepatocellular carcinoma, but these have not been observed as yet in dialysis patients. Myalgias associated

with elevated creatine phosphokinase levels have been noted in some dialysis patients on fluoxymesterone (147) and warfarin enhancement occurs.
Injectable androgens also cause side effects: in male patients priaprism, resulting in permanent impotence has been observed. Problems in women are hirsitism acne and coarsening of the features (148). It is pertinent that in a prospective study, 25% of dialysis patients could not continue on their androgens because of side effects (143). Therefore, androgens should not be administered routinely, but only to those patients with hematocrit values below 25% who are symptomatic from their anemia. The use of a recently described clonal assay utilizing a patient's own marrow cells may help to determine who will respond to androgens (149).

These drugs should be discontinued once a maximal response occurs, since elevated hematocrit levels may persist despite drug withdrawal.

Other possible stimulating agents. Oral cobaltous chloride has been shown to stimulate erythropoiesis in nondialyzed uremic patients and dialysis patients. Approximately 50% of patients will respond with a rise in hematocrit levels after 2 to 9 weeks of therapy (150). Some anephric patients also have responded. However, not all respond, and the response, if present, requires constant drug administration, and toxicity is appreciable. In addition to (reversible) gastrointestinal side effects many different toxic effects have been reported (nerve deafness, polyneuropathy, optic atrophy and others [151]).

Hypothyroidism occasionally occurs in dialysis patients, but no evidence of worsening of the anemia has been documented. Nevertheless, there are *in vitro* data indicating that T_3 and T_4 directly stimulate erythroid cells (of the rat) (152). On the other hand, a 4-week clinical trial of T_3 in four patients with stable chronic renal failure (not on dialysis) failed to improve the anemia (153).

Vitamin B_{12} deficiency has been reported in four dialysis patients, all of whom had decreased serum vitamin B_{12} levels and responded dramatically to replacement therapy (154). Other potential experimental ways to increase extrarenal ESF production or the direct stimulation of erythropoiesis recently have been reviewed (155).

Hypersplenism and/or osteitis fibrosa. Hypersplenism should be considered in any dialysis patient whose anemia worsens significantly after a period of relative stability and in whom iron stores are adequate. This is particularly true if there has been a history of liver disease, multiple transfusions, repeated exposures to hemolytic agents such as chloramine, or if severe osteitis fibrosa is present. The presence of an enlarged spleen by palpation and an isotopic scan should lead to appropriate studies of splenic sequestration.

Osteitis fibrosa without hypersplenism is probably more common than the reverse. At present there is no reliable way to predict whether parathyroidectomy will have a beneficial effect on the anemia. Immunoreactive PTH levels usually are elevated by at least 10-fold, as are levels in some non-responders, a factor suggesting that PTH is not an erythropoietic toxin per se. The extent of marrow fibrosis as seen on bone biopsy is the best single determinant as to whether parathyroidectomy will be of benefit, but quantitation of the fibrosis may be difficult (102).

Changing to peritoneal dialysis. There are many anecdotal instances that patients dialyzed peritoneally are less anemic than those treated by hemodialysis. Iron deficiency is common in the latter group, which may be part of the explanation. Several reports attest that chronic ambulatory peritoneal dialysis (CAPD) often is associated with higher hematocrit values than hemodialysis. Therefore, if technically feasible, CAPD should be considered if a patient's anemia is preventing the attainment of an acceptable quality of life.

Transfusions. If, despite the above therapeutic approaches, hypoxic symptoms persist, judical use of red cell transfusions is indicated. Only 1 unit, as packed red cells, should be given at a time in order to prevent volume overload, to minimize marrow suppressive effects, and because 1 unit is enough to improve tissue oxygenation unless there is marked blood loss. Recent evidence suggests that cadaveric, and to some extent related kidney transplant survival, are enhanced by previous red cell transfusions to the recipient (156). Transplant surgeons therefore are in favor of a more liberal transfusion policy for dialysis patients (157). Despite the statistical evidence (156), confirmed by most transplant centers, caution is urged before adopting an indiscriminate transfusion policy. Only a small number of dialysis patients are prospective renal transplant candidates. Prior transfusions to patients with aplastic anemia increases the incidence of marrow graft rejection from HLA-identical siblings (158), and the incidence of cytotoxic antibodies increases with frequent transfusions. Since white blood cell matching for the HLA-DR locus appears to improve cadaveric renal graft survival to the same extent as prior transfusions (159), the number of transfusions to improve graft survival and the accompanying risks may be reduced. These risks, which should always be considered before ordering a transfusion, include not only the non-fatal problems mentioned above, but also hepatitis, which can affect staff as well as patients and can even lead to fatalities (160). In addition, hemolytic reactions can occasionally occur (161).

BLEEDING ABNORMALITIES

Pathophysiology

Bleeding is a frequent complication of chronic renal failure and can be reduced or aggravated by dialysis. A qualitative defect in platelet function is the major abnormality caused by one or more uremic toxins, but the exact identity of these is unknown, although the dialyzable phenolic compounds and guandinosuccinic acid present in uremia inhibit platelets in vitro (162, 163 [see also Chapter 19]).

Platelets function by adhering initially to any traumatized endothelial subsurface. Platelet adhesion depends on the presence of the Von Willebrand factor. After adhesion, the hemostatic plug grows by the aggregation of more platelets to each other. Aggregation is promoted by the platelet binding of the agonists thrombin, epinephrine, collagen, ADP, and by the release of membrane phospholipid platelet factor 3. Following or during aggregation, platelet secretion or release of various membrane proteins, such as platelet factor 4 and β thromboglobulin occurs, as well as the activation of enzymatic processes that enhance the conversion of prothrombin to thrombin on the platelet surface, in turn allowing fibrinogen to be converted to fibrin. Detailed reviews of platelet physiology have recently been published (164, 165). (See also Chapter 10.)

The major clinical abnormality in uremia is a bleeding time prolonged over 3 to 4 times normal. The exact cause of this is not known, but the following abnormalities probably contribute: a defect in platelet adhesion, as shown *in vitro* (166), defective platelet aggregation by ADP, epinephrine and collagen by uremic plasma and guanidinosuccinic acid (163), and decreased availability of platelet factor 3 by phenolic compounds *in vitro* (30). Additional abnormalities develop as part of the hemodialysis procedure.

Beneficial effects of regular dialysis therapy

The bleeding time, usually exceeding 20 to 30 minutes in untreated uremic patients, typically shortens to within the normal range with repeated peritoneal dialysis (167), but not necessarily with conventional hemodialysis (167, 168). *In vitro* tests of platelet function disclose that platelet adhesiveness decreases when the plasma creatinine concentration rises above 530 µmol/l (6 mg/dl) and improves only slightly with twice-weekly hemodialysis (169) and peritoneal dialysis (170). Platelet aggregation improves only slightly with twice-weekly hemodialysis but returns to normal with peritoneal dialysis (170) and thrice-weekly hemodialysis that provides the same total amount of dialysis (12 m^2/h) per week as twice-weekly hemodialysis (171). Others also have shown normalization in platelet adhesiveness and aggregation by hemodialysis (172). The significance of normalization of these *in vitro* tests is not clear since bleeding times were not done. In one study of well hemodialyzed patients (18 m^2/h/wk), bleeding times were normal despite depressed *in vitro* platelet aggregation (173). Yet the clinical impression is that uremic bleeding is greatly reduced, if not eliminated, once repetitive hemo- or peritoneal dialysis is initiated. Of interest is that the bleeding time also can be transiently (up to 12 h) normalized by cryoprecipitate in uremic, non-dialyzed subjects (174).

Complications of the dialysis procedure

The only bleeding complication associated with peritoneal dialysis would be bleeding occurring during the insertion of the peritoneal catheter. This usually ceases spontaneously (175). There are several ways in which the hemodialysis procedure alters platelet function and coagulation. All current dialysis membranes, when exposed to blood, behave like traumatized endothelium, resulting in the initiation of platelet adhesion, aggregation, and ultimately fibrin deposition (see also Chapter 9). During this process platelet counts of patients will decrease transiently during dialysis (176) because of platelet consumption, and PF$_4$ and β-thromboglobulin levels increase due to platelet release (177). PF$_4$ has antiheparin activity which has been referred to as heparin neutralizing activity (HNA). Although heparinization during hemodialysis reduces the above platelet-membrane interactions, it does not prevent them, and it has been proposed that variable amounts of HNA secreted by the reacting platelets may account for the variable heparin requirements encountered in order to prevent thrombosis during dialysis (178, 179 [see also Chapter 10]). Recently, the infusion during hemodialysis of prostacyclin (prostaglandin I$_2$), an inhibitor of platelet activation secreted by vascular endothelium, has prevented the platelet-membrane reaction, as indicated by normalization of platelet and β-thromboglobulin levels (180). However, it is not yet appropriate for routine clinical use since hypotension easily occurs, especially with acetate dialysis (181), although this complication was not noted when first used in humans (180). This agent appears to be most promising, however, and if side effects can be reduced, it could eliminate the need for heparin and conceivably allow prolonged dialyzer re-use.

Because of increased thrombosis associated with vascular accesses, especially Teflon-Silastic arteriovenous cannulas, antithrombotic agents have been used with varying success. Warfarin and similar compounds help retard thrombotic episodes but increase the risk of bleeding because of their effects on the intrinsic clotting mechanism. Low doses of aspirin can reduce dialyzer thrombus formation (182), as well as AV cannula thrombosis (183). Platelet cyclo-oxygenase, an enzyme that activates thromboxane A$_2$ formation, one of the platelet aggregation mechanisms, is irreversibly inhibited by a single 200 mg dose of aspirin for 4 to 10 days (164). Sulfinpyrazone has also reduced AV shunt thromboses when given in a dose of 200 mg three times daily (184). Although this drug also inhibits platelet cyclo-oxygenase and decreases platelet aggregation *in vitro,* its *in vivo* mechanism is unknown, since it does not impair platelet function *in vivo* and no bleeding tendency is seen in patients taking this drug (164).

LEUKOCYTE PROBLEMS

Changes in chronic renal failure

There appear to be numerous secondary effects of renal failure on leukocyte kinetics and functions which can increase the susceptibility of dialysis patients to infections. Total leukocyte counts are often normal, and of the five major types of leukocytes only the circulating lymphocytes are reduced in number. They increase after months of hemodialysis, but not to normal levels (185).

Lymphoid atrophy probably contributes to decreased production of lymphocytes. These changes may be due to a deficiency in the thymic hormone thymosin that is responsible for these changes (186). As a result, the production of T and B cells is reduced, leading to a decrease in the recognition ability of the immunologic system (187). Although there is a deficiency in both T and B lymphocytes, there is a greater depletion in B cells in severe uremia. Both increase with dialysis, but only T cells return to normal levels (185).

The immunologic alterations in hemodialysis patients recently have been reviewed (188). Neutrophil function is also altered (189). The production of neutrophils, and the major functional aspects of neutrophils, i.e. the morphology, distribution, kinetic aspects and the phagocytic and bactericidal functions, all appear to be normal in hemodialysis patients. The major abnormality, however, is a defect in chemotaxis which is partially corrected by peritoneal, but not by hemodialysis (190, 191).

Effects of the dialysis procedure

The most striking effect of the hemodialysis procedure on leukocytes is the very rapid onset of neutropenia and monocytopenia that occurs within a few minutes after initiating hemodialysis (192–194). This is one of the most profound, yet asymptomatic, leukopenic events observed in humans and is thought to be the result of a blood or plasma-membrane interaction which stimulates leukocyte aggregation and agglutination. This reaction occurs with all dialyzer membranes, although minimally with the polyacrylonitrile membrane (89), but rarely whenever dialyzers are re-used or new dialyzers are substituted three hours after the reaction (195). Efforts to explain this phenomenon are still inconclusive. The release of some factor from cellophane activating the complement system, which in turn leads to neutrophil clumping and ultimately sequestration in the pulmonary vascular bed, has been suggested (87). This mechanism of complement-induced neutrophil aggregation has been proposed to account for the early hemodialysis-induced hypoxemia (87, 196 [see also Chapter 31]). However, as plausible as this seems, other investigators have not confirmed these findings or have concluded that there may be separate mechanisms which are responsible for these different events. Complement activation is not proportional to the neutropenia, since polyacrylonitrile membranes cause marked total complement activation with minimal neutropenia, whereas polycarbonate membranes are associated with the opposite effect (195).

There also is a divergence between the neutropenia and hypoxemia in that hypoxemia continues to occur with re-used dialyzers when neutrophil counts remain unchanged and ultrafiltration results in no changes in PAO_2 but induces neutropenia (197). Studies do suggest that neutrophil and monocyte aggregates sequester in the lungs of rabbits (87) and dogs (198), leading to leukostasis, but this reaction is transient and its clinical effects, if any, still are not well defined. The long term effect on pulmonary function needs clarification, although pulmonary fibrosis with calcinosis has been described (199). The effects on the immunological system are also unknown.

REFERENCES

1. Fried W: Erythropoietin and the kidney. *Nephron* 15:327, 1975.
2. Graber, SE, Krantz SB: Erythropoietin and the control of red cell production. *Annu Rev Med* 29:51, 1978
3. Krantz WB: Recent contributions to the mechanism of action and clinical relevance of erythropoietin. *J Lab Clin Med* 82:847, 1973
4. Fisher JW: Prostaglandins and kidney erythropoietin production. Editorial review. *Nephron* 25:53, 1980
5. Adamson JW, Eschbach JW, Finch CA: The kidney and erythropoiesis. *Am J Med* 44:725, 1968
6. Shaw AB: Haemolysis in chronic renal failure. *Br Med J* 2:213, 1967
7. McDermott FT, Galbraith AJ, Corlett RJ: Inhibition of cell proliferation in renal failure and its significance to the uraemic syndrome: A review. *Scott Med J* 20:317, 1973
8. Wallner SF, Vautrin RM: The anemia of chronic renal failure. Studies of iron transport in vitro. *J Lab Clin Med* 96:67, 1980
9. Naets JP, Heuse AF: Measurement of erythropoietic stimulating factor in anemic patients with or without renal disease. *J Lab Clin Med* 60:365, 1962
10. Caro J, Brown S, Miller O, Murray T, Erslev AJ: Erythropoietin levels in uremic nephric and anephric patients. *J Lab Clin Med* 93:449, 1979
11. Mirand EA, Murphy GP, Steeves RA, Groenewald JM, DeKlerk JN: Erythropoietin activity in anephric, allotransplanted, unilaterally nephrectomized and intact man. *J Lab Clin Med* 73:121, 1969
12. Fisher JW, Stuckey WJ, Lindholm DD, Abshire S: Extrarenal erythropoietin production. *Israel J Med Sci* 7:991, 1971
13. Finch CA, Deubelbeiss K, Cook JD, Eschbach JW, Harker LA, Funk DD, Marsaglia G, Hillman RS, Slichter S, Adamson JW, Ganzoni A, Giblett ER: Ferrokinetics in man. *Medicine* 49:17, 1970
14. Eschbach JW, Adamson JW, Cook JD: Disorders of red blood cell production in uremia. *Arch Intern Med* 126:812, 1970
15. Eschbach JW, Detter JC, Adamson JW. Physiologic studies in normal and uremic sheep. II. Changes in erythropoiesis and oxygen transport. *Kidney Int* 18:732, 1980
16. Radtke HW, Claussner A, Erbes PM, Scheuermann EH, Schoeppe W, Koch KM: Serum erythropoietin concentration in chronic renal failure: Relationship to degree of anemia and excretory renal function. *Blood* 54:877, 1979
17. Dagher FJ, Ramos E, Erslev AJ, Alongi SV, Karmi SA, Caro J: Are the native kidneys responsible for erythrocytosis in renal allorecipients? *Transplantation* 28:496, 1979
18. Stewart JH: Haemolytic anaemia in acute and chronic renal failure. *Q J Med* 36:85, 1967
19. Lieberman E, Heuser E, Donnell GN, Landing BH, Hammond GD: Hemolytic-uremic syndrome. Clinical and pathological considerations. *N Engl J Med* 275:227, 1966
20. Fisher JW: Mechanism of the anemia of chronic renal failure. *Nephron* 25:106, 1980
21. Zucker S, Lysik RM, Mohammad G. Erythropoiesis in chronic renal disease. *J Lab Clin Med* 88:528, 1976

22. Charles G, Lundin AP III, Manis T, Delano BG, Joshi T, Rao TKS, Friedman EA: Surprisingly high hematocrit during maintenance hemodialysis. *Kidney int* 19:144, 1981
23. Anagnostou A, Barone J, Kedo A, Fried W: Effect of erythropoietin therapy on the red cell volume of uraemic and non-uraemic rats. *Br J Haematol* 37:85, 1977
24. Van Stone JC, Max P: Effect of erythropoietin on anemia of peritoneally dialyzed anephric rats. *Kidney Int* 15:370, 1979
25. Eschbach JW, Adamson JW: Correction by erythropoietin therapy of the anemia of chronic renal failure in sheep. *Clin Res* 29:518A, 1981
26. Miyake T, Kung CK-H, Goldwasser E: Purification of human erythropoietin. *J Biol Chem* 252:5558, 1977
27. Garcia JF, Sherwood J, Goldwasser E: Radioimmunoassay of erythropoietin. *Blood Cells* 5:405, 1979
28. Kolk-Vegter AJ, Kolk AHJ: Some problems concerning the assay of erythropoietin using the haemagglutination inhibition kit. *Br J Haematol* 30:371, 1975
29. Lertora JJL, Dargon PA, Rege AB, Fisher JW: Studies on a radioimmunoassay for human erythropoietin. *J Lab Clin Med* 86:140, 1975
30. Horowitz HI: Uremic toxins and platelet function. *Arch Intern Med* 126:823, 1970
31. Castaldi PA, Rozenberg MC, Stewart JH: The bleeding disorder of uraemia. *Lancet* 2:66, 1966
32. Von Hartitzsch B, Carr D, Kjellstrand CM, Kerr DNS: Normal red cell survival in well-dialyzed patients. *Trans Am Soc Artif Intern Organs* 19:471, 1973
33. Eschbach JW Jr, Funk D, Adamson J, Kuhn I, Scribner BH, Finch CA: Erythropoiesis in patients with renal failure undergoing chronic dialysis. *N Engl J Med* 276:653, 1967
34. Eschbach JW, Korn D, Finch CA: ^{14}C cyanate as a tag for red cell survival in normal and uremic man. *J Lab Clin Med* 89:823, 1977
35. Blumberg A, Jarti HR: Red cell metabolism and haemolysis in patients on dialysis. *Proc Eur Dial Transpl Assoc* 9:91, 1972
36. Koch KM, Patya WD, Shaldon S, Werner E: Anemia of the regular hemodialysis patient and its treatment. *Nephron* 12:405, 1974
37. Müller-Wiefel DE, Sinn H, Gilli G, Schärer K: Hemolysis and blood loss in children with chronic renal failure. *Clin Nephrol* 8:481, 1977
38. Yen MC, Ball JH, Lowrie EG, Lazarus JM, Hampers CL, Merrill JP: The effect of androgens and dialysis on erythropoiesis in chronic renal failure. *Proc Dial Clin Transpl Forum* 3:33, 1973
39. Roxe DM, del Greco F, Hughes J, Krumlovsky F, Ghantous W, Ivanovich P, Quintanilla A, Salkin M, Stone NJ, Reins M: Hemodialysis vs peritoneal dialysis: Results of a 3-year prospective controlled study *Kidney Int* 19:341, 1981
40. Goldsmith HJ, Forbes A, Gyde OHB, Summerfield G: Hematologic aspects of continuous ambulatory peritoneal dialysis. *Continuous Ambulatory Peritoneal Dialysis* Proc Int Symp, Paris, nov 2 and 3 1970, edited by Legrain M, Amsterdam, Oxford, Princeton, Excerpta Medica, 1980, p 302
41. Madden MA, Zimmerman SW, Simpson DP: Longitudinal comparison of chronic intermittent and continuous ambulatory peritoneal dialysis. *Kidney Int* 19:153, 1981
42. Lindsay RM, Burton JA, Dargie HJ, Prentice CRM, Kennedy AC: Dialyzer blood loss. *Clin Nephrol* 1:24, 1973
43. Haskins D, Stevens AR Jr, Finch S, Finch CA: Iron metabolism. Iron stores in man as measured by phlebotomy. *J Clin Invest* 31:543, 1952
44. Fong TP, Smith EC, Thomas W Jr, Westerman MP: Diagnostic significance of bone marrow biopsy in chronic renal disease. *Nephron* 12:81, 1974
45. Miles LEM, Lipschitz DA, Bieber CP, Cook JD: Measurement of serum ferritin by a 2-site immunoradiometric assay. *Anal Biochem* 61:209, 1974
46. Mirahmadi KS, Wellington LP, Winer RL, Dabir-Vaziri N, Byer B, Gorman JT, Rosen SM: Serum ferritin level. Determinant of iron requirement in hemodialysis patients. *JAMA* 238:601, 1977
47. Bell JD, Kincaid WR, Morgan RG, Bunce III H, Alperin JB, Searles HE, Remmers AR Jr: Serum ferritin assay and bone-marrow iron stores in patients on maintenance hemodialysis. *Kidney Int* 17:237, 1980
48. Aljama P, Ward MK, Pierides AM, Eastham EJ, Ellis HA, Feest TG, Conceicao S, Kerr DNS: Serum ferritin concentration: A reliable guide to iron overload in uremic and hemodialyzed patients. *Clin Nephrol* 10:101, 1978.
49. Gokal R, Millard PR, Weatherall DJ, Callender STE, Ledingham G, Oliver DO: Iron metabolism in haemodialysis patients. *Q J Med* 158:369, 1979
50. Eschbach JW, Cook JD, Scribner BH, Finch CA: Iron balance in hemodialysis patients. *Ann Intern Med* 87:710, 1977
51. Hussein S, Prieto J, O'Shea M, Hoffbrand AV, Baillod RA, Moorhead JF: Serum ferritin assay and iron status in chronic renal failure and haemodialysis. *Br Med J* 1:546, 1975
52. Beallo R, Dallman PR, Schoenfeld PY, Humphreys MH: Serum ferritin and iron deficiency in patients on chronic hemodialysis. *Trans Am Soc Artif Intern Organs* 22:73, 1976
53. Dallman PR, Beutler E, Finch CA: Effects of iron deficiency exclusive of anaemia. *Br J Haematol* 40:179, 1978
54. Whitehead VM, Comty CH, Posen GA, Kaye M: Homeostasis of folic acid in patients undergoing maintenance hemodialysis. *N Engl J Med* 279:970, 1980
55. Hemmeløff Andersen KE: Folic acid status of patients with chronic renal failure maintained by dialysis. *Clin Nephrol* 8:510, 1977
56. Hampers CL, Streiff R, Nathan DG, Snyder D, Merrill JP: Megaloblastic hematopoiesis in uremia and in patients on long-term hemodialysis. *N Engl J Med* 276:551, 1967
57. Siddiqui J, Freeburger R, Freeman RM: Folic acid, hypersegmented polymorphonuclear leukocyte and the uremic syndrome. *Am J Clin Nutr* 23:11, 1970
58. Eichner ER, Paine CJ, Dickson VL, Hargrove MD Jr: Clinical and laboratory observations on serum folate-binding protein. *Blood* 46:599, 1975
59. Matter BJ, Pederson J, Psimenos G, Lindeman RD: Lethal copper intoxication in hemodialysis. *Trans Am Soc Artif Intern Organs* 15:309, 1969
60. Ivanovich P, Manzler A, Drake R: Acute hemolysis following hemodialysis. *Trans Am Soc Artif Intern Organs* 15:316, 1969
61. Manzler AD, Schreiner AW: Copper-induced acute hemolytic anemia. A new complication of hemodialysis. *Ann Intern Med* 73:409, 1970.
62. Boulard M, Blume K-G, Beutler E: The effect of copper on red cell enzyme activities. *J Clin Invest* 51:459, 1972
63. Yawata Y, Howe R, Jacob HS: Abnormal red cell metabolism causing hemolysis in uremia. A defect potentiated by tap water hemodialysis. *Ann Intern Med* 79:362, 1973
64. Eaton JW, Leida MN, Kjellstrand CM, Jacob HS: Oxidant-induced erythrocyte destruction in chronic renal disease. *Proc 12th Annu Contractors' Conf, Artif Kidney*

Program, NIAMDD, edited by Mackey BB NIH Publ No 81-1979, 1981, p 105
65. Higgins MR, Grace M, Ulan RA, Silverberg DS, Bettcher KB, Dossetor JB: Anemia in hemodialysis patients. Arch Intern Med 137:172, 1977
66. Neilan BA, Ehlers SM, Kolpin CF, Eaton JW: Prevention of chloramine-induced hemolysis in dialyzed patients. Clin Nephrol 10:105, 1978
67. Botella J, Traver JA, Sanz-Guajardo D, Torres MT, Sanjuan I, Zabala P: Chloramines, an aggravating factor in the anaemia of patients on regular dialysis treatment. Proc Eur Dial Transpl Assoc 14:192, 1977
68. Carlson DJ, Shapiro FL: Methemoglobinemia from well water nitrates: A complication of home dialysis. Ann Intern Med 73:757, 1970
69. Orringer EP, Mattern WD: Formaldehyde-induced hemolysis during chronic hemodialysis. N Engl J Med 294:1416, 1976
70. Howell ED, Perkins HA: Anti-N-like antibodies in the sera of patients undergoing chronic hemodialysis. Vox Sang 23:291, 1972
71. Shaldon S, Chevallet M, Maraoui M, Mion C: Dialysis associated autoantibodies. Proc Eur Dial Transpl Assoc 13:339, 1976
72. Kaehny WD, Miller GE, White WL: Relationship between dialyzer reuse and the presence of anti-N-like antibodies in chronic hemodialysis patients. Kidney Int 12:59, 1977
73. Koch KM, Fei U, Fassbinder W: Hemolysis and anemia in anti-N-like antibody positive hemodialysis patients. Trans Am Soc Artif Intern Organs 24:709, 1978
74. Fassbinder W, Pilar J, Scheuermann E, Koch M: Formaldehyde and the occurrence of anti-N-like cold agglutinins in RDT patients. Proc Eur Dial Transpl Assoc 13:333, 1976
75. Crosson JT, Moulds J, Comty CM, Polesky HF: A clinical study of anti-N_{DP} in the sera of patients in a large repetitive hemodialysis program. Kidney Int 10:463, 1976
76. Berkes SL, Kahn SI, Chazan JA, Garella S: Prolonged hemolysis from overheated dialysate. Ann Intern Med 82:363, 1975
77. Fortner RW, Nowakowski A, Carter CB, King LH Jr, Knepshield JH: Death due to overheated dialysate during dialysis. Ann Intern Med 73:443, 1970
78. Said R, Quintanilla A, Levin N, Ivanovich P: Acute hemolysis due to profound hyper-osmolality. A complication of hemodialysis. J Dial 1:447, 1977
79. Finch CA, Lenfant C: Oxygen transport in man. N Engl J Med 286:407, 1972
80. Neff MS, Kim KE, Persoff M, Onesti G, Schwartz C: Hemodynamics of uremic anemia. Circulation 43:876, 1971
81. Perutz MF: Haem-Haem interaction and the problem of allostery. Nature 228:726, 1970
82. Card RT, Brain MC: The 'anemia' of childhood. N Engl J Med 288:388, 1973
83. Blumberg A, Keller G: Oxygen consumption during maintenance hemodialysis. Nephron 23:276, 1979
84. Torrance JD, Milne FJ, Hurwitz SZ, Rabkin R: Changes in oxygen delivery during hemodialysis. Clin Nephrol 3:53, 1975
85. Ahmad S, Pagel M, Shen F, Vizzo J, Scribner BH: The role of hypoxemia in the expression of acetate intolerance. Abstracts Am Soc Nephrol 13:33A, 1980
86. Abu-Hamdan DK, Mahajan SK, Desai CW, Mueller B, Briggs WA, McDonald FD: Hypoxemia during bicarbonate dialysis. Abstracts Am Soc Nephrol 13:33 A, 1980
87. Craddock PR, Fehr J, Dalmasso AP, Brigham KL, Jacob HS: Hemodialysis leukopenia. Pulmonary vascular leukostasis resulting from complement activation by dialyzer cellophane membranes. J Clin Invest 59:879, 1979
88. Jacob AI, Gavellas G, Zarco R, Perez G, Bourgoignie JJ: Leukopenia, hypoxia, and complement function with different hemodialysis membranes. Kidney Int 18:505, 1980
89. Aljama P, Bird PAE, Ward MK, Feest TG, Walker W, Tanboga H, Sussman M, Kerr DNS: Haemodialysis-induced leucopenia and activation of complement: Effects of different membranes. Proc Eur Dial Transpl Assoc 15:144, 1978
90. Graefe U, Milutinovic J, Follette WC, Vizzo JE, Babb AL, Scribner BH: Less dialysis, induced morbidity and vascular instability with bicarbonate dialysate. Ann Intern Med 88:332, 1978
91. Tolchin N, Roberts JL, Hayashi J, Lewis EJ: Metabolic consequences of high mass-transfer hemodialysis. Kidney Int 11:366, 1977
92. Jones RH, Broadfield JB, Parsons V: Arterial hypoxemia during hemodialysis for acute renal failure in mechanically ventilated patients: Observations and mechanisms. Clin Nephrol 14:18, 1980
93. Hirszel P, Maher JF, Tempel GE, Mengel CE: Influence of peritoneal dialysis on factors affecting oxygen transport. Nephron 15:438, 1975
94. Stenzel KH, Cheigh JS, Sullivan JF, Tapia L, Riggio RR, Rubin AL: Clinical effects of bilateral nephrectomy. Am J Med 58:69, 1975
95. Kominami N, Lowrie EG, Ianhez LE, Skaren A, Hampers CL, Merrill JP, Lange RD: The effect of total nephrectomy on hematopoiesis in patients undergoing chronic hemodialysis. J Lab Clin Med 78:524, 1971
96. Laurent C, Wittek M, Vereerstraeten P, Toussaint C, Naets JP: Red cells life span, splenic sequestration and transfusions requirements in chronic renal failure treated by hemodialysis. Effects of bilateral nephrectomy. Clin Nephrol 2:35, 1974
97. Van Ypersele de Strihou C, Stragier A: Effect of bilateral nephrectomy on transfusion requirements of patients undergoing chronic dialysis. Lancet 2:705, 1969
98. Naets JP, Wittek M: Presence of erythropoietin in the plasma of one anephric patient. Blood 31:249, 1968
99. Avram MM, Alexis H, Rahman M, Son B, Iancu M: Decreased transfusional requirement following parathyroidectomy in long term hemodialysis. Abstracts Am Soc Nephrol 5:5, 1971
100. Shasha SM, Better OS, Winaver J, Chaimovitz C, Barzilai A, Erlik D: Improvement in the anemia of hemodialyzed patients following subtotal parathyroidectomy. Isr J Med Sci 14:328, 1978
101. Zingraff J, Drueke T, Marie P, Man NK, Jungers P, Bordier P: Anemia and secondary hyperparathyroidism. Arch Intern Med 138:1650, 1978
102. Barbour GL: Effect of parathyroidectomy on anemia in chronic renal failure. Arch Intern Med 139:889, 1979
103. Meytes D, Bogin E, Ma A, Dukes PP, Massry SG: Effect of parathyroid hormone in erythropoiesis. J Clin Invest 67:1263, 1981
104. Weinberg SG, Lubin A, Wiener S, Deoras MP, Ghose MK, Kopelman RC: Myelofibrosis and renal osteodystrophy. Am J Med 63:755, 1977
105. Gurney CW, Jacobson LO, Goldwasser E: The physiologic and clinical significance of erythropoietin. Ann Intern Med 49:363, 1958
106. Kopple JD, Swendseid ME: Evidence that histidine is an essential amino acid in normal and chronically uremic man. J Clin Invest 55:881, 1975
107. Giordano C, De Santo NG, Rinaldi S, Acone D, Esposito R, Gallo B: Histidine for treatment of uraemic anaemia.

Br Med J 4:714, 1973
108. Jontofsohn R, Heinze V, Katz N, Stuber U, Wilke H, Kluthe R: Histidine and iron supplementation in dialysis and pre-dialysis patients. Proc Eur Dial Transpl Assoc 11:391, 1974
109. Reeves RD, Barbour GL, Robertson CS, Crumb CK: Failure of histidine supplementation to improve anemia in chronic dialysis patients. Am J Clin Nutr 30:579, 1977
110. Bischel MD, Neiman RS, Berne TV, Telfer N, Lukes RJ, Barbour BH: Hypersplenism in the uremic hemodialyzed patient. Nephron 9:146, 1972
111. Hartley LCJ, Morgan TO, Innis MD, Clunie CJA: Splenectomy for anaemia in patients on regular haemodialysis. Lancet 2:1343, 1971
112. Ulan RA, Hill JR, Silverberg DS, Dawson ET, Dossetor JB: Erythrocyte survival and splenic sequestration in chronic dialysis patients. Abstracts Int Soc Nephrol 5:27, 1972
113. Rosenmund A, Binswanger U, Straub PW: Oxidative injury to erythrocytes, cell rigidity, and splenic hemolysis in hemodialyzed uremic patients. Ann Intern Med 82:460, 1975
114. Asaba H, Bergström J, Lundgren G, Sörbo B, Tranaeus A, Zachrisson L: Hypersequestration of ^{51}Cr-labelled erythrocytes as a criterion for splenectomy in regular hemodialysis patients. Clin Nephrol 8:304, 1977
115. Morgan T, Innes M, Ribush N: The management of the anaemia of patients on chronic haemodialysis. Med J Aust 1:848, 1972
116. Lichtman MA, Miller DR, Freeman RB: Erythrocyte adenosine triphosphate depletion during hypophosphatemia in a uremic subject. N Engl J Med 280:240, 1969
117. Jacob HS, Amsden T: Acute hemolytic anemia with rigid red cells in hypophosphatemia. N Engl J Med 285:1446, 1971
118. Baker LRI, Barnett MD, Brozovic B, Cattell WR, Ackrill P, McAlister J, Nimmon C: Hemosiderosis in a patient on regular hemodialysis: Treatment by desferrioxamine. Clin Nephrol 6:326, 1976
119. Pitts TO, Barbour GL: Hemosiderosis secondary to chronic parenteral iron therapy in maintenance hemodialysis patients. Nephron 22:316, 1978
120. Schaefer AI, Cheron RG, Dluhy R, Cooper B, Gleason RE, Soeldner JS, Bunn HF: Clinical consequences of acquired transfusional iron overload in adults. N Engl J Med 304:319, 1981
121. Bregman H, Winchester JF, Knepshield JH, Gelfand MC, Manz HJ, Schreiner GE: Iron-overload-associated myopathy in patients on maintenance haemodialysis: A histocompatibility-linked disorder. Lancet 2:882, 1980
122. Tisher CC, Barnett BMS, Finch CA, Scribner BH: Treatment of iron overload in patients with renal failure. Clin Sci 33:539, 1967
123. Kolk-Vegter AJ, Bosch E, van Leeuwen AM: Influence of serum hepatitis on haemoglobin level in patients on regular haemodialysis. Lancet 1:526, 1971
124. Coleman JC, Eastwood JB, Curtis JE, Fox RA, Edwards MS: Hepatitis and epidemic hepatitis associated antigen in a haemodialysis unit with observations on haemoglobin levels. Br J Urol 44:194, 1972
125. Simon P, Meyrier A, Tanquerel T, Ang K-S: Improvement of anaemia in haemodialysed patients after viral or toxic hepatic cytolysis. Br Med J 1:892, 1980
126. Brown S, Caro J, Erslev AJ, Murray TG: Spontaneous increase in erythropoietin and hematocrit value associated with transient liver enzyme abnormalities in an anephric patient undergoing hemodialysis. Am J Med 68:280, 1980

127. Goldberg AP, Hagberg JM, Delmez JA, Carney RM, McKevitt PM, Harter HR: Metabolic effects of exercise training in hemodialysis patients. Proc 12th Annu Contractors' Conf, Artif Kidney Program, NIAMDD, NIH Publ No 81-1979, 1981, edited by Mackey BB, p 7
128. Loge JP, Lange RD, Moore CV: Characterization of the anemia associated with chronic renal insufficiency. Am J Med 24:4, 1958
129. Rastogi SP, Padilla F, Boyd CM: Effect of aluminium hydroxide on iron absorption. Abstracts Am Soc Nephrol 8:21, 1975
130. Strickland ID, Chaput de Saintonge DM, Boulton FE, Francis B, Roubikova J, Water JI: The therapeutic equivalence of oral and intravenous iron in renal dialysis patients. Clin Nephrol 7:55, 1977
131. Parker PA, Izard MW, Maher JF: Therapy of iron deficiency anemia in patients on maintenance dialysis. Nephron 23:181, 1979
132. Hamstra RD, Block MH, Schocket AL: Intravenous iron dextran in clinical medicine. JAMA 243:1726, 1980
133. Kopple JD, Mercurio K, Blumenkrantz MJ, Jones MR, Tallos J, Roberts C, Card B, Saltzman R, Casciato DA, Swendseid ME: Daily requirement for pyridoxine supplements in chronic renal failure. Kidney Int 19:694, 1981
134. Eschbach JW, Adamson JW: Improvement in the anemia of chronic renal failure with fluoxymesterone. Ann Intern Med 78:527, 1973
135. De Gowin RL, Lavender AR, Forland M, Charleston D, Gottschalk A: Erythropoiesis and erythropoietin in patients with chronic renal failure treated with hemodialysis and testosterone. Ann Intern Med 72:913, 1970
136. Shaldon S, Koch KM, Oppermann F, Patyna WD: Testosterone therapy for anaemia in maintenance dialysis. Br Med J 3:212, 1971
137. Fried W, Jonasson O, Lang G, Schwartz F: The hematologic effect of androgen in uremic patients. Study of packed cell volume and erythropoietin response. Ann Intern Med 79:823, 1973
138. Williams JS, Stein JH, Ferris TF: Nandrolene decanoate therapy for patients receiving hemodialysis. Arch Intern Med 134:289, 1974
139. Hendler ED, Goffinet JA, Ross S, Longnecker RE, Bakovic V: Controlled study of androgen therapy in anemia of patients on maintenance hemodialysis. N Engl J Med 291:1046, 1974
140. von Hartitzsch B, Kerr DNS, Morley G, Marks B: Androgens in the anaemia of chronic renal failure. Nephron 18:13, 1977
141. Ball JH, Lowrie EG, Hampers CL, Merrill JP: Testosterone therapy in hemodialysis patients. Clin Nephrol 4:91, 1975
142. Mayer PP, Robinson BHB: Testosterone for anaemia in maintenance dialysis. Br Med J 2:373, 1971
143. Neff MS, Goldberg J, Slifkin RF, Eiser AR, Calamia V, Kaplan M, Baez A, Gupta S, Mattoo N: A comparison of androgens for anemia in patients on hemodialysis. N Engl J Med 304:871, 1981
144. Radtke HW, Erbes PM, Schippers E, Koch KM: Serum erythropoietin concentration in anephric patients. Nephron 22:361, 1978
145. Acchiardo SR, Black WD: Fluoxymesterone therapy in anemia of patients on maintenance hemodialysis: Comparison between patients with kidneys and anephric patients. J Dial 1:357, 1977
146. Singer JW, Adamson JW: Steroids and hematopoiesis. II. The effect of steroids on in vitro erythroid colony growth: Evidence for different target cells for different classes of steroids. J Cell Physiol 88:135, 1976
147. Ahmad S, Shen F, Pagel M, Goodman W: Accelerated

creatinine metabolism and elevated CPK with androgen therapy. *Proc Clin Dial Transpl Forum* 10:174, 1980
148. Editorial (Anonymous). Androgens in the anaemia of chronic renal failure. *Br Med J* 2:417, 1977
149. Kalmanti M, Martino J, Callahan M, Dainiak N: Use of a clonal assay system to predict therapeutic response to steroids in the anemia of chronic renal failure. *Kidney Int* 19:128, 1981
150. Curtis JR, Goode GC, Herrington J, Urdaneta LE: Possible cobalt toxicity in maintenance hemodialysis patients after treatment with cobaltous chloride: A study of blood and tissue cobalt concentrations in normal subjects and patients with terminal renal failure. *Clin Nephrol* 5:61, 1976
151. Editorial (anonymous): Cobalt in severe renal failure. *Lancet* 2:26, 1976
152. Malgor LA, Blanc CC, Klainer E, Irizar, Torales PR, Barrios L: Direct effects of thyroid hormones on bone marrow erythroid cells of rats. *Blood* 45:671, 1975
153. Ferrer J, Diez-Ewald M, Garcia R, Rubio L, Rodriguez-Iturbe B: Effects of triiodothyronine on the anemia of chronic renal failure. *Am J Hemat* 5:139, 1978
154. Bastow MD, Woods HF, Walls J: Persistent anemia associated with reduced serum vitamin B_{12} levels in patients undergoing regular hemodialysis therapy. *Clin Nephrol* 11:133, 1979
155. Fried W: Anemia in patients with chronic renal failure. *Int J Artif Organs* 3:62, 1980
156. Opelz G, Terasaki PI: Improvement of kidney-graft survival with increased numbers of blood transfusions. *N Engl J Med* 299:799, 1978
157. Vincenti F, Duca RM, Amend W, Perkins HA, Cochrum KC, Feduska NJ, Salvatierra O Jr: Immunologic factors determining survival of cadaver kidney transplants. *N Engl J Med* 299:793, 1978
158. Storb R, Thomas ED, Buckner CD, Clift RA, Deeg HJ, Fefer A, Goodell BW, Sale GE, Sanders JE, Singer J, Stewart P, Weiden PL: Marrow transplantation in thirty 'untransfused" patients with severe aplastic anemia. *Ann Intern Med* 92:30, 1980
159. Albrechtsen D, Bratlie A, Kiss E, Solheim BG, Thoresen AB, Wither N, Thorsby E: Significance of HLA matching in renal transplantation. *Transplantation* 28:280, 1979
160. Myhre BA: Fatalities from blood transfusion. *JAMA* 244:1333, 1980
161. Pineda AA, Brzica SM, Taswell HF: Hemolytic transfusion reaction: A recent experience in a large blood bank. *Mayo Clin Proc* 53:378, 1978
162. Horowitz HI, Stein IM, Cohen BD, White JG: Further studies on the platelet-inhibitory effect of guanidinosuccinic acid and its role in uremic bleeding. *Am J Med* 49:336, 1970
163. Rabiner SF, Molinas F: The role of phenol and phenolic acids on the thrombocytopathy and defective platelet aggregation of patients with renal failure. *Am J Med* 49:-346, 1970
164. Huebsch LB, Harker LA: Disorders of platelet function. *Western J Med* 134:109, 1981
165. Shattil SJ, Bennett JS: Platelets and their membranes in hemostasis: physiology and pathophysiology. *Ann Intern Med* 94:108, 1981
166. Salzman EW, Neri LL: Adhesiveness of blood platelets in uremia. *Thromb Diath Haemorrh* 15:84, 1966
167. Harker LA, Slichter SJ: The bleeding time as a screening test for evaluation of platelet function. *N Engl J Med* 287:155, 1972
168. Remuzzi G, Livio M, Marchiaro G, Mecca G, de Gaetano G: Bleeding in renal failure: Altered platelet function in chronic uremia only partially corrected by haemodialysis. *Nephron* 22:347, 1978
169. Lindsay RM, Moorthy AV, Koens F, Linton AL: Platelet function in dialyzed and non-dialyzed patients with chronic renal failure. *Clin Nephrol* 4:52, 1975
170. Lindsay RM, Friesen M, Koens F, Linton AL, Oreopoulos DG, de Veber G: Platelet function in patients on long term peritoneal dialysis. *Clin Nephrol* 6:335, 1976
171. Lindsay RM, Friesen M, Aronstam A, Andrus F, Clark WF, Linton AL: Improvement of platelet function by increased frequency of hemodialysis. *Clin Nephrol* 10:67, 1978
172. Jorenson KA, Ingeberg S: Platelets and platelet function in patients with chronic uremia on maintenance hemodialysis. *Nephron* 23:233, 1979
173. Wathen R, Smith M, Keshaviah P, Comty C, Shapiro F: Depressed in vitro aggregation of platelets of chronic hemodialysis patients: A role for cyclic amp. *Trans Am Soc Artif Int Organs* 21:320, 1975
174. Janson PA, Jubelirer SJ, Weinstein MJ, Deykin D: Treatment of the bleeding tendency in uremia with cryoprecipitate. *N Engl J Med* 303:1318, 1980
175. Tenckhoff H: *Chronic Peritoneal Dialysis Manual,* University of Washington, Seattle, Washington, 1974
176. Lindsay RM, Prentice CRM, Davidson JF, Burton JA, McNicol GP: Haemostatic changes during dialysis associated with thrombus formation on dialysis membranes. *Br Med J* 2:454, 1972
177. Rucinski B, Niewiarowski S, James P, Walz DA, Budzynski AZ: Antiheparin proteins secreted by human platelets. Purification, characterization, and radioimmunoassay. *Blood* 53:47, 1969.
178. Aronstam A, Dennis B, Friesen MJ, Clark WF, Linton AL, Lindsay RM: Heparin neutralizing activity in patients with renal disease on maintenance hemodialysis. *Thromb Haemost* 39:695, 1978
179. Lindsay RM: Variable heparin requirements during hemodialysis — Why? *asaio J* 3:81, 1980
180. Turney JH, Fewell MR, Williams LC, Parsons V, Weston MJ: Platelet protection and heparin sparing with prostacyclin during regular dialysis therapy. *Lancet* 2:219, 1980
181. Zusman RM, Rubin RH, Cato AE, Cocchetto DM, Crow JW, Tolkoff-Rubin N: Hemodialysis using prostacyclin instead of heparin as the sole antithrombotic agent. *N Engl J Med* 304:934, 1981
182. Lindsay RM, Ferguson D, Prentice CRM, Burton JA, McNicol GP: Reduction of thrombus formation on dialyser membranes by aspirin and RA 233. *Lancet* 2:1287, 1972
183. Harter HR, Burch JW, Majerus PW, Stanford N, Delmez JA, Anderson CB, Weerts C: Prevention of thrombosis in patients on hemodialysis by low-dose aspirin. *N Engl J Med* 301:577, 1979
184. Kaegi A, Pineo GF, Shimizu A, Trivedi H, Hirsh J, Gent M: Arteriovenous-shunt thrombosis. *N Engl J Med* 290:304, 1974
185. Hoy WE, Cestero RVM, Freeman RB: Deficiency of T and B lymphocytes in uremic subjects and partial improvement with maintenance hemodialysis. *Nephron* 20:182, 1978
186. Harris J, Sengar D, Rashid A, Hyslop D, Green L: Immunodeficiency in chronic uremia: Preliminary evidence for thymosin deficiency. *Transplantation* 20:176, 1975
187. Hosking CS, Atkins RC, Scott DF, Holdsworth SR, Fitzgerald MG, Shelton MJ: Immune and phagocytic functions in patients on maintenance dialysis and post-transplantation. *Clin Nephrol* 6:501, 1976
188. Goldblum SE, Reed WP: Host defenses and immunologic alterations associated with chronic hemodialysis. *Ann*

Intern Med 93:597, 1980
189. Dale DC: Neutrophils and the acute inflammatory response in chronic renal failure. Dial Transpl 8:314, 1979
190. Salont DJ, Glover A, Anderson R, Meyers AM, Rabkin R, Myburgh JA, Rabson AR: Depressed neutrophil chemotaxis in patients with chronic renal failure and after renal transplantations. J Lab Clin Med 88:536, 1976
191. Greene WH, Ray C, Mauer SM, Quie PG: The effect of hemodialysis on neutrophil chemotactic responsiveness. J Lab Clin Med 88:971, 1976
192. Kaplow LS, Goffinet JA: Profound neutropenia during the early phase of hemodialysis. JAMA 203:1135, 1968
193. Gral T, Schroth P, DePalma JR, Gordon A: Leukocyte dynamics with three types of hemodialyzers. Trans Am Soc Artif Intern Organs 15:45, 1969
194. Brubaker LH, Nolph KD: Mechanisms of recovery from neutropenia induced by hemodialysis. Blood 38:623, 1971
195. Savdie E, Bruce L, Vincent PC: Modified neutropenic response to re-used dialyzers in patients with chronic renal failure. Clin Nephrol 8:422, 1977
196. Jacob HS, Craddock PR, Hammerschmidt DE, Moldow CF: Complement-induced granulocyte aggregation. An unsuspected mechanism of disease. N Engl J Med 302:789, 1980
197. Dumler F, Levin NW: Unrelated effects of hemodialysis. Arch Intern Med 139:1103, 1979
198. Toren M, Goffinet JA, Kaplow LS: Pulmonary bed sequestration of neutrophils during hemodialysis. Blood 36:337, 1970
199. Conger JD, Hammond WS, Alfrey AC, Contiguglia SR, Stanford RE, Huffer WE: Pulmonary calcification in chronic dialysis patients: Clinical and pathologic studies. Ann Intern Med 83:330, 1975

33
HOST DEFENSES AND INFECTIOUS COMPLICATIONS IN MAINTENANCE HEMODIALYSIS PATIENTS

WILLIAM F. KEANE and LEOPOLDO R RAIJ

Introduction	646
Host defense mechanisms in uremia	646
Humoral immunity	646
Lymphocyte function	647
Polymorphonuclear cell functions	647
Mononuclear phagocytic system function	648
Response of the chronic hemodialysis patient to infection	648
Patient population	648
Mortality	648
Bacteremia in hemodialysis patients	649
Incidence	649
Infecting organisms	649
Mortality	650
Bacteremia secondary to access infection	650
Bacteremia source unknown	650
Bacteremia associated with a source of infection other than blood access device	650
Bacteriology	650
Treatment of bacteremic episodes	650
Other major infectious complications	651
Septic pulmonary emboli	651
Bacterial endocarditis	651
Osteomyelitis and septic arthritis	651
Polymicrobial bacteremia	651
Access infections	652
Systemic infections	653
Respiratory infections	653
Urinary tract infections	653
Unusual infections	653
Infections in patients with uremia secondary to rejection of a renal allograft	654
Summary	654
References	654

INTRODUCTION

Prior to the advent of chronic hemodialysis, infection was frequently a terminal or preterminal event in patients with end-stage renal failure. During the last decade, better hemodialysis techniques coupled with general advances in medical therapy have improved the prognosis (1–3). Nevertheless, infectious complications continue to be a major medical threat to patients receiving maintenance hemodialysis (4–10). It is unquestionable that the most common type of infections are those related to the blood access device. In this chapter we will review incidence and type of infectious complications that occur in patients undergoing chronic hemodialysis. It seems important to emphasize at the beginning that most of the infections seen in patients with severe renal failure can be accounted for by commonly occurring bacteria and not by unusual or opportunistic organisms. The repetitive exposure of these patients to infectious risk factors during hemodialysis appears of major importance in determining the infectious complications observed.

HOST DEFENSE MECHANISMS IN UREMIA

A delay in the rejection of skin and renal allografts has been demonstrated in uremic patients and experimental animals with uremia (11–13). Since these initial *in vivo* observations, many *in vitro* studies have been performed in an attempt to clarify the mechanisms of these phenomena. Table 1 summarizes the results of the various tests that have been utilized to define the alterations in the immunologic responsiveness of the uremic patient.

Table 1. Immunology of uremia.

	Result
Humoral and lymphocyte function	
Allograft rejection	↓
Antibody production	Normal
Lymphocyte counts	Normal–↓
Blastogenic response	Normal–↓
Interferon production	↓
Delayed hypersensitivity	↓
Polymorphonuclear cell function	
Chemotaxis	Normal–↓
Phagocytosis	Normal
Intracellular bacterial killing	Normal
Inflammatory response	Slightly ↓
Opsonic factors	Normal

Humoral immunity

Serum immunoglobulin A, G and M levels have been reported to be normal in uremic patients despite a slight reduction in the B lymphocyte population (11, 14, 15). Most studies have shown that humoral immunity is normal in uremic patients as evidenced by their response to a variety of antigens including O antigen of S. typhosa, influenza virus A and B, diphtheria toxoid, cytomegalovirus, pertussis and poliomyelitis (16-22). Hemodialysis patients vaccinated with pneumococcal capsular polysaccharide may have reduced but protective antibody responses (23-25). Of note, however, is the demonstration that uremic children develop a reduced antibody response to live attenuated virus vaccines (22). Finally, the development of a wide variety of autoantibodies has been observed in chronic hemodialysis patients (26-30). This corroborates that chronic hemodialysis patients have adequate capabilities for immunoglobulin and antibody formation.

Lymphocyte function

A moderate lymphopenia due to a decrease in both T and B lymphocytes has been commonly encountered in uremic patients, the mechanism of which is unclear (31-34). Hemodialysis partially corrects the decreased B-cell percentages found in uremic patients (35).

The blastogenic response of uremic lymphocytes to mitogens (i.e. phytohemagglutin) and specific antigens (i.e. PPD) has generally been near normal when studied in the presence of homologous or fetal calf serum (33, 36-38). However, a decreased response is observed when these lymphocytes are studied in uremic serum, a finding that suggests the absence of intrinsic cellular defects (15, 32, 39). Although the mixed lymphocyte culture test has been observed to be depressed by uremic serum, this seems to be related both to the presence of blocking antibodies induced by prior sensitization of the patients (33, 37) and to the uremic state (40). Recent experimental data have indicated that "middle molecule" substances as well as very low density lipoproteins, both increased in chronic renal insufficiency, may suppress the mixed lymphocyte reaction (40-42). Interferon production is depressed in patients with chronic uremia prior to or after the institution of dialysis (43). This defect is apparently due to a combination of plasma and lymphocyte factors.

Delayed hypersensitivity of both dialyzed and nondialyzed uremic patients, as measured by skin reactivity to a variety of antigens, has been found to be decreased (16, 31, 33, 38, 44, 45). However, many patients who are anergic to all tested antigens have a normal *in vitro* response to them indicating that the absence of reactivity is not necessarily due to a lack of antigen sensitive lymphocytes (38, 44). Patients treated with hemodialysis therapy for more than one year have more cutaneous anergy than patients undergoing less than one year of hemodialysis (44). The mechanism for this increasing incidence of skin anergy in hemodialysis patients is unknown. In this regard, serum inhibitors of chemotaxis have been associated with cutaneous anergy (46, 47). Recent studies have demonstrated a serum chemotactic inhibitor in hemodialysis patients which appears after initiation of maintenance hemodialysis (48). This inhibitor could play a role in the increasing incidence of cutaneous anergy in chronic hemodialysis patients.

In summary, suppression of many aspects of lymphocyte function has been observed in chronic hemodialysis patients. In general, this appears to result from suppressive effects of the uremic milieu. A long list of factors capable of interfering with lymphocyte function has emerged and includes nutritional status (49), toxic metabolites and serum chemical changes of uremia (33, 40), plasma cyclic AMP levels (50), thymosin deficiency (34), a reversible vitamin B6 coenzyme deficiency (51), and a variety of circulating cytotoxic antibodies (30). It is no wonder that hemodialysis itself is unable to correct completely all lymphocyte abnormalities observed in chronic uremic patients.

Polymorphonuclear cell functions

The inflammatory responsiveness of uremic patients not treated by hemodialysis has been studied utilizing the Rebuck skin window technique (29). The only abnormality demonstrated was a delay in the appearance and number of lymphocytes and macrophages at the site of the injury. A similar decrease in the inflammatory cell response has been noted following the injection of microcrystalline monosodium urate either intradermally or subcutaneously (53). In contrast, chronic hemodialysis patients have a normal inflammatory cell response when studied by the Rebuck skin window technique (54).

In vitro granulocyte locomotion is depressed in patients with renal failure, whether or not hemodialyzed (55-58). In some hemodialysis patients an intrinsic neutrophil chemotactic defect has also been observed (56). In addition, a serum chemotactic inhibitory factor against the C5 chemotactic fragment has been described in many maintenance hemodialysis patients (48). This factor was detected in patients serum only after three months of hemodialysis and probably resulted from the hemodialysis procedure itself. In this regard, hemodialysis membrane-granulocyte interactions which result in transient neutropenia are known to occur during the first hours of hemodialysis (59). Recent studies have suggested that activation of the alternative pathway of complement by hemodialysis membranes can generate C5 fragments (C5a) which can lead to granulocyte aggregation and granulocyte endothelial interactions. It is conceivable that this serum chemotactic inhibitor might play a protective role to modify C5a mediated leukocyte aggregation.

Most studies have shown that neutrophils from patients with chronic renal failure, conservatively managed or treated with maintenance hemodialysis, have normal *in vitro* phagocytosis and bactericidal activity in the presence of normal or uremic serum (60-62). In one study an initially depressed phagocytic function was correlated with elevated serum phosphate levels and subsequently corrected with reduction of serum phosphate concentrations to normal (63). In non-uremic and uremic patients with hyperparathyroidism abnormalities of neutrophil function have also been observed (64, 65).

However, no definite correlation between the measurement of any of the above mentioned *in vitro* abnormalities of granulocyte function, and the incidence of infection has been determined (48).

Mononuclear phagocytic system function

The mononuclear phagocytic system (MPS) includes resident macrophage cells in the liver and spleen. These cells are responsible for removal of a wide variety of substances from the blood including immune complexes and bacteria. These clearance functions are, in part, mediated by specific macrophage surface receptors for either the Fc fragment of immunoglobulin G or the C3b fragment of complement. The latter receptor appears important in the removal of certain bacteria and requires the presence of an intact complement system. No assessments of these important components of MPS function have been performed in patients with chronic uremia. However, clearance of microaggregated albumin by the liver, which does not depend on either of these surface receptors, appears unimpaired in chronic hemodialysis patients (66).

Using the Rebuck window technique a delay in mononuclear cell appearance and reduced phagocytosis of carbon particles has been observed in chronic uremic patients (67). These abnormalities reverted to normal after institution of hemodialysis therapy (67). However, despite this normalization, there remains a diminished mononuclear cell response to specific antigens such as dinitrochlorobenzene (54). The role that this reduced response to antigens may play in cutaneous anergy has not been explored.

In vitro studies have demonstrated that mononuclear cells obtained from chronic hemodialysis patients have normal locomotion and normal or slightly depressed phagocytic function (68, 69). However, uremic plasma contains a substance that suppresses these functions when tested with mononuclear cells from normal patients (70).

In summary, the overall conclusion reached in a wide variety of studies suggests that uremic patients do not have a specific deficiency that should markedly alter their capacity to cope with infections. To date, the main exception seems to be the relationship between a depressed interferon production and the high incidence of chronic hepatitis (71, 72) in patients undergoing hemodialysis and possibly, the frequent incidence of cytomegalovirus infection observed after renal transplantation (73). The recent speculation that malignancies may be found with a higher frequency in chronic uremic patients might also reflect an impairment in host defense mechanisms (74-78). Nonetheless, while there is a general clinical impression that uremic patients have an inherent increased susceptibility to infection, or a deficiency in their ability to recover from them, this has been difficult to document from the literature and in our own experience.

RESPONSE OF THE CHRONIC HEMODIALYSIS PATIENT TO INFECTION

Infection is usually associated with a two to three fold increase in basal metabolic energy requirements. In patients undergoing chronic hemodialysis who, at the same time, may have a marginal nutritional status, the increased metabolic demand created by an acute infectious process may have profound effects. Current indices of dialysis adequacy, such as serum creatinine and blood urea nitrogen concentrations, may not be reliable indicators of a hypercatabolic state in patients with concomitant nutritional deficiencies. The frequent onset of pericarditis after infection (79) or surgery (80) suggests that the routine dialytic regimen may be inadequate during these hypercatabolic episodes.

An increased incidence of infection has been observed in patients with protein-calorie malnutrition (Kwashiorkor syndrome) (81-83). Some chronic hemodialysis patients have evidence for chronic protein-calorie malnutrition (84) as well as deficiencies of a variety of co-factors which may impair host defense mechanisms. However, the role of the nutritional status of maintenance hemodialysis patients in their response to an infectious process has not been clearly defined. Inadequate caloric intake, accentuated by illness, and defects in intestinal absorption of amino acids together with dialyzer loss may all contribute to a relative protein-calorie deficiency (85-87 [see also chapter 27]). The recent development of parenteral hyperalimentation appears to be an important adjunctive therapy for patients with increased metabolic demands and its use may be considered early for severely ill chronic dialysis patients (88-91). In chronic dialysis patients with an infection, the febrile response as well as the polymorphonuclear leukocytosis appeared appropriate.

Infection itself may have a profound effect upon the dialysis procedure. In patients with severe infection, hypotension may develop during hemodialysis necessitating the use of plasma expanders or vasopressors. Finally, endotoxemia in the absence of clinical infection may also precipitate fever and hypotension in patients undergoing chronic hemodialysis (92-94).

PATIENT POPULATION

In order to achieve a comprehensive but brief overview of infections seen in patients with chronic uremia, treated by hemodialysis, we have divided these infections and their consequences into arbitrary but descriptive classifications. As a basis of comparison we have used our experience obtained from a retrospective analysis of the infectious complications seen in 445 patients during a 42 month period (8). Included in our study were only those patients who were accepted for chronic hemodialysis and received this therapy for a minimum of one month (8).

Mortality

Infection has been a leading cause of death in patients receiving regular dialysis treatment. Between 14% and 38% of all patient deaths have been attributed to this complication (4-10, 95). In our patient population during a 42 month period 111 of 445 (24.9%) died. In 22 patients (19.8%) infection was the primary cause of

Table 2. Association between primary site of infection and death.

	Pulmonary	Blood access device	Intra-abdominal	Urinary tract	Meningitis	Endo-carditis	Unknown
Source of infection causing death (22 patients)	5	5	5	4	2	1*	—
Source of infection contributing to death (14 patients)	8	2	1	2	—	—	1
Totals	13	7	6	6	2	1	1

* Two additional patients with endocarditis died. These patients had a simultaneous blood access device infection and are included in that category.

death. In an additional 14 patients (12.6%) infection was considered to be a contributory but not the primary factor in the demise of the patient. Infection either as a primary or as a contributory factor was responsible for 4.4 deaths/1000 treatment months. Deaths related to infection were more common in diabetic patients: 6.6 deaths/1000 treatment months, as compared to non-diabetic patients 4.2 deaths/1000 treatment months, (p<0.005). In addition, non-diabetic patients over 60 years of age also had a higher incidence of deaths related to infection than their younger counterparts (7.8 deaths vs. 1.4 deaths/1000 treatment months, p<0.005). However, this increased incidence of deaths in diabetic as well as older patients did not appear to be related to an enhanced susceptibility to die from a given infectious process but rather to the increased number of infections that occurred in both of these groups.

The sources of infection either causing or contributing to our patients demise are listed in Table 2. Blood access device and respiratory infections were the two most common sources. Bacteremia was detected in half of the patients whose primary cause of death was infection. The mean length of time that patients received hemodialysis treatment prior to their demise was 25 months (range 1 to 113 months). Over 60% of these patients were older than 60 years of age, reflecting the increasing number of elderly patients receiving hemodialysis treatment.

Bacteremia in hemodialysis patients

Despite considerable dialysis technological advances and the more frequent use of subcutaneous access devices, bacteremia continues to be a major problem in chronic hemodialysis patients. Indeed bacteremia has been reported in 10 to 20% of hemodialysis patients, a frequency not different from that reported 15 to 20 years ago (8–10). In our study, bacteremia was defined by one or more positive blood culture reports for bacteria which correlated with the clinical findings in the patient's records consistent with infection due to those organisms. Since bacteremia is a common complication in chronic hemodialysis patients, the importance of obtaining blood cultures during a febrile episode cannot be over emphasized.

Incidence

In our experience, bacteremia was documented 124 times in 91 patients (20.4%), an incidence of 15.3 episodes/1000 treatment months (8). Twelve patients had two bacteremic episodes and six patients had three or more episodes. The presenting symptoms observed in patients with bacteremia were not different than those in non-hemodialyzed patients and included fever, chills, leukocytosis and malaise. No relationship between etiology of renal disease and incidence of bacteremia could be defined except when patients were divided into two broad groups, diabetic and non-diabetic. There were 32.1 bacteremic episodes/1000 treatment months in the diabetic patients as compared to 13.2 episodes in the non-diabetic (p<0.01). A similar incidence of bacteremia (12.5 episodes/1000 treatment months) in chronic hemodialysis patients has also been recently reported by others (9).

Infecting organisms

Gram positive organisms continue to be the most common organism isolated from bacteremic episodes in he-

Table 3. Relationship between the bacteriology and site of infection in 124 bacteremic episodes.

	Access related bacteremia	Bacteremia source unknown	Bacteremia source other than access
Number of episodes	69 (55.7%)	20 (16.1%)	35 (28.2%)
Gram positive organisms	55	18	17
Staphylococcus aureus	32	4	1
Staphylococcus epidermidis	20	7	3
Streptococcus species	3	4	4
Diphtheroids	—	3	—
Bacillus species	—	—	3
Streptococcus pneumoniae	—	—	5
Clostridium perfringens	—	—	1
Gram negative organisms	14	2	18
Serratia marcescens	4	2	—
Pseudomonas aeruginosa	1	—	—
Escherichia coli	4	—	12
Klebsiella-Enterobacter	3	—	3
Proteus species	1	—	1
Achromobacter species	1	—	—
Listeria monocytogenes	—	—	2

modialysis patients (8–10, 96, 97). In our study, gram positive organisms were isolated in 72.6% of the bacteremic episodes while gram negative organisms were isolated in 27.4% (8). The single most common gram positive organism was *S. aureus* (Table 3). A similar preponderance of *S. aureus* has been observed in other studies of infection in chronic hemodialysis patients (9, 10, 96, 97).

Mortality
Sepsis continues to account for a 15 to 20% mortality in chronic dialysis patients (9, 10). In our study, 19 of 91 patients (20.9%) with bacteremia died, a frequency similar to that observed in nondialyzed patients in a large general hospital (98).

Bacteremia secondary to access infection
Despite the increased use of subcutaneous blood access device, vascular access continues to be the primary site of infection in over half of the bacteremic episodes (9, 10, 96, 97). In our experience, 56% of bacteremic episodes were secondary to an access infection and occurred in 60 patients, an incidence of 8.5 episodes/1000 treatment months. The incidence of bacteremia associated with access infection in diabetic patients was twice that seen in non-diabetic patients. Cannulas accounted for approximately 75% of the access related bacteremias. The remaining 25% were observed in patients with simple arterio-venous fistulas or bovine carotid arterio-venous fistulas. Mortality in confirmed access related bacteremia is approximately 10% in our study (8) and others (9, 10).

Bacteremia source unknown
In our experience, in 16% of bacteremic episodes clinical examination and cultures obtained from the blood access device failed to identify a local infection as the source of bacteremia. Most of these patients had either simple or bovine carotid arterio-venous fistulas, and the possibility that a small focus of infection was present cannot be excluded. The similarity in the bacteriology and clinical response of this group of patients to those with bacteremia related to access infections, suggest that the source was the blood access device in the majority patients. In addition, recent reports of gram negative bacteremias related to dialysis equipment and water supplies should alert us towards this etiology in patients without an obvious source of infection (99, 100).

Bacteremia associated with a source of infection other than blood access device
This group in our study represented 28% of all documented bacteremias, an incidence of 4.4 episodes/1000 treatment months (9). It should be noted that in none of these patients was previous renal transplantation contributory to these episodes. The gastrointestinal tract was the most frequent source accounting for 34% of these episodes, while the pulmonary and genitourinary systems were each considered the site of infection in 20% of them. In five of seven infections in which the urinary tract was considered the source of bacteremia, polycystic kidneys was the primary disease. The site of infection in the remaining 25% was varied.

Mortality in this group of patients was higher than we observed in access related bacteremia (8). Thirteen of the 27 patients (48%) died from their infection. The vast majority of these patients (77%) were older than 60 years. However, in elderly non-dialyzed patients, bacteremia is also associated with a high mortality (98). This would suggest that in our patients, the uremic state, per se, did not play an important role in the fatal outcome.

Bacteriology (Table 3)
In our study, 80% of isolates in access related bacteremic episodes were gram positive organisms. In patients in whom no definite access infection could be documented, but was suspected to be the source, gram positive organisms accounted for 90% of isolates and gram negative organism for 10%. It is unquestionable that *S. aureus* continues to be the most prevalent organism isolated in access related infections in our study and in others (–10). Recent epidemiologic data demonstrated that chronic hemodialysis patients have a threefold greater carriage rate of *S. aureus* than patients with chronic renal insufficiency not undergoing hemodialysis (101). In addition, a higher carriage rate of *S. aureus* has been observed in hemodialysis personnel and suggests that hemodialysis staff may represent the reservoir for *S. aureus* colonization (101).

In contrast to the two preceeding groups, in bacteremic episodes definitively unrelated to the blood access device, 57% of our isolates were gram negative organisms. *E. coli* was the most frequent gram negative organism isolated, and *S. pneumoniae* the most frequent gram positive organism (8).

Treatment of bacteremic episodes
Selection of antibiotics is dependent upon culture and sensitivity data. It is important to initiate prompt and appropriate antimicrobial therapy since delays in therapy may increase the risk of metastatic infections. Since *S. aureus* is the most frequent organism isolated, initiation of empiric antibiotic therapy should include an agent effective against this organism. The precise length of antibiotic therapy as well as the regimen most effective is difficult to determine. Usually in uncomplicated bacteremias clinical response with defervescence will occur within 48 to 96 hours. Treatment of uncomplicated bacteremias usually respond to approximately 14 to 21 days of antibiotic administration (102). In contrast, patients with evidence of endocarditis or metastatic infection usually require a minimum of 4 to 6 weeks of therapy.

The dosage of many antibiotics are modified by the uremic state (103) [see also chapter 39]). Dose adjustment in renal failure is dependent on the major pathway of elimination, the volume of distribution, plasma or biologic half-life and the extent of drug binding to plasma proteins (104). Drugs which are predominently excreted by the kidneys are profoundly influenced by reduced renal function and modifications of the dosing schedules are mandatory (104). In this regard, the availability of serum drug levels, particularly for the aminoglycoside antibiotics has improved the accuracy of dosing these agents and has reduced the frequency of severe toxic reactions.

Other major infectious complications

Included in this group are: septic pulmonary emboli, bacterial endocarditis, osteomyelitis, septic arthritis and polymicrobial bacteremia. In our experience, 45 episodes of these infectious complications were documented in 39 of 445 patients (8.8%) that received regular hemodialysis treatment.

Septic pulmonary emboli
In dialysis patients with chronic indwelling cannulas or subcutaneous fistulas subjected to repetitive needle puncture, the development of an infected thrombophlebitis or endarteritis associated with septic pulmonary emboli should not be unexpected. However, given the frequency of blood access device infections, this is clinically a rather uncommon complication. Previous reports, however, have emphasized that septic pulmonary emboli may develop even in the absence of obvious access infection (9, 105–107). The diagnosis of septic pulmonary emboli should be considered when fever, cough and pleuritic chest pain develop during the dialysis treatment. While antibiotic therapy has been successful even without removal of the blood access device (9, 106), our usual approach has been to remove it immediately while treating the systemic infection with appropriate antimicrobial therapy. Utilizing a combination of radiographic findings, pulmonary scintillation studies, suggestive clinical symptoms and positive blood cultures, an episode of septic pulmonary emboli was documented in seven of our patients (8). This represented an incidence of 0.7 episodes/1000 treatment months. In all episodes evidence for an associated infection of the blood access device was present, five of them were in cannulas and two in bovine carotid fistulas. *S. aureus* and *S. epidermidis* were the infecting organisms in three and two episodes, respectively, while *S. marcescens* and *E. coli* were the responsible organisms in each of the remaining two episodes. The combination of systemic antimicrobial therapy and removal of the access device was therapeutically successful in all patients for no deaths occurred in this group.

Bacterial endocarditis
Bacterial endocarditis in regularly dialyzed patients has been the subject of recent studies (108–113). Thirty-six episodes of endocarditis have been extensively reported in 35 patients treated by regular dialysis. *S. aureus* was the most frequently isolated organism and the cannula the commonest source of infection. The aortic valve was usually involved and eight patients underwent successful valve replacement. The outcome for this cumulative group could be determined in only 31 of the episodes and revealed a mortality of 55%. In our survey, there were nine episodes of endocarditis that occurred in nine patients, an incidence of 1.2 episodes/1000 treatment months. In five of nine episodes (56%), endocarditis was related to infection of the blood access device. *S. aureus* was the infecting organism in six of the cases (67%), *Listeria monocytogenes* in two and *Enterococci* in one. The aortic valve was involved in eight of the nine patients while mitral valvular involvement could only be documented in one patient. In six of nine patients antimicrobial therapy was effective and no recurrences have been observed. Three patients died as a consequence of an acute cerebral embolic event. *S. aureus* was the infecting organism in two of them and *Listeria* in one. In two patients prosthetic aortic valve replacement was also necessary because of the intractable cardiac failure. Both patients have done well without evidence of prosthetic valve endocarditis.

Osteomyelitis and septic arthritis
In 11 patients, we observed eight episodes of osteomyelitis and six episodes of septic arthritis, an overall incidence of 1.7 episodes/1000 treatment months (8). These complications were observed in the diabetic patients with an eight-fold higher incidence than in their nondiabetic counterparts (7.8 vs 1.0 episode/1000 treatment months, $p<0.01$). The blood access device was the origin of infection in eight cases (57.1%). *S. aureus* was isolated in 10 episodes, *S. epidermidis* in three and *S. marcescens* in two and *C. perfringens*, *Klebsiella enterobacter* group and *E. coli* were recovered each in one episode. In some patients with osteomyelitis, more than one organism was isolated from the culture of the bony lesion.

The diagnosis of osteomylitis still presents considerable difficulties. Nonspecific symptoms such as low grade fever, malaise and weight loss may dominate the clinical picture. The frequent lack of roentgenographic changes often delays correct diagnosis. In our previous reported experience, osteomyelitis was more common in vertebrae and ribs (114). In our current experience, the distal upper and lower extremities were the most frequent sites of infection (8). Therapeutically, long term antibiotics combined with early debridement of the osteomyelitic lesion was usually successful. However, in the diabetic patients, amputation of the affected limb was frequently necessary. All patients with osteomyelitis survived without development of chronic osteomyelitis.

In patients with septic arthritis the wrist, knee and shoulder were the commonest joints involved and *S. aureus* was the most frequent infecting organism. All patients responded to systemic antimicrobial therapy, and there have been no late sequelae.

Polymicrobial bacteremia
Polymicrobial bacteremia has been usually associated with malignancies or primary gastrointestinal diseases (115–117). Recent surveys have reported two or more bacteria responsible for 8.3% of bacteremic episodes in chronic hemodialysis patients (10). In 12% of our patients with bacteremia two or more microorganisms were isolated from the same blood sample (8). Fifteen episodes occurred in 12 patients, an incidence of 1.9/1000 treatment months. The site of infection and the

Table 4. Organisms and source of infection during polymicrobial bacteremia.

Recovered organisms	Source of infection	No. of times organisms isolated
S. aureus, α-Streptococcus	Blood access device	2
S. aureus, Diphtheroids	Blood access device	1
S. aureus, P. mirabilis	Blood access device	1
S. epidermidis, B. subtilis	Gastrointestinal	2
	Other sources	2
Enterococci, B. fragilis	Gastrointestinal	1
E. coli, S. pneumoniae	Pulmonary	1
E. coli, Fusobacterium	Gastrointestinal	1
E. coli, Bacteroides	Urinary tract	1
E. coli, Klebsiella-Enterobacter	Blood access device	1
E. coli, S. marcesens	Osteomyelitis	1
P. aeruginosa, Alcaligenes species	Gastrointestinal	1
Total		15

organisms isolated from the blood are listed in Table 4. Clinically no distinctive features aroused suspicion that a given infectious episode was caused by more than one type of bacteria. In two patients, recurrent episodes of polymicrobial bacteremia were documented, one patient with hepatic cirrhosis and inferior vena cava thrombosis had three episodes, and one patient with diabetes mellitus had two episodes. Mortality after polymicrobial bacteremia has been reported to be higher than that observed in single organism bacteremias, ranging from 35% to 70% (115–117). Three of our 12 patients (25%) with this complication died, a frequency only slightly higher than the mortality observed in single organism bacteremias.

Access infections

Infection and thrombosis continue to be major problems in the management of the arterio-venous shunts. The close association between these two events frequently makes it difficult to determine cause and effect. Local infection may precipitate episodes of clotting (118–121) which in turn may increase the risk of infection, sepsis and septic pulmonary emboli. Since the introduction of the simple subcutaneous arterio-venous fistulas (122) and the bovine carotid fistulas (123), the incidence of infection of the blood access device has been reduced considerably (124–140) but they continue to be the primary cause of staphylococcal bacteremia (8–10). However, cannulas continue to be used and remain a cause of major infectious complications in patients receiving chronic dialysis therapy (8, 141).

The usage of long term prophylactic antibiotics to reduce the frequency of access infection is controversial (142, 143). Since there is a wide spectrum of organisms that may cause access infection, it is improbable that one antibiotic will be effective against all organisms. In addition, the possibility of induction of resistant strains must be considered. Prophylactic vancomycin was used in one uncontrolled study of 25 patients (144).

S. aureus access infection was eliminated but there was an increase in infections caused by organisms from the *Klebsiella-Enterobacter* group. It may be reasonable to utilize antibiotics briefly prophylactically during manipulative procedures of the arterio-venous shunts, particularly following difficult declotting. In addition, short term antibiotic prophylaxis may be of value during procedures that are associated with transient bacteremias.

Infection of the blood access device as defined by presence of a local inflammatory reaction and positive culture obtained from the suppurative area accounted for 71% of all infectious complications seen in our hemodialysis patients, an incidence of 75.1 episodes/1000 treatment months (8). It should be emphasized that arteriovenous fistulas may in fact be the etiologic site of the bacteremia without evidence of definite local inflammatory changes (8–10). There was no significant difference in the incidence of access infections in the diabetic or non-diabetic patients (8). Hospitalization was considered necessary because of the severity of the infection in 19.3% of our patients. Bacteremia was detected in 64.5% of these patients and has been discussed in the section dealing with access related bacteremia. In those patients hospitalized, systemic antibiotics were usually administered. In addition, the access device was promptly removed in nearly 60% of these episodes. This high rate of access removal because of infection was predominantly the result of the frequent use of the Scribner shunt for blood access in our center during the early 1970s. We, as in other hemodialysis units, currently use primarily subcutaneous fistulas for blood access. In these situations, systemic antibiotics are usually effective in eradicating signs of infection. At times, surgical intervention for drainage of abscess, hematomas or resection of an aneurysmal dilation may be necessary. However routine ligation of a vascular access device that was likely a source of bacteremia does not appear warranted. Access devices infected with gram negative organism are usually resistant to antibiotic therapy and in our experience nearly 80% of accesses were removed. The bacteriology of access infections is listed in Table 5.

Table 5. Bacteriology of blood access device infections.

	Out patients	Hospitalized patients
Gram positive organisms	395 (83.5%)	85 (75.2%)
Staphylococcus epidermidis	166 (35.1%)	29 (25.7%)
Staphylococcus aureus	140 (29.7%)	51 (45.1%)
Streptococcus species	41 (8.6%)	5 (4.4%)
Diphtheroids	46 (9.8%)	—
Bacillus species	2 (0.4%)	—
Gram negative organisms	78 (16.5%)	28 (24.8%)
Klebsiella-enterobacter	33 (7.0%)	3 (2.7%)
Escherichia coli	17 (3.6%)	6 (5.3%)
Pseudomonas aeurginosa	17 (3.6%)	3 (2.7%)
Serratia marcescens	—	8 (7.0%)
Proteus species	4 (0.8%)	1 (0.9%)
Archromobacter species	2 (0.4%)	1 (0.9%)
Unspecified	5 (1.1%)	6 (5.3%)

Table 6. Summary of blood access device experience during 42 months.

Type of access	Number inserted (%)	Months of access utilization [a]	Mean access survival time (months)	Number of episodes of infections	Number of infections/ month of access utilization [b]
Cannula	397 (54.5)	3105	7.8	464	0.15
Simple fistula	180 (24.7)	2423	13.5	52	0.02
Bovine carotid fistula	128 (17.6)	2044	16.0	68	0.03
Other [b]	23 (3.2)	478	NA	2	NA
Totals	728	8050	–	586	–

[a] This represents actual number of months the access device was utilized for hemodialysis.
[b] This group includes saphenous vein fistulas, Sparks-mandril fistulas and other access devices not regularly used in the authors' center.

It is remarkable, that despite the current use of arteriovenous fistulas in chronic hemodialysis patients gram positive organisms, are still responsible for 70 to 80% of the bacterial isolates (8–10). In our past experience, the cannula system was the most frequent access utilized and accounted for 79% of blood access infections (Table 6). The cannula system was five and seven times more commonly infected than either the bovine carotid or simple fistulas, respectively. The lowest frequency of infection was seen in the simple fistulas, the second most commonly used access device. Patients with bovine carotid fistulas had a slightly higher incidence of infections than those with a simple fistula. This trend also has been reported in other studies (9, 135). Expanded polytetrafluoroethylene arterio-venous grafts have recently been introduced for blood access devices with moderate success (135–140). However as with the bovine carotid arterio-venous fistulas, infection appears to occur at a slightly higher rate than in simple fistulas (140).

Systemic infections

Respiratory infections
In our experience, there were 40 episodes of respiratory infections in 35 patients, an incidence of 5.7 episodes/1000 treatment months (8). S. pneumoniae was isolated in 50% of the patients admitted with a primary pneumonia in contrast to the frequent isolation of gram negative organisms in patients who developed pneumonia while in hospital. There was no difference in the frequency of this infection between diabetic and non-diabetic patients. Death occurred in 12% of patients admitted with pneumonia while 57% of those patients with a pneumonia acquired in the hospital eventually died (8). Chronic obstructive pulmonary disease and cardiac decompensation were commonly associated conditions in patients with respiratory infections. Few data are available regarding host defense mechanisms of the lung in hemodialysis patients (59). However, the altered nasopharyngeal flora seen in chronically ill and hospitalized patients (145), and the pathologic changes that occur in lungs of patients with uremia could all have a permissive role in pulmonary infections in chronic dialysis patients (146, 147).

Urinary tract infections
Bacteriuria has been reported to occur in 57.5% of chronic hemodialysis patients (148). However, the significance of this bacteriuria in these patients, who have minimal urinary outputs, is unknown. We documented 19 episodes of symptomatic urinary tract infections in 16 patients, an incidence of 2.3 episodes/1000 treatment months (8). Polycystic kidney disease was the underlying diagnosis in eight of these patients (50%). In five of them the clinical course was complicated by development of a perinephric abscess, refractory to systemic antibiotic therapy and necessitating surgical nephrectomy (8, 149). Three of these patients died post-operatively.

Unusual infections
During our 42 month survey only one patient became infected with a fungal organism (8). It was a patient with active Wegener's granulomatosis, receiving cyclophosphamide, who developed cryptococcal meningitis and subsequently died. Fungal infection of arteriovenous fistulas has been recently reported (150).

Tuberculosis in chronic dialysis patients has been observed to occur with a 10 fold greater incidence than in comparable non-uremic patients and has been reported to account for nearly 1% of mortality in chronic hemodialysis patients (151–156). Indeed, the insidious onset as well as the lack of diagnostic laboratory studies and clinical findings have frequently obscured the diagnosis. The unusual pulmonary presentation, frequent extrapulmonary involvement and isolation of atypical mycobacteria have characterized the course of the disease in chronic hemodialysis patients (151–156). However, prompt recognition and initiation of antituberculosis therapy appears to effectively erradicate this infection. Despite this apparent increased occurrence of tuberculosis, we have not observed a higher than expected incidence in our dialysis patients.

The increased frequency of infections with herpes virus in recipients of renal allografts is well known (20, 157–160). Higher than expected prevalence of cytomegalovirus or herpes virus has not been observed in chronic hemodialysis patients (20, 161, 162). However, transplanted kidneys from donors who have detectable circulating antibodies against herpes virus may serve as the source of these viral infections in recipients who do not have detectable viral antibody titers (163). Transmission of cytomegalovirus with a renal allograft has also been described (164).

Infections in patients with uremia secondary to rejection of a renal allograft

In patients undergoing rejection of a renal allograft it is difficult to define if uremia and hemodialysis have an additive role in increasing their susceptibility to infections. However, leukopenia and alterations in cellular and humoral immunity secondary to the high doses of immunosuppressive therapy used during acute rejection episodes seem important in increasing the risk to severe bacterial or opportunistic infections (165–169).

In contrast to chronic hemodialysis patients, gram negative bacteria are more frequently isolated from patients receiving "anti-rejection therapy". Urinary and pulmonary sources are the most common sites of infections (166, 167, 169). Viral and fungal infection are also responsible for the high morbidity and mortality seen in this selected group of patients (73, 168, 170). It should be underscored that the blood access device may serve as an important primary source of bacteremia in transplanted patients, that require hemodialysis (166). Mortality rate associated with serious infections in this group of patients has been approximately 35% (165, 169).

SUMMARY

Infection in patients with end-stage renal failure receiving maintenance hemodialysis therapy is a common cause of morbidity and mortality. The frequent, repetitive exposure of hemodialysis patients to potential infectious risk factors during the normal course of treatment is a unique medical situation. In fact, it is remarkable that serious infections do not occur more frequently. The blood access devices, particularly the cannulas, were (before the introduction of the AV fistula) major sources of infections in these patients. Enhanced susceptibility secondary to alterations in immune response induced by the uremic state per se seem to play a relatively minor role in determining type, incidence and outcome of these infectious complications. Although in our survey diabetic patients had an increased incidence of serious infections, we were unable to define any specific reason(s) for this observation, other than diabetes. However, severe peripheral vascular disease in these patients contributes to recurrent access problems, and may partially explain the higher frequency of serious access infections.

REFERENCES

1. Gross JB, Keane WF, McDonald AK: Survival and rehabilitation of patients on home hemodialysis. *Ann Intern Med* 78:341, 1973
2. Burton BT, Krueger KK, Bryan FA Jr: National registry of long-term dialysis patients. *JAMA* 218:718, 1971
3. Lewis EJ, Foster DM, de la Puente J, Scurlock C: Survival data for patients undergoing chronic intermittent hemodialysis. *Ann Intern Med* 70:311, 1969
4. Montgomerie JZ, Kalmanson GM, Guze LB: Renal failure and infection. *Medicine* 47:1, 1968
5. Blagg CR, Hickman RO, Eschbach JW, Scribner BH: Home hemodialysis: Six years experience. *N Engl J Med* 283:1126, 1970
6. Gurland HJ, Brunner FP, v Dehn H, Härlen H, Parsons FM, Schärer K: Combined report on regular dialysis and transplantation in Europe III, 1972. *Proc Eur Dial Transpl Assoc* 10:XVII, 1973
7. Lowrie EG, Lazarus JM, Mogelin AJ, Baily FL, Hampers CL, Wilson RE, Merrill JP: Survival of patients undergoing chronic hemodialysis and renal transplantation. *N Engl J Med* 288:863, 1973
8. Keane WF, Shapiro FL, Raij L: Incidence and type of infections occurring in 445 chronic hemodialysis patients. *Trans Am Soc Artif Intern Organ* 23:41, 1977
9. Dobkin JE, Miller MH, Steighigel NH: Septicemia in patients on chronic hemodialysis. *Ann Intern Med* 88:28, 1978
10. Nsouli KA, Lazarus JM, Schoenbaum SC, Gottlieb MN, Lowrie EG, Shocair M: Bacteremic infection in hemodialysis. *Arch Intern Med* 139:1255, 1979
11. Dammin GJ, Couch NP, Murray JE: Prolonged survival of skin homografts in uremia patients. *Ann NY Acad Sci* 64:967, 1957
12. Mannick JA, Powers JH, Mithoefer J, Ferrebee JW: Renal transplantation in azotemic dogs. *Surgery* 47:340, 1960
13. Morrison AB, Maness K, Tawes R: Skin homograft survival in chronic renal insufficiency. *Arch Pathol* 75:139, 1963
14. Casciani CU, DeSimone C, Bonini S: Immunological aspects of chronic uremia. *Kidney Int* 13 (Suppl 8):S49, 1978
15. Hosking CS, Atkins RC, Scott DR, Holdsworth SR, Fitzgerald MG, Shelton MJ: Immune and phagocytic functions in patients on maintenance hemodialysis and posttransplantation. *Clin Nephrol* 6:501, 1976
16. Wilson WEC, Kirkpatrick CH, Talmage DW: Suppression of immunologic responsiveness in uremia. *Ann Intern Med* 61:1, 1965
17. Jordan MC, Rousseau WE, Tegtmeier GE, Noble GR, Muth RG, Chin TDY: Immunogenicity of inactivated influenza virus vaccine in chronic renal failure. *Ann Intern Med* 79:790, 1973
18. Stoloff IL, Stout R, Myerson RM, Havens WP Jr: Production of antibody in patients with uremia. *N Engl J Med* 259:320, 1958
19. Spencer ES: Cytomegalovirus antibody in uremic patients prior to renal transplantation. *Scand J Infect Dis* 6:1, 1954
20. Naroqi S, Jackson GG, Jonasson O, Yamashiroya HM: Prospective study of prevalence, incidence and source of herpesvirus infections in patients with renal allografts. *J Infect Dis* 136:531, 1977
21. Osanloo EO, Berlin BS, Popli S, Ing TS, Cummings JE, Gandhi VC, Geis WP, Hano JE: Antibody response to influenza vaccination in patients with chronic renal failure. *Kidney Int* 14:614, 1978
22. Kleinknecht C, Margolis A, Bonnissol C, Gaiffe M, Sahyoun S, Broyer M: Serum antibodies before and after immunization in haemodialysed children. *Proc Eur Dial Transpl Assoc* 14:209, 1977
23. Friedman EA, Beyer MM, Hirsch SR, Schiffman G: Intact antibody response to pneumococcal capsular polysac-

charides in uremia and diabetes. *JAMA* 244:2310, 1980
24. Simberkoff MS, Schiffman G, Katz L, Spicehandler J, Moldover NH, Rahal JJ: Diminished radioimmunoassay antibody responses and opsonic titers in chronic hemodialysis patients. *Proc 11th Int Congr Chemotherapy and 19th Interscience Conf on Antimicrobial Agents and Chemotherapy.* Volume II, edited by Nelson JD and Gassi C, Washington, D.C., Am Soc Microbiol 1980, p 851
25. Dailey MP, Schiffman G, Piering WF, Hoffman RG, Rytel MW: Response of renal allograft recipents and dialysis patients to pneumococcal vaccine. *Proc 11th Int Congr Chemotherapy and 19th Interscience Conf on Antimicrobial Agents and Chemotherapy.* Volume II, edited by Nelson JD and Gassi C, Washington, DC, Am Soc Microbiol 1980, p 854
26. Crosson JT, Moulds J, Comty CM, Polesky HF: A clinical study of anti-N_{DP} in the sera of patients in a large repetitive hemodialysis program. *Kidney Int* 10:463, 1976
27. Kaehny WD, Miller GE, White WL: Relationship between dialyzer reuse and the presence of anti-N-like antibodies in chronic hemodialysis patients. *Kidney Int* 12:59, 1977
28. Howell ED, Perkins HA: Anti-N-like antibodies in the sera of patients undergoing chronic hemodialysis. *Vox Sang* 23:291, 1972
29. Nolph KD, Husted FC, Sharp GC, Siemsen AW: Antibodies to nuclear antigens in patients undergoing long-term hemodialysis. *Am J Med* 60:673, 1976
30. Ting A, Morris PJ: Reactivity of autolymphocytotoxic antibodies from dialysis patients with lymphocytes from chronic lymphocytic leukemia (CLL) patients. *Transplantation* 25:31, 1978
31. Kauffman CA, Manzler AD, Phair JP: Cell-Mediated immunity in patients on long-term haemodialysis. *Clin Exp Immunol* 22:54, 1975
32. Newberry WM, Sanford JP: Defective cellular immunity in renal failure: Depression of reactivity of lymphocytes to phytohemagglutinin by renal failure serum. *J Clin Invest* 50:1262, 1971
33. Touraine Jl, Touraine F, Revillard JP, Brochier J, Traeger J: T-Lymphocytes and serum inhibitors of cell-mediated immunity in renal insufficiency. *Nephron* 14:195, 1975
34. Harris J, Sengar D, Rashid A, Hyslop D, Green L, Goldstein Al: Immunodeficiency in chronic uremia. *Transplantation* 20:176, 1975
35. Hoy WE, Cestero RVM, Freeman RB: Deficiency of T and B lymphocytes in uremic subjects and partial improvement with maintenance hemodialysis. *Nephron* 20:182, 1978
36. Hurst KS, Saldanhar LF, Steinberg SM, Galen MA, Lowrie EG, Gagneux SA, Lazarus JM, Strom TB, Carpenter CB, Merrill JP: The effects of varying dialysis regimens on lymphocyte stimulation. *Trans Am Soc Artif Intern Organs* 21:329, 1975
37. Sengar D, Rashid A, Perelmutter L, Harris JE: Lymphocytotoxins and mixed leucocyte culture blocking factor activity in the plasma of uraemic patients undergoing haemodialysis. *Clin Exp Immunol* 20:249, 1975
38. Selroos O, Pasternack A, Virolainen M: Skin test sensitivity and antigen induced lymphocyte transformation in uraemia. *Clin Exp Immunol* 14:365, 1973
39. Kasakura S, Lowenstein L: The effect of uremic blood on mixed leukocyte reactions and on cultures of leukocytes with phytohemagglutinin. *Transplantation* 5:283, 1967
40. Fehrman I, Ringden O, Bergström J: MLC-blocking factions in uremic sera. *Clin Nephrol* 14:183, 1980
41. Raskova J, Morrison AB. Humoral inhibitors of the immune response in uremia. I. Effect of serum and of the supernatant of spleen cultures from uremic rats on the mixed lymphocyte reaction. *Lab Invest* 38:103, 1978
42. Raska K, Morrison AB, Raskova J: Humoral inhibitors of the immune response in uremia. III. The immunosuppressive factor of uremic rat serum is a very low density lipoprotein. *Lab Invest* 42:636, 1980
43. Sanders CV Jr, Luby JP, Sanford JP, Hull AR: Suppression of interferon responses in lymphocytes from patients with uremia. *J Lab Clin Med* 77:768, 1971
44. Sengar D, Rashid A, Harris J: In vitro cellular immunity and in vivo delayed hypersensitivity in uremic patients maintained on hemodialysis. *Int Arch Allergy Appl Immunol* 47:829, 1974
45. Bansal VK, Popli S, Pickering J, Ing TS, Hans JE: Protein calorie malnutrition and cutaneous anergy in hemodialysis maintained patients. *Am J Clin Nutr* 33:1608, 1980
46. Van Epps DE, Palmer DL, Williams RC: Characterization of serum inhibitors of neutrophil chemotaxis associated with anergy. *J Immunol* 113:189, 1974
47. Van Epps DE, Strickland RC, Williams RC: Inhibitors of leukocyte chemotaxis in alcoholic liver disease. *Am J Med* 59:200, 1975
48. Goldblum SE, van Epps DE, Reed WP: Serum inhibitor of C5 fragment-mediated polymorphonuclear leukocyte chemotaxis associated with chronic hemodialysis. *J Clin Invest* 64:255, 1979
49. Dreizen S: Nutrition and the immune response –a review. *Int J Vitam Nutr Res* 49:220, 1979
50. Hamet P, Stouder DA, Ginn HE, Hardman JG, Liddle GW: Studies of the elevated extracellular concentration of cyclic AMP in uremic man. *J Clin Invest* 56:339, 1975
51. Dobbelstein H, Korner WF, Mempel W, Grosse-Wilde H, Edel HH: Vitamin B_6 deficiency in uremia and its implications for the depression of immune responses. *Kidney Int* 5:223, 1974
52. Lang PA, Ritzmann SE, Merian FL, Lawrence MC, Levin WC, Gregory R: Cellular evolution in induced inflammation in uremic patients. *Tex Rep Biol Med* 24:107, 1966
53. Buchanan WW, Klinenberg JR, Seegmiller JE: The inflammatory response to injected microcrystalline monosodium urate in normal hyperuricemic, gouty and uremic subjects. *Arthritis Rheum* 8:361, 1965
54. Hanicki Z, Cichocki T, Komorowska Z, Sulowicz W, Smolenski O: Some aspects of cellular immunity in untreated and maintenance hemodialysis patients. *Nephron* 23:273, 1979
55. Baum J, Cestero RVM, Freeman RB: Chemotaxis of the polymorphonuclear leukocyte and delayed hypersensitivity in uremia. *Kidney Int* 7 (suppl 2):S147, 1975
56. Salant DJ, Glover AM, Anderson R, Meyers AM, Rabkin R, Myburgh JA, Robson AR: Depressed neutrophil chemotaxis in patients with chronic renal failure and after renal transplantation. *J Lab Clin Med* 88:536, 1976
57. Siriwatratananonta P, Sinsakul V, Stern K, Slavin RG: Defective chemotaxis in uremia. *J Lab Clin Med* 92:402, 1978
58. Greene WH, Ray C, Mauer SM, Quie PG: The effect of hemodialysis on neutrophil chemotactic responsiveness. *J Lab Clin Med* 88:971, 1976
59. Craddock PR, Fehr J, Dalmasso AP, Brigham KL, Jacob HS: Hemodialysis leukopenia: Pulmonary vascular leukostasis resulting from complement activation by dialyzer cellophane membranes. *J. Clin Invest* 59:879, 1977
60. Guckian JC, Karrh LR, Copeland JL, McCoy J: Phagocytosis by polymorphonuclear leukocytes in patients with renal faillure on chronic hemodialysis. *Tex Rep Biol Med* 29:193, 1971
61. Brogan TD: Phagocytosis by polymorphonuclear leucocytes from patients with renal failure. *Br Med J* 3:596, 1967

62. Chreitien JH, Garagusi VF: Phagocytosis and nitroblue tetrazolium reduction in uremia. *Experientia* 29:612, 1973
63. Hallgren R, Fjellstrom KE, Hokansson L, Vengi P: The serum-independent uptake of IgG-coated particles by polymorphonuclear leukocytes from uremic patients on regular dialysis treatment. *J Lab Clin Med* 94:277, 1979
64. Khan F, Khan AF, Papagaroufalis C, Marman J, Khan P, Evans HE: Reversible defect of neutrophil chemotaxis and random migration in primary hyperparathyroidism. *J Clin Endocrinol Metab* 48:582, 1979
65. Tuma SA, Martin RR, Mallette LE, Eknoyan G: Augmented polymorphonuclear chemiluminescence in patients with secondary hyperparathyroidism. *J Lab Clin Med* 97:291, 1981
66. Laknborg G, Berghim L, Ahlgren T, Groth CG, Lundgren G, Tillegard A: Reticuloendothelial function in human renal allograft recipients. *Transplantation* 28:111, 1979
67. Ringoir S, Van Looy L, Van de Heyning P, Leroux-Roels G: Impairment of phagocytic activity of macrophages as studied by the skin window test in patients on regular hemodialysis treatment. *Clin Nephrol* 4:234, 1975
68. Urbanitz D, Sieberth HG: Impaired phagocytic activity of human monocytes in respect to reduced antibacterial resistance in uremia. *Clin Nephrol* 75:13, 1975
69. Jorstad S, Viken KE: Inhibitory effects of plasma from uraemic patients on human mononuclear phagocytes cultures in vitro. *Acta Pathol Microbiol Scand* [C] 85:169, 1977
70. Jorstad S, Kvernes S: Uraemic toxins of high molecular weight inhibiting human mononuclear phagocytes cultured in vitro. *Acta Pathol Microbiol Scand* [C] 86:221, 1978
71. London WT, DiFiglia M, Sutnick AI, Blumberg BS: An epidemic of hepatitis in a chronic-hemodialysis unit. Australia antigen and differences in host response. *N Engl J Med* 281:571, 1969
72. Greenberg HB, Pollard RB, Lutwick LI, Gregory PB, Robinsin WS, Marigan TC: Human leukocyte interferon and hepatitis B virus infection. *N Engl J Med* 281:571, 1969
73. Lopez C, Simmons RL, Mauer SM, Najarian JS, Good RA: Association of renal allograft rejection with virus infections. *Am J Med* 56:280, 1974
74. Matas AJ, Simmons RL, Kjellstrand CM, Buselmeier TJ, Najarian JS: Increased incidence of malignancy during chronic renal failure. *Lancet* 1:883, 1975
75. Slifkin RF, Goldberg J, Neff MS, Baez A, Mattoo N, Gupta S: Malignancy in end-stage renal disease. *Trans Am Soc Artif Intern Organs* 23:34, 1977
76. Degaulet P. Reach I, Jacobs C: Cancer in patients on hemodialysis. *N Engl J Med* 300:1279, 1979
77. Herr HW, Engen DE, Hostetler J: Malignancy in uremia: Dialysis versus transplantation. *J Urol* 121:584, 1979
78. Hughsun MD, Hennigar GR, McManus JF: Atypical cysts, acquired renal cystic disease and renal cell tumors in end-stage dialysis kidneys. *Lab Invest* 42:475, 1980
79. Comty CM, Cohen SL, Shapiro FL: Pericarditis in chronic uremia and its sequels. *Ann Intern Med* 75:173, 1971.
80. Bailey GI, Hampers CL, Hager EB, Merrill JP: Uremic pericarditis: Clinical features and management. *Circulation* 38:582, 1968
81. Scrimshaw NS, Taylor CE, Gordon JE: Interactions of nutrition and infection. *WHO Monogr Ser* 57, 1978
82. Douglas SD, Schopfer K: Phagocyte function in protein-calorie malnutrition. *Clin Exp Immunol* 17:121, 1974
83. Schopfer K, Douglas SD: Neutrophil function in children with kwashiorkor. *J Lab Clin Med* 88:450, 1976
84. Guarnieri G, Ranieri F, Lipartiti T, Spangaro F, Giuntini D, Faccini L, Toigo G, Legnani F, Raimondi A, Campanacci L: Protein-calorie malnutrition in hemodialysis patients. *Int J Artif Organs* 3:143, 1980
85. Comty CM, Wathen RL, Shapiro FL: Protein metabolism in renal failure. *Urology* 1:528, 1973
86. Gulyassy PF, Aviram A, Peters JH: Evaluation of amino acid and protein requirements in chronic uremia. *Arch Intern Med* 126:855, 1970
87. Aviram A, Peters JH, Gulyassy PF: Dialysance of amino acid and related substances. *Nephron* 8:440, 1971
88. Dudrick SJ, MacFadyen BV, Van Buren CT, Ruberg RL, Maynard AT: Parenteral hyperalimentation: metabolic problems and solutions. *Ann Surg* 176:259, 1972
89. Dudrick SJ, Rhoads JE: Total intravenous feeding, *Sci Am* 226:73, 1972
90. Shils ME: Guidelines for total parenteral nutrition. *JAMA* 220:1721, 1972
91. Abel RM, Beck CH Jr, Abbott WM, Ryan JA Jr, Barnett GO, Fischer JE: Improved survival from acute renal failure after treatment with intravenous essential 1-amino acids and glucose. *N Engl J Med* 288:695, 1973
92. Robinson PJA, Rosen SM: Pyrexial reactions during haemodialysis. *Br Med J* 1:528, 1971
93. Raij L, Shapiro FL, Michael AF: Endotoxemia in febrile reactions during hemodialysis. *Kidney Int* 4:57, 1973
94. Hindman SH, Favero MS, Carson LA, Peterson NJ, Schonberger LB, Solano JT: Pyrogenic reactions during haemodialysis caused by extramural enodotoxin. *Lancet* 2:732, 1975
95. Siddiqui JY, Fitz AE, Lawton RL, Kirdendall WM: Causes of death in patients receiving long term hemodialysis. *JAMA* 212:1350, 1970
96. Latos DL, Stone WJ, Alford RH: Staphylococcus aureus bacteremia in hemodialysis patients. *J Dial* 1:399, 1977
97. Linnemann CC, McKee E, Laver MC: Staphylococcal infections in a hemodialysis unit. *Am J Med Sci* 276:67, 1978
98. McGowan JE, Barnes MW, Finland M: Bacteremia at the Boston City Hospital. Occurrence and mortality during 12 selected years (1935-1972), with special reference to hospital-acquired cases. *J Infect Dis* 132:316, 1975
99. Uman SJ, Johnson CE, Beirne GJ, Kunin CM: Pseudomonas aeruginosa bacteremia in a dialysis unit: I. Recognition of cases, epidemiologic studies and attempts at control. *Am J Med* 62:667, 1977
100. Kuehnel EG: Outbreak of pseudomonas cepacia bacteremia in a dialysis unit related to contaminated reused cells. *Clin Res* 23:466A, 1975
101. Kirmani N, Tuazon CU, Murray HW, Parrish AE, Sheagren JN: Staphylococcus aureus carriage rate of patients receiving long-term hemodialysis. *Arch Intern Med* 138:1657, 1978
102. Iannini PB, Crossley K: Therapy of staphylococcus aureus bacteremia associated with a removable focus of infection. *Ann Intern Med* 84:558, 1976
103. Bennett WM, Muther RS, Parker RA, Feig P, Morrison G, Golper TA, Singer I: Drug therapy in renal failure: dosing guidelines for adults. *Ann Intern Med* 93:62, 1980
104. Reidenberg MM, Drayer DE: Drug therapy in renal failure. *Annu Rev Pharmacol Toxicol* 20:45, 1980
105. Goodwin NJ, Gastronouvo JJ, Friedman EA: Recurrent septic pulmonary embolization complicating maintenance hemodialysis. *Ann Intern Med* 71:29, 1969
106. Levi J, Robson M, Rosenfeld JB: Septicaemia and pulmonary embolism complicating use of arteriovenous fistula in maintenance haemodialysis. *Lancet* 2:288, 1970
107. Shapiro FL, Messner RP, Smith HT: Satellite hemodialy-

sis. *Ann Intern Med* 69:673, 1968
108. Ribot S, Rothfeld D, Frankel HJ: Infectious endocarditis in maintenance hemodialysis. *Am J Med Sci,* 264:183, 1972
109. King LH Jr, Bradley KP, Shires DL Jr, Donohue JP, Glover JL: Bacterial endocarditis in chronic hemodialysis patients; a complication more common than previously suspected. *Surgery* 69:554, 1971
110. Ribot S, Gilbert L, Rothfeld EL, Parsonnet V, Jacobs MG: Bacterial endocarditis with pulmonary edema necessitating mitral valve replacement in a hemodialysis-dependent patient. *J Thorac Cardiovasc Surg* 62:59, 1971
111. Goodman JS, Crews HD, Ginn HE, Koenig MG: Bacterial endocarditis as a possible complication of chronic hemodialysis. *N Engl J Med* 280:876, 1969
112. Leonard A, Raij L, Shapiro FL: Infective endocarditis and access site infections in patients on hemodialysis. *Kidney Int* 4:407, 1973
113. Cross AD, Steigbigel RT: Infective endocarditis and access site infections in patients on hemodialysis. *Medicine* 55:453, 1976
114. Leonard A, Comty CM, Shapiro FL, Raij L: Osteomyelitis in hemodialysis patients. *Ann Intern Med* 78:651, 1973
115. Hochstein HD, Kirkham WR, Young VM: Recovery of more than one organism in septicemias. *N Engl J Med* 273:468, 1965.
116. Hermans PE, Washington JA: Polymicrobial bacteremia. *Ann Intern Med* 73:387, 1970
117. Bodey GP, Nies BA, Freireich EJ: Multiple organism septicemia in acute leukemia. *Arch Intern Med* 116:266, 1965
118. McIntosh CS, Petrie JC, Macleod M: Maintenance of Silastic-Teflon shunts for intermittent haemodialysis. *Br Med J* 4:717, 1969
119. Pendras JP, Smith MP: The Silastic-Teflon arterio-venous cannula. *Trans Am Soc Artif Intern Organs* 12:222, 1966
120. Haimov M: Vascular access for hemodialysis. *Surg Gynecol Obstet* 141:619, 1975
121. Kopp KF, Grossman DF, Frey J: The care and maintenance of the Scribner Teflon-Silastic shunt. Experience how to prevent infection. *Proc Eur Dial Transpl Assoc* 4:373, 1967
122. Brescia MJ, Cimino JE, Appel K, Hurwick BJ: Chronic hemodialysis, Using venipuncture and a surgically created arteriovenous fistula. *N Engl J Med* 275:1089, 1966
123. Chinitz J, Yokoyama T, Bower R, Swartz C: Self sealing prosthesis for arteriovenous fistula in man. *Trans Am Soc Artif Intern Organs* 18:452, 1972
124. Zerbino VR, Rice DA, Katz LA, Nidus BD: A six year clinical experience with arteriovenous fistulas and bypasses for hemodialysis. *Surgery* 76:1018, 1974
125. Lytton B, Goffinet JA, May CJ, Weiss RM: Experience with arteriovenous fistula in chronic hemodialysis. *J Urol* 104:512, 1967
126. Faris TD, Carey TA: Arteriovenous shunts for hemodialysis. *Am J Surg* 114:679, 1967
127. Byrne JP, Stevens LE, Weaver DH, Maxwell JG, Reemtsma K: Advantages of surgical arteriovenous fistulas for hemodialysis. *Arch Surg* 102:359, 1971
128. Ralston AJ, Harlow GR, Jones DM, Davis P: Infections of Scribner and Brescia arteriovenous shunts. *Br Med J* 3:408, 1971
129. Haimov M, Baez A, Neff M, Slifkin R: Complications of arteriovenous fistulas for hemodialysis. *Arch Surg* 110:708, 1975
130. VanderWerf BA, Rarrazzi LC, Katzman HA, Schild AF: Three year experience with bovine graft arteriovenous (A-V) fistulas in 100 patients. *Trans Am Soc Artif Intern Organs* 21:296, 1975
131. Merickel JH, Andersen RC, Knutson R, Lipschultz ML, Hitchcock CR: Bovine carotid artery shunts in vascular access surgery. Complications in the chronic hemodialysis patient. *Arch Surg* 109:245, 1974
132. Biggers JA, Remmers AR Jr, Glassford DM, Lindley JD, Sarles HE, Fish JC: Bovine graft fistulas in patients with vascular access problems receiving hemodialysis. *Surgery* 140:690, 1975
133. Yokoyama T, Bower R, Chinitz J, Schwartz A, Swartz C: Experience with 100 bovine arteriografts for maintenance hemodialysis. *Trans Am Soc Artif Intern Organs* 20:328, 1974
134. Kinnaert P, Vereerstraeten PJC, Toussaint CV and Gertruyden J: Nine years experience with internal arteriovenous fistulas for haemodialysis: A study of some factors influencing the results. *Br J Surg* 64:242, 1977
135. Mennes PA, Gilula LA, Anderson CB, Etheredge EE, Weerts C, Harter H: Complications associated with arteriovenous fistulas in patients undergoing chronic hemodialysis. *Arch Intern Med* 138:1117, 1978
136. Butler HG, Baker LD, Johnson JM: Vascular access for chronic hemodialysis: Polytetrafluoroethylene (PTFE) versus bovine heterograft. *Am J Surg* 134:791, 1977
137. Wellington JL: Expanded polytetrafluoroethylene prosthetic grafts for blood access in patients on dialysis. *Can J Surg* 21:420, 1978
138. Gross GF, Hayes JF: PTFE graft arteriovenous fistulae for hemodialysis access. *Am Surg* 45:748, 1979
139. Bhat DJ, Tellis VA, Kohlberg WI, Driscoll B, Veith FJ: Management of sepsis involving expanded polytetrafluoroethylene grafts for hemodialysis access. *Surgery* 87:445, 1980
140. Lilly L, Nghiem D, Mendez Picon G, Lee HM: Comparison between bovine heterograft and expanded PTFE grafts for dialysis access. *Am J Surg* 46:694, 1980
141. Kaslow RA, Zellner SR: Infection in patient on maintenance haemodialysis. *Lancet* 2:117, 1972
142. Martin AM, Clunie GJA, Tonkin RW, Robson JS: The aetiology and management of shunt infections in patients on intermittent haemodialysis. *Proc Eur Dial Transpl Assoc* 4:67, 1967
143. Dathan JR, Frankel RJ, Goodwin FJ, Marsh FP, Murray M, Thompson JM, Youngs GR: One year experience in a Ministry of Health dialysis centre. *Br Med J* 2:102, 1970
144. Morris AJ, Bilinsky RT: Prevention of staphylococcal shunt infections by continuous vancomycin prophylaxis. *Am J Med Sci* 261:88, 1971
145. Johanson WG, Pierce AK, Sanford JP: Changing pharyngeal bacterial flora of hospitalized patients. *N Engl J Med* 281:1137, 1969
146. Rackow EC, Fein IA, Sprung C, Groodman Rs: Uremic pulmonary edema. *Am J Med* 64:1084, 1978
147. Hopps HC, Wissler RW: Uremic pneumonitis. *Am J Pathol* 31:261, 1955.
148. Jadav DK, Sant SM, Acharya VN: Bacteriology of urinary tract infection in patients of renal failure undergoing dialysis. *J Postgrad Med* 23:10, 1977
149. Sweet R, Keane WF: Perinephric abscess in patients with polycystic kidney disease undergoing chronic hemodialysis. *Nephron* 23:237, 1979
150. Onorato IM, Axelrod JL, Lorch JA, Brensilver JM, Bokkenheuser V. Fungal infections of dialysis fistulae. *Ann Intern Med* 91:50, 1979
151. Pradhan RP, Katz LA, Nidus BD, Matalon R, Eisinger RP: Tuberculosis in dialyzed patients. *JAMA* 229:798, 1974

152. Papadimitriou M, Mimmos D, Metaxas P: Tuberculosis in patients on regular haemodialysis. *Nephron* 24:53, 1979
153. Andrew OT, Schoenfeld P, Hopewell PC, Humphreys M: Tuberculosis in patients with end-stage renal disease. *Am J Med* 68:59, 1980
154. Lundin AP, Adler AJ, Berlyne GM, Friedman EA: Tuberculosis in patients undergoing maintenance hemodialysis. *Am J Med* 67:597, 1979
155. Rutsky EA, Rostand SG: Mycobacteriosis in patients with chronic renal failure. *Arch Intern Med* 140:57, 1980
156. Sasaki S, Akiba T, Suenaga M, Tomura S, Yoshiyama N, Nakagawa S, Shoji T, Sasaoka T, Takeuchi J: Ten Years survey of dialysis associated tuberculosis. *Nephron* 24:141, 1979
157. Betts RF, Hanshaw JB: Cytomegalovirus in the compromised host. *Annu Rev Med* 28:103, 1977
158. Luby JP, Ramirz-Ronda C, Pinner S, Hull A, Vergne-Marini P: A longitudinal study of varicella-zoster virus infections in renal transplant recipients. *J Infect Dis* 135:659, 1977
159. Swuwansirikul S, Rao N, Dowling JN, Ho M: Primary and secondary cytomegalovirus infection. *Arch Intern Med* 137:1026, 1977
160. Chatterjee SN, Jordan GW: Prospective study of the prevalence and symptomatology of cytomegalovirus infection in renal transplant recipients. *Transplantation* 28:457, 1979
161. Betts RF, Cestero RV, Freeman RB, Douglas RG: Epidemiology of cytomegalovirus infection in end-stage renal disease. *J Med Virol* 4:89, 1979
162. Sexton DJ, Smith EW, Gutman RA, Helms MJ, Lang DJ: Cytomegalovirus infection and chronic hemodialysis. *Clin Nephrol* 11:3, 1979
163. Pass RF, Long WF, Whitley RJ, Sooney SJ, Diethelm AG, Reynolds DW, Alford CA: Productive infection with cytomegalovirus and herpes simplex virus in renal transplant recipients. Role of source of kidney. *J Infect Dis* 137:556, 1978
164. Betts RJ, Freeman RB, Douglas RG, Talley TE, Rundell B: Transmission of cytomegalovirus infection with renal allograft. *Kidney Int* 7:385, 1975
165. Anderson RJ, Schafer LA, Olin DB, Eickhoff TC: Infectious risk factors in the immunosuppressed host. *Am J Med* 54:452, 1973
166. Myerowitz RL, Medeiros AA, O'Brien TF: Bacterial infection in renal homotransplant recipients. *Am J Med* 53:308, 1972
167. Eickhoff TC, Olin DB, Anderson RJ, Schafer LA: Current problems and approaches to diagnosis of infection in renal transplant recipients. *Transplant Proc* 4:693, 1972
168. Burgos-Calderon R, Pankey GA, Figueroa JE: Infection in kidney transplantation. *Surgery* 70:334, 1971
169. Ahern MJ, Comite H, Andriole VT: Infectious complication associated with renal transplantation: An analysis of risk factors. *Yale J Biol Med* 51:513, 1978
170. Rifkind D, Marchioro TL, Schneck SA, Hill RB Jr: Systemic fungal infections complicating renal transplantation and immunosuppressive therapy. *Am J Med* 43:28, 1967

34

DIALYSIS ASSOCIATED HEPATITIS

SHEILA POLAKOFF

Introduction	659
Viral hepatitis	659
Epidemiology: general	659
Hepatitis type A	659
Hepatitis type B	660
Hepatitis Non-A, Non-B	661
Causal viruses and laboratory markers of infection	662
Hepatitis A virus	662
Hepatitis B virus	662
Hepatitis B surface antigen and antibody	662
HBsAg sub-types	662
Hepatitis B core antigen and its antibody	663
Hepatitis Be antigen and its antibody	663
DNA polymerase	663
Cell-mediated immune responses	663
Test methods for hepatitis B antigen/antibody systems	663
Hepatitis Non-A, Non-B agents	664
Clinical features	664
Fulminant hepatitis	664
Chronic hepatitis	664
Primary hepatocellular carcinoma	665
Other manifestations	665
Hepatitis in dialysis units	665
Background	665
Hepatitis A	666
Hepatitis B	666
Hepatitis Non-A, Non-B	666
Sources, routes and vehicles of infection	667
Cross-infection precautions	667
General procedures	668
Unit procedures	668
Staff	668
Samples for laboratory analysis	668
Unit supplies, equipment and catering	668
Unit cleaning	668
Means of control and prevention of hepatitis B infection	668
Detection and dialysis in isolation of infected patients	669
Passive immunisation	669
Active immunisation	670
Dialysis associated hepatitis in the future	671
Appendix: List of abbreviations	672
References	672

INTRODUCTION

Viral hepatitis is undoubtedly the most serious problem of infection associated with maintenance dialysis. Like many other infections it increases morbidity and mortality among patients but the feature that makes it unique among dialysis associated infections is its tendency to involve staff in dialysis units, in related hospital departments and also some of the general community in intimate contact with infected patients and staff. By chance dialysis units provide a situation that, among all others, is most ideally suited to the epidemic and endemic spread of some hepatitis viruses. The contributing features are best appreciated against the background of viral hepatitis in general.

VIRAL HEPATITIS

Epidemiology: general

During the past 50 years epidemiological and experimental studies have established hepatitis as a communicable disease of viral aetiology and have shown that the clinically indistinguishable illnesses are caused by more than one immunologically distinct hepatitis virus. A serological marker of one type of hepatitis virus infection was found in 1964 (1). Discoveries since then have made it possible to identify two types of hepatitis virus infections with certainty and, by exclusion, to recognise at least two other types.

Viral hepatitis is worldwide in distribution. In most countries acute hepatitis is a notifiable disease. Notifications are usually not differentiated by the type of causal virus and they are by no means complete in any country. In developed countries with temperate climates notification rates are low. Annual rates per 100,000 population reported for recent five year periods are 7 to 12 in the U.K. (2) and 26 to 30 in the USA (3). Rates in Eastern Europe are high, usually five times those of the USA (4). Case fatality rates are usually about 1%. Clinical hepatitis is much less common in underdeveloped countries.

Hepatitis type A
Hepatitis type A, or infectious hepatitis, is the most common type of acute hepatitis in Western Europe and North America. Studies made possible by the development of serological tests have confirmed long-established concepts of the epidemiology of the disease.

There appears to be no symptomless carrier state and no animal reservoir has been found. The incubation period ranges from 15 to 50 days. The virus circulates by spread from individuals in the incubation period and the early acute stage of the infection when the virus is excreted in the faeces. Spread is by the faecal-oral route either direct from person to person or via contaminated water, food or objects. Viraemia during the incubation period and the early acute illness is transient and blood spread is uncommon (5). Airborne transmission by droplets has been suggested but there is no clear evidence to support the hypothesis.

Infection with hepatitis A virus (HAV)* whether inapparent or clinical, is followed by sustained immunity to infection with the same type, though not to type B or other types. Infections in early childhood are usually inapparent. Where there is heavy exposure to faecal contamination early in life, immunity is usually acquired in childhood and clinical attacks are rare. As standards of hygiene and sanitation improve the age at exposure gradually increases. Clinical attacks become more common, first among older children and then among adults (6). At present, in most developed countries this stage has been reached and passed; the sources of infection in the community have decreased and only a small portion of young adults are immune (7).

Outbreaks arise in day nurseries or in residential institutions particularly those for the mentally subnormal. Sewage contaminated well water, food contaminated by infected food handlers or uncooked or inadequately cooked shellfish from sewage contaminated water, may lead to explosive outbreaks (8).

Although health service staff sometimes acquire HAV infections from patients in the course of institutional outbreaks or when tending individual patients, such as infants who are excreting the virus (9), HAV contributes little to hepatitis as an occupational hazard.

Hepatitis type B
This type of viral hepatitis was recognised when large outbreaks occurred among recipients of passive prophylaxis with pooled human serum or immunisation with a vaccine that contained human serum (10). The incubation period ranges from 6 weeks to 6 months, symptomless carriers of the virus form the reservoir of infection, spread is from blood to blood and there is no cross-immunity between the types (11, 12). The infection, initially termed serum or long-incubation hepatitis, is now known as type B. At first it was thought to be confined almost exclusively to developed countries with its spread dependent on medical procedures. After serological markers of hepatitis B virus (HBV) infection were discovered, their distribution in populations throughout the world revealed that it is far more common in tropical climates and that its circulation is independent of medical intervention (13).

HBV infection is least common in North West Europe and in North America, where 0.2 to 0.5% of the population are symptomless carriers and another 2 to 10% have evidence of active immunity from past infection, often without a history of hepatitis (14, 15). The infection is rare among children but HBV is responsible for about a quarter of acute hepatitis infections in adults.

The incidence is highest among young adult males. Though some of the patients have histories that indicate the source, e.g., blood transfusions, parenteral drug abuse, most do not. A high incidence among the sexually promiscuous, particularly homosexual males (16), and evidence of transmission to spouses indicates inapparent parenteral spread (17). Intimate contact provides opportunities for small amounts of serum to reach the circulation through minute abrasions of the skin or mucous membranes.

Although spouses of acute hepatitis patients are at high risk, other members of the household are rarely infected (18). Infection is more common among household contacts of carriers presumably due to accidental parenteral exposure at some time during a long period of infectivity (19).

Most HBV infections are sporadic; outbreaks caused by medical procedures in the past are prevented now by appropriate measures, e.g., the use of disposable needles and syringes and the exclusion of human serum from vaccines. The screening and exclusion of donors with evidence of HBV carriage has reduced transfusion associated hepatitis (TAH) type B (20) and some blood products are rendered HBV-free by heat treatment or cold ethanol fractionation (21). Apart from dialysis units which afford unique opportunities for the spread of HBV, outbreaks in hospitals are rare. Occasionally an unusual combination of circumstances in an oncology or intensive care unit has led to small clusters of infections (22).

Type B hepatitis is an occupational hazard for health service staff. The risk of acquiring infection is related to the opportunity for parenteral exposure to blood or blood products. The incidence of infection is highest among pathologists, surgeons and dentists. Staff with little or no direct exposure to patients or blood are at no greater risk than the general population (23).

There is a wide variation in the infectivity of blood. In the incubation period and early acute stage of hepatitis, serum usually contains so many virus particles that a trace is sufficient to cause infection. About one-fifth of symptomless carriers in the general population are highly infective but in the remainder, infectivity ranges from high to a low level at which even a large inoculum will not necessarily transmit infection (24). Certain groups of carriers tend to be highly infective, e.g., patients with abnormalities of immune response caused by inherent defects, disease or therapy (22, 25, 26). Staff accidentally exposed to the blood of such patients are at high risk of infection.

Spread of infection from staff to patients is uncommon. There are few reports of this type of transmission (27, 28). Usually, parenteral exposure of patients to staff can be prevented by appropriate precautions, e.g., occlusive covering of skin lesions and use of surgical gloves.

Endemic HBV infection is common in institutions for the mentally subnormal. Patients with Down's syndrome, particularly those admitted in infancy, tend to respond to HBV by becoming persistent symptomless and highly infective carriers. Other patients whose immune responses have been affected by therapy may res-

---
* See Appendix for abbreviations.

pond in this way. Infection may be transmitted by scratches or bites or indirectly via inanimate objects. As infection is spread from patient to patient the pool of carriers grows and the infection becomes endemic (25).

The part played in the circulation of HBV by vertical transmission from mother to child varies according to geographical situation and ethnic group. Women who are highly infective carriers of HBV or who develop acute HBV infections in the third trimester of pregnancy transmit the infection to their newborn by blood contamination at the time of birth. The infants usually develop persistent symptomless carriage, presumably because of the immaturity of their immune responses (29). In Caucasian populations however both acute HBV infections and the highly infective carrier state are uncommon and so HBV infection of the newborn is rare.

No animal reservoir has been found and there is no evidence in support of a route other than the parenteral, although this is often inapparent and may be indirect. Volunteers given large amounts of highly infective serum by mouth showed evidence of infection after protracted incubation periods but the virus probably reached the circulation through the mucosa (30). Markers of HBV infections are absent from faeces but, when sensitive test methods are used, they are sometimes found in normal body fluids (31, 32). These markers do not necessarily indicate the presence of whole virus particles. Infection has been transmitted experimentally to animals by large inoculations of saliva and semen (33). Extravasated serum in these fluids probably accounts for the presence of the virus. In general the role of body fluids in the spread of HBV seems small compared with that of blood.

HBV can survive for as long as a week in dried blood and contaminated inanimate objects may be involved in transmission (34). Spread of infection by inhalation of droplets containing HBV has been suggested but experimental transmission to a few susceptible animals by this route proved unsuccessful.

Insects such as bed bugs, cockroaches and mosquitoes may act as mechanical vectors of HBV infection. HBV markers can be found in some insect pools but there is no evidence of viral replication within the insects (35). No clear association between the prevalence of HBV markers in wild mosquitoes and in the populations of different areas was found (36).

The pattern of spread of HBV infection in high prevalence areas differs in several respects from that observed in low prevalence areas. In some parts of the world (e.g., tropical Africa, South East Asia), between 10 to 20% of adults have serological markers of HBV carriage and almost all the remainder have evidence of immunity from past infection, usually sub-clinical (37, 38). In these populations, vertical transmission from carrier mothers is common; its frequency is related not only to the prevalence of the carrier state but to the prevalence of high infectivity among carriers and this in turn is related to ethnic group. The highest rates are found among Chinese, then in descending order, African, Asian, Caucasian (29). The causes of these differences between races are not known but they are probably both genetic and environmental. There is a sex difference in response; males develop persistent carriage more often (39).

In high prevalence areas, children who are not infected at birth acquire the infection later and by adult life few susceptibles remain. In these populations morbidity and mortality rates from chronic liver disease and primary carcinoma of the liver are high, particularly among those with serological evidence of persistent HBV infection (40).

Hepatitis Non-A, Non-B

The existence of hepatitis viruses other than HAV and HBV was suggested by multiple attacks of acute hepatitis in drug abusers (41) and by TAH that was not type B. Newly available diagnostic serological tests for HAV infections show by exclusion that hepatitis is commonly caused by agents other than HAV, HBV, cytomegalovirus or Epstein-Barr virus. In the absence of specific identification, these infections have been termed non-A, non-B (NANB) hepatitis (42).

Experimental inoculation of chimpanzees confirms that transmissable agents cause NANB hepatitis (43). Accidental inoculation of a patient's blood caused acute hepatitis NANB in a nurse. Chimpanzees inoculated with serum from either the patient or the nurse developed hepatitis (44).

Cross-challenge experiments show that two immunologically distinct NANB agents are transmitted by transfusion of blood or blood products (45).

In the USA prospective studies of aminotransferase levels in patients after blood transfusion show that the incubation period of TAH NANB ranges from 14 to 91 days. The incidence after transfusion of 1 to 3 units of blood donated by volunteers is 5.4% of which one-third is clinical hepatitis. More than a quarter of TAH NANB infections progress to chronic hepatitis. The use of paid blood donors causes a five to six fold increase in the risk (46, 47). Though some similar studies in other countries are not strictly comparable the results confirm that TAH NANB is a world problem (48, 49).

Patients who require treatment with blood fractions that cannot be heat treated, e.g., anti-haemophilic factor concentrate, are at a particularly high risk of NANB infection (50).

NANB hepatitis is not restricted to TAH. It is responsible for sporadic cases of acute hepatitis where there is no known exposure. Among patients in hospital with acute hepatitis, NANB infection appears to be responsible for about a quarter in the USA but for a smaller portion in some European countries (51–53). Progression to chronic hepatitis appears to be less common in acute NANB hepatitis without a history of transfusion (54).

Evidence of a NANB agent with a non-parenteral route of spread has appeared recently. Two reports indicate that NANB infection was responsible for large outbreaks of hepatitis transmitted by sewage contaminated water. One of these had been regarded as a classic example of epidemic water borne infectious hepatitis, though the high attack rate in an adult population in which infectious hepatitis was hyperendemic had never been explained. Follow-up studies suggest that this type of NANB infection rarely causes chronic liver disease (55, 56).

Causal viruses and laboratory markers of infection

Hepatitis A virus
HAV is a RNA virus with a diameter of 27 nm. It is inactivated by ultra-violet irradiation, formalin or heating at 100 °C for five minutes, though it is partially resistant to 60 °C for one hour (57). Marmosets and chimpanzees are susceptible to infection. After experimental transmission they develop biochemical and histological, though rarely clinical, evidence of infection. During the incubation period and early acute stage of infection HAV can be found by electron-microscopy in the cytoplasm of hepatocytes and in faecal specimens (58).

In both experimental and natural infections, a short period of viraemia is succeeded, in the acute phase, by the development of antibody (anti-HAV). Anti-HAV immunoglobulin M (IgM) levels decline and usually disappear after a few months but anti-HAV immunoglobulin G (IgG) persists and confers solid immunity (59). A similar pattern is found in symptomless infections.

HAV does not appear to cause chronic liver disease (60).

Anti-HAV IgM tests are used for diagnosing present or recent infections. Tests for anti-HAV IgG are used for population studies.

Solid phase radio and enzyme immunoassay test methods are sensitive and specific (61).

Hepatitis B virus
Renewed research into hepatitis began with the discovery that an antigen, first detected in the serum of an Australian aborigine, was commonly found in serum hepatitis infections (62). This was termed the Australia antigen but later it was re-named the hepatitis B surface antigen (HBsAg).

HBV has not been grown in tissue culture but examination by electron-microscopy of serum containing HBsAg shows several types of particle, including a 42 nm spherical particle, the Dane particle, which is the complete virus (63). HBV consists of an inner core, containing DNA and a DNA polymerase, and an outer coat of HBsAg. HBsAg exists in the serum in other forms i.e. 22 nm spherical particles, long tubules and empty shells and these forms predominate over the Dane particles. The number of Dane particles per millilitre is variable but the average has been estimated as 10^5 (64).

Examination of liver tissue from patients with various types of HBV infections shows core particles (HBcAg) in the nuclei and HBsAg in the cytoplasm of hepatocytes (65).

HBV is destroyed by heat treatment. Boiling for one minute or heating for 10 h at 60 °C, previously considered adequate, have been shown insufficient for complete inactivation (66, 67).

HBV is a complex virus with several antigen/antibody systems and sub-types.

Hepatitis B surface antigen and antibody. The presence of HBsAg or its antibody (anti-HBs) indicates present or previous HBV infection. In most acute HBV infections HBsAg is found in the serum in the late incubation period, several weeks before the onset of jaundice, and in the early acute illness (30). Afterwards, HBsAg is usually cleared from the serum probably by cell-mediated immune mechanisms (68). Anti-HBs usually appears in the serum some weeks or months after HBsAg has disappeared and it persists with a slow decline in titre (69). In some patients HBsAg persists after recovery from acute illness; these patients often develop chronic liver disease (70).

Symptomless HBsAg carriers exist throughout the world. The underlying causes of HBsAg carriage by apparently healthy individuals exposed to HBV after infancy are uncertain but genetically determined defects of immune responses may be involved. Exposure to HBV in early infancy when immune responses are immature usually leads to persistent HBsAg carriage. In high prevalence areas it is common for HBsAg carriage to result from exposure to infected mothers at the time of birth (71). In low HBV prevalence areas, patients with deficient immune responses are at the greatest risk of developing symptomless HBsAg carriage after exposure to HBV (22, 25, 26).

Repeated observations of adult symptomless carriers show that more than half have consistently normal aminotransferase levels. In the remainder the levels fluctuate or remain slightly raised. Examination of liver biopsy specimens usually reveal either normal tissue, minor non-specific changes or mild diffuse hepatitis, but evidence of chronic active hepatitis is found in 4 to 20%, more often among those with raised aminotransferase levels. The results of prospective studies over 5 or more years differed; one group showed a marked increase in the evidence of liver disease with time, whereas in other studies there was little change (72–76). In high HBV prevalence areas HBsAg positive individuals in the population have the highest mortality rates. Among HBsAg positive men of 40 to 60 years in Taiwan the risk of developing primary liver carcinoma (PLC) is about 300 times that of HBsAg negative controls (77). In this population however, the greatly increased risk of cirrhosis and PLC is probably related to genetic and environmental influences and, in particular, to the acquisition of HBV infection in early infancy.

Anti-HBs in serum without HBsAg indicates recovery from infection and immunity. HBV reinfection of anti-HBs positive individuals is rare (78): when it occurs it may be due to waning immunity combined with an overwhelming infective dose. Anti-HBs is sometimes found in co-existence with HBsAg in the sera of carriers or patients with chronic liver disease (79). HBsAg/Anti-HBs complexes are often present in these cases.

HBsAg sub-types. HBsAg is a complex particle with multiple antigenic subspecificities (80). All specimens of HBsAg contain the group determinant a and generally at least two sub-determinants, usually either d or y and varients of w or r (81): d and y are usually mutually exclusive but they have been found together in a few specimens (82). Other sub-types exist (83) and the complete sub-type pattern is probably extremely complex. Sub-type patterns vary between populations throughout the world. Sub-type and virulence are not related (84) and the development of immunity appears to depend on the group determinant *a*. Sub-typing is useful in outbreak investigations because the sub-type of the source corresponds with those of secondary cases (85).

Hepatitis B core antigen (HBcAg) and its antibody (anti-HBc). A second antigen/antibody HBV system is contained in the Dane particle core (86). HBcAg is not found free in serum but anti-HBc is produced in response to virus replication in the liver. Anti-HBc appears in the acute phase of infection, usually when HBsAg is present in the serum. It precedes anti-HBs by weeks or months. Titres decline rapidly but anti-HBc usually persists long after recovery from an acute attack or in the sera of symptomless HBsAg carriers (87). Anti-HBc without HBsAg in serum may indicate continuing viral replication in the liver; blood that contains anti-HBc without other markers may transmit HBV infection (88), though probably only in a large dose such as a blood transfusion.

Occasionally it may be useful to distinguish, with a single HBsAg positive sample, an acute attack of hepatitis B from acute NANB infection with HBsAg carriage. Anti-HBc IgM levels, which are higher in acute than in persistent infections, may indicate the diagnosis (89).

Hepatitis Be antigen (HBeAg) and its antibody (anti-HBe). HBeAg and anti-HBe form a third HBV system (90). HBeAg is probably an integral part of the HBV core with an affinity for IgG but some findings suggest it is a host response to HBV (91).

HBeAg has three antigenic components, *e*1, *e*2 and *e*3. *e*1 appears to parallel total *e* activity but *e*2 and/or *e*3 are not always detectable in HBeAg positive sera (92).

In most acute HBV infections HBeAg appears early and disappears from the serum before biochemical abnormalities of liver function reach their peak (93): anti-HBe usually appears before clearance of HBsAg in acute self-limiting hepatitis (94).

HBeAg and anti-HBe are more useful as indicators of infectivity than as predictors of progression to chronic liver disease. HBeAg is found more often in chronic hepatitis whereas anti-HBe is found more often in HBsAg carriers with normal hepatic histology. HBeAg is positively and anti-HBe negatively correlated with HBcAg in hepatocyte nuclei and with high HBsAg titres in sera (95). In general HBeAg persistence long after the acute illness indicates progression to chronic liver disease but anti-HBe is not necessarily evidence of normal liver function as it is often found in chronic hepatitis (96). The HBeAg/anti-HBe system is a good indicator of the relative infectivity of HBsAg positive serum. HBeAg positive mothers usually transmit infection to their newborn whereas anti-HBe positive mothers rarely do (97). Accidental inoculation with HBeAg positive blood has a much greater risk of acute hepatitis than similar exposure to anti-HBe positive blood (26). Although anti-HBe positive serum is less likely to contain HBV it cannot be considered completely non-infectious. Chimpanzees have been infected by inoculation of anti-HBe positive serum (98). Some infants have been infected by anti-HBe positive mothers (99). Probably this is dose related. In the experimental transmission to chimpanzees the dose was large and the newborn is likely to be exposed to a large amount of maternal blood in terms of its body size.

HBeAg has been found in HBsAg negative sera. Four individuals had evidence of past HBV infections; all were anti-HBc positive and two were also anti-HBs positive. The significance of this finding in terms of the infectivity of HBsAg negative sera is not clear, as the other marker of infectivity – DNA polymerase – could not be found in the two sera examined (100).

DNA polymerase. The core of the Dane particle contains a DNA polymerase (101). DNA polymerase levels are highest in the late incubation period of acute HBV infection before biochemical evidence of hepatic dysfunction appears (102). High levels are also found in the sera of HBsAg carriers with large numbers of Dane particles in circulation. The presence of HBeAg and DNA polymerase are closely correlated and both indicate infectivity (103).

Cell-mediated immune responses. Cell-mediated immune responses, demonstrated by leucocyte migration inhibition tests in the convalescent stage of acute hepatitis B, appear to be involved in HBV clearance in acute attacks (104). Abnormal cellular responses to HBV infection are probably responsible for the development of chronic hepatitis or symptomless HBsAg carriage, though the mechanisms remain obscure. Several studies support the hypothesis that the chronic HBsAg carrier state results from poor T-lymphocyte recognition of the infective agent (105–107). A recent hypothesis proposes that the cellular immune response, via its suppressor T cell and cytotoxic effector cell functions, is the major pathogenic determinant of hepatocellular injury in viral hepatitis though there may be extrinsic modulation by the humoral immuno-regulatory system. The outcome of HBV infection depends on the balance in this system, which is influenced by several factors, including the underlying immunologic characteristics of the host (108).

Test methods for hepatitis B antigen/antibody systems. Detailed descriptions are given in WHO publications (109, 110).
1. HBsAg. Immunodiffusion (ID), counter immunoelectrophoresis (CIE), complement fixation (CF) and reversed passive latex inhibition have been replaced by highly sensitive and specific methods, i.e., radioimmunoassay (RIA), reversed passive haemagglutination (RPHA) and enzyme-linked immunosorbent assay (ELISA). RIA appears to be the most sensitive of the three.
2. Anti-HBs. The low prevalence of anti-HBs found in early studies reflected the lack of sensitivity of ID, CIE and CF methods. Passive haemagglutination (PH) and either solid phase RIA or radioimmuno-

precipitation reveal anti-HBs in the serum of most patients after recovery.
3. HBcAg and anti-HBc. Core antigen is not found free in serum but it is found in liver cell nuclei by various electronmicroscopy techniques. RIA methods are used for detection of anti-HBc. The tests, used at present for surveys and research, are not in general use for screening of, for example, blood donors.
4. HBeAg and anti-HBe. The ID and CIE methods first used were insensitive. With the RIA methods the proportion of sera positive for either HBeAg or anti-HBe have increased. HBsAg positive sera negative in both tests for HBeAg and anti-HBe are of intermediate infectivity.

Hepatitis Non-A, Non-B agents
Virus-like particles in the livers of patients with NANB infections or experimentally infected chimpanzees have been found (111–113), but there are as yet no serological tests for NANB agents. Despite several reports of the serological identification of antigen/antibody systems associated with NANB infection none has proved universally reproducible (114).

At present, diagnosis of NANB infection rests on clinical or biochemical evidence or both and the exclusion of HAV, HBV and other identifiable causal agents.

Identification of symptomless carriers of NANB infection among blood donors by means of aminotransferase tests has been investigated in the USA. A direct relationship was found between the aminotransferase levels of donors and the incidence of TAH NANB among recipients but most of the infections are transmitted by donors with normal levels (46, 47). Exclusion of donors with abnormal levels would prevent one-fifth of the infections. For a greater reduction some donors with levels within normal, at the upper end of the range, would have to be rejected. This might well cause difficulties for blood transfusion centres. Moreover aminotransferase screening on a large scale is costly. The most cogent argument in favour of such non-specific screening is the high prevalence of chronic liver diease associated with TAH NANB (115).

Cross-reactivity between HBeAg and a NANB antigen has been observed in Italy. Chimpanzees inoculated with serum containing this agent developed acute hepatitis B but a similar clinical illness developed in HBsAg carriers. It is suggested that this agent may be a defective HBV (116).

Clinical features

The similarity of acute viral hepatitis attacks make serological tests necessary to distinguish the causal agents.

Some clinical features, although not diagnostic, are associated with particular types. The onset is often abrupt in HAV infections, but it is usually insidious in the other types. Fever is more common in type A infection than in type B or NANB. HBV infections tend to be more severe but fulminant hepatitis may result from infection with any of the types (117).

In a typical acute attack there is a variable prodromal period before the onset of jaundice, during which gastrointestinal symptoms such as malaise, abdominal discomfort, anorexia, nausea and sometimes vomiting develop. Occasionally early symptoms are respiratory, particularly in HAV infections. Urticaria, skin rashes, angioneurotic oedema or polyarthritis may appear, particularly in HBV infections. Dark urine, and pale stools are usual. Pruritus may accompany jaundice. The liver is often enlarged and tender and there may be slight splenomegaly. Some patients remain anicteric throughout the illness. After a variable period, usually from one to four weeks, jaundice disappears and most patients recover within months of the onset (118).

The pathological lesion is similar in type A, B and NANB infections. The appearance is of hepatic cell necrosis and regeneration. In the early stages there is an inflammatory reaction with infiltration of lymphocytes, hyperplasia of Kupffer cells and bile stasis. Liver cells are swollen and necrotic. Later, signs of regeration appear. The appearance is similar in anicteric attacks (119).

Serum aminotransferase levels begin to rise before the onset of symptoms. The peak is variable but is usually within 500 to 5000 IU. Levels return to normal with clinical recovery but minor elevations may persist for some months. Peak levels are usually higher in HBV than in HAV or NANB infections. Serum bilirubin rises to a peak with the appearance of jaundice and decreases with recovery (53).

Fulminant hepatitis
A small portion of patients with acute icteric hepatitis, of any type, develop hepatic failure shortly after onset and only 20 to 25% survive (117).

Serological studies in fulminant HBV infections show accelerated responses in some patients i.e. swift loss of HBsAg and early appearance of anti-HBs (120).

In developing countries acute viral hepatitis in pregnancy, particularly in the third trimester, is often fulminant but this association is not found elsewhere (121).

The pathological appearance is one of massive hepatic necrosis. Clinically there is evidence of encephalopathy which in most cases progresses to coma and death. Sometimes hepatic failure may appear as late as a month or more after the onset of illness. Complications such as gastrointestinal haemorrhage, sepsis and cerebral oedema may contribute to the deaths in fulminant attacks (117).

Chronic hepatitis
Chronic hepatitis does not appear to result from HAV infections (60), but it appears to follow 5 to 10% of acute HBV infections (70, 122) and more than 10% of TAH NANB (46, 123). It seems less common after sporadic acute NANB infection and in one study all patients recovered without chronic sequelae (53, 124). Anicteric mild attacks of hepatitis are believed to progress to chronicity more often than severe infections (125).

Two forms of chronic hepatitis are recognised – persistent (CPH) and chronic active hepatitis (CAH). CPH represents delayed resolution of hepatic lesions, though eventually complete recovery ensues. CAH is a progressive disease with a variable course. In some cases hepatic necrosis and fibrosis is extensive and cirrhosis develops; in others fibrosis is not progressive (126). There may be long asymptomatic periods between exacerbations. Aminotransferase levels may be persistently raised or fluctuate. In acute HBV attacks HBsAg persistence six months after the onset suggests progression to chronic hepatitis (127). HBsAg positive CAH is less common in women (128). Immunosuppressive therapy increases the replication of HBV in patients with CAH type B (129).

Antiviral chemotherapy has been used to treat CAH type B. In a small controlled trial HBV replication appeared to be inhibited in some patients by adenine arabinoside (Ara-A) (129), but a controlled trial of human leucocyte interferon (HLI) showed no sustained effect on HBV replication (130). In a study in which controls were not randomly selected, Ara-A and HLI appeared to inhibit HBV replication and combined therapy was more effective than one agent alone (131). Large randomised controlled trials have been planned but results are not expected for some years (132).

Primary hepatocellular carcinoma
Primary hepatocellular carcinoma (PHC) is one of the most common malignant diseases in high HBV prevalence areas. Case control studies indicate a strong association between PHC and HBV infections (133–135). Large scale prospective studies of adult male populations in a high prevalence area show that the rate at which PHC developed was 300 times greater in the HBsAg positive group than in the HBsAg negative control group (77). Although PHC is less common in HBsAg negative individuals, its occurrence suggests that factors other than HBV are involved (136). The precise mechanism of the development of PHC is not clear but cirrhosis is a predisposing condition and the sequence is probably CAH, cirrhosis, PHC. In family studies the mothers of all HBsAg positive PHC patients were HBsAg positive, which suggests that early infection is critical in PHC development (137). Whether HBV infection is a primary carcinogen or a co-factor, the wide use of HBV vaccine in high prevalence areas is expected to reduce PHC incidence in the long term (40).

Other manifestations
HBV infection has been associated with a number of conditions which may accompany clinical hepatitis or occur with little or no evidence of liver involvement. In general, these manifestations are correlated with deposition of HBsAg/anti-HBs complexes in the blood vessels and other tissues. They include a serum sickness-like syndrome, polyarteritis nodosa, essential mixed cryoglobulinaemia, polymyalgia rheumatica, infantile papular acrodermatitis and glomerulonephritis (138–145).

HEPATITIS IN DIALYSIS UNITS

Background

Hepatitis appeared as a dialysis associated problem when maintenance dialysis was still in the pioneering stage and serological tests for hepatitis infection had not yet been developed. At that time some types of dialyser needed to be primed with blood for each dialysis and patients received frequent blood transfusions to correct anaemia. It was assumed that patients were usually infected directly from transfused blood and it was hoped that the hepatitis problem would be solved by keeping transfusions to a minimum and by introducing low blood volume dialysers that allowed a good wash back of blood. This hope proved unfounded; as the units grew in number and size reports of hepatitis increased (146–151).

There was a striking difference between staff and patients in the clinical evidence of infection; most patients appeared to have mild attacks whereas staff were usually acutely ill. Outbreaks differed also in the severity of infection. For example, in the UK, fatality rates were high in two outbreaks – 3 of 13 (23%) and 4 of 12 (33%) – but in four other outbreaks there were no deaths among 38 acutely ill staff (152–154). Infections among patients were more acute in outbreaks in which fatality rates among staff were high. It seemed possible that there were not only host differences between patients and staff in response to infection but also differences between the virulence of HBV strains.

Hepatitis was so common in dialysis units throughout the world by the nineteen seventies that the absence of hepatitis in a long established unit was more remarkable than an outbreak. Collaborative studies show that in 1973, for example, no less than 48% of 702 units in Europe reported hepatitis; 18% of 16,237 patients treated and 604 staff were infected during the year (155). The position in the USA was similar: a point prevalence study in 15 units in 1973 revealed HBsAg carriage in 16% of patients and 2% of staff. A further 34% of patients and 31% of staff had evidence of past infection. More than half of the home contacts of carrier patients had been infected (79).

Spread of infection to other hospital staff was common; those working in laboratories, where blood and tissue from patients were examined, and transplant teams were at high risk. The transfer of patients between units spread infection to previously unaffected units (146).

The case fatality rate in Europe in 1972 was 0.2% in dialysis patients and 2.4% among staff (156). The long term outcome of most of the infections in staff is difficult to assess but in general about 5% of acute HBV infections progress to CAH (70,122).

Means of control and prevention, developed over the years, have controlled the spread of HBV in some units but HBV infection remains endemic in many. The 1980 report from European centres shows that in 1978 more than 700 staff contracted viral hepatitis and it caused the death of 421 patients on renal replacement therapy. Although types of hepatitis infection were not differentiated, the report ascribes most of the infections to HBV (157).

Elimination of HBV infection from most blood transfusions has revealed a type NANB hepatitis problem (46, 47) which appears to exist in some dialysis units (158). NANB infection may spread within units by cross-infection and infections in patients frequently progress to chronic hepatitis (159).

Thus the great success of dialysis in maintaining the lives of patients who, without treatment, faced certain death has been and continues to be accompanied by serious viral hepatitis hazards.

Hepatitis A

Few outbreaks in dialysis units have been ascribed to HAV infection. Serological studies in 15 dialysis units in the USA showed anti-HAV prevalence rates among patients and staff no higher than would be expected in similar age and sex groups in the general population (160).

HAV infections may occur in patients and staff of dialysis units as they do in the general community and spread within the unit is possible. However, the apparent absence of a persistent carrier state suggests that HAV is unlikely to become established as an endemic infection in dialysis units.

Human normal immunoglobulin (ISG) affords effective protection against HAV infection (161).

Hepatitis B

HBV appears to be responsible for most dialysis associated hepatitis. The tendency of patients with chronic renal failure to become persistent HBsAg carriers is central to the problem. This tendency has been attributed to depression of cell-mediated immunity by uraemia. A study of dialysis unit patients showed that both persistent HBsAg carriers and patients without any evidence of past or present HBV infection had significantly decreased absolute numbers and functional T-lymphocytes. There was no significant difference between the number of T-lymphocytes in dialysis patients who had made a normal recovery from HBV infection and healthy control subjects (162). This suggests that the response of the individual patients infected in the same outbreak will depend on the severity of the uraemia. However other host factors influence the outcome; males develop persistent HBsAg carriage more often than females (163). Also differences in human histocompatibility antigens (164, 165) may play a part in addition to extrinsic factors such as the size and route of the infecting dose (166).

In general, more than half of the infected patients in dialysis units become persistent symptomless HBsAg carriers often without biochemical evidence of infection. The markers of high infectivity i.e. DNA polymerase, large numbers of Dane particles in circulation and HBeAg, are usually found in their serum (167). In a study of HBsAg carriage in patients, 74% in dialysis and transplantation units but only 28% in other hospital departments were HBeAg positive. These results were supported by differences in infection rates in staff. After accidental inoculation with HBsAg positive blood 22% of the dialysis unit staff but only 6% of the staff of other departments developed hepatitis B. When all staff were considered together, of those accidentally inoculated with HBeAg positive blood 30% had hepatitis B attacks and another 30% developed anti-HBs without symptoms; the corresponding rates for those inoculated with blood negative for both HBeAg and anti-HBe were 14% and 17%. None of nine similarly exposed to anti-HBe positive blood experienced hepatitis B but two had symptomless anti-HBs responses (26).

The evidence suggests that the admission of an HBeAg positive carrier patient to a dialysis unit free of HBV infection will cause cross-infection more readily than the admission of an anti-HBe positive carrier. But a large dose of anti-HBe positive blood may cause HBV infection. Since the persistence of HBeAg appears to depend on host response, and patients with chronic renal failure tend to develop persistent HBeAg, any secondary case may lead to widespread cross-infection in the unit.

In response to HBV infection, some dialysis unit patients experience either clinical hepatitis or a symptomless attack with transient HBsAg and recover with evidence of active immunity, i.e. anti-HBs, but a small number will have anti-HBc only. It has been suggested that anti-HBc as the only HBV marker in serum indicates some active replication of the virus which may be responsible for some TAH in recipients of HBsAg negative blood (168). However, patients with this sole marker have been dialysed in units for long periods without spread of HBV infection (169). When HBV particles are present in anti-HBc positive blood their number per millilitre is probably small. The difference between the ability of anti-HBc positive blood to cause infection in the two situations is probably dose related.

Immunosuppressive therapy tends to increase HBV replication and HBsAg positive patients with functioning transplants almost invariably remain positive (170). The emergency admission of patients for dialysis in transplant rejection episodes carries a higher risk of introducing the infection to a previously HBV-free unit than the admission of any other type of patient. Graft rejection however, particularly at an early stage, appears to be more common among patients with anti-HBs before transplantation than among HBsAg carriers. The most probable explanation is that immune responses sufficiently active to produce anti-HBs tend to cause graft rejection, but the fact that there was no excess early rejection by patients with anti-HBs when the graft donor was female suggested the possibility that y-linked histocompatibility antigens may influence the host response to both HBsAg and HLA antigens (171, 172).

Hepatitis Non-A, Non-B (NANB)

Serological tests to exclude HAV, HBV and other relevant virus infections indicate that other hepatitis agents cause TAH. This type of TAH often progresses to CAH. These agents appear to have the attributes necessary to cause dialysis associated hepatitis e.g. a symptomless carrier state and blood to blood spread (46, 47). In units with widespread HBV infection, NANB infection may well pass unnoticed but in HBV-free units, clusters of patients with abnormal aminotransferase levels have been observed. In the earliest of these outbreaks chronic liver disease developed later in 53% of the affected patients (159). Other clusters may be further examples of NANB infection (173) but similar episodes have been ascribed to other causes, e.g., drug therapy, toxic chemicals from dialysis tubing (174, 175). If the clusters observed in UK units are caused by NANB infections, the epidemiological pattern differs markedly from HBV in that none of the staff showed clinical evidence of hepatitis, few had abnormal aminotransferase levels and the abnormalities observed were slight.

Specific serological tests for NANB agents are necessary to define the nature and extent of these infections in dialysis units.

Sources, routes and vehicles of infection

Throughout the world, dialysis units are the only general hospital departments in which it is the rule rather than the exception for hepatitis to arise – often in explosive outbreaks – and to become endemic.

Man is the only reservoir of HBV. The staff of dialysis units do not differ from other hospital staff. The reason for the outbreaks must, therefore, be related to the patients and their treatment. At first, the known association between blood transfusion and hepatitis tended to obscure the fact that dialysis associated hepatitis is essentially a cross-infection problem.

Certainly, the infection may be introduced to a patient by a blood transfusion. However, the natural circulation of HBV infection in populations, combined with the tendency of uraemic patients to respond to HBV infection by developing symptomless carriage, will ensure that the proportion of HBsAg carriers among candidates for treatment in dialysis units will be larger than among the related population. This proportion may be increased by HBV infection that itself can cause glomerulonephritis and persistent HBsAg carriage (144, 145).

Dialysis unit patients normally live in the community and they may acquire the infection from outside the hospital at any time during intervals between treatment and introduce it to a unit previously free of HBV infection.

Sooner or later one of the patients in a dialysis unit will be a highly infective carrier. The opportunities for blood spread of the infection in a dialysis unit are obvious: the heparinised patients may haemorrhage from various sites, there may be blood spray during cannulation of an arterio-venous fistula and some blood spillage at the beginning and end of a dialysis session is common. Splashes of blood or less easily detected drops of serum may fall on exposed skin lesions of patients and on the clothes, bedding and equipment. HBsAg has been identified in swabs taken from many sites in a dialysis unit with endemic HBV infection (176).

Cross-infection between patients may result from shared equipment (177), by contamination of non-disposable venous pressure monitors (153), by blood splashes or by the transfer of infective material from contaminated objects to skin lesions or mucous membranes. Staff may inadvertently transmit infection from one patient to another via contaminated hands or clothes. Insects e.g. mosquitoes, bed-bugs, cockroaches may sometimes act as mechanical vehicles of infection (35, 36).

Airborne transmission has been postulated (178) but HBV is unlikely to spread by the airborne route in the same way as respiratory disease. Dialysis unit staff not in direct contact with patients, equipment or blood specimens are rarely infected (154). Furthermore, it is difficult to create blood aerosols under dialysis conditions (179).

The role of body fluids other than blood in the spread of dialysis associated hepatitis is not clear. High HBsAg titres have been found in ascitic fluid (180) which may be as highly infective as blood. Low HBsAg titres have been found in normal body fluids e.g. saliva, semen, sweat (32,181) but not in faeces or urine (31,182). Probably normal body fluids are not highly infective unless contaminated by serum and their role in the spread of HBV infection in dialysis units is small compared with that of blood.

Whatever the route of transmission, cross-infection between patients is the main factor in the creation of an outbreak. The HBsAg carrier patients form the reservoir of infection in the unit and the larger the reservoir the greater is the risk of infection of new patients or staff and of spread outside the unit.

Staff acquire infections by inoculation, contamination of cuts or abrasions or splashes into the eye or mouth. In a unit with hyperendemic infection staff may acquire infection but fail to remember any specific accident. The risk that staff incubating or symptomlessly carrying hepatitis B infection pose to patients is probably small (27). In dialysis unit outbreaks it is difficult to establish the origin, but whenever serological studies have made it possible, a patient has been shown to be the source (154). Although blood spread from patients to staff is common there are few opportunities for transmission of blood from staff to patients parenterally. It seems reasonable to assume that HBsAg carrier staff are unlikely to cause outbreaks in dialysis units but the possibility cannot be ruled out completely.

Little is known about the mode of spread of NANB agents in dialysis units but their role in TAH suggests that it may be similar to that of HBV.

Cross-infection precautions

Before serological tests for HBV infection became available, attempts to prevent the spread of hepatitis in dialysis units were based on the maintenance of good general hygienic standards, sterilisation and disinfection of equipment and the protection of staff by protective clothing, careful handling of potentially infective specimens and the observance of measures aimed at avoiding accidents (183).

With no means of identifying symptomless carriers among the patients being dialysed in open wards, the best that could be expected of these measures, if they were always observed, was that the spread of infection would be slowed down. Cross-infection precautions are time consuming and they are often overlooked when dramatic incidents occur during dialysis treatment. The danger of infection is greatest, for example, when there is a massive haemorrhage.

Serological tests for HBsAg and anti-HBs afford several methods of controlling and preventing dialysis associated hepatitis B. Nevertheless, there is no method or combination of methods likely to be effective enough to eliminate the need for the observance of adequate cross-infection precautions in dialysis units.

A general code of practice was formulated in the UK in 1972 but it is not mandatory (184). A summary of the recommendations aimed at the prevention of spread of any type of hepatitis infection is given below. The recommendations are now under review to take into account advances in treatment and improvements in equipment during the past ten years.

General procedures
1. Patients, known or suspected to be infective, are not admitted to the main unit but to an isolation area.
2. Staff are instructed in routine procedures initially and periodically.
3. A special book is kept to record the following accidents:
   a) a cut or other skin penetration caused by objects contaminated with blood, blood components or body fluids;
   b) blood contamination of broken skin surfaces;
   c) aspiration, ingestion or splashing of blood or other body fluids on to the face, lips or eyes: and
   d) extensive splashing of blood over large areas of body surface or clothing.

Unit procedures
1. Dialysing fluid supply units are restricted for use to the same group of patients. Each patient keeps to his own dialyser. Routines for disinfection of dialysers are clearly established. Disposables are discarded in plastic bags, sealed and incinerated.
2. A principal is present with an assistant (usually the patient) for each dialysis. Protective clothing is worn by staff and relatives in training.
3. Disposable water repellent squares are placed under shunts or fistulae.
4. On completion of dialysis the patient: Strips the bed, places items in disposable bags, puts on protective clothing, and takes the artificial kidney to the dismantling area to strip.
   If the patient is not well enough, staff wearing protective clothing undertake the procedures.
5. One member of staff wears protective clothing at all times in order to deal immediately with emergencies, e.g., haemorrhage.
6. Patients are encouraged to become as independent of assistance as possible and are fully instructed in unit techniques and procedures.
   Patients do not assist each other in assembling or dismantling equipment or enter the unit kitchen.
   Each patient has an individual thermometer, razor etc.

Staff
Staff observe the following routines in the dialysis unit:
They do not enter the unit with open sores or dermatitis.
They wear special unit dress while in the unit and wear protective clothing if contact with blood or body fluids of patients is possible or when in contact with equipment being assembled or stripped down.
Staff do not eat, drink or smoke in the treatment or equipment areas.

Samples for laboratory analyses
Staff wear protective clothing. Place a plastic sheet under the patient's arm. Discard the needle into a rigid container. Transfer blood from the syringe to a screw-capped container, avoiding external contamination. Place used equipment in containers for autclaving or incineration. Dilute any spilt blood with strong hypochlorite solution before wiping up. Place specimen containers in plastic bags, heat seal and attach self adhesive label. Place the request form outside the bag.

Unit supplies, equipment and catering
If disposable linen is not used, linen is doubly bagged and washed at 200°F (93°C) for 10 min.
All instruments, including those for return to the Central Sterile Supply Department, are soaked in disinfectant, e.g., 2% glutaraldehyde, after use.
Containers are not re-used.
Disposable utensils are used for all patients' meals.
Staff wash hands and put on clean gowns over unit dress before entering the kitchen.
Food is delivered to the unit in individual portions and passed through the hatch from the kitchen for distribution to patients.

Unit cleaning
Cleaning equipment is stored separately for the dialysis area.
The domestic assistant allocated to the dialysis area wears protective clothing while working there and removes it before entering the other areas.
Bed stations are cleaned after each dialysis session.
Machines, beds, lockers and floors are wiped with disinfectant, e.g., weak hypochlorite.
The breakdown and preparation area are separate.
The breakdown area is washed and disinfected after each session.
The preparation area is cleaned thoroughly daily and surfaces are wiped with disinfectant.
The patients' changing room is washed with disinfectant after each session.

Means of control and prevention of hepatitis B infection

When blood donations are screened by sensitive test methods, TAH type B is almost completely eliminated (185). This reduces the chance of introducing

HBV infection to dialysis units but neither prevents nor controls dialysis associated hepatitis B.

The three methods of preventing and controlling dialysis associated hepatitis are described in the order in which they became available:
1. Detection and dialysis in isolation of infected patients, combined with cross-infection precautions.
2. Passive immunisation.
3. Active immunisation.

Detection and dialysis in isolation of infected patients
The method originated in the UK where it has proved successful.

The main reason for the success of this control and prevention programme was its early institution before HBV infection had been introduced into most of the dialysis units in the UK.

In 1967 there were hepatitis outbreaks in only two of the 30 UK units. By collaboration between directors of two-thirds of the dialysis units and the Epidemiological Research Laboratory of the Public Health Laboratory Service (PHLS) a detailed epidemiological study was begun in 1968. In 1969, three new hepatitis outbreaks began; in July of the same year, however, HBsAg tests became available at the PHLS Virus Reference Laboratory. A pilot study of patients' sera showed that four of the five outbreaks were caused by HBV and, furthermore, that the admission of only one HBsAg carrier to a unit led to an outbreak (154). A retrospective study of stored sera confirmed the hypothesis that symptomless HBsAg carrier patients were responsible for the persistence of HBV infection in dialysis units (186).

These findings led to the development of a control programme for the infected units; this included HBsAg tests of sera taken from all patients in the units at weekly or two weekly intervals and the transfer of any infected patients to isolation for dialysis as soon as possible.

The control of existing outbreaks of a long incubation infection such as HBV could not be achieved quickly or easily. In outbreaks in which many persistent HBsAg carriers had been created, new dialysis patients required separate accomodation. Additional separate accommodation was necessary for previously exposed patients who required re-admission for emergency treatment as they might be either incubating the infection or were still susceptible.

Although these efforts were necessary to control existing outbreaks, it was clear that the specific laboratory tests could be put to better use to prevent outbreaks. Most UK units were free of HBV infection but, if new outbreaks were to arise at the rate observed in 1969, it could not be long before most of the units in the country would be infected.

If outbreaks could be prevented the risk of severe illness among staff would be reduced, the work of the unit could continue without interruption and a further pool of HBsAg carrier patients, potential future sources of infection, would not be created.

The prevention programme put into practice from January 1970 included the following:
1. HBsAg tests of candidates for treatment in the units.
2. Routine screening tests at regular intervals of sera from patients and staff for HBsAg and for abnormalities of liver function.
3. Acquisition of premises for dialysing a small number of patients in isolation.
4. Contingency plan of action when HBsAg was detected, i.e., adoption of the control programme until six months after the last time an infected patient was dialysed in the unit.
5. Cross-infection precautions at all times.

Staff candidates for work in the units who were found to be HBsAg carriers were routed to other departments, not so much to prevent infection in the units as to absolve them of suspicion in the event of an outbreak.

The control and prevention programme was undertaken informally as an extension of the existing survey. However, news of an outbreak with a high case fatality rate in a unit not participating in the survey (153) caused general concern and a national advisory group was formed in October 1970 to review the problem. This group reported in mid-1972 and all the features of the informal programme were included in the recommendations. Furthermore, by 1972 the effect of the informal programme was apparent; the incidence of HBV infection had decreased from 4.9% in 1970 to 1.4% in 1972 among patients and from 1.3% to 0.4% among staff (154, 187). By the end of 1973 any outbreaks were under control and all 33 units then included in the survey were free of HBV infection. The carrier pool was small, 41 (2%) of all patients dialysed in the units at any time (188).

At the end of 1979, the UK survey units remained free of HBV outbreaks (173).

In the past few years, reports from some units outside the UK show succesful results of the institution of similar programmes (189, 190).

Passive immunisation
Anti-HBs tests have made it possible to prepare immunoglobulin with high titres of anti-HBs from sera selected from normal blood donations or obtained by plasmapheresis of frequently transfused patients (191).

Experimental evidence of protection afforded by anti-HBs immunoglobulin (HBIG) was first demonstrated by studies made in an institution for the mentally subnormal in which HBV infection was endemic (192).

Two controlled trials among patients in dialysis units in Europe showed that HBIG conferred protection. In Belgium susceptible patients were given either HBIG or normal immunoglobulin (ISG). Two of the 15 patients in the HBIG group developed HBsAg which swiftly cleared; in the ISG group HBsAg appeared in the sera of 10 of the 14 patients and persisted in five (193). In France the control group did not receive ISG: none of the 15 patients who received HBIG became HBsAg positive, but in the control group HBsAg appeared in the sera of 10 of the 13 patients and persisted in 5 (194).

In a controlled trial of HBIG among dialysis unit staff in Sweden, in which the control group received ISG with a low anti-HBs titre, the incidence of HBV infection was similar in both groups. The clinical attack rate was

2.7%. An unselected untreated group observed during the same period experienced a much higher clinical attack rate of 10.4% (195). An earlier study made in an institution for the mentally subnormal in the USA showed similar results. The findings of both studies suggested that ISG with low anti-HBs titres conferred as much protection as HBIG. However, some serological studies afforded another explanation, i.e., that some batches of ISG act not by conferring passive immunity but by inducing active immunity. ISG produced from pools of donations not pre-screened for HBsAg may contain HBsAg/anti-HBs complexes that, during the Cohn cold ethanol process, may be distributed in the immunoglobulin fraction. These complexes, which would not be detected by testing for HBsAg and anti-HBs, are weak immunogens capable of inducing low levels of anti-HBs, particularly after repeated injections. Re-examination of specimens obtained in a trial confirmed this hypothesis; 36% of ISG recipients were found to have developed anti-HBs without hepatitis, HBsAg or anti-HBc, a response more compatible with immunisation by HBsAg than by infection. In addition, occult HBsAg in the form of immune complexes was found in the ISG used in the trial (196).

In four dialysis units with endemic HBV infection in France, staff were given HBIG at intervals of two weeks for four months, then every two months for eight months and afterwards every three months. None of the 90 who were followed up for 4 to 26 months developed HBV infection. The study did not include controls but of eight staff who did not receive HBIG three developed hepatitis B (197).

The only large multicentre trial of HBIG was made in the USA. New patients and staff were randomly allocated to receive high, intermediate titre HBIG or ISG with a low anti-HBs titre. The attack rate of 9% among patients who received high titre HBIG was lower than the rates in the other two groups (21% and 23%), and the attack rate among staff who received high titre HBIG was lower (7%), than that among the other two groups (11%). Nevertheless, the incidence among those receiving HBIG was higher than had been observed in other studies made in dialysis units (198). Trials of HBIG given to other high risk groups after exposure, i.e., the newborn of HBsAg and HBeAg positive mothers (199), staff after accidental inoculation with HBsAg positive material, showed a high protective efficacy (200). In one study however HBIG appeared not to protect but to prolong the incubation period. It was suggested that the fragmented anti-HBs, contained in the HBIG used, interfered with the neutralising activity of unfragmented anti-HBs also present (201). This may be the reason for the low protective efficacy of the HBIG used in the multicentre trial in dialysis units in the USA.

The evidence taken as a whole indicates that the routine use of HBIG reduces high rates of HBV infection among patients and staff of dialysis units but that this method used alone will not eliminate HBV infection completely; some patients will become infected and some will remain persistent carriers.

The use of HBIG to control HBV infection in dialysis units has some disadvantages. Doses need to be repeated at short intervals to maintain protection and this does not encourage passive-active immunity that would make further passive prophylaxis unnecessary. Although reactions to HBIG are mild and uncommon, repeated doses may lead to hypersensitivity. A few of the staff in France had to discontinue prophylaxis because of the appearance of adverse reactions after repeated doses (194).

In some countries HBIG is available after accidental inoculation or contamination of skin abrasions or mucous membranes with HBsAg positive material. The protection afforded by HBIG in these circumstances is not complete; about 1 to 2% of those given HBIG develop clinical hepatitis B (200). No effect of the interval from exposure to prophylaxis was demonstrated in trials of HBIG after accidental inoculations among staff. Although no effect of the interval from exposure to prophylaxis was demonstrated in trials when HBIG was given within a week of accidental inoculation of staff, it is nevertheless considered advisable to administer HBIG as soon as possible after accidental inoculation.

Active immunisation

Individuals with naturally acquired anti-HBs in their sera rarely develop hepatitis B after exposure (78). This suggested that vaccines that stimulate the active production of anti-HBs should protect against HBV infection.

It is not usually possible to develop a vaccine until the causal agent has been grown in tissue culture yet, despite the fact that HBV has not been propagated *in vitro*, hepatitis B vaccines have been produced and tested in the field by several groups. This unusual turn of events was initiated by experimental evidence that a diluted human serum, known to contain HBV, was not infective after heat treatment but it was immunogenic. One to three inoculations of the treated serum prevented or modified HBV infection in 69% of susceptible subjects challenged with the same serum, unheated, four to eight months later (202).

Crude heat treated serum is not a suitable substance for routine immunisation but the experiments suggested the possibility of producing a vaccine in an unconventional way by separating the non-infectious particles of HBsAg from the sera of carriers to obtain purified material that would stimulate active production of anti-HBs after injection. Several methods have been devised to extract HBsAg from serum and to render the end-product free from HBV.

The safety of a vaccine should be assessed before it is used for purposes other than experimental and the question of safety is of particular concern when a vaccine is derived from human serum. The possible dangers of these vaccines are that purification processes may fail to destroy HBV or other viruses that may be present in the serum and, furthermore, that possibly injurious host proteins may be retained in the final product together with HBsAg. The possibility of injurious host proteins in the vaccines seems remote as there have been no reports of untoward reactions to heated plasma fractions which must have contained HBsAg in the years before blood donations were routinely tested for HBsAg (203).

Animals can be used to monitor the vaccine. Chimpanzees are susceptible to HBV infection and the presence of HBV can be excluded by testing each batch of vaccine by inoculation of non-immune chimpanzees and monitoring them for evidence of active infection, i.e., HBsAg, anti-HBc, HBeAg and DNA polymerase. The presence of HAV can be monitored in chimpanzees or marmosets after inoculation (204). Although there are no laboratory tests for NANB agents, experiments with chimpanzees show that formalin treatment of vaccines will inactivate NANB agents (205).

Results of animal experiments indicate that the vaccines prepared were free of HBV, afforded effective protection against subsequent challenge with infective serum and cross-protection between HBV sub-types (206, 207).

The first field trial of HBV vaccine, made in a dialysis unit in France, did not include a randomly selected control group. Nevertheless the results showed that the vaccine was safe and suggested a high level of protection among patients and staff who respond by producing detectable anti-HBs. This was more common in staff (91%) than in patients (62%). Clinical hepatitis B and HBsAg appeared among those who did not develop anti-HBs responses at the same rate as they did in unvaccinated staff and patients (208).

A controlled trial was made in a large group of homosexual males in the USA. The vaccine used was a 1 ml 40 µg dose of HBsAg sub-type ad in an alum adjuvant. Three doses were given, the second one month and the third six months after the first. Adverse effects were mild and their incidence was similarly low in vaccine and placebo groups. The protective efficacy for all HBsAg positive infections was 88% and for clinical hepatitis B 92%. Those who did not develop anti-HBs in response to vaccination remained as susceptible as placebo recipients. Somewhat surprisingly, the failure to produce anti-HBs in response to vaccination did not appear to be associated with abnormal immune response to HBV infection; two vaccine recipients without detectable anti-HBs after three doses of vaccine acquired HBV infections and developed anti-HBs after recovery. An early reduction in the incidence of HBV infection in the vaccine group suggested that active immunisation might protect when given after exposure (209).

In controlled trials among susceptible staff and patients in dialysis units in France three doses of 1 ml, each continuing 5 µg of vaccine were given at monthly intervals. Adverse effects were mild and their incidence was similar in both vaccine and placebo groups. In response to vaccination 94% of staff but only 60% of patients developed anti-HBs. From two months after the beginning of the trial to the end of the year there were no HBV infections among staff recipients of vaccine but in the placebo group HBV infections continued. The protective efficacy for all HBsAg positive infections was 87%. Among patients the incidence of HBV infection was similar in both groups in the first two months of the trial; afterwards there were only two, both transient, in the vaccine group but there were 12 in the placebo group (210, 211). The overall protective efficacy for all HBsAg positive infections in patients appeared to be 54% but this estimate of vaccine efficacy is decreased by the inclusion of infections acquired before vaccination.

Studies of dialysis unit patients in the USA and France showed that women develop anti-HBs in response to vaccination more often than men do. Among patients in France, the anti-HBs response appeared to be age dependent; only 48% of those of 50 years or more but 80% of younger patients responded to vaccination (211, 212).

A large controlled trial of HBV vaccines in dialysis units in the USA is in progress and the results will be of interest. However, the evidence already available is sufficient to conclude that HBV vaccines can be expected to control and prevent dialysis associated HBV infection if immunisation is arranged to protect patients and staff before exposure in units with endemic HBV infection. This may be achieved by combining passive and active immunisation at the start of treatment or work in the units (213).

Investigations are being made of the possibilities of alternative HBV vaccines such as purified polypeptides, HBsAg synthesised by cell lines derived from primary liver carcinoma tissue or cloned in bacterial cells by recombinant DNA techniques or made of completely synthetic materials. None of these is available now.

Whatever vaccines are produced and however well vaccination programmes are arranged in dialysis units, an occasional failure must be expected. The protection afforded by anti-HBs actively acquired by natural means has been overcome occasionally (69, 78) and massive challenge doses given to chimpanzees will overcome the protection afforded by vaccination against smaller challenge doses (214).

In units in which HBV infection has been prevented by means other than immunisation, vaccination of patients and staff should be undertaken as an extra precaution rather than as an alternative method of prevention.

Dialysis associated hepatitis in the future

Most of the hepatitis observed in dialysis units throughout the world has been caused by HBV and immunisation can be expected to reduce type B infections to occasional sporadic events among those who have responded inadequately to vaccination. If the infection depended on HBV only, the era of widespread hepatitis in dialysis units would soon end. However, control of most TAH type B has revealed a high incidence of TAH NANB (46, 47). Some outbreaks appear to be caused by type NANB (159, 160) and retrospective studies suggest that both HBV and a NANB agent caused infections in an early outbreak with a high case fatality rate among staff (153, 215). It seems possible that NANB agents have been circulating in dialysis units with their effects obscured by HBV infection. Though NANB infections seemed of secondary importance in the past, they are now of particular interest as their nature and extent will dictate the size of the dialysis associated hepatitis problem in future.

The control of HBV infection will allow assessments of the incidence of clinical and sub-clinical NANB hepatitis and specific serological tests, when they become available, will indicate NANB infection rates. Meanwhile, though experience in any one country is not necessarily relevant to all, there is some evidence that NANB outbreaks, however widespread, are unlikely to be as dramatic as those caused by HBV. In the UK, observations of a large number of HBV-free units show an almost complete absence of any type of hepatitis among dialysis unit staff since the last HBV outbreak was controlled in 1973, although clustering of patients with raised aminotransferase levels is common (173). Whether the raised aminotransferase levels of patients are due to NANB infections or to other causes, it is clear that in the UK the removal of HBV infection from the units ended the excess hepatitis morbidity and mortality among staff. To patients, however, NANB infections may present a considerable risk; chronic hepatitis was a common outcome among affected patients in an outbreak ascribed to an NANB agent (160).

Possible means of reducing the risk of NANB infection of patients are similar to those considered for avoidance of HBV infection before HBsAg tests were developed, i.e., limitation of blood transfusions, use of ISG, observance of cross-infection precautions, isolation of affected patients.

The value of blood transfusion in improving the success of transplants precludes transfusion limitation, now that transplantation is the eventual aim for many dialysis patients (216). Aminotransferase testing of blood donors and rejection of those with levels above the midpoint of the normal range would reduce the introduction of NANB infection to dialysis units but, by analogy with the spread of HBV within units, seems unlikely to prevent it. Moreover, this type of non-specific screening presents considerable problems related to the management of blood donors.

ISG might afford either passive or active immunity to NANB infections if it contained either antibodies to NANB agents or antigen/antibody complexes that act as immunogens. However ISG has not conferred substantial protection against TAH NANB in the USA (123, 217) and frequently repeated doses given to patients in a dialysis unit did not control an outbreak of NANB hepatitis in the UK.

The observance of cross-infection precautions, which should be standard practice in all units, should help to limit cross-infection but without specific tests to detect symptomless NANB carriers for dialysis in isolation, spread to other patients may not be prevented in the long term.

The lack of specific tests to detect symptomless NANB carriers inhibits an effective isolation programme. Isolation of patients with raised aminotransferase levels will include patients without NANB infections and exclude infected patients whose levels may well remain within normal limits. Moreover, accommodation for dialysis in isolation of large numbers of patients is not available in most units.

The development of specific serological tests should, as with HBV infection, afford the key to control of any NANB infection in the units and lead eventually to the prevention of all dialysis associated hepatitis.

APPENDIX: LIST OF ABBREVIATIONS

Anti HAV	Antibody to hepatitis A virus
Anti HBc	Antibody to HB core antigen
Anti HBe	Antibody to HBe antigen
Anti HBs	Antibody to HB surface antigen
Ara-A	Adenine arabinoside
CAH	Chronic active hepatitis
CF	Complement fixation
CIE	Counter immunoelectrophoresis
CPH	Chronic persistent hepatitis
ELISA	Enzyme-linked immunosorbent assay
HAV	Hepatitis A virus
HBV	Hepatitis B virus
HBcAg	Hepatitis B core antigen
HBeAg	Hepatitis B e antigen
HBsAg	Hepatitis B surface antigen
HBIG	Anti HBs immunoglobulin
HLI	Human leukocyte interferon
ID	Immunodiffusion
ISG	Human normal immunoglobulin
NANB	Non-A, non-B hepatitis
PH	Passive haemagglutination
PHLS	Public Health Laboratory Service (UK)
PHC	Primary hepatocellular carcinoma
RIA	Radio immunoassay
RPHA	Reversed passive haemagglutination
TAH	Transfusion associated hepatitis

REFERENCES

1. Blumberg BS: Serum proteins and iso-precipitins. *Bull NY Acad Med* 40:377, 1964
2. On the State of the Public Health for the Year 1979. DHSS London, HMSO 1980 p 54
3. WHO Weekly Epidemiological Record. 52:253, 1977
4. Szmuness W, Prince AM: Epidemiologic patterns of viral hepatitis in Eastern Europe in the light of recent findings concerning the serum hepatitis antigen. *J. Infect Dis* 123:200, 1971
5. Mosley JW: Epidemiology of HAV infection. In: *Viral Hepatitis* edited by Vyas GN, Cohen SN, Schmid R, Philadelphia, Franklin Institute Press, 1978, p 85
6. McCollum RW: The natural history of hepatitis. *Bull NY Acad Med* 45:127, 1969
7. Szmuness W, Dienstag JL, Purcell RH: Distribution of antibody to hepatitis A antigen in urban adult population. *N Engl J Med* 295:755, 1976
8. Havens PW Jr, Paul JR: Infectious hepatitis and serum hepatitis. In: *Viral and Rickettsial Infections of Man*, edited by Horsfall FL, Tamm I, London, Pitman Medical, 1965, p 965
9. Orenstein WA, Wu E, Wilkins J, Robinson K, Francis DP, Timko N, Wayne R: Hospital-acquired hepatitis A: Report of an outbreak. *Pediatrics* 67:494, 1981
10. Wilson G: *The hazards of immunization*. London, The Athlone Press, University of London, 1967, p 111

11. Krugman S, Giles JP, Hammond J: Infectious hepatitis: evidence for two distinctive clinical epidemiological and immunological types of infection. *JAMA* 200:365, 1967
12. Murray R, Diefenbach WCL, Ratner F, Leone NC, Oliphant JW: Carriers of hepatitis virus in the blood and viral hepatitis in whole blood recipients. II. Confirmation of carrier state by transmission experiments in volunteers. *JAMA* 154:1072, 1954
13. WHO Tech. Rep. Ser. no. 512:1973
14. Tedder RS, Cameron CH, Wilson-Croome R, Howell DR, Colgrove A, Barbara JAJ: Contrast in patterns and frequency of antibodies to the surface, core and e antigens of hepatitis B virus in blood donors and homosexual patients. *J Med Virol* 6:323, 1980
15. Szmuness W, Harley EJ, Ikram H, Stevens CE: Sociodemographic aspects of the epidemiology of hepatitis B. In: *Viral Hepatitis* edited by Vyas GN, Cohen SN, Schmid R: Philadelphia, Franklin Institute Press, 1978, p 297
16. Stewart JS, Farrow LJ, Clifford RE, Lamb SGS, Coghill NF, Lindon RL, Sanderson IM, Dodd PA, Smith HG, Preece JW, Zuckerman AJ: A three year survey of viral hepatitis in West London. *Q J Med* XLVII (187):365, 1978
17. Szmuness W, Much MI, Prince AM, Hoofnagle JH, Cherubin CF, Harley EJ, Block GH: On the role of sexual behaviour in the spread of hepatitis B infection. *Ann Intern Med* 83:489, 1975
18. Koff RS, Slavin MM, Connelly LJD, Rosen DR: Contagiousness of acute hepatitis B. *Gastroenterology* 72:297, 1977
19. Perrillo RP, Gelb L, Campbell C, Wellington HW, Ellis FR, Overby L, Aach RD: Hepatitis e antigen, DNA polymerase activity and infection of household contacts with hepatitis B virus. *Gastroenterology* 76:1319, 1979
20. Hollinger FB, Weich J, Melnick JJ: A prospective study indicating that double-antibody radioimmunoassay reduces the incidence of post-transfusion hepatitis B. *N Engl J Med* 290:1104, 1974
21. Trepo C, Hantz O, Jacquier MF, Nenoz G, Cappel R, Trepo D: Different fates of hepatitis B virus markers during plasma fractionation. *Vox Sang* 45:143, 1978
22. Wands JR, Walker JA, Davis TT, Waterbury LA, Owens AH, Carpenter CCJ: Hepatitis B in an oncology unit. *N Engl J Med* 291:1371, 1974
23. Denes AE, Smith JL, Maynard JE, Doto IL, Berquist KR, Finkel AJ: Hepatitis B infection in physicians. *JAMA* 239:210, 1978
24. Magnius LO, Lindholm A, Lundin P, Iwarson S: A new antigen-antibody system. Clinical significance in long-term carriers of hepatitis B surface antigen. *JAMA* 231:356, 1975
25. Sutnick AI, London WT, Gerstley BJS, Cronkind MM, Blumberg BS: Anicteric hepatitis associated with Australia antigen occurrence in patients with Down's syndrome. *JAMA* 205:670, 1968
26. Grady GF, Gitnick GL, Prince AM, Kaplan MM, Fawaz KA, Vyas GN, Schmid R, Levitt MD, Galambos JT, Bynum TE, Senior JR, Akdamar K, Singleton JW, Clowdus BF, Steigman F, Aach RD, Schiff GM, Winkleman EL, Hersch T, Murphy BL, Hindman SH, Maynard JE: Relation of e antigen to infectivity of HBsAg positive inoculations among medical personnel. *Lancet* 2:492, 1976
27. Gerety RJ: Hepatitis B transmission between dental and medical workers and patients. *Ann Int Med* 95:229, 1981
28. Report of a Collaborative Study. Acute hepatitis B associated with gynaecological surgery. *Lancet* 1:1, 1980
29. Derso A, Boxall EH, Tarlow MJ, Flewett TH: Transmission of HBsAg from mother to infant in four ethnic groups. *Br Med J* 1:949, 1978
30. Krugman S, Giles JP: Viral hepatitis. New light on an old disease. *JAMA* 212:1019, 1970
31. Feinman SV, Berris B, Rebane A, Sinclair JC, Wilson S, Wrobel D: Failure to detect hepatitis B surface antigen (HBsAg) in feces of HBsAg positive persons. *J Infect Dis* 140:407, 1979
32. Heathcote J, Cameron CH, Dane DS: Hepatitis B antigen in saliva and semen. *Lancet* 1:71, 1974
33. Alter HJ, Purcell RH, Gerin JL, London WT, Kaplan PM, McAuliffe VJ, Wagner J, Holland PV: Transmission of hepatitis B to chimpanzees by hepatitis B surface antigen-positive saliva and semen. *Infect Immun* 16:928, 1977
34. Bond WW, Favero MS, Petersen NJ, Gravelle CR, Ebert JW, Maynard JE: Survival of hepatitis B virus after drying and storage for one week. *Lancet* 1:550, 1981
35. Leading article (Anonymous). Bedbugs, insects and hepatitis B. *Lancet* 2:752, 1979
36. Hawkes RA, Vale TG, Marshall JD: Contrasting seroepidemiology of Australia antigen and arbovirus antibodies in New Guinea. *Am J Epidemiol* 95:228, 1972
37. Gust ID, Dimitrakakis M, Zimmet P: Studies on hepatitis B surface antigen and antibody in Nauru. *Am J Trop Med Hyg* 27:1030, 1978
38. Tsuji T, Naito K, Tokuyama K, Okada T, Takata S, Shinohare T, Araki K, Equsa K, Nozaki H, Nagashina H, Kosaka K, Chen TC: An epidemiological study of viral hepatitis type B in Taichung, Taiwan. *Acta Med Okayama* 30:417, 1976
39. Blumberg BS, Sutnick AL, London WT, Melantin L: Sex distribution of Australia antigen. *Arch Intern Med* 130:227, 1972
40. Maupas P, Chiron J-P, Barin F, Coursaget P, Goudeau A: Efficacy of hepatitis B vaccine in prevention of early HBsAg carrier state in children. Controlled trial in an endemic area (Senegal). *Lancet* 1:289, 1981
41. Mosley JW: Hepatitis types B and non-B. Epidemiologic background. *JAMA* 233:967, 1975
42. Alter HJ, Holland PV, Purcell RH: The emerging pattern of post-transfusion hepatitis. *Am J Med Sci* 270:329, 1975
43. Hoofnagle JA, Gerety RJ, Tabor E, Feinstone SM, Barker LF, Purcell RH: Transmission of non-A, non-B hepatitis. *Ann Intern Med* 87:14, 1977
44. Tabor E, Gerety RJ, Drucker JA, Seeff LB, Hoofnagle JH, Jackson DR, April M, Barker LF, Pineda-Tamondong G: Transmission of non-A, non-B hepatitis from man to chimpanzee. *Lancet* 1:463, 1978
45. Bradley DW, Maynard JE, Cook EH, Ebert JW, Gravelle CR, Tsiquaye KN, Kessler H, Zuckerman AJ, Miller MF, Ling GM, Overby LR: Non-A/Non-B hepatitis in experimentally infected chimpanzees: Cross-challenge and electromicroscopic studies. *J Med Virol* 6:185, 1980
46. Aach RD, Lander JJ, Sherman LA, Miller WV, Kahn RA, Gitnick GL, Hollinger FB, Weich J, Szmuness W, Stevens CE, Kellner A, Weiner JM, Mosley JW: Transfusion-transmitted viruses: Interim analysis of hepatitis among transfused and non-transfused patients. In: *Viral Hepatitis* edited by Vyas GN, Cohen SN, Schmid R: Philadelphia Franklin Institute Press, 1978 p 383
47. Aach RD, Szmuness W, Mosley JW, Hollinger FB, Kahn R, Stevens CE, Edwards VM, Weich J: Serum alanine aminotransferase of donors in relation to the risk of non-A, non-B hepatitis in recipients. *N Engl J Med* 304:899, 1981
48. Report of a Medical Research Council Working Party. Post-transfusion hepatitis in a London hospital: results of

a two-year prospective study. *J Hyg (Camb)* 73:173, 1974
49. Iwarson S, Lindholm A, Norkrans G: Hepatitis B and non-A, non-B in a Swedish Blood Centre during 10 years of HBsAg screening. *Vox Sang* 39:79, 1980
50. Craske J, Dilling N, Stern D: An outbreak of hepatitis associated with intravenous injection of Factor VIII concentrate. *Lancet* 2:221, 1975
51. Dienstag JL, Alaama A, Mosley JW: Etiology of sporadic hepatitis B surface antigen-negative hepatitis. *Ann Intern Med* 87:1, 1977
52. Mathiesen LR, Papaevangelou G, Purcell RH, Grammatiloopoulos D, Contoyannis P, Wong D: Etiological characterization of hepatitis B surface antigen-negative hepatitis among adult patients in Athens, Greece. *J Clin Microbiol* 11:297, 1980
53. Kryger P, Aldershvile J, Christoffersen P, Hardt F, Juhl E, Mathiesen LR, Nielsen JO, Poulsen H: The Copenhagen hepatitis acuta programme. Acute non-A, non-B hepatitis. Clinical, epidemiological and histological characteristics. *Scand J Infect Dis* 12:165, 1980
54. Rakela J, Redeker AG: Chronic liver disease after acute non-A, non-B viral hepatitis. *Gastroenterology* 77:1200, 1979.
55. Khuroo MS, Saleem M, Teli MR, Sofi MA: Failure to detect chronic liver disease after epidemic non-A, non-B hepatitis. *Lancet* 2:97, 1980
56. Wong DC, Purcell RA, Sreenivasan MA, Prasad SR, Pavri KM: Epidemic and non-epidemic hepatitis in India: evidence for a non-A, non-B hepatitis. Viral aetiology. *Lancet* 2:876, 1980
57. Provost PJ, Hilleman MR: Propagation of human hepatitis A virus in cell culture in vitro. *Proc Soc Exp Biol Med* 160:213, 1979
58. Dienstag JL, Feinstone SM, Purcell RH, Hoofnagle JH, Barker LF, London WT, Popper H, Peterson JM, Kapikian AZ: Experimental infection of chimpanzees with hepatitis A virus. *J Infect Dis* 132:532, 1975
59. Bradley DW, Maynard JE, Hindman SH, Hornbech CL, Fields HA, McCaustland KA, Cook EH: Serodiagnosis of viral hepatitis A by radioimmunoassay. *J Clin Microbiol* 5:521, 1977
60. Mathiesen LR, Hardt F, Dietrichson O, Purcell RH, Wong D, Skinhøj P, Nielsen JO, Zoffman H, Iversen K: The Copenhagen hepatitis acuta programme. The role of acute hepatitis type A, B and non-A, non-B in the development of chronic active liver disease. *Scand J Gastroenterol* 15:49, 1980
61. Feinstone SM, Purcell RH: New methods for the serodiagnosis of hepatitis A. *Gastroenterology* 78:1092, 1980
62. Prince AM: An antigen detected in the blood during the incubation period of serum hepatitis. *Proc Natl Acad Sci USA* 60:814, 1968
63. Dane DS, Cameron CH, Briggs M: Virus-like particles in serum of patients with Australia-antigen associated hepatitis. *Lancet* 1:695, 1970
64. Almeida JD: Individual morphological variation seen in Australia antigen positive sera. *Am J Dis Child* 123:303, 1972
65. Huang SN: Hepatitis associated antigen hepatitis: an electron microscopic study of virus-like particles in liver cells. *Am J Pathol* 64:483, 1971
66. Krugman S, Overby LR, Mushahwar IK, Ling C-M, Frösner GG, Deinhardt F: Viral hepatitis type B. Studies on natural history and prevention re-examined. *N Engl J Med* 300:101, 1979
67. Shikata T, Karasawa T, Abo K, Takahashi T, Mayumi M, Oda T: Incomplete inactivation of hepatitis B virus after heat treatment at 60°C for 10 hours. *J Infect Dis* 138:242, 1978
68. Dudley FJ, Fox RA, Sherlock S: Cellular immunity and hepatitis-associated Australia antigen liver disease. *Lancet* 1:723, 1972
69. Barker LF, Peterson MR, Shulman NR, Murray R: Antibody responses in viral hepatitis, type B. *JAMA* 223:1005, 1973
70. Nielsen JO, Dietrichson O, Elling P, Christoffersen P: Incidence and meaning of persistence of Australia antigen in patients with acute viral hepatitis: development of chronic hepatitis. *N Engl J Med* 285:1157, 1971
71. Anderson KE, Stevens CE, Tsuai JJ, Lee W-C, Sun S-C, Beasley RP: Hepatitis B antigen in infants born to mothers with chronic hepatitis B antigenemia in Taiwan. *Am J Dis Child* 129:1389, 1975
72. Piccinino F, Manzillo G, Sagnelli E, Balestrieri GG, Maio G, Pasquale G, Felaco FM: The significance of the Australia antigen (HBsAg) persistent healthy carrier 'status': a long-term follow-up study of 34 cases. *Acta Hepatogastroenterol (Stuttg)* 25:171, 1978
73. Sampliner RE, Hamilton FA, Iserio A, Tabor E, Boitnott J: The liver histology and frequency of clearance of the hepatitis B surface antigen (HBsAg) in chronic carriers. *Am J Med Sci* 277:17, 1979
74. Reinicke V, Dybkjaer E, Poulsen H, Banke O, Lylloff K, Nordenfelt E: A study of Australia-antigen-positive blood donors and their recipients, with special reference to liver histology. *N Engl J Med* 286:867, 1972
75. de Franchis R, D'arminio A, Vecchi M, Ronchi G, del Ninno E, Parravicini A, Ferroni P, Zanetti AR: Chronic asymptomatic HBsAg carrier: histologic abnormalities and diagnostic and prognostic value of serologic markers of the HBV. *Gastroenterology* 79:521, 1980
76. Mazzor S, Szmuness W: Summary of Workshop. Chronic carriers of HBsAg. In *Viral hepatitis* edited by Vyas GN, Cohen SN, Schmid R: Philadelphia, Franklin Institute Press, 1978, p 661
77. Beasley RP, Hwang L-Y, Lin C-C, Chien CS: Hepatocellular carcinoma and hepatitis B Virus: a prospective study of 22 707 men in Taiwan. *Lancet* 2:1129, 1981
78. Grady GF, Lee VA: Hepatitis B. Immune globulin-prevention of hepatitis from accidental exposure among medical personnel. *N Engl J Med* 293:1067, 1975
79. Szmuness W, Prince AM, Grady GF, Mann MK, Levine RN, Friedman EA, Jacobs MJ, Josephson A, Ribot S, Shapiro FL, Stenzel KH, Suki WN, Vyas G: Hepatitis B infection: a point-prevalence study in 15 US hemodialysis centres. *JAMA* 227:901, 1974
80. Le Bouvier GL: The heterogeneity of Australia antigen. *J Infect Dis* 123:671, 1971
81. Bancroft WH, Mundon FK, Russell PK: Detection of additional antigenic determinants of hepatitis B antigen. *J Immunol* 109:842, 1972
82. Couroucé-Pauty AM, Drouet J, Kleinknecht D: Simultaneous occurrence in the same serum of hepatitis B surface antigen and antibody to hepatitis B surface antigen of different subtypes. *J Infect Dis* 140:975, 1979
83. Le Bouvier GL, Williams A: Serotypes of hepatitis B antigen (HBsAg): the problem of 'new' determinants, as exemplified by 't'. *Am J Med Sci* 270:165, 1975
84. Le Bouvier GL: Subtypes of hepatitis B antigen: clinical relevance? *Ann Intern Med* 79:894, 1973
85. Mosley JW, Edwards VM, Meihaus JE, Redeker AG: Subdeterminants d and y of hepatitis B antigen as epidemiological markers. *Am J Epidemiol* 95:529, 1974
86. Almeida JD, Rubenstein D, Stott EJ: New antigen-antibody system in Australia-antigen-positive hepatitis.

Lancet 2:1225, 1971
87. Hoofnagle JH, Gerety RJ, Ni LY, Barker LF: Antibody to hepatitis B core antigen: a sensitive indicator of persistent viral replication. *N Engl J Med* 290:1336, 1974
88. Hoofnagle JH, Gerety RJ, Barker LF: Antibody to hepatitis B core antigen. *Am J Med Sci* 270:179, 1975
89. Tedder RS, Wilson-Croome R: Detection by radioimmunoassay of IGM class antibody to hepatitis B core antigen. A comparison of two methods. *J Med Virol* 6:235, 1980
90. Magnius LO, Espmark JA: New specificities in Australia antigen positive sera distinct from the Le Bouvier determinants. *J Immunol* 109:1017, 1972
91. Katz D, Melnick JL, Hollinger FB: Characterization of HBeAg by physicochemical and immunochemical methods. *J Med Virol* 5:87, 1980
92. Trepo C, Hantz O, Vitvitski L, Chevallier P, Williams A, Lemaire JM, Sepetjian M: Heterogeneity and significance of HBeAg: characterization of a third specificity (e3). In: *Viral Hepatitis* edited by Vyas GN, Cohen SN, Schmid R: Philadelphia, Franklin Institute Press, 1978, p 203
93. Aldershvile J, Frösner GG, Nielsen JO, Hardt F, Deinhardt F, Skinhøj P: The Copenhagen hepatitis acuta programme. Hepatitis B e antigen and antibody measured by radioimmunoassay in acute hepatitis B surface antigen-positive hepatitis. *J Infect Dis* 141:293, 1980
94. Eleftheriou N, Thomas HC, Heathcote J, Sherlock S: Incidence and clinical significance of e antigen and antibody in acute and chronic liver disease. *Lancet* 2:1171, 1975
95. Trepo CG, Magnius LO, Schaefer RA, Prince AM: Detection of e antigen and antibody: correlations with hepatitis B surface and hepatitis B core antigens, liver disease and outcome in hepatitis B infections. *Gastroenterology* 71:804, 1976
96. Nielsen JO, Dietrichson O, Juhl E: Incidence and meaning of the e determinant among hepatitis B antigen positive patients with acute and chronic liver diseases. *Lancet* 2:913, 1974
97. Beasley RP, Trepo C, Stevens CE, Szmuness W: The e antigen and vertical transmission of hepatitis B surface antigen. *Am J Epidemiol* 105:94, 1977
98. Berquist KR, Maynard JE, Murphy BL: Infectivity of serum containing HBsAg and antibody to e antigen. *Lancet* 2:1026, 1976
99. Stevens CE, Neurath RA, Beasley RP, Szmuness W: HBeAg and anti-HBe detection by radioimmunoassay: correlation with vertical transmission of hepatitis B virus in Taiwan. *J Med Virol* 3:237, 1979
100. Tabor E, Ziegler JL, Gerety RJ: Hepatitis B e antigen in the absence of hepatitis B surface antigen. *J Infect Dis* 141:289, 1980
101. Kaplan PM, Greenman RL, Gerin JL, Purcell RH, Robinson WS: DNA polymerase associated with human hepatitis B antigen. *J Virol* 12:995, 1973
102. Kaplan PM, Gerin JL, Alter HJ: Hepatitis B — specific DNA polymerase activity during post-transfusion hepatitis. *Nature* 249:762, 1974
103. Nordenfelt E, Kjelten L: Dane particles, DNA polymerase and e antigen in two different categories of hepatitis B antigen carriers. *Intervirology* 5:225, 1975
104. Ibrahim AI, Vyas GN, Perkins HA: Immune response to hepatitis B surface antigen. *Infect Immun* 11:137, 1975
105. Dudley FJ, Guistino V, Sherlock S: Cell mediated immunity in patients positive for hepatitis-associated antigen. *Br Med J* 4:754, 1972
106. Guistino V, Dudley FJ, Sherlock S: Thymus dependent lymphocytic function in patients with hepatitis-associated antigens. *Lancet* 2:850, 1972
107. Newberry WH, Sanford JP: Defective cellular immunity in renal failure: depression of reactivity of lymphocytes to phytohemagglutination by renal failure serum. *J Clin Invest* 50:1262, 1971
108. Chisari FV, Routenberg JA, Anderson DS, Edgington TS: Cellular immune reactivity in HBV-induced liver disease. In: *Viral hepatitis* edited by Vyas GN, Cohen SN, Schmid R. Philadelphia, Franklin Institute Press, 1978, p 245
109. Report of a WHO Scientific Group: Laboratory methods for the detection of hepatitis B. Viral hepatitis. *WHO Tech Rep Ser* 570, 1975, p 12
110. Report of the WHO expert committee on viral hepatitis: Serological techniques for hepatitis B. *WHO Tech Rep Ser* 602, 1977, p 28
111. Bradley DW, Cook EM, Maynard JE, McCaustland KA, Ebert JW, Dolana GH, Petzel RA, Kantor RJ, Heilbrun A, Fields HA, Murphy BL: Experimental infection of chimpanzee with anti-hemophilic (factor VIII) materials: Recovery of virus-like particles associated with non-A, non-B hepatitis. *J Med Virol* 3:253, 1979
112. Yoshizawa H, Akahane Y, Itoh Y, Iwakiri S, Kitajima K, Morita M, Tanaka A, Nojiri T, Shimizu M, Miyakawa Y, Mayumi M: Virus like particles in a plasma fraction (fibrinogen) and in the circulation of apparently healthy blood donors capable of inducing non-A/non-B hepatitis in humans and chimpanzees. *Gastroenterology* 79:512, 1980
113. Hantz O, Vitvitski L, Trepo C: Non-A, Non-B hepatitis. Identification of hepatitis-B-like virus particles in serum and liver. *J Med Virol* 5:73, 1980
114. *WHO Weekly Epidem Rec* 55:249, 1980
115. Holland PV, Bancroft W, Zimmerman H: Post-transfusion viral hepatitis and the TTVS. *N Engl J Med* 304:1033, 1981
116. Rizzetto M, Hoyer B, Canese MG, Shih JW-K, Purcell RH, Gerin JL: Delta agent: association of delta antigen with hepatitis B surface antigen and RNA in serum of delta infected chimpanzees. *Proc Natl Acad Sci USA* 77:6144, 1980
117. Redeker AG: Clinical aspects of acute and chronic hepatitis. In: *Viral Hepatitis* edited by Vyas GN, Cohen SN, Schmid R. Philadelphia, Franklin Institute Press 1978, p 425
118. Sherlock S: Diseases of the Liver and Biliary system. Oxford, Edinburgh, Blackwell 1981, p 244
119. Weinbren K, Stirling GA: Pathology of viral hepatitis. *Br Med Bull* 28:125, 1972
120. Woolf IL, El Sheikh N, Cullens H, Lee WM, Eddleston ALWF, Williams R, Zuckerman AJ: Enhanced HBsAb production in pathogenesis of fulminant viral hepatitis type B. *Br Med J* 2:669, 1976
121. Aikat BK, Pandit VL, Gupta DA, Pal SR, Sengal S, Pathania AG, Chnuttani PN, Datta DV: Pathology and pathogenesis of fulminant hepatic failure — a review of 100 cases. *Indian J Med Res* 70:107, 1979
122. Redeker AG: Viral hepatitis: clinical aspects. *Am J Med Sci* 270:9, 1975
123. Knodell RG, Conrad ME, Ishak KG: Development of chronic liver disease after acute non-A, non-B post-transfusion hepatitis. *Gastroenterology* 72:902, 1977
124. Norkrans G, Frösner G, Hermodsson S, Iwarson S: Clinical epidemiological and prognostic aspects of hepatitis non-A, non-B - a comparison with hepatitis A and B. *Scand J Infect Dis* 11:259, 1979
125. Barker LF, Murray R: Acquisition of hepatitis associated antigen: clinical features in young adults. *JAMA* 216:1970, 1971
126. Popper H, Schaffner F: The vocabulary of chronic hepa-

titis. *N Engl J Med* 284:1154, 1971
127. Sherlock S: Predicting progression of acute type B hepatitis to chronicity. *Lancet* 2:354, 1976
128. Grady GF, Kaplan MM, Vyas GN: Antibody to hepatitis B core antigen in chronic hepatitis and primary biliary cirrhosis. *Gastroenterology* 72:590, 1977
129. Bassendine MF, Chadwick RG, Salmeron J, Shipton U, Thomas HC, Sherlock S: Adenine arabinoside therapy in HBsAg-positive chronic liver disease: a controlled study. *Gastroenterology* 80:1016, 1981
130. Weiman W, Heytink RA, Ten Kate FJP, Schalim SW, Masurel N, Shellekans H, Cantell K: Double-blind study of leucocyte interferon administration in chronic HBsAg positive hepatitis. *Lancet* 1:336, 1980
131. Merigan TC, Robinson WS: Antiviral therapy in HBV infection. In: *Viral Hepatitis* edited by Vyas GN, Cohen SN, Schmid R: Philadelphia, Franklin Institute Press, 1978, p 575
132. Scullard GH, Pollard RB, Smith JL, Sacks SL, Gregory PB, Robinson WS, Merigan TC: Antiviral treatment of chronic hepatitis B virus infection. I. Changes in viral markers with interferon combined with adenine arabinoside. *J Infect Dis* 143:772, 1981
133. Tabor E, Gerety RJ, Vogel CL, Bayley AC, Anthony PP, Chan CH, Barker LF: Hepatitis B virus infections and primary hepatocellular carcinoma. *J Natl Cancer Inst* 58:1197, 1977
134. Obata H, Hayashi N, Motoike Y, Aisainitsu T, Okuda H, Kobayashi S, Nishioka K: A prospective study on the development of hepatocellular carcinoma from liver cirrhosis with persistent hepatitis B virus infection. *Int J Cancer* 25:741, 1980
135. Trichopoulos D, Tabor E, Gerety RJ, Xirouchaki E, Sparros L, Munoz N, Linsell CA: Hepatitis B and primary hepatocellular carcinoma in a European population. *Lancet* 2:1217, 1978
136. Lutwick LI: Relation between aflatoxin hepatitis B virus and hepatocellular carcinoma. *Lancet* 1:755, 1979
137. Larouze B, London WT, Saimot G, Werner BG, Lustbader ED, Payet M, Blumberg BS: Host response to hepatitis B infection in patients with primary hepatic carcinoma and their families: a case/control study in Senegal, West Africa. *Lancet* 2:534, 1976
138. Drueke T, Barbanel C, Jungers P, Digeon M, Poisson M, Brivet F, Trecan G, Feldmann G, Crosnier J, Bach JF: Hepatitis B antigen-associated periarteritis nodosa in patients undergoing long-term hemodialysis. *Am J Med* 68:86, 1980
139. Gocke DJ: Extra-hepatic manifestations of viral hepatitis. *Am J Med Sci* 270:49, 1975
140. Trepo CG, Zuckerman AJ, Bird RC, Prince AM: The role of circulating B antigen/antibody immune complexes in the pathogenesis of vascular and hepatic manifestations in polyarteritis nodosa. *J Clin Pathol* 27:863, 1974
141. Levo Y, Gorevic PD, Kassab HJ, Zucher-Franklin D, Franklin EC: Association between hepatitis B virus and essential mixed cryoglobulinemia. *N Engl J Med* 296:1501, 1977
142. Bacon PA, Doherty SM, Zuckerman AJ: Hepatitis B antibody in polymyalgia rheumatica. *Lancet* 2:476, 1975
143. Gianotti F: Hepatitis B antigen in papular acrodermatitis in children. *Br Med J* 3:169, 1974
144. Combes B, Shorey J, Barrera A, Stastny P, Eigenbrodt EH, Hull AR, Carter NW: Glomerulonephritis with deposition of Australia antigen-antibody complexes in glomerular basement membrane. *Lancet* 2:234, 1971
145. Brzosko WJ, Krawczynski K, Nazarewicz T, Morzycka M, Nowoslawski A: Glomerulonephritis associated with hepatitis B surface antigen immune complexes in children. *Lancet* 2:477, 1974
146. Ringertz O, Nyström B: Viral hepatitis in connection with hemodialysis and kidney transplantation. *Scand J Urol Nephrol* 1:192, 1967
147. Jones PO, Goldsmith HJ, Wright FK, Roberts C, Watson DC: Viral hepatitis: a staff hazard in dialysis units. *Lancet* 1:835, 1967
148. London WT, DiFiglia M, Sutnick AI, Blumberg BS: An epidemic of hepatitis in a chronic hemodialysis unit. *N Engl J Med* 281:571, 1969
149. Eastwood JB, Curtis JR, Wing AJ, de Wardener HE: Hepatitis in a maintenance hemodialysis unit. *Ann Intern Med* 69:59, 1966
150. Knight AH, Fox RA, Baillod RA, Niazi SP, Sherlock S, Moorhead JF: Hepatitis associated antigen and antibody in haemodialysis patients and staff. *Br Med J* 3:603, 1970
151. Nordenfelt E, Lindholm T, Dahlquist E: A hepatitis epidemic in a dialysis unit: occurrence and persistence of Australia antigen among patients and staff. *Acta Pathol Microbiol Scand (B)* 78:692, 1970
152. *The Annual Report of the Chief Medical Officer of the Ministry of Health,* London, HMSO, 1965, p 46
153. Bone JM, Tonkin RW, Davison AM, Marmion BP, Robson JS: Outbreak of dialysis-associated hepatitis in Edinburgh, 1969-1970. *Proc Eur Dial Transpl Assoc* 8:189, 1971
154. Polakoff S, Cossart YE, Tillett HE: Hepatitis in dialysis units in the United Kingdom. *Br Med J* 3:94, 1972
155. Parsons FM, Brunner FP, Burck HC, Gräser W, Gurland HJ, Härlen H, Schärer K, Spies GW: Statistical report. *Proc Eur Dial Transpl Assoc* 11:53, 1974
156. Gurland HJ, Brunner FP, v Dehn H, Härlen H, Parsons FM, Schärer K: Combined report on regular dialysis and transplantation in Europe, III, 1972. *Proc Eur Dial Transpl Assoc* 10:XVII, 1973
157. Brynger H, Brunner FP, Chantler C, Donckerwolcke RA, Jacobs C, Kramer P, Selwood NH, Wing AJ: Combined report on regular dialysis and transplantation in Europe X 1979. *Proc Eur Dial Transpl Assoc* 1980, 17, 1980
158. Jacobs C, Broyer M, Brunner FP, Brynger H, Donkerwolcke RA, Kramer P, Selwood NH, Wing AJ, Blake PH: Combined report on regular dialysis and transplantation in Europe XI 1980. *Proc Eur Dial Transpl Assoc* 49, 1981
159. Galbraith RM, Portman B, Eddleston ALWF, Williams R, Gower PE: Chronic liver disease developing after outbreak of HBsAg-negative hepatitis in haemodialysis unit. *Lancet* 2:886, 1975
160. Szmuness W, Dienstag JL, Purcell RH, Prince AM, Stevens CE, Levine RW: Hepatitis type A and hemodialysis. *Ann Intern Med* 87:8, 1977
161. Seeff LB, Hoofnagle JH: Immunoprophylaxis of viral hepatitis. *Gastroenterology* 77:161, 1979
162. De Gast GC, Houwen B, van der Hem GK, The TH: T lymphocyte numbers and function and the course of hepatitis B in hemodialysis patients. *Infect Immun* 14:1138, 1976
163. London WT: Sex differences in response to hepatitis B virus, III. Responses to HBV and sex of donor and recipient in kidney and bone marrow transplantation. *Arthritis Rheum* 22:1267, 1979
164. Sengar DPS, McLeish WA, Sutherland M, Couture RA, Rashid A: Hepatitis B antigen (HBsAg) infection in a hemodialysis unit. I. HL-A8 and immune response to HBAg. *Can Med Assoc J* 112:968, 1975
165. Hillis WD, Hillis A, Bias WB, Walker WG: Association

of hepatitis B surface antigenemia with HLA locus B specificities. *New Engl J Med* 296:1310, 1977
166. Sengar DPS, Rashid A, McLeish WA, Harris JE, Couture RA, Sutherland M: Hepatitis B surface antigen (HBsAg) infection in a hemodialysis unit. II. Factors affecting host immune response to HBsAg. *Can Med Assoc J* 113:945, 1975
167. Arnold W, Hess G, Kösters W, Hütteroth TH, Meyer zum Büschenfelde KH: Hepatitis B-virus markers and immune complexes in HBsAg-positive patients on hemodialysis. *Acta Hepatogastroenterol* (Stuttg) 25:438, 1978
168. Hoofnagle JH, Seef LB, Bales ZB, Zimmerman HJ: Type B hepatitis after transfusion with blood containing antibody to hepatitis B core antigen. *N Engl J Med* 298:1379, 1978
169. Nagington J, Cossart YE, Cohen BJ: Re-activation of hepatitis B after transplantation operations. *Lancet* 1:558, 1977
170. Hillis WD, Hillis A, Walker WG: Hepatitis B surface antigenemia in renal transplant recipients. *JAMA* 242:329, 1979
171. London WT, Drew JS, Blumberg BS, Grossman RA, Lyons PJ: Association of graft survival with host response to hepatitis B infection in patients with kidney transplants. *N Engl J Med* 296:241, 1977
172. Stevens CE, Szmuness W, Zang EA: Hepatitis B virus markers and kidney transplant survival. Summary of workshop 8: HBV Markers (Part 2) Abstracts. In: *Viral Hepatitis Proceedings of the Third International Symposium,* edited by Szmuness W, Alter HJ, Maynard JE: Philadelphia, Franklin Institute Press, 1981, p 723
173. Polakoff S: Public Health Laboratory Service Survey: Hepatitis in dialysis units in the United Kingdom. *J Hyg (Camb)* 87:443, 1981
174. Simon P, Meyrier A, Menault M, Bombail D: Hepatitis non-A, non-B chez les hémodialysés: étiologie médicamenteuse. (Hepatitis non A, non B in haemodialysis patients: drug induced). *Nouv Presse Méd* 8:1186, 1979 (in French).
175. Neergaard J, Nielsen B, Faurby V, Christensen DH, Nielsen OF: Plasticizers in PVC and the occurrence of hepatitis in a haemodialysis unit. *Scand J Urol Nephrol* 5:141, 1971
176. Dankert J, Uitentuis J, Houwen B, Tegzess AM, van der Hem GK: Hepatitis B surface antigen in environmental samples from hemodialysis units. *J Infect Dis* 134:123, 1976
177. La Force FM, Nelson M: Air-rinsing after dialysis: a mode of transmission of hepatitis virus. *JAMA* 233:331, 1975
178. Almeida JD, Chisholm GD, Ku AI, MacGregor AB, Mackay DH, O'Donoghue EPN, Shackman R, Waterson AP: Possible airborne spread of serum hepatitis virus within a haemodialysis unit. *Lancet* 2:849, 1971
179. Medical Research Council Working Party of Subcommittee on Hepatitis Prevention in Renal and Associated Units: Experimental studies on environmental contamination with infected blood during haemodialysis. *J Hyg (Camb)* 74:133, 1975
180. Salo RJ, Salo AA, Fahlberg WJ, Ellzey JT: Hepatitis B surface antigen (HBsAg) in peritoneal fluid of HBsAg carriers undergoing peritoneal dialysis. *J Med Virol* 6:29, 1980
181. Teratar H, Kayhan B, Kes S, Karacadag S: HBAg in sweat. *Lancet* 2:461, 1974
182. Piazza M, Di Stasia G, Maio G, Marzano LA: Hepatitis B inhibitor in human faeces and intestinal mucosa. *Br Med J* 2:334, 1973
183. Public Health Laboratory Service: Infection risks of haemodialysis: some preventive aspects. *Br Med J* 3:454, 1968
184. Department of Health and Social Security: *Report of the Advisory Group on Hepatitis and the Treatment of Chronic Renal Failure 1970-1972.* London DHSS, 1972
185. Alter HJ, Purcell RH, Holland PV, Feinstone SM, Morrow AG, Monitsugu Y: Clinical and serological analysis of transfusion-associated hepatitis. *Lancet* 2:838, 1975
186. Turner GC, Bruce-White GB: SH antigen in haemodialysis-associated hepatitis. *Lancet* 2:121, 1969
187. Public Health Laboratory Service Survey: Decrease in the incidence of hepatitis in dialysis units associated with prevention programme. *Br Med J* 4:751, 1974
188. Public Health Laboratory Service: Hepatitis B in retreat from dialysis units in United Kingdom in 1973. *Br Med J* 1:1579, 1976
189. Postic B, Shreiner DP, Hanchett JE, Atchison RW: Containment of hepatitis B virus infection in a hemodialysis unit. *J Infect Dis* 138:884, 1978
190. Najem GR, Louria DB, Thind IS, Lavenham MA, Gocke MA, Gocke DJ, Baskin SE, Miller AM, Frankel HJ, Notkin J, Jacobs MG, Weiner B: Control of hepatitis B infection: The role of surveillance and an isolation hemodialysis center. *JAMA* 245:153, 1981
191. Surgenor DMacN, Chalmers TC, Conrad ME, Friedwald WT, Grady GF, Hamilton M, Mosley JW, Prince AM, Stengle JM: Clinical trials of hepatitis B immune globulin. *N Engl J Med* 293:1060, 1975
192. Krugman S, Giles JP, Hammond J: Viral hepatitis, type B (MS-2 strain): prevention with specific hepatitis B immune serum globulin. *JAMA* 218:1665, 1971
193. Desmyter J, Bradburne AF, Vermylen C, Daneels R, Beolaert J: Hepatitis B immunoglobulin in prevention of HBs antigenaemia in haemodialysis patients. *Lancet* 2:377, 1975
194. Kleinknecht D, Couroucé AM, Delons S, Naret C, Adhemar SP, Ciancioni C, Fermanian J: Prevention of hepatitis B in hemodialysis patients using hepatitis B immunoglobulin. *Clin Nephrol* 8:373, 1977
195. Iwarson S, Ahlmén J, Eriksson E, Hermodsson S, Kjellman H, Ljunggren C, Selander D: Hepatitis B immune globulin in prevention of hepatitis B among hospital staff members. *J Infect Dis* 135:473, 1977
196. Hoofnagle JH, Seef LB, Bales BZ, Wright EC, Zimmerman HJ: The Veterans Administration Cooperative Study Group. Passive-active immunity from hepatitis B immune globulin. *Ann Intern Med* 91:813, 1979
197. Couroucé-Pauty AM, Delons S, Soulier JP: Attempt to prevent hepatitis by using specific anti-HBs immunoglobulin. *Am J Med Sci* 270:375, 1975
198. Prince AM, Szmuness W, Mann MK, Vyas GN, Grady GF, Shapiro FL, Suki WN, Friedman EA, Avram MM, Stenzel KH: Hepatitis B immune globulin: Final report of a controlled multicentre trial of efficacy in prevention of dialysis-associated hepatitis. *J Infect Dis* 137:131, 1978
199. Reesink HW, Reerink-Brongers EE, Lafeber-Schut BJT, Kalshoren-Benschop J, Brummelhuis HGJ: Prevention of chronic HBsAg carrier state in infants of HBsAg-positive mothers by hepatitis B immunoglobulin. *Lancet* 2:436, 1979
200. Seeff LB, Wright EC, Zimmerman HJ, Alter HJ, Dietz AA, Felsher BF, Finkelstein JD, Garcia-Pont P, Gerin JL, Greenlee HB, Hamilton J, Holland PV, Kaplan PM, Kiernan T, Koff RS, Leevy CM, McAuliffe VJ, Nath N, Purcell RH, Schiff ER, Schwartz CC, Tamburro CH, Vlahcevic Z, Zemel R, Zimmon DS: Type B hepatitis after needlestick exposure: Prevention with hepatitis B immu-

noglobulin. *Ann Intern Med* 88:285, 1978
201. Grady GF, Lee VA, Prince AM, Gitnick GL, Fawaz KA, Vyas GN, Levitt MD, Senior JR, Galambos JT, Bynum TE, Singleton JW, Clowdus BF, Akdamar K, Aach RD, Winkleman EI, Schiff GM, Hersch T: Hepatitis B immune globulin for accidental exposures among medical personnel: final report of a multicentre controlled trial. *J Infect Dis* 138:625, 1978
202. Krugman S, Giles JP, Hammond J: Viral hepatitis, type B (MS-2 strain): studies on active immunization. *JAMA* 217:41, 1971
203. Redeker AG, Carpio NM, Gocke DJ: Increased anti-HBAg titres after administration of human protein solutions. *N Engl J Med* 287:102, 1972
204. Maynard JE, Krushak DH, Bradley DW, Berquist KP: Infectivity studies of hepatitis A and B in non-human primates. *Dev Biol Stand* 30:229, 1974
205. Tabor E, Gerety RJ: Inactivation of an agent of human non-A, non-B hepatitis by formalin. *J Infect Dis* 142:769, 1980
206. Hilleman MR, Buynak EB, Roehm RR, Tytell AA, Bertland AV, Lampson GP: Purified and inactivated human hepatitis B vaccine: Progress report. *Am J Med Sci* 270:401, 1975
207. Purcell RH, Gerin JL: Hepatitis B subunit vaccine: a preliminary report on safety and efficacy tests in chimpanzees. *Am J Med Sci* 270:395, 1975
208. Maupas P, Goudeau A, Coursaget P, Drucker J: Immunisation against hepatitis B in man. *Lancet* 1:1367, 1976
209. Szmuness W, Stevens CE, Harley EJ, Zang EA, Olesko WR, William DC, Sadovsky R, Morrison JM, Kellnar A: Hepatitis B vaccine. Demonstration of efficacy in a controlled clinical trial in a high-risk population in the United States. *N Engl J Med* 303:833, 1980
210. Crosnier J, Jungers P, Couroucé AM, Laplanche A, Benhamou E, Dagos F, Lacour B, Prunet P, Cerisier Y, Guersry P: Randomised placebo-controlled trial of hepatitis B Surface antigen vaccine in French haemodialysis units. I. Medical staff. *Lancet* 1:455, 1981
211. Crosnier J, Jungers P, Couroucé AM, Laplanche A, Benhamou E, Dagos F, Lacour B, Prunet P, Cerisier Y, Guesry P: Randomised placebo-controlled trial of hepatitis B surface antigen vaccine in French haemodialysis units. II. Haemodialysis patients. *Lancet* 1:797, 1981
212. Stevens CE, Szmuness W, Goodman AI, Wesely SA, Fotino M: Hepatitis B vaccine: immune responses in haemodialysis patients. *Lancet* 2:1211, 1980
213. Szmuness W, Stevens CE, Oleszo WR, Goodman A: Passive-active immunisation against hepatitis B: immunogenicity studies in adult Americans. *Lancet* 1:575, 1981
214. Prince AM, Hashimoto N, Neurath AR, Trepo C: Some considerations regarding active immunization with HBsAg. *Dev Biol Stand* 30:368, 1975
215. Marmion BP, Burrell CJ, Tonkin RW, Dickson J: Dialysis-associated hepatitis in Edinburgh; 1969–1978. *Reviews of Infectious Diseases* 4:619, 1982
216. Strom TB, Merrill JP: Hepatitis B, transfusions and renal transplantation. *N Engl J Med* 296:225, 1977
217. Kuhns WJ, Prince AM, Brotman B: A clinical and laboratory evaluation of immune serum globulin from donors with a history of hepatitis: attempted prevention of posttransfusion hepatitis. *Am J Med Sci* 272:255, 1976

35

RENAL OSTEODYSTROPHY AND MAINTENANCE DIALYSIS

JACK W. COBURN and FRANCISCO LLACH

Introduction	679
Vitamin D	679
Parathyroid Hormone	680
Pathogenesis	681
Secondary hyperparathyroidism	682
Phosphate retention	682
Abnormal vitamin D metabolism	682
Skeletal resistance to PTH	683
Altered renal degradation of PTH	683
Integration of pathogenic factors leading to secondary hyperparathyroidism	683
Defective mineralization of bone	683
Altered vitamin D metabolism	683
Hypophosphatemia	684
Altered metabolism and synthesis of collagen	684
Aluminum accumulation	684
Reduced plasma levels of parathyroid hormone	684
Histologic features of uremic bone disease	684
Techniques for bone biopsy	684
Osteitis fibrosa (fibro-osteoclasia)	687
Osteomalacia	688
Mixed skeletal lesion	688
Features of renal osteodystrophy	688
Symptoms and signs	688
Skeletal pain	688
Muscular weakness	688
Pruritus	689
Bone deformity and growth retardation	689
Fractures	689
Periarthritis	689
Tendon rupture	689
Calciphylaxis	689
Miscellaneous symptoms and signs	690
Biochemical features	690
Hyperphosphatemia	690
Hypophosphatemia	691
Hypocalcemia	692
Effect of hemodialysis on plasma Ca levels	692
Hypercalcemia	693
Hypermagnesemia	693
Plasma immunoreactive parathyroid hormone	694
Alkaline phosphatase, hydroxyproline and cyclic AMP	694
Radiographic features	694
Techniques	694
Subperiosteal erosions	694
Abnormalities of the skull	696
Periosteal neostosis	696
Alterations in growth zone	696
Osteosclerosis	697
Features of osteomalacia	697
Osteopenia	698
Bone mineral content	698
The Metacarpal Index	698
Scintiscan	698
Soft-tissue calcifications	698
Prevention and management	699
General management	699
Control of hyperphosphatemia	699
Calcium concentration in dialysis fluid	700
Oral calcium supplements	700
Dialysate magnesium	700
Fluoride-containing water	700
Aluminum-containing water	700
Heparin	700
Specific treatment	701
Vitamin D sterols	701
Treatment failure groups	702
Parathyroidectomy	703
Other treatments	705
Fractures	705
Extraskeletal calcifications	705
Acknowledgments	705
References	705

INTRODUCTION

In this discussion, the term 'renal osteodystrophy' will be used in a generic sense to include all the clinical syndromes of skeletal disease and altered calcium (Ca), phosphorus (P) homeostasis resulting from renal failure. The skeletal pathology can include osteitis fibrosa and other features of secondary hyperparathyroidism, osteomalacia, osteoporosis, osteosclerosis, and in children, retardation of growth. Emphasis will be placed on the manifestations of these syndromes that occur in patients on regular hemodialysis with a consideration of their pathogenesis, prevention and management.

Vitamin D

The term vitamin D is used to include vitamin D_3 or cholecalciferol, the naturally occurring sterol present in animals, and vitamin D_2 or ergocalciferol, a sterol generated through the ultraviolet irradiation of a plant precursor. Vitamin D_3 undergoes two step metabolism: first in the liver, where it is converted to 25-hydroxyvitamin $D_3 [25(OH)D_3]$ and the second in the kidney where the biologically active form, 1,25-dihydroxyvitamin $D_3 [1,25(OH)_2D_3]$ is produced (Figure 1). Thus, the kidney plays an important endocrine role by producing $1,25(OH)_2D_3$, the active hormone, from

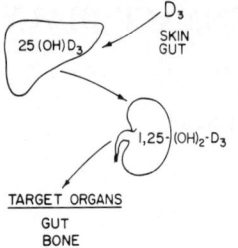

Figure 1. Schema showing the conversion of vitamin D₃ (D₃) to 25-hydroxyvitamin D₃ (25 (OH) D₃ or calciferol) in the liver and subsequently to 1,25 dihydroxyvitamin D₃ (1,25(OH)₂D₃) or calcitriol in the kidney.

25(OH)D₃.

Vitamin D₃ itself, is produced in the skin where ultraviolet irradiation converts 7 dehydrotachysterol to previtamin D, which, in turn, is converted to vitamin D (1). The latter leaves the skin attached to a specific, high affinity carrier-protein in plasma, an alpha₂-globulin (2). Cholecalciferol is carried to the liver where it is converted to 25(OH)D₃ (3). This conversion of vitamin D₃ to 25(OH)D₃ (or calcifediol) is not well regulated. The 25(OH)D₃, which is carried bound to the same vitamin D-binding protein, has a very slow turnover rate, i.e. t½ = 20 to 25 days, and it may represent a circulating, 'storage' form of vitamin D (4). The metabolic conversion of 25(OH)D₃ to 1,25(OH)₂D₃ (or calcitriol) in the proximal tubular cells is highly regulated; this conversion is closely controlled by various factors related to the need of the organism for Ca and P (5, 6). This last step is stimulated by low Ca diet and hypocalcemia, probably mediated via the action of parathyroid hormone (PTH), which is an important tropic factor for the bioactivation of vitamin D (7). The metabolic conversion to 1,25(OH)₂D₃ is also stimulated by a low P diet, and it may be augmented during certain physiologic events such as pregnancy, lactation, and growth, which are associated with increased needs for calcium (8, 9).

Calcitriol, is also bound to the vitamin-D-binding protein but with less affinity than is 25(OH)D₃; it is carried to several target tissues, including the intestine, bone, kidney and parathyroid glands (9, 10). Its best known action is on the intestine, where it enhances the active absorption of both calcium and phosphorus. It acts in the bone both to mobilize calcium, particularly in the presence of PTH, and to bring about the normal mineralization of osteoid. This may occur through the elevation of plasma Ca and P but also through a specific action on collagen metabolism. There are also cellular receptors for 1,25(OH)₂D₃ in the parathyroid glands, the pancreas, the kidneys and the salivary glands, although it's actions in these tissues are uncertain. Calcitriol may also have an action on striated muscle, although receptors have not been identified. Most evidence indicates that 1,25(OH)₂D₃ exerts its biological action in a manner similar to other steroid hormones (9, 10). Thus, the sterol is bound to a specific cytosolic receptor, the receptor-hormone complex is transported from the cell cytosol to the nucleus where it induces the synthesis of messenger RNA, which in turn may stimulate protein synthesis. The synthesis of one or more proteins, one of which may be calcium binding protein, facilitates the entry of calcium into the cell and induces its transepithelial transport. It is presumed that 1,25(OH)₂D₃ may act in a similar way on other target tissues.

In the absence of vitamin D, there is abnormally low intestinal absorption of Ca and, to a lesser extent, of P. This results in hypocalcemia, which leads to secondary hyperparathyroidism and hypophosphatemia. Also, there is impaired mineralization of osteoid (osteomalacia) and proximal myopathy, a prominent feature of vitamin D deficiency is usually present (11).

Another naturally occurring vitamin D sterol is 24,25 dihydroxyvitamin D₃(24,25(OH)₂D₃). This sterol is produced in the kidney, but perhaps also in the intestine and bone. The absence, or very low levels, of serum 24,25(OH)₂D₃ in anephric animals and humans (12) suggests that the kidney is primarily responsible for its generation. The biologic role of 24,25(OH)₂D₃ is controversial. Some data suggest that when given alone or in combination with calcitriol, 24,25(OH)₂D₃ may tend to lower plasma calcium (13) and to stimulate bone mineralization (14): other data suggest it may suppress PTH secretion (15). However, certain mammals may function well without 24,25(OH)₂D₃ (16). Further studies are needed to clarify the role of 24,25(OH)₂D₃ in man under physiologic circumstances and in pathologic states.

Parathyroid hormone

Parathyroid hormone is a single chain polypeptide of 84 amino acids, which is secreted in response to a fall in blood Ca and, to a lesser degree, by changes in the β-adrenergic system. Thus, there is a vital relationship between plasma Ca and PTH, and small changes in plasma Ca can influence hormonal secretion. Most changes in PTH occur as plasma Ca varies from 1.88 to 2.63 mmol/l (7.5 to 10.5 mg/dl [17]); changes in plasma Ca above or below this range have minor effects on PTH secretion (Figure 2). A small but important fraction of PTH secretion is not affected by the plasma Ca level; some basal PTH secretion has been demonstrated in the presence of substantial hypercalcemia (18). The β-adrenergic system, epinephrine and norepinephrine, can augment PTH secretion, and acute hypermagnesemia can suppress PTH secretion, at least transiently (19, 20).

The intact PTH molecule, with a molecular weight of 9500, is secreted into the blood; it undergoes rapid cleavage in the liver and kidney with the release of several fragments (21). There are several biologically inactive carboxy-terminal (C-terminal) fragments with molecular weights of approximately 7,000 which have a circulating half life of 15 to 60 min; the small biologically active, amino-terminal (N-terminal) fragment, with a molecular weight of 3500 to 4000, has a half life of only 4 to 5 min (22). The C-terminal fragments are removed from the circulation only by the kidney (23, 24); the N-terminal fragment is metabolized primarily by the skeleton (25). The circulating half-life of the C-terminal frag-

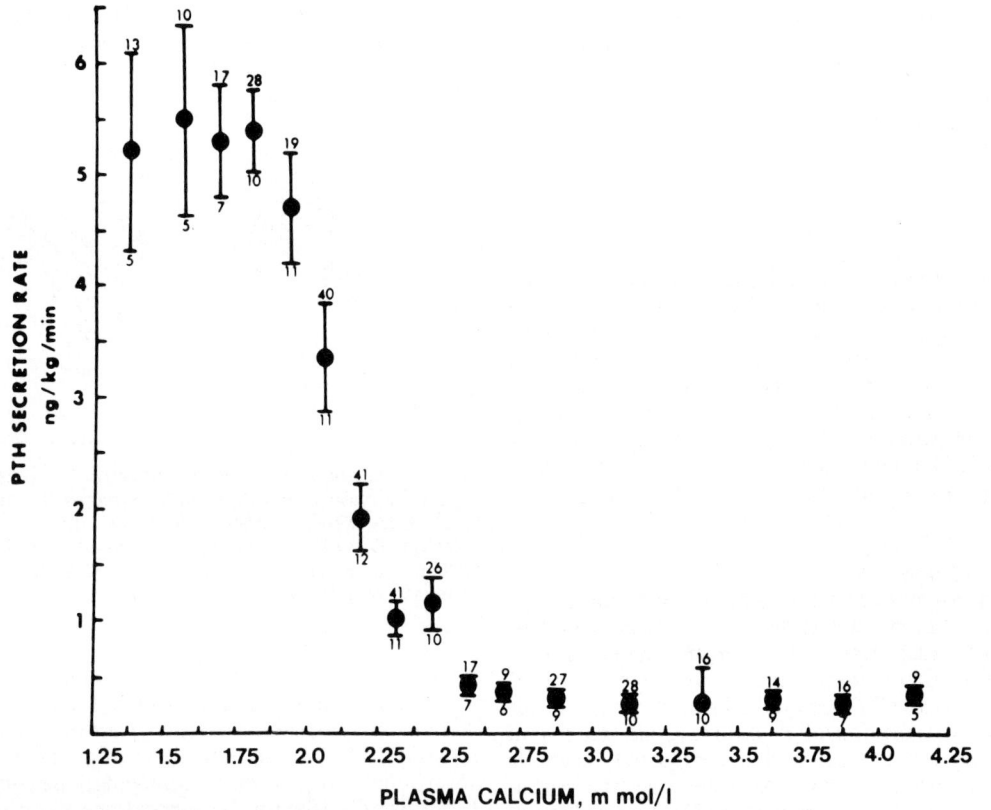

Figure 2. Secretory response of bovine parathyroid gland to changes in plasma Ca. The symbols and vertical bars indicate the secretory rate (mean ± SE). Note the sigmoidal nature of the relationship between secretory rate and plasma calcium concentration. (Modified after Mayer et al [17]).

(Ca: mmoles/l → mg/dl: multiply by 4
Ca: mmoles/l → mEq/l: multiply by 2)

ments is much longer than those of either the N-terminal fragment or intact PTH; thus, the blood level of C-terminal fragments is higher, and they are more often measured by available radioimmunossays. Because the kidney is the only organ capable of degrading the C-terminal fragments, patients with renal insufficiency commonly have very high serum levels of PTH as measured by C-terminal assays.

Parathyroid hormone acts on the kidney and bone via activation of an adenylate cyclase system. In the kidney, PTH inhibits the reabsorption of phosphate and stimulates the conversion of $25(OH)D_3$ to $1,25(OH)_2D_3$. With end stage renal failure, these biological actions becomes less important. In bone, PTH increases the conversion of mesenchymal cells to osteoclasts, increases bone resorption and activates osteoblasts. Hence, the effect of PTH is to increase bone resorption and formation, with an increase in bone turnover.

PATHOGENESIS

The striking skeletal abnormalities observed in advanced uremia are believed to have their origin early in

Table 1. Pathogenic factors in uremic bone disease.

A. *Hypocalcemia and secondary hyperparathyroidism*
 1. P retention with hyperphosphatemia
 2. Altered vitamin D metabolism
 3. Skeletal resistance to PTH
 4. Reduced degradation of PTH

B. *Defective skeletal mineralization*
 1. Abnormal collagen synthesis (vitamin D related?)
 2. Abnormal crystal growth and maturation
 3. Skeletal accumulation of aluminum
 4. Accumulation of skeletal Mg
 5. Accumulation of pyrophosphate
 6. Reduced carbonate content

C. *Other factors of uncertain or variable role*
 1. Heparin administration
 2. Acidosis
 3. Phosphate deficiency
 4. Skeletal accumulation of fluoride
 5. Absence of PTH
 6. Modification produced by therapy
  a. anticonvulsants
  b. parathyroidectomy
  c. vitamin D

the course of progressive renal disease. Since this chapter emphasizes features of advanced renal disease, these pathogenic events will be discussed only briefly (Table 1); the readers are referred elsewhere for detailed reviews (11, 26-29).

Secondary hyperparathyroidism

A decrease in the level of ionized Ca in plasma which leads to secretion of PTH and to parathyroid gland hyperplasia, occurs early in the course of renal insufficiency. As renal disease advances, hypocalcemia and parathyroid hyperplasia may become marked (30). The factors believed to lead to hypocalcemia include: 1) phosphate retention with hyperphosphatemia; 2) abnormal vitamin D metabolism, and 3) decreased skeletal response to the calcemic action of PTH.

Phosphate retention

It has been proposed that transient and even undetectable elevations in plasma P develop in early renal failure (31, 32). Such transient hyperphosphatemia may lower plasma Ca, thereby stimulating the parathyroid glands to increase PTH secretion. This, in turn, reduces the tubular reabsorption of P, returning plasma P and Ca levels toward normal and a new steady state is achieved. Observations that phosphate ingestion stimulates PTH secretion in normal man (33), that reduction in P intake in proportion to the decrease in GFR can largely prevent secondary hyperparathyroidism in experimental renal failure (32), and the finding that plasma PTH correlates positively with plasma P in uremia (34) support this view. However, plasma levels of both Ca and P may be reduced in patients with mild renal failure (35, 36), data that are inconsistent with this theory.

Overt hyperphosphatemia occurs only when renal function decreases below 25% of normal (30), and then it contributes to the degree of hypocalcemia and secondary hyperparathyroidism. Because of the importance of hyperphosphatemia, the factors which can contribute to an elevation in plasma P in end-stage renal disease (ESRD) are discussed in more detail below.

Abnormal vitamin D metabolism

Reduced metabolism of vitamin D to its active hormonal forms may also contribute to the development of hypocalcemia. Several lines of evidence support the view that vitamin D metabolism is abnormal in renal failure. There is diminished net intestinal absorption of Ca, which is unresponsive to doses of vitamin D that can cure nutritional rickets; there is defective skeletal mineralization (i.e., osteomalacia); and there is a failure to elevate plasma Ca normally following a standardized challenge with parathyroid hormone extract (PTE), which is also a feature of vitamin D deficiency.

The kidney is the only known site of the production of $1,25(OH)_2D_3$, the most active hormonal form of vitamin

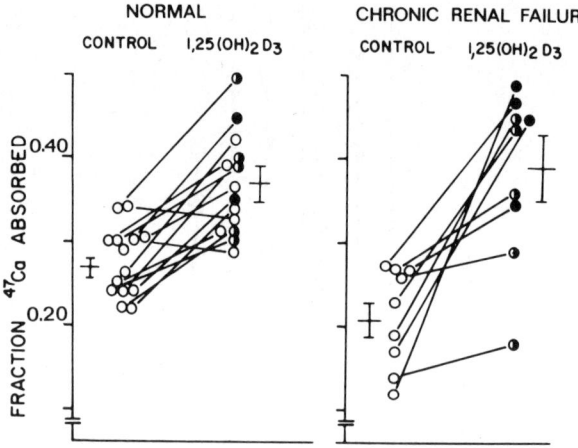

Figure 3. Changes in intestinal calcium absorption (^{47}Ca) in normal individuals and those with advanced chronic renal failure. Values were obtained before and after treatment with $1,25(OH)_2D_3$, 0.6 to 2.7 µg/day, for 7 to 10 days. The horizontal bars and brackets indicate mean ± SEM (Reprinted from Brickman et al [192] with permission).

in D. Observations in patients with end-stage renal failure that plasma levels of $1,25(OH)_2D_3$ are low (37), the failure of conversion of radiolabelled $25(OH)D_3$ to $1,25(OH)_2D_3$ (38), and the restoration of intestinal Ca absorption to normal following treatment with $1,25(OH)_2D_3$ (Figure 3), support the concept that the renal production of $1,25(OH)_2D_3$ is impaired in advanced renal failure (39, 40).

When in the course of progressive renal impairment, abnormal vitamin D metabolism develops is uncertain. Patients with serum creatinine levels below 220 µmol/l (2.5 mg/dl) exhibit normal gut Ca absorption (35), while those with greater azotemia have malabsorption of Ca. As renal disease progresses, this abnormality worsens, and intestinal Ca absorption decreases further in dialysis patients after bilateral nephrectomy (41). Such observations suggest that the diseased kidney generates only a small amount of $1,25(OH)_2D_3$.

Despite low plasma levels of $1,25(OH)_2D_3$ in most patients with advanced renal failure (37), osteomalacia is not invariably present. The explanation for this is unknown, but hyperphosphatemia may modify or ameliorate the mineralizing defect caused by a deficiency of $1,25(OH)_2D_3$

The mechanism for decreased production of $1,25(OH)_2D_3$ in renal failure is uncertain. A decrease in renal tissue mass could be the cause; also, it is possible that some metabolic consequence of uremia, i.e., P retention, acidosis, etc., could reduce the renal production of $1,25(OH)_2D_3$. The kidney is the primary organ responsible for generation of $24,25(OH)_2D_3$, a sterol which has been postulated to augment bone mineralization and which may have actions other than those of $1,25(OH)_2D_3$ (13). Serum levels of $24,25(OH)_2D_3$ are absent or undetectable in anephric humans (12).

A lack of the active form of vitamin D may have other consequences important in the pathogenesis of

Table 2. Consequences of lack of active forms of vitamin D.

A. *Intestine*
  1. Reduced Ca absorption
  2. Reduced P absorption

B. *Skeleton*
  1. Altered collagen synthesis
  2. Reduced responsiveness of bone to PTH
  3. Impaired mineralization
  4. Retarded growth

C. *Parathyroid*
  1. Impaired parathyroid suppression by elevated serum Ca (?)

D. *Muscle*
  1. Proximal myopathy

---

uremic bone disease (Table 2). Intestinal P absorption may be reduced in uremia, and $1,25(OH)_2D_3$ administration augments net intestinal absorption of P (42). Among the consequences of vitamin D deficiency on the skeleton is an alteration in the development of normal cross-linkages between collagen molecules, which may contribute to altered mineralization (43); a similar phenomenon may occur in uremia (44, 45). Presently, there is no agreement whether vitamin D stimulates mineralization directly or by its effect on the extracellular fluid Ca and P levels. The clinical observations in vitamin D deficiency that the skeleton remineralizes following vitamin D treatment, while plasma Ca and P remain unchanged, support a direct effect of vitamin D on bone mineralization. Impaired P absorption in patients with ESRD also may contribute to the development of osteomalacia.

Skeletal resistance to PTH
Patients with renal failure exhibit skeletal resistance to the calcium-mobilizing action of PTH, and such an abnormality is an important factor leading to hypocalcemia and secondary hyperparathyroidism (46, 47). The infusion of parathyroid extract to patients with mild and advanced renal insufficiency and to those undergoing dialysis fails to elevate plasma Ca to normal (48). This resistance to parathyroid extract is unrelated to the magnitude of hyperphosphatemia, hypocalcemia or the preinfusion plasma level of immunoreactive parathyroid-hormone (iPTH). Also, resistance to endogenous PTH can be shown (49). The reasons for this PTH resistance are unclear, but high concentrations of uremic metabolites (50), phosphate retention (47) or deficiency of $1,25(OH)_2D_3$ (51) may all play a role.

Altered renal degradation of PTH
The kidney plays a primary function in the degradation of PTH, particularly the C-terminal fragments (23, 24, 52). Patients with renal insufficiency have impaired degradation of these fragments, with their consequent accumulation in the circulation. Thus, the plasma levels of the C-terminal fragments which are measured with several currently available radioimmunoassays, are higher in dialysis patients than in patients with primary hyperparathyroidism. The metabolic clearance of the intact PTH molecule is also prolonged in dialysis patients, a factor which may contribute to prolonged action of PTH, aggravating the renal bone disease (28).

Integration of the pathogenic factors leading to secondary hyperparathyroidism
The relative roles of these factors in leading to hypocalcemia and secondary hyperparathyroidism in renal insufficiency are uncertain. Phosphate retention, which may occur in early renal failure, could impair the renal production of $1,25(OH)_2D_3$ (53) to provide yet another cause for hypocalcemia. Such a deficiency of $1,25(OH)_2D_3$ could reduce the calcemic response to PTH. Preliminary observations indicate that dietary P restriction in proportion to the reduction of GFR in patients with mild renal failure can raise the serum level of $1,25(OH)_2D_3$, enhance intestinal Ca absorption, reduce serum iPTH, and improve the calcemic response to PTH (54). In advanced renal failure, it is likely that hyperphosphatemia, *per se*, plays an important role in aggravating hypocalcemia and aggravating the secondary hyperparathyroidism.

Defective mineralization of bone

Defective mineralization or osteomalacia is another pathogenic process which can involve bone in patients with advanced renal failure. In contrast to secondary hyperparathyroidism which can be evaluated by measuring the plasma levels of iPTH, impaired mineralization or osteomalacia is not easy to detect. Moreover, the identification of the pathogenesis is less well understood.

Altered vitamin D metabolism
Since the plasma levels of $1,25(OH)_2D$ are markedly depressed in patients with advanced renal failure (55, 56), it is surprising that impaired mineralization is not observed more frequently in patients with end-stage uremia. Indeed, osteomalacia may be absent even in anephric patients (57). Factors which contribute to a low frequency of osteomalacia may be the presence of hyperphosphatemia and the normal levels of other vitamin D steroid, such as $25(OH)D_3$ or $24,25(OH)_2D_3$, which may contribute to normal bone mineralization (58, 59). The magnitude of sunlight exposure and supplementation of food with vitamin D in various parts of the world may account for differences in the incidence of osteomalacia seen in uremic patients from various renal units. Renal losses of $25(OH)D_3$ may be significant in patients with the nephrotic syndrome and marked proteinuria (60, 61) and may contribute to low plasma levels of $25(OH)D$ and to osteomalacia. A role of depressed generation of $24,25(OH)_2D_3$ in contributing to osteomalacia is possible but unproven. There is preliminary evidence that treatment with $24,25(OH)_2D_3$ plus $1,25(OH)_2D_3$ may result in bone mineralization of patients with osteomalacia (14) and that $24,25(OH)_2D_3$ can lower plasma Ca in contrast to the action of $1,25(OH)_2D_3$ (13); also, observations in animals suggest

that mineralization of bone is more normal with a combination of $1,25(OH)_2 D_3$ plus $24,25(OH)_2 D_3$ than with $1,25(OH)_2 D_3$, alone (59).

Hypophosphatemia
Subnormal levels of plasma phosphorus can contribute to impaired mineralization of bone; and in some reports there was a correlation between osteomalacia and a low plasma $Ca \times P$ product in patients with advanced renal failure and those undergoing dialysis (62). On the other hand, such a relationship has not been observed by others, and varying phosphate intake in different parts of the world may be an important factor leading to differing incidences of osteomalacia.

Altered metabolism and synthesis of collagen
The synthesis and maturation of collagen is abnormal in uremia and may contribute to impaired mineralization (43-45). Moreover, experimental evidence suggests that vitamin D may improve the maturation of collagen and enhance bone mineralization, observations suggesting that abnormal vitamin D metabolism could contribute to altered collagen metabolism (44, 45). Difficulties involved in the study of collagen metabolism in humans have limited such investigation to experimental animals.

Aluminum accumulation
Reports from certain geographic areas of the world, including the United Kingdom and parts of North America, suggest that osteomalacia is more prominent in areas where tap water with high levels of aluminum is used to prepare dialysis fluid (63, 64). Moreover, there is a strong association between osteomalacic bone disease and dialysis encephalopathy, an entity which is common in dialysis centers with aluminum-rich water (63, 65). Moreover, appropriate purification of water has resulted in marked reduction in the incidence of both the bone disease and the encephalopathy. Also, trabecular bone content of aluminum is strikingly elevated in dialysis patients with osteomalacia (66), and the parenteral administration of large quantities of aluminum to rats led to impaired mineralization of the endochondrial cartilage (67). The mechanisms for the accumulation of aluminum is unclear at times; thus, it may arise from aluminum-containing dialysate in some cases, while it is likely that aluminum is absorbed from the intestinal tract in others ([66] see also Chapters 41 and 42).

Reduced plasma levels of parathyroid hormone
One feature of uremic patients with osteomalacia is the finding of normal or even low levels of plasma iPTH (68); moreover, the osteomalacic syndrome may appear following total or sub-total parathyroidectomy (69, 70). The characteristics of this syndrome are low rates of bone apposition and turnover; these may occur as a result of the reduced levels of PTH. Thus, the degree of formation of the 'calcification front', an index of bone formation, was directly related to plasma iPTH levels in one study of dialysis patients (69). Although low levels of plasma iPTH can occur after parathyroidectomy, they are also seen in dialysis patients without parathyroid surgery. Also, patients with osteomalacia have plasma iPTH levels that do not increase during an acute hypocalcemic stimulus, adding further evidence for the presence of an abnormality in PTH secretion (71).

HISTOLOGIC FEATURES OF UREMIC BONE DISEASE

Techniques for bone biopsy

The study of bone itself, has evolved into a clinically useful tool for understanding the pathophysiologic processes involved and as a guide to the management of renal osteodystrophy. Under local anesthesia, a bone biopsy can easily and safely be obtained from the iliac crest. The sample, 5×20 mm, containing trabecular bone and both tables of cortices (72) is fixed in neutral formalin, then transferred to alcohol to prevent Ca loss, and embedded in a hard plastic, such as methacrylate. Thin sections of the undecalcified bone can be cut with a special microtome having a heavy steel blade. Uncalcified osteoid and calcified bone can be readily identified with such methods, unlike the specimen of bone prepared with the usual decalcification. Examples are shown in Figure 4.

In addition to the qualitative interpretation of the features of bone histology, a quantification of various features and bone dynamics with tetracycline labeling can increase the sensitivity of the method and aid in comparison of biopsy samples. One method utilizes a grid eye-piece placed in the microscope (73); the surfaces of trabecular bone which intersect the grid markings are identified as *forming* (i.e., with osteoblasts and osteoid), *resorbing* (with osteoclasts and Howship's lacunae) or

Figure 4. A. A representative bone biopsy from a patient with osteitis fibrosa. Distinctive features include large multi-nucleated osteoclasts located in a resorption cavity; osteoid covered with multiple columnar osteoblasts (orange color) and marked endosteal fibrosis (Goldner stain $\times 200$).
B. Unstained section of a bone biopsy of a patient with osteitis fibrosa after double tetracycline label. Note the presence of active mineralization and bone formation as evidenced by the uptake of tetracycline and the presence of a double label (yellow bands). The lack of well demarcated label lines demonstrates a disorganized and abnormal mineralization ($\times 200$).
C. A representative bone biopsy from a patient with osteomalacia. Characteristic features include broad osteoid seams (red color), lack of cellular activity, irregular scalloped interface between osteoid and mineralized bone (green color) and the absence of marrow fibrosis (Goldner stain $\times 200$).
D. Unstained section of a patient with osteomalacia after double tetracycline label. Note the marked decrease in tetracycline uptake evidencing the lack of mineralization. The osteoid seams appear as a lighter shade of green than the mineralized bone ($\times 200$).

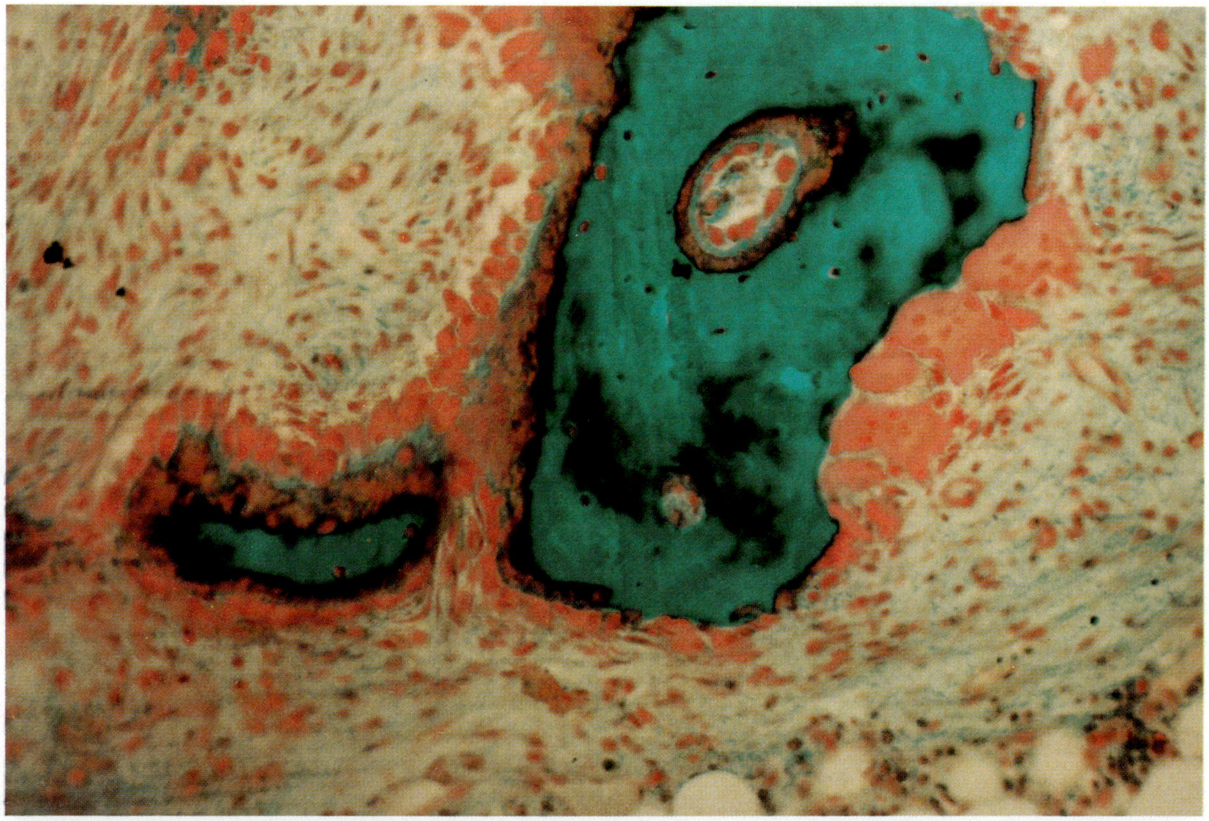

35: *Renal osteodystrophy and maintenance dialysis* 685

4A

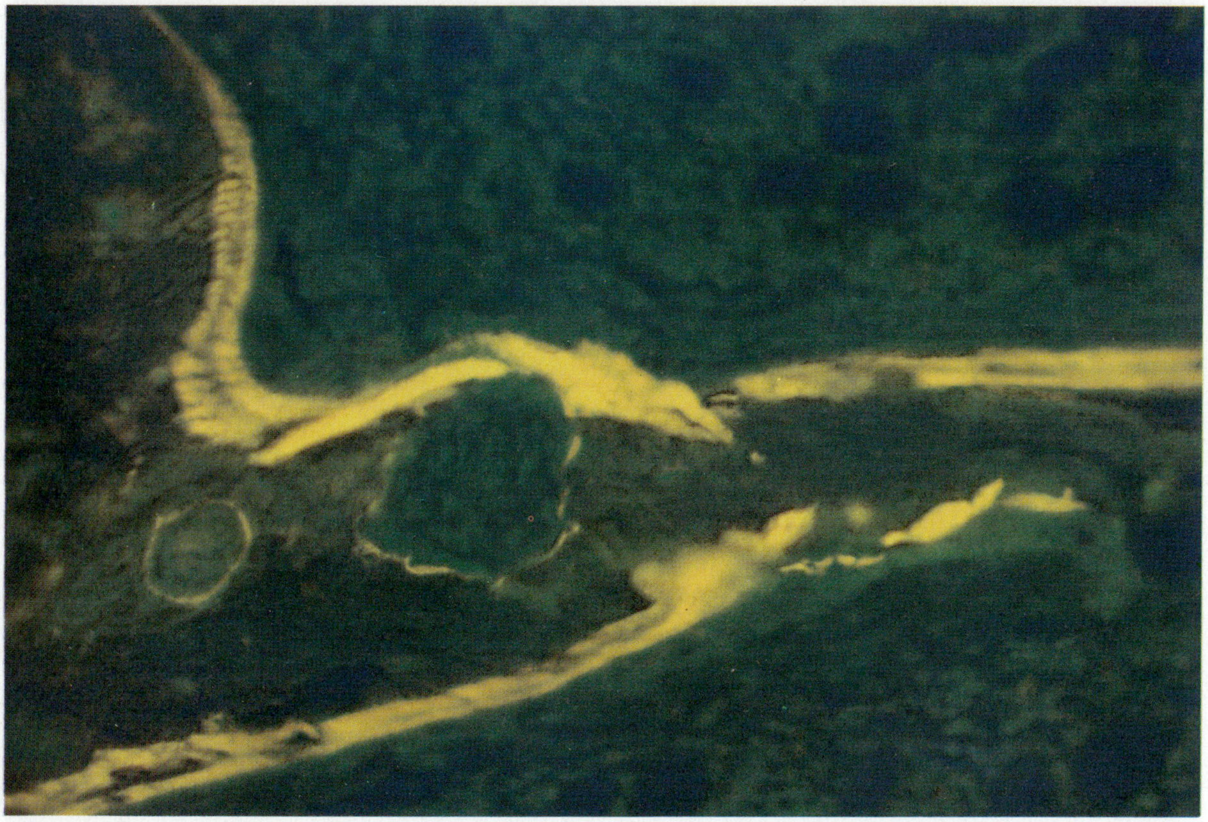

4B

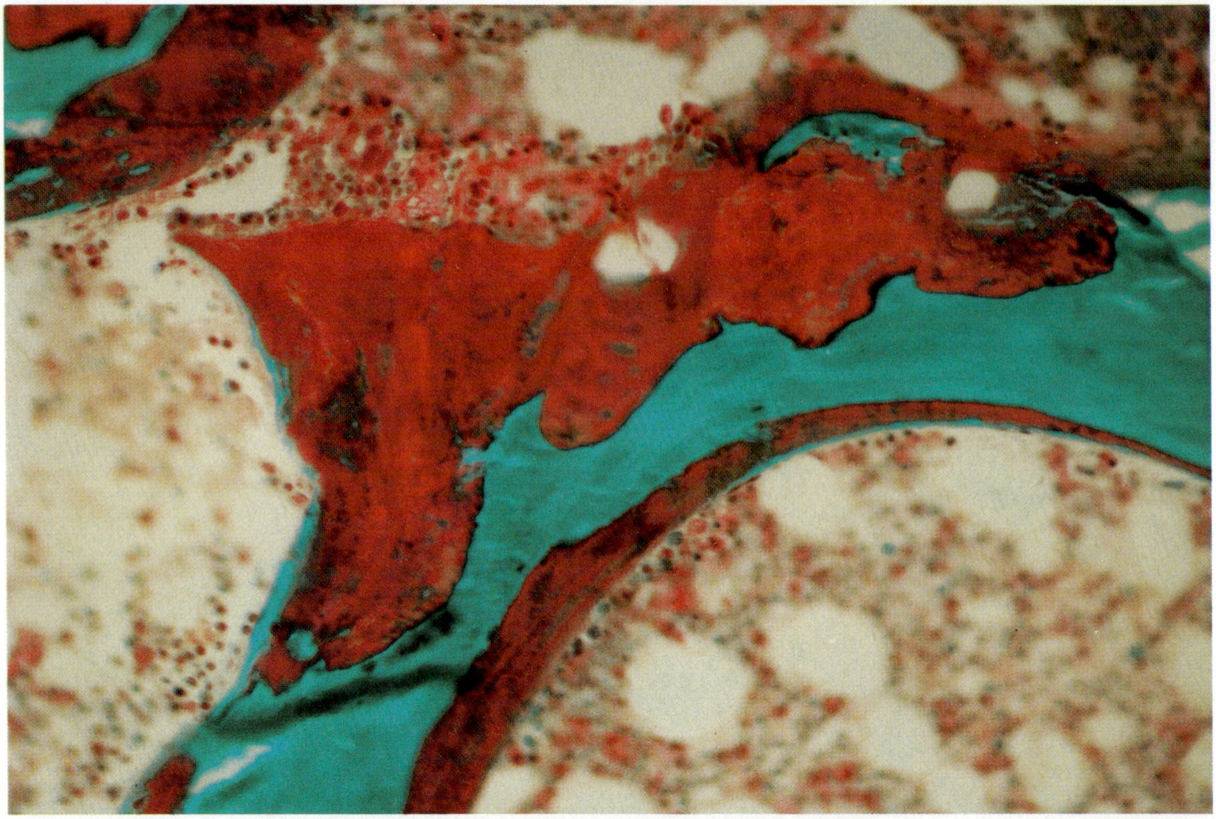

4

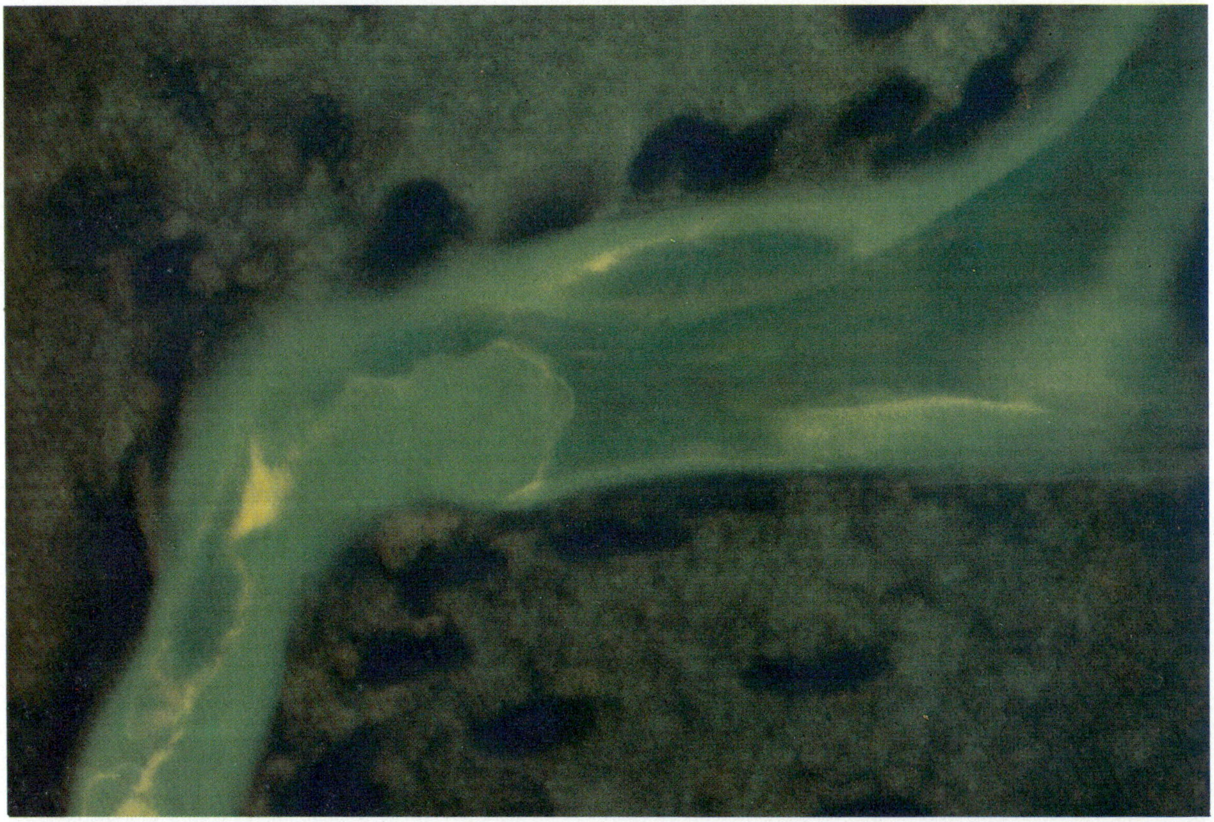

4

Osteitis fibrosa (fibro-osteoclasia)

Osteitis fibrosa, which presumably arises due to the high levels of PTH, is characterized by increased bone resorption and formation with a progressive increase in peritrabecular fibrosis. A greater fraction of trabecular bone surface is occupied by resorption cavities filled with osteoclasts (Howship's lacunae); also, increased numbers of osteoblasts overlie the newly formed unmineralized matrix of bone. As this process becomes severe, the narrow space is filled with fibrous tissue, creating typical 'osteitis fibrosa'. Double tetracycline labeling often reveals normal or increased bone turnover in patients with osteitis fibrosa (74).

Another feature of osteitis fibrosa is the alignment of collagen strands in an irregular, haphazard 'woven' pattern; this contrasts to the normal parallel alignment of strands of collagen aligned in a lamellar manner. This disorganized structure of collagen in 'woven' bone may lead to defective physical properties of bone in response to stress, and a greater amount of inferior, 'woven bone' may be required to maintain mechanical stability (76). This is shown schematically in Figure 6. Also, increased mineralization of large quantities of 'woven' bone may contribute to the osteosclerosis seen in uremia.

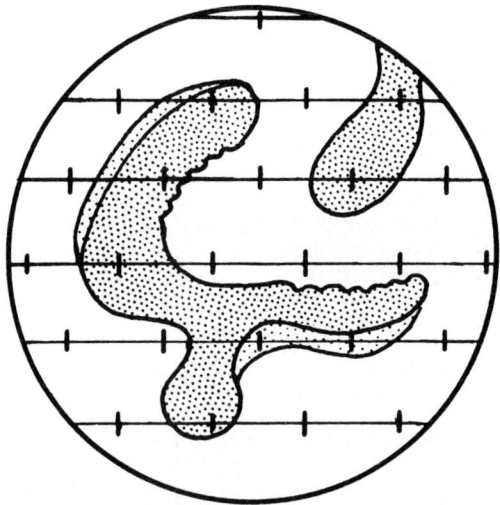

Figure 5. A diagram which shows a method for measuring bone dynamics using an integrating eye piece. Area measurements are utilized to derive volumes, with calcified bone (represented by dark stippling) showing six 'hits' and uncalcified bone (light stippling) showing two 'hits'. Length measurements are used to derive surface areas, with osteoid showing three intersections, resorbing surface, one intersection and resting surface showing 10 intersections. (Reproduced from Parfitt [72] with permission.)

resting (bone surface without cellular activity) (Figure 5). With another method, the microscopic image of bone is projected on a screen and each specific type of bone surface is traced with an electrical pencil attached to a computer and X-Y plotter (74). Quantitation of the surfaces occupied by active resorption, by formation, or by inactive bone can provide static information but may not provide data on the dynamics of bone formation, mineralization or resorption. Errors in static data may occur if the rate of metabolic activity varies (73); thus, the forming and resorbing surfaces could be twice normal, and yet skeletal dynamics can be normal if the activity of the osteoclasts and osteoblasts is reduced to half of normal. To obviate this problem, tetracycline, a fluorescent marker, which is incorporated into newly forming bone, is given on two separate occasions; this permits measurement of the rate of bone formation (75). In practice, the dynamics of trabecular bone are assessed after giving two separate doses of tetracycline, with the 'bone formation rate' quantitated as the distance between the two lines of fluorescence divided by the time between doses. By restricting each duration of labeling to 2 days, tetracycline toxicity is avoided.

The dynamics of turnover of trabecular bone differs from that of cortical bone, which is organized into units called osteons, which surround a Haversian canal. Cortical bone turnover involves sequential osteoclastic resorption within the Haversian canal, that is followed by osteoblastic formation. Also the numerous osteocytes, which are buried within the osteon, can participate in bone resorption through an 'osteocytic osteolysis'.

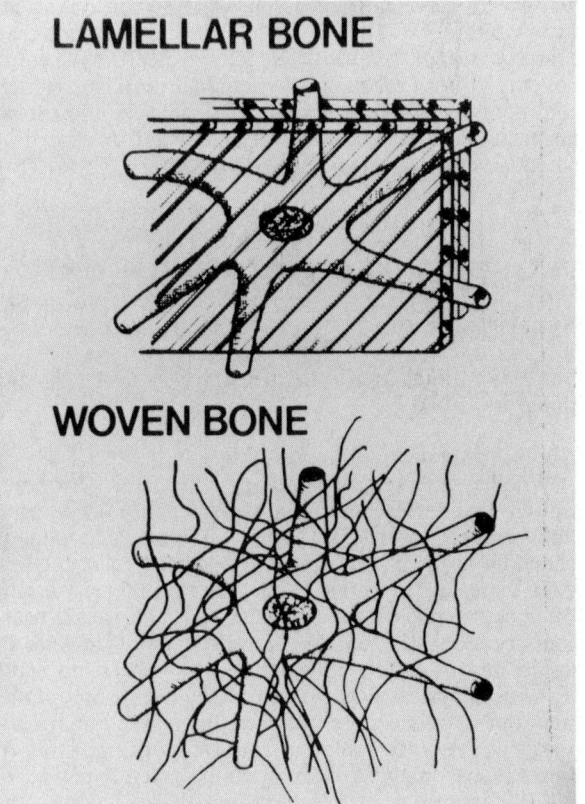

Figure 6. Schematic diagram showing the strain-sensitive properties of collagen about osteocytes in lamellar compared to woven bone. (Reproduced from Ritz et al [76], with permission).

Osteomalacia

Osteomalacia is characterized by an excess of unmineralized osteoid tissue, that arises from impaired mineralization of the protein matrix of bone. The major feature of osteomalacia is an increase in the width of unmineralized osteoid. This also occurs in osteitis fibrosa, however, due to the delay of mineralization of osteoid, which is formed so rapidly. Therefore, the use of tetracycline labeling to identify impaired mineralization rate is very useful in the identification of osteomalacia. Nonetheless, the criteria employed in the recognition of osteomalacia include: 1) the measurement of the width of osteoid seams; 2) the specific number of osteoid lamellae in these seams; 3) the extent to which bone surface is covered with osteoid; 4) the volume of osteoid expressed as a fraction of total bone surface and 5) a delayed rate of mineralization by tetracycline labeling (72, 73, 75).

Mixed skeletal lesion

Another sub-group of patients exhibit wide osteoid seams combined with typical features of osteitis fibrosa. Such skeletal lesions are somewhat more common in young patients, in those with hypocalcemia, and in patients who have not undergone dialysis or treatment with vitamin D (77). These histologic features may be characteristic of vitamin D deficiency itself, with components of both secondary hyperparathyroidism, which commonly occurs with vitamin D deficiency and osteomalacia. Plasma iPTH levels are significantly elevated in patients with this histologic lesion (66, 77).

Table 3. Symptoms and signs of renal osteodystrophy.

A. *Musculoskeletal system*
  1. Bone pain
  2. Fractures
  3. Acute pseudogout
  4. Calcific periarthritis
  5. Skeletal deformities
  6. Proximal myopathy
  7. Spontaneous tendon rupture
  8. Growth retardation
  9. Slipped epiphyses
  10. Tumoral calcification
B. *Cardiopulmonary system*
  1. Congestive heart failure
  2. Heart block
  3. Hypertension
C. *Ophthalmologic features*
  1. Corneal calcification (band keratopathy)
  2. Conjunctival calcification, with 'red' eye or 'white' eye.
D. *Dermatologic features*
  1. Pruritus
  2. Ischemic ulcers
  3. Cutaneous calcifications
E. *Metabolic, endocrine and hematological features*
  1. Insulin resistance
  2. Hypertriglyceridemia
  3. Impotence
  4. Menstrual abnormalities and/or sterility
  5. Anemia
  6. Pancytopenia
F. *Neurological features*
  1. Dialysis encephalopathy (Al)
  2. Peripheral neuropathy (?)
  3. Altered cognitive function
  4. Abnormal EEG (?)

FEATURES OF RENAL OSTEODYSTROPHY

Symptoms and signs

Some symptoms and signs of renal osteodystrophy are noted in Table 3.

Skeletal pain

Whether the skeletal pathology is secondary hyperparathyroidism or osteomalacia, skeletal pain may develop and progress to become totally disabling. The pain is generally vague and deep seated and may be in the low back, hips, legs or knees. It may vary in intensity and is often aggravated by gravitational stress and weight bearing; occasionally, the pain is localized about the knee or ankle, and its sudden appearance may suggest an acute arthritis. Physical findings are often absent. Symptoms may not correlate closely with radiographic abnormalities; patients with profound abnormalities on X-ray or bone biopsy may develop disability over a period of weeks to months to a degree that walking across the room is difficult. Low back pain may arise due to spontaneous vertebral collapse, and chest pain may be the first indication of a rib fracture occurring during a cough or sneeze.

Muscular weakness

An important symptom of renal osteodystrophy is muscular weakness. The evaluation of muscular strength is difficult, however, when bone pain is present. Weakness characteristically involves the proximal muscles. Initially, patients may note difficulty in climbing stairs or in rising from a sitting position; as the condition progresses, they may have difficulty in walking or in rising from a supine to a sitting position. The gait becomes waddling and resembles that of a penguin. The manifestations may be identical to those of vitamin D deficiency arising from other causes (78). Plasma levels of muscle enzymes, such as creatinine phosphokinase or aldolase, are generally normal; electromyography may reveal mild abnormalities suggesting a primary myopathy.

Ultrastructural abnormalities consist of diffuse degeneration of myofibrils characterized by streaming of Z-band material and loss of normal myosin-actin arrangement have been noted in such patients (79). A presumed role of vitamin D in producing such myopathy is suggested from the substantial improvement in muscle strength noted within a few days after administration of $1,25(OH)_2D_3$ (80) and by the reversal of the ultrastructural abnormalities following treatment with $25(OH)D_3$ (79).

Pruritus

A common symptom in patients with advanced renal failure is pruritus. It may improve or disappear after the initiation of adequate dialysis, but persists in some patients. Pruritus is especially common in uremic patients with overt secondary hyperparathyroidism and may improve or disappear after subtotal parathyroidectomy (81). The mechanism for the pruritus is unknown, but it may be related to a slightly high ionized plasma Ca in patients with overt secondary hyperparathyroidism (81). Pruritus may develop as a consequence of an elevation of plasma Ca from vitamin D overdosage, during a Ca infusion, or use of high Ca dialysate. Moreover, it may disappear following subtotal parathyroidectomy before there is a change in skin Ca content. The severe pruritus once frequent in dialysis populations is less common with the use of methods to prevent severe secondary hyperparathyroidism.

Bone deformities and growth retardation

In uremic children, deformities of bone include bowing of the tibia and femur and those due to slipped epiphysis (82) of the distal radius, distal ulna, and proximal femur. Thus, marked ulnar deviation of the hand can occur as a manifestation of a slipped epiphysis. The skeletal pathology associated with a slipped epiphysis is that of secondary hyperparathyroidism, and the radiolucent zone between the epiphyseal ossification center and metaphysis is caused by the accumulation of poorly mineralized woven bone and/or fibrous tissue (82); it does not arise from an excess of cartilage and chondrosteoid as occurs in vitamin D-deficiency rickets.

Retardation of growth is common in uremic children; the factors responsible for diminished growth in children, however, are far from clear. Growth impairment may be partly due to deficient caloric intake (83). Initiation of dialysis usually does not result in 'catch-up' growth, although improved growth has been reported after treatment with calcitriol (84).

Fractures

The syndrome 'dialysis osteopenia' with fractures has been reported from several centers in the United Kingdom (62, 63) and in North America (68). There is a strong association of this syndrome with the occurrence of dialysis encephalopathy and as many as 30% of dialysis patients may be afflicted in some units (63, 85). A high incidence has been reported in certain centers in North America (65), and a sporadic case may afflict a small fraction of patients (68). These patients have osteomalacia as the primary skeletal lesion; fractures which involve the axial skeleton, i.e., the ribs, vertebral bodies, hips, and even the long bones, are common. Such patients may develop scoliosis and substantial loss in height, and they may have profound disability. Dialysis encephalopathy, vitamin D resistant osteomalacia and muscular weakness have been correlated with aluminium accumulation. This chronic aluminum intoxication is attributed to uptake from the dialysis fluid and to a lesser extent from oral phosphate binders containing aluminum (see also Chapters 41 and 42).

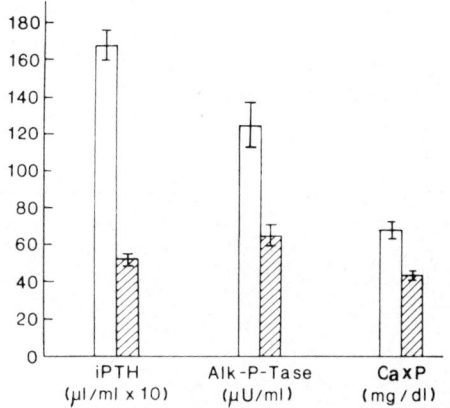

Figure 7. Values of iPTH, serum alkaline phosphatase and Ca × P observed in 12 patients with an acute monoarticular syndrome (open columns) compared with those of the other patients treated by dialysis (hatched columns). (Reproduced from Llach et al [86], with permission.)

Periarthritis

Acute pain, redness and swelling of the joints, periarticular structures, and/or tendon sheaths may occur in dialysis patients. This acute monoarticular syndrome may be indistinguishable from an acute arthritis; the joint fluid, if present, is clear without the presence of crystals, which distinguishes this syndrome from acute pseudogout or gouty arthritis. This syndrome probably reflects overt secondary hyperparathyroidism; and the afflicted patients have higher alkaline phosphatase levels, plasma Ca × P products and iPTH levels compared to other dialysis patients as shown in Figure 7 (86). Occasionally, calcium deposits can be seen radiographically about the affected joints. Synovial tissue biopsies may reveal crystals, which, when studied by x-ray defraction, are characteristic of hydroxyapatite. In general, this syndrome responds well to treatment with anti-inflammatory agents, such as phenylbutazone or indomethacin; also parathyroidectomy may lead to marked improvement.

Tendon rupture

An unusual but troublesome problem noted in dialysis patients is the spontaneous rupture of the tendon of the quadriceps muscle or of digits (87). Its cause is unclear, but its association with overt secondary hyperparathyroidism and a similar occurrence in primary hyperparathyroidism suggest that high levels of PTH may in some way, predispose to this lesion.

Calciphylaxis

This unusual syndrome is characterized by peripheral ischemic necrosis and vascular calcification; it may occur in patients with advanced chronic uremia, in dialysis patients, and in successful renal transplant recipients (88). These lesions are initially characterized by painful, violaceous mottling of the skin, followed by penetrating, progressive gangrenous ulcerations of the skin of the fingers, toes, and ankles, or fat and muscle of the thighs and/or buttocks (Figure 8). The lesions may

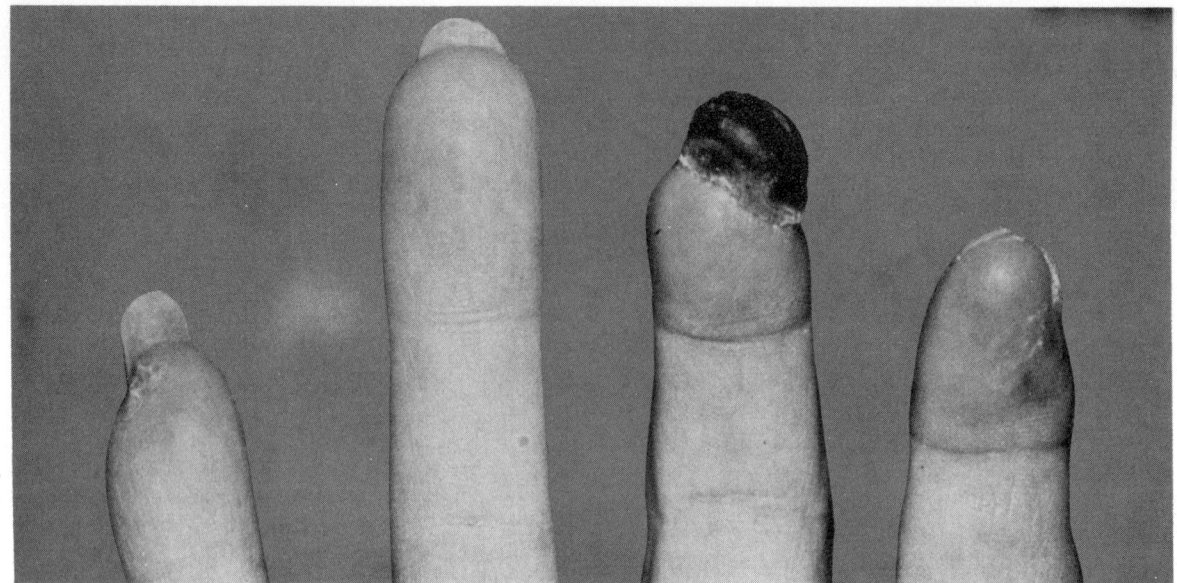

Figure 8. Ischemic necrosis involving the 2nd and 3rd digit of a uremic patient treated with maintenance hemodialysis. There was healing of the lesions following subtotal parathyroidectomy. (Case 3 from Gipstein et al [88].)

fail to heal and can contribute to the patients' death via secondary infection. Extensive calcification commonly involves the media of the arteries; most patients have a history of marked hyperphosphatemia and show bone erosions on X-ray and have elevated plasma iPTH levels. Control of plasma P may prevent but not heal these lesions. On the other hand, total healing of the lesions has followed subtotal parathyroidectomy, with striking improvement within 1 to 4 weeks, an observation suggesting that PTH levels may contribute to the pathogenesis of the syndrome (88). The similarity between these lesions and Selye's experimental syndrome, calciphylaxis (89), is striking. Because of the fulminant and even fatal course, subtotal parathyroidectomy should be considered when such lesions first appear.

Miscellaneous symptoms and signs
Certain other symptoms may be common in uremic patients with overt renal osteodystrophy and secondary hyperparathyroidism, although the reasons for these associations are unknown. Altered mental or central nervous system function is one such manifestation. Experimental evidence in dogs indicates that acute uremia leads to Ca accumulation with the brain; this is dependent on high PTH levels and is associated with EEG abnormalities (90). A clinical counterpart of this experimental syndrome may be suggested by sporadic improvement of encephalopathic symptoms following subtotal parathyroidectomy in a patient with overt secondary hyperparathyroidism (9). Recovery or marked improvement of long-standing impotence has been noted by some patients or their sexual partners after the reversal of secondary hyperparathyroidism (92).

The mechanisms whereby hyperparathyroidism may lead to these syndromes are unclear; PTH has certain catabolic actions; it may lead to insulin resistance (93) and may produce other metabolic events (94, 95) that add to uremic toxicity.

Biochemical features

The biochemical features of renal osteodystrophy are noted in Table 4.

Table 4. Biochemical features of renal osteodystrophy.

1. Hyperphosphatemia	9. Elevated plasma OH-proline
2. Hypocalcemia	10. Elevated plasma cyclic-AMP
3. Elevated alkaline phosphatase	11. Hypercalcemia
4. Hypermagnesemia	12. Hypophosphatemia
5. Elevated serum iPTH	13. Reduced calcitonin
6. Reduced plasma 1,25(OH)$_2$D	14. Elevated bone aluminum
7. Reduced plasma 24,25(OH)$_2$D$_3$	15. Elevated bone GLA protein
8. Increased Ca and Mg content of skin	

Hyperphosphatemia
Hyperphosphatemia is prevalent in most dialysis patients. Factors affecting plasma P levels in these patients are summarized in Table 5. Of these, the most important are dietary P intake and the ingestion of phosphate-binding gels. As dietary P increases, there is increased net absorption, although the fractional absorption of P may be slightly below normal in uremia (Figure 9). Results from metabolic balance studies indicate that alumi-

Table 5. Factors affecting serum phosphorus in patients undergoing dialysis.

1. Dietary P intake
2. Ingestion of phosphate-binding antacids
3. Skeletal responsiveness to plasma PTH
4. Degree of vitamin D deficiency and treatment with active vitamin D sterols
5. Frequency, duration and efficiency of dialysis
6. Ingestion of carbohydrate (transient effect)
7. Balance between degradation and synthesis of protoplasm
8. Rapid skeletal accretion (i.e. healing of osteomalacia or osteitis fibrosa)
9. Parenteral alimentation
10. Intake of large amounts of oral Ca supplements
11. Phosphate-containing enemas

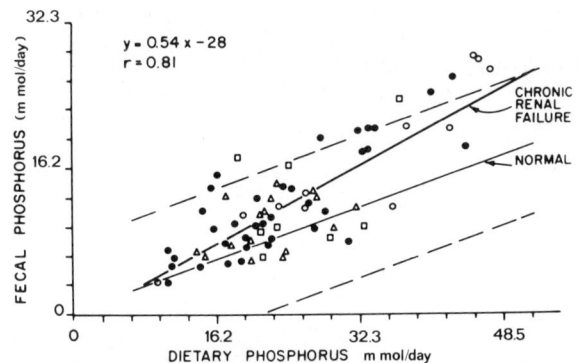

Figure 9. The relationship between fecal phosphorus excretion and the daily dietary intake of phosphorus in patients with end-stage renal failure. The regression line and confidence limits for normal values are included with the individual values for uremic patients. (Modified from Coburn et al [98])

(P [as phosphate] m mol → mg: multiply by 31)

num hydroxide gel, 75 to 200 ml/day, increases fecal phosphorus by 30 to 144% (96, 97). There is little relationship however, between the amount of aluminium hydroxide taken and either the net or relative increase in fecal P. When dietary P intake is below 1.0 g/day and aluminum hydroxide is taken, fecal P often exceeds dietary intake. However, when dietary P is increased to 2.0 g/day, fecal P is usually below dietary intake despite ingestion of the gels. Thus, a high phosphate diet can offset the effect of treatment with aluminum hydroxide or carbonate, emphasizing the need for modest dietary P restriction in combination with orally administered aluminum compounds. A schema showing quantitative relationship between dietary and fecal P and the influence of aluminum hydroxide is given in Figure 10 (98).

The active forms of vitamin D can increase the net absorption of P (Figure 11) and aggravate the hyperphosphatemia; particularly if the absorbed P remains in the extracellular fluid and is not deposited in bone (99, 100).

Patients with overt secondary hyperparathyroidism may have more hyperphosphatemia than those lacking this syndrome (101); there also may be a more rapid rebound of plasma P to high levels during the interdialytic interval in such patients. Presumably, this arises because bone resorption exceeds formation and there is a large pool size for P; a marked fall in plasma P often follows subtotal parathyroidectomy (101) or when secondary hyperparathyroidism is suppressed by an active form of vitamin D (100).

Hypophosphatemia

Occasional dialysis patients may exhibit normal or even low plasma P levels despite ingestion of a normal diet and no phosphate-binding gels (102, 103). Such patients probably have a markedly defective intestinal P

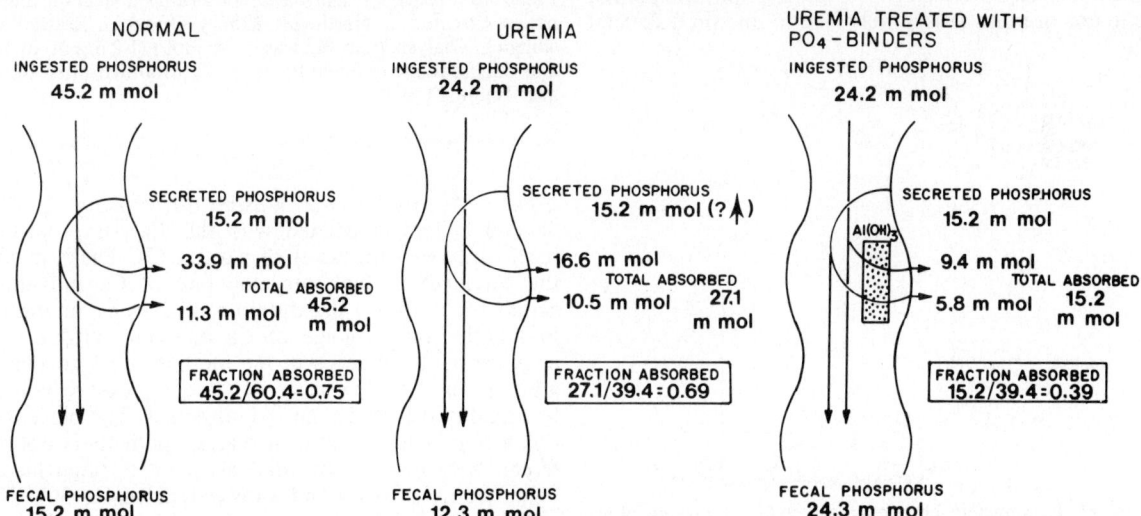

Figure 10. Schema showing approximate amount of phosphorus ingested, its fate in the intestine and the relative contribution of ingested and endogenously secreted phosphorus to total phosphorus lost in the feces. Representative values for a normal man are shown on the left; in the middle are those for a typical uremic patient; the effect of a phosphate-binding gel on phosphorus absorption in uremic patients is shown on the right. (Modified from Coburn et al [98])

(P [as phosphate] mmol → mg: multiply by 31)

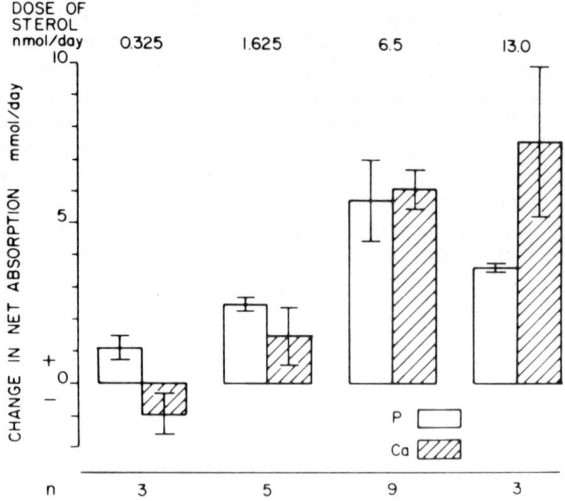

Figure 11. Changes in net absorption of calcium (Ca) and phosphorus (P) after varying daily doses of 1,25(OH)₂D₃ or 1 alpha (OH)D₃. Data in normal subjects and patients with end-stage renal failure are combined (mean±SEM). The doses of sterol correspond to 0.14, 0.68, 2.7 and 5 µg/day, respectively. (Modified after Coburn et al, with permission of the publisher [192]).

(Ca mmol → mg: multiply by 40.
P [as phosphate] m mol → mg: multiply by 31).

transport. Severe hypophosphatemia can also occur during rapid skeletal healing, whether the skeletal disorder is osteomalacia or osteitis fibrosa. In addition, the use of total parenteral nutrition solutions with amino acids and large amounts of glucose can cause hypophosphatemia.

The important pathogenic role of hyperphosphatemia in producing or aggravating secondary hyperparathyroidism has been stressed; however, hypophosphatemia, due to one or more causes, may lead to impaired skeletal

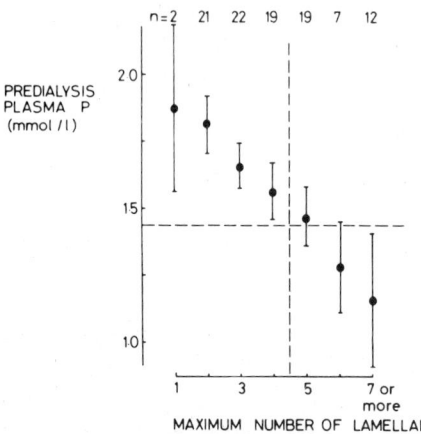

Figure 12. Relationship between mean value of plasma phosphorus (P) immediately prior to hemodialysis (±SEM) and the number of osteoid lamellae identified in bone biopsy in 102 dialysis patients. A horizontal line indicates the upper limit of the normal range. (From Kanis et al [62] slightly modified).

(P m mol/l → mg/dl: multiply by 3.1)

mineralization (Table 5). Thus, the severity of features of osteomalacia can correlate inversely with predialysis plasma P levels (Figure 12), an observation that underscores the need to avoid hypophosphatemia and phosphate depletion in dialysis patients.

Hypocalcemia
Reductions in total and ionized serum Ca are common in patients with advanced renal failure. Serum Ca levels below the normal range were noted in 40% of uremic patients; some showed marked hypocalcemia (30). With the initiation of regular hemodialysis, predialysis serum Ca levels increase and only a small number of patients remain or become hypocalcemic, although the mean values for a group of patients may be below normal (Figure 13). The reason for an increase in serum Ca during dialysis is unclear; it can occur despite use of a low dialysis fluid Ca of 1.25 mmol/l (2.5 mEq/l) and persistent hyperphosphatemia.

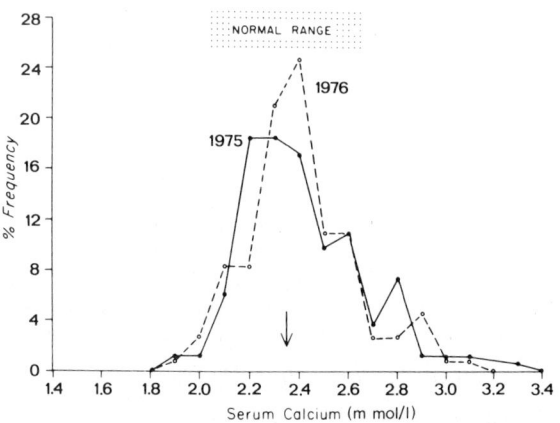

Figure 13. Frequency distribution of serum Ca level for dialysis patients treated at Northwest Kidney Center in Seattle, Washington. Dialysis fluid Mg was 0.5 m mol/l (1.2 mg/dl) in 1975 and 0.25 m mol/l (0,6 mg/dl) in 1976. (Modified after Burnell and Teubner [103])

(Ca m mol/l → mg/dl: multiply by 4)

Effect of hemodialysis on plasma Ca levels
Several factors associated with the dialysis procedure, itself, influence the level of plasma Ca. These include the Ca level in dialysate, the rate of Ca movement across the dialyzer, the duration of dialysis, alterations in kinetics of exchange of Ca between various body compartments, changes in the binding of Ca to plasma albumin, and the presence of Ca complexes which are less readily dialyzed than is ionized Ca. The percentage of Ca bound to albumin in dialysis patients is not different from normal, but dialysis patients often have a higher complexed Ca and a lower ionized Ca (30). With parallel plate dialyzers, the dialysance of Ca, calculated from the non-protein bound fraction in blood, was approximately 60 to 70% of that of urea (104). The total quantity of Ca transferred into a patient from dialysate can reach 17.5 to 27.5 mmol/l (700 to 1100 mg) during ten hours of dialysis (105) when dialysate Ca level ex-

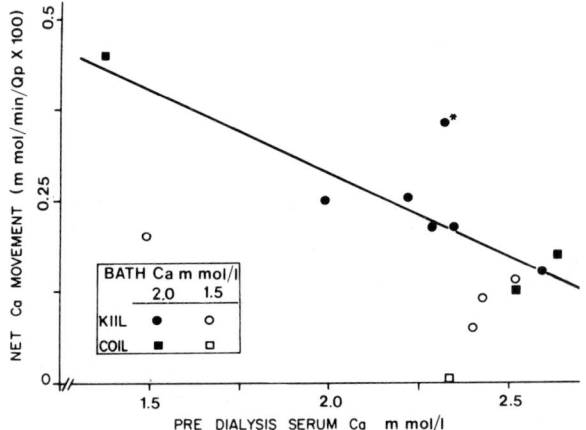

Figure 14. Net movement of Ca during hemodialysis, expressed as m mol/min per 100 ml plasma flow through the dialyzer. The movement is shown in relationship to predialysis serum Ca, the dialysis fluid Ca concentration and the type of dialyzer used. (Derived from data published by Mirahmadi et al [105])

(Ca m mol → mg: multiply by 40
Ca m mol/l → mg/dl: multiply by 4).

ceeds the plasma diffusible Ca by 0.4 to 0.5 mmol/l (0.8 to 1.0 mEq/l) (Figure 14).

Total plasma Ca often increases substantially during hemodialysis. This is due in large partly to an increase in plasma albumin induced by ultrafiltration and also to augmented protein-binding of Ca due to a rise in blood pH.

Studies with Ca electrodes show that during dialysis with a dialysate Ca of 1.25 mmol/l (2.5 mEq/l) ionized Ca falls even as total Ca increases (106). The increase in total serum Ca during dialysis with a dialysate Ca of 1.5 to 1.75 mmol/l (3.0 to 3.5 mEq/l) is associated with an acute rise in ionized Ca (106) and fall in plasma PTH (107).

Hypercalcemia

In patients undergoing treatment with hemodialysis hypercalcemia may appear spontaneously under at least two circumstances: 1) in conjunction with overt secondary hyperparathyroidism and 2) with osteomalacia. The former patients usually have radiographic signs of hyperparathyroidism with markedly elevated levels of serum iPTH (108). Such patients have been classified by some as having 'tertiary' hyperparathyroidism, and it has been implied that there is an autonomous secretion of PTH; however, plasma PTH levels usually decrease when plasma calcium is elevated. It seems that marked hyperplasia of the parathyroid glands is responsible for the continued secretion of the PTH excess. Parathyroidectomy is probably the most effective treatment for such patients.

Spontaneous hypercalcemia can also occur in patients with 'pure' osteomalacia (68, 70, 109). Such hypercalcemia is aggravated by low doses of vitamin D, high calcium intake, or the use of a high concentration of calcium (i.e. above 1.63 mmol/l [3.25 mEq/l]) in dialysis fluid (109). Parathyroidectomy is not indicated in these patients, and may even aggravate the condition (70). Hypercalcemia can also develop in dialysis patients in association with treatment with various forms of vitamin D, oral calcium supplements, and the long-term use of dialysis fluid containing 1.75 mmol/l (3.5 mEq/l) of calcium or above.

Hypermagnesemia

Hypermagnesemia is common in dialysis patients (30). The kidney plays a major role in regulating plasma Mg and body stores; the intestinal absorption of Mg is normal in patients with advanced renal failure (98). Thus, the occurence of hypermagnesemia is not surprising. The dietary intake of Mg in uremic patients ingesting a restricted protein diet is below normal, which may prevent hypermagnesemia in many patients. Abrupt and marked hypermagnesemia can develop, however, when Mg intake is increased by the ingestion of Mg containing laxatives or phosphate binding gels with added Mg oxide (71).

The level of Mg in the dialysis fluid also influences the serum magnesium levels in dialysis patients. In one center using a dialysis fluid Mg of 0.25 mmol/l (0.5 mEq/l), serum Mg ranged from 0.75 to 1.1 mmol/l (1.5 to 2.2 mEq/l), while serum levels were 1.25 to 2.25 mol/l (2.5 to 4.5 mEq/l) in other patients when dialysis fluid Mg of 0.75 mmol (1.5 mEq/l) was used (5). The effect of reducing dialysis fluid Mg from 0.5 mmol

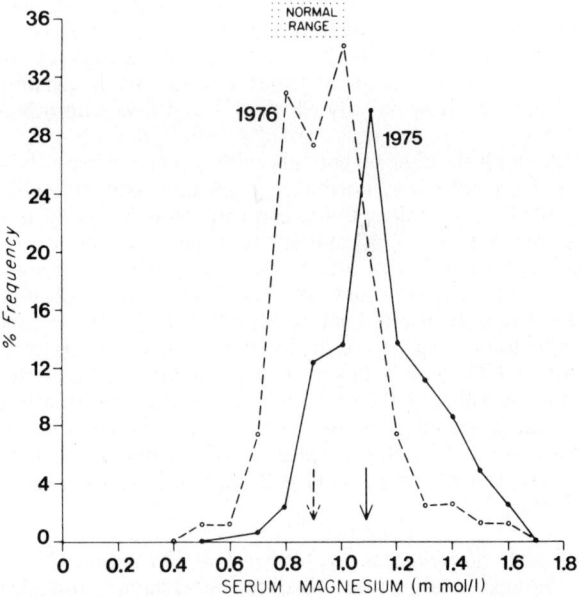

Figure 15. Frequency distribution of serum Mg levels in dialysis patients treated at the Northwest Kidney Center, Seattle, Washington. Dialysis fluid Mg concentration was 0,5 mmol/l in 1975 (N = 109) and 0.25 mmol/l in 1976 (N = 81). (Modified after Burnell and Teubner [103]).

(Mg mmol/l → mg/dl: multiply by 2,4)

to 0.25 mmol/l (1.0 mEq/l to 0.5 mEq/l) is shown in Figure 15 (103, see also Chapter 7).

Acute hypermagnesemia can suppress PTH secretion (20), raising the possibility that hypermagnesemia might diminish secondary hyperparathyroidism and, hence, be beneficial for dialysis patients. There are no data, however, to indicate that chronic hypermagnesemia has such an effect; this may reflect the fact that mild hypocalcemia is more effective in stimulating PTH secretion than is the suppressive action of hypermagnesemia (20).

Whether chronic hypermagnesemia is harmful or not in patients with ESRD is not clear. Long term hypermagnesemia may be associated with abnormal bone mineralization in uremia, and skeletal Mg is increased in association with hypermagnesemia (111). Alfrey et al. suggested that magnesium pyrophosphate, present in excess amounts in bone of uremic patients, may promote abnormal mineral turnover (112, 113). Moreover, Burnell and Teubner suggested that chemical characteristics of bone improve after dialysis fluid Mg is reduced and hypermagnesemia is prevented (110). Thus, prolonged and persistent hypermagnesemia is not desirable in patients undergoing dialysis.

Plasma immunoreactive parathyroid hormone
The plasma levels of iPTH are commonly elevated in dialysis patients, particularly when assayed with antisera directed toward the 'C-terminal' fragment. Assays utilizing 'intact' PTH or an 'N-terminal' antisera often show lesser degrees of elevation. Although significant correlations between plasma PTH and histomorphometric features of osteitis fibrosa have been reported in dialysis patients (114), such relationships have not been clearly established. Thus, some C-terminal assays report values that are 10 to 20 times normal, while plasma iPTH levels may be only elevated 3 to 4 fold with other assays.

A small number of patients with advanced renal failure may have low, normal or even undetectable levels of iPTH. Hypomagnesemia can cause low levels on occasion, but low or normal iPTH levels are common in uremic patients with osteomalacia and little or no evidence for osteitis fibrosa (68, 70). Serial levels of plasma iPTH may be useful for following the course of patients undergoing long-term dialysis. For a correct interpretation of PTH assays, however, it is essential to know the characteristics of the antisera and to have information on the correlation between levels of iPTH in uremic patients and biologic features of secondary hyperparathyroidism in patients with advanced renal insufficiency.

Alkaline phosphatase, hydroxyproline and cyclic AMP
Although total serum alkaline phosphatase includes isoenzymes arising from liver, intestine, kidney, and bone, its measurement can be a useful indicator of increased osteoblastic activity. An elevated serum alkaline phosphatase may occur with either osteitis fibrosa or osteomalacia, but markedly elevated levels may be more common in the former, with higher rates of bone turnover. Plasma alkaline phosphatase may be useful for monitoring therapy of skeletal disease with vitamin D compounds or calcium supplements (see Management). Since dialysis patients may have co-existing hepatic abnormalities, liver disease should be excluded as the cause of an elevated alkaline phosphatase.

An elevation of plasma hydroxyproline, both free and peptide bound, may provide an index for increased collagen turnover and bone resorption (115); others report that only the free hydroxyproline is useful (116). The hydroxyproline determination is cumbersome and not likely to become widely available. Plasma cyclic AMP is also elevated in the uremic patients; however, it does not correlate with the severity of secondary hyperparathyroidism (117). The bone gamma-carboxyglutamic acid (GLA) protein also may be elevated in patients with secondary hyperparathyroidism.

Other biochemical features associated with renal osteodystrophy and secondary hyperparathyroidism are noted in Table 4. The precise relationship of hypertriglyceridemia and insulin resistance (93-95), to altered divalent ion metabolism remains unclear.

Radiographic features

Techniques
The incidence of radiographic abnormalities of the skeleton varies considerably in different dialysis centers. This may reflect true differences related to patients' ages, the type of management, and the duration of dialysis. However, the radiographic techniques employed, the type of X-ray film used, and the interest of the radiologist may also account for differences (118). X-rays of bone, obtained utilizing standard film and developing procedures, result in films of poorer quality than those produced 20 years ago (119). Several techniques can increase the sensitivity of X-rays of the hand. The use of fine grain industrial film (i.e. Kodak M or mammography film), which is developed by manual rather than automatic film processing, the omission of screen or grid techniques, and magnification X-ray techniques add to the sensitivity (120). With conventional viewing, normal phalanges were noted in 67% of uremic patients, with only 8% manifesting marked subperiosteal resorption, while with magnification of the same films, only 26% were normal and 29% exhibited substantial resorption (120). With such magnification techniques, however, there is a danger of overreading and familiarity with normal variations is required.

Subperiosteal erosions
Certain radiographic features of renal osteodystrophy are listed in Table 6. Subperiosteal resorption or erosions are the most common specific features of secondary hyperparathyroidism. Erosions may occur in the phalanges, pelvis, distal ends of the clavicles, inferior surfaces of the ribs, femur, mandible and skull. The phalanges are the skeletal sites most accessible for careful radiographic evaluation. If appropriately sensitive techniques are applied, it is uncommon for erosions to be found elsewhere when the hands are normal (120). In its earliest form, resorption occurs on the radial surfaces

Table 6. Radiographic and other features of renal osteodystrophy.

A. Osteopenia (reduced density)
B. Skeletal features of secondary hyperparathyroidism
   1. Subperiosteal resorption
   2. Cortical striations
   3. Cyst formation (brown tumor)
   4. Slipped epiphysis
   5. Mottled ('salt and pepper') skull
   6. Periosteal new bone formation
C. Abnormal enchondral ossification
   1. Rickets-like lesion
   2. Slipped epiphysis
D. Osteosclerosis
E. Pseudofractures (Looser's zones)
F. Genu valgum
G. Protrusio acetabuli
H. Endosteal bone resorption (metacarpal index)
I. Vertebrae collapse (crush fracture)
J. Spontaneous rib fractures
K. Osteonecrosis (aseptic necrosis)
L. Soft tissue calcifications
   1. Periarticular calcification
   2. Tumoral calcifications
   3. Chondrocalcinosis
   4. Ocular calcification
   5. Cutaneous calcification
   6. Visceral calcification
      Pulmonary (perfusion-ventilation abnormality)
      Cardiac (conduction defect, congestive heart failure)
   7. Vascular calcification
      Medial
      Intimal
M. Reduced bone mineral content
   1. Photon absorptiometry
   2. Neutron activation
N. Abnormal skeletal scintiscan
   1. Increased uptake of $^{99}Tc^m$ polyphosphate
      Symmetrical in osteitis fibrosa
      Identification of fractures (osteomalacia)

of the middle phalanx of the second and/or third digit of the dominant hand (Figure 16). The tuft of the terminal phalanx commonly exhibits subperiosteal resorption (121). A detailed description of the progression of erosions of the middle phalanx is given elsewhere (117); Meema et al. (120) have documented the use and value of magnification of X-ray films particularly of the digits. With the use of careful techniques, subperiosteal resorption may occur in 40 to 50% of patients that show increased resorption on bone biopsy (120, 121). Also bone erosions are associated with higher serum iPTH levels in dialysis patients (Figure 17, [122]).

Cortical striations, resulting from enlarged Haversian canals (Figure 18), occur with secondary hyperparathyroidism and also with increased bone turnover due to other causes, i.e. primary hyperparathyroidism, hyperthyroidism, acromegaly, and during rapid growth (121). They usually occur in association with subperiosteal erosions (Figure 19). Cystic abnormalities of bone (i.e. brown tumors) develop in renal osteodystrophy less often than in primary hyperparathyroidism (123). Such lesions may be painful and when present in the mandible they can alter the configuration of the teeth. Almost invariably, subperiosteal erosions accompany cystic lesions. With healing, focal areas of sclerosis may appear.

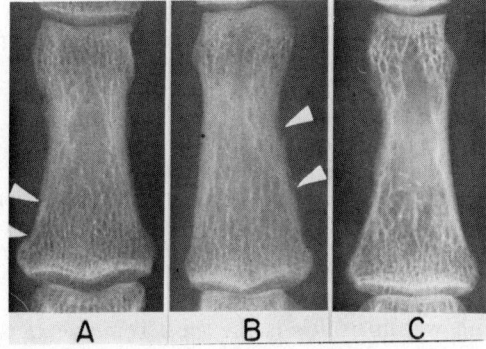

Figure 16. Appearance of subperiosteal erosions in 3 patients with renal osteodystrophy. A. There is an early saucer-shaped lesion with no overlying cortical bone on the lower radial shoulder (arrows). B. Moderately advanced erosion along the radial surface, but without an apparent break in the cortex (arrows). C. There is a cystic honeycomb appearance of the subperiosteal cortex (left). The erosions extend close to the distal interphalangeal joints (Reproduced from Parfitt [117] with permission).

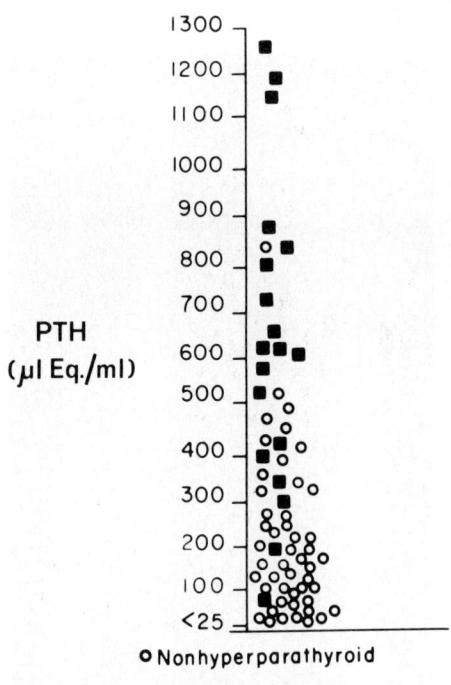

Figure 17. Levels of serum immunoreactive parathyroid hormone (PTH) in 71 dialysis patients. Those with clinically apparent secondary hyperparathyroidism (solid symbols) are compared to others lacking overt manifestations. The normal value for PTH is below 46 µl/Eq/ml. (Reproduced from Glassford et al [122] with permission.

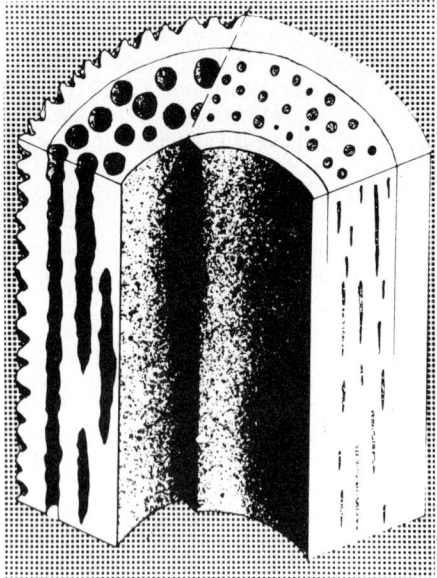

Figure 18. Diagrammatic representative of normal cortical bone (right) and that with secondary hyperparathyroidism (left) Erosive bone removal occurs at the endosteal, Haversian and periosteal surfaces. (Reprinted from Mehls et al [194] with permission of the publisher).

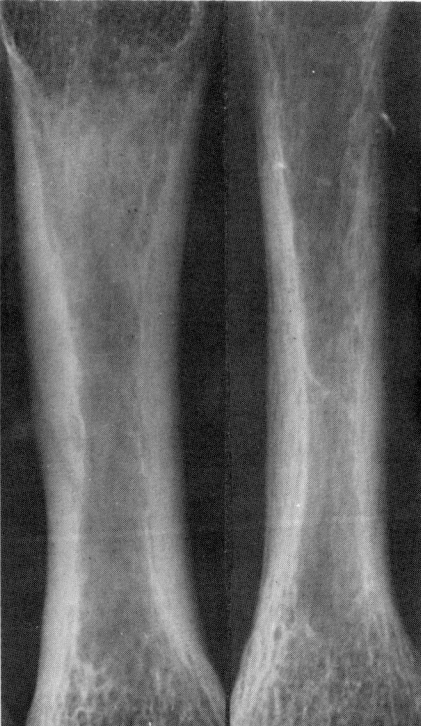

Figure 19. Left: cortical bone appears solid except for nutrient canal in the left cortex. Right: intracortical striations grade 3+ in a 30 year old female patient with end stage renal failure.

Abnormalities of the skull
Radiographic alterations of the skull have been divided into four types (124): 1) a diffuse 'ground-glass' appearance, with loss of sharp margins at the vascular grooves and diploic venous channels; 2) a diffuse mottled or granular appearance, which is most frequent and probably represents a network of enlarged resorption spaces within the tables of the skull; 3) focal lucent defects, 1 to 3 cm in diameter, which may be present with or without the 'ground-glass' or mottled appearance and 4) focal areas of sclerosis. These abnormalities may disappear completely after appropriate treatment (Figure 20).

Periosteal neostosis
Periosteal new bone formation, termed periosteal neostosis (125), can appear in 10% of dialysis patients in association with secondary hyperparathyroidism. This appears as a thin external layer of new bone separated from the original periosteum by a clear zone. Subsequently, the cortical bone may be thickened as the new bone is united with old. The most commonly involved sites are the metatarsals, pelvis, distal tibia and the hands. This abnormality can be confused with a calcified digital artery and with an artifact produced as a patient moves during radiography (117).

Alterations in growth zone
Abnormalities in the growth zone occur in children with secondary hyperparathyroidism or rickets. It may be difficult to separate true rickets from the 'rickets-like' abnormality of secondary hyperparathyroidism (117). Unlike true rickets, the lesion of hyperparathyroidism exhibits no widening of the physeal zone, and the irregularity of the metaphyseal lucent zone is very severe, extends laterally and blends with superiosteal resorption at the cortical junction (126). This lesion is more common in children over 10 years, while true rickets usually occurs before the age of 5. The radiolucent zone is caused by an accumulation of woven bone and/or fibrous tissue in a rickets-like lesion, whereas cartilage accumulates in vitamin D-deficiency rickets. The development of a slipped epiphysis is common in this rickets-like lesion. In a study by Mehls et al. (126), 10% of children with chronic renal failure had this lesion, while it was less common in children undergoing regular dialysis. A slipped epiphysis is often associated with pain or abnormal gait, but some patients are asymptomatic or have referred pain. The rickets-like lesion responds to treatment with vitamin D, probably due to suppression of secondary hyperparathyroidism.

Genu valgum which is the most common cause of adolescent knock knee, was found in over 10% of a series of patients with symptomatic renal osteodystrophy (117). Symptoms include difficulty in walking and pain. Other signs of rickets are often present, but the lesion can develop as a consequence of secondary hyperparathyroidism. Occasionally, the angulation is so great in weight-bearing joints that shearing of physeal plate may occur with partial slipping of the distal femoral epiphysis.

35: *Renal osteodystrophy and maintenance dialysis* 697

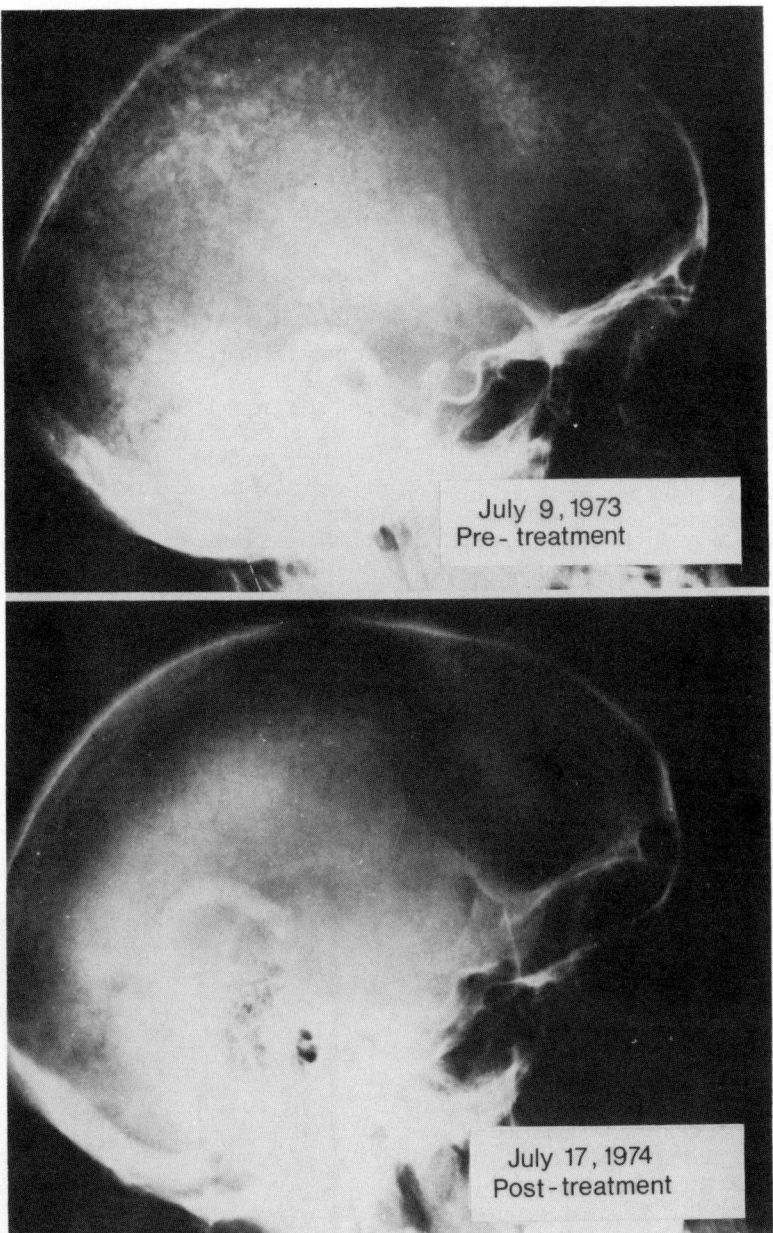

Figure 20. Radiographs of the skull in a dialysis patient with overt renal osteodystrophy. The upper X-ray was taken before, and the lower after 10 months of treatment with 1,25(OH)$_2$D$_3$.

Osteosclerosis
Osteosclerosis, a form of increased density of bone, may occur because of increased thickness and number of trabeculae in spongy bone. The vertebral bodies, pelvis, ribs, skull, and long bones are most commonly involved. It may be more common in young patients, particularly in those with radiographic evidence of hyperparathyroidism. In the spine this may produce the classic 'rugger jersey' appearance, with dense bands alternating with radiolucent zones. At times, osteosclerosis appears as narrow, dense sclerotic bands sharply demarcated from the rest of the vertebral body.

Features of osteomalacia
Special radiographic features of osteomalacia are rare in uremic patients. Pseudofractures or loosers zones are wide, straight radiolucent bands which abut upon the cortex perpendicular to the long axis of the bones. These are uncommon in our experience and were noted in less than 2% of dialysis patients in Germany (127), but they

occurred in 20% of Australian patients with symptomatic renal osteodystrophy (117). They occur in areas of the pelvis, clavicles, scapulae, and long bones that are subject to mechanical stress. Protrusio acetabuli, another feature of osteomalacia, is identified by a convex bulging of the pelvis overlying the acetabulum (128).

Aseptic necrosis (osteonecrosis) occasionally develops in dialysis patients (129), although it is much more common in renal transplant recipients; it has been attributed to marked secondary hyperparathyroidism.

Osteopenia

A radiographic decrease in bone density may be termed osteopenia; this can occur in dialysis patients due to either osteomalacia or osteoporosis. A syndrome termed, 'dialysis osteopenia', is characterized by reduced bone mass, bone pain, and/or fractures, which are out of proportion to radiographic evidence of osteomalacia or osteitis fibrosa. X-rays showed widened marrow cavities, i.e. increased endosteal resorption. The patients failed to improve after subtotal parathyroidectomy or receiving large doses of vitamin D; unfortunately, bone histology was not available. The clinical findings in these patients may resemble those of 'dialysis osteomalacia', described above, but the lack of histologic data does not permit classification of these patients (130).

Bone mineral content

Photon absorptiometry, total body Ca by neutron activation, and scintiscans of the skeleton are other noninvasive methods for evaluating the skeleton. Neutron activation may provide an accurate measure of total bone mineral content (131), but the expense and the scarcity of facilities limit its use. Photon absorptiometry measures mineral content by the transmission of gamma rays on photons through bone. It is more accurate than is the determination of density from X-ray film, however, its use is limited to measurements of cortical bone in the radius, ulna or phalanges. Bone mineral content can be reduced because of a lower volume of bone tissue, an increase in intracortical porosity from increased resorption spaces, or because mineralized bone is replaced by unmineralized osteoid or poorly mineralized woven bone (117). Photon absorptiometry does not distinguish between the causes of decreased density, and this technique is best combined with detailed radiography.

The Metacarpal Index

By measuring the dimensions of the cortex of the metacarpal bone on X-ray film, the 'Metacarpal Index' is obtained.

The metacarpal index is the ratio of cortical width to total bone width. Normal data are available for the second left metacarpal bone.

Increased net endosteal resorption has been reported in 28 to 40% of dialysis patients (117, 132).

With the use of a dialysis fluid Ca of 1.25 mmol/l (2.5 mEq/l) the metacarpal index fell 6% in dialysis patients while no change was observed in patients utilizing 1.75 mmol/l (3.5 mEq/l) as the dialysis fluid Ca concentration (133). Other data, however, show no correlation between such loss and other evidence of bone disease nor between the rate of bone loss and heparin dosage (134) (Vide infra).

Scintiscan

Bone scintigraphy, utilizing $^{99}Tc^m$ diphosphonate, is capable of detecting skeletal alterations in dialysis patients and is useful in following the response to treatment. The diphosphonate accumulates in areas of increased bone turnover and increased blood flow (135). The uptake of the diphosphonate may be related to abnormal collagen metabolism (136). Ølgaard et al. (137) noted abnormal scintigraphy in 90% of their dialysis patients, only 10% of whom had abnormal X-rays, suggesting that this method is more sensitive than radiography (Figure 21). The symmetrical uptake of diphosphonate throughout the skeleton can occur as a manifestation of osteitis fibrosa. The scintiscan may also be a sensitive method for detecting multiple fractures, even in the absence of radiographic evidence of such fractures, in patients with osteomalacia. Further refinements of the technique involve measurement of the kinetics and the plasma clearance of diphosphonate (136). It can be used for the detection of extraskeletal calcification in tissues such as the lung (138).

Soft-tissue calcifications

Soft-tissue calcifications of several distinct types are common in end-stage renal disease. An increase in the Ca × P product, the degree of secondary hyperparathyroidism, hypermagnesemia, alkalosis, and local tissue injury each predispose to their development (139). The

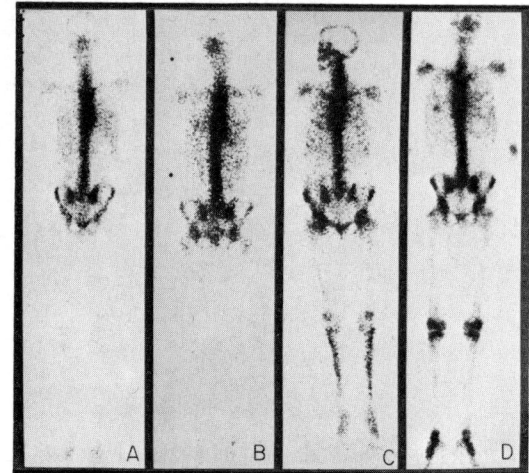

Figure 21. Skeletal scintigrams in a normal subject and patients with renal failure.
A. Grade 0, normal scintigram
B. Grade 1, scintigram showing abnormal uptake in the femoral heads with an extension to the femoral neck and trochanteric region
C. Grade 2, scintigram showing abnormal uptake in the femoral head and neck and in the proximal half of the tibial shaft
D. Grade 3, scintigram showing extensive uptake in the femoral head and marked uptake in femoral and tibial condyles, the tarsus and the proximal part of the metatarsus. (Reproduced from Ølgaard et al [137] with permission of the publisher.)

chemical and crystal composition of visceral calcifications was found to differ substantially from that observed in Ca deposits in periarticular, tumoral or vascular sites (140). The first variety is made up of amorphous microcrystals and has concentrations of Ca, Mg and P that resemble those of Ca whitlockite. Calcium deposits localized around the joints may consist of carbonate-containing apatite similar to that in bone; such crystals are more likely to induce inflammation than are amorphous microcrystals.

Calcifications may involve the sclera (band keratopathy), the conjunctiva, (see color plate in Chapter 38) the skin, where it can present as macular plaques, soft tissues about the joints, and periarticular sites or the joints themselves (chondrocalcinosis). Visceral calcification of the lungs or heart may have serious clinical consequences, e.g., myocardial calcifications may impair cardiac function or conduction and lead to congestive failure or heart block (141, 142) and pulmonary calcifications can be associated with perfusion-ventilation abnormalities (143).

Vascular calcifications can present in two major varieties: 1) intimal calcification, similar to that observed in atherosclerosis, is common in the aorta and large arteries and 2) medial calcification, a form more typical of uremia, involves the media of medium and large sized arteries (Figure 22); the lumen of the vessel is often patent, but surgery to establish a vascular access may be difficult. Because of rigidity of the involved vessel, pulses may be poorly palpable even when circulation is adequate. Medial calcifications may be associated with the syndrome, calciphylaxis, described above.

Soft-tissue calcifications are believed to be related to a high Ca × P product; they are common with secondary hyperparathyroidism. Parathyroid hormone may be a pathogenic factor, and Ca deposition in certain tissues such as joint, brain and heart, may relate directly to high PTH levels (144, 145). Dialysis patients with acute periarthritis have, as a group, higher levels of PTH than other dialysis patients (see Figure 7). For unexplained reasons, uremic children rarely develop soft tissue calcification (146).

PREVENTION AND MANAGEMENT

The general objectives of management that pertain to osteodystrophy in dialysis patients are to suppress secondary hyperparathyroidism, to produce normal mineralization of osteoid, to maintain blood concentrations of Ca, Mg and P near normal, and to prevent extraosseous calcification. Therapeutic considerations will be classified as general management, which apply to all dialysis patients, and specific treatment for problems arising in certain patients.

General management

The cornerstones of management include: 1) prevention of hyperphosphatemia by modest dietary P restriction and administration of aluminum hydroxide or aluminum carbonate; 2) dietary supplements of Ca; 3) and use of an appropriate Ca concentration in the dialysis fluid. In addition, hypermagnesemia should be prevented by avoiding foods or drugs containing excess Mg and by use of an appropriate Mg level in the dialysis solution. Fluoride and aluminum should be removed from tap water used for preparation of dialysis fluid by appropriate pretreatment (see Chapter 6).

The value of vitamin D for prophylaxis has not yet been established. Most children, however, undergoing dialysis eventually develop overt skeletal disease unless pharmacologic quantities of vitamin D are administered (147). Therefore, children should receive prophylactic treatment with active forms of vitamin D. Indications for parathyroidectomy and for treatment of overt bone disease with specific forms of vitamin D are discussed below.

Control of hyperphosphatemia
Factors that contribute to hyperphosphatemia in dialysis patients are noted in Table 5. In advanced uremia, dietary P intake in excess of 1 to 1.2 g (32 to 39 mmol)/day may lead to hyperphosphatemia despite the intake of substantial amounts of aluminum hydroxide. Modest dietary P restriction to 800-1000 mg (26-32 mmol)/day permits easier control of plasma P with aluminum hy-

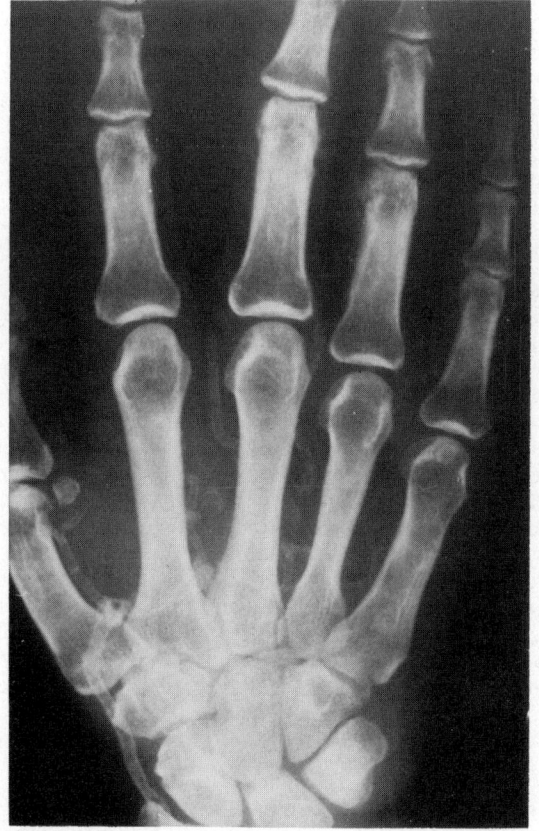

Figure 22. Radiograph showing marked calcification of the digital arteries; although intimal plaques may be present, the appearance is characteristic of extensive media calcification.

droxide or carbonate. It should be noted, however, that absorption of aluminum contained in phosphate binders may contribute to aluminum retention and toxicity.

With such treatment, several weeks may pass before plasma P falls, suggesting that P has been sequestered in bone and/or soft tissues (148). The reduction of plasma P toward normal is often associated with a small increase in plasma Ca and with a fall in plasma PTH and a reduced incidence of overt secondary hyperparathyroidism (149).

Secondary hyperparathyroidism may persist or progress in a substantial number of dialysis patients despite correction of hyperphosphatemia (80, 149, 150).

Calcium concentration in dialysis fluid
The use of dialysis solution containing 1.25 to 1.3 mmol/l (2.5 to 2.6 mEq/l) of Ca acutely decreases ionized Ca, which would aggravate secondary hyperparathyroidism, and most dialysis centers now utilize dialysis fluid with a Ca concentration of 1.5 to 1.75 mmol/l (3.0 to 3.5 mEq/l). An increase of Ca in the dialysis fluid from 1.25 to 1.50 mmol/l (2.5 to 3.0 mEq/l) decreased the incidence of overt skeletal disease (151), but it is not clear whether a further increase from 1.75 to 2.0 mmol/l (3.5 to 4.0 mEq/l) would produce any benefit. A transient postdialytic fall in plasma PTH was reported with the use of the higher dialysate Ca level, but predialysis PTH levels were unchanged (151). A stepwise increase of the Ca concentration in the dialysis solution from 1.13 to 1.5 mmol/l (2.25 to 3.0 mEq/l) and then to 1.75 mmol/l (3.5 mEq/l) did not affect pre-dialysis PTH nor the severity of bone disease (62). In another study (152), which compared a Ca concentration in the dialysis solution of 2.0 mmol/l (4.0 mEq/l) versus 1.75 mmol/l (3.5 mEq/l) only one of six patients showed a fall in plasma PTH and a decrease in bone resorption with the higher Ca concentration. Thus, current evidence indicates no benefit from the use of Ca concentrations in the dialysis fluid above 1.5 to 1.63 mmol/l (3.0 to 3.25 mEq/l) and there may be added risk of extraskeletal Ca deposition (153). (See also Chapter 7).

Oral calcium supplements
The diets ingested by dialysis patients often contain insufficient Ca to prevent a negative Ca balance (148, 154); a daily dietary Ca of 1.5 to 2.0 g/day (37.5 to 50 mmol/day) can prevent a negative balance. Thus, it seems reasonable to recommend dietary Ca supplements; calcium carbonate is palatable and least expensive, although other compounds may also be used. The oral administration of large amounts of Ca may suppress secondary hyperparathyroidism and improve bone mineral (155, 156), although the mineralization may be qualitatively abnormal (157).

Hypercalcemia may develop with use of oral Ca supplements (155, 156). When this occurs in conjunction with a markedly elevated plasma PTH and skeletal erosions, overt poorly suppressable hyperparathyroidism is likely, and subtotal parathyroidectomy may be indicated. Dietary Ca can be markedly reduced while an active form of vitamin D (i.e., 1,25(OH)$_2$D$_3$ or 1-alpha (OH)D$_3$) is given; such a regimen may suppress the secondary hyperparathyroidism and heal the skeletal disease without aggravating the hypercalcemia.

Dialysate magnesium
The use of a dialysis solution containing 0.25 mmol/l (0.5 mEq/l) of Mg, results in predialysis plasma Mg levels that approach normal (Figure 15); skeletal Mg may also fall in association with an improved chemical composition of bone (158). Medications containing Mg, such as laxatives and Mg-containing antacids, should be avoided.

Fluoride-containing water
The effect of using fluoride-containing tap water for preparation of dialysis solution is controversial (159). Normally excreted by the kidney, fluoride accumulates in the body, particularly in the bone, as kidney function deteriorates. This accumulation accelerates when fluoride containing water is used for preparing dialysis solution (160). A correlation of bone fluoride content and the duration of dialysis with both histologic and radiologic evidence of osteodystrophy has been noted (161). Moreover, a high incidence of overt bone disease was reduced after water purification was initiated with removal of fluoride and other substances from the dialysis fluid (162). Others have found that the use of fluoride-containing water does not worsen osteodystrophy provided that plasma Ca and P levels are adequately controlled (163). Nonetheless, pretreatment of water for dialysis fluid preparation is recommended when the tap water contains substantial quantities of fluoride (159 [see also Chapter 6]).

Aluminum-containing water
There is growing evidence that the presence of appreciable quantities of aluminum in the water utilized for preparing dialysis fluid is associated with a high incidence of osteomalacic bone disease (64, 66 [see chapters 7 and 42]). After institution of appropriate water-treatment and substantial reduction of its aluminum content, the incidence of such bone disease has been markedly reduced (64, 65). There is evidence that aluminum may accumulate in the bones of patients treated with dialysis (164, 165), and the aluminum content of bone is higher in patients with osteomalacia than with other types of bone disease (66). When a patient has fractures and bone histology reveals osteomalacia, the aluminum levels should be measured in city water and dialysis fluid, and appropriate methods of water-treatment should be initiated.

Heparin
Large doses of heparin can also impair bone mineralization (166, 167). With a shorter duration of dialysis treatments and reduced doses of heparin, however the total quantity of heparin given to dialysis patients is generally lower than that associated with such demineralization.

Specific treatment

Vitamin D sterols

A considerable number of dialysis patients develop progressive and disabling bone disease despite adherence to the management described above. Some exhibit evidence of secondary hyperparathyroidism, while others have osteomalacia. When the former develops, treatment with various forms of vitamin D, i.e., dihydrotachysterol (168), 25-hydroxyvitamin D_3 (169), 1-alpha-(OH)D_3 (170-172), or 1,25(OH)$_2D_3$ (80, 173, 174) and pharmacologic doses of vitamin D_2 itself (175), may produce clinical improvement, a return of X-rays toward normal, and amelioration of bone pathology. Also, elevated plasma levels of alkaline phosphatase and iPTH may fall (Figure 23). The decrease in plasma iPTH levels to normal during treatment despite only a slight increase in plasma Ca suggests that 1,25(OH)$_2D_3$ may facilitate the suppression of PTH secretion (Figure 24). Different forms and doses of vitamin D sterols are summarized in table 7.

During the first 1 to 2 months of treatment, serum P falls or remains unchanged (Figure 25) despite the increase in P absorption produced by the active forms of vitamin D (176), suggesting skeletal remineralization. Later, as the rate of mineralization slows, continued stimulation of intestinal absorption of Ca and P may produce hypercalcemia and hyperphosphatemia, which are readily reversed after discontinuation of the drug or reduction of the dose (Figure 26). Skeletal biopsies may show reduced fibrous tissue and improved mineralization (177), but bone histology rarely returns to normal.

Table 7. Forms and approximate doses of vitamin D sterols used for symptomatic renal osteodystrophy.

Sterol used	Daily dose
Vitamin D_2 [ergocalciferol]	0.25–5.0 mg *
Dihydrotachysterol	0.25–4.0 mg
Calcitriol [1,25-dihydroxyvitamin D_3, 1,25(OH)$_2D_3$]	0.20–1.0 μg
1 alpha-hydroxyvitamin D_3 [1-alpha-(OH)D_3]	1.0–2.0 μg
Calcifediol [25-hydroxyvitamin D_3, 25(OH)D_3]	20–50 μg

* Equivalent to 10,000 to 200,000 IU/day (1 IU = 0.025 μg).

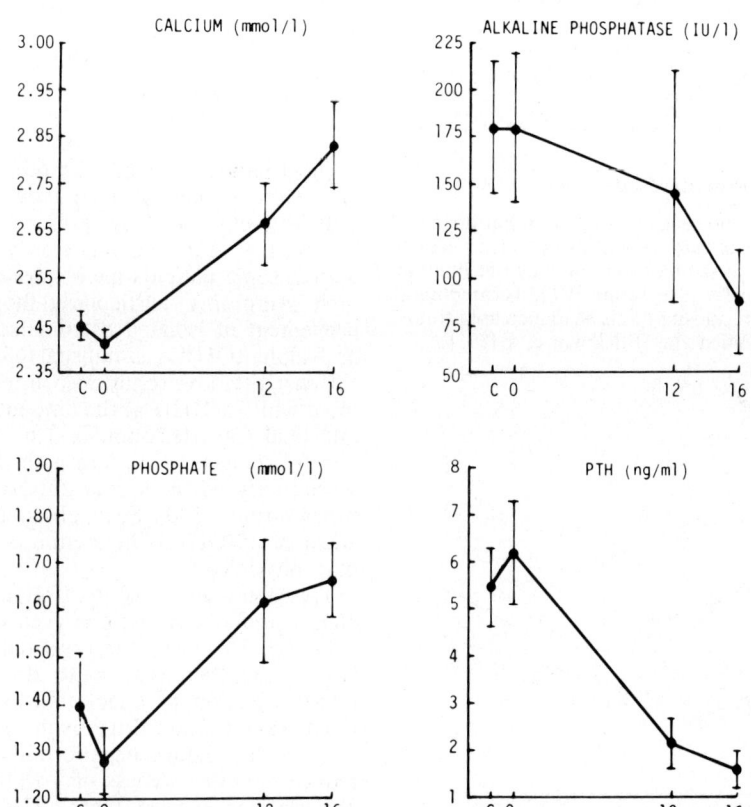

Figure 23. Mean values of plasma Ca, P, alkaline phosphatase, and serum immunoreactive PTH in 10 dialysis patients treated with 1-alpha-(OH)D_3 for 16 months. The initial dose was 1 μg/day, and the dose was adjusted in each patient during the trial. (Modified after Papapoulos et al [170])

(Conversion factors: Ca mmol/l → mg/dl: ×4
P (as phosphate): mmol/l → mg/dl: ×3.1)

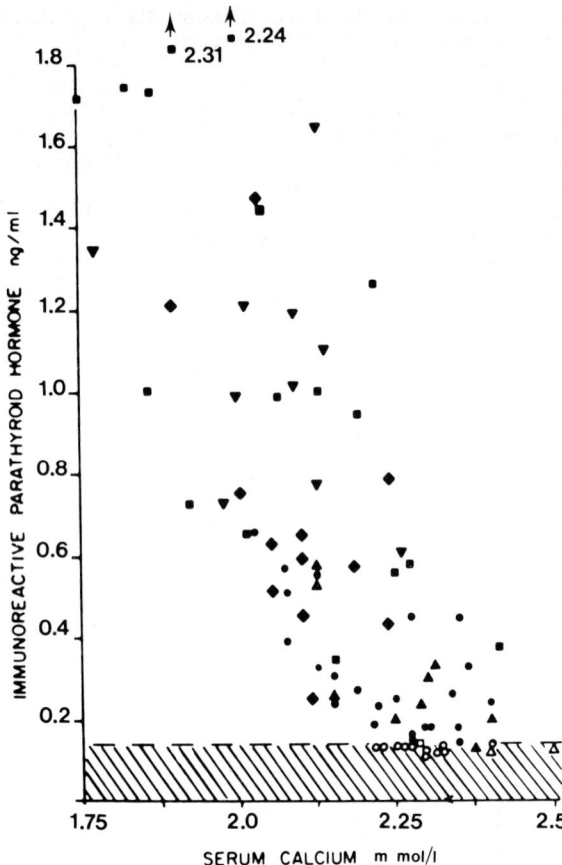

Figure 24. Levels of immunoreactive parathyroid hormone in 4 uremic patients with secondary hyperparathyroidism treated with 1,25(OH)$_2$D$_3$. Plasma samples were obtained at intervals of 4 to 7 days. As serum Ca rose, serum iPTH became undetectable even when serum calcium levels were increased from 2 to only 2.5 mmol/l (Modified after Brickman et al [195]).

(Conversion: Ca mmol/l → mg/dl: ×4)

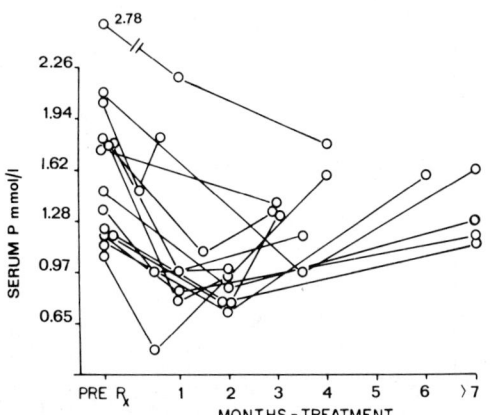

Figure 25. Representative values of serum phosphorus before and during treatment with 1,25(OH)$_2$D$_3$. The lowest values usually occurring at 1 to 2 months, and the final value during treatment are shown. (Data from Coburn et al [80]).

(Conversion: P (as phosphate) mmol/l → mg/dl: ×3.1)

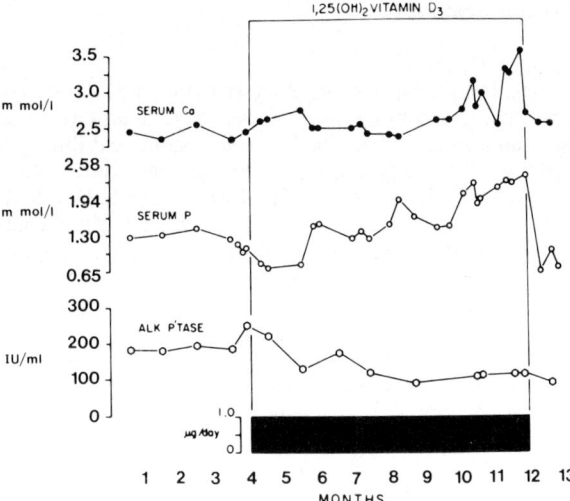

Figure 26. Treatment of renal osteodystrophy with 1,25(OH)$_2$D$_3$. Initially a decrease of serum P occurs suggesting remineralization of the skeleton.
Later when mineralization slows and stimulation of calcium and phosphate absorption continues, hypercalcemia and hyperphosphatemia may develop.
Both however, are rapidly reversed when the drug is discontinued or the dose is reduced.
(Adapted from Coburn et al [80])

(Conversion: Ca mmol/l → mg/dl: ×4
P [as phosphate] mmol/l → mg/dl: ×3.1)

Other patients treated with other vitamin D sterols do not improve their skeletal lesions (178). The widened osteoid seams, which are present in patients with mixed lesions, may improve only slowly during treatment. Although some patients have substantial improvement in their symptoms, particularly those of myopathy, improvement of isolated osteomalacia with 1,25(OH)$_2$D$_3$ or 1-alpha (OH)D$_3$ is unusual (68).

Renal osteodystrophy also improves following treatment with 25(OH)D$_3$; the amount required to stimulate intestinal Ca absorption is 3 to 4 fold that needed in normal subjects (179), and a therapeutic benefit is observed only when plasma 25(OH)D$_3$ levels are 2 to 3 times normal (180). Such observations suggest that the effect of 25(OH)D$_3$ in uremia is pharmacologic rather than physiologic.

Treatment with 1-alpha-(OH)D$_3$ produces beneficial effects similar to those observed with 1,25(OH)$_2$D$_3$ (80, 170-172). However, the dose required is 2 to 3 times larger. Also, there is a slightly slower onset of action and longer duration of effect following cessation of treatment (181). Certain drugs such as phenytoin or barbiturates, which induce hepatic microsomal enzymes, may reduce the effectiveness of 1-alpha-(OH)D$_3$ (182). Such observations suggest that 1,25(OH)$_2$D$_3$ may be preferred.

Treatment failure groups

There remains a group of patients who show little or no improvement of skeletal disease when treated with an active form of vitamin D (80, 170).

One subgroup of patients exhibits markedly elevated plasme iPTH levels and bone biopsy of such patients shows fibro-osteoclasia. Plasma Ca is either elevated or in the upper normal range before vitamin D treatment, and hypercalcemia develops within 1 to 2 weeks after treatment with 1,25(OH)$_2$D$_3$ or 1-alpha-(OH)D$_3$ (80, 170, 183). Such patients may have marked parathyroid hyperplasia which fails to regress with treatment; subtotal parathyroidectomy is probably indicated. Alternatively, rigid dietary Ca restriction and treatment with 1,25(OH)$_2$D$_3$ may be attempted.

A second subgroup who fail to improve following treatment with 1,25(OH)$_2$D$_3$ or 1-alpha-(OH)$_2$D$_3$ exhibit only osteomalacia. Plasma Ca levels may exceed 2.6 mmol/l (5.2 mEq/l) and plasma iPTH levels are usually low or normal. Treatment with vitamin D$_2$ in doses as low as 10,000 I.U./day, or calcitriol, 0.1 to 0.25 µg/day, may promptly cause hypercalcemia. The symptoms often do not improve, the alkaline phosphatase level remains elevated, and the bone disease does not heal (Figure 27). Thus, these patients have a defect in mineralization that is not corrected by calcitriol or by raising plasma Ca and P to normal levels or above. Preliminary observations suggest that certain patients may exhibit improvement in symptoms and improved mineralization of bone during treatment with a combination of 1,25(OH)$_2$D$_3$ plus 24,25(OH)$_2$D$_3$. In many patients, the tolerance for calcitriol, which previously caused hypercalcemia, was markedly increased during the concomitant administration of 24,25(OH)$_2$D$_3$ (184). Further observations are needed to substantiate their effects.

Parathyroidectomy

Many manifestations of secondary hyperparathyroidism regress following subtotal parathyroidectomy (150, 185, 186). However, the substantial improvement of patients with overt secondary hyperparathyroidism treated with vitamin D sterols has decreased the need for parathyroid surgery. Nevertheless, indications for parathyroidectomy still exist. Hypercalcemia, if associated with mental symptoms and severe hypertension, can be most quickly reversed following surgical management. However, hypercalcemia alone may not indicate the presence of parathyroid hyperplasia; this may occur with osteomalacia and normal iPTH levels and during treatment with vitamin D sterols, oral Ca supplements and the use of a high Ca in dialysis fluid. Therefore, evidence for secondary hyperparathyroidism, i.e. bone erosions and/or markedly elevated levels of plasma iPTH should be pre-

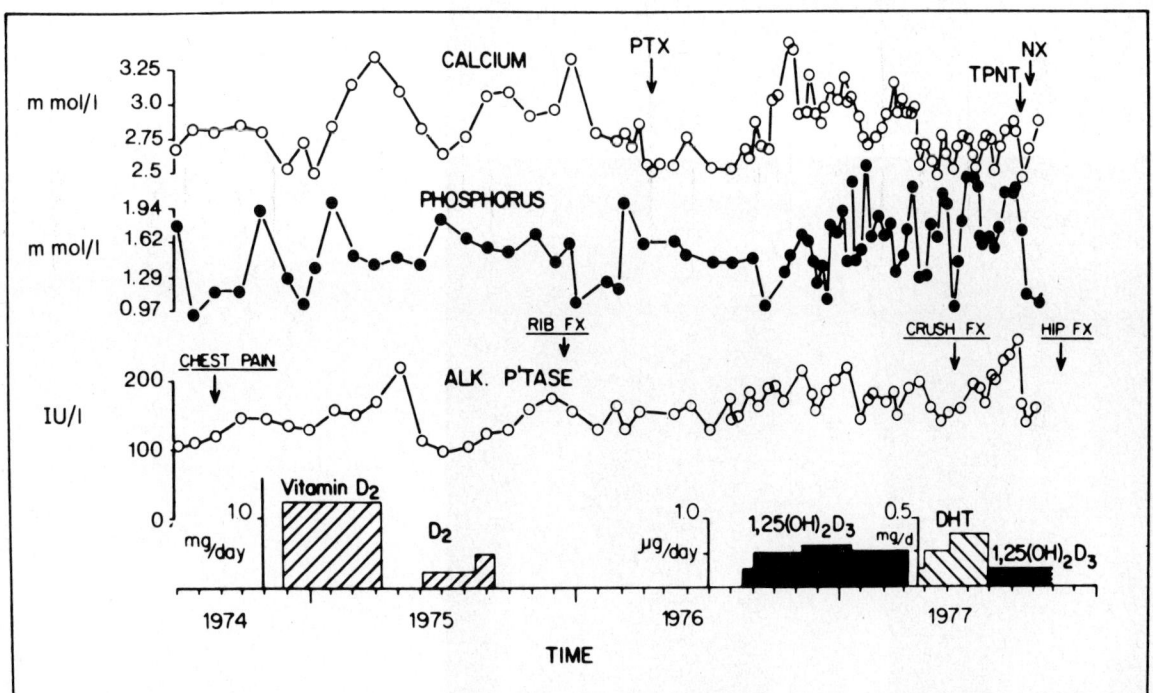

Figure 27. Course of a patient with dialysis osteomalacia. Symptomatic bone disease and marked skeletal demineralization developed after 2 years of home dialysis. Treatment with vitamin D$_2$, 50,000 IU/day or 10,000 IU/day resulted in hypercalcemia. Parathyroidectomy (PTX), performed because of progression of symptoms, resulted in no improvement. Subsequently, he received 1,25(OH)$_2$D$_3$ for 4 months with no change except that serum Ca increased. Adapted from Coburn et al [80] with permission.

FX = fracture
PTX = subtotal parathyroidectomy
TPNT = Transplant
NX = Nephrectomy

(Conversion: Ca mmol/l → mg/dl: ×4)

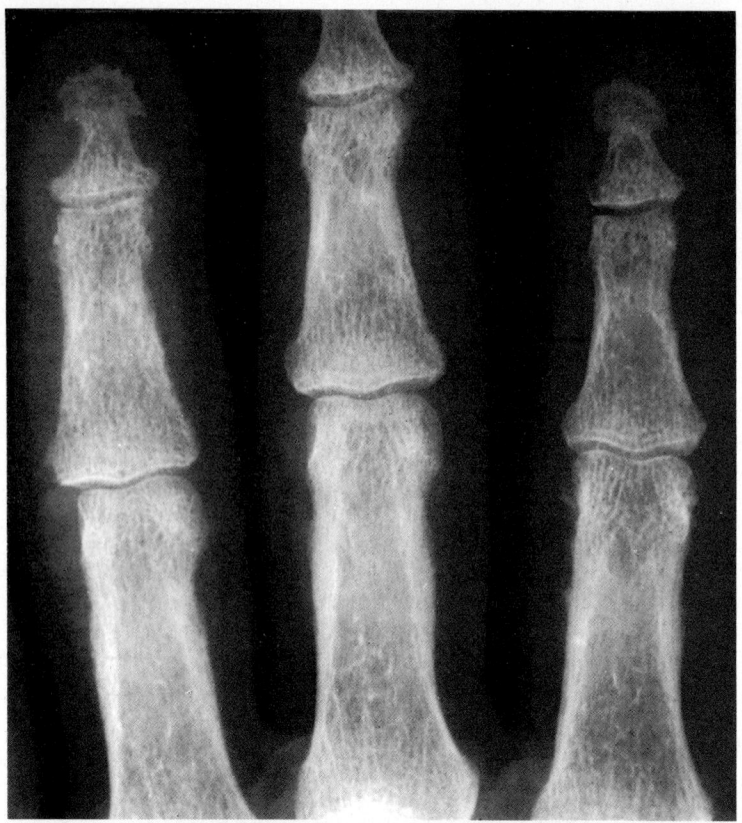
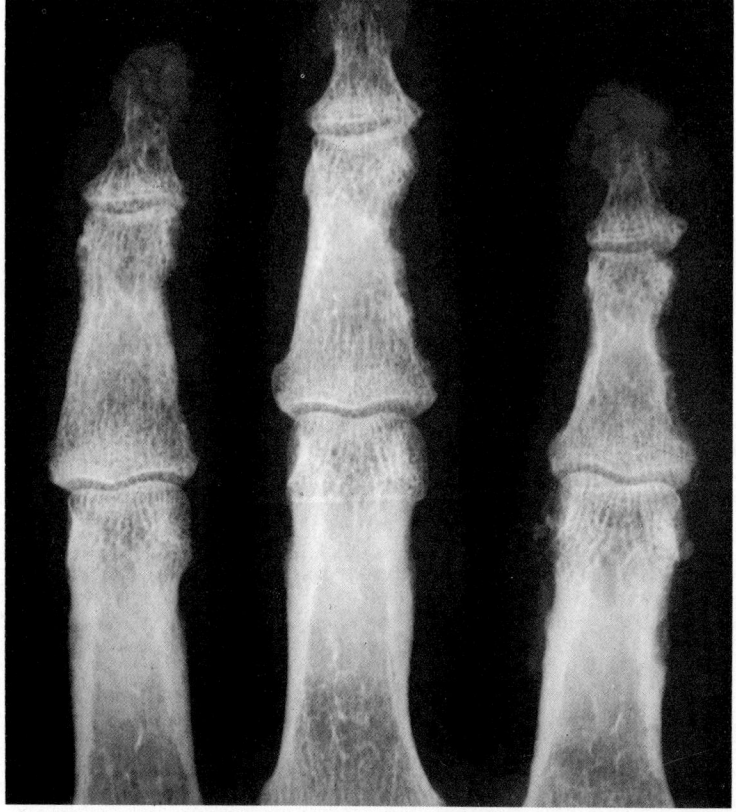

Figure 28. Extensive subperiosteal resorption involving the left hand of a 50 year old man with chronic end-stage renal failure. The resorptions, shown before parathyroidectomy (top), are characteristically more marked on the radial surfaces. Hemodialysis was initiated and sub-total parathyroidectomy was carried out. There was substantial symptomatic improvement; the X-ray (bottom), showing marked clearing of the erosions, was obtained 10 months later.

sent before a decision is made to undertake surgery. X-rays showing substantial improvement after subtotal parathyroidectomy are shown in Figure 28. In certain patients, severe osteomalacia may develop following parathyroidectomy (70). Thus, the total removal of the parathyroid glands may contribute to osteomalacia.

The appearance of ischemic skin ulcerations in association with marked vascular calcifications (calciphylaxis) is another indication for parathyroidectomy (88). Rarely, pruritus may be so severe that surgery should be considered, although it is unlikely to produce benefits in the absence of other manifestations of secondary hyperparathyroidism.

Whether to carry out total or subtotal parathyroidectomy is an important issue. The long-term management of surgically induced hypoparathyroidism in a dialysis patient is difficult; the hypocalcemia may be difficult to control and pharmacologic doses of vitamin D may lead to hypercalcemia. Moreover, as noted above, total parathyroidectomy may predispose to the development of isolated osteomalacia; for this reason, total parathyroidectomy is only rarely indicated.

During the post-operative period after parathyroidectomy, hypocalcemic tetany and convulsions may occur and lead to serious fractures. The most severe hypocalcemia developing during the post-operative period seems to correlate with the extent of osteoclastic activity and with the alkaline phosphatase level present in the preoperative bone biopsy (187). Such hypocalcemia occurs with the marked reduction of excess bone resorption and improved mineralization of the abnormal bone, i.e., the 'hungry bone' syndrome. Interestingly hypocalcemic seizures may not appear in such patients when plasma Ca is at the lowest value but are observed during the latter hours of hemodialysis or after dialysis, suggesting that hypocalcemia may predispose to central nervous system manifestations that are analogous to the 'dialysis disequilibrium' syndrome.

Other treatments

A beta-adrenergic modulation of PTH secretion has been shown (19), and preliminary data suggest that beta-adrenergic blockade with propranolol can lower serum PTH and alkaline phosphatase levels (188). Moreover, fewer radiographic features of renal osteodystrophy have been reported in dialysis patients receiving propranolol compared to patients not treated with this drug. The long-term treatment with propranolol has led to correction of hypercalcemia and a lowering of plasma PTH levels in certain patients with primary hyperparathyroidism (188). Further studies are needed to evaluate the role of this agent in the management of renal osteodystrophy.

Cimetidine has also been shown to suppress PTH levels in dialysis patients with normal plasma Ca (189).

Spontaneous hypercalcemia was successfully managed with cimetidine in two dialysis patients receiving this drug over a 6-month period (190).

The association of elevated plasma levels of calcitonin with a lower incidence of osteitis fibrosa in patients with high plasma PTH levels and knowledge that calcitonin can block certain effects of PTH on bone suggest that this hormone may be useful in the management of certain patients with severe secondary hyperparathyroidism.

Further trials with these agents are needed; their use should be limited to patients who are poor candidates for parathyroid surgery, for patients who have had recurrence of hyperparathyroidism after previous surgery, and for patients whose parathyroid tissue is believed to be in the thoracic cavity rather than in the neck.

Fractures

Spontaneous rib fractures, the most frequent fracture occurring in patients with renal osteodystrophy, may heal slowly over several months. Traumatic fractures of the long bones and femoral neck often have poor union, even after many months. When fractures occur in patients with secondary hyperparathyroidism, surgical repair should be delayed until the metabolic bone disease is treated appropriately. To avoid prolonged hypercalcemia, it is preferable that secondary hyperparathyroidism is treated with a short acting, active vitamin D sterol; parathyroidectomy should be reserved for the most urgent cases.

Extraskeletal calcification

Periarticular and tumoral calcifications often regress with control of hyperphosphatemia. However, vascular calcifications change only slowly if at all. Soft tissue calcifications have developed in association with vitamin D overdoses (191) but pharmacologic doses of vitamin D combined with prevention or correction of hyperphosphatemia may result in disappearance of vascular calcification (192).

ACKNOWLEDGMENTS

Some of the work described in the present chapter was supported by the Veterans Administration Research Funds from Wadsworth and Oklahoma City Veterans Administration Hospitals.

Figures 4A-4D are reproduced from color photomicrographs kindly provided by A. J. Felsenfeld M.D.

Figure 19 was kindly supplied by H. E. Meema, Toronto Western Hospital.

The secretarial assistance of Mrs. Alvia M. Woodfork is gratefully acknowledged.

REFERENCES

1. Holick MF, McNeil SC, MacLaughlin JA, Holick SA, Clark MB, Potts Jr JT: The physiologic implications of the formation of previtamin D₃ in skin. *Trans Assoc Am Physicians* 92:54, 1979
2. Haddad JG, Walgate J: Radioimmunoassay of the binding protein for vitamin D and its metabolites in human serum. *J Clin Invest* 58:1217, 1976
3. Ponchon G, DeLuca HF: The role of the liver in the metabolism of vitamin D. *J Clin Invest* 48:1273, 1969
4. Smith JE, Goodman DS: The turnover and transport of

vitamin D and of a polar metabolite with the properties of 25-hydroxycholecalciferol in human plasma. *J Clin Invest* 50:2159, 1971
5. Gray, RW Omdahl JL, Ghazarian JG, DeLuca HF: 35-hydroxycholecalciferol-1-hydroxylase. *J. Biol Chem* 247:7528, 1972
6. Midgett RJ, Spielvogel AM, Coburn JW, Norman AW: Studies of calciferol metabolism. VII. The renal production of the biologically active form of vitamin D, 1,25-dihydroxycholecalciferol; species, tissue and subcellular distribution. *J Clin Endocrinol* 36:1153, 1973
7. Hughes MR, Haussler MR, Wergedal J, Baylink DJ: Regulation of plasma 1 alpha, 25-dihydroxyvitamin D_3 by calcium and phosphate. *Clin Res* 23:323A, 1975
8. Pike JW, Toverud S, Baass A, McCain T, Haussler MR: Circulating 1 alpha, 25-$(OH)_2D$ during physiological states of calcium stress. In: *Vitamin D: Biochemical, Chemical and Clinical Aspects Related to Calcium metabolism,* edited by Norman AW, Schaefer K, Coburn JW, DeLuca HF, Fraser D, Grigoleit HG, and Herrath D v, Berlin, W de Gruyter, 1977, p 187
9. Haussler MR, McCain TA: Basic and clinical concepts related to vitamin D metabolism and action. *N Engl J Med* 297:974, 1041, 1977
10. DeLuca HF: Vitamin D endocrinology. *Ann Intern Med* 85:367, 1976
11. Levine BS, Coburn JW: Physiology of the vitamin D endocrine system and disorders of altered vitamin D metabolism. In: *Hormonal Function and the Kidney,* edited by Brenner BM, Stein JH, New York, Edinburgh, London, Churchill Livingstone, 1979, p 215
12. Horst L, Littledike ET, Gray RW, Napoli JL: Impaired 24, 25 dihydroxyvitamin D production in anephric man and pig. *J Clin Invest* 67:274, 1981
13. Llach F, Brickman AS, Singer FR, Coburn JW: 24, 25-dihydroxycholecalciferol, a vitamin D sterol with qualitatively unique effects in uremic man. *Metab Bone Dis Relat Res* 2:11, 1979
14. Hodsman AB, Wong EGC, Sherrard DJ, Brickman AS, Lee DBN, Singer FR, Norman AW, Coburn JW: Use of 24, 25-dihydroxyvitamin D_3 in dialysis osteomalacia; preliminary results. In: *Hormonal Control of Calcium Metabolism,* edited by Cohn DV, Talmage RV, Mathews JL. Amsterdam, Excerpta Medica, 1981, p 460
15. Henry HL, Taylor AN, Norman AW: Response of chick parathyroid glands to the vitamin D metabolites, 1, 25-dihydroxycholecalciferol and 24, 25-dihydroxycholecalciferol. *J Nutr* 107:1918, 1977
16. Tanaka Y, DeLuca HE: Biological activity of 24, 25-difluoro-25-hydro-vitamin D_3. *J Biol Chem* 254:7163, 1979
17. Mayer GP, Hurst JG: Sigmoidal relationship between parathyroid hormone secretion rate and plasma calcium concentration in calves. *Endocrinology* 102:1036, 1978
18. Mayer GP, Habener JF, Potts JF: Parathyroid hormone secretion: in vivo demonstration of a calcium-independent nonsuppressible component of secretion. *J. Clin Invest* 57:678, 1976
19. Mayer GP, Hurst JG, Barto JA, Keaton JA, Moore MP: Effect of epinephrine on parathyroid hormone secretion in calves. *Endocrinology* 104:1181, 1979
20. Habener JF, Potts JT Jr: Relative effectiveness of magnesium and calcium on the secretion and biosynthesis of parathyroid hormone in vitro. *Endocrinology* 98:197, 1976
21. Habener JF, Mayer GP, Dee PC, Potts JT Jr: Metabolism of amino- and carboxyl-sequence immunoactive parathyroid hormone in the bovine: Evidence for peripheral cleavage of hormone. *Metabolism* 25:285, 1976

22. Segre GV, Habener JF, Powel JF, Tregear GW, Potts JT Jr: Parathyroid hormone in human plasma. Immuno clinical characterization and biological indication. *J Clin Invest* 51:3163, 1972
23. Segre GV, Mall HD, Habener JF, Potts JT Jr: Metabolism of parathyroid hormone. Pathologic and clinical significance. *Am J Med* 56:774, 1974
24. Hruska KA, Kopelman R, Rutherford WE, Klahr S, Slatopolsky E: Metabolism of immunoreactive parathyroid hormone in the dog: The role of kidney and the effect of chronic renal disease. *J Clin Invest* 56:39, 1975
25. Martin KJ, Hruska K, Freitag JJ, Klahr S, Slatopolsky E: The peripheral metabolism of parathyroid hormone. *N Engl Med* 301:1092, 1979
26. Coburn JW, Slatopolsky E: Vitamin D, PTH and renal osteodystrophy. In: *The Kidney,* 2nd Edition, edited by Brenner BM, Rector FC Jr, Philadelphia, London, Toronto, WB Saunders Co, 1981, p 2213
27. Parfitt AM: The actions of parathyroid hormone on bone. Relation to bone remodeling and turnover, calcium homeostasis and metabolic bone disease. IV. The state of bones in uremic hyperparathyroidism. The mechanisms of skeletal resistance to PTH in renal failure and pseudo hypoparathyroidism and the role of PTH in osteoporosis, osteopetrosis and osteofluorosis. *Metabolism* 25:1157, 1976
28. Slatopolsky E, Hruska K, Martin K, Freitag J: Physiologic and metabolic effects of parathyroid hormone. In: *Hormonal Function and the Kidney,* edited by Brenner BM, Stein JH. New York, Edinburgh, Churchill Livingstone, London, 1979, p 169
29. Ritz E, Malluche HH, Krempien B, Mehls O: Calcium metabolism in renal failure. In: *Disorders of Mineral Metabolism.* Vol III, edited by Bronner F, Coburn JW, New York, Academic press, 1981, p 152
30. Coburn JR, Popovtzer MM, Massry SG, Kleeman CR: The physiochemical state and renal handling of divalent ions in chronic renal failure. *Arch Intern Med* 124:302, 1969
31. Slatopolsky ES, Caglar JP, Pennell DB, Taggart JM, Canterbury E, Reiss, Bricker NS: On the pathogenesis of hyperparathyroidism in chronic experimental insufficiency in the dog. *J Clin Invest* 50:492, 1971
32. Slatopolsky E, Cagler S, Gradowska L, Canterbury J, Reiss E, Bricker NS: On the prevention of secondary hyperparathyroidism in experimental chronic renal insufficiency using 'proportional reduction' of dietary phosphorus intake. *Kidney Int* 2:147, 1972
33. Reiss E, Cantebury JM, Bercovitz MA, Kaplan EL: The role of phosphate in the secretion of parathyroid hormone in man. *J Clin Invest* 49:2146, 1970
34. Fournier AE, Arnaud CD, Johnson WJ, Taylor WF, Goldsmith RS: Etiology of hyperparathyroidism and bone disease during chronic hemodialysis. II. Factors affecting serum immunoreactive parathyroid hormone. *J Clin Invest* 50:599, 1971
35. Coburn JW, Kopple MH, Brickman AS, Massry SG: Study of intestinal absorption of calcium in patients with renal failure *Kidney Int* 3:264, 1973
36. Llach F, Massry SG. Singer Fr, Kurokawa K, Kaye JH, Coburn JW: Skeletal resistance of endogenous parathyroid hormone in patients with early renal failure: A possible cause for secondary hyperparathyroidism. *J Clin Endocrinol Metab* 41:338, 1975
37. Haussler MR, Baylink DJ, Hughes MR, Brumbaugh PF, Wergedal JE, Shen FH, Nielsen RL, Counts SJ Bursac KM, McCain TA: The assay of 1-alpha-25-dihydroxyvitamin D_3; physiologic and pathologic modulation of circulating hormone levels. *Clin Endocrinol* 5:151S, 1976

38. Mawer EB, Backhouse J, Taylor CM: Failure of formation of 1, 25-dihydroxycholecalciferol in chronic renal insufficiency. *Lancet* 1:626, 1973
39. Brickman AS, Coburn JW, Norman AW: Effect of 1, 25-dihydroxycholecalciferol, the active metabolite of vitamin D, in uremic man. *N Engl J Med* 287:891, 1972
40. Brickman AS, Coburn JW, Massry SG, Norman AW: 1, 25-dihydroxyvitamin D₃ in normal man and patients with renal failure. *Ann Intern Med* 80:161, 1974
41. Oettinger CW, Merrill R, Blanton T, Briggs W: Reduced calcium absorption after nephrectomy in uremic patients. *N Engl J Med* 291:458, 1975
42. Brickman As, Hartenbower DL, Norman AW, Coburn JW: Actions of 1-alpha-hydroxyvitamin D₃ and 1, 25-dihydroxyvitamin D₃ on mineral metabolism in man. I. Effects on net absorption of phosphorus. *Am J Clin Nutr* 30:1064, 1977
43. Mechanic GL, Toverd SU, Ramp WK, Gonnerman WA: The effect of vitamin D on the structural cross links and maturation of chick bone collagen. *Biochim Biophys Acta* 393:419, 1975
44. Avioli LV: Collagen metabolism, uremia and bone. *Kidney Int* 4:105, 1973
45. Heidbreder E, Luke F, Heidland A: Collagen metabolism and mineralization of uremic bone-aspects of the molecular pathology of renal osteodystrophy. *Klin Wochenschr* 54:341, 1976
46. Massry SG, Stein R, Garty J: Skeletal resistance to the calcemic action of PTH in uremia; role of 1, 25(OH)₂D₃. *Kidney Int* 9:467, 1976
47. Somerville PJ, Kaye M: Evidence that resistance to the calcemic action of parathyroid hormone in rats with acute uremia is caused by phosphate retention. *Kidney Int* 16:552, 1979
48. Massry SG, Coburn JW, Lee DBN, Jowsey J, Kleeman CR: Skeletal resistance to parathyroid hormone in renal failure. *Ann Intern Med* 73:357, 1973
49. Llach F, Massry SG, Singer FR, Kurokawa K, Kaye JH, Coburn JW: Skeletal resistance to endogenous parathyroid hormone in patients with early renal failure: A possible cause for secondary hyperparathyroidism. *J Clin Endocrinol Metab* 41:338, 1975
50. Wills MR, Jenkins MV: The effect of uraemic metabolites on parathyroid extract induced bone resorption in vitro. *Clin Chim Acta* 73:121, 1976
51. Massry SG, Stein R, Garty J, Arieff AI, Coburn JW, Norman AW, Friedler RM: On the mechanisms of the skeletal resistance to the calcemic action of parathyroid hormone in uremia. Role of 1, 25(OH)₂D₃. *Kidney Int* 9:467, 1976
52. Martin KJ, Hruska KA, Lewis J, Anderson C, Slatopolsky E: The renal handling of parathyroid hormone: Role of peritubular uptake and glomerular filtration. *J Clin Invest* 60:808, 1977
53. Tanaka Y, DeLuca HF: The control of 25-hydroxyvitamin D metabolism by inorganic phosphorus. *Arch Biochem Biophys* 159:566, 1973
54. Llach F, Massry SG, Koffler A, Malluche HH, Singer FR, Brickman AS, Kurokawa K: Secondary hyperparathyroidism in early renal failure: Role of phosphate retention. *Kidney Int* 12:459, 1977
55. Brumbaugh PF, Haussler DH, Bressler R, Haussler MR: Radioreceptor assay for 1, 25-dihydroxyvitamin D₃. *Science* 183:1089. 1974
56. Eisman JS, Hamstra AJ, Kream BE, DeLuca HF: 1,25-dihydroxyvitamin D in biological fluids; a simplified and sensitive assay. *Science* 193:1021, 1976
57. Bordier PJ, Tun-Chot S, Eastwood JB, Fornier A, de Wardener HE: Lack of histological evidence of vitamin D abnormality in the bones of anephric patients. *Clin Sci* 44:33, 1973
58. Bordier P, Rasmussen H, Marie P, Miravet L, Gueris J, Ryckwaert A: Vitamin D metabolites and bone mineralization in man. *J Clin Endocrinol Metab* 46:284, 1978
59. Malluche HH, Henry H, Meyer-Sabellek W, Sherman D, Massry SG, Norman AW: Effects and interactions of 24, 25-dihydroxycholecalciferol and 1, 25-dihydroxycholecalciferol on bone. *Am J Physiol* 238:E294, 1980
60. Schmidt-Gayk H, Schmitt W, Grawunder C, Ritz E, Tschoepe W, Pietsch V, Andrassy K, Bouillon R: 25-hydroxyvitamin D in nephrotic syndrome. *Lancet* 2:105, 1977
61. Goldstein DA, Oda Y, Kurokawa K, Massry SG: Blood levels of 25-hydroxyvitamin D in nephrotic syndrome. Studies in 26 patients. *Ann Intern Med* 87:664, 1977
62. Kanis JA, Adams ND, Earnshaw M, Heyman G, Ledingham JGG, Oliver DO, Russell RG, Woods CG: Vitamin D, osteomalacia, and chronic renal failure. In: *Vitamin D: Biochemical, Chemical and Clinical Aspects Related to Calcium Metabolism,* edited by Norman AW, Schaefer K, Coburn JW, DeLuca HF, Fraser D, Grigoleit HG, Herrath D v, Berlin, W de Gruyter, 1977, p 671
63. Parkinson IS, Feest TG, Ward MK, Fawcett RWP, Kerr DNS: Fracturing dialysis osteodystrophy and dialysis osteomalacia encephalopathy; an epidemiological survey. *Lancet* 1:406, 1979
64. Ward MK, Feest TG, Allis HA, Parkinson IS, Kerr DNS: Osteomalacia dialysis osteodystrophy. Evidence for a waterborne aetiological agent, probably aluminium. *Lancet* 1:841, 1978
65. Pierides AM, Wedwards WG Jr, Cullum UX, McCall JT, Ellis HA: Hemodialysis encephalopathy with osteomalacic fractures and muscle weakness. *Kidney Int* 18:115, 1980
66. Hodsman AB Sherrard DJ, Alfrey AC, Ott S, Brickman AS, Miller NL, Maloney NA, Coburn JW: Bone aluminum and histomorphometric features of renal osteodystrophy. *J Clin Endocrinol Metab* 54:539, 1982
67. Ellis HA, McCarthy JH, Herrington J: Bone aluminum in haemodialysed patients and in rats injected with aluminum chloride: relationship to impaired bone mineralization. *J Clin Path* 32:832, 1979
68. Hodsman AB, Sherrard DJ, Wong EGC, Brickman AS, Lee DBN, Alfrey AC, Singer FR, Norman AW, Coburn JW: Vitamin D resistant osteomalacia in hemodialysis patients lacking secondary hyperparathyroidism: Description of the syndrome in 19 patients. *Ann Intern Med* 94:629, 1981
69. Teitelbaum SL, Bergfeld MA, Freitag J, Hruska KA, Slatopolsky E: Do parathyroid hormone and 1, 25-dihydroxyvitamin D modulate bone formation in uremia? *J Clin Endocrinol* 51:247, 1980
70. Felsenfeld AJ, Harrelson JM, Gutman RA: Post parathyroidectomy osteomalacia in uremic man. *Ann Intern Med* 96:27, 1982
71. Kraut JA, Shinaberger JH, Singer RR, Sherrard DJ, Saxton J, Hodsmann AB, Miller JH, Kurokawa K, Coburn JW: Reduced parathyroid response to acute hypo-calcemia in dialysis osteomalacia. *Clin Res* 29:102A, 1981
72. Parfitt AM: The quantitative approach to bone morphology. A critique of current methods and their interpretation. In: *Clinical Aspects of Metabolic Bone disease* edited by Frame B, Parfitt AM, Duncan H, Amsterdam, Excerpta Medica, 1973, p 86
73. Frost HM: The origin and nature of transient human bone remodeling dynamics. In: *Clinical Aspects of Metabolic Bone Disease* Edited by Frame B, Parfitt AM, Duncan H, Amsterdam, Excerpta Medica, 1973, p 124

74. Sherrard DJ, Baylink DJ, Wergedal JE, Maloney N: Quantitative histological studies on the pathogenesis of uremic bone disease. *J Clin Endocrinol* 39:119, 1974
75. Frost HM: Tetracycline-based histological analysis of bone remodeling. *Calcif Tissue Res* 3:211, 1969
76. Ritz E, Malluche HH, Krempien B, Mehls O: Bone histology in renal insufficiency. In: *Perspectives in Nephrology and Hypertension.* Edited by David DS, New York, John Wiley and Sons, 1977, p 197
77. Sherrard DJ, Coburn JW, Brickman AS, Singer FR, Maloney N: Skeletal response to treatment with 1, 25-dihydroxyvitamin D in renal failure. *Contrib Nephrol* 18:92, 1980
78. Schott GD, Wills MR: Muscle weakness in osteomalacia. *Lancet* 1:626, 1976
79. Schoenfeld PJ, Martin JH, Barnes B, Teitelbaum SL: Amelioration of myopathy with 25-hydroxyvitamin D_3 therapy (25(OH)D_3) in patients on chronic hemodialysis. *Third Workshop on Vitamin D, Book of Abstracts,* Asilomar, 1977, p 160
80. Coburn JW, Brickman AS, Sherrard DJ, Singer FR, Baylink DJ, Wong EGC, Massry SG, Norman AW: Clinical efficacy of 1,25-dihydroxyvitamin D_3 in renal osteodystrophy. In: *Vitamin D: Biochemical, Chemical, and Clinical Aspects Related to Calcium Metabolism,* edited by Norman AW, Schaefer K, Coburn JW, DeLuca HF, Fraser D, Grigoleit HG, Herrath D v, Berlin, W de Gruyter, 1977, p 657
81. Massry SG, Popovtzer MM, Coburn JW, Makoff DL, Maxwell MH, Kleeman CR: Intractable pruritus as a manifestation of secondary hyperparathyroidism in uremia. Disappearance of itching following subtotal parathyroidectomy. *N Engl J Med* 279:697, 1968
82. Mehls O, Ritz E, Burkhard K, Gilli G, Link W, Willich E, Schärer K: Slipped epiphysis in renal osteodystrophy. *Arch Dis Child* 50:545, 1975
83. Holliday MA: Calorie deficiency in children with uremia: Effect upon growth. *Pediatrics* 50:590, 1972
84. Chesney RW, Hamstra A, Jax DK, Mazess RB, DeLuca HF: Influence of long term oral 1,25-dihydroxyvitamin D in childhood renal osteodystrophy. *Contrib Nephrol* 18:55, 1980
85. Ellis HA, Pierides AM, Feest TG, Ward MK, Kerr DNS: Histopathology of renal osteodystrophy with particular reference to the effects of 1 alpha-hydroxyvitamin D_3 in patients treated by long term haemodialysis. *Clin Endocrinol* 7 (Suppl):31A, 1977
86. Llach F, Pederson J: Acute joint syndrome and maintenance hemodialysis. *Proc Clin Dial Transpl Forum* 9:17, 1979
87. Lotem M, Bernheim J, Conforty B: Spontaneous rupture of tendons: A complication of hemodialyzed patients treated for renal failure. *Nephron* 21:201, 1978
88. Gipstein RH, Coburn JW, Adams DA, Lee DBN, Parsa KP Sellers A, Suki WN, Massry SG: Calciphylaxis in man: A syndrome of tissue necrosis and vascular calcification in 11 patients with chronic renal disease. *Arch Intern Med* 136:1273, 1976
89. Selye H: *Calciphylaxis.* Chicago, University of Chicago Press, 1962
90. Arieff AI, Massry SG: Calcium metabolism of brain in acute renal failure. *J Clin Invest* 53:387, 1974
91. Ball JH, Butkus DE, Madison DS: Effect of subtotal parathyroidectomy on dialysis dementia. *Nephron* 18:151, 1977
92. Massry SG, Goldstein DA: The search for uremic toxin(s) 'X'. 'X' = PTH. *Clin Nephrol* 11:181, 1979
93. Amend WJ Jr, Steinberg SM, Lowrie EG, Lazarus JM, Soeldner JS, Hampers CL, Merrill JP: The influence of serum calcium and parathyroid hormone upon glucose metabolism in uremia. *J. Lab Clin Med* 86:435, 1975
94. Sinha TK, Thajchayapong P, Queener SF, Allen DO, Bell NH: On the lipolytic action of parathyroid hormone in man. *Metabolism* 25:251, 1976
95. Cantin M: Kidney, parathyroid hormone and lipemia. *Lab Invest* 14: 1691, 1965
96. Stanbury SW: The phosphate ion in chronic renal failure. In: *Phosphate Inorganique, Biologie et Physiopathologie* edited by Hioco DJ, Paris, International Symposium Sandoz, p 187, 1970
97. Clarkson EM, Luck VA, Hynson WV, Bailey RR, Eastwood JB, Woodhead JS, Clements VR, O'Riordan JLH, de Wardener HE: The effect of aluminium hydroxide on calcium, phosphorus and aluminium balances, the serum parathyroid hormone concentration and the aluminium content of bone in patients with chronic renal failure. *Clin Sci* 43:519, 1972
98. Coburn JW, Hartenbower, DL, Brickman AS, Massry SG, Kopple JD: Intestinal absorption of calcium, magnesium and phosphorus in chronic renal insufficiency. In: *Calcium Metabolism in Renal Failure and Nephrolithiasis* edited by David DS, New York, John Wiley & Sons, 1977, p 77
99. Brickman AS, Hartenbower DL, Norman AW, Coburn JW: Actions of 1 alpha-hydroxyvitamin D_3 and 1,25 dihydroxyvitamin D_3 on mineral metabolism in man. I. Effects on net absorption of phosphorus. *Am J Clin Nutr* 30:1064, 1977
100. Coburn JR, Brickman AS, Sherrard DJ, Singer FR, Baylink DJ, Wong EGC, Massry SG, Norman AW: Clinical efficacy of 1-25-dihydroxyvitamin D_3 in renal osteodystrophy. In: *Vitamin D: Biochemical Chemical and Clinical Aspects Related to Calcium Metabolism,* edited by Norman AW, Schaefer K, Coburn JW, DeLuca HF, Fraser D, Grigoleit HG, Herrath D v, Berlin, W. de Gruyter, 1977, p 657
101. Massry SG, Coburn JW, Popovtzer MM, Shinaberger JH, Maxwell MH, Kleeman CR: Secondary hyperparathyroidism in chronic renal failure: The clinical spectrum in uremia, during hemodialysis and after renal transplantation. *Arch Intern Med* 124:431, 1969
102. Shah S, Qruz C, Castillo W: Persistent hypophosphatemia in patients on chronic hemodialysis without phosphate binding gels. *Kidney Int* (Abstract) 10:526, 1976
103. Burnell JM, Teubner E: Effects of decreasing magnesium in patients with chronic renal failure. *Proc Clin Dial Transpl Forum* 5:191, 1976
104. Strong HF, Schatz BC, Shinaberger JH, Coburn JW: Measurement of dialysance and bi-directional fluxes of calcium in vivo using radiocalcium. *Trans Am Soc Artif Intern Organs* 17:108, 1971
105. Mirhamadi KS, Duffy BS, Shinaberger JH, Jowsey J, Massry SG, Coburn JW: A controlled evaluation of clinical and metabolic effects of dialysate calcium levels during regular dialysis. *Trans Am Soc Artif Intern Organs* 17:118, 1971
106. Ramen A, Chong YK, Sreenevasan GA: Effects of varying dialysate calcium concentration on the plasma calcium fractions in patients on dialysis. *Nephron* 16:181, 1976
107. Bouillon R, Verberckmoes R, Moor PD: Influence of dialysate calcium concentration and vitamin D on serum parathyroid hormone during repetitive dialysis. *Kidney Int* 7:422, 1975
108. Alvarez Ude F, Feest TG, Ward MK, Pierides AK, Ellis HA, Peart KM, Simpson W, Weightman D, Kerr DNS: Hemodialysis bone disease: Correlation between clinical, histologic and other findings. *Kidney Int* 16:68, 1978
109. Prior JC, Cameron EC, Ballan HS, Lirenman DS, Moriar-

ty MV, Price JDE: Experience with 1, 25-dihydroxycholecalciferol therapy in hemodialysis patients with progressive vitamin D_2-treated osteodystrophy. *Am J Med* 67:583, 1979
110. Burnell JM, Teubner E: Effects of decreasing magnesium in patients with chronic renal failure. *Proc Clin Dial Transpl Forum* 5:191, 1976
111. Alfrey AC, Miller NL, Butkus D: Evaluation of body magnesium stores. *J Lab Clin Med* 84:153, 1974
112. Alfrey AC, Solomons C, Ciricillo J, Miller NL: Extraosseous calcification. Evidence for abnormal pyrophosphate metabolism in uremia. *J Clin Invest* 57:692, 1976
113. Alfrey AC, Solomons CC: Bone pyrophosphate in uremia and its association with extraosseous calcification. *J Clin Invest* 57:700, 1976
114. Hruska KA, Teitelbaum SL, Kopelman R, Richardson CA, Miller P, Debman J, Martin K, Slatopolsky E: The predictability of the histological features of uremic bone disease by non-invasive technique. *Metab Bone Dis Relat Res* 1:39, 1978
115. Hart W, Duursma SA, Visser WJ, Njio LKF: The hydroxyproline content of plasma of patients with impaired renal function. *Clin Nephrol* 4:104, 1975
116. Hamet P, Stouder DA, Ginn HE, Hardman JG, Liddle GW: Studies of the elevated extra-cellular concentration of cyclic AMP in uremic man. *J Clin Invest* 56:339, 1975
117. Parfitt AM: Clinical and radiographic manifestations of renal osteodystrophy. In: *Calcium Metabolism in Renal Failure and Nephrolithiasis*, edited by David DS, New York, John Wiley & Sons, 1977, p 150
118. Meema HE, Schatz DL: Simple radiologic demonstration of cortical bone loss in thyrotoxicosis. *Radiology* 97:9, 1970
119. Dent CE, Harper CM, Philpot GR: The treatment of renal glomerular osteodystrophy. *Q J Med* 117:1, 1961
120. Meema HE, Rabinovich S, Meema S, Lloyd GJ, Oreopoulos DG: Improved radiological diagnosis of azotemic osteodystrophy. *Radiology* 102:1, 1972
121. Doyle FH: Radiological patterns of bone disease associated with renal glomerular failure in adults. *Br Med Bull* 28:220, 1972
122. Glassford DM, Remmers AR Jr, Sarles HE, Lindley JD, Scurry MT, Fish JC: Hyperparathyroidism in the maintenance dialysis patient. *Surg Gynec Obstet* 142:328, 1976
123. Craven JD: Renal glomerular osteodystrophy. *Clin Radiol* 15:210, 1964
124. Ellis K, Hochstim RJ: The skull in hyperparathyroid bone disease. *Am J Roentgenol* 83:732, 1960
125. Meema HE, Oreopoulos DG, Rabinovich S, Husdan H, Rapaport A: Periosteal new bone formation (periosteal neostasis) in renal osteodystrophy. *Radiology* 110:513, 1974
126. Mehls O, Ritz E, Burkhard K, Gilli G, Link W, Willich E, Schärer K: Slipped epiphysis in renal osteodystrophy. *Arch Dis Child* 50:545, 1975
127. Ritz E, Krempien B, Mehls O, Malluche H: Skeletal abnormalities in chronic renal insufficiency before and during maintenance hemodialysis. *Kidney Int* 4:116, 1973
128. Norfray J, Calenoff L, Del Greco F, Krumlovsky FA: Renal osteodystrophy in patients on hemodialysis as reflected in the bony pelvis. *Am J Roentgenol Radium Ther Nucl Med* 125:352, 1975
129. Bailey GL, Griffiths HJL, Mocelin AJ, Gundy DH, Hampers Cl, Merrill JP: Avascular necrosis of the femoral head in patients on chronic hemodialysis *Trans Am Soc Artif Intern Organs* 18:401, 1972
130. Parfitt AM, Massry SG, Winfield AC: Osteopenia and fractures occurring during maintenance hemodialysis. A 'new' form of renal osteoystrophy. *Clin Orthop* 87:287, 1972
131. Letteri JM, Cohn SH: Total body neutron activation; Analysis in the study of mineral homeostasis in chronic renal disease. In: *Calcium metabolism in Renal Failure and Nephrolithiasis*, Edited by David DS, New York, Hohn Wiley & Sons, 1977, p 249
132. Cochran M, Bulusu L, Horsman A, Stasiac L, Nordin BEC: Hypocalcemia and bone disease in chronic renal failure. *Nephron* 10:113, 1973
133. Bone JM, Davison AM, Robson JS: Role of dialysate calcium concentration in osteoporosis in patients on haemodialysis. *Lancet* 1:1047, 1972
134. Henderson RG, Russell RGG, Earnshaw MJ, Ledingham JGG, Oliver DO, Woods CG: Loss of metacarpal and iliac bone in chronic renal failure: Influence of haemodialysis, parathyroid activity, type of renal disease, physical activity and heparin consumption. *Clin Sci* 56:31F, 1979
135. Fleisch H, Russell RGG: Experimental clinical studies with pyrophosphate and diphosphonates. In: *Calcium Metabolism in Renal Failure and Nephrolithiasis*, edited by David DS, New York, John Wiley and Sons, 1977, p 293
136. Rosenthall L, Kaye M: Technetium-99m-pyrophosphate kinetics and imaging in metabolic bone disease. *J Nucl Med* 16:33, 1975
137. Ølgaard K, Heerfordt J, Madsen S: Scintigraphic skeletal changes in uremic patients on regular hemodialysis. *Nephron* 17:325, 1976
138. Davis BA, Poulose KP, Reba RC: Scanning for uremic pulmonary calcifications. *Ann Intern Med* 85:132, 1976
139. Massry SG, Coburn JW: Divalent ion metabolism and renal osteodystrophy. In: *Clinical Aspects of Uremia and Dialysis*, edited by Massry SG, Sellers AL, Spingfield, Ill, Charles C Thomas Co, 1976, p 304
140. Contiguglia SR, Alfrey AC, Miller NL, Runnells DE, LeGeros RZ: Nature of soft tissue calcification in uremia. *Kidney Int* 4:229, 1973
141. Dreher W, Shelp W: Atrioventricular block in a long term dialysis patient. Reversal after parathyroidectomy. *JAMA* 234:954, 1975
142. Schwartz KV: Heart block in renal failure and hypercalcemia. *JAMA* 235:1550, 1976
143. Conger JD, Hammond WS, Alfrey AC, Contiguglia SR, Standord RE, Huffer WE: Pulmonary calcification in chronic dialysis patients. Clinical and pathologic studies. *Ann Intern Med* 83:330, 1975
144. Arieff AI, Massry SG: Calcium metabolism of brain in acute renal failure. *J Clin Invest* 53:387, 1974
145. Kraikitpanitch S, Haygood CC, Baxter DJ, Yunice AA, Lindeman RD: Studies on the pathogenesis of myocardial calcification in azotemia. *Abstracts Am Soc Nephrol* 8:4, 1975
146. Ritz E, Mehls O, Bommer J, Schmidt-Gayk H Fiegel P, Reitinger H: Vascular calcification under maintenance hemodialysis. *Klin Wochenschr* 55:375, 1977
147. Kopple JD, Coburn JW: Metabolic studies of low protein diets in uremia. II. Calcium, phosphorus and magnesium. *Medicine* 52: 597, 1973
148. Goldsmith RS, Furszyfer J, Johnson WJ, Fournier AE, Arnaud CD: control of secondary hyperparathyroidism during long-term hemodialysis. *Am J Med* 50:692, 1971
149. Drueke T, Bordier PJ, Man NK, Jungers P, Mairie P: Effects of high dialysate calcium concentration on bone remodeling, serum biochemistry, and parathyroid hormone in patients with renal osteodystrophy. *Kidney Int*

11:267, 1977
150. Craven JD: Renal glomerular osteodystrophy. *Clin Radiol* 15:210, 1964
151. Randall RE Jr, Cohen MD, Spray CC Jr, Rossmeisl EC: Hypermagnesemia in renal failure. Etiology and toxic manifestations. *Ann Intern Med* 61:73, 1964
152. Clarkson EM, Eastwood JB, Koutsaimanis KG, de Wardener HE: Net absorption of calcium in patients with chronic renal failure. *Kidney Int* 3:258, 1973
153. Raman A, Chong YK, Sreenevasan GA: Effects of varying dialysate calcium concentrations on the plasma calcium fractions in patients on dialysis. *Nephron* 16:181, 1976
154. Clarkson EM, McDonald SJ, de Wardener HE: The effect of a high intake of calcium carbonate in normal subjects and patients with chronic renal failure. *Clin Sci* 30:425, 1966
155. Meyrier A, Marsac J, Richet G: The influence of a high calcium carbonate intake on bone disease in patients undergoing hemodialysis. *Kidney Int* 4:146, 1973
156. Eastwood JB, Bordier PJ, de Wardener HE: Some biochemical, histological, radiological and clinical features of renal osteodystrophy. *Kidney Int* 4:128, 1973
157. Rao TKS, Friedman EA: Fluoride and bone disease in uremia. *Kidney Int* 7:125, 1975
158. Strong HE, Schatz BC, Shinaberger JH, Coburn JW: Measurement of dialysance and bi-directional fluxes of calcium in vivo using radiocalcium. *Trans Am Soc Artif Intern Organs* 17:108, 1971
159. Taves D, Terry R, Smith FA, Gardner DE: Use of fluoridated water in long-term hemodialysis. *Arch Intern Med* 115:167, 1965
160. Posen GA, Marier JR, Jaworski ZF: Renal osteodystrophy in patients on long-term hemodialysis with fluoridated water. *Fluoride* 4:114, 1971
161. Siddiqui JY, Simpson W, Ellis HA, Kerr DNS: Serum fluoride in chronic renal failure. *Proc Eur Dial Transpl Assoc* 7:110, 1970
162. Oreopoulos DG, Taves DR, Rabinovich S, Meema HE, Murray T, Fenton SS, deVeber GA: Fluoride and dialysis osteodystrophy. Results of a double-blind study. *Trans Am Soc Artif Intern Organs* 20:203, 1974
163. Griffith GC, Nichols G Jr, Asher JD, Flanigan B: Heparin osteoporosis. *JAMA* 193:91, 1965
164. Maloney NA, Ott SM, Alfrey AC, Miller NL, Coburn JW, Sherrard DJ: Histological quantitation of aluminum in iliac bone from patients with renal failure. *J. Lab Clin Med* 99:206, 1982
165. Cournot-Witmer G, Zingraff J, Plachot JJ, Escaig F, Le Feure R, Boumati P, Bordeau A, Garabedian M, Galle P, Bourdon R, Drueke T, Balsan S: Aluminum localization in bone from hemodialyzed patients. Relationship to matrix mineralization. *Kidney Int* 20:375, 1981
166. Jaffe MD, Wellis PW III: Multiple fractures associated with long-term sodium heparin sodium heparin therapy. *JAMA* 193:158, 1965
167. Kaye M, Chatterjee G, Cohen GF, Sagar S: Arrest of hyperparathyroid bone disease with dihydrotachysterol in patients undergoing chronic hemodialysis. *Ann Intern Med* 73:225, 1970
168. Teitelbaum SL, Bone JM, Stein PM, Gilden JJ, Bates M, Boisseau VC, Avioli LV: Calciferol in chronic renal insufficiency. Skeletal response. *JAMA* 235:164, 1967
169. Chan JCM, Oldham SB, Holick MF: 1-alpha-hydroxyvitamin D_3 in chronic renal failure. A potent analogue of the kidney hormone, 1, 25-dihydroxycholecalciferol. *JAMA* 234:47, 1975
170. Papapoulos SE, Brownjohn AM, Goodwin FJ, Hately W, Marsh FP, O'Riordan JLH: The effect of 1-alpha-hydroxycholecalciferol on secondary hyperparathyroidism of chronic renal failure. In: *Vitamin D: Biochemical, Chemical and Clinical Aspects Related to Calcium Metabolism,* edited by Norman AW, Schaefer K, Coburn JW, DeLuca HF, Fraser D, Grigoleit HG. Herrath D v, Berlin, W de Gruyter, 1977, p 693
171. Kanis JA, Earnshaw M, Henderson GR, Heymen G, Ledingham JGG, Naik RB, Russell DO, Smith R, Wilkinson R, Woods CG: Correlation of clinical biochemical and skeletal responses to 1-alpha-hydroxycholecalciferol in renal bone disease. *Clin Endocrinol,* 1978
172. Brickman A, Sherrard DJ, Jowsey J, Singer FR, Baylink DJ, Maloney N, Massry SG, Norman AW, Coburn JW: 1, 25-Dihydroxycholecalciferol. Effect on skeletal lesions and plasma parathyroid hormone levels in uremic osteodystrophy. *Arch Intern Med* 134:883, 1974
173. Pierides M, Ward MK, Alvarez-Ude F, Ellis HA, Peart KM, Simpson W, Kerr DNS, Norman AW: Long-term therapy with 1, $25(OH)_2D_3$ in dialysis bone disease. *Proc Eur Dial Transpl Assoc* 12:237, 1976
174. Stanbury SW, Lumb GA: Metabolic studies of renal osteodystrophy: I. Calcium, Phosphorus and nitrogen metabolism in rickets, osteomalacia and hyperparathyroidism complicating chronic uremia and in the osteomalacia of the adult Fanconi syndrome. *Medicine* 41:1, 1962
175. Sherrard DJ, Coburn JW, Brickman AS, Baylink DJ, Norman AW, Maloney N: A histologic comparison of 1, $25(OH)_2$ vitamin D treatment with calcium supplementation in renal osteodystrophy. In: *Vitamin D: Biochemical, Chemical and Clinical Aspects related to Calcium Metabolism,* Edited by Norman AW, Schaefer K, Coburn JW, DeLuca HF, Fraser D, Grigoleit HG, Herrath D v, Berlin, W de Gruyter, 1977, p 719
176. Brickman AS, Hartenbower DL, Norman AW, Coburn JW: Actions of 1-alpha-hydroxyvitamin D_3 on mineral metabolism in man. 1. Effect on net absorption of phosphorus. *Am J Clin Nutr* 30:1064, 1977
177. Colodro IH, Brickman AS, Coburn JW: Effects of 25(OH) vitamin D_3 on intestinal absorption of calcium in normal and uremic man *Clin Res* 23:430, 1975
178. Kanis JA, Candy T, Earnshaw M, Henderson RG, Heynem G, Malk R, Russell RGG, Smith R, Woods CG: Treatment of renal bone disease with 1-alpha-hydroxylated derivatives of vitamin D_3. *Q J Med* 48:289, 1979
179. Recker RR, Schoenfeld P, Slatopolsky E: 25-hydroxyvitamin D in renal osteodystrophy. Results of a six center trial. In: *Vitamin D: Biochemical, Chemical and Clinical Aspects Related to Calcium Metabolism,* edited by Norman AW, Schaefer K, Coburn JW, DeLuca HE, Fraser D, Grigoleit HG, Herrath D v, Berlin, W de Gruyter, 1977, p 649
180. Brickman AS, Coburn JW, Friedman GR, Okamura WH, Massry SG, Norman AW: Comparison of effects of 1-alpha-hydroxyvitamin D_3 and 1, 25-dihydroxyvitamin D_3 in man. *J Clin Invest* 57:1540, 1976
181. Pierides AM, Kerr DNS, Ellis HA, Peart KM, O'Riordan JLH, DeLuca HF: 1-alpha-hydroxycholecalciferol in haemodialysis renal osteodystrophy. Adverse effects of anticonvulsant therapy. *Clin Nephrol* 5:189, 1976
182. Gordon HE, Coburn JW, Passaro E Jr: Surgical management of secondary hyperparathyroidism. *Arch Surg* 104:520, 1972
183. Regan RJ, Peacock M, Rosen SM, Robinson PJ, Horsman A: Effect of dialysate calcium concentration on bone disease in patients on hemodialysis. *Kidney Int* 10:246, 1976
184. Coburn JR, Wong EGC, Sherrard DJ, Brickman AS, Hodsman AB, Lee DBN, Singer FR, Norman AW: Use of 24, 25-dihydroxyvitamin D_3 in dialysis osteomalacia: Pre-

liminary results. *Clin Res*: 532A, 1980
185. David DS: Mineral and bone homeostasis in renal failure. Pathophysiology and management. In: *Calcium Metabolism in Renal Failure and Nephrolithiasis,* edited by David DS, New York, John Wiley & Sons, 1976, p 1
186. Wells SA Jr, Gunnells JC, Schneider AB, Sherwood LM: Transplantation of the parathyroid glands in man. Clinical indications and results. *Surgery* 78:34, 1975
187. Felsenfeld AJ, Gutman RA, Llach F, Harrelson JM, Wells SA: Postparathyroidectomy hypocalcemia as an accurate indicator of pre-parathyroidectomy bone histology in the uremic patient. *Mineral Electrolyte Metab* (in press)
188. Fournier A, Coeudet B, De Fremont JF, Gueris J, Caillens G, Desplan C, Calmette C, Moukhtar MS: Propranolol Therapy for secondary hyperparathyroidism in uremia. *Lancet* 2:50, 1978
189. Jacob AI, Lanier D, Canterbury J, Bourgoignie JJ: Reduction by cimetidine of serum parathyroid hormone levels in uremic patients. *N Eng J Med* 302:671, 1980
190. Sherwood JK, Ackroyd FW, Garua M: Effect of cimetidine on circulating parathyroid hormone in primary hyperparathyroidism *Lancet* 1:616, 1980
191. Verberckmoes R, Bouillon R, Krempien B: Disappearance of vascular calcifications during treatment of renal osteodystrophy. *Ann Intern Med* 82:529, 1975
192. Brickman AS, Coburn JW, Norman AW, Massry SG: Short-term effects of 1,25-dihydroxycholecalciferol on disordered calcium metabolism of renal failure. *Am J Med* 57:28, 1974
193. Coburn JW, Brickman AS, Hartenbower DL, Norman AW: Intestinal phosphate absorption in normal and uremic man: Effects of 1,25(OH)$_2$-vitamin D$_3$. In *Phosphate Metabolism,* edited by Massry SG, Ritz E, New York, Plenum Press, 1977, p 549
194. Mehls O, Ritz E, Krempien B, Willich E, Brommer J, Schärer K: Roentgenological signs in the skeleton of uremic children. An analysis of the anatomical principles underlying the roentgenological changes. *Pediatr Radiol* 1:183, 1973
195. Brickman AS, Jowsey J, Sherrard DJ, Friedman G, Singer FR, Baylink DJ, Maloney N, Massry SG, Norman AW, Coburn JW: Therapy with 1,25-dihydroxyvitamin D$_3$ in the management of renal osteodystrophy. In: *Vitamin D and Problems Related to Uremic Bone Disease,* Edited by Norman AW, Schaefer K, Grigoleit HG, Herrath D v, Ritz E: Berlin, W de Gruyter, 1975, p 241.

36
ENDOCRINE CHANGES IN PATIENTS ON CHRONIC DIALYSIS

JAMES P. KNOCHEL

Introduction	712
Growth hormone (somatotrophin)	713
Somatomedin	713
Adrenocortical trophic hormone (ACTH)	713
Melanotrophic hormone	713
Pituitary-gonadal hormones	713
Prolactin	713
Luteinizing hormone (LH)	714
Follicle stimulating hormone (FSH)	714
Luteinizing hormone releasing hormone (LHRH)	714
Testosterone	714
Pituitary-gonadal function in women	715
Thyroid function in uremia	715
Hypometabolism in uremia	716
Gastrin and other gastrointestinal hormones	717
Adrenocortical hormones	717
Cortisol (Hydrocortisone)	717
Aldosterone	718
Carbohydrate metabolism in uremia	718
Insulin metabolism	719
Hyperglucagonemia in uremia	720
Catecholamines	720
Antidiuretic hormone	720
Other peptides	721
References	721

INTRODUCTION

Patients with end-stage renal disease display a variety of endocrine disturbances. In some instances, clearly recognizable endocrinopathies occur. More commonly, evidence of endocrine dysfunction consists only of laboratory abnormalities. Many of these are not associated with apparent disease.

In recent years the development of new quantitative methods to assess endocrine function has progressed rapidly. Outstanding among these are a number of radioimmunoassay procedures which permit measurement of extremely low concentrations of certain hormones in body fluids. While such technological advances have improved our understanding of endocrine pathophysiology, one must be rigidly skeptical and alert for hasty conclusions based upon data derived from these exquisitely sensitive techniques.

There are at least nine clinically recognizable endocrine disturbances peculiar to the patient with end-stage renal disease. These include: 1) secondary hyperparathyroidism, 2) osteomalacia related to deranged cholecalciferol metabolism, 3) the complex of hyperreninemia, hyperaldosteronism and hypertension, 4) hyporeninemia, 5) hypoaldosteronism, 6) decreased erythropoietin production and red cell hypoplasia, 7) gynecomastia, 8) galactorrhea, and 9) gonadal atrophy or hypogonadism.

Although the pathophysiology of the foregoing disturbances is not completely understood, at least 10 abnormal processes may be considered to play a role. These are as follows. 1) Blunting of a specific hormonal effect. This is typified by insulin resistance. Its cause could be toxic interference, receptor dysfunction or actions of opposing hormones. 2) Synthesis of or secretion into the circulation of an abnormal molecular species of a hormone. This is exemplified by the increased fraction of circulating proinsulin in uremia. 3) Abnormal protein-binding of a hormone in plasma. This may be implicated in certain derangements of thyroid function in uremia. 4) Overproduction of a normal hormone in response to a physiologic stimulus incident to uremia. This is represented by overproduction of parathyroid hormone and disease of the skeleton. 5) Derangements of feed back control are observed, such as failure of follicle stimulating hormone to become elevated despite low levels of testosterone. 6) Diminished metabolism or degradation of a hormone. Many important peptide hormones are catabolized by the kidney. Accordingly, shrinkage of renal mass may permit their accumulation in plasma. This mechanism is partially responsible for accumulation of parathyroid hormone in uremia. 7) Diminished metabolism of a hormone at a peripheral tissue site other than the kidney, e.g. decreased conversion of thyroxin to triiodothyronine in peripheral tissues. 8) Increased metabolism or degradation of a hormone. Many hormones are metabolized in the liver. Arterial volume expansion in uremia may increase hepatic plasma flow and increased delivery of the hormone to the liver thereby may facilitate increased catabolism. 9) Hormonal deficiency directly related to the shrinkage of renal mass. For example, diminished production of renin or erythropoietin. 10) Deficiency of a hormone due to inadequate production of its trophic hormone e.g. hypoaldosteronism resulting from hyporeninemia in the anephric state.

Detailed discussions related to disturbances of renin and erythropoietin and of parathyroid hormone, vitamin D, will be found in Chapters 28, 32, 35. The remaining endocrine disorders, especially those of biochemical nature, will be covered in this chapter. Unfortunately, information on many important hormones remains incomplete.

GROWTH HORMONE (SOMATOTROPHIN)

Growth hormone levels are often elevated in renal failure (1). There is some evidence that the kidney plays an important role in degradation of growth hormone (2, 3). Thus, diminished renal mass may be responsible for its retention in renal failure. Normally, growth hormone concentration falls during hyperglycemia; in uremia, hyperglycemia may induce a paradoxical rise. Neither the elevated growth hormone levels nor the paradoxical rise with hyperglycemia improves after dialysis. Normal values reappear promptly, however, after successful renal transplantation. The functional significance of elevated growth hormone levels in uremia is unclear. They apparently do not play a role in uremic pseudodiabetes. Although administration of exogenous growth hormone may provoke nitrogen retention in patients with renal failure (4), it has not been ascertained whether this response can be correlated with initial levels of the hormone. Some have found that growth hormone may be more elevated in patients treated by chronic peritoneal dialysis than in those treated by hemodialysis (5). This could result from a greater degree of protein deficiency in those patients incident to protein losses across the peritoneum. Growth hormone levels are elevated in protein calorie malnutrition independent of renal disease. However, in patients undergoing chronic hemodialysis the levels do not fall when simply increasing dietary protein intake from 36 to 63 g per day (6). It is possible that difficulties with precise measurement of biologically normal growth hormone exist. Thus, the substance measured by immunoassay as growth hormone may not be the same as that measured in healthy plasma (7). Growth hormone levels in response to hemodialysis were reported to decrease, regardless of dialysis solution dextrose concentrations in adults (8). Growth-retarded children on chronic hemodialysis, whose growth hormone levels rose in response to insulin-hypoglycemia, show a decline if they are dialyzed against a dialysis solution containing dextrose (9). Such data, although not conclusive, suggest that failure of growth hormone secretion is probably not responsible for impairment of growth in uremic children.

SOMATOMEDIN

Somatomedin, originally called sulfation factor, is produced in peripheral tissues in response to growth hormone. It is probably responsible for linear growth. Levels in uremic children are generally below normal (10). Increased levels have been observed following successful hemodialysis therapy and this may correspond to increased growth velocity (11, 12). But current information does not permit a conclusion that increased somatomedin is responsible. Impaired growth in children with uremia is unequivocally multifactorial and is discussed in detail in Chapter 25. In contrast to the abnormally low values of somatomedin in uremic children, levels in adults with uremia may be significantly elevated (7). Recent reports suggest that bioassay techniques for estimation of somatomedin activity are unreliable in the presence of an elevated sulfate concentration in serum as occurs in uremia (13). Thus, the precise role of somatomedin in growth disturbances in uremia remains unsettled.

ADRENOCORTICAL TROPHIC HORMONE (ACTH)

This hormone has been measured by only one group of investigators in patients with chronic renal failure, receiving hemodialysis therapy (14). The levels were normal in most patients but slightly elevated in others. Such findings correspond to measurements by others on cortisol in chronic renal failure (*vide infra*).

MELANOTROPHIC HORMONE

Gilkes et al (14) and Smith and co-workers (15) reported substantial elevations of immunoreactive B-melanocyte-stimulating hormone in patients on chronic hemodialysis. The former group (14) contended that pigmentation of skin was greater in those patients whose melanotrophic hormone levels were highest. Two patients on peritoneal dialysis also had high values. In contrast to the report by Gilkes et al (14) the latter group (15) could not establish a relationship between melanotrophic hormone levels and intensity of pigmentation. In a second study, Smith and associates (16) showed that melanotrophic hormone levels became higher with increasing duration of dialysis treatment. It appeared that the hormone was not cleared by hemodialysis, that in most patients, its level corresponded to serum creatinine concentration and finally, that it became normal in patients who had undergone successful renal transplantation. The hormone is probably metabolized by the kidney. There is no proven function of this substance in man. Its relationship to pigmentation is uncertain.

PITUITARY-GONADAL HORMONES

Prolactin

Plasma prolactin levels are often elevated in endstage renal disease (17, 18). Its physiological role is to initiate and maintain lactation. This hormone is *not* responsible for gynecomastia. The kidneys apparently play a major role in metabolism of prolactin.

In normal subjects, administration of L-dopa stimulates release of prolactin-inhibitory factor (19). This response does not occur in uremic patients, thus suggesting either a defect in the normal feedback inhibitory pathways for prolactin release or possibly retention of an inactive abnormal species of prolactin in uremic plasma. The persistently elevated levels of prolactin could explain the inappropriate lactation sometimes observed in women with advanced chronic renal failure.

The most comprehensive study on the character of uremic hyperprolactinemia to date has been reported by Gomez and his co-workers (20). They studied 56 patients on chronic hemodialysis. They found that 11 of 15 women and 7 of 28 men had abnormally elevated levels. Thirteen patients treated with α-methyldopa for hypertension had considerably higher levels. This drug also increases prolactin levels in normal subjects (21). Dialysis did not lower prolactin levels in any of the patients. In men, they found a weak correlation between markedly elevated levels of prolactin and impotence. In women less than 45 years of age, estradiol levels were higher in those whose prolactin levels were normal. Galactorrhea was found in four women, receiving α-methyldopa. These four showed the highest prolactin levels observed among the female patients. Of great interest, plain skull films showed a normal sella turcica in all patients with elevated prolactin levels. However, tomography of the sella showed ballooning and blistering consistent with pituitary hyperplasia in those four patients whose prolactin levels were elevated and who also were on α-methyldopa. In contrast to the normally rapid rise and fall of prolactin levels following administration of luteinizing hormone releasing hormone and thyrotrophin-releasing hormone, prolactin levels in uremic patients underwent little if any change.

Gomez and his associates (20) also examined the effect of bromocriptine on prolactin levels. Bromocriptine is a dopamine receptor agonist that inhibits prolactin secretion in physiological states and in a variety of pathological conditions in which prolactin is elevated. In contrast to a number of hyperprolactinemic patients with normal renal function, a single dose of bromocriptine (2.5 mg) was markedly less effective, regardless whether the patients were treated with α-methyldopa or not. Nevertheless, a 6-week course of bromocriptine caused a substantial and significant reduction of prolactin levels. Of importance, the four women with galactorrhea showed persistence of this finding despite lowering (but not correction) of prolactin levels. No perceptible effects of bromocriptine were noted on sexual function in men who complained of impotence.

Luteinizing hormone (LH)

Luteinizing hormone is essential for ovulation, formation of the corpus luteum and stimulation of steroid hormone secretion by the corpus luteum. In the male, luteinizing hormone stimulates growth and secretory activity of the testicular interstitial (Leydig) cells.

Luteinizing hormone is elevated in chronic renal failure (22). It remains high and may rise even further after initiating hemodialysis therapy. Some have speculated (23) that this might be responsible for the development of gynecomastia which tends to appear shortly and transiently after initiating dialysis therapy in some male patients (24–26). Luteinizing hormone, like growth hormone, is also elevated in patients with protein calorie malnutrition. In the latter condition, gynecomastia may appear during refeeding and also be accompanied by tender enlargement of the testes. Testicular enlargement with pain has not been observed in hemodialysis patients with gynecomastia. Whether or not the elevated luteinizing hormone levels bear any relationship to gynecomastia is unsettled (27). It should be kept in mind that gynecomastia also may be a complication of α-methyldopa therapy for hypertension. Very high luteinizing hormone levels may persist after gynecomastia has resolved (23) and may also be seen in patients without gynecomastia (28).

Follicle stimulating hormone (FSH)

Follicle stimulating hormone is the pituitary hormone essential for the normal cyclic growth of the ovarian follicle. It stimulates spermatogenesis in the male. For optimal effect, it apparently requires the presence of luteinizing hormone.

Plasma levels of FSH in patients with end-stage renal disease are generally slightly less than normal (29). FSH levels tend to become normal after initiation of chronic hemodialysis therapy and in some circumstances may become exceptionally elevated. No definite significance can be attributed to these changes.

Luteinizing hormone releasing hormone (LHRH)

Distiller and his co-workers (29) studied the response to LHRH in 16 patients on chronic hemodialysis and chronic peritoneal dialysis. Two had gynecomastia. In all, the luteinizing hormone (LH) response to LHRH was abnormally high. They attributed this abnormality to decreased renal metabolism of LH. The FSH response to LHRH was moderately elevated in all patients. All patients who demonstrated increased basal FSH levels or increased response to LHRH had testicular atrophy. One patient with gynecomastia did not have appreciably elevated levels of either LH or FSH. Mean testosterone levels were low. This finding along with the exaggerated response of FSH to LHRH is compatible with primary Leydig cell dysfunction. Klinefelter's syndrome might be suspected in such patients. Eunuchoid proportions, nuclear bar bodies, or finding a XXY karyogram would help to identify the latter patients.

Testosterone

Uremia is often associated with decreased libido, impairment of potency and decreased spermatogenesis (27, 28). Although high LH levels have been correlated with low testosterone levels, this has not been a consistent finding. The low FSH levels in many patients (29) suggest a disturbance in hypothalmic-pituitary feedback mechanisms (22). Dialysis therapy may or may not improve libido, potency and spermatogenesis (27).

In seven uremic men studied before dialysis therapy, injection of chorionic gonadotrophin resulted in a sluggish increase of testosterone levels in plasma (30). The binding protein for testosterone was normal. Testosterone responsiveness increased following dialysis and this was not related to an increase in the binding protein. Since the abnormality in testosterone was correctable by dialysis, the authors proposed that in untreated patients a circulating toxin suppresses testosterone production. These findings may partially explain the reduced libido and potentia coeundi in uremia. Testosterone turnover is increased in uremia as a result of increased catabolism by the liver.

Ferraris and his co-workers (31) recently reported their findings in 31 young men with renal failure. In all, puberal development was delayed with respect to chronological age. In 9 patients not requiring hemodialysis (serum creatinine 220–710 µmol (2.5–8.0 mg/dl)) and 10 on hemodialysis, plasma testosterone was normal. Luteinizing hormone levels were normal. Plasma FSH levels were uniformly elevated except in patients who had been transplanted. When renal transplantation was performed and prednisone was administered, testosterone levels were abnormally low. The authors suggested that their findings could best be explained on the basis that Leydig cell function was normal and the pituitary hormone abnormalities reflected damaged germinal epithelium. The latter probably occurred very early in the course of renal insufficiency.

Average 24 h levels of several hormones in men whose age varied between 28 and 60 years were reported by Zumoff and his associates (32). Eight gave a history of impotence. Mean levels of LH, prolactin and cortisol were elevated. Adrenal androgen levels were depressed. The latter, in light of elevated cortisol, suggested a block in adrenal steroid biosynthesis, which had not been described previously. Preliminary studies suggested that hemodialysis did not improve these abnormalities. The investigators suggested that the enzyme C-17, 20-lyase, important in steroid biosynthesis in both adrenals and testes, could be defective and thus account for established abnormalities of testosterone production in uremia.

A potentially important cause of hypogonadism and impotence in patients on chronic hemodialysis may be zinc deficiency (33). Some evidence suggests that not only may zinc intake be deficient in such patients, but also losses of zinc may occur during hemodialysis with purified dialysis solution despite potential inward transport because of binding to dialyzer membranes and to plasma proteins (34). Symptoms and findings of zinc deficiency include anorexia, dysgusia, acrodermatitis, subungual white-speckling, alopecia, gonadal atrophy and impotence. Serum zinc concentrations are usually below normal (35). Although favorable responses to zinc have been reported, this is by no means proven. In malnourished patients with chronic renal failure, acrodermatitis, alopecia and wasting might also result from biotin deficiency or essential fatty acid deficiency (36).

Although priapism may occur in patients on chronic hemodialysis therapy, there is no existing evidence that it is the result of endocrine dysfunction.

Pituitary-gonadal function in women

Impaired fertility and either amenorrhea or menorrhagia are common in women with end-stage renal disease (37). After initiation of dialysis treatment menstruation may resume and ovulation may occur. Nevertheless, conception is rare and is generally followed by spontaneous abortion. In one series of 142 patients with chronic renal disease complicating pregnancy (38), there were no fetal survivals if the initial BUN was greater than 26 mg/dl (9.3 mmol/l of urea). Successful pregnancy in a woman on chronic hemodialysis has been reported by Unzelman et al (37). In this case, urinary excretion of estrogen rose between the 20th and 38th week suggesting normal fetoplacental function.

According to a recent statistical report of the European Dialysis and Transplant Registry, 14 successful pregnancies occurred in Europe in women on dialysis. All of them, however, had some residual renal function (39).

Swamy and his co-workers (40) studied 13 women on chronic hemodialysis. LH was uniformly elevated in all patients whether pre- or post-menopausal. FSH values were normal. However, neither FSH nor LH showed typical ovulatory spikes and pulsatile hormone release was lacking. Such findings indicate that hemodialysis does not correct the hypothalamic-pituitary-ovarian axis derangements in women with terminal renal failure.

THYROID FUNCTION IN UREMIA

Thyroid function in chronic renal disease has been examined by many workers. Some have reported biochemical evidence of hyperthyroidism and others evidence of hypothyroidism. Exophthalmos has been described in chronic dialysis patients but was not associated with other findings or definitive laboratory evidence of hyperthyroidism (41). Although the puffy appearance, pallor, and hypothermia of some patients with advanced renal disease might suggest myxedema, it would appear that uremia per se does not ordinarily induce important clinical disturbances of thyroid function. Thus, in most centers, clinically important thyroid disease appears to be no more common than in the general population. However, there seem to be certain geographic areas, viz, Salt Lake City, Utah, and Chicago, Illinois, USA, where goiter occurs in the majority of patients on chronic hemodialysis (42). Nevertheless, even there, frank hypothyroidism or myxedema appears to be highly unusual.

In chronic renal failure, plasma thyrotrophin (TSH) is normal (43). It rises slowly after administration of thyrotrophin-releasing hormone (TRH) and its rate of disappearance is markedly delayed. The normal kidney excretes about 25% of ^{14}C-labeled TRH during the first hour after administration (44). Even though the kidney is a major site for degradation of thyrotrophin, normal basal levels suggest that in patients with renal failure alternative sites are utilized or that thyrotrophin production is partially inhibited. Of unknown significance, growth hormone is released following injection of TRH in patients with renal failure but not in normal subjects.

In normal man, the kidney does not metabolize T_3 (triiodothyronine) or T_4 (thyroxine) in significant quantities. This probably explains why plasma levels of these hormones are either normal or low in most patients with endstage renal disease (45). Chronic renal failure patients usually show a normal or depressed T_3. Nevertheless, uremia is one chronic illness in which reverse T_3 tends to remain low despite a low T_3 (20). In most chronic wasting illnesses, in hypometabolism, malnutrition or starvation, T_3 falls but reverse T_3 becomes elevated. Lim and her associates (46) found that total T_3 levels were in the hypothyroid range in 80% of patients with chronic renal disease not on hemodialysis and in 43% of patients on hemodialysis. These investigators demonstrated a 50% reduction in extrathyroidal conversion of T_4 to T_3. They observed low normal values for T_4 that could not be completely explained by a low T_4-binding globulin. The free T_4 index was also slightly low. Rats with experimental chronic renal failure develop goiters which are dependent upon availability of iodine (47). Lim and her associates also studied chronically azotemic partially nephrectomized rats (48). They showed essentially the same serum values for T_4, T_3, and thyrotropin as those observed in patients with renal failure. In addition, they showed low tissue levels of T_3 and corresponding decreased activities of mitochondrial α-glycerophosphate dehydrogenase and cytosol malate dehydrogenase. Both enzyme activities are known to be depressed in hypothyroidism. Treatment of the animals with T_3 resulted in a substantial rise in the activities of both enzymes. They concluded that in rats with experimental renal failure, evidence for tissue hypothyroidism exists which is correctable by T_3 administration.

The thyroid status of patients on prolonged chronic hemodialysis may be considerably different from the status prevailing in untreated uremia. Ramirez and his associates (49) showed that 31 of 53 patients treated by chronic dialysis for an average period of 10 months developed enlargement of the thyroid gland to more than twice its normal size. Thyroid function studies showed low ^{131}I uptake, low thyroxine and normal triiodothyronine levels. Thyroxine binding globulin concentration was normal. They also found normal thyrotrophin levels. In more recent studies, the same investigators showed that administration of synthetic TRH was followed by a subnormal rise in thyrotrophin and thyroxine concentration (49).

Silverberg and his co-workers (50) examined thyroid function serially in 53 patients on chronic hemodialysis. In contrast to the findings by Ramirez and his associates, these investigators found evidence of goiter in only one of their 53 patients. Nevertheless, their laboratory findings were quite similar to those reported by Ramirez et al. In the studies by Silverberg, although TSH levels were low, radioactive iodine uptake rose after thyrotrophin injection suggesting a defect of pituitary secretion of thyrotrophin. Many patients complained of cold intolerance and dry skin. Ten whose serum thyroxine concentration and free thyroxine indices were low were treated with L-thyroxine. The response was equivocal. They considered the possibility that fluoride accumulating in plasma from fluoridated water interfered with thyroid function. Oddie, Flanigan, and Fisher (51) have reported normal serum thyroxine levels in patients undergoing chronic peritoneal dialysis. It should be mentioned that in contrast to hemodialysis, distilled water is used for preparation of dialysate for peritoneal dialysis.

Intravenous heparin may cause a marked rise in free thyroxine levels (52, 53) due to displacement of T_4 from thyroxine-binding protein. This effect may persist for 12 to 24 h. Some patients with paroxysmal atrial tachycardia apparently had elevated free thyroxine levels during their attacks (54). This suggested that the rise of free T_4 resulting from use of heparin during hemodialysis might induce tachycardia and (or) arrhythmias. Accordingly, administration of heparin to euthyroid patients on chronic hemodialysis resulted in an increase of free thyroxine concentration from three to eight times higher than control values. Triiodothyronine resin uptake also increased. Although arrhythmias did not occur, these observations suggest that liberation of free thyroxine during hemodialysis might favor development of arrhythmias in susceptible patients.

Finally, patients with uremia are unable to clear iodide (55), which leads to its retention (56). Elevation of plasma iodide as well as increase of the iodide pool suppresses radioiodine uptake. Depressed serum concentrations of T_3 and T_4 and increased resin uptake of T_3 suggest abnormalities of hormone binding (49). The abnormalities of TSH response to TRH are not easily explained. Although detectable TSH in plasma may be compatible with hypothyroidism, this is more likely the result of the dimished renal function, per se.

HYPOMETABOLISM IN UREMIA

Findings suggesting thyroid functional derangements in uremia can conceivably result from the metabolic effects of uremia, per se. Patients with advanced or severe uremia may be hypometabolic (57). In patients with severe azotemia, body temperature may be subnormal under basal conditions or normal in those who should have fever. Our own studies inferentially suggest that dialyzable uremic toxins may suppress sodium transport sufficiently to reduce transport-related oxygen utilization, hence heat production (57, 58). Compared to normal subjects on the same diet, respiratory quotients are abnormally low in patients with severe, untreated uremia. During the first days of conventional hemodialysis therapy, evidence may occur suggesting abnormally increased sodium transport activity (electrical hyperpolarization of muscle cells) (58), hypermetabolism, and elevation of the respiratory quotient equivalent to that noted in patients with hyperthyroidism. With continued hemodialysis therapy, the state of hypermetabolism resolves. It has been our contention, without proof, that hypometabolism in the untreated uremic and transient hypermetabolism in the uremic immediately after initiation of hemodialysis therapy may result from the presence and sudden reduction of circulating uremic toxins. Whether the associated metabolic states are related to corresponding alterations of thyroid function has not been examined.

GASTRIN AND OTHER GASTROINTESTINAL HORMONES

Korman and his associates (59) have shown that plasma gastrin concentration rises in proportion to plasma creatinine in chronic renal insufficiency. Gastrin is apparently metabolized by the kidney (60). Accordingly, the loss of functional renal mass would decrease its degradation and permit accumulation in plasma. Immunologically, the molecule that accumulates in uremic plasma appears to be identical to normal gastrin (61).

Although active peptic ulcer disease and gastric hyperacidity have frequently been observed in chronic hemodialysis patients (43, 44), there is a notable lack of correlation between basal acid secretion and plasma gastrin levels in such patients (59). In contrast, others have observed hypochlorhydria in uremia and postulated that this might stimulate gastrin production. However, appropriate correlation has not been made between these two events (27). It has also been suspected that gastrin release could be mediated by the associated hyperparathyroidism of uremia (62). Nevertheless, there is no evidence that parathyroid-hormone, *per se,* is responsible for gastrin release. Rather, hypercalcemia resulting from hyperparathyroidism would constitute a stimulus. Since patients with uremia not yet treated by dialysis are generally hypocalcemic, there appears to be no relationship between hyperparathyroidism and hypergastrinemia.

Besides gastrin and glucagon (to be discussed in the section on carbohydrate metabolism in uremia), information exists on 3 additional peptide hormones produced by the gut. These include cholecystokinin, gastric inhibitory polypeptide and secretin. Cholecystokinin is the peptide hormone released in response to ingestion of a fatty meal that induces contraction of the gallbladder. Gastric inhibitory polypeptide is produced in the intestinal mucosa. Ingestion of either protein, fat or carbohydrate stimulates its release. Independently of glucose, this peptide is probably one of the most powerful known stimulators for insulin secretion. Secretin is also produced in the small intestinal mucosa. Its major role is to increase exocrine secretory activity of the pancreas. Its most powerful stimulant is hydrochloric acid, followed in decreasing potency by protein, fat and glucose. Each of these hormones is a polypeptide and accordingly, each is degraded by the kidney (63-65). Predictably, in patients with renal failure, each is elevated in plasma in direct relationship to plasma creatinine concentration when the latter exceeds 3 mg/dl (265 µmol/l) (66). Hemodialysis appears to lower the plasma concentration of gastric inhibitory polypeptide but not that of cholecystokinin or glucagon (66). Hemodialysis may (67) or may not (66) lower gastrin levels. The possible significance of these derangements has not been determined.

ADRENOCORTICAL HORMONES

Cortisol (hydrocortisone)

This important hormone is conjugated in the liver to several metabolites collectively measurable as 17-hydroxycorticosteroids (17-OHCS). These products are normally excreted into the urine. Accordingly, in endstage renal disease, they accumulate in plasma in inverse proportion to the decline in glomerular filtration rate (68). Their concentration in plasma or daily excretion rates into the urine were formerly used to assess adrenal function inferentially. Estimation of 17-OHCS has been replaced by more reliable techniques to examine adrenal function, for example, measurement of plasma cortisol itself. Uremia, per se, does not appear to be associated with clinical disturbances of cortisol production. Cortisol levels in plasma are generally normal in patients on hemodialysis but moderately elevated levels have occasionally been observed (47). The latter observation may corresond to recent reports that impaired C-17,20-lyase activity in the adrenal cortex could be responsible for abnormally elevated mean 24 h cortisol levels (32). Following cortisol injection, plasma disappearance rates are prolonged (69, 70). The response of cortisol production to ACTH is normal (71, 72). Suppression of plasma cortisol following dexamethasone administration is also normal (71, 73). In correspondence to the usual finding that cortisol levels are normal plasma ACTH has also been reported to be normal (14).

Since the cortisol-binding protein (transcortin) is saturated when plasma cortisol concentration exceeds approximately 20 µg/dl, one would anticipate that any amount in plasma above this level would be dialyzable. In general, cortisol removal by dialysis is variable but the dialyzer clearance usually varies from 5 to 12 ml/min (70), representing a loss of about 0.1 to 0.4 mg during each dialysis. Since the total quantity of cortisol produced each day averages 20 to 30 mg, the quantity lost during dialysis is not of great significance (27). It should be kept in mind that cortisol levels may be substantially increased by medication with estrogen-derivatives due to an increase in protein binding. This does not cause clinical hypercorticism.

Adrenal insufficiency in the patient with endstage renal disease may be difficult to recognize. In our own experience, it has resulted from inadvertent removal of the adrenals in patients undergoing nephrectomy for unusually large polycystic kidneys and also after adrenal hemorrhage consequent to heparin use during dialysis. The potential occurrence of adrenal insufficiency should be kept in mind in patients who have previously received prolonged steroid therapy, those with infectious disease likely to involve the adrenals, amyloidosis and those who have previously received anticoagulation therapy. Possibly related to insulin resistance or to hyperglucagonemia, hypoglycemia has been unusual. The dominant manifestations have been chronic hypotension and more prominent weakness and hyperkalemia than usually observed in patients on dialysis. Its manifestations are subtle; the diagnosis may be readily proven by lack of responsiveness of plasma cortisol to ACTH.

Aldosterone

Of all the steroid hormones produced in the adrenal cortex, one of the most important in patients with end-stage renal disease is aldosterone. Some evidence suggests that aldosterone may be overproduced in uremia (74–76) as an adaptation to help prevent potassium intoxication (77) by promoting secretion of potassium into the bowel (78). Even in advanced renal disease, renin usually remains an important factor in the control of aldosterone production. In contrast, anephric patients show a virtual loss of plasma renin activity and often, a sharp decline in plasma aldosterone levels which do not increase after depletion of extracellular fluid volume (72). Although the precise factors controlling aldosterone production in anephric patients are incompletely settled, serum potassium concentration itself appears to be one of the most important. Thus, depression or elevation of plasma potassium will exert corresponding effects on aldosterone production.

The metabolic clearance rate (MCR) of aldosterone in patients on chronic dialysis may be increased in correspondence to the status of the circulatory volume (79). If volume expansion prevails along with a high cardiac output, as would exist in a patient with a large arteriovenous fistula (but not in a patient with an external Teflon-Silastic shunt) (80), the MCR would be increased. Except for some unusual influence, this implies that for a given volume of distribution and metabolic degradation of the hormone, production by the adrenal gland must necessarily proceed at a higher rate in order to maintain a normal concentration in plasma. Thus, in anephric patients who are hypokalemic, hypokalemia, per se, may explain why plasma aldosterone levels are low (72, 80, 81). In hypokalemic, anephric patients, administration of potassium and correction of plasma potassium concentration will increase plasma aldosterone levels.

Heparin in doses of 200 to 400 mg/day may diminish aldosterone production when given to a normal subject (82, 83). Whether or not smaller doses used in patients during hemodialysis have this effect has not been explored. It is conceivable that patients who become potassium deficient by dialysis against potassium-free solutions or other means might be more susceptible to inhibition of aldosterone production by heparin.

Aldosterone is dialyzable since it is of low molecular-weight (360) and only loosely bound to serum albumin (84–86). The quantity removed during a 7 h hemodialysis varies from 0.2 to 15.8 µg (84). This quantity is generally of no clinical importance and readily replaceable if normal aldosterone production is possible.

CARBOHYDRATE METABOLISM IN UREMIA

Patients with untreated uremia are often unable to metabolize glucose at a normal rate. Administered orally or intravenously, dextrose loads usually are not followed by pronounced hyperglycemia, but the decline to normal is delayed. Fasting hyperglycemia or ketosis is distinctly unusual. It is important to differentiate so called uremic pseudodiabetes from diabetes mellitus because of the serious implications associated with the latter diagnosis.

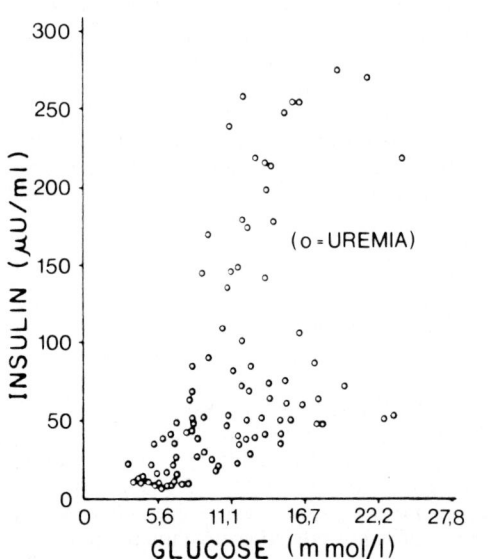

Figure 1. Comparison of immuno-reactive insulin and glucose in plasma during infusion of 10% dextrose at a rate of 1.5 g/min for 45 minutes in patients with end-stage renal failure (see text).
(Glucose mmol/l → mg/dl: multiply by 18).

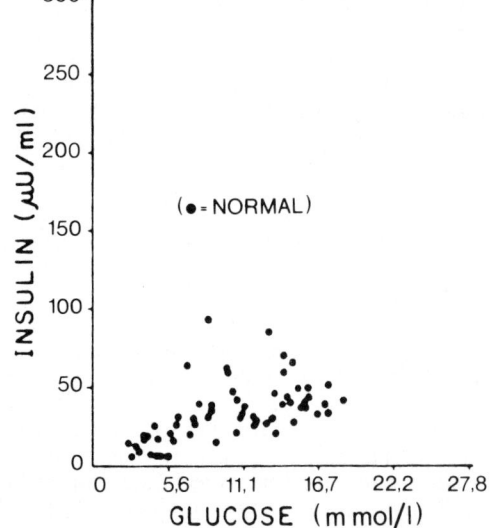

Figure 2. Comparison of immuno-reactive insulin and glucose in plasma during infusion of 10% dextrose at a rate of 1.5 g/min for 45 minutes in normal subjects (see text).

Insulin metabolism

The kidney plays a major role in the catabolism of insulin (87), which occurs within the proximal tubular cells. Although the capacity of the kidney to catabolize insulin decreases as renal mass diminishes, the fact that baseline serum concentrations of insulin remain normal or only become slightly elevated suggests that alternative catabolic sites gradually take over; these sites are probably in the liver.

Circulating immunoassayable insulin exists in two major fractions (88), one of small molecular weight which possesses strong hypoglycemic activity and another larger molecule, pro-insulin ('Big insulin') which has little activity. In patients with chronic renal failure, the proportion of proinsulin to insulin rises appreciably. The implications of the disturbed ratio of pro-insulin to insulin in renal failure suggest that the pool of circulating active hormone might actually be diminished.

Following administration of a dextrose load to patients with uremia, the peak insulin level in plasma is usually much higher for any given level of glucose than observed in normal subjects. This simple relationship is illustrated in Figures 1 and 2. Figures 3 and 4 show average values for insulin and glucose after a dextrose infusion in five patients before and after hemodialysis therapy (87). These data suggest that improvement was produced by dialysis. A study of uremic patients by Navalesi and co-workers (89) showed that the metabolic clearance rate (MCR) and delivery rate (DR) of insulin were reduced by approximately one-half. With the techniques used by these investigators it appeared that the estimated total body mass of insulin was increased. Following hemodialysis therapy, both MCR and DR became normal but the insulin mass did not change. They concluded that reduced insulin catabolism in uremia is the result of diminished functioning renal tissue associated with toxic depression of both insulin secretion and degradation.

Release of insulin in response to hyperglycemia is reduced in the face of a depressed ionized serum calcium concentration. Uremic hypocalcemia may thus reduce insulin release and be partially responsible for 'uremic pseudodiabetes'. Considerable work has been done to elucidate the role of calcium ions in insulin release from the β-cell (90). Glucose interferes with Ca extrusion, allows Ca concentration in the cell to rise and thereby insulin is released (91). Calcium extrusion from the cell is related to active sodium transport from the cell interior, since inhibition of sodium-transport ATPase (Na, K-activated, Mg-dependent ATPase) by ouabain blocks glucose-mediated insulin release. In addition, more recent studies have also identified a calcium-activated, Mg-dependent ATPase and an ATP-dependent calmodulin-stimulated calcium transport system in pancreatic islet cells of the rat (92).

The classical study demonstrating insulin resistance in uremia was reported by Westervelt (93). He compared the effects of insulin infusion into the brachial artery on the uptake of glucose, potassium and phosphate by the forearm. In normal subjects, insulin infused at a rate of 100 milliunits/kg/min for 45 min resulted in a glucose

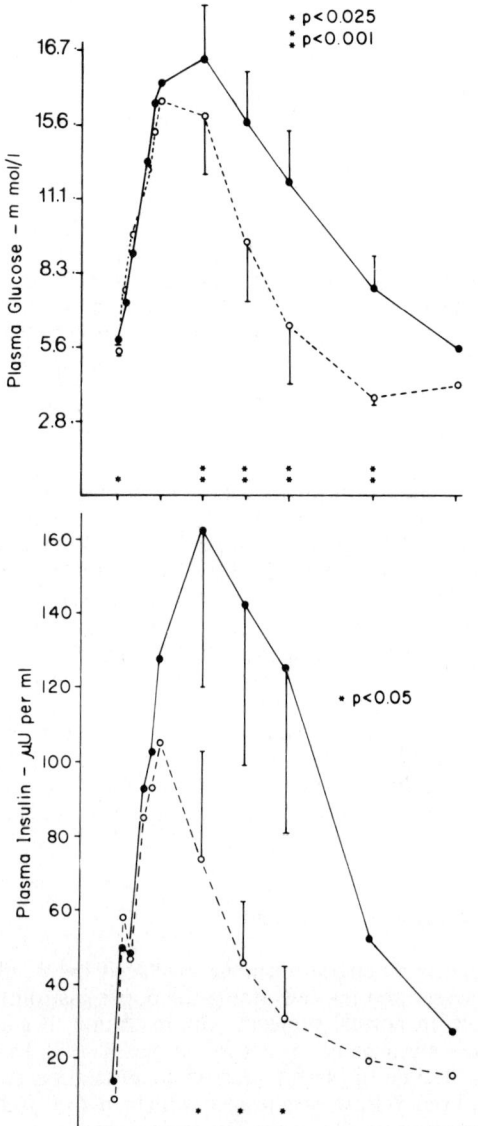

Figure 3a (top). Response of plasma glucose in five patients during dextrose infusion (1.5 g/min for 45 minutes) before hemodialysis (solid circles) and after 6 weeks of hemodialysis (open circles). Asterisk symbols represent significant differences by t analysis (see text).

(Glucose mmol/l → mg/dl: multiply by 18).

Figure 3b (bottom). Response of plasma insulin in five patients during dextrose infusion (1.5 g/min for 45 minutes) before hemodialysis (solid circles) and after 6 weeks of hemodialysis treatment (open circles). Asterisk symbols represent significant differences by t analysis (see text).

uptake of 8.3 µmol/min (149 µg/dl). In uremics, glucose uptake was only 1.6 µmol/min (28.8 µg/dl). Depressed values for lactate production were also observed. In correspondence with decreased glucose uptake in uremics, phosphorus uptake was also depressed, but interestingly, forearm uptake of potassium in response to insulin was normal. This probably reflects the independence of insulin mediated glucose and potassium uptake by skeletal muscle cells (94). Based upon such studies, it was postulated that an inhibitor of glucose metabolism is present in uremic serum. The improvement following dialysis therapy constituted the main evidence for such a hypothetical uremic toxin.

Potassium deficiency might decrease insulin production in response to hyperglycemia (95). We have shown that patients with end-stage renal disease may be modestly potassium deficient (96). Chronic dialysis therapy corrected the muscle potassium deficit as well as glucose intolerance. However, peak insulin levels in plasma during hyperglycemia were less after dialysis. Whether or not the hightly active species of insulin (small insulin) was secreted in greater quantities after dialysis has not been examined.

Carbohydrate utilization might be directly impaired by uremic serum. Such evidence has been obtained *in vitro* by studying glucose utilization by skeletal muscle (97). That metabolic acidosis also impairs glucose utilization has been reviewed by Relman (98).

It has been commonly observed that insulin requirements of patients with diabetes mellitus decline as they become uremic (87). Failure of the kidney to catabolize insulin may contribute to the decreased insulin requirement, but diminished caloric intake and energy metabolism also contribute. Most evidence indicates that the decreased insulin requirement results from a shrinkage of the functional body cellular mass occurring in chronic renal failure.

Hyperglucagonemia in uremia

Glucagon is a peptide hormone produced by α cells of the pancreas and the cells lining the upper gastrointestinal tract. In normal subjects, administration of glucose depresses glucagon concentration in plasma (99). In contrast, a decline of plasma glucose concentration stimulates a brisk release of glucagon which in turn induces glycogenolysis in the liver. The purpose of glucagon is therefore to aid in regulation of glucose concentration in plasma. Glucagon apparently stimulates gluconeogenesis in the liver.

Current evidence indicates that the kidney is a major catabolic site for glucagon (18, 100). Similar to insulin, the proximal tubular epithelium is the apparent site of glucagon catabolism. Accordingly, acute loss of renal function is associated with a prompt rise of plasma glucagon concentration (101, 102). In chronic renal failure, there is an apparent relationship between the degree of azotemia and the level of glucagon elevation (102). That glucagon is persistently elevated in patients with chronic renal failure (102) has been confirmed by several investigators (100, 101). Glucagon remains elevated even after adequate dialysis therapy, which stands in contrast to the relatively normal basal levels of insulin in patients under the same conditions (102). A large fraction of the retained glucagon, however, is a larger, relatively inactive molecule (101). The precise role or effect of hyperglucagonemia in uremia has not been ascertained. It does not seem to bear a precise relationship to glucose intolerance. It may exert a catabolic effect on body protein, thus stimulating gluconeogenesis from glucose precursors (amino acids) mobilized from skeletal muscle (87). Glucagon levels show a slight to moderate depression following induction of hyperglycemia in the uremic patient, but does not fall to normal values (102). Its plasma levels in uremic patients, as in normal subjects, rise moderately following administration of amino acids (102). Although glucose intolerance is improved following adequate hemodialysis therapy, glucagon levels remain elevated or even become higher (102). In contrast, glucagon levels fall to normal very rapidly following successful renal transplantation (103). Rejection of the transplanted kidney, even in the absence of a rise of serum creatinine concentrations, is associated with a pronounced rise of glucagon levels in plasma to values usually seen in patients with chronic renal disease. This response is considered to be similar to the glucagon elevations observed in inflammatory states (104).

CATECHOLAMINES

McGrath and co-workers (105) measured norepinephrine and epinephrine levels in 55 patients on chronic hemodialysis. Measurements were conducted on venous blood after being supine for 55 min. Norepinephrine levels were twice normal. Epinephrine levels were less than normal. In six anephric patients, norepinephrine levels were normal. Norepinephrine levels rose in response to head-up tilting.

ANTIDIURETIC HORMONE

The kidney is responsible for one third to one half of the metabolic clearance of vasopressin. Circulating vasopressin is not bound to plasma protein and, since its molecular mass is 1,084 daltons, it is freely filtered by the glomerulus. Clearance of arginine vasopressin (AVP) is nearly the same as the GFR. In the isolated perfused rat kidney, vasopressin clearance is more than twice the simultaneous value for GFR, indicating peritubular uptake. Besides the interaction of ADH with specific receptors at the contraluminal plasma membrane to produce its biological effect, there are abundant degradative enzymes in the tubular epithelium capable of destroying this peptide. For this reason, catabolism of ADH continues despite marked depression of GFR. In the studies by Rabkin and his associates (106), about 18% of the total AVP removed by the kidneys appeared in the urine, and fractional excretion was 38% of the filtered load. This suggests that about 20% of the filtered AVP was reabsorbed from the tubular lumen. Other peptide hormones, such as insulin, angiotensin II, and bradykinin are metabolized in the proximal tubule cells. Whether catabolism of ADH occurs at this site is unknown. However, the degradative enzymes shown to be capable of destroying ADH appear to be located in the distal tubular cell luminal membrane.

Only limited information is available on ADH levels in patients with renal failure. Unpublished studies by P. Vergne-Marini (University of Texas, Southwestern Medical School, Dallas, TX) have shown that normal values are 2.6 ± 2 pg/ml in hydrated subjects and 5.0 ± 1.0 pg/ml in dehydrated subjects. The mean predialysis value in 50 patients with chronic renal failure was 15.2 ± 1.0 pg/ml. Shimamoto and his co-workers also reported high values for plasma vasopressin in patients before and after hemodialysis (107).

OTHER PEPTIDES

Injected angiotensin II disappears rapidly from the circulation. When (^{14}C)-angiotensin II is infused into the distal tubule, nearly 95% appears in the urine as intact angiotensin II.

Bradykinin is metabolized by the kidney in a manner closely resembling that of angiotensin II. Micropuncture techniques were used to infuse ^{3}H-bradykinin in the rat tubule. When infused into the proximal tubule, 24% of the label was recovered from the urine, and 98% was recovered when infused into the distal tube. When infused into the proximal tubule, 85% of the label consisted of peptide fragments; when infused into the distal tubule, all radioactivity was found in intact bradykinin. It was concluded that the proximal tubular epithelium possesses peptidases capable of hydrolyzing bradykinin (57).

REFERENCES

1. Samaan NA, Freeman RM: Growth hormone levels in severe renal failure. *Metabolism* 19:102, 1970
2. Collipp PJ, Patrick JR, Goodheart C, Kaplan SA: Distribution of tritium-labelled human growth hormone in rats and guinea pigs. *Proc Soc Exp Biol Med* 121:173, 1966
3. Bala RM, Beck JC: Human growth hormone in urine. *J Clin Endocrinol Metab* 33:799, 1971
4. Bergström J, Fürst P, Josephson B, Noree LO: Factors affecting the nitrogen balance in chronic uremic patients receiving essential amino acids intravenously or by mouth. *Nutr Metab 14*:[Suppl] 62, 1972
5. Spitz I, Rubenstein AH, Bersohn I, Lawrence AM, Kirsteins L: The effect of dialysis on the carbohydrate intolerance of chronic renal failure. *Horm Metab Res* 2:86, 1970
6. Davidson MB, Fisher MB, Dabir-Vaziri N, Schaffer M: Effect of protein intake and dialysis on the abnormal growth hormone, glucose and insulin homeostasis in uremia. *Metabolism* 25:455, 1976
7. Bala RM, Ferguson, KA, Beck JC: Plasma biological and immunoreactive human growth hormone-like activity. *Endocrinology* 87:506, 1970
8. Hawkins DF, Strang F: Growth-hormone responses to haemodialysis. *Lancet* 1:1054, 1978
9. Ijaiya K, Bulla M, Roth B, Gladtke E, Schwenk A: Growth-hormone reponse to haemodialysis in children. *Lancet* 2:573, 1978
10. Lewy JE, New MI: Growth in children with renal failure. *Am J Med* 58:65, 1975
11. Saenger R, Wiedman E, Schwartz E, Korth-Schutz S, Lewy JE, Riggio RR, Rubin AL, Stenzel KH, New MI: Somatomedin and growth after renal transplantation. *Pediatr Res* 8:163, 1974
12. Pennisi AJ, Phillips LS, Uittenbogaart C, Ettenger RB, Malekyadeh MH, Fine RM: Nutritional intake, somatomedin activity and linear growth in children undergoing hemodialysis. *Abstracts Am Soc Nephrol* 9:37, 1976
13. Mehls O, Ritz E, Gilli G, Kreusser W: Growth in renal failure. *Nephron* 21:237, 1978
14. Gilkes JJH, Eady RAJ, Rees LH, Munro DD, Moorhead JF: Plasma immunoreactive melanotrophic hormones in patients on maintenance haemodialysis. *Br Med J* 1:656, 1975
15. Smith AG, Shuster S, Comaish JS, Plummer NA, Thody AJ, Alvarez-Ude F, Kerr DNS: Plasma immunoreactive B-melanocyte-stimulating hormone and skin pigmentation in chronic renal failure. *Br Med J* 1:658, 1975
16. Smith AG, Shuster S, Thody AJ, Alvarez-Ude F, Kerr DNS: Role of the kidney in regulating plasma immunoreactive beta-melanocyte-stimulating hormone. *Br Med J* 1:874, 1976
17. Marcovitz S, Friesen H: Regulation of proclatin secretion in man. *Clin Res* 19:773, 1971
18. LeFebvre P, Luyckx AS, Nizet A: Kidney function as a major factor regulating peripheral glucagon levels. *Diabetes* 23 [Suppl 1]:343, 1974
19. Turkington RW: Human prolactin. *Am J Med* 53:389, 1972
20. Gomez F, De La Cueva R, Wauters J, Lemarchand--Beraud T: Endocrine abnormalities in patients undergoing long-term hemodialysis. *Am J Med* 68:522, 1980
21. Steiner J, Cassar J, Mashiter K, Dawes I, Fraser TR, Breckenridge A: Effects of methyldopa on prolactin and growth hormone. *Br Med J* 1:1186, 1976
22. Guevara A, Vidt D, Hallbert MC, Zorn EM, Pohlman C, Weiland RC: Serum gonadotrophin and testosterone levels in uremic males undergoing intermittent dialysis. *Metabolism* 1:1062, 1969
23. Sawin CT, Longcope C, Schmitt GW, Ryan RJ: Blood levels of gonadotropins and gonadal hormones in gynecomastia associated with chronic hemodialysis. *J Clin Endocrinol Metab* 36:988, 1973
24. Lindsay RM, Briggs JD, Luke RG, Boyle IT, Kennedy AC: Gynaecomastia in chronic renal failure. *Br Med J* 4:779, 1967
25. Freeman RM, Lawton RL, Fearing MO: Gynecomastia: An endocrinologic complication of hemodialysis. *Ann Intern Med* 69:67, 1968
26. Schmitt GW, Shehadeh I, Sawin CT: Transient gynecomastia in chronic renal failure during chronic intermittent hemodialysis *Ann Intern Med* 69:73, 1968
27. Feldman HA, Singer I: Endocrinology and metabolism in uremia and dialysis: A clinical review. *Medicine* 54:345, 1974
28. Chen JC, Vidt DG, Zorn EM, Hallbert MC, Wieland RG: Pituitary-Leyding cell function in uremic males. *J Clin Endocrinol Metab* 31:14, 1970
29. Distiller LA, Morley JE, Sagel J, Pokroy MM, Robkin R: Pituitary-gonadal function in chronic renal failure: The effect of luteinizing hormonereleasing hormone and the influence of dialysis. *Metabolism* 24:711, 1975
30. Stewart-Bently M, Gans D, Horton R: Regulation of gon-

adal function in uremia. *Metabolism* 23:1065, 1974
31. Ferraris J, Saenger P, Levine L, New M, Pang S, Saxena BB, Lewy JE: Delayed puberty in males with chronic renal failure. *Kidney Int* 18:344, 1980
32. Zumoff B, Walter L, Rosenfeld RS, Strain JJ, Degen K, Strain GW, Levin J, Fukushima D: Subnormal plasma adrenal androgen levels in men with uremia. *J Clin Endocrinol Metab* 59:801, 1980
33. Antoniou LD, Shalhoub RJ: Zinc in the treatment of impotence in chronic renal failure. *Dial & Transpl* 7:912, 1978
34. Schreiner GE, Maher JF, Freeman RB, O'Connell JMB: Problems of hemodialysis. *Proc Int Congr Nephrol* Vol 3, edited by Becker EL, Basel, New York, E Karger, 1967, p 316
35. Mahler DJ, Walsh JR, Haynie GD: Magnesium, zinc, and copper in dialysis patients. *Am J Clin Pathol* 56:17, 1971
36. Riella MC, Broviac JW, Wells M, Scribner BH: Essential fatty acid deficiency in human adults during total parenteral nutrition. *Ann Intern Med* 83:786, 1975
37. Unzelman RF, Alderfer GR, Chojnacki RE: Pregnancy and chronic hemodialysis. *Trans Am Soc Artif Intern Organs* 19:144, 1974
38. Mackay EV: Pregnancy and renal disease. *Aust NZ J Obstet Gynaecol* 3:31, 1963
39. Brunner FP, Brynger H, Chantler C, Donckerwolcke RA, Hathway RA, Jacobs C, Selwood NH, Wing AJ: Combined report on regular dialysis and transplantation in Europe, IX, 1978. *Proc Eur Dial Transpl Assoc* 16:43, 1979
40. Swamy AP, Woolf PD, Cestero, RVM: Hypothalamic-pituitary-ovarian axis in uremic women. *J Lab Clin Med* 93:1066, 1979
41. Schmidt P, Strobaeus N, Prame G, Schittek F: Exophthalmos in chronic renal insufficiency. *Scand J Urol Nephrol* 5:146, 1971
42. Ramirez G, Jibiz W, Gutch CF, Bloomer HA, Siegler R, Kolff WJ: Thyroid abnormalities in renal failure. *Ann Intern Med* 79:500, 1973
43. Gonzales-Barcena D, Kastin AK, Schalch DS, Torres-Zamora M, Perrez-Pasten E, Kato A, Schally AV: Responses to thyrotropin-releasing hormone in patients with renal failure and after infusion in normal men. *J Clin Endocrinol Metab* 36:117, 1973
44. Redding TW, Schally AV: On the half-life of thyrotropin-releasing hormone in patients with renal failure and after infusion in normal men. *Neurendocrinology* 9:252, 1972
45. Fine A, Thomso RM, Jones JV, Murray RG, Tweedle A, Gray CE: The renal handling of insulin and thyroid hormones in normal man. *Clin Sci Mol Med* 50:435, 1975
46. Lim VS, Fang VS, Katz AI, Refetoff S: Thyroid dysfunction in chronic renal failure. *J Clin Invest* 60:522, 1977
47. Robertson BF, Prestwich S, Ramirez G, O'Neill W, Jubiz W: The role of iodine in the pathogenesis of thyroid enlargement in rats with chronic renal failure. *Endocrinology* 101:1272, 1977
48. Lim VS, Henriquez C, Seo H, Refetoff S, Martino E: Thyroid function in a uremic rat model. *J Clin Invest* 66:946, 1980
49. Ramirez G, O'Neill W Jr, Jubiz W, Bloomer HA: Thyroid dysfunction in uremia: Evidence for thyroid and hypophyseal abnormalities. *Ann Intern Med* 84:672, 1976
50. Silverberg DS, Ulan RA, Fawcett DM, Dossetor JB, Grace M, Bettcher K: Effects of chronic hemodialysis on thyroid function in chronic renal failure. *Can Med Assoc J* 109:282, 1973
51. Oddie TH, Flanigan WJ, Fisher DA: Iodine and thryoxine metabolism in anephric patients receiving chronic peritoneal dialysis. *J Clin Endocrinol Metab* 31:277, 1970
52. Hollander CS, Scott RL, Burgess JA, Rabinowitz D, Merimee JJ, Oppenheimer JH: Free fatty acid: a possible regulator of free thyroid hormone levels in man. *J Clin Endocrinol Metab* 27:1219, 1967
53. Hershman JM, Jones CM, Bailey AL: Reciprocal changes in serum thyrotropin and free thyroxine produced by heparin. *J Clin Endocrinol Metab* 34:574, 1972
54. Shatz DL: Serum free thyroxine and thyroxine binding protein studies in patients with supraventricular tachycardia. *J Clin Endocrinol Metab* 27:165, 1967
55. Bricker NS, Head CJ Jr: Observations on the renal clearance of I^{131}. *J Clin Invest* 34:1057, 1955
56. Koutras DA, Marketos FG, Rigopoulos GA, Malamos B: Iodine metabolism and chronic renal insufficiency. *Nephron* 9:55, 1972
57. Knochel JP, Seldin DW: The pathophysiology of uremia. In *The Kidney,* 2nd ed, Vol. II, edited by Brenner BM, Rector FC Jr, Philadelphia PA, London UK, Toronto Can, WB Saunders Company, 1980, p 2137
58. Cotton JR, Woodard T, Carter NW, Knochel JP: Resting skeletal muscle membrane potential as an index of uremic toxicity. *J Clin Invest* 63:501, 1979
59. Korman MC, Laver MC, Hansky J: Hypergastrinaemia in chronic renal failure. *Br Med J* 1:209, 1972
60. Clendinnen DG, Davidson WD, Lemmi CA. Jackson BM: Renal uptake and excretion of gastrin in the dog. *Gastroenterology* 58:935, 1970
61. Davidson WD, Corredor JS, Bassist L: A cause of fasting hypergastrinemia. *Clin Res* 19:390, 1971
62. Dent RI, James JH, Wang C, Deftos LJ, Talamo R, Fischer J: Hyperparathyroidism: Gastric acid secretion and gastrin. *Ann Surg* 176:360, 1972
63. Thompson JC, Fender HR, Ramus NI, Villar HV, Rayford PL: Cholecystokinin metabolism in man and dogs. *Ann Surg* 182:496, 1975
64. O'Dorisio TM, Sirinek KR, Mazzaferri EL, Cataland S: Renal effects on serum gastric inhibitory polypeptide (GIP). *Metabolism* 26:651, 1977
65. Curtis PH, Fender HR, Rayford PL, Thompson JC: Catabolism of secretin by the liver and kidney. *Surgery* 80:259, 1976
66. Owyang C, Miller LJ, DiMagno EP, Brennan LA, Go VLW: Gastrointestinal hormone profile in renal insufficiency. *Mayo Clin Proc* 54:769, 1979
67. Falcao HA, Wesdorp RIC, Fischer JE: Gastrin levels and gastric acid secretion in anephric patients and in patients with chronic and acute renal failure. *J Surg Res* 18:107, 1975
68. Englert E Jr, Brown H, Williamson DG, Wallach S, Simmons EL: Metabolism of free and conjugated 17-hydroxycorticosteroids in subjects with uremia. *J Clin Endocrinol Metab* 18:36, 1958
69. Bacon EG, Kenney FM, Murdaugh HV, Richards C: Prolonged serum half-life of cortisol in renal failure. *Johns Hopkins Med J* 132:127, 1973
70. Mishkin MS, Hsu JH, Walker WG, Bledsoe T: Studies on the episodic secretion of cortisol in uremic patients on hemodialysis. *John Hopkins Med J* 131:160, 1972
71. Barbour GL, Sevier BR: Adrenal responsiveness in chronic hemodialysis. *N Engl J Med* 290:1258, 1974
72. Weidmann P, Horton R, Maxwell MH, Franklin SS, Fichman M: Dynamic studies of aldosterone in anephric man. *Kidney Int* 4:289, 1973
73. Williams GH, Bailey GL, Hampers CL, Lauler DP, Merrill JP, Underwood RH, Blair-West JR, Coghlan JP,

Denton DA, Scoggings BA, Wright RD: Studies on the metabolism of aldosterone in chronic renal failure and anephric man. *Kidney Int* 4:289, 1973
74. Cope CL, Person J: Aldosterone secretion in several renal failure. *Clin Sci* 25:331, 1963
75. Corvol T, Bertagna X, Bedrossian J: Increased steroid metabolic clearance rate in anephric patients. *Acta Endocrinol* 75:756, 1974
76. Weidmann P, Maxwell MH, Lupu AN: Plasma aldosterone in terminal renal failure. *Ann Intern Med* 78:13, 1973
77. Alexander EA, Levinsky NG: An extrarenal mechanism of potassium adaptation. *J Clin Invest* 47:740, 1968
78. Hayes CP Jr, McLead ME, Robinson RR: An extrarenal mechanism for the maintenance of potassium balance in severe chronic renal failure. *Trans Assoc Am Physicians* 80:207, 1967
79. Reed VH, McCaa CS, Bower JD, McCaa RE: Effect of hemodialysis on metabolic clearance rate, plasma concentration and blood production rate of aldosterone in anephric man. *J Clin Endocrinol Metab* 36:773, 1973
80. Bayard F, Cooke CR, Tiller DJ, Beitins IZ, Kowarski A, Walker WG, Migeon CJ: The regulation of aldosterone secretion in anephric man. *J Clin Invest* 50:1585, 1971
81. McCaa RE, McCaa CS, Read VH, Bower JD: Influence of hemodialysis on plasma aldosterone concentration in nephrectomized patients. *Trans Am Soc Artif Intern Organs* 18:239, 1973
82. Bailey RE, Ford GC: The effect of heparin on sodium conservation and on the plasma concentration, the metabolic clearance and the secretion and excretion rates of aldosterone in normal subjects. *Acta Endocrinol* 60:249, 1969
83. Majoor CLH, Schlatmann RJAFM, Jansen AP, Preven H: Excretion pattern and mechanism of diuresis induced by heparin. *Clin Chem Acta* 5:591, 1960
84. Asbach HW, Vecsei P, Schuler HW, Gless KH: Serum and Dialysatespiegel von Corticosteroiden bei Langzeit-Hämodialyse (Concentrations of corticosteroids in serum and dialysate during longterm haemodialysis treatment). *Dtsch Med Wochenschr* 98:1958, 1973 (in German)
85. Deck KA, Siemon G, Sieberth HG, von Bayer H: Cortisolverlust und Plasma 11-Hydroxycorticosteroid Profil während der Hämodialyse (Loss of cortisol and plasma 11-hydroxy-corticosteroid profile during hemodialysis), *Verh Dtsch Ges Inn Med* 74:1195, 1968 (in German)
86. Read VH, Ott CE, Bower JD, McCaa RE, McCaa CS: Clearance of adrenocortical steroids by the artificial kidney. *Clin Res* 21:47, 1973
87. Knochel JP, Seldin DW: The pathophysiology of uremia. In: *The Kidney,* edited by Brenner BM, Rector FC Jr, Philadelphia PA, London, UK Toronto Can, WB Saunders Company, 1976, p 1448
88. Mako M, Block M, Starr J, Nielsen K, Friedman E, Rubenstein A: Proinsulin in chronic renal and hepatic failure; a reflection of the relative contribution of the liver and kidney to its metabolism. *Clin Res* 21:631, 1973
89. Navalesi R, Alessandro P, Silvia L, Donato L: Insulin metabolism in chronic uremia and in the anephric state. Effect of the dialytic treatment. *J Clin Endocrinol Metab* 40:70, 1973
90. Herchuelz A, Couturier E, Malaisse WJ: Regulation of calcium fluxes in pancreatic islets: glucose-induced calcium-calcium exchange. *Am J Physiol* 238:E96, 1980
91. Siegel EG, Wollheim CB, Renold AE, Sharp GWG: Evidence for the involvement of Na/Ca exchange in glucose-induced insulin release from rat pancreatic islets. *J Clin Invest* 66:996, 1980
92. Pershadsingh HA, McDaniel ML, Landt M, Bry CG, Lacy PE, McDonald JM: Ca^{2+}-activated ATPase and ATP-dependent calmodulin-stimulated Ca^{2+} transport in islet cell plasma membrane. *Nature* 288:492, 1980
93. Westervelt FB Jr: Insulin effect in uremia. *J Lab Clin Med* 74:79, 1969
94. Andres R, Baltzan MA, Cader G, Zierler KL: The effect of insulin on carbohydrate metabolism and on potassium in the forearm of man. *J Clin Invest* 41:108, 1962
95. Sagild U, Anderson V, Andreasen PB: Glucose tolerance and insulin responsiveness in experimental potassium depletion. *Acta Med Scand* 169:243, 1961
96. Bilbrey GL, Carter NW, White MG, Schilling JF, Knochel JP: Potassium deficiency in chronic renal failure. *Kidney int* 4:423, 1973
97. Dzúrik R, Krajči-Lazáry B: The effect of uremic serum on carbohydrate metabolism in rat diaphragm. *Experientia* 23:798, 1967
98. Relman AS: Metabolic consequences of acid-base disorders. *Kidney Int* 1:347, 1972
99. Unger RH: Glucagon physiology and pathophysiology. *N Engl J Med* 285:443, 1971
100. Sherwin RS, Basil C, Finkelstein FO, Fisher M, Black H, Hendler R, Felig P: Influence of uremia and hemodialysis on the turnover and metabolic effects of glucagon. *J Clin Invest* 57:722, 1975
101. Emmanouel DS, Jaspan JB, Kuku SF, Rubenstein AH, Katz AL: Pathogenesis and characterization of hyperglucagonemia in the uremic rat. *J Clin Invest* 58:1266, 1976
102. Bilbrey GL, Faloona GR, White MG, Knochel JP: Hyperglucagonemia of renal failure. *J Clin Invest* 53:841, 1974
103. Bilbrey GL, Faloona GR, White MG, Atkins C, Hull AR, Knochel JP: Hyperglucagonemia in uremia. Reversal by renal transplantation. *Ann Intern Med* 82:525, 1975
104. Lindsey A, Samteusanio F, Braten J, Faloona GR, Unger RH: Pancreatic alpha cell function in trauma. *JAMA* 227:757, 1974
105. McGrath BP, Ledingham JGG, Benedict CR: Catecholamines in peripheral venous plasma in patients on chronic haemodialysis. *Clin Sci Mol Med* 55:89, 1978
106. Rabkin R, Share L, Payne P, Young J, Crofton J: The handling of immunoreactive vasopressin by the isolated perfused rat kidney. *J Clin Invest* 63:6, 1979
107. Shimamoto K, Watarai I, Miyahara M: A study of plasma vasopressin in patients undergoing chronic hemodialysis. *J Clin Endocrinol Metab* 45:714, 1977

37

NEUROLOGICAL ASPECTS OF DIALYSIS PATIENTS

FRANS G.I. JENNEKENS and AAGJE JENNEKENS-SCHINKEL

Introduction	724
Cerebral disorders	724
Uraemic encephalopathy	724
Clinical picture	724
Laboratory investigations and pathology	725
Effect of dialysis; pathophysiology and pathogenesis	725
Encephalopathy due to electrolyte disturbances and acidosis	726
Sodium imbalance	726
Potassium imbalance	726
Metabolic acidosis	726
Calcium imbalance	726
Magnesium imbalance	727
Disequilibrium syndrome	727
Wernicke syndrome and drug induced encephalopathies	727
Cerebrovascular disorders in dialysis patients	727
Hypertensive encephalopathy	728
Multi-infarct dementia	728
Binswanger encephalopathy (subcortical arteriosclerotic encephalopathy (SAEL)	728
Transient ischaemic attacks (TIA); prevention of thrombotic stroke	729
Cerebral thrombosis and embolism	729
Intracerebral haemorrhage and subdural haematoma	729
Central nervous system infections	730
Management of epilepsy	730
Peripheral neuropathies	730
Uraemic polyneuropathy	730
Clinical features	730
Nerve conduction velocity	731
Neuropathy and the degree of renal insufficiency	731
Low protein, high calorie diet	731
The effect of maintenance dialysis	731
The effect of transplantation	732
Pathology and pathophysiology of uraemic polyneuropathy	732
Pathogenesis	732
Post vascular access neuropathy	734
Skeletal muscle disease	736
Psychological aspects	736
Neuropsychological considerations	736
Psychological stresses and coping mechanisms	737
References	738

INTRODUCTION

Neurological complications in dialysis patients are manifold and frequent. Some relate to the persistence of a minor degree of uraemia, others are complications of the dialysis procedure. A number of neurological disorders occur with relatively high frequency in patients requiring this form of therapy but are not related to uraemia nor to the methods used for treatment.

For practical reasons, the various neurological changes are discussed according to the location of the lesion. Dialysis encephalopathy will not be discussed; this subject is dealt with in detail in chapter 42.

CEREBRAL DISORDERS

Uraemic encephalopathy

The clinical syndrome of uraemic encephalopathy is presently observed only rarely on the hospital wards, owing to the efficiency of dialysis therapy.

When dialysis treatment is not initiated, the signs and symptoms of uraemic encephalopathy may remain subclinical for a long period of time provided that (a) renal function decreases gradually, (b) water and electrolyte balance is maintained, (c) blood pressure is kept within reasonable limits, (d) adequate food intake and protein restriction is observed and (e) iatrogenic intoxication is avoided. In some patients, however, renal insufficiency progresses rapidly and the course of the disease is complicated by unexpected or unavoidable factors. Encephalopathy in these patients is not necessarily due to 'uraemic intoxication' *per se* but to one or several other, often treatable conditions. It is often difficult to decide which manifestations result from uraemia and which from complicating disorders.

Clinical picture
The two main kinds of neurological changes to be distinguished in uraemic patients are those concerning complex mental functions and level of consciousness on the one hand and motor disturbances on the other hand. The initial neuropsychological changes involve decrease in alertness and attention span, inability to sustain attention and to concentrate on tasks. Patients become irritable or apathetic and incapable of performing their daily work. When the situation worsens, the sensorium becomes clouded and defects in orientation become apparent. Patients may be frightened and confused, and a delirious condition may develop. Often this can be attributed, however, to concomitant disturbances of electrolyte and water homeostasis. In the final stage, patients hardly react and become comatose (1).

The initial motor abnormality is *tremulousness*. This tremor is irregular in amplitude and has a frequency of 8 to 10 per second. It is only apparent during limb movements. The pathophysiology of this tremor is unknown. The second motor abnormality is called *asterixis* or flapping tremor. This phenomenon is not specific for uraemia but is also seen in other metabolic encephalopathies and occasionally in patients with focal brain lesions. Asterixis is caused by the inability to maintain a sustained position. When the hands are kept extended (or the feet dorsiflexed) a sudden interruption, lasting only a few moments, occurs, causing a downward flap. Electromyographic examination has shown that during this interruption there is electrical silence in the muscles involved which implies that the downward flap has to be attributed to a brief interruption of innervation (2). Malfunction of a hypothetical system concerned with maintenance of tonic postural contraction of muscle has been suggested as being responsible for the interruption (3). Bilateral and unilateral asterixis have been reported in patients with lesions localised in the mesodiencephalic region of the brain and in the parietal lobe (4, 5). *Myoclonus* is a third type of involuntary movement which develops in a late phase of uraemic encephalopathy. The term is used for twitchings occurring irregularly and asymmetrically in the limbs, trunk and head. At rest the muscle contractions are slight (fascicular) and cause no or only fine movements. During passive and/or active movements, and sometimes in response to sensory stimuli, the contractions become stronger and are better described as jerks. In occasional patients the movements may even appear as ballistic. There are no concomitant specific EEG abnormalities. Patients in this condition have a clouded sensorium and are often stuporous. The jerks disappear after intravenous administration of clonazepam (0.75-1 mg in adults). Chadwich and French (6) called attention to the fact that uraemic myoclonus as described here resembles action (or intention) myoclonus in postanoxic encephalopathy. It has been suggested that this myoclonus is mediated by a spino-bulbar-spinal reflex which is normally inhibited. The same authors point out that there is experimental evidence indicating that this type of myoclonus is caused by a functional disturbance of the reticular formation in the lower brain stem.

Generalised tonic and clonic convulsions are regularly seen in acute or advanced chonic renal failure. They are often indicative of non-uraemic complications as will be discussed later. In case of localised convulsions, focal brain lesions have to be considered. In the final stage patients are often mute and may be catatonic (7). The tendon reflexes may be brisk but in the terminal phase they are often diminished.

Laboratory investigations and pathological findings
The cerebrospinal fluid (CSF) pressure is not raised, and the CSF protein content is often only slightly elevated. The urea concentration is similar to that in serum. Pleocytosis has been reported previously but not in recent publications (8-11). Electro-encephalographic (EEG) changes develop concurrently with the clinical disorder and include disorganisation, slowing and loss of alpha frequency, diffuse slow wave bursts and specific paroxysmal discharges; the EEG equivalent of drowsiness is diffuse slowing (12, 13).

The classic study by Olsen (14) did not detect specific structural changes within the brain by light microscopy.

Effect of dialysis treatment; pathophysiology and pathogenesis
Little is definitely established about the pathophysiology and pathogenesis of uraemic encephalopathy. Several hypotheses have been introduced and rejected, others are being evaluated. Whatever the pathogenesis, the lesion(s) is (are) obviously rapidly reversible and therefore to a large extent functional and not structural. In this respect, the reaction to dialysis treatment and renal transplantation is instructive. Even when the clinical manifestations are severe, the whole syndrome clears up in a matter of days or weeks after the onset of adequate dialysis treatment. An equally rapid improvement of EEG abnormalities occurs (15). Increase of dialysis frequency from two to three times weekly is reflected in further improvement or normalisation of the EEG frequencies. Mild slowing of EEG waves which has been present for many months during dialysis treatment, may return to normal within 2 weeks following restoration of renal function by successful kidney transplantation (16).

Two differences between uraemic encephalopathy and polyneuropathy should be noted. Firstly, as mentioned before, structural changes in the central nervous system (CNS) have not been observed whilst structural changes in the peripheral nervous system (PNS) are frequent and have been demonstrated by many investigators. Secondly, in contrast to the encephalopathy, the peripheral neuropathy shows little immediately favourable reaction to dialysis treatment. This unresponsiveness cannot be explained by the presence of structural lesions, as the response to restoration of kidney function by successful transplantation is excellent. Clearly the lesions in the central and the peripheral nervous systems cannot be lumped together. Differences between the blood-brain barrier and the blood-nerve barrier may result in a better protection from structural injury of the CNS than of the PNS.

Brain metabolism has been shown to be reduced in uraemia (17, 18) possibly due to inhibition of cerebral enzyme activities by unknown uraemic toxins. Activity of sodium stimulated, potassium dependent ATP-ase in brain tissue of uraemic rats is depressed (19) and inhibition of many other cerebral enzymes by constituents of uraemic dialysates has been demonstrated (20). The nature of the putative uraemic toxins is still a matter of speculation and subject of intense investigation. (For comprehensive information the reader is referred to Chapter 19).

Organic acids retained and accumulated in the brain, may well be involved. In the past few years, much attention has also been given to the role of parathyroid hormone (PTH). Secondary hyperparathyroidism commonly accompanies renal failure. Plasma PTH levels have been reported to be raised even within 48 h of the onset of acute renal failure (21). According to Massry and Goldstein (22) excess PTH may adversely affect the function of the nervous system and other organs by (a) increasing the concentration of cellular calcium, (b) altering cellular membrane permeability, (c) inducing exaggerated stimulation of cyclic AMP, (d) causing deposition of calcium extracellularly with disruption of functional integrity, (e) other mechanisms. Experimental investigations have shown that the calcium content of brain tissue in acute uraemia is markedly raised and associated with slowing of EEG waves. Increase in calcium content and changes in EEG frequencies are prevented by parathyroidectomy before the induction of uraemia. Similar changes are provoked in normal animals by administration of parathyroid extract. Clinical observations supporting these experimental findings have been reported. Patients with elevated plasma PTH levels have indeed a raised calcium concentration of brain tissue (21, 23). Other studies of PTH are concerned with peripheral nerves and will be discussed in the section on uraemic polyneuropathy.

Encephalopathy due to electrolyte disturbances and acidosis

Sodium imbalance

Experimental investigations have shown that the brain is protected to some extent against osmolar shifts; slow osmolar changes are tolerated better than rapid shifts. Acute hypo-osmolality or hyponatraemia may cause brain oedema because osmolality of brain tissue remains high in comparison to plasma osmolality (24). Subacute or chronic experimental hyponatraemia causes only a mild increase in brain water content, the osmolality of brain and plasma remaining equal. The critical factor for encephalopathy is probably the accumulation of water in the cells in the brain (25).

A rapid fall in the plasma sodium level in patients to less than 130 mmol/l may cause neurological changes whilst a slow decrease need not become apparent neurologically until values of 120 mmol/l have been reached. There are many causes of hypo-osmolality and hyponatraemia in patients with renal failure, e.g. congestive heart failure, the nephrotic syndrome, impaired water excretion, excessive water ingestion, inappropriate fluid therapy or dialysis. The manifestations are non-specific and include headache, nausea, vomiting, drowsiness, muscle cramps, restless legs, asterixis, myoclonus, confusion, delirium, stupor and coma. Convulsions, either generalised or focal, are common. The CSF pressure is elevated and papilloedema may develop. The CSF protein is usually within normal limits.

Hypernatraemia and hyperosmolality cause brain shrinkage and are rare in patients with renal failure. They may occur accidentally during haemodialysis with high sodium dialysis fluid (see Chapter 31). Clinical manifestations include drowsiness, delirium, stupor or coma. Generalised or focal seizures and stroke-like motor deficits may occur (26).

Potassium imbalance

Potassium imbalance, either with hypo- or hyperkalaemia, causes neuromuscular and cardiac changes. Experimental investigations have elucidated that the mechanisms for potassium homeostasis in the CNS are highly efficient. This probably explains why potassium imbalance causes no clearly recognisable clinical manifestations of brain dysfunction (27).

Metabolic acidosis

Changes in pH have a profound effect on cellular metabolism and function. The brain is protected by several mechanisms against arterial pH changes (28). The acid-base balance in the brain is reflected in the pH of the CSF. The blood-CSF barrier offers little resistance against diffusion of CO_2 but is relatively impermeable to bicarbonate. The decrease in the plasma bicarbonate level in metabolic acidosis is not followed by a similar decrease in the CSF. The compensatory fall in PCO_2 of the blood occurs rapidly, however, the final effect of these two events resulting in a relatively stable pH of the CSF, which initially even may show a temporary rise.

Correction of metabolic acidosis by intravenous administration of sodium bicarbonate solution is followed by a rise of PCO_2 in blood and CSF. The rise of CSF bicarbonate is much slower, however, and results in a decrease of CSF pH which induces deterioration of brain function.

Chronic metabolic acidosis in advanced chronic renal failure resulting from retention of non volatile acids, does not cause clinically demonstrable effects on the central nervous system functions.

Rapidly developing severe metabolic acidosis, as occurs in acute renal failure, causes manifest hyperventilation and substantial loss of CO_2 from the blood and the CSF. This is likely to be one of the factors causing confusion, stupor and eventually coma. Uraemic patients with convulsions are usually moderately or severely acidotic (29).

Calcium imbalance

Calcium ions play important roles in numerous cellular processes. It is, therefore, not surprising that calcium imbalance results in functional disturbances of many organ systems including the nervous system. There is experimental evidence showing that the CSF calcium concentration remains relatively constant during alterations in plasma calcium concentration (30, 31). The homeostatic mechanisms involved, however, do not offer absolute protection. Following experimental parathyroidectomy CSF calcium concentration decreases over a period of several weeks. It is, therefore, likely that brief changes in plasma calcium concentration induce only slight responses in CSF calcium concentration. An exchange between CSS and brain calcium has been demonstrated.

The total plasma calcium level in renal failure is characteristically depressed. Both the protein bound fraction and the ultrafiltrable portion decrease. Nervous system manifestations of hypocalcaemia present themselves as tetany. Due to the protective action of the blood-brain barrier the CNS is, in general, less sensitive to hypocalcaemia than the PNS. The main signs of the CNS are generalised or focal seizures and mental changes; PNS manifestations include paraesthesias, muscle cramps, carpopedal spasms and laryngeal stridor. Trousseau's sign (carpal spasm within three minutes following inflation of a blood pressure cuff around the upper arm to above the systolic pressure) and the Chvostek sign (tapping on the facial nerve just in front of the ear elicits visible contractions in the facial musculature innervated by this nerve) may be positive. The chances of CNS manifestations of hypocalcaemia in uraemic patients are relatively small because the PTH levels are elevated and the calcium concentration in the brain is high (21, 23). Signs of peripheral nerve hyperexcitability are also observed only rarely, possibly because hypocalcaemia develops insidiously and peripheral nerve calcium concentrations remain relatively high (22).

Regardless of its cause, hypercalcaemic patients may present with such evidence of encephalopathy as impaired intellectual functioning, lethargy, confusion, hallucinations, delirium, stupor and coma (31, 32). Hypercalcaemia causes EEG changes strongly resembling those in other metabolic encephalopathies. Inappropriately high dialysate calcium concentrations in the dialysis fluid have been reported as the cause of hypercalcaemia in patients on maintenance dialysis (33). In addition to the changes already mentioned, these patients also developed dysarthria, myoclonic jerks and seizures.

Magnesium imbalance
Plasma magnesium levels are raised in severe chronic renal failure, usually without inducing any neurological manifestations (29, 34), but when magnesium levels increase to two to three times normal values drowsiness may develop. Levels of this magnitude may occur by excessive magnesium administration in patients with renal failure (34). Hypermagnesaemia affects the neuromuscular junction by inhibiting of acetylcholine release (29).

Disequilibrium syndrome

Manifestations of neurological dysfunction may become apparent during the course of a dialysis treatment, usually during its last hours or shortly thereafter (35). Mild symptoms such as headache, nausea and muscle cramps occur in many patients. More severe manifestations such as restlessness, confusion and generalised convulsions tend to develop during rapid dialysis, often in the early stages of the dialysis procedure. With the exception of the muscle cramps, the syndrome was originally attributed to a rapid decrease of plasma urea concentration, leaving the brain with a relatively high urea concentration. This osmotic gradient causes a shift of water into the brain inducing cerebral oedema and brain swelling. Results of animal investigations did not support, however, the hypothesis that the osmotic gradient had to be attributed to urea or electrolytes (36, 37). Subsequently, the syndrome was considered to result from an osmotic gradient of unidentified, osmotically active agents and to lowering of the pH of the CSF and the brain cell water (38). It was shown that during rapid dialysis of uraemic dogs the arterial pH rose slightly, whereas a fall was registered in brain and CSF pH. It has been suggested that organic acids accumulating during dialysis cause the decline in pH. These substances might be sufficiently osmotically active to cause brain swelling.

Prevention is possible by gradual correction of uraemia, particularly when initial blood urea concentrations are high. Intravenous use of osmotic agents like glycerol can reduce the osmolar shift and may prevent neurological manifestations (39).

Intracranial neurological disorders tend to worsen during dialysis. When a disequilibrium syndrome becomes apparent in a patient fully adapted to a dialysis programme, a complicating intracranial disorder or errors in the composition of the dialysis fluid should be considered.

Wernicke syndrome and drug induced encephalopathy

A Wernicke syndrome may develop after frequent vomiting in uraemic patients with restricted food intake (40). This syndrome is characterised by changes in ocular motility and ataxia. The ocular manifestations include nystagmus, abducens palsy or palsy of conjugate gaze. Ocular disturbances are almost a prerequisite for this diagnosis (41). The Wernicke syndrome is frequently associated with a Korsakoff psychosis. Such patients have a defective recent memory, are confused and tend to confabulate. The ocular disturbances and ataxia respond to high doses of thiamin. The effect on the mental symptoms is less favourable.

Administration of drugs normally excreted by the kidneys, may cause neurotoxic effects in patients with renal failure. Penicillin is a well-known example (42). In high doses it may cause myoclonus, hyperreflexia and coma. It has to be emphasised that similar manifestations occur in uraemic encephalopathy. (The reader is referred to Chapter 39 for further information).

Cerebrovascular disorders in dialysis patients

In the early seventies reports of causes of death in patients treated with maintenance dialysis showed a high prevalence of vascular disorders, in particular ischaemic heart disease and cerebrovascular accidents (43, 44). It was suggested that the life span of dialysed patients was limited by accelerated atherosclerosis (43). This seemed plausible in view of the large number of atherosclerotic risk factors in many of these patients, i.e. hypertension, hyperlipidaemia and hyperglycaemia. Continued investigations raised doubt about this pessimistic view. It was argued that insufficient allowance had been made for pre-existing morbid conditions (45, 46). When patients known to have diabetes mellitus, atherosclerosis or a long history of hypertension prior to initiation of maintenance dialysis were excluded, and the age factor was sufficiently accounted for, the death rate due to atherosclerotic vascular diseases in dialysed patients was not significantly higher than in matched control populations. The accelerated atherosclerosis hypothesis remains unproved (47).

Cerebral lesions resulting from vascular disorders have to be divided into two categories. The first category consists of diffuse or multifocal lesions or encephalopathies and the second comprises focal lesions. Among the diffuse lesions hypertensive encephalopathy is most frequent. Multi-infarct dementia and Binswanger encephalopathy may be present in occasional patients.

Hypertensive encephalopathy
Hypertensive encephalopathy is associated with severe hypertension either of primary or secondary origin, which usually has reached the malignant stage.

Patients with hypertensive encephalopathy commonly have renal lesions, but the syndrome has to be distinguished from uraemic encephalopathy.

Usually following an asymptomatic phase with moderate hypertension and proteinuria, patients develop an extremely high blood pressure (rarely less than 250/150 mm Hg) and neurological and ophthalmological changes become apparent (48), i.e. severe headache with nausea and vomiting, blurred vision, particularly during changes in posture, drowsiness, confusion or agitation. Patients may have generalised or focal convulsions and an occasional patient may display neck stiffness.

Ophthalmological investigation reveals papilloedema, retinal arteriolar abnormalities, 'cottonwool exudates' consisting of bundles of swollen axons (presumably resulting from ischaemia) and flame shaped haemorrhages localised in the nerve fibre layer of the retina. If therapy is unsuccessful, patients become unresponsive and comatose. The pressure of the CSF is raised and there may be a moderate rise in the CSF protein content. Some patients present evidence of persistent focal neurological lesions, but they do not belong to the basic manifestations of the syndrome. They are considered to be lesions, resulting from vascular damage and are due to either haemorrhage or thrombosis. If antihypertensive therapy is successful, the whole syndrome reverses rapidly with clearing of most manifestations within a day or two except for the focal changes.

The results of neuropathological investigations are of great interest. Apart from changes present in the brain of patients both with and without malignant hypertension, three characteristic abnormalities are observed: (a) fibrinoid necrosis in the walls of intracerebral arterioles and small arteries, sometimes associated with fibrin thrombi occluding the lumina and with extravascular deposits of fibrin, (b) focal or segmental changes in the walls of arterioles and small arteries consisting of fibrous thickening and hyalinisation and sometimes occlusion of the lumina, (c) microinfarcts, obviously associated with the vascular abnormalities described above (49).

As the clinical syndrome is entirely reversible, most authors attribute it to functional disturbances consisting of: (a) vasospasms, (b) segmental dilatation representing areas where muscular contractility of the vessel wall has been surmounted by high intraluminar pressures and (c) cerebral oedema (48). Changes in wall permeability of penetrating arterioles have been demonstrated within 90 seconds after onset of acute blood pressure elevation. For reasons unknown, small arteries and arterioles penetrating into the brain seem to be particularly liable to permeability changes localised at the level of the second and third cortical cell layers (50).

The predilection for changes in small vessels may be explained by the role these vessels have in autoregulation of cerebral blood flow. A rise in blood pressure is immediately followed by an increase in cerebrovascular resistance, localised mainly in the intracerebral small arteries. A breakdown of this auto-regulatory system occurring during hypertensive crises causes segmental dilatation of small vessels at sites where muscular contractility could not withstand intra-arterial blood pressure.

Multi-infarct dementia
The term dementia is used to describe a process of widespread decline of intellectual capacities. Multiple small infarcts ('état lacunaire') may underly dementia in patients with a history of hypertension (51). These infarcts are cavities of a few millimeters in diameter, localised around arterioles penetrating predominantly in the basal ganglia, thalamus, internal capsule, pons and cerebellum, and the semioval centre (52). They are believed to result from occlusion of the arteries supplying the area of the lacunae.

Vessel wall destruction, focal dilatation and deposition of fibrinoid and thrombotic material are observed at the point of occlusion (53). These changes have been ascribed to damage of the vessel wall by high intraluminar pressure (48, 52). Patients experience these recurrent infarctions as a process of steplike deterioration of intellectual and neurological functioning. The neurological changes comprise pseudobulbar palsy and other pyramidal signs, 'marché à petits pas', dysphagia and dysarthria.

Binswanger encephalopathy (subcortical arteriosclerotic encephalopathy (SAE))
Interest in this type of vascular encephalopathy has been recently revived by reports of diagnostically characteristic CT scan appearances (54, 55).

The SAE syndrome may develop in patients with a long history of hypertension or other disorders predisposing to vascular damage, e.g. diabetes mellitus (56-59). At middle age or in early senescence a slowly progressive dementia develops. There is loss of spontaneity, with sluggishness and perseveration. Aphasia, unilateral neglect or other neuropsychological defects are present. Memory loss is frequent but is not always predominant. At the same time, neurological manifestations of motor and sensory dysfunctions become apparent. Some of these may be due to cerebrovascular attacks but more often the neurological defects develop gradually in the course of many weeks or months. Periods of progression alternate with periods of stabilisation, lasting for months or years.

CSF pressure remains normal, the protein content is slightly elevated in some patients. CT scans show diffuse low attenuation in the white matter. Neuropathological investigations reveal diffuse and focal loss of brain tissue with gliosis in the subcortical areas. Other changes are similar to those in multi-infarct dementia. The white matter loss has been attributed to (a) focal ischaemia and (b) blood fluid transudation and oedema. The preferential localisation of the changes in the subcortical regions is unexplained. Some authors are convinced that there is no essential difference between Binswanger encephalopathy and multi-infarct dementia (60).

Transient ischaemic attacks (TIA); prevention of thrombotic stroke
Up to 80% of thrombotic strokes are preceded by transient or minor ischaemic attacks (TIA's), which are strong predictors of stroke and ischaemic heart disease (61, 62). TIA's deserve special attention because they offer an opportunity to prevent a disastrous cerebral lesion. Diagnosis of TIA's is not always easy, as they may be mimicked by many other disorders including focal epilepsy, syncope, Stokes Adams attacks, migraine and vertigo.

The physician usually does not have the opportunity to examine the patient during an attack. TIA's may last a few seconds to several hours, commonly 5 to 10 min. Some patients have many attacks but no strokes; in others a stroke may follow the first TIA within 1 to 7 days.

TIA's may be associated with a stenosis in any of the cerebral or cerebellar arteries. The clinical manifestations of the attack depend on which artery is involved. Attacks caused by stenosis in the carotid system produce contralateral weakness and paraesthesia, and ipsilateral visual disturbances. There may be aphasia when the hemisphere, which is dominant for speech, is involved. The visual disturbances are characterised by unilateral visual transient loss or blurring of the upper or lower half of one visual field (*amaurosis fugax*). Homonymous hemianopia may occur in TIA's either caused by a stenosis of the carotid artery or of the vertebrobasilar arterial systems. TIA's of the vertebrobasilar system are often particularly difficult to recognise. Strongly indicative of the latter are bilateral weakness, numbness or visual loss and alternating hemiparesis or hemisensory syndromes. Multiple TIA's on the basis of a local stenosis usually present a recurrent clinical pattern. This allows differentiation from recurrent cerebral emboli as these will lodge in different sites.

TIA's require immediate examination and treatment. Attacks may be successfully treated by antiplatelet agents or anticoagulants or by surgery or both. Thrombolytic agents have not as yet been proved to be effective. Special attention should be given to the vascular status in general, to cardiac abnormalities and the blood pressure. Multiple non-invasive diagnostic techniques are available for investigation of the carotid and vertebrobasilar systems (63). Most informative for the detection of a haemodynamically significant stenosis are (a) ophthalmodynamometry to measure the retinal artery pressure, (b) oculoplethysmography to determine whether ocular pulsations are delayed in comparison with pulsations of the ear lobe and (c) the Doppler effect to study arterial flow. Less severe stenoses without haemodynamic consequences are demonstrable by intravenous arteriography. Angiography is, of course, the most reliable method of obtaining information on the state of the extracranial and intracranial arteries, but it is an invasive technique and carries some risk. It should be performed only when surgical treatment is considered. In the large majority of patients, angiography will reveal stenosis or arteriosclerotic plaques either in the carotid or in the vertebrobasilar arteries (64). Protracted TIA's are often caused by emboli and frequently the arteries in these patients are patent (65, 66). Surgical management of arterial obstruction is considered justified if the combined risk of operative mortality and major morbidity is lower than 3%. The most effective surgical intervention is endarterectomy if a stenosis of the internal carotid artery in the region of the carotid sinus is present. Stenoses of the common carotid artery, the innominate and subclavian arteries are also suitable for surgery. Less beneficial are operations of stenotic processes at the origin of the vertebral artery.

Cerebral thrombosis and embolism
Although a *thrombotic stroke* may present as a single sudden attack, a gradual or a 'stuttering' progressive course during several hours or days is more common and this course may be diagnostically helpful. Onset or progress occur commonly during sleep or shortly after a-wakening.

The neurological picture is determined by the size and location of the infarct. When infarcts are large, cerebral oedema may develop which may be life-threatening. In these patients anti-oedema therapy is indicated and may be attempted with dexamethasone or with glycerol in doses of 50 g dissolved in 500 ml of 2.5% (427 mmol/l) saline solution given intravenously. Anticoagulants may be tried to arrest further evolution of the thrombotic process. Hypertension does not contra-indicate anticoagulant use if prothrombin activity is maintained at 25% or higher (67).

In *cerebral embolism* the embolic material is derived commonly from a thrombus in the heart or less frequently from a thrombus or an ulcerated atheromatous plaque in a carotid artery. The neurological defect appears suddenly, in a single attack. The brain region most commonly involved is the territory of the middle cerebral artery. A minority of the infarcts are haemorrhagic. The blood may reach the CSF but this is not usually the case. CT scans are helpful in demonstrating haemorrhagic infarcts. Administration of anticoagulants is advisable to prevent successive emboli. This therapy has however, to be delayed for several days if the infarct is haemorrhagic. To rule out this possibility CT scan and CSF investigations are necessary.

Intracerebral haemorrhage and subdural haematoma
The two main causes of nontraumatic intracranial haemorrhage are hypertension and anticoagulant therapy (68). Many dialysis patients have a long history of hypertension and periods of hypertension are not uncommon during maintenance dialysis. Systemic administration of heparin is necessary to carry out extracorporeal circulation and some patients are treated with warfarin or anti-platelet agents. It is clear, therefore, that

cerebral haemorrhage is a risk in patients treated with regular dialysis.

Hypertensive haemorrhages occur within the brain substance by ruptures of small penetrating arteries or arterioles with fibrinoid degeneration and micro-aneurysms. Extravasated blood forms an oval or roughly circular mass displacing and compressing adjacent brain tissue. Large haemorrhages may displace midline structures and vital centres may become compromised. Rupture or leakage through the cortical surface or into the ventricular system are common. The clinical picture is characterised by an abrupt onset and gradual or rapid evolution. CT scans accurately define and localise haemorrhages of 1.5 cm in diameter or larger, at least during the first two to three weeks after the onset of bleeding. During these weeks the X-ray absorption coefficient of the haematoma decreases and a phase will be entered in which the density is equal to that of the surrounding brain substance. If CT scanning is not possible, examination of the CSF is necessary for diagnosis. Usually the CSF will be bloody or xanthochromic. Apart from general medical care and anti-oedema treatment therapeutic possibilities are few. Surgical drainage of large intracerebral supratentorial haematoma is usually considered futile in the acute phase. In acute or subacute cerebellar haemorrhages surgical drainage is the treatment of choice when the haematoma is large (more than 3 cm) and brain stem dysfunction is not yet severe and has lasted 12 hours or less. In general the prognosis is poor in patients with large haemorrhages. When the haematoma is small, restitution of function is often better than in patients with ischaemic infarcts, because the brain tissue is often more displaced than destroyed by the haematoma.

Intracranial haemorrhages occurring during anticoagulant therapy are infrequent. They are usually localised in the subdural space (69-71). Subacute or chronic subdural haematomata may cause pseudodementia, drowsiness, confusion and mild hemiparesis. When the possibility of a haematoma in this location is considered, confirmation of the diagnosis is usually easy. The haematoma or hygroma may be visualised by CT scanning or arteriography. Exceptionally an epidural haematoma causing spinal cord compression with bilateral weakness of the legs and loss of sensibility in the lower limbs may occur in patients on anticoagulant therapy.

Central nervous system infections

Infections are a frequent complication in dialysis patients (see Chapter 33). Among these, intracranial infections are rare but often life threatening (72, 73).

Intracranial infections may develop insidiously and patients may have few clinical symptoms. In patients with unusually severe headaches, meningitis should be considered, signs of meningeal irritation (cervical rigidity and positive Kernig sign) should be sought and the cerebrospinal fluid should be examined. CT scanning is of great value in the diagnosis of brain abscesses. The presence of sources for a direct spread of infection to the meninges, particularly mastoïditis and infection of nasal air sinuses should be ruled out. Uncommon types of infections, such as fungal and cytomegalic virus infections, have been reported in patients treated with immunosuppressive drugs.

Management of epilepsy

Therapeutic management of pre-existent epilepsy has to be guided by routine assessment of anticonvulsant drug treatment (67). Renal failure may influence the response of anti-convulsants by altering the distribution, metabolism and clearance of the drugs. In patients with renal insufficiency the plasma protein binding of acidic drugs is decreased, whilst in basic drugs it is normal or decreased (74). The diminished protein binding is not, or only partly, due to decreased plasma protein concentrations. Several hypotheses have been put forward to explain this change in binding capacity of proteins. Either the binding capacity is inhibited competitively by uraemic toxins, or it is decreased by changes in properties of the proteins. The first hypothesis is the more likely since the impaired protein binding is reversible. It may be caused by organic acids known to be retained in renal insufficiency (75).

So far studies of anti-convulsants in uraemic patients have been limited mainly to phenytoin and valproic acid. It has been demonstrated that steady state total plasma concentrations of these drugs were lower in uraemia than in non-uraemic patients (76, 77). Due to decreased protein binding, however, the free concentrations were relatively high. A further decrease in protein binding of valproic acid was observed during haemodialysis. This is possibly related to the administration of heparin which activates lipoprotein lipase (77). As a result the serum level of non-esterified fatty acids increases and these compounds probably compete for binding sites with valproic acid.

Data presently available support the concept that no change in phenytoin and valproic acid dosages is required to treat epilepsy in uraemic patients. The lower steady state concentrations are compensated by higher free concentrations. Clinical experience is in conformity with this concept (see also Chapter 39).

PERIPHERAL NEUROPATHIES

Uraemic polyneuropathy

Polyneuropathy is one of the principal and most frequent neurological manifestations in chronic uraemia. At one time it was considered to be a potentially crippling disorder of patients on dialysis programmes, but it is now thought to be a calculable risk which can usually be prevented by early initiation of regular dialysis treatment. In a few patients, however, it may still cause serious problems.

Clinical features
Peripheral neuropathy is heralded by symptoms of dysfunction of lower motor neurones (LMN) or of primary

sensory neurones. Whether or not muscle cramps in renal failure patients belong to this category is still debated (78). Muscle cramps are recognised as early manifestations of LMN involvement in motor neurone disease (79) and many other neuropathies. They occur before the neurones have ceased to function, that is before muscle weakness occurs. Patients usually experience the cramps in the evening or late at night. The cramps are enhanced by preceding muscular exertion. Muscle cramps in chronic uraemia occur in a similar fashion.

The restless legs syndrome has been considered by some to be another early symptom of peripheral neuronal dysfunction in uraemic patients (80). In the evening or when in bed, patients experience a sensation of discomfort in the legs and feet and the urge to move the legs and to walk around. The syndrome has usually disappeared when clinical signs of neuropathy become apparent. The restless legs syndrome is, however, not a feature of LMN diseases and is absent in most other peripheral neuropathies. It has been reported in patients with a myoclonus syndrome. It responds favourably to clonazepam (0.5 mg at bedtime) in a similar way as action or intention myoclonus does. It is likely, therefore, that the site of origin is in the CNS (81).

When patients complain of paraesthesia (tingling or prickling) in the toes, feet or fingers, clinical signs of uraemic neuropathy are usually present and may be even severe (82). Burning feet occur only in a minority of patients (82, 83). Pain is absent in the early stages of neuropathy but may be prominent in advanced and severe neuropathy (84). Depressed or abolished ankle reflexes and impaired vibrational perception of the halluces are early and initially the only clinical signs of peripheral neuropathy (85). In a minority of patients neuropathy progresses further, particularly if regular dialysis treatment is unduly delayed. Atrophy and weakness of distal leg muscles may develop, as well as disturbance of all sensory modalities in a stocking-like distribution. Clinical signs of neuropathy in the upper limbs occur only in severe cases, which is in striking contrast to the changes in nerve conduction velocities (see below). As a rule, the peripheral autonomic system is involved concomitantly, but clinical manifestations of autonomic neuropathy remain the background (86). In chronic uraemia increased susceptibility of peripheral nerves to pressure has not been demonstrated. Children with end-stage renal failure usually present no clinical evidence of peripheral neuropathy (87, 88).

Nerve conduction velocity

Electrophysiological investigations of patients with chronic uraemia have demonstrated slowing of conduction in all peripheral nerves studied (89, 90). Slowing occurs to almost the same degree in motor and sensory nerve fibres and in nerves of upper and lower limbs. In uraemic patients without evidence of clinical neuropathy there is also a slight decrease in conduction velocity in comparison with normal controls. In the most severe cases conduction velocities may fall to 60 or 50% of the normal values (83, 91) (see also Chapter 20). According to Nielsen (92) there is no critical degree of slowing of conduction indicating whether clinical signs of neuropathy will appear. Serial measurements of the vibratory perception threshold are more suitable to evaluate the progression or recovery of uraemic neuropathy than nerve conduction studies (84, 93).

Neuropathy and the degree of renal insufficiency

Manifestations of clinical neuropathy are part of the terminal uraemic syndrome. In patients regularly controlled in outpatient departments, signs of neuropathy are generally lacking as long as the creatinine clearance exceeds 6 ml/min (82). Exceptions to this rule occur, however, and in these patients the possibility of a pre-existing neuropathy (induced, for instance, iatrogenically by treatment with nitrofurantoin or hydroxycholine derivatives) should be considered. It is only in a minority of patients that further decrease in renal function is complicated by weakness of distal lower limb muscles and disturbance of cutaneous sensation. In some patients this happens during a period of rapid exacerbation of chronic renal insufficiency. When it is possible to restore renal function to previous levels, the neuropathy persists and may now seem out of proportion to the degree of renal insufficiency (94).

Low protein, high calorie diet

Attempts have been made to prolong the non-dialysis period or the survival time of non-dialysable patients by prescribing low protein high calorie diets containing the minimal required amounts of essential amino-acids. As far as neuropathy is concerned, a satisfactory result was claimed with a diet containing 15 to 20 g of protein and a supplement of essential amino-acids and histidine (95). Patients on these diets have a low plasma urea/creatinine ratio. It is conceivable that the toxin(s) inducing uraemic neuropathy accumulate(s) in the body fluids concomitantly with urea.

The effect of maintenance dialysis

The decision as to when to start regular dialysis depends on a number of factors and is not always easy to make. As far as neuropathy is concerned depressed ankle reflexes and impaired vibrational sense are obviously not sufficient reasons but one should not wait until muscle weakness has developed. The dilemma is not solved by nerve conduction studies. There is no generally accepted degree of slowing that might serve as a criterion. In the late sixties and early seventies facilities for dialysis treatment were often insufficient and it was necessary to keep the patients as long as possible on a non-dialytic treatment regimen. Dialysis was often started during a period of rapid decline of renal function. When the patient had regained reasonable well being it sometimes became apparent that a severe neuropathy had developed. A timely start of regular dialysis prevents this complication. (The reader is also referred to Chapter 20.)

In spite of wide variations in dialysis techniques and schedules, there is general consensus as to the effect of regular dialysis on peripheral neuropathy. Once the first few weeks have elapsed, further worsening of the clinical neuropathy should not occur and stabilisation is the rule (84, 96, 97). The long-term effect (over many

of the ulnar nerve, numbness of the fifth and fourth finger and weakness of small hand muscles.

Severe nerve lesions, obviously due to ischaemia, were reported in patients with bovine graft fistulae in the upper arm between the brachial artery and the cephalic vein (144, 145).

SKELETAL MUSCLE DISEASE

Although loss in volume and power of proximal limb muscle in severe chronic uraemia is frequent, an incapacitating degree of proximal muscular weakness is rare. In general, muscular weakness is reversible by dialysis treatment and adequate food intake. However, a sustained rise in serum creatine kinase activity has been registered in 19% or more patients on maintenance dialysis programmes (146, 147). Histological studies have revealed a high frequency of mild myopathic changes in dialysis patients (148, 149).

Four causes of muscle weakness in patients with chronic renal failure have been reported in the literature.

1. *Muscular weakness may develop during periods of hypercatabolism.* Such weakness is located predominantly in the proximal muscles and other anterior compartment muscles of the lower limbs. The histopathology of this condition is characterised by type II fibre atrophy and is identical to the atrophy observed in cachexia (150).

2. *Muscular weakness which may be caused by secondary hyperparathyroidism.* A causal relationship between hyperparathyroidism and proximal limb muscle weakness is well established (151) and secondary hyperparathyroidism commonly accompanies renal failure. These patients often have bone pain. The muscle weakness is probably of neurogenic origin. There is atrophy of type II and to a lesser degree of type I fibres. In transverse sections the atrophic fibres are elongated in appearance, as in other cases of neurogenic muscular atrophy. The findings in electromyographic examinations are compatible with a neurogenic cause. Serum creatine kinase activity is usually not raised. Data on a possible correlation between proximal limb muscle weakness and the degree of secondary hyperparathyroidism in dialysis patients are not available.

3. *A possible cause of muscular weakness in dialysis patients is carnitine deficiency* (152). A substantial quantity of this small molecule (165 daltons) is lost during dialysis into the dialysate and a fall in plasma levels of 70% during dialysis has been demonstrated (153). The plasma levels are, however, restored within 6 to 8 h (154). Reports on carnitine concentrations in muscle are contradictory: they have been reported to be decreased by one group of authors (152) and found to be similar to those in a control group by other investigators (153). Storage of lipid droplets in type I fibres is considered to be the hallmark of myopathy caused by carnitine deficiency (155). No lipid storage has been found in skeletal muscle biopsies from dialysed patients (148, 149).

4. *A fourth cause of proximal limb muscle weakness is abnormal muscle iron deposition in patients who have inherited the 'haemachromatosis alleles'* (156). Iron overload in these patients is demonstrable by increased serum ferritin levels. The alleles for idiopathic haemachromatosis are linked to the antigens HLA – A3, B7 and B14.

An interesting observation of a completely different nature concerns a complication of the administration of high doses of carnitine to dialysis patients in order to lower hypertriglyceridaemia. Some of these patients developed a myasthenia-like syndrome (157). This effect is exerted by D, L-carnitine but not by L-carnitine. It has been suggested that D-carnitine blocks neuromuscular transmission by means of a hemicholinium-like blocking mechanism (158).

PSYCHOLOGICAL ASPECTS

Neuropsychological considerations

A complete neuropsychological assessment is a prerequisite of accurate evaluation of the impairment of complex mental functioning. In most dialysis patients cognitive efficiency suffers. Using intelligence tests, such as Wechsler's Adult Intelligence Scale, a deterioration of the total intelligence quotient (IQ) is found. This decline is partly due to slowness in performing the tests. In verbal tasks, requiring (over)learned knowledge, patients maintain their original level approximately. Performance IQ, as a measure of the ability to accomplish relatively new tasks under conditions of time pressure with a visuo-spatial component, deteriorates. Memory function is diminished particularly in registration, learning and reproduction of recently acquired data, the 'working memory' being more vulnerable than retrieval from long term memory store ('semantic memory'). A mild disturbance of language function may become manifest in the rather non-specific symptom of word finding difficulty. Written language may suffer from control errors (e.g. anticipations and perseverations). A clear-cut dyscalculia is seldom present. Patients may sometimes, however, lose grip of number structure, as becomes apparent in errors when writing dictated numbers. Gnosis and praxis are usually intact, although minor deviations may occur e.g. left-right mirroring and mild constructional disorders. Although patients are usually capable of sufficient mental tracking during examination, many of them complain of problems in concentration which increase demonstrably during the intervals between dialysis treatments (159). Irritability and restlessness are prominent during the last hours of dialysis, and have to be considered as manifestations of the disequilibrium syndrome (161). The total neuropsychological picture is seen in encephalopathies of different etiologies.

According to Teschan and coworkers (162) the adequacy of the dialysis treatment may be monitored by repeated neuropsychological measurements. Cognition-dependent indices vary directly with the degree of uraemia, choice reaction time and continuous performance tests being sensitive indices.

Psychological stresses and coping mechanisms

Almost invariably, chronic renal failure patients experience a variety of psychological stresses. Fear of death, loss of job satisfaction and sometimes loss or decrease of income, reduction in social status, uncertainty about the future, lack of stamina, changes in body image (dependency on apparatus), changed sexuality, problems in partner relationship and worry about additional medical problems are some of the factors that call for a thorough reappraisal of the patient's situation and of that of his family. Signs of hopelessness, lack of cooperation to treatment, feelings of inferiority are found among young patients without the prospect of kidney transplantation. Death acceptance seems to be somewhat more explicit in older patients, but generally patients in the extreme situation of chronic renal failure show a strong tendency to accept long-term treatment and to cooperate. Continuation of job responsibility appears to be an important factor in adaptation, which is more easily achieved, however, by those in higher educational and occupational groups. According to European figures derived in 1979 from a large dialysis population, only 35-40% of hospital dialysed patients were able to work full-time and actually did so (including return to full time housework). The home dialysis patients show far better rehabilitation figures: 62-68% were able to work and were working full-time (including return to full time house work) (see Table 1) (162).

Surprisingly, home dialysis treatment, although offering the patient not only better rehabilitation but also more freedom and a substantially better quality of life (and in addition is much less costly), is still rather unpopular in many countries (see also Chapter 43).

The practice of overnight dialysis, which was carried out in the early years of chronic dialysis and which has virtually disappeared from the hospital dialysis setting, is undoubtedly one of the factors contributing to the unsatisfactory rehabilitation figures for hospital dialysis patients. Daytime dialysis, thrice weekly, precludes full-time employment. The high unemployment rate in many countries may also influence the figures; finding a job has become increasingly difficult and many patients are forced to stay on sickness allowance, which certainly adds to their psychological discomfort.

Among the methods used by patients in coping with the stresses of dialysis treatment, denial has received much attention (163). Many patients tend to mask unintentionally those aspects of their life, which if perceived, would cause fear. In the psychological adaptation to chronic life-threatening illness this should be viewed as a normal, probably useful, mechanism.

Deaths resulting from non-adherence to the treatment have been reported by hospital staffs to be more than 400 times the incidence of suicide in the general population (164). Exsanguination, auto-intoxication and over-eating/over-drinking are judged to be major methods. Investigations reveal, however, that suicidal tendencies – although perhaps experienced subconsciously – are only seldom voiced. A very sensible approach is offered by the locus of control framework (165). As to control of behaviour, people may vary on a continuum ranging from internal to external positions. Those with an internal locus of control will perceive rewards and punishments as being direct consequences of their own behaviour. At the other end of the continuum are people with a purely external locus of control. They perceive events in their lives as occurring independently of their own actions. In their attempts to re-define their lives haemodialysis patients may adopt an external locus of control. By experiencing their actions and attitudes as of fortuitous importance, they place the sources of reinforcements outside themselves, thus attempting to reduce their part of the responsibility in the treatment programme and thereby alleviating fear.

The locus of control hypothesis implies an alternative view of 'suicidal behaviour' (163). Under external locus of control a discrepancy may develop between expectations of the social environment demanding cooperation and responsibility from the patient, and the patient's

Table 1. Rehabilitation of male and female dialysis patients in Europe, whose potential occupation was full time employment in 1979.

| | Number of patients | % of patients in each rehabilitation category ||||||
		1	2	3	4	5	6
Male							
Hospital dialysis	14, 278	35.7	20.6	13.2	14.5	14.2	1.9
Home dialysis	4, 261	62.1	13.0	8.2	10.0	6.2	0.4
Female							
Hospital dialysis	11, 037	39.6	29.7	7.9	8.1	12.9	2.0
Home dialysis	1, 756	67.5	20.4	4.0	2.9	5.2	0

1 = Able to work and working full time (including return to full time housework)
2 = Able to work and working part time (including return to part time housework)
3 = Able to work but no work available
4 = Able to work but not working: earning capacity less than social security benefits (State pension)
5 = Living at home, able to care for most personal needs (with variable amount of assistance)
6 = Unable to care for self (requires hospital care or equivalent at home)

From: Brynger et al (162), with permission of Pitman Medical, London, UK.

own feelings that his actions have only random effects. Eating enormous amounts of forbidden foods, for example, need not stem from suicidal tendencies but may be explained as an externalisation of the locus of control. Support strategies, such as behaviour modification procedures and psychotherapeutic interventions, should focus on developing a new feeling of responsibility.

It should be stressed, however, that it is not the psychotherapist who plays a central role in supporting the haemodialysis patient, but rather the dialysis staff (166). More flexibility in the arrangement of dialysis stations, more variation in individual and group-centred activities, wellplanned composition of the dialysis groups and regular group-centred support from the psychotherapist and others during the hours of dialysis should be considered (160). Sometimes a family-oriented crisis intervention approach may help the home-dialysis couple to re-adjust (167).

REFERENCES

1. Raskin NH, Fishman RA: Neurological disorders in renal failure (first of two parts). *N Engl J Med* 294:143, 1976
2. Leavitt S, Tyler HR: Studies in asterixis. *Arch Neurol* 10:370, 1964
3. Shahani BT, Young RR: Asterixis – a disorder of the neural mechanisms underlying sustained muscle contraction. In *The Motor System: Neurophysiology and Muscle Mechanisms*, edited by Shahani M, Amsterdam, Elsevier Scientific Publishing Company, 1976, chapter 7, p 301
4. Degos JD, Verroust J, Bouchareine A, Serdaru M, Barbizet J: Asterixis in focal brain lesions. *Arch Neurol* 36:705, 1979
5. Donat JR: Unilateral asterixis due to thalamic haemorrhage. *Neurology* 30:83, 1980
6. Chadwick D, French AT: Uraemic myoclonus: an example of reticular reflex myoclonus. *J Neurol Neurosurg Psychiatry* 42:52, 1979
7. Steinman TI, Yager HM: Catatonia in uremia. *Ann Intern Med* 89:74, 1978
8. Madonick MJ, Berke K, Schiffer I: Pleocytosis and meningeal signs in uremia: report on 62 cases. *Arch Neurol Psychiat* 64:431, 1950
9. Schreiner GE, Maher JF: *Uremia, Biochemistry, Pathogenesis and Treatment*. Springfield Ill, Charles C Thomas, 1961, p 256
10. Tyler HR: Neurologic disorders in renal failure. *Am J Med* 44:734, 1968
11. Jennekens FGI, Dorhout Mees EJ, Van der Most van Spijk D: Clinical aspects of uraemic polyneuropathy. *Nephron* 8:414, 1971
12. Jacob JC, Gloor P, Elwan H: Electroencephalographic changes in chronic renal failure. *Neurology* 15:419, 1965
13. Luyten JAFM, Storm van Leeuwen W, Jennekens FGI: EEG in uraemic patients with neuropathy. *Electroencephalogr Clin Neurophysiol* 28:423, 1970
14. Olsen S: The brain in uremia. *Acta Psychiatr Scand* 36 (Suppl 156):1, 1961
15. Kiley J, Hines O: Electroencephalographic evaluation of uremia, wave frequency evaluation on 40 uremic patients. *Arch Intern Med* 116:67, 1965
16. Kiley JE, Woodruff MW, Pratt KL: Evaluation of encephalopathy by EEG frequency analysis in chronic dialysis patients. *Clin Nephrol* 5:245, 1976
17. Heyman A, Patterson JL Jr, Jones RW Jr: Cerebral circulation and metabolism in uremia. *Circulation* 3:558, 1951
18. Scheinberg P: Effects of uraemia on cerebral blood flow and metabolism. *Neurology* 4:101, 1954
19. Minkoff L, Gaertner G, Darab M, Levin ML: Inhibition of brain sodium-potassium ATPase in uremic rats. *J Lab Clin Med* 80:71, 1972
20. Hicks JM, Young DS, Wootton IDP: The effects of uraemic blood constituents on certain cerebral enzymes. *Clin Chim Acta* 9:228, 1964
21. Cooper JD, Lasarowitz VC, Arieff AI: Neurodiagnostic abnormalities in patients with acute renal failure. Evidence for neurotoxicity of parathyroid hormone. *J Clin Invest* 61:1448, 1978
22. Massry SG, Goldstein DA: The search for uremic toxin(s) 'X'. 'X' = PTH. *Clin Nephrol* 11:181, 1979
23. Alfrey AC, Mishell JM, Burks J, Contiguglia SR, Rudolph H, Lewin E, Holmes JH: Syndrome of dyspraxia and multifocal seizures associated with chronic hemodialysis. *Trans Am Soc Artif Intern Organs* 18:257, 1972
24. Arieff AI, Llach F, Massry SG: Neurological manifestations and morbidity of hyponatremia: correlation with brain water and electrolytes. *Medicine* (Baltimore) 55:121, 1976
25. Fishman RA: Neurological manifestations of hyponatremia. In *Handbook of Clinical Neurology*, vol 28, edited by Vinken PJ and Bruyn GW, Amsterdam, North Holland Publishing Company, 1976, chapter 20, p 495
26. Plum F, Posner JB: *The Diagnosis of Stupor and Coma*. Third edition, Philadelphia PA, FA Davis Company, 1980, p 250
27. Reynolds EH: Neurological aspects of potassium imbalance. In *Handbook of Clinical Neurology*, vol 28, edited by Vinken PJ and Bruyn GW, Amsterdam, North Holland Publishing Company, 1976, chapter 18, p 463
28. Lockman L: Neurological aspects of acid-base metabolism. In *Handbook of Clinical Neurology*, vol 28, edited by Vinken PJ and Bruyn GW, Amsterdam, North Holland Publishing Company, 1976, chapter 21, p 507
29. Tyler HR: Neurological disorders in renal failure. In *Handbook of Clinical Neurology*, vol 27, edited by Vinken PJ and Bruyn GW, Amsterdam, North Holland Publishing Company, 1976, chapter 14, p 321
30. Bradbury M: *The Concept of a Blood-Brain Barrier*. New York, John Wiley and Sons, 1979
31. Davis FA, Schauf CL: Neurological manifestations of calcium imbalance. In *Handbook of Clinical Neurology*, vol 28, edited by Vinken PJ and Bruyn GW, Amsterdam, North Holland Publishing Company, 1976, chapter 22, p 527
32. Frame B: Neuromuscular manifestations of parathyroid disease. In *Handbook of Clinical Neurology*, vol 27, edited by Vinken PJ and Bruyn GW, Amsterdam, North Holland Publishing Company, 1976, chapter 13, p 283
33. Rivera-Vazquez AB, Noriega-Sánchez A, Ramírez-Gonzalez R, Martinez-Maldonado M: Acute hypercalcemia in haemodialysis patients: distinction from 'dialysis dementia'. *Nephron* 25:243, 1980
34. Durlach J: Neurological manifestations of magnesium imbalance. In *Handbook of Clinical Neurology*, vol 28, edited by Vinken PJ and Bruyn GW, Amsterdam, North Holland Publishing Company, 1976, chapter 23, p 545
35. Kennedy AC, Linton AL, Luke RG, Renfrew S, Dinwoodi A: The pathogenesis and prevention of cerebral dysfunction during dialysis. *Lancet* 1:790, 1964
36. Arieff AI, Massry SG, Barrientos A, Kleeman CR: Brain water and electrolyte metabolism in uremia: effects of slow and rapid hemodialysis. *Kidney Int* 4:177, 1973

37. Mann H, Stiller S: Elimination of sodium chloride as the cause of dialysis disequilibrium syndrome. *Kidney Int* 17:401, 1980 (Abstract)
38. Arieff AI, Guisado R, Massry SG, Lazarowitz VC: Central nervous system pH in uremia and the effect of hemodialysis. *J Clin Invest* 58:306, 1976
39. Arieff AI, Lazarowitz VC, Guisado R: Experimental dialysis disequilibrium syndrome: prevention with glycerol. *Kidney Int* 14:270, 1978
40. Faris AA: Wernicke's encephalopathy a complication of chronic hemodialysis. *Arch Neurol* 18:248, 1968
41. Victor M: The Wernicke Korsakoff syndrome. In *Handbook of Clinical Neurology*, vol 28, edited by Vinken PJ and Bruyn GW, Amsterdam, North Holland Publishing Company, 1976, chapter 9, p 243
42. Dukes MNG: *Meyler's Side Effects of Drugs*. Ninth edition, Amsterdam, Excerpta Medica, 1980, p 416
43. Lindner A, Charra B, Sherrard DJ, Scribner BH: Accelerated atherosclerosis and prolonged maintenance hemodialysis. *N Engl J Med* 290:697, 1974
44. Lazarus JM, Lowrie EG, Hampers CL, Merrill JP: Cardiovascular disease in uremic patients on hemodialysis. *Kidney Int* 7 (Suppl 2) S167, 1975
45. Burke JF Jr, Francos GC, Moore LL, Cho SY, Lasker N: Accelerated atherosclerosis in chronic dialysis: another look. *Nephron* 21:181, 1978
46. Rostand SG, Greter JC, Kirk KA, Rutsky EA, Andreoli TE: Ischemic heart disease in patients with uremia undergoing maintenance hemodialysis. *Kidney Int* 16:600, 1979
47. Lundin AP, Friedman EA: Vascular consequences of maintenance hemodialysis. An unproven case. *Nephron* 21:177, 1978
48. Dinsdale HB: Hypertension and the central nervous system. In *Current Neurology*, edited by Tyler HR and Dawson DM, Boston MA, Houghton Mifflin Professional Publishers, 1978, chapter 8, p 196
49. Chester EM, Agamanolis DP, Banker BQ, Victor M: Hypertensive encephalopathy: a clinicopathologic study of 20 cases. *Neurology* 28:928, 1978
50. Nag S, Robertson DM, Dinsdale HB: Cerebral cortical changes in acute experimental hypertension. An ultrastructural study. *Lab Invest* 36:150, 1977
51. Hachinsky VE, Lassen BA, Marshall J: Multi-infarct dementia. A cause of mental deterioration in the elderly. *Lancet* 2:207, 1974
52. Ross Russell RW: How does blood pressure cause stroke? *Lancet* 2:1283, 1975
53. Fisher CM: The arterial lesions underlying lacunes. *Acta Neuropathol* (Berl) 12:1, 1969
54. Rosenberg G, Kornfeld M, Stovring J, Bicknell JM: Subcortical arteriosclerotic encephalopathy (Binswanger): computerized tomography. *Neurology* 29:1102, 1979
55. Junck L, Herrick MK, Langston JW: CT scan in subcortical arteriosclerotic encephalopathy. *Neurology* 30:791, 1980
56. Olszewski J: Subcortical arteriosclerotic encephalopathy. *World Neurology* 3:359, 1962
57. Biemond A: On Binswanger's subcortical arteriosclerotic encephalopathy and the possibility of its clinical recognition. *Psychiatr Neurol Neurosurg* 73:413, 1970
58. Caplan LR, Schoene WC: Clinical features of subcortical arteriosclerotic encephalopathy. *Neurology* 28:1206, 1978
59. Editorial (anonymous): Binswanger's encephalopathy. *Lancet* 1:923, 1981
60. De Reuck J, Crevits L, De Coster W, Sieben G, van der Eecken H: Pathogenesis of Binswanger chronic progressive subcortical encephalopathy. *Neurology* 30:920, 1980
61. Reinmuth OM: Transient ischemic attacks. In *Current Neurology*, vol 1, edited by Tyler HR and Dawson DM, Boston MA, Houghton Mifflin Professional Publishers, 1978, chapter 7, p 166
62. Mohr JP, Fisher CM, Adams RD: Cerebrovascular diseases. In *Harrison's Principles of Internal Medicine*, edited by Isselbacher KJ, Adams RD, Braunwald E, Petersdorf RG, Wilson JD, New York, McGraw Hill Book Company, 9th Edn, 1980, chapter 365, p 1911
63. Leading article (anonymous): Carotid stenosis. *Lancet* 1:535, 1981
64. Toole JF, Yuson CP: Transient ischemic attacks with normal arteriograms. Serious or benign prognosis. *Ann Neurol* 1:100, 1977
65. Pessin MS, Duncan GW, Mohr JP, Poskanzer DC: Clinical and angiographic features of carotid transient ischemic attacks. *N Engl J Med* 296:358, 1977
66. Kostuk WJ, Boughner DR, Barnett HJM, Silver MD: Strokes: a complication of mitral-leaflet prolapse. *Lancet* 2:313, 1977
67. Calne DB: *Therapeutics in Neurology*, Oxford, Blackwell Scientific Publications, 2nd Edn, 1980, p 207
68. Caplan LR: Intracranial hemorrhage. In *Current Neurology*, edited by Tyler HR and Dawson DM, Boston, Houghton Mifflin Professional Publishers, 1979, chapter 12, p 185
69. Snyder M, Renaudin J: Intracranial hemorrhage associated with anticoagulation therapy. *Surg Neurol* 7:31, 1977
70. Bechar M, Lakke JPW, Van der Hem GK, Beks JWF, Penning L: Subdural hematoma during long term hemodialysis. *Arch Neurol* 26:513, 1972
71. Leonard A, Shapiro FL: Subdural hematoma in regularly hemodialyzed patients. *Ann Intern Med* 82:650, 1975
72. Keane WF, Shapiro FL, Ray L: Incidence and type of infections occurring in 445 hemodialysis patients. *Trans Am Soc Artif Intern Organs* 23:41, 1977
73. Nsouli KA, Lazarus JM, Schoenbaum SC, Gottlieb MN, Lowrie EG, Shocair M: Bacteremic infection in hemodialysis. *Arch Intern Med* 139:1255, 1979
74. Reidenberg MM: The binding of drugs to plasma proteins and the interpretation of measurements of plasma concentrations of drugs in patients with poor renal function. *Am J Med* 62:466, 1977
75. Depner T, Gulyassy PF, Stanfel DA, Jarrard EA: Plasma protein binding in uremia: extraction and characterization of an inhibitor. *Kidney Int* 18:86, 1980
76. Reynolds F, Jones NF, Zikoyanis PN, Smith SE: Salivary phenytoin concentrations in epilepsy and in chronic renal failure. *Lancet* 2:384, 1976
77. Bruni J, Wang LH, Marbury TC, Lee CS, Wilder BJ: Protein binding of valproic acid in uremic patients. *Neurology* 30:557, 1980
78. Asbury AK: Uremic neuropathy. In *Peripheral Neuropathy*, edited by Dyck PJ, Thomas PK, Lambert EH, Philadelphia PA, WB Saunders Company, 1975, chapter 48, p 982
79. Mulder DW: Motor neuron disease. In *Peripheral Neuropathy*, edited by Dyck PJ, Thomas PK, Lambert EH, Philadelphia PA, WB Saunders Company, 1975, chapter 38, p 759
80. Callaghan N: Restless legs syndrome in uremic neuropathy. *Neurology* 17:359, 1966
81. Boghen D: Successful treatment of restless legs with clonazepam. *Ann Neurol* 6:341, 1979
82. Jennekens FGI, Dorhout Mees EJ, Van der Most van

Spijk D: Uraemic polyneuropathy. Nephron 8:414, 1971
83. Nielsen VK: The peripheral nerve function in chronic renal failure. I Clinical symptoms and signs. *Acta Med Scand* 190:105, 1971
84. Nielsen VK: The peripheral nerve function in chronic renal failure. VII Longitudinal course during terminal renal failure and regular dialysis. *Acta Med Scand* 195:155, 1974
85. Nielsen VK: The peripheral nerve function in chronic renal failure. An analysis of the vibratory perception threshold. *Acta Med Scand* 191:287, 1972
86. Röckel A, Hennemann H, Sternagel-Haase A, Heidland A: Uraemic sympathetic neuropathy after haemodialysis and transplantation. *Eur J Clin Invest* 9:23, 1979
87. Mentser MI, Clay S, Malekzadeh MH, Pennisi AJ, Ettenger RB, Uittenbogaart CH, Fine RN: Peripheral motor nerve conduction velocities in children undergoing chronic hemodialysis. *Nephron* 22:337, 1978
88. Chan JC, Eng G: Long-Term hemodialysis and nerve conduction in children. *Pediat Res* 13:591, 1979
89. Nielsen VK: The peripheral nerve function in chronic renal failure. V Sensory and motor conduction velocity. *Acta Med Scand* 194:445, 1973
90. Van der Most van Spijk D, Hoogland RA, Dijkstra S: Conduction velocities compared and related to degrees of renal insufficiency. In *New Developments in Electromyography and Clinical Neurophysiology*, vol 28, edited by Desmedt JE, Basel, Karger, 1973, p 381
91. Tyler HR: Neurologic disorders in renal failure. *Am J Med* 44:734, 1968
92. Nielsen VK: The peripheral nerve function in chronic renal failure. VI The relationship between sensory and motor function and kidney function, azotemia, age, sex and clinical neuropathy. *Acta Med Scand* 194:455, 1973
93. Kominami N, Tyler HR, Hampers CL, Merrill JP: Variations in motor nerve conduction velocity in normal and uremic patients. *Arch Intern Med* 128:235, 1971
94. Dinn JJ, Crane DL: Schwann cell dysfunction in uraemia. *J Neurol Neurosurg Psychiatry* 33:605, 1970
95. Bergström J, Lindblom U, Norée LO: Preservation of peripheral nerve function in severe uraemia during treatment with low protein, high calorie diet and surplus of essential aminoacids. *Acta Med Scand* 51:99, 1975
96. Caccia MR, Mangili A, Mecca G, Ubiali E, Zanoni P: Effects of haemodialytic treatment on uremic polyneuropathy. *J Neurol* 217:123, 1977
97. Cadilhac J, Mion C, Duday H, Dapres G, Georgesco M: Motor nerve conduction velocities as an index of the efficiency of maintenance dialysis in patients with end-stage renal failure. In *Peripheral Neuropathies*, edited by Canal N, Pozza G, Amsterdam, Elsevier, North Holland Biomedical Press, 1978, p 211
98. Stanley E, Brown JC, Pryor JS: Altered peripheral nerve function resulting from haemodialysis. *J Neurol Neurosurg Psychiatry* 40:39, 1977
99. Edwards AE, Kopple JD, Kornfeld CM: Vibrotactile threshold in patients undergoing maintenance dialysis. *Arch Int Med* 132:706, 1973
100. Castaigne P, Cathala HP, Beaussart-Boulengé L, Petrover M: Effect of ischaemia on peripheral nerve function in patients with chronic renal failure undergoing dialysis treatment. *J Neurol Neurosurg Psychiatry* 35:631, 1972
101. Lowitzsch K, Göhring U, Hecking E, Köhler H: Refractory period, sensory conduction velocity and visual evoked potentials before and after haemodialysis. *J Neurol Neurosurg Psychiatry* 44:121, 1981
102. Dyck PJ, Johnson WJ, Lambert EH, O'Brien PC, Daube JR, Ovratt KF: Comparison of symptoms, chemistry and nerve function to assess adequacy of hemodialysis. *Neurology* 29:1361, 1979
103. Nielsen VK: The peripheral nerve function in chronic renal failure. A survey. *Acta Med Scand* Suppl 573:8, 1975
104. Ibraham MM, Crosland JM, Honigsberger L, Barnes AD, Dawson-Edwards P, Newman CE, Robinson BHB: Effect of renal transplantation on uraemic neuropathy. *Lancet* 2:739, 1974
105. Nielsen VK: The peripheral nerve function in chronic renal failure. IX Recovery after transplantation. Electrophysiological aspects (sensory and motor nerve conduction). *Acta Med Scand* 195:171, 1974
106. Oh SJ, Clements RS, Lee YW, Diethelm AG: Rapid improvement in nerve conduction velocity following renal transplantation. *Ann Neurol* 4:369, 1978
107. Nielsen VK: The peripheral nerve function in chronic renal failure. VII Recovery after renal transplantation. Clinical aspects. *Acta Med Scand* 195:163, 1974
108. Bolton CF: Electrophysiologic changes in uremic neuropathy after successful renal transplantation. *Neurology* 26:152, 1976
109. Asbury AK, Victor M, Adams RD: Uremic polyneuropathy. *Arch Neurol* 8:413, 1963
110. Forno L, Alston W: Uremic polyneuropathy. *Acta Neurol Scand* 43:640, 1967
111. Jennekens FGI, Dorhout Mees EJ, Van der Most van Spijk D: Nerve fibre degeneration in uraemic polyneuropathy. *Proc Eur Dial Transpl Ass* 6:191, 1969
112. Thomas PK, Hollinrake K, Lascelles RG, O'Sullivan DJ, Baillod RA, Moorhead JF, Mackenzie JC: The polyneuropathy of chronic renal failure. *Brain* 94:761, 1971
113. Dayan AD, Gardner-Thorpe C, Down PF, Gleadle RI: Peripheral neuropathy in uremia. *Neurology* 20:649, 1970
114. Dyck PJ, Johnson WJ, Lambert EH, O'Brien PC: Segmental demyelination secondary to axonal degeneration in uremic neuropathy. *Mayo Clin Proc* 46:400, 1971
115. Hansen S, Ballantyne JP: A quantitative electrophysiological study of uraemic neuropathy. *J Neurol Neurosurg Psychiatry* 41:128, 1978
116. Pekelharing CA, Winkler C: Mittheilung über die Beriberi (Communication on beriberi). *Dtsch Med Wochenschr* 13:845, 1887 (in German)
117. Babb AL, Popovich RP, Christopher TG, Scribner BH: The genesis of the square meter-hour hypothesis. *Trans Am Soc Artif Intern Organs* 17:81, 1971
118. Tenckhoff H, Shilipetar G, Boen ST: One year's experience with home peritoneal dialysis. *Trans Am Soc Artif Intern Organs* 11:11, 1968
119. Raskin NH, Fishman RA: Neurologic disorders in renal failure (Second of two parts). *N Engl J Med* 294:204, 1976
120. Merrill JP: The search for 'factor X'. *Clin Nephrol* 11:56, 1979
121. Baker LRI, Marshall RD: A reinvestigation of methylguanidine concentration in sera from normal and uraemic subjects. *Clin Sci* 41:563, 1971
122. Blumberg A, Esslen E, Bürgi W: Myoinositol – a uremic neurotoxin. *Nephron* 21:186, 1978
123. Sterzel RB, Semar M, Lonergan ET, Treser G, Lange K: Relationship of nervous tissue transketolase to the neuropathy in chronic uremia. *J Clin Invest* 50:2295, 1971
124. Kopple JD, Dirige OV, Jacob M, Wang M, Swenseid ME: Transketolase activity in red blood cells in chronic uremia. *Trans Am Soc Artif Intern Organs* 18:250, 1972
125. Dobbelstein H, Körner WF, Mempel W, Grosse-Wilde H,

Edel HH: Vitamin B6 deficiency in uraemia and its implication for the depression of immune responses. *Kidney Int* 5:233, 1974
126. Nielsen VK: Pathophysiological aspects of uraemic neuropathy. In *Peripheral Neuropathies*, edited by Canal N, Pozza G, Amsterdam, Elsevier/North Holland Biomedical Press, 1978, p 197
127. Goldstein DA, Chui LA, Massry SG: Effects of parathyroid hormone and uremia on peripheral nerve calcium and motor nerve conduction velocity. *J Clin Invest* 62:88, 1978
128. Avram MM, Iancu M, Morrow P, Feinfeld D, Huatuco A: Uremic syndrome in man: new evidence for parathormone as a multisystem neurotoxin. *Clin Nephrol* 11:59, 1979
129. Van Lis JMJ, Jennekens FGI, Veldman H: Calcium deposits in the perineurium and their relation to lipid accumulation. *J Neurol Sci* 43:367, 1979
130. Schaefer K, Offermann K, Von Herrath D, Schröter R, Stölzel R, Arntz HR: Failure to show a correlation between serum parathyroid hormone, nerve conduction velocity and serum lipids in hemodialysis patients. *Clin Nephrol* 14:81, 1980
131. Druecke T, Chkoff N, DiGiulo S, Zingraff J, Delons S, Man NK, Jungers P, Crosnier J: Absence of increased motor nerve conduction velocity after para-thyroidectomy in dialysis patients. *Kidney Int* 15:449, 1979 (abstract)
132. Venables GS, Cartlidge NEF: Brisk reflexes in the limbs of patients with arteriovenous fistulae. *Lancet* 1:143, 1981
133. Warren DJ, Otieno LS: Carpal tunnel syndrome in patients on intermittent haemodialysis. *Postgrad Med J* 51:450, 1975
134. Kumar S, Trivedi HL, Smith EKM: Carpal tunnel syndrome: a complication of arteriovenous fistula in hemodialysis patients. *Can Med Assoc J* 113:1070, 1975
135. Lindstedt E, Westling H: Effects of an antebrachial Cimino-Brescia arteriovenous fistula on the local circulation in the hand. *Scand J Urol Nephrol* 9:119, 1975
136. Bussell JA, Abbott JA, Lim RC: A radial steal syndrome with arteriovenous fistula for hemodialysis. *Ann Int Med* 75:387, 1971
137. Mancusi-Ungaro A, Cortes JJ, Spaltaro FD: Median carpal tunnel syndrome following a vascular shunt procedure in the forearm. *Plast Reconstr Surg* 57:96, 1976
138. Holtmann B, Anderson CB: Carpal tunnel syndrome following vascular shunts for haemodialysis. *Arch Surg* 112:65, 1977
139. Bosanac PR, Bilder B, Grunberg RW, Banach SF, Kintzel JE, Stephens HW: Post-permanent access neuropathy. *Trans Am Soc Artif Intern Organs* 23:162, 1977
140. Harding AE, LeFanu J: Carpal tunnel syndrome related to antebrachial Cimino-Brescia fistula. *J Neurol Neurosurg Psychiatry* 40:511, 1977
141. Hamilton DV, Evans DB, Henderson RG: Ulnar nerve lesion as complication of Cimino-Brescia arteriovenous fistula. *Lancet* 2:1137, 1980
142. Ahmad R, Raichura N: Ulnar nerve lesion as a complication of Cimino-Brescia arteriovenous fistula. *Lancet* 2:1381, 1980
143. Bailey RR, Lynn KL: Arteriovenous shunts and nerve damage. *Lancet* 1:211, 1981
144. Bolton CF, Driedger AA, Lindsay RM: Ischaemic neuropathy in uraemic patients caused by bovine arteriovenous shunt. *J Neurol Neurosurg Psychiatry* 42:810, 1979
145. Adams JP: Arteriovenous shunts and nerve damage. *Lancet* 1:211, 1981
146. Cohen IM, Griffiths J, Stone RA, Leach T: The creatine kinase profile of a maintenance hemodialysis population: a possible marker of uremic myopathy. *Clin Nephrol* 13:235, 1980
147. Galen RS: Creatine kinase isoenzyme BB in serum of renal disease patients. *Clin Chem* 22:120, 1976
148. Ahonen RE: Light microscopic study of striated muscle in uremia. *Acta Neuropathol* (Berl) 49:51, 1980
149. Ahonen RE: Striated muscle ultrastructure in uremic patients and in renal transplant recipients. *Acta Neuropathol* (Berl) 50:163, 1980
150. Jennekens FGI: Disuse, cachexia and ageing. In *Skeletal Muscle Pathology*, edited by Mastaglia FL and Walton Sir John, Edinburgh, London, New York, Churchill-Livingstone, Chapter 22, p 605
151. Bethlem J: *Myopathies*, 2nd Edn, Amsterdam, Elsevier/North Holland 1980, p 269
152. Böhmer T, Bergrem H, Eiklid K: Carnitine deficiency induced during intermittent haemodialysis for renal failure. *Lancet* 1:126, 1978
153. Mingardi G, Bizzi A, Cini M, Licini R, Mecca G, Garattini S: Carnitine balance in hemodialyzed patients. *Clin Nephrol* 13:269, 1980
154. Bizzi A, Cini M, Garattini S, Mingardi G, Licini R, Mecca G: L-carnitine addition to haemodialysis liquid prevents plasma carnitine deficiency during dialysis. *Lancet* 1:882, 1979
155. DiMauro S, Trevisan C, Hays A: Disorders of lipid metabolism in muscle. *Muscle Nerve* 3:369, 1980
156. Bregman H, Gelfand MC, Winchester JF, Manz HJ, Knepshield JH, Schreiner GE: Iron-overload-associated myopathy in patients on maintenance haemodialysis: a histocompatibility-linked disorder. *Lancet* 2:882, 1980
157. Bazzato G, Mezzina C, Ciman M, Guarnieri G: Myasthenia-like syndrome associated with carnitine in patients on long-term haemodialysis. *Lancet* 1:1041, 1979
158. Bazzato G, Coli U, Landini S, Mezzina C, Ciman M: Myasthenia-like syndrome after D, L- but not L-carnitine. *Lancet* 1:1209, 1981
159. West TPJ: A comparison of predialysis and postdialysis cognitive abilities. *Dial Transpl* 7:809, 1978
160. Van den Broek GPLA: *Een Prospectief Onderzoek naar de Mate van Angstloochening en de Invloed van Begeleiding bij Kunstnierpatiënten.* (Prospective Study of the Degree of Denial of Fear in Haemodialysis Patients. The Significance of Supportive Talks). M.D. thesis, University of Rotterdam, The Netherlands, 1980, p 116 (in Dutch)
161. Teschan PE, Ginn HE, Bourne JR, Ward JW: Neurobehavioral probes for adequacy of dialysis. *Trans Am Soc Artif Intern Organs* 23:556, 1977
162. Brynger H, Brunner FP, Chantler C, Donckerwolcke RA, Jacobs C, Kramer P, Selwood NH, Wing AJ: Combined report on regular dialysis and transplantation in Europe, X, 1979. *Proc Eur Dial Transpl Ass* 17:4, 1980
163. Goldstein AM, Reznikoff M: Suicide in chronic hemodialysis patients from an external locus of control framework. *Am J Psychiatry* 127:1204, 1971
164. Abram HS, Moore GL, Westervelt FB: Suicidal behavior in chronic dialysis patients. *Am J Psychiatry* 127:1199, 1971
165. Rotter JB: Generalized expectancies for internal vs external control of reinforcement. *Psychol Monograph* 80:1, 1966
166. Kaplan De-Nour A: Medical staff's attitudes and patients' rehabilitation. *Proc Eur Dial Transpl Assoc* 17:520, 1980
167. Levenbrug SB, Jenkins C, Wendorf DJ: Studies in family-oriented crisis intervention with hemodialysis patients. *Int J Psychiatry Med* 9:83, 1978

38
OPHTHALMOLOGICAL COMPLICATIONS ASSOCIATED WITH HAEMODIALYSIS

BETTINE C.P. POLAK

Visual complaints	742	Posterior segment	744
Anterior segment	743	Vascular changes	744
Conjunctival and corneal calcifications	743	Therapy-induced infections	746
Conjunctival haemorrhages	744	Fluorescence angiography	747
Lens opacities	744	Ocular changes in transplant patients	747
Intraocular pressure	744	References	748

VISUAL COMPLAINTS

Visual complaints are frequent, especially at the onset of chronic haemodialysis treatment. Many patients experience visual disturbances or headache, which are usually not due to a disequilibrium syndrome, causing a relative increase of intraocular pressure. In some patients these complaints do not disappear, returning during each individual dialysis session.

Lesions of the anterior segment such as limbal calcifications or limbal haemorrhages are generally asymptomatic. In the case of 'red eyes of renal failure' the patient may experience some itching of the irritated eyes due to deposition of calcium crystals in the superficial

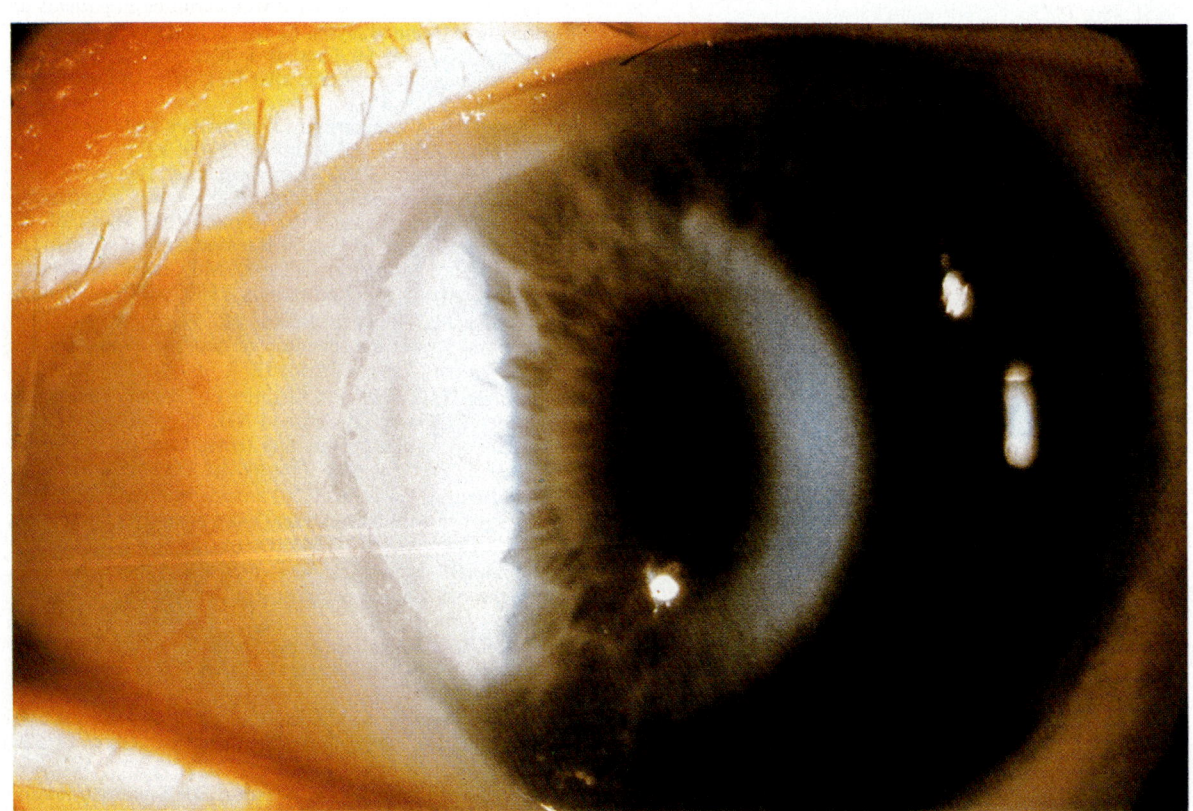

Figure 1. Slit-lamp picture of grade 3 calcification.

layers of the conjunctiva often in combination with an inadequate tear film. Lens opacities are uncommon in dialysis patients, and usually do not cause visual complaints. Retinal vascular accidents may occur in dialysis patients causing disturbances of visual acuity.

Visual complaints may be caused by therapy-induced eye infections, e.g. cytomegaloviral retinitis, but these infections are more frequent in transplanted patients due to immunosuppressive treatment.

ANTERIOR SEGMENT

Conjunctival and corneal calcifications

Corneal and conjunctival deposition of calcium salts, a frequent complication of chronic renal failure, usually occurs in the limbal area exposed by the interpalpebral fissure. This is thought to be due to the relatively high alkalinity, resulting from the diffusion of CO_2 from the exposed eye surface, which promotes the deposition of calcium salts if the $Ca \times PO_4$ product is elevated, especially in the presence of hyperphosphataemia. The latter is generally thought to be the main pathogenic factor involved in ocular calcification.

Ocular calcifications are usually asymptomatic although conjunctival irritation due to crystal deposition in the most superficial layers of the conjunctiva, better known as 'red eyes of renal failure' may occur. It seems probable that such conjunctival deposits in combination with an inadequate tear film are responsible for this phenomenon (1). Improvement has been noted after reduction of the $Ca \times PO_4$ product (2). Corneal calcification, however, usually does not regress after reduction of this product, whether achieved by diet and phosphate-binding antacids or adequate dialysis or both (3). Regression of corneal calcification may be observed when the $Ca \times PO_4$ product is reduced after parathyroidectomy and after kidney transplantation (4, 5).

Conjunctival and corneal calcifications can be evaluated by slit-lamp biomicroscopy and handlight examination, and are expressed in three grades of intensity:

Grade 0 No deposits
Grade 1 Conjunctival deposits, only visible with the slit-lamp
Grade 2 Conjunctival and strictly limbal deposits, visible with a hand light and the naked eye
Grade 3 Extensive conjunctival and corneal deposits, easily visible with diffuse illumination and the naked eye

Grade 3 calcification generally appears as white, coarse, superficial subepithelial deposits in the interpalpebral limbal region, both on the nasal and temporal sides.

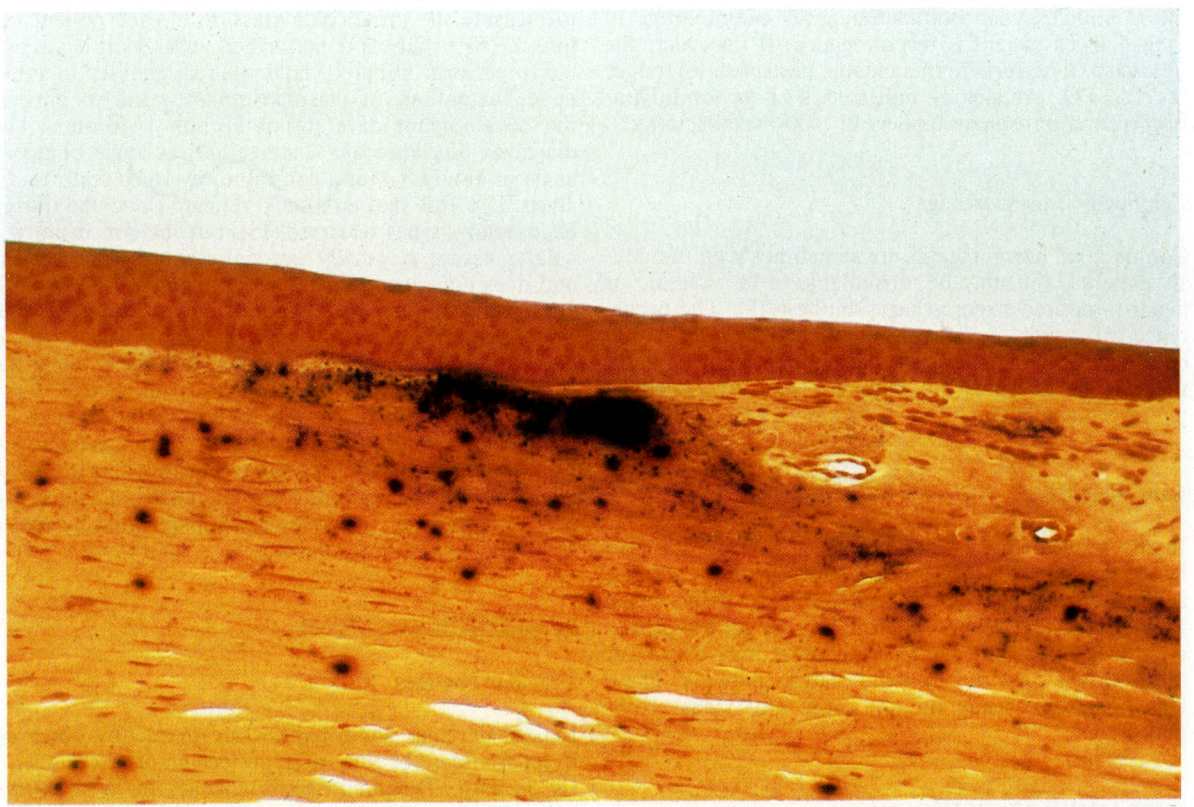

Figure 2. Histological section of the limbal area of the right eye of a 54 year-old patient with grade 3 calcification, deceased after 6 years of haemodialysis. Calcium deposits (black) in the limbal area are mainly located subepithelially, but also in the basal epithelial cells. Von Kossa's stain. Magnification 50×.

This extensive calcification can be distinguished from Vogt's limbus girdle as the calcification markedly extends into the cornea and conjunctiva (Figure 1). Histopathologically these deposits are seen in the limbal region, mainly subepithelial and to a lesser extent in the basal epithelial layers. Light microscopy shows deposition of Von Kossa positive material, indicating calcium-phosphate deposits (Figure 2).

Grade 2 calcification, however, cannot accurately be distinguished from Vogt's limbus girdle, since the absence of a clear cornea may occur in both conditions (6).

The incidence of pingueculae, histologically characterised by degeneration of elastic fibres, is significantly higher in dialysis patients than in healthy subjects (4). The high incidence of degenerative ocular lesions in the dialysed patients suggests that such lesions which are known to predispose to calcification, may promote calcification if the $Ca \times PO_4$ product is elevated. This suggests that both metastatic calcification as well as dystrophic factors contribute to the calciferous ocular lesions in dialysis patients.

Furthermore, ocular calcification correlates significantly with the duration of haemodialysis treatment and the patients' age (4).

Because conjunctival and corneal calcifications can be detected prior to calcifications elsewhere in the body and the presence of calcium deposits gives useful clinical information regular ophthalmological examination of each dialysis patient is recommended. It may alert the physician that certain therapeutic measures to reduce the $Ca \times PO_4$ product are indicated, such as administration of oral phosphate binders or parathyroidectomy.

Conjunctival haemorrhages

Conjunctival haemorrhages are sometimes seen in dialysis patients, and may be attributable to an uraemic or heparin-induced haemorrhagic diathesis (7). The occurrence of small limbal bleedings may indicate that changes in the technique of dialysis treatment or other therapeutic measures are required; they may also be merely coincidental.

Lens opacities

In dialysis patients only a few cases of lens opacities have been reported (8, 9). The development of cataracts has been attributed to hypocalcaemia in some cases. Previous long term corticosteroid therapy for the primary kidney disease or for graft rejection may also have induced lens opacities in some dialysis patients. These lens opacities usually do not cause any visual complaints.

INTRAOCULAR PRESSURE

Patients undergoing haemodialysis sometimes complain of headache, nausea and fatigue, developing a few hours after haemodialysis has begun and disappearing some time after haemodialysis is terminated. Sometimes these complaints develop in combination with a rise of intraocular pressure, associated with a simultaneous increase of cerebrospinal fluid pressure. Changes in intraocular pressure, however, develop during each haemodialysis as a consequence of a disequilibrium between aqueous and plasma. The rise of intraocular pressure has been attributed to a delayed clearance of urea from the aqueous as compared to rapid initial clearance from the blood (10). The blood-aqueous barrier acts as a semipermeable membrane, which explains the delayed removal of urea from the aqueous and the increase of intraocular pressure which rises concomitantly with the decrease of blood urea (11). The cerebrospinal fluid pressure rises concomitantly with the increase of intraocular pressure during haemodialysis. This is induced by a similar phenomenon caused by an increase of the blood-cerebrospinal fluid osmolar gradient. When the excess of urea from the aqueous diffuses into the plasma the intraocular pressure returns to normal. The urea-induced change in osmolarity can be counteracted by addition of dextrose to the dialysate (12). A gradual decrease of intraocular pressure could be demonstrated in patients who underwent dehydration by means of forced ultrafiltration without dialysis (4).

Because of the inevitable osmotically induced rise of intraocular pressure during each dialysis it is imperative to measure the intraocular pressure in each patient before the first dialysis is performed, whereas it is advisable to perform initially frequent short dialyses to avoid large fluctuations of plasmaosmolarity and to prevent the development of a disequilibrium syndrome. The diagnosis of glaucoma, whether narrow-angle or open-angle in nature, is not a contraindication to perform dialysis. It is true that an attack of acute glaucoma during haemodialysis has occurred (13), but the rise in intraocular pressure is usually not noticeable by the patient and does not cause subjective complaints. In cases with an antecedent increase of intraocular pressure or when glaucoma has occurred in relatives, short dialysis has to be carried out at least three times each week, while the increase of intraocular pressure can be mitigated by the addition of dextrose to the dialysis solution and by forced ultrafiltration. If a patient still develops an attack of glaucoma during dialysis treatment despite these measures, symptomatic therapy by means of miotic eye drops is indicated, if necessary, supplemented by use of a carbonic-anhydrase inhibitor.

POSTERIOR SEGMENT

Vascular changes

Retinal vascular abnormalities are frequently observed in renal disease because of hypertension or arteriosclerosis or both. The funduscopic changes in hypertensive and sclerotic retinopathy in association with renal disease have been evaluated by Scheie (14). Retinal vascular accidents, papilloedema, star-shaped macular oedema and spontaneous retinal haemorrhages may all occur

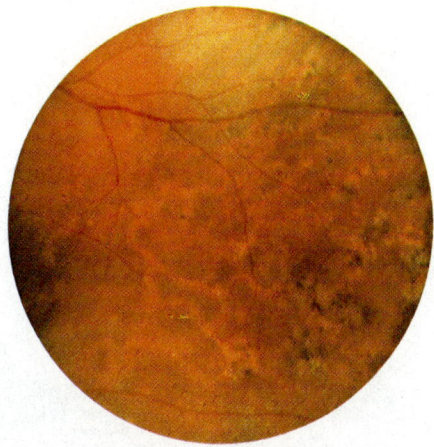

Figure 3. Funduscopic aspect of choroidal arteriosclerosis with yellow discolouration of choroidal vessels and small areas of pigment. Epithelial atrophy.

of arteriosclerosis of retinal and choroidal vessels, however, persist, sclerosis of the choroidal vessels being more pronounced (Figure 3).

Pigmentary disintegration of pigment epithelium and choroid may be secondary to metabolic disturbances due to insufficient circulation in the choroid, but differentiation between such lesions and cicatricial lesions of viral origin may be difficult. At histopathological examination the retinal arterioles show slight sclerosis, which is mostly confined to thickening of the media of the vessel walls (Figure 4). The choroidal arterial vessel walls, however, are found to be more sclerotic and thickened than the retinal vessel walls, and show mostly hyalinisation of the intima and occasional ruptures in the internal elastic membrane (Figure 5).

During regular dialysis treatment deterioration of diabetic retinopathy may occur, which has been attributed to iatrogenic (heparin-induced) haemorrhagic diathesis (15). To reduce the incidence of progressive visual impairment in diabetic patients with terminal renal failure early renal transplantation should be considered, since stabilisation of the diabetic retinopathy and visual acuity is seen after transplantation. Alternatively regular peritoneal dialysis which obviates the use of heparin is preferred by many clinicians instead of regular haemodialysis.

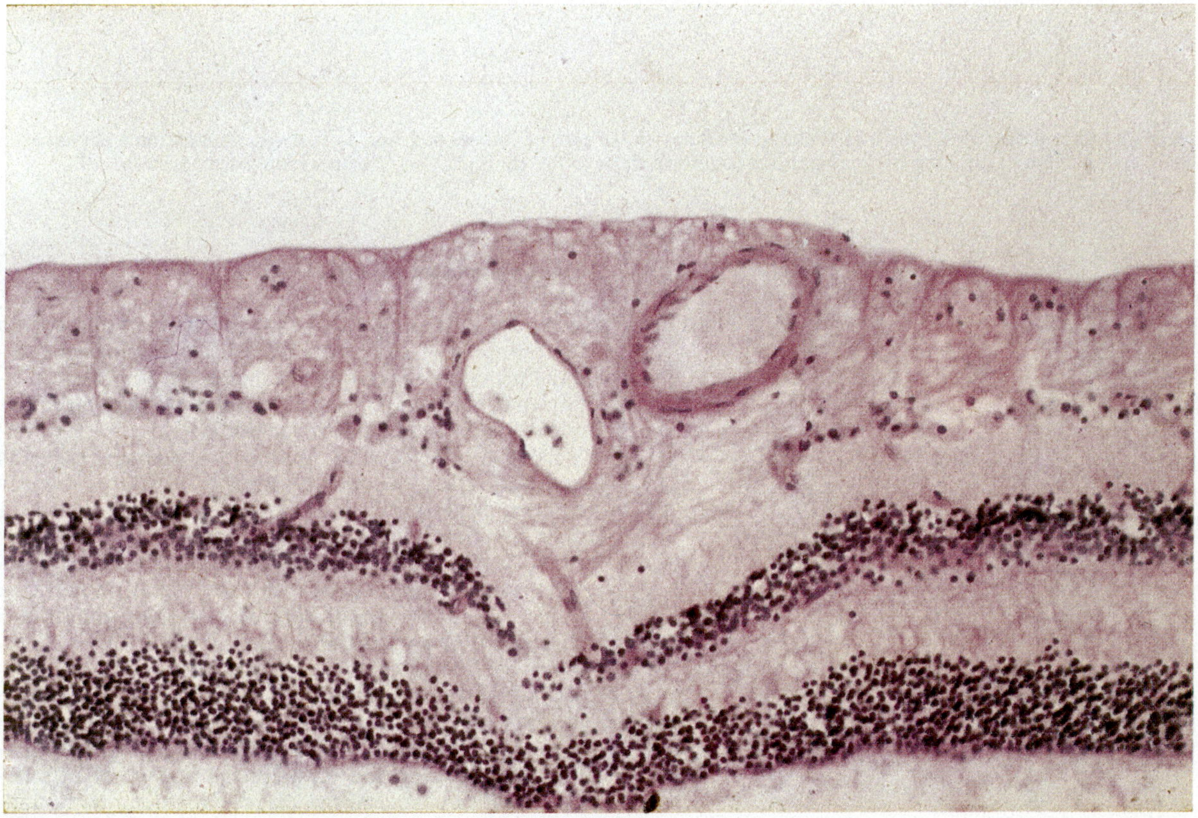

in dialysis patients. Signs of hypertensive vasculopathy may gradually decrease or even disappear if hypertension is controlled. Therefore funduscopy at regular intervals may offer important clinical information. The signs

Figure 4. Retinal arteriosclerosis in a 54 year-old woman, deceased after 6 years of haemodialysis same as in figure 2). Slight sclerosis of the retinal arterioles, mostly confined to thickening of the media of the vessel walls. H & E stain. Magnification 115×.

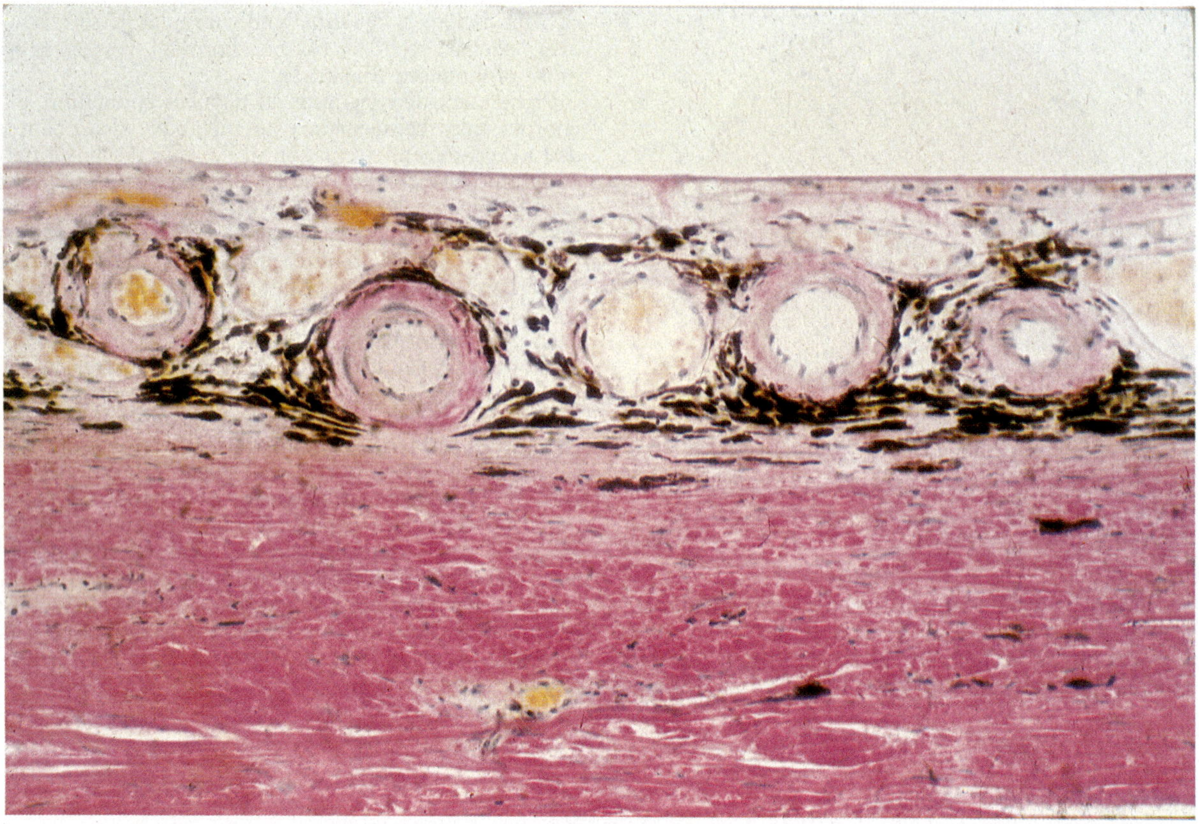

Figure 5. Choroidal arteriosclerosis, as observed at autopsy in all eyes of dialysis patients; 54 year-old woman (same patient as in figure 2 and figure 4). Striking thickening of the arteriolar walls of the choroid. Von Gieson's stain. Magnification 115×.

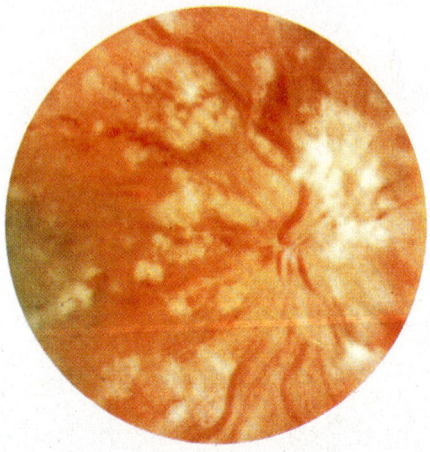

Figure 6. Presumably acute cytomegalic retinitis with the appearance of a retinal vascular accident. Hyperaemic optic disc, dilated veins, cotton-wool exudates and haemorrhages in the right eye of a 32-year old woman.

Therapy-induced infections

With the increasing numbers of haemodialysis patients the numbers of patients with positive serological reactions for cytomegalovirus has increased (16). This infection may occur in dialysis patients, but occurs more frequently after kidney transplantation.

Early cytomegaloviral retinitis lesions appear either as scattered areas of retinal necrosis or white granular patches, while the retinal vessels in the involved area may be sheathed and retinal haemorrhages may occur (17). The ophthalmoscopic appearance of cytomegalic retinitis is not specific and may be attributed to a retinal vascular accident because of similar appearance (Figure 6), or to vasculitis, giant cell ariitis or neoplasm (4). In the presence of funduscopic findings suggesting a necrotising retinitis, the diagnosis cytomegalic retinitis may be considered if the results of laboratory tests are positive. Only when histopathological examination demonstrates the intraretinal presence of cytomegalic inclusion bodies, the diagnosis is definitely established (Figure 7). There is no effective treatment for cytomegalic retinitis. Gammaglobulin and cytosine arabinoside have been used without effect, whereas the effect of high doses of steroids is debatable (18).

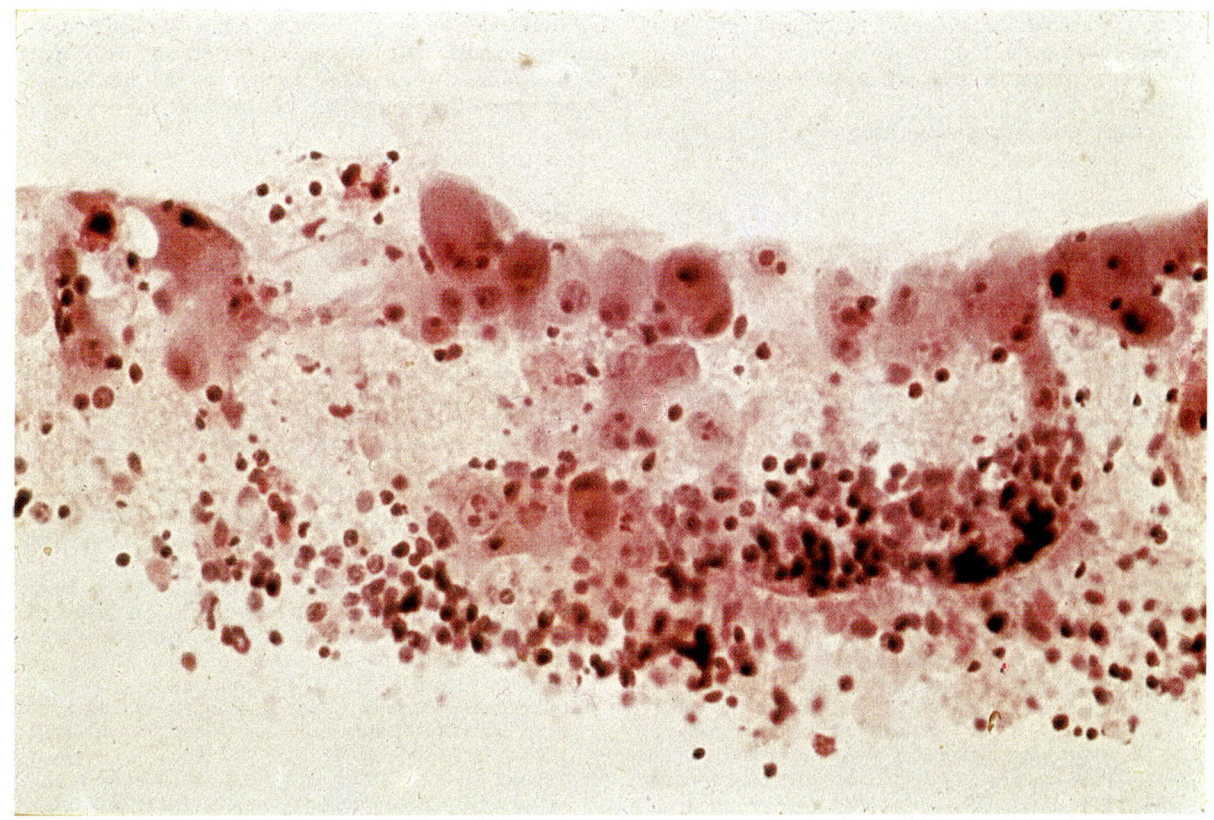

Figure 7. Cytomegaloviral inclusion bodies chorioretinitis. Circumscribed inflammation in equatorial retina and choroid in a 40-year old man. Large basophilic, partly multinucleated cells with inclusion bodies in nuclei and cytoplasm. Lymphocytic infiltration. Destruction of the retinal tissue. H & E stain. Magnification 93×.

Fluorescence angiography

The use of fluorescein in patients with terminal renal failure is not contraindicated because the dye (being water-soluble and having a small molecular mass [376 daltons]) is easily dialysable. Since fluorescence is maximal at normal blood pH and decreases when acidosis is present, the conditions for fluorescence are not optimal in patients with metabolic acidosis. Fluorescence, however, increases in anaemia, because haemoglobin absorbs fluorescein. Therefore, in dialysis patients, who are usually anaemic, the fluorographic pictures will show satisfactory contrast.

The remarkable fact that the choroidal sclerotic changes in dialysis patient dominate those of the retina is confirmed by fluorographic findings. In contrast to the normal fluorogram, where the choroidal filling precedes the retinal filling by 0.5 to 1.0 second, the choroidal and retinal filling occur simultaneously and sometimes the arterial filling even precedes the appearance of the choroidal fluorescence. The sclerotic thickening of the choroidal vessel walls and the subsequent narrowing of the lumen causes an increased flow resistance, retarding the flow through the choroidal vasculature, indicative of a choroidal perfusion disturbance in patients with renal function replacement therapy.

OCULAR CHANGES IN TRANSPLANT PATIENTS

Because the graft function and the normalisation of the $Ca \times PO_4$ product determine whether and when regression of corneal and conjunctival calcification occurs, regular slit-lamp examination may present clinical important information. The limbal calcifications usually do not change during the first post-transplant year.

Whereas lens opacities are uncommon during dialysis treatment, irreversible corticosteroid-induced posterior subcapsular cataracts are found in a high percentage of patients after renal transplantation. Glaucomatous visual-field defects may develop without subjective complaints, when blood pressure is reduced to normal. Regular control of the intraocular pressure is therefore also necessary after transplantation. Corticosteroid-induced ocular hypertension responds well to antiglaucomatous therapy.

Hypertensive vascular changes usually improve after

successful transplantation, but deterioration may occur if hypertension persists or recurs.

Infections are more frequent in immunosuppressed, transplanted patients.

Thorough funduscopy should be performed during febrile episodes or with the occurrence of visual complaints in transplanted patients to detect any early signs of infections. If present the findings of the ophthalmologist may offer important information to the clinician.

REFERENCES

1. Porter R, Crombie AL: Corneal and conjunctival calcification in chronic renal failure. *Br J Ophthalmol* 57:339, 1973
2. Berlyne GM, Shaw AB: Red eyes in renal failure. *Lancet* 1:4, 1967
3. Parfitt AM: Soft-tissue calcification in uremia. *Arch Intern Med* 124:544, 1969
4. Polak BCP: *Ophthalmological complications of haemodialysis and kidney transplantation.* MD Thesis, University of Leiden, the Netherlands. The Hague, Dr W Junk BV, 1980
5. Ehlers N, Kruse Hansen F, Hansen HE, Jensen OA: Corneo-conjunctival changes in uremia. Influence of renal allotransplantation. *Acta Ophthalmol* 50:83, 1972
6. Sugar HS, Kobernick S: The white limbus girdle of Vogt. *Am J Ophthalmol* 72:861, 1971
7. Pambor R, Pap I: Netzhautveränderungen unter der Hämodialyse (Retinal alterations during haemodialysis treatment). *Folia Ophthalmol* 2:114, 1977 (in German)
8. Junceda Avello J: Catarata estelar reversible (complicación de la dialisis extra-corporea) (Reversible stellate cataract complicating extracorporeal dialysis). *Arch Soc Oftalmol Hisp-Amer* 23:817, 1963 (in Spanish)
9. Koch HR, Siedek M, Wiekenmeier P, Metzler U: Katarakt bei intermittierender Hämodialyse (Cataract associated with intermittent haemodialysis). *Klin Monatsbl Augenheilkd* 168:346, 1976 (in German)
10. Gardner Watson A, Greenwood WR: Studies on the intraocular pressure during hemodialysis. *Can J Ophthalmol* 1:4, 1966
11. Galin MA, Davidson R, Pasmanik S: An osmotic comparison of urea and mannitol. *Am J Ophthal* 55:244, 1963
12. Pambor R, Lachlein L, Dahse P: Das Verhalten des intraokularen Druckes unter der Hämodialyse (The course of intraocular pressure during haemodialysis). *Folia Ophthalmol* 1:39, 1976 (in German)
13. Paul W, Bahlmann G: Chronische Hämodialyse und Augeninnendruck (Chronic haemodialysis and intraocular pressure). *Folia Ophthalmol* 1:43, 1976 (in German)
14. Scheie HG: Evaluation of ophthalmoscopic changes of hypertension and arteriolar sclerosis. *Arch Ophthalmol* 49:117, 1953
15. Jansen JLJ: Therapeutische mogelijkheden bij patiënten met terminale nierinsufficientie als gevolg van diabetische nefropathie (Therapeutic possibilities in patients with terminal renal failure from diabetic nephropathy). *Ned Tijdschr Geneeskd* 123:117, 1979 (in Dutch)
16. Coulson AA, Lucas ZJ, Condy M, Cohn R: An epidemic of cytomegalovirus disease in a renal transplant population. *West J Med* 120:1, 1974
17. Venecia de G, Zu Rhein GM, Pratt MV, Kisken W: Cytomegalic inclusion retinitis in an adult. *Arch Ophthalmol* 86:44, 1971
18. Carson S, Chatterjee SN: Cytomegalovirus retinitis: two cases occurring after renal transplantation. *Ann Ophthalmol* 10:275, 1978

39

PHARMACOLOGICAL ASPECTS OF RENAL FAILURE AND DIALYSIS

JOHN F. MAHER

Drugs and renal failure	749		*Tetracyclines*	766
Pharmacokinetics	749		*Polymyxins*	767
Biovailability	750		*Sulfonamides*	767
Distribution space	750		*Other antibiotics*	768
Protein binding	750		*Urinary antiseptics*	769
Elimination rate	751		*Tuberculostatic drugs*	769
Half life	751		*Fungicides*	770
Mechanisms of drug elimination	752		*Miscellaneous antimicrobials*	770
Renal handling of drugs	752		Cardiovascular drugs	770
Metabolic affects of drugs	752		*Digitalis glycosides*	770
End organ alterations	752		*Antihypertensives*	771
Adverse effects of drugs on the kidney	753		*β-adrenergic blockers*	773
Drug-dialysis interactions	754		*Diuretics*	773
Determinants of dialyzer clearances	754		*Antiarrhythmic agents*	774
Influence of dialysis of half life	755		*Other vasoactive drugs*	775
Depletion by dialysis	757		Sedatives, tranquilizers, and psychotherapeutic drugs	775
Metabolic effects of dialysis on drug action	757		Analgesics	777
Reverse dialysis and factors affecting unidirectional flux	757		Antirheumatic and anti-inflammatory drugs	778
Hemofiltration	757		Immunosuppressive and antineoplastic agents	778
Hemoperfusion	757		Hypoglycemic agents	779
Peritoneal dialysis	758		Anticonvulsants	780
Modification of drug dosage in renal failure	758		Vitamins	780
Specific drugs	760		Metals and chelates	781
Antimicrobials	760		Miscellaneous drugs	781
Aminoglycosides	760		Conclusions	782
Cephalosporins	762		Acknowledgement	782
Penicillins	764		References	783

Pharmacology considerations in patients with renal failure have become an area of increasing importance and expanding knowledge since such patients have been maintained by dialysis treatment. These considerations involve such topics as pharmacokinetics, nephrotoxicity, effects of drugs on elimination kinetics, dialysis of poisons, depletion of drugs by dialysis and dosage modifications. The abundant literature includes several recent reviews of these subjects (1-8).

DRUGS AND RENAL FAILURE

The high incidence of adverse drug reactions in uremic patients (1, 2, 9) is generally recognized and may be due to decreased elimination of the unchanged drug or of toxic metabolites, alterations in drug distribution or protein binding, drug associated metabolic loads, synergism of drug toxicity and metabolic abnormalities or possibly increased target organ susceptibility. In hospitalized patients, coexistent azotemia doubles the incidence of drug toxicity (10). The susceptibility may be even higher than recognized since toxicity can masquerade as uremia and toxic drugs are often avoided or given in lower dosage to patients with renal failure (11, 12).

Pharmacokinetics

Drugs are absorbed to various extents, distributed to body tissues where pharmacologic actions and toxic reactions take place and eliminated by one or more of several processes at various rates. Abnormalities in any of these factors may occur in uremia and be affected by dialysis. To avoid toxicity, guidelines can be followed, e.g. avoid unfamiliar drugs, verify maintenance doses or reduce dosage according to the decreased creatinine clearance. Pharmacokinetics in renal failure are often too complicated for crude guidelines to achieve non-toxic therapy, however. Physicians should not rely blindly on nomograms. Accordingly, some pharmacokinetic principles are outlined below and several reviews are recommended (1-4, 11-22).

Bioavailability

When administered orally, most drugs are incompletely absorbed or undergo some metabolic biotransformation during passage through the liver or both. The amount of the drug that reaches the left ventricle in its pharmacologically active form is the bioavailable drug, usually expressed as a fraction of that administered. This fraction varies according to the drug. It also varies according to the dose of a given drug because of saturation of first pass hepatic metabolic processes.

There has been little study of bioavailability of drugs in renal failure. Impaired absorption of calcium is well known, however. Antacids can bind not only phosphate, but iron as well (23), decreasing absorption. Moreover, changes in gastric pH accompanying uremia can decrease absorption by influencing non-ionic diffusion. Bioavailability of propanolol may be increased in patients with renal failure, possibly because of a decrease in first pass hepatic metabolism (13). Sulfonamide bioavailability is unchanged, but furosemide and pindolol absorption decrease (13). Coexistent heart failure, cirrhosis or gastrointestinal motility disorders can also affect bioavailability.

Distribution space

Once absorbed, a drug distributes into tissues in a fashion that is determined by lipophilicity and solubility characteristics and plasma and tissue binding affinities. The rate and extent of distribution vary according to physical properties of the drug. The distribution space of a drug is calculated as the amount of drug in the body at steady state divided by the steady state plasma concentration. After distribution equilibrium, the plasma concentration decreases as a function of the elimination rate. The plasma concentration that would occur at the moment of bolus injection, if distribution equilibrium occurred instantaneously, can be back calculated from the half life. This concentration can be used in the equation,

$$V = \frac{I}{p}$$

(volume equals quantity administered, divided by plasma concentration at time zero) to determine distribution volume. For unbound, water soluble solutes, the distribution space may be a value close to extracellular fluid volume or to total body water. Plasma protein binding decreases the apparent volume of distribution whereas tissue protein binding increases this value. Lipid soluble solutes often have high apparent volumes of distribution due to sequestration in tissues, including body fat (Figure 1).

By knowing the distribution volume of a given drug, its clearance can be considered in relation to this volume. Even if the clearance is a high absolute value, should it be a low fraction of the distribution volume, the plasma concentration will be expected to decline slowly. For example, chlorpromazine clearance is 600 ml/min but the distribution volume exceeds 1400 l, so the half life is about 30 h.

The removal rate by dialysis may be so rapid that it exceeds the intercompartmental transfer rate (24). This results in a transient rapid decline in the plasma concen-

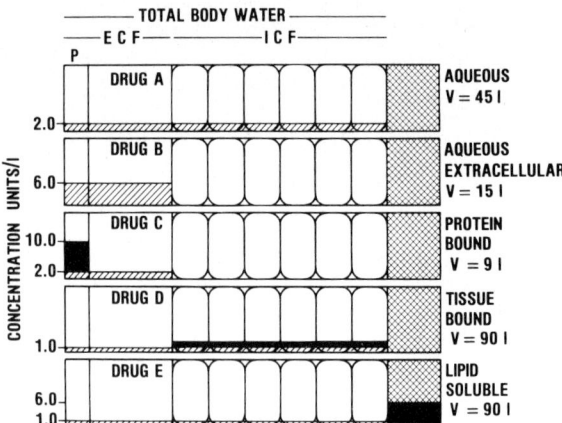

Figure 1. Net infusion of the same quantity of a solute yields different plasma concentrations because solutes distribute differently. A: total body water distribution, unbound; B: extracellular, unbound, C: extracellular with plasma protein binding, D: total body water with tissue protein binding, E: preferential distribution in body fat.

tration followed by an increment, as equilibrium is slowly reestablished (25).

For many drugs it is known that both pharmacologic and toxic effects correlate with the concentration at the site of action. This can be the concentration in interstitial fluid at the cell surface and usually equals the concentration in plasma water. Yet, because many drugs circulate bound to plasma or tissue proteins or both, the plasma water concentrations are lower than those of plasma or tissues (Figure 1).

Protein binding

A portion of most drugs normally binds to albumin or other plasma proteins. Such protein binding limits the concentration in the compartments that induce pharmacologic and toxic effects and ordinarily restricts the quantity available for elimination (Figure 1). In general, the more protein binding and the larger the distribution space of a drug, the lower is the plasma water concentration for a given quantity administered, but the longer is the pharmacologic effect because the large reservoir outside of plasma water prolongs the elimination.

Decreased plasma protein binding of many drugs occurs in uremia (18, 19, 26, 27) as listed in Table 1. The decrease in binding increases the fraction filtered, so removal rate may not decrease as rapidly as the decline in renal function. For drugs that are eliminated by extrarenal routes, such as phenytoin and diazepam, a greater fraction of free drug is delivered, for example to the liver, so the removal rate is faster than normal. Removal by hemodialysis is less impeded when protein binding is lower, so dialyzer clearances may be higher than in normal subjects. The distribution space increases when plasma protein binding is impaired and after a single dose therapeutic and toxic effects may be greater

Table 1. Renal failure decreases protein binding of these drugs.

1. Cephalosporins	5. Penicillins
Cefazolin	Cloxacillin
Cefotixin	Dicloxacillin
Cephalexin	Nafcillin
Cephalothin	Penicillin G
2. Cardiac glycosides	6. Clofibrate
Digoxin	7. Diazepam
Digitoxin	8. Diazoxide
3. Sulfonamides	9. Doxycycline
Sulfadiazine	10. Furosemide
Sulfamethazole	11. Hippurate
Sulfamethoxazole	12. Insulin
Sulfisoxazole	13. Phenylbutazone
4. Barbiturates	14. Phenytoin
Amobarbital	15. Salicylates
Pentobarbital	16. Thyroxine
Thiopental	17. Triamterene
	18. Valproic Acid
	19. Warfarin

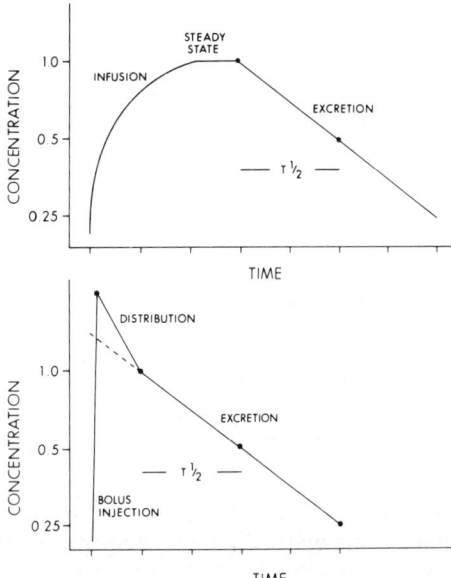

Figure 2. Plasma concentrations achieve steady state equilibrium during continuous infusion (upper half). Infused solute (minus that excreted) divided by steady state concentration equals distribution. After cessation of the infusion, plasma concentrations decrease exponentially. Plasma levels decrease by 50% in the interval, T ½. With rapid ('bolus') injection, plasma levels are higher and decline more rapidly until the solute has distributed and then decrease exponentially. The plasma concentration projected to time zero can be used to estimate solute distribution.

than normal because of the higher plasma water concentration.

The decrease in protein binding is due, at least in part, to competition for the binding site by a retained metabolite. The binding inhibitor is dialyzable, water soluble, heat stable and extractable in acid pH by organic solvents or by charcoal (28–30). On the other hand, the decreased binding of phenytoin does not correct with extensive *in vivo* dialysis, suggesting a change in protein composition in uremia (31).

In the case of digoxin, tissue protein binding decreases in uremia, which reduces the distribution space considerably (32). Therefore, because the distribution space is smaller, the plasma half life would be expected to be shorter. Because the dominant mechanism of elimination, renal clearance, is also markedly decreased the half life is increased, nevertheless.

Elimination rate
The elimination rate (mass per unit time) is usually corrected for plasma concentration and expressed as clearance. The plasma (drug) clearance is the sum of all mechanisms of elimination and is expressed as volume/time, customarily milliliters/minute. Solutes may be eliminated by a single route or concurrently by several routes. If the plasma clearance is predominantly renal, the dose of the drug in question must be reduced considerably, should severe renal failure develop.

When the plasma clearance per unit time is a high fraction of the distribution volume, the plasma concentration will decline rapidly. Conversely with a low fractional clearance due either to a low absolute clearance or a high volume of distribution, the plasma level will decline slowly. Since the rate of decline of the plasma concentration correlates directly with the plasma clearance, any decrease in this rate in uremic patients will be determined by the fractional decrease in total clearance that results from renal failure. Conversely, the additional clearance by dialysis considered as a fraction of the total clearance, rather than as an absolute value, defines the augmentation attributed to dialysis.

Half life
The biologic half life is the time interval required to eliminate half of the body burden or of the administered dose of a drug. It can be expressed by the formula:

$$T\,1/2 = \frac{0.693}{r}$$

where r is the elimination rate constant. Following steady state conditions, e.g. at cessation of a continuous infusion that has reached equilibrium, the biologic half life equals the interval required for the plasma concentration to decrease by 50%. After a single bolus dose, however, disappearance from plasma is determined by a combination of distribution and elimination. During the distributive phase, the plasma concentration declines faster than the true elimination half life (Figure 2), so the elimination half life or β can only be determined in the post distributive phase. Nevertheless, as the plasma half life is an easily determined and conveniently obtained variable, it is popularly used and related to clearance by:

$$T\,1/2 = \frac{0.693 \times V}{C}$$

where V is the apparent volume of distribution and C is the plasma clearance. The symbol CL is also frequently used to signify clearance.

By this formula, it can be appreciated that the half life increases, i.e. drugs persist in plasma, as clearance decreases. The extent of prolongation of the half life in renal failure is a good guideline for the necessary lengthening of the dosing interval for such patients.

Mechanisms of drug elimination

Drugs may be excreted unchanged by the kidney, skin or bowel, or if volatile, by the lung. Many drugs are lipid soluble allowing their penetration into cells. This increases the distribution space, thereby decreasing the fraction in circulation, thus limiting the quantity available for excretion by mechanisms involving ultrafiltration or diffusion which are effective for elimination of water soluble compounds. Biotransformation in tissues such as the liver promotes elimination of many compounds. Metabolic processes that biotransform drugs are oxidations, reductions, hydrolyses, acetylations and conjugations, such as esterifications, e.g. with sulfate or synthesis of a glycine or glucuronide compound. Such biotransformed compounds are usually more water soluble and thus readily excreted by the kidney and their pharmacologic activity or toxicity may be more pronounced, the same, less or nonexistent. Renal failure often results in retention of such drug metabolites and biotransformation may be decreased, unchanged or even increased in uremia (1).

Renal handling of drugs

Renal elimination of drugs may occur by several possible mechanisms (33). A few substances, such as mannitol or iothalamate are only filtered by the glomerulus and are neither secreted nor reabsorbed and not synthesized or degraded. Their renal clearance equals that of inulin and closely approximates glomerular filtration rate under all circumstances. Renal handling of most drugs has not been thoroughly studied, however, and cannot be assumed to equal the filtration rate. Some high molecular weight solutes such as insulin, glucagon and other hormones are removed by the kidney, by molecular biotransformation during the reabsorptive process after filtration. When glomerular filtration rate declines, the rate of such removal decreases (34, 35). The excretion of such drugs as salicylates involves combined glomerular filtration and passive tubular reabsorption. With nephron loss, fractional reabsorption may decrease so the drug clearance decreases less than glomerular filtration does. Passive reabsorption may involve simple diffusion gradients, as exemplified by urea. Reabsorption by nonionic diffusion also may occur as a function of pH, since ionized solutes are poorly reabsorbed unlike the unionized fraction. Excretion of passively reabsorbed solutes is also flow dependent, correlating with urinary volume as well as glomerular filtration rate. Since active transport is the mechanism whereby such drugs as mercurials and bromide are reabsorbed, their excretion is maintained despite marked reduction in glomerular filtration if fractional reabsorption decreases. The renal tubule also actively secretes many drugs, such as penicillins and cephalosporins. This is the major mechanism of renal excretion of highly protein bound, poorly filterable solutes. With those drugs for which maximal tubular transport considerably exceeds therapeutic concentrations, nephron loss and decreased glomerular filtration may correlate poorly with the excretory rate, which is limited mostly by the renal blood flow rate. Whenever possible, the drug clearance should be determined rather than assumed to be a constant fraction of the residual glomerular filtration rate.

Metabolic effects of drugs

Whether eliminated normally or not, certain drugs have important metabolic effects influencing renal excretion. This may result from the drug composition itself. For example, the magnesium content of antacids may accumulate causing hypermagnesemic coma. A metabolic product of a drug may cause complications such as paraldehyde induced acidosis. An effect on metabolism, such as the antianabolic effect of tetracyclines, may aggravate azotemia. Drugs that are anionic salts such as the penicillins can affect mineral and acid base balance by renal excretion of the nonreabsorbable anion or alternatively by metabolism of the anion. An influence on a hormonal or renal mechanism, e.g. controlling water elimination, may result from drugs such as lithium or chlorpropamide. Table 2 lists some drugs with important metabolic effects.

End organ alterations

Because renal failure has important effects on the sites of therapeutic or toxic action, alterations in end organ response to drugs may occur. For drugs that affect the

Table 2. Examples of drug induced metabolic abnormalities.

Hyperkalemia: Salt substitutes, Penicillin G, Spironolactone, Triamterene, Mannitol
Hypermagnesemia: Antacids, Laxatives
Hypercalcemia: Antacids, Thiazides, Hydroxylated Vitamin D
High sodium load: Kayexalate, Carbenicillin, Ampicillin, Cephalothin
Azotemia: Ammonium Chloride, Urethane, Tetracyclines, Adrenal corticosteroids
Acidosis: Phenformin, Paraldehyde, Nitrofurantoin, Methenamine mandelate, Ammonium chloride, Acetazolamide, Isoniazid
Alkalosis: Absorbable antacids, Carbenicillin, Large doses of Penicillin G, Viomycin
Water retention: Acetaminophen, Chlorpropamide, Clofibrate, Cyclophosphamide, Indomethacin, Phenylbutazone, Vincristine
Water loss: Demeclocycline, Lithium, Fluoride anesthetics
Nephrotic syndrome: Oxazoladines, Heavy metals, Chelates, Probenecid, Tolbutamide, Captopril

urinary tract, two modified responses occur. With a decreased nephron mass, the response to diuretics will be quantitatively less at any given dose although the fractional change in salt and water excretion may be higher than occurs in health. Limited responsiveness can lead to the use of higher doses, thereby increasing the incidence of toxicity (36). Decreased excretion of certain antibiotics not only leads to higher plasma concentrations, but also lower urinary concentrations, with which therapeutic response of urinary infection correlates (37). Accordingly, the drug may achieve toxicity without therapeutic effectiveness.

Uremic gastritis can contribute to the frequency of nausea and vomiting complicating therapy in uremic patients (12). The high ammonia content of gastrointestinal fluid in uremic patients, secondary to degradation of increased lumenal urea, will be reduced as bacterial urease decreases with antibiotic therapy. This lowers gastric pH, and thereby can affect drug absorption and induce peptic ulcers. In selected renal failure patients, antacid therapy may be required during antibiotic treatment. Increased susceptibility to peptic ulceration may relate more to other factors such as high concentrations of gastrin in uremic patients, however. The factors that affect the gastric mucosa increase the possibility of drug induced gastrointestinal hemorrhage in uremic patients when drugs such as salicylates are used.

Dermal drug reactions are frequent in patients with renal failure, may be misinterpreted as uremic dermatitis, may exaggerate uremic pruritus and often lead to excoriation and hemorrhage. Whether trace metal accumulation contributes to the greyish dermal discoloration that some dialyzed patients acquire is uncertain.

Myocardial irritability in uremic patients (38) is often aggravated by direct action of drugs like digitalis. Acute increases in plasma ionized calcium or potassium depletion complicating laxative or diuretic therapy may augment this risk.

Central nervous system depressants may cause or aggravate lethargy or coma in uremic patients not only because of drug accumulation, but also because of increased susceptibility. Thiopental anesthesia, the short duration of which is due to the fact that this lipid soluble barbiturate promptly distributes out of plasma into body fat, is prolonged in renal failure (39). Because urea facilitates the transport of dyes into the central nervous system, it may be anticipated that drug narcosis may be exaggerated in uremic patients. The demonstrated alteration in the blood cerebrospinal fluid barrier in uremic patients (40) may also contribute to higher cerebral concentrations of drugs or toxins that can cause central nervous system depression, easily misinterpreted as uremia.

ADVERSE EFFECTS OF DRUGS ON THE KIDNEY

Nephrotoxicity, a clinically important problem of remarkably high frequency, is a particular hazard for patients with preexisting renal disease (41–43). Careful surveillance and prevention may delay the progression of chronic renal failure to end-stage anuria. Explanations for the increased vulnerability of the kidney to toxins relative to other organs include the high renal blood flow rate and oxygen consumption, considerable enzyme activity, the large epithelial surface area, tubular transcellular transport mechanisms that often involve uncoupling of toxins from protein ligands and the interstitial and intratubular concentration gradients established by the countercurrent multiplication system (6).

Direct tubular damage may occur from heavy metals, for example from retention of bismuth, mercurial, antimony or iron compounds used therapeutically. When organic mercurial excretion is decreased because of preexisting renal disease, increased metabolic conversion to inorganic toxic products occurs potentially aggravating renal failure. Toxic tubular injury now most frequently occurs as a complication of antibiotic therapy, notably with the aminoglycosides. Other important classes of drugs causing nephrotoxicity are the organic iodides, hemolysins such as quinine and pigment producers such as phenazopyridine. The decrement in renal function may be irreversible and misinterpreted as progression of the underlying disease. Tubular injury from such toxins as gold or mercury may chronically release renal tubular epithelial cell antigens, an immunologic reaction to which causes membranous nephropathy.

Another type of nephrotoxicity is the papillary necrosis that follows prolonged ingestion of high doses of mixed analgesics (44). Accumulation of the phenacetin metabolite, N-acetyl-p-aminophenol, in the renal medulla and papilla may lead to oxidant injury aggravated by salicylate induced uncoupling of oxidative phosphorylation and inhibition of prostaglandin synthetase. Renal function deteriorates as abusive analgesic intake persists and may stabilize or improve with cessation of ingestion (45). Even after advanced irreversible disease has occurred, analgesic abuse should be avoided because of the risk of uroepithelial malignancy (46).

Acute hypersensitivity interstitial nephritis is often preceded by exposure to drugs including penicillins, sulfonamides, cephalosporins, phenytoin, para-aminosalicyclic acid, phenedione, polymyxin, antipyrine, rifampin, allopurinol, phenylbutazone, furosemide and non-steroidal anti-inflammatory agents (47, 48). Nephrotic syndrome may also occur with hypersensitivity to such drugs as the oxazolidine anticonvulsants, chelates, non-steroidal anti-inflammatory drugs, captopril, or probenicid. Less frequently, drug hypersensitivity may cause an acute renal angiitis or glomerulonephritis.

Obstructive uropathy may result from precipitation of a drug such as methotrexate or sulfonamide crystals, from a metabolite such as oxalate derived from methoxyflurane, or from drug induced uricosuria. The crystals of 2,8 dioxyadenine, a poorly soluble metabolite of adenine, used in blood preservative solutions can also precipitate inducing renal injury (Peck C (Uniformed Services University of the Health Services, Bethesda, MD): Personal communication). Methysergide therapy of migraine headaches may be complicated by retroperitoneal fibrosis causing periureteral obstruction. Alternatively, drugs may lead to interstitial calcification in the kidney as exemplified by the milk-alkali syndrome and hypervitaminosis D.

Indirect mechanisms potentially causing nephrotoxicity are the hemodynamic effects of hypotension, for example, complicating antihypertensive therapy or extracellular fluid depletion due to diuretic or laxative excess. Similarly, potassium depletion complicating drug therapy may cause tubular injury. A precipitous fall in renal blood flow can occur when prostaglandin synthetase is inhibited by such drugs as aspirin or indomethacin in patients that depend on prostaglandin medicated vasodilation to offset vasoconstrictor effects of angiotensin or catecholamines (49).

The importance of nephrotoxicity in patients with preexisting renal disease is magnified by a potentially higher incidence as human exposure to an array of biologically active compounds increases. Radiation nephritis is another by-product of scientific progress. Some forms of nephrotoxicity can be prevented by quantitatively decreasing or eliminating exposure. Further, the recognition of the association of renal damage and of nephrotoxin exposure in an individual can lead to reversibility of functional and histologic changes upon removal of the toxin or discontinuation of exposure. Correction of toxic nephropathy may thus delay or obviate the need of such therapeutic procedures as dialysis and hemofiltration or may allow easier management of advanced renal failure by preserving some residual function.

DRUG-DIALYSIS INTERACTIONS

The interactions of drugs and dialysis include depletion of therapeutic concentrations when dialysis is undertaken for such purposes as therapy of renal failure, therapeutic removal of drug excess by dialysis, effects of drugs on dialysis kinetics and effects of dialysis induced metabolic alterations on pharmacologic activity. There are marked differences between the removal rates of drugs by hemodialysis, hemofiltration, hemoperfusion and peritoneal dialysis.

Determinants of dialyzer clearances

During dialysis, solutes are removed from blood by diffusion through the semipermeable dialysis membrane along chemical concentration gradients. The removal process, customarily expressed as a clearance, varies inversely with the square root of molecular size or approximately of molecular weight (50). Because the molecular size of drugs varies, so does the clearance for any species of dialyzer. Thus, clearances must be measured or at least the clearance should be predicted based on the known physical properties of the drug. The relation of dialyzer clearance to molecular weight is illustrated in Figure 3. As molecular size increases, the resistance to diffusive transport of solutes contributed by the dialysate becomes less important and membrane resistance becomes the more important impediment to diffusive transport (51). The trend toward more permeable membranes and improved blood flow geometry with thinner blood films should result in increased clearances of high molecular weight drugs as new dialyzers are developed.

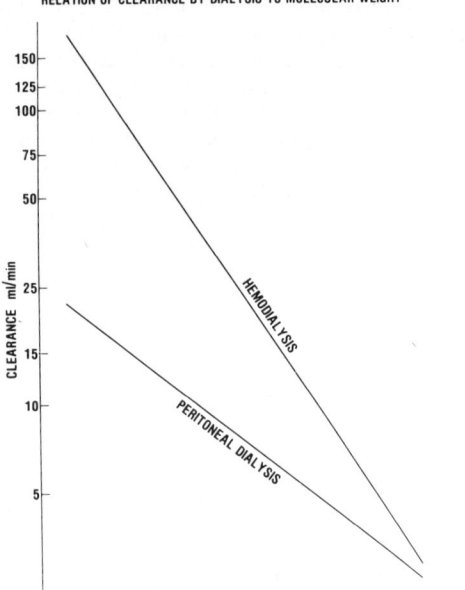

Figure 3. Clearance by hemodialysis or peritoneal dialysis is illustrated as inversely proportional to the square root of solute molecular weight.

Further, ultrafiltration does not discriminate according to molecular size until membrane permeability limitation is reached. Thus, ultrafiltration becomes a mechanism for solute removal of increasing importance as solute size increases (52). Hemofiltration should also result in high clearances of high molecular weight drugs.

In vitro measurements of dialyzer clearance often translate poorly into the transport characteristics during clinical dialysis. Solute diffusion and filtration occur from plasma water. Accordingly, protein binding limits solute transport unless equilibration is rapid between the free and bound moieties (Figure 4). *In vitro* studies using plasma as the perfusate offsets this error somewhat. The use of blood flow rates in clearance calculations assumes that plasma concentrations equal whole blood concentrations and that diffusion from cells occurs readily during dialysis. These assumptions have not been proved for most solutes and the evidence favors diffusion predominantly from plasma water during extracorporeal transit (53). It is customary to measure the extraction rate of a solute from plasma and multiply that value by the flow rate of whole blood through the dialyzer. The error in such a calculation (54) is not as critical with most pertinent endogenous metabolites as it is with drugs. The validity of the clearance can be verified by measuring the quantity recovered in the dialysate and dividing by the plasma concentration. Increased protein concentration and hematocrit also affect viscosity, and therefore, hydrostatic pressure and ultrafiltration rates, but decrease the water fraction of plasma or of whole blood. Protein-solute binding is often highly dependent on plasma protein concentrations or solute concentra-

39: *Pharmacological aspects of renal failure and dialysis* 755

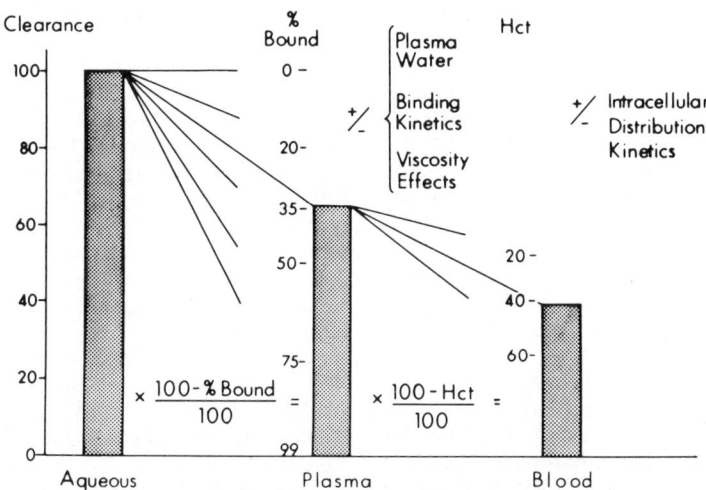

Figure 4. Compared to dialyzer aqueous (*in vitro*) clearances, the clearances, during clinical dialysis are lower because of protein binding and red blood cells limiting solute delivery to the membrane. (Reprinted from Maher [58] with permission).

tion and cannot be regarded as a constant fraction when these parameters vary. While a trace metal like tin is bound far below saturation at physiologic concentrations, remaining almost completely protein bound despite a three fold decrease in protein concentration or a one hundred fold increase in tin concentration (55), other solutes like iodide demonstrate saturation of the binding at low concentrations. Accordingly, the plasma clearance increases as iodide concentration increases (56). Recently, the clearance of several barbiturates has been inversely correlated with the fractional protein binding (Figure 5), while slight variations in molecular weight did not noticeably affect clearance (57). The low peritoneal clearance of digoxin is also explained in part by protein binding. Corrected to plasma water concentration, the removal rate is more appropriate for the molecular size (58). For highly bound solutes, influx during dialysis may proceed at a high rate, while efflux is impeded (50, 55).

As a general guideline, those solutes that are excreted by glomerular filtration will have high dialyzer clearances. However, renal elimination often interposes tubular transport, after ultrafiltration, and therefore does not necessarily correlate with dialyzer clearance. For example, the dialyzer rapidly clears bromide, but slowly clears phenolsulfophtalein a large, slowly diffusible solute. In contrast, the renal tubule reabsorbs bromide almost completely, but renal excretion of phenolsulfophthalein is rapid because of tubular secretion. When measurements are not available, hemodialyzer clearance can be very crudely estimated by dividing the square root of the molecular weight into 1200 ml/min and multiplying the product by the unbound fraction of the drug. With intermittent peritoneal dialysis, the clearance will be about 12% that of hemodialysis but somewhat higher for larger solutes because of the higher permeability of the peritoneum (50).

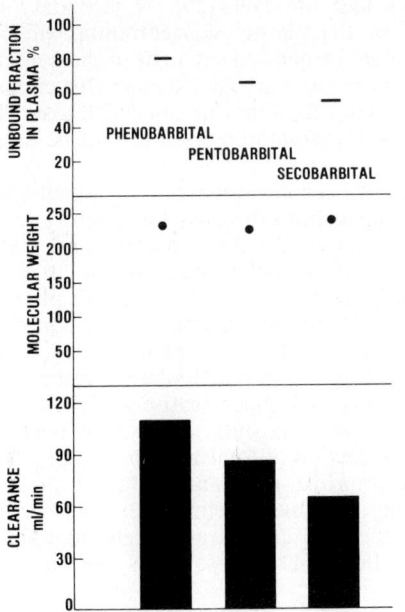

Figure 5. The clearance of three barbiturates differs not because of differing molecular weights, but because of varying degrees of protein binding.

Influence of dialysis of half life

Clearance is simply a removal rate corrected for the plasma concentration. In order to assess the effect of dialysis on the biologic half life of a drug, the dialyzer clearance must be considered in relation to the distribution volume. At any given clearance the half life will correlate directly with the distribution volume. But endogenous clearance of plasma continues during dialysis, so the effect of dialysis on total plasma clearance must be assessed. Provided that intercompartmental transfer is sufficiently rapid that concentration disequilibrium does not occur, i.e. the distribution space remains constant during dialysis, and that dialysis does not affect the endogenous clearance by renal and extrarenal routes, the fractional increment in clearance should predict the change in half life. For example, doubling the total body clearance decreases the half life by 50%. Drugs and toxins have been considered dialyzable if the procedure removes a high fraction of the body burden of a drug in a reasonable period of time, but poorly dialyzable if a low fraction is removed (8, 16). Such guidelines are helpful, but by ignoring the concurrent endogenous clearance, may overestimate or underestimate the contribution of dialysis. For example, hemodialysis adds considerably to the removal rate and significantly decreases the half life of the slowly metabolized methanol but it changes the declining plasma concentration slope of the rapidly metabolized ethanol only slightly despite comparable dialyzer clearance (59). By contrast, a low dialyzer clearance may add considerably to the physiologic removal rate under conditions that impede the normal mechanism of elimination, for example, dialyzer removal of aminoglycosides from the anuric patient.

In relating dialyzer clearance to the physiologic clearance, the effect of the drug itself on its own elimination must be considered. Comparisons of the half life during shock and dialysis with half life data obtained on healthy subjects exposed to low drug concentrations are often meaningless. Similarly, dialyzer removal rates of toxins from uremic patients should not be compared to physiologic data from normal individuals. To illustrate, the plasma half life of glutethimide in intoxicated patients is prolonged with shock. It also increases as the plasma concentration increases, independent of changes in blood pressure, consistent with a rate limited metabolic degradation (60). Accordingly, dialysis adds less to the relatively rapid removal rate at low plasma concentrations than to the slower removal rate at high levels since dialyzer clearance is not concentration dependent, unlike metabolic clearance. Clearances of a given solute in uremic patients may be higher than those achieved in normal subjects because of decreased protein binding and because anemia increases the fraction of plasma in extracorporeal circulation.

Dialyzer clearance must also be related to the changes in the total body clearance achieved by other therapeutic modalities. While patients mildly intoxicated from long acting barbiturates may respond to forced diuresis, those with severe intoxication and circulatory insufficiency or those with advanced renal failure have a less salutary response to forced diuresis. Dialysis may improve considerably the half life and clinical course of such patients (61). Similarly, the high dialyzer clearance of bromide may be an unnecessary addition to the removal rate of intoxicated, otherwise normal, subjects (62), whereas those unresponsive to diuretics or intolerant of salt loading, as occurs with heart failure or end stage renal disease, have a prolonged predialysis half life that improves considerably with dialysis.

The distribution volume of a solute is a determinant of the fraction of the body burden removed by dialysis. For solutes such as digoxin, propoxyphene or glutethimide, the distribution space is very large due to such factors as tissue binding or a high lipid partition coefficient. Although the dialyzer clearance may be high, the low fraction of body digoxin in plasma means that little is presented to the dialysis membrane. Unless there is rapid equilibration between plasma and tissue stores, it is fallacious to expect that enhanced removal, by using lipid or protein in the dialysate or by charcoal or resin hemoperfusion, will change materially the removal from tissue reservoirs. Indeed, it has been shown that even a rapidly diffusible solute like bromide is removed from plasma faster than equilibration occurs with such extravascular bromide as that found in cerebrospinal fluid (63).

The clinical effects of a drug correlate with concentrations in a particular extravascular compartment. This concentration will bear a constant relationship with plasma concentrations except after an acute load is administered or after a process of rapid elimination is initiated. If distribution into plasma keeps pace with the removal rate, the plasma concentration will continue to reflect pharmacologic or toxic manifestations. When equilibration does not keep pace, the plasma concentration decreases rapidly during the procedure, suggesting therapeutic success. But the clinical response may be less than anticipated and an inappropriately small distribution volume is estimated using either the formula: amount removed/delta plasma concentration or: plasma clearance x half life/0.693 (25). A secondary rebound increment in the plasma concentration will occur as there has been a smaller decrement in the concentration within the extravascular space. Under this circumstance an accurate half life cannot be calculated from clearance data because the volume cleared cannot be determined precisely.

Dialysis has been criticized as a therapeutic modality for some intoxications, because the quantity removed is a small fraction of the dose ingested and presumably absorbed and thus of the body burden. It is assumed that the entire body burden of the drug is pharmacologically active. There are examples to the contrary, however, such as thiopental, the pharmacologic and toxic actions of which correlate with plasma, rather than body fat concentration (64). Such reasoning would also incorrectly argue that therapeutic removal of potassium expressed as a fraction of total body potassium is low and could not improve potassium intoxication clinically, contradicting the obvious clinical experience. In which space does the drug concentration determine therapeutic and toxic effects? For most drugs the answer is unknown.

In the final analysis, the most important parameter by which to judge the effect of dialytic removal of a drug may be the clinical response, often difficult to quantify accurately.

Table 3. Drugs that usually require supplemental doses post dialysis.

Aminoglycosides: Amikacin, Gentamicin, Kanamycin, Netilmicin, Streptomycin, Tobramycin
Cephalosporins: Cephacetrile, Cefadroxil, Cefamandole, Cefazolin, Cefotixin, Cefuroxim, Cephalexin, Cephalothin
Penicillins: Amoxicillin, Ampicillin, Azlocillin, Carbenicillin, Penicillin G
Other Antibiotics: Chloramphenicol, Cycloserine, Ethambutol, Flucytosine, Fosfomycin, Isoniazid, Sulfonamides, Trimethoprim
Vasoactive Drugs: Aminophylline, Methyldopa, Procainamide, Quinidine
Immunosuppressive Drugs: Azathioprine, Cyclophosphamide, 5-Fluorouracil, Methylprednisolone
Vitamins: Ascorbic Acid, Folic Acid, Pyridoxine, Thiamin
Miscellaneous: Salicylates, Barbital, Phenobarbital, Lithium

Depletion by dialysis

When patients undergo repetitive dialysis for therapy of renal failure, depletion of drugs, such as antibiotics, and of physiologic solutes, such as vitamins and amino acids, may occur. Drug assay methods may have insufficient sensitivity to detect therapeutic concentrations accurately rather than toxic concentrations. Moreover, the clincial considerations for determining insufficient therapy are often less accurate than clinical signs of toxicity. Depletion of water soluble vitamins has been recognized (65), however, and removal of such drugs as antibiotics has been documented. Based on the available data, the drugs frequently used in patients with renal failure and removed sufficiently rapidly by dialysis, that supplemental therapy may be required, are listed in Table 3. Whenever possible, serum concentrations should be measured to guide replacement therapy.

Metabolic effects of dialysis on drug action

Dialysis may affect profoundly the pharmacologic activity of a drug despite changing the serum concentration only slightly. The frequently recognized and extensively studied example of this effect is the precipitation or aggravation of digitalis intoxication during dialysis as hyperkalemia, hypocalcemia, hyponatremia and acidosis are corrected. Whether metabolic alterations of dialysis affect the activity of other drugs is largely unknown. Changes in osmolality, pH, protein, urea or glucose concentrations can influence pharmacologic activity. Because there are many drug interactions, lowering the concentration of one drug can affect the action of another poorly dialyzable drug. For example, decreasing quinidine concentrations by dialysis may affect digoxin concentrations and pharmacodynamics. Moreover, improvement by dialysis of such lesions as uremic colitis may decrease the toxicity that ensues from a given excess of a specific drug.

Reverse dialysis and factors affecting unidirectional flux

Transport by diffusion during dialysis should occur at the same rate from plasma water to dialysate as in the opposite direction. Ultrafiltration, a more important transport mechanism for large solutes, will increase net flux in the direction of filtration. As the unidirectional flux is a function of concentration gradients, solutes added to or contaminating dialysate may manifest higher influx than efflux, if protein bound in plasma. Rapid binding of solutes to plasma proteins decreases plasma water concentrations, maintaining influx gradients, while measured efflux from plasma is decreased by protein binding. Preferential distribution into tissue, if rapid, also maintains influx gradients, whereas slow equilibration with a tissue pool limits efflux as well as decreasing more rapidly the influx gradient. The binding of trace metals and drug to hemodialysis membranes (66, 67) can favor inward transport, contribute to solute removal and create errors in calculations of transport kinetics. Special considerations apply to peritoneal dialysis. Solutes can accumulate in dialysate not only from plasma water but also from adjacent tissue as exemplified by fatty acids which are generated locally and enter peritoneal fluid directly, rather than via circulating blood (68). Moreover, because hepatic clearance rates may exceed absorptive rates from the peritoneum, it is possible to add, locally, drugs with potential systemic toxicity without achieving measurable concentrations in the systemic circulation (69).

Hemofiltration

Recently, hemofiltration has been developed as an alternative to hemodialysis for the treatment of uremia (70), and because simultaneous filtration-dialysis is often poorly tolerated hemodynamically, sequential filtration-dialysis has been introduced as a procedural variant (71). Unlike dialysis, the transport by hemofiltration does not discriminate by molecular size (until sieving occurs). Hence, the clearances of larger solutes can be much higher than occurs with hemodialysis. The considerable loss of large peptide hormones by hemofiltration (72) attests to this. Although there has been virtually no study of pharmacokinetics during hemofiltration, clearances should be predictable. With the post-dilution technique, clearances should approximate the rate of ultrafiltration multiplied by the unbound fraction in plasma for all but the largest of drugs, e.g. vancomycin, which may be sieved somewhat. Predilution may allow some diffusion of drugs from erythrocytes or transfer from plasma protein to plasma water, so the clearance may be slightly higher than half the ultrafiltration rate corrected for binding.

Hemoperfusion

Cleansing of blood by direct perfusion through columns of sorbents or exchange resins has gained considerable popularity recently, especially for removal of drugs and poisons (73–75). Because of direct contact of plasma with the sorbent (except for an ultrathin highly porous coating), extraction rates and consequently clearances are very high. Often the sorbent has a higher binding affinity for a drug than plasma proteins have, so the clearance of many drugs approaches the blood or plasma flow rate despite protein binding. As hemoperfusion proceeds, however, the sorbent approaches saturation and the extraction rate declines. Nevertheless, hemoperfusion is an effective method of removing many protein bound drugs rapidly. Despite the high clearance, the clinical results may not be favorable and the mortality may remain high, because of the large distribution spaces and the low intercompartmental transfer rates, tissue binding and unavoidable delays in initiating treatment (75, 76). Nevertheless, it is prudent to be aware of the capability of this technique to remove poisons and drugs. Amberlite resin perfusion removes nonpolar drugs better than polar compounds and charcoal perfusion clears each type of drug equally well (77).

Another technique of detoxification recently described is an on line plasma separator from which plasma perfuses a device wherein toxins diffuse into a channel containing cofactors and enzymes and detoxified solutes then diffuse back into circulation (78). Because uremia is characterized by a non dialyzable inhibitor of the enzyme thiopurine-methyl-transferase (79), which is involved in the metabolism of 6-mercaptopurine, azathioprine and 6-thioguanine, such a system could be useful in selected uremic patients should they become so intoxicated.

Peritoneal dialysis

It is naive to consider the peritoneum inert like hemodialyzer membranes. Although solute removal occurs predominantly by diffusion along electrochemical gradients as with extracorporeal hemodialysis there are several important transport differences (80–82). Convection contributes fractionally more to total mass transport, and membrane permeability is higher, so that relatively higher transport rates of large solutes occur. Blood and dialysate flow rates are much lower than with hemodialysis, however. Diffusion equilibrium isn't reached within an hour, even for the smallest solutes, so predictably maximal clearances are below 30 ml/min. Moreover, the diffusion barrier is living and its ionic charges restrict somewhat the passage of charged solutes. Lithium, phosphate and potassium transport rates are slower than predicted by solute size (50) and transport of cationic or anionic drugs such as penicillins should also be impeded. The diffusion barrier and the blood flow rate respond to pathologic, physiologic and pharmacologic influences. Numerous drugs, hormones and prostaglandins can alter transport kinetics both in patients with normal and abnormal vasculature (83). In general transport can be augmented when drugs are instilled locally, e.g. nitroprusside, selectively dilate the splanchnic vasculature, e.g. glucagon, or correct abnormal systemic hemodynamics, e.g. dipyridamole (84, 85). Transport can also be augmented by increasing convection, by increasing the osmotic gradient (86), raising capillary hydrostatic pressure (87) or increasing the hydraulic permeability of the capillary, e.g. with secretin (88). Augmentation of the transport of specific drugs may be increased by adding appropriate agents such as chelates, albumin, tris buffer or lipid (83). In addition to the intentional use of drugs to accelerate transport, the physician must be aware that drugs used for other purposes can influence mesenteric blood flow and peritoneal transport rates. For example, the vasoconstrictor norepinephrine given intravenously significantly decreases peritoneal transport rates (87). In contrast, intravenous dopamine in high doses increases transport by virtue of adrenergic receptor-mediated somatic vasoconstriction raising perfusion pressure and dopaminergic receptor-mediated splanchnic vasodilation.

Recognition of the limited value of high dialysate flow rates led to the development of continuous ambulatory peritoneal dialysis, wherein small solutes reach virtual concentration equilibrium between plasma and dialysate before the fluid is replaced (89). Since dialysate flow rate averages about 8 ml/min, clearances do not exceed that value. Except for the rare drug with a very low elimination rate, such low transport rates during continuous peritoneal dialysis will not add significantly to the total plasma clearance.

MODIFICATION OF DRUG DOSAGE IN RENAL FAILURE

The margin of safety in therapeutics is the range between the effective dose or plasma concentration and the one that induces toxic reactions. For some drugs there is considerable latitude between these levels. For example, the dose of penicillin that results in neuromuscular toxicity may be as much as several hundred times the minimal effective dose. Unless massive dosage is used, for example to treat endocarditis, the dose calculation need not be precise. On the other hand, the cardiac glycosides have a narrow margin of safety. Unless the dosage is calculated carefully, plasma concentrations may be too low to achieve the desired effect or so high as to cause dose related toxicity.

In adjusting dosage for patients with renal failure, usually the initial loading dose needs little or no reduction from the normal. A few notable exceptions include digoxin and morphine because of changes in distribution

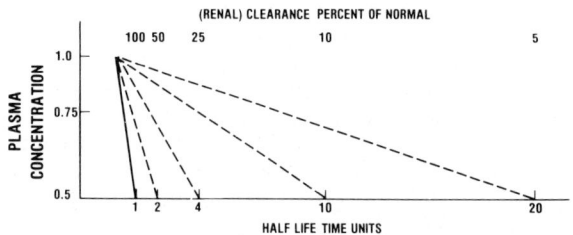

Figure 6. The half life in time units (e.g. hours) increases as an inverse function of renal clearance expressed as percent of normal, so plasma concentrations decline more gradually.

39: Pharmacological aspects of renal failure and dialysis

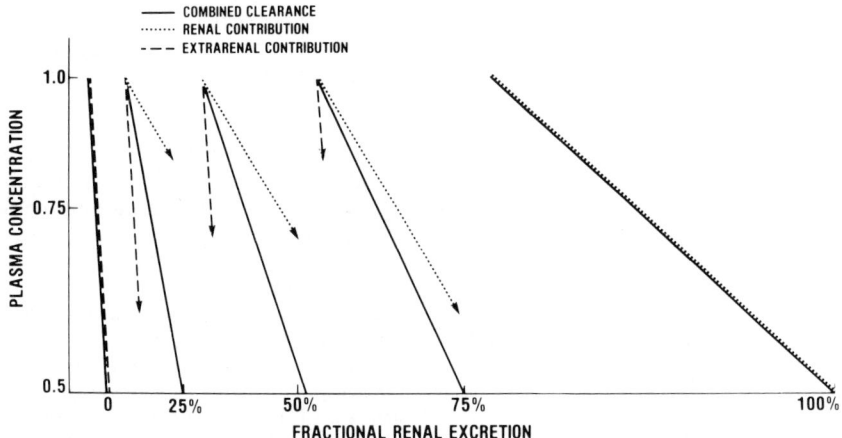

Figure 7. At any given level of impaired renal function, the rate of decrease of plasma concentration of a solute depends on the fraction eliminated by the kidney. When the renal contribution to total elimination is low, plasma concentrations may decrease rapidly despite renal failure. For solutes that depend mostly on renal excretion, elimination is very prolonged with renal failure.

volume and sensitivity. After the initial dose achieves the peak plasma concentration, the plasma level will decrease more slowly, i.e., the half life will be prolonged in proportion to the severity of renal failure as reflected by the increase in the plasma creatinine concentration or the decrease in glomerular filtration rate (Figure 6). It must be stressed that with renal failure the serum creatinine, when increasing, underestimates the severity of renal functional loss because it has not reached equilibrium concentration. The prolonged half life means that the plasma concentration will be higher than usual when the next dose is due.

A marked reduction in dosage will be required when the kidney is the only route of excretion of a drug and renal failure is severe. Obviously, the half life of those drugs eliminated predominantly by extrarenal routes will be affected little by renal failure and intermediate effects will result when elimination is partially renal (Figure 7). The fractional elimination by the kidney (the renal clearance as a fraction of total plasma clearance) determines the extent of dosage adjustment required in renal failure. This is the predominant basis whereby drugs are categorized as requiring little or no dosage modification in renal failure, modest adjustment or marked reduction.

Administration of the usual maintenance dose to a patient when the half life is prolonged by renal failure results in accumulation of the drug in plasma because the concentration is higher when the subsequent dose is added (Figure 8). The plasma concentration will eventually reach a level almost as many times higher than normal as the half life is prolonged and that high equilibrium concentration will be approached after about five half lives.

Therapeutic concentrations can be maintained by administering a lower dose at the usual interval or the usual dose at a prolonged interval. Because it is often

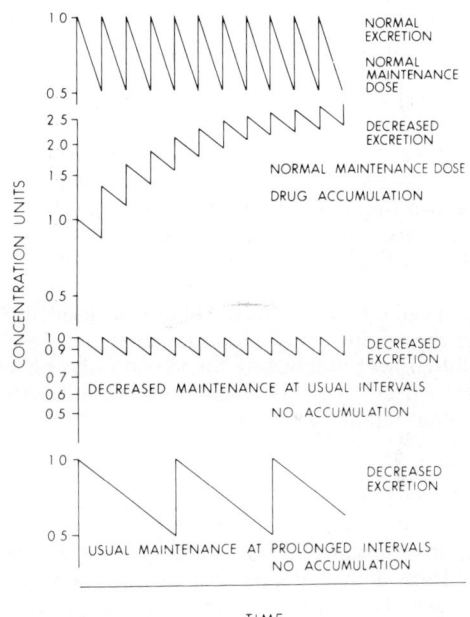

Figure 8. Repetitive administration of half the dose of a drug after half has been eliminated maintains appropriate concentrations. With slower elimination, the usual maintenance dose causes drug accumulation, while acceptable concentrations can be achieved with lower maintenance dosage or longer dosing intervals.

difficult to fractionate the dose, it is customary to increase the dosing interval. Moreover, it has been shown that fractionation of aminoglycoside dosage results in more toxicity than administering the same total maintenance dose at prolonged intervals (90). Nevertheless, prolongation of the dosing interval to longer than 48 h may allow concentrations to fall to suboptimal levels and remain so for too long a duration.

Obviously when renal failure is severe or when combined with hepatic failure, doses must be calculated most carefully. Unless clearance values for the specific drug are available, dosage reduction can be guided by the formula (91):

$$\text{Patient's dose} = \text{Normal dose} \times \frac{FE(C-1)+1}{1}$$

where FE is the fraction of the drug elimination normally contributed by renal excretion, and C is the patient's creatinine clearance as a fraction of the normal. The dosing interval may be calculated by the inverse equation:

$$\text{Patient's dosing interval} =$$
$$= \text{Normal interval} \times \frac{1}{FE(C-1)+1}$$

For example, with a drug excreted 80% by the kidney and clearance reduced to 10% of normal, the dosing interval should be $1/0.8(0.1-1)+1$ or $1/0.28$ times the normal interval.

Because of the potential inaccuracies in dosage calculations, recommendations for drug therapy of renal patients include (92):
1. Restrict drug use in renal failure patients to definite indications.
2. If established, follow a previously determined regimen for dosage of a given drug in renal failure.
3. A rough estimate of the proper dose may be calculated by formulae that use an assay of renal function factored by the renal contribution to normal elimination.
4. When available, drug assay should be used for periodic measurements of blood levels.
5. Careful clinical monitoring for toxicity and pharmacologic effectiveness is mandatory for all patients with renal failure.

SPECIFIC DRUGS

Given these problems in the interpretation of interactions of drugs with dialyzers and with disturbances of normal pathways of elimination in renal failure and methods for calculating dosage adjustments, we can consider the available knowledge about specific compounds.

Antimicrobials

Nephrotoxicity has become a major complication of antibiotic therapy, particularly in patients with underlying renal failure (6). Often antibiotic nephrotoxicity is misinterpreted as infection or, conversely, is incriminated when hemodynamic effects of infection or pyelonephritis decrease renal function. The frequency, severity and mechanism of nephrotoxicity arising from different antibiotics varies considerably. Many have a narrow margin of safety and, since most are excreted by the kidney, their accumulation in renal failure can increase toxicity. Unfortunately, at any plasma level, the urinary concentration is lower when renal function is impaired so that treatment of urinary tract infection may be less effective when blood levels are necessarily maintained below the toxic range (37). On the other hand, the diffusion of a toxic antibiotic across a dialysis membrane can decrease plasma concentrations below toxic and even below therapeutic levels.

Aminoglycosides

The aminoglycoside antibiotics are noted for their nephrotoxicity and ototoxicity. Neomycin is the most nephrotoxic and streptomycin is the least toxic of this class of drugs. The aminoglycosides are filtered at the glomerulus and a variable fraction is reabsorbed by proximal tubules, leading to renal cortical accumulation and proximal tubular injury manifested by tubular transport abnormalities and depression of glomerular filtration rate (93). Nephrotoxicity is more likely with advancing age, prior renal dysfunction or exposure to other nephrotoxins and follows renal cortical accumulation of the aminoglycosides, from which the elimination half life is normally several days (94). The high incidence of hearing loss among patients with chronic renal failure may relate, in part, to exposure to ototoxins, of which aminoglycosides are most notorious (95). Aminoglycoside toxicity also includes a myasthenic syndrome due to neuromuscular blockade associated with impaired release of acetylcholine. This toxicity is more frequent in those with renal failure, is correctable by calcium administration, and often presents as a respiratory arrest after anesthesia (96).

Streptomycin, when first introduced, sometimes caused proteinuria, cylindruria, decreased urea clearance and, rarely, tubular necrosis (97). Such nephrotoxicity has been abolished by purification of the drug. Ototoxicity, a function of the dose and inversely of renal excretion, improves as dialysis decreases blood levels of streptomycin by more than 50% (98). Elimination is predominantly renal, by glomerular filtration, and the maintenance dose must be reduced substantially (Table 4) from the normal 0.5 g (0.86 mmol) every 12 h as renal failure prolongs the half life (3, 19). Dialyzer clearance exceeds 40 ml/min (99) reducing the half life sufficiently to warrant a supplemental dose after dialysis. In Table 4, the notation, add 4 (mg/kg), indicates the dose to be added, after dialysis, to the usual dose for the anephric patient.

Neomycin, like other aminoglycosides, is poorly absorbed and can be used orally or by local application with relative impunity. When absorbed, it is very toxic, causing vestibular damage, deafness and proximal tubular necrosis. High dosage, enhanced absorption or impaired renal excretion contribute to the toxicity that sometimes complicates oral use, causing anuria and a high mortality rate (100). Hemodialysis removes neomycin rapidly enough (Table 4) to be useful in the treatment of inadvertent systemic administration of neomycin (101).

Table 4. Aminoglycoside pharmacokinetics.

Drug (mol. wt)	% Bound in plasma	% Renal elimination	Distribution volume (l/kg)	Clearance (ml/min) Normal / Anephric / Hemodial.	Half-life (h) Normal / Anephric / Hemodial	Dose (mg/kg) Normal / Anephric / Hemodial.
Amikacin (586)	4	98	0.20	85 / 1.6 / 20	2.0 / 60 / 5.0	5/8 h / 2/24 h / Add 4*
Dibekacin (452)	—	High	0.20	96 / 4.3 / 80	2.3 / 42 / 3.7	— / — / —
Gentamicin (543)	<10	>90	0.28	90 / 2.0 / 30	2.2 / 50 / 7.0	1.0–1.5/8 h / 0.5–1.0/72 h / Add 0.7
Kanamycin (441)	0	90	0.24	78 / 4.0 / 30	2.5 / 55 / 6.0	5/8 h / 4/72 h / Add 4
Neomycin (615)	—	High	—	— / — / 44	2.0 / 24 / 9.0	(Oral only) 15/8 h / Avoid / -
Netilmicin (475)	—	High	0.22	70 / — / 35	2.5 / 40 / 6.0	1.0–1.5/8 h / 0.7/72 h / Add 0.7
Paromomycin (616)	—	—	—	— / — / —	2.0 / 40 / —	10/8 h orally / — / —
Sisomycin (448)	0	High	0.22	— / — / —	3.0 / 40 / —	— / — / —
Streptomycin (582)	35	60–90	0.26	80 / — / 42	2.3 / 70 / 5.0	10/12 h / 7/72 h / Add 4
Tobramycin (468)	10	90	0.25	79 / — / 32	2.2 / 55 / 5.0	1.0–1.5/8 h / 1.2/72 h / Add 0.5

* Dose to be added (mg/kg) after dialysis to the usual dose for the anephric patient.

Kanamycin sulfate was found to be an effective aminoglycoside antibiotic with a broader antibacterial spectrum than streptomycin, but its use was complicated by proteinuria, microhematuria, granular or hyaline cylindruria, and azotemia in 10 to 20% of patients at a dosage of 25 to 50 mg (57–113 µmol)/kg/day (102). Prolonged use, for example in chemotherapy of tuberculosis, usually causes proteinuria and cylindruria after 15 mg (34 µmol)/kg/day and oliguric renal failure occurs in about 10% of patients so treated. Overt ototoxicity is infrequent and, like nephrotoxicity, is dose related. Kanamycin accumulates both in the renal cortex and in the middle ear, from which sites it is slowly eliminated (103). Because kanamycin is eliminated predominantly by the kidney, it accumulates in body fluids of patients with renal failure and the dose must be reduced substantially (Table 4). The half life in hours may be roughly estimated by multiplying the serum creatinine concentration (mg/dl) by 3 (104). Hemodialysis removes kanamycin rapidly enough that a supplemental dose is required thereafter (105), while peritoneal clearance is 5 to 8 ml/min which reduces the half life to about 16 h (106, 107). Supplemental doses of 100 mg (225 µmol) may be given daily during peritoneal dialysis if the plasma concentration decreases to 1 µg/ml (2 µmol/l) or less.

Gentamicin was introduced as a potentially safer, alternative aminoglycoside with a wider antibacterial spectrum. Unfortunately, the incidence of nephrotoxicity is comparable to that of kanamycin. Nephrotoxicity, characterized by decreased glomerular filtration and proteinuria and often preceded by saluresis and enzymuria, occurs in 10 to 30% of patients receiving 2.0 mg (4 µmol)/kg daily for more than one week (108–110). Proximal tubular necrosis with acute renal failure occurs occasionally, particularly after prolonged high doses, with preexisting renal disease, advanced age, prior methoxyflurane anesthesia, furosemide induced salt depletion or during concurrent therapy with cephalosporins (110, 111). Elimination, which is predominantly renal, decreases as the glomerular filtration rate declines so that the half life in hours is approximately 4 times the equilibrium plasma creatinine concentration (mg/dl) (112, 113). Unless dosage is reduced substantially in patients with end-stage renal disease, a 30% incidence of vestibular toxicity occurs, correlating with duration of treatment and total dose (114). Although the dose should not raise the peak plasma concentration above 10 µg/ml (22 µmol/l) (115), nephrotoxicity correlates more with the minimal (predose) concentration, which should be kept below 2 µg/ml (4 µmol/l) by appropriate spacing of doses (90, 116). When plasma concentrations are higher, as many as one third of patients develop overt nephrotoxicity. Hemodialysis shortens the half life considerably (Table 4) so toxicity is lessened and supplemental doses are required to maintain therapeutic concentrations (112, 117). Binding of gentamicin amino groups to sulfite radicals of the polyacrylonitrile membrane of the dialyzer can augment the removal rate during the beginning of dialysis (68). With hemoperfusion, clearances exceed 100 ml/min and the half life is reduced to the normal value of about 2 h (118). The peritoneal clearance is 4 ml/min/M^2, which reduces the half life to about 20 h (119).

Amikacin is a semisynthetic kanamycin derivative that appears to be somewhat less toxic but is also eliminated predominantly by the kidney, thereby requiring dosage reduction in patients with renal failure (Table 4). Nephrotoxicity and ototoxicity occur in about 9% and 5%, respectively, of patients treated with amikacin, increasing in incidence with the same risk factors as for other aminoglycosides (120). The prolonged half life in patients with renal failure is decreased considerably by hemodialysis (121, 122) which affects the normal elimination half life only slightly (123). During peritoneal dialysis, the half life is about 20 h (121, 122).

Tobramycin has antimicrobial activity and pharmacokinetic properties similar to those of gentamicin, but the incidence of nephrotoxicity appears to be lower. Renal failure prolongs the half life, which correlates with plasma creatinine concentration (124). Hemodialysis removes tobramycin sufficiently rapidly to decrease the half life almost to normal (Table 4), so the reduced dosage used for uremic patients must be supplemented after dialysis (124, 125). The clearance of tobramycin by peritoneal dialysis is about 10 ml/min (half of the urea clearance) which reduces the half life to 16 h (126).

Paromomycin is an ambecidal aminoglycoside that is used orally. It is poorly absorbed but accumulates in patients with renal failure (Table 4). Dosage adjustments for renal failure and dialysis pharmacokinetics have not been defined precisely (127).

Newer aminoglycosides include *sisomicin,* a gentamicin derivative that has pharmacokinetics comparable to it (128), but may be less toxic. The half life of sisomicin is prolonged in renal failure (Table 4) and the drug is removed by hemodialysis (129). *Netilmicin,* n-ethyl sisomicin, is a semisynthetic aminoglycoside that appears to be even less toxic (130). The elimination rate is about 60% of the glomerular filtration rate (Table 4) and the half life in hours is approximately 3 times the serum creatinine concentration (mg/dl) (131, 132). Hemodialysis removes netilmicin fast enough to lower the half life substantially (131, 132). *Dibekacin,* 3′, 4′ dideoxykanamycin is also eliminated at a rate proportional to the glomerular filtration rate (133, 134). With renal failure, the distribution volume of dibekacin increases. Nevertheless, hemodialysis lowers the half life almost to normal. *Verdamicin* is a new broad spectrum aminoglycoside, the pharmacokinetics and toxicity of which have not been precisely defined (135). *Lividomycin,* which has not had much clinical use, accumulates in renal failure, the half life increasing from 2 to 44 h (136). Dialysis pharmacokinetics have not been defined.

Cephalosporins

As a group, the cephalosporins have a broad antibacterial spectrum, are chemically similar to the penicillins, and are excreted predominantly by the kidney, by filtration and secretion (137). A rapid succession of new semisynthetic cephalosporin analogues have been developed during the past decade. Dose-related renal tubular injury occurs frequently with *cephaloridine,* which accumulates in patients with renal failure (138), whereas the normal renal clearance of 100 ml/min rapidly depletes plasma concentrations (139). Since hemodialysis decreases the serum half life almost to normal (Table 5), plasma concentrations will fall below the therapeutic range and remain so unless supplemented post dialysis (140). Peritoneal dialysis decreases serum half life to 7 h (141). The drug should be avoided in those with preexisting renal insufficiency because of the risk of further renal impairment. In anephric patients, however, it could be acceptable.

Cephalothin clearance is quite high, due mostly to secretion by the kidney since a large fraction of plasma cephalothin is protein bound (137, 139). After the normal dose of 1000 mg (2.5 mmol) intramuscularly, the peak plasma concentration of about 20 µg/ml (50 µmol/l) declines rapidly (137). With severe renal failure, cephalothin persists in plasma despite the high extrarenal clearance (Table 5) but the half life is reduced only to 6 h by peritoneal dialysis and to 3 h by hemodialysis (139, 141, 142). The low clearances by dialysis can be explained by protein binding, which is nevertheless, decreased in uremic patients (18). Hemoperfusion achieves clearances as high as 150 ml/min (118). Very high plasma concentrations of cephalothin can cause myoclonic seizures. Cephalothin can cause reversible acute renal failure (143) but verification of the diagnosis can be difficult amid the many other potential causes of renal impairment in severely ill patients. Increased susceptibility to cephalothin nephrotoxicity should be anticipated in patients who receive excessive dosage (over 6.0 g (15 mmol/day), who have preexisting renal impairment, the elderly, those who suffer from intercurrent cephalosporin or penicillin sensitivity or those treated concurrently with other potential toxins or with potent diuretics such as furosemide or ethacrynic acid (137, 144, 145). By blocking tubular secretion, probenecid can be protective to the kidney, but will cause greater accumulation in plasma (146).

Cefazolin reaches higher peak plasma concentrations than cephalothin, has a smaller distribution space and a longer half life, in part because it is more highly bound to plasma proteins (137). Renal excretion is largely by secretion and bactericidal urinary concentrations can be maintained despite moderate renal failure (147). Cefazolin accumulates in plasma of patients with renal fail-

39: Pharmacological aspects of renal failure and dialysis

Table 5. Cephalosporin pharmacokinetics.

Drug (mol. wt.)	% Bound in plasma	% Renal elimination	Distribution volume (l/kg)	Clearance (ml/min) Normal / Anephric / Hemodial.	Half-life (h) Normal / Anephric / Hemodial.	Dose (mg/kg) Normal / Anephric / Post-Hemodial.
Cephalothin (396)	70	52	0.25	450 / — / —	0.6 / 12 / 3	15/8 h / 15/24 h / Add 7*
Cephaloridine (416)	30	85	0.23	150 / — / —	1.3 / 20 / 4	15/8 h / 7/48 h / Add 7
Cephalexin (347)	15	96	0.28	250 / — / —	0.8 / 30 / 5	15/6 h / 7/24 h / Add 7
Cefazolin (445)	90	90	0.13	60 / — / —	2.0 / 35 / 5	15/8 h / 4/24 h / Add 6
Cephapirin (445)	50	49	0.18	300 / — / —	0.7 / 2.5 / 1.8	15/6 h / 15/12 h / Add 3
Cephradine (349)	10	86	0.30	360 / — / —	0.9 / 15 / —	7/6 h / Reduce / —
Cefaclor (367)	—	About half	0.33	— / — / 41	0.7 / 2.4 / 1.6	15/6 h / 15/12 h / Add 4
Cefamandole (485)	70	96	0.21	200 / — / 25	0.9 / 14 / 5	30/8 h / 15/24 h / Add 10
Cefoxitin (426)	73	78	0.16	390 / — / —	1.0 / 18 / 4	30/8 h / 15/24 h / Add 9

* See note to Table 4.

ure (Table 5), as the half life in hours is approximately 3 times the serum creatinine concentration (mg/dl) (148-151). Hemodialysis reduces the half life considerably (148, 149). Despite only a modest reduction of protein binding in patients with renal failure, binding is markedly decreased during hemodialysis (152).

Cephalexin is effective orally, achieving plasma concentrations of almost 20 µg/ml (60 µmol/l) with standard dosage (137). Thereafter, plasma concentrations decline rapidly but elimination is almost entirely renal, so cephalexin accumulates in patients with renal failure (16, 139, 142, 151). The prolonged half life of cephalexin in uremic patients (Table 5) is reduced by hemodialysis (139). Nephrotoxicity can occur with high plasma concentrations of cephalexin (153).

Cefoxitin is a semisynthetic cephamycin derivative that may have antibacterial properties exceeding those of its predecessors (137). It is normally rapidly cleared by the kidney (154) and accumulates in patients with renal failure (Table 5) but not as much as anticipated because decreased protein binding of cefoxitin in uremia augments hepatic clearance (19, 155). Although decreased binding should increase the clearance by dialysis, the distribution volume increases considerably with renal failure (156). Nevertheless, the half life of cefoxitin decreases substantially with hemodialysis (8).

Cefamandole is another new cephalosporin that is particularly effective against certain gram negative organisms. Despite considerable protein binding, it normally has a short half life (Table 5) and depends mostly on renal elimination (19, 157, 158). The prolonged half life of cefamandole in patients with renal failure is reduced substantially by hemodialysis but only lowered to 7.2 h by peritoneal dialysis (157, 159).

Cephapirin has a short half life (Table 5) that increases only modestly with renal failure since a considerable fraction of its elimination is extrarenal (19, 137). The half life is reduced only minimally by hemodialysis, presumably because a high fraction is protein bound (160).

Cephradine is almost completely absorbed after oral administration, is rapidly cleared, mostly by the kidney (Table 5) and accumulates in patients with renal failure (19, 161). Because of minimal protein binding, it should be rapidly cleared by hemodialysis.

Cefaclor has the advantages that it is rapidly absorbed

from the gastrointestinal tract and fractional elimination by the kidney is less than that of other cephalosporins (Table 5), so that accumulation in patients with renal failure is only minimal (162–164). Removal of cefaclor by hemodialysis is not rapid, presumably because of protein binding (162, 163).

Cefadroxil (363 daltons), another new cephalosporin, is a derivative of cephalexin. It is well absorbed from the gastrointestinal tract, distributed in 0.3 l/kg and eliminated almost exclusively by the kidney at a clearance of 170 ml/min (165). The normal half life is 1.4 h, increasing to 25 h with renal failure but is reduced to 4 h by hemodialysis. The usual dose of cefadroxil, 15 mg (40 µmol)/kg/12 h, should be reduced to 7 mg/kg/24 h with renal failure, and 10 mg/kg should be given after dialysis.

Cephaloglycin (405 daltons) is also effective orally, but absorption is poor and the drug has largely been replaced. Nevertheless, as excretion is mostly renal, it accumulates in patients with renal failure (166). *Cephacetrile* (361 daltons) has a half life of less than an hour after parenteral use (137). With renal failure, the half life increases to 26 h and it decreases with hemodialysis to about 2 h. The recommended dose of cephacetrile, 15 mg (40 µmol)/kg/8 h, should be reduced to 7 mg/kg/24 h in uremic patients, but a supplement of 10 mg/kg should be given after dialysis. Accumulation in plasma can cause a reversible encephalopathy that improves with hemodialysis (167). *Ceftezole* (462 daltons) is distributed in about 0.2 l/kg has low fractional binding, predominant excretion by the kidney at a clearance of 220 ml/min and a normal half life of 0.6 h that increases to 11 h with renal failure (168). *Ceforanide* is administered parenterally and has a normal half life of 3 h. With renal failure, the half life increases to 19 h but it is reduced to 5 h by hemodialysis despite 80% protein binding of the drug (169). The normal clearance of ceforanide is 46 ml/min but the distribution volume is only 0.17 l/kg. *Cefmetazole* is a new cephamycin derivative that is eliminated mostly (70%) by the kidney with a renal clearance of 110 ml/min (170). Its distribution volume, 0.19 l/kg, is unaffected by renal failure, which prolongs the half life from 0.8 h to 15 h (170). *Cefoperazone* is a new cephalosporin that is cleared from plasma at a rate of 74 ml/min, mostly by extrarenal routes (171). Because 89% of cefoperazone is protein bound, plasma concentrations should not be greatly influenced by dialysis. *Cephanone* is cleared from plasma at 56 ml/min, 95% of which occurs by renal excretion (151). In plasma, 88% of the drug is bound and its distribution volume is 0.18 l/kg. The normal elimination half life is 2.5 h. *Cefuroxim*, distributed in a volume of about 0.25 l/kg, has a normal half life of 1.1 h, which increases to 15 h with renal failure. Accordingly, the usual dose of cefuroxim, 20 mg/kg/8 h, should be reduced to 7 mg/kg/24 h in patients with renal failure. Hemodialysis reduces the half life to about 3 h, so a supplement of 7 mg/kg should be given after dialysis. *Cefotaxime* has a large distribution volume (about 0.47 l/kg) but a half life of only 1.2 h, which increases to 2.5 h with renal failure and is not reduced appreciably by hemodialysis despite measurable removal (172). With renal failure, the dose should be reduced from 30 mg/kg/12 h to about 10 mg/kg/12 h.

Penicillins

The penicillins are antibiotics of choice for many infections. An infrequent but serious complication of penicillin therapy is acute hypersensitivity interstitial nephritis. Patients often manifest skin rash, eosinophilia, hematuria, leukocyturia (including eosinophiluria), proteinuria, cylindruria, enlarged tender kidneys and impaired renal function with or without oliguria (173). Interstitial accumulation of mononuclear cells and eosinophils accompanies an intense immune response at the tubular basement membrane to a penicilloyl haptene (173). Although the lesion does not depend on the dose or elimination rate, it is seen more often with higher doses and with the synthetic penicillins, methicillin and ampicillin (174, 175). Because recovery is so gradual despite drug withdrawal, adrenal corticosteroid therapy is recommended in the acute phase (175). Patients may lose residual renal function for a prolonged period. Acute hypersensitivity angiitis and glomerulonephritis may also complicate penicillin therapy (176).

An increased incidence of hypersensitivity skin reactions, but not of gastrointestinal toxicity, complicates penicillin therapy when renal failure preexists (177). Massive dosage, especially with concurrent probenecid therapy blocking renal tubular secretion or with antecedent renal failure may be complicated by neurotoxicity with myoclonic seizures and coma (178). The potassium content of penicillin G, 1.7 mEq/million units can be potentially toxic. Alternatively, sodium retention with resultant fluid overload may result from massive doses of the sodium salts of penicillin, (1.7 mEq/million units), ampicillin (3 mEq/g) or carbenicillin or ticarcillin (5 mEq/g). High doses of penicillins can also impair hemostasis by inducing abnormalities of platelet function and a heparin-like effect (179).

Penicillin G is excreted mostly unchanged by the kidney by filtration and secretion at a clearance approaching renal plasma flow. The phenoxy-methyl derivative, *penicillin V*, is better absorbed, but bioavailability is not known to be impaired in uremia. After absorption, the drugs are loosely bound to albumin, distributed in a large volume and rapidly eliminated (Table 6). Renal failure prolongs the half life substantially, but unless massive doses are used, e.g. for septicemia, dosage adjustment need not be very precise because of the wide margin of safety (11, 92, 161). When the dose exceeds 20 million units daily (1.6 million units equals one gram), or considerably less in patients with renal failure, penicillin can cause lethargy, coma, multifocal myoclonus or eleptiform seizures (166). Abnormalities in the blood cerebrospinal fluid barrier in uremia (40) which normally maintains a 20:1 penicillin gradient can contribute to this abnormality which is responsive to hemodialysis. About 30% of absorbed penicillin can be removed by hemodialysis (180) and a supplemental dose can be required thereafter. Little is removed by peritoneal dialysis, however. Charcoal hemoperfusion can achieve a penicillin clearance of 140 ml/min. Combined with hemodialysis, hemoperfusion is superior to dialysis, alone,

Table 6. Penicillin pharmacokinetics.

Drug (mol. wt.)	% Bound in plasma	% Renal elimination	Distribution volume (l/kg)	Clearance (ml/min) Normal / Anephric / Hemodial.	Half-life (h) Normal / Anephric / Hemodial.	Dose (mg/kg) Normal / Anephric / Post-Hemodial.
Penicillin (356)	60	80	0.33	420 / 36 / 40	0.5 / 12 / 4.0	5-100/8 h / 1-5/12 h / Add 1-10*
Ampicillin (349)	20	90	0.24	270 / – / 30	1.2 / 14 / 5.0	7/6 h / 4/6 h / Add 5
Amoxicillin (365)	18	52	0.34	370 / – / –	1.2 / 12 / 4.0	10/8 h / 7/12 h / Add 7
Azlocillin (–)	–	65	0.23	180 / – / –	0.9 / 5.7 / 2.5	15/8 h / 7/12 h / Add 7
Carbenicillin (378)	50	90	0.15	100 / 11 / 50	1.2 / 20 / 8.0	50/4 h / 30/12 h / Add 15
Cloxacillin (436)	90	67	0.15	150 / – / –	0.5 / 1.2 / –	7/6 h / 7/8 h / Add 0.5
Dicloxacillin (470)	95	60	0.14	110 / – / –	0.7 / 1.2 / –	4/6 h / Unchanged / Unchanged
Floxacillin (454)	–	71	0.13	120 / – / –	0.8 / 2.8 / 2.8	15/8 h / 7/24 h / Unchanged
Methicillin (402)	40	88	0.31	425 / – / –	0.5 / 4.0 / –	15/6 h / 7/12 h / Add 3
Nafcillin (436)	90	25	0.70	410 / – / 14	0.8 / 2.0 / 2.0	7/6 h / 7/6 h / Unchanged

* See note to Table 4.

for treatment of penicillin intoxication (181). *Sulbenicillin*, a sulfabenzyl penicillin, (414 daltons), is also rapidly eliminated by the kidney. With renal failure, the half life increases from 0.5 h to 7 h so the usual dose of one gram should be given every 12 h rather than every 6 h (182).

Ampicillin is a readily absorbed broad spectrum penicillin that causes hypersensitivity reactions, including interstitial nephritis, more often than penicillin G. Because ampicillin elimination is predominantly by the kidney (Table 6), the normal short half life increases substantially in patients with renal failure (3, 16, 180, 183). Accordingly, the dose should be decreased in uremic patients to avoid ampicillin neurotoxicity. Hemodialysis removes ampicillin sufficiently rapidly to decrease the half life so that dosage should be supplemented after dialysis (16, 184). Peritoneal dialysis does not affect plasma ampicillin concentrations or half life appreciably (185), although ampicillin absorption across the peritoneum has been demonstrated (186).

Amoxicillin is closely related chemically and pharmacologically to ampicillin. Pharmacokinetic parameters in health, with renal failure and during hemodialysis (Table 6) are also similar for these two amino-penicillins (166, 187, 188) except that because of better absorption from the gastrointestinal tract, amoxicillin reaches higher peak plasma concentrations and a greater fraction is eliminated by the liver.

Hetacillin is also a chemical modification of ampicillin to which it is metabolized (166). Accordingly, the pharmacokinetics of this well-absorbed drug become those of ampicillin. *Privampicillin* is another ester of ampicillin with enhanced absorption and comparable pharmacokinetics after metabolic conversion. Other similar semisynthetic aminopenicillins are *bacampicillin*, *talampicillin*, *epicillin* and *cyclacillin* (166).

Methicillin is a semisynthetic penicillinase resitant penicillin, administered parenterally because of poor gastrointestinal absorption. It is rapidly eliminated (Table 6) mostly by the kidney (16, 189), requiring modest dosage reduction in patients with renal failure. Hemodialysis reduces the half life only slightly so supplementation after dialysis can be minimal, if any, and peritoneal dialysis does not alter elimination kinetics appreciably. Methicillin has caused acute interstitial nephritis (173, 190, 191) more often than other penicillins. As many as 17% of patients given high doses of methicillin develop detectable renal abnormalities. Restoration of renal function is more likely and occurs more rapidly with prednisone therapy (191) and occasionally methicillin induced renal failure is so severe as to require hemodialysis (191, 192).

Nafcillin is a semisynthetic penicillinase resistant penicillin that is partially absorbed after oral administration (166). Its elimination is mostly extrarenal (Table 6) and as it is highly protein bound and distributed in a large volume, the elimination kinetics are not appreciably affected by dialysis (193). Metabolism of large doses of sodium nafcillin may induce metabolic alkalosis.

Oxacillin is an oral, semisynthetic penicillinase resistant penicillin. Oxacillin and 3 other isoxazolyl penicillins, *cloxacillin, dicloxacillin,* and *floxacillin* are eliminated rapidly both by renal excretion and hepatic degradation (Table 6). The dose must be modified only slightly, if at all, in patients with renal failure (194-197). Since each of these penicillins is highly protein bound, little removal occurs with hemodialysis and supplemental doses are not required (180, 185, 194, 196, 197). Removal by peritoneal dialysis is also minimal. Although protein binding decreases considerably in uremic patients, the distribution volumes of cloxacillin and dicloxacillin increase substantially so that the low clearances by dialysis do not decrease the half lives appreciably. Oxacillin has caused hypersensitivity interstitial nephritis (198) and neurotoxicity (199).

Carbenicillin, a synthetic penicillin particularly effective against Pseudomonas species, is distributed in a small volume and in plasma, about half is protein bound (200). Excretion is rapid and predominantly renal (Table 6) and in uremic patients, the plasma half life increases substantially (19, 180, 201). As hepatic degradation contributes to the elimination, combined renal and hepatic failure prolongs the half life even longer (to 24 h). To avoid neurotoxicity, the dosage should be decreased and the dosing interval increased to 12 h with oliguria and to 24 h with associated hepatic failure (200). Hemodialysis decreases the half life by about 50% and a dosage supplement is required after dialysis, while the peritoneal clearance of 6 to 7 ml/min affects the half life somewhat less (200–203). In patients retaining salt, the sodium content of carbenicillin can contribute to fluid overload. Large doses in sodium restricted patients can cause hypokalemic alkalosis because the carbenicillin anion is poorly reabsorbed by the tubule, promoting potassium and hydrogen ion loss (204). Massive doses of penicillin can cause the same problem (205). High plasma concentrations of carbenicillin can also cause neurotoxicity (206), hepatotoxicity (207) and abnormalities of coagulation (179, 208), including platelet dysfunction, impaired conversion of fibrinogen to fibrin and heparin-like activity. Carbenicillin is administered parenterally. *Carbenicillin indanyl* is an ester that is rapidly absorbed from the small intestine and is hydrolyzed to carbenicillin and thereafter has the same pharmacokinetics (209). Absorption of an oral dose is somewhat delayed in uremic patients but a higher peak plasma concentration is reached since the half life is prolonged considerably. Hemodialysis reduces the half life of the absorbed carbenicillin by about 50%.

Ticarcillin is a semisynthetic penicillin with pharmacologic properties similar to carbenicillin but greater bacterial activity (210-213). Because dosage is lower, less toxicity is anticipated. Nevertheless, renal failure prolongs the half life sufficiently (212, 213) to warrant dosage reduction to avoid neurotoxicity (214). Hemodialysis removes ticarcillin rapidly enough to justify post dialysis supplementation, but the peritoneal clearance of 6 ml/min only reduces the half life to 9 h.

Azlocillin is an acylureido penicillin that resembles carbenicillin, pharmacologically. It is normally rapidly eliminated by the kidney (Table 6) so it is retained in renal failure (215, 216). Hemodialysis removes 30 to 45% of administered azlocillin, reducing the half life substantially (215, 216). Thus, dosage must be reduced in uremic patients and a supplement is required after dialysis.

Mezlocillin is another new, extended-spectrum penicillin that is pharmacologically similar to carbenicillin but is a more potent antibacterial (166). It is normally eliminated rapidly by renal and extrarenal mechanisms although the latter may demonstrate saturation at high plasma concentrations. Because mezlocillin elimination decreases with renal failure, the half life is prolonged and modest reduction of the dose is required (217–220). Hemodialysis decreases the half life, sufficiently to warrant a supplemental dose, thereafter (217–219), whereas during peritoneal dialysis the half life is about 3 h and little or no supplementation is required (218, 219).

Other extended-spectrum penicillins include the piperazine derivative, *piperacillin* which is very effective against Pseudomonas species and other gram negative organisms. The normal half life of 1.4 h increases only to 2.1 h with renal failure and is reduced to normal by hemodialysis which removes about half of an administered dose in 4 h (221). *Mecillinam,* the first of the amidinopenicillins has bactericidal effects against a variety of gram negative organisms, but not Pseudomonas. The normal plasma clearance of about 340 ml/min yields a half life of 0.8 h which increases to 3.4 h as the clearance decreases to 70 ml/min in patients with renal failure (222). In patients with renal failure treated by hemodialysis, the elimination rate of mecillinam is approximately doubled, so the half life decreases by 50%.

Tetracyclines

The tetracyclines are broad-spectrum bacteriostatic agents that should be avoided, when possible, in patients with renal failure because their antianabolic effects considerably increase azotemia, negative nitrogen balance, acidosis and serum phosphate and their gastrointestinal toxicity frequently induces fluid and electrolyte depletion with attendant decrements in renal function (223-225). There is little evidence of direct nephrotoxicity, although massive doses of *tetracycline* infused acutely decrease inulin and PAH clearances (226). *Demeclocycline,* which impairs renal conservation of water, by

Table 7. Tetracycline pharmacokinetics.

Drug	Mol. wt.	% bound in plasma	Distribution volume (l/kg)	% renal excretion	Half-life (h) normal	Half-life (h) anephric
Chlortetracycline	479	60	1.5	15	6.0	8.0
Demeclocycline	465	75	1.8	20	13	70
Doxycycline	444	85	1.4	40	18	21
Methacycline	442	80	1.0	50	12	—
Minocycline	458	75	—	10	16	24
Oxytetracycline	460	30	1.9	30	9.0	60
Tetracycline	444	55	1.3	50	8.0	70

inhibiting cyclic AMP action and release (227), causes reversible renal failure, especially in cirrhotic patients, without inducing overt extracellular volume depletion (228, 229). *Doxycycline* appears to be the least likely of these drugs to aggravate azotemia (230). Outdated tetracyclines are degraded to anhydro-metabolites that can cause a reversible Fanconi syndrome (231).

The tetracyclines are bound in plasma to a variable extent, have large distribution volumes and rather long elimination half lives in health (Table 7). *Chlortetracycline* and *minocycline* have the lowest fractional elimination by the kidney. Only modest retention of minocycline and doxycycline occur in plasma of patients with renal failure (230, 232–234) and little dosage modification, if any, is needed to avoid excessive plasma concentrations. Nevertheless, toxicity may occur even when the dose has been adjusted (235). The half lives of demeclocycline, *oxytetracycline* and tetracycline are prolonged substantially in uremic patients (161). *Methacycline* also is excreted in large part by the kidney. Hemodialyzer clearances of most tetracyclines exceed 20 ml/min (236) but, because of the large distribution spaces, the half-lives remain long, decreasing by only 10 to 25% (225). Binding of doxycycline to dialysis membranes can contribute to the removal during the procedure (67). Hemoperfusion should achieve higher clearances than hemodialysis but elimination would nevertheless be slow because of the large distribution volume. Peritoneal clearance of tetracycline is only about 5 ml/min, which does not reduce plasma concentrations appreciably. Considerable absorption can occur from dialysis fluid, however (106, 237).

Polymyxins

Renal and neural toxicity are major drawbacks to therapy with polymyxins, a group of polypeptide antibiotics of which *polymyxin B* may be the least toxic. Although toxicity is negligible at doses below 2 mg (2 μmol)/kg/day, higher doses or impaired excretion cause tubular degeneration and necrosis, proteinuria, cylindruria, azotemia and abnormalities of tubular transport (238). Polymyxin B (1200 daltons) is excreted predominantly by the kidney without metabolic change (239). Severe renal failure prolongs the half life from 4 to 36 h (Table 8) and the dose must be decreased from 0.8 mg/kg/8 h to 0.8 mg (0.7 μmol)/kg every 3 to 4 days (3). The extent of protein binding of polymyxin B is controversial, but dialysis removes very little of this large solute, nevertheless, and dosage supplementation after dialysis is not warranted.

Table 8. Miscellaneous antimicrobials: half lives (hours).

Drug	Normal	Anephric	Hemodialysis
Colistimethate	4.0	15	Slight decrease
Polymyxin B	4.0	36	Unchanged
Sulfadiazine	10	22	11
Sulfisoxazole	6.0	12	6
Sulfamethoxazole	11	14	7
Chloramphenicol	2.7	3.6	Slight decrease
Clindamycin	3.1	3.7	Unchanged
Lincomycin	5.0	10	Unchanged
Erythromycin	1.6	4.5	Unchanged
Vancomycin	6.0	200	Unchanged
Fosfomycin	1.5	12	2.0

Sodium *colistimethate* was introduced with the expectations of greater safety than polymyxin B with which it has a comparable molecular size, antibacterial spectrum and pharmacokinetics. Toxicity at therapeutic blood levels of 5 to 10 μg/ml (4 to 8 μmol/l) is not well established. But renal failure is a serious complication that occurs with higher levels, which are especially likely in the elderly, those with preexisting renal impairment or after high doses (240–243). Neuromuscular blockade, potentially causing apnea, is also more frequent with antecedent renal disease (96, 243). *Colistin*, which has been shown to be identical to polymyxin E, is excreted unchanged by the kidney. Accordingly, the plasma half life increases from about 4 to 15 h with severe renal failure (Table 8) and the dose must be decreased from the normal 2.5 mg (2 μmol)/kg every 12 h to 2.0 mg/kg or less every 72 h (244). Despite more than 75% protein binding, hemodialysis accelerates the disappearance rate from plasma somewhat and peritoneal clearances are less than 10 ml/min, influencing the half life insufficiently to recommend a dosage supplement, thereafter (245–247). Occasionally, acute hypersensitivity interstitial nephritis has complicated therapy with the polymyxins (248).

Sulfonamides

Most sulfonamides (249–314 daltons) are well absorbed from the gastrointestinal tract (70 to 100%), are highly bound to plasma proteins (50-90%) and distributed in volumes ranging from 0.15 to 0.6 l/kg (19). Elimination is predominantly renal, both of the free sulfonamide and after acetylation to the more active, less soluble metabolite (1). The renal clearance of sulfonamides ranges from about 20 to 30 ml/min and is increased by alkalinization of the urine (19). Renal failure decreases the elimination rate considerably, prolonging the half lives (e.g. *sulfisoxazole* from about 6 to 12 h, *sulfadiazine* from 10 to 22 h, *sulfamethizole* from 8 to 18 h and *sulfamethoxazole* from 11 to 14 h), thereby increasing concentrations in plasma (1, 18, 19, 249-252). Persistence of free sulfonamide in plasma (partly due to some impairment of acetylation rate [253, 254]) allows increased availability for conversion to the acetylated form, which is normally fractionally bound to a greater extent. Nevertheless, protein binding of sulfonamides decreases in patients with renal failure (27, 255, 256). Appropriate dosage of sulfonamides for uremic patients has not been precisely defined, but should be reduced to about 25% of normal (8). Sulfonamides are removed by hemodialysis (257). The hemodialyzer clearance of about 20 ml/min decreases the prolonged half life (Table 8) by about 50% (249, 250) and dialysis increases the impaired protein binding of sulfonamides toward normal (256).

Nephrotoxicity is a serious adverse reaction to sulfonamides that was very frequent before the development of more soluble congeners, sulfonamide mixtures and alternative antibiotics (258). After high dosage, especially with acidosis or dehydration, characteristic sulfonamide crystals may be identified in the urinary sediment or distal tubule, often accompanied by tubular degeneration and necrosis and interstitial edema. Sulfonamides may also impair renal function by acute hypersensitivity interstitial nephritis, focal or diffuse granulomatous nephritis or tubular necrosis without demonstrable crystallization (259). Rarely, sulfonamide derivatives such as acetazolamide have also crystallized in the urinary tract (260). Deterioration in renal function with azotemia and tubular necrosis has also occurred with *cotrimoxazole,* a preparation of sulfamethoxazole and trimethoprim (261). Interstitial fibrosis with irreversible renal failure can occur with this combination or reversible acute interstitial nephritis can develop (262).

Other antibiotics

Chloramphenicol (323 daltons) is eliminated in part by renal excretion of the unchanged drug, but mostly by hepatic conjugation to the glucuronide and renal excretion of this conjugate. With renal failure, protein binding of chloramphenicol, normally about 55% (16, 19), decreases slightly but significantly, an abnormality that dialysis corrects (263). The distribution space of chloramphenicol is about 0.9 l/kg. Nevertheless, because of rapid hepatic elimination the half life is only 2.7 h, only increasing to 3.6 h in uremic patients (Table 8), but persisting much longer in those with hepatic failure (264). The glucuronide conjugate persists in uremic patients with a half life of about 100 h. This metabolite is not known to contribute to hematologic toxicity, but the bone marrow in uremic patients is more susceptible to inhibition. Nevertheless, therapeutic concentrations can only be achieved in uremic patients with full doses of chloramphenicol. With hepatic failure the dose must be reduced or the drug avoided. The clearance of chloramphenicol by hemodialysis is about 50 ml/min which affects the half life only slightly in uremic patients but, by doubling the elimination rate decreases the half life considerably in those with combined renal and hepatic failure (265). Hemoperfusion rapidly removed chloramphenicol from an inadvertently intoxicated child (266).

Clindamycin (425 daltons), an especially useful drug for anaerobic infections, is about 95% bound in plasma and distributed in a volume of 0.66 l/kg from which it is rapidly cleared, mostly by the liver (19). The half life in plasma is prolonged only slightly by renal failure (18, 267) and is unaffected by dialysis which removes negligible amounts of clindamycin (Table 8). The clearance by hemoperfusion ranges from 55 to 125 ml/min (119).

Lincomycin, a less preferred analogue of clindamycin, is not as active an antibiotic and has more side effects, but a similar antibacterial spectrum and pharmacokinetics. Lincomycin (407 daltons) is highly protein bound and eliminated mostly by hepatic metabolism. Renal failure prolongs the half life from 5 to 10 h and removal by dialysis is so minimal that plasma concentrations do not change appreciably (268).

Erythromycin, a rather large solute (734 daltons), is moderately well absorbed from the gastrointestinal tract, about 70% protein bound in plasma and distributed in a volume of 0.7 l/kg (19). Elimination is mostly by the liver and the half life is prolonged only moderately in patients with renal failure (Table 8) from the normal value of 1.6 h (18, 269). The effect of dialysis on plasma erythromycin concentrations has not been studied systematically but should be minimal because of the large molecular size, the high fractional protein binding and the high distribution volume which even increases in uremia. No dosage adjustment is recommended in uremic patients but erythromycin may cause ototoxicity (270), and acute interstitial nephritis (48).

Vancomycin (about 1800 daltons) is an antistaphylococcal antibiotic that is about 10% protein bound in plasma and slowly distributes into a volume of about 0.6 l/kg. Elimination is almost exclusively renal at 50 to 80% of the filtration rate (19). Vancomycin accumulates in plasma in patients with renal failure as the half life is prolonged from 6 to 200 h and negligible amounts of this large solute are removed by hemodialysis (271-273). Accordingly, the dose should be decreased in uremic patients from the normal 1.0 g (about 600 µmol) every 12 h to 1.0 g every 7 days and no supplement is warranted after dialysis. Even though transport across the peritoneum is measurable, the half life is not reduced very much by peritoneal dialysis (274). Overdosage of vancomycin can cause direct nephrotoxicity and ototoxicity.

Very little *novobiocin* is excreted unchanged by the kidney and dialysis is not known to decrease appreciably the plasma concentration of this antibiotic (613 daltons) so no dosage modification is recommended for uremic patients (1).

Fosfomycin, a broad spectrum antistaphylococcal antibiotic, is retained in renal failure (Table 8) and removed by hemodialysis (275). The dose should be decreased from 1.0 g every 6 h to 1.0 g every 24 h and a supplement of 800 mg should be given after hemodialysis.

Bacitracin (1411 daltons), is so nephrotoxic that its use is restricted to local application. If absorbed, this large poorly dialyzable solute is excreted mostly by the kidney at a clearance normally of 100 ml/min (276).

Urinary antiseptics
Treatment of urinary tract infections with *nitrofurantoin* is less efficacious as renal failure decreases the normally high renal excretion and thus urinary concentration. Peripheral neuropathy and metabolic acidosis are complications that make it preferable to avoid nitrofurantoin in patients with renal failure (277). Although 60% protein bound in plasma, dialysance of nitrofurantoin, (238 daltons), approaches 80 ml/min (56). *Nalidixic acid,* (232 daltons) highly protein bound and eliminated by both hepatic metabolism and renal excretion, persists in plasma of uremic patients. Therapeutic efficacy of nalidixic acid diminishes with renal failure, side effects are more frequent, metabolic acidosis may be aggravated and dialytic removal has not been studied (278). Similarly, *methenamine mandelate,* (292 daltons), normally rapidly excreted by the kidney with a half life in plasma of 3 to 6 h (8) also presumably accumulates in renal failure. As it may exaggerate metabolic acidosis, *mandelamine* should be avoided in uremic patients. Dialysis pharmacokinetics have not been studied. *Phenazopyridine* (Pyridium) is potentially nephrotoxic (279). Its elimination is delayed in renal failure and it should be avoided when possible in uremic patients. *Cinoxacin* is a synthetic organic compound used for the treatment of urinary tract infections. The normal half life of 1.6 h increases to 12 h when the creatinine clearance is below 20 ml/min, consistent with decreased urinary concentrations and efficacy in uremia (280).

Tuberculostatic drugs
Because of long-term use, excessive accumulation of tuberculostatic drugs may induce chronic toxicity. *Isoniazid* (137 daltons), is minimally bound in plasma (Table 9), distributed in a large volume and excreted in the urine at a clearance of about 40 ml/min, partly unchanged, but mostly after acetylation (281). The acetylation rate varies among patients as genetically determined, and also as influenced by hepatic function. Thus, the normal half life varies from about 3 to 8 h. Renal failure prolongs the half life to about 4 to 9 h, so the dose should be 200 mg (1.5 mmol) daily (1–3). Excessive dosage can be removed by hemodialysis, which doubles the elimination rate, by peritoneal dialysis or hemoperfusion (282–285). After dialysis, a supplemental dose of about 3 mg (22 µmol)/kg should be given (285). *Rifampin,* a large solute (823 daltons), is distributed in a large volume and is highly bound to plasma proteins (Table 9). Only a small fraction is eliminated by the kidney. Neither renal failure nor dialysis affect elimination kinetics sufficiently to warrant dosage modification (1, 19, 92). Acute hypersensitivity interstitial nephritis may occur, especially with intermittent rifampin therapy (286). This lesion may be insidious in onset and follow a prolonged course terminating with interstitial fibrosis (287). Rifampin can also induce digoxin and digitoxin metabolism, decreasing plasma levels and precipitating heart failure (288). *Ethambutol* (204 daltons) is minimally protein bound, but also distributed in a large volume (Table 9). It is excreted mostly unchanged by the kidney at a clearance exceeding 400 ml/min (289). With renal failure, the half life is prolonged and the dose should be reduced. Hemodialyzer clearance is about 50 ml/min which decreases the half life in uremic patients to about 5 h, requiring a dosage supplement of about 5 mg (25 µmol)/kg after dialysis. Since most *cycloserine* is excreted unchanged by the kidney, dosage reduction is advised in uremic patients if the drug must be used (1). This minimally bound, small drug (102 daltons) should be removed rapidly by dialysis. Overdosage has been successfully treated by peritoneal dialysis, with removal of 17% of the ingested dose (290). *Para-aminosalicylate* is excreted mostly by the kidney, partly unchanged and partly after acetylation or glycine conjugation. With renal failure, the half life, normally one hour, is prolonged to about 20 h and although some free para-aminosalicylate is removed by dialysis, the dose should not exceed 2 g/day (2, 3). *Pyrazinamide* is excreted predominantly by the kidney, so dosage reduction is advisable in uremic patients, whereas *ethionamide* elimination is mostly extrarenal (291). *Viomycin* is also eliminated mostly into the urine (129) but pharmacokinetics of each of these drugs during renal failure or dialysis have not been studied in detail. Both viomycin and *capreomycin* are potentially nephrotoxic (129).

Table 9. Pharmacokinetics of tuberculostatic drugs.

Drug	% bound in plasma	Distribution volume (l/kg)	% renal excretion	Half life (h) normal	Half life (h) anephric	Dose (mg/kg) normal	Dose (mg/kg) anephric
Isoniazid	<10	0.7	15*	5.0	6.0	4.0/24 h	3.0/24 h
Rifampin	80	1.6	16	3.0	4.0	9/24 h	9/24 h
Ethambutol	20	1.1	80	3.0	9.0	20/24 h	5/72 h
P-Aminosalicylate	–	0.6	80	1.0	20	150/24 h	Avoid
Cycloserine	<10	0.6	65	–	–	4/12 h	–

* After acetylation most isoniazid is excreted in the urine.

Fungicides

Antifungal therapy with the insoluble polyene antibiotic, *amphotericin B,* is often limited by dose dependent and potentially reversible nephrotoxicity, characterized by cylindruria, decreased renal blood flow and filtration rate, tubular acidosis, tubular necrosis and interstitial calcification (292-294). While the kidney eliminates only a small fraction of amphotericin B and preexisting renal failure does not demand dosage reduction, the development of azotemia is an indication to discontinue the drug or decrease the dose. Salt depletion aggravates the fall in renal blood flow and filtration rate induced by amphotericin B while sodium loading attenuates it (295). Amphotericin B has a very large distribution space (4.0 l/kg), slow intercompartmental transfer and a normal half life of several days (8). Negligible amounts of amphotericin B (about 1,000 daltons and 90% protein bound in plasma) are removed by dialysis (296).

Eliminated largely unchanged by the kidney at a clearance about two thirds that of creatinine, *5-fluorocytosine* (129 daltons) is distributed in a volume of 0.6 l/kg and only about 5% is bound in plasma (297, 298). Renal failure prolongs the half life from about 5 to 100 h (8, 298), increasing the likelihood of bone marrow suppression and hepatotoxicity. In uremic patients, the dosage must be decreased from 35 mg (270 µmol)/kg every 6 h to about 5 mg (40 µmol)/kg/24 h and the patient must be monitored carefully for toxicity. Hemodialysis achieves clearances of 55 to 113 ml/min (125) and decreases plasma concentrations sufficiently to recommend a maintenance dosage of 20 mg (150 µmol) after each dialysis (296, 298). *Miconazole* is an imidazole fungicide that is more than 90% bound in plasma and is eliminated mostly by the liver, so the normal half life of about 24 h does not change appreciably in uremic patients (299). Protein binding should inhibit removal by dialysis.

Miscellaneous antimicrobials

Chloroquin (320 daltons) is 55% bound in plasma and highly bound in tissue. It is normally slowly eliminated from a large volume by biotransformation and partly unchanged by the kidney at a clearance approximately half that of creatinine and has a plasma half life of several days. The chloroquin clearance decreases when creatinine clearance does, but short courses of therapy for acute malaria do not require dosage modification (1,300). With a glomerular filtration rate below 30 ml/min, prolonged treatment should be avoided, if possible, and dosage should be limited to 100 mg (300 µmol)/day for the first two weeks and 50 mg daily thereafter (300). *Chloroguanide,* a smaller molecule, is also bound in plasma but considerably less in tissue. Accordingly, renal excretion of the unchanged drug, which accounts for 40 to 60% of elimination normally decreases plasma concentrations to negligible levels within 24 h, raising the possibility of slowed elimination in uremic patients (301). *Pyrimethamine* (249 daltons) has a renal clearance of about 3 ml/min and a plasma half life of 4 to 6 days (302). The effect of renal failure and of dialysis on its pharmacokinetics needs further study. *Trimethoprim* is rapidly absorbed, is about 50% protein bound, and is distributed in tissue in a volume of 1.5 l/kg (8). About half of trimethoprim (290 daltons) is eliminated by the kidney at a clearance of 200 ml/min. The normal half life of 12 h increases to 24 h in uremic patients (18, 252). *Primaquine* (259 daltons) is rapidly biotransformed, little of the unchanged drug normally appearing in the urine. The hemolytic effect on sensitive erythrocytes and the antimalarial effect depend on the metabolite, the elimination kinetics of which need to be studied in uremic and hemodialysis patients (303). After virtually complete absorption, *quinine* (324 daltons) binds to plasma proteins (70%) and distributes into cells. Largely biotransformed by hepatic hydroxylation, less than 5% of quinine is excreted unchanged by the kidney (303). The half life of 4 to 6 h probably is unaffected by renal failure and little, if any, dose modification is required. Dose related toxicity includes hemolysis and tubular necrosis (304). Peritoneal clearance of quinine is 8 ml/min or less, below the normal renal clearance and much lower than achieved by hemodialysis *in vitro* (305). Quinine amblyopia improves with dialysis despite only modest reduction in plasma quinine concentrations (306).

Dapsone (248 daltons), a sulfone used for therapy of leprosy, is distributed throughout body water and is about 50% bound in plasma (291). Since about 70% of excretion is renal, dosage reduction has been recommended for uremic patients (92). Other drugs used for leprosy include *sulfoxane,* a substituted dapsone, and *amithiozone,* a thiosemicarbazone, both of which are likely to be retained in renal failure and *clofazimine,* a phenazine congener that has a large distribution volume and a long half life and is less likely to be affected by impaired renal function. Dialysis pharmacokinetics of these drugs need to be studied.

Pentamidine (593 daltons), which is effective against Pneumocystis carinii, disappears rapidly from plasma into tissues where it persists for months (8). Because excretion is at least partially renal, modest dosage reduction is recommended with concurrent severe renal failure and nephrotoxicity is a potential complication (307).

Amantidine, an antiviral agent, is eliminated by the kidney, normally at a clearance of about 400 ml/min from a very large distribution space with a resultant half life in plasma of about 15 h (308). It accumulates in patients with renal failure and can cause cardiac arrhythmias and neuropsychiatric toxicity (309). Hemodialysis clears amantidine at 67 ml/min, reducing the extremely prolonged half life in uremic patients to about 24 h (310).

Thiabendazole, used for treatment of strongyloidiasis is rapidly metabolized by the liver, so its elimination is unimpaired in uremic patients, but the hydroxymetabolite may accumulate causing vomiting (311). Removal of both thiabendazole and its metabolite by hemodialysis is minimal and dosage adjustment is not advised except that it is preferred to keep therapeutic courses brief.

Cardiovascular drugs

Digitalis glycosides

Digitalis toxicity is a frequent and serious problem,

especially in patients with renal failure. Whenever possible, the therapeutic emphasis in dialysis patients should be on control of salt and water balance by restriction of intake and removal of excess by dialysis so that digitalis can be avoided or used in modest dosage.

Ouabain (585 daltons) is rapidly excreted by the normal kidney and the plasma half life, normally 14 h (Table 10), increases to 60 h in anuric patients (312, 313). Little, if any, is bound in plasma and the distribution space is large. About 15% of a dose can be eliminated by dialysis. In contrast, *digitalis* (powdered leaf) is excreted more slowly, but like ouabain, is retained in renal failure increasing the likelihood of intoxication.

Digitoxin and digoxin have been studied more extensively, and because of shorter half lives than digitalis and greater understanding of their kinetics, are preferred in patients with renal failure (314, 315).

Digoxin (781 daltons) is well absorbed, about 25% protein bound in plasma and distributed in a large volume, equivalent to about 9 l/kg because of considerable binding in tissue. Absorption is slower in uremic patients but higher plasma concentrations are obtained because tissue binding decreases with renal failure or hyperkalemia, reducing the volume of distribution by about 50% (32, 316). For this reason a full loading dose of digoxin can be hazardous and a dose of 100 μg (13 nmol)/kg has been recommended (317). Excretion is primarily by the kidney as unchanged digoxin at a clearance close to that of creatinine (314, 318). Digoxin half life (Table 10) increases from 42 h to 120 h with advanced renal failure (18, 19). There is also evidence that digoxin is partially reabsorbed and that excretion is flow rate dependent at low rates of urine flow (319). Optimal serum digoxin concentrations are 0.5 to 2.0 ng/ml (0.7 to 2.6 nmol/l). While toxicity may occur at these concentrations in association with such metabolic abnormalities as hypercalcemia and hypokalemia, toxicity is much more frequent with levels above 3.0 ng/ml (314). The maintenance dose for uremic patients should be reduced to about one third of the usual. There are, however, considerable individual differences among uremic patients in digoxin bioavailability, distribution volume, clearance and sensitivity and patients must be monitored carefully (320). Because of the narrow margin of safety, the dose should be calculated carefully and serum concentrations assayed. The maintenance dose may be calculated from the equation, $\mu g/kg/day = 0.06\, Ccr + 1.3$ (318). The creatinine clearance (Ccr) should not be assumed to be a simple reciprocal of serum creatinine concentration in the elderly, in those with decreased lean body mass or in dialyzed patients. Although digoxin traverses dialysis membranes, clearances of only 10 to 20 ml/min do not affect the elimination half life appreciably (although plasma levels may decrease transiently), supplemental dosage should not be given and potassium removal by dialysis may precipitate digitalis intoxication (321, 322). Digoxin clearances of 50 to 100 ml/min have been achieved by hemoperfusion decreasing the half life (323–325), but only a small fraction of the absorbed drug is removed and the observed clinical improvement may relate to other factors. During continuous ambulatory peritoneal dialysis, peritoneal digoxin clearance is 2.0 ml/min, which is much less than the endogenous removal rate (326).

Digitoxin (765 daltons) is almost completely absorbed and is extensively metabolized by hepatic microsomal enzymes. The kidney excretes mostly cardioinactive metabolites and only about 10% unchanged digitoxin. Optimal serum concentrations are 10 to 35 ng/ml (15 to 50 nmol/l) and toxicity is usually associated with concentrations above 40 ng/ml (318). The volume of distribution of this lipophilic drug is about 0.5 l/kg (19). Renal failure prolongs the half life only slightly (Table 10) from about 150 to 170 h (18, 19, 327). Accordingly, the dose requires little reduction in uremic patients (about 70% of the usual maintenance of 0.1 to 0.2 mg/day) but maximal loading doses may be hazardous. With severe coexistent liver failure, the dose of digitoxin must be reduced further. The metabolism of digitoxin may be accelerated by drugs such as phenobarbital and rifampin that induce microsomal enzymes (288). As digitoxin is about 90% protein bound in plasma, little is removed by dialysis. The long half life, even in patients with normal elimination rates, portends a prolonged episode of digitalis intoxication, once it occurs. Hemoperfusion, however, can double the elimination rate of experimentally intoxicated dogs and may be useful clinically (328).

Antihypertensives

In uremic patients, hypertension is a frequent problem, often responsibe to dietary sodium restriction, diuretics, and dialysis. Whereas excessive salt depletion may precipitate reversible uremia in patients with preterminal renal failure, once terminal oliguria occurs, therapy of hypertension must stress control of sodium balance. Some patients only respond after hemofiltration, continuous ambulatory peritoneal dialysis or use of potent antihypertensive drugs, which should not substitute for

Table 10. Half lives of cardiovascular drugs (hours).

Drug	Normal	Anephric	Hemodialysis
Ouabain	14	60	Slight decrease
Digoxin	42	120	Unchanged
Digitoxin	150	170	Unchanged
Reserpine	72	+	Unchanged
Hydralazine	2.5	+	Unchanged
Prazosin	3	3	–
Clonidine	12	40	15
Minoxidil	4	4	–
Propranolol	3.5	3.5	3.5
Sotalol	5	50	7
Practolol	9	60	14
Acebutolol	4	4	Decreased
Atenolol	6	75	6
Metoprolol	4	4	–
Thiazides	2	6	–
Furosemide	0.5	3	Slight decrease
Amiloride	6	100	–
Lidocaine	2	2	–
Procainamide	3	13	6
Quinidine	7	9	Slight decrease
Disopyramide	6	12	–

sodium hemeostasis, and should be titrated carefully against blood pressure.

Reserpine therapy may be complicated by bradycardia, peptic ulceration, nasal congestion, depression, diarrhea and extrapyramidal disturbances. Partially absorbed, reserpine is distributed in a large volume including body fat. It rapidly depletes catecholamines. Reserpine is eliminated partially unchanged by the kidney and partially after metabolic hydrolysis (329). The plasma half life, normally 48 to 96 h, increases non-linearly as creatinine clearance decreases and little reserpine (609 daltons) should be removed by dialysis because of the large size of the molecule and the large distribution volume (Table 10).

Hydralazine, a peripheral vasodilator, may cause tachycardia, headache, neuropathy, anemia, retroperitoneal fibrosis (330) and a lupus like syndrome. Peak plasma concentrations of hydralazine may exceed 1 µg/ml normally and a small fraction of the drug is excreted into the urine within 24 h, while most of it undergoes hepatic acetylation (331, 332). Hydralazine is about 85% protein bound in plasma, distributes in a volume of 1.6 l/kg and has an elimination half life (Table 10) of about 2.5 h, only minimally affected by the acetylation rate (19). Increased plasma concentrations in uremic patients (332) may represent a retained metabolite. The effects of dialysis on pharmacokinetics of this small solute (160 daltons) are largely unknown.

Prazosin, also a peripheral vasodilator, is about 92% bound in plasma, and distributes in a volume of 0.6 l/kg (19, 333). The elimination half life of about 3 h, is not changed meaningfully in patients with renal failure (Table 10), because less than 1.0% is excreted by the kidney. The blood pressure response may be augmented in patients with renal failure in association with increased bioavailability, higher peak plasma concentrations and a change in the distribution volume (334). Because of the high fractional protein binding, little prazosin (382 daltons) should be removed by dialysis.

Methyldopa is excreted predominantly by the kidney, but most of the drug is first conjugated by the liver to the ortho-methyl sulfate (335). Less than half of an oral dose is absorbed, normally, and peak plasma levels occur in 3 to 6 h. The distribution space of α-methyldopa is about 0.4 l/kg and elimination is biphasic with elimination half lives of about 2 h and 6 h. As renal failure decreases the excretion rate, plasma methyldopa persists (336), but the rate of hepatic conjugation increases. Toxicity includes drowsiness, impotence, hemolytic anemia, hepatic dysfunction and retroperitoneal fibrosis. Dialysis removes 30 to 40% of an administered dose of methyldopa (211 daltons) at a dialysance one third that of urea (337).

Clonidine, an imidazoline derivative, also lowers blood pressure by altering central nervous sympathetic activity. The drug is well absorbed, about 30% bound in plasma and distributed in a large volume, about 3 l/kg (8, 19). More than half of administered clonidine is excreted by the kidney and the removal rate, normally about 200 ml/min, correlates with creatinine clearance (338). The normal half life of about 12 h increases (Table 10) to about 40 h with severe renal failure (8, 338, 339). The clearance of clonidine (230 daltons) by hemodialysis averages about 40 ml/min which removes 5% of an administered dose but decreases the half life to 15 h. Only minimal reduction of the maintenance dose is advised for uremic patients.

Guanfacine is an antihypertensive with properties similar to clonidine. Although excreted predominantly by the kidney, renal failure does not result in retention of the drug because the metabolic clearance rate increases in uremic patients (340).

Guanethidine (198 daltons), a potent postganglionic blocker, is excreted partly unchanged, but mostly after hepatic metabolism. The renal clearance is 300 ml/min, but the normal half life of guanethidine is several days, consistent with a large distribution space (341). Although small amounts of the drug persist for days because of tissue uptake, urinary excretion appears to be an important pathway for elimination of guanethidine, the side effects of which include postural hypotension, bradycardia, impotence, diarrhea, and nasal congestion. Dialysis kinetics of this small solute have not been studied.

Since elimination of *hexamethonium,* a ganglionic blocker, is mostly renal at a clearance approximating that of inulin, retention would be anticipated in uremic patients and dosage reduction required (342). Similarly *mecamylamine* excretion by the kidney is decreased with renal failure and blood pressure should be titrated with lower doses (343). *Tetraethylammonium* is rapidly and quantitatively eliminated by the kidney by secretion via the organic base pathway. Caution is advised in treating uremic patients since the elimination rate is delayed (344).

Plasma clearance of *minoxidil,* a potent vasodilator, approaches 600 ml/min, most of which is by hepatic glucuronide conjugation (345). The distribution volume approaches 3 l/kg and the drug half life in plasma is 4 h. Little unchanged minoxidil appears in the urine, and accumulation is not expected in uremic patients. The remarkably potent antihypertensive effect of minoxidil is sometimes accompanied by unanticipated improvement in renal function that justifies its use in severe hypertension. The effect of dialysis on plasma minoxidil (212 daltons) is unknown. Side effects include salt retention, hypertrichosis and an increased incidence of pericardial effusion (346).

After a peak therapeutic *diazoxide* concentration of 20 µg/ml (90 µmol/l), 95% of which is protein bound, and distribution into a volume of 0.25 l/kg the half life in plasma is about 24 h (347). The potent vasodilator effect of this salt retaining thiazide correlates with the unbound fraction. About 30% of renal excretion is as the unchanged drug at a clearance of 25 ml/min, while the metabolites are cleared at 100 ml/min. Uremia does not change the half life appreciably, but decreases the bound fraction to 85% while the pharmacologic activity of a given blood level or dose is not increased (348). Despite the protein binding, the clearance by hemodialysis is 25 ml/min and peritoneal dialysis shortens the half life (349).

Nitroprusside is eliminated by metabolism, but the metabolite, thiocyanate depends on renal elimination, can cause psychosis and hypothyroidism and is rapidly removed by dialysis (350). When given systemically, nitroprusside does not preferentially dilate the mesenteric vasculature or increase peritoneal clearances, but it does when administered intraperitoneally (83, 84).

It is not known whether pharmacokinetics of the angiotensin antagonists, *saralasin* or *captopril,* or the α-adrenergic blocking agents *phenoxybenzamine* or *phentolamine* are affected by renal disease. Saralasin, the competitive antagonist of angiotension, does distinguish renin mediated hypertensive patients despite renal failure, however, predicting the therapeutic response to surgery (351). Captopril, which inhibits peptidyl dipeptidase, the enzyme important in the synthesis of angiotensin II and the degradation of bradykinin has a potent antihypertensive action but can induce proteinuria (352), reversible renal failure (353) and a serum sickness like syndrome with membranous glomerulopathy (354).

β-adrenergic blockers

β-adrenergic blocking agents are useful in the treatment of hypertension, angina pectoris and cardiac arrythmias. *Propranolol* (259 daltons), the prototype, undergoes first pass hepatic metabolism, which may be reduced in uremia, and is then about 93% bound in plasma and distributed in a volume of more than 3.5 l/kg (8, 19). Hepatic clearance of 800 ml/min biotransforms propranolol to 4-hydroxypropranolol, napthoxylactic acid and unidentified metabolites (355, 356). The half life in plasma, normally 3.5 h, is not prolonged by renal failure (Table 10), but the metabolites persist at very high concentrations with a half life of 120 h (356, 357). Hemodialysis clears propranolol at 15% of the urea clearance which doesn't reduce the half life, but the metabolites are cleared rapidly by dialysis, reducing the half life to 5 h (339, 355). A recent report notes that cimetidine, which decreases hepatic blood flow, reduces the elimination rate of propranolol by about 30% (358).

Other nonselective β-adrenergic blockers include *Nadolol* (307 daltons) the elimination of which correlates with glomerular filtration rate and which is removed by hemodialysis (359). *Pindolol,* about 50% bound in plasma and distributed in a volume of 2 l/kg, is normally cleared at 540 ml/min, half of which is by the kidney (360). Its half life is not appreciably prolonged in patients with renal failure. *Sotalol* elimination is predominantly renal and correlates with creatinine clearance (361). With renal failure, its half life increases from about 5 h to 50 h (Table 10) but it is reduced by hemodialysis to 7 h (359, 361, 362). Because of the large distribution volume, plasma concentrations increase after dialysis. The half life of *timolol* (5 h) is not prolonged by renal failure (359).

Practolol, the prototype of the cardioselective β-adrenergic blockers, depends on renal elimination. The normal half life of 9 h increases to about 60 h with severe renal failure (Table 10) but it is reduced to 14 h by hemodialysis (363). Fractional binding in plasma is low and the distribution space is high. A new β blocker, *acebutolol* is minimally protein bound, distributed in a volume of 1.2 l/kg, and eliminated mostly by biotransformation to an N-acetylmetabolite (19, 364). Renal failure does not increase the half life, normally about 4 h (Table 10), but prolongs the half life of its metabolite. Hemodialysis clears acebutolol at a rate of about 42 ml/min, decreasing the half life of both the drug and its metabolite (364). *Atenolol* is distributed in a volume close to 1.0 l/kg and eliminated predominantly by the kidney at a clearance approaching that of creatinine (365). The elimination half life increases from 6 h to about 75 h when renal failure occurs (Table 10) and the dose must be decreased to about 25% of the usual 100 mg (0.4 mmol)/d (339, 365, 366). Hemodialysis reduces the half life to about 7 h, so supplemental dosage is needed thereafter (339, 366). Atenolol and other β-adrenergic blocking agents can cause retroperitoneal fibrosis (367). *Metoprolol* (253 daltons) is about 13% bound in plasma, distributes in a volume of 4.2 l/kg and is eliminated by α-hydroxylation (19). The half life of 4 h is not increased by renal failure (Table 10) which does prolong the half life of the hydroxy metabolite to 72 h or longer (339, 368). Hemodialysis reduces the half life of the metabolite to 5 h. The elimination half lives of several other β blockers, (*bufuralol, labetalol* and *tolamolol*) are not appreciably lengthened by renal failure.

Diuretics

As renal failure progresses, potent diuretics become less effective, most agents are clinically ineffective and the risk of drug toxicity increases. *Mannitol* is distributed extracellularly and cleared by glomerular filtration. In renal failure, the half life of mannitol increases considerably, prolonging the expansion of extracellular fluid volume, potentially precipitating heart failure, and little osmotic diuresis ensues. In anephric patients, the plasma clearance of mannitol is only 2 ml/min (369).

Since aminophylline, a combination of two small solutes, *theophylline* and ethylenediamine, is eliminated mainly by hepatic oxidation, the half life, normally 9 h, should not increase in uremia (19). Renal clearance is only 2 ml/min. Because theophylline is rapidly removed by peritoneal dialysis, hemodialysis or hemoperfusion, supplemental dosage may be required after these procedures to maintain therapeutic concentrations (370–375). At plasma levels above 35 μg/ml (225 μmol/l) hepatic oxidation is saturated and the half life is prolonged (376). In intoxicated patients hemoperfusion lowers the half life from 50 h to 4 h (374, 375). *Dyphylline* (dihydroxypropyltheophylline) is eliminated predominantly by the kidney, so the half life, normally 2 h, increases to 12 h in uremic patients. The clearance by hemodialysis is 109 ml/min, which lowers the half life to 4.5 h (377).

Organic *mercurials* are bound in tissue, particularly renal tubular cells, and rapidly excreted by the kidney. With renal failure, the half life increases from the normal 2 to 3 h to more than 24 h and with preexisting renal insufficiency, mercurials should be avoided (8). Acute renal failure is more apt to occur when mercurial diuretics are given to patients with preexisting renal impairment or following frequent parenteral or prolonged oral administration (378). Shortly after a massive dose, sufficient mercury may be in circulation that slow dialytic removal may contribute significantly to the impaired total elimination rate.

After nearly complete gastrointestinal absorption, *acetazolamide* (222 daltons) is highly protein bound in plasma, tightly bound in tissues to carbonic anhydrase and rapidly excreted by the kidney (1). Nevertheless, the clearance by hemodialysis is 22 ml/min (379). *Thiazides,* distributed extracellularly and 20 to 80% bound in plasma, are excreted unchanged by the kidney within a few hours by filtration and secretion. Patients with heart failure or impaired renal function excrete thiazides more slowly, prolonging the half life from about 2 h to 6 h (1, 8, 19). An extrarenal effect of thiazides may be potentiation of parathyroid hormone activity increasing serum calcium and magnesium in maintenance dialysis patients (380). Most thiazide complications, however, are either those of diuresis or related to hypersensitivity, e.g., acute interstitial nephritis (48, 381). Despite renal failure, *ethacrynic acid* may induce saluresis, but often only after high doses with attendant ototoxicity, hyperuricemia and gastrointestinal disturbances (36, 382, 383). Elimination of ethacrynic acid at a half life of about 3 h is partly hepatic and partly renal. This highly bound drug is secreted by the organic acid pathway after which some pH dependent back diffusion occurs. High doses of either *metolazone* or *furosemide* can also induce a clinically effective diuresis despite severe renal failure (384, 385). More than 90% of furosemide is bound in plasma. It is distributed in a volume about 30% of body weight, is excreted by the kidney at a clearance close to that of creatinine and is retained in renal failure and cirrhosis (386, 387). Toxicity includes gastrointestinal disturbances, hyperuricemia, hyperglycemia, and deafness (383). Acute interstitial nephritis has rarely been attributed to furosemide or thiazides (388). Potent diuretics influence tubular transport of toxins and can precipitate acute renal failure by aggravating renal ischemia secondary to extracellular volume depletion. The new uricosuric saluretic, *ticrynafen* has induced renal failure frequently, due to tubular degeneration, interstitial nephritis or acute uric acid precipitation (389–391). With renal failure the aldosterone antagonist, *spironolactone,* is less effective but the risk of hyperkalemia is increased (92). Spironolactone is rapidly biotransformed by the liver to active metabolites that may be retained in renal failure (392). *Triamterene* also may cause hyperkalemia. Normally, this drug is about 50% bound in plasma, distributes in a volume of 2.5 l/kg and is eliminated mostly by metabolism and to a lesser extent by the kidney by filtration and secretion (393). The metabolites may be pharmacologically active. Triamterene can induce immune hemolytic anemia with reversible oliguric renal failure (394). *Amiloride* elimination correlates with creatinine clearance. Renal failure prolongs the half life from 6 h to over 100 h (395). There are no data on the effect of dialysis on plasma concentrations of most diuretics, although protein binding obviously limits the diffusion of most of these drugs.

Antiarrythmic agents
Lidocaine is eliminated almost entirely by the liver. Renal failure does not alter the distribution volume (1.5 l/kg), protein binding in plasma (50%), or elimination half life (2 h) and no change in dosage is required (8, 19, 396, 397). Heart failure decreases both the distribution volume and the clearance, so peak concentrations are higher, but the half life is not prolonged. The hemodialyzer clearance of 10 to 20 ml/min is insufficient to warrant dosage adjustment (398).

Procainamide (272 daltons) is well absorbed and distributes rapidly to tissues where it is bound. About 20% is bound in plasma and the distribution volume is about 2.0 l/kg (8, 19, 399). Therapeutic plasma concentrations are 4 to 8 µg/ml (15 to 30 µmol/l). Elimination is partly by acetylation at a genetically determined rate and partly by renal excretion of the unchanged drug (399). Nonrenal clearance in slow acetylators is 240 ml/min and in fast acetylators is 350 ml/min, while renal clearance is normally 370 ml/min, regardless of the acetylator type (19, 400). Renal failure increases the half life to 10 to 16 h from the normal 2.5 to 3.5 h and the dosing interval should be increased to 12 to 24 h from the usual 4 to 6 h or the drug should be avoided (8, 400–402). The N-acetyl metabolite is pharmacologically active, depends highly on renal elimination and is retained in renal failure as the half life increases from 6 to 41 h (400, 403). The hemodialyzer clearance is about 60 ml/min for both procainamide and its metabolite which reduces the half life to about 6 h, justifying a small supplement, thereafter (402–404).

Oral *quinidine* is almost completely absorbed and in plasma 70 to 80% is bound at therapeutic concentrations of 2 to 5 µg/ml (6 to 15 µmol/l). Quinidine (324 daltons) distributes in a large volume (2.5 l/kg) because of binding by tissue proteins (8, 19). Elimination occurs by hydroxylation with a half life of 7 h which is not appreciably prolonged by renal failure, (Table 10), but excretion of the metabolites is delayed (405). Intoxication with quinidine, manifesting resistant shock has been treated by hemodialysis which achieves a clearance of 20 ml/min, reduces plasma concentrations by 25%, shortens the half life slightly and induces clinical improvement (406). Because hypokalemia protects against quinidine intoxication, low potassium dialysate is recommended.

Disopyramide (340 daltons), a well absorbed antiarrhythmic drug, distributes in a volume approaching 1.0 l/kg. Plasma protein binding correlates inversely with drug concentration and is about 30% at therapeutic plasma levels of 3 µg/ml (9 µmol/l) (19). Elimination occurs by the kidney, both as unchanged drug and as the dealkylated metabolite. The elimination half life correlates with creatinine clearance, increasing from 6 h to more than 12 h with renal failure (407). Neither hemodialysis nor hemoperfusion lower the half life appreciably, so no further dosage adjustment is needed (408, 409). The clearance by resin hemoperfusion (108 ml/min) is sufficient to improve hemodynamics and electrocardiographic abnormalities complicating acute intoxication, however (410).

Bretylium, an adrenergic neuronal blocker, that has potent anti-arrhythmic action, is excreted mostly unchanged by the kidney with a half life of 7 to 10 h (411). In uremic patients the half life is prolonged to about

30 h but decreases to 13 h with hemodialysis (412). Other antiarrhythmic β-adrenergic blockers are discussed above and phenytoin is discussed in the anticonvulsant section.

Other vasoactive drugs
Neither *isosorbide* dinitrate nor *nitroglycerin* depend on the kidney for elimination (19). *Amphetamine, ephedrine* and *phentermine* are partially excreted unchanged and partially metabolized (1). Accumulation of these drugs may occur in patients with renal failure, but other sympathomimetic amines are largely metabolized. More than half of *neostigmine* is excreted by the kidney and renal failure prolongs the half life from 1.3 h to 3.0 h (413). *Tolazoline* also is rapidly excreted by the kidney via the organic base secretory pathway (414). Dosage reduction should be indicated in uremic patients.

Sedatives, tranquilizers, and psychotherapeutic drugs

Barbiturates that have increased duration of activity have lower fractional protein binding and lipid solubility and higher renal excretion and dialyzer clearances (61). *Barbital* (184 daltons) is not concentrated in body fat, is only 5% bound in plasma and is excreted predominantly by the kidney at a clearance well below the filtration rate due to passive back diffusion. It may accumulate in uremic patients (415). Renal excretion of *phenobarbital* (232 daltons) also occurs by filtration with pH dependent back diffusion, and accounts for 25% of its elimination, increasing with alkaline osmotic diuresis to a maximum of 17 ml/min (416). The remainder is inactivated by hepatic microsomal enzymes. In plasma about 20% of phenobarbital is protein bound at therapeutic concentrations. Because of a lipid partition coefficient of 3:1, the distribution space is about 0.9 l/kg (19). The half life in intoxicated patients is about 24 h (Table 11). It is longer with low doses, probably because a higher fraction is bound. Retention of phenobarbital may aggravate uremic lethargy and coma and if used in patients with renal failure, the dose should be decreased and the patient monitored for oversedation (12). Peritoneal clearance of phenobarbital is 5 to 10 ml/min, but increases by as much as 30 percent with addition of an alkaline buffer or protein to the dialysate (417). Intraperitoneal furosemide increases peritoneal clearance of phenobarbital from 6 to 16 ml/min (418). Hemodialyzer clearances exceeding 50 ml/min improve acute intoxication but at low plasma concentrations higher fractional binding may limit depletion (61). In contrast to these barbiturates, *thiopental* is ultrashort acting, because its very high lipid partition coefficient causes rapid distribution out of plasma. Although eliminated by metabolism rather than by renal excretion, thiopental narcosis is prolonged by uremia (39). *Secobarbital* and *pentobarbital*, preferentially distributed in body fat and about 40 and 30% bound in plasma, are short acting and eliminated predominantly by hepatic biotransformation (419). Protein binding of pentobarbital decreases when renal failure occurs (420). Clearances of secobarbital and of pentobarbital by forced diuresis and peritoneal dialysis do not exceed 5 ml/min despite alkaline, osmotic diuresis or intraperitoneal alkali or albumin and the half lives are affected only slightly (61, 421). Hemodialyzer clearances above 30 ml/min decrease the half life of severely intoxicated patients from 35 to 20 h (61). *Amobarbital* and *butabarbital* are intermediate in their elimination rates by dialysis, protein binding, lipid partition and duration of action. Lipid soluble barbiturates may be cleared more rapidly by hemoperfusion through charcoal or resin columns (422–425).

The benzodiazepines, *chlordiazepoxide* (300 daltons) and *diazepam* (285 daltons) are more than 95% bound in plasma and biotransformed by the liver. Chlordiazepoxide distributes into a volume of 0.3 l/kg and diazepam into 1.1 l/kg (19). In uremic patients, protein binding of diazepam decreases, which may increase its pharmacologic effect (426). Benzodiazepine pharmacokinetics are complex with active metabolites excreted by the kidney and half lives of about 10 h (chlordiazepoxide) and 30 h (diazepam), but the drugs are generally well tolerated by uremic patients (1, 16, 427, 428). Although some removal occurs with dialysis, pharmacokinetics have not been studied in detail (429). *Lorazepam* and *oxazepam* are also highly protein bound and are eliminated by conjugation to metabolites that are inactive, unlike the other benzodiazepams (16, 19). *Flurazepam* has a large distribution volume and depends only partly on renal elimination (8). Nevertheless, a metabolic encephalopathy can occur from retention of a poorly dialyzable metabolite in uremic patients treated with the usual dose (430).

Chloral hydrate circulates about 50% bound to plasma protein and is biotransformed to trichlorethanol, an active metabolite eliminated by the liver and the kidney with a half life of about 8 h (431). Overdosage responds clinically to dialysis, which achieves trichlorethanol clearances above 150 ml/min, decreasing the plasma half life to less than 4 h (432). Hemodialysis clears chloral hydrate at 120 ml/min, decreasing the half life from 35 h to 6 h (433) and chloral hydrate is also removed rapidly by hemoperfusion (434).

Normally, *ethchlorvynol* (145 daltons), about 40% protein bound in plasma and distributed in a volume of

Table 11. Half lives of miscellaneous drugs (hours).

Drug	Normal	Anephric	Hemodialysis
Phenobarbital	24	60	9
Bromide	24	—	2
Lithium	22	40	6
Corticosteroids	2	4	Slight decrease
Cyclophosphamide	6	+	2.5
Methotrexate	2	+	Unchanged
Chlorpropamide	30	200	Slight decrease
Phenytoin	24	8	Slight decrease
Propylthiouracil	17	50	—
Methimazole	2	9	—
Organic iodides	1	30	4
Clofibrate	17	100	—
Cimetidine	1.9	4.3	2.5

4 l/kg, is eliminated slowly (half life about 30 h) by hepatic metabolism and to a lesser extent by renal clearance of 23 ml/min (8). Peritoneal clearances of 19 ml/min and hemodialyzer clearances of 64 ml/min decrease the ethchlorvynol half life to less than 24 h (435). Resin hemoperfusion achieves clearances above 200 ml/min and decreases the half life to about 4 h (436–438). Although extraction by the resin is nearly complete, removal is limited by the large distribution volume and slow intercompartmental transfer (438).

Glutethimide, about 50% bound in plasma and eliminated mostly by hepatic metabolism, has a very high lipid partition coefficient and thus a large distribution volume (about 3 l/kg). It should not be retained in renal failure and is removed slowly by forced diuresis or peritoneal dialysis (60, 439). Its half life is longer with higher plasma glutethimide levels than at therapeutic concentrations because of saturation kinetics (60). Hemodialyzer clearances of glutethimide (217 daltons) may exceed 90 ml/min decreasing the plasma half life from 40 h to 15 h (60, 439). Clearances of 120 to 200 ml/min can be achieved by hemoperfusion (424, 425, 440–442).

Meprobamate is readily absorbed from the gastrointestinal tract, distributes relatively uniformly throughout the body, is about 20% bound in plasma and is excreted predominantly by the liver (8). Only 20% of meprobamate is excreted unchanged by the kidney at a clearance below 40 ml/min. Forced diuresis may increase the clearance. Some degree of drug retention should be anticipated with renal failure, but only modest reduction of the dose is required. As peritoneal clearance of meprobamate (218 daltons) approaches 20 ml/min and dialysance using a coil hemodialyzer may exceed 100 ml/min, severe intoxication with meprobamate may improve with dialysis (443, 444). With hemoperfusion, clearances exceed 100 ml/min (425, 442).

Less than 3% of *methyprylon* is excreted unchanged, and renal clearance remains below 10 ml/min despite forced diuresis. Thus, retention of methyprylon is not anticipated with renal failure nor would major modification of dosage seem necessary. Acute intoxication with methyprylon (183 daltons) may improve with dialysis as peritoneal clearances of 15 to 20 ml/min and hemodialyzer clearances of 80 ml/min may be achieved (445, 446). With severe intoxication, the half life is longer because of saturation kinetics or shock (447). Hemoperfusion can clear methyprylon at 50 to 160 ml/min (425, 440, 442).

Methaqualone intoxication also responds to charcoal hemoperfusion (440, 442) which achieves clearances of about 200 ml/min or to dialysis which achieves a peritoneal clearance of 7.5 ml/min and a hemodialyzer clearance of 23 ml/min (448). Methaqualone is about 80% bound in plasma, distributes in a volume of about 6 l/kg and is eliminated mostly by the liver (8, 16).

Ethinamate intoxication has been successfully treated by hemodialysis, but the pharmacokinetics need further study (449). It is normally eliminated by hepatic metabolism.

Although clinical improvement has accompanied dialysis for *paraldehyde* intoxication, this may have resulted from correction of the metabolic acidosis (450). Some paraldehyde (132 daltons) is eliminated unchanged by the lung but most is metabolized by the liver. Uremia increases susceptibility to paraldehyde acidosis.

The phenothiazines include such drugs as *promethazine, chlorpromazine, triflupromazine, prochlorperazine, perphenazine,* and *thioridazine.* After absorption of an unpredictable fraction, phenothiazines avidly bind to plasma proteins and rapidly distribute to all body tissues, and because of marked lipophilicity, have distribution volumes as high as 20 l/kg (8, 19). They are slowly eliminated by metabolism. Although renal elimination is minimal, uremic patients may be more susceptible to phenothiazine toxicity, including extrapyramidal myoclonus and toxic psychosis (1, 451). Because of avid tissue binding, phenothiazine removal by dialysis or hemoperfusion has a negligible effect on half life.

Imipramine, nortriptyline, and *amitriptyline* are dibenzazepine compounds that also avidly bind to plasma proteins, are very lipophilic and distribute into spaces of 10 l/kg or more and then eliminated primarily by hepatic metabolism with half lives over 12 h (8, 19). Dialysis removes minimal amounts of dibenzazepines (452, 453) and despite high clearances by hemoperfusion, only a small fraction is removed from the large distribution volume (77, 434, 454, 455). Nevertheless, clinical improvement may occur.

Monoamine oxidase inhibitors include *phenelzine, pargyline, tranylcypromine, isocarboxazid* and *nialamide.* Their pharmacologic effects persist after the drugs or their active metabolites are eliminated. Retention of these drugs does not occur with renal failure and although clinical improvement has occurred with dialysis, there are no pharmacokinetic data to provide a basis for such therapy (7).

Sodium *bromide,* distributed in extracellular fluid and normally excreted by the kidney at a clearance below 2 ml/min, accumulates when sodium is retained as in heart failure, nephrotic syndrome or cirrhosis, potentially causing a toxic psychosis. The normal half life in plasma may exceed 24 h (Table 11) and it is not prolonged by renal failure until oliguria occurs. Saline diuresis decreases the half life of bromide to about 12 h and with potent diuretics, clearances may reach 14 ml/min, decreasing the half life to below 6 h (62). The peritoneal clearance of bromide is 14 ml/min and the hemodialyzer clearance exceeds 100 ml/min, decreasing the half life to below 2 h, faster than distribution equilibrium occurs (62, 63).

Lithium salts, in popular psychotherapeutic use, have a narrow margin of safety, potentially causing neuromuscular irritability and distal tubular necrosis when plasma concentrations exceed 2.0 mmol/l (6, 456). Dose dependent nephrogenic diabetes insipidus is attributed to inhibition of vasopressin stimulated water transport at a site biochemically proximal to that of cyclic AMP (457). Lithium excretion by the kidney, at a clearance of 15 to 25 ml/min, occurs by filtration with proximal tubular reabsorption. It is increased by osmotic diuresis, acetazolamide or bicarbonate therapy. Chronic lithium therapy can induce irreversible renal failure with chronic interstitial nephritis, tubular atrophy and medullary fibrosis (458). Lithium accumulates in renal failure (Table 11) causing toxic coma, which improves with hemodialysis, decreasing the half life from over 40 h to less than 6 h (459). Peritoneal clearances of lithium of 13 to 15 ml/min can exceed renal clearances and reduce the half life to 14 h (460). Lithium can be efficaciously and safely used in maintenance hemodialysis patients by following pharmacokinetic principles (461, 462).

Analgesics

Salicylates are small solutes (137 to 180 daltons) distributed in a volume of 0.15 l/kg and as much as 50% bound in plasma (19). The kidney excretes unchanged salicylates and the metabolites, salicyluric acid, salicylic phenolic and acyl glucuronides and gentisic acid. The excretion of free salicylate is increased when the urine is rendered alkaline. Plasma salicylate at any given dose is higher with a decreased glomerular filtration rate or decreased proximal tubular secretion due either to renal disease or competitive inhibition. Plasma protein binding decreases with high salicylate concentrations, hypoproteinemia or renal failure (463). Major clinical signs of salicylate intoxication include tinnitus, acid base disturbances, gastric ulceration, bleeding tendencies, central nervous system depression and nephrotoxicity, manifested by renal tubular cyturia, hematuria, leukocyturia and, rarely, tubular necrosis or papillary necrosis (6). Only a small fraction of patients with salicylate intoxication (i.e. following massive overdosage, those with plasma concentrations above 80 mg/dl (58 mmol/l), with concurrent disease or clinical deterioration) should be considered for dialysis (63). Hemodialyzer clearance exceeds 100 ml/min decreasing the plasma half life in intoxicated patients from about 16 h to 4 h (464). Comparable clearances are achieved by hemoperfusion (424, 425). Peritoneal clearances are much lower but increase with the addition of an alkaline buffer or albumin to the dialysate, and are sufficient to improve clinical intoxication (465). Maintenance of plasma concentrations in the therapeutic range in uremic patients requires dosage reduction but susceptibility to toxicity is high, nevertheless. Because salicylates inhibit prostaglandin synthetase, they can depress renal blood flow in patients with congestive heart failure, lupus erythematosus or other conditions that lead to stimulation of the renin angiotensin system and compensatory prostaglandin mediated renal vasodilatation (18).

Diflunisal, a recently introduced difluorophenyl salicylate, is normally more than 99% protein bound in plasma. Uremia decreases the binding to 54%, because of a lower association constant and competitive binding, an abnormality that hemodialysis corrects (466).

Phenacetin and its major metabolite, *acetaminophen* (paracetamol), are rapidly absorbed, only minimally bound to plasma proteins and readily diffuse into a volume of 0.9 l/kg (8, 16). Chronic high dosage is associated with papillary necrosis and chronic interstitial nephritis and, acutely, acetaminophen may cause hepatic necrosis (6, 44, 467). Analgesic nephropathy accounts for 3 to 20% of patients requiring regular dialysis for end-stage renal disease and may be complicated by uroepithelial malignancy (468, 469). These small solutes are cleared by hemodialysis at more than 100 ml/min, decreasing the plasma half life below that of conventional therapy (470, 471). Peritoneal clearances are only 3 ml/min (472). The half life of acetaminophen in normals and anephric patients is about 2.5 h as hepatic clearance of 330 ml/min yields the conjugates acetaminophen glucuronide and acetaminophen sulfate which accumulate in uremic plasma (473). Hemodialysis clears acetaminophen at 80% of urea clearance and the metabolites at 50 to 70% of urea clearance, yet dosage does not have to be modified during or after dialysis because the rapid hepatic removal predominates. Hemoperfusion clearances of 120 ml/min decrease to 30 ml/min with saturation of the charcoal column but the procedure decreases the half life (474), may be the most efficient method for rapid removal of acetaminophen (424), and can lower the incidence of hepatic abnormalities when patients are seen too late after ingestion (15 h) for N-acetylcysteine to be effective (475).

Propoxyphene is eliminated mainly by hepatic metabolism. In anephric patients, first pass metabolism is decreased, raising peak plasma concentrations, but the terminal half life is not increased (476). Hepatic clearance normally is about 800 ml/min and the half life is about 12 h (8, 476). Overdosage can cause coma and respiratory arrest, responsive to narcotic antagonists. In anuric patients with plasma concentrations in the therapeutic range, the clearance by hemodialysis is only 7 ml/min while the metabolite, norpropoxyphene, is cleared at 16 ml/min (476). With acute intoxication, however, hemodialyzer clearance may exceed 100 ml/min, possibly because the fraction bound to protein is lower, and peritoneal clearance is 8 ml/min (477). Nevertheless, because of the very large volume of distribution (10 to 25 l/kg), less than 10% of ingested propoxyphene (339 daltons and 80% protein bound) is recovered in dialysate.

The half life of *antipyrine* is significantly shorter in uremic patients (7.3 h) than in normal subjects (13.2 h), a paradox that is explained by induction of hepatic metabolism as the volume of distribution remains unchanged (478).

Pentazocine rapidly disappears from plasma by oxidation and conjugation in the liver (479). The half life is 2 to 3 h, dosage modification is not required in uremic patients and dialysis pharmacokinetics await study.

The *opiates* rapidly distribute in a large tissue volume and then are removed by dealkylation and hydrolysis in the liver and excreted in the urine (480). About 35% of *morphine* is bound in plasma, the distribution volume is 3 l/kg and the half life is 3 h (19). Most opiate excretion is as glucuronides, while about 10% appears in the urine, unchanged, by filtration and secretion at an increasing rate as the urine is acidified. Although opiates are not retained in uremic patients, there may be increased sensitivity to standard dosage. Blood levels can be decreased by dialysis, but pharmacokinetics require further study (481). About 10% of *meperidine* is excreted in the urine unchanged, while most of the drug undergoes rapid hepatic degradation to normeperidine which can induce convulsions (482). *Methadone* can be used in patients on dialysis without complications. It is about 85% protein bound in plasma and is eliminated by hepatic biotransformation (483).

Antirheumatic and anti-inflammatory drugs

Well absorbed, *indomethacin* is eliminated predominantly by hepatic biotransformation (19). Some indomethacin undergoes enterohepatic recycling and renal excretion. Renal excretion of indomethacin decreases with blockade of tubular secretion or renal failure. The half life, normally 2 to 3 h, does not increase, and dosage modification is not required in uremic patients, however. Dialysis should not remove much indomethacin (357 daltons) because about 90% is bound in plasma. Indomethacin can cause severe hyperkalemia, renal ischemia, nephrotic syndrome and interstitial nephritis with irreversible renal failure (19, 484–486).

Phenylbutazone is well absorbed and more than 95% bound in plasma. It is eliminated slowly by hepatic metabolism. With renal failure, protein binding of phenylbutazone decreases and the half life, normally 70 h, decreases slightly (487). Binding is still sufficient to inhibit removal by dialysis, however. Inhibition of prostaglandin synthetase with acute renal failure and serious hypersensitivity reactions including acute interstitial nephritis may complicate therapy (488, 489). Hemoperfusion rapidly removes phenylbutazone reducing the half life to 6 h (490).

Ibuprofen, naproxen and *fenoprofen* are propionic acid derivatives. Such nonsteroidal anti-inflammatory agents inhibit prostaglandin synthetase and can reduce renal function (49). Ibuprofen is 99% protein bound and is eliminated by metabolism with a half life of about 2 h (491). Neither accumulation in renal failure nor removal by dialysis would be likely but pharmacokinetics need further study. Naproxen is also 99% protein bound and is eliminated partly by metabolism and partly by renal excretion of the unchanged drug with a half life of about 15 h (491). The half life is not prolonged by renal failure nor decreased by hemodialysis, so dosage adjustments are not required (492, 493). Fenoprofen, which is eliminated mostly by metabolism, has caused nephrotic syndrome and reversible renal failure (494). Fenbufen also is biotransformed and its elimination half life of 11 h is not prolonged by renal failure (495). *Mefanamic acid* is a potent nonsteroidal anti-inflammatory agent that inhibits prostaglandin synthetase activity and has induced acute renal failure (496). About 90% of mefanamic acid, is protein bound in plasma and the half life, normally 4 h, is not prolonged by renal failure nor decreased by hemodialysis which achieves clearances of only 8 to 16 ml/min (497).

Colchicine is rapidly absorbed and distributes into a very large volume from which about 20% is excreted into the urine unchanged and the rest undergoes metabolism. The half life is about 2 h and does not increase with renal failure (8, 92). Gastrointestinal irritation may preclude high doses or prolonged use in renal failure. Dialysis pharmacokinetics need study, but colchicine is removed by hemoperfusion, although little clinical benefit ensues (75).

Gold salts, often effective antirheumatic drugs, are excreted slowly, mainly by the kidney, augmented by such chelates as penicillamine and dimercaprol. Almost completely protein bound in plasma, little removal by dialysis should be anticipated and accumulation would be likely in patients with renal failure. Toxicity includes cutaneous hypersensitivity reactions, bone marrow depression and nephrotoxicity, heralded by proteinuria and microhematuria, potentially leading to nephrotic syndrome or acute renal failure (498).

Probenecid, by blocking active tubular reabsorption (large doses), causes uricosuria. This effect and blockade of secretion of such organic acids as uric acid (by small doses) and penicillin, quantitatively decrease as renal failure progresses. About 80% protein bound in plasma, the half life of probenecid (285 daltons) in plasma is between 6 to 12 h with most of the elimination by extrarenal metabolism (8). Toxicity includes recurring nephrotic syndrome and chronic renal failure (499).

Sulfinpyrazone (404 daltons), a uricosuric and antiplatelet aggregating agent, is highly protein bound in plasma, and eliminated mostly by renal secretion. The half life increases from about 2.5 h to 9.5 h with severe renal failure, and it is not appreciably affected by hemodialysis (500). Sulfinpyrazone can cause acute interstitial nephritis (41).

Allopurinol (135 daltons) is rapidly metabolized to oxipurinol (alloxanthine) thereby inhibiting xanthine oxidase. Oxipurinol is excreted by the kidney with a plasma half life of 28 h (501). Accumulation of this metabolite occurs with renal failure and the dose should not exceed 300 mg (22 mmol)/day. As neither solute is protein bound, removal by dialysis is anticipated. Allopurinol can cause acute interstitial nephritis (41). It also delays elimination of azathioprine.

Immunosuppressive and antineoplastic agents

Adrenal corticosteroids are well absorbed and more than 90% protein bound in plasma. Elimination occurs by hepatic metabolism with renal excretion of inactive metabolites. Half lives are 0.5 to 4 h. Neither renal failure nor dialysis appear to affect the half lives appreciably (table 11). Hemodialyzer clearances are less than 20 ml/min, but dialysis removes cortisol metabolites (502, 503).

Azathioprine is well absorbed and distributed in total body water with about 30% protein binding in plasma. It is cleaved nonenzymatically to 6-mercaptopurine and oxidized (8). Renal failure decreases the rate of elimination of azathioprine metabolites but does not modify biologic activity, probably because very rapid metabolic inactivation of the biologically active metabolites limits the duration of activity (504). The dose does not have to be decreased as renal function declines. The incidence, precocity and duration of leukopenia is unaffected by renal failure and immunosuppressive activity also remains unchanged despite inhibition of thiopurine methyl transferase, the enzyme pertinent to metabolic disposition (79). Nevertheless, other considerations often warrant dosage reduction when renal failure occurs. High doses of 6-mercaptopurine may cause crystalluria and hematuria (505). Concurrent allopurinol therapy delays elimination of the purine analogs, e.g. azathioprine, because of the inhibition of xanthine oxidase. The dialyzer clearance of azathioprine is close to the uric acid clearance and the half life in plasma during dialysis is 4 h, only slightly below the normal value (506).

Cyclophosphamide distributes into a volume of about 0.5 l/kg and is less than 20% protein bound in plasma (8). About 90% of cyclophosphamide is biotransformed in the liver. One or more of the metabolites may function as an alkylating agent (507). Cyclophosphamide impairs free water clearance, but is not nephrotoxic. Hemorrhagic cystitis is attributed to the excretion of a metabolite. With renal failure the half life increases moderately (to 6.5 h) favoring avoidance of the drug or substantial dosage reduction with careful hematologic monitoring (508). Hemodialysis clears cyclophosphamide (261 daltons) at 104 ml/min, reducing the half life (Table 11) to about 2.5 h (508–510). Other alkylating agents such as *chlorambucil, mechlorethamine, melphalan* and *busulfan* have undergone less study in renal failure, but disappear rapidly from plasma by metabolism with half lifes of less than 2 h. It is not likely that their plasma concentrations would be influenced appreciably by dialysis or renal failure.

The nitrosoureas include *streptozocin* and *methyl CCNU* (semustine) which do not depend on renal elimination but their metabolites may have prolonged half lives in uremic patients. Streptozocin can cause reversible proximal tubular injury and renal failure (511) while treatment with methyl CCNU can be followed by progressive renal atrophy, interstitial fibrosis and renal failure (512).

The pyrimidine analogs *5-fluorouracil* and *cytosine arabinoside* are rapidly distributed and biotransformed. Renal failure does not influence their metabolic rate and, normally, little unchanged drug appears in the urine. Hemodialysis removes 37% of the 5-fluorouracil (130 daltons) that perfuses the dialyzer allowing safe regional chemotherapy perfusion, but probably affects systemic therapy considerably less because of the larger distribution volume (510).

Methotrexate is about 50% bound to plasma proteins and distributes in a volume of about 0.5 l/kg (8, 19). This folic acid analog is eliminated from plasma with a half life of about 2 h, mainly by renal excretion (513). Plasma accumulation occurs in uremic patients, but dosage modification to achieve a normal plasma concentration is complicated by the fact that plasma protein binding decreases, increasing the biologically active fraction (514). Renal failure prolongs the half life, considerably. It is not decreased by hemodialysis or peritoneal dialysis, which achieve clearances of 37 and 5 ml/min, respectively (515, 516). Hemoperfusion, especially with uncoated charcoal, achieves higher clearances but delayed intercompartmental transfer causes postperfusion rebound increments (517). In addition to bone marrow suppression, toxicity may include acute tubular necrosis (516, 518).

With renal failure, *bleomycin* is eliminated more slowly (half life exceeds 20 h) and there is no measurable removal by hemodialysis (519). Its normal half life is less than 10 h. *Doxorubicin* distributes in a very large volume and is rapidly eliminated, mostly by hepatic metabolism (8). This antineoplastic antibiotic has caused progressive glomerular lesions, tubular atrophy, interstitial nephritis and renal failure (520). Care must be taken in administering these drugs since necrosis of the hand can result from retrograde flow in an arteriovenous fistula (521). Hemoperfusion clears doxorubicin at 43 ml/min which doubles the elimination rate in animals and, *in vitro, daunorubicin* is adsorbed sufficiently by carbon to consider hemoperfusion for the treatment of clinical toxicity (522).

Dose dependent nephrotoxicity is the major hazard limiting the use of the potent antitumor agent *cis-platinum* (523, 524). More than 90% of cis-platinum in plasma is protein bound, so hemodialysis removes very little and although only a portion of its elimination occurs via the urine, renal failure prolongs the half life from about 60 h to 240 h (525).

Hypoglycemic agents

Insulin metabolism is discussed extensively in Chapter 36. Resistance to insulin characterizes renal failure, but since the elimination rate decreases by as much as 50% and body mass and caloric intake may decrease, dosage reduction is often required. Hemodialysis does not affect the elimination rate of insulin (34, 526). Insulin is absorbed from peritoneal dialysis fluid, allowing control of carbohydrate metabolism in diabetic patients, despite the high load of glucose (527).

The sulfonylureas and biguanides are hypoglycemic agents to which uremic patients have increased sensitivity. *Tolbutamide*, a sulfonylurea, is about 90% protein bound in plasma and eliminated with a half life of 5 h by oxidation to inactive metabolites normally excreted by the kidney (528). As neither renal failure nor dialysis affect plasma concentrations significantly, it is the preferred oral hypoglycemic for uremic patients. The metabolites of *tolazamide* and *acetohexamide* cause hypoglycemia and are excreted by the kidney. *Chlorpropamide,* about 90% protein bound in plasma, is slowly excreted, unchanged, by the kidney (528). Renal failure prolongs the half life from 35 h to as long as 200 h. Delayed excretion correlates better with loss of tubular function than with glomerular filtration, and the half life increases with concurrent therapy with drugs such as probenecid, chloramphenicol and probably to a lesser extent, allopurinol and clofibrate (529). Severe recurrent hypoglycemic coma has complicated renal retention of chlorpropamide (530). As plasma protein binding decreases with increased concentrations of chlorpropamide, dialysis can contribute to removal of excessive dosage (531). Chlorpropamide may induce water retention with hyponatremia and reversible and reproducible features of the syndrome of inappropriate antidiuretic hormone secretion (532).

The biguanides, *buforman* and *phenformin* have normal half lives of 2 to 3 h. They are excreted into the urine unchanged and faster in alkaline urine, although phenformin is in part metabolized (533). Phenformin should be avoided in uremic patients not only because of potential retention in plasma, but also because of the increased tendency to lactic acidosis. Although little phenformin is removed by dialysis, lactic acidosis can be improved (534, 535).

Anticonvulsants

Phenytoin (diphenylhydantoin) is eliminated mostly by oxidation followed by conjugation of the metabolite with glucuronic acid and subsequent renal excretion of the conjugate. Phenytoin is about 90% protein bound in plasma, distributes in a volume of 0.64 l/kg and has an elimination half life that is concentration dependent but averages 24 h (19). Renal failure decreases the protein binding to about 65% which has been attributed both to a compositional change in plasma proteins in uremia and to competitive binding by a uremic metabolite (31, 536, 537). At any given dose, less protein binding allows greater distribution to sites of action and metabolism. Accordingly, the half life decreases in renal failure to about 8 h (Table 11). No dosage modification is recommended and phenytoin is usually well tolerated in uremic patients. Conjugated 4-hydroxyphenytoin is retained in the plasma of uremic patients (538). Osteomalacia may complicate chronic use and acute interstitial nephritis is a potential hazard (47, 539). Decreased protein binding allows a dialyzer clearance of about 12 ml/min in uremic patients but only a small fraction is removed from the large distribution volume and the half life is 15 h (540). Both peritoneal dialysis and hemodialysis have been clinically effective in treating massive overdosages of phenytoin (541, 542) despite low clearances (23% of peritoneal dialysate flow rate (543) and 31 ml/min (544) by hemodialysis). At high plasma concentrations the half life increases because of saturation kinetics, so these clearances and those achieved by carbon hemoperfusion (12 to 48 ml/min) lower the half life (545).

Liver injury increases the potency and duration of action of the oxazolidine anticonvulsants, *trimethadione* and *paramethadione*, but nephrectomy prolongs and potentiates only paramethadione activity in the rat (546). Hypersensitivity to the oxazolidines may be manifested by the nephrotic syndrome with minimal glomerular changes (547).

Valproic acid is an anticonvulsant that is normally about 80% protein bound in plasma, distributes in a volume of about 0.78 l/kg and is eliminated by β oxidation with a half life of 13 h (19, 548). Renal failure decreases the concentration dependent protein binding to about 70% but does not delay the elimination nor does the hemodialyzer clearance of 23 ml/min accelerate it, so dosage adjustment is not necessary (548).

Carbamazepine, an anticonvulsant, also used for treatment of trigeminal neuralgia, has caused reversible acute renal failure (549). It is normally eliminated slowly and the clearance by hemodialysis (54 ml/min) can exceed endogenous plasma clearance (28 ml/min) despite 70% protein binding in plasma (550).

Vitamins

Nutrition in uremic patients, which is discussed in Chapter 27, usually includes vitamin supplementation. The fat soluble *vitamin A*, which is degraded metabolically, circulates bound to protein and is extensively stored in tissues, notably the liver. In renal failure, plasma vitamin A increases from 1.4 to 3.6 µmol/l (65, 551), although vitamin A is normally absent in urine and only appears coincident with proteinuria. The increment in vitamin A levels correlates with increases in plasma cholesterol and triglycerides, does not decrease with discontinuation of dietary supplements and is reduced only minimally by hemodialysis (552, 553). As discussed in greater detail in Chapter 35, *vitamin D* is converted by the kidney to the metabolically active form, 1,25 dihydroxycholecalciferol. Accordingly, vitamin D resistance occurs in renal failure, causing hypocalcemic osteodystrophy. Because of this vitamin D resistance and awareness that overdosage of vitamin D can precipitate or aggravate renal failure (554, 555), vitamin D has been used cautiously in uremic patients. The availability of 1,25 dihydroxycholecalciferol and potent analogues has been valuable for adjunctive treatment of renal osteodystrophy but can cause hypercalcemia and further deterioration of renal function (556, 557).

Thiamin, a water soluble B vitamin, is stored in tissues and metabolically degraded, appearing in the urine only when tissue depots are saturated. Plasma concentrations increase slightly with renal failure and decrease with hemodialysis but only by about 10% because of protein binding (558). Nevertheless, unless supplemented, maintenance dialysis patients may have low plasma concentrations (65). About 10% of *riboflavin* is excreted into the urine and the metabolic fate of the remainder is unknown. Plasma riboflavin concentrations increase significantly with renal failure and dialyzer clearance is about 25% of urea clearance (559). With adequate dietary intake, supplements should not be required after dialysis. *Nicotinic acid* and *nicotinamide* are eliminated mainly by metabolism, but the kidney contributes more importantly to elimination when very high doses are given. Plasma levels decrease minimally with dialysis and may be decreased in uremic patients (560). *Pyridoxine,* a small solute is eliminated metabolically. Deficiency of pyridoxine in uremic patients can manifest decreased erythrocyte transaminase activity, diminished reactivity of lymphocytes and neuropathy (65, 561). Dialysis pharmacokinetics have not been studied thoroughly. *Pantothenic acid* is excreted primarily by the kidney. Elevated plasma concentrations in uremic patients are decreased by about 30% by dialysis (561). As *biotin* is also excreted by the kidney, increased plasma concentrations may occur with renal failure (561). Plasma concentrations change minimally with dialysis, but kinetics have not been studied extensively. *Folic acid* is partially bound in plasma and at low concentrations, little appears in urine. High plasma concentrations are mainly excreted by the kidney. Maintenance dialysis patients may become depleted as the dialyzer clearance can exceed 50 ml/min, but tissue storage limits removal and plasma concentrations usually remain above 7 ng/ml (16 nmol/l) (562, 563). Peritoneal dialysis can also induce folate depletion (564). *Cyanocobalamin* is stored in the liver, is excreted by the kidney, and is cleared very slowly by dialysis because of its large size and partial protein binding (560). Hemofiltration can remove it more rapidly. Dietary vitamin B_{12} should keep most patients from deficiency, maintaining plasma concentrations between 200 and 900 pg/ml (150 and 660 pmol/l). *Ascorbic acid* is mostly metabolized, but high doses are excreted by the kidney. One of the metabolites, oxalate may accumulate in tissues of uremic patients, including kidney, potentially accelerating renal failure (565). As dialysis decreases plasma ascorbic acid by about 40%, supplements may be required (566). Maintenance dialysis patients may have low plasma *vitamin E* concentrations (65).

Metals and chelates

Pharmacokinetics of organic gold salts, platinum and mercury have been discussed under antirheumatics, antineoplastics and diuretics, respectively. *Iron,* which may gain access to the circulation from dialysate (66), is removed to a greater extent as blood is lost leading to iron deficiency, discussed in detail in Chapter 32. Oral iron is satisfactorily absorbed in uremic patients and can improve iron deficiency anemia (23, 567). Parenteral iron dextran also repletes iron stores but may not be utilized as well and can be followed by hemosiderosis (23, 568). The treatment of renal osteodystrophy (Chapter 35) with *aluminum* hydroxide phosphate binding gels can lead to hyperaluminumemia (569), one of the trace metal abnormalities discussed in Chapters 41 and 42. Contamination of dialysate water, however, is usually the predominant source of aluminum, the protein binding of which inhibits removal by dialysis (570). Chelation with desferrioxamine can augment removal of aluminum by dialysis, however (571). *Phosphate* depletion may result from excessive use of these oral sorbents leading not only to osteomalacia, but also to an encephalopathy, possibly also related to aluminum intoxication (572, 573). The *magnesium* content of antacids and of laxatives also may accumulate, leading to an encephalopathy. *Cobalt* toxicity may occur in maintenance dialysis patients treated with cobaltous chloride and this metal, normally eliminated by the kidney, should be avoided in uremic patients (574). Organic *antimonials* are also excreted primarily by the kidney and may accumulate in patients with renal failure when treated for protozoal infections (575). *Arsenicals* and *bismuth* preparations are not only dangerous in patients with renal disease because of their retention, but also because of potential nephrotoxicity aggravating renal failure (6). In general, protein binding limits removal of metals during hemodialysis but they may enter the blood from the dialysate (55, 576). With the addition of a chelate, the complexed metals may diffuse out of blood, usually slowly, but often faster than the removal rate by the injured kidney (236, 577). Although measurable quantities of $^{67}gallium$-citrate are found in hemodialysate, removal rates are low and do not interfere with imaging techniques (578).

Chelating agents tightly bind metal ions and these metallocomplexes are excreted unchanged by the kidney. Renal failure impairs their therapeutic effectiveness. *Dimercaprol* binds those metals that have affinity for sulfhydryl groups. It accumulates in patients with renal failure, potentially causing hypoglycemia and can be removed slowly by dialysis (579). Excreted by both glomerular filtration and tubular secretion, *calcium disodium edetate* should accumulate in renal failure patients and can cause nephrotoxicity related at least partly to transtubular transport of the dissociable metallocomplexes (580). *Penicillamine,* rapidly excreted into the urine, effectively binds such metals as copper, lead and mercury and potentially accumulates in renal failure. Hypersensitivity toxic reactions include nephrotic syndrome (581, 582). Dialysance of *diethylenetriaminepentaacetic acid,* exceeding 40 ml/min, provides a mechanism for treating hemosiderosis in uremic patients (125, 236). *Desferrioxamine,* another iron chelate, is also excreted by the kidney and should be removed slowly by dialysis. Desferrioxamine has induced acute renal failure (583).

Miscellaneous drugs

Neither heparin nor the oral anticoagulants are removed by dialysis. *Heparin,* more than 8,000 daltons and extensively protein bound, is eliminated by enzymatic degradation with a half life of less than 2 h, and is unaffected by renal failure (8, 19). *Bishydroxycoumarin* is more than 99% bound in plasma and eliminated by hepatic metabolism. Renal failure does not prolong the effect on prothrombin time (584). Sodium *warfarin,* which is about 97% protein bound in plasma, is eliminated slowly, by metabolism, with a normal half life of about 40 h (8, 19). Protein binding decreases with renal failure and the half life may be somewhat shorter. *Phenindione* therapy is occasionally complicated by sensitivity reactions including severe dermatitis, leukocytosis, proteinuria, edema and tubular necrosis (585). Caution is advised with the use of oral anticoagulants, not because of increased responsiveness, but because of the bleeding diathesis and lesions of uremia (586).

Antiplatelet aggregating agents, including *dipyridamole* and *prostacyclin,* have been used to maintain shunt patency, reduce heparin dose or eliminate it or augment peritoneal transport rates (85, 587, 588). Their pharmacokinetics are not appreciably influenced by uremia or by dialysis. (The half life of prostacyclin is only 3 to 5 min.) *Ticlopidine,* another inhibitor of platelet aggregation, decreases thrombotic episodes in arteriovenous shunts and grafts increasing urea clearance (589).

Since *propylthiouracil* is excreted in part by the kidney, the half life is prolonged from about 17 h to about 50 h and dosage should be reduced (92). Dialysis kinetics have not been studied. *Methimazole* is also partly excreted by the kidney and partly metabolized. Dosage reduction is recommended as renal failure prolongs the half life (Table 11) from 2 to 9 h (1, 92).

Iodide is excreted by the kidney by filtration and reabsorption in competition with thyroidal uptake (590). Because protein binding is minimal with high dosage, dialysis is an effective mechanism of iodide removal. The iodinated radiographic contrast media normally excreted by the kidney, with half lives of less than an hour (Table 11), accumulate in patients with renal failure as the half life is prolonged to about 30 h (591). Hemodialysis decreases the half life to 4 h. Hemodialyzer clearances exceed 50% of urea clearances and peritoneal clearance is 7 ml/min (592, 593). Nephrotoxicity, the most important complication of radiographic studies with iodides, occurs with a variety of contrast media and is a function of the structural configuration of the organic iodide, the percentage of iodine, the dose used and the site of injection (594–596). Care should be taken to avoid dehydration or manipulations that decrease renal blood flow prior to iodide radiography, particularly in those with preexisting impairment of renal function. Acute renal failure, a recognized complication of infusion pyelography, can easily be misinterpreted as natural progression of the underlying renal disease.

The kidney excretes *clofibrate* (242 daltons), in part unchanged, and also after hepatic conjugation. As the half life increases from 17 h to 100 h with renal failure, significant dosage reduction is mandatory (591, 598). Removal of clofibrate by dialysis is limited by 95% protein binding, which decreases somewhat in uremic patients. The dose should be lowered from 1.5 to 2.0 g/day to 1.0 to 1.5 g (4 to 6 mmol) per week to avoid toxicity including ataxia, muscle weakness, gastrointestinal disturbances and increased creatinine phosphokinase, while maintaining the lipid lowering effect (597, 598). Acute interstitial nephritis with renal failure also may complicate therapy (599).

Gallamine is a muscle relaxant eliminated almost exclusively by the kidney. It should be avoided in patients with renal failure as neuromuscular blockade due to gallamine will be prolonged, but it can be removed by dialysis which achieves a clearance of only 13 ml/min but reduces plasma levels by 61% (600, 601). Preexisting renal functional impairment may predispose to further loss of renal function due to the toxic effects of the fluorinated anesthetics, *enflurane* and *methoxyflurane* (602). Up to 50% of *atropine* is excreted by the kidney and caution is advised when atropine is used in uremic patients (603). Hemodialysis also clears *dimethyltubocurarine* and *alcuronium* at about 20 ml/min, reducing plasma concentrations by more than 50% (601). A detailed discussion of anesthesia for renal failure patients is given in Chapter 40.

Cimetidine (252 daltons), a reversible competitive antagonist of histamine H_2 receptor action, is excreted mostly by the kidney. About 20% of cimetidine is protein bound in plasma and the distribution volume is 2.1 l/kg (19). With renal failure, the elimination half life increases from 1.9 h to 4.3 h (Table 11) as the elimination rate correlates with creatinine clearance (604, 605). Cimetidine increases plasma creatinine concentrations possibly by decreasing secretion but does not decrease glomerular filtration rate or other parameters of renal function (606, 607). In uremic patients, cimetidine dosage must be reduced to 300 mg (1.2 mmol)/12 h, half of the usual dose, to prevent toxicity consisting of drowsiness, dizziness, confusion, flushing, sweating, diarrhea, muscular pain and rash (608), symptoms that can mimic uremia. Cimetidine decreases hepatic blood flow, impairing metabolism of drugs such as diazepam, antipyrine and propranolol (358, 609). Cimetidine also reversibly lowers circulating levels of immunoreactive parathyroid hormone without affecting serum concentrations of calcium, phosphorus or magnesium (610). Hemodialysis clears cimetidine at 30 to 40 ml/min, reducing the half life to 2.5 h (605, 606) and reducing plasma concentrations by about 70% (608). Peritoneal clearance of cimetidine ranges from 3 to 10 ml/min, insufficient to affect pharmacokinetics appreciably (611, 612), but hemoperfusion clears cimetidine at 85 ml/min which compares with the normal elimination rate of 350 ml/min and with a clearance of 130 ml/min when renal failure occurs (612).

CONCLUSIONS

In choosing a drug for the uremic patient, it is preferable, when possible, to select one that normally does not depend primarily on renal excretion, one that is little affected by changes in plasma protein binding, distribution volume or receptor sensitivity and one that is not complicated by active or toxic metabolites (359). For example, diazepam is preferable to barbiturates, alkylating agents are preferable to methotrexate and synthetic penicillins are preferable to tetracyclines and aminoglycosides.

Pharmacokinetic principles must be followed in caring for uremic patients. The physician who must rely blindly on nomograms and 'cookbook' style guidelines to adjust dosage in the treatment of renal disease has no business administering potentially toxic drugs to patients with impaired renal function (22).

ACKNOWLEDGEMENT

The opinions and assertions contained herein are the private views of the author and should not be construed as official or as necessarily reflecting the views of the Uniformed Services University of the Health Sciences or Department of Defense. There is no objection to publication. Because data are acquired rapidly in this field the reader is advised to check package inserts and current literature for pertinent new findings.

The author appreciates the helpful suggestions of Dr. Thomas Gibson (Northwestern University, Chicago, IL) and those of Dr. Carl Peck (USUHS, Bethesda, MD) in revising the chapter from the first edition. The extensive and excellent secretarial assistance of Mrs. Barbara Fitzgerald is greatly appreciated.

REFERENCES

1. Reidenberg MM: *Renal Function and Drug Action.* Philadelphia, WB Saunders Co, 1971
2. Fabre J, Balant L, Chavaz A: Recent drug management advances in renal insufficiency. *Adv Nephrol* 4:223, 1974
3. Whelton A: Antibacterial chemotherapy in renal insufficiency. A review. *Antibiot Chemother* 18:1, 1974
4. Dedrick RL: Pharmacokinetic and pharmacodynamic considerations for chronic hemodialysis. *Kidney Int* 7 (Suppl 2):S7, 1975
5. Kerr DNS, Dettli L, Rawlins M, Leber HW, Maddocks J: Drug metabolism in chronic renal failure. *Proc Eur Dial Transpl Assoc* 13:597, 1976
6. Maher JF: Toxic and irradiation nephropathies in *Strauss and Welt's Diseases of the Kidney,* Edited by Earley LE, Gottschalk CW, Boston, Little, Brown and Co, 1979, p 1431
7. Winchester JF, Gelfand MC, Knepshield JH, Schreiner GE: Dialysis and hemoperfusion of poisons and drugs – update. *Trans Am Soc Artif Intern Organs* 23:762, 1977
8. Bennett WM, Muther RS, Parker RA, Feig P, Morrison G, Golper TA, Singer I: Drug therapy in renal failure: dosing guidelines for adults. *Ann Intern Med* 93:62, 286, 1980
9. Richet G, deNovales EL, Verroust P: Drug intoxication and neurological episodes in chronic renal failure. *Br Med J* 2:394, 1970
10. Smith JW, Seidl LG, Cluff LE: Studies on the epidemiology of adverse drug reaction. V. Clinical factors influencing susceptibility. *Ann Intern Med* 65:629, 1966
11. Cutler RE, Christopher TG, Forrey AW, Blair AD: Modification of drug therapy in chronic dialysis patients. *Kidney Int* 7 (Suppl 2):S16, 1975
12. Schreiner GE, Maher JF: *Uremia: Biochemistry, Pathogenesis and Treatment.* Springield IL, Charles C Thomas Co, 1961
13. Atkinson AJ Jr, Kushner W: Clinical pharmacokinetics. *Annu Rev Pharmacol Toxicol* 19:105, 1979
14. Gibson TP: Effect of renal disease on pharmacokinetics and bioavailability. *Proc Conf Chr Renal Dis, NIH* (in press)
15. Talki S, Gambertoglio JG, Honda DH, Tozer TN: Pharmacokinetic evaluation of hemodialysis in acute drug overdose. *J Pharmacokinet Biopharm* 6:427, 1978
16. Gibson TP, Nelson HA: Drug kinetics and artificial kidneys. *Clin Pharmacokinet* 2:403, 1977
17. Bennett WM: Drugs and the kidney in *Contemporary Nephrology,* edited by Klahr S, Massry SG, New York, London, Plenum Med Book Co, 1981, p 657
18. Welling PG, Craig WA: Pharmacokinetics in disease states modifying renal function in *The Effect of Disease States on Pharmacokinetics,* edited by Benet LZ, Washington, Am Pharm Assoc Acad Pharm Sci, 1976, p 155
19. Benet LZ, Sheiner LB: Design and optimization of dosage regimens; pharmacokinetic data in *The Pharmacological Basis of Therapeutics,* edited by Gilman AG, Goodman LS, Gilman A, 6th edn, New York, MacMillan Publ Co, 1980, p 1675
20. Dettli L: Drug dosage in renal disease. *Clin Pharmacokinet* 1:126, 1976
21. Fabre J, Balant L: Renal failure, drug pharmacokinetics and drug action. *Clin Pharmacokinet* 1:99, 1976
22. Levy G: Pharmacokinetics in renal disease. *Am J Med* 62:461, 1977
23. Parker PA, Izard MW, Maher JF: Therapy of iron deficiency in patients on maintenance dialysis. *Nephron* 23:181, 1979
24. Schindhelm K, Skalsky M, Mahoney JF, Farrell PC: Creatinine transfer between interstitial and intracellular fluid: a comparison between normal and uremic subjects. *asaio J* 2:25, 1979
25. Maher JF: Interrelation of hemoperfusion, plasma clearance and half life in *Artificial Kidney, Artificial Liver and Artificial Cells,* edited by Chang TMS, New York and London, Plenum Press, 1978, p 297
26. Boobis SW: Alteration of plasma albumin in relation to decreased drug binding in uremia. *Clin Pharmacol Ther* 22:147, 1977
27. Reidenberg MM: The binding of drugs to plasma proteins and the interpretation of measurements of plasma concentrations of drugs in patients with poor renal function. *Am J Med* 62:467, 1977
28. Lichtenwalner DM, Suh B, Lorber B, Rudnick MR, Craig WA: Partial purification and characterization of the drug-binding-defect inducer in uremia. *J Lab Clin Med* 97:72, 1981
29. Depner TA, Gulyassy PF: Plasma protein binding in uremia: extraction and characterization of an inhibitor. *Kidney Int* 18:86, 1980
30. Bowmer CJ, Lindup WE: Investigation of the drug-binding defect in plasma from rats with glycerol-induced acute renal failure. *J Pharmacol Exp Ther* 210:440, 1979
31. Reidenberg MM, Odar-Cederlöf I, von Bahr C, Borga ML, Sjoqvist F: Protein binding of diphenylhydantoin and desmethylimipramine in plasma from patients with poor renal function. *N Engl J Med* 285:264, 1971
32. Jusko WJ, Weintraub M: Myocardial distribution of digoxin and renal function. *Clin Pharmacol Ther* 16:449, 1974
33. Weiner IM: Mechanisms of drug absorption and excretion. *Annu Rev Pharmacol* 7:39, 1967
34. Navalesi R, Pilo A, Lenzi S, Donato L: Insulin metabolism in chronic uremia and in the anephric state: effect of the dialytic treatment. *J Clin Endocrinol Metab* 40:70, 1975
35. Emmanuel DS, Lindheimer MD, Katz AI: Uremia in rats with normal kidneys: a model for the study of renal function in a uremic environment. *Kidney Int* 11:209, 1977
36. Maher JF, Schreiner GE: Studies on ethacrynic acid in patients with refractory edema. *Ann Intern Med* 62:15, 1965
37. Kunin CM: Limitations upon the use of antibiotics imposed by renal insufficiency. *Modern Treatment* 7:355, 1970
38. Bailey GL, Hampers CL, Merrill JP: Reversible cardiomyopathy in uremia. *Trans Am Soc Artif Intern Organs* 13:263, 1967
39. Richards RK, Taylor JD, Kueter KE: Effect of nephrectomy on the duration of sleep following the administration of thiopental and hexobarbital. *J Pharmacol Exp Ther* 108:461, 1953
40. Freeman RB, Sheff MF, Maher JF, Schreiner GE: The blood-cerebrospinal fluid barrier in uremia. *Ann Intern Med* 56:233, 1962
41. Roxe DM: Toxic nephropathy from diagnostic and therapeutic agents. Review and commentary. *Am J Med* 69:759, 1980
42. Schreiner GE: Drug related nephropathy. *Contrib Nephrol* 10:30, 1978
43. Lee HA: Drug related disease and the kidney. *Br Med J* 1:104, 1979
44. Dawborn JD, Fairley KF, Kincaid-Smith P, King WE: The association of peptic ulceration, chronic renal disease and analgesic abuse. *Q J Med* 35:69, 1966
45. Nanra RS, Fairley KF, Kincaid-Smith P: Recovery of renal function in patients with analgesic nephropathy.

Aust Ann Med 19:195, 1970
46. Gonwa TA, Corbett WT, Schey HM, Buckalew VM Jr: Analgesic associated nephropathy and transitional cell carcinoma of the urinary tract. Ann Intern Med 93:249, 1980
47. Heptinstall RH: Interstitial nephritis: a brief review. Am J Path 83:214, 1976
48. Linton AL, Clark WF, Driedger AA, Turnbull DI, Lindsay RM: Acute interstitial nephritis due to drugs. Review of the literature with a report of nine cases. Ann Intern Med 93:735, 1980
49. Kimberly RP, Bowden RE, Keiser HR, Plotz PH: Reduction of renal function by newer nonsteroidal anti-inflammatory drugs. Am J Med 64:804, 1978
50. Lasrich M, Maher JM, Hirszel P, Maher JF: Correlation of peritoneal transport rates with molecular weight: a method for predicting clearances. asaio J 2:107, 1979
51. Colton CK, Smith KA, Merrill EW, Farrell PC: Permeability studies with cellulosic membranes. J Biomed Mater Res 5:459, 1971
52. Nolph KD, Nothum RJ, Maher JF: Ultrafiltration: a mechanism for removal of intermediate molecular weight substances in coil dialyzers. Kidney Int 6:55, 1974
53. Nolph KD, Bass OE, Maher JF: Acute effects of hemodialysis on removal of intracellular solutes. Trans Am Soc Artif Inter Organs 20:622, 1974
54. Bass OE, Nolph KD, Maher JF: Dialysance and clearance measurements during clinical dialysis – a plea for standardization. J Lab Clin Med 86:378, 1975
55. Maher JF, Montero G, Chieffo S: Tin protein binding kinetics in normal and uremic plasma and its effect on dialysis fluxes. Trans Am Soc Artif Inter Organs 22:149, 1976
56. Maher JF, Schreiner GE, Marc-Aurele J: Methodologic problems associated with in vitro measurements of dialysance. Trans Am Soc Artif Intern Organs 5:120, 1959
57. Maher JF: Selective dialysis for removal of large solutes, a reappraisal. Kidney Int 7 (Suppl 3):S361, 1975
58. Maher JF: Principles of dialysis and dialysis of drugs. Am J Med 62:475, 1977
59. Marc-Aurele J, Schreiner GE: The dialysance of ethanol and methanol: a proposed method for the treatment of massive intoxication by ethyl or methyl alcohol. J Clin Invest 39:892, 1960
60. Maher JF: Determinants of serum half life of glutethimide in intoxicated patients. J Pharmacol Exp Therap 174:450, 1970
61. Setter JG, Freeman RB, Maher JF, Schreiner GE: Factors influencing the dialysis of barbiturates. Trans Am Soc Artif Intern Organs 10:340, 1964
62. Schmitt GW, Maher JF, Schreiner GE: Ethacrynic acid enhanced bromuresis. A comparison with peritoneal and hemodialysis. J Lab Clin Med 68:913, 1966
63. Schreiner GE: The role of hemodialysis (artificial kidney) in acute poisoning. Arch Intern Med 102:896, 1958
64. Brodie BB, Bernstein E, Mark LC: The role of body fat in limiting the duration of action of thiopental. J Pharmacol Exp Therap 105:421, 1952
65. Kopple JD, Swenseid ME: Vitamin nutrition in patients undergoing maintenance hemodialysis. Kidney Int 7 (Suppl 2):S79, 1975
66. Maher JF, Freeman RB, Schmitt G, Schreiner GE: Adherence of metals to cellophane and removal by whole blood. A mechanism for solute transport during hemodialysis. Trans Am Soc Artif Intern Organs 11:104, 1965
67. Rumpf KW, Rieger J, Ansorg R, Doht B, Scheler F: Binding of antibiotics by dialysis membranes and its clinical relevance. Proc Eur Dial Transpl Assoc 14:607, 1977
68. Maher JF, Hirszel P, Hohnadel DC, Abraham J, Lasrich M: Fatty acid removal during peritoneal dialysis: mechanisms, rates and significance. asaio J 1:8, 1978
69. Dedrick RL, Myers CE, Bungay PM, De Vita VT Jr: Pharmacokinetic rationale for peritoneal drug administration in the treatment of ovarian cancer. Cancer Treat Rep 62:1, 1978
70. Henderson LW: Hemofiltration. Kidney Int 13 (Suppl 8):S145, 1978
71. Bergström J, Asaba H, Fürst P, Oulès R: Dialysis, ultrafiltration and blood pressure. Proc Eur Dial Transpl Assoc 13:293, 1977
72. Kramer P, Matthaei D, Fuchs C, Arnold R, Ebert R, McIntosh C, Schauder P, Schwinn G, Scheler F, Ludwig H, Spittelu G: Assessment of hormone loss through hemofiltration. Artif Organs 2:128, 1978
73. Chang TMS: Hemoperfusion alone and in series with ultrafiltration or dialysis for uremia, poisoning and liver failure. Kidney Int 10, (Suppl 7):S305, 1976
74. Rosenbaum JL, Kramer MS, Raja R, Winsten S, Dalal F: Hemoperfusion for acute drug intoxication. Kidney Int 10 (Suppl 7):S341, 1976
75. Bismuth C, Conso F, Wattel F, Gosselin B, Lambert H, Genestal M: Coated activated charcoal hemoperfusion. Experience of French antipoison centers in 60 cases. Vet Hum Toxicol 2:81, 1979
76. Farrell PC: Acute drug intoxication and extracorporeal intervention. asaio J 3:39, 1980
77. Pond S, Rosenberg J, Benowitz NL, Takki S: Pharmacokinetics of haemoperfusion for drug overdose. Clin Pharmacokin 4:329, 1979
78. Sofer S, Wills RA, Van Wie BJ: A model enzymic extracorporeal detoxification system. Artif Organs 3:147, 1979
79. Pazmiño P, Sladek SL, Weinshilboum RM: Thiol S-methylation in uremia: Erythrocyte enzyme activities and plasma inhibitors. Clin Pharmacol Ther 28:356, 1980
80. Nolph KD, Popovich RP, Ghods AJ, Twardowski ZJ: Determinants of low clearances of small solutes during peritoneal dialysis. Kidney Int 13:117, 1978
81. Nolph KD: The first hemodialyzer. asaio J 1:2, 1978
82. Maher JF: Characteristics of peritoneal transport: physiological and clinical implications. Miner Electrolyte Metab 5:201, 1981
83. Maher JF: Peritoneal transport rates: mechanisms, limitations and methods for augmentation. Kidney Int 18 (Suppl 10):S117, 1980
84. Nolph KD, Ghods AJ, Brown PA, Twardowski ZJ: Effects of intraperitoneal nitroprusside on peritoneal clearances in man with variations of dose, frequency of administration and dwell times. Nephron 24:114, 1979
85. Maher JF, Hirszel P, Lasrich M: An experimental model for study of pharmacologic and hormonal influences on peritoneal dialysis. Contrib Nephrol 17:131, 1979
86. Zelman A, Gisser D, Whittam PJ, Parsons RH, Schuyler R: Augmentation of peritoneal dialysis efficiency with programmed hyper/hypo-osmotic dialysates. Trans Am Soc Artif Intern Organs 23:203, 1977
87. Hirszel P, Lasrich M, Maher JF: Augmentation of peritoneal mass transport by dopamine. Comparison with norepinephrine and evaluation of pharmacologic mechanisms. J Lab Clin Med 94:747, 1979
88. Maher JF, Hirszel P, Lasrich M: Effects of gastrointestinal hormones on transport by peritoneal dialysis. Kidney Int 16:130, 1979
89. Popovich RP, Moncrief JW, Nolph KD, Ghods AJ, Twardowski ZJ, Pyle WK: Continuous ambulatory peritoneal dialysis. Ann Intern Med 88:449, 1978
90. Bennett WM, Plamp CE, Gilbert DN, Parker RA, Porter

GA: The influence of dosage regimen on experimental gentamicin nephrotoxicity: dissociation of peak serum levels from renal failure. *J Infect Dis* 140:576, 1979
91. Tozer TN: Nomogram for modification of dosage regimens in patients with chronic renal function impairment. *J Pharmacokinet Biopharm* 2:13, 1974
92. Anderson RJ, Gambertoglio JG, Schrier RW: *Fate of drugs in renal failure,* in The Kidney, edited by Brenner BM, Rector FC Jr Philadelphia, WB Saunders Co 1976, p 1911
93. Kaloyanides GJ, Pastoriza-Munoz E: Aminoglycoside nephrotoxicity. *Kidney Int* 18:571, 1980
94. Cronin RE: Aminoglycoside nephrotoxicity: pathogenesis and prevention. *Clin Nephrol* 11:251, 1979
95. Henrich WL, Thompson P, Bergström G, Lum SM: Effect of dialysis on hearing acuity. *Nephron* 18:348, 1977
96. McQuillen MP, Cantor HE, O'Rourke JR: Myasthenic syndromes associated with antibiotics. *Arch Neurol* 18:402, 1968
97. McDermott W: Toxicity of streptomycin. *Am J Med* 2:491, 1947
98. Edwards KDG, Whyte HM: Streptomycin poisoning in renal failure. *Br Med J* 1:753, 1959
99. Goodwin NJ, Thomson GE, Friedman EA: Antituberculous therapy during maintenance hemodialysis. *Abstracts Am Soc Nephrol* 1:25, 1967
100. De Beukelaer MM, Travis LB, Dodge WF, Guerra FA: Deafness and acute tubular necrosis following parenteral administration of neomycin. *Am J Dis Child* 121:250, 1971
101. Krumlovsky FA, Emmerman J, Parker RH. Wisgerhof M, Del Greco F: Dialysis in treatment of neomycin overdosage. *Ann Intern Med* 76:443, 1972
102. Yow EM, Abu-Nasser H: Kanamycin: A reevaluation after three years experience, in *2nd Int Symposium Chemother* edited by Kuemmerle HP, Basel, S Karger, 1963, p 148
103. Toyoda Y, Tachibana M: Tissue levels of kanamycin in correlation with oto and nephrotoxicity. *Acta Otolaryngol (Stockh)* 86:9, 1978
104. Cutler RE, Orme BM: Correlation of serum creatinine concentration and kanamycin half life. *JAMA* 209:539, 1969
105. Danish M, Schultz R, Jusko WJ: Pharmacokinetics of gentamicin and kanamycin during hemodialysis. *Antimicrob Agents Chemother* 6:841, 1974
106. Greenberg PA, Sanford JP: Removal and absorption of antibiotics in patients with renal failure undergoing peritoneal dialysis. Tetracycline, chloramphenicol, kanamycin and colistimethate. *Ann Intern Med* 66:465, 1967
107. Atkins RC, Mion C, Despaux E, Van-Hai N, Julien C, Mion H: Peritoneal transfer of kanamycin and its use in peritoneal dialysis. *Kidney Int* 3:391, 1973
108. Wilfert JN, Burke JP, Bloomer HA, Smith CB: Renal insufficiency associated with gentamicin therapy. *J Infect Dis* 124:S148, 1971
109. Luft FC, Patel V, Yum MN, Patel B, Kleit SA: Experimental aminoglycoside nephrotoxicity. *J Lab Clin Med* 86:213, 1975
110. Milman N: Renal failure associated with gentamicin therapy. *Acta Med Scand* 196:87, 1974
111. Gary NE, Buzzeo L, Salaki J, Eisinger RP: Gentamicin-associated acute renal failure. *Arch Intern Med* 136:1101, 1976
112. Christopher TG, Korn D, Blair AD, Forrey AW, O'Neill MA, Cutler RE: Gentamicin pharmacokinetics during hemodialysis. *Kidney Int* 3:38, 1974
113. McHenry MC, Gavan TL, Gifford RW, Guerkink NA, Van Ommen RA, Town MA, Wagner JG: Gentamicin dosages for renal insufficiency. Adjustments based on endogneous creatinine clearance and serum creatinine concentration. *Ann Intern Med* 74:192, 1971
114. Gailiunas P, Dominguez-Moreno M, Lazarus JM, Lowrie EG, Gottlieb MN, Merrill JP: Vestibular toxicity of gentamicin. Incidence in patients receiving long-term hemodialysis therapy. *Arch Intern Med* 138:1621, 1978
115. Dahlgren JG, Anderson ET, Hewitt WL: Gentamicin blood levels: a guide to nephrotoxicity. *Antimicrob Agents Chemother* 8:58, 1975
116. Hull JH, Sarubbi FA: Gentamicin serum concentrations: pharmacokinetic predictions. *Ann Intern Med* 85:183, 1976
117. Letourneau-Saheb L, Lapierre L, Daigneault R, Prud'Homme M, St-Louis G, Sirois G: Gentamicin pharmacokinetics during hemodialysis in patients suffering from chronic renal failure. *Int J Clin Pharmacol Biopharm* 15:116, 1977
118. Rosenbaum JL, Levine J, Falk B, Raja R, Kramer MS: Effect of hemoperfusion on clearance of gentamicin, cephalothin and clindamycin from plasma of normal dogs. *J Infect Dis* 136:801, 1977
119. Jusko WJ, Balia T, Kim KH, Gerbachy LM, Yaffe SJ: Pharmacodynamics of gentamicin during peritoneal dialysis in children. *Kidney Int* 9:430, 1976
120. Lane AZ, Wright GE, Blair DC: Ototoxicity and nephrotoxicity of amikacin. An overview of phase II and phase III experience in the United States. *Am J Med* 62:911, 1977
121. Regeur L, Golding H, Jensen H, Kaupmann JP: Pharmacokinetics of amikacin during hemodialysis and peritoneal dialysis. *Antimicrob Agents Chemother* 11:214, 1977
122. Madhavan T, Yaremchuk K, Levin N, Pohlad D, Burch K, Fisher E, Cox F, Quinn EL: Effect of renal failure and dialysis on the serum concentration of the aminoglycoside amikacin. *Antimicrob Agents Chemother* 10:464, 1976
123. Ho PWL. Pien FD, Kominami N: Massive amikacin 'overdose'. *Ann Intern Med* 91:227, 1979
124. Pechere J, Dugal R: Pharmacokinetics of intravenously administered tobramycin in normal volunteers and in renal-impaired and hemodialyzed patients. *J Infect Dis* 134:S118, 1976
125. Christopher TG, Blair AD, Forrey AW, Cutler RE: Hemodialyzer clearances of gentamicin, kanamycin, tobramycin, amikacin, ethambutol, procainamide and flucytosine with a technique for planning therapy. *J Pharmacokinet Biopharm* 4:427, 1976
126. Malacoff RF, Finkelstein FD, Andriole VT: Effect of peritoneal dialysis on serum levels of tobramycin and clindamycin. *Antimicrob Agents Chemother* 8:574, 1975
127. Navarini A, Montanari A, Bruschi G, Rossi E, Borghetti A, Migone L: The kinetics of aminosidine in renal patients with different degrees of renal failure. *Clin Nephrol* 4:23, 1975
128. Rodriguez V, Bodey GP, Valdivieso M, Feld R: Clinical pharmacology of sisomycin. *Antimicrob Agents Chemother* 7:38, 1975
129. Appel GV, Neu HC: The nephrotoxicity of antimicrobial agents, *N Engl J Med* 296:663, 1977
130. Luft FC, Block R, Sloan RS, Yum MN, Costello R, Maxwell DR: Comparative nephrotoxicity of aminoglycoside antibiotics in rats. *J Infect Dis* 138:541, 1978
131. Pechere J, Dugal R, Pechere M: Pharmacokinetics of netilmicin in renal insufficiency and hemodialysis. *Clin Pharmacokin* 3:395, 1978
132. Luft FC, Brannon DR, Stropes LL, Costello RJ, Sloan RS, Maxwell DR: Pharmacokinetics of netilmicin in patients

with renal impairment and in patients on dialysis. *Antimicrob Agents Chemother* 14:403, 1978
133. Leroy A, Humbert G, Fillastre JP: Pharmacokinetics of dibekacin in normal subjects and in patients with renal failure. *J Antimicrob Chemother* 6:113, 1980
134. Campillo JA, Lanao JM, Dominguez-Gil A, Rubio F, Martin A: Disposition of dibekacin in patients undergoing haemodialysis. *Eur J Clin Pharmacol* 18:347, 1980
135. Weinstein MJ, Wagman GH, Marquez JA, Testa RT, Waitz JA: Verdamycin, a new broad spectrum aminoglycoside antibiotic. *Antimicrob Agents Chemother* 7:246, 1975
136. Fillastre JP, Humbert G, Daufresne MF, Dubois D, Leroy A: Pharmacodynamics of lividomycin in renal failure. *Proc Eur Dial Transpl Assoc* 10:547, 1973
137. Moellering RC Jr, Swartz MN: The newer cephalosporins. *N Engl J Med* 294:24, 1976
138. Benner EJ: Cephaloridine and the kidneys. *J Infect Dis* 122:104, 1970
139. Kirby WMM, deMaine JB, Serrill WS: Pharmacokinetics of the cephalosporings in healthy volunteers and uremic patients. *Postgrad Med J* 47:S41, 1971
140. Curtis JR, Marshall MJ: Cephaloridine serum levels in patients on maintenance haemodialysis. *Br Med J* 2:149, 1970
141. Perkins RL, Smith EM, Saslow S: Cephalothin and cephaloridine: comparative pharmacodynamics in chronic uremia. *Am J Med Sci* 257:116, 1969
142. Craig WA, Welling PG, Jackson TC, Kunin CM: Pharmacology of cephazolin and other cephalosporins in patients with renal insufficiency. *J Infect Dis* 128:S347, 1973
143. Engle JE, Drago J, Charlin B, Schoolwerth AC: Reversible acute renal failure after cephalothin. *Ann Intern Med* 83:222, 1975
144. Linton AL, Bailey R, Turnbull DI: Relative nephrotoxicity of cephalosporin antibiotics in an animal model. *Can Med Assoc J* 107:414, 1972
145. Carling PC, Idelson BA, Casano A, Alexander EA, McCabe WR: Nephrotoxicity associated with cephalothin administration. *Arch Intern Med* 135:797, 1975
146. Tune BM, Wu KY, Longerbeam DF, Kempson RL: Transport and toxicity of cephaloridine in the kidney. Effect of furosemide, p-aminohippurate and saline diuresis. *J Pharmacol Exp Ther* 202:472, 1977
147. Eastwood JB, Gower PPE, Curtis JR: The serum half life and urine concentrations of cefazolin sodium in patients with terminal renal failure: effect of haemodialysis. *Scott Med J* 20:240, 1975
148. Hiner LB, Baluarte J, Polinsky MS, Gruskin AB: Cefazolin in children with renal insufficiency. *J Pediat* 96:335, 1980
149. Brogard JM, Pinget M, Brandt C, Lavillaureix J: Pharmacokinetics of cefazolin in patients with renal failure; special reference to hemodialysis. *J Clin Pharmacol* 17:225, 1977
150. Levinson ME, Levinson SP, Ries K, Kaye D: Pharmacology of cefazolin in patients with normal and abnormal renal function. *J Infect Dis* 128:S354, 1973
151. Kirby WMM, Regamy C: Pharmacokinetics of cefazolin compared with four other cephalosporins. *J Infect Dis* 128:S341, 1973
152. Greene DS, Tice AD: Effect of hemodialysis on cefazolin protein binding. *J Pharm Sci* 66:1508, 1977
153. Verma S, Kieff E: Cephalexin related nephropathy. *JAMA* 234:618, 1975
154. Humbert G, Fillastre JP, Leroy A, Godin M, Van Winzum C: Pharmacokinetics of cefoxitin in normal subjects and in patients with renal insufficiency. *Rev Infect Dis* 1:118, 1979
155. Sasano H, Fujimato T, Une T, Tachizawa H, Ogawa H: Cefoxitin, a semi-synthetic cephamycin antibiotic. Metabolism in rats with renal insufficiency. *Arzneim Forsch* 28:1596, 1978
156. Garcia MJ, Dominguez-Gil A, Tabernero JM, Bondia Román A, Pharmacokinetics of cefoxitin in patients undergoing hemodialysis, *Int J Clin Pharmacol Biopharm* 17:366, 1979
157. Gambertoglio JG, Aziz NS, Len ET, Grausz H, Naughton JL, Benet LZ: Cefamandole kinetics in uremic patients undergoing hemodialysis. *Clin Pharmacol Ther* 26:592, 1979
158. Brogard JM, Kopferschmitt J, Spach MO, Grudet O, Lavellaureix J: Cephamandole pharmacokinetics and dosage adjustments in relation to renal function. *J Clin Pharmacol* 19:366, 1979
159. Ahern MJ, Finkelstein FO, Andriole VT: Pharmacokinetics of cephamandole in patients undergoing hemodialysis and peritoneal dialysis. *Antimicrob Agents Chemother* 10:457, 1976
160. McCloskey RV, Terry HE, McCracken AW, Sweeney MJ, Forland MF: Effect of hemodialysis and renal failure on serum and urine concentrations of cephapirin sodium. *Antimicrob Agents Chemother* 1:90, 1972
161. Bryan CS, Stone WJ: Antimicrobial dosage in renal failure: a unifying nomogram. *Clin Nephrol* 7:81, 1977
162. Berman SJ, Boughton WH, Sugihara JG, Wong EGC, Sato MM, Siemsen AW: Pharmacokinetics of cefaclor in patients with end-stage renal disease and during hemodialysis. *Antimicrob Agents Chemother* 14:281, 1978
163. Gartenberg G, Meyers BR, Hirschman SZ, Srulevitch E: Pharmacokinetics of cefaclor in patients with stable renal impairment and patients undergoing hemodialysis. *J Antimicrob Chemother* 5:465, 1979
164. Spyker DA, Thomas BL, Sande MA, Bolton WK: Pharmacokinetics of cefaclor and cephalexin: dosage nomograms for impaired renal function. *Antimicrob Agents Chemother* 14:172, 1978
165. Humbert G, Leroy A, Fillastre JP, Godin M: Pharmacokinetics of cefadroxil in normal subjects and in patients with renal insufficiency *Chemotherapy* 25:189, 1979
166. Mandell GL, Sande MA: Antimicrobial agents: Penicillins and cephalosporins in *The Pharmacologic Basis of Therapeutics,* Edited by Gilman AG, Goodman LS, Gilman AS, 6th edn., New York. MacMillan Publ Co 1980, p 1126
167. Heinecke G, Höffler MJ, Finke K: Reversible encephalopathy following cephacetrile therapy in high doses in a patient on chronic intermittent hemodialysis. *Clin Nephrol* 5:45, 1976
168. Ohkawa M, Kuroda K: Pharmacokinetics of ceftezole in patients with normal and impaired renal function. *Chemotherapy* 26:242, 1980
169. Hess JR, Berman SJ, Boughton WH, Sugihara JG, Musgrave JE, Wong EGC, Siemsen AM: Pharmacokinetics of ceforanide in patients with end-stage renal disease on hemodialysis. *Antimicrob Agents Chemother* 17:251, 1980
170. Ohkawa M, Orito M, Sugata T, Shimamura M, Sawaki M, Nakashita E, Kuroda K, Sasahara K: Pharmacokinetics of cephmetazole in normal subjects and in patients with impaired renal function. *Antimicrob Agents Chemother* 18:386, 1980
171. Balant L, Dayer P, Rudhardt M, Allaz AF, Fabre J: Cefoperazone: pharmacokinetics in humans with normal and impaired renal function and pharmacokinetics in rats. *Clin Ther* 3:50, 1980
172. Chodos J, Francke EL, Saltzman M, Neu HC: Pharmacokinetics of intravenous cefotaxime in patients undergoing chronic hemodialysis. *Ther Drug Monitor* 3:71, 1981

173. Baldwin DS, Levine BB, McCluskey RT, Gallo GR: Renal failure and interstitial nephritis due to penicillin and methicillin. *N Engl J Med* 279:1245, 1968
174. Tannenberg AM, Wicher KJ, Rose NR: Ampicillin nephropathy. *JAMA* 218:449, 1971
175. Woodroffe AJ, Thomson NM, Meadows R, Lawrence JR: Nephropathy associated with methicillin administration. *Aust NZ J Med* 4:256, 1974
176. Schrier RW, Bulger RJ, Van Ardsel PP Jr: Nephropathy associated with penicillin and homologues. *Ann Intern Med* 64:116, 1966
177. Tourkantonis A, Friedrich H, Heinze V: Ampicillin-Nebenwirkungen bei Patienten mit Niereninsuffizienz. *Med Klin* 66:1154, 1971
178. Bloomer HA, Barton LJ, Maddock RK Jr: Penicillin incuded encephalopathy in uremic patients. *JAMA* 200:121, 1967
179. Andrassy K, Ritz E: Penicillin and hemostasis. *Cardiov Med* 2:604, 1977
180. Barza M, Weinstein L: Pharmacokinetics of the penicillins in man: *Clin Pharmacokin* 1:297, 1976
181. Wickerts CJ, Asaba H, Gunnarson B, Bygdeman S, Bergström J: Combined carbon haemoperfusion and haemodialysis in treatment of penicillin intoxication. *Br Med J* 1:1254, 1980
182. Montanari A, Borghi L, Canali M, Coruzzi P, Novarini A, Borghetti A: The influence of renal function on the elimination kinetics of sulbenicillin in man. *Int J Clin Pharmacol Ther Toxicol* 18:225, 1980
183. Kunin CM, Finkelberg Z: Oral cephalexin and ampicillin: antimicrobial activity, recovery in urine and persistence in blood of uremic patients. *Ann Intern Med* 72:349, 1970
184. Jusko WJ, Lewis GP, Schmitt GW: Ampicillin and hetacillin pharmacokinetics in normal and anephric subjects. *Clin Pharmacol Ther* 14:90, 1973
185. Reudy J: Effects of peritoneal dialysis on physiologic disposition of oxacillin, ampicillin and tetracycline in patients with renal disease. *Can Med Assoc J* 94:257, 1966
186. Bulger RJ, Bennett JV, Boen ST: Intraperitoneal administration of broad-spectrum antibiotics in patients with renal failure. *JAMA* 194:1198, 1965
187. Francke EL, Appel GB, Neu HC: Kinetics of intravenous amoxillin in patients on long-term dialysis. *Clin Pharmacol Ther* 26:31, 1979
188. Humbert G, Spyker DA, Fillastre JP, Leroy A: Pharmacokinetics of amoxillin: dosage nomogram for patients with impaired renal function. *Antimicrob Agents Chemother* 15:28, 1979
189. Bulger RJ, Lindholm DD, Murray JS, Kirby WMM: Effect of uremia on methicillin and oxacillin blood levels. *JAMA* 187:319, 1964
190. Nolan CM, Abernathy RS: Nephropathy associated with methicillin therapy. Prevalence and determinants in patients with staphylococcal bacteremia. *Arch Intern Med* 137:997, 1977
191. Galpin JE, Shinaberger JH, Stanley TM, Blumenkrantz MJ, Bayer AS, Friedman GS, Montgomerie JZ, Guze LB, Coburn JW, Glassock RJ: Acute interstitial nephritis due to methicillin. *Am J Med* 65:756, 1978
192. Platia EV, Whelton PK: Severe methicillin-induced renal failure treated with hemodialysis. *Johns Hopkins Med J* 142:152, 1978
193. Rudnick M, Morrison G, Walker B, Singer I: Renal failure, hemodialysis and nafcillin kinetics. *Clin Pharmacol Ther* 20:413, 1977
194. Nauta EH, Mattie H: Pharmacokinetics of flucloxacillin and cloxacillin in healthy subjects and patients on chronic intermittent haemodialysis. *Br J Clin Pharmacol* 2:111, 1975
195. Rosenblatt JE, Kind AC, Brodie JL, Kirby WMM: Mechanisms responsible for the blood level differences of isoxazolyl penicillins. *Arch Intern Med* 121:345, 1968
196. McCloskey RV, Hayes CP: Plasma levels of dicloxacillin in oliguric patients and the effect of hemodialysis. *Antimicrob Agents Chemother* 7:770, 1967
197. Oe PL, Simonian S, Verhoef J: Pharmacokinetics of the new penicillins: amoxycillin and flucloxacillin in patients with terminal renal failure undergoing hemodialysis. *Chemotherapy* 19:279, 1973
198. Tillman DB, Oill PA, Guze LB: Oxacillin nephritis. *Arch Intern Med* 140:552, 1980
199. Malone AJ Jr, Field S, Rosman J, Shermerdiak WP: Neurotoxic reaction to oxacillin. *N Engl J Med* 296:453, 1977
200. Hoffman TA, Cestero R, Bullock WE: Pharmacodynamics of carbenicillin in hepatic and renal failure. *Ann Intern Med* 73:173, 1970
201. Latos DL, Bryan CS, Stone WJ: Carbenicillin therapy in patients with normal and impaired renal function. *Clin Pharmacol Ther* 17:692, 1975
202. Johny M, Derrington AW, Lawrence JR, Clapp KH: Carbenicillin therapy in renal failure. *Med J Aust* 2:681, 1969
203. Eastwood JB, Curtis JR: Carbenicillin administration in patients with severe renal failure. *Br Med J* 1:486, 1968
204. Klastersky J, Vanderkelen B, Daneau N, Mathieu M: Carbenicillin and hypokalemia. *Ann Intern Med* 78:774, 1973
205. Brunner FP, Frick PG: Hypokalemia, metabolic alkalosis and hypernatremia due to massive penicillin therapy. *Br Med J* 4:550, 1968
206. Whelton A, Carter CG, Garth MA: Carbenicillin-induced acidosis and seizures. *JAMA* 218:1942, 1971
207. Wilson FM, Belamaric J, Lauter CB, Lerner AM: Anicteric carbenicillin hepatitis. *JAMA* 232:818, 1975
208. Brown CH III, Natelson EA, Bradshaw MW, Williams TW Jr, Alfrey CP Jr: The hemostatic defect produced by carbenicillin. *N Engl J Med* 291:265, 1974
209. Bailey RR, Eastwood JB, Vaughan RB: The pharmacokinetics of an oral form of carbenicillin in patients with renal failure. *Postgrad Med J* 48:422, 1972
210. Libke RD, Clarke JT, Ralph ED, Luthy RP, Kirby WMM: Ticarcillin vs carbenicillin: clinical pharmacokinetics. *Clin Pharmacol Ther* 17:441, 1975
211. Parry MF, Neu HC: Pharmacokinetics of ticarcillin in patients with abnormal renal function. *J Infect Dis* 133:46, 1976
212. Davies M, Morgan JR, Anand C: Administration of ticarcillin to patients with severe renal failure. *Chemotherapy* 20:339, 1974
213. Wise R, Reeves DS, Parker AS: Administration of ticarcillin, a new antipseudomonal antibiotic in patients undergoing dialysis. *Antimicrob Agents Chemother* 5:119, 1974
214. Kallay MC, Tabechian H, Riley GR, Chessin LN: Neurotoxicity due to ticarcillin in patients with renal failure. *Lancet* 1:608, 1979
215. Aletta JM, Francke EF, Neu HC: Intravenous azlocillin kinetics in patients on long-term hemodialysis. *Clin Pharmacol Ther* 27:563, 1980
216. Leroy A, Humbert G, Godin M, Fillastre JP: Pharmacokinetics of azlocillin in subjects with normal and impaired renal function. *Antimicrob Agents Chemother* 17:344, 1980
217. Kosmidis J, Doundoulaki P, Stathakis C, Zerefos N, Bounia A, Daikos GK: Elimination kinetics of mezlocillin in

normal and impaired renal function including effects of dialysis. *Arzneim Forsch* 29:1960, 1978
218. Francke E, Mehta S, Neu HC, Appel GB: Kinetics of intravenous mezlocillin in chronic hemodialysis patients. *Clin Pharmacol Ther* 26:228, 1979
219. Kampf D, Schurig R, Weihermüller K, Förster D: Effects of impaired renal function, hemodialysis and peritoneal dialysis on the pharmacokinetics of mezlocillin. *Antimicrob Agents Chemother* 18:81, 1980
220. Aronoff GR, Sloan RS, Luft FC, Nelson RL, Maxwell DR, Kleit SA: Mezlocillin pharmacokinetics in renal impairment. *Clin Pharmacol Ther* 28:523, 1980
221. Francke EL, Appel GB, Neu HC: Pharmacokinetics of intravenous piperacillin in patients undergoing chronic hemodialysis. *Antimicrob Agents Chemother* 16:788, 1979
222. Bailey K, Cruickshank JG, Bisson PG, Radford BL: Mecillinam in patients on hemodialysis. *Br J Clin Pharmacol* 10:177, 1980
223. Shils ME: Renal disease and the metabolic effects of tetracycline. *Ann Intern Med* 58:489, 1963
224. Orr LH Jr, Rudisill E Jr, Brodkin R, Hamilton RW: Exacerbation of renal failure associated with doxycycline. *Arch Intern Med* 138:793, 1978
225. Morgan T, Ribush N: The effect of oxytetracycline and doxycycline on protein metabolism. *Med J Aust* 1:55, 1972
226. Clausen G, Nagy Z, Szaloy L, Aukland K: Mechanisms in acute oliguric renal failure induced by tetracycline infusion. *Scand J Clin Lab Invest* 35:625, 1975
227. Singer I, Rotenberg D: Demeclocycline induced nephrogenic diabetes insipidus. In vivo and in vitro studies. *Ann Intern Med* 79:679, 1973
228. Carrilho F, Bosch J, Arroyo V, Mas A, Viver J, Rodes J: Renal failure associated with demeclocycline in cirrhosis. *Ann Intern Med* 87:195, 1977
229. Oster JR, Epstein M, Ulano HB: Deterioration of renal function with demeclocycline administration. *Curr Ther Res* 20:794, 1976
230. Stenback O, Myhre E, Berdal BD: The effect of doxycycline on renal function in patients with advanced renal insufficiency. *Scand J Infect Dis* 5:199, 1973
231. Frimpter GW, Timpanelli AE, Eisenmenger WJ, Stein HS, Ehrlich LI: Reversible 'Fanconi Syndrome' caused by degraded tetracycline. *JAMA* 184:111, 1963
232. Lee P, Crutch ER, Morrison RBI: Doxycycline: studies in normal subjects and patients with renal failure. *NZ Med J* 75:355, 1972
233. Allen JC: Minocycline. *Ann Intern Med* 85:482, 1976
234. Heaney D, Eknoyan G: Minocycline and doxycycline kinetics in renal failure. *Clin Pharmacol Ther* 24:233, 1978
235. George CRP, Guiness NDG, Lark DJ, Evans RA: Minocycline toxicity in renal failure. *Med J Aust* 1:640, 1973
236. Maher JF, Freeman RB, Setter JG, Rubin M, Schreiner GE: Dialysance studies of varied solutes and biochemical changes during hemodialysis. *Trans Am Soc Artif Intern Organs* 10:332, 1964
237. Rose HD, Roth DA, Koch ML: Serum tetracycline levels during peritoneal dialysis. *Am J Med Sci* 250:66, 1965
238. Yow EM, Moyer JH, Smith CP: Toxicity of polymyxin B. II. Human studies with particular reference to evaluation of renal function. *Arch Intern Med* 92:248, 1953
239. Hoeprich PD: The polymyxins. *Med Clin North Am* 54:1257, 1970
240. Adler S, Segal DP: Non-oliguric renal failure secondary to sodium colistimethate: a report of four cases. *Am J Med Sci* 262:109, 1971
241. Brunfitt W, Black M, Williams JD: Colistin in pseudomonas pyocyanea infections and its effect on renal function. *Br J Urol* 38:495, 1966
242. Koch-Weser J, Sidel VW, Federman EB, Kanarek P, Finer DC, Eaton AE: Adverse effects of sodium colistimethate. *Ann Intern Med* 72:857, 1970
243. Wolinsky E, Hines JD: Neurotoxic and nephrotoxic effects of colistin in patients with renal disease. *N Engl J Med* 266:759, 1962
244. MacKay DN, Kaye D: Serum concentrations of colistin in patients with normal and impaired renal function. *N Engl J Med* 270:394, 1964
245. Curtis JR, Eastwood JB: Colistin sulfomethate sodium administration in the presence of severe renal failure and during haemodialysis and peritoneal dialysis. *Br Med J* 1:484, 1968
246. Goodwin NJ, Friedman EA: The effects of renal impairment, peritoneal dialysis and hemodialysis on sodium colistimethate levels. *Ann Intern Med* 68:984, 1968
247. Swick HM, Maxwell E, Charache P, Levin S: Peritoneal dialysis in colistin intoxication. Report of a case. *J Pediatr* 74:976, 1969
248. Beirne GJ, Hansing CE, Octaviano GN, Burns RO: Acute renal failure caused by hypersensitivity to polymyxin B sulfate. *JAMA* 202:62, 1967
249. Baethke R, Golde G, Gahl G: Sulfamethoxazole/trimethoprim: pharmacokinetic studies in patients with chronic renal failure. *Eur J Clin Pharmacol* 4:233, 1972
250. Adam WR, Dawborn JK: Urinary excretion and plasma levels of sulfonamides in patients with renal impairment. *Australas Ann Med* 3:250, 1970
251. Welling PG, Craig WA, Amidon GL, Kunin CM: Pharmacokinetics of trimethoprim and sulfamethoxazole in patients with renal failure. *J Infect Dis* 128:S556, 1973
252. Bergan T, Brodwall EK, Vik-Mo H, Anstad U: Pharmacokinetics of sulfadiazine, sulfamethoxazole and trimethoprim in patients with varying renal function. *Infection* 7 (Suppl 4):S382, 1979
253. Fine A, Sumner D: Alteration of hepatic acetylation in uraemia. *Proc Eur Dial Transpl Assoc* 11:433, 1974
254. Reidenberg MM, Kostenbauder H, Adams WP: Rate of drug metabolism in obese volunteers before and during starvation and in azotemic patients. *Metabolism* 18:209, 1969
255. Anton AH: The effect of disease, drugs and dilution on the binding of sulfonamides in human plasma. *Clin Pharmacol Ther* 9:561, 1968
256. Kawamura T, Yagi N, Sugawara H, Yamahata K, Takada M: Efficacy of hemodialysis and the effects of certain displacing agents on plasma protein binding of sulfamethoxazole and sulfaphenazole in patients with chronic renal failure. *Chem Pharm Bull* (Tokyo) 28:268, 1980
257. Skimming LH, Knies PT, Anthony MA, Melerango ES: Hemolytic anemia caused by sulfamethoxypyridazine. Report of a case successfully treated by hemodialysis. *Ohio State Med J* 57:280, 1961
258. Weinstein L, Madoff MA, Samet CM: The sulfonamides. *N Engl J Med* 263:793, 1960
259. Lehr D: Clinical toxicity of sulfonamides *Ann NY Acad Sci* 69:417, 1957
260. Glushein AS, Fisher ER: Renal lesions of sulfonamide type after treatment with acetazolamide (Diamox). *JAMA* 160:204, 1956
261. Kalowski S, Nanra RS, Mathew TH, Kincaid-Smith P: Deterioration in renal function in association with co-trimoxazole therapy. *Prog Biochem Pharmacol* 9:129, 1974
262. Smith EJ, Light JA, Filo RS, Yum N: Interstitial nephritis

caused by trimethoprim-sulfamethoxazole in renal transplant recipients. *JAMA* 244:360, 1980
263. Grafnetterova J, Vodrážka Z, Jandova D, Schück O, Tomášek R, Lachmanová J: The binding of chloramphenicol to serum proteins in patients with chronic renal insufficiency. *Clin Nephrol* 6:448, 1976
264. Kunin CM, Glasko AJ, Finland M: Persistence of antibiotics in blood of patients with acute renal failure. II Chloramphenicol and its metabolic products in the blood of patients with severe renal disease or hepatic cirrhosis. *J Clin Invest* 38:1498, 1959
265. Slaughter RL, Cerra FB, Koup JR: Effect of hemodialysis on total body clearance of chloramphenicol. *Am J Hosp Pharm* 37:1083, 1980
266. Mauer SM, Chavers BM, Kjellstrand CM: Treatment of an infant with severe chloramphenicol intoxication using charcoal-column hemoperfusion. *J Pediat* 96:136, 1980
267. Peddie BA, Dann E, Bailey RR: The effect of impairment of renal function and dialysis on the serum and urine levels of clindamycin. *Aust NZ J Med* 5:198, 1975
268. Reinarz JA, McIntosh DA: Lincomycin excretion in patients with normal renal function, severe azotemia and with hemodialysis and peritoneal dialysis. *Antimicrob Agents Chemother* 5:232, 1965
269. Kunin CM, Finland M: Persistence of antibiotics in the blood of patients with acute renal failure. III Penicillin, streptomycin, erythromycin and kanamycin. *J Clin Invest* 38:1509, 1958
270. Mery A, Kanfer A: Ototoxicity of erythromycin in patients with renal insufficiency. *N Engl J Med* 301:944, 1979
271. Lindholm DD, Murray JS: Persistence of vancomycin in the blood during renal failure and its treatment by hemodialysis. *N Engl J Med* 274:1047, 1966
272. Nielsen HE, Hansen HE, Korsager B, Skov PE: Renal excretion of vancomycin in kidney disease. *Acta Med Scand* 197:261, 1975
273. Eykyn S, Phillips I, Evans J: Vancomycin for staphylococcal shunt site infections in patients on regular hemodialysis. *Br Med J* 3:80, 1970
274. Ayus JC, Eneas JF, Tong TG, Benowitz NL, Schoenfeld PY, Hadley KL, Becker CE, Humphreys MH: Peritoneal clearance and total body elimination of vancomycin during chronic intermittent peritoneal dialysis. *Clin Nephrol* 11:129, 1979
275. Revert L, Lopez J, Pons J, Olag T: Fosfomycin in patients subjected to periodic hemodialysis. *Chemotherapy* 23 (Suppl 1):204, 1977
276. Zintel HA, Ma RA, Nichols AC, Ellis H: The absorption, distribution, excretion, and toxicity of bacitracin in man. *Am J Med Sci* 218:439, 1949
277. Felts JH, Hayes DM, Gergen JA, Toole JF: Neural, hematologic and bacteriologic effects of nitrofurantoin in renal insufficiency. *Am J Med* 51:331, 1971
278. Adam WR, Dawborn JK: Plasma levels and urinary excretion of nalidixic acid in patients with renal failure. *Aust NZ J Med* 2:126, 1971
279. Alano FA, Webster GD: Acute renal failure and pigmentation due to phenazopyridine (Pyridium). *Ann Intern Med* 72:89, 1970
280. Szwed JJ, Brannon DE, Sloan RS, Luft FC: Pharmacokinetics of cinoxacin in patients with renal failure. *J Antimicrob Chemother* 4:451, 1978
281. Jenne JW, Beggs WH: Correlation of *in vitro* and *in vivo* kinetics with clinical use of isoniazid, ethambutol and rifampin. *Am Rev Respir Dis* 107:1013, 1973
282. Hagstam KE, Lindholm T: Treatment of exogenous poisoning with special regard to the need for artificial kidney in severe complicated cases. *Acta Med Scand* 175:507, 1964
283. Cocco AE, Pazourek LJ: Acute isoniazid intoxication-management by peritoneal dialysis. *N Engl J Med* 269:852, 1963
284. Königshausen T, Altrogge G, Hein D, Grabansee B, Putter D: Hemodialysis and hemoperfusion in the treatment of most severe INH-poisoning. *Vet Hum Toxicol* 21:12, 1979
285. Gold CH, Buchanan N, Tringham V, Viljoen M, Strickwold B, Moodley GP: Isoniazid pharmacokinetics in patients in chronic renal failure. *Clin Nephrol* 6:365, 1976
286. Campese VM, Marzullo F, Schema FP, Coratelli P: Acute renal failure during intermittent rifampicin therapy. *Nephron* 10:256, 1973
287. Bansal VK, Bennett D, Molnar Z: Prolonged renal failure after rifampin. *Am Rev Respir Dis* 116:137, 1977
288. Novi C, Bissoli F, Simonati V, Volpini T, Baroli A, Vignati G: Rifampin and digoxin: possible drug interaction in a dialysis patient *JAMA* 244:2521, 1980
289. Christopher TG, Blair A, Forrey A, Cutler RE: Kinetics of ethambutol elimination in renal disease. *Proc Clin Dial Transpl Forum* 3:96, 1973
290. Atkins R, Cutting CJ, Mackintosh TF: Acute poisoning by cycloserine. *Br Med J* 1:907, 1965
291. Mandell GL, Sande MA: Antimicrobial agents: drugs used in the chemotherapy of tuberculosis and leprosy in *The Pharmacologic Basis of Therapeutics,* edited by Gilman AG, Goodman LS, Gilman A, 6th edn, New York, MacMillan Publ Co, 1980, p 1200
292. Butler WT, Bennett JE, Alling DW, Wertlake PT, Utz JP, Hill GJ: Nephrotoxicity of amphotericin B. *Ann Intern Med* 61:175, 1964
293. McCurdy DK, Frederic M, Elkinton JR: Renal tubular acidosis due to amphotericin B. *N Engl J Med* 278:124, 1968
294. Burgess JL, Birchall R: Nephrotoxicity of amphotericin B with emphasis on changes in tubular function. *Am J Med* 53:77, 1972
295. Gerkins JF, Branch RA: The influence of sodium status and furosemide on canine acute amphotericin B nephrotoxicity. *J Pharmacol Exp Ther* 214:306, 1980
296. Block ER, Bennett JE, Levoti LG, Klein WJ, MacGregor RR, Henderson L: Flucytosine and amphotericin B: Hemodialysis effects on the plasma concentration and clearance. *Ann Intern Med* 80:613, 1974
297. Dawborn JK, Page MD, Schiavone JD: Use of 5-fluorocytosine in patients with impaired renal function. *Br Med J* 3:382, 1973
298. Rault RM, Hulme B, Davies RR: 5-Fluorocytosine treatment of candidiasis on a patient receiving regular hemodialysis. *Clin Nephrol* 3:225, 1973
299. Stevens DA, Levine HB, Deresinski SC: Miconazole in coccidioidomycosis. II. Therapeutic and pharmacologic studies in man. *Am J Med* 60:199, 1976
300. Fabre J, de Freudenreich J, Duckert A, Pitton JS, Rudhardt M, Virieux C: Influence of renal insufficiency on the excretion of chloroquin, phenobarbital, phenothiazines and methacycline. *Helv Med Acta* 33:307, 1967
301. Smith CC, Ihrig J, Menne R: Antimalarial activity and metabolism of biguanides. *Am J Trop Med Hyg* 10:694, 1961
302. Smith CC, Ihrig J: Persistent excretion of pyrimethamine following oral administration. *Am J Trop Med Hyg* 8:60, 1959
303. Rollo IM: Drugs used in the chemotherapy of malaria, in *The Pharmacological Basis of Therapeutics,* edited by Gilman AG, Goodman LS, Gilman A, 6th edn, New

York, MacMillan Publ Co 1980, p 1038
304. Lang PA, Jones CC: Acute renal failure precipitated by quinine sulfate in early pregnancy. JAMA 188:464, 1964
305. Donadio JV, Whelton A, Gilliland PF, Cirksena WJ: Peritoneal dialysis in quinidine intoxication. JAMA 204:274, 1968
306. Floyd M, Hill AVL, Ormston BJ, Menzies R, Porter R: Quinine amblyopia treated by hemodialysis. Clin Nephrol 2:44, 1974
307. Walzer PD, Perl DP, Krogstad DJ, Rawson PG, Schultz MG: Pneumocystis carinii pneumonia in the United States. Epidemiologic, diagnostic and clinical features. Ann Intern Med 80:83, 1974
308. Aoki FY, Sitar DS, Ogilvie RI: Amantidine kinetics in healthy young subjects after long-term dosing. Clin Pharmacol Ther 26:729, 1979
309. Ing TS, Daugirdas JT, Soung LS, Klawans HL, Mahurkar SD, Hayashi JA, Geis WP, Hano JE: Toxic effects of amantadine in patients with renal failure. Can Med Assoc J 120:695, 1979
310. Soung L, Ing TS, Daugirdas JT, Wu M, Gandhi VC, Ivanovich PT, Hano JE, Viol GW: Amantadine pharmacokinetics in hemodialysis patients. Ann Intern Med 93:46, 1980
311. Schumaker JD, Band JD, Lensmeyer GL, Craig WA: Thiabendazole treatment of severe strongyloidiasis in a hemodialyzed patient. Ann Intern Med 89:644, 1978
312. Selden R, Haynie G: Ouabain plasma level kinetics and removal by dialysis in chronic renal failure. A study in fourteen patients. Ann Intern Med 83:15, 1975
313. Kramer P, Horenkamp J, Quellhorst E, Scheler F: Elimination von H^3-g-Strophanthin durch Hämodialyse. (Removal of H^3-g-strophantidin by hemodialysis) Klin Wochenschr 48:148, 1970 (in German)
314. Doherty JE: Digitalis glycosides. Pharmacokinetics and their clinical implications. Ann Intern Med 79:229, 1973
315. Finkelstein FO, Goffinet JA, Hendler ED, Lindenbaum J: Pharmacokinetics of digoxin and digitoxin in patients undergoing hemodialysis. Am J Med 58:525, 1975
316. Ohnhaus EE, Vozeh S, Neusch E: Absolute bioavailability of digoxin in chronic renal failure. Clin Nephrol 11:302, 1979
317. Gault MH, Churchill DN, Kalra J: Loading dose of digoxin in renal failure. Br J Clin Pharmacol 9:593, 1980
318. Gault MH, Jeffrey JR, Chiruto E, Ward LL: Studies of digoxin dosage, kinetics and serum concentrations in renal failure and review of the literature. Nephron 17:161, 1976
319. Halkin H, Skeiner LB, Peck CC, Melman KL: Determinants of renal clearance of digoxin. Clin Pharmacol Ther 17:385, 1975
320. van der Vijgh WJF, Oe PL: Pharmacokinetic aspects of digoxin in patients with terminal renal failure. IV. Clinical implications of own observations with a recent review of literature. Int J Clin Pharmacol Biopharm 16:540, 1978
321. Ackerman GL, Doherty JE, Flanigan WJ: Peritoneal dialysis and hemodialysis of tritiated digoxin. Ann Intern Med 67:718, 1967
322. van der Vijgh WJF, Oe PL: Pharmacokinetic aspects of digoxin in patients with terminal renal failure. II. On hemodialysis. Int J Clin Pharmacol Biopharm 15:255, 1977
323. Carvallo A, Ramirez B, Honig H, Knepshield J, Schreiner GE, Gelfand MC: Treatment of digitalis intoxication by charcoal hemoperfusion. Trans Am Soc Artif Intern Organs 22:718, 1976
324. Gibson TP, Lucas SV, Nelson HA, Atkinson AJ Jr, Okita GT, Ivanovich P: Hemoperfusion removal of digoxin from dogs. J Lab Clin Med 91:673, 1978
325. Smiley JW, March NM, Del Guercio ET: Hemoperfusion in the management of digoxin toxicity. JAMA 240:2736, 1978
326. Pancorbo S, Comty C: Digoxin pharmacokinetics in continuous peritoneal dialysis. Ann Intern Med 93:639, 1980
327. Jeliffe RW, Buell J, Kalaba R, Sridhar R, Rockwell R, Wagner JG: An improved method of digitoxin therapy. Ann Intern Med 72:453, 1970
328. Shah G, Nelson HA, Atkinson AJ Jr, Okita GT, Ivanovich P, Gibson TP: Effect of hemoperfusion on the pharmacokinetics of digitoxin in dogs. J Lab Clin Med 93:370, 1979
329. Zsotér TT, Johnson GE, DeVeber GA, Paul H: Excretion and metabolism of reserpine in renal failure. Clin Pharmacol Ther 14:325, 1973
330. Curtis JR: Drug-induced renal disease. Drugs 18:377, 1979
331. Zak SB, Bartlett MF, Wagner WE, Gilleron TG, Lucas G: Disposition of hydralazine in man and a specific method for its determination in biological fluids. J Pharm Sci 63:225, 1974
332. Koch-Weser J: Hydralazine. N Engl J Med 295:320, 1976
333. Lowenthal DT, Hobbs D, Affrime MB, Twomey TM, Martinez EW, Onesti G: Prazosin kinetics and effectiveness in renal failure. Clin Pharmacol Ther 27:779, 1980
334. Stokes GS, Monaghan JC, Frost GW, MacCarthy ED: Responsiveness to prazosin in renal failure. Clin Sci Mol Med 57 (Suppl 5):383S, 1979
335. Buks RP, Beck JL, Speth OC, Smith JL, Trenner NR, Cannon PJ, Laragh JH: The metabolism of methyldopa in hypertensive human subjects. J Pharmacol Exp Ther 143:205, 1964
336. Myhre E, Brodwall EK, Stenback O, Hansen T: Plasma turnover of methyldopa in advanced renal failure. Acta Med Scand 191:343, 1972
337. Yeh BK, Dayton PG, Waters WC III: Removal of alpha-methyldopa (Aldomet) in man by dialysis. Proc Soc Exp Biol Med 135:840, 1970
338. Hulter HN, Licht JH, Ilnicki LP, Singh S: Clinical efficacy and pharmacokinetics of clonidine in hemodialysis and renal insufficiency J Lab Clin Med 94:223, 1979
339. Niedermayer W, Seiler KU, Wasserman O: Pharmacokinetics of antihypertensive drugs (atenolol, metoprolol, propranolol and clonidine) and their metabolites during intermittent haemodialysis in humans. Proc Eur Dial Transpl Assoc 15:607, 1978
340. Kirch W, Kohler H, Braun W, Gizycki C: The influence of renal function on plasma concentration, urinary excretion and antihypertensive effects of guanfacine. Clin Pharmacokinet 5:476, 1980
341. McMartin C, Randel RK, Vinter J, Allan BR, Humberstone M, Leishman AWD, Sandler G, Thirkettle JL: The fate of guanethidine in two hypertensive patients. Clin Pharmacol Ther 11:423, 1970
342. Young IM, de Wardener HE, Miles BE: Mechanism of renal excretion of methonium compounds. Br Med J 2:1500, 1951
343. Milne MD, Rowe GG, Somers K, Muehrcke RC, Crawford MA: Observations on the pharmacology of mecamylamine. Clin Sci 16:599, 1957
344. Rennick BR, Moe GK, Lyons RH, Hoobler SW, Neligh R: Absorption and renal excretion of the tetraethylammonium ion. J Pharmacol Exp Ther 91:210, 1947
345. Gottlieb TB, Thomas RC, Chidsey CA: Pharmacokinetic

studies of minoxidil. *Clin Pharmacol Ther* 13:436, 1972
346. Zarate A, Gelfand MC, Horton JD, Winchester JF, Gottlieb MJ, Lazarus JM, Schreiner GE: Pericardial effusion associated with minoxidil therapy in dialyzed patients. *Int J Artif Organs* 3:15, 1980
347. Pruitt AW, Faraj BA, Dayton PG: Metabolism of diazoxide in man and experimental animals. *J Pharmacol Exp Ther* 188:248, 1974
348. Pohl JEF, Thurston H: Use of diazoxide in hypertension with renal failure. *Br Med J* 4:142, 1971
349. Sellers RM, Koch-Weser J: Protein binding and vascular activity of diazoxide. *N Engl J Med* 281:1141, 1969
350. Danzig LE: Dynamics of thiocyanate dialysis. The artificial kidney in the therapy of thiocyanate intoxication. *N Engl J Med* 252:49, 1955
351. Lifschitz MD, Kirschenbaum MA, Rosenblatt SG, Gibney R: Effect of saralasin in hypertensive patients on chronic hemodialysis. *Ann Intern Med* 88:23, 1978
352. Case DB, Atlas SA, Mouradian JA, Fishman RA, Sherman RL, Laragh JH: Proteinuria during long term captopril therapy. *JAMA* 244:346, 1980
353. Farrow PR, Wilkinson R: Reversible renal failure during treatment with captopril. *Br Med J* 2:1680, 1979
354. Hoorntje SJ, Weening JJ, Kallenburg CGM, Prins EJL, Donker AJM: Serum-sickness-like syndrome with membranous glomerulopathy in patient on captopril. *Lancet* 2:1297, 1979
355. Lowenthal DT, Briggs WA, Gibson TP, Nelson H, Cirksena WJ: Pharmacokinetics of oral propranolol in chronic renal disease. *Clin Pharmacol Ther* 16:761, 1974
356. Thomson FD, Joekes AM, Foulkes DM: Pharmacokinetics of propranolol in renal failure. *Br Med J* 2:434, 1972
357. Stone WJ, Walle T: Massive propranolol metabolite retention during maintenance hemodialysis. *Clin Pharmacol Ther* 28:449, 1980
358. Feely J, Wilkinson JR, Wood AJJ: Reduction of liver blood flow and propranolol metabolism by cimetidine. *N Engl J Med* 304:692, 1981
359. Fabre J, Fox HM, Dayer P, Balant L: Differences in kinetic properties of drugs: implications as to the selection of a particular drug for use in patients with renal failure with special emphasis on antibiotics and β-adrenoceptor blocking agents. *Clin Pharmacokinet* 5:441, 1980
360. Safar LE, Chau NP, Levenson JA, Simon AC, Weiss YA: Pharmacokinetics of intravenous and oral pindolol in hypertensive patients with chronic renal failure. *Clin Sci Mol Med* 55:275S, 1978
361. Berglund G, Descaps R, Thomis JA: Pharmacokinetics of sotalol after chronic administration to patients with renal insufficiency. *Eur J Clin Pharmacol* 18:321, 1980
362. Tjandramaga TB, Thomas J, Verbeek R, Verbesselt R, Verberkmoes R, De Schepper PJ: The effect of end-stage renal failure and haemodialysis on the elimination kinetics of sotalol. *Br J Clin Pharmacol* 3:259, 1976
363. Harvengt C, Desager JP, Muschart JM, Tjandramaga TVM, Verbuck R, Verberkmoes R: Influence of hemodialysis on the half life of practolol in patients with severe renal failure. *J Clin Pharmacol* 15:605, 1975
364. Roux A, Aubert P, Guedon J, Flouvat B: Pharmacokinetics of acebutolol in patients with all grades of renal failure. *Eur J Clin Pharmacol* 17:339, 1980
365. McAinsh J, Holmes BF, Smith S, Hood D, Warren D: Atenolol kinetics in renal failure. *Clin Pharmacol Ther* 28:302, 1980
366. Domart M, Goupil A, Baglin A: Pharmacokinetics of atenolol in patients with terminal renal failure and influence of haemodialysis. *Br J Clin Pharmacol* 9:379, 1980

367. McCluskey DR, Donaldson RA, McGeown MG: Oxyprenolol and retroperitoneal fibrosis. *Br Med J* 2:1459, 1980
368. Seiler KU, Schuster KJ, Meyer GF, Niedermayer W, Wasserman O: The pharmacokinetics of metroprolol and its metabolites in dialysis patients. *Clin Pharmacokin* 5:192, 1980
369. Young TK, Lee SC, Tai LN: Mannitol absorption and excretion in uremic patients regularly treated with gastrointestinal perfusion. *Nephron* 25:112, 1980
370. Weinberger M, Hendeles L: Role of dialysis in the management and prevention of theophylline toxicity. *Dev Pharmacol Ther* 1:26, 1980
371. Lawyer C, Aitchison J, Sutton J, Bennett W: Treatment of theophylline neurotoxicity with resin hemoperfusion. *Ann Intern Med* 88:516, 1978
372. Maher JF, Cassetta M, Shea C, Hohnadel DC: Transperitoneal theophylline flux and peritoneal permeability. *Nephron* 20:18, 1978
373. Levy G, Gibson TP, Whitman W, Procknal J: Hemodialysis clearances of theophylline. *JAMA* 237:1466, 1977
374. Lee CS, Marbury TC, Perrin JH, Fuller TJ: Hemodialysis of theophylline in uremic patients. *J Clin Pharmacol* 19:219, 1979
375. Russo ME: Management of theophylline intoxication with charcoal hemoperfusion. *N Engl J Med* 300:24, 1979
376. Miceli JN, Clay B, Fleischmann LE, Sarnaik AP, Aronow R, Done AK: Pharmacokinetics of severe theophylline intoxication managed by peritoneal dialysis. *Dev Pharmacol Ther* 1:16, 1980
377. Lee CSC, Wang LH, Majeske BL, Marbury TC: Pharmacokinetics of dyphylline elimination by uremic patients. *J Pharmacol Exp Ther* 217:340, 1980
378. Freeman RB, Maher JF, Schreiner GE, Mostofi FK: Renal tubular necrosis due to nephrotoxicity of organic mercurial diuretics. *Ann Intern Med* 57:34, 1962
379. Vaziri ND, Saiki J, Barton CH, Rajudin M, Ness RL: Hemodialyzability of acetazolamide. *South Med J* 73:422, 1980
380. Koppel MH, Massry SG, Shinaberger JH, Hartenbower DL, Coburn JW: Thiazide-induced rise in serum calcium and magnesium in patients on maintenance hemodialysis. *Ann Intern Med* 72:895, 1970
381. Magil A, Baloon HS, Cameron EC, Rae A: Acute interstitial nephritis associated with thiazide diuretics. Clinical and pathologic observations in three cases. *Am J Med* 69:939, 1980
382. Cannon PJ, Ames RP, Laragh JH: Methylene butyrylphenoxyacetic acid. Novel and potent natriuretic and diuretic agent. *JAMA* 185:854, 1963
383. Levin NW: Furosemide and ethacrynic acid in renal insufficiency. *Med Clin North Am* 55:107, 1971
384. Dargie HJ, Allison MEM, Kennedy AC, Gray MJB: High dosage metolazone in chronic renal failure. *Br Med J* 4:196, 1972
385. Gregory LF Jr, Durrett RR, Robinson RR, Clapp JR: The short term effect of furosemide on electrolyte and water excretion in patients with severe renal disease. *Arch Intern Med* 125:69, 1970
386. Huang CM, Atkinson AJ, Levin M, Levin NW, Quentanilla A: Pharmacokinetics of furosemide in advanced renal failure. *Clin Pharmacol Ther* 16:659, 1974
387. Beermann B, Dalén E, Lindstrom B: Elimination of furosemide in healthy subjects and in those with renal failure. *Clin Pharmacol Ther* 22:70, 1977
388. Lyons H, Pin VW, Cortell S, Cohen JJ, Harrington JT: Allergic interstitial nephritis causing reversible renal failure in four patients with idiopathic nephrotic syndrome.

N Engl J Med 288:124, 1973
389. Cohen LH, Norby LH, Champion C, Spargo B: Acute renal failure from ticrynafen. *N Engl J Med* 301:1180, 1979
390. McLain DA, Garriga FJ, Kantor OS: Adverse reactions associated with ticrynafen use. *JAMA* 243:763, 1980
391. Paddack GL, Wahl RC, Holman RE, Schorr WJ, Lacher RW: Acute renal failure associated with ticrynafen. *JAMA* 243:764, 1980
392. Karim A, Zagarella J, Hribar J, Dooley M: Spironolactone I. Disposition and metabolism. *Clin Pharmacol Ther* 19:158, 1976
393. Pruitt AW, Dayton PG, Steinhorst J: Fate of triamterene in man. *Clin Res* 22:77A, 1974
394. Takahashi H, Tsukada T: Triamterene-induced haemolytic anemia with acute intravascular haemolysis and acute renal failure. *Scand J Haematol* 23:169, 1979
395. George CF: Amiloride handling in renal failure. *Br J Clin Pharmacol* 9:94, 1980
396. Thomson PD, Melmon KL, Richardson JA, Cohn K, Steinbrunn W, Cudihee R, Rowland M: Lidocaine pharmacokinetics in advanced heart failure, liver disease and renal failure in humans. *Ann Intern Med* 78:499, 1973
397. Collinsworth KA, Strong JM, Atkinson AJ Jr, Winkle RA, Perlroth F, Harrison DC: Pharmacokinetics and metabolism of lidocaine in patients with renal failure. *Clin Pharmacol Ther* 18:59, 1975
398. Vaziri ND, Saiki JK, Hughes W: Clearance of lidocaine by hemodialysis. *South Med J* 72:1567, 1979
399. Koch-Weser J: Pharmacokinetics of procainamide in man. *Ann NY Acad Sci* 179:301, 1979
400. Gibson TP, Atkinson AJ Jr, Matusik E, Nelson LD, Briggs WA: Kinetics of procainamide and N-acetylprocainamide in renal failure. *Kidney Int* 12:422, 1977
401. Goicoechea FJ, Bischel MD, Jelliffe RF: Kinetics of procainamide in anuric patients undergoing hemodialysis. *Proc Clin Dial Transpl Forum* 3:92, 1973
402. Nattel S, Ogilvie RI, Kreeft J, Sitar DS, Graham DN, Rangno RE, Dufresne LR, Barre PE: Procainamide acetylation and disposition in dialysis patients. *Clin Invest Med* 2:5, 1979
403. Stec GP, Atkinson AJ Jr, Nevin MJ, Thenot JP, Ruo TI, Gibson TP, Ivanovich P, Del Greco F: N-acetylprocainamide pharmacokinetics in functionally anephric patients before and after perturbation by hemodialysis. *Clin Pharmacol Ther* 26:618, 1979
404. Atkinson AJ, Krumlovsky FA, Huang CM, Del Greco F: Hemodialysis for severe procainamide toxicity. Clinical and pharmacokinetic observations. *Clin Pharmacol Ther* 20:585, 1976
405. Kessler KM, Lowenthal DT, Warner H, Gibson T, Briggs W, Reidenberg MM: Quinidine elimination in patients with congestive heart failure or poor renal function. *N Engl J Med* 290:706, 1974
406. Woie L, Øyri A: Quinidine intoxication treated with hemodialysis. *Acta Med Scand* 195:237, 1974
407. Johnston A, Henry JA, Warrington SJ, Hamer NAJ: Pharmacokinetics of oral diisopyramide phosphate in patients with renal impairment. *Br J Clin Pharmacol* 10:245, 1980
408. Sevka MJ, Matthews SJ, Nightingale CH, Izard MW, Fieldman A, Chow MSS: Diisopyramide hemodialysis and kinetics in patients requiring long-term hemodialysis. *Clin Pharmacol Ther* 29:322, 1981
409. Holt DW, Helliwell M, O'Keefe B, Hayler AM, Marshall CB, Cook G: Successful management of serious diisopyramide poisoning. *Postgrad Med J* 56:256, 1980
410. Gosselin B, Mathieu D, Chopin C, Wattel F, Depuis B, Haguenoer JM, Desprez M: Acute intoxication with diisopyramide: clinical and experimental study by hemoperfusion on Amberlite XAD 4 resin. *Clin Toxicol* 17:439, 1980
411. Heissenbuttel RH, Bigger JT Jr: Bretylium tosylate: a newly available antiarrythmic drug for ventricular arrhythmias. *Ann Intern Med* 91:229, 1979
412. Adir J, Harang PK, Josselson J, Sadler JH: Pharmacokinetics of bretylium in renal insufficiency. *N Engl J Med* 300:1390, 1979
413. Cronnelly R, Stanski DR, Miller RD, Sheiner LB, Sohn YJ: Renal function and the pharmacokinetics of neostigmine in anesthetized man. *Anesthesiology* 51:222, 1979
414. Weiner N: Drugs that inhibit adrenergic nerves and block adrenergic receptors, in *The Pharmacological Basis of Therapeutics*, Edited by Gilman AG, Goodman LS, Gilman A, 6th edn, New York, MacMillan Publ Co, 1980, p 176
415. Cameron JS, Toseland PA, Read JF, Bewick M, Ogg CS, Ellis FG: Accumulation of barbitone in patients on regular haemodialysis. *Lancet* 1:912, 1970
416. Myschetsky A, Lassen NA: Urea induced osmotic diuresis and alkalinization of urine in acute barbiturate intoxication. *JAMA* 185:936, 1963
417. Campion DS, North JD: Effect of protein binding of barbiturates on their rate of removal during peritoneal dialysis. *J Lab Clin Med* 66:549, 1965
418. Exaire E, Treviño-Becerra A, Monteon F: An overview of treatment with peritoneal dialysis in drug poisoning. *Contrib Nephrol* 17:39, 1979
419. Goldbaum LR, Smith PK: The interaction of barbiturates with serum albumin and its possible relation to their disposition and pharmacologic actions. *J Pharmacol Exp Ther* 111:197, 1954
420. Ehrnebo M, Odar-Cederlöf I: Binding of amobarbital, pentobarbital and diphenylhydantoin to blood cells and plasma proteins in healthy volunteers and uraemic patients. *Eur J Clin Pharmacol* 8:445, 1975
421. Knochel JP, Barry KG: THAM dialysis; an experimental method to study diffusion of certain weak acids in vivo II. Secobarbital. *J Lab Clin Med* 65:361, 1965
422. Yatzidis H, Oreopoulos D, Triantaphyllidis D, Voudiclari S, Tsaparas N, Gavras C, Stavroulaki A: Treatment of severe barbiturate poisoning. *Lancet* 2:216, 1965
423. Rosenbaum JL, Kramer MS, Raja R: Resin hemoperfusion for acute drug intoxication. *Arch Intern Med* 136:263, 1976
424. Gelfand MC, Winchester JF, Knepshield JH, Hanson KM, Cohan SL, Strauss BS, Geoly KL, Kennedy AC, Schreiner GE: Treatment of severe drug overdosage with charcoal hemoperfusion. *Trans Am Soc Artif Intern Organs* 23:599, 1977
425. Koffler A, Bernstein M, LaSette A, Massry SG: Fixed-bed charcoal hemoperfusion. Treatment of drug overdose. *Arch Intern Med* 138:1691, 1978
426. Kangas L, Kanto J, Forsström J, Iisalo E: The protein binding of diazepam and N demethyldiazepam in patients with poor renal function. *Clin Nephrol* 5:114, 1976
427. DeSilva JAF. Koechlin BA, Bader G: Blood level distribution patterns of diazepam and its major metabolite in man. *J Pharm Sci* 55:692, 1966
428. Randall LO: Pharmacology of chlordiazepoxide (Librium). *Dis Nerv Syst* 22:7, 1961
429. Cruz IA, Kramer NC, Parrish AE: Hemodialysis in chlordiazepoxide toxicity. *JAMA* 202:438, 1967
430. Taclob L, Needle M: Drug induced encephalopathy in patients on maintenance hemodialysis. *Lancet* 2:704, 1976
431. Breimer DD: Clinical pharmacokinetics of hypnotics. *Clin Pharmacokinet* 2:93, 1977

432. Vazari ND, Kumar KP, Mirahamadi K, Rosen SM: Hemodialysis in treatment of chloral hydrate poisoning. *South Med J* 70:377, 1977
433. Stalker NE, Gambertoglio JG, Fukumitsu CJ, Naughton JL, Benet LZ: Acute massive chloral hydrate intoxication treated with hemodialysis. *J Clin Pharmacol* 18:136, 1978
434. Heath A, Wickström I, Ahlmen J: Hemoperfusion in tricyclic antidepressant poisoning. *Lancet* 1:155, 1980
435. Teehan BP, Maher JF, Carey JJH, Flynn PD, Schreiner GE: Acute ethchlorvynol (Placidyl ®) intoxication. *Ann Intern Med* 72:875, 1970
436. Lynn RI, Honig CL, Jatlow PI, Kliger AS: Resin hemoperfusion for treatment of ethchlorvynol overdose. *Ann Intern Med* 91:549, 1979
437. Zmuda MJ: Resin hemoperfusion in dogs intoxicated with ethchlorvynol (Placidyl ®). *Kidney Int* 17:303, 1980
438. Benowitz N, Abolin C, Tozer T, Rosenberg J, Rogers W, Pond S, Schoenfeld P, Humphries M: Resin hemoperfusion in ethchlorvynol overdose. *Clin Pharmacol Ther* 27:236, 1980
439. De Myttenaere M, Schoenfeld L, Maher JF: Treatment of glutethimide poisoning; a comparison of forced diuresis and dialysis. *JAMA* 203:885, 1968
440. Chang TMS, Coffey JD, Lister C, Taroy E, Stark A: Methaqualone, methyprylon and glutethimide clearance by the ACAC microcapsule artificial kidney. In vitro and in patients with acute intoxication. *Trans Am Soc Artif Intern Organs* 19:87, 1973
441. De Myttenaere MH, Maher JF, Schreiner GE: Hemoperfusion through a charcoal column for glutethimide poisoning. *Trans Am Soc Artif Intern Organs* 13:190, 1967
442. Rosenbaum JL, Kramer MS, Raja RM: Amberlite hemoperfusion in the treatment of acute drug intoxication. *Int J Artif Organs* 2:316, 1979
443. Maddock RK, Bloomer HA: Meprobamate overdosage; evaluation of severity and methods of treatment. *JAMA* 201:999, 1967
444. Lobo PI, Spyler D, Surratt P, Westervelt FB Jr: Use of hemodialysis in meprobamate overdosage. *Clin Nephrol* 7:73, 1977
445. Yudis M, Swartz C, Onesti G, Ramirez O, Snyder D, Brest A: Hemodialysis for methyprylon (Noludar) poisoning. *Ann Intern Med* 68:1301, 1968
446. Mandelbaum JM, Simon NM: Severe methyprylon (Noludar) intoxication treated by hemodialysis. *JAMA* 216:139, 1971
447. Pancorbo AS, Palagi PA, Piecoro JJ, Wilson HD: Hemodialysis in methyprylon overdose; some pharmacokinetic considerations. *JAMA* 237:470, 1977
448. Proudfoot AT, Noble J, Nimmo J, Brown SS, Cameron JC: Peritoneal dialysis and haemodialysis in methaqualone (Mandrax) poisoning. *Scott Med J* 13:232, 1968
449. Langecker H, Neuhaus G, Ibe K, Kessel M: Ein Suicid-Versuch mit Valamin mit einem Beitrag zur elimination und Therapie (A suicide attempt with Valmid with a contribution to removal and therapy). *Arch Toxicol* 19:293, 1962 (in German)
450. Gutman RA, Burnell JM, Solak F: Paraldehyde acidosis. *Am J Med* 42:455, 1967
451. Berger M, White J, Travis LB, Browhard BH, Cunningham RJ III, Patnode R, Petrusick T: Toxic psychosis due to cyproheptadine in a child on hemodialysis: a case report. *Clin Nephrol* 7:43, 1977
452. Hawthorne JW, Marcus AM, Kaye M: Management of massive imprimine overdosage with mannitol and artificial dialysis. *N Engl J Med* 268:33, 1963
453. Oreopoulos DG, Lal S: Recovery from massive amitriptyline overdosage. *Lancet* 2:221, 1968
454. Trafford JAP, Jones RH, Evans R, Sharp P, Sharpstone P, Cook J: Haemoperfusion with R-004 amberlite resin for treating acute poisoning. *Br Med J* 2:1453, 1977
455. Winchester JF, Gelfand MC, Tilstone WJ: Hemoperfusion in drug intoxication: clinical and laboratory aspects. *Drug Metab Rev* 8:69, 1978
456. Davis JM, Fann WE: Lithium. *Annu Rev Pharmacol* 11:285, 1971
457. Singer I, Rotenberg D: Mechanisms of lithium action. *N Engl J Med* 289:254, 1973
458. Hansen HE, Hestbech J, Sorensen JL, Norgaard K, Heilskov J, Amdisen A: Chronic interstitial nephropathy in patient on long-term lithium treatment. *Q J Med* 48:577, 1979
459. Amdisen A, Skjoldborg: Haemodialysis for lithium poisoning. *Lancet* 2:213, 1969
460. Wilson JHP, Danker AJM, Van der Hem GK, Wientjes J: Peritoneal dialysis for lithium poisoning. *Br J Med* 2:749, 1971
461. Procci WR: Mania during maintenance hemodialysis successfully treated with oral lithium carbonate. *J Nerv Ment Dis* 164:355, 1977
462. Port F, Kroll PD, Rosenzweig J: Lithium therapy during maintenance hemodialysis. *Psychosomatics* 20:130, 1979
463. Borga O, Odar-Cederlöf I, Ringberger V, Norlin A: Protein binding of salicylate in uremic and normal plasma. *Clin Pharmacol Ther* 20:464, 1976
464. Schreiner GE, Maher JF, Argy WP Jr, Siegel L: Extracorporeal and peritoneal dialysis of drugs, in *Concepts in Biochemical Pharmacology, Handbook of Experimental Pharmacology*, edited by Brodie BB, Gillette JR, Vol 28, Berlin, Springer-Verlag, 1971
465. Summitt RL, Etteldorf JN: Salicylate intoxication in children; experience with peritoneal dialysis and alkalinization of the urine. *J Pediatr* 64:803, 1964
466. Verbeek RK, De Schepper PJ: Influence of chronic renal failure and hemodialysis on diflusinal plasma protein binding. *Clin Pharmacol Ther* 27:628, 1980
467. Boyer TD, Rouff SL: Acetaminophen induced hepatic necrosis and renal failure. *JAMA* 218:440, 1971
468. Bengtsson U, Johansson S, Angervall L: Malignancies of the urinary tract and their relation to analgesic abuse. *Kidney Int* 13:107, 1978
469. Gonwa TA, Hamilton RW, Buckalew VM Jr: Chronic renal failure and end stage renal disease in northwest North Carolina. Importance of analgesic associated nephropathy. *Arch Intern Med* 141:462, 1981
470. Faird NR, Glynn JP, Kerr DNS: Haemodialysis in paracetamol self-poisoning. *Lancet* 2:396, 1972
471. Marbury TC, Wang LH, Lee CS: Hemodialysis of acetaminophen in uremic patients. *Int J Artif Organs* 3:263, 1980
472. Maclean D, Peters DJ, Brown RAG, MacCathie M, Baines GF, Robertson PGC: Treatment of acute paracetamol poisoning. *Lancet* 2:849, 1968
473. Øie S, Lowenthal DT, Briggs WA, Levy G: Effect of hemodialysis on kinetics of acetaminophen elimination by anephric patients. *Clin Pharmacol Ther* 18:680, 1975
474. Rigby RJ, Thomson NM, Parkin GW, Cheung TPF: The treatment of paracetamol overdose with charcoal haemoperfusion and cysteamine. *Med J Austr* 1:396, 1978
475. Winchester JF, Gelfand MC, Helliwell M, Vale JA, Goulding R, Schreiner GE: Extracorporeal treatment of salicylate or acetaminophen poisoning – is there a role: *Arch Intern Med* 141:370, 1981
476. Giacomini KM, Gibson TP, Levy G: Effect of hemodialysis on propoxyphene and norpropoxyphene concentrations in blood of anephric patients. *Clin Pharmacol Ther* 27:508, 1980

477. Gary NE, Maher JF, De Myttenaere MH, Liggero SH, Scott KG, Matusiak W, Schreiner GE: Acute propoxyphene hydrochloride intoxication. *Arch Intern Med* 121:453, 1968
478. Maddocks JL, Wake CJ, Harber MJ: The plasma half life of antipyrine in chronic uraemic and normal subjects. *Br J Clin Pharmacol* 2:339, 1975
479. Berkowitz B: Influence of plasma levels and metabolism on pharmacological activity: pentazocine. *Ann NY Acad Sci* 179:269, 1971
480. Way EL, Adler TK: The pharmacologic implications of the fate of morphine and its surrogates. *Pharmacol Rev* 12:383, 1960
481. Zabinska K, Smólenski O, Hanicki Z, Bogdal J, Paczek Z, Wiernikowski A, Hirszel P: Ostre zatrucia leczone dialysa. (Severe intoxications treated with dialysis.) *Przegl Lek* 23:717, 1967 (in Polish)
482. Szeto HH, Inturrisi CE, Houde R, Saal S, Cheigh J, Reidenberg MM: Accumulation of normeperidine, an active metabolite of meperidine in patients with renal failure or cancer. *Ann Intern Med* 86:738, 1977
483. Glazer WM, Cohn GL: Methadone maintenance in a patient on chronic hemodialysis. *Am J Psych* 134:931, 1977
484. MacCarthy EP, Frost GW, Stokes GS: Indomethacin-induced hyperkalemia. *Med J Aust* 1:550, 1979
485. Kleinknecht C, Broyer M, Gubler MC, Palcoux JB: Irreversible renal failure after indomethacin in steroid resistant nephrosis. *N Engl J Med* 302:691, 1980
486. Gary NE, Dodelson R, Eisinger RP: Indomethacin-associated acute renal failure. *Am J Med* 69:135, 1980
487. Held H, Enderle C: Elimination and serum protein binding of phenylbutazone in patients with renal insufficiency. *Clin Nephrol* 6:388, 1976
488. Lipsett MB, Goldman R: Phenylbutazone toxicity; report of a case of acute renal failure. *Ann Intern Med* 41:1075, 1954
489. Kimberly RP, Brandstetter RD: Exacerbation of phenylbutazone related renal failure by indomethacin. *Arch Intern Med* 138:1711, 1978
490. Strong JE, Wilson J, Douglas JF, Coppel DL: Phenylbutazone self-poisoning treated by charcoal haemoperfusion. *Anaesthesia* 34:1038, 1979
491. Flower RJ, Moncada S, Vane JR: Analgesic-antipyretics and anti-inflammatory agents; drugs employed in the treatment of gout, in *The Pharmacological Basis of Therapeutics,* edited by Gilman AG, Goodman LS, Gilman A, 6th edn, New York, MacMillan Publ Co, 1980, p 682
492. Anttila M, Haataja M, Kasanen A: Pharmacokinetics of naproxen in subjects with normal and impaired renal function. *Eur J Clin Pharmacol* 18:263, 1980
493. Weber SS, Troutman WG, Trujeque L: Effect of hemodialysis on plasma naproxen concentration. *Am J Hosp Pharm* 36:1567, 1979
494. Curt GA, Kaldany A, Whitley LG, Crosson AW, Rolla A, Merino MJ, D'Elia JA: Reversible rapidly progressive renal failure with nephrotic syndrome due to fenoprofen calcium. *Ann Intern Med* 92:72, 1980
495. Rogers HJ, Savitsky JP, Glenn B, Spector RG: Kinetics of single doses of fenbufen in patients with renal insufficiency. *Clin Pharmacol Ther* 29:74, 1981
496. Robertson CE, Ford MJ, Van Someren V, Dlugolecka M, Prescott LF: Mefenamic acid nephropathy. *Lancet* 2:232, 1980
497. Wang LH, Lee CS, Marbury TC: Hemodialysis of mefenamic acid in uremic patients. *Am J Hosp Pharm* 37:956, 1980
498. Silverberg DS, Kidd EG, Shnitka TK, Ulan RA: Gold nephropathy. A clinical and pathologic study. *Arthritis Rheum* 13:812, 1970
499. Scott JJ, O'Brien PK: Probenecid, nephrotic syndrome and renal failure. *Ann Rheum Dis* 27:249, 1968
500. Bern M, Cavaliere BM, Lucas G: Plasma levels and effects of sulfinpyrazone in patients requiring chronic hemodialysis. *J Clin Pharmacol* 20:107, 1980
501. Elion GB, Yu T, Gutman AB, Hitchings GH: Renal clearance of oxipurinol, the chief metabolite of allopurinol. *Am J Med* 45:69, 1968
502. Sherlock HE, Letteri JM: Effect of hemodialysis on methylprednisolone plasma levels. *Nephron* 18:208, 1977
503. Deck KA, Fischer B, Hillen H: Studies on cortisol metabolism during haemodialysis in man. *Eur J Clin Invest* 9:203, 1979
504. Bach JF, Dardenne M: The metabolism of azathioprine in renal failure. *Transplantation* 12:253, 1971
505. Duttera MJ, Carolla RL, Gallelli JF, Gullion DS, Leim DE, Henderson ES: Hematuria and crystalluria after high dose 6-mercaptopurine administration. *N Engl J Med* 287:292, 1972
506. Schusziarra V, Ziekursch V, Schlamp R, Siemensen HC: Pharmacokinetics of azathioprine under haemodialysis. *Int J Clin Pharmacol Biopharm* 14:298, 1976
507. Cohen JL, Jao JY, Jusko WJ: Pharmacokinetics of cyclophosphamide in man. *Br J Pharmacol* 43:677, 1971
508. Wang LH, Lee CS, Majeske BL, Marbury TC: Clearance and recovery calculations in hemodialysis: application to plasma, red blood cell and dialysate measurements for cyclophosphamide. *Clin Pharmacol Ther* 29:365, 1981
509. Milsted RAV, Jarman N: Haemodialysis during cyclophosphamide treatment. *Br Med J* 1:820, 1978
510. Galletti PM, Pasqualino A, Geering RG: Hemodialysis in cancer chemotherapy. *Trans Am Soc Artif Intern Organs* 12:20, 1966
511. Holt S, Naysmith S, Reid J, Buist TAS: Hazards of hepatic artery infusion of streptozocin. *Scott Med J* 24:163, 1979
512. Harmon WE, Cohen HJ, Schneeberger EE, Grupe WE: Chronic renal failure in children treated with methyl CCNU. *N Engl J Med* 300:1200, 1979
513. Henderson ES, Adamson RH, Oliverio VT: The metabolic fate of tritiated methotrexate. II. Absorption and excretion in man. *Cancer Res* 25:1018, 1965
514. Bryan CW, Henry P: Methotrexate clearance in rats with impaired renal function. *Clin Res* 21:817, 1973
515. Hande KR, Balow JE, Drake JC, Rosenberg SA, Chabner BA: Methotrexate and hemodialysis. *Ann Intern Med* 87:495, 1977
516. Ahmad S, Shen F, Bleyer WAL: Methotrexate induced renal failure and ineffectiveness of peritoneal dialysis. *Arch Intern Med* 138:1146, 1978
517. Gibson TP, Reich SD, Krumlovsky FA, Ivanovich P: Hemoperfusion for methotrexate removal. *Clin Pharmacol Ther* 23:351, 1978
518. Condit PT, Chanes RE, Joel W: Renal toxicity of methotrexate. *Cancer* 28:126, 1969
519. Crooke ST, Luft F, Broughton A, Strong J, Casson K, Einhorn L: Bleomycin serum pharmacokinetics as determined by radioimmunoassay and a micro-biologic assay in a patient with compromised renal function. *Cancer* 39:1430, 1977
520. Burke JF, Laucius F, Brodovsky HS, Soriano RZ: Doxorubicin hydrochloride-associated renal failure. *Arch Intern Med* 137:385, 1977
521. Dragon LH, Braine HG: Necrosis of the hand after daunorubicin infusion distal to an arteriovenous fistula. *Ann Intern Med* 91:58, 1979
522. Winchester JF, Rahman A, Tilstone WJ, Bregman H, Mortensen LM, Gelfand MC, Schein PS, Schreiner GE:

Will hemoperfusion be useful for cancer chemotherapeutic drug removal? *Clin Toxicol* 17:557, 1980
523. Madias NE, Harrington JT: Platinum nephrotoxicity. *Am J Med* 65:307, 1978
524. Dentino M, Luft FC, Yum MN, Williams SD, Einhorn LH: Long term effect of cis-diammine-dichloride platinum (CDDP) on renal function and structure in man. *Cancer* 41:1274, 1978
525. Prestayko AW, Luft FC, Einhorn L, Crooke ST: Cisplaten pharmacokinetics in a patient with renal dysfunction. *Med Pediatr Oncol* 5:183, 1978
526. Fuss M, Bergans A, Brauman H, Toussaint C, Vereerstraeten P, Franckson M, Corvilain J: ^{125}-I-insulin metabolism in chronic renal failure treated by renal transplantation. *Kidney Int* 5:372, 1974
527. Shapiro DJ, Blumenkrantz MJ, Levin SR, Coburn JW: Absorption and action of insulin added to peritoneal dialysate in dogs. *Nephron* 22:174, 1977
528. Smith DL, Vecchio TI, Forist AA: Metabolism of antidiabetic sulfonylureas in man. *Metabolism* 14:229, 1965
529. Petitpierre B, Perrin L, Rudhardt M, Herrera A, Fabre J: Behaviour of chlorpropamide in renal insufficiency and under the effect of associated drug therapy. *Int J Clin Pharmacol* 6:120, 1972
530. Rothfield EL, Crews AH Jr, Ribot S, Bernstein A: Severe hypoglycemia. Result of renal retention of chlorpropamide. *Arch Intern Med* 115:468, 1965
531. Graw RG, Clarke RR: Chlorpropamide intoxication – treatment with peritoneal dialysis. *Pediatrics* 45:106, 1970
532. Weissman PN, Shenkman L, Gregerman RJ: Chlorpropamide induced hyponatremia. Drug induced inappropriate antidiuretic-hormone activity. *N Engl J Med* 284:65, 1971
533. Beckman R: The fate of biguanides in man. *Ann NY Acad Sci* 14:820, 1968
534. Ewy G, Pabico RC, Maher JF, Mintz DH: Lactic acidosis associated with phenformin therapy and localized tissue hypoxia. Report of a case treated by hemodialysis. *Ann Intern Med* 59:878, 1963
535. Tobin M, Mookerjee BK: Hemodialysis for phenformin associated lactic acidosis. *J Dial* 2:273, 1979
536. Letteri JM, Mellk H, Louis S, Kutt H, Durante P, Glazko A: Diphenylhydantoin metabolism in uremia. *N Engl J Med* 285:648, 1971
537. Steele WH, Lawrence JR, Elliott HL, Whiting B: Alterations of phenytoin protein binding with in vivo haemodialysis in dialysis encephalopathy. *Eur J Clin Pharmacol* 15:69, 1979
538. Borgå O, Hoppel C, Odar-Cederlöf I, Garle M: Plasma levels and renal excretion of phenytoin and its metabolites in patients with renal failure. *Clin Pharmacol Ther* 26:306, 1979
539. Agarwal BN, Cabebe FG, Hoffman BI: Diphenylhydantoin-induced acute renal failure. *Nephron* 18:249, 1977
540. Martin E, Gambertoglio JG, Adler DS, Tozer TN, Roman LA, Grausz H: Removal of phenytoin by hemodialysis in uremic patients. *JAMA* 238:1750, 1977
541. Tenckhoff H, Sherrard DJ, Hickman RO: Acute diphenylhydantoin intoxication. *Am J Dis Child* 116:422, 1968
542. Thiel GB, Richter RW, Powell MR, Doolan PD: Acute Dilantin poisoning. *Neurology* 11:138, 1961
543. Czajka PA, Anderson WH, Christoph RA, Banner W Jr: A pharmacokinetic evaluation of peritoneal dialysis for phenytoin intoxication. *J Clin Pharmacol* 20:565, 1980
544. Rubinger D, Levy M, Roll D, Czaczkes JW: Inefficiency of haemodialysis in acute phenytoin intoxication. *Br J Clin Pharmacol* 7:405, 1979

545. Baehler RW, Work J, Smith W, Dominic JA: Charcoal hemoperfusion in the therapy for methsuximide and phenytoin overdose. *Arch Intern Med* 140:1466, 1980
546. Swinyard EA, Schiffman DO, Goodman LS: Effects of liver injury and nephrectomy on the anticonvulsant activity of oxazolidine-2,4-diones. *J Pharmacol Exp Ther* 105:365, 1952
547. Bergstrand A, Bergstrand CG, Engstrom N, Herrlin KM: Renal histology during treatment with oxazolidine-diones (trimethadione, ethadione and paramethadione). *Pediatrics* 30:601, 1962
548. Marbury TC, Lee CS, Bruni J, Wilder BJ: Hemodialysis of valproic acid in uremic patients. *Dial Transpl* 9:961, 1980
549. Nicholls DP, Yasin M: Acute renal failure from carbamazepine. *Br Med J* 4:490, 1972
550. Lee CS, Wang LH, Marbury TC, Bruni J, Perchalski RJ: Hemodialysis clearance and total body elimination of carbamazepine during chronic hemodialysis. *Clin Toxicol* 17:429, 1980
551. Werb R, Clark WR, Lindsay RM, Jones EOP, Linton AL: Serum vitamin A levels and associated abnormalities in patients on regular dialysis treatment. *Clin Nephrol* 12:63, 1979
552. Ellis S, DePalma J, Cheng A, Capozzalo P, Dombeck D, Discala VA: Vitamin A supplements in hemodialysis patients. *Nephron* 26:215, 1980
553. Gotloib L, Sklan D, Mines M: Hemodialysis; effect on plasma levels of vitamin A and carotenoid. *JAMA* 239:751, 1978
554. Chaplin H Jr, Clark LD, Ropes MW: Vitamin D intoxication. *Am J Med Sci* 221:269, 1951
555. Nolph KD, Stoltz M, Maher JF: Calcium free peritoneal dialysis. Treatment of vitamin D intoxication. *Arch Intern Med* 128:809, 1971
556. Berl T, Berns AS, Huffer WE, Hammill K, Alfrey AC, Arnaud CD, Schrier RW: 1,25 dihydroxycholecalciferol effects in chronic dialysis. A double-blind controlled study. *Ann Intern Med* 88:774, 1978
557. Christiansen C, Rodbro P, Christensen MS, Hartnack B, Transbol I: Deterioration of renal function during treatment of chronic renal failure with 1,25 dihydroxycholecalciferol. *Lancet* 2:700, 1978
558. Niwa T, Ito T, Matsui E: Plasma thiamine levels with hemodialysis. *JAMA* 218:885, 1971
559. Ito T, Niwa T, Matsui E: Vitamin B_2 and vitamin E in long-term hemodialysis. *JAMA* 217:699, 1971
560. Lasker N, Harvey A, Baker H: Vitamin levels in hemodialysis and intermittent peritoneal dialysis. *Trans Am Soc Artif Intern Organs* 9:51, 1963
561. Dobbelstein H, Korner WF, Mempel W, Grosse-Wilde H, Edel HH: Vitamin B_6 deficiency in uremia and its implications for the depression of immune responses. *Kidney Int* 5:233, 1974
562. Whitehead VM, Comty CH, Posen GA, Kaye M: Homeostasis of folic acid in patients undergoing maintenance hemodialysis. *N Engl J Med* 279:970, 1968
563. Skoutakis VA, Acchiardo SR, Meyer MC, Hatch FE: Folic acid dosage for chronic hemodialysis patients. *Clin Pharmacol Ther* 18:200, 1975
564. Watson AJS, Lawler E, Keogh JAB: Acute folate deficiency during peritoneal dialysis. *Br Med J* 2:1608, 1980
565. Reznik VM, Griswold WR, Brams MR, Mendoza SA: Does high dose ascorbic acid accelerate renal failure? *N Engl J Med* 302:1418, 1980
566. Sullivan JF, Eisenstein AB, Mottola OM, Mittal AK: The effect of dialysis on plasma and tissue levels of vitamin C. *Trans Am Soc Artif Intern Organs* 18:277, 1972
567. Eschbach JW, Cook JD, Scribner BH, Finch CA: Iron

balance in hemodialysis patients. *Ann Intern Med* 87:710, 1977
568. Ali M, Fayemi O, Rigolosi R. Frascino J, Marsden T, Malcolm D: Hemosiderosis in hemodialysis patients; an autopsy study of 50 cases. *JAMA* 244:343, 1980
569. Berlyne GM, Ben Ari J, Pest D, Weinberger J, Stern M, Gilmore GR, Levine R: Hyperaluminaemia from aluminium resins in renal failure. *Lancet* 2:494, 1970
570. Kaehny WD, Alfrey AC, Holman RE, Shorr WJ: Aluminum transfer during hemodialysis. *Kidney Int* 12:361, 1977
571. Ackrill P, Ralston AJ, Day JP, Hodge KC: Successful removal of aluminium from a patient with dialysis encephalopathy *Lancet* 2:692, 1980
572. Pierides AM, Ward MK, Kerr DNS: Haemodialysis encephalopathy; possible role of phosphate depletion. *Lancet* 1:1234, 1976
573. Alfrey AC, Le Gendre GR, Kaehny WD: The dialysis encephalopathy syndrome. Possible aluminum intoxication. *N Engl J Med* 294:184, 1976
574. Curtis JR, Goode GC, Herrington J, Urdaneta LE: Possible cobalt toxicity in maintenance hemodialysis patients after treatment with cobaltous chloride: a study of blood and tissue cobalt concentration in normal subjects and patients with terminal renal failure. *Clin Nephrol* 5:61, 1976
575. Rees PH, Keating MI, Kager PA, Hockmeyer WT: Renal clearance of pentavalent antimony (sodium stibogluconate). *Lancet* 2:226, 1980
576. Salvadeo A, Minola C, Segagni S, Villa S: Trace metal changes in dialysis fluid and blood of patients on hemodialysis. *Int J Artif Organs* 2:17, 1979
577. Gilberson A, Vaziri ND, Mirahamadi K, Rosen SM: Hemodialysis of acute arsenic intoxication with transient renal failure. *Arch Int Med* 136:1303, 1976
578. Marlette JM, Ma KW, Shafer RB: Effect of hemodialysis on gallium-67-citrate scanning. *Clin Nucl Med* 5:401, 1980
579. Doolan PD, Hess WC, Kyle LH: Acute renal insufficiency due to bichloride of mercury. Observations on gastrointestinal hemorrhage and BAL therapy. *N Engl J Med* 249:273, 1953
580. Foremen H, Finnegan C, Lushbaugh CC: Nephrotoxic hazard from uncontrolled edathamil calcium disodium therapy. *JAMA* 160:1042, 1956
581. Felts JH, King JS, Boyce WH: Nephrotic syndrome after treatment with D-penicillamine. *Lancet* 1:53, 1968
582. Ross JH, McGinty F, Brewer DG: Penicillamine nephropathy. *Nephron* 26:184, 1980
583. Batey R, Scott J, Jain S, Sherlock S: Acute renal insufficiency occurring during intravenous desferrioxamine therapy. *Scand J Haematol* 22:277, 1979
584. Sacho JJ, Henderson RR: Use of bishydroxycoumarin (Dicoumarol) in the presence of impaired renal function. *JAMA* 148:839, 1952
585. Wright JS: Phenindione sensitivity with leukaemoid reaction and hepatorenal damage. *Postgrad Med J* 46:452, 1970
586. O'Reilly RA, Aggler PM: Determinants of the response to oral anticoagulant drugs in man. *Pharmacol Rev* 22:35, 1970
587. Turney JH, Williams LC, Fenwell MR, Parsons V, Weston MJ: Platelet protection and heparin sparing with prostacyclin during regular dialysis therapy. *Lancet* 2:219, 1980
588. Zusman RM, Rubin RH, Cato AE, Cocchetto DM, Crow JM, Tolkoff-Rubin N: Hemodialysis using prostacyclin instead of heparin as the sole antithrombotic agent. *N Engl J Med* 304:934, 1981
589. Kobayashi K, Maeda K, Koshikawa S, Kawaguchi Y, Shimizu N, Naito C: Antithrombotic therapy with ticlopidine in chronic renal failure patients on maintenance hemodialysis – a multicenter collaborative double-blind study. *Thromb Res* 20:255, 1980
590. Bricker NS, Hlad CJ: Observations on the renal clearance of I^{131}. *J Clin Invest* 34:1057, 1955
591. Hansson R, Lindholm T: Elimination of hypaque (sodium-3,5 diacetamido-2,4,6triiodobenzoate) and the effect of hemodialysis in anuria. A clinical study and an experimental investigation on rabbits. *Acta Med Scand* 174:611, 1963
592. Bahlmann J, Krüskemper HL: Elimination of iodine containing contrast media by haemodialysis. *Nephron* 10:250, 1973
593. Ackrill P, McIntosh CS, Nimmon C, Baker LRI, Cattell WR: A comparison of the clearance of urographic contrast medium (sodium diatrizoate) by peritoneal and haemodialysis. *Clin Sci Mol Med* 50:69, 1976
594. Byrd L, Sherman RL: Radiocontrast-induced acute renal failure: a clinical and pathophysiologic review. *Medicine* 58:270, 1979
595. Mudge GH: Nephrotoxicity of urographic radiocontrast drugs. *Kidney Int* 18:540, 1980
596. Swartz RD, Rubin JE, Leeming BW, Silva P: Renal failure following major angiography. *Am J Med* 65:31, 1978
597. Goldberg AP, Sherrard DJ, Haas LB, Brunzell JD: Control of clofibrate toxicity in uremic hypertriglyceridemia. *Clin Pharmacol Ther* 21:317, 1977
598. Gugler R, Kürten JW, Jensen CJ, Klehr U, Hartlapp J: Clofibrate disposition in renal failure and acute and chronic liver disease. *Eur J Clin Pharmacol* 15:341, 1979
599. Cumming A: Acute renal failure and interstitial nephritis after clofibrate treatment. *Br Med J* 2:1529, 1980
600. Singer MM, Dutton R, Way WL: Untoward results of gallamine administration during bilateral nephrectomy: treatment with haemodialysis. *Br J Anaesth* 43:404, 1971
601. Cozantis D, Haapenen E: Studies on muscle relaxants during haemodialysis. *Acta Anaesthesiol Scand* 23:225, 1979
602. Sievenpiper TS, Rice SA, McClendon F, Kosek JC, Mazze RI: Renal effects of enflurance anesthesia in Fischer 344 rats with preexisting renal insufficiency. *J Pharmacol Exp Ther* 211:36, 1979
603. Gosselin RE, Gabourel JD, Wills JH: Fate of atropine in man. *Clin Pharmacol Ther* 1:597, 1960
604. Bjaeldager PAL, Jensen JB, Larsen NE, Hvidberg EF: Elimination of oral cimetidine in chronic renal failure and during haemodialysis. *Br J Clin Pharmacol* 9:585, 1980
605. Larsson R, Bodemar G, Norlander B: Oral absorption of cimetidine and its clearance in patients with renal failure. *Eur J Clin Pharmacol* 15:153, 1979
606. Ma KW, Brown DC, Masler DS, Silvis SE: Effects of renal failure on blood levels of cimetidine. *Gastroenterology* 74:473, 1978
607. Larsson R, Bodemar G, Kagedal B, Walan A: The effects of cimetidine (Tagamet ®) on renal function in patients with renal failure. *Acta Med Scand* 208:27, 1980
608. Jones RH, Lewin MR, Parsons V: Therapeutic effect of cimetidine in patients undergoing haemodialysis. *Br Med J* 1:650, 1979
609. Klotz U, Reimann I: Delayed clearance of diazepam due to cimetidine. *N Engl J Med* 302:1012, 1980
610. Jacob AI, Lanier D, Canterbury J, Bourgoinie JJ: Reduction by cimetidine of serum parathyroid hormone levels in uremic patients. *N Engl J Med* 302:671, 1980

611. Vaziri ND, Ness RL, Barton CH: Peritoneal dialysis clearance of cimetidine. *Am J Gastroenterol* 71:572, 1979
612. Pizzella KM, Moore MC, Schultz RW, Walshe J, Schentag JJ: Removal of cimetidine by peritoneal dialysis, hemodialysis and charcoal hemoperfusion. *Ther Drug Monitor* 2:273, 1980

40

ANAESTHESIA AND MAJOR SURGERY IN PATIENTS WITH RENAL FAILURE

K. BRIAN SLAWSON

Introduction	798
Factors influencing anaesthesia	798
Anaemia	798
Acidosis	798
Potassium	799
Other fluid and electrolyte disturbances	799
Hypertension	799
Drugs used in anaesthesia	799
Intravenous induction agents	799
Inhalational agents	799
Chloroform and ether	799
Cyclopropane	799
Halothane	799
Methoxyflurane	799
Enflurane	799
Trichloroethylene	799
Neuroleptanaesthesia	800
Muscle relaxants	800
Suxamethonium	800
Gallamine	800
Tubocurarine	800
Pancuronium	800
Vecuronium	800
Atracurium	800
Spinal and epidural analgesia	800
The conduct of anaesthesia	801
Pre-operative preparation	801
Induction	801
Maintenance	801
Intravenous infusions	801
Monitoring	801
Post-operative sedation	801
Precautions	801
Conclusions	802
References	802

INTRODUCTION

Patients who suffer from chronic renal failure and require major surgery, whether for renal transplantation, for bilateral nephrectomy or for conditions unrelated to the kidney disease, present the anaesthetist with a unique series of problems. Fortunately, their health has usually been improved by dialysis; indeed, they are often in much better general condition than before their initial dialysis when relatively minor preliminary procedures, such as the creation of arterio-venous fistulae or shunts, had to be carried out.

Uraemic patients suffer anaemia, acidosis, hyperkalaemia, other fluid and electrolyte disorders and hypertension; the latter may be further complicated by drugs given in an attempt to control it. Efficient dialysis may be expected to correct many of these abnormalities, but leads to a loss of platelets, haemoglobin, serum enzymes and vitamins; hypertension may not always be fully controlled. Fortunately, the patient often adapts to these disorders and other metabolic disturbances.

FACTORS INFLUENCING ANAESTHESIA

Anaemia

The haemoglobin level is reduced in chronic renal failure, and patients have been presented in the past for anaesthesia and surgery with a haemoglobin level as low as 4.0 g/dl. The anaemia is normochromic and normocytic and is due partly to haemolysis and partly to diminished haemopoiesis in subjects lacking erythropoietin, with the loss of blood and folic acid mentioned above (1).

It has now been shown that blood transfusion given before renal transplantation may improve subsequent graft survival (2) and so patients presenting for operation in the future are unlikely to be so anaemic as in the past, when transfusion was believed disadvantageous.

It is possible to take advantage of the fact that chronically anaemic patients tolerate anaesthesia surprisingly well (3), whilst agreeing that this practice is undesirable in most instances (4). It is most important, therefore, that oxygenation, tissue perfusion and blood pressure be maintained at all times (5).

Acidosis

Fortunately dialysis usually corrects the metabolic acidosis found in the uraemic patient, as this disorder may complicate anaesthesia in several ways. The dissociation curve of haemoglobin is shifted to the left, and the muscle relaxant effect of depolarising agents such as suxamethonium and decamethonium is antagonised, while that of pancuronium (a non-depolarising relaxant) is potentiated, apparently due to changes in transmembrane potential (6).

Patients hyperventilate in order to compensate for their acidosis; general anaesthesia depresses ventilation (7), and this may result in an increase in PCO_2, a fall in blood pH and a possible rise in plasma potassium (8), which may cause cardiac arrhythmias (9). Many feel that the anaesthetised patient should be hyperventilated, but it has been suggested that it is more important to ensure a normal plasma potassium concentration before commencing anaesthesia.

Potassium

Plasma potassium is frequently raised in renal failure; if above 7 mmol/l electrocardiographic changes are common, and ventricular tachycardia or fibrillation may possibly occur (See Chapter 19). It is preferable to delay an operation long enough to reduce the plasma potassium to below 5 mmol/l and any subsequent rise should be minimised by avoiding hypoventilation (see above), transfusion of old or cold whole blood (9), or the use of suxamethonium to produce muscular relaxation (11, 12). Should an emergency operation be required, there is usually time for at least a short period of haemodialysis; failing that a cation exchange resin (Resonium A) may be administered orally unless anaesthesia is imminent, when the resin may be given more safely rectally. It will then not act for about three hours but intravenous dextrose (50 ml of a 50% solution) together with 20 units of soluble insulin will give control within 20 to 30 min. This intravenous regimen may also be useful during the course of anaesthesia if electrocardiographic evidence of hyperkalaemia is observed, in the shape of tall, peaked, tent-like T-waves (followed, if untreated, by ST depression and eventual atrioventricular block [See Chapters 19 and 26]).

The electrocardiogram should start to revert to normal in about ten minutes; the plasma potassium will be at a minimum in one hour and the effect will normally last for 3 to 4 h. The anaesthetist must be aware of the possible hazard of acute hyperkalaemia following release of the vascular clamps after transplantation of kidneys perfused with Collins' solution.

Other fluid and electrolyte disturbances

Haemodialysis may dehydrate patients and, during general anaesthesia in such circumstances, there will be difficulty in stabilising the blood pressure; central venous pressure measurement can be used to monitor correction of the defect. Anaesthetic management in general is much easier in patients with near normal plasma sodium concentrations than in subjects less well prepared (14). Derangement of calcium or magnesium balance may lead to difficulty in achieving or reversing muscular relaxation with drugs acting at the neuromuscular junction.

Hypertension

In some patients efficient dialysis controls hypertension, but others will still be receiving hypotensive drug therapy when they are presented for anaesthesia and surgery. Some workers have suggested that these agents be withdrawn prior to anaesthesia, but this can be unwise, as the patient may then be exposed to all the hazards of hypertension. It has been shown that the risks of anaesthesia are increased in uncontrolled hypertension (15), and that treatment with beta-adrenergic blockers helps to protect the patient against blood pressure rises, tachycardia, dysrhythmias and myocardial ischaemia (16).

DRUGS USED IN ANAESTHESIA

Intravenous induction agents

While an inhalational induction may be considered necessary for some extremely ill patients, for the great majority intravenous agents will be satisfactory, provided that a smaller than normal dose is given slowly (17). In hypertensive subjects, it may be that thiopentone is safer than methohexitone, propanidid or diazepam (18). Althesin, while safe (19), has a very brief duration of action which is not advantageous for major surgical procedures.

Inhalational agents

Chloroform and ether
These are nephrotoxic (20, 21), and the latter is, like cyclopropane, inflammable and cannot be used with diathermy.

Cyclopropane
This may be most useful in severely ill patients, as it can be administered with a high oxygen concentration and cardiac output is well maintained during its use (22).

Halothane
Probably the most widely used volatile agent is halothane and its successful use is noted in several published series (3, 23). One possible disadvantage is that it may lower cardiac output and blood pressure (24). It is not a good analgesic unless used in a concentration of at least 0.35% (25).

Methoxyflurane
Despite its apparent nephrotoxicity methoxyflurane (26) is probably not precluded from use in the absence of renal function, but a transplanted kidney would obviously be put at risk if this agent was used at or after transplantation. Low concentrations (0.3 to 0.5%) may be harmless (27), but there is a danger that metabolites, oxalate and fluoride (28), may cause oxalosis and stone formation, renal damage with polyuria and even affect the retina (29).

Enflurane
This may be nephrotoxic (30, 31), but isoflurane probably has no effect on renal function (32).

Trichloroethylene
This is an excellent analgesic and its use is not commonly associated with changes in blood pressure and pulse rate (33), although Strunin (34) felt that it could. It may

also cause cardiac arrhythmias. In the presence of beta-adrenergic blocking drugs, trichloroethylene anaesthesia may be accompanied by an impaired response to haemorrhage (35), as the combination causes direct depression of myocardial performance. Its use for longer than two hours has been known for many years to give prolonged post-operative sedation since it is partly metabolised to trichloroethanol, a sedative (36). As trichloroethylene is normally excreted in the urine recovery will be prolonged if renal function is impaired.

Neuroleptanaesthesia

There are reports of the use of droperidol and fentanyl anaesthesia for operations on patients with poor renal function (37), and also for renal transplantation (38), because neuroleptanaesthesia has little effect on the cardiovascular system in general (18, 39) and on renal blood flow in particular (40).

Muscle relaxants

Animal experiments suggest that the acidosis of patients with renal failure may antagonise the action of depolarising muscle relaxants (suxamethonium and decamethonium) and potentiate a non-depolarising block.

Suxamethonium
It is possible that dialysis may remove pseudocholinesterase from the plasma (41) and early workers feared that there might be prolonged apnoea if suxamethonium was employed to provide muscular relaxation (42). This has proved unfounded (22, 23, 34). In view of the fact that its administration is commonly associated with raised plasma potassium levels (11, 12, 43, 44) in patients already liable to such an abnormality by reason of their primary disability and their tissue catabolism (45, 46), it is probably unwise to give this drug except when rapid complete muscular relaxation is necessary for safe tracheal intubation in the presence of a full stomach (3). Suxamethonium has been shown to lower the renal blood flow in dogs (47) (not yet confirmed in man) and this is yet another reason for avoiding the drug.

A single dose of suxamethonium may be justified where rapid, easy intubation is necessary for a patient with a full stomach, for the rise of plasma potassium after such a single dose may be no more than in normal patients (45-50). Recently it has been suggested that hexafluorenium may be used safely to prolong the action of suxamethonium without ill effects in patients with renal failure (51), or that it would be safer to substitute suxethonium in these cases (52).

Gallamine
This highly ionised drug is dependent on the kidney for its elimination (53). Nevertheless in a series of 17 patients with chronic renal failure the action of gallamine was successfully reversed (54). Noteworthy is the case of a patient in whom gallamine was used during exploration of a transplanted kidney; the relaxation was only reversed three days later by dialysis (55). Obviously the use of this drug should be avoided.

Tubocurarine
This agent has been used successfully in many patients with chronic renal failure (3, 23) although occasional difficulty has been experienced in reversing its effects (14). The acidosis may limit and oppose the antagonist effect of physostigmine (56) and it has been suggested that pyridostigmine be used instead of physostigmine. The dose of relaxant required should be reduced by using an inhalational rather than a narcotic supplement to nitrous oxide anaesthesia (55). The safety of this drug appears to be due to the fact that, in the presence of renal failure, the liver has a greatly increased capacity to secrete tubocurarine into the bile, providing an alternative excretory pathway is not available for gallamine (58).

Administration of furosemide or mannitol to encourage early function of a transplanted kidney may, either by redistributing curare or by a direct effect on the neuromuscular junction, enhance blockade at that junction (59), whereas azathiaprine has been held to antagonise curariform block (60), possibly by inhibiting phosphodiesterase.

Pancuronium
This non-depolarising agent is now widely used to provide muscular relaxation for all types of major surgery, as it does not tend to lower blood pressure (61) or renal blood flow (62), and the onset of muscular paralysis is rapid (63). As with tubocurarine and other similar agents, its excretion is slow in renal disease (64), possibly due to some central redistribution, but reversal of its effects is usually readily accomplished. Again, this drug is eliminated to a varying but significant degree by the liver (65).

The only sure way to assess the adequacy of reversal of non-depolarising blockade is by the use of peripheral nerve stimulation (66).

Vecuronium
This new non-depolarising muscle relaxant may be an important new drug, as it has a rapid onset of action, a much shorter elimination half-life than pancuronium, and no cardiovascular side-effects (67). Repeated doses do not lead to a prolonged duration of effect, and studies in the cat suggest that the absence of renal function has less effect on neuromuscular blockade than is the case with pancuronium (68).

Atracurium is another newly introduced non-depolarising muscle relaxant. It may prove to be suitable for use in renal failure, since it undergoes enzyme-independent 'Hofmann elimination' to pharmacologically inactive products, and so its breakdown is dependent on neither renal nor hepatic function (78).

SPINAL AND EPIDURAL ANALGESIA

Renal transplants are placed extraperitoneally in the lower abdomen, so that adequate analgesia by these techniques need not be accompanied by the hypotension of high blockade (69, 70). In a recent series it was found that four of five patients given an epidural anaesthetic had to be given a general anaesthetic in addition but spinal anaesthesia was satisfactory, being accompanied by minimal hypotension (71). The patients needed no intubation or muscular relaxant drugs and were awake and reactive early post-operatively. Since uraemic patients may bleed unduly there is a danger of epidural haematoma and nerve root compression (72); in addition patients given regional analgesics frequently need heavy sedation or general anaesthesia to control distress or restlessness (3, 23).

Operations can be carried out in the upper abdomen in patients with no renal function under spinal or epidural analgesia provided blood pressure is maintained by fluid infusion or administration of vasopressors, any unwanted effect on renal vasculature being irrelevant in such cases.

THE CONDUCT OF ANAESTHESIA

Pre-operative preparation

Patients requiring emergency operations may have full stomachs, which must be aspirated or onward passage encouraged by giving metoclopramide (10 mg intramuscularly). Emergency haemodialysis may be necessary and in this case regional is preferable to systemic heparinisation (see Chapter 10); in either case a full screening of the clotting system is an essential preliminary to the operation.

Many premedicant drugs have been used. Barbiturates are probably best avoided as they may not be excreted for a long time, and in any case relieve apprehension less well than diazepam (73). Pain must be treated with an effective analgesic, remembering to adjust the dose to body weight. Atropine should be administered to protect against vagal effects of orotracheal intubation but can, of course, be injected intravenously at the time of induction.

Induction

As previously mentioned inhalation induction commonly with cyclopropane, is employed if indicated by the severity of the patient's condition, but in cases with renal failure under control by dialysis an intravenous induction, preferably with thiopentone, may be used following pre-oxygenation. Further protection against vagal stimulation on intubation can be provided by spraying the trachea with a local analgesic (74).

Maintenance

Hyperventilation with nitrous oxide and oxygen with a volatile supplement following muscular relaxation with d-tubocurarine or pancuronium is probably the technique of choice. The safest procedure is probably the one with which the anaesthetist is most familiar for,... 'patients of this type need not present a difficult challenge to the anaesthetist, but a high standard of practice is important...', and no particular anaesthetic technique has become associated with failure of a transplanted kidney in man (24). Halothane and nitrous oxide had no effect on rejection in mice and dogs (75). That there may, however, be a favourable effect is suggested by the finding that urethane facilitated graft survival in neonatal mice (76), and one might expect that anaesthesia, by an action on immune mechanisms, has such an influence.

Intravenous infusions

These patients must not be overtransfused, and unless they are hypovolaemic, infusion should be limited to 10 ml/kg/24 h (23). Meticulous haemostasis will limit the need for blood transfusion; if this becomes necessary the use of warmed, washed, fresh red cells will limit any untoward effects such as high infused potassium levels, cooling and unwanted immunological complications. If the operation is for renal transplantation, the kidney will function better if presented with a fluid load post-operatively, but monitoring of central venous pressure is then important to provide control over the fluid administration.

Monitoring

Central venous and arterial pressures should be carefully recorded, and electrocardiographic monitoring will give early warning of a rise in plasma potassium concentration, which is commonly seen post-operatively. Since reversal of muscle relaxants may on occasion be difficult or 'recurarisation' occasionally occurs (57), use of a nerve stimulator will give valuable information at the end of a procedure.

Post-operative sedation

For post-operative pain, all the common analgesic sedatives have been used, but it must be remembered that the dose should be adjusted according to body weight and drugs only prescribed when needed, and not routinely, for their action may be prolonged (77) or modified in the absence of renal function (see also Chapter 39.) Restlessness unaccompanied by pain may be treated by small intravenous increments of diazepam.

Precautions

Patients such as these readily acquire infections and great care must be taken not to introduce pathogens. Endotracheal tubes must therefore be sterile and the technique of injection and setting up infusions should be meticulous. Any patient treated for renal failure is a possible carrier of hepatitis B virus and all staff should take appropriate precautions, wearing hat, mask, goggles, gown and gloves whenever they are in intimate contact with a patient or his secretions (See Chapter 34).

CONCLUSIONS

Patients with chronic renal failure are poor anaesthetic risks but efficient haemodialysis and antihypertensive therapy will improve the prognosis. A variety of anaesthetic techniques have been used and the key to success is careful choice of agents and meticulous attention to detail.

REFERENCES

1. Smith BH: Anaesthetic problems of renal transplantation. *Proc R Soc Lond* [Biol] 66:918, 1973
2. Proud G: Blood transfusion and organ transplantation. *Ann R Coll Surg Engl* 62:271, 1980
3. Samuel JR, Powell D: Renal transplantation: anaesthetic experience of 100 cases. *Anaesthesia* 25:165, 1970
4. Gillies IDS: Anaemia and anaesthesia. *Br J Anaest* 46:589, 1974
5. Nunn JF, Freeman J: Problems of oxygenation and oxygen transport in anaesthesia. *Anaesthesia* 19:120, 1964
6. Crul-Sluijter EJ, Crul JF: Acidosis and neuromuscular blockade *Acta Anaesthesiol Scand* 18:224, 1974
7. Fourcade HE, Larson CP, Hickey RF, Bahlman SH, Eger EI: Effects of time on ventilation during halothane and cyclopropane anesthesia. *Anesthesiology* 36:83, 1972
8. Goggin MJ, Joekes AM: Gas exchange in renal failure. I: Dangers of hyperkalaemia during anaesthesia. *Br Med J* 2:244, 1971
9. Compamanes CI, Boyan CP, Belville JW, Howland WS: Cardiac conduction disturbances during anesthesia in the uremic patient. *Anesth Analg (Cleve)* 38:283, 1959
10. Maizels M: Phosphate, base and hemolysis in stored blood. *Q J Exp Physiol* 32:143, 1943
11. Paton WDM: Mode of action of neuromuscular blocking drugs. *Br J. Anaesth* 28:470, 1956
12. List WF: Serum Potassium changes during induction of anaesthesia. *Br J Anaesth* 39:480, 1967
13. Hirshman CA, Edelstein G: Intraoperative hyperkalaemia and cardiac arrests during renal transplantation in an insulin-dependent diabetic patient. *Anesthesiology* 51:161, 1979
14. Katz J, Kountz SL, Cohn R: Anesthetic considerations for renal transplant. *Anesth Analg (Cleve)* 46:609, 1967
15. Prys-Roberts C, Meloche R, Foëx P: Studies of anaesthesia in relation to hypertension. I: Cardiovascular responses of treated and untreated patients. *Br J Anaesth* 43:122, 1971
16. Prys-Roberts C, Foëx P, Biro GP, Roberts JG: Studies of anaesthesia in relation to hypertension. V: Adrenergic beta-receptor blockade. *Br J Anaesth* 45:671, 1973
17. Dundee JW, Richards RK: Effect of azotemia upon the action of intravenous barbiturate anesthesia. *Anesthesiology* 15:333, 1954
18. Prys-Roberts C, Greene LT, Meloche R, Foëx P: Studies of anaesthesia in relation to hypertension. II: Haemodynamic consequences of induction and endotracheal intubation. *Br J Anaesth* 43:531, 1971
19. Coleman AJ, Downing JW, Leary WP, Moyes DG, Styles M: The immediate cardiovascular effects of Althesin (Glaxo CT 1341), a steroid induction agent, and thiopentone in man. *Anaesthesia* 27:373, 1972
20. Jacobsen E, Christiansen AH, Lunding M: The role of the anaesthetist in the management of acute renal failure. *Br J Anaesth* 40:442, 1968
21. Rosenmann E, Dishon T, Durst A, Boss JH: Kidney and liver damage following anaesthesia with ether and pentobarbitone. *Br J Anaesth* 44:465, 1972
22. Hansen DD, Fernandes A, Skousted P, Berry P: Cyclopropane anaesthesia for renal transplantation. *Br J Anaesth* 44:584, 1972
23. Aldrete JA, Daniel W, O'Higgins JW, Homatas J, Starzl TE: Analysis of anesthetic-related morbidity in human recipients of renal homografts. *Anesth Analg (Cleve)* 50:321, 1971
24. Logan DA, Howie HB, Crawford J: Anaesthesia and renal transplantation. *Br J Anaesth* 46:69, 1974
25. Houghton IT, Cronin M, Redfern PA, Utting JE: The analgesic effect of halothane. *Br J Anaesth* 45:1105, 1973
26. Mazze RI, Cousins MJ, Kosek JC: Dose-related methoxyflurane nephrotoxicity in rats. *Anesthesiology* 36:571, 1972
27. Robertson GS, Hamilton WFD: Methoxyflurane and renal function. *Br J Anaesth* 45:55, 1973
28. Van Dyke RA, Wood CL: Metabolism of methoxyflurane. *Anesthesiology* 39:613, 1973
29. Bullock JD, Albert DM: Generalised oxalosis with retinal involvement following methoxyflurane anesthesia. *Anesthesiology* 41:296, 1974
30. Loehning RW, Mazze RI: Possible nephrotoxicity from enflurane in a patient with severe renal disease. *Anesthesiology* 40:203, 1974
31. Eichhorn JH, Hedley-Whyte J, Steinman TI, Kaufmann JM, Laasberg LH: Renal failure following enflurane anesthesia. *Anesthesiology* 45:557, 1976
32. Mazze RI, Cousins MJ, Barr GA: Renal effects and metabolism of isoflurane in man. *Anesthesiology* 40:536, 1974
33. Buchan AS, Bauld HW: Blood gas changes during trichloroethylene and intravenous pethidine anaesthesia. *Br J Anaesth* 45:93, 1973
34. Strunin L: Some aspects of anaesthesia for renal homotransplantation. *Br J Anaesth* 38:812, 1966
35. Roberts JG, Foëx P, Clarke TNS, Bennett MJ, Saner CA: Haemodynamic interactions of high-dose propranolol pretreatment and anaesthesia in the dog. *Br J Anaesth* 48:411, 1976
36. Greene NM: A new aspect of the metabolism of halothane. *Anesthesiology* 44:191, 1976
37. Trudnowski RJ, Mostert IW, Hobika GH, Rico R: Neuroleptanalgesia for patients with kidney malfunction. *Anesth Analg (Cleve)* 50:679, 1971
38. Monks PS, Lumley J: Anaesthetic aspects of renal transplantation. *Ann R Coll Surg Engl* 50:354, 1972
39. Zauder HL, Del Guercio LRM, Feins N, Barton N, Wellman S: Hemodynamics during neuroleptanalgesia. *Anesthesiology* 26:266, 1965
40. Gorman HM, Craythorne NWB: The effects of a new neuroleptanalgesia agent on renal function in man. *Acta Anaesthesiol Scand* [Suppl] 24:111, 1966
41. Holmes JH, Nakamoto S, Sawyer KC: Changes in blood composition before and after dialysis with the Kolff twin coil Kidney. *Trans Am Soc Artif Intern Organs* 4:16, 1958
42. Le Vine DS, Virtue RW: Anaesthetic agents and techniques for renal homotransplants. *Can Anaesth Soc J* 11:425, 1964
43. Roth F, Wüthrich H: The clinical importance of hyperkalaemia following suxamethonium administration. *Br J Anaesth* 41:311, 1969
44. Powell JN: Suxamethonium induced hyperkalaemia in a uraemic patient. *Br J Anaesth* 42:806, 1970
45. Striker TW, Morrow AG: Effect of succinylcholine on the level of serum potassium in man. *Anesthesiology* 29:214, 1968

46. List WF: Succinylcholine induced cardiac arrhythmias. *Anesth Analg (Cleve)* 50:361, 1971
47. Leighton KM: Studies on the effects of succinylcholine upon the circulation of the anaesthetised dog. *Can Anaesth J* 18:100, 1971
48. Koide M, Waud BE: Serum potassium concentrations after succinylcholine in patients with renal failure. *Anesthesiology* 36:142, 1972
49. Miller RD, Way WL, Hamilton WK, Layzer B: Succinylcholine-induced hyperkalemia in patients with renal failure? *Anesthesiology* 36:138, 1972
50. Walton JD, Farman JV: Suxamethonium, potassium and renal failure. *Anaesthesia* 28:626, 1973
51. Kleine JW, Moesker A: Hexafluorenium and renal failure. *Br J Anaesth* 48:713, 1976
52. Day S: Plasma potassium changes following suxamethonium and suxethonium in normal patients and in patients in renal failure. *Br J Anaesth* 48:1011, 1976
53. Prescott LF: Mechanisms of renal excretion of drugs. *Br J Anaesth* 44:246, 1972
54. White RD, De Weerd JH, Dawson B: Gallamine in anesthesia for patients with chronic renal failure undergoing bilateral nephrectomy. *Anesth Analg (Cleve)* 50:11, 1971
55. Churchill-Davidson HC, Way WL, De Jong RH: The muscle relaxants and renal excretion. *Anesthesiology* 28:540, 1967
56. Miller RD, Van Nyhuis LS, Eger EI, Way WL: The effect of acid-base balance on neostigmine antagonism of d-tubocurarine-induced neuromuscular blockade. *Anesthesiology* 42:377, 1975
57. Miller RD, Cullen DJ: Renal failure and post-operative respiratory failure: recurarisation? *Br J Anaesth* 48:253, 1976
58. Cohen EN, Brewer HW, Smith D: The metabolism and elimination of d-tubocurarine-H^3. *Anesthesiology* 28:309, 1967
59. Miller RD, Sohn YJ, Matteo RS: Enhancement of d-tubocurarine blockade by diuretics in man. *Anesthesiology* 45:442, 1976
60. Dretchen KL, Morgenroth VH III, Standaert EG, Walts LF: Azothiaprine: effects on neuromuscular transmission. *Anesthesiology* 45:604, 1976
61. Lee D, Johnson DL: Effect of d-tubocurarine and anaesthesia upon cardiac output in normal and histamine-depleted dogs. *Can Anaesth Soc J* 18:157, 1971
62. Leighton KM, Koth B, Bruce C: Pancuronium and renal perfusion. *Can Anaesth Soc J* 21:131, 1974
63. Baird WLM, Reid AM: The neuromuscular blocking properties of a new steroid compound, pancuronium bromide. *Br J Anaesth* 39:775, 1967
64. McLeod K, Watson MJ, Rawlings MD: Pharmacokinetics of pancuronium in patients with normal and impaired renal function. *Br J Anaesth* 48:341, 1976
65. Agoston S, Vermeer GA, Kersten VW, Meijer DKF: The fate of pancuronium in man. *Acta Anaesthesiol Scand* 17:267, 1973
66. Geha DG, Blitt CD, Moon BJ: Prolonged neuromuscular blockade with pancuronium in the presence of acute renal failure *Anesth Analg (Cleve)* 55:343, 1976
67. Norman J, Bowman WC: Symposium on Org NC 45. *Br J Anaesth* 53:15, 1980
68. Durant NN, Houwertjes MC, Agoston S: Renal elimination of Org-NC 45 and pancuronium. *Anesthesiology* 51:5266, 1979
69. Vandam LD, Harrison JH, Murray JE, Merrill JP: Anesthetic aspects of renal homotransplantation in man. *Anesthesiology* 23:783, 1962
70. Wyant GM: The anaesthetist looks at tissue transplantation: three years experience with kidney transplants. *Can Anaesth Soc J* 14:255, 1967
71. Linke CL, Merin RG: A regional anesthetic approach for renal transplantation. *Anesth Analg (Cleve)* 55:69, 1976
72. Löfström B: Anaesthetic problems in renal transplantation. *Scand J Urol Nephrol* 1:161, 1967
73. Dundee JW, Nair SG, Assaf RAE, Clarke RSJ, Kernohan SM: Pentobarbitone premedication for anaesthesia. *Anaesthesia* 31:1025, 1976
74. Stoelting PK, Peterson C: Circulatory changes during anesthetic induction. *Anesth Analg (Cleve)* 55:77, 1976
75. Duncan PG, Cullen BF: Anesthesia and immunology. *Anesthesiology* 45:522, 1976
76. Bruce DL, Wingard DW: The effects of anesthesia on transplant rejection. *Anesthesiology* 30:235, 1969
77. Don HF, Dieppa EA, Taylor P: Narcotic analgesics in anuric patients. *Anesthesiology* 42:745, 1975
78. Hunter JM, Jones RS, Uttingg JE: Use of the muscle relaxant atracurium in anephric patients: preliminary communication. *Jroy Soc Med* 75:336, 1987

41

TRACE METALS AND REGULAR DIALYSIS

ALLEN C. ALFREY and W. RODMAN SMYTHE

Introduction	804	Acute intoxication	807
Evaluation of body trace elements	804	Chronic intoxication and depletion	807
Tissue trace elements in uremia	805	Summary	808
Mechanisms of trace element disturbances	805	References	809
Physiological consequences of trace element disorders	807		

INTRODUCTION

Although the emphasis on identifying uremic toxins has centered around organic compounds, it is now apparent that inorganic solutes also may be responsible for some of the symptomatology of the uremic state. The importance of such electrolyte disturbances as the cardiac and neuromuscular effect of hyperkalemia and hypermagnesemia, the extraskeletal calcification caused by hyperphosphatemia and hypertension induced by excess body sodium and water have been studied repeatedly. However, little attention has been directed toward trace element disturbances and their physiological consequences in dialyzed uremic patients.

A number of considerations suggest that trace element disturbances might occur in dialyzed uremic patients. As renal function declines retention of certain trace elements, normally excreted by the kidneys, may occur. With proteinuria those elements which are protein bound might be excreted in increased amounts in the urine. As a result of the disturbances in vitamin D metabolism the gastrointestinal absorption of some trace elements may also be affected. Finally, the dialysis procedure, *per se*, could appreciably alter the body burden of trace elements in that some may be removed, whereas others present as contaminants in the dialysate could be transferred to the patient.

EVALUATION OF BODY TRACE ELEMENTS

During the past decade analytical methods for trace element measurements have improved markedly. The more laborious and less sensitive colorimetric and gravimetric methods have largely been replaced by neutron activation analysis, x-ray fluorescence, flame and flameless atomic absorption techniques and more recently inductively coupled plasma emission spectroscopy. The ideal method for the determination of trace elements in biological specimens should be applicable to small sample sizes, have minimal preparatory steps and have adequate sensitivity and specificity for the element in question. Another consideration in regard to selecting the appropriate analytical technique is whether a single element or multiple elements in a biological sample require analysis. For single element analysis the two commonly available systems are atomic absorption spectrophotometry and flameless atomic absorption spectrophotometry. For multiple elemental analyses neutron activation analysis, x-ray fluorescence, electron microprobe analysis and inductively coupled plasma emission spectroscopy have largely replaced emission spectroscopy because of improved sensitivity and marked reduction or elimination of interferences. Although these methodologies have been simplified and their sensitivity has improved, erroneous conclusions may be made if the investigator is not familiar with limitations of the methodology.

Another difficult problem in evaluating trace element disturbances is determining which tissue or fluid reflects satisfactorily the body burden of the trace element in question. Mertz (1) has divided tissues into four categories.

The *first group* included regulatory sites or tissues responsible for *maintaining homeostasis* by regulating absorption or excretion of an element, such as the thyroid for iodide and the intestinal mucosa for iron.

The *second group* consists of tissues where the element under study has an *essential biological function* e.g. for those elements which are essential cofactors of enzymes in specific organs or tissue. An example is zinc in carbonic anhydrase present in erythrocytes. Because of strong regulatory mechanisms, trace elements in such tissues may remain normal in concentration despite total body depletion of the element in question. Thus, these tissues would not be good indicators of the body status of certain trace elements.

The third group is comprised of tissues involved in trace element *storage and transport*. Storage tissues, such as the bone marrow for iron, may sensitively reflect alterations in body stores of certain trace elements. Although blood serum and plasma are the most frequently analyzed samples, results may be difficult to interpret, e.g. when elements are stored. Plasma trace element concentrations may be misleading when: 1) recently absorbed elements are transported to target organs, transiently elevating plasma concentrations, 2) the plasma is not in equilibration with important tissue stores, and 3) binding proteins are reduced, e.g. such conditions as cirrhosis and the nephrotic syndrome, with spurious lowering of the plasma concentrations of protein bound trace elements.

The fourth group of tissues are *the sequestering tissues.* This group consists of the lungs, the kidneys, parts of the reticulo-endothelial system, nails, hair and the stratum corneum of the skin. These tissues can be used as indices of chronic exposure. Hair is especially useful for certain elements such as mercury and arsenic (in case of intoxication) and zinc and chromium (in case of deficiency).

TISSUE TRACE ELEMENTS IN UREMIA

Tissue trace element profiles have now been well characterized in both dialyzed and non-dialyzed uremic patients (2). A number of trace element disturbances have been identified. These can be divided into three groups. The first group represents a similar disturbance in multiple tissues documenting an alteration in the total body burden of that element. Six elements belong to this group. Total body aluminum, tin, zinc and strontium are increased whereas total body rubidium is decreased in dialyzed and non-dialyzed uremic patients. Total body bromine is decreased only in dialyzed uremic patients.

The second group of disturbances represents elements that may be increased or reduced in some tissues, whereas they are either normal or affected in the opposite direction in other tissues. Examples of this alteration are the increased liver and spleen iron concentration in dialyzed uremic patients and the increased copper concentration in lungs associated with a reduced copper concentration in heart of both dialyzed and non-dialyzed uremic patients (2).

The third disturbance in trace elements would appear to be a translocation of an element from one organ to another. Two elements that fall into this group are cadmium and molybdenum both of which are reduced in the diseased kidneys and increased in the liver.

Of the remaining essential elements, tissue selenium levels have been found to be normal in uremic patients (2). Iodine stores would seem to be adequate in most uremic patients as estimated by normal thyroid function (See Chapter 36). Silicon has been found to be increased in spleen and liver in patients with chronic renal failure (3). Bone fluoride has been found to be increased in patients who have been exposed to dialysate contaminated with fluoride (4 [See Chapters 7 and 35]). Blood vanadium levels have been reported to be both normal (5) and increased (6) in uremic patients.

Plasma nickel has been found to be decreased in patients with chronic renal failure (7). This is felt to be a consequence of reduced nickel plasmin, an a-macroglobulin. Inadequate information is available on the status of three other essential elements: chromium, cobalt and manganese, in uremic patients.

Of the non-essential elements, blood arsenic has been reported to be ten times higher in uremic patients as compared to normal controls (8, 9). Tissue stores of lead (2, 3) and mercury (2) appear to be normal in most uremic patients. Uranium has been found to be increased in several dialyzed uremic patients (10). The most likely source for this perturbation is uranium contamination present in some water supplies.

MECHANISMS OF TRACE ELEMENT DISTURBANCES

It would appear that most trace element disturbances that occur in uremic patients are a result of uremia, *per se,* and not the dialysis procedure since most elemental disturbances are shared by dialyzed and non-dialyzed uremic patients (2). However the severity of the disturbance tends to be greater in the dialyzed patients. For most elements this presumably occurs as a result of the longer duration of uremia in the dialyzed patient.

As a result of loss of renal function strontium (11) and tin (12) which depend on the kidney for elimination are probably retained accounting for the increased body burden of these elements.

Another mechanism for some trace element disturbances is a translocation from one tissue to another in uremia. Normally kidney cadmium content is considerably greater than other tissues. However, which chronic renal insufficiency the cadmium content in the kidney decreases to extremely low levels possibly as a consequence of reduction in binding proteins (metallothionine) in this diseased organ (12). The failure of the diseased kidney to bind and excrete cadmium may result in its displacement to the liver. A similar mechanism is proposed for the reduced renal content and increased hepatic content of molybdenum found in uremic patients.

Similarly the high tissue zinc levels may also be a result of a translocation since muscle (2) and plasma (13, 14) zinc concentrations tend to be low in association with the increased zinc levels in other tissues.

The most difficult trace element alteration to understand is rubidium depletion. It has largely been assumed that rubidium metabolism is similar to potassium metabolism. However, rubidium depletion in non-dialyzed uremic patients is far in excess of potassium depletion which may or may not be present. Thus, it would appear that in association with loss of renal function, rubidium excretion is somehow enhanced.

Other mechanisms of trace element disturbances are medications given to uremic patients and the dialysis procedure. The amount of increased total body aluminum found in some non-dialyzed uremic patients cannot be ascribed to the retention of the small amount of aluminum normally absorbed and excreted. A more likely explanation is retention of aluminum, because of loss of renal function, after absorption of aluminum from phosphate binding gels commonly administered to these patients. Aluminum has been shown to be absorbed from these aluminum containing phosphate binding gels (15-17). In 13 normal subjects urinary aluminum excretion increased from a mean of ·16 to

806 Allen C Alfrey and W Rodman Smythe

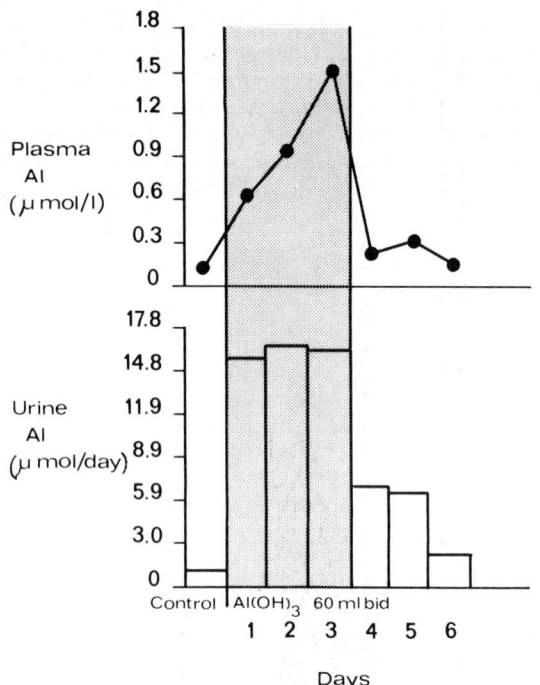

Figure 1. Plasma and urine aluminum concentrations in a control subject who received oral aluminum hydroxide for three days.

(Conversion SI units [μmol/l or μmol/day] → conventional units: multiply by 27 [= μg/l or μg/day])

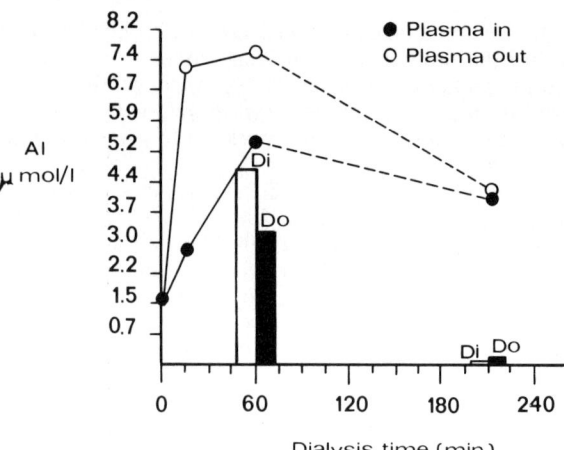

Figure 2. Aluminum concentrations of plasma and dialysate during hemodialysis of one patient. Di and Do refer to dialysis fluid entering or leaving the dialyzer. Filtered tap water was used to prepare the dialysate during the initial 60 min of study; water treated by reverse osmosis was used thereafter. Reprinted from Kidney International [19] with permission. (Slightly modified).

(Conversion SI units [μmol/l or μmol/day] → conventional units: multiply by 27 [= μg/l or μg/day])

259 μg/day (0.6 to 9.6 μmol) during the time the individuals ingested 60 ml of Al(OH)$_3$, twice daily. The changes in plasma concentration and urinary excretion of aluminum in one patient ingesting Al(OH)$_3$ (120 mg/day [4.4 mmol/day]) is shown in Figure 1. Although the increase in urinary aluminum seems small, if excretion was prevented because of renal failure, in one year's time this would result in an increase in the total body burden of aluminum of approximately 94 mg (3.5 mmol). Since the normal total body aluminum content is probably less than 30 mg (1.1 mmol) this would represent a major increase in total body aluminum.

A second source of aluminum in dialyzed uremic patients is aluminum contaminated dialysate. Aluminum has been shown to cross the dialyzing membrane readily (18, 19). In addition aluminum is bound in plasma to a non-dialyzable constituent, most likely a protein, therefore virtually any aluminum contamination present in the dialysate acts as an effective gradient from the dialysate to the blood (18, 19). Furthermore, because of plasma binding of aluminum even when dialysate aluminum content is negligible, aluminum is not removed from plasma. The effect of aluminum contamination of dialysate on plasma aluminum levels is shown in Figure 2. It can be appreciated that plasma aluminum levels rapidly increase during the first hour when dialysis was performed with aluminum contaminated dialysate. However, following removal of aluminum from the dialysate, aluminum was not extracted from plasma as de-

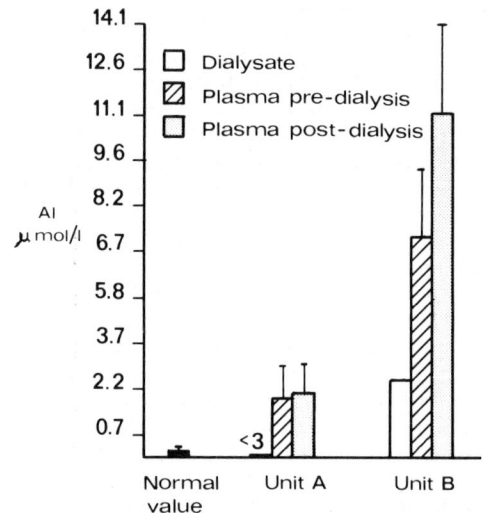

Figure 3. Plasma aluminum concentrations in a control population and two groups of dialyzed uremic patients. Patients in Unit A had been maintained on low aluminum dialysate whereas Unit B had inadequate water treatment and aluminum contaminated dialysis fluid.

(Conversion SI units [μmol/l or μmol/day] → conventional units: multiply by 27 [= μg/l or μg/day])

termined by measuring post-dialyzer dialysate and plasma aluminum levels. Another study carried out in patients from two dialysis units, one having aluminum free dialysate and the second having aluminum contaminated dialysate further supports the transfer of aluminum from dialysate to plasma (19). In those receiving dialysis with aluminum free dialysate plasma aluminum levels, although elevated, were less than values found in patients dialyzed with aluminum contaminated dialysate. In contrast to the latter group where post-dialysis plasma aluminum values were significantly higher than pre-dialysis values there was little differences between pre- and post-dialysis plasma aluminum levels in the former group of patients (Figure 3). If the concentration of aluminum in dialysis fluid is less than that of plasma water some removal of aluminum can occur gradually (see also chapters 6, 7 and 42).

The dialysis procedure also tends to intensify rubidium depletion and creates the bromide deficiency which is found only in dialyzed uremic patients (2). Provided that the concentration of these elements in dialysis fluid is low enough, as is usual, they will be extracted by the hemodialyzer and removed. This contrasts with normal renal handling which results in conservation of these elements by tubular reabsorption as occurs, for example with chloride. Otherwise the dialysis procedure could not be incriminated in the production of any of the other chronic trace element disturbances found in uremic patients (2). The only trace element disturbance improved by dialysis is cadmium excess.

PHYSIOLOGICAL CONSEQUENCES OF TRACE ELEMENT DISORDERS

Acute intoxication

A number of accidental intoxications have been described in dialyzed uremic patients. These have resulted from unexpected trace element contamination of the dialysate resulting from either the dialysis equipment or improper water treatment. To date, no naturally occurring trace element in water supplies has induced any acute toxicity. One patient, on home dialysis in Australia, had attacks of nausea, vomiting and fever during dialysis. Water used for the preparation of the dialysate was stored in a galvanized tank and the patient was subsequently shown to have high plasma and erythrocyte zinc concentrations (20). The symptoms were alleviated by performing dialysis using properly pretreated water. Acute copper intoxication characterized by hemolysis, leukocytosis, metabolic acidosis and gastrointestinal symptoms has been described in a number of dialysis patients (21–25, [See also Chapter 32]). It was subsequently shown that copper was leached from copper tubing in the delivery system. Most of these intoxications occurred when the anion exchange column became depleted rendering the water acidic. We recently had the opportunity of studying a group of patients who experienced headache, dizziness, nausea and vomiting during dialysis. High nickel levels were present in the plasma of these patients and the dialysate. The source of the nickel was found to be a stainless steel heating unit used to warm the water after reverse osmosis treatment (26).

A common factor in these acute intoxications is that the elements involved, copper, zinc and nickel, are all bound to large plasma molecules. Thus, virtually any concentration of these elements in the dialysate would result in their transfer to the patient. It might be anticipated that under certain conditions other elements used in plasticizers or alloys such as mercury, iron, cadmium, tin and chromium could also be introduced into the dialysate and transferred to the patient, resulting in acute or chronic intoxication.

Acute fluoride intoxication occurred in one group of dialysis patients as a consequence of a malfunction in a municipal water treatment facility which increased the fluoride content of the water 50 times normal. All patients developed gastrointestinal symptoms and one patient died of a cardiac arrest (27).

Chronic intoxication and depletion

It is much more difficult to determine what chronic toxicity might result from trace element disturbances in dialyzed uremic patients. It should be appreciated that trace element disturbances in dialyzed uremic patients have not been fully characterized. In addition, geographical variations could also occur. Listed in Table 1 are some of the well established trace element alterations found in uremic patients and some of the clinical consequences that may be associated with these disturbances.

Table 1. Trace element disturbances in uremic patients.

Trace element	Possible clinical importance
Increased tissue burden	
Aluminum	Prophyria cutanea tarda
	Dialysis dementia
	Osteomalacia
Fluoride	Osteomalacia
Molybdenum	Gout
Silicon	Unknown
Cadmium	Zinc deficiency
Strontium	Reduced $1,25(OH)_2D_3$
Tin	Impairment of drug and toxin metabolism
Zinc	Unknown
Decreased tissue burden	
Bromide	Unknown
Rubidium	Impairment of neurological function

Probably the strongest evidence to date suggesting that trace elements may be responsible for some of the symptomatology in chronic dialysis patients is the association between aluminum excess and dialysis dementia. It was initially shown in 1976 that patients with this syndrome had significantly higher brain gray matter aluminum levels than dialysis patients who died of other causes (28). Subsequently, other investigators have con-

RJ, Owen R: Pulmonary fibrosis and encephalopathy associated with the inhalation of aluminum dust. *Br J Ind Med* 19:282, 1975
37. Crapper DR, Krishman SS, Dalton AJ: Brain aluminum distribution in Alzheimer's disease and experimental neurofibrillary degeneration. *Science* 180:511, 1973.
38. Pierides AM, Edwards WG Jr, Cullum UX Jr, McCall JT, Ellis HA: Hemodialysis encephalopathy with osteomalacic fractures and muscle weakness. *Kidney Int* 18:115, 1980
39. Hodsman AB, Sherrard DJ, Brickman AS, Alfrey AC, Goodman WG, Maloney N, Lee DBN, Coburn JW: Bone aluminum in osteomalacic renal osteodystrophy correlation with excess osteoid. *Abstracts Soc Nephrol* 13:20A, 1980
40. Disler P, Day R, Pascoe M, Blekkenhorst G, Eales L: The role of aluminum in dialysis related porphyria cutanea tarda. *Abstracts Int Soc Nephrol* 8:252, 1981
41. Posen GA, Taves Dr, Marier JR, Jaworski ZF: Renal osteodystrophy in long-term hemodialysis with fluoridated water. *Abstracts Am Soc Nephrol* 2:51, 1968
42. Omdahl JL, DeLuca HF: Strontium induced rickets: metabolic basis. *Science* 174:949, 1971
43. Piscator M: The chronic toxicity of cadmium. In: *Trace Elements in Human Health and Disease,* edited by Prasad AS, New York, Academic Press, 2, 1976, p 431
44. Brook AC, Johnston DG, Ward MK, Watson MJ, Cook DB, Kerr DN: Absence of a therapeutic effect of zinc in the sexual dysfunction of haemodialysed patients. *Lancet* 2:618, 1980
45. Vallee BL, Ulmer DD: Biochemical effects of mercury, cadmium and lead. *Annu Rev Biochem* 41:91, 1972
46. Hammer DI, Colucci AV, Hasselblad V, Williams ME, Pinkerton C: Cadmium and lead in autopsy tissues. *J Occup Med* 151:956, 1973
47. Piscator M, Lind B: Cadmium, zinc, copper and lead in human renal cortex. *Arch Environ Health* 24:425, 1972
48. Cousins RJ, Barber AK, Trout JR: Cadmium toxicity in growing swine. *J Nutr* 103:964, 1973
49. Vigliani EC: The biopathology of cadmium. *Am Ind Hyg Assoc J* 30:329, 1969
50. Stoner HB, Barner JM, Duff JI: Studies on the toxicity of alkyl tin compounds. *Br J Pharmacol* 10:16, 1955
51. Alajouanine T, Derobert L, Thieffry S: Etude clinique d'ensemble de 210 cas d'intoxication par les sels organiques d'etain. (Clinical study of 210 cases of intoxication by organic tin compounds). *Rev Neurol (Paris)* 98:85, 1973
52. Kappas A, Maines MD: Tin: a potent inducer of heme oxygenase in kidney. *Science* 192:60, 1976
53. Stiefel EJ: Proposed molecular mechanism for the action of molybdenum in enzymes: coupled proton and electron transfers. *Proc Natl Acad Sci USA* 70:988, 1973
54. Higgins ES, Reichert DA, Westerfeld WW: Molybdate deficiency and tungstate inhibition studies. *J Nutr* 59:539, 1956
55. Bosshardt DK, Huff JS, Barner RH: Effect of bromine on chick growth. *Proc Soc Exp Biol Med* 92:219, 1956
56. Huff JW, Bosshardt DK, Miller OP, Barner RH: A nutritional requirement for bromine. *Proc Soc Exp Biol Med* 92:216, 1956
57. Carroll BJ, Sharp PT: Rubidium and lithium: opposite effects on amine-mediated excitement. *Science* 172:1355, 1971
58. Fieve RR, Meltzer H, Dunner DL, Levitt M, Mendlewicz J, Thomas A: Rubidium: biochemical, behavioral and metabolic studies in humans. *Am J Psychiatry* 130:55, 1973
59. Hopkins LL Jr, Mohr HE: Vanadium as an essential nutrient. *Fed Proc* 33:1773, 1974
60. Levine RA, Steeten DHP, Doisy RJ: Effect of oral chromium supplementation on the glucose tolerance test in the elderly. *Metabolism* 17:114, 1968
61. O'Dell BL: Biochemistry and physiology of copper in vetebrates. In: *Trace Elements in Human Health and Disease,* edited by Prasad AS, New York, Academic Press, 1, 1976, p 391
62. Russell JE, Avioli LV: Effect of progressive end-stage renal insufficiency on bone mineral-collagen maturation. *Kidney Int 7 (suppl 2)*:S97, 1975

42

ALUMINIUM TOXICITY IN RENAL FAILURE

MICHAEL K. WARD and IAN S. PARKINSON

Introduction	811	Dialysis fluid aluminium	813
Dialysis encephalopathy	811	Oral administration of aluminium	816
Vitamin D resistant osteomalacia	812	Treatment of aluminium toxicity	817
Non-specific toxicity syndrome	812	Summary	817
Aluminium accumulation in renal failure	812	References	817

INTRODUCTION

Aluminium is found in very low concentrations in blood and tissues in the normal population (1–5). As exposure is inevitable, because it is the commonest metal in the earth's crust, there must exist an effective barrier to the accumulation of aluminium in the normal human.

Although originally thought to be of little biological significance in man, there is growing evidence that aluminium accumulates in humans with chronic renal failure where it can cause three toxic syndromes – *dialysis encephalopathy, vitamin D resistant osteomalacia* and a *non-specific toxicity syndrome*. The evidence for this is reviewed.

DIALYSIS ENCEPHALOPATHY

A distinctive clinical syndrome first described by Alfrey and colleagues in 1972 (6) has now been described in the majority of countries where haemodialysis is performed in the management of end-stage renal failure. The syndrome has been documented in 17 out of 22 countries reporting to the European Dialysis and Transplant Association Registry (7, 8) and appears in reports from Australia (9) and the United States of America (10–14). The syndrome has been termed dialysis dementia, or more correctly dialysis encephalopathy as dementia may be a late feature. The clinical syndrome was originally described in patients undergoing haemodialysis for the management of end-stage renal failure, but has now been reported in one patient treated by peritoneal dialysis (15) and in children (16, 17) and adults (18, 19) with renal failure prior to the initiation of regular dialysis.

The presenting symptoms are often subtle changes in personality, reduction in short term memory, slurring or stuttering of speech – often occuring initially towards the end of a haemodialysis session. Myoclonic spasms of the muscles of the face, arms, legs and trunk may become a major problem. Hallucinations with frank psychotic behaviour and major seizures often lead to progressive intellectual impairment and global dementia (6, 9–12, 20–22). Symptoms and signs may first appear after successful renal transplantation (23, 24). Early reports indicated that the syndrome progressed to death from suicide, aspiration pneumonia from disorganised pharyngeal function or cessation of therapy (14, 20). The speech disorder, myoclonic spasms and seizures can be controlled by diazepam or clonazepam (25, 26), although these drugs have no influence on the eventual outcome of the disease (9, 14, 20, 25, 26). Formal assessment of speech (27), intellectual function (28) and the finding of a characteristic electroencephalogram (EEG) may indicate the earliest manifestations of the syndrome before clinical features become obvious (11). A distinctive pattern of episodic bursts of spiky, high voltage activity on a background of slow-wave activity has been described on EEG tracings (Figure 1) in most patients affected by the syndrome and may precede clinical features (6, 11, 20, 29–33).

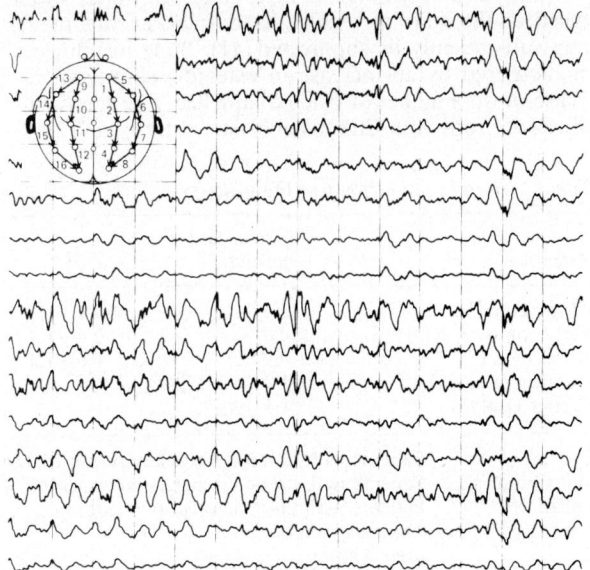

Figure 1. The EEG shows a characteristic pattern of episodic bursts of spiky, high voltage activity on a background of slow-wave activity in a patient with dialysis encephalopathy.

No specific pathologic features have been found on macroscopic examination of the brain of patients who died of the syndrome (20, 32). On microscopic examination cortical cell loss, neuronal loss and degeneration was observed with a marked increase in the size and the number of astrocytes in the cerebral cortex and the brain stem. There was a striking loss of Purkinje cells in the cerebellum (20). Other workers, however found no microscopic abnormalities (34). Using electron microprobe analysis, micro-crystals of aluminium phosphate have been found in the lysosomes of brain neurones (35). Altered CSF dynamics with low pressure hydrocephalus have been reported (30).

VITAMIN D RESISTANT OSTEOMALACIA

Several centres have reported the clinical association of dialysis encephalopathy with osteomalacic or fracturing renal osteodystrophy (1, 12, 20, 21, 36). This bone syndrome is characterised by progressive bone pain which is initially noted in the lower limbs, especially on weight bearing, and later spreads to involve back, ribs and upper limbs. Proximal myopathy, giving rise to difficulty in climbing stairs, may progress to marked generalised weakness, confining the patient to a wheelchair (37, 38). The osteomalacic syndrome may develop either without evidence of encephalopathy or several months or years before encephalopathic features present as well as in conjunction with encephalopathy.

Multiple pathological fractures are seen on skeletal radiology often with little evidence of active secondary hyperparathyroidism (39). Biochemically, serum alkaline phosphatase is usually within or just above the normal range, with reduction in the bone isoenzyme fraction (40).

Parathyroid hormone (PTH) concentrations, often raised at the start of regular haemodialysis treatment, may subsequently be suppressed (41). Bone histology is characterised by an increase in osteoid volume, an increase in the number of osteoid lamellae, a reduced calcification front with little osteoblastic activity and little evidence of active osteitis fibrosa although there may be evidence of previously active osteitis fibrosa (12, 42–44).

This osteomalacic syndrome fails to respond to vitamin D therapy with dihydrotachysterol, 1 α-hydroxycholecalciferol or 1.25 dihydroxycholecalciferol (41, 42). Treatment with 1 α-hydroxycholecalciferol often resulted in troublesome hypercalcaemia.

To assess whether phosphate depletion was an aetiological factor Feest and colleagues (45) undertook a prospective trial with phosphate enriched dialysis fluid in association with 1 α-hydroxycholecalciferol, without a positive response.

This vitamin D resistant osteomalacia appears similar to that described in other reports of osteomalacic renal bone disease (1, 34, 46–50).

NON-SPECIFIC TOXICITY SYNDROME

A microcytic hypochromic anaemia has been reported in association with the neurological and bone syndrome (51). This anaemia is reversible following installation of appropriate water treatment. In addition, much of the 'non-specific' symptomatology, including anaemia, cardiac failure, weight loss and general ill-health seen in dialysis populations where encephalopathy and bone disease have occurred may be part of a generalised aluminium toxicity syndrome (1).

ALUMINIUM ACCUMULATION IN RENAL FAILURE

Despite the warnings of Berlyne and colleagues in 1970 (52) of the potentially toxic consequences of aluminium accumulation in patients with chronic renal failure and the demonstration of increased aluminium content of bone in patients on haemodialysis in 1972 (53), it was not until 1976 that aluminium accumulation was implicated as the cause of dialysis encephalopathy. In that year Alfrey and colleagues (36) showed a striking

Table 1. Aluminium content of brain (μg/g).

Reference	Control tissue (normal)	CFR	Haemodialysis	DES	Method
Alfrey et al (54)	2.4 ± 1.3	4.1 ± 1.7	8.5 ± 3.5	24.5 ± 9.9	FAAS 1
McDermott et al (2)	4.0	2.4 ± 1.4	5.1 ± 2.8	20.4 ± 1.6	FAAS 1
Arieff et al (53)	0.9 ± 2	6.6 ± 1.5	3.8 ± 0.8	12.4 ± 4.9	FAAS 1
Flendrig et al (21)	11.9 ± 6.1–17.8	–	12.1 (4.4–19.8)	90.8 (36–142)	NAA 2
Cartier et al (3)	1.5 ± 0.9	–	–	5.5 ± 1.6	FAAS 1

CRF: Patients with chronic renal failure not dialysed
Haemodialysis: Patients with chronic renal failure haemodialysed without encephalopathy
DES: Patients with encephalopathic syndrome
1: Brain grey-matter
2: Mixed brain
FAAS: Flameless atomic absorption spectrophotometry
NAA: Neutron activation analysis
SI conversion: μg/g → μmol/g: divide by 27
μg/g → nmol/g: multiply with 37

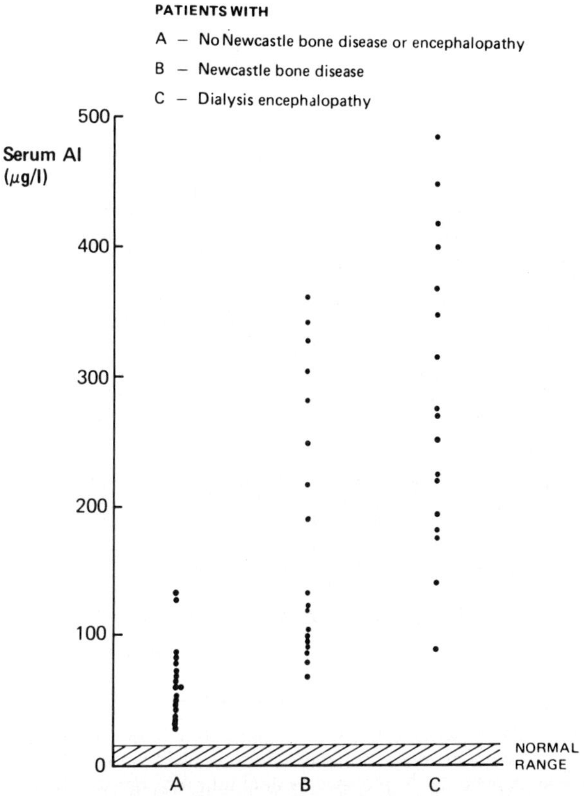

42: Aluminium toxicity

for the development of vitamin D resistant osteomalacia and a number of other, non-specific, symptoms.

Dialysis fluid aluminium

The major source of aluminium accumulation leading to these syndromes in haemodialysed patients is aluminium contamination of the water supply used to prepare the dialysis fluid. Aluminium in water is either naturally occurring or added in variable quantities as a flocculating agent to clarify the water as part of the preparation of water for domestic use.

Considerable elevation of the serum aluminium concentration is seen during haemodialysis when dialysis fluid is contaminated with aluminium (61–64) (Figure 3). Even at low dialysis fluid aluminium concentrations, a slight rise in the serum aluminium concentration can occur through aluminium transfer across the dialysis membrane against a concentration gradient due to plasma protein binding (65) and as a result of haemoconcentration subsequent to ultrafiltration (Figure 3).

The most direct evidence of aluminium toxicity from aluminium-contaminated dialysis fluid comes from the report by Flendrig and colleagues (21) of the accidental contamination of the water supply used to prepare dia-

Figure 2. There is a significant increase in serum aluminium concentration in haemodialysed patients with vitamin D resistant osteomalacia (Newcastle bone disease) and patients with dialysis encephalopathy syndrome.

(SI conversion: µg/l → µmol/l: divide by 27)

elevation of the aluminium content of bone, muscle and the grey matter of brain in patients on haemodialysis in the Denver area. The fact that brain grey-matter aluminium concentrations were higher in all patients with dialysis encephalopathy than in any of the other dialysis patients or controls led Alfrey and colleagues to propose that the encephalopathy syndrome was due to aluminium intoxication.

The striking elevation of brain grey-matter aluminium content in patients with dialysis encephalopathy has now been confirmed by other groups (2, 3, 21, 54, 55) (Table 1), as has the raised bone aluminium content in association with the osteomalacic syndrome (42, 56); moreover, a vitamin D resistant osteomalacic syndrome has been reported in rats following intraperitoneal administration of aluminium (44). Although serum aluminium concentration reflects recent exposure and not the total body aluminium burden, a striking association between serum aluminium, encephalopathy and vitamin D resistant osteomalacia has been found in Newcastle (Figure 2) and other centres (57, 58). Although other aetiological agents have been considered (reviewed by Bone (59) and Lang and Henry (60)), aluminium toxicity is now firmly implicated as the cause of dialysis encephalopathy and is probably a major factor responsible

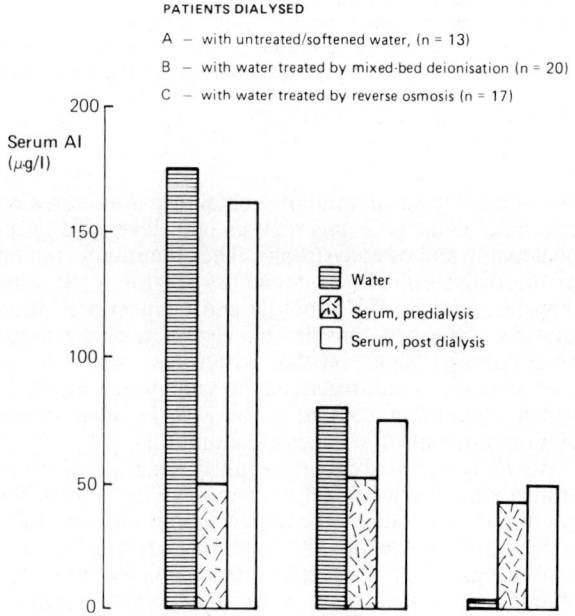

Figure 3. Considerable increase in serum aluminium concentration occurs during dialysis when patients are haemodialysed against untreated water containing aluminium. Mixed-bed deionisation partially reduces the aluminium in the raw water but fails to prevent the rise in serum aluminium concentration during dialysis. Reverse osmosis effectively removes aluminium from the water used for dialysis, although serum aluminium concentration rises slightly due to haemoconcentration subsequent to ultrafiltration.

(SI conversion: µg/l → µmol/l: divide by 27)

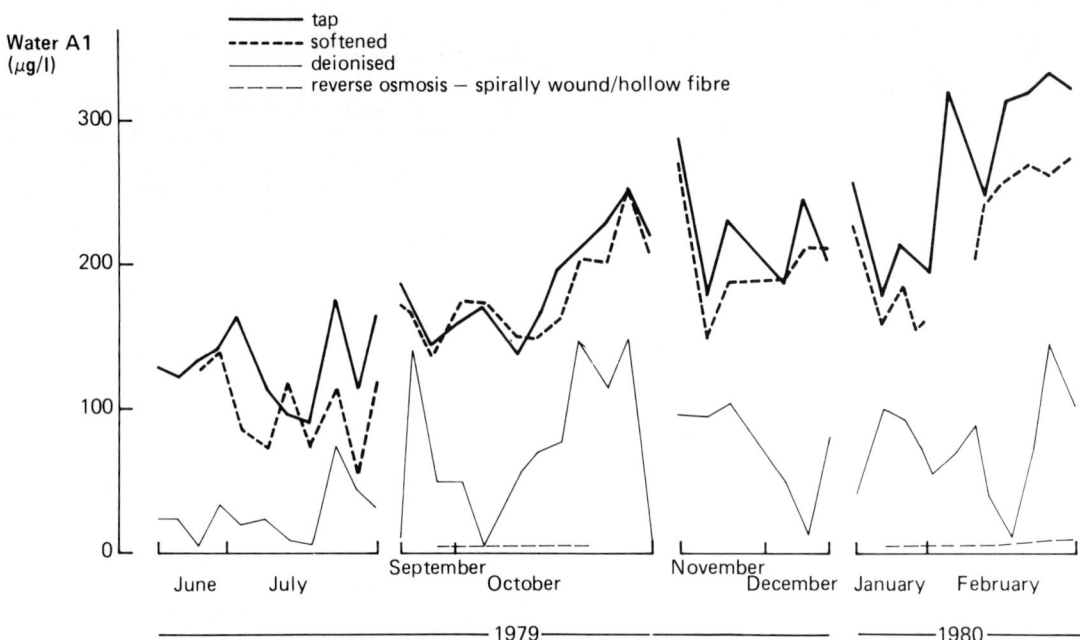

Figure 4. Aluminium sulphate is added in variable concentrations to the Newcastle tap water supply as a flocculating agent, resulting in a considerable week to week variation in tap water aluminium content. Water softeners fail to remove aluminium from the water source. Mixed bed deionisation gives an erratic performance, depending on the species of aluminium present. Reverse osmosis consistently removes aluminium from the water supply.

(SI conversion: µg/l → µmol: divide by 27)

lysis fluid by an aluminium containing anti-corrosion electrode. Patients in this dialysis unit developed encephalopathy and osteodystrophy. The aluminium content of the dialysis fluid was found to be grossly elevated (approx. 1000 µg/l [37 µmol/l]) and neutron activation analysis confirmed considerable elevation of the tissue aluminium content. Neither syndrome was seen in another dialysis unit receiving the same water supply in which aluminium contamination was avoided (water aluminium content < 60 µg/l [2.2 µmol/l]).

An 18 centre study in the United Kingdom demonstrated a highly significant rank correlation between the aluminium content of the water supply and the incidence of encepalopathy and fracturing osteomalacic osteodystrophy (63). This close association between the aluminium content of the water supply and encephalopathy and fracturing or osteomalacic osteodystrophy also appeared in reports from Sheffield, U.K. (37), Glasgow, U.K. (1), the United States (12, 64), France (3) and in a study undertaken by the Registry of the European Dialysis and Transplant Association (8).

The association between dialysis water aluminium, aluminium accumulation and the development of encephalopathic and bone syndromes is strong enough to warrant immediate efforts to reduce the aluminium content of the dialysis water supply by water treatment. A 'safe' dialysis fluid aluminium concentration has not been determined but it is certainly below 50 µg/l (1.9 µmol/l) (63) and is more likely to be below 20 µg/l (0.7 µmol/l) (62, 63, 65) (see also chapters 2, 6 and 7).

The aluminium content of raw tap water comes from two sources; 'naturally occurring' from rocks and soils and from aluminium sulphate added by water authorities as a coagulant to remove colour and turbidity. The physico-chemistry of aluminium in water is complex, with the total content and speciation varying from supply to supply and from week to week in the same supply due to the varying quantities of aluminium sulphate added and the influence of rainfall and drought (Figure 4). The solubility of aluminium (and dialysability) is dependent on the pH (67) (Figure 5), speciation and complex formation and therefore the ability of ion exchange resins to remove aluminium is dependent on the other components of the supply (Figure 6). The physico-chemistry of aluminium in water is such that aluminium is not effectively removed by water softening plants (47, 48) (Figure 4) and in water supplies where the total content of aluminium varies substantially and where pH and chemical composition are conducive to the formation of insoluble aluminium species, aluminium may not be removed effectively by mixed bed deionisers (68) (Figure 4). The most consistently effective method of removing aluminium of all species is reverse osmosis (68) (Figure 4). In order to prescribe an

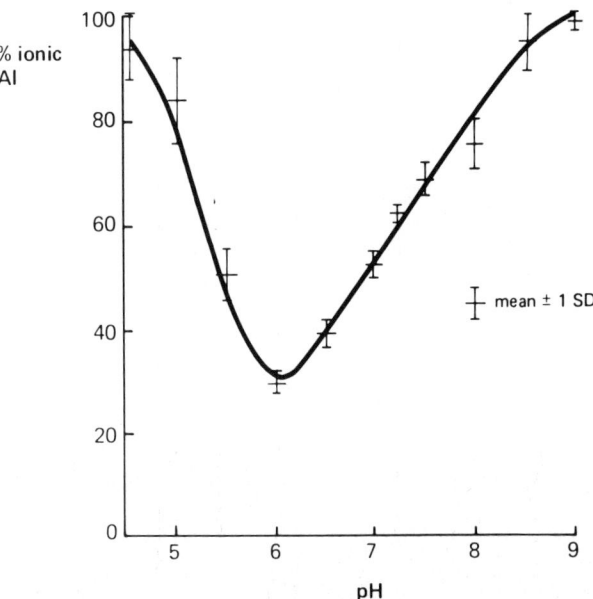

Figure 5. Effect of pH on the proportion of ionic aluminium in Newcastle raw water (four samples). This figure demonstrates that pH has a considerable effect on the proportion of ionic to non-ionic aluminium in tap water.

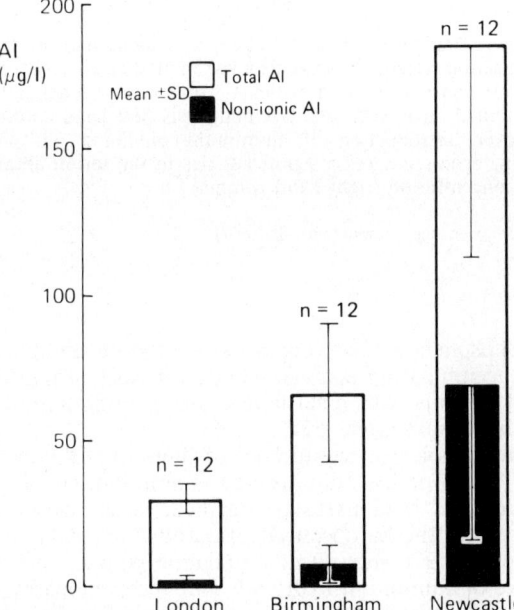

Figure 6. There is considerable variation in the aluminium content and its speciation in different water supplies. This is illustrated for London, Birmingham and Newcastle, U.K.

(SI conversion: µg/l → µmol/l: divide by 27)

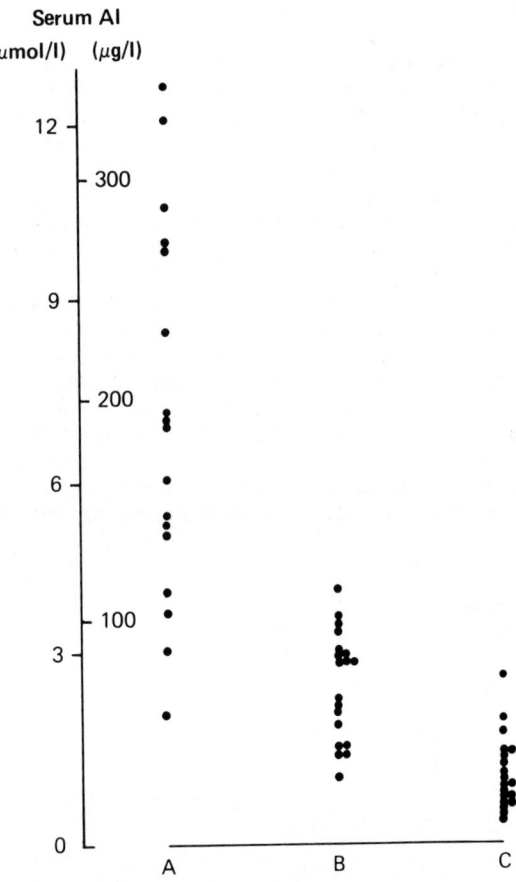

A Patients dialysed with softened water
B Patients dialysed with deionised water
C Patients dialysed with reverse osmosis treated water

Figure 7. The introduction of effective water treatment for a water supply containing a significant amount of aluminium can prevent the rise in serum aluminium concentration seen with untreated or softened water.

appropriate water treatment to remove aluminium (see also Chapter 6), it is necessary to know the total aluminium content of the water supply over several months and the proportion of the total content that is not removed by mixed bed deionisers (due to non-ionic chemical speciation or complexes) so that the most effective water treatment apparatus can be prescribed for that water supply. Some water supplies will require filters and reverse osmosis. Others may need deionisation in addition to achieve a dialysis fluid concentration of aluminium below 20 µg/l (0.7 µmol/l). Other water supplies may only require mixed-bed deionisation.

Installation of appropriate water treatment apparatus to remove aluminium has reduced the patients' exposure to aluminium. This is reflected in a substantial reduction in pre-dialysis serum aluminium concentration (Figure 7) and an absence of further incidences of both encephalopathy and osteodystrophy (12, 57) in centres that have reported the syndromes, although long-term follow up from some centres is still awaited.

Oral administration of aluminium

Although the gastrointestinal tract provides an absorption barrier to aluminium in the normal individual, recent evidence indicates that in times of oral aluminium loading, aluminium is absorbed, leading to increased renal aluminium excretion (5).

There is a small but highly significant elevation of serum aluminium concentration in non-dialysed patients with chronic renal failure not taking aluminium-containing phosphate binding agents (Figure 8). This is presumably a reflection of reduced renal excretion of absorbed dietary aluminium due to impaired renal function. A further marked elevation of serum aluminium concentration occurs in non-dialysed patients with chronic renal failure consuming aluminium-containing phosphate binding agents (18, 69, 70), (Figure 8). A similar elevation of serum aluminium content is found in patients maintained on haemodialysis with appropriate water treatment who are consuming aluminium-contain-

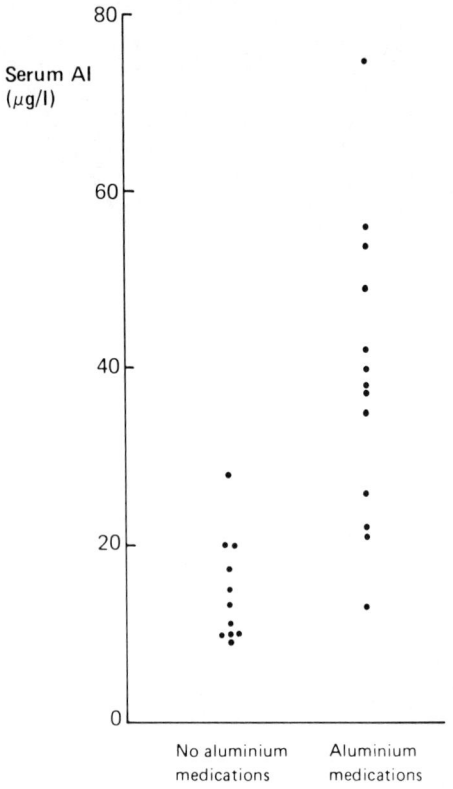

Figure 9. Using water treated by reverse osmosis and polishing deionisation effectively prevents a rise in predialysis serum aluminium concentration in patients with chronic renal failure maintained on intermittent haemodialysis (left hand column). However, introduction of aluminium-containing phosphate binding agents induces a significant rise in the serum aluminium concentration (right hand column).

(SI conversion: µg/l → µmol/l: divide by 27)

ing phosphate binders (Figure 9), and significant aluminium accumulation takes place in the tissues of non-dialysed patients with renal failure due to oral aluminium administration alone (55).

The pathological significance of aluminium accumulation from orally administered aluminium-containing medications remains to be clarified. A survey by the Registry of the European Dialysis and Transplant Association in 1976 showed no correlation between the oral intake of aluminium hydroxide and encephalopathy (7). However, the development of encephalopathic syndromes have been described in children (16) and adults (19) taking aluminium-containing phosphate binding agents in renal failure. In one child, the brain aluminium content was grossly elevated (17). Marsden and colleagues (18) have reported the development of an encephalopathic and osteomalacic syndrome similar to that seen in patients on haemodialysis in an adult with chronic renal failure taking oral aluminium-containing phosphate binding agents for several years and found

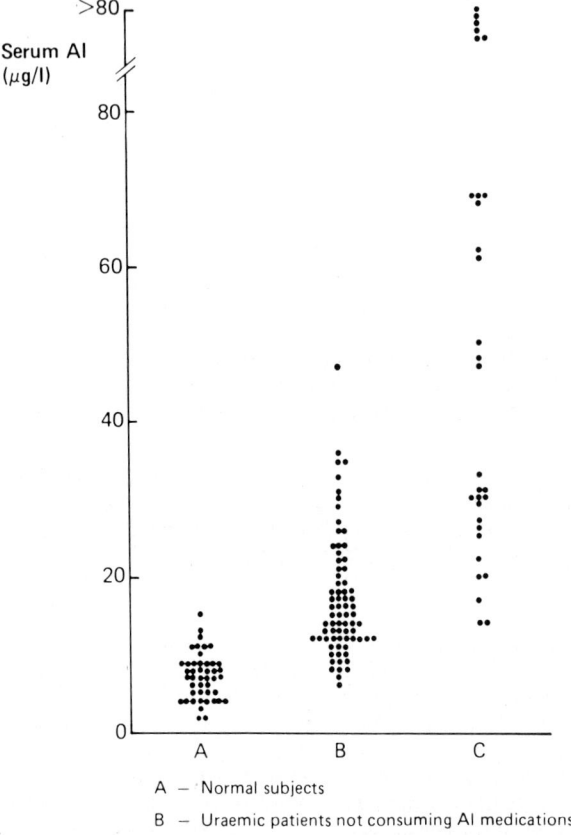

Figure 8. Serum aluminium concentration is significantly greater in patients with chronic renal failure *before the initiation* of haemodialysis than in normal subjects. Patients with chronic renal failure consuming aluminium-containing phosphate binding agents have a further striking elevation of serum aluminium concentration.

SI conversion: µg/l → µmol/l: divide by 27)

significant elevation of the bone content of aluminium. One report documents the recurrence of encephalopathic features after reintroduction of oral aluminium-containing phosphate binding agents in patients who had developed encephalopathic symptoms and who had improved when adequate water treatment was used to prepare dialysis fluid and aluminium-containing phosphate binders had been withdrawn (71). Others document improvement following withdrawal of aluminium medications alone (72, 73).

Treatment of aluminium toxicity

Many reports (20-22, 33,74) suggest that the prognosis is uniformly poor. However, early recognition of the syndromes with elimination of aluminium in the dialysis fluid and withdrawal of oral aluminium or successful renal transplantation has been shown to stabilise or significantly improve the clinical features (2, 64, 72, 75, 76). Significant aluminium removal has been achieved by reduction of dialysis fluid aluminium concentration (77) and by administration of the chelating agent, desferrioxamine (78, 79). It has been demonstrated that a dialysis fluid aluminium concentration of less than 14 µg/l (0.5 µmol/l) is required to promote transfer of aluminium from plasma to dialysis fluid (80).

SUMMARY

A considerable amount of evidence now suggests that aluminium accumulation in uraemic man is responsible for the development of dialysis encephalopathy, vitamin D resistant osteomalacia, microcytic anaemia and 'non-specific' ill health. The major source of aluminium is the water used to prepare dialysis fluid. This aluminium toxicity syndrome can be prevented by adequate pretreatment of water used for preparation of dialysate. Care is needed in the choice of water treatment because of the different aluminium species present in different supplies. Monitoring of treated water aluminium content is recommended. Aluminium accumulation also occurs from oral administration of aluminium containing medications, although the potential toxicity from this route needs clarification. Administration of aluminium-containing phosphate binding agents should therefore be undertaken with caution and not regarded as safe. It would seem important for the pharmaceutical industry to develop a non-aluminium-containing phosphate binding agent for use in uraemic man.

REFERENCES

1. Elliott HL, Dryburgh F, Fell GS, Sabet S, McDougall AI: Aluminium toxicity during regular haemodialysis. *Br Med J* 1:1101, 1978
2. McDermott JR, Smith AI, Ward MK, Parkinson IS, Kerr DNS: Brain aluminium concentration in dialysis encephalopathy. *Lancet* 1:901,1978
3. Cartier F, Allain P, Gary J, Chatel M, Menault F, Pecker S: Myoclonic encephalopathy in dialysis. *Nouv Presse Méd* 7:97, 1978
4. Zumkley H, Bertram HP, Lison A, Knoll O, Losse H: Aluminium, zinc and copper concentrations in plasma in chronic renal insufficiency. *Clin Nephrol* 12:18,1979
5. Kaehny WD, Hegg AP, Alfrey AC: Gastrointestinal absorption of aluminum from aluminum containing antacids. *N Engl J Med* 296:1389, 1977
6. Alfrey AC, Mishell JM, Burks J, Contiguglia SR, Rudolph H, Lewin E, Holmes JH: Syndrome of dyspraxia and multifocal seizures associated with chronic hemodialysis. *Trans Am Soc Artif Intern Organs* 18:257, 1972
7. Jacobs C, Brunner FP, Chantler C, Donckerwolcke RA, Gurland HJ, Hathway RA, Selwood NH., Wing AJ. Combined report on regular dialysis and transplantation in Europe, VII, 1976. *Proc Eur Dial Transpl Assoc* 14:51, 1977
8. Wing AJ, Brunner FP, Brynger H, Chantler C, Donckerwolcke RA, Gurland HJ, Jacobs C, Kramer P, Selwood NH: Dialysis dementia in Europe. *Lancet* 2:190, 1980
9. Barratt LJ, Lawrence JR: Dialysis associated dementia. *Aust NZ J Med* 5:62, 1975
10. Chokroverty S, Bruetman ME, Berger V, Reyes MG: Progressive dialytic encephalopathy. *J Neurol Neurosurg Psychiatry* 29:411, 1976
11. Mahurkar SD, Dhar SK, Salta R, Meyer L, Smith EC, Dunea G: Dialysis dementia. *Lancet* 1:1417, 1973
12. Pierides AM, Edwards WG, Cullum UX, McCall JT, Ellis HA: Hemodialysis encephalopathy with osteomalacic fractures and muscle weakness. *Kidney Int* 18:115, 1980
13. Rozas VV, Port FK, Easterling RE: An outbreak of dialysis dementia due to aluminum in the dialysate. *J Dial* 2:459, 1978
14. Burks J, Alfrey AC, Huddlestone J, Norenberg MD, Lewin E: A fatal encephalopathy in chronic haemodialysis patients. *Lancet* 1:764, 1976
15. Smith DB, Lewis JA, Burks JS, Alfrey AC: Dialysis encephalopathy in peritoneal dialysis. *JAMA* 244:365, 1980
16. Baluarte HJ, Gruskin AB, Hiner LB, Foley CM, Grover WD: Encephalopathy in children with chronic renal failure. *Proc Clin Dial Transpl Forum* 7:95, 1977
17. Nathan E, Pedersen SE: Dialysis encephalopathy in a non-dialyzed uraemic boy treated with aluminium hydroxide orally. *Acta Paediatr Scand* 69:793, 1980
18. Marsden SNE, Parkinson IS, Ward MK, Ellis HA, Kerr DNS: Evidence of aluminium accumulation in renal failure. *Proc Eur Dial Transpl Assoc* 16:588, 1979
19. Mehta RP: Encephalopathy in chronic renal failure appearing before the start of dialysis. *Can Med Assoc J* 120:1112, 1979
20. Ward MK, Pierides AM, Fawcett P, Shaw DA, Perry RH, Tomlinson BE, Kerr DNS: Dialysis encephalopathy syndrome. *Proc Eur Dial Transpl Assoc* 13:348, 1976
21. Flendrig JA, Kruis H, Das HA: Aluminium intoxication: The cause of dialysis dementia? *Proc Eur Dial Transpl Assoc* 13:355, 1976
22. Madison DP, Baehr ET, Bazell M, Hartmen RW, Mahurkar SD, Dunea G: Communicative and cognitive deterioration in dialysis dementia: two case studies. *J Speech Hear Disord* 42:238, 1977
23. Davison AM, Giles GR: The effect of transplantation on dialysis dementia. *Proc Eur Dial Transpl Assoc* 16:407, 1979
24. Platts MM, Moorhead PJ, Grech P: Dialysis dementia. *Lancet* 2:159, 1973
25. Snider WD, DeMaria AA, Mann JD: Diazepam and dialysis encephalopathy. *Neurology* 29:414, 1979

26. Trauner DA, Clayman M: Dialysis encephalopathy treated with Clonazepam. *Ann Neurol* 6:555, 1979
27. Ackrill P, Barron J, Whitley S, Horn AC, Ralston AJ. A new approach to the early detection of dialysis encephalopathy. *Proc Eur Dial Transpl Assoc* 16:659, 1979
28. English A, Savage RD, Britton PG, Ward MK, Kerr DNS. Intellectual impairment in chronic renal failure. *Br Med J* 1:888, 1978
29. Nadel AM, Wilson WP: Dialysis encephalopathy: a possible seizure disorder. *Neurology* 26:1130, 1976
30. Mahurkar SD, Meyers L, Cohen J, Komath RU, Dunea G. Encephalographic and radionuclide studies in dialysis dementia. *Kidney Int* 13:306, 1978
31. Chui HC, Damasio AR: Progressive dialysis encephalopathy. *J Neurol* 222:145, 1980
32. Dewberry FL, McKenney TD, Stone WJ. The dialysis dementia syndrome. *asaio J* 3:102, 1980
33. Sabouraud O, Chatel M, Menault F, Peron JD, Cartier F, Garré M, Gary J, Pecker S: Progressive myoclonic encephalopathy of dialysis. *Rev Neurol (Paris)* 134:575, 1978
34. Mahurkar SD, Smith EC, Mamdani BH, Dunea G: Dialysis dementia – The Chicago experience. *J Dial* 2: 447, 1978
35. Galle P, Chatel M, Berry JP, Menault F: Encephalopathie myoclonique progressive des dialyses (Progressive myoclonic encephalopathy in dialysis patients). *Nouv Presse Med* 8:4091, 1978 (in French)
36. Alfrey AC, LeGendre GR, Kaehny WD: The dialysis encephalopathy syndrome: possible aluminum intoxication. *N Engl J Med* 294:184, 1976
37. Platts MM, Goode GC, Hislop JS. Composition of the domestic water supply and the incidence of fractures and encephalopathy in patients on home dialysis. *Br Med J* 2:657, 1977
38. Alvarez-Ude F, Feest TG, Ward MK, Pierides AM, Ellis HA, Peart KM, Simpson W, Weightman D, Kerr DNS: Hemodialysis bone disease: Correlation between clinical, histological and other features. *Kidney Int* 14:68, 1978
39. Simpson W, Ellis HA, Kerr DNS, McElroy M, McNay RA, Peart KM: Bone disease in long term haemodialysis: a correlation between radiological and histological abnormalities: *Br J Rad* 49:105, 1976
40. Pierides AM, Skillen AW, Ellis HA. Serum alkaline phosphatase in azotemic and hemodialysis osteodystrophy. *J Lab Clin Med* 93:899, 1979
41. Pierides AM, Simpson W, Ward MK, Ellis HA, Dewar JH, Kerr DNS: Variable response to long term 1-alphahydroxycholecalciferol in heamodialysis osteodystrophy. *Lancet* 1:1092, 1976
42. Ellis HA, Pierides AM, Feest TG, Ward MK, Kerr DNS: Histopathology of renal osteodystrophy with particular reference to the effects of 1α-hydroxyvitamin D_3 in patients treated by long-term haemodialysis. *Clin Endocrinol (Oxf)* 7 (suppl):30S, 1977
43. Ellis HA: Metabolic bone disease. In: *Recent Advances in Histopathology,* Edited by Anthony PP and MacSween RNM, Edinburgh, London, New York Churchill-Livingstone, 1981, p 185
44. Ellis HA, McCarthy JH, Herrington J: Bone aluminium in haemodialysed patients and in rats injected with aluminium chloride. *J Clin Pathol* 32:832, 1979
45. Feest TG, Ward MK, Ellis HA, Aljama P, Kerr DNS: Osteomalacic dialysis osteodystrophy: a trial of phosphate-enriched dialysis fluid. *Br Med J* 1:18, 1978
46. Hodsman AB, Sherrard DJ, Wong EGC, Brickman AS, Lee DBM, Alfrey AC, Singer FR, Norman AW, Coburn JW: Vitamin D resistant osteomalacia in hemodialysis patients lacking secondary hyperparathyroidism. *Ann Intern Med* 94:629, 1981
47. Coburn JW, Sherrard DJ, Brickman AS, Wong EGC, Norman AW, Singer FR: Skeletal mineralising defect in dialysis patients. *Contrib Nephrol* 18:172, 1980
48. Posen GA, Gray DC, Jaworski ZF, Couture R, Rashid A: Comparison of renal osteodystrophy in patients dialysed with deionised and non-deionised water. *Trans Am Soc Artif Intern Organs* 18:405, 1972
49. Kanis JA, Candy T, Earnshaw M, Henderson RG, Hegon G, Naik R., Russell RGG, Smith R, Woods CG: Treatment of renal osteodystrophy with 1 alphahydroxylated derivatives of vitamin D_3. *Q J Med* 48:289, 1979
50. Cameron EC, Prior JC, Ballon HS: Haemodialysis patients with a unique mineralizing defect unresponsive to 1, 25-dihydroxycholecalciferol. *Contrib Nephrol* 18:162, 1980
51. Short AIK, Winney RJ, Robson JS. Reversible microcytic hypochromic anaemia in dialysis patients due to aluminium intoxication. *Proc Eur Dial Transpl Assoc* 17:226, 1980
52. Berlyne GM, Ben-Ari J, Pest D, Weinberger J, Stern M, Gilmore GR, Levine R: Hyperaluminaemia from aluminium resins in renal failure. *Lancet* 2:494, 1970
53. Parsons V, Davies C, Goode C, Ogg C, Siddiqui J: Aluminium in bone from patients with renal failure. *Br Med J* 4:273, 1971
54. Arieff AI, Cooper JD, Armstrong D, Lazarowitz VC: Dementia, renal failure and brain aluminum. *Ann Intern Med* 90:741, 1979
55. Alfrey AC, Hegg A, Crasswell P: Metabolism and toxicity of aluminum in renal failure. *Am J Clin Nutr* 33:1509, 1980
56. Cournot-Witmer G, Zingraff J, Bourdon R, Drueke T, Balsan S: Aluminium and dialysis bone disease. *Lancet* 2:795, 1979
57. Elliott HL, Macdougall AI: Aluminium studies in dialysis encephalopathy. *Proc Eur Dial Transpl Ass* 15:157, 1978
58. Ward MK, Feest FG, Ellis HA, Parkinson IS, Kerr DNS, Herrington J, Goode GL: Osteomalacic dialysis osteodystrophy: evidence for a water-borne aetiological agent, probably aluminium. *Lancet* 1:841, 1978
59. Bone I: Progressive dialysis encephalopathy. In: *Dialysis Review,* edited by Davison AM, Tunbridge Wells UK Pitman Medical, 1978, p 216
60. Lang SM, Henry AC: The pathogenesis of dialysis dementia, *J Dial* 3:277, 1979
61. Kovalchik MT, Kaehny WD, Hegg AP, Jackson JT, Alfrey AC: Aluminum kinetics during hemodialysis. *J Lab Clin Med* 92:712, 1978
62. Allain P, Thebaud HE, Dupouet L, Coville P, Pisant M, Spiesser J, Alquier P: Aluminium, manganese, cadmium, lead, copper, zinc in chronic haemodialysis patients before and after dialysis. *Nouv Presse Méd* 7:92, 1978
63. Parkinson IS, Ward MK, Feest TG, Fawcett RWP, Kerr DNS: Fracturing dialysis osteodystrophy and dialysis encephalopathy: an epidemiological survey. *Lancet* 1:406, 1979
64. Dunea G, Mahurkar SD, Mamdani B, Smith EC: Role of aluminum in dialysis dementia. *Ann Intern Med* 88:502, 1978
65. Kaehny WD, Alfrey AC, Holman RE, Shorr WJ. Aluminum transfer during hemodialysis. *Kidney Int* 12:361, 1977
66. Sorenson JRJ, Campbell IR, Tepper LB, Lingg RD: Aluminum in the environment and human health. *Environ Health Perspect* 8:3, 1974
67. Gacek EM, Babb AL, Uvelli DA, Fry DL, Scribner BH. Dialysis dementia: the role of dialysate pH in altering the dialyzability of aluminum. *Trans Am Soc Artif Intern Organs* 25:409, 1979
68. Parkinson IS, Beckett A, Ward MK, Feest TG, Hoenich N,

Strong A, Kerr DNS: Aluminium: removal from water supplies. *Proc Eur Dial Transpl Assoc* 15:586, 1978
69. Kovarik J, Graf H, Meisinger V, Stummvoll HK, Wolf A. Influence of phosphate binders on serum aluminum levels in patients on chronic hemodialysis. *Miner Electrolyte Metab* 2:242, 1979
70. Boukari M, Rottembourg J, Jaudon MC, Clavel JP, Legrain M, Galli A: Influence de la prise prolongée de gels d'aluminium sur les taux sériques d'aluminium chez les patients atteints d'insufficance rénale chronique (Influence of long term intake of aluminium gels on the serum aluminium concentrations in patients with chronic renal failure). *Nouv Presse Méd* 7:85, 1978 (in French)
71. Masselot JP, Adhemar JP, Jaudon MC, Kleinknecht D, Galli A: Reversible dialysis encephalopathy: role for aluminium containing gels. *Lancet* 2:1386, 1978
72. Poisson M, Marshaly R, Lebkiri B: Dialysis encephalopathy: recovery after interruption of aluminium intake. *Br Med J* 2:1610, 1978
73. Buge A, Poisson M, Masson S, Bleibel JM, Mashaly R, Jaudon MC, Lafforgue B, Lebkiri B, Raymond P: Reversible dialysis encephalopathy after discontinuing oral aluminium. *Nouv Presse Méd* 8:2729, 1979
74. Mattern WD, Krigman MR, Blythe WB: Failure of successful renal transplantation to reverse the dialysis-associated encephalopathy syndrome. *Clin Nephrol* 7:275, 1977
75. Sullivan PA, Murnaghan DJ, Callaghan N: Dialysis dementia: recovery after transplantation. *Br Med J* 2:740, 1977
76. Platts MM, Anostassiades E: Dialysis encephalopathy precipitating factors and improvement in prognosis. *Clin Nephrol* 15:223, 1981
77. Graf H, Stummvoll HK, Meisinger V, Wolf A, Pingerra WF: Aluminum removal by hemodialysis. *Kidney Int* 19:587, 1981
78. Ackrill P, Ralston AJ, Day JP, Hodge KC: Successful removal of aluminium from patient with dialysis encephalopathy. *Lancet* 2:692, 1980
79. Arze RS, Parkinson IS, Cartlidge NEF, Britton P, Ward MK: Reversal of aluminium dialysis encephalopathy after desferrioxamine treatment. *Lancet* 2:1116, 1981
80. Hodge KC, Day JP, O'Hara M, Ackrill P, Ralston AJ: Critical concentrations of aluminium in water used for dialysis. *Lancet* 2:802, 1981

43

PLANNING, DEVELOPING AND OPERATING A DIALYSIS PROGRAMME

ANTHONY J.F. d'APICE, NAPIER M. THOMSON, WALTER F. HEALE and
PRISCILLA S. KINCAID-SMITH

Introduction	820
Basic data required for planning	821
Funding	821
Input rate and population size	821
Rate of exit from dialysis	821
Nature of patient population	822
Population distribution	822
Philosophy and policy	822
Relationship with transplantation	822
Dialysis options	822
Self-help	823
Structure	823
National Dialysis-Transplantation Committee	823
Regions	823
Core units	823
Organisation	823
Staffing	823
Facilities	824
Size and number of core units	824
Patient management	824
Peripheral units	825
Satellite dialysis	825
Self-care dialysis	825
Home dialysis	825
Holiday dialysis	825
Hepatitis B antigen positive unit	825
Paediatric unit	826
Interrelationships	826
Regions	826
Core units	826
Peripheral units	826
Medical management	826
Ancillary services	826
Education	826
Staff	826
Patients	827
Patient and staff dialysis societies	827
Community	827
Research	827
Quality control and record keeping	827
Cost and funding of dialysis	828
Comparative costing	828
Summary	828
Acknowledgement	829
References	829

INTRODUCTION

Nephrology did not emerge as a major clinical specialty until dialysis and transplantation were introduced. Initially, dialysis was a laborious procedure performed in a few hospitals by doctors with cumbersome equipment and involving considerable risk to the patient who was selected by a rigorous vetting procedure from the many with end-stage renal failure. Today, the word dialysis, is almost a generic term for several different freely available procedures which can be performed by the patients themselves in almost any location. The evolution of dialysis is still continuing and has wrought major changes to the specialty of nephrology whose face has come more and more to resemble that of its magic procedure.

The success of dialysis has itself created problems which are more political than medical. There are the ever increasing number of patients on dialysis and the even more rapidly increasing cost of managing them. Figure 1 shows the steadily increasing number of patients in Australia (population 14 million). While the number and distribution of patients is different from that in many other countries the rate of increase is similar to that in most developed countries.

In comparison Figure 2 shows the figures from Europe between 1972 and 1980 (1).

The two critical determinants of the number of patients on dialysis are the rate of entry, which reflects predominantly the level of the economy and the health policy of the country and the rate of exit, which is influenced by the rate of transplantation, and mortality. Experience indicates that the number of patients will

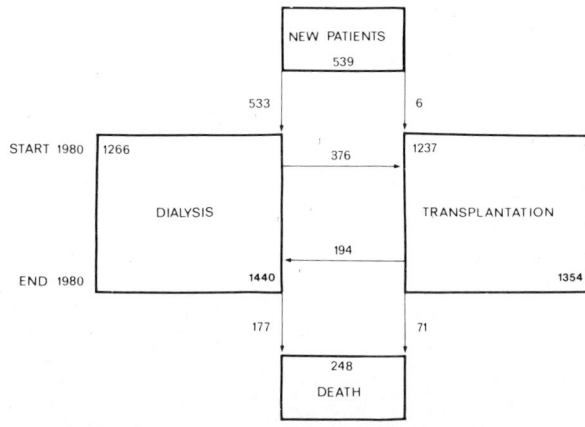

Figure 1. Flow chart of dialysis/transplantation, Australia 1980 (population 14 mill.). (Data from the Australian and New Zealand Dialysis and Transplant Registry).

43: Planning, developing and operating a dialysis programme   821

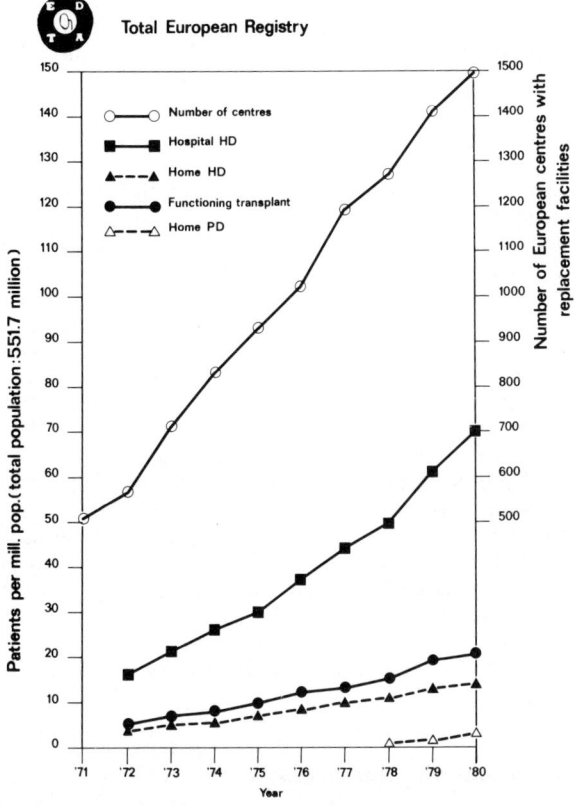

Figure 2. Number of patients (per mill. population) on different treatment for end stage renal disease in Europe on 31 December 1972-1980. Chart includes increase of numbers of European centres 1972-1980.

continue to increase, because restriction of entry is generally considered unacceptable and despite considerable effort in many countries, the rate of transplantation remains far behind the level that is needed. Consequently, the only available solution appears to be a reduction of the cost of dialysis. Cost containment has been a major driving force in the trend toward self dialysis. This is resulting in yet another step in the evolution of dialysis – today a substantial number of patients in many countries are dialysing at home or in limited care centres and fewer are being dialysed in high cost hospital based dialysis units.

The plan of a regional dialysis programme discussed in this chapter emphasises the decentralisation of dialysis which is dependent on a much greater degree of patient involvement in his own care than has been traditional.

BASIC DATA REQUIRED FOR PLANNING

The basic data required to plan a regional dialysis programme are listed in Table 1.

Table 1. Basic data required for planning a regional dialysis programme.

1. Funding
2. End-stage renal failure acceptance rate
3. Population size and demography
4. Nature of patient population
5. Availability of transplantation

Funding

The cost of a regional dialysis programme and methods of funding the service will be discussed in a later section. However, the level of funding and its future security are vital pieces of information in planning the programme because these ultimately determine the number of patients that can be treated and consequently whether any restrictions need be imposed on entry.

Input rate and population size

Assuming that financial restrictions have not imposed a restriction on the number of patients that can be treated, the input rate in most developed countries is 30 to 50 per million of population per year. Predictions of population size can be obtained from the Government Statistitian. If financial restrictions limit the number of patients that can be treated, it is probably best to design arbitrary selection criteria so that the input rate is appropriate to the situation and constant. Since such arbitrary criteria are necessary because of political decisions, they should be formally endorsed and promulgated by the funding authority.

The other source of patients is re-entry after failed transplantation, the rate depending on the age and size of the transplant programme and its success rate. The annual re-entry rate in Australia is approximately 40% of the annual transplant rate or 10% of total number of transplant patients.

Rate of exit from dialysis

Figure 1 is a flow chart of entry and exit to and from dialysis and transplantation in Australia in 1980. This figure serves to illustrate two points of importance. Firstly, the only exits from dialysis are death or transplantation. The annual dialysis death rate is approximately 35% of the annual entry rate or 11% of all patients dialysed during the year. Both figures will vary depending on the age of the dialysis programme (and its patients). Secondly, the rate of transplantation is the only adjustable factor other than the entry rate. The flow chart shows that the number of dialysis patients in Australia increased by 14% during 1980. Without transplantation, it would have increased by about 30%. On a larger scale, the effect of variable entry and transplant rates can be seen from the annual statistical reports of the European Dialysis and Transplant Association. An exaggerated example is the comparison of the number of patients on dialysis in Australia and Japan. The entry rates are similar, but in Australia the transplant rate is 22/million/year compared to a negligible rate in Japan and as a result Japan has approximately 235 dialysis patients per million compared to 88 per million in Australia.

Thus, it is obvious that the availability of a transplantation programme and its level of activity are critical components of the equation.

Nature of the patient population

Paediatric patients present special problems. They are ideally dialysed at home, under the supervision of a paediatric nephrology unit. However, unless the population of the region is very large, the number of paediatric patients will be too few to justify a separate dialysis service. The paediatric referral rate and the ages of those referred varies markedly depending on the attitudes of the local paediatricians.

Hepatitis-B antigen (HBsAg) positive patients are another special group (see also Chapter 34). Attitudes about how to manage this problem vary from taking virtually no precautions, particularly in an area with a high HBsAg carriage rate, to complete isolation of all HBsAg positive patients. Many compromise 'solutions' have arisen largely for pragmatic reasons. The opportunity to manage the problem optimally presents when planning a new regional dialysis programme and it is the authors' view that total separation of HBsAg antigen positive and negative patients should be achieved. This is particularly important in countries where the HBsAg carriage rate is low, because the immunity rate will also be low. The separation can be most effectively made by testing all new referrals, whether as ward or clinic patients, with immediate transfer of those found to be HBsAg antigen positive.

If an arbitrary selection policy must be employed for fiscal reasons, one can expect that the patient population will be younger and healthier. This will influence the relative proportions that will be best managed by different dialysis modalities and at different sites. The main effect will be reduction in the numbers of patients who can only be managed by hospital based centre dialysis. Conversely, even in the presence of a restrictive selection policy, the passage of time will generate an increasing number of ageing or medically unfit patients, who cannot reasonably be transplanted and who will require hospital based centre dialysis.

Population distribution

The distribution of the population throughout the region will influence the structure of the programme and siting of facilities. Patients in isolated areas can only be managed by home dialysis. Self-care dialysis units of variable size, even single patient units, can be established in community health centres, country hospitals etc. Larger self-care units can be sited throughout the suburban areas of large cities to reduce the travelling time of patients. The location of major centre dialysis units is dependent on existing hospitals and the population distribution may have changed since they were built.

PHILOSOPHY AND POLICY

Every dialysis programme has a basic philosophy, although it is usually not so developed as to be more than a series of policies which reflect an unstated and often unformed philosophy. In the main, the philosophy depends on the personalities of the dominant staff and the pressures exerted by the patient load and financial considerations. An example is the variance of policy about dialyser reusage (see Chapter 15). One group justifies a vigorous reuse policy on the grounds of fiscal responsibility, while the other justifies single use on ground of patient safety and comfort and staff time.

In planning a new regional dialysis programme one has the opportunity to develop a philosphy and put it into practice through a series of policies. The final product will inevitably be a compromise between what is felt to be ideal and what can practically be offered as a result of various restrictions. Probably the most difficult area, which will influence the programme to the greatest extent is the selection of patients (discussed in Chapter 44).

Relationship with transplantation

Despite the marked variations in practice, there is no doubt in the authors' minds that successful transplantation should be the ultimate aim for nearly all patients. This subject is discussed in Chapter 44. Clearly, the decision about transplantation will have major implications for the dialysis programme, particularly in relation to the number of patients that have to be catered for and the rate of growth of the programme. The relationship between dialysis and transplantation can either be an association between physically separate, separately staffed programmes or a fully integrated programme. One of the main advantages of the latter, is the integration of the staff, so that patients are cared for by the same staff and in the same place from presentation for the rest of their lives. At a practical level, integration assists in optimal preparation for transplantation. Probably the only circumstance where a definite policy not to transplant any patients should be persued, would be when the mortality rate or success rate of the particular transplant service are unacceptable.

Dialysis options

Should a regional dialysis service offer, or have available, all currently employed modes of dialysis at a variety of locations? The options are: haemodialysis (including haemofiltration), intermittent peritoneal dialysis either at home, or in a self care centre or in a centre dialysis unit or continuous ambulatory peritoneal dialysis (CAPD). The answer is probably in the affirmative, although the final role of CAPD has not yet been fully established. There is no doubt that haemodialysis remains unchallenged as the major form of dialysis and consequently in planning a regional dialysis programme one is primarily concerned with provision of this form of treatment at a variety of sites.

Dialysis is commenced as an in-hospital form of treatment and later extended into the home and still later into self-care centres. The increasing number of dialysis patients makes it impossible to provide dialysis exclusively in hospital centre dialysis units. The role of the hospital dialysis centre is changing quickly from being the site at which most patients are managed to being the back-up system for a large home and self-care based programme.

Self-help

Historically, dialysis was a procedure which doctors and nurses performed on patients who had a purely passive role themselves. The changes in the sites at which dialysis is performed have been necessarily accompanied by an increase in patient participation in their own dialysis. The level of patient participation can vary from complete self-dialysis at home to none in a hospital based unit. Because of the need for patient mobility between the various sites of dialysis, it is ideal to aim at maximum patient participation from the start of each patient's dialysis career.

STRUCTURE

This section will describe a tiered structure of a regional dialysis programme and the interrelationship of its components.

National Dialysis-Transplantation Committee

The purpose of such a committee should be to define broad policies in relation to dialysis and transplantation and to provide expert opinion on problem areas. A major role is as a lobbyist with government authorities. A National Dialysis-Transplantation Registry, as described later, is a natural component. Such a committee should represent a medical viewpoint and consequently its membership should represent the medical personnel involved in dialysis and transplantation in each of the regions of the country. In Australia, this committee is formed under the auspices of the Kidney Foundation and Nephrology Society.

Examples of areas of activity of a National Dialysis-Transplantation Committee are inter-region organ sharing schemes, organ retrieval programmes, publication of educational material, and interaction with National Standards Associations in relation to standards for dialysis-associated equipment and water purification policy.

Regions

The formation of regions within a country will usually be decided by pre-existing political or other organisational boundaries, and thus they will often differ markedly in size. In Australia, the geopolitical boundaries of the states define the regions whose populations vary from 0.25 to 5 million. Each region contains a variable number of major dialysis or dialysis-transplantation facilities – core units – based on major hospitals. The core units are independent and relate to one another and to regional funding authorities through Regional Dialysis-Transplantation Committees. The population drainage areas of each core unit may be fixed by the health authority or be more flexible as in Australia, allowing some degree of competition between core units.

Core units

Dialysis should not be viewed in isolation from nephrology or transplantation. Consequently, core dialysis units should be an integral part, together with transplantation, of general nephrology services. This does not mean that hospital based dialysis should be the basic method providing dialysis. Indeed, the core unit should function only as a new patient entry point, acute dialysis service and support system for both transplantation and a decentralised maintenance dialysis service.

Organisation

The core unit should be the smallest part of the dialysis service but control the activities of all the physically or numerically larger peripheral units. Probably the most important organisational aspect is designing the staff structure so that medical, nursing and paramedical staff have a broad exposure to all aspects of nephrology, including transplantation, while having their major responsibility in a particular component. This can be achieved by dual responsibility and (or) rotation of staff. A disadvantage of having staff permanently committed to one mode of treatment or one type of patient is a narrowing of knowledge and perspective which is often evident in their management of patients.

The components of a core unit will be the in-hospital haemodialysis service, the in-hospital peritoneal dialysis training service, the machine maintenance service and the administration of the core attached peripheral units.

Staffing

The medical staff needs should be viewed in the context of an integrated dialyis-transplant-general nephrology service. The need for the dialysis component is approximately 1 full-time nephrologist and one junior medical officer per 50 maintenance dialysis patients. This allocation allows some time for other activities, such as research.

Staff requirements in the core haemodialysis unit are high as it provides acute haemodialysis and dialysis of new patients and patients who are unable to self-dialyse or have superimposed acute medical problems. The patient-to-staff ratio should not exceed 2:1. This ratio does not include staff used for administration, record keeping and staff training.

Technical staff requirements vary depending on the type of machinery e.g. central delivery systems, single patient units, etc. The technical staff will cover the whole dialysis service including the home dialysis and self-care units. Two technicians can manage the machinery of about 120 dialysis patients. Hospitals and health authorities are notoriously reluctant to provide adequate administrative assistance to dialysis services. Despite this reluctance, dialysis has a large business component because of the large staff number and high cost of the technology. A dialysis service maintaining 100 patients requires one senior administrator and two clerks. This level of staffing is cost efficient because of savings that can be made in purchasing and stock control.

Facilities

The dialysis programme should be able to offer home haemodialysis, home peritoneal dialysis (both intermittent and continuous ambulatory), self-care haemodialysis, acute haemodialysis and peritoneal dialysis, holiday dialysis and rarely permanent in-hospital haemodialysis. The role of the core unit is largely in dialysis of new patients, acute renal failure, problem patients and providing the medical management, administration, staff training, paramedical services and technical services for the whole programme. Special facilities include a machine workshop and a vehicle for visiting home dialysis patients and peripheral units. A central computer for patient records and programme administration should be available.

Size and number of core units

The various factors which influence the size of a regional dialysis programme have been discussed previously. The size of the individual core units will depend on their number and distribution and on whether their drainage areas are regulated. In the authors' view, the upper limit for maximal efficiency of each individual programme within a region is likely to be about 250 patients. If this is accepted, several other observations can be made. Firstly, it is unwise to allow one programme to progress alone toward this size, because once it reaches this size it can only stagnate. In any dialysis programme there are always a proportion of patients who by passage of time or by the ravages of failed transplantation become untransplantable and (or) hospital dialysis dependent. The number of these dependent patients increases progressively with time. Once a unit stops growing, the proportion of dependent patients will increase markedly, the transplant rate will fall and finally the programme will collapse onto its base – the in-hospital dialysis unit. It is better to develop two or more units simultaneously or only a few years apart so that the growth of each is less rapid.

In the initial planning of the region, the number of core units and the timing of their commencement should be decided. The size of the core dialysis units should be designed initially to suit the final need and not the immediate requirement only. Expansion of a hospital-based facility is often impossible after the original structure has been designed. Generous allocation of space is essential to allow future growth. The initial plans need not include all the plumbing and water purification plant necessary at some future date, but should not be such as to prevent expansion or modification of the basic technology.

A core unit haemodialysis facility should allow space for 10 to 12 haemodialysis chairs. Allowing three dialyses per patient per week and two shifts per day, this facility will cope with 40 to 48 patients. The size of the core unit haemodialysis facility determines the size of the total dialysis population that can be supported in peripheral facilities and at home. A 10 station centre unit can support about 250 patients in toto. It is worth re-emphasising that as a dialysis programme ages, it generates a steadily increasing number of dependent patients and consequently the size of the dialysis population outside the hospital centre cannot be expanded beyond its capacity to support them.

A further consideration in the relationship between the size of the hospital centre and the total dialysis population is the balance of the various modalities by which the non-hospital patients are managed. For example, CAPD is an attractive method of managing a large number of patients without need for expensive facilities. However, an epidemic of multiple antibiotic resistant staphylococcal peritonitis can quickly produce chaos, unless the hospital dialysis facility can cope with the sudden influx of patients. At present, it would seem wise to restrict the size of a peritoneal dialysis programme to approximately one-third of the total dialysis population.

Patient management

It is important to make it clear to patients who are acceptable candidates for entry into the programme, that there are a few ground rules, the observance of which is essential for their entry and their continued treatment. Some nephrologists view this attitude as inappropriate and unnecessarily authoritarian, although they have usually not run a dialysis-transplant service. Unfortunately, it is sometimes necessary to insist that patients follow these rules because their failure to do so can jeopardise the management of other patients or waste valuable resources such as donor kidneys. Thus, it is essential to educate patients about the way the system works.

The day-to-day management of the patients is best conducted by the dialysis nursing staff with doctors intervening only when problems develop. The aim is to make dialysis a self-care procedure, with nursing or technical assistance if necessary and medical management by out-patient visits only, except in urgent situations.

Peripheral units

The majority of patients will be dialysed outside the hospital after a short period of adjustment to dialysis. Several possible sites and levels of staffing are possible.

Satellite dialysis
This type of dialysis service is a small scale or geographically remote replica of a hospital dialysis unit. The necessity for such units depends on the geographic distribution of core units and the total dialysis population. For example, a city with a population of 100,000 situated 100 miles (approximately 160 km) from the nearest core unit, would not warrant a full dialysis-transplant service, but may require a small, fully-staffed dialysis service. This type of unit is not a low staff/patient ratio service and can be optimally used by siting it in a general hospital where it can provide acute dialysis and be used as a home dialysis training facility. The control of such units should be by a core unit and they should not be fully independent. This can be achieved by medical staff joint appointments and rotation of staff in both directions, even if only for short periods, to allow continuing education. Transplantation should be performed at the core unit.

Self-care dialysis
This form of self-help dialysis is particularly appropriate for those in whom home dialysis is difficult or impossible for social reasons such as an unsatisfactory home environment or lack of an assistant. The aim is to provide a place where patients can dialyse themselves with minimal assistance and supervision. As in home dialysis, the patient is responsible for his own dialysis. These units have an optimal size of 10 stations (40 patients) and can be managed very easily by two staff per shift. This staff level is necessary for industrial reasons, patient confidence and mutual support, but may exceed that dictated by the work load alone. This allows patient training to be conducted at the self-care centres. These centres are able to be 'personalised' and made much more attractive and less clinical than a hospital dialysis unit and are popular with patients. The amount of patient time per dialysis and the capital and maintenance cost can be reduced by using a central delivery system.

The cost of self-care dialysis is comparable to home dialysis and is much less expensive than hospital based dialysis. These units can be sited in relation to patient demography and the facilities can be shared by several core units. The management should be shared through the core unit to which it primarily relates and the staff should rotate through the parent unit.

Smaller self-care units of one or two stations are suitable for medium sized towns and can be staffed by part-time workers who are trained in the core unit and regularly spend a few weeks in the core unit. The capital cost of such mini-units is usually no more than that involved in establishing a single patient on home dialysis because they can be sited in district hospitals or community centres.

Home dialysis
The majority of patients on dialysis can be managed either by home dialysis or in self-care centres. The popularity of home dialysis varies from country to country and seems to be in inverse proportion to the financial reward for institutional dialysis. This form of dialysis can, as is often emphasised by its opponents, place some stress on domestic relationships, but is most often satisfactory, provided there is adequate space and family support. The peripheral unit to which home dialysis patients relate is the home dialysis training centre. This may be physically associated with the hospital centre, a self-care unit, or may be totally separate. A large home training facility can provide its service to several core units but final management should remain with one core unit.

In designing a home dialysis training unit, provision should be made for several two bedroom appartments in which patients who live a long distance away can be accomodated during the training period.

Holiday dialysis
One of the advantages of transplantation is the fact that patients can go on holidays. The provision of holiday dialysis facilities extends this advantage to dialysis patients. The authors' patients have used the Redy (Sorb)-system dialysis machine (see Chapter 17), temporary CAPD and caravans equipped with dialysis machines in addition to visitor status dialysis, to enable them to have a holiday. One major disadvantage of international travel is that holiday dialysis often comes at an exorbitant price in foreign countries and may not be covered by home country health insurance. Dialysis holiday homes, established by patient interest groups, provide excellent holiday facilities for the patient and his whole family. Service clobs are often willing to sponsor the establishment of those facilities. In Australia, most units are happy to accept visitors for dialysis provided they are HBsAg negative.

Hepatitis B antigen positive unit
The answer to the question of how to manage HBsAg positive patients varies depending on the prevalence of antigenaemia in the population (see also chapter 34). In most developed countries, hepatitis B antigenaemia is uncommon (< 1% of the population), and consequently the level of immunity is low. The major concern is accidental infection of staff. One statisfactory approach is to transfer all antigen positive patients to a special hepatitis unit. This should be backed by a high level of awareness, bordering on paranoia, in core units. It is our practice to test all new nephrology patients for hepatitis B antigenaemia at their first visit whether this involves hospital admission or a clinic visit. All staff, including domestic staff, and all dialysis patients are tested monthly. HBsAg

positive staff are not employed in the dialysis area, and any patient found to be positive is transferred to a special unit which serves six core units. These patients are only returned to the core units when they are HBs antibody positive or persistently antigen negative. Transplantation of antigen positive patients is performed at the special unit. Staff from positive units should not rotate through core units.

Many units manage the problem satisfactorily by less drastic measures. However, in all circumstances, the most effective method of protection of the staff is a high level of awareness and treating all blood contaminated articles as though they were HBsAg positive.

Recently an efficient antihepatitis B vaccine has become available (see Chapter 34).

Paediatric unit
Opinion and practice vary on whether children should be managed in essentially adult dialysis-transplant services or whether they should be managed in special paediatric facilities (see also chapter 25). The deciding factors will often be the size of the region and the attitudes of the paediatric nephrologists about acceptance of children into end-stage renal failure programmes. These factors will decide the size of paediatric patient population. A small patient population would not justify a separate paediatric facility as the quality of the care is likely to be lower, unless there are enough patients to provide continuing experience and activity for the staff. However, if the population is sufficiently large, a paediatric service is justified because of the special needs and problems of children which may be less well understood or overlooked in a predominantly adult dialysis-transplant unit. An intermediate sized paediatric patient population can be managed in a paediatric hospital by staff rotated frequently through an adult core unit to maintain dialysis experience and expertise. Joint medical staff appointments can help overcome many patient management problems.

Interrelationships

Regions
The major areas of interaction between regional dialysis programmes are in relation to organ sharing schemes, patient transfers and holiday dialysis. The value of a National Dialysis-Transplant Committee in policy definition and interacting with government has been discussed.

Core units
Within a regional programme, close co-operation between core units is highly desirable. Such co-operation should be sought at all levels. A regional dialysis-transplant committee representing each core unit is a useful method of co-ordinating all facilities such as the HBsAg positive units, home dialysis training units, holiday units, satellite and self-care units. In most cases these should be under the control of one core unit with access available to other units. Standardisation of dialysis machinery and disposables throughout a region is desirable

and facilitates patient transfer. It is also particularly useful in price negotiations for supply of consumables, such as dialysers, lines, and dialysis fluid concentrate, which can be put up for tender to supply the whole region.

Sharing of experience should also be encouraged by regular inter-unit meetings at a nursing and technical level. Such meetings can result in standardisation of dialysis techniques throughout the region without it being imposed in an authoritarian fashion.

Each unit should develop an area of particular interest and expertise. Co-ordination of these special interests results in a valuable broad range of expertise being available in the region. Brief rotation of selected senior nursing and technical staff through other core units may also be of value.

Peripheral units
The desirability of rotation of staff of peripheral units through the core unit has been discussed. This prevents the staff and patients in peripheral units from becoming isolated and allows continuing staff education. Patient movement between dialysis facilities should be flexible. It is often valuable to allow home dialysis patients several weeks dialysis in a self-care centre each year to give their helper a holiday from duty.

Medical management
There is a tendency for dialysis patients and sometimes their whole families, to use the dialysis medical staff for all their medical needs. This can be unwittingly fostered by both the family practitioners and the nephrologists. Adequate communication usually overcomes the problem, particularly if the family doctor, who has probably never seen a dialysis patient before, is given a clear understanding of the process and is asked to contact the nephrologist whenever the patient is seen, particularly if any change in therapy is contemplated. The major role must remain with the nephrologist, who should see the patient, even if long distances are involved, at least once every 3 months.

Ancillary services
Each patient requires the services of a variable number of councillors, dieticians, social workers, psychiatrists and clergy. In most cases the need for these services for an individual patient must be perceived by the nephrologist, and their involvement initiated and co-ordinated by him. Local community social workers and welfare agencies can often be of considerable assistance and their activities are most easily co-ordinated by the family practitioner in consultation with the nephrologist. Often a valuable local support system can be established for the patient and is particularly necessary if he is dialysing at home and is a long distance from the core unit.

EDUCATION

Staff

The quality of any dialysis service will ultimately depend on the quality of the staff training. The key person is the Staff Educator who must be a practical rather than a theoretical educator. New nursing staff should ideally have been fully trained as nephrology nurses before commencing special dialysis training. The training period should include rotation through various peripheral units including the home dialysis training centre and a self-care dialysis unit. The bulk of the training should be practical and the trainees should be supernumerary during most of the training period.

Compulsory refresher courses, particularly for peripheral unit staff rotating through the core unit, should be run at regular intervals. In addition, the Staff Educator should monitor all staff at their work at least once a year.

Patients

Patient education should begin well before they commence dialysis. Self help, self control and co-operation are the main lessons which patients find most difficult to accept. On the other hand, from the patients' point of view, learning about their illness, its implications and how to cope with their fear of dialysis and the unknown, are the most important areas.

Patient education should be structured towards self dialysis, which can usually be achieved within a few months at most. Education, commenced before dialysis began, should be repeated after commencement and stabilisation. The education should stress that dialysis is only one phase of management of their illness and that successful transplantation is the ultimate aim.

Patient and staff dialysis societies

Both patients and staff should be encouraged to form regional or national societies. Patient dialysis associations provide considerable support and education for the members and can overcome many of the problems which the patient accepts as insoluble or doesn't discuss with the medical and nursing staff. It is desirable that patient associations should have an interested 'medical adviser', who can often clear up common misconceptions and so prevent these societies functioning like labour unions.

Dialysis nurses and technicians should be encouraged to form a scientific society and form links with the National Nephrology Society. These societies play an important role in continuing education in the same way as medical scientific societies.

Community

Education of the community is mainly concerned with preventive medical aspects (e.g. the dangers of analgesic abuse) and the value of kidney transplantation. There is little doubt that a high level of community awareness about transplantation results in a lower refusal rate when relatives are approached for permission for cadaveric renal donation.

RESEARCH

In planning a regional dialysis programme, research should be regarded as an integral part of the programme. Each core unit should develop and maintain an active research programme in its area of special interest and expertise. Dialysis is often viewed as purely a business or service commitment. However, the quality of the service will depend in part on the academic interest and activity in the scientific aspects of chronic renal failure and its management.

In planning the programme, research should be given a high priority and this should be implemented by employing sufficient medical, nursing and technical staff and allocating sufficient space so that research is possible. However, the most important aspect is to make proven research ability a high priority when selecting the medical staff, particularly the directors of core units. A closely co-operating group of core units within a National or Regional Dialysis Programme is able to undertake collaborative controlled trials which would be impossible or unduly prolonged in single units.

QUALITY CONTROL AND RECORD KEEPING

These aspects of a dialysis programme are closely linked. Units which have poor records usually have poor quality control and are likely to have poor results – if these could be assessed.

Medical records are one of the neglected areas of many hospitals and the very large, often massive amount of data, generated by a nephrology-dialysis-transplant service overwhelms their systems. Unless the hospital's medical record system is exceptional, it is worthwhile establishing partially independent record systems in each core unit. These should cover all patients in the dialysis-transplant programme. It is virtually impossible to reorganise the past records of a large ongoing programme. However in planning a new programme, proper record keeping with a rapid retrieval, integration and analysis system should be given a high priority. These specifications can only be met by computerisation. The hardware needed for such a system is not excessive, although the soft ware and more particularly the operator costs may appear expensive. When these are related to the cost of dialysing one patient for one year, they assume much less daunting proportions. Peripheral units should be linked to the core unit computer system, otherwise much of the data will never be recorded.

Adequate, accessible, analysable records form the basis of any quality control system. Each core unit should regularly analyse its results and subject them to peer review.

Each country should have a National Dialysis and Transplant Registry and health funding authorities should insist on complete data returns as a condition of funding, if co-operation cannot be obtained on a voluntary basis. The Australian-New Zealand Dialysis Transplant Registry is an outstanding example with complete registration and data return on all patients who have ever entered dialysis-transplant programmes. This body of data is thus unique in being unselected. It provides a firm data base for predictions of future needs, quality control and peer review and provides answers to many scientific questions. New questions should be asked prospectively to examine new areas of interest as retrospective returns may be inaccurate or incomplete.

COST AND FUNDING OF DIALYSIS

The question of the cost of management of end-stage renal failure, particularly by dialysis, has been mentioned in different contexts in previous sections of this chapter. Most doctors hate thinking about it and most health administrators seem to think of nothing else. The rapid escalation of the costs of health care and social welfare during the last two decades have resulted in these two areas of government spending being particular targets for Treasury inspired pruning or no growth policies in most developed countries. The health administrators are given a static or shrinking budget to administer. At the same time, there has been a trend toward favourable treatment of community based and low technology programmes. This is obviously at the expense of dreaded high technology programmes of which dialysis is the archtype. Proven new high technology programmes, such as cardiac transplantation, face a bleak outlook. In contrast, dialysis is established; its problem is one of progressive expansion and consequent increasing cost. The attack of health administrators is to minimise this growth and given the incentive they will undoubtedly succeed.

What can be done about this prospect? A vigorous and emotional doctor-patient campaign for more funds may delay the day of reckoning, but eventually the cost issue must be faced by both doctors and patients. The alternatives are limited; either reduce the per dialysis cost so that more patients can be dialysed for the same total cost or continue the status quo in which most patients are receiving high cost institutional dialysis and restrict entry to dialysis by arbitrary criteria. There is no doubt that both approaches, either separately or together, are being taken in different countries.

If the view exposed in Chapter 44 is accepted, namely that all medically suitable patients should be accepted for dialysis, then the future trend in the management of end-stage renal failure will be toward those treatment modalities which are the least expensive. The approach to planning a new regional dialysis programme outlined in this chapter is based on the belief that high quality management can be provided by a programme which is based on the less expensive forms of treatment, namely transplantation and home and self-care dialysis.

Comparative costing

Table 2 shows the approximate relative costs of various methods of managing end-stage renal failure. The actual

Table 2. Comparative annual maintenance cost of different methods of managing end-stage renal failure.

	Relative cost $
Hospital haemodialysis	1.00
Home haemodialysis (single pass)	0.30
Home haemodialysis (dialysate regeneration)	0.40
Self-care haemodialysis	0.35
Home intermittent peritoneal dialysis	0.90
Cadaveric transplantation – 1st year	0.60
Cadaveric transplantation – subsequent years	0.10

costs vary considerably from country to country and with time, although the relative cost appear to remain fairly constant (2, 3). Continuous ambulatory peritoneal dialysis has not been included in the table because the cost is highly variable depending on the amount of time spent in hospital as a result of peritonitis.

It is obvious that hospital based haemodialysis and intermittent automated home peritoneal dialysis are expensive ways of managing end-stage renal failure compared to transplantation and home and self-care haemodialysis.

SUMMARY

The major current and future problem in providing management for end-stage renal failure is one of escalating numbers of patients and cost. Consequently, both currently established and new regional dialysis programmes must be modified or planned to provide the service economically and be capable of expansion. Both of these requirements are best met by a programme in which the majority of patients are managed by transplantation and limited care or home dialysis. Hospital based facilities should remain reserved for new patients' induction and management of problem patients.

Thus, most patients will dialyse themselves, decreasing cost by reducing staff requirements, and at the same time increasing the patients benefit by greater independence. The effective management of such a decentralised dialysis programme requires a high level of communication and clearly defined relationships between the various components of the programme.

It should be emphasised that, without a plan of organisation of centralised management, situations may arise wherein optimal treatment is not provided to the patients. For instance, personal biases and economic incentives among uncontrolled competing physicians can cause inequities in patient care with limited options favouring institutional dialysis, imbalance of facilities, higher expenditures and impediments to co-operative clinical research.

ACKNOWLEDGEMENT

Figure 2 has been modified slightly from the EDTA Registry Report, XI, 1981 and is reproduced by kind permission of the Editors of the Proceedings of the EDTA, published by Pitman, London, UK.

REFERENCES

1. Broyer M, Brunner FP, Brynger H, Donckerwolcke RA, Jacobs C, Kramer P, Selwood NH, Wing AJ, Blake PH: Combined report on regular dialysis and transplantation in Europe, XI 1980 (and preceding years). *Proc Eur Dial Transpl Assoc* 18:2, 1981
2. Siemsen AW, Coad RJ, Wong EGC, Sugihara JG, Musgrave JE, Basilio R: Economic impact of an integrated approach to hemodialysis and dialyzer reuse. *Dial Transpl* 9:933, 1980
3. Mahony JF, Kachel G: Comparative costs of dialysis. In: *Peritoneal Dialysis,* edited by Atkins RC, Thomson NM, Farrell PC, Edinburgh, London, Churchill-Livingstone, 1981, p 418

44
SELECTION OF PATIENTS AND THE INTEGRATION BETWEEN DIALYSIS AND TRANSPLANTATION, THE QUALITY OF LIFE OF THE PATIENTS

TIMOTHY H. MATHEW, ANTHONY J.F. d'APICE, PRISCILLA S. KINCAID-SMITH

Introduction 830
Selection of patients 830
    Factors applying when dialysis availability is unrestricted 831
        Expected quality of life 831
        Age 831
        Compliance 831
    Additional factors applying when dialysis availability is inadequate 831
        Vascular status 831
        Ability to self dialyse 832
        Likelihood of transplantation 832
Practical problems related to selection 833
    The Right to Reject 833
    'Who makes the decision?' 833
    Patient involvement in decisions 833
    The option of no active treatment 834
    Ideal versus the practical 834
    Individual versus the Group 834
    Local versus regional policies 834
Integration of dialysis and transplantation 834
Quality of life 835
References 836

INTRODUCTION

The selection of patients for treatment in a renal replacement programme is based on multiple factors which include medical and social aspects and the availability of facilities. Where facilities are not a restricting factor, only a small percentage of patients referred for treatment need be refused (1). Few countries have demonstrated a capacity or willingness to put unrestricted resources at the disposal of nephrologists. Thus, attention from the outset has been paid to efficient utilisation of available facilities. In Australia an early decision was taken to promote cadaver transplantation actively. It soon became apparent that, for optimal therapy to be offered to all patients, a combination or 'integration' of dialysis and transplantation was necessary (2) and that this could be based on an attempt to find a successful transplant for all medically suitable candidates (1). This approach, now practiced widely in Australia and elsewhere, is believed to make maximum use of facilities while providing patients with the best possible quality of life.

SELECTION OF PATIENTS

The problem of selection of patients is easily dismissed as a non issue in those countries where adequate facilities exist and refusal for treatment needs to be made only on medical grounds. It is cogent to remember, however, that only in USA, Canada, Australia, Japan and in some parts of Europe, are more than 20 patients/million/year accepted for active treatment. In those countries with a reduced acceptance rate, age (3) and available funds are the greatest discriminants.

The original criteria used by the Seattle Medical Advisory Committee appear 20 years later, still provide a reasonable basis for selection on medical grounds when some limitation is necessary. In conformity with these criteria stable adults under the age of 45 were acceptable with no irreversible cardiovascular disease who cooperated well with treatment. Undoubtedly criteria similar to these are still in use in many countries. The Seattle plan of having a second lay committee to rank priority for treatment among those deemed medically suitable was initially followed in many units but was progressively abandoned in the late 1960's (4). The view that if limitation is necessary a 'first come, first served' method as the one most ethically feasible has been advanced (5) and, in practice, is that mostly followed by physicians who are forced to act as 'gatekeepers'.

In practice selection for treatment means selection for dialysis treatment as it is seldom possible and is usually undesirable to transplant a patient without prior dialysis. Further, as there are no absolute contraindications to long term dialysis and as dialysis is the backbone of a treatment programme, selection for the programme is

Table 1. Factors influencing acceptance onto treatment programme.

Adequate facilities available	*Inadequate facilities available*
Quality of life expected	Quality of life expected
Age	Age
Compliance (e.g. psychosis)	Compliance (e.g. psychosis)
	Vascular status
	Ability to self dialyse
	— home/satellite
	Likelihood of transplantation
	— live donor source
	— cadaver donor source

primarily a selection onto dialysis. Once accepted for dialysis, choices must be made regarding type of dialysis, the timing of transplantation and source of kidney donor. Even where adequate facilities exist to dialyse allcomers, refusal of treatment is sometimes in the best overall interest of the patient. Specific factors influencing the selection procedure are summarised in Table 1. As hospital dialysis space is frequently the major restriction, patients who can be seen as only transiently requiring dialysis in hospital may be favoured.

Factors applying when dialysis availability is unrestricted

Expected quality of life

The predicted quality of life on the renal replacement programme is the overriding consideration in any medically based decision to refuse acceptance onto a programme. All factors, physical and mental affect the quality of life achievable by an individual. Assessment is sometimes easy. The 78 year old widow immobilised by a stroke and dependent on nursing support for existence would be accepted onto very few programmes and in fact may not even be referred to a nephrologist despite advanced renal failure. Conversely assessment may be very difficult as in the case of a 55 year old single epileptic man with no family support with a record of non-compliance, alcoholism and depression. Experience has shown such patients tend to do poorly but this is not wholly predictable. The reasonable decision is to commence a trial of dialysis and to assess progress. It is not easy to withraw therapy but it can be done.

The quality of life achieved on dialysis was recently assessed in a large multi-centre study in the USA. Physical activity and employment status were surveyed. Only 60% of non-diabetic patients and 23% of diabetic patients were capable of doing more than caring for themselves. Data, such as these can be interpreted variously but for some the conclusion will be that the quality of life achieved cannot justify the stress for the patient and the cost for the community (6).

Age

As in most medical conditions the risk of treatment by dialysis or transplantation rises with increasing age. This has been clearly shown by the European and Australian Registries (3, 7) (Table 2). The marked difference in survival over the age of 60 has led to a general reluctance to accept patients of this age for transplantation. It is widely believed, however, that it is the apparent age of the patient and not the calendar age which should be the real discriminant. In practice 25% of patients aged 60-69 presenting to Australian units in 1975-78 were transplanted by the end of 1979 compared to 65% of the 30-39 year age group.

There is no absolute age limit to acceptance onto a dialysis programme. The expected quality of life and apparent age should weigh more heavily than the calendar age though in most countries it is rare for patients over 70 years to be accepted. Recently in countries with no limit to available facilities (e.g. USA) there has been a tendency to offer dialysis to all comers including the bedridden aged. This is unlikely to be seen in the long term as justifiable utilisation of the health dollar and can be criticised in human terms as well. Dialysis should not differ from other areas in medicine in this regard. A serious potential danger is that if physicians are not seen to be using appropriate discretion in treatment decisions, funds may be reduced arbitrarily and young patients who are otherwise medically fit may then have to be denied active treatment.

Age, therefore, has already been shown to be a major discriminant of success in both dialysis and transplantation. It may be used either as absolute indication of non-acceptability for the 60-70$^+$ yr group or as a means of selection in the presence of restricted facilities.

Compliance

Occasionally patients who are manifestly psychotic or have a past history of psychosis present with chronic renal failure. They pose a difficult problem and are often deemed unsuitable for either dialysis or transplantation. The over-riding consideration is whether they will comply with the restrictions and therapies needed for successful dialysis treatment and transplantation. Endogenous depression (particularly if previously severe enough to necessitate hospitalisation) is in our experience an indication of a likely poor outcome especially should stresses occur during treatment. The use of steroid drugs post-transplantation may also accentuate an otherwise compensated or latent psychosis and this must be considered before commitment to transplantation.

Additional factors applying when dialysis availability is inadequate

Vascular status

Atherosclerosis with the occlusion of major arteries poses technical difficulties for both haemodialysis and transplantation. Atherosclerosis is common in patients (particularly diabetics) presenting for treatment who also may have a past history of myocardial infarction or stroke (8). It is seldom necessary to refuse treatment to a patient on vascular grounds alone unless organ damage secondary to ischaemia is severe and incapacitating. Vascular access for haemodialysis can almost always be obtained. If necessary a graft (e.g. umbilical vein) can be performed from a large artery to a large vein. In the

Table 2. Patient survival, effect of age at time of acceptance.

Age	Percent survival at 5 years	
	Transplant	Dialysis
20-29	92	93
40-49	80	86
60-69	49	79

Data from A. & N.Z. Dialysis and Transplantation Registry 1975-1978.

difficult case, peritoneal dialysis provides a plausible alternative.

Atheroma of the pelvic vessels may provide difficulties to the transplant surgeon, but it is usually possible to establish blood flow even if operative disobliteration of the iliac vessels prior to transplant insertion is necessary.

With restricted facilities established vascular disease at presentation may well be used as a discriminating factor. Atherosclerotic complications are the major cause of death on a renal replacement programme particularly with dialysis (3). However, it is common experience that patients, even with gross atheroma at multiple sites, may continue satisfactorily on dialysis for up to 10 years with no new major vascular events. Accordingly, refusal for the individual patient with atheroma is fraught with possible injustice.

Ability to self dialyse
In the face of restricted facilities the ability to self dialyse makes dialysis at home or in a non-hospital satellite (limited care) unit possible. The two advantages of this are the lower cost (estimated at 1/3 to 1/2 the cost of hospital dialysis) and the avoidance of overcrowding in the hospital unit which will always have a finite limit of space (9).

The percentage of patients capable of home dialysis is at least 50% (7) and up to an additional 20 to 30% can cope with limited assistance in a satellite centre. This leaves only a small number of patients dependent long term on a hospital unit. Although hospital units can theoretically be run on a low staff: patient ratio and practice self care, it is virtually impossible to do so. With the easy availability of doctors, the mixture of sick and well patients and the accummulated hard core of dependent patients all mitigating against self-care, those patients who can self dialyse feel penalised for doing so and motivation to continue soon diminishes.

In the Australian experience the ability and motivation to home dialyse is found more commonly in the educated and upper income groups. This relates to suitable space at home and the availability of a partner who has the time to assist in the procedure. An important aspect of the success of Australian home dialysis has been the provision by the Government of all hardware and the disposables free of charge to all patients, moreover no renal physician has been dependent on dialysis fees for his basic income. Accordingly, both patients and physicians have not had any financial barrier to contend with in deciding whether to do dialysis at home.

The geographical isolation of country patients has been another factor encouraging a number of patients to dialyse at home. When faced with the alternative of moving house and job to a major city the majority of patients find the motivation to proceed with home dialysis.

The willingness or ability to self dialyse then is an important factor in selection of patients onto restricted programmes. In Australia, it appears that up to 80% of all patients (if offered the right circumstances i.e. the option of home or satellite dialysis) can self dialyse. This percentage might be even higher when the full impact of continuous ambulatory peritoneal dialysis (CAPD) with its simplicity is felt (see Chapters 21, 22 and 23). Accordingly this criterion alone will not frequently result in refusal.

Likelihood of transplantation
Apart from non-hospital dialysis or death, transplantation offers the only exit from hospital dialysis. Greater experience has increased our ability to assess the likelihood of transplantation candidacy. The Australian Registry has recently examined this and Table 3 summarises the findings. Some of the restrictions are absolute, e.g. a recent diagnosis of malignancy, but others are relative, e.g. age. In a competitive situation even the relative contra-indications may be used as a reason for refusal. Patients with a high degree of sensitisation to HLA are extremely difficult to transplant successfully and may become effectively untransplantable. This impediment is not always apparent prior to starting dialysis and may in fact be induced whilst on dialysis consequent upon blood transfusion. With the present wide acceptance of deliberate transfusion as a means of increasing graft success rates, it is likely that increasing numbers of highly sensitised patients which cannot be transplanted will accummulate and will block available dialysis facilities.

Table 3. Likelihood of cadaver transplantation.

		Percent
No restriction		39
Restriction		
Serological		18
Medical		13
— coronary artery dis.	5	
— lung disease	5	
— malignancy	3	
— technical	3	
Age deemed too high		19
Patient disinclination		11

Data from A. & N.Z. Dialysis and Transplant Registry (7).

The waiting time for a transplant depends on the pool size and the cadaver donor procurement rate. In Australia the median wait for a first cadaver graft had increased from 6 months in 1973 to 8 months in 1979, which is a relatively short wait by world standards (10). In this setting with cadaver transplantation being actively promoted, 85% of patients in one series were maintained on a functioning graft 4 years from commencement on the programme (1).

There is hope that in the future we can select from a given group of medically fit patients, those with a high chance of graft success. At the moment some advantage is gained by good matching at the HLA, A, B and DR loci. The future may see refinements to matching techniques and better means of early testing of intrinsic immune reactivity (e.g. by DNCB reaction). As the case is strong to use the scarce resource of cadaver kidneys in those patients with a higher chance of success it is possible that an early accurate assessment of the likelihood of graft success could be made and thus an effective selection barrier for transplantation be created.

Regional, national and international swapping schemes already exist in order to achieve better tissue matching. The future is likely to see even more kidneys exchanged as the benefit of matching (particularly on the DR locus) becomes more apparent and as storage techniques are improved and simplified.

In the selection of patients to maximise graft success rates due regard must be paid to the risk run by the patient. Mortality rates have declined in recent years but are still too high. It is in this area that great discretion and judgement is needed. The temptation to 'give it a go' in the hope that a successful graft will cure underlying problems is not compatible with a maximum graft success rate. Similarly the pressure to use a kidney locally 'to build up the numbers' or because 'it is ours as we procured it' often means that the kidney is not offered to the best recipient and consequently the overall graft success rate will suffer.

The availability of a live related donor over-rides these considerations. This was a major factor determining acceptance for any treatment in USA a decade ago. In Australia and Europe, 11 and 12% respectively of all transplants in 1979 were from a living related source. It is believed unlikely that this percentage can rise substantially if one haplotype matching or better is demanded, for at least in Australia determined efforts have already been made to maximise the live donor rate.

Factors mitigating against a successful transplant include a previous history of early graft rejection and the diagnosis 'malignant' focal glomerulosclerosis as the original cause of kidney failure. Focal glomerulosclerosis frequently recurs in a graft and may cause early graft failure (7). In both these situations the reduced chance of graft success provides a relative contraindication to future grafting.

If transplant likelihood is assessed as low or negative, long term dialysis becomes the only available therapy and in this situation the pressure on a patient to dialyse in a non-hospital based setting is likely to be even more intense.

Practical problems related to selection

The Right to Reject

A philosophy has developed in some areas that dialysis physicians have no 'right' to reject any patient asking for dialysis. The situation surely should be not different with dialysis than it is with other areas of medical therapy. Physicians do have the right and indeed the responsibility to offer therapy only when it is indicated and when in their judgement it is in the best interests of the patient (11). Cancer surgery is not offered to patients with wide spread malignancy. Dialysis therapy should not be offered to patients in whom therapy will prolong misery and suffering and indeed may create extra burden. Failure to exhibit reasonable responsibility in these matters will surely in the long run adversely affect the attitude of the community to the provision of dialysis facilities. Either guidelines will be set up for physicians to follow or more likely there will be an overall financial cut-back which will force dialysis physicians to make these judgements.

'Who makes te decision?'

The responsibility for refusal rests on the shoulders of the caring physician. This responsibility may be delegated to others (e.g. to a special advisory committee) but this seldom happens presently. When definite medical contra-indications to acceptance onto dialysis exist, e.g. 75 year old with wide spread cancer, this decision must be communicated and explained in a conventional manner. If the decision is because of lack of dialysis facilities for a medically suitable person then this should be clearly explained to all involved including the hospital administration. If the refusal is based on a mixture of medical and social reasons then the whole caring team should be consulted, a second opinion sought if necessary, and the patient and his family should be involved in the decision making process. The final decision should be seen to rest with the physician. If the relatives are made to feel it was their decision it is difficult to avoid later feelings of guilt and anxiety.

Patient involvement in decisions

The attitudes of previous generations which regarded medical decisions as 'law' and recognised little need or right for the patient to be involved in any decisions have largely been replaced. 'Consumerism' first came to USA but is now being felt in all countries to a variable degree. There is now no question that patients should always be involved in making decisions particularly those of a negative sort which may involve their own life and death. It is up to the medical profession to accommodate itself to this approach.

While an occasional patient refuses to accept the idea of treatment by dialysis or transplantation, it is remarkable how few patients maintain the stance of refusing treatment when the chips are finally down. Quite frequently the 'not for me' attitude will be exhibited for many months. This form of denial is effective in allowing a temporary escape from the reality of impending treatment and should not be mistaken by the caring team as a definitive decision. Only rarely in our experience will the refusal be persistent and if it is those patients are usually so severely depressed that their mental state would preclude successful treatment even if they were accepted.

It is rare, as noted above, for the decision not to proceed with active therapy to be a point of disagreement between the patient or his relatives and the doctor. If a negative decision is made due to restricted facilities in a medically suitable candidate, then the doctor must make this clear and in doing so remove himself from any position of blame for the situation. If disagreement about medical suitability does arise, then second opinions should be sought. If doubt continues, a trial of therapy would usually be commenced with a definite time scale announced. To deny dialysis therapy on medical grounds where reasonable doubt exists is not different to denying other types of medical care. In such a process a doctor may well place himself in legal jeopardy.

The Australian experience for the last decade where there has been no appreciable restriction on dialysis facilities has been that in the small number of cases justifying refusal on medical grounds the relatives and patient usually understood the medical logic and agreed with the suggested course of action.

The option of no active treatment
In some patients a trial of dialysis will have been undertaken and after some time has elapsed it will be evident that continuation of dialysis is not in the patient's best interest. An example of this may be the patient with diffuse vascular disease of his legs who is having severe rest pain necessitating narcotic analgesia and who is so confused with cerebro-vascular disease that his life is vegetative. Similarly when a transplant has failed (usually after some years of function) it may be deemed unwise by both patient and doctor for dialysis to be reinstituted. In these situations involving cessation of therapy, it is crucial for the team to be aware of the decision and for any dissenting views to be discussed and resolved. The full support and understanding of the caring team is needed. It takes only one dissenting voice to create in the relatives a great amount of anxiety and doubt with later guilt feelings.

Death from uraemia usually involves increasing confusion and a gradual lapse into unconsciousness. From this point of view uraemia is not the worst way to die and usually involves no pain. It is important to assiduously avoid fluid overload with the consequent suffering from pulmonary oedema.

Ideal versus the practical
As in most areas of medicine the final decision will be a compromise of the ideal and the practical. For example it may be necessary to perform peritoneal dialysis as a holding manoeuvre until the blood access develops to a usable stage. It may be necessary to use hospital dialysis for some weeks waiting for a place in the home training programme. One area where experience has taught us not to compromise is that of doing transplantation to get 'out of trouble'. Transplantation results will only be good if patients are optimally fit at the time of transplantation and all factors are operating in their favour. To rush into a transplant because of transient difficulties with dialysis brings with it a lower transplant success rate and this can jeopardise the patient's safety and bring the transplant programme into disrepute. It is extraordinarily seldom for a dialysis patient in a competent dialysis programme to genuinely need an urgent transplant. Further sites for access are always available and perhaps apart from dialysis dementia or neuropathy all problems on dialysis may be solved by more and better dialysis and time. Thus transplanting out of trouble should be a rare event and arguably should not be allowed to occur.

Individual versus the Group
In the complex matter of caring for chronic renal failure patients one must constantly bear in mind the very visible and potential long lasting results of any decisions. The wrong decision will easily put fuel on the fire of those mounting a case against widespread availability of dialysis and it is easy to do the overall group a grave disadvantage. It is our belief that the majority of patients are advantaged both in terms of numbers, treatment and the quality of life obtained with the organisation of a well integrated programme of dialysis and transplantation. Very few patients will have to be refused from such a programme which if based on active cadaver transplantation will provide the best and cheapest result for most people. In this situation it may be necessary to restrict numbers of patients using permanent hospital dialysis on the grounds that such space is finite and blocking it long term must reduce the through-put. This problem becomes increasingly uncommon as adequate satellite facilities with limited staffing arrangements, and consequently operating on a low cost basis, are made available.

Local versus regional policies
It is easy for various hospitals within a city or region to develop different beliefs and philosophies regarding suitability of patients for dialysis. In this situation patients may be referred or find their own way to other units if they are displeased with the decisions of the first. Whilst recognising the desirability of competition in order to avoid a monopoly situation it is, however, meaningless if such policies cannot be coordinated on a regional basis. Otherwise all that happens is that one hospital puts more patients on dialysis than the other. It, therefore, seems highly desirable for hospitals within a region to resolve policy differences and apply them uniformly. The same can be argued at a national level for the mobile populations in America, Europe and Australia soon find their way to the point of least resistance if that is necessary for their perceived advantage.

INTEGRATION OF DIALYSIS AND TRANSPLANTATION

Integration of dialysis and transplant programmes was first reported in 1970 (8) and was put into practice in many areas soon thereafter (1, 2). By integration it is meant that the two treatments, dialysis and transplantation, are regarded as complementary and not competitive, with patients progressing from one treatment to the other and back as medically indicated from time to time.

For integration to be applied successfully it is necessary to have both modalities of treatment readily available and for the caring physician to feel a commitment to both treatments. This occurs most easily when the dialysis physician is also involved in the transplant programme. If the transplant programme is run by a surgical team and nephrology (dialysis) physicians are excluded from any meaningful involvement, barriers develop and attitudes are created against transplantation. This can lead to a dichotomy – the path which patients follow being determined by the initial referral and having nothing necessarily to do with the real needs of the patient. This division is accentuated if some patients are returned to the dialysis physician's care after graft failure in a weakened wasted condition (as is sometimes difficult to avoid) and all the patients grafted successfully are never seen again, except by the surgical team (12).

In all Australian cities integrated programmes exist and in most of these the nephrologist is in effective control of both treatments. This does not necessarily impinge on or weaken the traditional surgical role and responsibility. It is a combined team effort with various degrees of involvement for physicians and surgeons. The crucial point is that the physician is not excluded from significant interaction with the transplant team. This makes it easier for the physician to maintain a positive attitude regarding transplantation and to reflect this to his patients.

One essential feature in running a full scale integrated programme is to have available all modalities and sufficient locations of dialysis so that the therapeutic regimen can be tailored for each patient. This allows the best preparation for transplantation. The transplant programme must have a reasonable availability of cadaver kidneys; if the average wait for a cadaver transplant is 5 years it can hardly be said that the programme is integrated.

The integrated approach provides flexibility in management and should allow both therapies to be practiced successfully to the benefit of the patients. Transplantation can be offered when the patient is ready and fit and the return to dialysis can occur at an optimal time if the graft is failing. To time these events to the patient's greatest advantage requires all options to be freely available and requires the right judgements to be made. The flexibility allows either medical or social pressures to be accommodated. In Australia the decision by a patient to stay on dialysis and to refuse transplantation would usually bring with it firm pressure to dialyse out of hospital, usually at home.

It can be seen that the integrated approach allows better tailoring of the ideal programme for the individual but it also has advantage for the community. As integration tends to maximise the rate of transplantation (through increased motivation of physicians and the patients) and as the cost of transplantation is significantly lower than dialysis, there accrues a large cost benefit. Another advantage is the appreciable increase in rehabilitation of patients post-transplant with the consequent increase in positive contribution to society.

The cadaver donor procurement rate is also affected by an integrated approach. If a transplant programme is well supported by all nephrologists and is successful, non-renal physicians and surgeons in charge of potential donors are much more likely to initiate appropriate action than if the reverse is true. This will lead to an increased referral of donors and a consequent improvement in the supply of kidneys.

Whilst integration is most easily achieved within one institution there is no reason why an integrated programme cannot involve several dialysis units feeding one transplant unit. In this situation good communications are paramount with regular contact occurring with all physicians so that there is a definite feeling of involvement. The essential point is that the dialysis physician must have a meaningful participation in the transplant programme.

Patients must have an explanation of this integration of therapies and will usually find it plausible and reassuring. This is particularly so if continuity of care occurs and the patient is not made to feel totally passive. With an integrated programme the decisions can be taken with only one aim in mind: what is the best for the individual patient.

In summary an integrated approach to dialysis and transplantation allows patients assess to the treatment option which is best for them at any point in time. It prevents the isolation of dialysis from transplantation which if it exists may adversely affect both areas with consequent reduction in the quality of patient care. Integration by maximising transplantation, also allows a greater number of patients to be treated at a lower and more acceptable cost to the community.

QUALITY OF LIFE

The quality of life of the chronic dialysis patients is reviewed elsewhere in this book (see Chapter 45) but it is appropriate at this point to make mention of it as it effects the selection of patients and organisation of a combined programme of dialysis and transplantation. Brief mention was made above, of quality of life as an issue which should be considered in the selection of all patients.

Experience through the years has revealed the remarkable adaptability of patients to their various burdens and difficulties. The instinct for survival is strong in most people and life styles, ambitions and ideas are all capable of great modifications given sufficient stress. Frequently, patients will say they do not want to continue with treatment and life unless 'life can be lived to the fullest'. Yet only a few months later they will accept a life style which has many restrictions. When dialysis facilities have been available without restriction there has been a tendency for physicians to avoid denying therapy and to leave such decisions to patients themselves. This may result in the continuation of dialysis in situations where, by any criteria, life can only be said to be miserable for the patient and all those around him. The instinct for survival is so strong that seldom will a patient or his family initiate what amounts to public suicide or the voluntary suggestion of treatment withdrawal. Here, the dialysis physician should exhibit his responsibility and the right to intervene. As noted above the patient and family will seldom disagree with decisions made by an experienced dialysis physician and which are explained fully to them. There can come a point where continuation of dialysis is unwarranted and the dialysis physician's identification of this point and his assistance to the family at this time is usually seen as being positive. In between the two ends of the spectrum there is a grey zone and here much difficulty may ensue. A trial of dialysis, with given goals of accomplishment and time, is useful in these situations and is preferable to a dogmatic negative decision being taken on uncertain grounds.

Objective assessment of the quality of life is extraordinarily difficult and superficial questionnaires particularly involving assessments made by others may be quite misleading. Despite these difficulties, the Australia and New Zealand Registry has, for some years, asked physicians to rank rehabilitation of all patients on dialysis and transplantation. The pattern through the last decade has been a consistent one and is shown below.

Table 4. Rehabilitation of patients on dialysis and transplantation.

	On dialysis Percent	With functioning transplant Percent
Fulltime work	43	73
Part time work	17	10
Able to work but unemployed	4	2
Able to work but retired (>60 yrs)	8	3
Total able to work	72	88
Unwilling to work	8	3
Medically unfit to work	17	9
Dialysis schedule precludes work	3	—
Total unable or unwilling	28	12

Assessment of 1254 dialysis patients and 1224 patients with a functioning transplant at 31 October 1979 from A. & N.Z. Dialysis and Transplant Registry (7).

This assessment has been criticised for being 'work orientated'. Nevertheless it continues to provide health administrators, politicians and the community with a tangible measure as to the success of the programmes. The data shown in Table 4 are similar to the European data (3). A substantially better rehabilitation rate in patients with a functioning transplant (88% classified able to work) is achieved compared to patients on dialysis (72% classified able to work). Almost twice as many on dialysis are classified medically unfit to work. These figures do not take account of the difference in mean ages between the groups and as with all figures comparing dialysis and transplantation suffer from the bias which usually results in the transplantation of the fitter patients away from dialysis. Despite these precautions the data confirm the strong clinical impression that the general degree of rehabilitation post-transplant tends to exceed that on dialysis. This degree of rehabilitation is highly desirable to justify the large expenditure of public money on renal replacement programmes. If the situation in USA is accurately reflected in the multicentre study of Gutman (6) many may conclude that an adjustment of fund allocation must be made or that guidelines for acceptance onto dialysis should be established.

Both the European and Australian data show a better rehabilitation rate for home dialysis compared to hospital dialysis, but to a degree this reflects the younger and fitter patient population dialysed at home. In the European experience there is very little difference between the home dialysis patient potential for employment and that of transplanted patients.

It must be remembered that our best available measures of the quality of life at this time are subjective. It is therefore desirable to use great caution in making any judgements on this basis. Predicting adjustment to dialysis and quality of life obtainable is fraught with difficulty. Many patients who create initial concern to the caring team about their ability to cope and to achieve a reasonable quality of life on dialysis survive happily and with a positive life many years later. While there is no 'correct' figure, an appropriate patient rejection rate for the 1980's, in a situation where dialysis facilities are not restricted, should be somewhere between 1 and 10%. If any unit is refusing to accept more than 10% of patients offered to it for dialysis, then the guidelines being used should be carefully reassessed. Confirmation that one is making right judgements may come from having the occasional failure. If all patients started on dialysis do well, then it seems likely that some patients are being refused unnecessarily. The occasional failure and necessity to withdraw therapy will show that judgement (while not perfect) is erring on the preferred side giving patients the benefit of the doubt.

REFERENCES

1. Mathew TH, Marshall VC, Vikraman P, Hill AVL, Johnson W, McOmish D, Morris PJ, Kincaid-Smith P: Integrated programme of dialysis and renal transplantation. *Lancet* 2:137, 1975
2. Clunie GJA, Hartley LCJ, Ribush NT, Emmerson BT, Morgan TO: An integrated service for the treatment of irreversible renal failure *Med J Aust* 2:403, 1971
3. Brynger H, Brunner FP, Chantler C, Donckerwolcke RA, Jacobs C, Kramer P, Selwood NH, Wing AJ, Blake PH: Combined Report on Regular Dialysis and Transplantation in Europe, X, 1979. *Proc Eur Dial Transpl Ass* 17:2, 1980
4. Katz AH, Proctor DM: Social psychological characteristics of patients receiving hemodialysis in treatment for chronic renal failure. *Kidney Disease Control Program.* Public Health Service Publication U.S.A. July 1969
5. Abrams HS: Psychiatry and prolongation of life. *Medical, Moral and Legal Concerns,* Proc Conf on Energy, edited by Siemsen AW, Greifer I, Honolulu HI, St. Francis Hospital, 1976
6. Gutman TA, Stead WW, Robinson RR: Physical activity and employment status of patients on maintenance dialysis. *New Engl J Med* 304:309, 1981
7. Disney APS, Correll R: Report of the Australia and New Zealand Combined Dialysis and Transplant Registry. *Med J Aust* 1:117, 1981
8. Lindner A, Charra B, Sherrard DJ, Scribner BH: Accelerated atherosclerosis in prolonged maintenance dialysis. *New Engl J Med* 290:697, 1974
9. Mahony J: Cost analysis of dialysis alternatives. In *Peritoneal dialysis,* edited by Atkins RC, Thomson NM, Farrell PC, Churchill-Livingstone, Edinburgh, London, 1981, p 418
10. *Third Annual Report of the Australia and New Zealand Dialysis and Transplant Registry.* Edited by Disney APS, Adelaide, SA, The Queen Elizabeth Hospital, 1980, p 24
11. Inglefinger RJ: Arrogance. *New Engl J Med* 303:1507, 1980
12. De Palma J: Guest Editorial, *Dial Transpl* 4 (nr 5):6, 1975

45

THE QUALITY OF LIFE OF THE CHRONIC DIALYSIS PATIENT

H. EARL GINN and PAUL E. TESCHAN

'For mere living is not a good, but living well. Accordingly, the wise man will live as long as he ought, not as long as he can... He always reflects concerning the quality, and not the quantity, of his life. As soon as there are many events in his life that give him trouble and disturb his mind, he sets himself free... It is not a question of dying earlier or later, but of dying well or ill. And dying well means escape from the danger of living ill.'

Seneca, *'On Suicide'* (1)

Introduction	837	The psychosocial dimension	840
Malfunction of the brain and nerves in uremia	838	Sexual dysfunction	841
The psychological dimension	838	Obstacles to rehabilitation	842
Psychological reaction to dialysis	838	Conclusion	842
Management of the medical regimen	839	References	842

INTRODUCTION

In the course of everyday living, people become ill and society maintains a prescribed set of expectations dealing with the person as a patient. It is assumed that the patient will be exempt from normal social obligations and from the responsibility of his own state, that he will be somewhat helpless and dependent on others, and finally, that he will either get better and be cured or get worse and die. Many life-extending technological advances in modern medicine have created a departure from this classical 'image of the ill' and, simultaneously, have introduced complex personal stresses for patients as well as ethical, moral, legal, theological, social and financial questions for health professionals and society.

During the course of his illness, the patient with chronic renal disease usually experiences at least one crisis episode that requires his admission to a hospital for acute care. Most often such an episode occurs when his kidney function fails to the extent that it will no longer sustain life. At this point, he is comfortably in compliance with society's expectations and is accepted as free from normal functioning. The immediate questions are: should he be accepted for long term treatment of terminal renal disease, and, if so, who should pay for it? To some extent the sick person is subjected to medical, psychological, social and financial scrutiny. From a medical standpoint we wish to determine whether there exist other imminently lethal complications or catastrophic debilities. Will our treating this particular person permit him to maintain the dignity of his individuality? The general public, certainly the patient, expects of us a high degree of care and caution, and in no sense does he wish to be used for purposes other than those of benefit to him.

The psychological and social queries are concerned with an overview as to whether or not the patient and his family can cope with the many aspects of a rather complicated and costly therapeutic regimen and what measures might be brought to bear to lessen this burden. That financial considerations should even enter our decisions of whether or not to treat patients with end-stage kidney disease disturbs our idealistic sentiments. Unlike the acutely ill, who either get worse and die or get properly treated and cured, these patients confront the prospect that they must cooperate continuously, for an indefinite time, with treatment that is costly in terms of time, thought, effort (their own and others) and money. Tragically, some patients conclude that their only real options are death or a heavily burdened and precarious life.

This chapter will consider the consequences of renal failure in the patients' daily living, specifically when treated by intermittent dialysis. The patients' struggles to cope with their disease, with our therapeutic regimen and technology, changes in self image and expectations for the future and society's image of them must evoke in us a sense of awe and admiration as well as our empathy, our compassion, our resolve to make the treatment more effective and less burdensome and our affirmation of the further options for quality of life which the treatment makes possible.

To attempt an assessment of the quality of these people's lives we must first understand the nature of the sickness, called uremia, that attends kidney failure. Most of the symptoms of uremia, especially those that impair the patients' clinical well-being and their effective personal and social functioning are mediated by the nervous system (2-6, reviewed in Chapter 37). They primarily reflect impairments in cognition, consciousness, neuromuscular function and in such control functions as the regulation of blood pressure and body temperature. They may be improved and controlled by dialysis treatment. Actually all of the body's organ systems are affected by failure of the kidneys, but few of those other abnormalities produce symptoms which impede the daily living of most patients or symptoms that are much affected by dialysis treatment.

For patients with renal failure the relief of symptoms and chemical restoration by dialysis are necessary, but by no means sufficient for satisfactory living. Even though we can, by competent medical care, including dialysis, restore the chemical environment of the brain and other body cells virtually to normal, at least as indicated by conventional chemical measurements, and also can demonstrate objectively that the nervous system's function is normal, a significant number of patients do not yet exhibit normal activity in daily living. Hence, in addition to 'medical' concerns for the proper function of patients' body machinery we must consider and contribute to at least two further ingredients in patients' adaptation to life with renal failure and dialysis, namely what we will call the psychological and the psychosocial dimensions. The attitude of health care professionals toward patients' future prospects impacts on both of these domains.

MALFUNCTION OF THE BRAIN AND NERVES IN UREMIA

It is useful to begin by considering the major, disabling symptoms of uremia. A characteristic of kidney failure is that it usually grows more severe as time progresses, more rapidly in some patients than in others. Patients' physicians, friends and family will notice this trend as the characteristic symptoms and impaired functions of uremia appear and disappear, wax and wane, while they gradually progress in a lengthening and broadening array (2-6). These symptoms include a sense of sluggishness, easy fatigue on exertion, insomnia and daytime drowsiness, itching, decreased appetite, impaired ability to focus attention or to perform mental arithmetic or to express ideas in more than simple language, erratic memory, slurred speech, vague headaches, waning sexual interest and potentia, restlessness, emotional irritability and withdrawal, nausea, vomiting, lowered body temperature and sensations of coldness; muscle twitching, muscle jerks and cramps, 'restless legs', 'burning feet', hiccoughs, flapping tremor of the palm and fingers held in extension, paranoid and compulsive personality changes; bizarre behavior, anxiety, disorientation, confusion, hallucinations, muttering and mumbling speech, neck stiffness resembling meningitis, inability to speak, deafness, jerking eye movements, numbness of extremities, dizziness, lurching and stumbling in attempts to walk, and variable paralyses. Unless competent and timely treatment intervenes at some point in this sequence, torpor (with occasional episodes of alertness), coma and convulsions will occur, the terminal events before the patient dies. Indeed, that was the story of every patient with advanced chronic renal failure prior to 1960 and the modern era of maintenance dialysis and renal transplantation. Clearly these symptoms characterize and define the clinical uremic syndrome and reflect disordered function of the nervous system. They are also reversed and controlled by dialysis and transplantation and are recognized clinical indications for dialysis (5-11).

THE PSYCHOLOGICAL DIMENSION

In early studies of changes in the behavior of uremic patients, psychologists and psychiatrists used conventional descriptors of mental illnesses (neuroses and psychoses) or of organic nervous disorders. For example, Baker and Knutsen (10) classified uremic patients' psychiatric manifestations as: 1) asthenic, 2) acute delirious, 3) schizophrenic, 4) depressed, 5) manic and 6) paranoid. Locke et al (11) described early functional symptoms which include lassitude, lethargy, disinterest and irritability, to be followed later by more 'organic' disorders of disorientation, confusion, misinterpretation of environmental stimuli and agitation. Other studies (12, 13) also emphasize cognitive and behavioral abnormalities reflecting activated defenses against the threat of serious illness. It is worth noting, however, that patients and families may notice these behavior changes before initial medical advice is sought and the diagnosis and its implications are revealed.

Psychological reaction to dialysis

When patients enter dialysis programs, they often traverse phases of adjustment as described especially by Abram (14) and by Reichsman and Levy (15). *Phase 1: The pretreatment period.* Patients display the symptoms listed above to a varying extent and uniformly experience grief over loss of health and threat of death. *Phase 2: The initiation of dialysis which produces a shift toward physiological equilibrium.* The patient 'returns from the dead', but with continued apathy, varying degrees of uremic drowsiness and torpor, euphoria (perhaps due to the 'reprieve'), increased anxiety, depression and helplessness which is often fostered by the hospital and environment. *Phase 3:* Convalescence, 'return to the living'. Patients may remain physically weak and anxious, with lingering headaches and vomiting, and experience loss of libido, depression and emerging dependent-independent responsibilities. *Phase 4: Struggle for normalcy.* Patients encounter problems of changed life styles within the constraints of diet, medications, dialysis and complications of treatment.

Once the patient who is maintained by dialysis reaches a stabilized medical status he usually has a clear and conscious awareness of marked improvement, physical and emotional. This is accompanied by a marked emergence of 'joie de vivre', confidence and hope (15). During this stage most patients temporarily accept their intense dependency upon the machine, the procedure, and the professional staff, with few if any expressions of displeasure. Psychological difficulty is created by the contradiction that the patient feels better but that he is not and probably cannot be cured. It is the concept of perpetual treatment without cure that induces conflict in the patient, since he is neither dying nor is he returned to society 'healed'.

The patient is sent out of the protected environment of the hospital wherein dependency and helplessness is the accepted, even fostered mode of behavior, into his once routine world with a handful of contradictory messages. He is told to lead a normal life but to be sure to take his medications on schedule and not to incorporate too much protein, salt, potassium or fluid into his diet. He is told to return to work but that he dare not miss any of the thrice weekly dialysis treatments. He is reminded continuously not to fixate on his illness, yet he is repeatedly made aware of his somewhat less than desirable sexual potency and a lingering lethargy that may seriously affect his ability to perform adequately at his job. The patient may become discouraged by what he perceives as impossible expectations by his family and professional staff members. Often well meaning but poorly guided medical personnel, spouses and (or) employers either underestimate his physical limitations and push him beyond his capabilities or they pamper him to a point that he is thoroughly convinced he can do nothing.

According to revised societal expectations, since the public is paying for a large part of the treatment costs, the patient with end-stage renal disease is not sick. Unless severely impaired he is expected to perform routine tasks, pick up his job where he left it at the time of hospitalization, and return to his home to resume his former obligations. For most patients, on the other hand, every aspect of life is altered by the dependence on dialysis that would preclude what society defines as a 'healthy' existence. It is this marginality between illness and health that is to a great extent responsible for the manifestations of inner turmoil that become visible to his family and associates.

In normal living, day-to-day stress is coped with by such adaptive or defensive devices as eating, the use of tobacco, tranquilizers and alcohol, by physical exercise, or in sexual outlets. The patient with chronic renal failure is denied many of these normal means of coping. The sexual outlet may be blunted by the loss of libido which accompanies chronic renal failure. Nevertheless, another manifestation of anxiety, a reaction to the stress of dialysis, is the occurrence of concealed or unconcealed masturbation (15) in many patients, mostly male but occasionally female as well, during the early months of dialysis. Unconcealed masturbation tends to be enormously disconcerting to dialysis personnel as well as to other in-center patients. It seems to be primarily related to the patient's anxiety toward the dialysis procedure, which they initially perceive as being a highly dangerous procedure that is completely out of their control. This manifestation of anxiety can be avoided or relieved by distracting the patient with games or, much better, by teaching patients the dialysis procedure and relinquishing control of the procedure to them, i.e., by self-care.

Psychopersonal problems are not limited to patients. Spouses' reactions to dialysis treatment in centers and at home include feelings of deprivation and hostility attributed to tensions over the enormous expenses, loss of opportunities for professional advancement, decreased sexual interest and ability, relatives' refusal to donate kidneys, emotional disturbances in one or more of the children, and patient's regressive, childlike, demanding and self-centered behavior (16). Wives of patients are often distressed by the change in dominance roles.

Reactions and behaviors on the part of dialysis unit staff may also influence patients significantly (17). For example, staff members may harbor guilt concerning decisions for selection and non-selection of patients. Differences of professional opinion concerning the medical regimen or choice and timing of dialysis or transplantation may add a further devastating dimension to the patients' experience (18).

In view of these important factors, DeNour (19) questioned whether patients on maintenance dialysis really achieved emotional equilibrium, by what mechanisms, and at what price. Patients regularly employed denial of illness, displacement, isolation of affect, projection, and reaction-formation. The cost of these defenses included superficial emotional relationships and limited interest in 'outside' people and events.

Management of the medical regimen

The medical problems encountered by dialysis patients are elaborated in this book and elsewhere. The basic medical regimen recommended for all dialysis patients is designed to avoid such medical problems and thereby to improve their quality of health and life. Treatment requires frequent dialysis to remove metabolic waste products and to control fluid volume, water soluble vitamins to replace those lost during dialysis, some dietary restrictions in protein, salt, potassium and fluid to reduce chemical electrolyte and volume loads, iron and sometimes androgens to relieve anemia, and phosphate binders to prevent secondary hyperparathyroidism. Yet one of the most frustrating aspects of patient care is that of non-compliance with the medical regimen. This refers to the person who appears for his dialysis either overloaded with fluid, even to the extent of congestive heart failure, or with plasma chemical concentrations significantly out of line, indicating some variety of dietary abuse or medication omissions. Why does a patient fail to comply? Is this simply denial of his illness? Is he acting out aggressive behavior or manifesting a suicidal tendency? Does he resolve, to some degree, his psychological stress by maintaining himself in the sick role? His behavior certainly attracts considerable attention from the medical and paramedical staff.

Regimen management may not seem a problem of much magnitude for it is either followed by obedient and sensible patients or ignored at their peril. Indeed, physicians and other health personnel tend to regard patients who do not carry out the prescribed regimens as not only foolish but as downright uncooperative. The issue may not be one of willfulness, stupidity, or even medical ignorance. The issue may be primarily that patients must continue to manage their daily existences under specific sets of financial and social conditions. Their chronic illness and the associated regimens only complicate – and are secondary to – their daily management problems. Indeed, medical regimens may present even more difficulties than the symptoms themselves. In that regard every regimen is actually or potentially on trial. Regimens are judged either on the basis of efficiency or legitimacy or both. Hence, they will be adopted and adhered to only under certain conditions, such as: 1) there is an initial or continuing trust in the physician or whoever else prescribes the regimen; 2) no rival supersedes the physician in his legitimating; 3) there is awareness that the regimen works either to control symptoms or the disease or both; 4) no distressing, frightening side effects appear; 5) the side effects are outweighed by symptom relief or by sufficient fear of the disease itself; 6) there is a relative noninterference with important daily activities, either of the patient or of people around him; 7) the regimen's perceived good effects are not outweighed by a negative impact on the patient's sense of identity (20).

Such evaluations are not just made once and for all but are made continually if not continuously. Patients, and to some extent their families, should learn the purpose of the regimen and how to administer it. Reinforcement and an awareness of the influence of the various aspects of the regimen on specific chemistries are necessary to assure continued adherence. Certain side effects, particularly constipation secondary to aluminum hydroxide gels must be forewarned, and prevented with stool softeners and laxatives.

Learning to operate the dialysis equipment is more complex and may initially provoke much anxiety. Extensively trained personnel who are dedicated to the procedure are essential for a successful self-care training program.

THE PSYCHOSOCIAL DIMENSION

We must learn more about and become more effective in the larger domain where the patient lives his life, his 'social, interactive existence': the domain of family, friends, employers, and if he is lucky, that of wise and skillful social workers, the domain which exists beyond the province of physicians and nurses concerned with patients' chemical and corporeal health and skilled in the supporting technologies of dialysis and psychiatry. Objective, 'outcome' measures in that domain are needed, as is continuous feedback to those concerned with patients' orientation, training and treatment and to those concerned with developing supportive family and community relationships.

The remarkable fact is that few efforts have been reported to assess patients' actual performance in the 'open systems of daily living', i.e., in practical life situations – without medical treatment, under medical management alone, during maintenance dialysis or following transplantation. A wide consensus concerning acceptable degrees of rehabilitation might be expected among staffs of dialysis and transplant centers after more than a decade of experience with maintenance dialysis, particularly since 'rehabilitation' is the announced object of the treatment. But most professional teams are more directly occupied with control of symptoms – patients' complaints – than with the other facets of patients' lives. Still, functional rehabilitation, perhaps the ultimate outcome measure of adequate management and dialysis, is apparently only indirectly and imperfectly related to the existence of the uremic symptoms: i.e., what a patient does may or may not relate precisely to the level of symptom-control which his treatment achieves for him.

Several studies bear on this point and should be reviewed. In their early experience with maintenance dialysis in patients with chronic renal failure, Scribner and colleagues defined rehabilitation as the patient's ability to perform his usual work comfortably. This criterion was met in 5 of the original 8 hospital-center-based patients (21), in 9 of 11 community center-based patients (22, 23), and in 73 of 175 patients cumulated through 1969 by the community dialysis center (24) including patients undertaking dialysis at home among the more recent patient groups. Recently, Scribner used an Activity Index, a scored daily inventory of time actually spent at each of several levels of activity or energy expenditure. This among other measures is employed to compare various dialysis treatment schedules. However, Gombos et al (25) in 1964 were the first to use performance evaluations according to a graded set of objective criteria in patients treated by dialysis. As shown in Table 1, each class (Able to Work, Unable to Work, Hospital or Home Care) was divided into groups representing further degrees of disability. In their series, all four patients progressed from class III to class I during the year's treatment, but dialyses at increasing frequency

Table 1. Evaluation criteria: effect of dialysis on performance.

Class	Group
I. Able to work; no special care	A. Normal B. Minor symptoms C. Signs and symptoms
II. Unable to work; lives at home; needs care	A. Self-care B. Occasional help with self-care C. Requires much help and frequent medical care
III. Hospital care or home-equivalent	A. Disabled; specialized care B. Severely disabled; hospitalized C. Moribund

were required to maintain class I status. A somewhat similar rehabilitation grading has also been adopted by the Registry of European Dialysis and Transplant Association. Use of such criteria is helpful in assessing both individuals and groups of patients.

In 1967-68, Friedman et al (26) studied the psychosocial adjustment of 20 patients to hospital-center-based maintenance dialysis before and during dialysis therapy. They recorded: 1) the number of days of hospitalization required for shunt care and other problems; 2) the time in hours allocated during each week to work, sleep, dialysis and non-specific free time; 3) annual income; and 4) 'social adjustment', which was graded 1 to 4 in three areas (a) compliance and acceptance of treatment regimen including the diet, (b) response and achievement in constructive activity, and (c) maturity and extent of interpersonal relationships. These assessments revealed significant problems: hospitalization averaged 28 days per year; dietary compliance was poor or erratic; and 6 of the 11 patients who were gainfully employed reported reduced income.

Goldberg et al (27) studied 25 patients undergoing center-based hemodialysis while awaiting renal transplantation. He investigated several elements of vocational adjustment: 1) work patterns, hours per week, job stability, occupational status, activities and responsibilities at work; 2) work values, vocational plans and interests and educational plans before and during dialysis treatment; and 3) home responsibilities and activities of daily living. The results were that even with expectations for transplantation, only 7 of the 25 patients remained productive: 6 of the 15 women as homemakers and one of the 10 men (none of the women) in gainful employment. Vocational interests, work values and educational plans were maintained, but vocational planning was deflected after dialysis was begun and vocational aspirations before dialysis did not predict for 'vocational adjustment' during dialysis.

A questionnaire-interview study of 102 patients treated by or trained for home dialysis at our Nashville dialysis clinic (28) yielded data that were not altogether encouraging. Full time employment for men dropped from 70 to 13%; for women from 38% to zero. Women tended to become homemakers (3.7 to 52%). Patients became 'medically retired': men from 9 to 48%, women from 2 to 22%. Unemployment trebled (5 to 15%). Differing levels of motivation were found to overcome the problem of finding jobs which fit the dialysis schedule. The 41 patients receiving dialysis at home succeeded better than those treated at the center: 54% of home dialysis patients were in full or part-time employment compared with 31% of center-based patients.

The European rehabilitation figures, dating from 1978 (29), were somewhat better: 37% of the male and 39% of the female hospital dialysis patients were in full employment, whereas 20% of the males and 31% of the females performed part time work. Among the home dialysis patients, 64% of the males and 66% of the females worked full time and 12% and 19% of these groups worked part time (See also Chapters 37/final section and 47). Although over half the patients reported only minor symptoms of their disease or none at all, an astonishing 12% of patients interviewed found life to be 'unacceptable and meaningless'.

Human beings are a vital composite of interrelating biological, psychological, and social forces. Anyone who has worked consistently with patients who have renal disease knows that it is often difficult to assess the level of actual physical discomfort and at times next to impossible to separate the physiological variables from the psychological and psychosocial ones. The human problem we confront in the chronic dialysis patient may be understood in the interrelated set: brain-mind-behavior, as illustrated by the following questions: is the patient with kidney failure apathetic and listless because his brain and muscles and viscera don't work and don't feel well, or is he apathetic and listless because he has little hope that anything he ventures in his environment – including his work – will result in a satisfying outcome? Are impotence and diminished frequency of sexual intercourse to be understood as disordered function of the autonomic nervous system, as a result of declining general health, as expressions of hopelessness and eroded self-esteem or as a result of the patient's perception that his relationship with his spouse has changed?

SEXUAL DYSFUNCTION

Several studies have indicated that sexual dysfunction is a common symptom for patients, especially males, with end-stage renal failure (30-41). The conclusions from the majority of these reports, however, were based on data provided by the patients through personal interviews and or questionnaires. Factors such as a patient's physical condition, presence of severe anemia, systemic disease or other organ dysfunction, frequency and adequacy of the dialytic therapy, treatment with medications that affect sexual function, or the effect of aging were not taken into consideration in most studies.

Recently, Procci and colleagues (42) reported results on patients wherein conditions interfering with potency, such as diabetes mellitus or treatment with medications that affect sexual function were excluded. Dialytic therapy consisted of three dialyses of five hours each per week. They also evaluated the role of chronic illness, age, and depression in the sexual dysfunction experienced by these patients. Nocturnal penile tumescence (NPT) and frequency of intercourse were indices of sexual potency. Results demonstrated that about half of the patients with renal failure had erectile dysfunction and reported a significant decline in the frequency of intercourse. On the other hand, some of their dialysis patients between 18 and 39 years of age reported a frequency of intercourse of 20 times per month. Patients with other chronic disease but normal renal function did not report a significant decline in frequency of intercourse, and only a few complained of erectile difficulty. The incidence of mild and major depression in their patients with renal failure was 43%, with 16% having major depression and 27% a mild depression. There were, however, no significant differences in complaints of erectile difficulty or the frequency of intercourse among depressed and non-depressed patients. Similarly, the presence or absence of depression was not associated with differences in the frequency of sexual intercourse in patients with other chronic illness. Almost half of their patients with uremia had abnormally low NPT, indicating that organic causes may be responsible for their sexual dysfunction. There was a significant and direct correlation between NPT and frequency of intercourse ($r = 0.68$, $P<0.01$).

The personal view of Oberley (43) who is both a dialysis patient and physician is that some of the uremic toxins may reduce sex drive in the male after a prolonged period between dialyses, and certainly the fatigue associated with a lowered hematocrit will have an occasional effect on the libido.

For dialysis patients, who do not have systemic disease or other organ dysfunction and who do not require medications which cause impotency, sexual dysfunction is not an invariable consequence. Despite physical and psychological limitations, many dialysis patients can have relatively normal sex lives. To some extent, the presence or absence of sexual dysfunction may prove to be an indicator of adequacy of dialysis.

OBSTACLES TO REHABILITATION

Our treatment in the medical sphere including dialysis and transplatation serves to create a favorable chemical environment for the functioning cells of the nervous system and the rest of the patient's body. Available data suggest that analogous treatment in the psychosocial sphere is needed to create a similarly favorable environment for the functioning whole-organisms, the patients whom we serve. Some of the major obstacles to the progress and development which these ideas call for are:

Obstacle 1. The mistaken assumption that current methods of dialysis and transplantation, along with other medical and psychosocial management, are established, settled and accepted technics. The data herein reviewed, together with the fact that renal transplantation remains a relatively infrequent option, support just the opposite conclusion, i.e., that current practice can in no way be considered an established, settled or accepted format. The admixture of ignorance, burdens and risks is too great for that. However, the danger of prematurely accepting current technology is already evidenced in the US by reducing funding of the research needed to improve these methods further. Ironically that danger will grow because of the enormous prestige and pressure of billion-dollar financing for current treatment systems.

Obstacle 2. Our continuing reliance on subjective, narrative, anecdotal descriptions of the uremic sickness in patients, their reaction to dialysis, the effect of dialysis in their lives and their level of rehabilitation. Obviously a change to objective, quantitative measurement is essential. This is a platitude for any health professional who thinks in terms of quality assurance or for anyone at all who considers cost-benefit relationships.

Obstacle 3. The danger that some of the conventional, historical concepts and practices of 'vocational rehabilitation' will impede and impair comprehensive and intelligent assistance to patients with end-stage renal disease. Instead, vocational rehabilitation as a particular component of patients' total social behavior will depend upon the integrity and health of the entire set: behavior-mind-brain in the whole person.

Obstacle 4. The danger that many of us, drawn from various backgrounds, experience and training and with different current responsibilities, will fail to realize how truly complex and interrelated the patient's problems are. His disease, treatment, rehabilitation, and administrative and financial support should all be considered. The danger lies in the failure to recognize that no one's skill, profession or office is equipped to understand and to deal with all of the issues at stake.

CONCLUSION

So we are engaged in an enormous, exciting and anxious enterprise. Let us be reminded that the cause for the anxiety is real: in all of these complexities, the patients, whom we all seek to serve, can get hurt if any of us loses track of human and medical reality and makes a wrong move. On the other hand, with a concerted effort to obtain the information and to develop the methods which we now lack, and with well-orchestrated, cooperative action, our patients may indeed 'have life, and have it more abundantly' (44).

REFERENCES

1. *Seneca,* Epistulae Morales. 'On Suicide', in *Moral Problems in Medicine,* edited by Gorowitx S, Englewood Cliffs, Prentice-Hall, 1976
2. Tyler HR: Neurological disorders seen in the uremic patient. *Arch Intern Med* 126:781, 1970
3. Bright R: Cases and observations, illustrative of renal disease accompanied by the secretion of albuminous urine. *Guy's Hosp Rep* 1:338, 1836
4. Bradley SE: *The Pathologic Physiology of Uremia in Chronic Bright's Disease.* Springfield IL, Charles C Thomas, 1948
5. Schreiner GE: Mental and personality changes in the uremic syndrome. *Med Ann DC* 28:316, 1959
6. Schreiner GE, Maher JF: *Uremia: Biochemistry, Pathogenesis and Treatment.* Springfield IL, Charles C Thomas, 1961
7. Teschan PE: EEG and other neurophysiological abnormalities in uremia. *Kidney Int* 7 (suppl 2):S210. 1975
8. Ginn HE: Neurobehavioral dysfunction in uremia. *Kidney Int* 7 (suppl 2):S217, 1975
9. Ginn HE, Teschan PE: The nervous system in uremia. In: *Clinical Aspects of Uremia and Dialysis,* edited by Massry SG, Sellers AL, Springfield IL, Charles C Thomas, 1976
10. Baker AB, Knutson J: Psychiatric aspects of uremia. *Am J Psychiatry* 102:683, 1946
11. Locke S, Merrill JP, Tyler HR: Neurologic complications of acute uremia. *Arch Intern Med* 108:519, 1961
12. Abram HS: The psychiatrist, the treatment of CRF and the prolongation of life. II. *Am J Psychiatry* 126:157, 1969
13. Greenberg RP, Davis G, Massey R: The psychological eva-

luation of patients for a kidney transplant and hemodialysis program. *Am J Psychiatry* 130:274, 1973
14. Abram HS: The psychiatrist, the treatment of chronic renal failure and the prolongation of life. *Am J Psychiatry* 124:1351, 1968
15. Reichsman F, Levy NB: Problems in adaptation to maintenance hemodialysis – a four year study of 25 patients. *Arch Intern Med* 130:859, 1972
16. Shambaugh PW, Hampers CL, Bailey GL, Snyder D, Merrill JP: Hemodialysis in the home – emotional impact on the spouse. *Trans Am Soc Artif Intern Organs* 13:41, 1967
17. DeNour AK, Czaczkes JW: Emotional problems and reactions of the medical team in a chronic haemodialysis unit. *Lancet* 2:987, 1968
18. Calland C: Iatrogenic problems in end-stage renal failure. *N Engl J Med* 287:334, 1972
19. DeNour AK, Shaltiel J, Czaczkes JW: Emotional reactions of patients on chronic hemodialysis. *Psychosom Med* 30:521, 1968
20. Strauss AL: *Chronic Illness and the quality of Life,* St Louis MO, Mosby, 1975
21. Hegstrom RM, Murray JS, Pendras JP, Burnell JM, Scribner BH: Two years' experience with periodic hemodialysis in the treatment of chronic uremia. *Trans Am Soc Artif Intern Organs* 8:266, 1962
22. Murray JS, Pendras JP, Lindholm DD, Erickson RV: 25 months' experience in the treatment of chronic uremia at an out patient community hemodialysis center. *Trans Am Soc Artif Intern Organs* 10:19, 1964
23. Lindholm DD Burnell JM, Murray JS: Experience in the treatment of chronic uremia in an outpatient community hemodialysis center. *Trans Am Soc Artif Intern Organs* 9:3, 1963
24. Pendras JP, Pollard TL: Eight Years' experience with a community dialysis center: The Northwest Kidney Center. *Trans Am Soc Artif Intern Organs* 16:77, 1970
25. Gombos EA, Lee TH, Horton MR, Cummings JW: One years' experience with an intermittent dialysis program. *Ann Intern Med* 61:462, 1964
26. Friedman EA, Goodwin NJ, Chaudry L: Psychosocial adjustment to maintenance hemodialysis. *NY State J Med* 70:629, 1970
27. Goldberg RT, Bigwood AW, Donaldson WH: Vocational adjustment, interests, work values, and careers plans of patients awaiting renal transplantation. *Scand J Rehabil Med* 4:170, 1972
28. Burns S, Johnson HK: Rehabilitation potential of a dialysis versus a transplant population. *Dial Transpl* 5 (No 6):54, 1976
29. Brunner FP, Brynger H, Chantler C, Donckerwolcke RA, Hathway RA, Jacobs C, Selwood NH, Wing AJ: Combined report on regular dialysis and transplantation in Europe, IX, 1978. *Proc Eur Dial Transpl Assoc* 16:44, 1979
30. Panel: Living or dying adaptation to hemodialysis in *Living or Dying: Adaptation to Hemodialysis,* edited by Levy NB, Springfield IL, Charles C Thomas 1974
31. Friedman EA, Goodwin NJ, Chaudhry L: Psychological adjustment of family to maintenance hemodialysis. Part II. *NY State J Med* 70:767, 1970
32. Levy NB: Sexual adjustment to maintenance hemodialysis and renal transplantation: National survey by questionnaire. Preliminary report. *Trans Am Soc Artif Intern Organs* 19:138, 1973
33. Foster FG, Cohn GL, McHegney FP: Psychological factors and individual survival on chronic renal hemodialysis: a two year follow-up. Part I. *Psychosom Med* 35:64, 1973
34. Levy NB: The quality of life on maintenance haemodialysis. *Lancet* 1:1328, 1975
35. Abram HS, Hester LR, Sheridan WF, Epstein G: Sexual functioning in patients with chronic renal failure. *J Nerv Ment Dis* 160:220, 1975
36. Sherman FP: Impotence in patients with chronic renal failure on dialysis: its frequency and etiology. *Fertil Steril* 26:221, 1975
37. Salvatierra O, Fortmann JL, Belzer FO: Sexual function in males before and after renal transplantation. *Urology* 5:64, 1975
38. Bommer J, Tschope W, Ritz E, Andrassy K: Sexual behavior of hemodialyzed patients. *Clin Nephrol* 6:315, 1976
39. Steele TE, Finkelstein SM, Finkelstein FO: Hemodialysis patients and spouses: marital discord, sexual problems and depression. *J Nerv Ment Dis* 162:225, 1976
40. Milne JF, Golden JS, Fibus L: Sexual dysfunction in renal failure: a survey of chronic hemodialysis patients. *Int J Psychiatry Med* 8:335, 1977-78
41. Kaplan DeNour A: Hemodialysis: Sexual functioning. *Psychosomatics* 19:229, 1978
42. Procci WR, Goldstein DA, Adelstein J, and Massry SG: Sexual dysfunction in the male patient with uremia: a reappraisal. *Kidney Int* 19:317, 1981
43. Oberley TD: Sexual problems in kidney patients: acknowledging the individual. *Dial Transpl* 9:906, 1980
44. *The Holy Bible,* John 10:10

46

THE SOCIAL IMPACT OF CHRONIC MAINTENANCE HEMODIALYSIS

RICHARD B. FREEMAN

Introduction	844
Historical outline	844
Dialysis treatment and the 'quality of life'	845
Impact on the immediate environment	845
The surrounding environment	845
Politics and medicine	846
Economics, restricted resources and reality	846
Innovation	847
Quality of life	847
Advances in technology	847
Transplantation	847
Administrative costs	848
Prevention	848
Summary	848
References	848

INTRODUCTION

This treatise is an attempt to examine an expensive, well-defined program of therapy that serves a relatively small segment of the population. It is intended to look beyond daily affairs, unencumbered by details of administration, patient care and teaching. It is justified as a response to those who recognize that traditional legal, economic, and moral systems have been outstripped by advances in medical technology and call for a continuous open forum on the subject (1). The purpose is to continue the dialogue on problems that transcend the purview of individual professions and disciplines, and develop systemic analyses that will enhance knowledge, understanding, and optimize utilization of resources.

HISTORICAL OUTLINE

The treatment of patients with end-stage renal disease became possible because a group of dedicated physicians recognized, synthesized and applied advances in disparate fields of technology. Repetitive hemodialysis became realistic because of the availability of reliable hemodialysis equipment and the capability of implanting permanent, low-thrombogenic cannulae which allowed repeated access to the circulation (2). In the early 1960's it was demonstrated unequivocally that patients could be kept alive when treated with maintenance hemodialysis and that these individuals were capable of conducting most of their normal activities. Later, a lively debate developed over the exact 'quality of life' restored or maintained in these patients, and over the wisdom of spending large sums of money to treat all acceptable candidates. To state the issues another way, there was (and still is) considerable doubt that hemodialysis was a mode of therapy that could restore dignified life to patients with end-stage renal disease. Even if there was some success in the latter, there was serious concern as to whether public and private funds could, or should, be expended at the risk of compromising the pursuit of other scientific and social goals.

Organ transplantation paralleled the evolution of dialysis as a means of treatment of patients with terminal renal failure. Again, the combination of advances in surgical technique and organ preservation, the development of immunosuppressive drugs, and dialysis were responsible for reasonable success. Usually, the 'quality of life' was more satisfactory following successful transplantation, but the morbidity and mortality were higher than in maintenance hemodialysis patients.

After vigorous debate over the issues, a landmark decision, the Gottschalk Report, pronounced in 1967 dialysis and transplantation as accepted forms of therapy (3). A national program supported by the United States Government was recommended to extend care to all patients in whom treatment was indicated. Five years later, the US Congress extended medicare benefits to virtually all Americans by enacting Public Law 92-603.

These two modalities of therapy, chronic dialysis and transplantation, have now been organized into routine treatment procedures in most of the developed countries of the world. Worldwide, there are over 100,000 patients on maintenance dialysis and 50,000 who have received a renal transplant. New treatments have been developed over the past 5 years the future of which is somewhat uncertain. These include intermittent peritoneal dialysis, chronic ambulatory peritoneal dialysis and hemofiltration. For purposes of simplicity, these will all be referred to as dialysis in the remainder of this discussion.

Now, 15 years after the Gottschalk Report and a similar conclusion of the Ministry of Health in England also dating from 1967, there is, perhaps, a perspective about 'quality of life', the economic impact, restrictions in resources, and other problems that remain to be resolved.

The subjects to be addressed here will begin with the individual patient and extent concentrically into the immediate and surrounding environments of the patient and into society.

A discussion of this sort becomes confusing as expressed by Ballantine (4):

'Services rendered by physicians do not now seem to be considered in the context of the relief of pain and suffering and prolongation of useful life, but rather in terms of its economic effect on the Gross National Product and the enrichment of physicians, and as an issue by which politicians gain or lose favor with their constituents. To achieve fame and favor by attempts to halt the rising costs of medical care, politicians, medical economists and others are, by subterfuge and the use of fuzzy language, causing situations that will deny beneficial medical and surgical procedures to the public, or make access to them so difficult that both the patient and the physician give up.'

Some may not agree with all statements or concepts presented here, nor should they because they represent a set of circumstances as viewed by a single observer.

DIALYSIS TREATMENT AND THE 'QUALITY OF LIFE'

The literature that addresses the degree of success achieved in the treatment of patients on maintenance dialysis is filled with clichés. For example: 'half-way technology', as applied to patients with end stage renal disease, may be viewed as a means of 'extending life', with a very poor 'cost-benefit ratio', because the 'quality of life' is often a 'prolongation of the process of dying', filled with stress.

Exactly what is the 'quality of life' of those whose treatment is so very expensive? In the most basic analysis, if asked whether they would prefer to be dead or alive, the vast majority answer alive, of course! Would they like to feel better and be more productive? Certainly, but then so would most of us. Clearly, individuals who are dependent on machines and schedules, restricted to diets, and have an impressive array of aberrations in their metabolic functions, including abnormal cerebral functions, will be unlikely to be as content as a comparable healthy population.

Success of treatment has commonly been measured by the degree of rehabilitation achieved which is equated to productive work in society or in the home. About one third of our chronic dialysis patients can be considered fully rehabilitated, another third work part-time or are legitimately retired because of age, and the remaining third are medically retired because of significant disabilities. (See also Chapter 37, final section and Chapters 45 and 47.) Preoccupation with the physical status and productivity limits our perspective of the total patient. Circumstances of treatment programs are not always conducive to psychological rehabilitation. The atmosphere in which hemodialysis is conducted is often detrimental: patients are sometimes placed in mass production lines, given rigid diets, belittled when they fail to follow prescribed programs, and made to feel dependent on the personnel or the system or both. This discourages the patient from moving into a new lifestyle imposed by his situation.

The key to successful rehabilitation is achieving or restoring a state of personal dignity to the patient. Dignity must be developed to the degree where the individual has achieved what Ericson (5) calls *integrity*. Although Ericson's definition of this term encompasses a very broad concept, it is quite applicable to anyone threatened with a terminal illness or one who becomes dependent on other people or artificial devices. In adapting, the individual must accept this own life and lifestyle irrespective of other's standards. The goal is the realization and acceptance that this one life is significant and there is no substitute for this particular life and lifestyle. If achieved, the individual becomes less fearful of all physical and economic threats, and approves of himself as a being, significant to society.

Ericson cites data that the inability to do this is signified by disgust and despair. 'Fate is not accepted' and displeasure is hidden behind a show of disgust or contemptuous displeasure with particular institutions and particular people – a disgust and displeasure which signifies the individual's contempt of himself (5). Persons with this disposition can be found in all parts of society but they can be found quite easily in any chronic dialysis program. The frequency of rehabilitation in terms of dignity achieved is not measured by the accumulation of a few statistics on a population of thousands but by intensive, open-ended interviews to gain insight to the patient's view of himself.

IMPACT ON THE IMMEDIATE ENVIRONMENT

The immediate environment is defined as the people with whom the patient has most contact when not undergoing dialysis. It includes families, friends, and employers. It is in this area where there is a great paucity of information of the impact of this particular treatment program. What are the pressures on families? Anecdotal instances of families rallying to support the patient are well-known, but how long does this last and how frequent is it? What are the pressures and long term effects on the spouse, parents, and children of these patients? What about the pressures on potential transplant donors? What economic burdens are incurred that do not show in official treatment costs?

To reiterate, there is very little information available in this area other than anecdotes. But, it may be that we will discover that those in the immediate environment carry burdens that, on balance, weight the impact toward a total detrimental rather than a beneficial effect.

THE SURROUNDING ENVIRONMENT

This is defined as the community in which the patient lives, including the medical personnel and institutions that are delivering care. It is well-known that personnel caring for dialysis patients are at risk of developing hepatitis and perhaps other diseases. Some develop restricting attachments to patients. There have been a number of instances where nurses or technicians have married patients. What causes friction between many patients and some personnel? What are the rights of the individuals who are treating these people? Is the judgment of professionals sufficient to terminate treatment in those who become total invalids? Can one honor a will or contract signed at a time of desperation which supersedes another agreement signed under more pleasant circumstances? Exactly what are the legal implications of terminating life support systems when all are in agreement that therapy should be withdrawn? Unfortunately, there is little help from the Quinlan and Saikewicz cases which are notable recent examples of this medicolegal problem (6). The Storar and Eichner (Brother Fox) cases do not clarify the legal problems either, though some guidelines resulted. Apparently, an individual judged to be mentally competent can make a decision to have extraordinary treatments withheld. Preceding statements made by the patient to this effect are admissible as solid evidence (Brother Fox). On the other hand, patient's advocates do not have the right to decide whether an incompetent individual should have treatment withheld or withdrawn (Storar [7]). The judiciary arm of our society is trained to settle controversies between two parties and is ill equipped to settle issues of this type. Courts can claim no special competence to reach an ultimate decision because they must depend on not only medical data, but also on theological tenets and perceptions of human values which defy classification and calibration. In fact, physicians and patients, together with patient's families, theologians and others have been making these kinds of decisions for years with no apparent harm to society. Intervention by government policies is quite another matter which will be addressed below.

POLITICS AND MEDICINE

In 1965 the United States Government extended health insurance benefits to individuals over the age of 65 and to the indigent. Systems of socialized health care were already underway in many countries in the world at that time. However, with the medicare and medicaid legislation in the United States there came regulations for compliance of institutions for reimbursement for services rendered. In that single stroke of legislation the authority of physicians moved away from medical professionals toward political professionnals. The end-stage renal disease benefits were simply an extension of this system with further regulations. The legislation enacting this program was fuzzy in language, but the regulations that followed narrowed the capabilities of the professionals to individualize care and added a bureaucracy to a system already too cumbersome. Granted, the end-stage renal disease program is viewed by many as an 'experiment' in the treatment of catastrophic illness (8), but will adequate information be derived to judge whether or not the program is a success? And what if it is not a success? What then? And who will define the criteria by which a judgment is made? The United States is woefully negligent in compiling data and should look to Europeans for an example of how meaningful information is gathered and analyzed (i.e. the annual reports of the European Dialysis and Transplant Association Registry).

ECONOMICS, RESTRICTED RESOURCES AND REALITY

The original estimate of the cost of the United States program was 250 million dollars for the first year which was expected to escalate and to level off at about 1.0 billion* dollars at the end of the 10 years (8). An estimate of the number of patients who would require maintenance dialysis was made, based on 12 years of experience of an organized network program in the Rochester, NY, area. Eventually the number of new patients entering the program would equal the number leaving either by death or successful transplantation. Equilibrium will be reached in 1992 when 632 patients per million population will need treatment. Based on the experience to date about 500 patients/million will be treated in dialysis centers (9). The cost will exceed 1.7 billion dollars and could reach 3 billion depending on policies, accounting practices and inflation (10).

Now, in terms of a cost-benefit ratio analysis, this treatment program can only be viewed as dismal from the administration level. Of course, the individual patient and physician are not so interested in cost benefit ratios, particularly in clear-cut situations where treatment maintains life, and non-treatment means certain death. The Gottschalk report stated that cost-effectiveness was meaningless in this situation 'because of the difficulty of putting a value on human life' (3). But when actual figures, based on experience, reach astronomical levels, there are second thoughts. Some old questions have been resurrected as well as startling new ones. To be blunt, there are two primary economic issues: is it worth it now? And the second: can we afford this treatment program in an age that is different than the 1960's?

The fact remains, however, that chronic dialysis programs exist in virtually all communities in the Western world. Data from Europe show a clear correlation between the numbers of patients on treatment and the per capita gross national product of individual countries (11). Thus, the trend is clear. This treatment program must be viewed in the context of priorities for social programs in each country. In those faced with high rates of death from starvation or perinatal mortality, treatment of renal failure will be relatively low on a priority scale. But, change in social priorities may not be perceived easily, nor may established practices be changed quickly. The dilemma may be best put into focus by comparing the penal system in the US with treatment programs for renal failure. There are about 85,000 persons sentenced to life terms for murder in federal and state maximum security facilities. The cost per year is between $ 75,000 to $ 80,000 per convict per year. Time Magazine (23 March, 1981) reports that the

---

* The American billion is 10^9.

cost of incarceration in the US is 4 billion dollars and increasing exponentially.

The figures speak for themselves. Dialysis and transplantation are realities. More data are desperately needed both for treatment of chronic renal failure but also for the cost of other programs. How much does it cost to maintain persons in nursing homes, mental institutions and the like? What are the rates of rehabilitation? Who will interpret the data? In the past, when the state has dictated changes in priorities without consultation and action from responsible professionals, values and ethics have become distorted.

INNOVATION

As stated, there is no argument that if the value of human life is removed from the discussion for theoretic purposes, a cost-effectiveness analysis would have dreadful results. But the history of medicine, science and technology is replete with examples of settling thorny issues by addressing problems and purposefully setting about to resolve them. The following are some possibilities of reducing costs and improving the results of dialysis treatment.

Quality of life

The atmosphere of maintenance dialysis units must be changed. The patients are not typical hospital patients nor should they be viewed as such. They are people in limbo, neither sick nor well, terminal nor curable. They will benefit from more positive attitudes of the staff to bring them closer to a state of integrity as defined previously. A positive attitude of the staff can have a significant effect on the degree of satisfaction that the patient has with himself (12). Too often, patients are chastized for not following diet orders, adhering to medication schedules, etc. Support and therapy can be delivered in a positive manner without resorting to condescending orders.

In retrospect, the location of maintenance dialysis facilities should not have been placed in hospital space. Hospital space is simply too expensive and undoubtedly has a negative effect on the psychology of the patient. However, the construction of facilities designed to 'mass produce' hemodialysis, though intended to reduce costs, is not conducive to maintain the privacy of the individual. Free standing units have been very successful and should probably be expanded to meet the needs of the treatment of stable chronic dialysis patients. But the design of the units should be more cheerful and flexible to allow privacy. The facilities should be constructed so that renovation into other useful space could be accomplished at a minimum cost should the number of patients with chronic renal failure decline. The institutionalization concept of the treatment of these individuals should be avoided!

Motivation of physicians and patients to perform home dialysis has been disappointing. The reasons for this are complex, but they include the psychological pressures that are placed on both the patient and the family, economic constraints, attitudes of the staff of individual treatment centers, and limitations for physical renovation in living areas such as apartments and rural areas.

In addition, the intellectual capacity of some patients and the supporting family are not sufficient to carry out the necessary procedures. The goal of moving 50% of maintenance dialysis patients to the home has been suggested, but the actual experience indicates that only 11 to 14% of patients will do home dialysis. Of course, more patients could be home-trained if that is made the only available option. Is this an infringement on the right of the patient to choose his therapy? How much stress is placed on the supporting home dialysis family? (See also Chapters 24 and 43).

Advances in technology

Reduction in costs by improvements in hardware and simplification of treatment would seem to be a realistic possibility and a desirable goal. Despite considerable government funding over the past decade it is fair to state that there have been no major advances in the technology of dialysis except for the development of the subcutaneous fistula and vein grafts. Others are developing (resins for removal of toxins, direct hemoperfusion through resins and other materials, chronic ambulatory peritoneal dialysis, hemofiltration) but their effectiveness remains to be proven in routine treatment. Practically all of these 'advances' have been made in the private sector without program oriented government support. Some have been innovations created in laboratories in private institutions or by private industry. The latter is now sufficiently developed and competitive that further technologic developments might best be left to the private sector. However, the sponsorship of biomedical research should not be reduced. Creative projects have been crucial in clarifying biochemical and physiologic derangements in patients with renal failure and there has been a sizeable spinoff benefiting other areas in medicine.

Transplantation

After early experience which might be termed experimental, the success of renal transplantation has improved only slightly over the past decade except that deaths due to complications of immunosuppressive therapy have been reduced. A scientific breakthrough in the selective control of the rejection process would have a remarkable impact on treatment of end-stage renal disease. Obviously successful transplant patients would be moved out of the dialysis pool with no need for the repetitive expensive treatments with the artificial kidney. And, depending on the degree of success in function of the allograft and control of side effects of the drugs, the patients are restored to a more natural life-style.

Logically, a heavy investment in research directed at controlling the rejection reaction seems indicated. Even if there was a breakthrough obtained in this field, there will still be difficulty in acquiring suitable kidneys for transplantation unless some major legal definitions are clarified. The necessity to challenge certain tenets by court trial is too inefficient to evolve a suitable set of codes that can be developed in a deliberate manner. The process is further constrained by the inability of the most expert medical teams to arrive at a suitable definition of death and the indications for termination of systems for life support. Again, responsible professionals must take the lead in clarifying these issues.

Administrative costs

When the process of delivery of care becomes subject to legislative controls, a program may become fossilized by regulations and rigid codes, all of which require rather large bureaucracies to monitor, control, and disperse resources. The cost of maintaining a staff within the bureaucracy makes the price higher. To the physician and often the patient, the necessity to deal with overlapping politico-administrative authorities, and with the layers of regulations becomes stifling. It is counter productive to the evolution of knowledge, sensitivity, and understanding through experiences with specific individuals. If there is one lesson to be learned from the dialysis program, it should be that there must be more efficient planning in the development of delivery of resources and retrieval of detailed data from pilot studies before support is extended to large scale treatment programs.

PREVENTION

The analogy of treatment of chronic renal failure by dialysis to pre-vaccine poliomyelitis treatment techniques and to tuberculosis hospitals, all now obsolete and all of which cost large amounts of money, does not hold when one considers the numbers and diversity of diseases that may lead to renal failure. All major registries are in virtual agreement on the incidence of specific categories of diseases that cause terminal renal failure (11, 13, 14). Inspection of these figures gives little hope for primary or secondary prevention. Over 50% of patients who arrive at the point of requiring dialysis or transplantation have one or another type of immune disorder of the kidney. Many windows have been opened by researchers into the mechanisms whereby these diseases occur, but the present state of the field is exemplified by the fact that practically all of these disorders are referred to in terms of the pathological description of the kidney tissue or the clinical course of the patient. Too few, in fact, very few, are designated by the etiologic agent or agents or events that initiate and perpetuate the disorder. And, of course, without knowledge of the specific cause, preventive or therapeutic measures are nothing more than blind trial and error. It is crucial, however, that the few leads that exist regarding the pathogenesis of immune diseases of the kidney be followed intensely in the research setting.

Infections of the kidney, once thought to be a major cause of end-stage renal disease, account for only 7 to 23% of cases, and at least half of these are perpetuated by an underlying predisposing cause to chronic infection (15-18). Hypertension is one bright area for prevention if organized screening, compliance and education are promoted successfully. Nevertheless, the potentials are not optimistic for an early reduction in the numbers of new patients requiring treatment for end-stage renal failure each year by application of preventive measures. Hopefully, this assessment of the potentials for prevention will be modified by current and future investigational activities.

SUMMARY

In summary, the experiences with the treatment of patients with end-stage renal disease have been examined in the context of the changing interactions between the medical profession and society. The reality of the success of this treatment, at least a partial success, must be recognized. However, confusion continues over quantitation of the total benefits to the patient, family, supporting professional and non-professional personnel, and the conservation of resources. Whatever the outcome of further studies, present experience indicates that it will be erroneous to assume that more harm than good will result from continuation of this program. The most serious error would be to divert all or large investments from investigations in this and other areas of study in order to support only the delivery of services. Most organizations invest a percentage of a service budget into research and development.

Solutions to the biomedical, social, ethical, and legal problems will only be found through further inquiry.

REFERENCES

1. Bennett IL Jr: Technology as a shaping force. *Daedalus* 106(nr 1):125, 1977
2. Scribner BH, Buri R, Caner JEA, Hegstrom R, Burnell JM: The treatment of chronic uremia by means of intermittent hemodialysis: a preliminary report. *Trans Am Soc Artif Intern Organs* 6:114, 1960
3. Gottschalk CW: *Report of the Committee on Chronic Kidney Disease, Bureau of the Budget.* US Government Printing Office, 1967
4. Ballantine HT Jr: Medical care and the English language. *N Engl J Med* 295:1012, 1976
5. Eriscon EH: *Identity: Youth and Crisis.* New York, WW Norton & Co, Inc, 1968
6. Collester DG Jr: The Quinlan case and the problems of the right to die. *Rutgers Law Rev* 30(2):304, 1977
7. Court of Appeals Opinions in 'Right to Die' cases. *New York Law J.* April, 1981
8. Report of Subcommittee on Health and Subcommittee on Oversight, Committee on Ways and Means. US House of Representatives. *Background Information in Kidney Dis-*

ease benefits Under Medicare. US Government Printing Office (June 24), 1975
9. Cestero RVM, Jacobs MO, Freeman RB: A regional end-stage renal disease program: Twelve years experience. *Ann Intern Med* 93:494, 1980
10. Cummings NB: *Data Book Fiscal Year 1976. Research In Kidney and Urinary Tract Diseases,* Bethesda MD, National Institutes of Health, 1977, p 4
11. Wing AJ, Brunner FP, Brynger H, Chantler C, Donckerwolcke RA, Gurland HJ, Hathway RA, Jacobs C: Combined report on regular dialysis and transplantation in Europe, VIII, 1977 *Proc Eur Dial Transpl Assoc* 15:3, 1978
12. De-Nour AK, Czaczkes JW, Lilos P: A study of chronic hemodialysis teams: Difference in opinions and expectations. *J Chron Dis* 25:441, 1972
13. Brunner FP, Giesecke B, Gurland HJ, Jacobs C, Parsons FM, Schärer K, Seyffart G, Spies G, Wing AJ: Combined report on regular dialysis and transplantation in Europe V, 1974. *Proc Eur Dial Transpl Assoc* 12:3, 1975
14. The 12th report of the human transplant registry. *JAMA* 233:787, 1975
15. Sanford JP: Urinary tract symptoms and infections. *Annu Rev Med* 26:485, 1975
16. Bullen M, Kincaid-Smith P: Asymptomatic pregnancy bacteriuria: A follow-up study 4-7 years after delivery. In: *Renal Infection and Renal Scarring,* edited by Kincaid-Smith P, Fairley KF, Melbourne, Mercedes Publishing Services, 1970, p 33
17. Gower PE: A long term study of renal function in patients with radiological pyelonephritis and other allied radiological lesions. In: *Urinary Tract Infection,* edited by Brumfitt W, Asscher AW, London, Oxford Medical Publications, 1972, p 74
18. Freeman RB, Smith WM, Richardson JA: Long term therapy for chronic bacteriuria in men. US Public Health Service Study. *Ann Intern Med* 83:133, 1975

47

COMPARATIVE REVIEW BETWEEN DIALYSIS AND TRANSPLANTATION

ANTONY J. WING, FELIX P. BRUNNER, HANS O.A. BRYNGER, CLAUDE JACOBS and PETER KRAMER

Expansion of facilities	850
Evolution of national programmes	850
Japan	850
United States of America	851
Europe	853
Contribution of CAPD	854
Rates of acceptance of new patients and of transplantation	854
Economic constraint on national programmes	855
Evolution of dialysis strategies	855
Methods of treatment	855
Dialysis schedules	856
Geographical variation in age structure and primary renal disease	856
Age of patients	857
Distribution of primary renal disease	858
Comparative survival statistics	859
Survival as related to the method of treatment	860
Survival as related to age at start of treatment	861
Survival as related to primary renal disease	861
Factors affecting graft survival	862
Prognostic factors independent of transplantation immunology	862
Age	862
Primary renal disease	862
Hepatitis B	862
Rehabilitation status at time of transplantation	863
Quality of cadaveric kidneys	863
Prognostic factors related to transplantation immunology	863
Living related donor transplantation	863
Cadaveric transplantation	863
ABO matching, sex and race	863
HLA matching	863
Cytotoxic antibodies	863
Pregnancy	864
Blood transfusion	864
Time on dialysis before transplantation	864
Splenectomy	864
Bilateral nephrectomy	864
Re-transplantation	864
Causes of death	864
Death rates	864
Myocardial ischaemia	865
Cerebrovascular accident	865
Malignancy	865
All causes	866
Quality of life	866
Rehabilitation	866
Hospitalisation	867
Disabling bone disease	867
Conclusions	868
Acknowledgements	868
References	868

EXPANSION OF FACILITIES

In 1976, we estimated that the global total of patients who owed their lives to an artificial kidney machine was 64,000 (1). By the close of 1980, there were approximately 150,000 patients alive on regular haemodialysis therapy, 37% of them in the USA, 33% in Europe, 24% in Japan and 6% in other countries. Functioning renal transplants gave life to approximately 37,000 patients, 49% of whom were in the USA, 35% in Europe and 16% in other countries. Continuous ambulatory peritoneal dialysis (CAPD), a treatment modality not available at the time of our last review in 1976 (1), supported around 7,000 patients. It, therefore, appears possible that by the time these words appear in print, the number of patients alive on renal replacement therapy worldwide will be approaching one quarter of a million.

Information was collected for a world-wide survey (2) to 31st December 1979 and numbers of patients on treatment per million population at that date are shown according to country in Table 1. Fairly comprehensive data was available for 37 countries, 31 of which returned individual patient questionnaires to the Registry of the European Dialysis and Transplant Association (EDTA). A combined patient Registry recorded activity in Australia and New Zealand (3); South African patients were also registered individually with the EDTA Registry pending the establishment of an independent registry. Reports from Canada (4) and Japan (Odaka M, 1981, personal communication) were based on centre questionnaires, and information from the USA came through the reports to Congress of the Health Care Financing Administration (5). Some preliminary information has been collected in Brazil (6).

Evolution of national programmes

Japan
Japan treated 286 patients per million population on 31st December 1979, out of a total population of 114.9 million, the largest per capita number in any country (7). Almost all of these patients were treated by hospital haemodialysis and the rapid growth during the past 10 years in the hospital haemodialysis programme in Japan is shown in Figure 1. This figure also shows that this rapid

Table 1. Numbers of patients alive on treatment per million population on 31st December 1979. The total (*) includes patients known to be on treatment but whose mode of therapy was uncertain. Some figures were estimated (x) and those for Australia and New Zealand are at 30th April 1980 (+).

Country	Peritoneal dialysis	Haemodialysis	(% home)	Functioning transplant	Total *
Japan	2 x	278	(<1%)	6	286
USA	8	207	(13%)	68 x	283
Switzerland	10	132	(23%)	74	221
Belgium	6	134	(7%)	60	206
Israel	14	150	(12%)	31	201
Canada	27	84	(33%)	78	189
France	8	150	(17%)	23	188
Australia +	14	80	(45%)	91	185
Denmark	10	75	(23%)	91	181
Luxembourg	0	122	(0)	2	164
Fed Rep Germany	3	137	(21%)	14	161
Italy	4	137	(12%)	12	158
Sweden	8	64	(22%)	71	149
Netherlands	1	95	(9%)	47	148
New Zealand +	6	62	(52%)	67	135
Austria	<1	91	(7%)	25	119
Finland	5	32	(3%)	77	118
Norway	3	29	(4%)	80	117
Spain	3	99	(6%)	8	114
UK	4	57	(64%)	48	111
Greece	1	61	(<1%)	8	77
Iceland	0	30	(0)	45	77
Ireland	1	36	(33%)	31	69
German Dem Rep	1	37	(0)	16	56
Yugoslavia	<1	42	(0%)	4	50
Czechoslovakia	<1	28	(<1%)	7	36
South Africa	2	15	(11%)	9	26
Bulgaria	0	20	(0)	1	22
Cyprus	0	5	(0)	10	21
Brazil	2	13	(0)	5 x	20
Hungary	<1	13	(0)	4	18
Portugal	<1	14	(1%)	<1	15
Poland	1	10	(0)	2	14
Lebanon	0	11	(0)	0	11
Tunisia	0	8	(0)	0	9
Turkey	<1	2	(0)	1	3
Egypt	0	1	(2%)	0	1

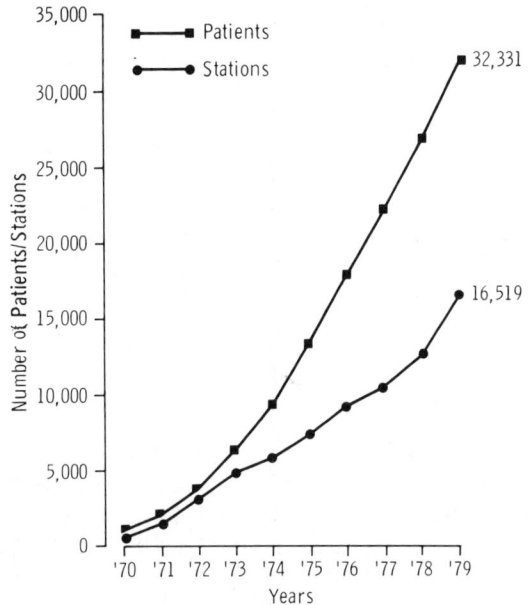

Figure 1. Numbers of chronic dialysis patients and of stations in Japan, 1970-1979.

growth has been made possible by expansion of facilities so that at the end of 1979 there were 144 treatment stations per million population. Over 12,000 staff, including 935 doctors and 6,792 nurses were directly committed to the care of these patients (Odaka M, 1981, personal communication).

United States of America

In the USA transplantation has made a more significant contribution and we estimate that between 35,000 and 38,000 grafts were performed between 1960 and 1980. The proportion of live related donors has always been higher than in Europe and was 29% in 1976 (8). Allowing for the greater success with live donors compared to cadavers, a generous estimate suggests that there were 18,000 patients in the USA alive with functioning grafts at the close of 1980.

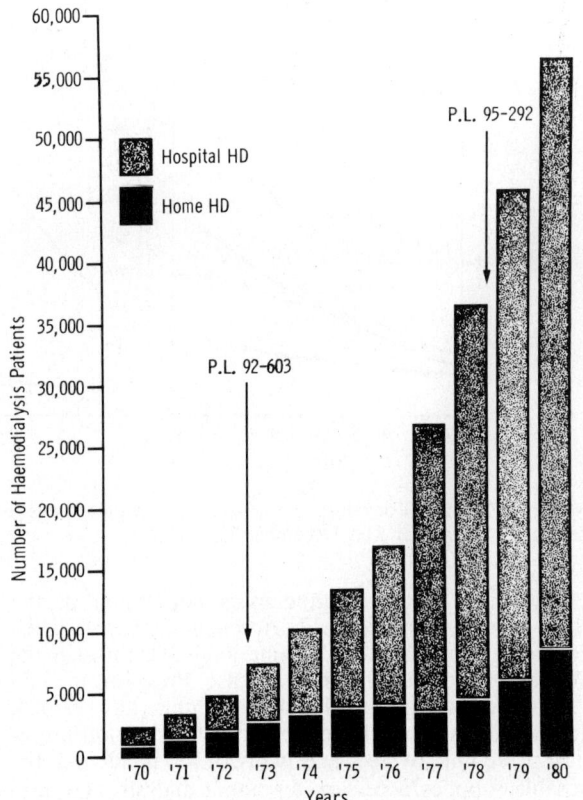

Figure 2. Growth of haemodialysis in USA, 1970-1980, showing the diminishing contribution of home dialysis and the dates of relevant public laws (P.L.).

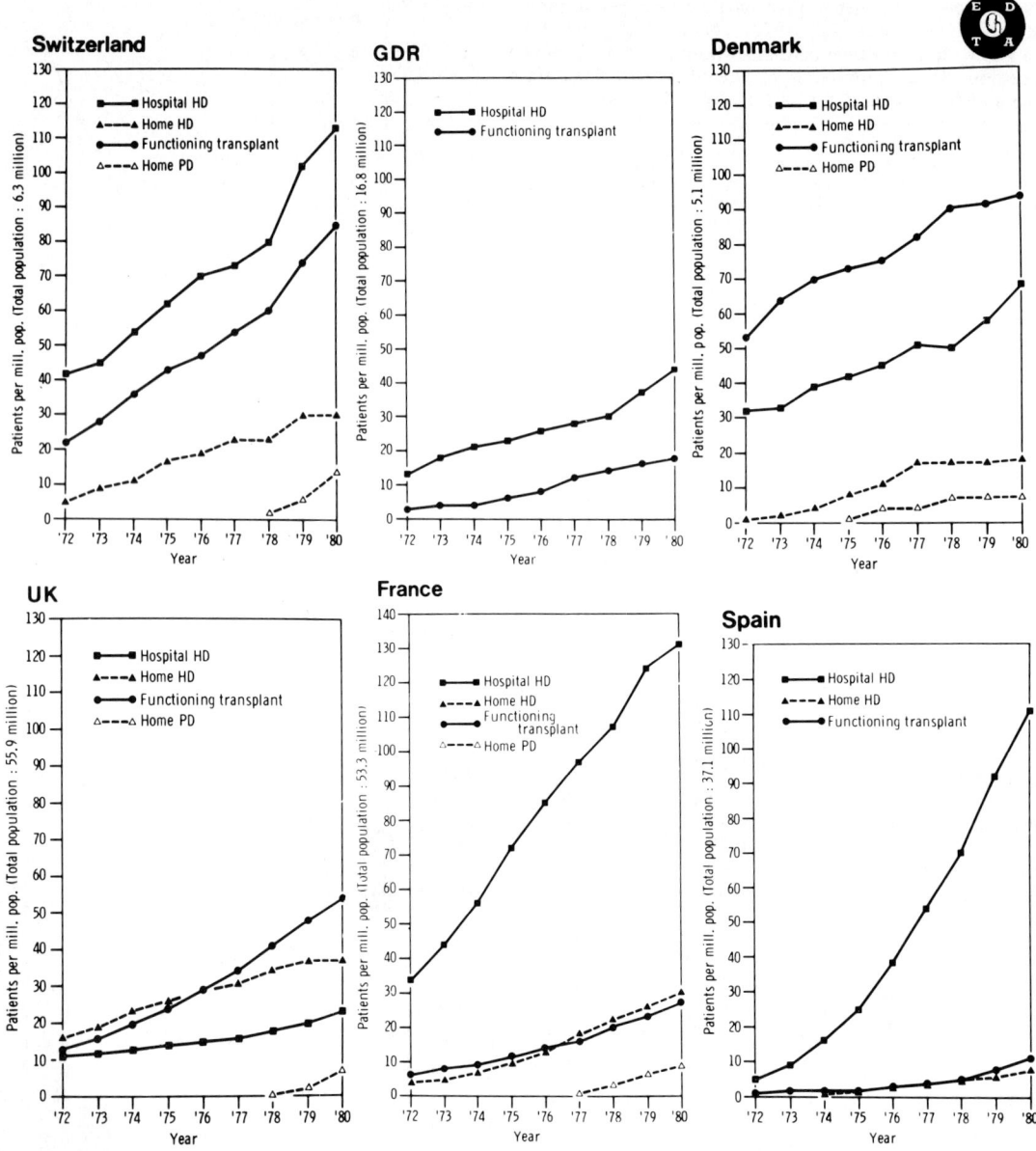

Figure 3. Patterns of development of treatment programmes in six European countries. Number of patients per million of population are shown for 31st December 1972-1980.

Expansion of the haemodialysis population in the USA is shown in Figure 2. Acceleration began when Federal funds started to become available through the Medicare End Stage Renal Disease Program in July 1973. Under the original legislation, Public Law 92-603, home dialysis support services furnished by non-physicians were not covered, and many of the incidental disposable supplies necessary for home dialysis were also not covered. A decline in the proportion of patients treated by home dialysis then occurred from 40% in 1972 to 12% in 1978. Burton and Hirschman (8) suggested that other factors were involved: the motivation of the physician to steer the patient to one mode of treatment or the other and the patient's own choice between the responsibility of self treatment and having the work done by trained staff in a dialysis centre. Public Law 95-292 was enacted on 1st October 1978 to remove the disincentives to home dialysis by defining coverage in terms of the procedure rather than the treatment setting and by waiving the waiting period necessary to establish entitlement to Medicare benefits (5).

The extension of Medicare benefits had other effects on the demography of the patient population in the USA. Evans and colleagues (9) have recently compared the social and demographic profiles of patients who commenced treatment in 1967 with those who started in 1978. Age distribution shifted so that the proportion of patients aged 55 years and older increased from 7% in 1967 to 45% in 1978. The 1978 sample showed a larger proportion who had low educational achievement and broken marriages and who were unemployed or financially disadvantaged. The percentage of blacks increased fivefold and they constituted 24% of the end stage renal disease population in 1978, compared to 11% of the general population. Thus, Medicare has brought about important advances in the access to medical services, although treatment is by no means equally distributed throughout the USA (10). However, the escalation of costs has become a topic of frequent debate as annual Federal Government expenditure on dialysis and transplantation rose from $242 million in 1974 to exceed $1 billion* in 1979 and is predicted to pass $3 billion by 1984 (9).

Europe
The EDTA Registry (11) has recently compared the patterns of development of treatment programmes in six countries (Figure 3). On 31st December 1980, the European country with the highest treatment rate was Switzerland with 260 patients per million population from a total population of 6.3 million. Numbers of Swiss patients on hospital haemodialysis, home haemodialysis, alive with a functioning transplant and on home peritoneal dialysis have been increasing in parallel during the years 1972 to 1980. What, therefore, appears to be a balanced and integrated programme was delivered by a total of 31 centres, 5.1 for every million of population – a high concentration of facilities in comparison with other European countries.

An interesting contrast is made by the German Democratic Republic (GDR) with a total population of 16.8 million and 65 patients per million population on treatment where only two modes of therapy, hospital haemodialysis and transplantation, were practiced. The parallel increase in patients on these two treatments suggests that they were geared together and that most patients commencing dialysis were selected as suitable for transplantation. Denmark, like Sweden, Norway and Finland, has relied on renal transplantation since the early years and in all these countries the numbers of patients alive with a functioning transplant have been greater than those on any other form of therapy. Fifty per cent of all living Danish patients owed their survival to functioning grafts at the end of 1980. One unusual aspect of the Danish programme is that the rate of acceptance of new patients has remained fairly constant throughout the years 1972 to 1979, whereas in other countries it has risen progressively.

In the United Kingdom (UK) hospital haemodialysis has been limited by tight budgetry controls over expansion of services which have kept the number of centres down to one per million population. The dialysis population has, therefore, been expanded by using home haemodialysis to treat two thirds of the patients. However, for the last three years, the number of patients alive with a functioning graft has exceeded even those on home haemodialysis and the transplanted group of patients continues to grow more rapidly.

In France, the hospital haemodialysis programme based on 3.4 centres per million population has raced ahead of other treatments. Home haemodialysis and renal transplantation have made smaller contributions and home peritoneal dialysis has only recently come into the picture. The scene in the other large Western European countries is similar with even less contributed by transplantation and home dialysis. In the Federal Republic of Germany (FRG), 109 patients per million population were on hospital haemodialysis in 3.5 centres per million population, but the other treatments combined supported only 43 patients per million. Italy had 121 patients per million population on hospital haemodialysis in 3.5 centres per million, but only 29 patients per million on other modes of therapy. Spain provides the most extreme example of a hospital haemodialysis programme unsupported by other modes of treatment. There were 92 patients per million population on hospital haemodialysis in 2.9 centres per million population, but only 15 patients per million on other treatments. These countries must be considered at present to have unbalanced programmes, but there is sufficient investment in haemodialysis facilities to ensure a large patient base from which to develop other modes of therapy. Their present picture is not dissimilar from the American scene and it is interesting to reflect on the similarities for health financing, based to a greater or lesser degree on reimbursement or insurance. All of these

Table 2. Numbers of patients on CAPD on 30th June 1981.

Country	Patients	Per million population
Australia	154	10.7
Belgium	145	14.6
Canada	699	29.5
Denmark	55	10.8
Fed Rep Germany	212	3.5
Finland	51	10.6
France	545	10.2
Israel	67	17.6
Italy	563	9.9
Japan	41	0.4
Mexico	50	0.7
Netherlands	47	3.4
New Zealand	54	16.9
Norway	17	4.1
Puerto Rico	43	12.6
South Africa	64	2.2
Spain	123	3.3
Sweden	117	14.1
Switzerland	120	19.0
UK	662	11.9
USA	4,096	18.6
Venezuela	59	4.1
Others	19	—
Total	8,003	—

---
* The American billion is 10^9.

countries are currently implementing legislation or other constraints in order to restrain this costly deployment of medical resources. The contrasting graphs for the GDR, Denmark and the UK are the product of planned medical development and controlled expenditure.

Contribution of CAPD

The number of patients on CAPD on 30th June 1981 is shown in Table 2. Over 4,000 patients were on this treatment in the USA, 2,734 in Europe (including Israel) and 1,165 in the remaining countries, amongst whom it is interesting to note activity in CAPD in some South American countries.

CAPD has been the fastest growing mode of dialysis in Canada since 1977, matching the rate of growth in the number of patients alive with a functioning transplant. In the UK, 83% of centres offering haemodialysis had also commenced CAPD by the end of 1980, resulting in rapid expansion in the number of patients treated in 1980 and early 1981. One factor speeding the deployment of CAPD may have been the reduction in transplantation activity (Figure 4) following unfortunate publicity concerning 'brain death' (12 [TV programme 'Panorama', October 13, 1980]) and the ethical pressure

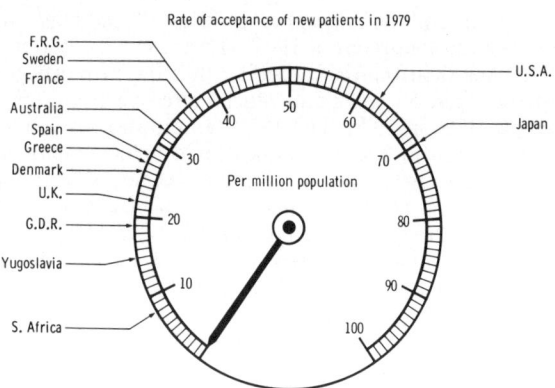

Figure 5. Comparison of rate of acceptance of new patients in different countries (1979).

on British nephrologists to select patients for their limited facilities (13). Now that the limitations of CAPD are becoming more clear (11), it appears predictable that the large number of patients on CAPD in the UK in 1981 will present a considerable embarrassment to the limited facilities for hospital haemodialysis as the 'dropouts' from CAPD need alternative modes of therapy.

Rates of acceptance of new patients and of transplantation

The rate of acceptance of new patients in 1979 was highest in Japan and the USA where it was twice that of most Western European countries and three times that of the UK (Figure 5). It is hoped that the high acceptance rate in Belgium (48 per million population) and Switzerland (40 per million) may be less necessary when measures taken to prevent the renal consequences of analgesic abuse take effect. The acceptance rate in Canada, for many years similar to that in Western Europe, is thought to have approached 40 patients per million in 1979 because of more liberal selection policies encouraged by CAPD (4). The acceptance rate in the United Kingdom was well below all reliable estimates of need, which indicates that at least 40 patients per million require therapy (14). Figure 6 compares the age specific

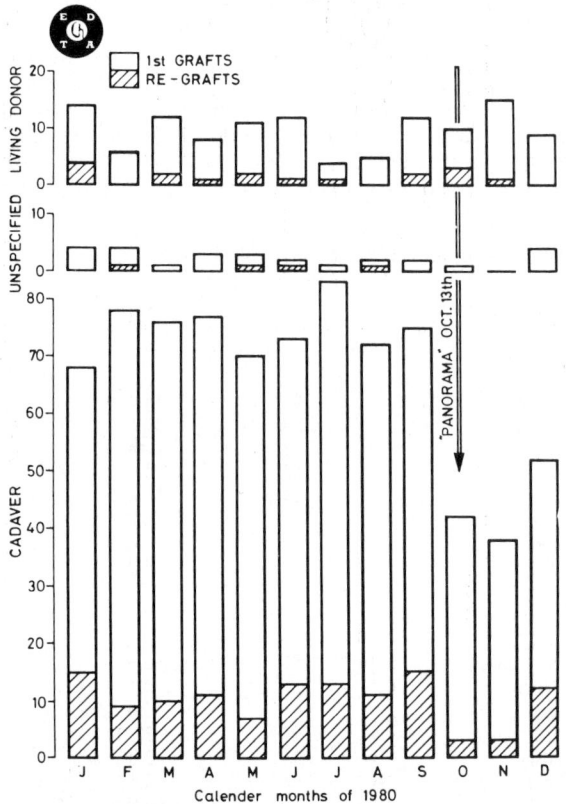

Figure 4. Monthly transplants in UK during 1980. Numbers are shown separately for grafts from live donors, unspecified donors and from cadavers. The monthly cadaver transplant rate fell from an average of 75 in January-September to 41 in October-December and preliminary data for January-October 1981 indicates that the rate has not yet been restored.

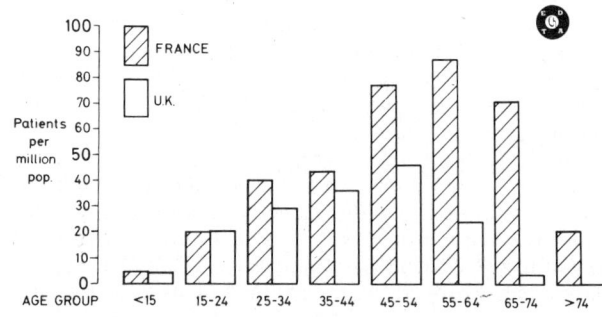

Figure 6. Comparison of age specific acceptance rates for patients in UK and France (1978).

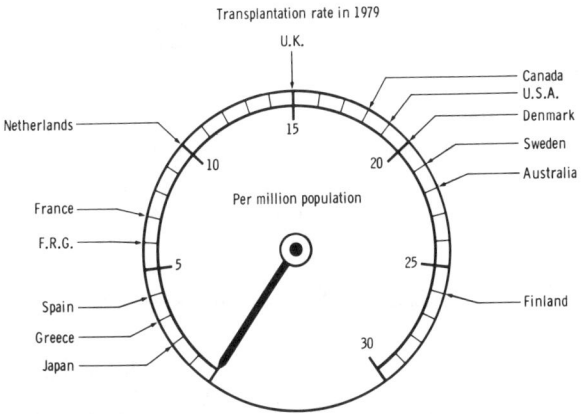

Figure 7. Comparison of rate of transplantation in different countries (1979).

20 per million population, and in the USA, where it was not far short at 19.5 per million population (Figure 7). Ireland, the UK, Belgium and Israel also had active programmes but there is obviously real opportunity for other countries to increase their transplantation rate and some of these are in the upper part of Table 1, that is, they have a large stock of dialysis patients as potential recipients.

Economic constraint on national programmes

Achievements of different countries in treating end stage renal failure are shown in relation to their economic productivity in Figure 8 (11). Data on gross national products was provided by the World Bank (16). The numbers of patients on all treatments combined (Table 1) correlate significantly with the per capita gross national products (GNP) expressed in US dollars. Switzerland, Sweden and the FRG provide treatment for rather fewer patients than their respective gross national products would seem able to support. This could indicate that these countries have less pressing clinical demand for these treatments than Japan, Israel and Italy, which otherwise appear to accord greater priority to the use of resources for this expensive endeavour. The intercept of the regression line, at US $2,700, suggests that it is difficult, or possibly even inappropriate for countries with a gross national product lower than this to put many patients on treatment. Three quarters of the world's population live in countries with a per capita gross national product of less than US $2,700.

acceptance rates in the UK and France. Using WHO population statistics, acceptance rates in 1978 are expressed per million of population in different age groups. The exclusion of older patients from treatment in the UK is clearly not due to differences in population age structure. It rather demonstrates implicit rationing (15) operating through resource constraints which have limited the number of centres to one per million population. The mechanism of the rationing of facilities is not a deliberate or formally agreed selection policy, so much as a low referral rate from colleagues who are anxious to protect their patients from the arousal of false hope.

Transplantation rates were highest in Finland, Scandinavian and Australasian countries, where they exceeded

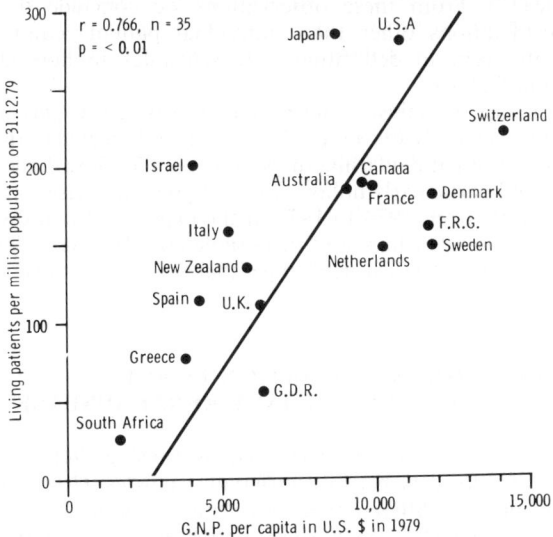

Figure 8. Correlation between number of patients alive on treatment for end stage renal failure (ESRF) and per capita gross national product (GNP). Eighteen countries are named in the figure but the regression was performed with data from 35 countries.

EVOLUTION OF DIALYSIS STRATEGIES

Methods of treatment

Expansion of facilities has been based on a growing number of centres and on the diversification of treatment modalities offered by these centres. The pattern of commencement of different modes of treatment in European centres during the last 18 years is shown in Figure 9. This figure is compounded mostly from activity in the five largest West European nations, the FRG, France, Italy, Spain and the UK (11). Expansion of hospital haemodialysis was maximal in the late 1960's and early 1970's and thereafter declined, especially during the last three years. Growth of hospital haemodialysis in the UK was restricted during the 1970's; but continued in France, the FRG and Italy and was a more recent phenomenon in Spain. The number of centres which performed renal transplantation has been growing steadily by rather less than 20 per year since 1966. Intermittent peritoneal dialysis began to spread in 1977 but was immediately overtaken by the soaring growth in centres which started CAPD, notably in the United Kingdom and France, during the past few years. Commencement of new haemofiltration facilities since 1976 was particularly striking in the FRG, and to a lesser extend in France. In 1980, 227 centres claimed to have used hae-

Table 3. Age distribution of all living patients according to mode of therapy on 31st December 1979.

Mode of therapy	Average age	% of patients aged			
		0–14	15–34	35–54	55+
Hospital HD	47.8	1.4	19.7	44.1	34.9
Home HD	43.8	1.0	23.9	55.4	19.8
Hospital PD	53.6	2.6	11.3	34.5	51.6
Home PD	59.2	2.6	9.1	32.7	55.7
Functioning CAD	38.9	2.7	36.7	49.6	11.0
Functioning LD	33.6	4.4	53.8	37.9	3.8

CAD = Cadaver graft.
LD = Living donor graft.

The age distribution at the time of transplantation in 3,475 American and 12,217 European patients is compared in Figure 13. The American patients tend to be younger at transplantation. This probably owes much to the wider use of living donor grafts in the USA, and both the differences in donors and younger age of recipients would be expected to result in better overall graft survival in the USA compared to Europe.

In Europe, the patient population has increased in age due to the acceptance of a greater proportion of older patients in recent, compared to earlier, years (Figure 14). Furthermore, the age distribution in patients on different modes of therapy was not the same (Table 3). Patients treated by peritoneal dialysis were older and those with functioning grafts younger than those on haemodialysis. These important demographic differences should be recalled when comparisons are made between various groups of patients and methods of treatment.

Distribution of primary renal diseases

Table 4 shows some interesting differences in the distribution of primary renal diseases recorded in Australia, Europe, Japan and the USA. The comparison must not be pressed too hard because of assumptions made in equating the different code structures. New patients commencing treatment in 1979 were used for the first three areas, but for the USA the whole file was used and unfortunately, a diagnosis was recorded in only 49% of American patients and it may be dangerous to assume that the distribution of primary renal diseases in those with no diagnosis recorded is the same as in those with a diagnosis. Distribution of primary renal diseases in various countries or regions of Europe is shown in Table 5.

Glomerulonephritis dominated the diagnosis of Japanese patients, possibly because of a lower rate of diagnosis of pyelonephritis/interstitial nephritis.

Analgesic or drug nephropathy caused one in five cases of end stage renal failure in Australia and it occurred with a similar frequency in Switzerland and Belgium, but the high proportions in these small countries are lost in the overall European average of 3.5% of cases. The percentage of patients with analgesic or drug nephropathy decreased from 7% in 1974 to 3% in 1979 in Scandinavian countries where legislation to restrict the sale of phenacetin containing drugs and other analgesics was introduced two decades ago. The condition was not coded for in the Japanese Registry and, although coded in the American data, was not frequently recognised in USA.

Cystic kidney disease accounted for 9% of patients in Australia, Europe and the USA. The very low propor-

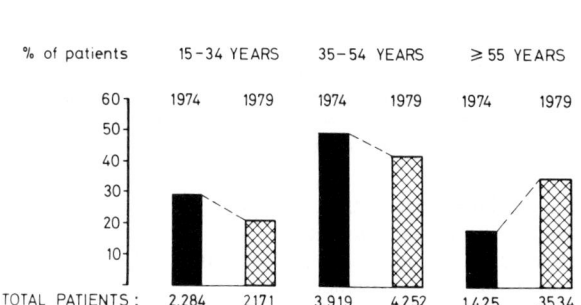

Figure 14. Age distribution of patients starting renal replacement therapy in Europe in 1974 and 1979.

Table 4. Distribution of main primary renal diseases in Australia, Europe, Japan and USA. Analysis of new (1979) patients in Australia, Europe and Japan; of total file for USA where only 49% had a diagnosis recorded (PRD = Primary Renal Disease).

	New patients in 1979			USA All patients on file (Only 49% had PRD recorded)
	Australia	Europe	Japan	
Total patients	463	10,229	7,523	31,276
Glomerulonephritis	35%	30%	71%	30%
Pyelonephritis	7%	21%	3%	13%
Analgesic/drug nephropathy	19%	3%	(Not coded)	1%
Cystic kidney disease	9%	9%	2%	9%
Hypertension/reno-vascular	5%	8%	4%	22%
Diabetic nephropathy	4%	7%	9%	14%
Other PRD	21%	22%	11%	11%

Table 5. Geographical distribution of primary renal diseases, per cent of all patients accepted for replacement therapy in 1979 in European countries. Figures between ( ) refer to 1974. 'Benelux' includes Belgium, Netherlands and Luxembourg and 'Scandinavia' includes Finland with the Nordic countries.

PRD	Benelux	Scandinavia	France	F.R.G.	Italy	Spain	Switzerland	UK	Whole registry
CRF, aetiology uncertain	8.8 (1.1)	3.4 (1.0)	11.4 (4.0)	13.4 (1.5)	12.5 (3.5)	19.5 (5.6)	9.8 (1.0)	13.9 (1.9)	11.1 (2.4)
GN	25.0 (40.3)	30.5 (36.6)	24.8 (35.4)	26.6 (39.0)	31.8 (55.8)	25.8 (49.6)	21.1 (31.3)	31.1 (46.0)	30.7 (45.2)
PN interstitial N	15.3 (13.7)	16.2 (19.0)	17.8 (17.1)	26.2 (29.0)	23.1 (17.0)	18.4 (16.0)	17.5 (20.9)	13.9 (17.3)	21.2 (19.6)
Drug nephropathy	13.4 (11.0)	3.4 (6.9)	1.6 (1.7)	5.0 (4.9)	1.0 (1.0)	0.4 (0.3)	17.5 (19.9)	1.2 (1.4)	3.5 (3.5)
Cystic kidney disease	10.1 (13.5)	11.6 (12.3)	11.7 (9.2)	7.3 (8.5)	7.3 (7.3)	10.0 (6.4)	11.9 (7.0)	12.1 (10.0)	9.2 (9.0)
Heredo-familial	3.1 (2.7)	1.5 (3.1)	4.3 (7.2)	1.6 (3.2)	2.3 (1.2)	3.1 (5.6)	0.5 (6.5)	3.1 (3.5)	2.5 (3.5)
Renal vascular disease	8.2 (4.6)	6.1 (4.5)	12.4 (11.5)	4.8 (2.8)	8.9 (4.7)	9.9 (8.1)	4.6 (2.5)	14.1 (7.0)	7.6 (5.3)
Multi-system diseases	12.4 (4.6)	24.2 (11.7)	11.6 (5.9)	12.1 (5.7)	9.2 (2.7)	7.8 (2.5)	11.3 (5.5)	8.3 (4.8)	10.8 (5.0)
Other	3.8 (8.5)	2.9 (4.8)	4.3 (8.1)	3.0 (5.4)	3.9 (6.8)	4.9 (5.9)	5.7 (5.5)	2.2 (8.2)	3.4 (6.6)

PRD = primary renal disease.
CRF = chronic renal failure.
GN = glomerulonephritis.
PN = pyelonephritis.
Multisystem diseases include diabetes.

tion (2%) in Japan seems less than could be accounted for by the dilutional effect of the high frequency of glomerulonephritis. We have suggested (17) that cystic kidney disease is more common in Northern European countries compared to Southern European countries and there may be some real geographical difference in the frequency of this, the most prevalent congenital renal disease.

End stage renal failure due to hypertension or renovascular disease contributed one in five American patients. This may reflect the high incidence of hypertensive reno-vascular disease in American blacks and (or) the older age of the patients in the USA.

The frequency with which diabetic nephropathy was recorded on different Registries probably owes most to differences in selection policies. In Europe, the number of new patients with diabetes taken on to treatment has increased steadily, and it almost doubled between 1977 and 1980. In 1980, the 847 patients with diabetic nephropathy represented 7.2% of all reported patients commencing treatment for end stage renal disease, according to the EDTA Registry (11). The highest percentages were noted in Northern European countries with 28% in Finland, 19% in Sweden and 12% in Norway. A recent estimate of the proportion of diabetics starting treatment in the USA is 20-25%. The increase in the number of patients undergoing treatment for end stage diabetic nephropathy appears surprising in view of the pessimistic statements issued in the early 1970's about the results of treating diabetic patients with dialysis. By the end of 1980, 60.9% of the diabetic patients in Europe were treated by hospital haemodialysis, and very few were on home dialysis (3.7%). Peritoneal dialysis was quite popular for diabetics with an almost equal proportion of patients being treated by intermittent peritoneal dialysis (9.9%) and CAPD (10.1%). Functioning transplants kept 15.4% alive. The proportion of first cadaver grafts given to diabetics increased in the late seventies but wide geographical differences persist (11). Few diabetics were transplanted in France and the UK, whereas many diabetics were being transplanted in the Scandinavian countries as long ago as 1974 and 1975. In 1980, diabetics accounted for 14.5% of first grafts in Norway, for 18.7% in Sweden and 23.5% of the first grafts performed in Finland.

COMPARATIVE SURVIVAL STATISTICS

The life-table method for calculation of patient survival rates was first used in American cancer research programmes (18-21). The method was applied to dialysis patients in 1969 (22) and used to compare dialysed and transplanted patients in 1970 (23). At that time and in subsequent years, many investigators published data for relatively small patient groups from single centres (24-29). These and many further analyses of small numbers of patients differed in results as well as conclusions. Unfortunately, the life-table method has often been used uncritically and applied to unallowably small patient samples. If results are to be meaningful from an actuarial point of view, the group from which survival rates are calculated must include at least 20 deaths and cumulated survival statistics must not be extended beyond the time interval with the last death. The advantage of survival calculations based on a single centre is that patient selection criteria are likely to be more uniform than in a combined study. However, not only patient selection

Table 6. Per cent actuarial survival according to age groups for different methods of treatment, EDTA Registry (17).

Method of treatment / Age groups	Total registry up to 1979 Sample size	5 yr %	10 yr %	Starting each treatment 1977–79 Sample size	1 yr %	2 yr %	3 yr %
Centre haemodialysis							
15–34	20,425	66	54	6,305	91	84	80
35–44	15,828	58	40	5,271	88	80	73
45–54	18,010	50	27	6,989	88	79	71
55–64	10,953	41	18	5,452	85	73	64
65+	4,448	27	—	2,982	78	61	51
Home haemodialysis							
15–34	3,802	82	73	1,235	98	95	93
35–44	3,091	77	53	1,072	96	92	91
45–54	3,019	68	43	1,209	95	90	87
55–64	1,153	57	—	596	94	87	78
After first CAD graft							
15–34	6,525	69	55	2,364	89	86	83
35–44	4,268	56	42	1,577	84	77	72
45–54	3,461	46	30	1,244	75	67	65
55–64	951	33	19	406	66	58	50
After first LD graft							
15–34	1,547	73	63	474	92	88	85
35–44	428	67	54	145	93	91	—

CAD = Cadaver graft.
LD = Living donor graft.

criteria but also bias regarding a wide variety of factors, may be more uniform. What would appear to be right for one centre may then be wrong for others. The so called 'centre effect' was studied in the United Kingdom where delivery of health care through its National Health Service can be assumed to be more uniform and consistent than in other countries. Nevertheless, death rates for patients on any form of therapy varied more than three fold between centres, and first cadaveric graft survival at 2 years ranged from 82% in the 'best' to 20% in the 'worst' centre (30).

For these reasons the following discussion has been restricted mainly to survival calculations of the EDTA Registry, which by now is the only large international venture of collecting and providing data on patients with end stage renal disease on combined treatment programmes by any form of dialysis and renal transplantation. Table 6 summarises 1 to 3 year survival figures for patients commencing treatment between 1977 to 1979 as well as 5 and 10 year survival for all patients registered since the beginning of the EDTA Registry in 1964 up to the end of 1979 (17). It should be noted that many patients with end stage renal disease, who have survived beyond the 10 year mark, have benefited from integrated treatment of dialysis and transplantation. At the end of 1979 there were more than 3,000 patients on the files of the EDTA Registry who had lived longer than 10 years on renal replacement therapy (11). Forty per cent were treated by dialysis alone, but transplantation contributed to the survival of 60% of these living patients and 14% were transplanted more than once. Fifteen per cent had a graft that had been functioning for more than 10 years.

Three major factors, method of treatment, age at start of treatment and to some extent primary renal disease, determine patient survival and are discussed below. Sex appears not to have any influence (31), despite a different distribution of primary renal diseases between male and female patients with end stage renal disease.

Survival as related to the method of treatment

Survival for patients on home haemodialysis has usually been found superior to survival on hospital haemodialysis and survival with a living donor transplant better than with a cadaveric transplant. However, this kind of comparison must be unfair to the different methods, since the groups of patients undergoing these different types of treatment are far from comparable or randomised or carrying similar risk factors for dying. Patient groups on dialysis and with transplants may differ because of the availability of, and the policy regarding recipient selection for renal transplantation. Active transplantation of low risk patients may remove good risk patients from the haemodialysis group leaving the poor risk patients on dialysis. On the other hand, there may be selection of poor risk patients for the transplanted group if transplantation is used as a way of no return for patients doing extremely poorly on dialysis.

Selection of patients is partly the reason for better

results observed in the home dialysed group. Clinical selection criteria include absence of 'high risk' medical complications, good nutrition and social conditions plus, usually, a well motivated partner. Further selection occurs because of the mortality of the early months of dialysis in the hospital required for stabilising and training before patients commence home dialysis. Deaths during this period count as death on hospital dialysis and effectively select out some of the high risk patients from entering home dialysis programmes. Social, psychological or medical reasons compelling home patients to return to hospital dialysis might also select out a group at higher risk of dying. The EDTA Registry has therefore adopted the convention of including this group within the home haemodialysis population for survival calculations and death supervening after an unlimited time of hospital haemodialysis following home haemodialysis has been considered as death in the home haemodialysis group.

The varying contribution of home dialysis to different national programmes and the economic factors and practical problems which have determined its role have been discussed above. In the UK, where two thirds of all dialysed patients are treated at home, the survival rate for home dialysis is below the European average, suggesting that selection of British patients for this mode of treatment is dictated more by economic than medical considerations.

For renal transplantation, survival calculations must distinguish between patient and graft survival. Patient survival is defined as the period beginning with the day of the transplant operation until either the day of the death of the patient or the conclusion of the period of observation. This may include periods of dialysis or re-transplant after the first transplant has ceased to function. Graft survival is defined as the period beginning with the day of the transplant until either transplant failure (including death with functioning transplant) or the conclusion of the period of observation.

Until recently, peritoneal dialysis has been used as a definitive form of treatment for a small number of patients only, the majority of them concentrated in a few centres with specialised interest in this form of treatment. With the advent of CAPD a dramatic increase in the use of the peritoneum as dialysis membrane has occurred. One group of Canadian authors have proposed that up to 50% of patients with end stage renal failure might be suitable candidates for CAPD (32). Little can be said about patient survival on CAPD as compared to other methods of treatment since patients of advanced age and those with haemodynamic instability, ischaemic heart disease and diabetes have been started preferentially on CAPD by many centres (11). Nevertheless, actuarial one year survival on CAPD started in 1978 to 1979 as treatment of first choice was similar to that on hospital haemodialysis with $87 \pm 4\%$ for 130 patients in the age group 55 to 64 years and $81 \pm 3\%$ for 401 patients older than 65 years on the EDTA Registry files.

Some centres have attempted to compare survival rates of their dialysis patients with those treated in an integrated programme of dialysis and renal transplantation (33). For the integrated treatment group, survival calculations began with commencement of dialysis, regardless of the length of wait for a transplant. Another approach to compare survivals with different methods of treatment is to calculate the mean waiting time for a transplant and to correct the transplant survival rate to begin at this time (34).

Survival as related to age at start of treatment

Age at start of treatment plays a decisive role in determining survival on all forms of dialysis as well as for living donor and cadaver transplantation (Table 6). Survival rates become significantly worse with increasing age at commencement of the relevant therapy. Thus, there was a 15% difference in 3 year survival of the age group 15 to 34 years compared to that of 55 to 64 years, both for home and hospital haemodialysis patients, and of over 30% for recipients of first cadaver transplants (17). Because of this fact, patients more than 55 years of age are not considered as candidates for transplantation in some centres.

Survival as related to primary renal disease

Survival rates in dialysed and transplanted patients cannot be compared for different primary renal diseases unless the groups compared are homogeneous with respect to age and other 'high risk' factors, such as hypertension. Roberts (35) has analysed the survivals achieved in 1063 patients trained for home dialysis between 1967 and 1973. Sex ratio and distribution of renal diseases among the patients were comparable to those found in other large series and no significant differences in age existed between the groups of patients with various renal diseases, except for those with polycystic kidneys whose average age was slightly higher. No differences in survival rates were found when the patients with glomerulonephritis, pyelonephritis and polycystic renal disease were compared with each other. All these patients tended to have a longer survival than did patients with hypertensive, diabetic and other systemic renal disease. However, European centre dialysis patients aged 45 to 54 years with polycystic renal disease (36) were shown to have better survival rates than those achieved by all dialysed patients of the same age group (74% versus 62% at 3 years). No difference in survival rates was found for polycystic patients after renal transplantation when compared to an age-matched group of transplanted patients with other renal diseases. Since transplantation in patients with polycystic kidneys produced average survival, whereas dialysis results were strikingly better than average, it was suggested (36) that particularly cogent reasons would be necessary to advise transplantation in patients with polycystic kidney disease.

Knowledge of survival rates in patients with renal failure secondary to metabolic and systemic diseases is gaining importance as a sharp increase in their proportion among patients with end stage renal disease has occurred during the last decade. Average survival for patients with diabetic nephropathy (irrespective of age) was 63% at 1 year, 40% at 2 years and 32% at 3 years after start of hospital dialysis, compared to 87%, 77% and 69% of all patients on file of the EDTA Registry between 1976 and 1980 (11). Similarly poor survival for diabetic patients was recorded by an American group in 1976 (37). Patient survival of the younger group of diabetics after cadaveric transplantation was 55% at 1 and 44% at 3 years between 1976 and 1980. However, the selected recipients of living related donor transplants achieved much higher patient survival, approaching 80% at 3 years (11).

Rarer systemic diseases which have increased in frequency according to the EDTA Registry include amyloidosis with 1.4%, lupus erythematosus with 1.4% of females and 0.3% of males and haemolytic uraemic syndrome with 0.4% of new patients in 1979 (17). Two years after start of hospital dialysis, survival rate for patients with lupus was 23% worse than average and 10% worse for those with amyloidosis (36). Less than 50% of patients with myeloma survived 1 year (17). Long term survivals were often observed after renal transplantation in patients with lupus, amyloidosis and cystinosis. In contrast, survival rates were extremely poor in patients with oxalosis, whether treated by dialysis or transplantation (38-40).

Factors affecting graft survival

Worldwide and European comprehensive statistics showed a slight improvement in cadaver graft survival up to the late sixties (41, 42). Thereafter, patient survival rates continued to rise slowly or plateaued but, in contrast, graft survival rates fell slowly but unrelentingly for both living related donor and cadaveric transplants (31, 36, 41, 43-45). Terasaki and colleagues (45) explained this deterioration by suggesting that an increasing number of non-transfused patients had been receiving transplants. Since 1976, many transplant centres, at least in Europe, have changed their transfusion policy, now refusing transplantation in non-transfused recipients. Concomitantly, results of both patient and graft survival have improved steadily during the last few years (17).

Prognostic factors independent of transplantation immunology

Age
The impact of age on results of transplantation was delineated in the 1975 EDTA Report (36). The number of grafts lost due to rejection was similar in all age groups. It was the frequency of non-immunological complications including death with a functioning graft, that increased in parallel with rising age. First year graft survival was 71% in children, compared to 48% in the 55 to 64 year old recipients of first cadaveric grafts from 1977 to 1979. Therefore, comparison of graft survival statistics requires that groups compared are matched for age at the time of transplantation.

Primary renal diasease
Primary renal disease may recur in the transplanted kidney and compromise graft survival. This is particularly true for oxalosis which, in the absence of special precautions (46), almost invariably leads to rapid destruction of the graft. Amyloid deposition has been observed in renal transplants of patients with amyloidosis but did not appear to affect graft function. In familial Mediterranian fever, amyloid deposition in the graft might be preventable by colchicine prophylaxis (47). Alport's disease, medullary cystic disease, gout, cystinosis and Fabry's disease have not recurred in renal transplants (39, 48). However, transplantation of patients with Fabry's disease is not recommended because they appear to succumb frequently and precociously to infectious and cardiovascular complications (49). Kidneys grafted into diabetic patients have been shown to develop changes of diabetic nephropathy, of which the earliest feature was afferent and efferent arteriolar hyalinosis, but this did not adversely affect graft survival (50). The relatively low graft survival in diabetic patients is largely due to the high frequency of lethal infectious and cardiovascular complications. Diabetics aged 20 to 45 years had a 2 year first cadaver graft survival of 41% which was lower than the 46% in non-diabetic recipients aged 55 to 64 years at the time of transplantation from 1978 to 1980. Living donor grafts in diabetics have done extremely well with 82% surviving at 1 year (11).

Glomerulonephritis does recur quite often (51-53) but is rare among the causes of graft failure (31, 36, 42-44) except in monozygotic twin grafts (54). According to the EDTA Registry, 3 of 34 grafts between monozygotic twins were lost due to recurrence of glomerulonephritis (17). Dense deposit disease (52, 53) appears to recur almost invariably. Anti-glomerular basement membrane (GBM) antibody-induced glomerulonephritis often recurs in the graft, particularly when transplantation is performed before disappearance of anti-GBM-activity in the recipient's serum (55). The nephrotic syndrome associated with focal glomerulosclerosis (51-53) may reappear immediately at transplantation (53, 56). Congenital nephrotic syndrome appears to be curable by transplantation (57). Although rapid loss of graft function has been observed in cases of recurrent glomerulonephritis with the nephrotic syndrome (58), glomerular disease of any form should, in general, not be viewed as a contraindication to transplantation.

Patients with bilateral diffuse renal cortical necrosis were reported to reject transplants almost invariably and often hyperacutely (59). A recent report of successful transplantation in four out of five cases suggests that females with cortical necrosis should not be denied transplantation (60).

Hepatitis B
Toussaint and colleagues (61) reported better than average graft survival in hepatitis B antigen carriers, because antibody response in these individuals is poor. This could not be confirmed by the 1977 EDTA analysis (34)

(which appeared to be in agreement with London and colleagues (62)), which indicated that patients who actively form antibodies against HBAg also stage a more vigorous attack against renal transplants and thus have a higher rate of graft failure by rejection. Pirson and colleagues (63) stressed the high mortality of HBAg positive patients due to hepatic failure 3 to 5 years after transplantation.

Rehabilitation status at the time of transplantation
The rehabilitation status of a patient may be used as a measure to a certain extent of his physical fitness and thus of his ability to withstand the increased stress post transplantation. Indeed, recipients unable to work at the time of transplantation with a first cadaveric graft exhibit a graft survival which is markedly shorter than that of the fitter recipients who were considered able to work (17, 34, 64).

Quality of cadaveric kidneys
That rising donor age would be associated with decreasing cadaveric graft survival (65) is probably not true. Early graft failure rate of cadaveric kidneys from donors older than 50 years was slightly, though not significantly, greater and the failure rate after three months identical to that of grafts from younger donors used in the UK between 1978 and 1980 (30). No correlation has been found between length of warm and cold ischaemia times and graft survival (30, 66). Also simple flushing and cold storage and the more complicated machine preservation techniques have yielded organs of similar quality (30, 66, 67). It appears, therefore, that current evaluation of viability is adequate. Adverse effects on graft survival of anatomical peculiarities such as multiple renal arteries, veins and ureters have not been studied extensively but may be of prognostic significance.

Prognostic factors related to transplantation immunology

Living related donor transplantation
The best survival prognosis is given by HLA identical sibling grafts. These grafts do, in the long run, almost as well as grafts from identical twins, which cannot be rejected but often develop recurrence of glomerulonephritis leading to graft failure (52, 64). HLA identity can be proven by serotyping for the HLA A, B and Dr-antigens as well as by performing a mixed lymphocyte culture. Graft survival in HLA A and B identical sibling donor transplants is currently – at least in transfused recipients (68) – above 90% at one year. Grafts with identity for one haplotype only (which is the case for all parent-child donor-recipient pairs) have a first year survival rate approaching 80% (17). Living donor grafts differing for both haplotypes are rarely performed (17). Recipients of one haplotype identical grafts with a low mixed lymphocyte culture stimulation index also have a first year graft survival approaching 90%, whereas those with a high stimulation index may not do better than recipients of cadaveric transplants (69, 70).

Pretreatment of one haplotype identical recipients with blood transfusions from non-related blood donors (71) or with donor-specific blood transfusions in those recipients with a high mixed lymphocyte culture stimulation index (70) appears to promote excellent graft survival unless cytotoxic antibodies are generated against the prospective donor.

Cadaveric transplantation
ABO matching, sex and race. The last Report of the Human Renal Transplant Registry (72) failed to show that A-recipients retain O-kidneys less well than A-kidneys (73, 74). If there is a difference in graft prognosis between ABO compatible and ABO identical grafts, it must, therefore, be small. The majority of ABO incompatible grafts probably have undergone rapid rejection. However, blood group A_2-kidneys can be transplanted successfully into blood group O-recipients (75). Red cell incompatibilities aside from ABO groups appear to have a marginal effect on graft prognosis (66) with the possible exception of the Lewis antigen system (76). The suggestion of the London transplant group that male kidneys appear to survive better than average in female recipients while female kidneys do worse in female recipients (77) was disproven by a larger British analysis (72). Graft survival in negro and oriental recipients as well as that of negro and oriental kidneys in caucasian recipients does not seem to be lower (78, 79). Previous reports to the contrary (66, 80) find an explanation in the so-called centre effect (78).

HLA matching. According to the most recent and comprehensive international analysis (66), no convincing overall difference in first cadaveric graft survival could be demonstrated between any combination of highly matched, unmatched or highly mismatched groups at the HLA A, B, and Dr locus. Nevertheless, relatively small differences appear to exist in certain patient groups. Thus, male recipients of blood group A, B, and AB, but not females, have better graft survival with increasing matching grade at the HLA A and B locus. By contrast, male recipients of blood group O and female recipients do not seem to profit from a close HLA A and B match (66, 73, 81, 82). The value of Dr matching remains controversial. That first cadaveric grafts well matched at the Dr locus do better (83-85) has not been confirmed by the international co-operative study, with the exception of non-transfused recipients whose otherwise poor graft survival might be improved to the level of that seen in poly-transfused recipients (66, 85).

Cytotoxic antibodies. There is no doubt that hyperacute rejection is often associated with preformed cytotoxic antibodies against HLA determinants. Many observers found lower graft survival in antibody positive recipients, particularly in those having a broad spectrum of antibodies causing cytotoxicity in over 50% of random lymphocyte donors (86-90). However, Opelz and colleagues (68) found no difference in graft survival comparing groups of recipients without antibodies to those with antibodies reacting against 6 to 50% or even against 51 to 90% of a random panel. Only the relatively small group of recipients with lymphocytotoxins reacting against over 90% of random lymphocyte donors had significantly decreased first cadaveric graft survival. Furthermore, there appears to be a large difference according to whether immunisation leads to persistent antibody formation or to transient antibody formation. Only those recipients with persistently detectable antibodies against over 50% of a random panel showed decreased graft survival (68).

Not all lymphocytotoxic antibodies are deleterious for a prospective graft. Grafts performed in the presence of antibodies directed against donor B lymphocytes or even against both T and B lymphocytes may have similar success rates to those in recipients without donor specific antibodies prior to transplantation (91).

Pregnancy. Pregnancy is a well known cause of cytotoxic antibody formation but does not influence subsequent graft prognosis (42, 43, 66).

Blood transfusion. Blood transfusion may transmit hepatitis and other infections or possibly oncogenic viruses apart from inducing cytotoxic antibodies. For these reasons, nephrologists and immunologists likewise had endeavoured to keep blood transfusion to an absolute minimum in patients on dialysis and awaiting transplantation. Increasing success in managing prospective transplant recipients without blood transfusion was held responsible for decreasing graft survival rates up to the early seventies (45, 92). The majority of worldwide retrospective and rarely prospective analyses of graft survival in relation to pre-transplant blood transfusion as well as animal studies have led to the conclusion that pre-transplant blood transfusion is beneficial for renal transplantation (93, 94) and many centres now refuse to operate on non-transfused patients. Some controversy remains about the optimal number of transfusions necessary to obtain a maximal enhancing effect in prospective recipients. A positive correlation has been found between the number of pre-transplant transfusions and subsequent graft survival by international analysis (66, 94), while a single unit of leucocyte poor blood according to a Dutch prospective study (95) or two units of leucocyte poor blood according to a Swedish study (96) has been all that was needed to obtain excellent graft survival. The enhancing effect of blood transfusions cannot be achieved by frozen blood (94, 97) or leucocyte free blood (95).

Time on dialysis before transplantation. According to the 1976 EDTA analysis (64), first cadaveric grafts survived better if the recipients had been dialysed for more than 2 years as compared to those dialysed for 1 to 2 years or for less than 1 year in particular. Prolonged dialysis was associated with a lower rate of graft loss by rejection. The whole explanation for this 'dialysis effect' on subsequent graft survival appears to be the increased number of blood transfusions or the decreased number of non-transfused recipients (66), and the change in transfusion policy of many European centres is probably the reason that the effect of prolonged time on dialysis on subsequent graft survival is disappearing (17).

Splenectomy. According to the Minnesota experience, splenectomy might improve cadaveric graft survival but not patient survival (98), confirming a trend shown by the last analysis of the Human Renal Transplant Registry (74). However, if death with a functioning graft is included as a cause of graft failure, no difference in first cadaveric graft survival comparing splenectomised to other recipients has been obtained in the UK (30). Most centres do not perform splenectomy in preparation for transplantation in view of the frequency of subsequent infectious and thromboembolic complications.

Bilateral nephrectomy. The Human Renal Transplant Registry twice published statistics on graft survival with or without bilateral removal of the patient's own kidneys and both times showed slightly superior outcome in the nephrectomy group (41, 99). This was particularly significant for polycystic renal disease (41). Nevertheless, it would be entirely wrong to fall back into the bad habit of performing routine bilateral nephrectomy in every transplant candidate. Firstly, there is some mortality for this operation which might reduce the number of high risk transplant candidates entering the nephrectomised group. Secondly, the most compelling explanation for the small difference in graft survival (55% in nephrectomised versus 50% in non-nephrectomised patients one year after a cadaveric graft, irrespective of primary renal disease [41]) was probably the need for blood transfusion which is higher amongst anephric patients.

Re-transplantation. Good agreement has been reached by a number of studies concerning the factors determining the prognosis of re-transplants. Average graft survival rates for second transplants (living related donor or cadaveric) have usually been found slightly lower than for first transplants and drastically reduced for third and fourth grafts (17, 31, 36, 42-44, 100, 101). However, second cadaveric grafts showed highly significantly better survival than the first grafts in the same recipient group (101). Bad prognostic signs for re-transplants are early loss by rejection of the previous graft (34, 64, 100-104) and the formation of cytotoxic antibodies after a failed graft (100-103). That repetition of two or more of the same HLA A or B mismatches would adversely affect second graft survival (100) has not been confirmed by a more recent and expanded analysis (101), but close HLA A and B matching appears to be of importance in recipients of re-transplants who have cytotoxic antibodies (87, 100, 102). Re-grafts fully matched at the Dr locus may do better than Dr mismatched re-grafts (66). Excellent graft survival has been obtained in second grafts when the first graft functioned for more than one year (34, 64, 100-102), and also in third grafts when the second graft functioned for more than 1 year (101).

CAUSES OF DEATH

Death rates

We have introduced the calculation of death rates using actuarial methods (105) in order to compare the relative

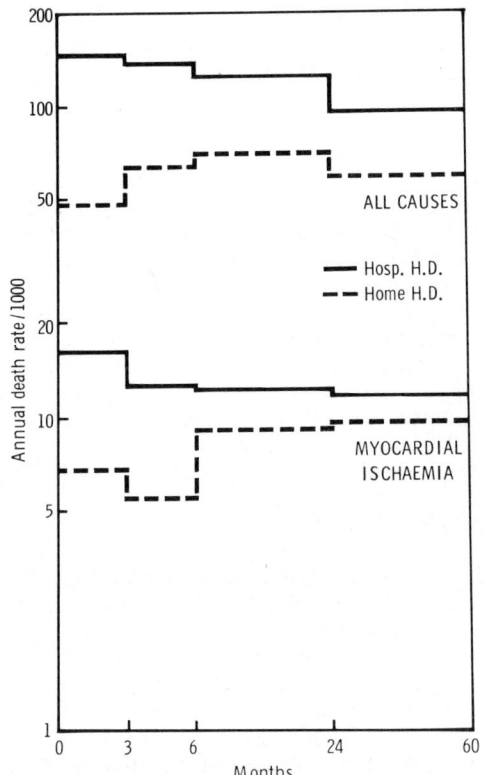

Figure 15. Annual death rates per 1000 patients on haemodialysis due to all causes and due to myocardial ischaemia in the age group 35-54 years, according to time on treatment.

risks of different causes of death in dialysis and transplant patients with the risks in the general population and at different times after commencing treatment.

Myocardial ischaemia
Figure 15 shows annual death rates related to time on dialysis in patients aged 35 to 54 years. More than one tenth of the total death rate was accounted for by myocardial ischaemia and infarction. This cause of death had almost the same rate in home dialysis patients as in hospital dialysis patients, except that the rate was higher during the early months of hospital haemodialysis compared to the lower rate during the early months of dialysis in the home. Death rate remained stable with time on treatment.

Figure 16 shows the same death rates in recipients of a first cadaver graft. Death rate due to all causes was high for the first 6 months, but thereafter fell below the death rate in dialysis patients (Figure 15). Death rate due to myocardial ischaemia was high initially, but stabilised 6 months after transplantation to a rate similar to that in dialysis patients and, because it remained constant, was responsible for an increasing proportion of the diminishing overall death rate in the later period.

The death rate due to myocardial ischaemia did not accelerate during treatment in either dialysed patients, as suggested by Lindner and colleagues (106), or in

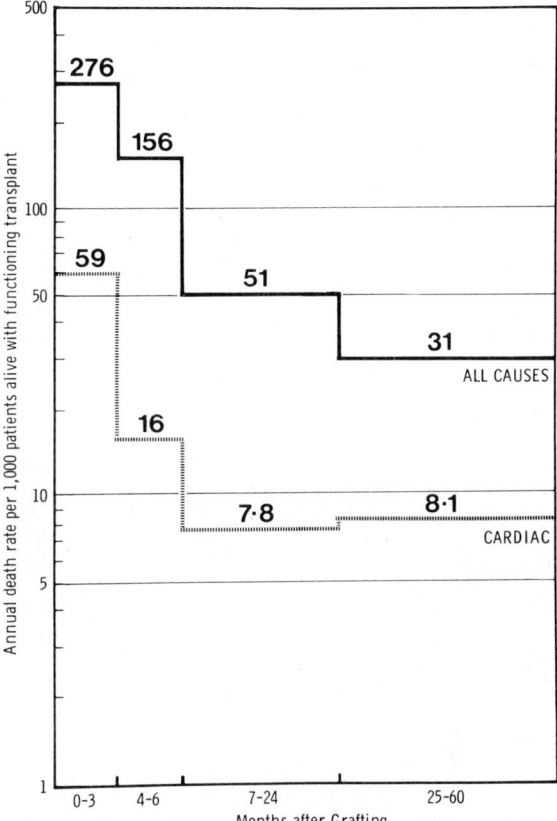

Figure 16. Annual death rates with functioning first cadaver graft due to all causes and cardiac causes according to time after transplantation.

transplanted patients. However, comparison of the death rate due to myocardial ischaemia and infarction in all patients on renal replacement therapy in 1978 with that of a control population impressively demonstrates the high death rate due to coronary disease in renal patients. While renal patients over 55 years had a death rate of some 10 times that of the general population, coronary deaths were some 150 times more frequent in younger renal patients aged 15 to 34 years (105).

Cerebrovascular accident
Compared to the population of France, where cerebrovascular accident was intermediately frequent as a cause of death, patients on renal replacement therapy older than 55 years had a death rate from cerebrovascular accident which was some 20 times, those aged 35 to 54 years some 50 times and those aged 15 to 34 years some 250 times higher than the general population (105).

Malignancy
Death rate in dialysis patients aged 55 years or more due to malignant disease, excluding that possibly induced by immunosuppressive therapy, was stable around 10 per 1,000 during the first 5 years of hospital dialysis. Death rate due to malignancies in patients on hospital haemo-

Table 7. Death rates per 1000 hospital haemodialysis patients of all ages at risk according to cause of death.

Causes of death	1977	1978	1979
Myocardial ischemia and infarction	12.3	11.9	13.5
Cardiac failure or arrest	36.6	34.9	30.3
Cerebro-vascular accident	17.0	13.9	15.1
All cardiac and vascular causes	71.0	66.2	63.2
Hyperkalaemia	4.2	4.8	5.3
Septicaemia	8.4	7.6	7.9
All infectious causes	17.2	15.7	14.6
Suicide and/or refusal of treatment	2.2	2.3	2.3
Cachexia	3.8	4.7	4.7
Malignant disease *not* induced by immunosuppressive therapy	4.2	6.4	6.0
Dementia	3.3	2.9	2.9
Other causes	11.3	12.9	11.6
Cause of death uncertain/not determined	–	0.4	3.6
All causes of death	117.2	116.3	114.2

dialysis in all countries reached some three to six times that of cancer in the general population of England and Wales in comparable age groups (105).

Malignant disease, possibly induced by immunosuppressive therapy, in patients with functioning first cadaver transplants caused a low death rate in the first 3 months, but by 6 months rose to 2.3 per 1,000. This death rate remained stable indicating that malignant disease in relation to other causes of death became an increasingly important killer of patients alive with a functioning transplant during the later periods. After 2 years, 1 in every 14 deaths in patients with a functioning graft was due to malignant disease possibly induced by immunosuppressive therapy (105, 107).

All causes

Tables 7 and 8 summarise the death rate analyses which we have carried out for hospital haemodialysis and transplant patients in each of the years 1977 to 1979 (17, 105). Death rates have decreased in both treatment categories despite increasing age of the patient populations and have been notably reduced in the transplant recipients, particularly by a reduction in death rate due to infectious causes. These results reflect improvements in patient care and it is particularly encouraging that this can be shown on pooled results for all European countries as well as in a seven centre study recently reported from the USA (108).

QUALITY OF LIFE

Results of dialysis and transplantation have been assessed not only according to survival achieved but also by the quality of life enjoyed by the patients. Cost effective analysis of expensive medical endeavour seems likely to require such an audit in any competition for scarce medical resources. The EDTA Registry has developed a simple methodology to quantitate patients' quality of life. We have collected information on rehabilitation to work, hospitalisation and disabling bone disease (17).

Rehabilitation

The patients' work status was linked to the potential occupation expected if he or she was healthy. Thus, patients whose rehabilitation target was full time education, housework, or retirement were excluded from the analysis. Table 9 compares rehabilitation in male and female patients and on different modes of treatment. Over 80% of males on home dialysis or with functioning grafts had a potential occupation of full time employment. A smaller percentage of men on hospital haemodialysis (66%) and of all female patients had full time employment recorded as their potential occupation. Amongst those with this rehabilitation target, the distribution of rehabilitation status was similar in male and female patients on the same treatment. Hospital haemodialysis interfered with the performance of full time work, although many patients managed part time work.

Rehabilitation status was compared for haemodialysis and transplanted patients in different countries. A high proportion of patients worked full time in Italy, Portugal, Israel and Spain and this suggests that dialysis schedules were arranged to suit working hours in these countries. Suitable part time work seems to be most easily obtained in the GDR, Switzerland, Finland, Czechoslovakia and Poland. Work was not available for more than 15% of patients who were fit enough for it in Greece, the UK, Bulgaria, the Netherlands, the FRG and Hungary.

Table 8. Death rates per 1000 recipients with functioning first cadaver grafts at risk according to cause of death.

Causes of death	1977	1978	1979
Myocardial ischaemia and infarction	7.7	5.7	5.2
Cardiac failure or attest	4.8	4.3	4.0
Cerebro-vascular accident	3.0	2.8	5.0
All cardiac and vascular causes	19.5	14.6	16.7
Septicaemia	8.1	8.3	4.4
All infectious causes	24.1	17.0	12.3
Gastro intestinal haemorrhage	1.4	2.3	1.3
Malignant disease possibly induced by immunosuppressive therapy	1.8	2.5	1.3
Other identified causes	8.6	9.6	8.4
Cause of death uncertain not determined	–	0.2	0.8
All causes of death	55.4	46.2	40.8

Table 9. Rehabilitation of male and female patients whose potential occupation was full time employment ('Category 2').

Mode of treatment	Number of patients	% patients with potential occupation ('Category 2')	\% patients in each rehabilitation category					
			1	2	3	4	5	6
Male								
Hospital dialysis	14,278	65.5	35.7	20.6	13.2	14.5	14.2	1.9
Home dialysis	4,261	81.5	62.1	13.0	8.2	10.0	6.2	0.4
Living donor transplant	730	85.1	81.5	3.6	3.4	5.4	5.8	0.2
Cadaver donor transplant	3,526	85.1	66.9	12.6	7.1	6.9	6.0	0.4
Female								
Hospital dialysis	11,037	26.8	39.6	29.7	7.9	8.1	12.9	2.0
Home dialysis	1,756	33.2	67.5	20.4	4.0	2.9	5.2	0
Living donor transplant	348	53.4	82.8	6.1	3.7	1.8	5.5	0
Cadaver donor transplant	2,263	44.5	67.0	17.9	6.0	3.1	5.2	0.9

1 = Able to work and working full time (including return to full time housework).
2 = Able to work and working part time (including return to part time housework).
3 = Able to work but not working: no work available.
4 = Able to work but not working: earning capacity less than social security benefits, e.g. State pension.
5 = Unable to work: living at home, able to care for most personal needs (variable amount of assistance required).
6 = Unable to care for self: requires hospital care or equivalent at home.

More than 25% of patients, able to work, had an earning capacity below social security benefits or state sickness pension in Yugoslavia, Bulgaria, Hungary and Czechoslovakia (17). This analysis is therefore not only an assessment of the patient's fitness but also of local employment and sickness payments under the different economic and social conditions of European countries.

Hospitalisation

Replies about hospitalisation were coded according to whether the patient was hospitalised for a total of more than 3 months, less than 3 months or definitely never hospitalised. Results in the age group 35 to 54 years are shown in Figure 17. In both patient groups approximately 9% of the patients were hospitalised more than 3 months during the first year of treatment, after that the proportion of patients who required lengthy hospitalisation was smaller in the transplanted group. Patients who returned to hospital haemodialysis after failure of their graft were particularly likely to have more than 3 months' hospitalisation at this critical juncture in their management (17).

Disabling bone disease

Analysis of disabling bone disease compared patients on hospital haemodialysis with patients alive with a functioning first cadaver graft who received no more than 1 year pre-transplant dialysis (Figure 18). In both groups the proportion with disabling bone disease increased with length of treatment, and after 5 years 14% of the

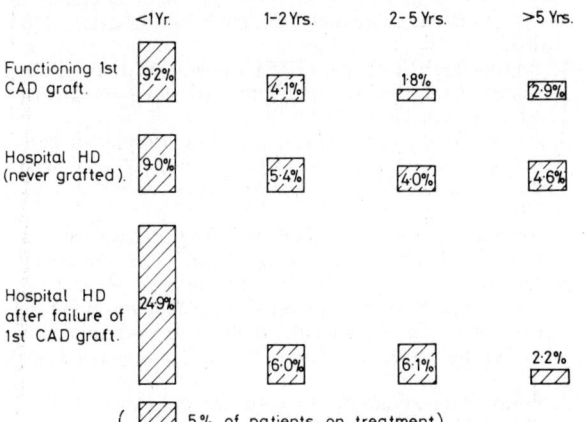

Figure 17. Hospitalisation for more than three months (excluding admission for routine dialysis, routine post-transplant check or research) in 1979 according to mode and length of treatment in patients aged 35-54 years.

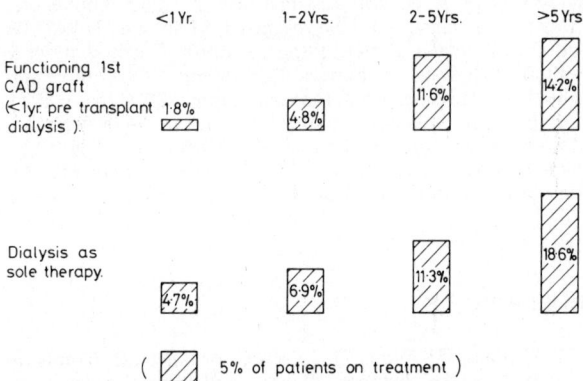

Figure 18. Disabling bone disease (bone pain requiring regular analgesics, fracture(s), major deformity, aseptic necrosis and slipped epiphysis) in 1979 according to mode and length of treatment.

successfully transplanted and 19% of the dialysed patients suffered with this complication (17). Control of bone disease is crucial to the well being of longer term survivors (11).

CONCLUSIONS

There is widespread concern to record activity in dialysis and transplantation and this appears to be felt, not only by doctors practising in the field but also by politicians, health care planners, patient activist groups and editors of medical journals. Demographic analyses on pooled data collected by central Registries have shown that national programmes are developing along different lines. The impact of CAPD is beginning to be felt. Economic factors have overriding importance.

The age distribution of patients varies and there are apparent differences in the distribution of primary renal diseases, some of which may represent true geographical variations while others may be due either to differences in diagnostic fashions or in the availability of facilities.

Patient and graft survival has improved in recent years. Death rates due to all causes have fallen, particularly those due to infections. Quality of life as measured by rehabilitation to work, hospitalisation and prevalence of disabling bone disease appears acceptable but has not improved and a regular percentage of patients have a poor quality of life.

Haemodialysis in hospital and home, peritoneal dialysis and transplantation are complementary forms of treatment. The trend is to offer all treatments in an integrated programme (see also Chapter 43). The choice for any particular individual patient will be governed by what is available as well as by the results given in this chapter. Long term survivors who have been treated for more than 10 years have mostly received mixed treatment (11). The appropriate mode of treatment for a patient may change with altered medical or domestic circumstances. With increased awareness of the prospects and problems, patients may be expected to make their own request for changes in treatment.

ACKNOWLEDGEMENTS

Figures 3, 8, 9, 10, 11, 14, 15, 16, 17, 18 and Tables 4, 6, 7 and 10 have been reproduced from Reports of the EDTA Registry published by Pitman Medical, London with the permission of the Editor, Dr. B. H. B. Robinson.

Figure 1 and Table 1 have been reproduced from Recent Advances in Renal Disease II, Editors N.F. Jones and D.K. Peters, with the permission of the Editor and the publishers, Churchill Livingstone, Edinburgh, London.

The authors gratefully acknowledge the courtesey of Messrs. Travenol Ltd, UK, who provided the figures for Table 2.

We particularly thank the doctors and their staff who have completed EDTA Registry questionnaires. Information from countries reporting to other organisations was provided by Dr. T. Mathew, (Adelaide, South Australia), (Australia and New Zealand), Dr. A. G. S. Shimizu, Associate Professor, McMaster University, St. Joseph's Hospital, Hamilton, Ontario (Canada), Prof. T. Inou, Director, Registry for Japanese Transplantation, Surgical Dept. of Medical Research Inst. of Tokyo University, School of Medicine, 4-6-1 Shiroganedai, Minatoku, Tokyo 108 and Dr. M. Odaka, Director, Reg. for Japan. Haemodialysis & Peritoneal Dialysis, 2nd Surgical Department, Chiba University School of Medicine, 1-8-1 Inohana, Chiba 280 (Japan), Prof. K. I. Furman, Medical School, University of Witwatersrand, Hospital Street, Johannesburg (South Africa), Dr. C. R. Blagg (North West Kidney Center, Seattle, U.S.A.) and Ms. M. McMullan (Health Care Financing Administration, U.S.A.).

REFERENCES

1. Gurland HJ, Wing AJ, Jacobs C, Brunner FP: Comparative review between dialysis and transplantation. In *Replacement of Renal Function by Dialysis,* edited by Drukker W Parsons FM, Maher JF, The Hague, Boston, London, Martinus Nijhoff, 1978, p 663
2. Wing AJ, Selwood NH: Registry data, a collaborative exercise. *Proc 8th Int Congr Nephrol (Athens).* Edited by Zurukzoglu W, Papadimitriou M, Pyrpasopoulos M, Sion M, Zamboulis, Basel, New York, Karger 1981, p 571
3. Mathew TH: *Third Report of the Australian and New Zealand combined dialysis and transplant registry,* Adelaide, Australia, 1981
4. Shimizu A: Dialysis in Canada today. *Int J Artif Organs* 4:41, 1981
5. Health Care Financing Administration (Baltimore, Md): End stage renal disease: *Second Annual Report to Congress,* Department of Health and Human Services, USA, 1980
6. Ianhez LE, Aguiar JA, Ajzen H, Fo FS, Knijnik R: Tratamento do paciento renal cronico terminal en Brasil (Treatment of patients with terminal chronic renal failure in Brazil). *J Bras Nefrol* 1:43, 1979 (in Spanish)
7. Wing AJ, Selwood NH: Achievements and problems in the treatment of end stage renal failure. In: *Recent Advances in Renal Disease,* II, edited by Jones NF and Peters DK, London, Edinburgh, Churchill Livingstone, p 103, 1982
8. Burton BT, Hirschman GH: Demographic analysis: End stage renal disease and its treatment in the United States. *Clin Nephrol* 11:47, 1979
9. Evans RW, Blagg CR, Bryan FA: Implications for health care policy – a social and demographic profile of hemodialysis patients in the United States. *JAMA* 245:487, 1981
10. Relman AS, Rennie D: Treatment of end-stage renal disease: free but not equal. *N Engl J Med* 303:996, 1980
11. Jacobs C, Broyer M, Brunner FP, Brynger H, Donckerwolcke RA, Kramer P, Selwood NH, Wing AJ, Blake PH: Combined report on regular dialysis and transplantation in Europe, 1980, XI. *Proc Eur Dial Transpl Assoc* 18:2, 1981
12. Editorial (anonymous): An appalling panorama. *Br Med J* 281:1028, 1980
13. Parsons V, Lock P: Triage and the patient with renal failure. *J Med Ethics* 6:173, 1980
14. Laing W: Renal failure; a priority in health? *Office of Health Economics,* 162 Regent Street, London No 62, 1978

15. Mechanik D: Approaches to controlling the costs of medical care. *N Engl J Med* 298:249, 1978
16. World Bank Atlas, *World Bank* 1818 H Street N.W. Washington D.C. 20433, 1980
17. Brynger H, Brunner FP, Chantler C, Donckerwolcke RA. Jacobs C. Kramer P, Selwood NH, Wing AJ: Combined report on regular dialysis and transplantation in Europe, X, 1979. *Proc Eur Dial Transpl Assoc* 17:2, 1980
18. Berkson J, Gagie RP: Calculation of survival rates for cancer. *Proc Staff Meet Mayo Clin* 25:270, 1950
19. Cutler SJ, Ederer F: Maximum utilization of the life table method in analyzing survival. *J Chronic Dis* 8:699, 1958
20. Ederer F, Axtell LM, Cutler SJ: The relative survival rate: a statistical methodology. *Natl Cancer Inst Monogr* 6:101, 1961
21. Merrell M, Shulman LE: Determination of prognosis in chronic disease, illustrated by systemic lupus erythematosus. *J Chronic Dis* 1:12, 1955
22. Lewis EJ,. Foster DM, de la Puente J, Scurlock C: Survival data for patients undergoing chronic intermittent hemodialysis. *Ann Intern Med* 70:311, 1969
23. Gurland HJ, Härlen H, Henze H, Spoek MG: Intermittent dialysis and renal transplantation in Europe: Survival rates. *Proc Eur Dial Transpl Assoc* 7:20, 1970
24. Calne RY, Shackman R, Nolan B, Petrie J, Woodruff M: Results of kidney transplantation. *Lancet* 1:671, 1970
25. Cameron JS, Ellis FG, Ogg CS, Bewick M, Boulton-Jones M, Robinson RO, Harrison J: A comparison of mortality and rehabilitation in regular dialysis and transplantation. *Proc Eur Dial Transpl Assoc* 7:25, 1970
26. Moorhead JF, Baillod RA, Hopewell JP, Knight AJ, Crockett RE, Fernando ON, Varghese Z: Survival rates of patients treated by home and hospital dialysis and cadaveric renal transplantation. *Br Med J* 4:83, 1970
27. Gross JB, Keane WF, McDonald AK: Survival and rehabilitation of patients on home hemodialysis: five years' experience. *Ann Intern Med* 78:341, 1973
28. Sweatman AJ, Baillod RA, Moorhead JF: Comparison of home dialysis and other treatments for chronic renal failure. *Practitioner* 212:56, 1974
29. Lowrie EG, Lazarus JM, Mocelin AJ: Survival of patients undergoing chronic hemodialysis and renal transplantation. *N Engl J Med* 288:863, 1973
30. UK Transplant Service, Southmead Rd., Bristol UK, *Annual Report* 1980
31. Brunner FP, Giesecke B, Gurland HJ, Jacobs C, Parsons FM, Schärer K, Seyffart G, Spies G, Wing AJ: Combined report on regular dialysis and transplantation in Europe, V, 1974. *Proc Eur Dial Transpl Assoc* 12:3, 1976
32. Fenton SSA, Cattran DC, Allan AF, Rutledge P, Ampil M, Dadson J, Locking H, Smith SD, Wilson DR: Initial experience with continuous ambulatory peritoneal dialysis. *Artif Organs* 3:206, 1979
33. Mathew TH, Marshall VC, Vikraman P, Hill AVL, Johnson W, McOmish D, Morris PJ, Kincaid-Smith P: Integrated programme of dialysis and renal transplantation. *Lancet* 2:137, 1975
34. Wing AJ, Brunner FP, Brynger H, Chantler C, Donckerwolcke RZ, Gurland HJ, Hathway RA, Jacobs C, Selwood NH: Combined report on regular dialysis and transplantation in Europe, VIII, 1977. *Proc Eur Dial Transpl Assoc* 15:3, 1978
35. Roberts JL: Analysis and outcome of 1,063 patients trained for home hemodialysis. *Kidney Int* 9:363, 1976
36. Gurland HJ, Brunner FP, Chantler C, Jacobs C, Schärer K, Selwood NH, Spies G, Wing AJ: Combined report on regular dialysis and transplantation in Europe, VI, 1975. *Proc Eur Dial Transpl Assoc* 13:2, 1976
37. Comty CM, Kjellsen D, Shapiro FL: A re-assessment of the prognosis of diabetic patients treated by chronic dialysis therapy. *Trans Am Soc Artif Intern Org* 22:404, 1976
38. Jacobs C, Rottembourg J, Reach I, Legrain M: Treatment of terminal renal failure due to oxalosis: case report and results of a co-operative study of 14 patients. *Proc Eur Dial Transpl Assoc* 11:359, 1974
39. Barnes BA, Bergan JJ, Braun WE, Fraumeni JF Jr, Kountz SL, Mickey MR, Rubin AL, Simmons RL, Stevens LE, Wilson RE: Renal transplantation in congenital and metabolic diseases. A report from the ASC/NIH renal transplant registry. *JAMA* 232:148, 1975
40. Donckerwolcke RA, Chantler C, Broyer M, Brunner FP, Brynger H, Jacobs C, Kramer P, Selwood NH, Wing AJ: Combined report on regular dialysis and transplantation of children in Europe. *Proc Eur Dial Transpl Assoc* 17:87, 1980
41. Barnes BA, Bergan JJ, Braun WE, Fraumeni JF Jr, Kountz SL, Mickey MR, Rubin AL, Simmons RL, Stevens LE, Wilson RE: The twelfth report of the human renal transplant registry. *JAMA* 233:787, 1975
42. Brunner FP, Gurland HJ, Härlen H, Schärer K, Parsons FM: Combined report on regular dialysis and transplantation in Europe, II, 1971. *Proc Eur Dial Transpl Assoc* 9:3, 1972
43. Gurland HJ, Brunner FP, v. Dehn H, Härlen H, Parsons FM, Schärer K: Combined report on regular dialysis and transplantations in Europe, III, 1972. *Proc Eur Dial Transpl Assoc* 10:XVI, 1973
44. Parsons FM, Brunner FP, Burck HC, Gräser W, Gurland HJ, Härlen H, Schärer K, Spies GW: Statistical report IV, 1973. *Proc Eur Dial Transpl Assoc* 11:3, 1974
45. Terasaki PI, Opelz G, Mickey MR: Analysis of yearly kidney transplant survival rates. *Transplant Proc* 8:139, 1976
46. Morgan JM, Hartley MW, Miller AC, Diethelm A: Successful renal transplantation in hyperoxaluria. *Arch Surg.* 109:430, 1974
47. Jacob ET, Bar-Nathan N, Shapira Z, Gafni J: Renal transplantation in the amyloidosis of familial mediterranean fever. *Arch Intern Med* 139:1135, 1979
48. Spence MW, MacKinnon KE, Burgess JK, d'Entremont DM, Belitsky P, Lannon SG, MacDonald AS: Failure to correct the metabolic defect by renal allotransplantation in Fabry's disease. *Ann Intern Med* 84:13, 1976
49. Maizel SE, Simmons RL, Kjellstrand C, Fryd DS: Ten-year experience in renal transplantation for Fabry's disease. *Transplant Proc* 13:57, 1981
50. Mauer SM, Barbosa J, Vernier RL, Kjellstrand CM, Buselmeier TJ, Simmons RL, Najarian JS, Goet FC: Development of diabetic vascular lesions in normal kidneys transplanted into patients with diabetes mellitus. *N Engl J Med* 295:916, 1976
51. Dixon FJ, McPhaul JJ, Lerner R: Recurrence of glomerulonephritis in the transplanted kidney. *Arch Intern Med* 123:554, 1969
52. Hamburger J, Berger J, Hinglais N, Descamps B: New insights into the pathogenesis of glomerulonephritis afforded by the study of renal allografts. *Clin Nephrol* 1:3, 1973
53. Mathew TH, Mathews DC, Hobbs JB, Kincaid-Smith P: Glomerular lesions after renal transplantation. *Am J Med* 59:177, 1975
54. Glassock RJ, Feldman D, Reynolds ES, Dammin GJ, Merrill JP: Human renal isografts: a clinical and pathological analysis. *Medicine* 47:411, 1968
55. Wilson CB, Dixon FJ: Anti-glomerular basement membrane antibody-induced glomerulonephritis. *Kidney Int.*

3:74, 1973

56. Hoyer JR, Raij L, Vernier RL, Simmons RL, Najarian JS, Michael AF: Recurrence of idiopathic nephrotic syndrome after renal transplantation. *Lancet* 2:343, 1972
57. Hoyer JR, Mauer SM, Kjellstrand CM, Buselmeier TJ, Simmons RL, Michael AF, Najarian JS, Vernier RL: Successful renal transplantation in 3 children with congenital nephrotic syndrome. *Lancet* 1:1410, 1976
58. Cheigh JS, Mouradian J, Susin M, Stubenbord WT, Tapia L, Riggio RR, Stenzel KH, Rubin AL: Kidney transplant nephrotic syndrome: relationship between allograft histopathology and natural course. *Kidney Int* 18:358, 1980
59. Gelfand MC, Friedman EA: Prognosis of renal allotransplants in patients with bilateral renal cortical necrosis. *Transplantation* 10:442, 1970
60. Silke B, Spenser S, Hanson S, Carmody M, O'Dwyer WF: Renal transplantation in cortical necrosis of pregnancy. *Dial Transpl* 9:1023, 1980
61. Toussaint C, Thiry C, Kinnaert P, Clinet G, Vereerstraeten P, Van Geertruyden P: Prognostic significance of hepatitis B antigenemia in kidney transplantation. *Nephron* 17:335, 1976
62. London WT, Drew JS, Blumberg BS, Grossman RA, Lyons PJ: Association of graft survival with host response to hepatitis B infection in patients with kidney transplants. *N Engl J Med* 296:241, 1977
63. Pirson Y, Alexandre GPJ, van Ypersele de Strihou C: Role of HBs antigenaemia in liver disease after renal transplantation. *Proc Eur Dial Transpl Assoc* 13:193, 1976
64. Jacobs C, Brunner FP, Chantler C, Donckerwolcke RA, Gurland HJ, Hathway RA, Selwood NH, Wing AJ: Combined Report on dialysis and transplantation in Europe, VIII, 1976. *Proc Eur Dial Transpl Assoc* 14:3, 1977
65. Darmady EM: Transplantation and the ageing kidney. *Lancet* 2:1046, 1974
66. Opelz G, Terasaki PI: Study of histocomptability in renal transplantation. *Transplantation* 33:87, 1982
67. Blohmé I, Brynger H: Clinical kidney preservation with Sacks' solution. *Scand J Urol Nephrol* (Suppl) 54:81, 1980
68. Opelz G, Mickey MR, Terasaki PI: Blood transfusions and kidney transplants: remaining controversies. *Transplant Proc* 13:136, 1981
69. Cochrum KC, Salvatierra O Jr, Perkins JA, Belzer FO: MLC testing in renal transplantation. *Transplant Proc* 7 (suppl 1):659, 1975
70. Salvatierra O Jr, Amend W, Vincenti F, Potter D, Cochrum KC, Hopper S, Hanes D, Iwaki J, Opelz W, Terasaki PI, Duca R, Feduska NJ: Pretreatment with donorspecific blood transfusions in related recipients with high MLC. *Transplant Proc* 13:142, 1981
71. Brynger H, Frisk B, Larsson O, Sandberg L: Planned third-party transfusions prior to first transplantations from living related donors. *Scand J Urol Nephrol* (Suppl) 64, 152, 1981
72. Barnes BA, Bergan JJ, Braun WE, Fraumeni JF Jr, Kountz SL, Mickey MR, Rubin AL, Simmons RL, Stevens LE, Wilson RE: The 13th report of the human renal transplant registry. *Transplant Proc* 9:9, 1977
73. National Organ Matching Service, Southmead Rd., Bristol, UK, *Annual Report* 1975-1976
74. National Organ Matching Service, Southmead Rd., Bristol, UK, *Annual Report* 1977-1978
75. Brynger H, Blohmé L, Lindholm A, Samuelsson B, Rydberg L, Sandberg L: Transplantation of cadaver kidneys from blood group A, donors to 'O' recipients. *Transplant Proc* 14:195, 1982
76. Lenhard V, Roelcke D, Dreikorn K, Wernet P, Muller G, Wilms H, Halbfass HJ, Gumbel B, Albert FW, Ewald RW, Sprenger-Klasen I, Fischer M, Goldmann SF: Significance of Lewis and HLA system in kidney transplantation: a multicenter study in Germany. *Transplant Proc* 13:930, 1981
77. Festenstein H, Sachs JA, Paris AM, Pegrum GD, Moorhead JF: Influence of HL-A matching and blood-transfusion on outcome of 502 London Transplant group renalgraft recipients. *Lancet* 1:157, 1976
78. Perdue ST, Terasaki PI: Analysis of interracial variation in transplant and patient survival. *Transplantation* 34:75, 1982
79. McDonald JC, Vaughan W, Filo RS, Mendez Picon G, Niblack G, Spees EK, Williams GM: Cadaver donor renal transplantation by centers of the south eastern organ procurement foundation. *Ann Surg* 193:1, 1981
80. Opelz G, Mickey MR, Terasaki PI: Influence of race on kidney transplant survival. *Transplant Proc* 9:137, 1977
81. UK Transplant *Annual Report*, Southmead Rd., Bristol, UK 1978-1979
82. Opelz G, Terasaki PI: Influence of sex on histocompatibility matching in renal transplantation. *Lancet* 2:419, 1977
83. Ting A, Morris PJ: Matching for B-cell antigens of the HLA-Dr series in cadaver renal transplantation. *Lancet* 1:575, 1978
84. Persijn GG, Gabb BW, van Leeuwen A, Nagtegaal A, Hoogeboom J, van Rood JJ: Matching for HLA antigens of A, B, and Dr loci in renal transplantation by Eurotransplant. *Lancet* 1:1278, 1978
85. Moen T, Albrechtsen D, Flatmark A, Jakobsen A, Jervell J, Halvorsen S, Solheim BG, Thorsby E: Importance of HLA-Dr matching in cadaveric renal transplantation. *N Engl J Med* 303:850, 1980
86. Opelz G, Mickey MR, Terasaki PI: HL-A and kidney transplants: re-examination. *Transplantation* 17:371, 1974
87. van Hooff JP, Schippers HMA, van der Steen GJ, van Rood JJ: Efficacy of HL-A matching in Eurotransplant. *Lancet* 2:1385, 1972
88. Oliver RTD, Sachs JA, Festenstein H, Pegrum GD, Moorhead JF: Influence of HL-A matching antigenic strength and immune responsiveness on outcome of 349 cadaver renal grafts. *Lancet* 2:1381, 1972
89. Dausset J, Hors J, Busson M, Festenstein H, Oliver RTD, Paris AMI, Sachs JA: Serologically defined HL-A antigens and long-term survival of cadaver kidney transplants. *N Engl J Med* 290:979, 1974
90. Stenzel KH, Whitsell JC, Cheigh JS, Riggio RR, Stubenbord WT, Sullivan JF, Rubin AL, Fotino M: Effects of HL-A matching and immune responsiveness on cadaver kidney graft survival. *Transplant Proc* 6:89, 1974
91. Morris PJ, Ting A: The crossmatch in renal transplantation. *Tissue Antigens* 17:75. 1981
92. Opelz G, Sengard DPS, Mickey MR, Terasaki PI: Effect of blood transfusions on subsequent kidney transplants. *Transplant Proc* 5:253, 1973
93. Van Es AA, Balner H: Effect of pretansplant transfusions on kidney allograft survival. *Transplant Proc* 9:127, 1979
94. Opelz G, Terasaki PI: Dominant effect of transfusions on kidney graft survival. *Transplantation* 29:153, 1980
95. Persijn GG, Lansbergen Q, Cohen B, Van Leeuwen A, D'Amaro J, Parleviet J, Van Rood JJ: Two major factors influencing kidney graft survival in Eurotransplant: HLA-Dr matching and blood transfusion(s). *Transplant Proc* 13:150, 1981
96. Frisk B, Brynger H, Wedel N, Sandberg L: Blood transfusion in cadaveric renal transplant patients – a prospective

study. *Scand J Urol Nephrol* (Suppl) 64:100, 1981
97. Opelz G, Terasaki PI: Poor kidney- transplant survival in recipients with frozen blood transfusions or no transfusions. *Lancet* 2:696, 1974
98. Fryd DS, Sutherland DER, Simmons RL, Ferguson RM, Kjellstrand CM, Najarian JS: Results of a prospective randomized study on the effect of splenectomy versus no splenectomy in renal transplant patients. *Transplant Proc* 13:48, 1981
99. Advisory committee to the renal transplant registry: The 10th Report of the human renal transplant registry. *JAMA* 221:1495, 1972
100. Opelz G, Terasaki PI: Recipient selection for renal re-transplantation *Transplantation* 21:488, 1976
101. Opelz G, Terasaki PI: Absence of immunization effect in human kidney re-transplantation. *N Engl J Med* 299:369, 1978
102. Claes G, Gustavsson A, Heidemann M: Outcome of renal re-transplantation. *Proc Eur Dial Transpl Assoc* 13:152, 1976
103. Freier DT, Haines RF, Rosenzweig J, Neiderhuber J, Konnak J, Turcotte JG: Sequential renal transplants: some surgical and immunological implications on management of the first homograft. *Surgery* 79:262, 1976
104. Casali R, Simmons RL, Ferguson RM, Mauer SM, Kjellstrand CM, Buselmeier TJ, Najarian JS: Factors related to success or failure of second renal transplants. *Ann Surg* 184:145, 1976
105. Brunner FP, Brynger H, Chantler C, Donckerwolcke RA, Hathway RA, Jacobs C, Selwood NH, Wing AJ: Combined report on dialysis and transplantation in Europe, IX, 1978. *Proc Eur Dial Transpl Assoc* 16:3, 1979
106. Lindner A, Charra B, Sherrard DJ, Scribner BH: Accelerated atherosclerosis in prolonged maintenance hemodialysis. *N Engl J Med* 290:6, 1974
107. Jacobs C, Brunner FP, Brynger H, Chantler C, Donckerwolcke RA, Hathway RA, Kramer P, Selwood NH, Wing AJ: Malignant diseases in patients treated by dialysis and transplantation in Europe. *Transplant Proc* 8:729, 1981
108. Belzer FO, Corry R, Diethelm A, Mendez R, Salvatierra O, Tilney N, Cerrilli J: Current results and expectations of renal transplantation. *JAMA* 246:330, 1981

48

PLASMA EXCHANGE: PRINCIPLES AND PRACTICE

ANDREW J. REES

Introduction	872
Technique of plasma exchange	872
Methods of separation	873
Centrifugation	873
Plasma filtration	873
Techniques for specific removal of toxic macromolecules	873
Anticoagulation	873
Vascular access	873
Replacement solutions	874
Plasma protein fraction	874
Freeze dried plasma	874
Fresh frozen plasma	874
Hazards of plasma exchange	874
Electrolyte disturbance	874
Expansion of intravascular volume	874
Infection	874
Effects of plasma exchange	874
Immunoglobulins	875
Inflammatory mediators	875
Effect on circulating antigen-antibody complexes	875
Concomitant immunosuppressive therapy	875
Use of plasma exchange in management of renal disease	876
Background	876
Antiglomerular basement membrane mediated nephritis	876
Background	876
Results	876
Control of anti-GBM antibody synthesis	876
Clinical response	877
Renal function	877
Pulmonary haemorrhage	877
Relapses	877
Deaths	877
Summary	877
Crescentic nephritis not due to antiglomerular basement membrane antibody	877
Background	877
Results	878
Cryoglobulinaemia	878
Systemic lupus erythematosus	878
Renal transplantation	879
Thrombotic thrombocytopenic purpura	880
Use of plasma exchange in other diseases	880
Conclusion	880
References	880

INTRODUCTION

Plasmapheresis was introduced to increase the harvest of plasma from blood donors and soon after to remove myeloma protein from patients with hyperviscosity syndromes (1, 2). Originally units of blood were collected from patients and centrifuged individually, the packed cells being then reinfused together with crystalloid solutions. With this technique a maximum of 1 to 2 l of plasma could be removed on each occasion. Later the development of automated methods for cell separation, capable of removing 3 to 4 l of plasma at a single session, made it feasible for the first time to use plasma exchange in the treatment of severe immunologically mediated disease.

The rationale for such treatment was the removal of autoantibodies, pathogenic immune complexes and inflammatory mediators, and the attraction was the rapidity with which this could be achieved, perhaps before conventional drug treatment could be effective. Additionally it is now clear that plasma exchange has a profound effect on the rate of antibody synthesis and the clearance of immune complexes. It can also be used to restore deficient plasma factors.

Two questions must be asked of any new treatment; firstly, whether it works and secondly, what its effectiveness is in relation to more conventional treatment. It has to be conceded that for plasma exchange there has been great difficulty in answering these questions. One problem is that plasma exchange has frequently been used in conjunction with immunosuppressive drugs and often it has been used to treat rare or fulminant diseases. These are the circumstances in which conventional controlled clinical trials are least effective and presently the value of plasma exchange has only been assessed by detailed monitoring of individual patients, collection of results from small groups of patients and by unsatisfactory comparison with historical controls. Although it is impossible to make a definitive statement about the place of plasma exchange in renal disease none-the-less some conclusions can be made.

TECHNIQUE OF PLASMA EXCHANGE

Manual plasma separation has been replaced by automated methods using either centrifugation or filtration through large pore membranes. These have the great advantage that 2 to 4 l exchanges can be completed in under 2 h with little discomfort to the patient. Even so they do bring attendent problems: the need for a skilled operator to avoid rapid changes of plasma volume, vascular access capable of withstanding blood flows of more than 100 ml per minute, and large supplies of replacement fluid. It is the last of these that has been most troublesome and the daily cost and supply of 4 l of plasma or plasma substitute has limited the application of plasma exchange. One way round this problem is to remove the toxic macromolecules specifically whilst reinfusing the rest of the patient's plasma. Satisfactory systems, however, are not generally available although removal of IgG by its affinity for staphylococcal protein A (3) or specific antibody by affinity columns (4) and more recently double membrane separations (5) and cryoseparation (6, 7) have been described.

Methods of separation *

Separation of plasma from cells is achieved either by centrifugation or by filtration through membranes with exclusion coefficients in excess of 1 million daltons (8–10). Available evidence suggests there is little to choose between the efficacy of the different methods.

Centrifugation

Three different centrifugal systems have been extensively used and others will be available soon. The Aminco Celltrifuge and IBM 2997 systems are similar. Blood is drawn into a centrifuge bowl from which plasma can be withdrawn separately from leucocytes, platelets and erythrocytes. Thus during plasma exchange the cellular components are reinfused continuously together with replacement fluid whilst the patient's plasma is discarded. These systems are efficient and have small extracorporeal volumes but capital costs are relatively high and the machines are rather cumbersome.

The other centrifugal system, Haemonetics Model 30, is simpler and is semicontinuous. Blood is pumped into the centrifuge bowl and the plasma withdrawn until the bowl is filled with packed cells which are then returned to the patient before the bowl is filled again. This prolongs the duration of exchange and also increases the extracorporeal volume particularly of packed cells which can cause symptoms in severely anaemic patients with a haemoglobin concentration below 8 g/dl. The main advantages of the Haemonetics system is its robustness and portability which means it can be readily moved to the intensive care unit or bedside.

Plasma filtration

Initial experience with plasma filters rapidly demonstrated their simplicity and efficiency. They need no complex equipment, just blood pumps and arterial and venous pressure monitors (9). The Asahi PF01 has been widely tested but may be replaced by the more recently introduced PF02 (now known as the HI05). Both have cellulose diacetate hollow fibre membranes of 0.5 µm pore size housed in a dialyser casing. The PFO2 has a smaller surface area (0.5 m^2 compared to 0.65 m^2) but because of its thinner membrane (75 µm compared to 160 µm) has better performance and excludes molecules larger than 2 to 3 million daltons (11).

Both devices work best with a blood-flow rate between 70 and 150 ml/min and with transmembrane pressures less than 50 mm Hg. Pressures above 100 mm Hg are liable to cause haemolysis. At the start of exchange the filtrate line should be clamped and then released very slowly to avoid the pores becoming clogged with protein. Even when this is done there is a tendency for the efficiency of the PFO1 to diminish with time but this is not evident with the PFO2.

The great advantage of membrane filters is their simplicity and the lack of capital outlay. But they are expensive and cannot be reused.

There is likely to be little difference in the therapeutic effects of the PFO2 and centrifugal plasma exchange and the choice of separation technique should be dictated by local facilities.

Techniques for specific removal of toxic macromolecules

Various systems have been described for more specific removal of toxic macromolecules such as IgG (3), specific antibody (4), and molecules greater than 100,000 daltons (5, 6). These abolish the need for large volumes of plasma replacement fluid as the patient's own albumin may be returned. However, insufficient experience using these techniques has been reported yet to allow useful comment.

Anticoagulation

Anticoagulants are needed to maintain the extracorporeal circuit irrespective of which technique is used. Heparin and acid citrate dextrose (ACD) have both been used and are equally effective. We routinely use heparin, giving an initial dose of 2,000 U and thereafter a continuous infusion throughout the separation. When ACD is used it must be in the B form because the higher citrate content of ACD-A may cause cardiac arrhythmias (12). The anticoagulants have relatively little systemic effect as they are largely removed with the plasma. This is just as well because platelets are consumed to some extent by all plasma exchange procedures and intrinsic coagulation factors are removed (13, 14).

Vascular access

Initially we used arterio-venous shunts for vascular access in most patients but the high incidence of shunt infections in these immunosuppressed patients having daily exchanges led us to abandon this practice wherever possible. We now use either the antecubital veins or, when this is not possible, insert catheters into the inferior or superior vena cava.

---

* Terminology: *Plasma separation* refers to any technique for separating blood into plasma and cells; *plasmapheresis* refers to removal of plasma and its replacement with crystalloid; *plasma exchange* is used when replacement is made with a protein containing solution.

Replacement solutions

The application of plasma exchange has been limited considerably by the need for large volumes of plasma as replacement fluid and it remains to be tested whether the present attempts to circumvent this problem will be successful. Replacement fluids for large volume exchanges should have a high oncotic pressure for substitution of crystalloid for plasma (that is plasmapheresis) is liable to be complicated acutely by the development of oedema. Similarly the use of large volumes of synthetic substitutes such as dextran or hydroxystarch (Haemocel) should be avoided. The most commonly used replacement fluids in plasma exchange are plasma protein fraction (PPF), freeze dried plasma, and fresh frozen plasma (FFP).

Plasma protein fraction
PPF is essentially a 5% solution of albumin prepared by Cohn fractionation. It contains no immunoglobulins, complement or procoagulants and cannot transmit hepatitis. Some preparations, although not those available in the United Kingdom, contain a bradykinin like substance which has been blamed for hypotension in some patients during exchange. PPF has a very low risk of transfusion reactions (we haven't seen one in over 2,000 exchanges) and most of the unwanted effects are caused by its electrolyte content. PPF has a high sodium concentration (often 150 to 160 mmol/l) together with low potassium and calcium concentrations and some preparations are alkaline because of a high citrate and low chloride concentration (15, 16).

Freeze dried plasma
Freeze dried plasma has also been used as replacement fluid. It contains immunoglobulin but like PPF has few biologically active mediators. Its sodium and potassium content are similar to plasma. Its use in exchange cannot be recommended because of the unacceptably high incidence of transfusion reactions and the risk of hepatitis.

Fresh frozen plasma
FFP also carries a risk of transfusion reactions and of hepatitis. It can be useful, though, in specific circumstances as a source of biologically active mediators such as complement, procoagulants and other less defined substances necessary for the control of coagulation and inflammation. We regularly infuse 2 units of FFP at the end of a 4 l plasma exchange in patients who have had a recent biopsy or are at risk from haemorrhage. The indications for using FFP as the only replacement fluid are more speculative: it may be advantageous to restore complement concentrations to normal in patients with genetic deficiencies (17), it has been suggested that patients with systemic lupus erythematosus (SLE) have a more prolonged remission after plasma exchange using FFP than after exchanges using PPF (18). In some patients with thrombotic thrombocytopenic purpura, infusions of large volumes of FFP, made possible by plasma exchange, can restore the normal capacity of endothelial cells to produce prostacyclin (19, 20). Whether these effects are important is still uncertain (19, 20). Finally, there is a danger of aggravating injury when fresh complement is infused into patients whose plasma contains activating factors such as cryoglobulins.

HAZARDS OF PLASMA EXCHANGE

In an experienced unit the hazards associated with plasma exchange are few. It shares in common with all extracorporeal circuits the necessity for accurate control of plasma volume, the danger of air embolism and the risks of anticoagulation. In addition there are a few specific complications that should be avoided.

Electrolyte disturbance

In the early days of plasma exchange there were numerous reports of acute hypocalcaemia and hypokalaemia due to infusions of large volumes of albumin solution deficient in these cations. This can be prevented easily by the addition of calcium chloride (0.45 mmol) and potassium chloride (1.4 mmol) to each unit (400 ml) of PPF. In patients with renal failure metabolic alkalosis caused by infusion of high citrate/low chloride containing solution can be prevented by use of a more appropriate solution (15). Sodium overload has been less frequently commented on but, given the average sodium concentrations of PPF as about 150 mmol/l, a 4 l exchange will impose an obligatory sodium load of 50 to 60 mmol. Patients with renal failure may need intensive dialysis to maintain a correct sodium balance.

Expansion of intravascular volume

In addition to the effect of sodium loading, expansion of intravascular volume will accompany an abrupt increase in plasma albumin brought about by plasma exchange. This is a particularly troublesome cause of hypertension in nephrotic children so in these patients we routinely reduce the albumin concentration of replacement fluids by diluting with 5% dextrose.

Infection

It is difficult to quantitate the risk of infection in patients receiving plasma exchange. Arterio-venous shunt infections were very common when used for vascular access. Prevention of intercurrent infection is very important because it may provoke a relapse of the underlying disease (21), therefore we avoid the use of arterio-venous shunts wherever possible. With this proviso plasma exchange by itself probably confers little additional risk of infection (22), but any effect of immunosuppressive drugs may be magnified (23).

EFFECTS OF PLASMA EXCHANGE

There is little uniformity in the intensity with which plasma exchange has been practiced, partly because of the constraints imposed by the cost and supply of replacement fluids. In some diseases, such as those mediated by autoantibodies to glomerular basement membrane (anti GBM disease) and cryoglobulins, the dose of exchange can be tailored to control the titre of the pathogenic molecules. More commonly ignorance of what these molecules are, or the inability to measure them, dictates that the intensity of treatment must rest on assumptions about the mechanism of injury and predicted rates of removal of antibody molecules, immune complexes and inflammatory mediators.

The extent of removal of macromolecules depends on their intravascular/extravascular distribution, their reequilibration after plasma exchange and their resynthesis time. For example, single 2 and 4 l plasma exchanges will remove about 70% and 90% respectively of an intravascular substance such as IgM compared to 50% and 70% respectively of IgG of which less than half is present within the circulation (13). There are probably no practical consequences dependent on rates of reequilibration, but differing rates of resynthesis have a marked effect. Plasma concentrations of immunoglobulins (13) and complement (13, 24) can be maintained at less than 30% of normal by repeated plasma exchange whilst a protein with a much greater synthesis rate, such as the acute phase C-reactive protein, is barely affected by the most vigorous regimen of exchanges.

Resynthesis rates of individual proteins vary depending on the circumstances; infections or other causes of acute inflammation increase the synthesis of many proteins including complement, fibrinogen and immunoglobulin as well as that of classical acute phase proteins. Similarly immunosuppressive drugs have a general effect and reduce synthesis of many proteins. The effect of plasma exchange on specific proteins will now be considered.

Immunoglobulins

As described in the preceding section a single 4 l plasma exchange will remove about 60% of the total IgG from an adult man and by inference a similar proportion of specific antibody. By repeated plasma exchange, the serum concentrations of IgG, IgM and IgA can be maintained well below the normal range. Hypoglobulinaemia is prolonged for months after repeated plasma exchange (25, 26) in some healthy subjects but more usually concentrations return to normal within a few weeks. The rate of resynthesis may be delayed by concomitant administration of immunosuppressive drugs.

The synthesis rate of immunoglobulins is merely the average for all individual antibody molecules, which will vary considerably. This disparity has been extensively studied in patients with anti-GBM disease in which repeated exchanges, sufficient to produce very low IgG concentrations, may have a trivial effect on anti-GBM antibody titres (27), unless immunosuppressive drugs are given concomitantly, perhaps because removal of specific antibody may increase resynthesis.

In practice the rebound of antibody titre to higher than pre-exchange values as reported in experimental animals after primary immunisation (28, 29), has not been a problem. The concomitant use of immunosuppressive drugs is probably the main reason for this. In fact they may act synergistically with plasma exchange to selectively 'switch-off' vigorous antibody responses (30). There is also evidence that plasma exchange may qualitatively affect antibody production and change the isotypes of IgG produced (31).

Inflammatory mediators

Most inflammatory mediators have both intravascular and extravascular distribution and a high synthesis capacity. Nevertheless repeated plasma exchange will reduce concentrations of complement components C3, C4 and factor B (13, 24).

Similarly concentrations of other procoagulants are drastically reduced (13, 14). Fresh frozen plasma can be used instead of PPF to maintain their concentrations within the normal range.

Effect on circulating antigen-antibody complexes

Although antigen-antibody complexes undoubtedly cause injury in experimental models of nephritis it remains controversial whether deposition of circulating complexes or their formation in situ is the more important. Although there is no direct evidence for the pathogenicity of immune complexes detected in serum from patients with glomerulonephritis, they may be readily removed by plasma exchange. It is also possible that their formation is limited by concurrent removal of constituent antibody and antigen. More interesting is the observation that plasma exchange may enhance endogenous clearance of immune complexes. Small volume plasma exchange, without other treatment, frequently has a greater effect on the immune complex titre than can be explained by mere physical removal (32, 33). The suggestion of improved endogenous clearance is supported by the observation that titres of immune complexes continue to fall after the end of an exchange (33). This may be due to the effect of plasma exchange on reticuloendothelial function (RES). Defective RES function, assessed by splenic clearance of IgG coated autologous erythrocytes, is common in patients with severe systemic lupus erythematosus or systemic vasculitis (33, 34) and is rapidly and selectively improved by plasma exchange (33).

Concomitant immunosuppressive therapy

Except when used for experimental purposes, such as defining the effect of plasma exchange on splenic function, plasma exchange has rarely been used as the single component of therapy. Although it complicates the interpretation of results there are sound theoretical reasons for combining plasma exchange with immunosuppressive drugs. In antibody mediated diseases they limit antibody synthesis (35) and there is some evidence that the combination of intensive plasma exchange and immunosuppressive drugs result in a premature switch off of antibody formation (30). The case for combined therapy is less clear in putative immune complex disease. Nevertheless, we have generally used a regimen of prednisolone 60 mg/day, cyclophosphamide 3 mg/kg/day (scaled down to the nearest 50 mg) and azathioprine 1 mg/kg/day (scaled down to the nearest 50 mg). Azathioprine is omitted in patients over 55 years of age. The dose of steroids has been reduced rapidly, generally to less than 20 mg/day within one month.

USE OF PLASMA EXCHANGE IN MANAGEMENT OF RENAL DISEASE

Background

The use of therapeutic plasma exchange will always be limited by expense and because it is cumbersome. It will have to offer substantial advantages before it can be accepted generally as treatment for a particular disease. Many enthusiastic reports imply that it does just this but in only a few circumstances is the case already established. When used as part of a multiple treatment for crescentic nephritis it is usually easy to identify an effect of the treatment as a whole but much more difficult to define the effects of individual components of the regimen. This is a very difficult area for conventional controlled clinical trials which are at their weakest when assessing rare, severe and potentially heterogeneous conditions. Besides the problem of accumulating enough patients it may prove impossible to match the study groups sufficiently for meaningful comparisons to be made. Multicentre trials have been advocated as a way round these difficulties but inevitably these introduce fresh variables and it is to be doubted whether even they will answer the question of how to treat the most severely affected patients.

It is even more difficult to determine any effect on diseases, such as chronic nephritis, which evolve over many years. The problem of designing an appropriate treatment regimen without knowledge of the precise pathogenesis or having suitable ways to monitor disease activity seems insuperable. This, together with the duration of therapy required before an anticipated effect occurs, should be sufficient to deter most investigators from the use of plasma exchange in these circumstances.

It may occasionally be rational to use plasma exchange as a purely experimental tool to define the importance of plasma factors in the generation of disease. This has been best illustrated by studies in patients with myasthenia gravis which finally established the pathogenicity of antibodies to acetylcholine receptors (36). Subsequently plasma exchange has found a small but definite place in the management of myasthenia gravis (37, 38). An example of plasma exchange used for this purpose in nephrology is the investigation of circulating permeability factors in the nephrotic syndrome. In patients who have focal segmental sclerosis immediate proteinuria after transplantation has been modified by exchange in some patients (39).

Antiglomerular basement membrane mediated nephritis

Background
The pathogenicity of anti-GBM antibodies is established (40) and they are a rare cause of glomerulonephritis. Typically, this has a rapidly progressive course accompanied by irreversible renal failure which develops in days or weeks; less commonly the nephritis may be indolent (41). Between a half and three quarters of patients also have pulmonary haemorrhage (Goodpastures syndrome). Diagnosis is made by characteristic linear staining of immunofluorescent preparations of renal biopsies and by measurement of anti-GBM antibodies in serum by radioimmunoassay (42, 43). Untreated the outlook is dismal and Wilson and Dixon (44) reported that none of 39 untreated patients with severe disease and only 1 of 29 treated with steroids and cytotoxic drugs retained renal function.

Results
It is against this background that results with plasma exchange must be judged. We originally reported improvement in renal function in a small series of patients treated by intensive plasma exchange (45) and have now treated a total of 41 patients. Usually daily 4 l plasma exchanges are continued for 14 days or until evidence of disease activity has subsided. These exchanges are combined with prednisolone, cyclophosphamide and azathioprine in doses described in the preceding section. Patients are monitored by repeated measurement of circulating anti-GBM antibodies and by indices of renal and pulmonary injury.

Control of anti-GBM antibody synthesis
Titres of anti-GBM antibodies fell in every patient after introduction of this regimen. In some patients they became permanently undetectable in less than 3 weeks (30). There are other reports on the effect of plasma exchange on anti-GBM antibodies (27, 46–49). Reduction in antibody titre may occur in an occasional patient with immunosuppressive drugs alone (44), and occasionally with small volume plasma exchange, but immediate control can only be achieved in the majority when intensive plasma exchange is combined with immunosuppressive drugs.

Although anti-GBM antibody synthesis is self limiting the rapidity with which it was terminated in our patients was surprising and was probably directly related to plasma exchange. When a group of clinically similar patients, matched for initial antibody titre, for the amount of immunosuppressive drugs they received and differing only in the intensity of plasma exchange, were compared, antibody switch off occurred significantly more rapidly in patients who had more than 12 exchanges compared to those in whom exchanges were less intensive (30). The reason for this more rapid switch off is not known. The simplest explanation is that removal of antibody by exchange provoked proliferation of antibody forming cells and rendered them more susceptible to cytotoxic drugs. However, it is possible to speculate about other mechanisms such as an effect of removal of GBM-antigen or of wholesale removal of antibody on the immunological network (50).

Clinical response

Renal function. Unsurprisingly the response to treatment with the plasma exchange regimen depends on the severity of the initial injury. None of 19 patients who had severe oliguria (urine volume less than 400 ml/24 h) had a worthwhile improvement in renal function. The prognosis in those patients whose plasma creatinine concentration was greater than 600 µmol/l (6.8 mg/dl) was also poor; only one of the five regained useful renal function. By contrast 15 of 17 patients with a plasma creatinine concentration below 600 µmol/l improved even when the creatinine level was rising rapidly (30). Subsequent follow up of up to 7 years showed renal function had deteriorated in only two, both of whom had developed hypertension with slowly progressive renal failure but without the reappearance of circulating anti-GBM antibodies.

Pulmonary haemorrhage. Thirty three patients had pulmonary haemorrhage but when plasma exchange was introduced it was rapidly controlled in 29. It continued in the remaining four patients, each of whom was infected and required positive pressure ventilation. Infection can severely exacerbate pulmonary and renal injury in anti-GBM disease (21).

Relapses. Some patients have had pulmonary or renal relapses after the start of treatment; 22 of 30 relapses were immediately associated with intercurrent infection, most frequently of the arterio-venous shunt. Fluid overload can also cause relapse of pulmonary haemorrhage (21) which is of practical importance because of the obligatory sodium load that occurs with plasma exchange.

Deaths. Fifteen of the 41 patients have died, 7, each of whom was anuric, during the initial period of hospitalisation and 8 subsequently. Four of the early deaths were caused by uncontrolled pulmonary haemorrhage, one died following a myocardial infarction and two died when dialysis support was withdrawn from patients not considered suitable for long term treatment. Two late deaths were from pulmonary haemorrhage in regular dialysis patients not treated by plasma exchange in other hospitals, two were from infection and four from complications of dialysis or transplantation.

A number of case reports of patients with anti-GBM disease have been reported as well as a few small series – none of more than five patients. These results, although difficult to interpret, are broadly similar to our own. Immediate improvement of renal function, related to starting plasma exchange with immunosuppressive drugs, has been reported (46–55) always in patients with some residual renal function and usually with plasma creatinine concentrations less than 600 µmol/l (6,8 mg/dl). Failure to improve has also been reported (27, 47, 48, 54, 56), always in patients who were either anuric or who had plasma creatinine concentrations above 800 µmol/l (9.0 mg/dl), when immunosuppressive therapy and plasma exchange were started.

Summary

There are no controlled studies of the use of plasma exchange in the management of anti-GBM disease but the dismal prognosis in untreated patients makes possible some assessment of the present results. Anti-GBM antibodies are responsible for injury in this form of glomerulonephritis and, untreated, the antibodies slowly disappear but usually after complete destruction of the kidneys has developed; this may occur within 24 h in patients with the most aggressive disease. Although immunosuppressive drugs alone may hasten the disappearance of anti-GBM antibodies the only reliable way to reduce rapidly the titre of these antibodies is by daily 4 l plasma exchanges combined with immunosuppressive drugs. We would strongly advocate this treatment, instituted as an emergency, in all patients with anti-GBM disease when renal function is rapidly declining. The improvement that occurred in 15 of 16 patients, and the results of others, support this approach. We would advocate a similar policy in patients with this syndrome with severe pulmonary haemorrhage combined with measures to remove fluid. The position is much less clear for patients who are already anuric; their renal function is unlikely to improve but they remain at risk from pulmonary haemorrhage and cannot be transplanted before anti-GBM antibodies have disappeared from the circulation; plasma exchange with immunosuppression may hasten this. Nor can definite conclusions be drawn about the small number of patients with anti-GBM disease and stable renal function. Some of these may deteriorate abruptly, particularly if they develop infections, others may have truly indolent disease. Without treatment most of these patients will develop renal failure and so treatment with immunosuppressive drugs alone or with plasma exchange is reasonable.

What is the duration of treatment? We have shown that intensive plasma exchange continued for 14 days results in more rapid switch off of anti-GBM antibody synthesis than less intensive exchanges. Using this regimen anti-GBM antibody is undetectable in less than 2 months, and we have been able to discontinue immunosuppression. Return of antibody is very rare after it has become undetectable.

Crescentic nephritis not due to antiglomerular basement membrane antibody

Background

Crescentic nephritis without anti-GBM antibodies is often associated with systemic disease such as polyarteritis, Wegener's granulomatosis and Henoch-Schönlein purpura; other patients have had streptococcal infection and some have visceral abscesses. Occasionally a crescentic phase is superimposed on underlying chronic glomerulonephritis (57). Most cases are presumed to be due to immune complex deposition in glomeruli although direct evidence for this is lacking and immune complexes are found in serum by conventional tests in only a half to two thirds of patients. Interpretation of the results of treatment with plasma exchange in this group is much more difficult than in anti-GBM disease because a proportion, maybe most, respond to treatment with immunosuppressive therapy alone.

Results

We have treated 37 patients with crescentic nephritis without anti-GBM antibodies and not associated with previous chronic glomerulonephritis using the same regimen described for anti-GBM disease. Circulating immune complexes were detected in 19 by fluid phase Clq binding assay but generally these correlated poorly with disease activity. Immune complexes disappeared rapidly after the introduction of plasma exchange and were consistently absent, thereafter.

Seventeen of the 37 patients were oligo-anuric or were on dialysis when treatment was started; 3 died within 9 days, 3 had no improvement in renal function and the remaining 11 improved sufficiently to come off dialysis. Of eight patients with plasma creatinine concentrations above 600 µmol/l (6.8 mg/dl) but not on dialysis when treatment started, one continued to deteriorate whilst the remaining seven improved with four maintaining plasma creatinine concentrations less than 250 µmol/l (2.8 mg/dl). Irrespective of initial improvement a total of 13 patients have died, 7 during the initial hospitalisation and 6 later. Early deaths were usually caused by systemic disease or infection; two of six late deaths were also caused by infection, two died from uraemia, and one each died from myocardial infarction and a cerebrovascular accident. Others have reported similarly favourable renal responses to regimens of immunosuppression combined with plasma exchange (54, 58–61). Although we have shown that plasma exchange alone is very effective for cutaneous vasculitis we have not evaluated its effect in isolation for systemic vasculitis with nephritis and there must remain considerable uncertainty whether plasma exchange confers additional benefit to immunosuppressive drug therapy alone.

It is clear that crescentic nephritis has a much better renal prognosis when not associated with anti-GBM antibodies. The part that plasma exchange plays in this improvement is, however, unclear. We are currently conducting a controlled trial of immunosuppression with prednisolone, cyclophosphamide and azathioprine compared with immunosuppression and plasma exchange. Before results of this or other trials are known it seems reasonable to reserve plasma exchange for the most severely ill patients or those in whom there are strong contraindications to steroids or cytotoxic drugs.

Cryoglobulinaemia

One of the early indications for plasmapheresis was the treatment of hyperviscosity syndrome associated with myeloma and Waldenström's macroglobulinaemia (1, 2); thus the treatment of cryoglobulinaemia was a logical extension (62). Cryoglobulins are cold precipitable complexes of rheumatoid factor and immunoglobulins that frequently cause intense activation of the classical complement pathway. They have been categorised into three types (62). Types I and II contain monoclonal rheumatoid factors (usually IgM); Type I cryoglobulins react with themselves and Type II with polyclonal IgG. They are frequently associated with vascular purpura, glomerulonephritis, peripheral neuropathy and other manifestations of immune complex disease. Type III contain polyclonal rheumatoid factors and polyclonal IgG and may be found in low concentration in many autoallergic and infective diseases.

Two approaches to treatment have been adopted in a small number of patients (62–70). Some patients have had plasma exchange combined with cytotoxic drugs whilst others have been treated by intermittent plasma exchange alone. The response to plasma exchange alone is variable; some patients regenerate cryoglobulin very slowly after removal by plasma exchange (63, 64), whilst in others there is a rapid return of cryoglobulins which can only be controlled by concurrent treatment with cytotoxic drugs. Symptomatic improvement, particularly the control of arthralgia, purpura and digital vasculitis together with some improvement in renal function, usually follows plasma exchange but peripheral neuropathy usually responds poorly, if at all. In some patients substantial clinical benefit can be gained without complete loss of the cryoglobulin which may be due to the fact that the temperature at which cryoglobulins precipitate is concentration dependent (70); at low concentrations they precipitate at lower temperatures and may be less pathogenic. Presently it is reasonable to treat patients with essential cryoglobulinaemia, unassociated with overt lymphoproliferative disease, either with a cytotoxic drug such as cyclophosphamide, chlorambucil or melphalan and to add intermittent plasma exchange only if drug therapy does not control disease activity. The alternative is to start treatment with plasma exchange and only add immunosuppressive drugs if the exchanges have to be performed unacceptably frequently to control the disease. The decision as to which approach to use will probably be governed by the risks of cytotoxic drugs to an individual patient. One last practical point must be made about plasma exchange in patients with cryoglobulinaemia. Most patients with cryoglobulinaemia have very low concentrations of the complement components C2 and C4 which may limit inflammation (71). FFP given as part of plasma exchange supplies complement which may be consumed to increase injury.

Systemic lupus erythematosus

SLE is an autoimmune disease characterised by circulating autoantibodies to double stranded DNA and injury to many organs including skin, joints, kidneys, lungs and brain. Some features are mediated directly by autoantibodies but most result from widespread deposition of immune complexes which are often found in high titres in these patients. The course and severity of SLE are very variable and in most patients symptoms can be controlled by non steroidal anti-inflammatory drugs together with small doses of steroids. There remain a small number of patients, particularly those with renal disease, who need more aggressive therapy including immunosuppressive drugs. Verrier Jones and colleagues (32) first used plasma exchange in these patients and have subsequently accumulated the largest reported experience (72, 73). Generally they used less intensive plasma exchange than that described for the treatment of crescentic glomerulonephritis: three to four 2 l exchanges for PPF in the first week followed by 1 to 2 exchanges in succeeding weeks. There was a clinical and immunological improvement in 8 out of 14 patients after the introduction of plasma exchange, either as the sole treatment or without change in previous steroid therapy; 3 did not respond and the results were uninterpretable in a further 3 patients.

A striking finding however was the reduction in titre of circulating immune complexes which was much greater than could be explained by physical removal, which suggested enhanced endogenous clearance. Frank and colleagues (34) have demonstrated impaired reticuloendothelial function in patients with active SLE and Lockwood and colleagues (33) have shown that this defect is rapidly reversed by plasma exchange.

Our own experience in the use of plasma exchange in the management of SLE has been restricted to patients with fulminant disease; particularly those who had failed to respond to high dose steroids and cytotoxic drugs. Each of 10 patients treated with daily 4 l exchanges had diffuse lupus nephritis and renal failure, in addition 3 had severe cerebral lupus and 2 had extensive pulmonary vasculitis. There was an improvement in four out of five patients treated after failure of steroid therapy and in three out of four in whom treatment with plasma exchange and steroids were started concurrently. Others have also suggested a beneficial effect of plasma exchange in severe lupus nephritis (54, 60).

A different approach using regular small volume plasma exchanges has been used by Clark and colleagues (74) in patients with renal lupus in an attempt to minimise the dose of steroids. Preliminary results of this controlled (though not 'blinded') clinical trial are inconclusive.

The choice of replacement fluid for patients with SLE is also controversial. Moran and coworkers (18) reported additional benefits of FFP over PPF which is theoretically attractive as many patients with SLE have functional complement deficiencies which could impair the way they metabolise immune complexes (75). Further, Young and colleagues (17) have reported a sustained improvement of features of immune complex disease in a patient with C1q deficiency.

In this relatively small experience, plasma exchange is associated with definite though temporary improvement of symptoms and signs in a high proportion of patients with SLE; the important question, as yet unanswered, is whether it has additional benefits over conventional therapy. Most patients can be adequately treated by non steroidal anti-inflammatory drugs and steroids. On present evidence it is unlikely that plasma exchange will be preferred for these patients but it may be a useful adjunct for those who need high doses of steroids or cytotoxic drugs. More evidence is needed to settle this point and it is to be hoped that this will be provided by controlled trials. Apart from such a study it seems best to reserve therapeutic (as opposed to experimental) plasma exchange as an adjunct to conventional therapy in patients with fulminant disease.

Renal transplantation

Although renal transplantation is generally accepted as an effective treatment for chronic renal failure nearly all patients have at least one rejection episode and 30% to 40% of kidneys are lost from rejection within a year of transplantation. Most rejection episodes are thought to be initiated by cytotoxic T cells and respond to treatment with prednisolone. But there is gathering evidence that antibodies to alloantigens are also involved (76). Attempts to remove such alloantibodies provides the rationale for the use of plasma exchange. Initial reports were encouraging; Cardella and colleagues (77) described improvement after treatment with two to eight 4 l plasma exchanges in six of eight rejection episodes unresponsive to high dose steroids. Subsequently, however, all but two of these grafts failed. Further uncontrolled reports have been equally inconclusive (78-83) and Power and colleagues (83) have questioned the need for further trials after successive episodes of rejection had failed to improve. Preliminary results from three controlled studies have already been reported and with small numbers of patients none have shown significant benefit from plasma exchange. In two there was a trend toward worse results in the plasma exchanged group (84, 85), whilst in the third (86) the trend favours plasma exchange. These results do not present a convincing case for plasma exchange in unselected episodes of transplant rejection and exclude a substantial benefit from plasma exchange in most.

Before this conclusion can be accepted two points must be satisfied: firstly protection from alloantibody mediated injury by plasma exchange necessitates choosing a regimen that controls antibody titres *before* unrepairable injury has taken place, and secondly if anything other than a temporary improvement is to be made, concomitant drug therapy must be given to terminate antibody synthesis. It is probable that neither of these conditions would be satisfied by the plasma exchange regimens used thus far; they have generally not been intensive enough to control a vigorous antibody response, indeed titres of cytotoxic antibodies have not been controlled in some of the patients already reported. Similarly concomitant drug therapy has been much more suited to suppression of cell mediated immunity than that of antibody synthesis where cyclophosphamide would be much more appropriate (35). However it is unlikely that a place for plasma exchange, if any, will be defined until rapid quantitative techniques are available for measuring alloantibodies.

Thrombotic thrombocytopenic purpura

Haemolytic uraemic syndrome (HUS), post partum renal failure and thrombotic thrombocytopenic purpura (TTP) have a number of common features including microangiopathic haemolytic anaemia and renal failure. Their pathogenesis is unknown but is likely to be heterogeneous. Recent attention has focused on the role of factor(s) necessary for generation of prostacyclin present in normal plasma but absent in HUS (19, 20). Thus far about 48 patients with TTP or HUS have been treated with plasma exchange (87–92); 34 were said to have improved although concomitant therapy in all but two makes the role of plasma exchange difficult to interpret. There is some evidence that plasma exchange for TTP corrects impaired prostacyclin synthesis in these patients; Remuzzi and coworkers (19) reported the restoration in the capacity of patients plasma to sustain synthesis of prostacyclin after 31 plasma exchanges for TTP in two patients, whilst Machin reported that after plasma exchange there was an increase to normal in the concentration of 6-keto-PGF_1, the stable metabolite of prostacyclin (20). Whether these results are of therapeutic as opposed to investigative interest remains to be determined. Presently it is reasonable to treat patients with microangiopathic haemolytic anaemia by plasma exchange using FFP for replacement fluid.

USE OF PLASMA EXCHANGE IN OTHER DISEASES

Plasma exchange has been used in the management of many non-renal diseases, in some instances to remove antibody or immune complexes and in others to overcome metabolic defects. The use of plasma exchange in these diseases has recently been comprehensively reviewed (8, 30) and an extensive list of references on plasma exchange has been assembled (93). Presently plasma exchange has a definite place in the management of severe myasthenia gravis, Guillain-Barré syndrome, pemphigus, exopthalmic Graves disease and diabetes mellitus with anti-receptor antibodies, as well as in hyperviscosity syndrome and in rare individuals with homozygous type II hypercholesterolaemia. Its use in other non renal diseases is speculative.

CONCLUSION

Although a vast literature of case reports surrounds the use of plasma exchange in the management of autoimmune and inflammatory diseases its place cannot yet be defined with confidence. Many of the reports are far too uncritical; but equally uncritical is the call for randomised controlled clinical trials in every circumstance for which the use of plasma exchange is contemplated. It must be recognised that conventional techniques of controlled trials are not applicable to certain types of disease and are not necessary in others; diabetes mellitus due to autoantibodies to insulin receptors is an extreme example. Only a handful of such patients have been described and plasma exchange with reduction of autoantibody titre results in prompt amelioration of their diabetes (94). In these circumstances a controlled trial is clearly unnecessary and anyway precluded by the scarcity of patients. This approach is only applicable when effector molecules of a particular disease are known and can be measured. In nephrology only anti-GBM antibodies and cryoglobulins fulfill these criteria and in neither case is the evidence clear cut. More definite conclusions about the use of plasma exchange will only be made by careful observations on individual patients together with the selective use of controlled trials.

REFERENCES

1. Adams WS, Blahd WH, Bassett SM: A method of human plasmapheresis. *Proc Soc Exp Biol Med* 80:377, 1952
2. Soloman A, Fahey JL: Plasmapheresis therapy in macroglobulinemia. *Ann Intern Med* 58:789, 1963
3. Ray PK, Idiculla A, Rhoads JR JE, Besa E, Bassatt JG, Cooper DR: Immunoadsorption of IgG molecules from the plasma of multiple myeloma and autoimmune hemolytic anemia patients. *Plasma Therapy* 1:11, 1980
4. Terman DS, Buffaloe G, Sullivan M, Mattioli C, Tilquist R, Ayus JC: Extracorporeal immunoadsorption: initial experience in human systemic lupus erythematosus. *Lancet* 2:824, 1979
5. Agishi T, Kaneko I, Hasuo Y, Hayasaka T, Sanaka K, Ota M, Abe T, Ono T, Kawai S, Yamane K: Double filtration plasmapheresis. *Trans Am Soc Artif Intern Organs* 26:406, 1980
6. Malchesky PS, Asanuma Y, Zawicki I, Blumenstein M, Calabrese L, Kyo A, Krakauer R, Nosé Y: On-line separation of macromolecules by membrane filtration with cryogelatin. In: *Plasma Exchange. Plasmapheresis – Plasmaseparation,* Edited by Sieberth HG, Stuttgart (FRG), New York, Schattauer, 1980, p 134
7. McLeod BC, Sassetti RJ: Plasmapheresis with return of cryoglobulin-depleted autologous plasma (cryoglobulinpheresis) in cryoglobulinemia. *Blood* 55:866, 1980
8. Pinching AJ: Plasma exchange in immunologically mediated disease. In: *Recent Advances in Clinical Immunology 2* edited by Thompson RA, Edinburgh, London, Melbourne, New York, ChurchillLivingstone, 1980, p 313
9. Smith JW, Wysenbeek AJ, Krakauer RS: Plasmaseparation I: membrane filtration methods. *Plasma Therapy* 2:53, 1981
10. McLeod BC: Technical aspects of therapeutic plasmapheresis: *Plasma Therapy* 1:43, 1979
11. Yamazaki Z, Inoue N, Fujimori Y, Takahama T, Wada T, Oda T, Ide K, Kataoka K, Fujisaki Y: Biocompatibility of plasma separator of an improved cellulose acetate hollow fiber. In: *Plasma Exchange. Plasmapheresis – Plasmaseparation,* edited by Sieberth HG, Stuttgart (FRG), New York, Schattauer, 1980, p 45
12. Cardella CJ, Uldale PR, Sutton DMC, Katz A, Harding M, DeVeberg A, Cook GT: Effects and complications of intensive plasma exchange for treatment of transplant rejection. In: *Plasma Exchange. Plasmapheresis – Plasmaseparation,* edited by Sieberth HG, Stuttgart (FRG), New York, Schattauer, 1980, p 247

13. Lockwood CM, Pussell B, Wilson CB, Peters DK: Plasma exchange in nephritis. *Adv Nephrol* 8:383, 1979
14. Keller AJ, Urbaniak SJ: Intensive plasma exchange on the cell separator: effects on serum immunoglobulins and complement components. *Br J Haematol* 38:531, 1978
15. Rahilly GT, Berl T: Severe metabolic alkalosis caused by administration of plasma protein fractions in end-stage renal failure. *N Engl J Med* 301:824, 1979
16. Watson DK, Penny AF, Marschall RW, Robinson EA: Citrate induced hypocalcaemia during cell separation. *Br J Haematol* 44:503, 1980
17. Young DW, Thomson RA, Mackie PH: Plasmapheresis in hereditary angioneurotic edema and systemic lupus erythematosus. *Arch Intern Med* 140: 127, 1980
18. Moran CJ, Parry HF, Mowbray J, Richards JDM, Goldstone AH: Plasmapheresis in systemic lupus erythematosus. *Br Med J* 1:1573, 1977
19. Remuzzi G, Misiani R, Marchesi D, Livio M, Mecca G, De Gaetano G, Donati MB: Treatment of the hemolytic uremic syndrome with plasma. *Clin Nephrol* 12:279, 1979
20. Machin SJ: Plasma 6-keto-PGF_1 levels after plasma exchange in thrombotic thrombocytopenic purpura. *Lancet* 1:661, 1980
21. Rees AJ, Lockwood CM, Peters DK: Enhanced allergic tissue injury in Goodpastures syndrome by intercurrent infection. *Br Med J* 2:723, 1977
22. Cohen J, Pinching AJ, Rees AJ, Peters DK: Infection and immunosuppression: a study of the infective complications in 75 patients with immunologically mediated disease. *Q J Med* 201:1, 1982
23. Wing EJ, Bruns FJ, Fraley DS, Segal DP, Adler S: Infectious complications of plasmapheresis in rapidly progressive nephritis. *JAMA* 244:2423, 1980
24. Keller AJ, Chirnside A, Urbaniak SJ: Coagulation abnormalities produced by plasma exchange on the cell separator with special reference to fibrinogen and platelet levels. *Br J Haematol* 42:543, 1979
25. Kliman A, Carbone PP, Gaydos LA, Freireich FJ: Effects of intensive plasmapheresis on normal blood donors. *Blood* 23:647, 1964
26. Friedman BA, Schork MA, Mocniak JL, Oberman HA: Short-term and long-term effects of plasmapheresis on serum proteins and immunoglobulins. *Transfusion* 15:467, 1975
27. Swainson CP, Robson JS, Urbaniak SJ, Keller AJ, May AB: Treatment of Goodpasture's disease by plasma exchange and immunosuppression. *Clin Exp Immunol* 32:233, 1978
28. Urh JW, Müller G: Regulatory effect of antibody on the immune response. *Adv Immunol* 8:81, 1969
29. Bystryn JC, Schenken I, Uhr JHW: A model for regulation of antibody synthesis by serum antibody. In: *Progress in Immunology,* edited by Amos DB, New York, Academic Press, 1971, p 630
30. Lockwood CM, Pusey CD, Rees AJ, Peters DK: Plasma exchange in the treatment of immune complex disease. In: *Clinics in Immunology and Allergy,* edited by Fauci, AS, London, W.B. Saunders Co. Ltd., 1981, p 433
31. Garelli S, Mosconi L, Valbonesi M, Schieppati G, Navassa G: Plasma exchange for a haemolytic crisis due to autoimmune haemolytic anaemia of the IgG warm type. *Blut* 41:387, 1980
32. Jones JV, Bucknall RC, Cumming RH, Asplin CM, Fraser ID, Bothamley J, Davis P, Hamblin TJ: Plasmapheresis in the management of acute systemic lupus erythematosus? *Lancet* 1:709, 1976
33. Lockwood CM, Worlledge S, Nicholas A, Cotton CH, Peters DK: Reversal of impaired splenic function in patients with nephritis or vasculitis (or both) by plasma exchange. *N Engl J Med* 300:524, 1979
34. Frank MM, Hamburger MI, Lawley TJ, Kimberley RD, Plotz PH: Defective reticulo-endothelial system Fc-receptor function in systemic lupus erythematosus. *N Engl J Med* 300:518, 1979
35. Rees AJ, Lockwood CM: Clinical aspects of immunosuppression. In: *Clinic Aspects of immunology,* edited by Lachman PJ, Peters DK, Oxford, Edinburgh, Blackwell 1982, p 507
36. Pinching AJ, Peters DK, Newson-Davis J: Remission of myasthenia gravis following plasma-exchange. *Lancet* 2:1373, 1976
37. Newson-Davis J, Vincent A, Wilson SG, Ward CHD: Long-term effects of repeated plasma exchange in myasthenia gravis. *Lancet* 1:464, 1979
38. Dau PC, Lindstrom JM, Cassel ChK, Denys EH, Shev EE, Spliter LE: Plasmapheresis and immunosuppressive drug therapy in myasthenia gravis. *N Engl J Med* 297:1134, 1977
39. Willassen Y: Reduction of proteinuria following plasma exchange in recurrent renal allograft glomerulosclerosis. *Kidney Int* (Abstract) 61:669, 1982
40. Lerner RA, Glassock RJ, Dixon FJ: The role of antiglomerular basement membrane antibody in the pathogenesis of human glomerulonephritis. *J Exp Med* 126:989, 1967
41. Rees AJ, Lockwood CM, Peters DK: Nephritis due to antibodies to GBM. In: *Progress in Glomerulonephritis,* edited by Kincaid-Smith P, D'Apice AJF, Atkins RJ, New York, John Wiley, 1980, p 348
42. Wilson CB, Dixon FJ: Anti-glomerular basement membrane antibody-induced glomerulonephritis. *Kidney Int* 3:74, 1973
43. Lockwood CM, Amos N, Peters DK: Goodpasture's syndrome: radio-immunoassay for measurement of circulating anti-GBM antibodies. *Kidney Int* 16:93A, 1979
44. Wilson CB, Dixon FJ: The renal response to immunological injury. In: *The Kidney,* edited by Brenner BM, Rector FC, 2nd edn Philadelphia, London, Toronto, Saunders, 1981, p 1237
45. Lockwood CM, Rees AJ, Pearson TA, Evans DJ, Peters DK, Wilson CB: Immunosuppression and plasma exchange in the treatment of Goodpasture's syndrome. *Lancet* 1:711, 1976
46. Rossen RD, Duffy J, McCredie KB, Reisberg MA, Sharp JT, Hersh EM, Eknoyan G, Suki WN: Treatment of Goodpasture's syndrome with cyclophosphamide, prednisone and plasma exchange transfusions. *Clin Exp Immunol* 24:218, 1976
47. Johnson JP, Whitman W, Briggs WA, Wilson CB: Plasmapheresis and immunosuppressive agents in antibasement membrane antibody-induced Goodpasture's syndrome. *Am J Med* 64:354, 1978
48. Briggs WA, Johnson JP, Teichman S: Antiglomerular basement membrane antibody-mediated glomerulonephritis and Goodpasture's syndrome. *Medicine* (Baltimore) 58:348, 1979
49. Walker RG, D'Apice AJF, Becker GJ, Kincaid-Smith P, Crasswell PWT: Plasmapheresis in Goodpasture's syndrome with renal failure. *Med J Aust* 1:875, 1977
50. Jerne NK: Towards a network theory of the immune response. *Ann Immunol* (Paris) 125C:373, 1974
51. Erickson SB, Kurtz SB, Donadio JV, Holley KE, Pineda AA: Use of combined plasmapheresis and immunosuppression in the treatment of Goodpasture's syndrome. *Mayo Clin Proc* 54:714, 1979
52. Espinosa-Mel'Endez E, Forbes RD, Hollomby DJ, Ahuja

DJ, Katz MG: Goodpasture's syndrome treated with plasmapheresis. Report of a case. *Arch Intern Med* 140:542, 1980
53. Rosenblatt SG, Knight W, Bannayan GA, Wilson CB, Stein JH: Treatment of Goodpasture's syndrome with plasmapheresis. *Am J Med* 66:689, 1979
54. McKenzie PE, Taylor AE, Woodroffe AJ, Seymour AE, Chan YL, Clarkson AR: Plasmapheresis in glomerulonephritis. *Clin Nephrol* 12:97, 1979
55. Bruns FJ, Stachura I, Adler S, Segel DP: Effect of early plasmapheresis and immunosuppressive therapy on natural history of antiglomerular basement membrane glomerulonephritis. *Arch Intern Med* 139:372, 1979
56. McLeish KR, Maxwell DR, Luft FC: Failure of plasma exchange and immunosuppression to improve renal function in Goodpasture's syndrome. *Clin Nephrol* 10:71, 1978
57. Cameron JS: The natural history of glomerulonephritis. In: *Renal Disease*, edited by Black DAK, Jones NF, Oxford, Edinburgh, Blackwell, 1979, p 329
58. Asaba M, Rekola S, Bergstrand A, Wassermann H, Bergström J: Clinical trial of plasma exchange with a membrane filter in treatment of crescentic glomerulonephritis. *Clin Nephrol* 14:60, 1980
59. Becker GJ, d'Apice AJF, Walker RG, Kincaid-Smith P: Plasmapheresis in the treatment of glomerulonephritis. *Med J Aust* 2:693, 1977
60. Russ GR, D'Apice AJF: Plasma exchange and immunosuppression in crescentic glomerulonephritis. *Proc 8th Congr Nephrol (Athens)* edited by Zurukzoglu W, Papadimitriou M, Pyrpasopoulos M, Sion M, Zamboulis C, Basel, Karger, 1981, p 667
61. Ravnskov U, Dahlbäck O, Messeter L: Treatment of glomerulonephritis with drainage of the thoracic duct and plasmapheresis. *Acta Med Scand* 202:489, 1977
62. Brouet JC, Clauvel JP, Denou F, Klein M, Seligman M: Biological and clinical significance of cryoglobulins. *Am J Med* 57:775, 1974
63. Berkman EM, Orlin EB: The use of plasmapheresis and partial plasma exchange in the management of patients with cryoglobulinaemia. *Transfusion* 20:171, 1980
64. Pusey CD, Schifferli JA, Lockwood CM, Peters DK: Use of plasma exchange in the management of mixed essential cryoglobulinaemia. *Artif Organs* 5(Suppl):183, 1981
65. Clark RAF, Long JC: Case records of the Massachusetts General Hospital: Painful cold induced skin lesions and lymphadenopathy in a young man. *N Engl J Med* 300:610, 1979
66. Geltner D, Koln RW, Gorevic P, Franklin EC: The effect of combination therapy (steroids, immunosuppression and plasmapheresis) on five mixed cryoglobulinaemia patients with renal neurological and vascular involvement. *Arthritis Rheum* 22:1146, 1981
67. Valbonesi M, Garelli S, Mosconi L, Montani F, Camerone G: Plasma exchange and combined immunosuppressive therapy in the management of severe renal damage due to immune complex disease. *Plasma Therapy* 2:139, 1981
68. Bombardieri S, Maggiore Q, L'Abbate A, Bartolomeo F, Feni C: Plasma exchange in essential mixed cryoglobulinaemia. *Plasma Therapy* 2:101, 1981
69. Houwert DA, Hene RJ, Struyvenberg A, Kater L: Effects of plasmapheresis, corticosteroids and cyclophosphamide in essential mixed polyclonal cryoglobulinaemia associated with glomerulonephritis. In: *Plasma Exchange. Plasmapheresis - Plasmaseparation*, edited by Sieberth HG, Stuttgart (FRG), New York Schattauer, 1980, p 179
70. Lockwood CM: Lymphoma, cryoglobulinaemia and renal disease. *Kidney Int* 16:522, 1979
71. Tarentino A, Arelli A, Costantino A, De Vecchi A, Monti G, Massaro L: Serum Complement in essential mixed cryoglobulinaemia. *Clin Exp Immunol* 32:77, 1978
72. Jones JV, Cumming RH, Bacon PA, Evers J, Fraser ID, Bothamley J, Tribe CR, Davis P, Hughes GRV: Evidence for a therapeutic effect of plasmapheresis in patients with systemic lupus erythematosus. *Q J Med* 192:555, 1979
73. Jones JV, Robinson MF, Parciany RK, Layfer LF, McLeod B: Therapeutic plasmapheresis in systemic lupus erythematosus. *Arthritis Rheum* 24:1113, 1981
74. Clark WF, Lindsey RM, Chodirker WB, Cattran DC, Linton AL: Elective plasmapheresis in SLE nephritis: pilot for a controlled prospective study. *Abstracts Am Soc Nephrol* 928:1979
75. Schifferli J, Woo P, Peters DK: Complement mediated inhibition of immune precipitation. I. Role of the classical and alternative pathways. *Clin Exp Immunol* 47:555, 1982
76. Paul LC, Van Es LA, Van Rood JJ, Van Leeuwen A, De La Rivière GB, de Graeff J: Antibodies directed against antigens or endothelium of peritubular capillaries in patients with rejecting renal allografts. *Transplantation* 27:175, 1979
77. Cardella CJ, Sutton D, Uldall PR, DeVeber GA: Intensive plasma exchange and renal-transplantation rejection. *Lancet* 1:264, 1977
78. Disney A, Taylor H, Norman J, Fazzalari R, Pugsley D, Mathew T: Plasmapheresis in renal transplantation. *Aust NZ J Med* 8:227, 1978
79. Naik RB Ashlin R, Wilson C, Smith DS, Lee HA, Slapak M: The role of plasmapheresis in renal transplantation. *Clin Nephrol* 11:245, 1979
80. Rifle G, Chalopin JM, Turc JM, Guigner F, Vialtel P, Dechelette E, Chenais F, Cordonnier D: Plasmapheresis in the treatment of renal allograft rejections. *Transplant Proc* 11:20, 1979
81. Allan TL, Briggs JD, Cumming RLC, Hogg RB, Junor BJR, Sawers AH: Plasma exchange in renal transplant rejection. In: *Plasma Exchange. Plasmapheresis - Plasmaseparation*, edited by Sieberth HG, Stuttgart (FRG), New York, Schattauer, 1980, p 247
82. Oto K, Toma H, Takahashi K, Hayasaka Y, Agishi T, Ito K: Plasma exchange for treatment of renal allograft rejection. In: *Plasma Exchange. Plasmapheresis - Plasmaseparation*, edited by Sieberth HG, Stuttgart (FRG), New York, Schattauer, 1980, p 257
83. Power D, Nicholas A, Muirhead N, MacLeod AM, Engeset J, Catto GRD, Edward N: Plasma exchange in acute allograft rejection: is a controlled trial really necessary? *Transplantation* 32:162, 1981
84. Allen NH, Slapak M, Lee HA: Plasma exchange in renal allograft rejection. In: *Therapeutic Plasma Exchange*, edited by Gurland HJ, Heinze V, Lee MA, Berlin, Springer Verlag, 1981, p 175
85. Kirubakaran C, Disney APS, Norman J, Paysley DJ, Matthew TH: A controlled trial of plasmapheresis in the treatment of renal allograft rejection. *Transplantation* 32:164, 1981
86. Cardella CJ, Sutton DMC, Katz A, Uldall PR, Harding M, Cook GT, De Veber GA: Plasma exchange in renal transplantation. *Proc 8th Int Congr Nephrol Athens* edited by Zurukzoglu W, Papadimitriou M, Pyrpasopoulos M, Sion M, Zamboulis C, Basel, Karger, 1981, p 681
87. Yang C, Nussbaum M, Park H: Thrombotic thrombocytopenic purpura in early pregnancy. *Acta Haematol* 62:112, 1979
88. Taft EG: Thrombotic thrombocytopenic purpura and dose of plasma exchange. *Blood* 54:842, 1979

89. Ryan PF, Cooper IA, Firkin BG: Plasmapheresis in the treatment of thrombotic thrombocytopenic purpura: a report of five cases. *Med J Aust* 1:69, 1979
90. McLeod B, Wu KK, Knopse WH: Plasmapheresis in thrombotic thrombocytopenic purpura. *Arch Intern Med* 140:1059, 1980
91. Richmond JM, D'Apice AJF, Whitworth JA, Kincaid-Smith P: Thrombotic thrombocytopenic purpura and anuria: response to plasma exchange. *Aust NZ J Med* 10:48, 1980
92. Myers T: Thrombotic thrombocytopenic purpura: combined treatment with plasmapheresis and antiplatelet agents. *Ann Intern Med* 92:149, 1980
93. *Therapeutic Plasma Exchange,* edited by Gurland HJ, Heinze V, Lee MA, Berlin, Springer Verlag 1981
94. Muggeo M, Flier JS, Abrams RA, Harrison LC, Deisseroth AB, Kahn CR: Treatment by plasma exchange of a patient with autoantibodies to the insulin receptor. *N Engl J Med* 300:477, 1979

DIALYSIS AND HAEMOFILTRATION FOR NON-RENAL CONDITIONS

HANS J. GURLAND, PETER KRAMER, NORBERT NEDOPIL, FRANK M. PARSONS, WALTER SAMTLEBEN, NEVILLE H. SELWOOD and ANTONY J. WING

Introduction	884
Psoriasis	884
Initial hypothesis	884
Pathogenesis of psoriasis	884
Natural history of psoriasis	885
Possible therapeutic mechanisms of dialysis	885
Removal of substances	885
Side effects of heparin and non-specific dialysis effects	885
Interference of dialysis procedure with immunity	886
Results of dialysis in patients with psoriasis	886
Non-uraemic patients	886
Patients with end stage renal failure	887
Transplanted patients	888
Other modes of treatment	888
Conclusions	888
Schizophrenia	888
Initial hypotheses	888
Early use of blood purification in schizophrenia	888
Recently published experiences	888
Questionnaire survey	889
The possible role of β-endorphin	891
Conclusions	891
Cancer	891
Initial hypothesis	891
Dialysis induced potassium and magnesium depletion	891
References	893

INTRODUCTION

In recent years haemodialysis and related 'blood purification procedures' have been used experimentally for the treatment of a number of different conditions not related to each other and unrelated to renal failure and uraemia, such as psoriasis, schizophrenia and metastasing cancer.

In this chapter the basic considerations for this treatment are discussed briefly.

PSORIASIS

Initial hypothesis

Psoriasis affects approximately 1 to 3% of the population. Conventional treatments include topical steroids, tar, a combination of tar and ultraviolet light of B wavelength, or, more recently PUVA therapy which is a combination of Psoralens with ultraviolet light of A wavelength. In very severe cases antimetabolites, e.g., methotrexate, have been used with success, but due to adverse side effects this therapy has not found widespread application.

In 1967, Russian workers reported on the use of haemodialysis treatment in chronic skin disease (1). This included two patients with psoriasis resistant to topical treatment who responded to dialysis therapy. In 1976, McEvoy and Kelly (2) reported a patient with psoriasis who had developed end stage renal failure. Local treatment of the skin lesions was only partially effective. Following the third haemodialysis the psoriasis began to clear. One year after starting dialysis treatment a successful renal transplantation was performed and one year later he was still free of psoriatic lesions. Stimulated by this report more than 70 papers have been published generally confirming amelioration of the psoriatic condition in dialysed patients with and without renal failure.

Pathogenesis of psoriasis

Psoriasis is a multifactorial disease with a genetic background. Although both dominant and recessive modes of inheritance have been proposed, it is more likely that the disease is caused by both environmental and genetic factors. An increased association of psoriasis with certain HLA-antigens (B13, B17, B37) has been described (3, 4). Cell mediated mechanisms may be involved.

Two autoantibodies may be involved in the immunopathology of psoriasis.
1. Stratum corneum (SC) antibody is detectable in sera of healthy persons, but it does not react with this antigen because of the dermoepithelial barrier. In psoriatics the normal barrier created by lymphoid cells and polymorphonuclear (PMN) leucocytes may be disturbed and antigen – antibody – complement interaction may follow (5).
2. Anti-basal cell nuclear antibodies have been demonstrated on the cell membranes of circulating lymphoid cells and PMN leucocytes only in patients with psoriasis, but free antibody is not present in the circulation. Locally recruited lymphoid cells and PMN leucocytes may release the antibodies from the cell membranes. Binding to antigenic receptors on the membranes of the basal cells in the dermis induces a

shift of resting basal cells into the proliferating pool. This rapid proliferation is followed by a derangement of keratinisation (6).

A decrease in circulating T-cells in psoriasis has also been reported by several authors but this finding is not disease specific (7–10). There is also an inverse correlation between T-cells and disease activity. The responsiveness to non-specific mitogens of the T-cells is also disturbed (9).

Other factors that have been suggested as interfering with the proliferation of the basal cells include prostaglandins, cyclic AMP, abnormal glucose 6-phosphate dehydrogenase activity, increased heparin precipitable cryofibrinogen, and psychological factors (11).

An alternative immune mechanism has been proposed by Gelfant (12). He demonstrated that the epidermal germinating layer is composed of cycling cells which are actively moving through a cell cycle and non-cycling cells which are blocked in G1 and G2 phase of the cycle. The release of the non-cycling cells into the proliferative pool may result in an increased epidermal cell proliferation. It was postulated that a 'psoriasis factor' accumulates in the body fluids and that this, together with environmental and genetic factors, may trigger the hyperproliferation of the basal cell layer.

Dalen and colleagues (13) demonstrated virus-like material in 13 patients with psoriasis which was not detectable in 20 healthy controls. The T-cell deficit in psoriasis could be due to a viral infection.

Natural history of psoriasis

Psoriasis is a disease with a variable cyclical course. The rate of remissions in unselected cases is about 30% whereas placebo treated patients show an improvement or remission in 20 to 55% (14). Spontaneous recurrence occurs in 65 to 75% of patients during the first year following clearing of lesions with conventional or PUVA therapy (15). Because of this unpredictable natural course, it is difficult to assess the effect of a new therapy such as dialysis. There are, however, several theoretical mechanisms through which dialysis might exert an influence on the skin disease.

Possible therapeutic mechanisms of dialysis

The following hypotheses exist:
a) Removal of substances responsible for epidermal cell proliferation;
b) Side effects of heparin and non-specific effects of the dialysis procedure;
c) Interference by dialysis with cellular and humoral immune mechanisms involved in epidermal cell growth regulation.

Removal of substances
If a 'psoriasis factor' is involved in psoriasis (12) several mechanisms might explain its accumulation despite normal renal function (16, 17): large solutes cannot pass through the glomerular filter; small solutes may be rejected by virtue of the electrostatic characteristics of the glomerular filter; finally, small solutes may be filtered through the glomerulus and then be reabsorbed actively by the renal tubules. Small solutes can be removed effectively by haemodialysis (upper limit 5,000 daltons), peritoneal dialysis (20,000 daltons), haemofiltration (10,000 daltons), and haemoperfusion (dependent on protein binding and chemical affinity) whereas larger molecules can be removed from the circulation only by plasmapheresis.

Investigating serum and dialysate from psoriasis patients by column chromatography, Mastrangelo and colleagues (18) found a 1,000 dalton substance which decreased after dialysis. However, Chen and co-workers (16) could not demonstrate stimulation of DNA synthesis in cultured skin by a 10% ultrafiltrate from psoriasis patients. Maeda and colleagues (19) passed blood through a dialyser without using dialysis fluid and reported no clinical improvement. Polyamines (i.e. spermine and spermidine, 155 and 202 daltons respectively) have been found to be elevated in the blood of psoriasis patients, but their role is unclear (20) and their dialysance unknown.

Holzmann and colleagues (21) claimed that dehydroepiandrosterone (DHEA) deficiency was a pathogenetic factor in psoriasis. Free DHEA was reduced in patients with end stage renal failure and after haemodialysis the levels returned to normal.

Haemodialysis removes certain factors from normal as well as uraemic plasma which are essential for DNA synthesis as shown by studies of ^{14}C-thymidine incorporation in transforming lymphocytes (22), and reduction of such factors could explain a therapeutic effect of dialysis (23). Reduced folate levels occur in dialysis patients and this could interfere with DNA synthesis in a similar manner to that produced by methotrexate (11).

Side effects of heparin and non-specific dialytic effects
Clearance of psoriasis following systemic heparinization has been observed by several clinicians (24–26), and it has been suggested that the anticoagulant is the active agent in dialysis and cardiopulmonary bypass (27). In contrast to haemodialysis no heparin (or only small doses) is given in peritoneal dialysis (28), and only a small amount is absorbed from the peritoneum (29, 30). A few groups used heparin alone and compared its effect with haemodialysis: heparin given for 20 days had no favourable effect (18). In a sham dialysis group, heparin did not improve psoriasis (31).

Another possible mechanism concerns the depressed intracellular levels of cyclic nucleotides (cyclic AMP and cyclic GMP) which cause increased epidermal proliferation. Dialysis can lead to prostaglandin liberation from platelets, thus stimulating cyclic AMP formation and suppressing epidermal hyperproliferation (11).

The effects of dialysis on persons with normal renal function are (32): decrease in plasma concentration of small solutes (urea, uric acid, phosphate), reduction of plasma levels of some enzymes (SGOT, LDH), net removal of fluid and electrolytes depending on the composition of the dialysis fluid and an increase of total CO_2 following bicarbonate generation due to uptake of acetate or lactate. Some investigators tried to exclude these non-specific changes caused by dialysis. Uric acid added to the dialysis fluid did not alter the clearance of the skin lesions, and no difference was observed when bicarbonate was used instead of acetate in the dialysis fluid (18).

Interference of dialysis procedure with immunity
The accumulation of PMN leucocytes in the psoriatic epidermis is a constant feature of this disease and therefore the effect of dialysis on PMN leucocytes must be considered. PMN leucocytes and lymphocytes form infiltrates in psoriatic skin lesions (MUNRO microabscesses) and some of these cells could also be carriers of immunoglobulins and autoantibodies against stratum corneum antigen (33). Accumulation of PMN leucocytes may be enhanced by chemo-attractants such as immune complexes and complement cleavage products and also by an increased chemotaxis in psoriasis (34).

Glinsky and colleagues (33) reported that during 3 to 4 weeks of continuous ambulatory peritoneal dialysis (CAPD) [2.0 l dialysis fluid 5 times a day] a total loss of 42 to 280×10^9 (mean 108×10^9) PMN leucocytes into the dialysate occured. The same group suggested that removal of PMN leucocytes might reduce enzymatic damage to the stratum corneum by serine proteinase activity (35).

Neutrophil function is also affected by haemodialysis using cellulose membranes because the complement system is activated and large amounts of the chemotactic factor C5a are generated (36). This seems to be responsible for leucopenia through neutrophil sequestration in the lungs and also impairs recovery of leucocyte function (37) (see also Chapters 31 and 32). Furthermore, leucocyte chemotaxis is depressed by haemodialysis which has been explained by the loss of reactive C5a – receptors on the surface of the PMN leucocytes (38).

Complement activation has also been observed during cardiopulmonary bypass oxygenation (39, 40) and this might be relevant to the clearance of psoriasis in a single patient 6 weeks after cardiopulmonary bypass (27).

Polyacrylonitrile (PA) membrane dialysers can also activate complement without causing significant leucopenia (41). PA membranes seemed to clear psoriatic skin lesions even more rapidly than dialysis using cellulose membranes (18).

Results of dialysis in patients with psoriasis

Non-uraemic patients
Case reports on 140 psoriasis patients without renal failure treated by extracorporeal blood purification procedures have been published (Table 1, [1, 4, 18, 19, 28, 29, 31, 32, 42–50]). Most of the patients were treated by haemodialysis or peritoneal dialysis. However, duration and frequency of treatment were generally different from the regimens used in end stage renal failure. In a few cases only one session was performed and it is therefore difficult to assess the efficacy of treatment. It appeared that in the group of patients treated with a 'large dose' of dialysis therapy the fraction of responders was higher than in the 'low dose' group. For example, Mastrangelo and co-workers (18) dialysed 18 patients two or three times a week until the disappearance of the skin lesions and observed a successful outcome in all patients. On the other hand, Nissenson and co-workers (31) dialysed four patients for 6 hours on 4 consecutive days followed by a 4 day course of sham dialysis 4 weeks later. Three other patients were sham treated before haemodialysis was performed. This crossover study failed to demonstrate any benefit from dialysis. Other case reports were conflicting: in some cases a single treatment was reported as being effective, whereas in others no improvement was seen despite prolonged dialysis therapy.

Data from 93 centres were collected by the EDTA Registry in a special survey (51, 52). This collaborative study included 49 psoriatic patients with normal renal function, some of whom may overlap with the case reports quoted above. The effect of dialysis on psoriasis was assessed through three criteria – the doctor's general impression, each patient's personal opinion, and by objective data concerning the severity of skin lesions and the frequency and average duration of exacerbations. Adequate objective data were recorded for 27 of the psoriatic patients with normal renal function and 17 of these improved both according to objective criteria and patients' personal opinion (Figure 1). This is only marginally better than the remission rates observed in placebo treated patients (14) and most of the patients had been on dialysis for less than one year. Furthermore, the possibility of bias was raised by the fact that almost half of these patients were treated by doctors who held the opinion that dialysis was definitely useful in some cases

Table 1. Application of blood purification systems in psoriatics without renal failure.

Mode of therapy	Number of patients	Partial/ complete remission	No change	Relapse after therapy	Reference
Peritoneal dialysis	50	39	11	10	28, 29, 32, 42–45
Haemodialysis	60	47	13	6	1, 4, 18, 31, 46–49
Haemofiltration	22	13	9	–	19, 48, 50
Haemoperfusion	6	6	–	–	19
Sham dialysis	2	–	2	–	48

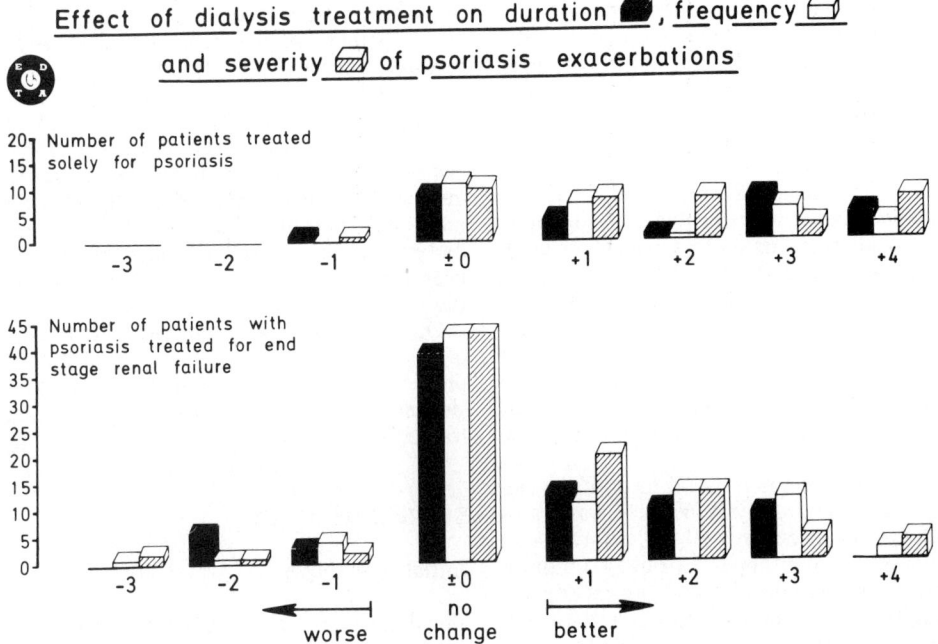

Figure 1. Effect of dialysis on duration, frequency and severity or exacerbations of psoriasis in 27 non-uraemic patients and 76 patients with end stage renal failure. Data collected by the E.D.T.A. Registry (52). (Reproduced by permission of the Editor of Clinical Nephrology).

of psoriasis. The authors were not able to conclude that these pooled observations presented evidence that dialysis benefited non-uraemic psoriatic patients (52).

Patients with end stage renal failure
Case reports on 33 patients with psoriasis and end stage renal failure have been published (Table 2, [2, 16, 23, 29, 43, 46, 53–66]). Twenty-six patients were treated by haemodialysis, six by peritoneal dialysis, and one by haemofiltration. An improvement of the psoriasis was reported in 13 of the 26 patients treated by haemodialysis, all six patients treated by peritoneal dialysis and the one treated by haemofiltration. Amongst those treated by haemodialysis were seven in whom the skin disease remained unchanged, six in whom it worsened and three in whom it relapsed. Four patients have been reported in whom psoriasis developed *de novo* between 4 and 10 years after commencement of haemodialysis (54, 56, 59, 64). In another patient psoriasis, which had been cured before the development of end stage renal failure, relapsed after initiation of dialysis (62).

The EDTA Registry, with 35,001 patients on haemodialysis and 839 patients on peritoneal dialysis in 1978 predicted that between 300 and 600 patients with end stage renal failure would have a history of psoriasis. Data on 97 psoriatic patients with end stage renal failure were collected in the special survey referred to above (51, 52). Less than one quarter of these were treated by doctors who held the opinion that dialysis was definitely useful. Only 2 of these patients were treated by peritoneal dialysis, the remaining 95 received haemodialysis, and most of the patients had been dialysed for more than 1 year. Adequate objective criteria were obtained from 76 of the patients and changes in objective criteria showed good correspondance with patients' personal opinion. At least 20% of patients experienced a definite long term improvement (Figure 1) which is twice as good as the spontaneous long term remission rate (14) and the authors of this report con-

Table 2. Effect of renal replacement therapy on psoriasis in uraemic patients.

Mode of therapy	Number of patients	Partial/ complete remission	No change	Worsened	Relapse despite therapy	Reference
Peritoneal dialysis	6	6	—	—	—	16, 23, 29, 53–55
Haemodialysis	26	13	7	6	3	2, 16, 43, 46 54, 56–65
Haemofiltration	1	1	—	—	—	66

clude that some benefit was demonstrated in the psoriatic patients with uraemia (52). Obviously, no control study on the long term effect of uraemia uninfluenced by dialysis is possible.

Transplanted patients
Reports on eight transplanted patients with a history of psoriasis have been published (2, 11, 23, 55, 57, 60). Seven patients were treated with regular dialysis before transplantation. In all these patients a partial or complete remission of the skin disease was observed during the weeks after dialysis was started. In two patients a relapse of the psoriasis occurred a few weeks after successful transplantation. A few months to 7 years after successful kidney transplantation five of the seven patients were still free of the original skin disease. All the patients received steroids and azathioprine for immunosuppression.

The eighth patient seemed to respond to immunosuppressive therapy but not to dialysis (60). He was transplanted without having been on dialysis before. After the operation his psoriasis disappeared but two months later he developed chronic rejection and regular dialysis treatment was initiated. During this period, without immunosuppressive therapy, psoriatic skin lesions reappeared. They disappeared again after a second transplantation was performed. Four months later the second graft was rejected and upon reinstitution of dialysis the psoriasis relapsed.

Other modes of treatment
Anecdotal reports on procedures related to dialysis have been published:
1. In 1978 MacAuley (24) recommended heparin for treatment of psoriasis. In the same year Wilson (25) described two psoriatic patients who improved dramatically following administration of heparin for ischaemic heart disease.
2. In one patient psoriasis disappeared 6 weeks after heart surgery requiring cardiopulmonary bypass oxygenation. During this procedure heparin is used and, as with haemodialysis, an initial drop of white blood cells is common. An improvement of arthropathy was also observed in this patient (27).
3. Rasmussen (67) observed disappearance of skin lesions in a young patient who was hospitalised to commence dialysis treatment of end stage renal disease. Dialysis was only 'threatened' but never performed.
4. Remission of psoriasis was also observed in a patient with myasthenia treated by plasmapheresis and azathioprine. On cessation of plasmapheresis the lesions returned despite continued immunosuppression (68).

All these case reports must be placed alongside the results achieved with topical steroids, PUVA therapy, cytotoxic drugs, and retinoids (69).

Conclusions

Several hypotheses exist for a mechanism whereby dialysis could interfere with the hyperproliferative process in psoriasis. Published results of the treatment by dialysis and other blood purification systems justify further research, particularly to determine which patients should be selected and which method of treatment is most effective. The cost and other disadvantages of dialysis should not be overlooked, but must be weighed against the long term side effects of the systemic treatment applied in severe cases of psoriasis, e.g. from treatment with methotrexate. The discomfort associated with dialysis is usually well tolerated by patients who have been heavily burdened physically and psychologically by the disabling forms of the disease.

On the other hand it is obvious that dialysis treatment of severe psoriasis has to be carried out exclusively by physicians experienced in the technique of routine dialysis and other 'blood purification methods' and their trained co-workers.

SCHIZOPHRENIA

Initial hypotheses

The diagnosis of schizophrenia, a disease affecting about 1% of the population, is based on subjective symptomalogy and cannot be confirmed by physical findings or laboratory tests. Even though this mental disorder is relatively common, its pathological basis is still unknown. At least four hypotheses concerning specific toxins or biochemical pathways have been discussed in the literature:
1. Imbalance between dopamine and other neurotransmitter substances in the brain,
2. Elevated levels of a circulating copper-containing 'psychotogenic' globulin ('taraxein'),
3. Elevated levels of endorphins, especially β-leucine^5-endorphin, a 3,300 dalton substance,
4. Alteration of catecholamine metabolism.

None of these hypotheses has been validated.

Early use of blood purification in schizophrenia

'Exchange transfusion' was tried for the first time in the year 1670 and reportedly performed for the treatment of a schizophrenic patient. After blood-letting, an equivalent volume of calf blood was transfused to the patient whose schizophrenic symptoms decreased thereafter (70).

In 1938, Reiter (71) performed exchange transfusion in three acute catatonic schizophrenics and reported abatement of the disease in all three cases. In contrast, no change was observed in a patient who suffered from chronic schizophrenia. As a result of his successes, Reiter believed that acute schizophrenia was caused by endogenous intoxication.

Recently published experiences

Haemodialysis for the treatment of schizophrenia was first employed in 1960 by Thoelen and co-workers (72, 73) who used the therapy in four patients suffering from the catatonic form of schizophrenia. Three patients showed a good response. The fact that dialysis in the early sixties was a hazardous and very expensive procedure might explain why this application lay dormant for the next 17 years. It was not until 1977 that Wagemaker and Cade (74) published their striking report on the treatment of schizophrenia by haemodialysis. They observed a remission in five out of six schizophrenics. Palmour and Ervin (75) reported that the plasma and dialysate of some of these patients contained large amounts of β-leucine[5]-endorphin, an opiate-like peptide not detectable in the plasma of healthy subjects.

These findings attracted wide attention and generated much speculation. Several others were prompted to embark on studies of their own to evaluate the effect of dialysis in schizophrenia. However, no common guidelines existed. To overcome this difficulty, Hippius and associates (76) in a joint effort with 36 psychiatrists and nephrologists set up the 'Recommendations for the Evaluation of Possible Therapeutic Effects of Blood Purification Methods in Chronic Schizophrenic Patients' in 1978. This was not intended to serve as a uniformly fixed protocol but rather to give important guidelines including patient selection, concomitant drug treatment, duration and frequency of treatment as well as evaluation of the response.

A multicentre study was never achieved but numerous publications dealing with the subject followed. Methodology varied widely, as did the quality of the data and the degree of adherence to the Hippius guidelines. Twenty-nine centres in fact, reported their experiences of dialysis and other blood purification systems in schizophrenic patients without renal failure and these are recorded in Table 3 (77-96) and Table 4 (97-102). Of a total of 239 patients treated, 32 (13%) were withdrawn ('dropouts'), marked improvement was reported in 68 patients (33%) and some improvement in 34 patients (16%). Five reports were published on the effect of dialysis therapy in schizophrenia in uraemic patients. Of 58 patients eight (14%) showed an improvement of their mental condition (Table 5) (103-107).

Questionnaire survey

Nedopil and co-workers (108), with the support of the Registry of the EDTA, have recently completed a project to evaluate more systematically the possible efficacy of this detoxication treatment. Of 1,090 European renal units replying to the Registry in 1978, 82 indicated that they had treated schizophrenics by blood purification methods. Specially designed questionnaires were sent to these centres and also to 13 others in North America. The survey was designed to answer the following questions:

1. Were the experimental treatments in the different research centres comparable?
2. Were there systematic changes during treatment as a consequence of the detoxication therapy?

Table 3. Application of haemodialysis in schizophrenic patients without renal disease.

Author	Number of patients	Dropouts	Marked improvement	Some improvement
Bond 1979 (77)	21*	7	5*	—
Cohen 1979 (78)	11	1	3	—
Drori 1979 (79)	5	—	1	1
Emrich 1979 (80)	3	—	—	—
Escobar 1978 (81)	1	—	—	1
Hombrouckxs 1979 (82)	5	—	1	—
Horikawa 1979 (83)	4	—	3	1
James 1980 (84)	4	—	1	1
Lamperi 1979 (85)	5	1	2	2
Malek-Ahmadi 1980 (86)	6	—	—	3
Meurice 1980 (87)	1	—	—	—
Neumann 1981 (88)	4	—	—	—
Pitts 1980 (89)	7	—	1	6
Pozzessere 1979 (90)	4	—	4	—
Schulz 1981 (91)	8*	—	—	—
Sidorowicz 1980 (92)	4	—	—	—
Splendiani 1981 (93)	27	9	11	—
Thölen (Feer) 1960 (72)	5	—	1	2
Vanherweghem 1979 (94)	7*	—	5*	—
Wagemaker & Cade 1982 (**)	36	5	18	6
Weddington 1977 (95)	1	—	—	—
Westile 1979 (96)	8	3	—	—
Total	177	26	56	23

* Double blind studies with controls. Data refer only to actively dialysed patients.
** H Wagemaker, B Cade, The J. Hillis Miller Health Center, Univ. of Florida, Gainesville, USA (Personal communication to the authors, 1982).

Table 4. Application of other blood purification systems in schizophrenic patients without renal failure.

Author	Number of patients	Dropouts	Marked improvement	Some improvement
A) *Haemoperfusion or haemodialysis and haemoperfusion*				
Kinney 1979 (**)	6*	—	4*	—
Luzhnikov 1980 (97)	9	—	1	8
Nedopil 1979 (98)	10	3	2	—
Sjöstedt 1979 (99)	13	3	—	3
B) *Haemofiltration*				
Kolff and Stephen 1979 (100)	4	—	1	—
Seidel 1981 (101)	12	—	2	—
C) *Continuous ambulatory peritoneal dialysis (CAPD)*				
Drori 1979 (79)	5	—	—	—
Sichel 1981 (102)	3	—	2	—
Total	62	6	12	11

* Double blind studies with controls. Data refer only to actively dialysed patients.
** MJ Kinney, Marshall Univ. School of Medicine, Huntington, West Virginia, USA (Personal communication to the authors, 1979).

Table 5. Effect of renal replacement therapy on schizophrenia in uraemic patients.

Author	Number of patients	Improved
Ferris 1977 (103)	1	—
Hariprasad 1981 (104)	2	—
Kroll 1978 (105)	2	—
Levy 1977 (106)	3	—
Port 1978 (107)	50	8
Total	58	8

3. Would it be possible to identify subgroups of patients who responded more favourably to the treatment than did others?

Out of a total of 95 centres, 39 (41%) replied (35 from Europe representing 100 patients and 4 from the USA representing 46 patients). There is considerable overlap – 98 entries – between these patients and those in Tables 3 and 4. The number of patients treated in the different centres varied from 1 to 35 patients per centre. Only five centres had more than 10 patients.

Evaluation of the questionnaires (contingency table analysis using the chi square test) showed, rather disappointingly, a wide variation in patient selection criteria (age, diagnosis) and treatment protocols (neuroleptics, mode of treatment) from centre to centre. This made meaningful comparison almost impossible. The response to treatment was also significantly different from one centre to another. The total success rates for the European and the American centres are given in Table 6. From the responses it was calculated that the maximal therapeutic effect was observed between the third and sixth week of treatment with most patients receiving their maximal improvement during the sixth week. Fifty-six % of patients showing improvement achieved no further benefit after this point of time. In attempting to identify variables which could predict the outcome of treatment, and thus define a subgroup of patients who would respond to blood purification treatment, all other survey data were tested against the item 'success of treatment' by contingency table analysis. Neither sex nor age nor the duration of the disease before onset of treatment nor diagnostic categories had any significance regarding the reported outcome. The same was true for

Table 6. Treatment of schizophrenic patients with 'blood purification' methods *: Results from questionnaire survey.

		Patients without renal disease				Renal patients		
	N	N	Dropouts	Marked improvement	Some improvement	N	Marked improvement	Some improvement
All patients	146	131	10 (7%)	40 (30%)	32 (25%)	15	3 (20%)	4 (27%)
European patients	100	85	8 (9%)	14 (17%)	18 (21%)	15	3 (20%)	4 (27%)
American patients	46	46	2 (4%)	26 (57%)	14 (30%)	—	—	—

N = Number of patients.
* Haemodialysis, haemoperfusion, haemodialysis + haemoperfusion, haemofiltration or CAPD (continuous ambulatory peritoneal dialysis) (See text and Table 4).

the mode of treatment, the frequency of treatment sessions and the equipment used.

The possible role of β-endorphin

Wagemaker and Cade (74) first speculated that a polypeptide accumulated in the serum of schizophrenics and that its removal by haemodialysis accounted for the observed improvement of the patient.

β-endorphin is an opiate-like polypeptide with a molecular mass of about 3,300 daltons which is usually synthesised in the hypophysis. Palmour and Ervin (75) reported that β-leucine^5-endorphin, a variant of the naturally occuring β-methionine^5-endorphin, was detectable in the dialysate of schizophrenics. They suggested that abnormal levels of this endorphin in schizophrenics might be due to a renal dysfunction with increased tubular reabsorption. Under this condition, haemodialysis would be more effective than the normal kidney in removing this low molecular weight peptide from the circulation.

Other authors, however, failed to confirm Palmour and Ervin's results or to confirm their speculations. Lewis and colleagues (109) were unable to detect β-leucine^5-endorphin in the haemofiltrate of two patients. James and colleagues (84) failed to find either the abnormal or the naturally occuring endorphin in the filtrate of one schizophrenic. Höllt and colleagues (110) found that endorphin plasma levels were within the normal range at the beginning of treatment, but were elevated at the end of a haemoperfusion session. They also demonstrated that β-endorphin could not be cleared from plasma by sorbent membranes used either for dialysis or haemoperfusion. On balance then, the causative role of β-endorphin in schizophrenia has been disputed in the majority of relevant publications.

Conclusions

There seems little doubt that many schizophrenic patients treated by haemodialysis will undergo at least temporary improvement. The problem relates to interpretation: are the benefits really a consequence of toxin removal during haemodialysis or are they largely artefactual? During haemodialysis the patients are subjected to awesome (to them) machinery; they are told that impurities are being washed from their blood; and they receive almost unheard of attention (in some cases a doctor was in attendance during the whole treatment session). Given the psychosomatic basis of the disease and the patient's desire for improvement, the placebo effect must be very strong and, in the view of many investigators, probably accounts for the perceived improvements. This view is further supported by:
1. The extremely modest improvement rate seen in the dialysis of schizophrenic uraemic patients for whom dialysis has become routine and who receive no special attention from doctors and staff (Table 5).
2. The results of sham studies, such as those of Vanherweghem and co-workers (94) which showed no significant difference between schizophrenics treated on sham and real dialysis.

It is impossible, on the basis of current results, to recommend that dialysis therapy be widely applied to the treatment of schizophrenia nor is it justified to consider the matter closed. Given the increasing evidence for the biochemical aetiology of mental illness and the ever increasing potency of extracorporeal dialysis therapy, continued careful and innovative research seems to be warranted.

CANCER

Initial hypothesis

Following ureterosigmoidostomy and total cystectomy for carcinoma many examples of 'spontaneous regression' of bladder tumour were recorded (reviewed by Everson and Cole [111] who defined 'spontaneous regression' as not necessarily progressing 'to complete disappearance of tumor, nor that spontaneous regression is synonymous with cure'). It was suggested that this regression occurred when a urinary carcinogen, necessary for tumour growth, was diverted into the colon. Additional information questioned this theory and further observations suggested that an asymptomatic biochemical imbalance, induced by the ureterosigmoidostomy, might be contributory, the most likely imbalance being a potassium and magnesium depletion (112). Profound regression was observed in two patients, who had a carcinoma of bladder and breast respectively, when a potassium and magnesium depletion was induced by dietary manipulation. Not surprisingly, magnesium depletion is difficult to achieve in the human for Fitzgerald and Fourman (113) removed only 45.8 mEq and 51 mEq (22.9 and 25.5 mmol respectively) in two normal subjects using dietary manipulations for 3 to 4 weeks. The dietary method of inducing a depletion in patients with cancer was found to be unreliable and had to be abandoned.

Dialysis induced potassium and magnesium depletion

Haemodialysis, using a magnesium free dialysis fluid, readily removes magnesium (see also the magnesium section of Chapter 7) but in order to achieve a total body depletion of magnesium a low magnesium diet is essential. Total body potassium depletion can be obtained using haemodialysis and/or cation exchange resins given orally.

Considerable regression of many different types of tumours was noted in a preliminary communication (112). Histologically the regression took the form of liquefaction or fibrosis of both primary and secondary tumours. During the depletion plasma magnesium and potassium concentrations fell to 0.3 mmol/l (0.6 mEq/l) and 3.0 mmol/l respectively without symptoms (114). The most profound feature was the apparent depressant action on tumour activity so that there was a rapid return, and continued maintenance, of clinical well-being. For instance, in sensitive tumours, pain arising from bone-metastases usually disappeared after the first or second haemodialysis. Furthermore resistance to infection seemed to be unimpaired in the depleted subject as bone marrow activity appeared to remain normal.

In the rat, subjected to depletion of potassium and/or magnesium, there was a significant retardation in growth of two transplantable tumours (115). The greatest retardation (85%) occurred in the combined depletion of potassium and magnesium. In the observations on the rat the change in intracellular cation concentration in normal and tumour cells during the depletion was quite dissimilar. This suggested that malignant cells have 'lost' the ability to withstand an extracellular deficit of potassium and magnesium, possibly becoming extremely acidotic leading to self-destruction.

Patient acceptance of haemodialysis and the unpalatable low magnesium diet was, understandably, poor. Maintenance of vascular access, in the presence of normal renal function, was precarious and all too frequently the procedure had to be abandoned. Few patients could take the diet orally so it had to be given by nasogastric drip. These difficulties with vascular access and diet prevented any long term assessment even though it was estimated that up to 90% of sensitive tumours could be eradicated in two 3 weekly depletion courses separated by a 3 week interval on normal diet without dialysis.

Later the dietary problem was overcome following the observation that sodium cellulose phosphate, 30 g per day, given with food trapped all dietary magnesium in the gut (FM Parsons and BEC Nordin, General Infirmary at Leeds, U.K. unpublished data). This allowed a normal dietary intake although it is important to make sure that the patient is taking sufficient food, particularly calories, to prevent a negative protein balance.

Earlier experience with intermittent peritoneal dialysis using a Trocath were unfavourable due to the development of adhesions and white thrombi (112). Even so, it was decided to apply a CAPD protocol to the investigation using heparinised potassium and magnesium free dialysis fluid (116). The first patient treated is illustrated in Figure 2. She had had a recurrence of a carcinoma of breast with bone metastases requiring continuous morphine to relieve pain. On starting dialysis she took a normal diet with 30 g sodium cellulose phosphate daily and 2 l of magnesium and potassium free peritoneal dialysis fluid was used for the first four days, with a 6 h dwell time. The plasma magnesium and potassium concentrations fell from 0.76 mmol/l (1.52 mEq/l) to 0.23 mmol/l (0.46 mEq/l) and 3.2 to 2.5 mmol/l respectively. On the fourth day of treatment all bone pain had ceased and the return to clinical well being was profound; she even queried the necessity to stay in hospital. The dialysis schedule was then charged to a dwell time of 12 h, the plasma magnesium concentration falling to 0.15 mmol/l by the 10th day. Dialysis was then stopped and the plasma magnesium concentration started to rise despite the continued administration of sodium cellulose phosphate (see Figure 2). At three weeks she commenced a course of cytotoxic therapy but in a much better clinical state than before the induction of the cation depletion. A further course of cytotoxic therapy was given a month later. Two years later a local recurrence in the right hip was treated by high energy radia-

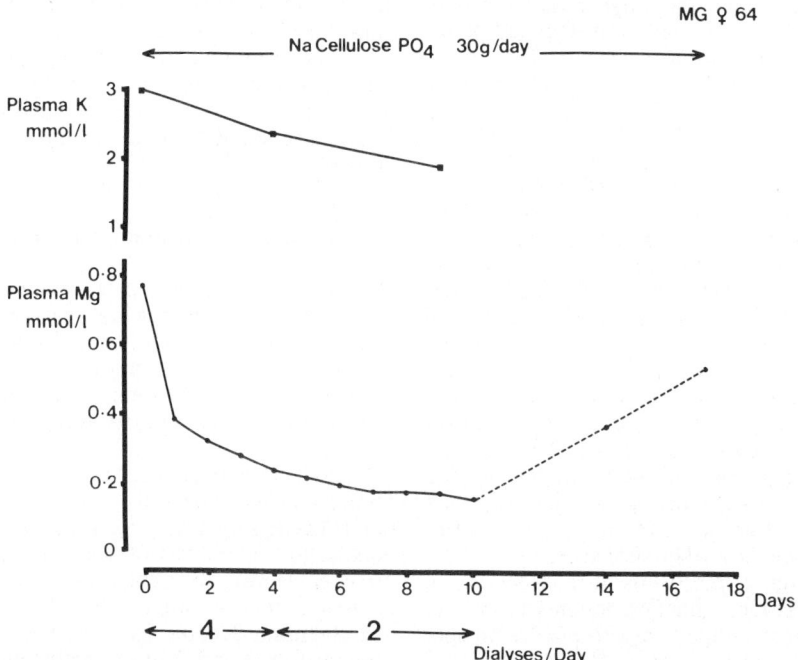

Figure 2. Induction of magnesium and potassium depletion in a patient with carcinomatosis using peritoneal dialysis and oral sodium cellulose phosphate.

tion with prompt symptomatic relief. She is now alive 3 years after commencing the depletion regimen.

More recently two further patients have been treated, one with metastases following bilateral mastectomy for carcinoma, and the other with metastases 8 years after an anterior resection of colon for carcinoma. Both failed to respond but previously both had received high energy radiation. A similar finding was recorded in an earlier patient who developed widespread metastases after excision of a carcinoma of the breast. Two further patients, with metastases from a carcinoma of cervix and osteogenic sarcoma respectively, also failed to respond to the cation depletion after previous radiotherapy and chemotherapy (Dr A.G. Hocken, Otago Hospital, Dunedin, N.Z., personal communication). Currently it would seem unwise to use the cation depletion in patients who have previously received irradiation (and, possibly, chemotherapy).

Although profound regression, supported by histological findings, has been shown to occur in many types of malignant tumours no controlled trial has been possible. The main difficulty in persuing the investigation has been the lack of suitable patients for nearly all cancer patients are referred to oncologists who enter them into a controlled trial, usually for chemotherapy. There is an understandable reluctance to subject patients to a new and unproven form of therapy. This is unfortunate for some of the results have been spectacularly successful and probably as good as, if not superior, to conventional therapy. Certainly, despite all the difficulties, the investigations should continue.

REFERENCES

1. Rakhmanov VA, Petekaev NS, Sorokine MI, Cilingradi EK, Konstantinov AV: Experience with dialysis in the treatment of chronic skin diseases *Sov Med* 30, 6:23, 1967 (in Russian)
2. McEvoy J, Kelly AMT: Psoriatic clearance during haemodialysis. *Ulster Med J* 45:76, 1976
3. Svejgaard A, Staub Nielsen S, Svejgaard E, Kissmeyer Nielsen F, Hjortshøj A, Zachariae H: HLA in psoriasis vulgaris and in pustular psoriasis. Population and family studies. *Br J Dermatol* 91:145, 1974
4. Sprenger-Klasen I, Franz HE, Rodermund OE: Besserung der Psoriasis durch Hämodialyse (Amelioration of psoriasis by haemodialysis). *Dtsch Med Wochenschr* 105:925, 1980 (in German)
5. Krogh HK: Antibodies in human sera to stratum corneum. *Int Arch Allergy Appl Immunol* 36:415, 1969
6. Cormane RH: Immunopathology of psoriasis. *Arch Dermatol Res* 270:201, 1981
7. Cormane RH, Hunyadi J, Hamerlinck F: Méchanismes immunologiques du psoriasis (Immunological mechanisms in psoriasis). *Ann Dermatol Syphiligr* 103:567, 1976 (in French)
8. Guilhou JJ, Clot J, Meynadier J, Charmasson E, Dardenne M, Brochier J: Immunological aspects of psoriasis. II. Dissociated impairment of thymus-dependent lymphocytes. *Br J Dermatol* 95:295, 1976
9. Sauder DN, Bailin PL, Sundeen J, Krakauer RS: Suppressor cell function in psoriasis. *Arch Dermatol* 116:51, 1980
10. Rosenfeld J, Shohat B, Halevy J, Boner G, Feuerman J: Effect of peritoneal dialysis for psoriasis on cell mediated immunity. *Abstracts Eur Dial Transpl Assoc* 16:79, 1979
11. Buselmeier TJ, Nelson RS, Bentley CR, Dungey RK, Kjellstrand CM: Dialysis treatment of psoriasis. *Dial Transpl* 8:568, 1979
12. Gelfant S: The cell cycle in psoriasis. A reappraisal. *Br J Dermatol* 95:577, 1976
13. Dalen A, Hellgren L, Iversen OJ, Vincent J: Presence of retrovirus in psoriasis. *J Invest Dermatol* 74:450, 1980 (Abstract)
14. Braun-Falco O: Übersicht über neue Behandlungsverfahren der Psoriasis vulgaris (Vitamin D$_2$, Folsäure, Milchsäure u.a.). (Survey of new treatment procedures for psoriasis vulgaris [Vitamin D$_2$, folic acid, lactic acid etc.]). *Therapiewoche* 13:180, 1963 (in German)
15. Henseler T, Hoenigsmann H, Wolf K, Christophers E: Oral 8-methoxypsaralen photochemotherapy of psoriasis. The European PUVA study: a co-operative study among 18 European centres. *Lancet* 1:853, 1981
16. Chen WT, Hu CH, Schiltz JR, Nakamoto S: In search of 'psoriasis factor(s)': A new approach by extracorporeal treatment. *Artif Organs* 2:203, 1978
17. Bohrer MP, Baylis C, Humes D, Glassock RJ, Robertson CR, Brenner BM: Permselectivity of the glomerular capillary wall. *J Clin Invest* 61:72, 1978
18. Mastrangelo F, Lamperi S, Buoncristiani U, Binazzi M, Carrozzi S, Rizzelli S: About the mechanism of the dialytic effect on psoriasis. *(Abstracts) Eur Dial Transpl Assoc* 17:67, 1980
19. Maeda K, Saito A, Kawaguchi S, Niwa T, Sezaki R, Kobayashi K, Asado H, Yamamoto Y, Ohta K: Psoriasis treatment with direct hemoperfusion. In: *Hemoperfusion, Kidney and Liver Support and Detoxification,* edited by Sideman S, Chang TMS, Washington, New York, London, Hemisphere Publ Corp 1980, p 349
20. Proctor MS, Fletcher HV, Shukla JB, Rennert OM: Elevated spermidine and spermine level in the blood of psoriasis patients. *J Invest Dermatol* 65:409, 1975
21. Holzmann H, Benes P, Morsches B, Matthaei D, Stöhr L: Psoriasis und Hämodialyse (Psoriasis and haemodialysis). *Dtsch Med Wochenschr* 106:1245, 1981 (in German)
22. Gombos EA, Jefferson DM, Bhat JG: Effect of haemodialysis on immune response. *Proc Eur Dial Transpl Assoc* 11:367, 1975
23. Muston H, Conceicao S: Remission of psoriasis during haemodialysis. *Br Med J* 1:480, 1978
24. MacAuley JC: Dialysis and psoriasis. *Ann Intern Med* 89:430, 1978
25. Wilson LM: Dialysis and psoriasis. *Ann Intern Med* 88:842, 1978
26. Bauer J: Heparin-Calcium und Psoriasis vulgaris. (Heparin-calcium and psoriasis vulgaris) *Dtsch Med Wochenschr* 106:318, 1981 (in German)
27. Buselmeier TJ, Cantieri JS, Dahl MV, Nelson RS, Baumgaertner JC, Bentley CR, Goltz RW: Clearing of psoriasis after cardiac surgery requring cardiopulmonary bypass oxygentation: a corollary to clearance after dialysis? *Br J Dermatol* 100:311, 1979
28. Halevy S, Halevy J, Boner G, Rosenfeld JB, Feuerman EJ: Dialysis therapy for psoriasis. *Arch Dermatol* 117:69, 1981
29. Twardowski ZJ, Nolph KD, Rubin J, Anderson PC: Peritoneal dialysis for psoriasis. An uncontrolled study.

Ann Intern Med 88:351, 1978
30. Nolph KD, Rubin J, Anderson PC: Dialysis and psoriasis. Ann Intern Med 89:285, 1978
31. Nissenson AR, Rapaport M, Gordon A, Narins RG: Hemodialysis in the treatment of psoriasis. Ann Intern Med 91:218, 1979
32. Anderson PC: Dialysis for psoriasis. Artif Organs 2:202, 1978
33. Glinsky W, Jablonska S, Imiela J, Nosarzewski J, Jarzabek-Chorzelska M, Haftek M, Obalek S: Continuous peritoneal dialysis for treatment of psoriasis. I. Depletion of PMNL as a possible factor for clearing of psoriatic lesions. Arch Dermatol Res 265:337, 1979
34. Christophers E, Schröder JM: Neutrophile Granulozytenchemotaxis und Psoriasis (Chemotaxis of neutrophile granulocytes and psoriasis) Hautarzt 32:558, 1981 (in German)
35. Glinsky W, Jablonska S, Jarzabek-Chorzelska M, Zarebska Z, Imiela J: Continuous peritoneal dialysis for treatment of psoriasis. II. Destruction of stratum corneum with peritoneal PMNL serine proteinase. Arch Dermatol Res 266:83, 1979
36. Craddock PR, Hammerschmidt D, White JG, Dalmasso AP, Jacobs HS: Complement (C5a)-induced granulocyte aggregation in vitro. J Clin Invest 60:260, 1977
37. Buselmeier TJ, Cantieri JS: Remission of psoriasis during haemodialysis. Br Med J 2:1139, 1978
38. Greene WH, Ray C, Mauer M, Quie PG: The effect of haemodialysis on neutrophil chemotactic responsiveness. J Lab Clin Med 88:671, 1976
39. Jacob HS: Granulocyte-complement interaction. Arch Intern Med 138:416, 1978
40. Chenoweth DE, Cooper SW, Hugli TE, Stewart RW, Blackstone EE, Kirklin JW: Complement activation during cardiopulmonary bypass. N Engl J Med 304:498, 1981
41. Aljama P, Brown P, Turner P, Ward MK, Kerr DNS: Haemodialysis-triggered asthma. Br Med J 2:251, 1978
42. Glinsky W, Zarebska Z, Jablonska S, Imiela J, Nosarzewski J: The activity of polymorphonuclear leukocyte neutral proteinases and their inhibitors in patients with psoriasis treated with a continuous peritoneal dialysis. J Invest Dermatol 75:481, 1980
43. Göring HD, Thieler H, Güldner G, Schmidt U: Peritonealdialysebehandlung bei Psoriasis vulgaris (Treatment of psoriasis vulgaris with peritoneal dialysis). Hautarzt 32:173, 1981 (in German)
44. Rose I: Dialysis for psoriasis Can Med Assoc J 120:1209, 1979
45. Ülkü U, Önen K, Erek E, Savaskan H, Katogvan A, Serdengecti K: Peritoneal dialysis in psoriatic patients. (Abstracts) 8th Int Congr Nephrol (Athens), 1981, p 413
46. Buselmeier TJ, Kjellstrand CM, Dahl MV, Cantieri JS, Nelson RS, Burgdorf WC, Bentley CR, Najarian JS, Goltz RW: Treatment of psoriasis with dialysis. Proc Eur Dial Transpl Assoc 15:171, 1978
47. Caglar S, Akkaya S, Koleman F, Yasavul U, Tasdemir I: Treatment of psoriasis with dialysis, Kidney Int 19:103, 1981 (abstract)
48. Chugh KS, Kumar B, Pareek SK, Kher V, Shingal PC, Lal M, Sharma L: Evaluation of dialytic therapy in psoriasis. A controlled study. (Abstracts) 8th Int Congr Nephrol (Athens), 1981, p 379
49. Hanicki Z: Some aspects of dialytic treatment of psoriasis. Preliminary report. In: Proceedings of the Second Prague Symposium on Chronic Renal Failure 1979, edited by Válek A, Lund, Gambro AB, 1980, p 195
50. Nakamoto S, Paganini E, Steck W, Bailin P: Psoriasis treated with extracorporeal device. (Abstracts) 8th Int Congr Nephrol (Athens), 421, 1981
51. Brynger H, Brunner FP, Chantler C, Donckerwolcke RA, Jacobs C, Kramer P, Selwood NH, Wing AJ: Combined report on regular dialysis and transplantation in Europe, X, 1979. Proc Eur Dial Transpl Assoc 17:3, 1980
52. Kramer P, Brunner FP, Brynger H, Chantler C, Donckerwolcke RA, Jacobs C, Selwood NH, Wing AJ: Dialysis treatment and psoriasis in Europe. Clin Nephrol 18:62, 1982
53. Foulard M: Rémission d'un psoriasis sous dialyse péritonéale et hémodialyse (Remission of psoriasis with peritoneal dialysis and haemodialysis) Soc Franc Pédiat 1978, p 376 (in French)
54. Giordano C, De Santo NG, Capodicasa G, Cirillo D, Cicchetti T, Senatore R, Damiano M, Fortunato G: Which dialysis for psoriasis in the uremic-psoriatic patients? (Abstracts) Eur Dial Transpl Assoc 16:32, 1979
55. Son BT, Baguio MS: Dialysis and psoriasis Ann Intern Med 88:842, 1978
56. Breathnach SM, Boon NA, Black MM, Jones NF, Wing AJ: Psoriasis developing during dialysis. Br Med J 1:236, 1979
57. Brunner F: Treatment of psoriasis with dialysis (discussion remark). Proc Eur Dial Transpl Assoc 15:176, 1978
58. Farr MJ: Treatment of psoriasis with dialysis (discussion remark). Proc Eur Dial Transpl Assoc 15:176, 1978
59. Friedman EA, Delano BG: Psoriasis developing de novo during hemodialysis. Ann Intern Med 90:132, 1979
60. Graf H, Wolf A, Stummvoll HK: Dialysis and psoriasis. Ann Intern Med 90:994, 1979
61. Gurland HJ, Samtleben W: Is blood purification suitable for an effective cure of psoriasis?: In: Proceedings of the Second Prague Symposium on Chronic Renal Failure 1979, edited by Válek A, Lund, Gambro AB, 1980, p 190
62. Klinkmann H.: Treatment of psoriasis with dialysis (discussion remark). Proc Eur Dial Transpl Assoc 15:176, 1978
63. Perez GO, Oster JR, Vaamonde CA, Halprin KM: Psoriasis during hemodialysis. Ann Intern Med 90:858, 1979
64. Peserico A: Development of psoriasis during dialysis. Arch Dermatol 115:1169, 1979
65. Shimkus EM, Malygina TA, Kalenkovich NI: Hemodialysis for psoriasis in patients treated conservatively without success Vestn Dermatol Venerol 44:69, 1970 (in Russian)
66. Kramer P: Dialysis for psoriasis patients (discussion remark). Proc 11th Annu Contractors' Conf Art Kidney Progr NIAMDD, edited by Markey BB, DHEW Publication NO (NIH) 79-1442, 1978, p 217
67. Rasmussen JE: Clearing of psoriasis after threatened dialysis? Arch Dermatol 116:752, 1980
68. Dau PC: Remission of psoriasis during plasmapheresis therapy Arch Dermatol 115:1171, 1979
69. Smith JG: Psoriasis and dialysis. JAMA 241:1376, 1979
70. Philipp M: Hämodialyse und die Idee der Blutreinigung in der Schizophreniebehandlung (Haemodialsysis and the idea of purification of the blood in the therapy of schizophrenia) Fortschr Neurol Psychiatr 47:36, 1979 (in German)
71. Reiter PJ: Untersuchungen zur Bedeutung der Intoxikationstheorie bei der Dementia praecox mit besonderer Berücksichtigung der Versuche mit Totaltransfusionen (Investigations concerning the hypothesis of intoxication in dementia praecox with special attention to exchange transfusions) Z Gesamte Neurol Psychiat 160:598, 1938 (in German)
72. Thölen H, Stricker E, Feer H, Massine MA, Staub H: Über die Anwendung der künstlichen Niere bei Schizoph-

renie und Myasthenia gravis. (On the application of the artificial kidney for schizophrenia and myasthenia gravis) *Dtsch Med Wochenschr* 85:1012, 1960 (in German)
73. Feer H, Thölen H, Massini MA, Staub H: Hemodialysis in schizophrenia. *Compr Psychiatry* 1:338, 1960
74. Wagemaker H, Cade R: The use of hemodialysis in chronic schizophrenia. *Am J Psychiatry* 134:684, 1977
75. Palmour RM, Ervin FR: Biochemical and physiological characterization of a peptide from the hemodialysate of psychotic patients. *Psychopharmacol Bull* 15:21, 1979
76. Hippius H, Matussek N, Nedopil N, Strauss A, v. Zerssen GD, Emrich H, Kolff WJ, Gurland HJ: Recommendations for the evaluation of possible therapeutic effects of blood purification methods in chronic schizophrenic patients. *Artif Organs* (Suppl) 3:104, 1979
77. Bond IK, Elek HK, Jansen B, Linton PG, Fenton SSA: Preliminary report of a double blind study on the effect of hemodialysis on schizophrenic symptomatology. *Proc Eur Soc Artif Organs* 6:137, 1979
78. Cohen IM, Scheiber SC, Novak R, Reisine T, Yamamura HI: Hemodialysis in schizophrenia. *Kidney Int* 16:914, 1979 (abstract)
79. Drori JB, Weinstein R, Weis T: The effect of continuous ambulatory peritoneal dialysis in chronic schizophrenia. *Psychopharmacol Bull* 15:17, 1979
80. Emrich HM, Kissling W, Fischler M, v Zerssen GD, Riedhammer H, Edel HH: Hemodialysis in schizophrenia: three failures with chronic patients. *Am J Psychiatry* 136:1095, 1979
81. Escobar JI, Codd EE, Byrne WL: Endorphins and schizophrenia. *Proc VII Latin American Congr Pharmacol*, Sao Paulo, 1978
82. Hombrouckx R, Bollengier L: Hemodialysis as treatment for chronic schizophrenia. *(Abstracts) Europ Dial Transpl Assoc* 16:40, 1979
83. Horikawa N, Iwai K, Shibati S, Ota K, Sanaka T: Treatment of schizophrenics with hemodialysis. *Artif Organs* (Suppl), vol 3:162, 1979
84. James NM, Hearn MTW: Hemodialysis, endorphins, and schizophrenia. *Am J Psychiatry* 137:488, 1980
85. Lamperi S, Carozzi S, Trasforini D, Barocci S, Loeb C, Roccatagliata G, Maffini M: Preliminary results of hemodialytic treatment in subjects with chronic schizophrenia. *Minerva Nefrol* 26:109, 1979
86. Malek-Ahmadi P, Sorkin MI, Callen KE, Davis D, Davis LG: Hemodialysis and schizophrenia: A double blind study. *South Med J* 73:873, 1980
87. Meurice E, Godon JP, Mathieu F: Therapeutic trials in schizophrenia with dialysis. *Acta Psychiatr Belg* 80:436, 1980
88. Neumann NU, Graske TP. Zur Hämodialysebehandlung schizophrener Psychosen (On haemodialysis treatment of schizophrenic psychoses) Paper given at: Bayerischer Nervenärztetag Günzburg (FRG), Oct. 1979 (in German [not published])
89. Pitts F: cited by Fogelson DL, Marder SR, Van Putten T: Dialysis for schizophrenia: Review of clinical trials and implications for further research. *Am J Psychiatry* 137:5, 1980
90. Pozzessere G, Liguori N, Marasco M, Spadaro M, Pierelli F, Cappello G, Botti M, Morocutti C, Casciani C.: Hemodialysis treatment in chronic schizophrenia: Preliminary report. *Artif Organs* (Suppl) 3:36, 1919
91. Schulz SC, Balow JE, Flye MW, Bunney WE: Dialysis in schizophrenia: A double-blind evaluation. *Science* 211:1066, 1981
92. Sidorowicz S, Firko M, Wasik A, Szewczyk Z, Szepietowski HD, Weyde W: Hemodialysis in chronic schizophrenia. *Acta Psychiatr Scand* 61:223, 1980
93. Splendiani G: Hemodialysis in schizophrenia. *Proc Eur Soc Artif Organs* 8:187, 1981
94. Vanherweghem JL, Linkowski P, Jadot C, Mendlewicz J: Hemodialysis in schizophrenia: A double blind study. – Preliminary report. *Proc Eur Dial Transpl Ass* 16:148, 1979
95. Weddington WW: Can dialysis help the chronic schizophrenic? (letter). *Am J Psychiatry* 134:1310, 1977
96. Westlie L, Haug J, Hage G: Hemodialysis and schizophrenia. *Artif Organs* (Suppl) 3:160, 1979
97. Luzhnikow EA, Churkin EA, Gorbunova NA, Kostomarova LG: Test in treatment of schizophrenia by the method of detoxification hemosorption. *Zh Nevropatol Psikhiatr* 80:103, 1980 (in Russian)
98. Nedopil N, Dieterle D, Matussek N, Hippius H, Gurland HJ, Hillebrand G: Blutreinigung bei chronisch schizophrenen Patienten (Purification of the blood in chronic schizophrenic patients) *Nervenarzt* 51:123, 1980 (in German)
99. Sjöstedt L, Franzen G, Rorsman B, Lindholm T, Thysell H, Heinegard D, Terenius L, Wahlström A: Hemodialysis in chronic schizophrenia: A negative report. *Artif Organs* (Suppl), vol 3:155, 1979
100. Kolff WJ, Stephen RL: cited in Fogelson DL, Marder SR, Van Putten T: Dialysis for schizophrenia. Review of clinical trials and implications for further research. *Am J Psychiatry* 137:5, 1980
101. Seidel M, Ernst K, Lindenau K: Zum Stand der extrakorporalen Detoxikationsverfahren als Therapiemethoden der Schizophrenie. (The present state of extracorporeal detoxification therapy for schizophrenia) *Psychiatr Neurol Med Psychol* (Leipz) 33:705, 1981 (in German)
102. Sichel JP, Baldauf A, Horber M, Wasser P, Marichal JF, Faller B: La dialyse péritonéale continue ambulatoire chez les schizophrènes (Expérimentation dans trois cas). (Continuous ambulatory peritoneal dialysis in schizophrenics [a trial in three cases]) *Encephale* 7:129, 1981 (in French)
103. Ferris GN: Can dialysis help the chronic schizophrenic? *Am J Psychiatry* 134:1310, 1977
104. Hariprasad MK, Nadler IM, Eisinger RP: Hemodialysis for uremic schizophrenics: No psychiatric improvement. *J Clin Psychiatry* 42:5, 1981
105. Kroll P, Port FK, Silk KR: Hemodialysis and schizophrenia. A negative report. *J Nerv Ment Dis* 166:291, 1978
106. Levy NB: Can dialysis help the chronic schizophrenics? *Am J Psychiatry* 134:1311, 1977
107. Port FK, Kroll PD, Swartz PD: The effect of hemodialysis on schizophrenia: A survey of patients with renal failure. *Am J Psychiatry* 135:743, 1978
108. Nedopil N, Dieterle D, Gurland HJ, Koepcke W, Wing AJ, Selwood NA: Detoxication treatment in chronic schizophrenia. Results from a survey. *Artificial Organs* (in press)
109. Lewis RB, Gerber LD, Stein S, Stephen RL, Grosser BI, Velick S, Udenfriend S: On β_H-Leu^5-endorphin and schizophrenia. *Arch Gen Psychiatry* 36:237, 1979
110. Höllt V, Hillebrand G, Schmidt B, Gurland HJ: Endorphins in schizophrenia: hemodialysis/hemoperfusion are ineffective in clearing β-Leu^5-endorphin and β-endorphin from human plasma. *Pharmakopsychiatr Neuropsychopharmakol* 12:339, 1979
111. Everson TC, Cole WH: Spontaneous regression of cancer of the urinary bladder. In: *Spontaneous Regression of Cancer* Philadelphia WB Saunders, 1966, p 320
112. Parsons FM, Anderson CK, Clark PB, Edwards GF, Ahmad S, Hetherington C, Young GA: Regression of malignant tumours in magnesium and potassium depletion induced by diet and haemodialysis. *Lancet* 1:243, 1974

113. Fitzgerald MG, Fourman P: An experimental study of magnesium deficiency in man. *Clin Sci* 15:635, 1956
114. Burman ND, Parsons FM: Hyperalimentation in the treatment of advanced carcinoma with induced magnesium and potassium depletion. *S Afr Med J* 50:1695, 1976
115. Young GA, Parsons FM: The effects of dietary deficiencies of magnesium and potassium on the growth and chemistry of transplanted tumours and host tissues in the rat. *Eur J Cancer* 13:103, 1977
116. Mills FH, Sheldon DM, Parsons FM: Magnesium deficiency produced by peritoneal dialysis as an adjunct to cancer therapy. *Med J Aust* 2:145, 1979

INDEX OF SUBJECTS

AAMI standards for dialysis water 144, 161
Abdominal pain
    Copper intoxication 615
    Digoxin mesenteric vasoconstriction 632
    Hepatitis 664
    Peritoneal dialysis, complicating 460, 470, 476
    Peritonitis indicator 471
    Retroperitoneal hematoma 621
Abel, John Jacob 3-6, 107
Abortions causing acute renal failure 541
Absorbent 341
Absorption of drugs 750
ACAC hemoperfusion system 309, 313
Accelerated hypertension, see Malignant
Acebutolol 773
Acetaminophen 315, 753, 777
Acetate 72-74, 157, 158, 334
    Anion gap induced by 158
    Buffer anion for peritoneal dialysis 417
    Dialysance 157
    Dialysis fluid 28, 35, 64, 65, 72, 77, 157, 158, 324, 334, 552
    Dialysis fluid, hypoxia 633
    Distribution volume 74
    Flux 77
    Hemodynamic effects 238, 251, 614
    Hemofiltration diluting fluid 267
    Kinetics 72, 73, 334
    Kinetics in Redy-sorb system 334
    Lipid metabolism, effect 158, 589, 615
    Peritoneal dialysis fluid concentration 464, 465
    Plasma concentration 72, 158
    Release from zirconium phosphate 331
    Transport during hemodialysis 158
Acetate intolerance 158, 162
Acetate metabolism 35, 71-73, 77, 157, 158, 556, 614
Acetate toxicity 35, 158, 334, 528, 581, 615
Acetazolamide 774
Acetic acid, dialyzer sterilant, reuse 292
Acetoacetate, plasma, and dialysis fluid dextrose 160
Acetohexamide 779
Acetoin 367
Acetoper 292, 293
Acetylation 752
Acetylcholine, magnesium inhibition 727
Acetylcholine receptor antibodies 876
Acetyl-coenzyme A 552, 556
N-acetylprocainamide 774
N-acetyltryptophan 366
Acid (see hydrogen ion) 71
Acid-base balance 65, 71-77
    In renal failure 357, 358
    Redy-sorb system 331, 332
Acid citrate dextrose 873
Acidosis 71, 77, 159
    Adverse effects 615
    Anesthesia, effect on 798
    Bone, effect on 158
    Cerebrospinal fluid response 726
    Clinical and metabolic effects 357
    Dialysis disequilibrium, contribution to 393
    Dialysis effect 358
    Dialysis indication, acute renal failure 550
    Drug induced 769, 776
    Drug intoxication, complicating, dialysis for 315
    Glucose utilization, impaired 720
    Hyperchloremia, peritoneal dialysis 416
    Hyperkalemia, aggravating 357, 544
    Hypokalemia after correction 552
    Incomplete correction with acetate 615
    Intracellular 612
    Lipid metabolism, effect on 590
    Muscle relaxant effects 798, 800
    Neurological effects 726
    Parathyroid hormone, effect on 358
    Persistent, after peritoneal dialysis 475
    Persistent, with Redy dialysis 334, 335
    Physostigmine effect, limited 800
    Redy-sorb system dialysis correcting 334, 335
    Sorbent effect on dialysate causing 335
    Tendon degeneration cause 624
    Treatment in children 516
Acrocyanosis, cold dialysis fluid causing 476
Acrodermatitis 665, 715
Actin 364
Activated carbons for hemoperfusion 306, 307
Activity index 394, 840
Activity restriction by AV shunt 175
Acute renal failure 536-568
    Cause of death 542, 543
    Children 515-519
    Complications 516, 548-550
    Dialysis in children 517-519
    Dialysis requirement 515, 537
    Duration 559
    Endocrine-metabolic abnormalities 549
    Etiology 537
    Hemodialysis 21, 152, 550-556
    Hemofiltration 267, 271, 556
    Hyperalimentation 548, 570
    Incidence 537
    Irreversible 559
    Mortality 536, 541-543, 558
    Mortality, effect of catabolic rate 542
    Mortality, effect of precipitating cause 541, 542
    Nutrition 547, 548, 569
    Pathogenesis 539, 540
    Peritoneal dialysis 415, 416, 423, 476, 550, 556-558
    Pharmacokinetics 548
    Post-obstetrical 541, 558
    Post-surgical 541, 542, 549, 558
    Precipitating factors 515
    Prognosis 541, 542, 559
    Residual dysfunction 559
    Survival, improving 558
    Treatment 423, 540, 541, 543-560
    Urinary abnormalities 539
    See also Renal failure, Uremia
Acute tubular necrosis, see Tubular necrosis 536-568
Adaptation to dialysis 737
Adenine arabinoside therapy of hepatitis 665
Adenine nucleotides, release from platelets 191, 201, 205
Adenosine nucleotide, stimulating platelet adhesion 190, 214
Adenosine triphosphatase, see ATPase

Adenosine triphosphate, see ATP
Adenyl cyclase 212, 372
Adequacy of dialysis 62, 393, 394
Adhesion of blood on surfaces 186
Adipic acid 367
Adolescents, dialysis for 495
ADP, platelet aggregation stimulator 639
Adrenal cortical function in uremia 717, 718
Adrenal corticosteroid 717
    Cataracts 744
    Pharmacokinetics 778
    Treatment of air embolism 619
Adrenal insufficiency in uremic patients 717
Adrenal steroid biosynthesis 715
β adrenergic blocker 528, 532, 555, 578, 773
    Hyperparathyroidism treatment 705
    Hypertension treatment 578
    Hypoglycemia complicating 621, 622
    Impaired response to hemorrhage 800
    Pharmacokinetics 773
β adrenergic stimulus of parathyroid hormone 680
Adrenocortical trophic hormone 713
Adsorbent 306, 307, 323, 341
Adsorption 306, 307
    Characteristics of carbon 306
    Chemical 307
    Coagulation factors 308
    Hemoperfusion, effect of sorbent coating 307
    Proteins to artificial surfaces 186, 187, 214
    Role of diffusion 306
Adsorptive filters 146
Affinity columns for antibody removal 873
Age
    Dialysis patients 399, 853, 857
    Dialysis risk factor 831
    Hemodialysis acceptance 854, 855
    Influence on dialysis treatment 494, 495
    Ocular calcification correlation 744
    Recovery from acute renal failure, effect 559
    Survival effect 525, 542, 861
    Transplant risk factor 831, 862
Air bubble, blood leak detector interference 234
Air bubble transit, measuring blood flow 121, 122, 226
Air detector 228-230, 619
Air embolism 163, 229, 230, 235, 238, 543, 618-620
    Causes 618
    Consequences 618, 619
    Critical volume 230, 618
    Home hemodialysis 509
    Plasma exchange hazard 874
    Prevention 619, 620
    Treatment 619
Air entry in hemodialyzer, causes 229
Air rinse, hemodialyzer 288
Air transport, dialysate to blood 235
β alanyl histidine 364
Alarms 224, 228, 229
Albumin
    Artificial surfaces, coating 188, 194
    Drug binding 750
    Hypotension treatment 554, 582
    Intraperitoneal, for drug removal 477
    Plasma, decreased with peritoneal dialysis 479
    Plasma, nutritional assessment 569
    Plasma osmolality, contribution to 246, 247
    Plasma volume expansion during dialysis 554
    Pressor effect during dialysis 537, 554
    Sieving coefficient 256, 552

    Transport into peritoneum 256, 444, 446
Alcuronium 782
Aldehyde oxidase 808
Alditol in uremic serum 367
Aldolase 688
Aldonolactone in uremic serum 367
Aldose in uremic serum 367
Aldosterone 581, 718
Aliphatic amines 364, 365
Alkaline phosphatase 694
    Aluminum osteomalacia 812
    Liver disease, increase 694
    Osteoblastic activity indicator 694
    Periarthritis, increased in 689
    Plasma elevation, with Redy-system dialysis 335
    Sulfate retention, correlation 358, 701
    Vitamin D therapy, effects 694
Alkalosis, complicating peritoneal dialysis 475
Alkalosis, plasma exchange complication 874
Alkylating agents 773
Alkyltetramethylammonium bromide 290
Allen-Brown arteriovenous shunt 173
Alloantibody, plasmapheresis removal 879
Allogenic vein graft 179
Allopurinol 778, 779
Alport's syndrome 862
Althesin 799
Alumina, adsorption of phosphate by 323
Aluminum 233, 805-808, 811-819
    Absorption from phosphate binders 700, 816
    Accumulation 700, 812, 816
    Bicarbonate effects in dialysis fluid 337
    Body content 805, 813
    Brain content 39, 812, 813
    Charcoal contamination 336
    Dialysis encephalopathy 807, 808, 811, 816
    Dialysis fluid content 336, 337, 806, 813, 814
    Dialysis fluid, safe concentration 337
    Diffusion 337
    Measurement, sensitivity of 336
    Osteomalacia 808, 812, 813
    Peritoneal dialysis fluid contaminant 464
    Pharmacokinetics 781
    Phosphate binders 143, 348, 805, 806, 816, 817
    Plasma concentration 806, 816
    Redy-sorb system 336-338
    Removal from water 814
    Sorbents contaminant 468
    Transport during dialysis 39, 337, 806, 813
    Water content 39, 143, 161, 523
    Water for dialysis solution 700, 814, 815
    Zirconium phosphate absorption of 337
Aluminum hydroxide gel, peptic ulcer prevention 546
Aluminum hydroxide gel, phosphate binder 158, 270, 690, 691
Aluminum intoxication 38, 39, 142, 689, 806-808, 811-819
    Encephalopathy 808, 811, 812, 816
    Metabolic effcts 335
    Osteomalacia 684
    Redy-sorb system 337, 338
    Treatment 817
Aluminum oxide content of sorbent cartridge 336, 337
Aluminum silicate, dialysate regeneration, for 324
Alwall, Nils 17, 18, 107
Alzheimer's disease 808
Amanita phalloides intoxication 315, 316
Amantidine 770
Amaurosis fugax 729

Amberlite sorbent for hemoperfusion 306, 307, 758
American Society for Artificial Internal Organs 31
Amikacin 761, 762
Amiloride 774
Amines, in renal failure 364-366
Amino acid 363
    Absorption, impaired, in uremia 648
    Bound, in renal failure 364
    Branched chain, imbalance in renal failure 364
    Charcoal adsorption 330
    Dextrose free hemodialysis, loss with 159
    Energy source 90
    Essential, decreased in renal failure 363
    Hemofiltration removal of 267
    Hemoperfusion removal of 311
    Hepatic encephalopathy abnormalities 317
    Middle molecule components 369
    Muscle transport in uremia 355
    Peritoneal dialysis fluid additive 464, 465
    Peritoneal dialysis removal 469, 573
    Plasma concentration, during dialysis 159
    Supplementation 469, 529, 548, 569
    Treatment of acute renal failure 541
    Uremic abnormalities 363, 526
Amino acid acylase 366
Amino acid conjugates 363, 364
4 aminobenzoic acid 366
Aminoglycoside 760-762
    Clearance, hemodialyzer versus renal 756
    Dialysis 760-762
    Intraperitoneal for peritonitis 473, 474
    Nephrotoxicity 540, 753, 760-762
    Ototoxicity 760-762
    Pharmacokinetics 760-762
4-amino-5-imidazole carboxamide 363
β-aminoisobutyric acid 364
Aminolevulinic acid dehydrase inhibition 371
Aminophylline 605, 773
Aminopyrine demethylation, inhibition 360
Aminotransferase 662, 664, 665, 672
Amithiozone 770
Amitriptylline 776
Amitriptylline intoxication, hemoperfusion for 315, 316
Ammonia 66
    Binding to oxystarch 345
    Chloramine precursor 632
    In regenerated dialysate 329
Ammonia intoxication, dialysate regeneration 331, 335
Ammonium chloride 71
Ammonium ion, Redy system, kinetics 324, 329, 331, 333
Amobarbital 775
Amoxicillin 765
Amphetamine 775
Amphotericin B 473, 474, 770
Ampicillin 765
Amyloidosis 401, 604, 862
Anabolic steroids 526, 548, 605
Analgesic 777, 801
Analgesic nephropathy 753, 777, 858
Anaphylactoid purpura 538
Anaphylaxis causing tubular necrosis 540
Ancrod 211, 216
Androgen
    Effect on lipid metabolism 589
    Side effects 637
    Treatment of uremic anemia 397, 637
Anemia 630-638
    Acute renal failure 549

Aluminum intoxication 812
Anesthesia risk 798
Assessment, in renal failure 397
Cardiac effects 602, 605, 606
Children treated by maintenance dialysis 527, 528, 530
Chloramine induced 143, 528
Compensating adjustments 633
Dialysis adequacy, correlation 371, 394
Hemodialysis aggravated 133, 631-633
Hemodynamic effects 602, 603
Histidine deficiency 635
Hyperparathyroidism aggravating 634
Infection aggravating 635
Methylguanidine induced 362
Nephrectomy aggravating 581, 634
Parathyroid hormone induced 373
Pathogenesis, in renal failure 397
Polyamine induced 366
Refractory, treatment 637
Sympathetic tone, effect on 577
Treatment 636-638
Uremic 335, 573, 630
Zinc, hemolysis 144
Anergy in hemodialysis patients 647
Anesthesia 798-803
    Acidosis effect 798
    Anemia, influence on 798
    Blood pressure effects 799
    Drugs 799-802
    Induction 801
    Potassium, effect on 799
    Regional blockade 800, 801
    Risk factors, uremia 798, 799
Aneurysm, angioaccess 178, 181
Angina 399, 602
Angioaccess for dialysis 21-23, 34, 171-185
    Acute renal failure 518, 551
    Anticoagulants for 639
    Atherosclerosis 831
    Children 182, 183, 510, 521, 531
    Choice for chronic use 392
    Diabetic patients 400
    Emergency 171, 392
    Exhaustion of sites 175
    Femoral artery jump graft 183
    Femoral vein 21, 34, 172, 173, 392
    Graft materials 179
    Hemodynamic stress in children 522
    Heroin addicts 402
    Home hemodialysis, for 497, 498
    Hybrid devices 183
    Implantation site 179, 180
    Infection 175, 177, 181, 650, 652, 653
    Ischemia complicating 175, 181
    Maturation 392
    Neuropathy 734
    New approaches 183
    Obese patients 171
    Planning 171, 172
    Saphenous vein 18, 179, 392
    Shuntless 183
    Temporary 171, 172
    Timing surgery 392, 531
    See also Arteriovenous
Angioaccess for plasmapheresis 873
Angiography
    Angioaccess implantation 180
    Cerebral 620, 729

Angiography (*continued*)
    Coronary 604, 605
    Fluorescence, ocular 747
    Retroperitoneal hematoma 621
Angioplasty, transluminal 174
Angiotensin 576, 578, 721
Angiotensin antagonist 396
Angiotensin inhibitor 576, 578
Angiotensinogen 578
1,5-anhydroglucitol 367
Anion gap, plasma due to acetate 158
Ankle reflexes, impaired, neuropathy 731
Anorexia
    Children with chronic renal failure 529
    Hepatitis 664
    Impeding protein repletion 571
    Intensive dialysis, causing 529
    Methylguanidine induced 362
    Peritoneal dialysis 470, 479
    Polyamine induced 366
    Uremic 354
Antacid, magnesium source 700
Antiarrhythmic agents 774, 775
Anti-basal cell nuclear antibody 884
Antibiotic 760-770
    Acute renal failure, use 558
    Decay in peritoneal dialysis fluid 465
    Gastrointestinal pH effect 753
    Nephrotoxicity 760-762
    Peritoneal dialysis fluid additive 465, 473, 557, 558
    Peritoneal transfer rate 474
    Peritonitis 473, 474
    Pharmacokinetics 760-770
    Prophylactic, for angioaccess infection 652
    Treatment of bacteremia 650, 651
    Urinary levels, renal failure 753
Antibody, hepatitis virus 662
Antibody synthesis, effect of plasma exchange 872, 875
Antibody titer, rebound after plasmapheresis 875
Anticoagulation 208, 209, 214-216
    Acute renal failure, dialysis risk 543
    Angioaccess thrombosis prevention 216
    Bleeding complicating 620, 621, 634, 729
    Cerebral ischemia treatment 729
    Hemodialysis 187, 208, 209, 214-216, 553
    Hemodialysis, monitoring 207
    Home dialysis use 499
    Plasmapheresis 873, 874
    Risk-benefit ratio 537, 538
    See also Heparin
Anticonvulsant 613, 730, 780
Antidiuretic hormone 720, 721
Antigen antibody complexes, see Immune complexes
Anti-glomerular basement membrane antibody, plasmapheresis 875-877
Anti-hepatitis A antibody 662
Anti-hepatitis B core antibody 663, 664, 666
Anti-hepatitis B e antibody 663, 664, 666
Anti-hepatitis B surface antibody 662, 663, 666
Anti-hepatitis B surface immunoglobulin 669, 670
Antihistamine, pruritus treatment 622
Antihypertensive agents 771-773
    Anesthesia interaction 799
    Hemodialysis hypotension contributor 555
    Home dialysis patients 499
Antimalarial hemolysis 635
Antimony 753, 781
Anti-N antibodies 299, 625, 633

Antiplasmin 210, 211, 550
Antiplatelet agents 187, 192, 211-214, 217
    Angioaccess, use for 175, 181, 216
    Cerebral ischemia treatment 729
    Side effects 213
Antipyrine 777
Antithrombin III 203, 208
Anxiety 838
    Allayed by simplicity of CAPD 495
    Control and prevention, children on dialysis 530
    Home dialysis, patient and family 495
Aortic valve disease 606, 651
Apathy, uremia 724
Aphasia 728, 729
Apheresis, see Plasmapheresis 872-883
Apolipoprotein, cofactor abnormalities 589
Apoprotein composition of lipoprotein 588
Aprotenin 210
Arachidonic acid 205, 212, 557
Arginase, lysine inhibition, low urea synthesis 360
Arginine 361
Arginosuccinate lyase 360
Aromatic amine 365
Aromatic amino acid 366
Aromatic compound in uremia 367
Arrythmia 606, 607
    Acute renal failure 549
    Cause of death, dialysis patients 596
    Citrate induced 873
    Dialysis disequilibrium 612
    Electrolyte abnormalities causing 606, 607
    Hemodialysis complication 543, 555
    High incidence during hemodialysis and digoxin 399
    Hypotension cause 613
    Myocardial calcification 604
    Pericarditis induced 598, 599
    Peritoneal dialysis complication 475, 476, 558
    Potassium relationship 544, 606
    Renal failure 397
    Thyroxine precipitating 716
    Trichloroethylene 799, 800
Arsenic 142, 144, 805
Arterial blood line 225
Arterial jump graft 183
Arterial steal syndrome 177, 181, 734
Arteriovenous fistula 31, 35, 43, 171, 172, 176-179
    Aneurysm and pseudoaneurysm complicating 178
    Blood flow rates 603
    Children 521
    Complications 177-179, 603
    Congestive heart failure complicating 179, 397, 522, 603
    Hemodynamic effects 603
    Home dialysis use 498
    Infection 177, 652
    Ischemia from 177
    Location 176
    Maturation 171, 392
    Metabolic clearance rate effects 718
    Peripheral nerve effects 734
    Prosthetic, see Graft 179-181
    Stenosis 177
    Technical considerations 176, 177
    Thrombosis 177
    Venous hypertension from 177
Arteriovenous shunt 21-23, 28, 31, 34, 43, 173-175
    Acute renal failure 551
    Anticoagulant use for 216, 217
    Blood flow rates 603

Arteriovenous shunt (*continued*)
    Children 518, 521, 551
    Complications 174, 175
    Hemorrhage 175
    Home dialysis use 498
    Infection 175, 652, 873, 874
    Psychological problems 175
    Restriction of activity 175
    Skin erosion 175
    Technical considerations 173, 174
    Teflon-Silastic 22, 173, 217
    Use until fistula matures 392
Arteriovenous ultrafiltration, spontaneous 272
Arthritis, complicating hemodialysis 624
Artificial kidney, see Hemodialyzer 4
Artificial surface 186-191, 193
Arvin 211
Aryl acid 366
Ascites
    Extracorporeal dialysis of 401
    Hemodialysis complication 401
    Hypotension cause 581, 582
    Peritoneal dialysis complication 476
    Peritoneal lavage treatment 412
Ascitic fluid, hepatitis B surface antigen 667
Ascorbic acid 632, 781
Asellus aquaticus 144
Asepsis, peritoneal catheter care 458, 461
Aseptic necrosis of bone 698
β aspartylglycine 364
Aspiration pneumonia, complicating peritoneal dialysis 475
Aspirin 187, 192, 212, 213, 215, 217, 777
    Anticoagulant for angioaccess 639
    Hemoperfusion anticoagulant 308
Asterixis 364, 725, 726
Asthenia 838
Asthma, hemodialysis membrane sensitivity 625
Ataxia 727
Atelectasis, complicating peritoneal dialysis 475, 558
Atenolol 773
Atherosclerosis 37, 591-593
    Accelerated 591-593, 727
    Cause of death, dialysis patients 595
    Chronic hemodialysis patients 591-593, 595
    Hypertension predisposing to 575
    Long-term survivors of hemodialysis 398, 399
    Medical selection for dialysis 831
    Pathogenesis 206, 591-593
Atherosclerotic heart disease, risk factors 398, 399, 591, 604
Atherosclerotic retinopathy 744
Atomic absorption spectrophotometry 804
ATP, effect of guanidinosuccinic acid 362
ATP, erythrocyte 632
ATPase, see also sodium, magnesium, and calcium 355, 356
    Inhibition in uremia 355, 719, 725, 734
    Middle molecule inhibition 372
    Phenol inhibition 366, 367
Atropine 470, 782, 801
Australia antigen 662
Autoantibody, removal by plasmapheresis 872
Autogenous vein graft 179
Autoimmune hemolysis 635
Autonomic nervous system 251
    Pathogenesis of hypertension 576, 577
Autonomic neuropathy, see Neuropathy
Axonal degeneration 732
Azathioprine 778, 779
    Curare antagonist 800
    Metabolism 758
    Plasmapheresis, use with 875, 876
Azelaic acid 367
Azlocillin 766
Azotemia, aggravated by tetracycline 752, 766

Babb-Grimsrud miniature artificial kidney cell 99
Bacampicillin 765
Bacitracin 769
Back flux 258
Back pain 297, 479, 620, 688
Bacteremia, complicating hemodialysis 509, 649-652
Bacteria, removal by complement and phagocyte 648
Bacterial contamination of hemodialyzer 135
Bacterial contamination, peritoneal dialysis fluid 465
Bacterial endocarditis 605, 606, 651
    Cause of death, dialysis patients 596
    Evaluation 397
    Heroin addicts 402
    Treatment 397
Bacterial endotoxin, contaminating hemodialysis system 293, 299
Bacterial filters for peritoneal dialysis fluid 466
Bacterial flora, intestinal, pathogenesis of uremia 355
Bacterial sepsis, causing tubular necrosis 540
Bactericidal activity, neutrophil in uremia 648
Bacteriologic contamination, hemodialysis systems 293
Bacteriologic control in reprocessing hemodialyzers 292, 293
Bacteriology of bacteremia 650
Bacteriuria 653
Bacteroides peritonitis 472
Band keratopathy 699, 742, 743
Barbital 775
Barbiturate 775
    Intoxication, hemoperfusion for 315, 316
    Pharmacokinetics 775
    Preanesthetic use 801
    Protein binding limiting transport 755
    Removal by diuresis versus dialysis 756
    Vitamin D metabolic interference 702
Baroreceptors 251
    Control of renin secretion 576
    Dysfunction causing hypertension 577, 603
    Dysfunction causing hypotension 581
Basal cell proliferation 885
Base equivalents 78
Basic platelet reaction 205, 211
Behavior, uremia 364, 838, 839
Behavior control, dialysis patients 737
Benzalkonium chloride 292
Benzodiazepine 581, 775
Benzoic acid 366
Benzylammonium chloride 290
Betadine 293, 458, 461, 468
Bicarbonate 63, 71, 77
    Administration to children 516
    Buffer anion for pediatric dialysis 519
    Buffer anion for peritoneal dialysis 417, 517
    Cerebrospinal fluid flux 726
    Depletion, by buffering retained acid 357
    Dialysis fluid 28, 35, 72, 75, 77, 148, 158, 159, 552
    Dialysis fluid, advantages 615
    Dialysis fluid, control of blood pressure 576, 582
    Dialysis fluid delivery system 162
    Dialysis fluid, hypoxia 633
    Distribution volume 75
    Effects on aluminum in dialysis fluid 337
    Hazard in dialysis fluid of Redy 337, 338

Index of subjects

Bicarbonate (*continued*)
    Hemofiltration diluting fluid 267
    Hyperkalemia treatment 545
    Kinetics 75
    Mass balance 77
    Plasma concentration 75, 88
    Redy-sorb system, kinetics 329, 331, 335
    Regeneration by acetate 158
    Renal tubular reabsorption 358
    Short dialysis, effect on 395
    Stability in dialysate, regenerated 329
    Transport 63, 64, 75, 77
Bilirubin, increased in hepatitis 664
Binswanger encephalopathy 728
Bioassay of uremic toxin 355
Bioavailability of drugs 750
Biocompatibility of new and reused dialyzers 297
Biocompatibility of sorbents 306, 308, 313
Biological reactors 325
Biotin 715, 780
Biotransformation 752
Bis(2-ethylhexyl)phthalate leaching 625
Bishydroxycoumarin 781
Bismuth 753, 781
Bladder catheter, hazards in acute renal failure 545
Bladder perforation, peritoneal access risk 460
Blastogenic response to mitogens 647
Bleeding 638, 639
    Acute renal failure, complicating 543
    Anticoagulation complication 639
    Dialysis adequacy correlation 394, 631
    Increased, in elderly patients 399
    Peritoneal dialysis complication 459, 462, 518
    Urea associated 360
    Uremic 213, 355, 634, 639
Bleeding patient, peritoneal dialysis preference 477
Bleeding time 207, 639
Bleomycin 779
Blindness, see Vision 400
Blood
    Adherence to protein adsorbed on surfaces 186
    Coagulation system 186
    Interactions with artificial surfaces 187-190
    Polymer compatibility 194
    Residual in hemodialyzer 133, 134
    Residual volume after hemoperfusion 308
    Storage between dialyses 286
    Water 59
Blood access device, see Angioaccess 171
Blood-cerebrospinal fluid barrier 726, 753
Blood flow 6, 191
Blood flow meter 226
Blood flow path, resistance 250
Blood flow rate 55, 57, 59, 225, 226, 553
    Effect on clearances 125
    Effect on ultrafiltration rate 259
    Hemodialysis in children 521
    Measurement 120-122
    Peritoneal capillary 445, 452
    Splanchnic 445
Blood flow recirculation 123, 394
Blood leak detector 234, 235, 239
Blood leak, hemodialyzer 615
Blood loss
    Chronic renal failure 634
    Contribution to anemia 631
    Hemodialysis 132, 528, 573, 631
    Home dialysis, prevention 499

Blood-membrane interactions 131, 132, 555, 556
Blood pressure 575-587
    Acetate effect 158, 238
    Control, in chronic dialysis patients 575-587
    Extracorporeal 226-228, 238, 239
    Hemodialysis, response to 11, 268-276
    Hemofiltration response 268-270
    Infants and children 515
    Monitoring during pediatric hemodialysis 518
    Monitoring, perioperative 801
    Osmotic disequilibrium, effect on 272
    Relation to hydration 246
    Ultrafiltration 239
    See also Hypertension, Hypotension
Blood pump 17, 19, 122, 225
    Causing hemolysis 225, 632
    Effect on extracorporeal blood pressure 227
    Flow rate 225
    Mechanisms of action 225
    Peristaltic roller 225
Blood resistance, hemodialyzer transport 55, 120
Blood resistance, transport, peritoneal dialysis 441
Blood transfusion
    Children, increased need 527
    Elderly, increased need 399
    Erythropoiesis suppression 634, 635
    Hypotension, treatment of 582
    Indications 397, 636, 638
    Iron overload cause 635
    Kidney transplant survival 638, 672, 798, 832, 863, 864
    Long-term hemodialysis survival effect 399
    Perioperative 801
    Post nephrectomy, increased need 634
    Risks 638
    Sickle cell anemia and hemodialysis 402
Blood tubing clamp 230
Blood viscosity, effect on blood flow resistance 130
Blood volume 250
    Child's, calculation of 516
    Extracorporeal 226, 521, 551, 582
Body base 74
Body surface area vs dialyzer membrane area 522
Body temperature, uremia 716
Body weight
    Dry 239, 240, 250, 531
    Monitoring 239, 240, 522, 543
    Relation to hydration 239
    Relative 569
Bohr effect 633
Bone, see also Osteodystrophy
    Abnormalities in growth zone 696
    Aluminum 700, 813
    Aseptic necrosis 527
    Cystic abnormalities 695
    Fluoride 696
    Vitamin D action 680
Bone age, nutritional assessment 569
Bone biopsy 527, 684
Bone collagen turnover 364
Bone deformities, osteodystrophy 526, 689
Bone formation rate 687
Bone gammacarboxyglutamic acid protein 694
Bone histology, osteodystrophy 684-688
Bone marrow
    Androgen stimulation 637
    Hypoproliferation without erythropoietin 630
    Inhibition 362, 371, 373
    Iron granules in reticuloendothelium 631

Index of subjects 903

Bone marrow fibrosis, hyperparathyroidism 634, 638
Bone mineral content 698
Bone mineralization 683, 694, 700
Bone pain 736, 812
Bone turnover, ostitis fibrosa 687, 695
Boron release from Redy system 336
Bovine carotid artery graft 35, 179
Bradycardia 362, 470
Bradykinin 578, 721, 874
Brain
    Abnormalities, acute renal failure 549
    Aluminum content 812, 813
    Calcium, increased 690
    Idiogenic osmoles, dialysis disequilibrium 393
    Osmolality 612
    Pathology, dialysis encephalopathy 812
    Response to dialysis 838
    Uremia, structure 725
    Vascular disease 727-730
Brain abscess 730
Brain metabolism 725
Breath, uremic, methylamines in 365
Brescia-Cimino arteriovenous fistula 31, 176-179
Bretylium 774, 775
Bromide 776, 807
    Body content 805
    Depletion 808
    Elimination 752, 755, 756
    Pharmacokinetics 756, 776
    Psychosis 776
Bromocriptine inhibition of prolactin secretion 714
Broviack catheter 551
Buffer 74-78
Buffer anion, dialysis fluid 465
Buffer anion, hemofiltration diluting fluid 267, 552
Buformin 779, 780
Bufuralol 773
Bulk of flow of water 243, 244
BUN, see Urea
Burning feet 731
Burns, causing renal ischemia 540
Bursitis, uremic 624
Buselmeier shunt 34, 173
Busulfan 779
Butabarbital 775
2,3 butylene glycol 367

Cadaverine 365
Cadmium 144, 148, 805, 807, 808
Calcifediol 680
Calcification 698, 699
    Arterial 689, 690
    Ocular 742-744
    Renal 753
    Soft tissue 526, 698, 699, 705
Calciphylaxis 689, 690, 705
Calcitonin 549, 705
Calcitriol 680
Calcium 153
    Aggravation of digitalis intoxicity 753
    Body content 155, 698
    Brain, in uremia 549, 690, 726
    Cation exchange, in dialysate regeneration 324, 330
    Content of water supply 154
    Dialysance 692
    Dialysis fluid 143, 153-155, 527, 552, 692, 693, 700
    Gastrointestinal reabsorption 154, 155
    Hemodialysis, effect on plasma 692, 693
    Hemofiltration, influence on 267, 270
    Hemoperfusion, removal by 308
    Hyperkalemia treatment 545, 546
    Ionized, plasma concentration 552
    Metabolism, renal failure 372
    Mitochondrial transport 355, 361
    Muscle relaxant effect 799
    Omission from peritoneal dialysis fluid 417
    Oral supplements 700
    Peripheral nerve concentration 734
    Peripheral vascular resistance, effect 577
    Peritoneal dialysis fluid concentration 464, 465
    Plasma, abnormal and osteodystrophy 398
    Plasma, acute renal failure 549
    Plasma, monitoring during vitamin D therapy 527
    Platelet release reaction transmitter 205
    Precipitation in alkaline solution 153
    Redy-sorb system 330, 334
    Response to parathyroid hormone 682, 683
    Transport during dialysis 154, 692
    Ultrafilterable fraction in plasma 154
    Ultrafiltration, removal by 154, 248
    Water softening, removal by 145
Calcium balance 154, 155
Calcium carbonate supplements 700
Calcium intake, uremic children 516, 527
Calcium-phosphorus product
    Long-term survival 398
    Ocular calcification 742-744
    Periarthritis 689
    Soft tissue calcification 604, 699
Caloric requirement, renal failure 547, 572
Canavaninosuccinic acid 362
Cancer
    Cause of death 865, 866
    Dialysis for 891-893
    Regression after electrolyte depletion 891-893
    Underlying polymicrobial bacteremia 651
Cancer chemotherapeutic, hemoperfusion removal 318
Candida peritonitis 472
Capacitance air detector 230
Capillaries, peritoneal transport 441
Capreomycin 769
Captopril 576, 773
    Pharmacokinetics 773
    Toxicity 579, 753
    Treatment of hypertension 396, 528, 578-580
Carbamazepine 780
Carbamylation reactions, urea induced 360
Carbenicillin 765, 766
Carbohydrate, dietary and hyperlipidemia 590
Carbohydrate metabolism in uremia 718-720
Carbon
    Activated, requirements for clinical hemoperfusion 306, 307
    Affinity for ions 323
    Contaminant toxicity, hemoperfusion 308, 336
    Sorbent material 306, 307, 323, 341
Carbon dioxide 63, 64, 71
    Excretion 65, 76
    Kinetics with Redy-sorb system 331, 332
    Removal by hemodialysis 556, 623, 633
    Transport 63, 65
Carbon dioxide content 64
Carbon dioxide generation 65
Carbonic anhydrase inhibitor, glaucoma treatment 744
3 Carboxyanthralinic acid 366
Cardiac arrhythmia, see Arrhythmia

Index of subjects

Cardiac complications of regular dialysis 595-610
Cardiac dysfunction, iron overload 636
Cardiac failure, see Heart failure 602
Cardiac function, impaired in children 528
Cardiac output
    Baroreceptor response 251
    Effects of uremia 359, 360
    Increased, with arteriovenous fistula 179, 528
Cardiac tamponade 397, 596, 599, 601
Cardiomyopathy 602
Cardiorespiratory effects of peritoneal dialysis 470, 558
Cardiotoxicity, uremic metabolites 362, 372
Cardiovascular complications, acute renal failure 549
Cardiovascular complications of hemodialysis 528
Cardiovascular complications of peritoneal dialysis 475
Cardiovascular disease
    Morbidity in renal failure 398, 399, 591
    Polyamine induction hypothesis 365
    Preference for peritoneal dialysis 477
Cardiovascular drugs 770-775
Cardiovascular stability with peritoneal dialysis 478
Cardiovascular symptoms, uremic 354
Carnitine
    Deficiency, hyperlipemia 365, 589
    Deficiency, muscle weakness 736
    Excess 736
    Plasma level in renal failure 365
    Removal by hemodialysis 365, 589, 736
Carnosine 364
Carotenoids 372
Carpal tunnel syndrome 398, 624, 734
Carpopedal spasm 727
Catabolism, increasing nutritional requirements 569
Cataract 744, 747
Catecholamine
    Abnormal metabolism, schizophrenia 888
    Control of renin secretion 576
    Plasma level, dialysis patients 238, 269, 528, 720
    Plasma level response to hemofiltration 269
    Pressor effect 576
    Response to ultrafiltration 238, 251, 614
Catheter, see Peritoneal catheter 458-464
Cation exchange, in dialysate regeneration 329
Cation, total osmotically active 79
Cefaclor 763, 764
Cefadroxil 763, 764
Cefamandole 763
Cefazolin 762, 763
Cefmetazole 764
Cefoperazone 764
Ceforanide 764
Cefotaxime 764
Cefoxitin 763
Ceftezole 764
Cefuroxim 764
Cell growth, ribonuclease inhibition 373
Cell membrane permeability, uremia 726
Celloidin 3, 7
Cellophane 12, 19, 26, 32, 98, 107
Cellular respiration, inhibition in uremia 359
Cellular solute, distortion of clearance calculation 261
Cellulose, oxidized, oral use 344-347
Cellulose acetate membrane 102, 103, 146, 252
Cellulose diacetate hollow fiber membranes 873
Cellulose membranes 97, 98, 252
Centrifugation, plasma exchange 872, 873
Cephacetrile 764
Cephalexin 763

Cephaloglycin 764
Cephaloridine 762, 763
Cephalosporin 762-764
    Hemolysis 635
    Nephrotoxicity 540, 762
    Pharmacokinetics 762-764
    Renal elimination 752, 763
Cephalothin
    Intraperitoneal 465, 473, 474
    Pharmacokinetics 762, 763
Cephanone 764
Cephapirin 763
Cephradine 763
Cerebral depression, phenol induced 366
Cerebral edema
    Cerebral vascular disease 729
    Dialysis disequilibrium 612, 727
    Hemodialysis complication 543, 555, 633
    Hepatitis complication 664
    Malignant hypertension 728
    Water intoxication 726
Cerebral embolism 729
Cerebral hemorrhage 543, 729
Cerebral thrombosis 729
Cerebrospinal fluid
    Acidosis 612, 726
    Binswanger encephalopathy 729
    Hyponatremia 726
    Intracranial bleeding 730
    Malignant hypertension 728
    Myoinositol levels 367
    pH changes during dialysis 612
    Phenols 366
    Uremia 725
Cerebrospinal fluid pressure, dialysis disequilibrium 393, 61 744
Cerebrovascular accident 727-730, 865
Ceruloplasmin 632
Cetylpyridinium chloride 290
Charcoal
    Adsorption 35, 36, 344
    Adsorption of essential solutes 307, 308
    Dialysate regeneration 323, 324, 330
    Encapsulation, reducing side effects 308
    Hemoperfusion, for 306, 307, 758
    Lipid binding 344, 348-350
    Oral 344
    Oral, treatment of hyperlipemia 349, 350
    Pruritus treatment 622
    Side effects of oral 344
Charcoal hemoperfusion 344
    Drug intoxication, for 314, 315
    Hepatic encephalopathy, for 316-318
Chelating agents 342
Chelation, iron removal with hemodialysis 636
Chemisorbents 307
Chemoreceptor, control of renin secretion 576
Chemotaxis, uremia, impaired 640, 647
Chemotherapy, cancer response after electrolyte loss 893
Chest pain 297, 651, 688
    Differential diagnosis 599
    Pericarditis causing 598
Children 514-535
    Acute renal failure 515-519
    Angioaccess 521, 531
    Cardiac causes of death 528
    Chronic renal failure 519-533
    Dialysis 514-535, 826

Index of subjects 905

Children (*continued*)
  Energy requirements, chronic renal failure 528, 529
  Hemodialysis 294, 295, 514-535
  Hemodialysis, practical aspects 531-533
  Hemodialyzer, choice of 532
  Home dialysis 494, 495, 512
  Peritoneal dialysis 477, 480, 481
  Psychologic stress of hemodialysis 529, 530
  Renal failure treatment centers 520
  Survival with chronic renal failure 524
Chloral hydrate 517, 775
Chlorambucil 779, 878
Chloramines 143, 145, 146, 528, 617, 632
Chloramphenicol 768
Chlordiazepoxide 775
Chloride
  Dialysis fluid 148, 158, 159, 464, 553
  Plasma concentration 148, 159
  Release from zirconium phosphate 331
Chlorine, chloramine precursor 632
Chlorine dioxide 292
2-Chloroethanol toxicity 625
Chloroform 799
Chloroguanide 770
Chloroquin 770
Chlorpromazine 516, 517, 750, 776
Chlorpropamide 752, 779
Chlortetracycline 767
Choice reaction time 364, 736
Cholecalcifererol 679, 680
Cholecystokinin 717
Cholestasis, fluoxymesterone 637
Cholesterol emboli 559
Cholesterol, plasma level
  Dialysis fluid dextrose, relation to 160
  Dietary effect on 572
  Hemofiltration, response to 271
  Lipoprotein cholesterol relationship 590
  Lowering by charcoal 349, 350
  Uremic patients 588
Cholestyramine, pruritus treatment 622
Choline 364, 365
Chorionic gonadotrophin 715
Choroidal vasculature 745, 747
Chromatography
  High-pressure liquid 369
  Ion exchange 369
  Middle molecule assay 280, 281, 369
Chromium 805, 807, 808
Chromium, radioactive labelled erythrocytes 133, 134
Chronic active hepatitis 664, 666
Chronic hepatitis 661-664
Chronic obstructive pulmonary disease, pneumonia complicating 653
Chronic persistent hepatitis 664
Chronic renal failure, see Renal failure
Chvostek sign 727
Chylous peritoneal dialysate 445
Cimetidine 705, 773, 782
Cinoxacin 769
Cirrhosis, hepatic 581, 665, 750
Cis-platinum 779
Citrate, arrhythmia induced by 873
Citrulline 364
Cleaning hemodialyzer for reuse 289-292
Clearance 57, 59-61, 122, 253
  Blood flow effects 125
  Calculation 123, 124
  Calculation distortion 123, 261, 449, 754
  Calculation, hemofiltration 123, 261
  Calculation, sequential dialysis and ultrafiltration 123
  Convective, urea 254
  Determinants 125-127
  Dialysis fluid flow rate effect 125, 127, 331, 421
  Dialyzer, fraction of total 751
  Diffusive 58
  Distribution volume relationship 751
  Drugs 751
  Half life, inverse relationship 751, 752, 755, 756
  Hematocrit effect 125, 260
  Hemodialysis and hemofiltration comparison 283
  Hemofiltration, by 256, 259-261, 266
  Intracellular solute trapping, effect on 450
  In vitro 754
  Membrane characteristics effect 126, 127
  Middle molecules, dialyzer 126, 127
  Middle molecules, renal 370
  Peritoneal dialysis 254, 429, 430, 442, 443
  Renal, fraction of total 751
  Restriction by protein binding 449
  Reused dialyzers 288, 295, 296
  Small solutes, by hemofiltration 268
  Temperature effects 125
  Ultrafiltration effects 125
  Urea 21
Clindamycin 175, 768
Clinitest, assay for formaldehyde 295, 300, 336, 633
Clofazimine 770
Clofibrate 590, 782
Clonazepam 725, 731, 811
Clonidine 396, 579
Clostridium peritonitis 472
Clotrimazole 546
Clotting time 70, 207
Cloxacillin 765, 766
Coagulation
  Activation by erythrocyte-surface adhesion 190
  Acute renal failure, abnormalities 550
  Effect of leukocyte adherence 189
  Hemoperfusion abnormalities, hepatic encephalopathy 317
  Penicillin induced abnormalities 764, 766
Coagulation cascade, enhanced by platelet factor 188
Coagulation factors, adsorption of 308
Coagulation factors, extracorporeal activation 186, 187
Coagulation system 186, 187
  Extrinsic 202, 206
  Intrinsic pathway 187, 202
Coagulation tests 206, 207
Cobalt 638, 781, 805
Cognition 736, 820
Coil hemodialyzer, see also Hemodialyzer 18, 111-114, 551
Colchicine 778
Cold agglutinins, underheated dialysate 233
Colistimethate 767
Colitis, uremic 354
Collagen
  β Aspartylglycine source 364
  Cross linkages, effect of vitamin D 683
  Irregular alignment, ostitis fibrosa 687
  Platelet aggregation stimulator 639
  Uremic abnormalities 684
Collagen membranes 100
Collagen metabolism, vitamin D action 680
Coma
  Acidosis 726

Coma (*continued*)
   Air embolism 618
   Dialysis disequilibrium 612
   Drug induced 753
   Hypercalcemia 727
   Hyperosmolar non-ketonic 400, 464, 475
   Penicillin neurotoxicity 727, 764
   Uremic 354
   Water intoxication 356, 726
Community support of home dialysis 510
Comonomers 100
Complement
   Activation by hemodialysis 132, 252, 555, 592, 647, 886
   Depletion, cryoglobulinemia 878
   Fresh frozen plasma component 874
   Plasmapheresis and resynthesis 875
   Removal of bacteria 648
   Role in leukopenia complicating hemodialysis 189, 214, 640
   Serum, nutritional assessment 569, 571
Complement fixation, hepatitis virus 663
Complement system 186
Complexing agent 342
Compliance
   Dialysis selection criterion 831
   Dialyzer blood compartment 129, 130
   Dietary, increased in elderly patients 399
   Medical regimen 839-841
Compression chamber, treatment of air embolism 619
Computer for record keeping 827
Computerized tomography, subdural hematoma 620
Concanavilin A 885
Concentration
   Average of plasma 87
   Change, affecting clearance calculation 449
   Drug effect correlation 756
   Intercompartmental difference 88
   Plasma, decay of 69, 751
   Rebound increase after dialysis 85, 756
   Solute, determinants during hemodialysis 394
   Solute, in plasma water 249
   Solute, in ultrafiltrate 245
Concentration equilibrium 69
Concentration gradient 54, 55, 57-59, 122, 245
   Across semipermeable membrane 242
   Peritoneal, increased by ultrafiltration 448
Concentration polarization 100, 128, 255, 258
   Effect on ultrafiltration rate 258, 282
Conductivity monitor, dialysate regeneration 326
Conductivity monitoring, dialysis solution 232
Confabulation 727
Confusion 356
   Acidosis 726
   Acute renal failure 549
   Dialysis disequilibrium 727
   Hypercalcemia 727
   Hyponatremia 726
   Intracranial bleeding 730
   Korsakoff psychosis 727
   Malignant hypertension 728
   Mental, pericarditis sign 598
Congestive heart failure, see Heart 397
Conjugation, biotransformation process 752
Conjunctival calcification 699, 742-744
Conjunctival hemorrhage 744
Conservative treatment versus dialysis 17, 423
Contamination of tap water 142-144
Continuous ambulatory peritoneal dialysis 432-435, 468, 469, 479, 480
   Acute renal failure 476, 557
   Advantages 432, 433, 495, 497
   Anemia improved by 638
   Children 495, 524
   Clinical and biochemical results 479
   Complications 524
   Cost 433
   Disadvantages 433
   Drug removal 758
   Enthusiasm for 433, 458
   Exchange frequency 479
   Expansion of use 854
   Future role in treatment of uremia 434, 435
   Home dialysis 497
   Hypotensive patient 582
   Middle molecule removal 370, 433
   Nutrition 573
   Patient population 873, 874
   Peritonitis complicating 433, 480, 524
   Protein intake and exchange volume 479
   Protein loss 433
   Sodium intake 573
   Survival 479, 861
   Technical evolution 432
   Technique survival 479
   Training 501
   Urea clearance 433
Continuous cyclic peritoneal dialysis 434, 469
Continuous flow peritoneal dialysis 415, 418
Continuous hemofiltration 556
Continuous performance test 394, 736
Convection 36, 58-61, 253-256, 281
   Albumin in peritoneal dialysis 256
   Contribution to solute transport 244, 253
   Impact on diffusion in peritoneal dialysis 254-256
   Peritoneal dialysis, electrolyte removal 448, 449
   Peritoneal dialysis, transport contribution 254, 428, 444, 448, 758
   Sodium transport by 333
   Transport, relation to solute size 252
Converting enzyme 576, 578
Convulsions
   Acidosis 726
   Acute renal failure 516, 549
   Air embolism 618
   Children 516, 522, 533
   Dialysis encephalopathy 596, 811
   Hemodialysis complication 522, 533, 612, 633
   Hypocalcemia 705, 726, 727
   Malignant hypertension 728
   Methylguanidine induced 362
   Penicillin 764
   Peritoneal dialysis complication 475
   Treatment 613, 730
   Uremic 354, 725
   Water intoxication 356, 726
Copolymer membrane 100, 101, 103
Copper 233, 805
   Binding by zirconium oxide 326
   Body stores 808
   Hemolysis 528, 601, 632, 807
   Intoxication 143, 144, 807
   Leaching from pipes 143, 632, 807
   Plasma levels 529
   Release from Redy-sorb system 336
   Tap water, in 143, 144, 161
Cornea, calcification 742-744
Coronary angiography 604, 605
Coronary artery disease, hemodialysis patients 591, 595, 865

Coronary bypass surgery, hemodialysis patients 399
Corpus luteum 714
Cortical bone turnover 687
Cortical necrosis, renal
    Causing acute renal failure 537, 559
    In children 515, 520
    Survival 862
Cortisol 715
    Hemodialysis removal 717
    Plasma level in renal failure 526, 717
Cortisone, plasma level response to hemofiltration 270
Cost of dialysis 433, 828, 844, 846
Cotrimoxazole 768
Cough, septic pulmonary emboli 651
Coumadin 175, 216
Coumarin derivatives 187, 209, 213, 216, 217
Counter immunoelectrophoresis 663
Coxsackievirus, pericarditis 598
C-reactive protein, plasmapheresis 875
Creatine 361, 362
Creatine ketolase 736
Creatine kinase 736
Creatinine 361
    Adsorption by carbon 323, 330, 344
    Hemoperfusion removal of 308-310
    Intestinal fluid content 343
    Methylguanidine precursor 361
    Monomethylamine precursor 365
    Plasma concentration 34, 68, 78
    Plasma level and initiation of dialysis 531, 550
    Plasma, predictor of plasmapheresis response 877
    Removal by regenerated dialysate 323
    Toxicity 361
    Transport by intestinal perfusion 342, 343
Creatinine clearance 67, 68
    Dialysis fluid flow rate effect 331
    Endogenous, correlation with uremic symptoms 392
    Endogenous, hemodialysis initiation 391, 392
    Hemodialyzer reuse, effect of 288
    Measurement 478
    Overall 478
Creatinine generation 68, 78
Creatinine metabolism 361
Creatinine phosphokinase 688
Crescentic nephritis, see Glomerulonephritis 877
p-Cresol 366, 367
Cryoglobulin, plasma exchange 874, 875
Cryoglobulinemia 665, 878
Cryoseparation 873
Cuff erosion, peritoneal catheter 462
Cuprophane 24, 32, 34, 98
    Dialysis effect on uremic neuropathy 271
    Hydraulic permeability 253, 276
    Sensitivity, asthma 625
    Sieving coefficient 247, 252, 281
    Solute permeability 276, 279
Cyanate, urea derivative 360
Cyanide, urea derivative 360
Cyanocobalamin, see Vitamin B_{12} 781
Cyanosis 619, 632
Cyclacillin 765
Cyclers, see peritoneal dialysis fluid 419, 421, 466
Cyclic AMP 363, 885
    Abnormal stimulation, uremia 726
    Hemodialysis effect on 363
    Impaired lymphocyte function 647
    Mechanism of plasma increase 363
    Plasma level, in renal failure 363, 694
    Platelet 211

Cyclophosphamide 779
    Cryoglobulinemia treatment 878
    Plasmapheresis, use with 876
Cyclopropane 799, 801
Cycloserine 769
Cystathionine, accumulation in renal failure 364
Cysteine, accumulation in renal failure 364
Cystic fibrosis, peritoneal dialysis 479
Cystinosis, survival 862
Cytomegalovirus infection 653, 654
    Immunosuppressed patient 730
    Kidney transplants 648, 654
    Pericarditis cause 598, 620
    Retina 743, 746
Cytosine arabinoside 779
Cytosol malate dehydrogenase 716
Cytosolic receptor for vitamin D 680
Cytotoxic drug, cryoglobulinemia 878
Cytotoxic drug, psoriasis treatment 884, 888

Dacron felt cuff of peritoneal catheter 460-462
Dane particles 40, 663, 666
Dapsone 770
Daunorubicin 779
Deaeration of dialysis fluid 125, 163, 164, 229, 232, 234, 235, 332, 618
Deafness, see Ototoxicity 624
Deane's prosthesis for peritoneal access 459
Decamethonium 798, 800
Degassing dialysis fluid: see Deaeration
Dehydration 540, 613
Dehydroepiandrosterone 885
Dehydrotachysterol 680
Deionizer 145
Deionizer exhaustion, copper contamination 632
Delayed hypersensitivity, decreased in uremia 647
Delerium 724, 726, 727, 838
Demeclocycline 766, 767
Dementia 728
Demyelination 732
Dependency, dialysis patients 839, 845
Dependent variable 88, 91
Depletion by dialysis 757
Depression
    Dialysis selection criterion 831
    Reserpine 772
    Uremia 838
Dermal drug reactions 753
Desferrioxamine 781, 817
Detergents for hemodialyzer reuse 290
Detoxification, extracorporeal, enzyme 758
Dexamethasone, cerebral edema treatment 729
Dextran, peritoneal osmotic agent 416, 464
Dextran treatment of air embolism 619
Dextrose
    Absorption from peritoneal fluid 421, 433
    Anhydrous 247
    Carmelization in dialysis fluid 465
    Charcoal absorption 330
    Deterioration of osmotic effect 254, 464
    Dialysis fluid 148, 149, 151, 159, 160, 555
    Disequilibrium prevention and treatment 393, 613, 744
    Energy source 90
    Gradients along peritoneal membrane 449
    Hyperkalemia treatment 545, 546
    Lipid metabolism effect 160, 590
    Metabolic effects of dialysis fluid content 159, 160
    Monohydrate 247
    Osmolar contribution in dialysis fluid 127, 243, 247

Index of subjects

Dextrose (*continued*)
    Osmotic agent for peritoneal dialysis 252, 464
    Peritoneal fluid concentration 416, 464, 470, 517, 557
    Transport during hemodialysis 159
    See also Glucose
Diabetes insipidus, lithium, nephrogenic 776
Diabetes mellitus 400
    Atherosclerosis risk 591, 604, 727
    Antireceptor antibodies, plasmapheresis 880
    Binswanger encephalopathy risk 728
    Hemodialysis high risk group 400
    Infection complicating 649, 651
    Pericarditis complicating 598
    Reduced peritoneal clearance 444
Diabetic nephropathy
    Peritoneal dialysis for 480
    Protein malnutrition 573
    Survival 862
    Treatment modes 859
Diabetic retinopathy 744, 745
Diafiltration 265
Dia-flo membranes 100
Dialysance 55, 57-61, 114, 122-124, 253
    Blood flow relationship 124
    Diffusive 57-60
    Peritoneal dialysis 442
    Rhône-Poulenc hemodialyzer 276
Dialysate
    Bacterial growth 135, 144, 235
    Middle molecule content 280
    Pressure drop in transit 131
    Pressure monitoring 233
    Resistance to transport 32, 55, 136
    Unstirred layers, impeding transport 255, 256
    See also Dialysis fluid
Dialysate circuit, hemodialyzer, monitoring 230-236
Dialysate mixing, peritoneal dialysis 255
Dialysate pressure 227, 231
Dialysate regeneration 323-340
    Acid base balance 331, 332
    Aluminum, bicarbonate interactions 337
    Clinical experience 335
    Dialysis fluid flow rate effect 331
    Economics 335
    Electrochemical methods 325
    History of development 323-325
    Hypercapnia complicating 332
    Indications for use 335
    Practical aspects 326-338
    Sodium kinetics 333, 334
    Urea load effect 331
Dialysis 3
    Acceptance rate 830, 836, 854
    Acidosis correction 358
    Acute renal failure 517-519, 550-556
    Adaption phase, nutrition 570
    Adaption, psychologic 737
    Adequacy of 62, 279, 393, 394
    Age distribution of patients 853, 857
    Aliphatic amine removal 364
    Anemia, treatment of 636
    Antagonism against 834
    Blood pressure control 575-587
    Carnitine removal 736
    Children 515-535, 822, 826
    Chronic renal failure 15, 24-28
    Cost 29, 41, 42, 158, 341, 828
    Cost containment 821, 828
    Criticism of 17
    Delayed by minoxidil therapy 580
    Dependency 839, 845
    Depletion caused by 757
    Discontinuation 393, 834, 846
    Dose response, psoriasis 886
    Drugs 760-782
    Drugs, fractional removal 756
    Duration, effect on transplant outcome 864
    Efficiency related to middle molecule levels 370
    Electrolyte depletion 892
    Environmental impact 840, 845, 846
    Ethical issues 393
    Evolution 820, 821
    Family support 845
    Fractional clearance of distribution volume 756
    Frequency 70, 120
    Funding 821, 828, 846
    Geographical distribution 42, 341, 850-855
    Governmental regulations 846
    Gross national product correlation 855
    Half-life, influence on 755, 756
    Holidays 825
    Home, see Home hemodialysis 28-31, 493-513
    Hospitalization rates 867
    Immediate for chronic renal failure 392
    Inadequate, clinical picture 479, 597
    Indications in acute renal failure 550
    Infrequent 395, 396
    Intestinal 341-343
    Invention of 3
    Late initiation inhibiting rehabilitation 391
    Medical management of patients 396-398, 324, 826
    Medical selection 837
    Medicolegal aspects 846
    Metabolic effects on drug action 757
    Methods 855
    Methods to improve 558
    Middle molecule removal 370
    Mortality rate 821, 864-866
    National programs, evolution 850-853
    National standards 823
    Neurological complications 724-741
    Neurological response 838
    Neuropathy, prevention and treatment 731, 732
    Nutrition 569-574
    Overnight, unattended 493
    Patient flux 821
    Patient population characteristics 822
    Pediatric facilities 520-522, 826
    Pericarditis, need for increased 600
    Pharmacological aspects 749-797
    Platelet function improvement 631, 639
    Portable 479
    Postponement by dietary restriction 392
    Program planning 820-829
    Program policy 822
    Protein binding, effect on 363
    Psoriasis 38, 318, 884-888
    Psychological stress 736-738, 838, 839
    Psychosocial aspects 840, 841
    Quality control 827
    Quality of life 837-843
    Record keeping 827
    Reduced efficiency and protein intake 394
    Regional organization 823, 834
    Regional programs 826
    Removal impeded by slow intercompartmental transfer 84, 750
    Requirement for acute renal failure 537

Dialysis 3 (*continued*)
  Research need 847
  Schedules 33, 34, 532, 856
  Schizophrenia 41, 318, 888-891
  Selection criteria 28, 821, 822, 830-834
  Self care 494, 495, 825
  Sham 886, 891
  Slow, to prevent disequilibrium 613
  Socioeconomic aspects 41, 42
  Sodium balance 79, 80
  Survival 859-861
  Technological advances 3-35, 414-434, 847
  Temporary methods 834
  Terminally ill patients, ethics 393
  Trace metal abnormalities 804-810
  Transplantation, integration with 822, 830, 834, 835
  Traveling capability 335
  Treatment options 822
  Vitamin requirements 572, 573
  Water balance 79, 80
  Wearable system 458
  See also Hemodialysis, Peritoneal
Dialysis associated hepatitis 659-678
Dialysis dementia, see Dialysis encephalopathy 142, 811
Dialysis disequilibrium 120, 271, 393, 475, 551, 555, 612, 613, 727, 736
  Children 518-522
  Differential diagnosis 612, 613, 620
  Electroencephalogram 612
  Home dialysis, avoiding 499
  Pathogenesis 393, 612, 727
  Prevention and treatment 393, 555, 613, 727
  Prevention by reducing clearance 553
  Relation to osmolality changes 120, 150, 151
Dialysis encephalopathy 38, 39, 142, 348, 811, 816
  Aluminum relationship 337, 807, 808, 811, 816
  Clinical aspects 811
  Epidemiology 811
Dialysis facilities 823, 824
  Availability 831
  Center interaction 826
  Core units 823
  Education 827
  Organization of services 823
  Research 827
  Size and number of core units 824
  Staffing 823, 824
Dialysis fluid 148-170
  Acetate 28, 35, 64, 65, 72, 157, 158, 324, 615
  Aluminum 337, 806, 813, 814
  Analysis 162
  Bicarbonate 28, 35, 72, 77, 148, 158, 552, 615
  Buffer anion 552, 633
  Calcium 143, 148, 153-155, 527, 692, 693, 700
  Central supply system 28
  Chloride 148, 553
  Concurrent flow 56
  Composition, acute renal failure 551
  Concentrate 28, 161, 162, 231
  Conductivity monitoring 232
  Constituting 161
  Copper contamination 143, 144
  Counter current flow 19, 24, 56
  Deaeration 125, 163, 164, 229, 232, 234, 236, 332
  Delivery systems 28, 35, 162, 163, 231, 235, 236, 278
  Dextrose 148, 149, 151, 159, 160, 552
  Dextrose-free 159
  Electrical resistance 232
  Flow 21, 24
  Flow path 28, 32, 113, 115, 135
  Flow rate 55, 57, 59, 111, 127, 225, 234, 331
  Flow resistance 130
  Fluoride 143, 160
  Hypotonic causing hemolysis 633
  Magnesium 143, 148, 155-157, 552, 693, 700
  Mixing 161
  Modified composition for regeneration 324, 333
  Monitoring composition 232
  Negative pressure 163
  Nitrate 143
  Osmolality, dextrose contribution 243
  Overheated causing hemolysis 233
  pH effects on aluminum kinetics 337
  Potassium 148, 152, 153, 552, 606
  Preparation 231, 232, 498
  Proportioning pump 232, 332, 426
  Proportioning systems 162, 163, 232
  Recirculation 114, 122, 162
  Redy-sorb system, acetate for 334
  Replenishing fixed volume 148
  Reuse 35
  Sodium 78, 81, 82, 144, 148-152, 232, 551, 552
  Sodium concentration for Redy system 333, 334
  Sorbent adsorption of sodium 335
  Sterilization 235, 236
  Tank supply system 161
  Temperature monitoring 232, 233
  Trace metal contamination 142-144
  Turbulent flow 7
  Underheated, precipitating cold agglutinins 233
  Volume 162, 323
  See also Dialysate
Dialysis fluid delivery system 235, 236
Dialysis index 33, 368, 370, 394, 522
Dialysis membrane 97-105
Dialyzer, see also Hemodialyzer
  Hoop 3, 5
Diamine oxidase 362, 365
Diaphragm, displacement, peritoneal dialysis 465
Diarrhea, methylguanidine induced 362
Diarrhea therapy see Gastrointestinal lavage 343
Diazepam 775, 799
  Convulsions treatment 533, 615
  Dialysis encephalopathy treatment 811
  Disequilibrium treatment 613
  Perioperative use 801
  Peritoneal dialysis premedication 517
  Protein binding 750
Diazoxide 516, 533, 580, 772
Dibekacin 762
Dicloxacillin 765, 766
Diet, see Nutrition 569-574
  Children 528, 529, 531
  Diabetic patient treated by hemodialysis 400
  Hyperlipemia treatment 590
  Low protein 394, 571
  Protein, effects 362
Diet log assay of dialysis adequacy 394
Diethylenetriaminepentaacetic acid 781
Diffusion 3, 36, 54, 55, 58, 243
  Contribution to solute transport 253
  Convection effect on peritoneal dialysis 254
  Effect of solute size 98
  Enhancement by dialysate mixing 255
  Into sorbents 306
  Non-ionic and peritoneal dialysis 443

Diffusion (*continued*)
    Peritoneal dialysis, rate determinants 442
Diffusivity 54, 55
Diflunisal 777
Digitalis 770, 771
    Electrolyte effects on 753
    Margin of safety 758
    Need for potassium in dialysis fluid 464, 552, 555
    Pericarditis use 599, 600
    Pharmacokinetics 771
    Treatment of heart failure 605
Digitalis toxicity 770, 771
    Acute renal failure complication 543
    Electrolyte effects 753, 757
    Peritoneal dialysis complication 475
    Risk of lowering potassium 616
Digitoxin 771
    Pharmacokinetics 363, 771
    Removal by hemoperfusion 315, 316, 771
    Toxicity 771
Digoxin 771
    Abdominal pain complicating 617
    Arrhythmia during dialysis 399
    Distribution volume 756, 771
    Heart failure treatment 397
    Increased use in elderly 399
    Loading dose 758
    Pharmacokinetics 771
    Quinidine interactions 757
    Removal by hemoperfusion 315, 316
    Tissue protein binding 751, 771
    Toxicity 771
Dihydroxybenzoic acid 366
1,25-Dihydroxyvitamin D_3 679, 680, 682, 683, 780
    Decreased plasma levels 683
    Growth retardation treatment 689
    Myopathy of osteodystrophy treatment 688
    Osteodystrophy treatment 398, 527, 701
    Parathyroid suppression by 700
    Production 679, 680, 682
    Resistance, aluminum intoxication 812
24,25-Dihydroxyvitamin D_3 680, 682
    Impaired production 683
    Use for vitamin D treatment failures 703
Diluting fluid for hemofiltration 257, 267
    Composition 267, 281
    Site of infusion 266, 267
    Volume 267, 281
Dimercaprol 781
Dimethyladipic acid 367
Dimethylamine 365
Dimethyltubocuranine 782
Dinitrochlorobenzene 648
Dioctyl sodium succinate 454
Dipeptide 364
Diphenylhydantoin, see Phenytoin 363
Diphenylmethane diisocyanate, antibodies to 625
2,3-Diphosphoglycerate 633
    Decrease with hypophosphatemia 635
    Erythrocyte, peritoneal dialysis effects 470
Diphosphonate 698
Dipyridamole
    Antiplatelet effect 181, 187, 192, 212, 213
    Arteriovenous shunt patency 175, 217
    Peritoneal dialysis fluid additive 557, 758
    Pharmacokinetics 781
Disc catheter for peritoneal dialysis 461
Discalculia 736
Disequilibrium, see Dialysis disequilibrium 612, 613

Disinfection
    Dialysis fluid delivery system 235, 236
    Hemodialysis equipment 292, 498
    Hepatitis prophylaxis 668
    Peritoneal dialysis tubing 458, 461, 468
Disopyramide 774
Distribution coefficient, transcellular 259
Distribution equilibrium 750
Distribution kinetics, transcellular 262
Distribution volume, see Volume
Diuretic
    Acute renal failure treatment 540
    Decreased response, renal failure 753
    Hypertension treatment 577
    Peritoneal transport effect 454
    Pharmacokinetics 773, 774
    Potassium depletion cause 753
DNA polymerase 663, 666
Donnan effects 57, 59, 61, 80, 159, 248, 261, 553
Donnan factor 58, 59, 80, 81
Dopa carboxylase inhibition 365
Dopamine 541, 557, 758
Dopamine β hydroxylase 252
    Blood pressure correlation 396, 577, 582
    Marker for sympathetic activity 577
    Plasma, after ultrafiltration 251, 577
Doppler effect 226
Doppler technique, blood flow measurement 603, 729
Dosing interval related to half life 752
Doxorubicin 779
Doxycycline 767
Drainage, peritoneal dialysate, inadequate 460, 462, 557, 558
Droperidol 800
Drowsiness, hypermagnesemic 727
Drug
    Accumulation in renal failure 548, 759
    Adverse reactions 749
    Anesthesia 799-801
    Cardiovascular 770-775
    Concentration correlation with effect 756
    Depletion by dialysis 757
    Distribution volume 315, 750
    Dosage reduction, renal failure 758-760
    Dosing interval 759, 760
    End organ response, renal failure 752, 753
    Fractional removal by dialysis 756
    Fractional renal excretion 756
    Hemofiltration clearance 757
    Hemoperfusion, elimination by 315
    Impotence 841
    Intercompartmental transfer 315
    Interference with middle molecule assay 370
    Lipid metabolism, effects on 589, 590
    Loading dose 758, 759
    Margin of safety 758
    Metabolic effects 752
    Metabolic effects of dialysis on 757
    Peritoneal dialysis efficiency augmentation 428, 429
    Peritoneal transport, effects on 758
    Protein binding in uremia 360, 363, 750
    Renal elimination 752
    Renal failure modifications 749-797
    See also Specific drugs
Drug elimination rate 751
Drug intoxication
    Hemodialysis for 314, 756
    Hemoperfusion treatment of 314-316, 758
    Simulating uremia 753
Drug metabolism, urea interference 360

Drug nephrotoxicity 753
Dry body weight 239, 240, 250
Dying, prolongation of 845
Dyphylline 773
Dysgeusia 715, 808
Dyspnea due to air embolism 619

Echocardiogram
    Long term hemodialysis survivors 399
    Myocardial assessment 528, 604
    Pericardial effusion diagnosis 597, 599, 600
    Pericarditis evaluation 397, 598
Echogram, retroperitoneal hematoma 621
Echovirus pericarditis 598
Edema
    Plasmapheresis complication 874
    Response to ultrafiltration 272
EDTA registry 846, 860, 866, 887, 889
Education
    Children on dialysis 530
    Community 827
    Dialysis staff 826, 827
    Patients 827
Elastase, to clean dialyzer 291
Elderly patient
    Hemodialysis treatment 399, 495
    Infection, higher incidence 649
    Morbidity 399
    Peritoneal dialysis preference 477, 481
Electrical hazards of dialysis equipment 236
Electrical resistance of dialysate 232
Electrical shock from hemodialyzer 236
Electrocardiogram
    Hyperkalemia 357, 544-546, 799
    Monitoring digitalized patient 620
    Pericarditis evaluation 397
Electroencephalogram
    Adequacy of dialysis assay 394
    Dialysis disequilibrium 612
    Dialysis encephalopathy 811
    Hypercalcemia 690, 727
    Parathyroid hormone induced abnormality 373
    Rubidium 808
    Subdural hematoma 620
    Trimethylamine effects 364
    Uremia 725, 726
Electrochemical degradation of organic compounds 325
Electrokinetic charge of artificial surface 191
Electrolysis, dialysate regeneration method 325
Electrolyte
    Concentrations in ultrafiltrate 248
    Effect of charge on transport 248
    Effect of dissociation on osmolality 244
    Kinetics, dialysate regeneration 324
Electrolyte abnormalities
    Peritoneal dialysis effects 416
    Plasma exchange 874
    Resin hemoperfusion induced 308
    Uremia 356-358
Electromagnetic blood flow meter 121, 181, 226
Electromyogram
    Asterixis 725
    Hemoperfusion improvement of 313
    Hyperparathyroidism 736
    Myopathy of osteodystrophy 688
Electron microprobe analysis 804
Electronic blood pressure manometer 228
Electrophoresis, middle molecule separation 369

Elimination rate constant 751
Elimination rate, drugs 751
Emboli, particle, by hemoperfusion 307, 309
Emboli, thrombi on artificial surfaces 187, 190
Emission spectroscopy 804
Emotional response, hemodialysis of children 530
Employment, dialysis patients 831, 841, 866
Encapsulation, reducing hemoperfusion side effects 308, 313
Encephalopathy
    Aluminum 807, 808, 811
    Binswanger 728
    Electrolyte imbalance 726
    Hypercalcemia 690, 727
    Hypermagnesemia 781
    Hyponatremia 726
    Hypotonic dialysis fluid 633
    Tin 808
    Uremic 724-726
Enclosed sack blood pressure monitor 228
Endarterectomy, cerebral vascular disease 729
Endarteritis, septic pulmonary emboli 651
Endocarditis, see Bacterial endocarditis 397
Endocrine abnormalities
    Acute renal failure 549
    Causing uremic symptoms 354
    Children treated by chronic dialysis 525, 526
    Iron overload induced 636
    Uremic 712-723
β Endorphin 41, 318, 891
Endosteal reabsorption 698
Endothelial cell injury and atherosclerosis 591
Endotoxemia 540, 617, 618, 648
Endotoxin contamination of hemodialyzer 135, 293, 299
End-stage renal disease, see Renal failure
Energy intake 90
Energy requirements, children with renal failure 516, 528 529
Enflurane 782, 799
Enterocolitis, uremic 354
Environmental impact of dialysis 840, 845, 846
Enzymatic hydrolysis of urea 325
Enzyme
    Detoxification 758
    Inhibition 360, 361, 365, 372
    Uremic abnormalities 355
Eosinophilia 472, 473, 625
Ephedrine 775
Epicillin 765
Epidermal cell proliferation 885
Epidermal DNA synthesis 885
Epidural anesthesia 800
Epidural hematoma 730
Epilepsy 730
Epinephrine 639, 720
Epiphysiolysis, osteodystrophy in children 526
Epiphysis, slipped, osteodystrophy 689, 696
Epsilon aminocaproic acid 209, 210
Equilibration, erythrocyte and plasma water 262
Equilibrium concentration, peritoneal dialysate 421
Equilibrium plasma concentration 69
Equipment, home dialysis 505-508
Ergocalciferol 679
Erythrocyte
    Adherence to artificial surfaces 190
    ADP decrease with hypophosphatemia 635
    Anion concentration 59
    Damage by hemodialysis 131
    Damage by shear stress 190, 191
    Globin synthesis, methylguanidine inhibition 362

Erythrocyte (*continued*)
    Mechanical trauma 632
    Mechanisms of injury 632
    Middle molecule content 370
    Osmolar injury 632
    Osmotic fragility, middle molecule increase 371
    Oxidant injury 632
    Proliferation and maturation inhibition 361
    Radiolabelled to measure dialyzer residue 133, 134
    Rheologic factors and platelet interactions 191
    Solute equilibration with plasma water 262
    Solute uptake, phenolic inhibition 367
    Thermal injury 632, 633
    Transcellular membrane flux 261
Erythrocyte glycolysis, inhibition 632
Erythrocyte survival 630, 631, 635
Erythroid proliferation, uremic depression 630
Erythromycin 768
Erythropoiesis
    Bioassay of uremic toxin 355
    Decreased, renal failure 634
    Hepatitis, increased 636
    Histidine dependence 635
    Improved by hemodialysis 631
    Middle molecule inhibition 371
    Parathyroid hormone inhibition 634
    Renal dependency 630
    Stimulated by hypoxia 634
    Suppression by blood transfusion 634
Erythropoietin
    Androgen stimulation 637
    Assay 631
    Decreased, post nephrectomy 634
    Decreased production, renal failure 549, 630
    Extrarenal production 630, 634
    Increased plasma levels, hepatitis 636
    Inhibitors, uremic 631
    Plasma levels, renal failure 630
Escherichia coli bacteremia 650
Esterification 752
Ethacrynic acid 540, 577, 774
Ethambutol 769
Ethanol intoxication, hemodialysis for 315, 756
Ethchlorvynol 315, 316, 775, 776
Ether 799
Ethinimate 776
Ethionamide 769
Ethylamine 365
Ethylene diamine tetraacetic acid 291, 781
Ethylene glycol intoxication 315
Ethylene oxide metabolite toxicity 625
European Dialysis and Transplant Association 31
Exchange transfusion, schizophrenia treatment 888
Exercise, treatment of anemia 636
Exercise treatment of hypertriglyceridemia 591
Exit site infection, peritoneal catheter 460, 462
Exogenous intoxication
    Hemofiltration treatment 271
    Hemoperfusion for 314-316
    Peritoneal dialysis for 477
Exophthalmos 715
Extracellular fluid sequestration 540
Extracellular fluid volume
    Contraction, muscle cramps 623
    Expansion causing hypertension 603
    Response to hemodialysis 269
    Response to hemofiltration 269
Extracorporeal blood circuit monitoring 225-230

Extracorporeal blood volume 226, 521, 551, 582
Extracorporeal thrombogenesis 186-200
Extravascular fluid mobilization 252
Eye abnormalities in hemodialysis patients 742-748

Fabry's disease 862
Fail safe concept and hemodialysis 223
Familial Mediterranean fever 401, 862
Family stress, hemodialysis 839, 847
Family support, dialysis patient 845
Fat, dietary and hyperlipemia 590
Fatigue, uremic symptom 354
Fatty acid 365, 470, 589, 715, 757
Febrile response, uremic patients 648
Fecal nitrogen, oral sorbent effect 346
Femoral vein angioaccess 21, 34, 172, 173, 392, 518, 551, 582
Fenbufen 778
Fenoprofen 778
Fentanyl 800
Ferritin 528, 631, 636, 637, 731
Ferrokinetic studies 635
Fever 617, 618
    Bacterial endocarditis 606
    Infection complicating hemodialysis 649
    Osteomyelitis 651
    Overheated dialysis fluid 618
    Pericarditis sign 598
    Septic pulmonary emboli 651
    Zinc intoxication 807
Fiber bundle volume, reused dialyzers 288
Fibrin 206, 210
Fibrin degradation products 206
Fibrinogen 206, 211, 216
    Depletion by hemoperfusion 309
    In peritoneal dialysate 445
    Interaction at blood-artificial surface interface 187, 188
    Plasma level increase due to methylguanidine 362
    Release from platelets 201
Fibrinolysis 203, 210, 211
    Bioassay of uremic toxin 355
    Methylguanidine inhibition 362
    Uremic inhibition 355
Fibrinolytic agents 175, 209, 210
Fibrinolytic system 186, 202, 203, 206, 209, 210
Fibrinolytic therapy 210, 217
Fibrinopeptide A 206
Fibroblast proliferation 355, 372
Fibro-osteoclasia 703
Fick's law 54
Filter, water treatment 146
Filtration for plasma exchange 872, 873
Filtration fraction, hemofiltration 261, 282
Financial status effect on home dialysis 497
First order process 63
First pass metabolism 750
Fistula see Arteriovenous fistula 175-179
Flameless spectrophotometric analysis 336
Flow meter 121, 234
Floxacillin 766
Fluid
    Diluting, for hemofiltration 266, 267
    Excess 371, 543
    Extravascular, mobilization 252
    Intercompartmental transfer rate 250, 269
    Replacement for plasma exchange 874
    Restriction 529, 571
Fluid balance see also Water balance 516

Index of subjects 913

Fluid balance (continued)
  Hemofiltration 267, 281
  Monitoring body weight 543
  Perioperative 801
  Peritoneal dialysis in children 517
  Sequestered fluid effect 543
Fluid film boundary layers 136
Fluorescence angiography 747
Fluoride
  Accumulation 700
  Acute intoxication 807
  Bone 160
  Dialysis fluid 143, 160
  Parathyroid hormone interaction 160
  Osteodystrophy 143, 160, 700, 808
  Thyroid function, interference with 716
  Water for dialysis solution 160, 700
5-Fluorocytosine 474, 770
5-Fluorouracil 779
Fluoxymesterone 637
Flurazepam 775
Flux 54, 56-60
  Backward 258
  Convective 58
  Diffusive 58
  Fluid 57, 242, 245, 258
  Net, contribution of ultrafiltration 757
  Per unit area 55
  Relation to gradient 58, 59
  Solute 57, 245
  Transcellular 261
  Unidirectional 757
  Uptake from peritoneal fluid 246
  Water relative to solute 245
Foam in extracorporeal circuit 229
Focal glomerulosclerosis 833, 862
Folate 355, 632, 885
Folic acid 397, 632, 780, 781
Follicle stimulating hormone 526, 714, 715
Formaldehyde 104, 109, 146, 235, 236, 286, 300, 336
  Antimicrobial effect 295
  Anti-N antibodies cause 299, 625
  Detection 236, 295
  Flushing from stored dialyzer 295, 299
  Hemodialyzer sterilant for reuse 292, 293, 498
  Peritoneal dialysis equipment disinfection 467
  Reversible binding to dialysis membrane 295
  Toxicity 236, 299, 632, 633
Fosfomycin 769
Fourier's law 54
Fracture of bone
  Hypocalcemic tetany 705
  Osteodystrophy 689, 812
  Treatment 705
Freeze dried plasma 874
Fresh frozen plasma 874
Friedreich's ataxia 732
Fructose, osmotic agent 416, 464, 613
Fungal infection 465, 546, 653
Fungal peritonitis 472, 474
Fungicide 770
Furosemide 540, 577, 774
  Acute renal failure treatment 540, 541
  Hypertension treatment 577
  Interference with middle molecule assay 370
  Intraperitoneal effect on sodium transport 558
  Pharmacokinetics 577, 774
  Predisposition to gentamicin nephrotoxicity 761

  Pulmonary edema, treatment 544
  Toxicity 577, 774, 800

Gait, abnormal, osteodystrophy 688, 696
Galactorrhea, hyperprolactinemia 714
Gallamine 782, 800
Gallium 781
Gangrene 175, 177, 479, 689
Ganter, G. 413, 414
Gastric acidity in uremia 717
Gastric inhibitory peptide 270, 717
Gastric lavage, treatment of uremia 342
Gastric pH, effect on drug absorption 750
Gastrin 270, 549, 717, 753
Gastritis, uremic 354, 549
Gastrointestinal bleeding 620
  Acute renal failure 543
  Complicating hepatitis 664
  Hemodialysis and liver disease 401
  Prevention 546, 547
  Salicylates 753
Gastrointestinal complications, acute renal failure 546, 547, 549
Gastrointestinal lavage 343
Gastrointestinal motility and drug bioavailability 750
Gastrointestinal perfusion, see Intestinal 341
Gastrointestinal symptoms, uremia 354
Gastrointestinal tract, bacteremia source 650, 651
Gastrointestinal tract, urea degradation 359
Gel filtration 369
Gelatin, osmotic agent 416, 464
Gentamicin 465, 473, 761
Genu valgum 696
Gibbs Donnan effect, see Donnan effect
Glaucoma 744-747
Globin synthesis, inhibition 371
Glomerular filtration rate, see Creatinine
  Infants and children 514
  Measurement 478
Glomerulonephritis
  Anti-GBM mediated 876
  Cause of renal failure 537, 858
  Complicating hepatitis 665
  Cryoglobulinemia 878
  Immune complexes 878
  Rapidly progressive, plasmapheresis 877, 878
  Recurrence after transplant 862
  Research need, to prevent 848
  Therapeutic trials 876
Glossitis 354
Glucagon 720
  Peritoneal clearance effects 453, 557, 758
  Renal elimination 752
Glucokinase inhibition 372
Gluconeogenesis 160, 366, 373, 720
β_2 Glucoprotein 372
Glucose 719, 720
  Effect on plasma osmolality 79
  Peripheral uptake in uremia 719
  Plasma level, dialysis 475, 480, 552
  Removal by hemoperfusion 308
  See also Dextrose
Glucose intolerance, uremia induced 360-362, 366
Glucose metabolism, bioassay of uremic toxin 355
Glucose-6-phosphate dehydrogenase 363, 372
Glucose transport, polyamine inhibition 365
Glucose uptake by cell, inhibition 360

Glucose utilization 362, 372, 719, 720
Glucoronic acid 367
Glucuronide 369
Glutamic acid 612
Glutamic acid carboxylase 365
Glutamic acid decarboxylase 365
Glutaraldehyde, hemodialyzer sterilant 292, 293
Glutethemide 315, 316, 756, 776
Glyceraldehyde 3-phosphate dehydrogenase 632
Glycerol
    Cerebral edema, prevention 726, 729
    Dialysis fluid 151, 152, 393
    Maintenance of plasma osmolality 555, 613
α Glycerophosphate 716
Glycine amidinotransferase 362
Glycogenolysis 720
Glycolysis, inhibition 367, 632
Glycolytic enzyme 632
Glyoxylate-glycolate 358
Gnosis 736
Goiter 715, 716
Gold 753, 778
Goldberg catheter 425
Gonads, atrophy 715
Goodpasture's syndrome 537, 876, 877
Gottschalk Report 844
Gouty nephropathy 477
Governmental regulation of dialysis 846
Gradient, concentration 54-59
Gradient ion exchange chromatography 369
Gradient pressure 57
Graft arteriovenous fistula 171, 172, 179-182
    Complications 180-182
    Infection 181
    Technical considerations 179, 180
    Thrombosis 181
    Venous obstruction 181
Graham, Thomas 3, 4
Grief 838
Growth
    Children, treated by dialysis 523-526, 529
    Children treated by CAPD 524
    Inhibition by branched chain amino acid imbalance 364
    Malnutrition impeding 569
    Osteodystrophy retarding 689
    Retardation, vitamin D treatment 689
    Stimulation of vitamin D 680
Growth hormone 713
    Hemofiltration, plasma level response 270
    Hemoperfusion removal of 311
    Plasma level in renal failure 526
Guanethidine 579, 772
Guanfacine 772
Guanidine 361
    Adsorption 323, 344
    Hemoperfusion removal of 308, 310
    Measurement 361
    Platelet dysfunction, induced by 550
    Renal failure effects 361-363
    Retention in renal failure 361
    Toxicity 361
Guanidinoacetic acid 362
Guanidinobutyric acid 362
Guanidinoproprionic acid 363
Guanidinosuccinic acid 362, 638
Guillain-Barre syndrome 880
Gynecomastia 713, 714

Haas, Georg 5, 7-11, 107
Hageman factor 202
Hales, Stephen 410-412
Half life 751, 752
    Clearance relationship 755, 756
    Distribution volume relationship 756, 758
    Dosing interval relationship 752
    Drug, correlation with creatinine 759
    Effect of fractional renal elimination 759
    Influence of dialysis 755, 756
Half-way technology 845
Hallucinations, dialysis encephalopathy 811
Halothane 799, 801
Hantzsch test 236, 295, 300
Hard water syndrome 143, 145, 146, 157, 617
Haversian canals 695
Headache
    Dialysis disequilibrium 612, 727
    Hemodialysis complication 271
    Hemofiltration complication 271
    Hydralazine 772
    Hyponatremia 726
    Intracranial infection 730
    Malignant hypertension 728
    Nickel intoxication 807
    Subdural hematoma 620
    Urea induced 360
Hearing loss, complicating hemodialysis 624
Heart block, myocardial calcification 699
Heart disease, dialysis patients 528, 591, 595-610
Heart failure 397, 599-605
    Angioaccess complication 175, 179, 182, 522, 603
    Cause of death, dialysis patients 528, 595
    Causes in dialysis patients 603
    Causing prerenal failure 538
    Diabetes mellitus, hemodialysis 400
    Differentiation from pericarditis 599
    Evaluation 397
    Hemodialysis intolerance 605
    High output 397
    Hypotension cause 613
    Impaired bioavailability of drugs 750
    Intractable 479, 543
    Myocardial calcification 604, 699
    Pathogenesis 602-604
    Pericarditis complication 599, 600
    Pneumonia complicating 653
    Treatment 397, 604
Heart murmur 606
Heat exchanger, deaeration method 164
Heat exchanger, for dialysis fluid 233
Heat production, uremia 716
Heat sterilization of dialysis fluid 235
Heavy metal, nephrotoxicity 753
Hela cell, bioassay of uremic toxin 355
Hemachromatosis 636, 736
Hemagglutination, hepatitis antibody 663
Hematocrit
    Assay of adequacy of dialysis 394
    Blood flow resistance effect 130
    Effect on whole blood clearance 260
    Increase with peritoneal dialysis 478, 479, 524, 631
    Maintenance in acute renal failure 548, 549
    Relation to hydration 246
Hematologic problems of dialysis patients 630-645
Hematoma 181, 620, 621
Hemodiafiltration 256, 272

Hemodialysis 391-409
  Acute renal failure 13, 16, 21, 152, 518, 519, 550-556
  Adequacy, assessment of 393, 394
  Administrative costs 848
  Advantages, acute renal failure 550
  Age specific acceptance rates 855
  Aldosterone removal 718
  Aluminum transport kinetics 333, 807, 813
  Aminoglycoside 760-762
  Amyloidosis 401
  Anemia 527, 528, 631-633
  Anergy induced by 647
  Anesthesia 798-803
  Anticoagulation for 208, 209, 214-216
  Atherosclerotic heart disease patients 399
  Bacteremia complicating 649, 650
  Behavior control 737
  Biochemical complications 615-617
  Bleeding complications 639
  Blood components, damage to 131, 132
  Blood loss 528, 573, 631
  Blood pressure response 11, 268-270
  Calcium, plasma, effect on 692, 693
  Cardiovascular complications 528, 595-610
  Carnitine removal 365
  Catecholamine response to 269
  Cephalosporins 762-764
  Children, patient monitoring 532
  Choline removal 365
  Chronic renal failure in children 520-522
  Clearance, compared to hemofiltration 283
  Clearance determinants 754
  Clinical aspects 391-409
  Complement activation 132, 886
  Complications 522, 530, 553, 611-629
  Complications of first treatment 393
  Coronary bypass patients 399
  Cortisol removal 717
  Cost 844, 846, 847, 853
  Creatinine clearance, endogenous and initiation 391, 392
  Cyclic AMP removal 363
  Demographics 850-855
  Dermatologic abnormalities 622
  Diabetes mellitus 400
  Digoxin 771
  Disadvantages, acute renal failure 550
  Drug intoxication treatment 315
  Early phase of maintenance 393
  Elderly patients 399
  Emotional reaction 839
  Equipment 106-141, 223, 511
  Erythrocyte survival improvement 631
  Erythropoiesis improved by 631
  Evolution 844, 855
  Extracellular fluid volume response 269
  Family stress 839
  First animal 3
  First patient experiences 7, 16, 27, 28
  Frequency of treatments 395, 396, 553
  Geographical variation in age 854, 856, 857
  Glucagon, effect on 720
  Glucose metabolism effects 720
  Growth hormone response 713
  Hematocrit of patients 631
  Hemodynamic changes 603
  Hemofiltration, combined with 118, 272
  Hemoperfusion, combined with 119, 310, 313
  Heparin free 192, 194
  Hepatic encephalopathy, for 316, 317
  Hepatitis complicating 659, 665-672
  Heroin addicts 402
  High risk patients 399-402
  History 3-52
  Home, see Home hemodialysis 493-513
  Hospital 823, 847, 853, 855, 867
  Hours necessary for adequacy 368, 394
  Hypotension complicating 250-252, 613-615
  Hypoxia 555, 640
  Inadequacy correlated with neuropathy 368
  Indole removal 366
  Infectious complications 223, 648-653
  Infrequent, disadvantages 395
  Initial use 393
  Initiation, acute renal failure 553
  Initiation of maintenance 391-393
  Intensive causing anorexia 529
  Intolerance, heart failure 605
  Intoxication, exogenous, treatment for 314
  Large solute clearance 256
  Leukopenia induced by 131, 132, 640
  Lipid metabolism, effect on 589, 596
  Liver disease complicating uremia 401
  Long-term survivors 398, 399
  Lupus erythematosus 400
  Maintenance, for chronic renal failure 391-409
  Management, in children 522
  Membrane permeability less than peritoneum 421
  Membrane permeability related to neuropathy 368
  Membrane surface needed for adequacy 368, 394
  Middle molecule removal 33, 34
  Mobility during 323, 324
  Monitoring 223-241
  Morbidity 35, 82, 158, 159, 395
  Mortality rates 391
  Multiple myeloma 400, 401
  Myoinositol removal 367
  Neuropathy complicating 732
  Nutritional aspects, chronic 570-573
  Ocular calcification and duration 744
  Opthalmological complications 742-748
  Overnight, unattended 493
  Oxalic acid removal 367
  Oxygenation, effect on 132
  Patient flux 511, 846
  Patient population 846, 850
  Penicillin 764-766
  Percentage of patients at home 494
  Peripheral resistance during 269
  Peritoneal dialysis, versus, acute 423, 556
  Phenol removal 366
  Placebo effect 891
  Planning maintenance treatment 392
  Platelet, effects on 131, 639
  Portable systems 35
  Potassium removal 616
  Practical aspects 391-409
  Practical guide for children 531-533
  Preferential use 477, 556
  Pregnancy complicating 402
  Preparation of water for 142-147
  Privacy of individual 847
  Professional staff reactions 839
  Protein binding, effect on 730
  Protein binding, impeding solute removal 750
  Psychologic stress 529, 530
  Psychosocial problems in children 529

Hemodialysis (*continued*)
  Pulmonary function 623
  Pyridine metabolites, effect on 363
  Rapid, complications 612
  Rehabilitation 500
  Safety of 223, 611
  Salicylate 777
  Schedules 393-396, 522, 856
  Schizophrenia treatment 41, 318, 888-891
  Scleroderma 400
  Selection of patients 830-836
  Shortage of facilities 493, 494
  Sickle cell anemia complicating 402
  Single, adequacy of 394
  Single needle 122, 237, 238, 551
  Slow, to avoid hypotension 614
  Social impact 844-849
  Solute concentration determinants 394
  Somatomedin response 713
  Survival 391, 860, 861
  Technical problems 13, 223
  Technique in children 518, 531, 532
  Thrombus formation during 187, 214
  Thyroid function effects 716
  Timing initiation and survival 391
  Transplant interrelation 853
  Uremia progression after late initiation 391
  Venesection for heart failure 605
  Worldwide patient population 391
  Years of treatment and middle molecules 370
Hemodialysis system
  Bacterial contamination 293, 294
  Standards for water quality 144
Hemodialyzer 106-141
  Abel's 4
  Bacterial contamination 135
  Blood compartment compliance 129, 130, 522
  Blood distribution 110, 115, 120, 131
  Blood flow resistance 21, 24, 109, 111, 113, 117, 130
  Blood leak 133, 233, 615
  Blood loss 132
  Blood pressure drop across 130
  Blood residue 133, 134
  Blood volume 21, 26, 107, 110, 114, 117, 119, 120, 129
  Cell volume of hollow fiber 288
  Choice 107, 135, 521, 532, 551
  Cleaning 289-292
  Clearance 61, 122, 125, 234
  Coil 18-21, 29, 32, 111-114, 125, 286
  Cost 135
  Design 107, 135
  Dialysate flow distribution 131
  Disposable 109-116
  Efficiency 55
  Electrical hazards 236
  Flushing 295
  High permeability membranes 118
  Hollow fiber 32, 107, 114-118, 125
  Home dialysis considerations 498
  Hydrostatic pressure 127
  Kiil 24-27, 32, 55, 108
  Kolff's 12-14, 16, 107
  Large surface area 116
  Leachables 135
  Maintenance, home dialysis 508-510
  Membrane permeability 55
  Membrane surface area 120, 521, 522
  Membrane support 108, 110
  Parallel flow 17, 19, 24-27, 32
  Pediatric 119, 521
  Performance measurement 120
  Plate 17, 24-27, 32, 107-111, 125, 286
  Portable 323, 324, 326, 396
  Priming volume 129
  Priming with saline or blood 518, 522
  Pyrogenic reactions 108, 135
  Recirculating single pass 113, 122
  Requirements of ideal 106
  Rinsing blood compartment 134
  Rotating drum 12-14, 16, 17
  Safety, monitoring of 134, 236, 237
  Skeggs-Leonards 19, 24, 107
  Sorbent 118
  Sterilization 114
  Storage, refrigerated between dialyses 286
  Technology, impact of middle molecule hypothesis 368
  Thrombogenicity 116, 131, 133
  Transport: mechanisms 54
  Transportation 335
  Urea clearance 553
  Vortex mixing 136
Hemodialyzer reuse 189, 194, 286-304
  Bacteriologic control in reprocessing 292, 293, 300
  Biocompatibility 297
  Cell volume measurement 300
  Cleaning procedures 289, 292
  Clearance 288, 295, 296
  Complications 298-300
  Cosmetic appearance 298
  Demographics 287
  Device evaluation 300
  Equipment for processing 300
  Evolution of technique 287
  Fiber bundle volume 288, 296
  Flushing stored dialyzer 301
  Functional studies 295, 296
  History 286, 287
  Home dialysis 498
  Immunologic complications 299
  Infectious complications 299
  Labeling control 300
  Morbidity 297
  Motivation for technical development 286
  Patient survival 296
  Practical aspects 300
  Preparation for subsequent use 295, 301
  Process and quality control 300-302
  Processing 287, 288
  Rationale 286, 287
  Records maintenance 301
  Reprocessing 292, 300
  Rhône Poulenc dialyzer 277
  Rinsing of dialyzer 288
  Sterilization 292-295
  Storage of dialyzer 288, 301
  Surface area and clearance 296
  Technical complications 299
  Tubing 295
  Ultrafiltration rate and clearance 296
Hemodynamic effects of peritoneal dialysis 470
Hemodynamic effects of ultrafiltration 251, 252
Hemofiltrate, regeneration by electro-oxidation 325
Hemofiltration 2, 36, 118, 242-274, 757
  Acute renal failure 267, 271, 556
  Balance of fluid flow rates 118
  Blood pressure response 268-270, 577

Index of subjects 917

Hemofiltration (continued)
  Calcium balance 267
  Catecholamine response to 269
  Chronic renal failure 267
  Clearance 123, 256, 261, 268
  Clearance, compared to hemodialysis 283
  Clearance, effect of diluting site 259, 266
  Clinical aspects 267-272, 283
  Continuous 556
  Diluting fluid 257, 259, 267
  Diluting fluid composition 267, 281
  Diluting fluid, site of infusion 259, 266, 267
  Disequilibrium incidence 271
  Duration of treatments 267
  Exogenous intoxication treated by 271
  Extracellular fluid volume response 269
  Fluid balance 81, 267, 281
  Heart failure, treatment 605
  Hemodialysis, combined with 118, 272
  Hemodynamic effects 268
  High flux membranes for 265
  Hormone levels, response to 270
  Hypertension treatment 396, 582
  Hypotension during 268
  Indications 267
  Lipid metabolism, effect on 271
  Mass balance calculation 259, 260
  Mass transfer characteristics 281
  Membranes 257, 265, 266
  Middle molecule removal 268
  Mineral metabolism, effect on 270
  Muscle cramps complicating 271
  Patient population 855, 856
  Peptide hormone removal 757
  Peripheral resistance during 269
  Phosphate removal 270, 284
  Polyacrylonitrile membrane for 281
  Principle of 242-246, 252-254, 256-262, 265
  Rhône-Poulenc hemodialyzer for 281
  Sodium balance 267
  Sodium flux during 81
  Solute removal 118
  Sorbent regeneration of filtrate 267
  Sterility of system 271
  Technical aspects 265-267
  Tolerance 269
  Urea removal 267
Hemoglobin, affinity for oxygen 470, 633, 798
Hemoglobin carbamylation 360
Hemoglobinemia, acute renal failure 540
Hemoglobin synthesis, inhibition 371, 630
Hemolysis 632, 633, 635
  Aliphatic amine induced 365
  Anti N-antibody 299, 625, 633
  Autoimmune 635
  Blood pump induced 225, 632
  Chloramine induced 143, 528, 617, 632
  Copper induced 143, 528, 617, 632, 807
  Drugs 635
  Formaldehyde 633
  Guanidine induced 362, 363
  Hemodialysis complication 555
  Hemoperfusion complication 309
  Hypersplenism 635
  Hypoosmolar 616, 633
  Hypophosphatemia 635
  Methyldopa 772
  Methylguanidine induced 362

  Middle molecule induced 371
  Nitrate induced 528, 617, 632
  Overheated dialysate 233, 618, 633
  Plasma filtration complication 873
  Quinine induced 770
Hemolysis test 104
Hemolytic uremic syndrome 520, 528, 537, 880
Hemoperfusion 2, 35, 305-322, 757, 758
  Adsorption of coagulation factors 308
  Adsorption of essential solutes 307, 308
  Amino acid removal 311
  Carbon contaminant toxicity 308
  Carbon, removal of uremic toxins 308-311
  Clinical requirements 306, 307
  Competitive adsorption of solutes 311
  Device comparison 313
  Digitalis intoxication 316, 771
  Drug intoxication treated by 314-316
  Future developments 319
  Hematologic effects 309
  Hemodialysis, with, for uremia 119, 310, 313
  Hemofiltration, with, for uremia 313
  Hepatic encephalopathy 316-318
  History 308-310
  Hormone adsorption 307, 308, 311
  Hybrid devices 314
  Immunoabsorption by 318, 319
  Middle molecule removal 307, 310, 370
  Particle embolization 307, 309
  Platelet aggregate causing hypotension 308
  Principle 305-308
  Psoriasis treatment 318
  Pyrogen reactions 308
  Removal of anticancer drugs 318
  Residual blood volume 308
  Resins for 306, 307
  Schizophrenia treatment 318
  Side effects 307 309
  Solute spectrum adsorbed 307
  Sorbent encapsulation reducing side effects 308, 313
  Sorbents used 306, 307
  Thrombocytopenia complicating 315
  Trace metal adsorption 307, 308
  Urea removal, limited 310
  Uremia treated by 308-313
Hemopericardium 606, 620
Hemorrhage
  Arteriovenous shunt 175
  β blockade impairing response 800
  Causing hypotension 615
  Cerebral 729
  Conjunctival 744
  Hemodialysis complication 620, 621
  Home hemodialysis 509
  Intradermal 621
  Prevention 615
  Pulmonary 877
Hemostasis 201-207
  After percutaneous angioaccess 173
  Localization 204
Hemostatic response to vascular injury 201, 202
Hemothorax 621
Hemoultrafiltration 256
Henoch Schönlein purpura 877
Heparin 7, 8, 10, 11, 70, 107, 208-210
  Aldosterone suppression 718
  Anticoagulant effect 208, 217
  Antithrombin III enhancement 203

Heparin (*continued*)
    Attachment to membranes 133
    Binding to artificial surfaces 187, 192, 193
    Bleeding complications 214
    Bone mineralization impairment 700
    Composition 208
    Continuous hemofiltration, dose 556
    Desorption 193
    Dosage 208, 217, 218
    Dose, effect of platelet function 214
    Electronegative charge 208
    Elimination constant 70
    Hemodialysis anticoagulant 187, 190, 191, 208, 209, 214, 519, 522, 553, 556
    Home dialysis use 499
    Infusion 218, 219, 225, 229, 230, 619
    Intraperitoneal for peritonitis 473
    Kinetics 214
    Lipid metabolism, effect on 590
    Low dose infusion 215, 216, 400, 553, 620
    Mechanism of action 208
    Minimal dose 215
    Neutralization by platelet factor *4* 189, 190, 214, 639
    Pericarditis, contribution to 598
    Peritoneal dialysis fluid additive 459, 465, 517, 557
    Pharmacokinetics 781
    Plasmapheresis 873
    Platelets, effect on 208, 214
    Priapism complicating 623
    Prostacyclin, interactions with 190, 193, 215
    Protein binding of drugs, effect on 730
    Psoriasis treatment 885
    Rebound 216
    Regional use, for dialysis 215, 216, 553, 801
    Requirements 131, 215
    Sensitivity 71
    Surface bonding, effect on permeability 193
    Thyroxine displacement from protein 716
    Treatment of air embolism 619
    Variable dose requirements 214, 215, 639
Heparin-antithrombin III complex 206
Heparin neutralizing activity 214, 215
Heparin profile 215
Hepatic blood flow, cimetidine decrease 782
Hepatic clearance of peritoneal absorbate 757
Hepatic dysfunction, iron overload 636
Hepatic encephalopathy 316-318, 477
Hepatic friction rub 624
Hepatitis 659-678
    Active immunization 670, 671
    Blood transfusion risk 668
    Chronic 661-664
    Detection 669
    Disinfection procedures 668
    Epidemiology 659
    Erythropoiesis, increased 666
    Fluoxymesterone 637
    Fulminant 664
    Hemodialysis complication, history 665
    Hemodialyzer reuse, association 299
    Home dialysis, decreased incidence 479, 497
    Incidence in dialysis units 665
    Infectivity 663
    Interferon production, depressed 648
    Isolation of patients 669, 672, 822, 826
    Mortality 665
    Passive immunization 669, 670
    Precautions against spread 667-669, 672, 825, 826
    Prevention 672
    Risk of plasma exchange 874
    Transmission 226, 660, 661
    Transplant, influence on 862, 863
    Vaccine 41, 670, 671
    Viral 39-41, 659-678
Hepatitis A 659, 660, 666
    Transmission 660
    Virus 662
Hepatitis B 660, 661
    Dialysis associated hepatitis 665-667
    Incidence 660
    Prevention 660, 668, 669, 801
    Transmission 660, 661, 666, 667
    Virus 662, 663, 666
Hepatitis B core antigen 662-664
Hepatitis B e antigen 663, 664, 666
Hepatitis B surface antigen 662-666
    Assay 663
    Subtypes 662
    Testing 669
Hepatitis non A, non B 661, 664, 666, 671, 672
Hernia, complicating peritoneal dialysis 476, 479
Heroin addicts, hemodialysis 402
Herpes virus infection 653, 654
Hetacillin 765
Hexamethonium 772
Hexokinase inhibition 632
Hexosemonophosphate shunt 635
Hickman catheters 551
Hiccup, uremic 354
High density lipoprotein 588
High pressure liquid chromatography 369
Hippuric acid 355, 366
Hirsutism 580, 637
Hirudin 3, 7, 8, 10
Histaminase 362
Histamine enhanced peritoneal transport 444
Histidine 364
    Deficiency, anemia 373, 635
    Intake and dietary protein 635
    Supplementation 397, 573
    Treatment of anemia 637
Holiday dialysis 825
Hollow fiber hemodialyzer 55, 114-116, 551
    Comparison with peritoneal dialysis 450-452
    Flushing for reuse 301
    Storage procedure 301
    Plasma filtration 873
Home dialysis 493-513, 825
    Adolescents, special consideration 495
    Availability 494
    Children 494, 495, 512
    Community support 510
    Elderly patients 495
    Medical management 508, 509
    Patient selection 494-497
    Role of local physician 509
    Supplies, disposable 510
    Psychological stress 423
    Social worker role 510
Home hemodialysis 28-31, 493-513
    Advantages 497, 510, 511, 522, 737
    Age considerations 494, 495
    Angioaccess 497, 498
    Anticoagulation 499
    Anxiety of patient 495
    Areas remote from dialysis center 510
    Blood loss, prevention 499
    Children 495, 496, 522

Home hemodialysis (*continued*)
   Determinants 832
   Dialysis fluid preparation 498
   Disequilibrium, avoiding 499
   Disruption of household 495
   Distance from home to dialysis center 497
   Equipment 505-508
   Equipment cleaning and sterilization 498
   Equipment lifespan 511
   Failures 511, 512
   Family stress 847
   Financial status affecting 497
   First experiences 493
   Hemodialyzers for 498
   Hepatitis incidence, decreased 479, 497
   Home adaptations 505-508, 523
   Hospitalization of patient 511
   Household accommodation 497
   Household assessment 505
   Hypertension, control of 499
   Hypotension, dangers 498
   Intelligence influencing 497, 832, 847
   Learning ability 496
   Maintenance of equipment and supplies 508-510
   Marital status, effects 495
   Monitoring 498
   Motivation 493, 494
   Partner participation 495, 499, 500
   Patient flux 511
   Personalized treatment 497
   Physical impairment prolonging training 500
   Physician motivation 847, 852
   Psychological aspects 499, 523
   Rehabilitation 510, 523
   Responsible person 499, 500
   Retraining 510
   Selecting the room 505, 506
   Selection criterion for dialysis 832
   Self care 499, 500
   Single patient considerations 495
   Storage space 507, 508
   Survival rates 510, 522, 860, 861
   Teacher characteristics 501
   Teaching methods 501, 502
   Technical and medical aspects 497-499
   Technical service 509, 510
   Training 500-505
   Training capacity of center 511
   Transfer to the home 505
   Ultrafiltration control and dangers 498, 499
   Updating dialysis technique 510
   Venepuncture training 504
   Water preparation for dialysis 498
   Water supply 505, 523
Home peritoneal dialysis 423, 479, 495, 497
Homeostasis 66
Homocysteine 364, 395
Homonymous hemianopsia 729
Homovanillic acid 366
Hormone 712-723
   Adsorption by hemoperfusion 307, 308, 311
   Effects on peritoneal transport 758
   Plasma levels, response to hemofiltration 270
Hospital hemodialysis 853, 855
Hospitalization rates, dialysis patients 841, 867
Host defense mechanisms, impaired 646-648
Howship's lacunae 684, 687
Humoral immunity, uremia 646, 647

Hungry bone syndrome 689
Hydralazine 516, 532, 580, 772
Hydration, relation to blood pressure 239, 246
Hydraulic permeability 248, 253
Hydraulic pressure, effect on hemodialyzer ultrafiltration 245
Hydraulic pressure gradient 242, 244
Hydrogen ion 63, 64, 71
   Balance 74
   Buffering 357, 358
   Cation exchange in dialysate regeneration 329
   Concentration control in dialysis fluid 324
   Generation 71, 72, 75, 77, 88
   Homeostasis in renal failure 357, 358
   Intracellular and oxygen affinity 633
   Intracellular, uremia 358
   Kinetics with Redy-sorb system 331, 332
   Metabolic sources 357
   Mobilization 75
   Peritoneal fluid concentration 443
   Renal excretion 76, 77, 358
   Skeletal buffering in renal failure 358
   Turnover rate 358
Hydrogen peroxide, hemodialyzer cleaning 290
Hydrolysis, biotransformation method 752
Hydrops fetalis, peritoneal dialysis for 477
Hydrostatic pressure ultrafiltration 149, 226, 244
Hydrostatic transmembrane pressure gradient 127, 242, 244
Hydrothorax complicating peritoneal dialysis 475, 524
4-Hydroxybenzoic acid 366
β-Hydroxybutyrate and dialysis fluid dextrose 160
17-Hydroxycorticosteroid 717
Hydroxylysine 364
Hydroxyphenolic acid 367
Hydroxyphenylacetic acid 367
p-Hydroxyphenylalaninic acid 366
2-Hydroxyphenylic acid 366
4-Hydroxyphenyllactic acid 367
Hydroxyproline 364
5-Hydroxytryptamine 366
3-Hydroxytyramine 365
1 α Hydroxyvitamin D_3 527, 700-702
25-Hydroxyvitamin D_3 679, 680
   Renal loss in nephrotic syndrome 683
   Treatment of osteodystrophy 701, 702
Hyperalimentation 547
   Acute renal failure 541, 547, 548, 570
   Complications 547, 548
   Fluid composition 548
   Metabolic instability nutrition 537, 648
Hyperbilirubinemia, peritoneal dialysis for 477
Hypercalcemia 154, 693
   Arrhythmia cause 606
   Calcium supplements causing 700
   Encephalopathy 727
   Gastric acid stimulant 717
   Hard water syndrome 617
   Hemodialysis complication 509, 617
   Nephrotoxic acute renal failure 540
   Parathyroidectomy indication 703
   Pathogenesis in uremic patients 693
   Peritoneal dialysis for 477
   Pruritus 622, 689
   Vitamin D treatment complication 527, 701, 780
   See also Calcium
Hypercapnia complicating dialysate regeneration 332
Hypercatabolism, acute renal failure determinant 542, 736
Hyperchloremic acidosis complicating peritoneal dialysis 249, 416

Hypercholesterolemia 526
Hypergammaglobulinemia 399
Hyperglycemia
    Cerebral complications of rapid correction 518
    Growth hormone paradoxical response 713
    Peritoneal dialysis complication 433, 475, 518, 558
    Uremia 549, 718
    See also Dextrose, Glucose
Hyperkalemia 152, 153, 544, 726
    Acidosis potentiating 357, 544
    Acute renal failure 543-546
    Adrenal insufficiency 717
    Anephric patient, increased risk 581
    Anesthetic risk 799
    Arrhythmia cause 606
    Cause of death, dialysis patients 596
    Causes 356, 357
    Children, increased frequency 522
    Dialysis indication, acute renal failure 550
    Electrocardiographic effects 357, 799
    Hemodialysis, complicating 616
    Indomethacin 778
    Ion exchange resins, control by 348
    Muscle relaxant induced 800
    Overheated dialysis fluid 618, 633
    Peritoneal dialysis, complicating 475
    Toxicity 357
    Treatment 516, 545, 546, 799
    See also Potassium
Hyperlipidemia 588-594
    Frequency in uremic patients 588
    Pathogenesis 589, 590
    Predisposing to atherosclerosis 591
    Treatment 590-591
Hypermagnesemia 156, 552, 693
    Bone mineralization abnormality 694
    Causes 693
    Drug induced 752
    Encephalopathy 727
    Hard water syndrome 617
    Hemodialysis complication 617
    Parathyroid hormone suppression 680, 694
    Prevention 699
    See also Magnesium
Hypermetabolism, hemodialysis induced 716
Hypernatremia 616
    After dialysis 151, 159
    After peritoneal dialysis 249, 448, 464, 470, 475, 518, 558
    Causes 616
    Consequences 616
    Encephalopathy 726
    From water softening 145
    Treatment 249, 516, 552, 616
    See also Sodium
Hyperosmolality complicating hemodialysis 616
Hyperosmolar non-ketotic coma 400, 464, 475
Hyperparathyroidism 37, 682, 683
    Anemia, aggravation of 634, 638
    Bone turnover, increased 695
    Calcium supplements suppressing 700
    Children 526
    Cyclic AMP level, indicator of 363
    Dialysis fluid calcium relationship 153, 154, 700
    Encephalopathy 690
    Gastric acid secretory effects 717
    Hypercalcemia cause 693
    Hyperphosphatemia relationship 691
    Insulin resistance 690, 694
    Muscular weakness 736
    Neutrophil function 647
    Pathogenesis in renal failure 682, 683
    Periarthritis due to 689
    Pericarditis association 598
    Periosteal neostosis 696
    Persistent despite phosphate control 700
    Pruritus 622, 689
    Soft tissue calcification 699
    Tendon degeneration cause 624, 689
    Tertiary 693
    Treatment 703, 705
    Vitamin D metabolites, effect of 527
    See also Parathyroid hormone
Hyperphosphatemia
    Acute renal failure 552
    Causes 690, 699
    Hyperparathyroidism relationship 692
    Lowering plasma calcium 682
    Pathogenesis of calciphylaxis 690
    Need for low dialysis fluid calcium 552
    Osteomalacia, effect on 682, 683
    Phagocytosis depression 648
    Prevention 699
    Vitamin D treatment complication 701
    See also Phosphate
Hypersplenism 528, 635, 638
Hypertension 575-581
    Anesthesia interactions 799
    Atherosclerosis predisposition 575, 591, 727
    Binswanger encephalopathy risk 728
    Cause of renal failure 859
    Cerebral hemorrhage risk 729
    Children 528
    Convulsions, cause in children 516
    Dialysis resistant 575
    Drug therapy 771-773
    Hard water syndrome 157, 617
    Home dialysis, control of 499
    Incidence 575
    Malignant 580, 728
    Malignant, decreased peritoneal clearance 444
    Malignant, treatment 580
    Nephrectomy, bilateral for 396, 400, 522, 528, 575, 581, 603, 605
    Nervous system role in pathogenesis 576
    Pathogenesis 396, 573-577
    Plasma exchange complication 874
    Redy-sorb system dialysis, control of 333
    Renin dependent 270, 396, 529, 576, 578
    Survival, long term hemodialysis, effect 398
    Treatment 396, 532, 577-581, 771-773
    Treatment, preventing uremia 580, 848
    Ultrafiltration, effect on 269, 270
    Venous from arteriovenous fistula 177
    Volume dependent 239, 269, 396, 529, 575, 576, 603
Hypertensive encephalopathy 728
Hypertensive retinopathy 744
Hyperthyroidism 715, 880
Hypertrichosis, minoxidil 772
Hypertriglyceridemia 588
    Clofibrate treatment 590
    Complicating CAPD 433, 479
    Exercise treatment 591
    Hemofiltration, response to 271
    Osteodystrophy sign 694
    Uremia 526
    Vanadium deficiency 808
    See also Triglyceride
Hyperuricemia, see Uric acid 363, 477, 540

Hyperviscosity, plasmapheresis 878, 880
Hypervolemia, peritoneal dialysis complication 475
Hypoalbuminemia complicating dialysis 401, 524
Hypocalcemia
    Arrhythmia cause 606
    Children 516
    Dialysate regeneration complication 324
    Hypotension associated 582
    Incidence in uremia 692
    Insulin release impaired by 719
    Parathyroid stimulation 680, 682
    Pathogenesis 682, 683
    Plasma exchange complication 874
    Postparathyroidectomy 705
    Tetany 726
    Vitamin D stimulation 680
    See also Calcium
Hypochlorite, see Sodium hypochlorite
Hypoglycemia 621, 622
    Adrenal insufficiency 717
    After dialysis 159
    Contribution to dialysis disequilibrium 393, 612
    Insulin after peritoneal dialysis 475
    Peritoneal dialysis for 477
    See also Dextrose, Glucose
Hypoglycemic agents 213, 779
Hypogonadism 714, 715
Hypokalemia
    Aldosterone suppression in anephric 718
    Correction of acidosis inducing 552
    Digitalis toxicity aggravated 753
    Hemodialysis complication 616, 617, 726
    Indication for potassium in dialysis fluid 465
    Peritoneal dialysis complication 475, 558
    Plasma exchange complication 874
    See also Potassium
Hypokalemic alkalosis, penicillin induced 752, 764, 766
Hypomagnesemia, see also Magnesium 552, 606, 694
Hypometabolism 716
Hyponatremia
    Causes 615, 616, 726
    Dialysis complication 509, 552, 615, 616
    Dialysis disequilibrium cause 393, 612
    Encephalopathy 726
    Renal failure complication 356, 516, 549
    Sorbent effect on dialysate causing 335
    Stimulation of renin release 576
    See also Water intoxication, Sodium
Hypoosmolality 616, 623, 726
Hypophosphatemia 552, 553
    Aluminum hydroxide side effect 547
    Causes 691
    Hemolysis 635
    Skeletal mineralization impaired 692
    See also Phosphate
Hypoplasia of kidneys 519, 520
Hypoproteinemia complicating peritoneal dialysis 524
Hypotension 581, 582, 613-615
    Acetate induced 238, 251, 614
    Adrenal insufficiency 717
    After nephrectomy 581
    Anesthetic interactions 799
    Arrhythmia cause 606
    Consequences 575
    Differential diagnosis 599
    Drug induced 754
    Effect on drug removal 756
    Excessive ultrafiltration 613

Guanethidine 772
Hemodialysis complication 238, 250-252, 268, 528, 543, 551-555, 599, 600, 613-615
Hemodialysis with liver disease 401
Hemofiltration, during 268, 556
Hemoperfusion induced 308
Hemorrhage induced 615
Home hemodialysis 498, 509
Infection causing 648
Middle molecule induced 372
Pathogenesis 581, 582
Pericarditis induced 598, 600
Peritoneal clearance decreased by 444
Peritoneal dialysis complication 444, 470, 475, 558
Plasma exchange complication 874
Prerenal failure cause 538
Prevention during dialysis 613
Slow hemodialysis, treatment 614
Sodium and fluid depletion 613
Symptoms 613
Treatment 533, 582, 613
Hypothermia 477, 518
Hypothyroidism 638, 715, 773
Hypovolemia
    Hemodialysis complication 528, 554, 623
    Hypotension, cause of 581
    In children, causing ischemia 515, 516
    Peritoneal dialysis complication 475
Hypoxia
    Acetate in dialysis fluid 158, 552
    Hemodialysis complication 132, 252, 555, 556, 633, 640
    Independent of leukocyte-membrane effects 623, 640
    Stimulating erythropoiesis 634

Ibuprofen 778
Idiogenic osmoles, cerebral, disequilibrium 393, 612
Ileus, peritoneal catheter induced 462
Ileus, peritonitis complication 471
Illness, societal expectations 837
Imipramine 776
Immune complex
    Endothelial injury 592
    Glomerulonephritis 878
    Hemoperfusion removal 318
    Lupus erythematosus 879
    Plasmapheresis removal 872, 875, 878
Immune response
    Hepatitis B virus 663
    Impaired, uremia 543, 548, 646
Immune system impairment 355, 366, 369, 371, 547, 548
Immunization for hepatitis 41, 669-671
Immunoabsorption by hemoperfusion 318, 319
Immunodiffusion, hepatitis virus 663
Immunoglobulin removal 476, 875
Immunoglobulin synthesis 647, 875
Immunoglobulin A, plasmapheresis removal 875
Immunoglobulin G, plasmapheresis removal 873, 875
Immunoglobulin M, plasma exchange 875
Immunosuppression, aggravation of hepatitis B 666
Immunosuppressive drug
    Cryoglobulinemia treatment 878
    Glomerulonephritis treatment 878
    Infection complicating use 654, 873
    Lupus erythematosus treatment 879
    Plasma exchange, use with 875, 876
    Risk-benefit ratio 537, 538
Impotence 714, 715, 841, 842
    Cause 841

Index of subjects

Impotence (continued)
    Diabetes mellitus 841
    Drug induced 772, 841
    Hyperprolactinemia 714
    Zinc deficiency 715, 808
Inanedione anticoagulants 209
Independent variable 88, 91
Indican 366
Indole 308, 311, 366
Indole acetic acid 366
Indomethacin 778
    Antiplatelet agent 212
    Periarthritis treatment 689
    Pericarditis treatment 397, 601
    Persistent abdominal pain treatment 470
    Prostaglandin synthetase inhibitor 577
Indoxyl 366
Infancy, metabolism and physiology 514, 515
Infection 646-658
    Acute renal failure cause 541
    Acute renal failure, risk in 549
    Anemia due to 635
    Angioaccess 175, 177, 181, 652, 653, 873, 874
    Cause of death, acute renal failure 542, 543, 558
    Diabetic patients, higher incidence 649
    Diagnostic problems, acute renal failure 549
    Elderly, higher incidence 399, 649
    Hemodialysis complication 230, 617, 648-653
    Hemodialysis patients 646-658
    Hemodialyser reuse complication 299
    Hypotension due to 648
    Intracranial 730
    Malnutrition predisposing 648
    Metabolic response 648
    Mortality 648-650
    Nutritional requirements increasing 569
    Perioperative 801
    Peritoneal catheter, around 460, 462
    Prophylaxis 545, 546, 549
    Renal failure complication 646-658
    Sources 649
Infectious hepatitis 659, 660
Inflammation, effects on peritoneal permeability 446
Inflammatory mediators, plasma exchange effects 872, 875
Influenza virus pericarditis 598
Infusion pump 230, 326
Ingestible sorbents, see Sorbents 341-353
Inorganic solute, abnormalities in uremia 356-358
Insomnia 621
Insulin
    Decreased production, potassium deficiency 720
    Dextrose free dialysis, plasma response 159
    Hemofiltration, plasma response 270
    Hemoperfusion removal of 311
    Hyperkalemia treatment 545, 546
    Impaired release, renal failure 719
    Lipid metabolism, effect on 589
    Peritoneal dialysis, use 465, 475, 480, 518, 558
    Pharmacokinetics 779
    Renal elimination 752
    Renal failure, effects on 719, 720
    Requirements, uremic diabetic patients 720
    Response to glucose 719
Insulin metabolism 719, 720
Insulin resistance 549, 690, 694, 712, 719
Insulinase inhibition by indoles 366
Intelligence, home dialysis, influence on 497, 847
Intelligence quotient 736
Intercellular channels of peritoneum 441, 444

Intercompartmental transfer rate 252, 315, 750, 756, 758
Intercompartmental transport coefficient 84
Interferon production, suppressed 647, 648
Interferon treatment of hepatitis 665
Intermittent peritoneal dialysis, see Peritoneal 418, 468
Interstitial fluid composition 148
Interstitial fluid drug concentration 750
Interstitial nephritis, acute causing renal failure 537, 538
Interstitial nephritis, acute drug hypersensitivity 753, 764, 765, 767, 769, 778
Interstitium, mesothelial 440
Intestinal absorption of calcium 680, 682
Intestinal absorption of phosphate 683
Intestinal flora, pathogenesis of uremia 355, 364
Intestinal fluid composition 343
Intestinal motility effect on peritoneal transport 412
Intestinal perforation complicating peritoneal dialysis 459, 462, 474, 518, 557
Intestinal perfusion 341-343
    Clinical results 342, 343
    Creatinine transport 342, 343
    Effect on hypertension 342
    Effect on plasma creatinine 342
    Transport determinants 342, 343
    Urea transport 342, 343
    Uric acid transport 342, 343
Intestine, aliphatic amine source 364
Intoxication, drug 314-316
Intraabdominal pressure, peritoneal dialysis 470
Intracellular amino acids 364
Intracellular fluid flux during hemofiltration 269
Intracellular pH in uremia 358
Intracellular trapping effect on clearance 450
Intracranial infection 730
Intradermal test 104
Intraocular pressure 742, 744
Intravascular catheter, infection complicating 545, 546
Inulin
    Clearance 248, 288, 752
    Sieving coefficient 248
    Transmittance coefficient 281
    Transport by hemodialysis 248
Iodide retention in uremia 716, 753, 755, 782
Iodinated radiocontrast material 476, 540
Iodine disinfection of peritoneum 458, 461, 473
Ion exchange chromatography 369
Ion exchange materials 341, 348
Ion exchange resin for hyperkalemia 153, 306, 307, 324, 348
Ionic charge effect on transport 248, 449
Iothalamate clearance 752
Iron 781
    Abnormalities in uremia 805
    Absorption 637
    Balance 636, 637
    Loss, hemodialysis 631
    Nephrotoxicity 753
    Overload 528, 635, 636, 736
    Removal by chelation and hemodialysis 636
    Repletion 391, 637
    Requirements, patients treated by dialysis 573
    Serum, correlation with iron stores 637
    Serum levels 631
    Stores 631
    Supplements, danger of excess 528
    Tap water 144
    Uptake, bone marrow, inhibition 362, 371
Iron deficiency 631, 637
    Chronic renal failure 634
    Consequences 631

Iron dextran 781
  Complications of use 637
  Treatment of anemia 635, 637
Irritability 724, 725
Ischemia
  Cerebral 729
  Renal, precipitation tubular necrosis 540
  Vascular response 577
Ischemic heart disease 591, 603
Ischemic necrosis, calciphylaxis 689, 690
Isocarboxazid 776
Isocyanate 360
Isoflurane 799
Isolated heart test 104
Isolation of hepatitis patients 669, 672
Isolations of patient from hemodialyzer alarm 225
Isoleucine 364
Isoniazid 474, 769
Isorbide dinitrate 605, 775
Isotachophoresis 369
Isotonic peritoneal dialysis solution 247

Jaundice, hepatitis causing 664
Jehovah's witness, peritoneal dialysis for 477
Jugular vein angioaccess in children 518
Juxtaglomerular apparatus 576, 578
Juxtamedullary nephrons in infants 514

Kanamycin 761
Katchalsky cell 99
Ketoacidosis 77
Ketoconazole 474
Kidney
  Artificial, see Hemodialyzer 4
  Endocrine function 712
  Maturation 514, 515
  Residual function 33, 67, 78, 87
Kidney transplant 847
  ABO matching 863
  Age related survival 831
  Blood transfusion effect 638, 672, 798, 832, 863, 864
  Cadaveric 863
  Candidacy 832
  Cytomegalovirus infection 648, 654
  Cytotoxic antibodies 863, 864
  Dialysis duration effect 864
  Hemodialysis interrelation 853
  Hepatitis influence on 862, 863
  HLA matching 832, 863
  Infection complicating rejection 654
  Integration with dialysis 822, 830, 834, 835
  Living related donors 863
  Mortality 844, 864-866
  Nephrectomy, bilateral, effect on outcome 864
  Neuropathy improvement 732
  Ocular abnormalities after 747
  Organ procurement 833
  Peritoneal dialysis interrelation 480
  Plasma exchange for 879
  Psoriasis, effect on 888
  Quality of life 844
  Rate 821, 822, 850, 855
  Rehabilitation 863
  Research need 847
  Restrictions 832
  Second grafts 864

  Selection of patients 830-834
  Splenectomy effect 864
  Survival 860, 861-864
  Viral infection complicating 653, 654
  Waiting interval 832
Kiil hemodialyzer 24-27, 32, 55, 108
  Preparation for use 286
  Reuse 286
Kinetic modelling 61
Kinetics of middle molecule transport 84-88
Kinin system 186
Kolff, Willem 5, 12-17, 107, 342
Korsakoff psychosis 727
Krebs-Henseleit urea cycle 359
Kwashiorkor syndrome 648
Kynurenate 366

Labetalol 773
Lactate, buffer anion for dialysis 289, 417, 465
Lactate intolerance 558
Lactate production 719
Lactation 680, 713
Lactic acid 76, 465
Lactic dehydrogenase inhibition 355, 360, 367, 369, 372
Lactobacillus casei assay 632
Lange calipers 569
Laryngeal stridor 727
Law of conservation of mass 63
Laxative toxicity 700, 753
Leachables 104, 134, 135, 143, 144, 299, 625
Lead
  Body content 805
  Dialysis fluid content 144
  Intoxication in dialysis patients 617
Leak, blood from dialyzer 133, 615
Leakage, peritoneal dialysis fluid 418, 460, 462, 518, 524
Lecithin 364
Leeches 5
Lens opacities 744
Leonard-Bluemle cell 99
Lethargy, drug induced 753
Leucine 364
Leukocyte
  Adherence to artificial surfaces 186, 189, 190, 214
  Chemotaxis 640, 647, 886
  Involvement in psoriasis 884, 886
  Pulmonary sequestration 132, 158, 252, 555, 623, 633
  Removal, peritoneal dialysis 886
  Response to infection, acute renal failure 549
  Response to polyacrylonitrile membrane 276
Leukocyte count in peritoneal dialysate 445, 471
Leukocyte function
  Dialysis inadequacy indicator 394
  Inhibition of 366, 371, 373
Leukocyte migration inhibition test 663
Leukocyte reactivity on exposure to artificial surfaces 187
Leukocytosis, infection complicating hemodialysis 649
Leukopenia
  Effect of membrane type 131
  Induced by hemodialysis 131, 189, 214, 252, 555, 623, 640, 647
Leydig cells 714, 715
Libido, decreased, uremia 714, 715
Lidocaine 622, 774
Light chain, removal by peritoneal dialysis 401
Light chain disease, dialysis experience 401
Limulus amebocyte lysate test 300

Lincomycin 768
Lipase, hepatic 589
Lipid
    Acetate incorporation into 615
    Catabolism 589
    Plasma lowering by charcoal 349, 350
    Plasma, nutritional assessment 569
Lipid abnormalities 37, 588-591
    Carnitine associated 365
    Hemodialysis effect on 589, 590
    Hemofiltration effect on 271
    Treatment 590, 591
Lipid solubility effect on peritoneal transport 450
Lipid soluble drugs, hemoperfusion 314
Lipochrome 372
Lipolysis, uremic toxin bioassay 355
Lipolytic activity post heparin 589
Lipophilicity effect on drug distribution 750
Lipoprotein 37
    Assessing changes with treatment 590
    Cholesterol content 596
    Composition 588
    High density, plasma 588
    Infiltration of injured endothelium 592
    Low density, plasma 588
    Smooth muscle cell proliferation 592
    Very low density, plasma 588
Lipoprotein lipase 37, 589
    Basal adipose tissue activity 589
    Inhibition in uremia 355
    Middle molecule inhibition 372
Liquid membrane capsules 347, 348
Lithium 752, 758, 776, 777, 808
Liver carcinoma, primary 662, 665
Liver disease hemodialysis experience 401
Liver dysfunction, alkaline phosphatase increase 694
Liver hematoma, subcapsular 621
Lividomycin 762
Locust bean gum 347
Log kill function of sterilant 292
Looser's zones 697
Lorazepam 775
Lung, bacteremia source 650
Lupus erythematosus
    Cardiac involvement 604
    Causing acute renal failure 538
    Decreased peritoneal clearance 444
    Hemodialysis experience 400
    Hemolysis 635
    Hydralazine induced 772
    Immunoabsorption treatment 319
    Plasma exchange 874, 878, 879
    Survival 862
    Treatment 879
Luteinizing hormone 550, 714, 715
Luteinizing hormone releasing hormone 714
Lymphatics, peritoneal transport 441, 445
Lymphoceles 182
Lymphocyte DNA synthesis 362
Lymphocyte function in uremia 647
Lymphocyte transformation, uremic toxin bioassay 355
Lymphoid atrophy 639, 640
Lymphopenia 639, 647
Lysine depletion 589
Lysine reduction of urea synthesis 360
Lysozyme 373
Lysyl oxidase 808

Macroglobulinemia, plasmapheresis 878
Macromolecule removal by plasmapheresis 873, 875
Macrophage surface receptors 648
Macroporous resin for hemoperfusion 307
Magnesium 358
    Brain content, acute renal failure 549
    Depletion, cancer regression with 891-893
    Dialysate regeneration, addition for 329, 334
    Dialysis fluid 143, 155-157, 552, 693, 700
    Dialysis fluid, low, for pruritus 622
    Drug sources 348, 547, 766, 781
    Hemodialysis removal of 156
    Kinetics in Redy-sorb system 334
    Muscle relaxant effects 799
    Osteodystrophy, relation to 156, 157
    Peritoneal dialysis fluid concentration 464, 465
    Plasma concentration 155, 157
    Plasma protein binding 155
    Removal by water softening 145
    Sodium cellulose phosphate removal of 892
    Toxicity 156, 547
Maintenance hemodialysis, see Hemodialysis 391-409
Malaise due to infection 649, 651, 664
Malayan pit viper venom 211
Malic dehydrogenase 367
Malignancy, see Cancer
Malignant hypertension 580, 728
Malnutrition
    Acute renal failure, prognosis 543
    Children with chronic renal failure 526
    Growth hormone increase 713
    Growth retardation cause 689
    Increased infection, with 648
    Luteinizing hormone increase 714
    Lymphocyte function impairment 647
    Middle molecule correlation 371
    Morbidity 569
    Peritoneal dialysis complication 476
    Prevention 547, 548, 569-571
    Somatomedin, effect on 526
    Thyroid function effects 716
Manganese 144, 799
Mania 838
Mannitol
    Elevated concentrations in uremia 367
    Infusion to maintain plasma osmolality 151, 152, 533, 555, 614
    Neuromuscular junction effect 800
    Osmotic agent for peritoneal dialysis 252
    Pharmacokinetics 773
    Pressor effect during dialysis 552
    Prevention of dialysis disequilibrium 393, 533, 553, 555, 613
    Renal elimination 752
    Treatment of acute renal failure 540, 541
    Volume expansion 614
Manometer
    Electric, blood pressure 228
    Measurement of dialysate pressure 233
    Mechanical, blood pressure 227
Maple syrup urine disease 477
Marker solutes 61
Mass balance 54, 57, 61-66, 70, 259, 260
Mass balance equation 62, 64-66, 70, 74, 77
Mass conservation, law of 63
Mass transfer coefficient 54, 55, 124, 442, 474, 481
Mass transfer rate, peritoneal dialysis 442

Mass transfer resistance, calculation 253
Mass transport 54, 55, 57, 97
    Contributions of convection and diffusion 248, 253, 254
    Hemofiltration, limited by sieving 281
    Peritoneal, impeded by dialysate 255, 256
    Kinetic analysis 60, 421
    Solute size effect 60, 61
    Urea 60
Mass transport resistance 55, 256
Mathematical model of dialysis 62, 63, 65
Mecamylamine 772
Mechanical blood pressure manometer 227
Mechanical trauma to erythrocytes 632
Mechlorethamine 779
Mecillinam 766
Meclofenamate 212
Median nerve compression 734
Mediators, inflammatory, plasma exchange 875
Medicare and medicaid legislation 846, 852
Medicolegal aspects of dialysis 846
Medullary cystic disease 862
Mefanamic acid 778
Megakaryocyte 204
Melanotrophic hormone 713
Melphalan 779, 878
Membrane 97-105
    Allergy to 135
    Area 60, 242, 256
    Cellulose 97, 98, 252
    Cellulose acetate 102, 103, 146, 252
    Cellulose, binding heparin to 193
    Characteristics affecting ultrafiltration 129
    Characterization 259
    Collagen 100
    Composition, effect on thrombus formation 214
    Copolymer 100, 101
    Cuprophane 24, 98, 247
    Diaflow 100
    Diffusive resistance 55, 225
    Endothelial monolayer coating 194
    Geometry effect on thrombus formation 214
    Hemodialysis 97-105
    Hemofiltration 36, 257, 265, 266
    High permeability 118
    Hydraulic permeability 114, 127, 128, 248, 259
    Leak 133, 233, 615
    Leukocyte interaction 131, 555
    Non-cellulosic 99
    Nucleopore 102
    Nylon epoxy 102
    Permselectivity 98, 99, 137
    Polyacrylonitrile 34, 102, 114, 118, 252, 275-277, 279
    Polyaminoacid 100
    Polyelectrolyte 99
    Polemethacrylate 118
    Polypeptide 100, 103
    Polysulfone 114, 247
    Polyvinyl alcohol 99
    Polyvinylpyrrolidine 99
    Pores 97, 98, 243
    Porosity 98, 99, 102
    Protein coating 259
    Protein interaction, reused dialyzers 298
    Radiation grafted 102
    Resistance to transport 55
    Reverse osmosis 145
    Rupture 239
    Selective permeability 98, 137
    Sieving 259
    Sieving coefficients 247
    Sorbent 103
    Stearic hindrance to transport 245
    Sterilization 104, 135
    Support geometry 32, 108, 110, 135
    Surface coating 128
    Synthesis 99
    Tolerance of transmembrane pressure 281
    Toxicity 252
    Trace metal binding 757
    Trace metal content 135
    Ultrafiltration characteristics 118
    Ultrathin 103
    Variability 129
Membrane filters 873
Membrane permeability 55, 103, 114, 245, 256, 265
    Cell, increased by urea 360
    Determinant of clearance 126, 127
    Peritoneum versus hemodialyzer 421
    Short dialysis relationship 395
Membrane separation, plasmapheresis 873
Membrane transport, cellular, uremic effects 355, 367
Memory loss 732, 736
Meningitis 730
Menstruation 715
Mental concentration 364, 724
Mental confusion 356, 598, 599
Meperidine 777
Meprobamate 315, 316, 776
6-Mercaptopurine 758, 779
Mercurial diuretic 752, 773
Mercury 750, 752, 753
Mesenteric blood flow 758
Mesentery, visceral 440, 441
Mesothelium 440, 441, 444, 449
    Metabolism affecting transport 448
    Permeability 448
    Pore area 448
    Transport resistance 446, 452
Metabolic complications of peritoneal dialysis 475, 558
Metabolic degradation, rate limited 756
Metabolic effects of drugs 752
Metabolic process 63, 355
Metabolism, intermediary, uremic effects 355, 549
Metabolite, toxic synergism of combinations 359
Metacarpal index 698
Metalloenzymes 808
Metallothionine 805
Methacrylate membrane encapsulation of sorbent 308, 313
Methacycline 767
Methadone 778
Methanol intoxication 315, 756
Methaqualone 315, 316, 344, 776
Methemoglobinemia 144, 632
Methenamine mandelate 769
Methicillin 765, 766
Methimazole 781, 782
Methohexitone 799
Methotrexate 779
Methoxyflurane 559, 753, 782, 799
Methyladipic acid 367
Methylamine 365
Methyl CCNU 779
α Methyldopa 772
    Cause of hypotension 555
    Gynecomastia complicating 714
    Hemolysis 635

α Methyldopa (*continued*)
    Hyperprolactinemia complicating 714
    Interference with middle molecule assay 370
    Pharmacokinetics 579, 772
    Toxicity 579
    Treatment of hypertension 579
Methylguanidine 361, 362
    Creatinine metabolite 361
    Excretion 361
    Intracellular accumulation 361
    Methylamine contamination 365
    Neuropathy induced by 362, 734
    Production 361
    Toxicity 362
Methylhistidine 364
Methylhydantoin 361
N-Methyl-2-pyridone-5-carboxylic acid 363
N-Methyl-2-pyridone-5-formamidoacetic acid 363
Methyprylon 776
Methysergide nephrotoxicity 753
Metoclopramide 801
Metolazone 774
Metoprolol 396, 773
Mevalonate-5-phosphate-kinase 367
Mevalonate-5-pyrophosphate decarboxylase 367
Mezlocillin 766
Miconazole 474, 770
β_2-Microglobulin 372
Microsomal enzyme, drug induction 702
Middle molecule 368-372
    Accumulation 83, 279, 370
    Amino acid composition 369
    Assay, interference by drugs 376
    CAPD removal of 433
    Carbohydrate component 369
    Characterization 280, 281, 368, 369
    Clearance, hemodialyzer 126, 127, 331
    Clearance, renal 370
    Clinical effects 371, 589
    Dialysate, identification in 280
    Dialysis index correlation 370
    Dialysis technique correlation 370
    Elimination 370
    Erythrocyte concentration 370
    Generation rate 370
    Hemodialysis removal 33, 34, 126, 279, 370
    Hemodialysis years of treatment correlation 370
    Hemofiltration removal 267, 268
    Hemoperfusion removal 307, 310, 319, 370
    Inadequate dialysis indicator 394
    Identification 33, 34, 280, 281, 369
    Isolation and characterization 368
    Kinetics of transport 83-88
    Molecular size 370
    Molecular structure 369
    Neuropathy pathogenesis 732
    Peptide characterization 369
    Peptide containing spermidine 365
    Pericarditis pathogenesis 597
    Permeation of peritoneum 279
    Plasma level in uremia 370
    Removal by convection 257
    Removal, comparison of hemofiltration and dialysis 284
    Residual renal function correlation 370
    Separation techniques 369
    Suppression of mixed lymphocyte reaction 647
    Toxicity 33, 34, 84, 279, 371, 372
    Transport resistance 279
    Urinary levels in uremia 370
Middle molecule hypothesis 32, 33, 116, 126, 279, 368
Military experience, acute renal failure 542
Millipore filter sterilization 425
Minocycline 767
Minoxidil 396, 528, 580, 581, 772
Mitochondrial metabolism, uremic toxin bioassay 355
Mitochondrial respiration inhibition 360, 361, 372
Mitogen response 647, 885
Mixed lymphocyte reaction 371, 647
Model, mathematical of dialysis 62, 63, 65
Molecular interaction, sieving effect 449
Molecular mass 61, 370
Molecular size, dialyzer clearance determinant 754
Molecular structure of middle molecules 369
Molybdenum 805, 808
Monitor 223-241
    Functional testing 237
    Hemodialysis 223-241
    Home dialysis considerations 498
    Isolation from blood 228
    Minimal system 236, 237
    Specificity 224
Monitoring 223-241
    Blood leaks 234, 235, 239
    Dialysate circuit of hemodialyzer 230-236
    Dialysate pressure 231, 233
    Dialysis fluid composition 232
    Dialysis fluid conductivity 232
    Dialysis fluid flow rate 234
    Dialysis fluid temperature 232, 233
    Electrical safety of hemodialyzer 236
    Extracorporeal blood circuit 225-233
    Fluid balance during ultrafiltration 267
    Hemodialysis in children 518
    Medical problems in dialysis patients 223, 239, 396-398
    Requirements for ideal system 224
    Single needle hemodialysis 237, 238
    Ultrafiltration 272
N-Monoacetylcysteine 364
Monoamine oxidase inhibition 360, 365
Monoamine oxidase inhibitors 776
Monocytopenia complicating hemodialysis 640
Monomethylamine 361, 365
Mononuclear phagocyte 648
Morbidity
    Elderly patients 399
    Hours of dialysis correlation 395
    Reused dialyzers 297
    Transplant recipient 844
Morphine 758, 777
Mortality
    Acute renal failure 536, 541-543, 558
    Anti-GBM disease 876, 877
    Bacteremia 650
    Cardiovascular, dialysis patients 528, 595
    Cardiovascular risk factors 591
    Chronic renal failure in children 525
    Chronic renal failure, nutrition effect 571, 572
    Diabetes mellitus, hemodialysis treatment 400
    Dialysis 391, 821, 864-866
    Elderly patients, increased 399
    Hepatitis 665
    Infection causing 648-650
    Transplant recipient 844, 864-866
Motor nerve conduction, see Nerve 398
Multi-infarct dementia 728
Multiple myeloma

Multiple myeloma (*continued*)
    Hemodialysis experience 400, 401
    Peritoneal dialysis for 476
    Plasmapheresis 872, 878
    Survival 862
Munro Microabscesses 886
Muscle atrophy, peripheral neuropathy 731
Muscle cramps
    Complicating hemodialysis 35, 78, 250, 271
    Dialysis disequilibrium 727
    Hypocalcemia 727
    Hyponatremia 726
    Low sodium dialysis 576
    Peripheral neuropathy 731
Muscle mass 78, 569
Muscle membrane potential 394
Muscle potassium 357
Muscle relaxant 798-800
Muscle sodium 356
Muscle weakness 354, 356, 736
    Aluminum intoxication 689
    Osteodystrophy 688
    Peripheral neuropathy 731
Myalgia 637
Myasthenia 736, 760
Myasthenia gravis, plasmapheresis 876, 880
Myelofibrosis, hyperparathyroidism 634
Myocardial calcification 604, 699
Myocardial infarction
    Acute renal failure, prognosis 543
    Causing death 866
    Differentiation from pericarditis 599
    Treatment 605
Myocardial irritability 753
Myocarditis complicating pericarditis 599
Myocardium
    Effect of acetate 158
    Oxygen extraction in uremia 359
Myoclonus
    Acute renal failure 549
    Aliphatic amine correlation 364
    Dialysis encephalopathy 811
    Drug induced 727, 762, 764, 776
    Hyponatremia 726
    Peripheral neuropathy 731
    Uremic 725
Myoglobinemic acute renal failure 540
Myoinositol
    Cerebrospinal fluid levels 367
    Hemodialysis removal 367
    Hemoperfusion removal 311
    Metabolism 367
    Neurotoxicity 367, 734
    Plasma levels 367
    Vitamin B complex component 367
Myopathy
    Aluminum osteodystrophy 812
    Iron overload 636, 736
    Osteodystrophy 688
    Proximal, vitamin D deficiency 680, 688
    Treatment with vitamin D 702
Myosin 364
Myxedema 715

Nadolol 773
Nafcillin 465, 765, 766
Nalidixic acid 769
Nandrolone decanoate 397, 637
Naproxen 212, 778
Natriuretic hormone 356, 372
Necheles, Heinrich 5, 7, 414
Negative pressure deaeration 163, 235
Negative pressure, generation of 233
Neomycin 760, 761
Neostigmine 775
Nephrectomy, bilateral
    Anemia aggravated by 634
    Dialysis ascites 401
    Effect on transplant outcome 864
    Erythropoietin deficiency 634
    Hormonal consequences 581
    Hypertension treatment 396, 400, 522, 528, 575, 581, 603, 605
    Hypoalbuminemia 401
    Scleroderma 400
Nephrotic syndrome, drug induced 753
Nephrotoxicity 753
    Amphotericin B 770
    Aminoglycoside 760-762
    Analgesic 777
    Cephalosporin 762
    Iodide 782
    Methoxyflurane 799
    Polymyxins 767
    Precipitating acute renal failure 540
    Sulfonamide 768
    Vancomycin 768
Nerve action potential 732
Nerve compression 734
Nerve conduction velocity 398, 731, 734
    Assay of dialysis adequacy 394
    Delay by myoinositol 367
    Hemofiltration effect on 271
    Hemoperfusion improvement of 313
    Middle molecule impairment of 371
    Parathyroid hormone effect 373
    Polyacrylonitrile, short dialysis 279
Nerve fiber degeneration 732
Nerve function, single dialysis effect 732
Nerve, peripheral, calcium content 734
Nervous system, pathogenesis of hypertension 576, 577
Netilmicin 762
Neurologic abnormalities 354, 724-741, 838
Neuropathy, autonomic 731
    Blood pressure effect 555, 577, 581, 582
    Diabetic, effect of peritoneal dialysis 480
    Hemodynamic effects 251
    Impeding fluid removal 400
    Methylguanidine induced 362
    Vitamin deficiency, inducing hypotension 582
Neuropathy, peripheral 354, 730-735
    Angioaccess related 734
    Clinical features 730, 731
    Cobalt induced 638
    Correlation with severity of uremia 731
    Dialysis membrane surface correlation 368
    Dialysis, prevention and treatment 731, 732
    Dialysis time correlation 368
    Evaluation 397, 398
    Hemofiltration response 271
    Hydralazine induced 580, 772
    Inadequate dialysis indicator 368, 394
    Kidney transplant improving 732
    Membrane permeability effect 271
    Middle molecule correlation 83, 84, 279-281, 371, 732
    Nitrofurantoin 769

928 Index of subjects

Neuropathy (continued)
    Pathogenesis 732, 733
    Pathology 732
    Peritoneal dialysis association 421, 471, 732
    Plasma choline correlation 365
    Polyacrylonitrile response 281
    Polyamine induced 365, 366
    Residual function relationship 368
    Short dialysis relationship 395
    Sorbitol associated 367
    Symptoms 398
    Treatment 398
    Uremic 33, 354, 730-735
Neurotoxicity
    Penicillin 727, 764
    Phenol induced 366
    Polymyxins 767
    Reserpine 772
Neurotoxin, middle molecule 369, 371
Neurotransmitter imbalance, schizophrenia 888
Neutron activation analysis 804
Neutropenia, hemodialysis, see Leukopenia 640, 647
Neutrophil function in uremia 640, 647
Neutrophil locomotion 647
New dialyzer syndrome 297, 625
Nialamide 776
Nickel 617, 805, 807
Nicoladoni-Branham sign 603
Nicotinamide 780
Nicotinamide-adenine dinucleotide 632
Nicotinic acid 780
Nitrate 143, 161, 528, 617, 632
Nitrate reductase 808
Nitrofurantoin 731, 769
Nitrogen balance 66, 68, 471, 552
Nitrogen utilization, impaired 364
Nitrogenase 808
Nitrogenous wastes, adsorption of 323, 330
Nitroglycerin 605, 775
Nitroprusside increased peritoneal transport 429, 444, 446, 453, 557, 580, 760, 773
Nitrosourea 779
Nitrous oxide 801
Nocturnal penile tumescence 841, 842
Non-ionic diffusion 750
Non-steroidal anti-inflammatory drugs 212, 778
Norepinephrine 720
    Decreased peritoneal transport 758
    Synthesis and degradation 252
    Transport inhibition by methylguanidine 362
Normeperidine 778
Norpropoxyphene 777
Nortriptyline 315, 316, 776
Novobiocin 768
Nucleic acid metabolites 363
Nucleopore membranes 102
Nutrition 68, 89, 90, 569-574
    Assessment 569
    Children with renal failure 516, 528
    Chronic renal failure 363, 570-573
    Continuous ambulatory peritoneal dialysis 573
    Diabetic patient treated by dialysis 573
    Increased requirements in children 522
    Index of dialysis adequacy 394
    Maintenance hemodialysis 570-573
    Parenteral 474, 570
    Requirements, acute renal failure 569
Nylon/epoxy membranes 102

Nystagmus 727
Nystatin 546

Obese patients, angioaccess 171
Obesity complicating CAPD 479
Obstruction, peritoneal catheter 418, 460, 462
Obstructive uropathy, drug induced 753
Ocular abnormalities, transplant patients 747
Ocular motility abnormalities 727
Oculoplethysmography 729
Oedema, see Edema
Oliguria, acute, prognostic sign 542
Oncotic pressure and capillary ultrafiltration 245, 246, 252
Ophthalmodynamometry 729
Ophthalmological complications of hemodialysis 742-748
Opiate 581, 777
Optic atrophy, cobalt induced 638
Oral contraceptives and atherosclerosis 591
Oral sorbents 341, 343-350
Oreopoulos catheter 425, 461
Organ procurement 833, 835
Organic acid, intracerebral accumulation 725, 727
Organic acid methylates 367
Organic acid removal by hemoperfusion 308, 311
Organic anions 77
Organic compound accumulation in uremia 358-374
Organic compound, electrochemical degradation 325
Organic ion, renal transport inhibition 366
Org-NC 45 800
Osmolality 242
    Disequilibrium during dialysis 150, 151, 612
    Dissociated electrolytes, effect 244
    Maintenance by mannitol 614
    Peritoneal dialysis fluid 252, 453
    Plasma 151, 356
    Plasma lowering causing symptoms 151, 528, 555
    Plasma reduction inducing hypovolemia 554, 555
    Rate of change related to hypotension 614
    Sodium contribution to plasma 152
    Urea effect on 152
Osmolar injury to erythrocytes 632
Osmoles, idiogenic, cerebral and disequilibrium 393
Osmosis 146
Osmotic agent for peritoneal dialysis 252, 416, 417
Osmotic disequilibrium, blood pressure effects 272
Osmotic effects on vascular volume 250, 251
Osmotic force across peritoneum, components 246
Osmotic gradient
    Dialysis disequilibrium 727
    Intraocular pressure change 744
    Peritoneal 247, 254
Osmotic presssure 128, 146
Osmotic transmembrane pressure gradient 127, 242, 244, 245
Osteitis fibrosa 687
    Alkaline phosphatase increase 694
    Anemia aggravated by 634, 638
    Uremic children 526
Osteoblast 684, 688
Osteoblastic activity and alkaline phosphatase 694
Osteoclast 684, 688, 705
Osteodystrophy 37, 38, 355, 398, 679-711
    Acidosis, effect of 158, 358
    Aggravated by nephrectomy 581
    Aluminum 684, 812
    Calcium in dialysis fluid relationship 154, 155, 465, 700
    Children 526, 527
    Clinical features 688
    Disabling 867, 868

Osteodystrophy (*continued*)
    Duration of hemodialysis correlation 399
    Evaluation 398
    Fluoride relationship 143, 160, 700
    Growth retardation cause 526
    Magnesium relationship 155-157
    Parathyroid hormone role 372, 681, 682
    Pathogenesis 358, 681-684
    Peritoneal dialysis, occurrence with 479
    Prevention and management 699-705
    Radiographic features 694-699
    Sorbent dialysis relationship 335
    Sulfate, possible pathogenetic role 358
    Treatment 398, 702
Osteoid
    Increase, aluminum osteodystrophy 812
    Unmineralized in osteomalacia 688
Osteomalacia 38, 39, 683, 684, 688
    Aluminum toxicity 337, 684, 689, 700, 808, 812
    Decreased parathyroid response 684
    Fluoride 808
    Hyperphosphatemia, effect of 682, 683
    Low parathyroid hormone levels 694
    Phenytoin 780
    Radiographic features 697, 698
    Uremic children 526
    Vitamin D deficiency 680, 682
    Vitamin D metabolites, effect of 527
    Vitamin D treatment failures 703
Osteomyelitis 651
Osteonecrosis 698
Osteopenia 689, 698
Osteosclerosis 687, 697
Ototoxicity 624
    Aminoglycoside 760-762
    Antibiotic 760-762, 768
    Cobalt 638
    Diuretic 577, 774
Ouabain 771
Outflow pressure 250
Ovarian follicle 714
Overall creatinine clearance 478
Overall mass transfer coefficient 54, 55, 59, 60
Overdialysis 33
Overheated dialysate causing hemolysis 233, 618
Ovulation 714
Oxacillin 462, 765, 766
Oxalic acid 367
Oxalosis 862
Oxazepam 775
Oxazolidine anticonvulsant 753, 780
Oxidant 753
    Binding by zirconium oxide 326
    Dialysate regeneration method 325
    Erythrocyte injury 632
    Hemolysis 635
Oxidation
    Cerebral, inhibition 365, 366
    Drug biotransformation process 752
Oxidative phosphorylation 753
Oxidized starch, see Oxystarch
Oxipurinol 778
Oxycellulose, oral use 307, 344-346
Oxygen
    Concentration decrease, hemodialysis 633
    Myocardial extraction in uremia 359
    Supplementation during hemodialysis 556
    Treatment of air embolism 619
    Treatment of heart failure 605

Oxygen consumption, cerebral 360, 361, 367
Oxygen dissociation curve 633, 798
Oxygen saturation 555, 556
Oxygen transport 470, 633
Oxymetholone 637
Oxystarch
    Ammonia binding 345
    Dialysate regeneration, for 324
    Oral, raising fecal nitrogen 346
    Oral use 307, 344-346
    Potassium removal by oral 346
    Urea removal by 345, 346
Oxytetracycline 767

Pain, peripheral neuropathic 731
Pain, peritoneal see Abdominal pain 460, 470
Palmer catheter 425
Pancreatic ATPase inhibition 362
Pancreatic secretion 362
Pancreatitis
    Acute renal failure, prognosis 543
    Causing renal ischemia 540
    Peritoneal lavage 477
    Uremic 354
Pancuronium 798, 800, 801
Pantothenic acid 780
Papillary necrosis, analgesic nephropathy 537, 753, 777
Papilledema 728, 744
Para-aminosalicylate 769
Paracetamol, see Acetaminophen 777
Paradoxical pulse 599
Paraldehyde 752, 776
Parallel plate hemodialyzer 17, 24-27, 32, 107-111, 125, 286, 551
Paramethadione 780
Paranoia 838
Paraquat intoxication 315, 316
Parathyroid gland, autotransplantation 527
Parathyroid hormone 680, 681
    Action 681
    Aluminum osteodystrophy 812
    Assay 694
    Calcemic response 683
    Cimetidine decrease 782
    Control with CAPD 524
    C-terminal fragment 694
    Dialysis fluid calcium effect 154, 155
    Erythropoiesis inhibitor 634
    Fluoride interrelationship 160
    Hemofiltration, plasma level response 270
    Magnesium relationship 155-157, 694
    Metabolic clearance 680, 681, 683
    Neurotoxicity 734
    N-terminal assay 694
    Pathogenesis of calciphylaxis 690
    Peak 7 level correlation 370
    Phosphate retention stimulating 682
    Plasma level increase 694
    Plasma level, low 684, 694
    Reduction by phosphate restriction 527
    Renal acidosis, effect on 358
    Renal failure, kinetics 372
    Response to hypocalcemia 680
    Response to vitamin D 701
    Skeletal resistance 683
    Stimuli of secretion 680
    Toxicity in uremia 372, 373
    Trophic factor for vitamin D 680
    Uremic encephalopathy 725

Parathyroid hypertrophy 37
Parathyroidectomy
    Adverse effects 705
    Anemia, improvement of 397, 634
    Calciphylaxis treatment 690
    Dialysis fluid calcium after 155
    Hypercalcemia indicating 693, 700, 703
    Osteitis fibrosa treatment 398, 527
    Osteomalacia after 684
    Periarthritis treatment 689
    Regression of calcification 743
Paresthesia 398, 727, 731
Pargyline 776
Paromomycin 761, 762
Partial thromboplastin time 71, 206, 207
Particle embolization, hemoperfusion 307, 309
Particulate matter contaminating stored dialyzer 295
Patient education 827
Patient monitoring 239
Patient selection, home hemodialysis 494-497
Peak 7 369, 370
    Composition of components 369
    Generation rate 370
    Parathyroid hormone correlation 370
    Removal by hemoperfusion 310
Peak b 280, 281, 369
Peak 7c, composition 369
Pediatric dialysis 514-535
Pediatric dialysis unit 826
Pediatric hemodialyzer 119
Pemphigus 880
Penicillamine 781
Penicillin 764-766
    Hemolysis 757
    Hypokalemic alkalosis 752
    Interstitial nephritis 764-766
    Margin of safety 758
    Neurotoxicity 727, 758, 764, 766
    Peritoneal dialysis fluid additive 465, 473
    Pharmacokinetics 765
    Renal elimination 752
    Toxicity 764-766
Penicillin G 764, 765
Penicillin V 764
Pentamadine 770
Pentazocine 777
Pentobarbital 613, 775
Peptic ulcer 543, 546, 547, 717, 753, 772
Peptide
    Characterization of middle molecules 369
    Isolation techniques 369
    Kinetics 85, 86
    Plasma isolates in uremia 34, 368
    Toxic 83
Peptide hormone 373
    Hemofiltration removal 757
    Renal degradation 373, 717, 720
Peracetic acid 292
Percutaneous venous access 172, 173
Perforation of viscus complicating peritoneal dialysis 459, 460, 462, 518, 557
Performance evaluation 840
Perfusion, intestinal 341-343
Periarthritis 689, 699
Periarticular calcification 699
Pericardial effusion 596-599, 620
    Cause of hypotension 581
    Hemorrhagic 620
    Minoxidil associated 580, 772

Pericardial fibrosis 596
Pericardial friction rub 598, 599
Pericardiectomy 601
Pericardiocentesis 397, 601, 621
Pericarditis 596-601
    Acute renal failure 549
    Children, despite adequate dialysis 522
    Clinical evaluation 397
    Clinical features 598
    Complications 599
    Constrictive 596, 600
    Diabetic patient, higher incidence 598
    Differential diagnosis 599
    Fluid overload precipitating 598
    Hemoperfusion improvement of 311
    Hyperparathyroidism association 598
    Inadequate dialysis 597
    Incidence 596
    Increased dialysis for 600
    Infectious 598
    Low incidence with peritoneal dialysis 478
    Middle molecule correlation 371, 597
    Mortality 597
    Pathogenesis 597
    Treatment 397, 600, 601
    Uric acid concentration correlation 363
    Viral 598, 620
Perinephric abscess 653
Periodic peritoneal dialysis 468
Periosteal neostosis 696
Peripheral neuropathy, see Neuropathy 397, 398
Peripheral vascular resistance
    Acetate effect on 158, 236, 552
    Anemia effect on 602, 603
    Baroreceptor response 251
    Causes of increased 577
    Response to dialysis 269
    Response to hemofiltration 269
    Response to ultrafiltration 236, 251
Peritoneal access, see Peritoneal catheter 458-464
Peritoneal adhesions complicating peritonitis 471, 481
Peritoneal blood flow rate 445, 452
    Drug induced increase 428, 429, 453
    Measurement 445
Peritoneal Capillary 441
    Basement membrane 441
    Cell wall charge restricting transport 449
    Endothelial resistance to transport 448, 452
    Endothelium 441
    Intercellular channels 444
    Permeability 446
    Permeability increase with vasodilation 446
    Pore area 451
    Precapillary sphincter control 451
    Proximal site of ultrafiltration 448
    Source of solutes transported to dialysate 443-445
    Surface area increase with vasodilation 446, 453
Peritoneal catheter 418-420, 424, 425, 458-464
    Acute renal failure 556
    Complications of insertion 459, 460, 462-464
    Cuff erosion 462
    Disc type 461
    Dual 418, 443
    Encasement by adhesions 462
    Indwelling plastic conduit for 422
    Insertion 458-461, 517, 523, 556
    Malfunction 462
    Malposition 462
    Obstruction 418, 460, 462, 474, 518, 524, 558

Index of subjects 931

Peritoneal catheter (continued)
   Pediatric 517, 523
   Permanent 424, 425, 460-464
   Permanent, care of 461
   Removal 463, 474
   Replacement 464
   Revision 463
   Stylet 419, 420, 458-460
   Subcutaneous 461
   Subcutaneous tunnel infection 462
   Survival 464
   Technical evolution 418, 419
   Temporary 419
   Tenckhoff 424, 425
Peritoneal cavity
   Access 418, 419, 422, 424, 425, 458-464
   Access by repeated puncture 422, 423
   Access, Deane's prosthesis 459
   Access via indwelling plastic conduits 422
   Iodine flush disinfection 473
Peritoneal clearance 254, 442, 443
   Carbon dioxide gas 445
   Decrease after peritonitis 481, 518
   Determinants 442, 443
   Dialysate mixing, enhancing 447
   Dialysis fluid flow rate effect 427, 428, 431, 443
   Dioctyl sodium sulfosuccinate effects 454
   Diuretic effects 454
   Fluid dwell time effect 428
   Fluid recirculation, increase by 429
   Glucagon effects 453
   Hyperosmolar fluid increase 444
   Hypotension decreasing 444
   Instantaneous 442
   Limitation by dialysis fluid flow rate 443, 451
   Maximal 758
   Mean per exchange 442
   Methods to increase 427-431, 443, 444, 477, 758
   pH effects 443
   Pharmacologic enhancement 428, 429, 557, 758
   Reciprocating technique increasing 430
   Temperature effects 412, 428, 443
   Ultrafiltration increasing 448
   Urea 415, 428, 443, 445, 479
   Vascular disease decreasing 444
   Vasoactive drug effects 444, 445, 453
   Volume of dialysis fluid effects 427, 443
Peritoneal dialysate
   Cloudy, indicator of peritonitis 471
   Cultures, recommended procedures 471
   Drainage 419
   Eosinophilia 472, 473
   Fibrinogen 445
   Gram staining 471
   Inadequate drainage 460, 462
   Leukocyte count 445, 471
   Lymphocytosis 472
   Protein 256
   Sorbent regeneration 431, 432, 443, 468
   Stagnant fluid films 255, 256, 441, 447
   See also Peritoneal dialysis fluid
Peritoneal dialysis 33, 246-249, 252, 254, 410-492, 758
   Acute renal failure 415, 416, 476, 517, 518, 550, 556-558
   Advantages 481
   Amino acid losses 469, 573
   Anemia improved by 638
   Antibiotic, additive 465, 473
   Antibiotic transfer rates 474
   Barrier to transport 441
   Cardiopulmonary complications 470, 558
   Cardiovascular complications 475
   Channeling fluid with dual catheter 443
   Children 480, 517, 518, 523
   Chronic renal failure 426, 476, 478, 523
   Chronic use, feasibility demonstrated 423
   Clinical aspects 458-492
   Closed circuit disconnections and peritonitis 433
   Closed circuit systems 465
   Closed dialysate delivery, sterility 467
   Comparison with hollow fiber dialyzer 450, 451
   Complications 416, 423, 470-475, 517, 518, 524, 557, 558
   Conservative treatment, versus 423
   Continuous ambulatory, see Continuous 432, 468, 469
   Continuous cyclic 434, 469
   Continuous lavage technique 414-418, 443
   Continuous versus intermittent 480
   Contraindications 477, 556
   Convective mass transport 254, 256, 448, 449
   Conversion to hemodialysis, reasons 479, 480
   Criticism of early use 414
   Demographics of use 426
   Dialysis fluid flow rate 442, 443
   Diffusion, determinants of rate 442
   Disadvantage 550, 557
   Early clinical experience 414-416
   Efficiency, assessment of 442
   Efficiency, loss of 481, 518
   Efficiency, see also Peritoneal clearance 427, 442, 443
   Electrolyte abnormalities 416
   Exchange cycles 468
   Exogenous intoxications 477
   First human 414
   First successful chronic use 422
   Future 434, 435, 480, 481
   Gastrointestinal side effects 470
   Hematocrit 631
   Hemodialysis, versus, acute 423
   Hemodynamic side effects 470
   High flow rate automated 468
   History 410-439
   Home, intermittent 423, 479
   Hyperchloremic acidosis complicating 416
   Hypotensive patient 582
   Inadequate, clinical picture 479
   Indications 476, 477, 480, 481
   Inefficiency 471, 474, 518
   Inferior vena caval pressure 470
   Intermittent 419, 426, 427, 468, 478, 479
   Intermittent, clinical results 478
   Intermittent, duration of treatment 427, 478, 517
   Intermittent, dwell time 419, 517
   Intermittent lavage, first 415
   Intermittent, manual technique 467
   Intermittent, survival rates 479
   Intermittent, technique survival 479
   Intraabdominal pressure 470
   Invention 410, 411
   In vitro simulation 447
   Light chain removal 401
   Lipid soluble substances 450
   Mass transfer rate 442
   Mass transport kinetics 421
   Metabolic complications 469, 470, 475, 558
   Microbial contamination opportunities 468
   Middle molecules, effect on 83, 370
   Neurological complications 475

932 *Index of subjects*

Peritoneal dialysis (*continued*)
    Neuropathy, low incidence of 421, 732
    Osmotic gradient deterioration 254
    Osmotic ultrafiltration 246, 252
    Oxygen transport effects 470
    Pain complicating 471
    Pathways for solute movement 441
    Pericarditis treatment 600
    Pharmacologic influences 758
    Potassium transport 444
    Practical aspects 457-492
    Preferential use 434, 476, 550, 556, 620, 745
    Procedure 468, 469
    Prolonging anephric dog survival 415
    Protein loss 444, 469, 573
    Pulmonary complications 475
    Reciprocating 430, 443, 468
    Recirculation 429, 468
    Resistance to solute transport 441, 446
    Resorption affected by intestinal motility 412
    Routes of contamination 471
    Schedules 478
    Semicontinuous fluid flow 430, 431, 468
    Side effects 469, 470
    Solute removal, calculation of 442
    Sterile technique 468, 473
    Technical aspects 458-469, 523
    Technical progress for chronic use 419-423, 434, 457, 458
    Transplantation interrelation 480
    Transport increased by convection 428
    Ultrafiltrate source 443, 444
    Ultrafiltration rate 252
    Use while awaiting angioaccess maturation 392
    See also Dialysis, Peritoneal clearance
Peritoneal dialysis equipment 465-468
Peritoneal dialysis fluid
    Acetate as buffer anion 417, 464, 465
    Amino acid additive 465
    Automatic cyclers 425, 465, 466
    Bicarbonate as buffer anion 465
    Buffer anion 417, 465
    Calcium concentration 464, 465
    Channeling with continuous flow 418
    Chloride concentration 464
    Closed system circuit 417, 425, 426
    Cold, complications of 476
    Composition 415-417, 464, 465, 517, 556, 557
    Concentrated solutions 465
    Concentration equilibrium 421
    Cyclers 465-467
    Delivery system 465-467
    Dextrose absorption 421
    Dextrose concentration 416, 464, 470
    Distribution, effect on efficiency 443
    Dwell time 419, 428
    Extravasation into abdominal wall 518
    Flow rate 468
    Flow rate determining clearance 421, 442, 443, 451
    Flow rate-urea clearance correlation 428, 452
    Flow rates with recirculation 429
    Glass bottles 465
    Heparin, additive 459
    High flow rate 431
    Hypertonic increasing clearance 444
    Infusion technique 417, 419
    Isotonic 247
    Lactate as buffer anion 417, 464, 465
    Leakage 418, 460, 462, 518, 524
    Magnesium concentration 464, 465
    Microbial contamination 465
    Optimal flow rate 421
    Original composition 415
    Osmolality 252
    Osmolality effect on interstitium 453
    Osmotic agents 252, 416, 417, 464
    Overheated 476
    Plastic bags 465, 468
    Potassium concentration 464, 465
    Preparation 425, 426, 466, 467
    Prolonged dwell 432
    Proportioning system 425, 426
    Protein added, increasing clearance 443
    Recycling machine 419, 421
    Sodium concentration 416, 464, 465, 470, 481
    Sterilization 425, 432, 465
    Storage 465
    Volume 468, 517, 549
    See also Peritoneal dialysate
Peritoneal dialysis machine, automated 421, 422, 424-426, 466
Peritoneal dialysis system, semiautomated 419, 421
Peritoneal fibrosis 524
Peritoneal interstitium 441, 444
    Effect of dialysis fluid osmolality 453
    Hydration 453
    Resistance to transport 446, 447, 452
Peritoneal lavage 410, 412
    Peritonitis treatment 473
    See Peritoneal dialysis
Peritoneal lymphatics 441, 445
Peritoneal membrane
    Area 248, 256
    Deterioration 481
    Permeability coefficients 442
Peritoneal permeability 246, 247, 256, 413, 441
    Bidirectional, early studies 413
    Drug induced increase 428, 429
    Inflammation affecting 413, 446
    Vasodilator effect 445
    Venular 446
Peritoneal surface area 440
Peritoneo-venous shunt 582
Peritoneum
    Anatomy 440-442
    Blood supply 440
    Diffusion, early studies 412
    Fluid absorption 414
    Fluid transfer, early studies 412
    Parietal 440
    Permeability, exceeding hemodialyzer membranes 421
    Physiology 412
    Recognition as semipermeable membrane 412
    Relative contributions, parietal and visceral 440
    Sclerotic thickening 481
    Visceral 440, 441
Peritonitis 470-475, 524
    Antibiotics, intraperitoneal 473, 474
    Antibiotics, prophylactic 473
    Bacterial contamination of disconnected circuit 419, 433
    Catheter obstruction cause 474
    Chronic plastic 481
    Closed system, decreased incidence 467
    Complicating CAPD 433, 469, 524
    Consequences 422, 471, 474
    Diagnosis 471, 558
    Discouraging use of peritoneal dialysis 422, 457

Index of subjects 933

Peritonitis (*continued*)
    Endogenous source 471
    Fungal 472, 474
    Heparin, intraperitoneal, treatment 473
    Home dialysis, management 509
    Inadequate dialysis after 481, 517, 518, 524
    Incidence 473
    Indication for catheter removal 474
    Infectious 472
    Lavage treatment 473
    Parenteral nutrition for 474
    Perforated viscus 474, 557
    Peritoneal dialysis associated 470-475, 558
    Prevention 473
    Prognosis 474
    Protein loss exaggerated 471, 573
    Reduced ultrafiltration after 474
    Sterile 472, 473
    Treatment 473, 474
    Tuberculous 472, 474
Permeability, hydraulic 248
Permeability, peritoneal versus hemodialyzer membrane 421
Perphenazine 776
pH, see Hydrogen ion concentration
Phagocyte, mononuclear, uremic toxin bioassay 355
Phagocytosis, neutrophil in uremia 647
Pharmacokinetic modeling, hemoperfusion effect on 314
Pharmacokinetics 749-752
Pharmacological aspects of dialysis 749-797
Phenacetin 753, 777
Phenazopyridine 753, 769
Phenelzine 776
Phenformin 779, 780
Phenindione 781
Phenobarbital 209, 344, 477, 775
Phenol
    Adsorption by carbon 323, 330, 344
    Assay method 366
    Hemoperfusion removal of 308, 310
    Inhibition of platelet factor *3* 639
    Toxicity 366, 367
Phenolic Acid 366, 367
Phenolsulfophthalein 755
Phenothiazine 209, 315, 549, 555, 581, 776
Phenoxybenzamine 580, 773
Phentermine 775
Phentolamine 580, 773
N-Phenylacetyl-α-aminoglutaramide 368
Phenylalanine hydroxylase inhibition 355
Phenylalanine, phenol precursor 366
Phenylalanine/tyrosine ratio 363, 364
Phenylbutazone 209, 212, 689, 778
Phenylethylamine 365
Phenylglucuronide 367
Phenyllactic acid 367
Phenytoin 780
    Folate antagonist 632
    Pharmacokinetics 780
    Protein binding 363, 730, 750, 780
    Treatment of convulsions 730
    Treatment of disequilibrium 613
    Vitamin D metabolic interference 702
Pheochromocytoma 576
Phosphate 358, 682
    Adsorption 323
    Control of plasma, improving anemia 634
    Control with CAPD 479, 524
    Depletion 781
    Dialysis fluid additive 553
    Dietary 691, 699
    2,3-DPG determinant 633
    Effect on progression of renal failure 358
    Erythrocyte, in uremia 355
    Fecal 691
    Hemofiltration effect on 270, 284
    Homeostasis and renal failure 358
    Intestinal fluid content 343
    Metabolism in renal failure 372
    Parathyroid hormone, effect on 358
    Peritoneal clearance 758
    Plasma level, acute renal failure 549
    Plasma, reduction by diet and binders 699, 700
    Plasma, removal by regenerated dialysate 323
    Release from bone with acidosis 158
    Response of plasma to vitamin D 701
    Restriction, control of hyperparathyroidism 527
    Retention 682, 683
    Vitamin D interaction 680, 691
    Zirconium oxide binding 330
Phosphate binders 348
    Aluminum source 699, 805, 816, 817
    Treatment of renal osteodystrophy 527
Phosphocreatine 361
Phosphoenolpyruvatecarboxykinase 366
Phosphofructokinase inhibition 632
Phosphorylation, bioassay of uremic toxin 355
Photocell air detector 229
Photon absorptiometry 698
Phthalic anhydride, antibodies to 625
Physical activity, children on dialysis 530
Physostigmine 800
Phytohemagglutinin 647
Pigmentation 355, 713
Pillow blood pressure manometer 228
Pimelic acid 367
Pindolol 773
Pingueculae 744
Piperacillin 766
Pituitary function in uremia 712-715
Pituitary hormone survival relationship 399
Pivampicillin 765
Plasma 874
    Frozen 874
    Greenish, copper intoxication 632
    Middle molecule identification in 280
Plasma clearance 751
Plasma exchange, see Plasmapheresis 2, 36, 872-883
    Anti-GBM disease 876, 877
    Definition 873
    Effects 874, 875
    Hazards 874
    Kidney transplant 879
    Lupus erythematosus 878, 879
    Management of renal disease 876-880
    Prostacyclin synthesis, effect on 880
    Replacement fluids 874
    Technique 872-874
    Thrombotic thrombocytopenic purpura 880
Plasma filtration 873
Plasmapheresis 36, 37, 872-883
    Cryoglobulinemia 878
    Definition 873
    Hyperviscosity 878, 880
    Immune complex removal 878
    Psoriasis 888
    Rapidly progressive glomerulonephritis 877, 878
    Risk-benefit ratio 537, 538
Plasma protein-artificial surface interaction 187, 188

934 *Index of subjects*

Plasma protein fraction 874
Plasma separation 873
Plasma separator 758
Plasma water
    Drug concentration 750
    Solute concentration 249, 259
    Solute equilibration with erythrocyte 262
    Volume, fractional 249
Plasmin 203, 206, 212
Plasminogen 203, 209-211
Plasminogen activator 203, 209, 210, 212
Plasticizers 135, 625
Platelet
    Activated 203
    Contraction inhibitors 212
    Count 204, 207, 555, 639
    Cyclo-oxygenase 212, 639
    Damage 131, 132, 191, 192
    Depletion, sorbent induced 308, 309
    Disappearance 204
    Dysfunction 213, 214, 550, 620, 638, 639
    Energy metabolism and methylguanidine 362
    Interaction with membrane 214
    Morphology 205
    Production 204
    Reactivity, exposure to artificial surfaces 187
    Role in pathogenesis of atherosclerosis 206
    Shape change 205
    Survival 213, 217
    Turnover 204
Platelet activating factor 188, 191
Platelet actomysin 206
Platelet adherence
    To artificial surfaces 187, 188, 190, 191, 217
    To artificial surfaces, inhibition 194, 217
    To polyacrylonitrile membrane 276
    To proteins adsorbed on surfaces 186, 188
Platelet adhesion 201, 214, 638, 639
    Effect of drugs 211
    Inhibition by surface coating with albumin 188, 193
    Stimulated by adenosine nucleotides 190
    Uremic abnormality 631, 638, 639
Platelet aggregation 189-191, 202, 205, 208, 214
    Effect of leukocytes adherent to surfaces 189
    Hemoperfusion induced 308
    Heparin enhancement 214
    Inhibition 217, 360, 362, 363, 366, 371, 639
    Stimuli 639
    Uremic abnormality 639
Platelet aggregometry 208
Platelet factor *3* 188, 631, 639
Platelet factor *4* 189, 190, 201, 208, 214, 215, 639
    Contribution to atherosclerosis 592
    Increase during hemodialysis 639
    Inhibition by guanidinosuccinic acid 362
Platelet function
    Bioassay of uremic toxin 355
    Effect of dialysis 213, 631, 639
    Effect on heparin activity 214, 215
    Improved with peritoneal dialysis 478
    Inhibition of 211
    Tests of 207
Platelet injury, rheologic factors 190
Platelet membrane interaction with reaction inducer 205
Platelet release reaction 188, 190, 191, 201, 205, 206, 211, 212
Pleural dialysis 558
Pleural effusion 599, 621

Pneumococcal antigen, immune response 647
Pneumococcal bacteremia 650
Pneumonia 544, 546, 558
Pneumonitis, uremic 602
Pneumoperitoneum 476
Poisoning, see Exogenous intoxication
Polyacrylonitrile membrane 34, 102, 114, 118, 247, 252, 275-277, 279
    Biocompatibility 276, 283
    Blood cell reaction to 276
    Hemodialysis for hepatic encephalopathy 317
    Hemofiltration 281
    High permeability for short dialysis 279
    Hydraulic permeability 276, 277
    Mass transfer characteristics, with hemofiltration 281
    Middle molecule transport 279
    Permeability 275, 276
    Psoriasis, dialysis 886
    Sieving coefficient 281
    Thrombogenicity 276
    Transport effect on uremic neuropathy 271
    Ultrafiltration rate 282
Polyaldehyde oral sorbents 307, 344-347
Polyamine 365, 885
Polyamine conjugates 365
Polyarteritis nodosa 665, 877
Polycystic kidney disease 653, 858, 859, 861
Polymer
    Blood compatibility 194
    Coating of sorbent 307
    Surface binding by heparin 192, 193
    Water soluble 99
Polymicrobial bacteremia 651, 652
Polymyalgia rheumatica complicating hepatitis 665
Polymyxin B 768
Polypeptide 368, 373
Polypeptide membranes 100, 103
Polysulfone membranes 103, 283
Polytetra-fluoro-ethylene grafts 35, 179
Polyuric acute renal failure 538
Polyvinyl chloride leaching 625
Polyvinylpyrrolidone 99
Porphobilinogen synthesis inhibition 371
Porphyria cutanea tarda 622, 808
Portable suitcase kidney 396
Possilian flow 244
Postdilution hemofiltration 259
Potassium 152, 356, 357
    Accumulation in renal failure 356, 357
    Addition for dialysis regeneration 330, 334
    Balance 153
    Body content 78, 79, 153
    Cation exchange in dialysate regeneration 329
    Deficiency decreasing insulin production 720
    Depletion and cancer regression 891-893
    Dialysis fluid 148, 152, 153, 552, 606
    Dialysis fluid concentration and digoxin 399
    Dialysis induced depletion 891, 892
    Distribution into cells 153
    Drug induced depletion 754
    Erythrocyte concentration 153
    Fecal excretion 357, 718
    Hemodialysis transport 248
    Intracellular level and arrhythmia 606
    Intake 153, 516, 573
    Muscle, in renal failure 152, 357
    Omission from peritoneal dialysis fluid 517
    Peritoneal dialysis fluid concentration 417, 464, 465, 557

Index of subjects 935

Potassium (*continued*)
 Peritoneal transport 444, 758
 Peritoneal ultrafiltrate concentration 444
 pH effect on distribution 153, 617
 Plasma concentration 152, 153, 356, 357
 Radioactive 153
 Redy-sorb system kinetics 334
 Removal by hemodialysis 616
 Removal by ion exchange resins 348
 Removal by oral oxystarch 346
 Removal from dialysate by ion exchange 324
 Renal excretion 357
 Toxicity correlation with concentration 357, 756
Povidone iodine disinfection 458, 461, 473
Practolol 773
Praxis 736
Prazosin 579, 772
Predilution hemofiltration 259
Prednisone 537, 538, 601, 876
Pregnancy, hemodialysis management 402, 715
Prerenal failure, differential diagnosis 538, 539
Pressure
 Cerebrospinal fluid 744
 Hydraulic 242
 Intraabdominal, during peritoneal dialysis 470
 Intraocular 742, 744
 Osmotic 242
 Relation to deaeration 163
 Transmembrane 226, 227
 Venous outflow 250
Pressure gradient 57
 Osmotic, peritoneal 254
Pressure monitor
 Accuracy 228
 Alarms 228
 Dialysate 233
 Hemodialyzer blood circuit 226-229
Prevention of uremia 848
Priapism 623, 638, 715
Primaquine 770
Probenecid 753, 778
Procainamide 774
Prochlorperazine 776
Procoagulants 202
 Circulating inhibitors 202
 Fresh frozen plasma component 874
 Interaction at blood-artificial surface interface 187
 Plasmapheresis removal 875
 Synthesis 204
 Tests of function 206
Progressive systemic sclerosis 400
Proinsulin 712, 719
Prolactin 713, 715
Promethazine 776
Propanidid 799
Prophylactic antibiotics for angioaccess 652
Propionic acidemia 477
Proportioning pumps 232, 234
Propoxyphene 756, 777
Propranolol 578, 773
 Anginal treatment 605
 Delayed metabolism, cimetidine 782
 Hyperparathyroidism treatment 705
 Hypertension treatment 396, 578, 579
 Hypoglycemia complicating 621, 622
 Lipid metabolism effect 589
 Pharmacokinetics 579, 773
 Toxicity 579
Propylthiouracil 781

Prostacyclin 192-194, 206, 212, 217
 Hemodialysis anticoagulant 192, 215, 216, 553, 639
 Hemolytic uremic syndrome 880
 Hemoperfusion anticoagulant 308, 317
 Heparin sparing effect 215
 Hemorrhage complicating hemodialysis 620
 Increased in acute renal failure 550
 Interactions with heparin 190, 194, 215
 Pharmacokinetics 781
 Synthesis after plasma exchange 874, 880
Prostaglandin
 Pathogenesis of hypertension 577
 Peritoneal transport effects 557, 758
 Release during hemodialysis 555
 Role in renal ischemia 540
 Use with hemodialysis 133
Prostaglandin E_2 192
Prostaglandin synthetase inhibition 753, 778
Prosthetic arteriovenous fistula 179-182
Prosthetic shunt, see Arteriovenous 173-175
Protamine sulfate 215, 216, 230
Protein
 Adsorption to artificial surfaces 186, 187, 190, 191, 194, 214
 CAPD losses 433
 Composition, dietary 569
 Composition, influence on platelet adhesion 188
 Concentration polarization 258
 Denaturation after surface adsorption 187
 Dietary, effects of 355, 362
 Dietary, hematopoiesis 632, 635
 Elimination, impaired in uremia 373
 Interaction with reused membrane 298
 Perfusate, effect on ultrafiltration 129, 257
 Peritoneal dialysate 256, 469, 524, 573
 Peritoneal dialysis fluid additive 443
 Peritonitis induced loss 446, 471
 Plasma concentration 61, 81, 127, 129
 Plasma concentration, nutritional assay 569
 Plasma, oncotic effects 127, 243, 251
 Plasma, volume fraction 249
 Repletion 571
 Restriction preventing neuropathy 731
 Supplementation 469
 Synthesis 355, 360
 Turnover 359, 526
Protein binding
 Distribution volume effect 750
 Drugs 356, 730, 750, 751
 Effect on directional flux 757
 Hormones 712
 Improvement after dialysis 363
 Reduced in uremia 363, 730, 750
 Saturation 755
 Solute, restricting transport 449, 750, 754
Protein bound drugs, hemoperfusion 314
Protein catabolic rate 62, 66, 88-90
 Caloric intake effect 548
 Dialysis fluid dextrose effect 160
 Redy dialysis adequacy relationship 331
Protein catabolism 65, 72, 77, 355, 720
Protein intake 65, 66
 Anemia treatment 636
 Children with renal failure 516, 529
 Chronic renal failure, recommended 572
 Determinant of number of CAPD exchanges 479
 Recommendation for children on CAPD 524
 Restricted, renal failure 569
 Survival, renal failure correlation 571, 572

Protein malnutrition 469, 571, 573
Proteolytic enzymes to clean dialyzer 291
Prothrombin time 206, 209, 213
Protrusio acetabuli 698
Pruritus 355, 622, 753
    Hemoperfusion improvement 313
    Hyperparathyroidism 689
    Jaundice 664
    Methylguanidine induced 362
    Parathyroidectomy indication 705
    Treatment 622
    Urea induced 360
Pseudoaneurysm complicating angioaccess 181
Pseudodiabetes, uremic 718
Pseudogout 624
Pseudomonas peritonitis 472
Pseudouridine 363
Psoriasis 884-888
    Chemical cause 885
    Dialysis for 41, 318, 884-888
    Hemoperfusion for 318
    Heparin treatment 885, 888
    Kidney transplant, after 888
    Non-uremic patients 886, 887
    Onset after hemodialysis 887
    Pathophysiology 885
    Peritoneal dialysis for 477, 886
    Plasmapheresis 888
    Treatment modes 884, 888
    Uremic patients 887
Psychological aspects of dialysis 499, 736-738, 838, 839
Psychological aspects of uremia 838
Psychological characteristics long-term survivors 399
Psychological problems of arteriovenous shunt 175
Psychological stress of dialysis 529, 530, 737, 738, 839
Psychosis
    Bromide intoxication 776
    Complicating hemodialysis 555
    Dialysis encephalopathy 811
    Dialysis selection criterion 831
    Phenothiazine 776
    Thiocyanate 772, 773
Psychosocial aspects of dialysis 529, 840, 841, 845, 846
Pubertal development 526
Pulmonary capillary permeability 602
Pulmonary complications, acute renal failure 549
Pulmonary complications, peritoneal dialysis 475
Pulmonary edema 544
Pulmonary emboli 174
    Acute renal failure, prognosis 543
    Pulmonary edema, differential 544
    Septic 651
Pulmonary function
    Effect of hemodialysis 132, 623
    Long term dialysis survivors 399
    Peritoneal dialysis effect 470
Pulmonary hemorrhage 877
Pulmonary insufficiency, peritoneal dialysis contraindication 477
Pulmonary sequestration of leukocytes 633
Purine metabolites 363
Purulent pericarditis 598, 599, 601
Putrescine 365
Pyelography for urinary obstruction 538
Pyelonephritis 545, 848
Pyrethins 144
Pyridine metabolites 363
Pyridostigmine 800
Pyridoxal phosphate deficiency 734

Pyridoxine 580, 780
Pyrimethamine 770
Pyrizinamide 769
Pyrogen in dialysis fluid 325
Pyrogen reaction
    Hemodialysis 135, 144, 146, 601
    Hemoperfusion induced 308
    Home hemodialysis 498, 509
    Prevention 602
    Reused dialyzers 298
    Stored dialyzers 286
    Treatment 602
Pyrogen test 104
Pyruvate, increased plasma levels 160, 367
Pyruvatekinase inhibition 372, 632

Quadriceps tendon rupture 607, 689
Quality control, dialysis 827
Quality of life 835, 837-843, 866, 867
    Anticipated, dialysis selection criterion 831
    Dialysis patients 837-845, 847
    Effect of staff attitudes 847
    Transplant recipient 844
Quinidine 397, 399, 753, 757, 774
Quinine 606, 770

Race track for measuring blood flow rate 121, 122, 226
Rachitic cartilage bioassay 355
Radiation grafted membranes 102
Radioimmunoassay, hepatitis virus 663
Radiotherapy, cancer response 893
Rebound plasma concentration after dialysis 85, 756
Rebuck skin window technique 647, 648
Reciprocating peritoneal dialysis 430, 443, 468
Recirculating dialysis system, see Redy 326-340
Recirculating single pass dialyzer 113, 122, 231
Recirculation of blood through dialyzer 394
Recirculation peritoneal dialysis 429, 468
Record keeping for dialysis 827
Red blood cell, see Erythrocyte
Reduction, drug biotransformation 752
Redy-sorb system 35, 326-340
    Acid base balance 331, 332
    Acidosis correction 334, 335
    Aluminum content of cartridge 336-338
    Cation kinetics 334
    Clinical experience 335
    Dialysis of patient with low urea 335
    Economics 335
    Indications for use 335
    Long term results 335
    Monitors 326, 335
    Practical aspects 330-338
    Sodium kinetics 333
    Sulfate accumulation 358
    Toxicologic studies 336
Reflection coefficient 245, 247
Regeneration of dialysate 323-340
Regeneration peritoneal dialysis 431, 432
Regional dialysis programs 826
Regional heparinization 215, 216, 553, 620
Registry, dialysis and transplant patients 827
Rehabilitation 500, 737, 831, 840, 841, 845, 866, 867
    Children treated by dialysis 523, 530, 531
    Home dialysis 510, 523
    Inhibited by late dialysis 391
    Kidney transplant 863
    Obstacles to 842
    Osteodystrophy impeding 867, 868

Rejection coefficient 245, 247
Relative cell 99
Renal blood flow 576, 754
Renal cortical necrosis, see Cortical
Renal disease, type affecting survival 861
Renal failure
    Acid base homeostasis 357, 358
    Age, effect on treatment mode 858
    Amines 364-366
    Amino acid abnormalities 363
    Anemia 573, 630-638
    Anesthesia 798-803
    Aromatic amines 365
    Bleeding 638, 639
    Carnitine, plasma 365
    Causes 858, 859
    Children 519-533
    Choline, plasma 365
    Chronic, reversal of 393
    Creatinine homeostasis 361
    Cyclic AMP increase in plasma 363
    Drug dosage modification 758-760
    End organ response to drugs 752, 753
    Endocrine abnormalities in children 825, 826
    Hemofiltration treatment 267
    Hemoperfusion treatment 308-313
    Indoles 366
    Infection 646-658
    Leukocyte, effects on 639, 640
    Lipochromes 372
    Magnesium metabolism 358
    Mineral metabolism 372
    Nutrition 363, 569-574
    Myoinositol levels 367
    Peritoneal dialysis for 423, 426, 476-478
    Pharmacological aspects 749-797
    Phosphate homeostasis 358
    Potassium homeostasis 356, 357, 682
    Prevention 848
    Progression rate of chronic 392
    Severity correlated with drug half life 759
    Severity correlation, vitamin D abnormalities 682
    Sodium homeostasis 356
    Survival 525, 571, 572
    Survival without dialysis 392
    Treatment facilities needed for children 520
    See also Acute, Chronic, Uremia
Renal functional recovery, acute renal failure 548, 558
Renal functional recovery with minoxidil therapy 580
Renal function, residual 33, 67, 78, 87
    Effect on dialysis need 478
    Middle molecule correlation 370
    Relation to neuropathy 368
    Short dialysis tolerance 394
Renal ischemia 540
Renal rickets, see Osteodystrophy 679-711
Renal transplant, see Kidney transplant
Renal vein thrombosis 515
Renin 578
    Aldosterone, control of 581, 718
    Control of secretion 576
    Hypertension pathogenesis 270, 529, 576, 578
    Physiology 578
    Role in renal ischemia 540
    Unresponsiveness during hemodialysis 528
Reptilase time 206
Research component of dialysis facility 827
Reserpine 579, 772

Resins for hemoperfusion 306, 307
Resin hemoperfusion for drug intoxication 314
Resistance
    Blood 250
    Blood flow in dialyzer 109, 111, 113, 130
    Mesothelial transport 448, 452
    Peritoneal dialysis transport 446-448, 452
    Stagnant fluid films 447, 451
Respiratory infection 653
Respiratory quotient 716
Restlessness 621
Restless leg syndrome 731
Reticuloendothelial blockade, infectious 635
Reticuloendothelial function, plasmapheresis effect on 875
Retina, vascular abnormalities, malignant hypertension 728
Retinal-binding protein 373
Retinitis, cytomegalovirus 743, 746
Retinoids, psoriasis treatment 888
Retinopathy 481, 744, 745
Retroperitoneal fibrosis 753, 772
Retroperitoneal hematoma 173, 621
Reuse, see Hemodialyzer reuse 286
Reverse dialysis 757
Reverse osmosis 145, 146, 161
    Aluminum removal 814
    Peritoneal dialysis fluid preparation 425, 426, 466, 467
    Water preparation for home dialysis 498
Reye's syndrome 477
Rhabdomyolysis 549
Rhodial system 275-285
Rhône-Poulenc hemodialyzer 238, 275-285
    Blood flow resistance 276
    Characteristics and performance 276
    Dialysis fluid delivery system 278
    Hemofiltration by 281
    Pediatric use 518
    Reuse 277
    Ultrafiltration 277, 279
    Volume of blood compartment 276
Rib fracture, osteodystrophy 688
Riboflavin 780
Ribonuclease 373
Rifampin 474, 769
Rinsing hemodialyzer for reuse 288
RNA synthesis, induction by vitamin D 680
Rotating dialysis cell 99
RP 6 dialyzer, see Rhône-Poulenc hemodialyzer 275
Rubidium 805, 807, 808
Rugger jersey appearance of bone 697

Salicylates 209, 212, 215, 216, 777
    Gastrointestinal hemorrhage 753
    Interference with middle molecule assay 370
    Intoxication 315, 316, 477, 777
    Pharmacokinetics 777
    Renal elimination 752, 777
Salivary flow, reduced by methylguanidine 362
Salt, see Sodium 356
Saphenous vein grafts 35, 179
Saralasin 396, 576, 578, 773
Sarcosine 361, 364
Satellite dialysis 825
Schizophrenia
    Hemodialysis treatment 41, 318, 888-891
    Hemoperfusion treatment 318
    Pathogenesis 888
    Psychosomatic aspects 891
    Uremia 838

Index of subjects

Schooling, children treated by dialysis 530
Schwann cells 732
Scintiscan of skeleton 698
Scleroderma 400, 444
Scribner, Belding 22-24, 28, 29, 32
Secobarbital 344, 775
Secretin 717, 758
Sedative 775
    Intoxication 314, 315
    Pharmacokinetics 775
    Postoperative use 801
Sediment filters 146
Seizures, see Convulsions
Seldinger technique, angioaccess 172, 518
Selection of patients 830
    Dialysis and transplantation 830-834, 837
    Medical criteria 830, 831
    Patient involvement in decision 833
    Refusal of candidates 833
Selenium 805
Self dialysis 823, 825, 832
Sella turcica abnormalities, hyperprolactinemia 714
Septic arthritis 651
Septicemia
    Acute renal failure, prevalence 545
    Hemodialysis hypotension cause 555, 613
    Hepatitis complication 664
    Staphylococcal, in heroin addicts 402
    See also Bacteremia 649
Septic pulmonary emboli 651
Sequential ultrafiltration and dialysis 35, 151, 238, 239, 251, 265, 272, 528, 553, 582, 614
Sequestering agent 342
Serotonin in renal failure 366
Serotonin release from platelets 191, 201, 205, 214
Serum sickness complicating hepatitis 665
Servo-control system, fluid proportioning 232
Sexual dysfunction 841, 842
Shaldon catheter 21, 172
Sham dialysis 886, 891
Shear stress 190, 191
Sherry hypothesis 211
Short dialysis 33, 117, 152, 279, 394, 395
    Adequacy of 279
    Adverse effects 395
    Bicarbonate, effect on 395
    Children at home 512
    Exchangeable body sodium relationship 395
    Membrane permeability relationship 279, 395
    Precautions required 395
    Prevention of intraocular pressure rise 744
    Residual renal function, importance of 394
    Technical requirements 395
Shunt, see Arteriovenous shunt 173-175
Sick cell syndrome 355
Sickle cell anemia 402, 635
Side effects impairing treatment compliance 840
Sieving, peritoneal ultrafiltration 448, 449
Sieving coefficient 245, 247, 249, 252, 259
    Albumin 256
    Correlation with molecular size 259
    Cuprophane 281
    Inulin 248
    Limiting solute transport 281
    Measurement 248
    Polyacrylonitrile membrane 281
Sieving effect 244
Silicon 805

Single needle hemodialysis 122, 237, 238, 551
    Diasadvantages 238
    Indications 238
    Intermittent blood pump 238
    Monitoring 237, 238
    Principle 237
Single needle hemodialysis systems 122, 237, 238
Single pass delivery, hemodialysis fluid 231
Sisomicin 761, 762
Skatole 366
Skatoxyl 366
Skeletal mineralization, impaired, hypophosphatemia 692
Skeletal pain 688
Skeleton
    Maturation, children on chronic dialysis 526
    Pathology, renal osteodystrophy 679, 685, 686, 688
    Radiographic abnormalities, osteodystrophy 694
    Resistance to parathyroid hormone 518
    Response to vitamin D 701
    Scintiscan 698
Skin
    Abnormalities, dialysis patients 355, 622
    Erosion by arteriovenous shunt 175
    Flushing, copper intoxication 632
    Hemorrhage 621
    Ulcerations, hyperparathyroidism 705
Skin fold thickness, nutritional assay 569
Skull, radiographic abnormalities, osteodystrophy 696
Smoking, effect on long term survival 398
Smoking, predisposition to atherosclerosis 591
Snake bite 541
Social impact of hemodialysis 844-849
Social worker 510, 826
Sodium
    Accumulation complicating peritoneal dialysis 416
    Addition by water softening 145
    Analysis 15
    Blood pressure stability during ultrafiltration 556, 614
    Body content 334
    Cation exchange in dialysate regeneration 329
    Concentration gradient 80, 149
    Convective transport 149, 248, 333
    Depletion causing hypotension 613
    Dialysis fluid 78, 80, 81, 144, 148-152, 232, 551, 552
    Dialysis fluid concentration for Redy system 333, 334
    Distribution volume 75
    Equilibration during peritoneal dialysis 464
    Excess, plasma exchange complication 874
    Exchangeable body content 78, 79, 82, 395
    Flux, hemodialysis 78, 80, 81, 248
    Flux, hemofiltration 78, 81
    Fractional tubular reabsorption 373
    Hypertonic, hemodialyzer disinfectant 292
    Infusion to treat hypotension 582, 613
    Intake 516, 573
    Intracellular, in uremia 355, 356
    Kinetics 79, 82
    Kinetics with dialysate regeneration 333
    Muscle, in renal failure 356
    Osmolar contribution to plasma 152
    Pathogenesis of hypertension 529, 576
    Peripheral vascular resistance effect 577
    Peritoneal dialysis fluid 416, 464, 470
    Peritoneal ultrafiltrate concentration 448
    Plasma concentration 79, 80, 82, 151
    Plasma protein fraction concentration 874
    Prevention of disequilibrium 613
    Redy-sorb system effect on plasma level 334

Sodium (*continued*)
    Removal by peritoneal dialysis 464
    Removing during dialysis 80, 149
    Renal excretion by failing kidney 356, 362
    Renal wasting 356
    Restriction, treatment of hypertension 396, 577
    Retention, adaptation to 356
    Retention, renal failure 356
    Sorption from dialysis fluid 335
    Tap water concentration 144
    Tonicity indicator in plasma 356
    Transport 362, 367, 372, 716, 734
    Treatment of muscle cramps 623
    Tubular reabsorption and renal failure 356
    Wasting in infancy 514
Sodium balance
    Determinants in Redy-sorb system 333
    During hemofiltration 267
    Urea correlation in dialysate regeneration 331, 333
Sodium bicarbonate, see Bicarbonate
Sodium bisulfite in peritoneal dialysis fluid 464
Sodium cellulose phosphate 892
Sodium dodecyl cholate 281
Sodium dodecyl sulphate 281
Sodium hydroxide in peritoneal dialysis fluid 465
Sodium hypochlorite 236, 275, 277, 286, 289
Sodium polystyrene sulfonate 348
Sodium, potassium ATPase 356, 371
Sodium pump, electrogenic, in uremia 355
Solute accumulation 60
Solute concentration, determinants during dialysis 394
Solute concentration in ultrafiltrate 245
Solute flux, relative to water flux 245
Solute kinetic modelling 61
Solute transport, stearic hindrance by membrane 245
Solutes, marker 61
Solvent drag 244, 443
Somatomedin B 270, 526, 713
Somatotrophin 713
Sonogram, see Echo 621
Sorbent 305-308
    Biocompatibility 305, 306, 341-353
    Coating, effect on solute adsorption 307
    Depletion of platelets 308
    Encapsulation 306, 308
    Hemoperfusion use 306, 307
    Oral use 341, 343-350
    Regeneration of dialysate 323-330
    Regeneration of hemofiltrate 267
    Regeneration of peritoneal dialysate 431, 432, 443, 468
    Saturation 758
    Types 306, 307, 341, 342
    Uses 341
Sorbent cartridge 326-329
    Aluminum content 336-338
    Functions 326
Sorbent hemoperfusion, see Hemoperfusion 305-322
Sorbent membranes 103
Sorbent system, animal testing 325
Sorbitol 35, 36
    Increased concentration in uremia 367
    Peritoneal dialysis osmotic agent 252, 464
    Treatment of pulmonary edema 544
    Use with aluminum hydroxide 547
Sorb system, see Redy 35, 326-338
Sore thumb syndrome 177
Sorption, see Adsorption 306, 307
Sotalol 773

Speech abnormalities, dialysis disequilibrium 811
Spermatogenesis 714
Spermidine 365
Spermine 365, 885
Spiegler equation 245
Spinal anesthesia 800
Spironolactone 774
Splanchnic blood flow rate 445
Splenectomy, effect on transplant outcome 864
Splenomegaly 634, 635
Square meter-hour hypothesis 32, 33, 116, 368
Stagnant fluid film resistance 447
Standards for hemodialysis equipment 223
Standards for water purity 144, 161
Staphylococcal peritonitis 472, 474
Staphylococcal septic arthritis 624
Staphylococcus aureus
    Bacteremia 650
    Endocarditis 651
    Osteomyelitis 651
    Septic pulmonary emboli 651
Starch, oxidized, oral use 344-346
Staverman's reflection coefficient 245, 247
Steal syndrome 177, 181, 734
Stearic hindrance by membrane to solute transport 245
Sterilant 292, 293
Sterile peritonitis 472
Sterility 292, 293
Sterilization of dialysis solution 235, 236
Sterilization of hemodialyzer for reuse 292-295
Stomatitis, uremic 354
Storage of coil dialyzer 286
Storage of hemodialyzer for reuse 288
Stratum corneum antibody 884
Streptokinase 203, 209, 210, 217, 460
Streptomycin 760, 761
Streptozotocin 779
Stress of dialysis 839
Stress test, cardiac and long term dialysis survival 398, 399
Stroke 729, 730
Strontium 144, 805, 808
Stupor, uremic 354
Stylet catheter 458-460
    Complications of insertion 459, 460
    Implantation 458, 459
    Indications 458
    Peritoneal dialysis 419, 458-460
    Positioning 459
Subclavian vein angioaccess 173, 518, 551
    Complications 551
    While awaiting fistula maturation 392
    Subcutaneous tunnel, peritoneal catheter 460, 462
Subdural hematoma 620, 729
Subperiosteal erosions 694, 695
Substitution fluid, hemofiltration 266, 267, 281
Subxiphoid window 601
Succinate oxidation, inhibition 365
Succinic acid 367
Suicide 737
    Arteriovenous shunt disconnection 175
    Dialysis encephalopathy 811
Sulbencillin 765
Sulfadiazine 767, 768
Sulfamethazole 768
Sulfamethoxazole 767, 768
Sulfate
    Increased, effects 358
    Metabolic effects 335

Sulfate (continued)
    Metabolic origin 358
    Plasma, increased with Redy-sorb system 330
    Retention in renal failure 358, 713
    Tap water 144
    Toxicity 144
Sulfinpyrazone 187, 192, 209, 212, 213, 216, 217, 778
    Anticoagulant for angioaccess 639
    For hemoperfusion 308
Sulfisoxazole 767, 768
Sulfite oxidase 808
Sulfonamide
    Hemolysis 635
    Pharmacokinetics 767, 768
    Protein binding, decreased 363
    Toxicity 15, 16, 768
Sulfoxane 770
Suloctodil 192
Supplies, disposable, home dialysis 510
Surface, artificial
    Binding by heparin 192, 193
    Coating with albumin 188, 194
    Electrokinetic charge 191
    Protein adsorption 186, 187
Surgery
    Coronary artery disease 605
    Pericarditis treatment 601
    Precipitating acute renal failure 540-542, 549
    Preparation 801
    Treatment of heart failure 604
Survival 859-861
    Acute renal failure 558
    Age effect 525
    Cardiovascular risk factors 591
    Children with chronic renal failure 525
    Chronic renal failure, nutrition effect 571, 572
    Continuous ambulatory peritoneal dialysis 479
    Hemodialysis 860, 861
    Home hemodialysis 510, 522, 860
    Kidney transplant 862-864
    Long term hemodialysis treatment 398, 399
    Patient with reused dialyzers 296
    Peritoneal dialysis 479, 862
    Primary renal disease effect 861
    Related to treatment method 860
    Timing initiation of hemodialysis 391
Suxamethonium 798, 800
Sympathetic control of renin release 576
Sympathetic neuropathy, see Neuropathy, autonomic
Sympathetic tone, blood pressure effect 577
Synergism, metabolite combinations causing uremia 359
Synovial fluid, osteodystrophy 689
Synthesis, biotransformation mode 752
Synthesis rate of proteins after plasmapheresis 875
Systemic lupus erythematosus, see Lupus 400, 879
Systemic toxicity test 104

Talampicillin 765
Taraxein 888
Taste, relation to zinc 808
Taurine 364
Taurocyamine 362
Temperature
    Central/peripheral gradient indicating vasoconstriction 518
    Dialysis fluid, monitoring 232, 233
    Effect on conductivity monitoring 232
    Effect on peritoneal transport 412, 428, 443

    Effect on ultrafiltration rate 129
    Relation to deaeration 163, 164, 235
Tenckhoff catheter 424, 425, 460-464
    Advantages 458
    Care of 461
    Implantation 460, 461
Tendon reflex asymmetry, angioaccess induced 734
Tendon rupture, spontaneous 624, 689
Teprotide 576, 578
Terminating dialysis treatment 846
Terra sigillata 343
Testes abnormalities with malnutrition 714
Testosterone 226, 714, 715
Testosterone enanthate treatment of anemia 397, 637
Tetany, hypocalcemic 705, 726
Tetracycline 766, 767
    Antianabolic effect 752, 766
    Fluorescent labelling of bone 684-687
Tetraethylammonium 772
Theophylline 370, 773
Thermal erythrocyte injury 632, 633
Thermostat for dialysis fluid 233, 618
Thiabendazole 770
Thiamin 732, 780
    Deficiency 602, 732
    Removal by dialysis 732
    Treatment of Korsakoff psychosis 727
Thiazide 577, 589, 774
Thin film dialysis cell 99
Thiocyanate 360, 580, 772, 773
6-Thioguanine 758
Thiopental 613, 753, 756, 775, 799, 801
Thiopurine methyl transferase inhibition 355, 758, 778
Thioridazine 776
Thirst
    After dialysis 151, 152
    Exaggerated in diabetic patients 400
    Peritoneal dialysis side effect 464, 470, 478
Thomas shunt 34, 173
Threonine in renal failure 364
Thrombin
    Action on fibrinogen 202, 211
    Adsorption to artificial surfaces 187
    Amplification of platelet aggregation 202, 205, 639
    Formation 186, 189
Thrombin time 206
Thrombocytopenia 204, 555
Thromboembolism prevention 190, 192
Thrombogenesis, extracorporeal 186-200
β Thromboglobulin 208, 639
Thrombolytic agent treatment of cerebral ischemia 729
Thrombophlebitis, infected, embolus to lung 651
Thromboplastic substances released from erythrocytes 190
Thromboresistant surfaces 193
Thrombosenin 206
Thrombosis of angioaccess 174, 177, 181
Thrombotic thrombocytopenic purpura 874, 880
Thromboxane 188, 191, 201, 205, 206, 212
Thrombus formation 202
    Membrane characteristics, effect on 214
    On artificial surfaces 186-188, 191, 214
    Prevention 188, 191-194
    Rheological factors in extracorporeal circuit 186
    Role of platelets in extracorporeal circuit 187, 214
Thymidine kinase inhibition 355
Thymidine uptake by bone marrow, inhibition 371
Thymosin deficiency 640, 647
Thyroid function in uremic patients 526, 712, 715, 716

Thyroid stimulating hormone 270, 526, 715, 716
Thyrotropin releasing hormone 715, 716
Thyroxine 715, 716
    Hemoperfusion removal of 311
    Plasma level response to hemofiltration 270
Thyroxine binding globulin 716
Ticarcillin 766
Ticlopidine 781
Ticrynafen 774
Timolol 773
Tin 805, 807, 808
    Body content 805
    Dialysis fluid 144
    Protein binding 755
Tissue culture toxicity tests 104
T-lymphocyte 663, 885
Tobramycin 761, 762
Tolamolol 773
Tolazamide 779
Tolazoline 557, 775
Tolbutamide 779
Toronto Western Hospital catheter 425, 461
Total body water 249
Toxin, uremic 354-390
Trabecular bone turnover 687
Trace element 781, 804-810
    Abnormalities 804-810
    Accumulation 144, 358, 753
    Acute intoxication 807
    Adsorption by hemoperfusion 307, 308
    Analysis 804
    Binding to membranes 757
    Biological half life 142
    Body stores 805
    Dialysis fluid contamination 142-144
    Mechanisms of abnormalities 805
    Pharmacokinetics 804
    Plasma protein binding 142
    Release from Redy-sorb system 336
    Tissue distribution 804, 805
    Zirconium oxide binding 326
Trace metal content of membranes 135
Trade-off hypothesis 372
Training for home dialysis 500-505
Tranquilizer 315, 775-777
Transamidation producing guanidinosuccinic acid 362
Transcellular transport across erythrocyte 261
Transcortin 717
Transferrin, plasma, nutritional assessment 569, 571
Transfusion reaction, risk of plasma exchange 874
Transient ischemic attacks 729
Transketolase inhibition in uremia 355, 362, 734
Transluminal angioplasty 174, 181
Transmembrane pressure 233, 234
    Blood compartment pressure relationship 250
    Effect on ultrafiltration rate 128, 239, 257, 282
    Estimated from venous outflow pressure 250
    Gradient 127, 257
    Membrane tolerance 281
    Plasma filtration 873
Transplant rejection, delay in uremia 646
Transplantation, see Kidney transplant
Transport
    Abnormal, in uremia 355
    Bicarbonate 63, 75
    Carbon dioxide 63, 65
    Carbonic acid 63
    Intercompartmental 84
    Mechanisms 54, 97
    Organic ion, renal 366
    Resistance, dialysis 754
    Resistance, peritoneal dialysis 446-448, 451, 452
    Solute, by ultrafiltration 252
Tranylcypromine 776
Trauma, acute renal failure, survival 542
Travelling and dialysis treatment 335
Treatment, stress on patient 839, 840
Tremor, uremic 725
Trendelenburg position, treatment of air embolism 619
Triamcinolone, pericarditis treatment 397, 601
Triamterene 774
Trichlorethanol 315, 316, 775, 800
Trichlorethylene 799, 800
Tricyclic drug intoxication 315, 316
Triflupromazine 776
Triglyceride 37, 588
    Cholesterol relationship 590
    Dietary effects 572
    Hemofiltration effect on plasma 271
    Plasma lowering by charcoal 349, 350
    Relation to dialysis fluid dextrose 160
    Removal 589
    Transport 588
Triiodothyronine 715, 716
Trimethadione 780
Trimethephan 580
Trimethoprim 770
Trimethoprim-sulfamethoxazole 474
Trimethylamine 364
Trousseau's sign 727
Trypsin release from platelets 205
Tryptamine 366
Tryptophan 363, 366
Tryptophan hydroxylase 366
Tryptophan pyrrolase 366
Tuberculosis 653
Tuberculostatic drugs 769
Tuberculous pericarditis 601
Tuberculous peritonitis 472, 474
Tubocuranine 800, 801
Tubular necrosis
    Clinical course 558, 559
    Differential diagnosis 538, 539
    Drug induced 753
    Precipitating factors 540-542
    Prognosis 541-543
    See also Acute renal failure 536-568
Tunnel infections, peritoneal catheter 462
Tunnel, subcutaneous for Tenckhoff catheter 460
Twitching 354, 356, 364, 725
Tyramine 365
Tyrosine 364

Ulnar nerve 734
Ultrafiltrate
    Electrolyte concentration 248
    Flux rate 259
    Path during peritoneal dialysis 449
    Peritoneal, reabsorption 464
    Peritoneal, source 444
    Replacement of fluid volume 257
    Solute concentration 245, 249, 257, 259
    Urea concentration 257
    Volume 249, 281
Ultrafiltration 11, 18, 19, 35, 61, 242-274
    Calcium removal 154

942 Index of subjects

Ultrafiltration (*continued*)
    Capacity, loss with CAPD 480
    Clinical application 249, 265-274
    Combined with dialysis with regenerated fluid 324
    Congestive heart failure treatment 397
    Determinants 242
    Distorting mass transfer resistance calculation 253
    Donnan effect limiting cation removal 553
    Edema treatment 227
    Electrolyte transport in peritoneal dialysis 448, 449
    Excessive 240, 509, 613
    Hemodialysis in children 518
    Hemodynamic effects 238, 251, 252
    Home dialysis, dangers and control 498, 499
    Hydrostatic pressure induced 149, 159, 244, 281, 449
    Hypertension treatment 239, 269, 270, 396, 528
    Increasing peritoneal transport 444, 448
    Intolerance caused by pericarditis 598
    Isolated 238
    Limited, in children 522
    Middle molecule clearance, effect on 127
    Monitoring in children 522, 532
    Negative pressure 163
    Obligatory 250
    Osmotic, peritoneal 246, 464
    Osmotic, sieving effects 449
    Peritoneal, osmotic, causing hypernatremia 464
    Peritoneal, proximal capillary site 448
    Principle of 242-249, 252-262, 265
    Reduced after peritonitis 474
    Rhône-Poulenc hemodialyzer 277, 279
    Sequential, preceding dialysis 35, 151, 238, 239, 251, 522, 528, 553, 614
    Sodium balance, effect on 80, 149
    Solute transport effects 59, 60, 86, 252, 757
    Spontaneous arteriovenous 272
    Tolerance of 151, 152, 238, 250-252, 269, 614
Ultrafiltration coefficient 57, 59, 128
Ultrafiltration rate 59, 78, 82, 102, 103, 109, 114, 127, 250
    Blood flow rate effect on 259
    Blood pressure effect on 250, 614
    Capillary bed, determinants of 245
    Control of 234
    Factors affecting 257
    Hemodialyzer, determinants 129, 245
    Maximal 248
    Measurement 239, 240, 250
    Membrane area effect 259
    Per unit area of membrane 242, 265
    Peritoneal dialysis 252
    Peritoneal, decrease with time 254
    Peritoneal, patient variability 252
    Plasma protein effect 129, 258
    Polyacrylonitrile membrane 282
    Redy-sorb system, measurement 326
    Temperature effect 129
    Transmembrane pressure effect 128, 226, 227
Ultrasonic air detector 230
Ultrasonic blood flow meter 121, 226
Ultrasonography, diagnosis of urinary obstruction 538
Ultraviolet light irradiation producing vitamin D 680
Ultraviolet light sterilization 432, 466
Ultraviolet phototherapy of psoriasis 622, 884
Umbilical vein graft 179
Umbilical vessels, newborn angioaccess 521
Underdialysis, clinical picture 479
Uranium 805
Urate 363

Urea 71, 359
    Accumulation 66, 70
    Adsorption by locust bean gum 347
    Adsorption, restricted 323, 324, 331
    Antipyretic effect 549
    Appearance, see Urea generation 548
    Charcoal adsorption capacity 344
    Concentration disequilibrium 393, 612
    Convective clearance 254
    Degradation by bacterial urease in gut 359
    Dialysate regeneration problems 323-325, 331
    Dialyzer clearance 19
    Distribution volume 66, 68, 70
    Effect of adding to dialysis fluid 360
    Effect on sodium balance in Redy-sorb 331, 333
    Effect on transport into brain 753
    Enzymatic hydrolysis 325
    Hemofiltration removal of 267, 268, 556
    Hemoperfusion removal of 310, 319
    Hydrolysis in Redy-sorb system 326, 329
    Increased by hypercatabolism of malnutrition 528
    Inhibition of protein binding of drugs 360
    Intercompartmental flux 612
    Insterstitial fluid content 343
    In vitro studies of toxicity 360
    Kinetics 68, 550
    Liquid membrane capsule, removal by 347, 348
    Low, dialysis with Redy-sorb system 335
    Osmotic effect 152, 247, 359
    Oxystarch affinity 345
    Plasma-aqueous humor disequilibrium 744
    Plasma concentration 66-68, 70, 359-361
    Plasma level, risk of disequilibrium 548, 613
    Potentiation of toxins 360
    Prevention of disequilibrium 613
    Removal by dialysis 3, 12, 15, 67, 68
    Removal from dialysate, methods 324, 325
    Role as uremic toxin 359, 360
    Synthesis 359
    Toxic effects 359, 360
    Transport across intestinal wall 355
Urea clearance 67, 68
    Continuous ambulatory peritoneal dialysis 433, 479
    Dialysis fluid flow rate effect 331
    Hemodialysis 553
    Hemodialyzer reuse, effect on 288
    Hemofiltration 283
    Intestinal perfusion 342, 343
    Peritoneal dialysis 443, 445, 452
Urea generation rate 65-68, 70, 88, 89, 268
    Acute renal failure 542, 548
    Correlation with protein catabolism 359
    Determinant of number of CAPD exchanges 479
    Effect of plasma urea concentration 360
    Effect on dialysate regeneration efficiency 331
    Nutritional assessment method 569
Urea nitrogen 65
    Hemodialysis effect on plasma level 550
    Plasma level indicating dialysis 550
    Turnover 359
Urease 347
    Dialysate regeneration ingredient 324-326
    Stabilization by zirconium oxide 326
Uremia 1, 7, 8, 15, 16, 33, 61, 65, 354-390
    Acidosis 357, 358
    Aliphatic amines 364, 365
    Aromatic Amines 365
    Bleeding tendency 213, 638, 639

Uremia (*continued*)
    Breath, methylamines causing odor 365
    Carbohydrate levels, abnormal 367
    Carbohydrate metabolism 718-720
    Cardiomyopathy 602
    Cardiovascular symptoms 355
    Cell metabolism 355
    Cellular respiration inhibition 359
    Clinical description 354
    Collagen abnormalities 684
    Convulsions cause 516
    Correlation with plasma solute levels 358, 359, 368
    Delayed hypersensitivity 647
    Dermal changes 355, 753
    Drug binding impairment 750
    Drug intoxication, simulating 749
    Electrolyte abnormalities 356-358
    Encephalopathy 724-726
    Endocrine abnormalities 712-723
    Enzyme abnormalities 355
    Evaluation of patient for dialysis 837
    Gastrointestinal lavage treatment 343
    Gastrointestinal symptoms 354, 753
    Growth retardation 526
    Hematologic consequences 355, 630-645
    Hemoperfusion treatment 308-313
    High molecular weight toxins 373
    Homeostatic adaptation to sodium excess 356
    Host defense mechanisms 646-648
    Immunologic responsiveness 355, 646, 647
    Indoles 366
    Integrated therapeutic approach 835
    Intestinal perfusion treatment 342, 343
    Lack of correlation with guanidinosuccinic acid 362
    Locust bean gum treatment 347
    Lymphocytes 640, 647
    Malnutrition resembling 476
    Metabolic effects 355
    Neurological complications 279, 354, 724-741, 838
    Neutrophils 640, 647
    Oral charcoal treatment 344
    Organic compound accumulation 358-374
    Osteodystrophy 355, 679-711
    Oxystarch treatment 346
    Pathogenesis 355
    Patient coping with 837
    Peptides 368
    Phenols 366, 367
    Platelet dysfunction 213, 214, 638, 639
    Pneumonitis 602
    Polyamines 365, 366
    Polypeptides 368, 373
    Prevention 355, 848
    Progression despite hemodialysis 391
    Protein binding abnormality 363, 750
    Protein toxins 373
    Psychological aspects 838
    Pyridine metabolites 363
    Relation to protein intake 355
    Reversible 355
    Symptom correlation with creatinine clearance 392
    Symptoms, middle molecule correlation 371
    Thyroid function 715-717
    Trace element abnormalities 358, 804-810
    Trade-off hypothesis 372
    Transport abnormalities 355
    Treatment 305, 306, 355
    Treatment options 392
    Water metabolism abnormalities 356
    See also Renal Failure, Acute, Chronic
Uremic toxin 83, 354-390
    Bacterial flora of intestine producing 355
    Bioassay 355
    Criteria for relevance 358, 359
    Hemoperfusion removal 308-310
    Inorganic solutes 356-361
    In vitro testing 359
    Protein catabolism derivation 355
    Search for 354
    Synergism of several compounds 359
Ureterosigmoidostomy, regression of cancer 891
Urethane 801
Uric acid 363
    Adsorption by carbon 323, 330, 344
    Hemoperfusion removal of 308-310
    Impairment of renal function 549
    Intestinal fluid content 343
    Plasma concentration and pericarditis 363
    Plasma concentration in renal failure 363, 549
    Plasma, removal by regenerated dialysate 323
    Toxicity 363
    Transport by intestinal perfusion 342, 343
Uricolysis 363
Urinary antiseptic 769
Urinary sediment in acute renal failure 539
Urinary tract, bacteremia source 650
Urinary tract infection 545, 653
Urinary tract obstruction 516, 537, 538
Urine
    Chemical composition in tubular necrosis 539
    Creatinine concentration 67
    Sodium concentration in renal failure 539
    Urea concentration 67
    Volume 67, 538, 542
Uroepithelial malignancy 753
Urokinase 203, 209, 210

Valine 364
Valine/glycine ratio 363
Valproic acid 730, 780
Vanadium 356, 805, 808
Vancomycin 175, 768
    Angioaccess infection 652
    Membrane sieving 757
    Peritoneal catheter wound infection 462
    Peritonitis treatment 474
Van't Hoff's law of osmotic pressure 244, 245
Vascular abnormalities, malignant hypertension 728
Vascular access, see Angioaccess 171
Vascular calcification 690, 699
Vascular instability 615
Vascular volume 250, 251
Vasculitis 444, 538
Vasoactive amine
    Blood pressure maintenance during ultrafiltration 605
    Loss during hemodialysis 555
    Platelet release during hemoperfusion 308
    Treatment of hemodialysis hypotension 555, 582
Vasoconstriction 251, 518
Vasoconstrictor decrease of peritoneal clearance 444, 453
Vasodilation increasing peritoneal permeability 428, 429, 444-446, 453, 557
Vasopressin, see Antidiuretic hormone 720
Venom, snake, anticoagulant use 211
Venous access, percutaneous 172, 173

Index of subjects

Venous blood line of dialyzer 225
Venous obstruction of graft AV fistula 181
Venous outflow pressure from hemodialyzer 227, 250
Venous pressure
    Decreased in prerenal failure 538
    Deviation in pericarditis 599, 600
    Increase excessive ultrafiltration 613
    Increase from fistula 177, 181, 734
    Monitoring 518, 544, 600
Venous tubing occlusion 229
Ventilation anesthesia, effect of acidosis 798
Ventilation, depression by hemodialysis CO_2 loss 623, 624
Ventriculogram, radionuclide, cardiac evaluation 604
Venturi orifice for dialysis fluid proportioning 232
Verdamicin 762
Vertebral collapse from osteodystrophy 688
Very low density lipoprotein 588
Vibratory sense, dialysis effect 732
Vibration sense, impaired, neuropathy 731
Vibratory threshold test 398
Viomycin 769
Viral antigen, immune response in uremia 646, 647
Viral hepatitis, see Hepatitis 659-678
Viral infection 653, 654
Viral pericarditis 598, 620
Viremia, hepatitis A 662
Visceral calcification 699
Vision
    Abnormalities, cerebral ischemia 729
    Dialysis disequilibrium blurring 612
    Hemodialysis induced abnormalities 742-748
    Loss, diabetic patients, hemodialysis related 400
    Malignant hypertension blurring 728
Vital capacity, effect of peritoneal dialysis 470
Vitamin 780, 781
    Deficiency inducing hypotension 582
    Removal by dialysis 572, 573, 757
    Requirements, chronic dialysis 572, 573
Vitamin A 573, 780
Vitamin B complex, see individual vitamins
Vitamin B_{12} 781
    Clearance by hemofiltration 283
    Deficiency 638
    Repletion 397
Vitamin C 632, 781
Vitamin D 37, 38, 154, 155, 679, 680, 780
    Actions 680
    Anemia improvement with 634
    Deficiency, consequences 683
    Hypercalcemia complicating 693
    Impaired metabolism 682
    Intestinal calcium absorption effect 155
    Metabolism 38, 679, 680
    Need to monitor plasma calcium with therapy 527
    Osteodystrophy treatment 526, 527, 701
    Phosphate absorption effect 691
    Prevention of osteodystrophy 696, 699
    Resistance, aluminum osteodystrophy 812
    Toxicity 155, 398
    Treatment decreasing parathyroidectomy need 703
    Treatment failure 702, 703
    Treatment of hypocalcemia after parathyroidectomy 705
Vitamin D_3 679
Vitamin E 781
Vitamin K 209
Vividiffusion apparatus 4
Vocational adjustment 841
Vogt's limbus girdle 744

Volume
    Extracellular fluid 78, 239, 269
    Extracorporeal, plasmapheresis technique 873
    Fluid, dependent hypertension 269, 270
    Intracellular fluid 78
    Intravascular expansion, plasma exchange 874
    Vascular, depletion 250, 251
    Vascular, repletion 250, 252
Volume of distribution
    Acetate 74
    Bicarbonate 75
    Drugs 315, 750
    Effect on half life 750, 756, 758
    Effect on solute removal 449
    Protein binding influence on 750
    Relation to dialyzer clearance 756
    Sodium 78
    Urea 68
Volumetric pump for fluid balance in hemofiltration 281, 282
Vomiting
    Complicating peritoneal dialysis 470
    Copper intoxication 632
    Dialysis disequilibrium 612
    Hepatitis 664
    Hyponatremia 726
    Malignant hypertension 728
    Methylguanidine induced 362
    Trace metal intoxication 807
    Urea induced 360
    Uremic 354

Waldenstrom's macroglobulinemia 878
Warfarin 209, 216, 639, 781
Warrick, Christopher 410, 412
Water 142
    Aluminum 700, 813, 814
    Bacterial contamination 161
    Balance 516, 752
    Bulk flow 243, 244, 448
    Calcium 154
    Chlorination 143
    Contaminants of tap 142-144, 161
    Distribution, determinants 79
    Fluoride 160, 700
    Flux, relative to solute flux 245
    Hardness 143
    Intake, chronic dialysis patient 573
    Intoxication 356, 549, 633
    Loss in infancy 515
    Low pH of 144
    Metabolism, uremic abnormalities 356
    Monitoring of quality 146
    Particulate matter in 144, 146
    Plasma, volume fraction 259
    Preparation for hemodialysis 142-147, 498, 523
    Purification standards 142, 823
    Quality standards for dialyzer reuse 300
    Quality standards for hemodialysis 144
    Removal during dialysis 149
    Removal, ineffectiveness of hemoperfusion 311
    Supply for home dialysis 505, 523
    Total body 69, 78, 239, 249, 250
    Transcellular movement in peritoneal dialysis 449
    Transcompartmental flux 79
    Transport 57
    Treatment methods 145, 146
Water softener 145